Volume 4

Pediatric Orthopedics

SECOND EDITION

Volume 4

Pediatric Orthopedics

SECOND EDITION

MIHRAN O. TACHDJIAN, M.S., M.D.
Professor of Orthopedic Surgery,
Northwestern University Medical School
Attending Orthopedic Surgeon and Former Head
Division of Orthopedics
Children's Memorial Hospital
Chicago, Illinois

1990
W.B. SAUNDERS COMPANY
Harcourt Brace Jovanovich, Inc.
Philadelphia ■ London ■ Toronto ■ Montreal ■ Sydney ■ Tokyo

W. B. SAUNDERS COMPANY
Harcourt Brace Jovanovich, Inc.

Independence Square West
Philadelphia, PA 19106

Library of Congress Cataloging-in-Publication Data

Tachdjian, Mihran O.

Pediatric orthopedics.

Includes bibliographies and index.

1. Pediatric orthopedia. I. Title. [DNLM: 1. Orthopedics—in infancy & childhood. WS 270 T117p]

RD732.3.C48T33 1990 617′.3 87–13006

ISBN 0–7216–8726–1 (set)

Listed here is the latest translated edition of this book together with the language of the translation and the publisher.

Spanish (*1st Edition*)–Nueva Editorial Interamericana S.A. de C.V., Mexico 4 D.F., Mexico

Editor: Edward H. Wickland, Jr.
Developmental Editor: Kathleen McCullough
Designer: Bill Donnelly
Production Manager: Bill Preston
Manuscript Editors: Ruth Barker, Constance Burton, Tina Rebane
Mechanical Artist: Karen Giacomucci
Illustration Coordinator: Peg Shaw
Indexer: Julie Schwager

Volume 1 ISBN 0–7216–8722–9
Volume 2 ISBN 0–7216–8723–7
Volume 3 ISBN 0–7216–8724–5
Volume 4 ISBN 0–7216–8727–X
Pediatric Orthopedics Complete Set ISBN 0–7216–8726–1

Last digit is the print number: 9 8 7 6 5 4 3 2

Dedicated With Love to
My Wife
Vivian B. Tachdjian

Preface

During the past 18 years, great strides have been made in pediatric orthopedics. A new edition of this book is long overdue. The gestation period of such an *Arbeit* has been prolonged because of the tremendous amount of labor involved in writing a single-author book. The objectives and format of the textbook have not changed from the first edition. I have attempted to present a thorough and comprehensive treatise on the affections of the neuromusculoskeletal system in children.

I have expressed my preferred methods of treatment and surgical procedure based upon my personal experience and the privilege of association with the leaders in pediatric orthopedics throughout the world who have participated in the faculty of the Pediatric Orthopedic International Seminars, which I have directed annually since 1972. The names of the faculty appear in the acknowledgments in the following pages.

The illustrations and operative plates are all original; the majority represent the superb artistry of Mr. Ernest Beck, to whom I am greatly indebted. I also wish to acknowledge Miss Patricia Piescinski for her beautiful drawings.

I wish to thank the entire staff of the W.B. Saunders Company, particularly Miss Ruth Barker, Mr. Albert Meier, Mrs. Kathleen McCullough, and Mr. Edward H. Wickland, Jr.

I would also like to express my gratitude to Mrs. Mikie Boroughf, who assisted in the preparation of this book.

A question frequently posed to me over the years has been, "How do you write such an extensive book?" Every word has been handwritten in my illegible handwriting, readable only by Mrs. Lynn Ridings, without whose assistance and editorial support this work would not have been possible.

MIHRAN O. TACHDJIAN, M.D.

Acknowledgments

I would like to give special thanks to the following people for their help in writing certain sections of this book: Ellen Chadwick, M.D., and Stanford Shulman, M.D.—infectious diseases; Ramiro Hernandez, M.D.—CT scan of the hip; James Donaldson, M.D.—ultrasonography in congenital dislocation of the hip; Andrew Poznanski, M.D.—assistance in imaging findings in various skeletal disorders, especially bone dysplasias; Steven Hall, M.D.—orthopedic aspects of pediatric anesthesia; David McLone, M.D., and Thomas Naidich, M.D.—neurosurgical aspects of myelomeningocele and spinal dysraphism; Dror Paley, M.D.—Ilizarov limb lengthening; George Simons, M.D.—complications of talipes equinovarus; David H. Sutherland, M.D.—gait; and Mary Weck, R.P.T.—physical therapy for cerebral palsy.

I also wish to express my gratitude to the members of the faculty of the Pediatric Orthopedic International Seminars over the past 18 years.

Robert Abrams, M.D.
James Aronson, M.D.
Marc Asher, M.D.
R. Kirklin Ashley, M.D.
Henry H. Banks, M.D.
Riad Barmada, M.D.
Melvin H. Becker, M.D.
Henri Bensahel, M.D.
Anthony Bianco, M.D.
Eugene E. Bleck, M.D.
Prof. Alexander Bliskunov
Walter P. Blount, M.D.
J. Richard Bowen, M.D.
David W. Boyer, M.D.
Robert Bright, M.D.
Prof. Dieter Buck-Gramcko
Wilton H. Bunch, M.D.
Aloysio Campos da Paz, Jr., M.D.
S. Terry Canale, M.D.
Henri Carlioz, M.D.
Nils Carstam, M.D.
Prof. Robert Cattaneo
Mr. Anthony Catterall, F.R.C.S.
Prof. Paul L. Chigot
Eldon G. Chuinard, M.D.
Robert G. Chuinard, M.D.
Stanley M.K. Chung, M.D.
Sherman S. Coleman, M.D.
Mr. Christopher L. Colton, F.R.C.S.
Clinton L. Compere, M.D.
James J. Conway, M.D.
Henry R. Cowell, M.D.
Alvin H. Crawford, M.D.
Burr H. Curtis, M.D.
Prof. George Dall, F.R.C.S.
Prof. G. DeBastiani
Prof. Julio dePablos
Luciano Dias, M.D.
Harold M. Dick, M.D.
Alain Dimeglio, M.D.
James Donaldson, M.D.
John Dorst, M.D.
James Drennan, M.D.
Denis S. Drummond, M.D.

Prof. Jean Dubousset
Mr. Denis M. Dunn, F.R.C.S.
Peter M. Dunn, M.D.
Robert E. Eilert, M.D.
Richard E. Eppright, M.D.
John J. Fahey, M.D.
Albert B. Ferguson, Jr., M.D.
J. William Fielding, M.D.
Mr. John Fixsen, F.R.C.S.
Victor Frankel, M.D.
Nicholas Giannestras, M.D.
Prof. Alain Gilbert
J. Leonard Goldner, M.D.
Neil E. Green, M.D.
William T. Green, M.D.
Paul P. Griffin, M.D.
Donald Gunn, M.D.
John E. Hall, M.D.
Judith G. Hall, M.D.
John E. Handelsman, M.D.
Robert Hensinger, M.D.
Ramiro Hernandez, M.D.
Charles Herndon, M.D.
John A. Herring, M.D.
M. Mark Hoffer, M.D.
Walter A. Hoyt, Jr., M.D.
Mr. J. Rowland Hughes, F.R.C.S.
Prof. Sean P. F. Hughes
Prof. Gabriel Abramovich Ilizarov
Roshen Irani, M.D.
Francois Iselin, M.D.
Preston James, M.D.
Prof. Lutz F.H. Jani
Ali Kalamchi, M.D.
William J. Kane, M.D.
Buni'chiro Kawamura, M.D.
Theodore E. Keats, M.D.
Armen S. Kelikian, M.D.
Hampar Kelikian, M.D.
Mr. J.A. Kenwright, F.R.C.S.
Ara Y. Ketenjian, M.D.
Eugene Kilgore, M.D.
Richard E. King, M.D.
Prof. Predrag Klisiç
Steven Kopits, M.D.
Warren G. Kramer, M.D.
Mr. Douglas Lamb, F.R.C.S.
Prof. Anders F. Langenskiöld
Loren Larsen, M.D.
Franco Lavini, M.D.
Richard E. Lindseth, M.D.
Mr. George Lloyd-Roberts, F.R.C.S.
John E. Lonstein, M.D.
Wood Lovell, M.D.
G. Dean MacEwen, M.D.
John B. McGinty, M.D.
Douglas W. McKay, M.D.
Mr. Brian McKibbin, F.R.C.S.
David McLone, M.D.
John E. Madewell, M.D.
Roger A. Mann, M.D.
Prof. P.G. Marchetti
Prof. S. Matsuno
Peter L. Meehan, M.D.
Malcolm B. Menelaus, M.D.
Michael Michelson, M.D.
Lee W. Milford, M.D.
Edward A. Millar, M.D.
Mr. George P. Mitchell, F.R.C.S.
Prof. Giorgio Monticelli
Raymond T. Morrissy, M.D.
Colin F. Moseley, M.D.
Alf S. Nachemson, M.D.
Ann Nachemson, M.D.
John J. Niebauer, M.D.
John A. Ogden, M.D.
Michael B. Ozonoff, M.D.
Lauren M. Pachman, M.D.
Dror Paley, M.D.
Arsen Pankovich, M.D.
Arthur M. Pappas, M.D.
Klausdieter Parsch, M.D.
Sir Dennis Paterson
Hamlet A. Peterson, M.D.
Guillermo de Velasco Polo, M.D.
Ignacio V. Ponseti, M.D.
Melvin Post, M.D.
Jean-Gabriel Pous, M.D.
Andrew K. Poznanski, M.D.
Charles T. Price, M.D.
Mercer Rang, M.D.
Mr. A.H.C. Ratliff, F.R.C.S.
Inge Reimann, M.D.
L. Renzi-Brivio, M.D.
B. Lawrence Riggs, M.D.
Veijo A. Ritsila, M.D.
John M. Roberts, M.D.
Charles Rockwood, M.D.
Robert B. Salter, M.D.
Robert L. Samilson, M.D.
Shahan K. Sarrafian, M.D.
Michael F. Schafer, M.D.
William L. Schey, M.D.
Keith Schroeder, M.D.
Mr. W.J.W. Sharrard, F.R.C.S.
Stanford T. Shulman, M.D.
Robert S. Siffert, M.D.
Michael A. Simon, M.D.
George W. Simons, M.D.
Clement B. Sledge, M.D.
Wayne O. Southwick, M.D.
Donald P. Speer, M.D.
Prof. Renato Spinelli
Jurgen Spranger, M.D.
Lynn T. Staheli, M.D.
Stanko Stanisavljevic, M.D.
Herbert H. Stark, M.D.
Howard Steel, M.D.
David H. Stulberg, M.D.
Y. Sugioka, M.D.
David H. Sutherland, M.D.
Alfred B. Swanson, M.D.
Prof. W. Taillard
David J. Thompson, M.D.
Georges R. Thuilleux, M.D.
Dietrich Tonnis, M.D.

Levon K. Topouzian, M.D.
Miguel Ferrer Torrelles, M.D.
Prof. Naoichi Tsuyama
Prof. Raoul Tubiana
Vincent J. Turco, M.D.
Prof. M.V. Volkov
Prof. Heinz Wagner
Prof. Isidor Wasserstein
R.S. Watanabe, M.D
Hugh G. Watts, M.D.
Prof. B.G. Weber
Stuart L. Weinstein, M.D
Prof. S. L. Weissman
Dennis R. Wenger, M.D.
G. Wilbur Westin, M.D.
Harvey White, M.D.
Mr. Peter Williams, F.R.C.S.
John C. Wilson, M.D.
Robert Winter, M.D.
Miss Ruth Wynne-Davies, F.R.C.S.
Yasuo Yamauchi, M.D.
Prof. Eduardo Zancolli
Seymour Zimbler, M.D.

Preface to the First Edition

This work was undertaken upon the invitation of its publisher and begun with interest and great personal involvement that have never faltered. Now that its manuscript is complete, I must seize the occasion of this prefatory statement to answer the reader's natural question: Why was it done?

I began with the perhaps-simplistic idea of providing a detailed technical presentation of surgical treatment of disorders of the neuromuscular and skeletal systems in children. I intended to write primarily for the orthopedic surgeon but I hoped also to interest physicians and surgeons of other specialties involved in the care of children.

I had no sooner set out on what proved a long and tortuous path than I began to appreciate that one cannot describe the techniques of surgery without considering also the biological principles of surgery, the dynamics of trauma, and the rationale for surgical intervention. That rationale is itself dependent upon knowledge of neuromuscular physiology and of the biomechanics of motion. One cannot speak of the management of disorder or of the amelioration of congenital defect without understanding disease process and the genesis of musculoskeletal anomaly. The surgeon who operates well performs not only with skill but also with reason; and that reason rests upon a diagnostic acumen fortified by physical examination, pathology, radiology and accurate classification. Similarly, the evaluation of surgery cannot be set out without attention to its possible complications and its aftercare.

On reflection, I realize the project I have undertaken is more ambitious than I had originally envisioned. And so I have written a long and complex book. Its very length and complexity must mean occasional omission and even error. I have tried to guard against them by citing for each important statement significant findings from the vast literature of pediatric orthopedics; but the opinions I have expressed concerning preferred methods of treatment and surgical procedure arise from personal experience and from the privilege of having learned and worked at fine teaching centers.

In another and perhaps more important way I have departed from original intent. I decided to omit chapters on the hand and on orthotics and prosthetics in the conviction that these highly individual subjects should be treated intensively and thoroughly in separate monographs.

I wish to express gratitude to John Dusseau, Editor of the W. B. Saunders Company, for the confidence he invested in me. Without his support, advice, and encouragement, this work would have been impossible.

I wish to express thanks also to the Trust Under Will of Helen Fay Hunter–Crippled Children's Fund, and to Mr. Carl A. Pfau and the Harris Trust and Savings Bank Trustees for their generous support.

The kind indulgence of the Board of Directors of Children's Memorial Hospital in allowing me the necessary time to complete this work is greatly appreciated. I also wish to thank certain of my professional colleagues and members of the orthopedic staff for their sincere cooperation during preparation of this manuscript.

With the exception of a few that have been reproduced from other works, the illustrations and operative plates are all original. The majority represent the superb artistry of Mr. Ernest Beck, to whom I am greatly indebted. I also wish to thank medical artists Wesley Bloom, Jean McConnell, Diane Nelson, and Laurel Schaubert. The diligent work of Miss Helen Silver and Mr. John Kelley of the Photography Department, Children's Memorial Hospital, must be particularly acknowledged.

The entire staff of W. B. Saunders Company, particularly Miss Ruth Barker and Mr. Raymond Kersey, are to be commended for their meticulous work during the preparation and production of the printed book.

Finally, I wish to thank Miss Eleanor Lynn Schreiner, who, in her role as my personal editor, has prepared and finalized the entire manuscript as it has been written during the past four years. Without her assistance and meticulous attention to clarity, this task would have been difficult, if not impossible, to achieve. For her unselfish dedication I shall always be grateful.

I shall conclude in the hope that if the reader learns as much from reading as the writer has from writing this monograph, its attendant trouble and trial will have been amply repaid in the better care of children.

MIHRAN O. TACHDJIAN

Contents

VOLUME 1

2

VOLUME 2

3

VOLUME 3

5

VOLUME 4

7

8

Volume 4

7. The Foot and Leg

General Considerations

INTRODUCTION

The human foot has the dual function of supporting the body in stance and propelling it in gait. It consists of three major parts: (1) the hindfoot, which includes the talus, the calcaneus, and the navicular bone; (2) the midfoot, which contains the cuneiform and the cuboid bones; and (3) the forefoot, which is made up of the metatarsals and the phalanges. Some anatomists include the navicular among the bones of the midfoot.

Architecturally, the skeletal components of the foot form a longitudinal arch, the function of which is to provide a resilient spring during locomotion. This longitudinal arch, highest medially at the midtarsal joint and shallow laterally, where it is limited by the lateral border of the foot that lies flat on the floor, is maintained by the structure and relationship of the bony parts, by the ligaments, and by the muscle tone of the four long plantar muscles—the posterior tibial, flexor digitorum longus, flexor hallucis longus, and peroneus longus.

Articulating in a complex system of multiplaned synovial joints, the components of the foot form a functional unit capable of the complex motions of flexion, rotation, inversion, eversion, and translation. For description and discussion of the mechanics of the human foot, the reader is referred to the cited literature.[1–38]

References

1. Barnett, C. H., and Napier, J. R.: The axis of rotation of ankle joint in man. Its importance upon the form of the talus and the mobility of the fibula. J. Anat., *86*:1, 1952.
2. Basmajian, J. V.: Electromyography of postural muscle. *In* Evans, F. G. (ed.): Biomechanical Studies of the Musculoskeletal System. Springfield, Ill., Charles C Thomas, 1961, pp. 136–160.
3. Basmajian, J. V.: Human locomotion. *In* Muscles Alive: Their Functions Revealed by Electromyography. 3rd Ed. Baltimore, Williams & Wilkins, 1974, pp. 205–252.
4. Brunnstrom, S.: Ankle and foot. *In* Clinical Kinesiology. 3rd Ed. Philadelphia, F. A. Davis, 1972, pp. 197–224.
5. Cordier, G.: Etude statigraphique de l'architecture de la voute plantaire. Ann. Anat. Pathol. (Paris), *16*:376, 1939–1940.
6. Elftman, H.: A cinematic study of the distribution of pressure in the human foot. Anat. Rec., *59*:481, 1934.
7. Elftman, H.: The function of muscles in locomotion. Am. J. Physiol., *125*:357, 1939.
8. Elftman, H.: The transverse tarsal joint and its control. Clin. Orthop., *16*:41, 1960.
9. Elftman, H., and Manter, J. T.: The axes of the human foot. Science, *80*:484, 1934.
10. Gardner, G. M., and Murray, M. P.: A method of measuring the duration of foot-floor contact during walking. Phys. Ther., *55*:751, 1975.
11. Grundy, M., Tosh, P. A., McLeish, R. D., and Smidt, L.: An investigation of the centers of pressure under the foot while walking. J. Bone Joint Surg., *57-B*:98, 1975.
12. Hall, M. C.: The trabecular patterns of the normal foot. Clin. Orthop., *16*:15, 1960.
13. Hall, M. C.: The Locomotor System Functional Anatomy. Springfield, Ill., Charles C Thomas, 1965.

14. Hicks, J. H.: Mechanics of the foot. J. Anat., *87*:345, 1953.
15. Hiss, J. M.: Foot in motion. *In* Functional Foot Disorders. Los Angeles, Univ. Pub. Co., 1937, pp. 35–52.
16. Houtz, S. J., and Walsh, F. P.: Electromyographic analysis of the function of the muscle acting on the ankle during weight-bearing with special reference to the triceps surae. J. Bone Joint Surg., *41-A*:1469, 1959.
17. Howorth, B.: Dynamic posture in relation to the foot. Clin. Orthop., *16*:74, 1960.
18. Huson, H. H., and Walker, P. S.: Stabilizing mechanisms of the loaded and unloaded knee joint. J. Bone Joint Surg., *58-A*:87, 1976.
19. Hutton, W. C., Stott, J. R. R., and Stokes, I. A. F.: The mechanics of the foot. *In* Klenerman, L. (ed.): The Foot and Its Disorders. Oxford, Blackwell Scientific Publications, 1976, pp. 30–48.
20. Inman, V. T.: The Joints of the Ankle. Baltimore, Williams & Wilkins, 1976.
21. Kaplan, E. B.: Some principles of anatomy and kinesiology in stabilization operation of the foot. Clin. Orthop., *34*:7, 1964.
22. Klenerman, L.: Functional anatomy. *In* Klenerman, L. (ed.): The Foot and Its Disorders. Oxford, Blackwell Scientific Publications, 1976, pp. 19–29.
23. Lambert, K.: The weight bearing function of the fibula. J. Bone Joint Surg., *53-A*:507, 1971.
24. Lapidus, P. W.: Subtalar joint. Its anatomy and mechanics. Bull. Hosp. Jt. Dis., *16*:179, 1955.
25. Levens, A. S., Inman, V. T., and Blosser, J. A.: Transverse rotation of the segments of the lower extremity in locomotion. J. Bone Joint Surg., *30-A*:859, 1948.
26. Mann, R. A.: Biomechanics of the foot. *In* American Academy of Orthopedic Surgeons: Atlas of Orthotics. Biomechanical Principles and Applications. St. Louis, Mosby, 1975, pp. 257–266.
27. Mann, R. A., and Inman, V. T: Phasic activity of intrinsic muscles of the foot. J. Bone Joint Surg., *46-A*:469, 1964.
28. Manter, J. T.: Movements of the subtalar and transverse tarsal joints. Anat. Rec., *80*:397, 1941.
29. Morris, J. M.: Biomechanics of the foot and ankle. Clin. Orthop., *122*:10, 1977.
30. Murray, M. P., Guten, G. N., Baldwin, J. M., and Gardner, G. M.: A comparision of plantar flexion torque with and without the triceps surae. Acta Orthop. Scand., *47*:122, 1976.
31. Sammarco, G. J., Burstein, A. H., and Frankel, V. H.: Biomechanics of the ankle: A kinematic study. Proceedings, American Orthopedic Foot Society. Orthop. Clin. North Am., *4*:75, 1973.
32. Sarrafian, S.: Anatomy of the Foot and Ankle. Philadelphia, Lippincott, 1983.
33. Scranton, P. E., McMaster, J. H., and Kelly, E.: Dynamic fibular function. A new concept. Clin. Orthop., *118*:76, 1976.
34. Weinert, C. R., Jr., McMaster, J. H., and Ferguson, R.: Dynamic function of the human fibula. Am. J. Anat., *138*:145, 1973.
35. Weinert, C. R., Jr., McMaster, J. H., Scranton, P. E., Jr., and Ferguson, R. J.: Human fibular dynamics. *In* Bateman, J. E. (ed.): Foot Science. Philadelphia, Saunders, 1976, pp. 1–6.
36. Weseley, M. S., Koval, R., and Kleiger, B.: Roentgen measurement of ankle flexion-extension motion. Clin. Orthop., *65*:167, 1969.
37. Wright, D. G., and Rennels, D. C.: A study of the elastic properties of plantar fascia. J. Bone Joint Surg., *46-A*:482, 1964.
38. Zitzlsperger, S.: The mechanics of the foot based on the concept of the skeleton as a statically indeterminated space framework. Clin. Orthop., *16*:47, 1960.

DEVELOPMENT AND OSSIFICATION OF THE FOOT AND LEG

The embryonic period, comprising the first seven postovulatory weeks, is the stage of organogenesis. The lower limb bud first appears in embryos of four postovulatory weeks (3 to 6 mm. crown-rump length) as a minute bud that elongates and develops in a proximal to distal direction. The foot is first seen at four and a half weeks. Soon afterward three or four digital prolongations can be observed.[1–5]

The tarsus is first distinguished as a condensed mesenchyme at five to six weeks (9 to 14 mm. crown-rump length). A few days later (at 12 to 21 mm.) chondrification begins in the center of each blastemal element. The individual bones of the foot chondrify in a definite sequence, the second to fourth metatarsals first, followed by the cuboid and fifth metatarsal. The navicular bone is the last tarsal element to chondrify. In the digits chondrification proceeds in a proximal to distal direction, with the distal phalanx of the little toe last to chondrify. By the end of the embryonic period the form and arrangement of the bony elements of the foot resemble those of an adult (Fig. 7–1). Although ossification of the foot does not occur during the embryonic period proper, the synovial joints begin to develop as "interzones" between the various elements. Thus, in considering the pathogenesis of congenital malformations of the feet, it is important to keep in mind that their structure and skeletal components are determined prior to the seventh postovulatory week of intrauterine life. Gardner, Gray, and O'Rahilly noted cartilaginous fusion between the talus and calcaneus in a 28-mm. crown-rump–length embryo, as shown in Figure 7–2; partial fusion between the lateral cuneiform, calcaneus, and cuboid bones in one embryo; and symphalangism of the middle and distal phalanges of the little toe in another embryo. A bipartite medial cuneiform bone was found in both feet of an 18-mm. embryo. Accessory tarsal cartilages were not found in the embryonic foot. The digital sesamoids may chondrify as early as seven weeks, with distribution and frequency very similar to those of the adult.[3]

Vascular invasion of the tarsus, heralding the approach of ossification, first begins in the talus. Vascular channels in the cartilaginous anlage of the talus can be seen at a length of 43 mm. and are constantly present at 78 mm. The vessels in the canals originate principally from the arteries of the sinus tarsi and the tarsal canal; it

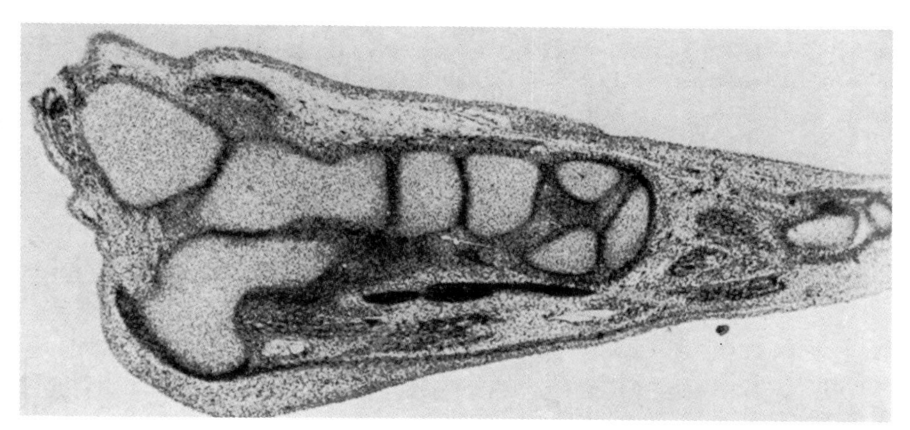

FIGURE 7–1. Sagittal section of the right foot in a 26-mm. crown to rump–length embryo.

The fibula is at the upper left, then the talus, and the calcaneus is at the lower left. × 41. (From Gardner, E., Gray, D. J., and O'Rahilly, R.: The prenatal development of the skeleton and joints of the human foot. J. Bone Joint Surg., *41*:856, 1959. Reprinted by permission.)

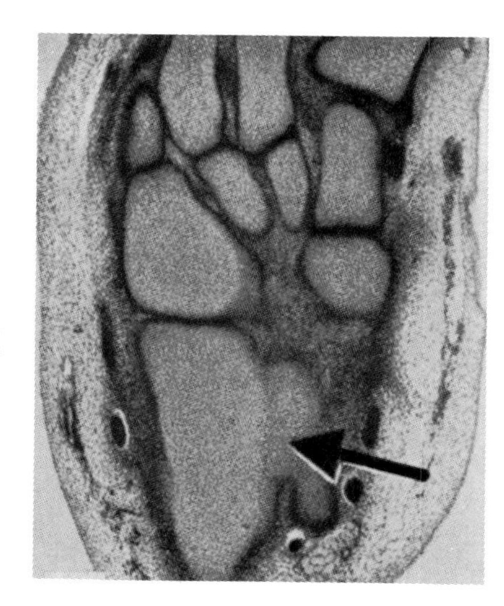

FIGURE 7–2. Horizontal section of the right foot in a 28-mm. embryo.

Note the cartilaginous fusion between the talus *(arrow)* and the os calcis. × 41. (From Gardner, E., Gray, D. J., and O'Rahilly, R.: The prenatal development of the skeleton and joints of the human foot. J. Bone Joint Surg., *41-A*:856, 1959. Reprinted by permission.)

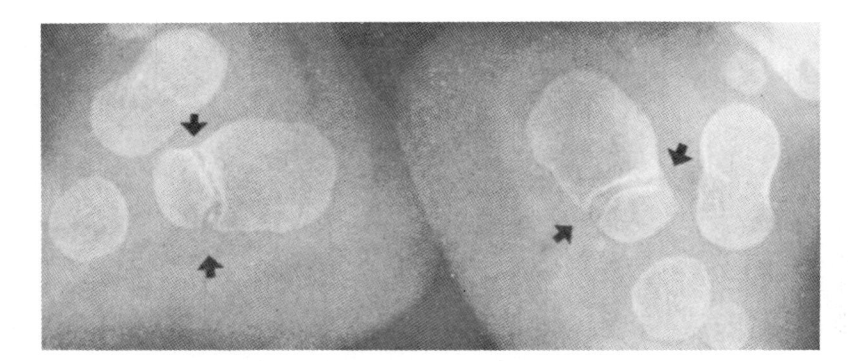

FIGURE 7–3. Two centers of ossification in the body of the calcaneus in a 20-month-old infant.

The cartilaginous line of radiolucency separating the two ossific centers should not be mistaken for a fracture. (From Caffey, J., et al.: Pediatric X-ray Diagnosis, 7th Ed., Vol 2, p. 1064. Copyright © 1978, Year Book Medical Publishers, Inc., Chicago. Reprinted by permission.)

should be noted that these vessels are the principal source of blood supply to the talus in the adult. The vascular invasion then proceeds in the calcaneus, navicular, cuboid, cuneiforms, metatarsals, and phalanges.

Ossification in the foot first begins in the tips of the distal phalanges and then advances proximally. Soon after, periosteal bone collars are formed around the metatarsal shafts, and later around the proximal and middle phalanges, in that sequential order.

The calcaneus is the first of the tarsal bones to begin ossification; its primary ossific center appears between the first and sixth fetal months. Occasionally the body of the calcaneus appears to have two centers (Fig. 7–3). The apophysis of the os calcis begins to ossify at four to six years of age in girls, and at five to nine years in boys; it fuses with the body of the calcaneus toward 16 years in the female and 20 years in the male. The talus is the second tarsal bone to ossify, usually about the eighth fetal month. Ossification of the cuboid bone takes place at or near birth, but it may be delayed until 21 days of age. In the tarsus, at birth, the primary centers of ossification of the calcaneus, talus, and cuboid bone are usually present. The average age for ossification of the lateral cuneiform bone is 4 to 20 months; for the medial cuneiform, two years; and for the intermediate cuneiform, three years. The navicular ossifies between the second and fifth years (Figs. 7–4 and 7–5).

The primary centers of ossification of the second and third metatarsals appear at the ninth week of fetal life, whereas those of the fourth and fifth metatarsals appear at the tenth week. The secondary centers of ossification arise at the epiphyses, which are distally located; they are visible between three and four years of age, appearing in a variable order. The epiphyses of the lateral four metatarsals fuse with the diaphyses between the ages of 16 and 18 years. The primary ossific center of the first metatarsal is visible at the twelfth week of fetal life, and the secondary center for the epiphysis (located proximally) appears between three and four years; it fuses with the diaphysis at between 16 and 18 years.

The cartilaginous sesamoids can be distinguished early in the fetal period—between 30 and 45 mm. The ossification of the medial and lateral sesamoids of the big toe usually takes place between 12 and 14 years of age, but sometimes as early as 8 years. The sesamoids of the second and fifth toes are not constant; if present they ossify late, after 15 years of age.

The tibia and fibula can be seen as mesenchymal condensations at the fifth week (about 11 to 13.5 mm.). Soon chondrification commences. At this early stage the fibula is in contact with the calcaneus. At the eighth week the malleoli chondrify. The primary center of ossification of the tibia appears at the ninth week of intrauterine life. Toward the eighth or ninth month of fetal life, the proximal epiphysis of the tibia begins to ossify; the ossific center of the distal tibial epiphysis does not appear until between the sixth and tenth months of postnatal life. The medial malleolus begins to ossify at seven years in girls and at eight years in boys (Fig. 7–6). The proximal tibial tubercle begins to ossify between 7 and 11 years. In the fibula the primary center of ossification appears at the tenth week of fetal life. The distal epiphysis appears between the eleventh and eighteenth postnatal months, and the upper epiphysis begins to ossify between two and five years. Both the upper and lower epiphyses fuse with the diaphysis between 18 and 22 years of age.

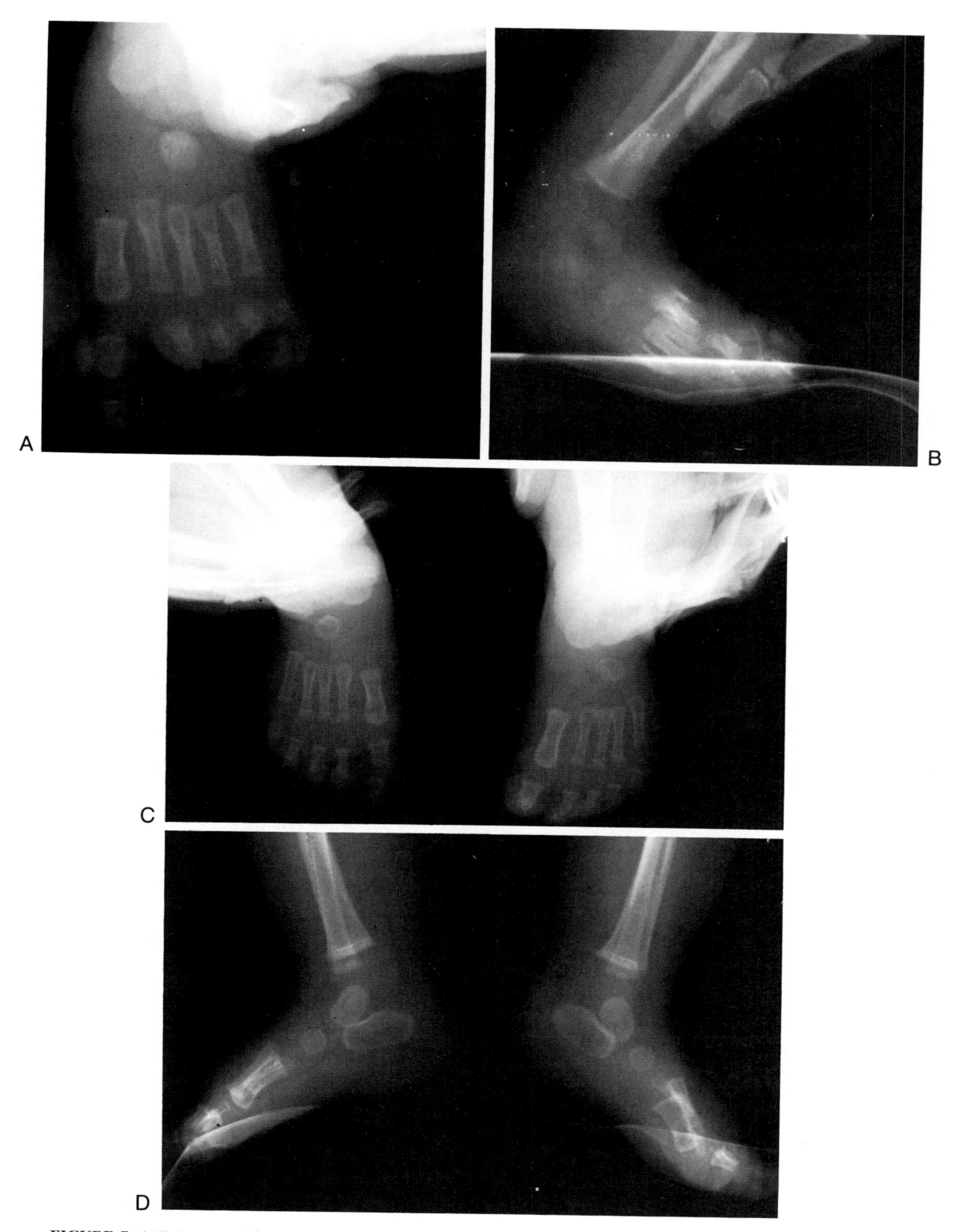

FIGURE 7–4. Primary ossification centers of the calcaneus, talus, and cuboid bones seen in radiograms at birth.
A and **B.** Anteroposterior and lateral projections of right foot.
C and **D.** Anteroposterior and lateral radiograms of the feet at seven months of age.

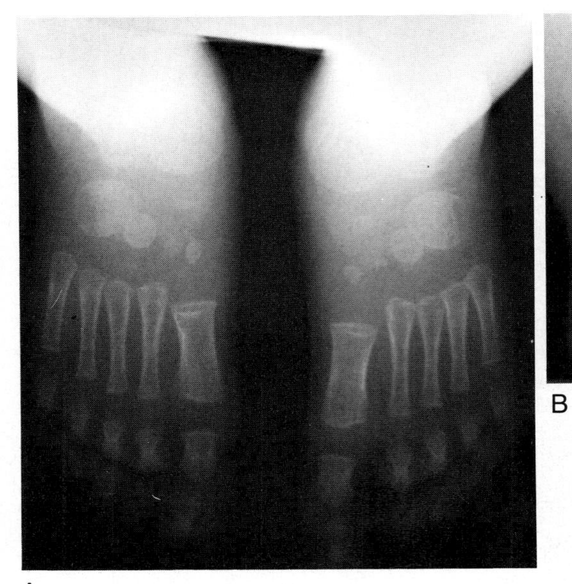

A

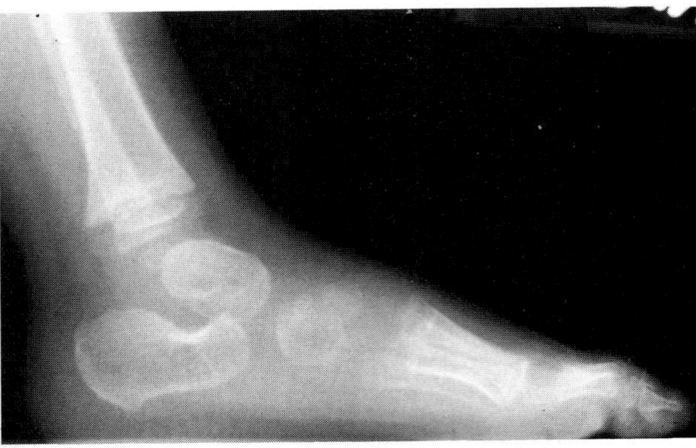

B

FIGURE 7–5. Ossification of the tarsal bones and metatarsals in a three-year-old-boy.

A. Anteroposterior radiogram of both feet.
B. Lateral radiogram of right foot. Note that the medial and intermediate cuneiform and navicular bones are ossified.

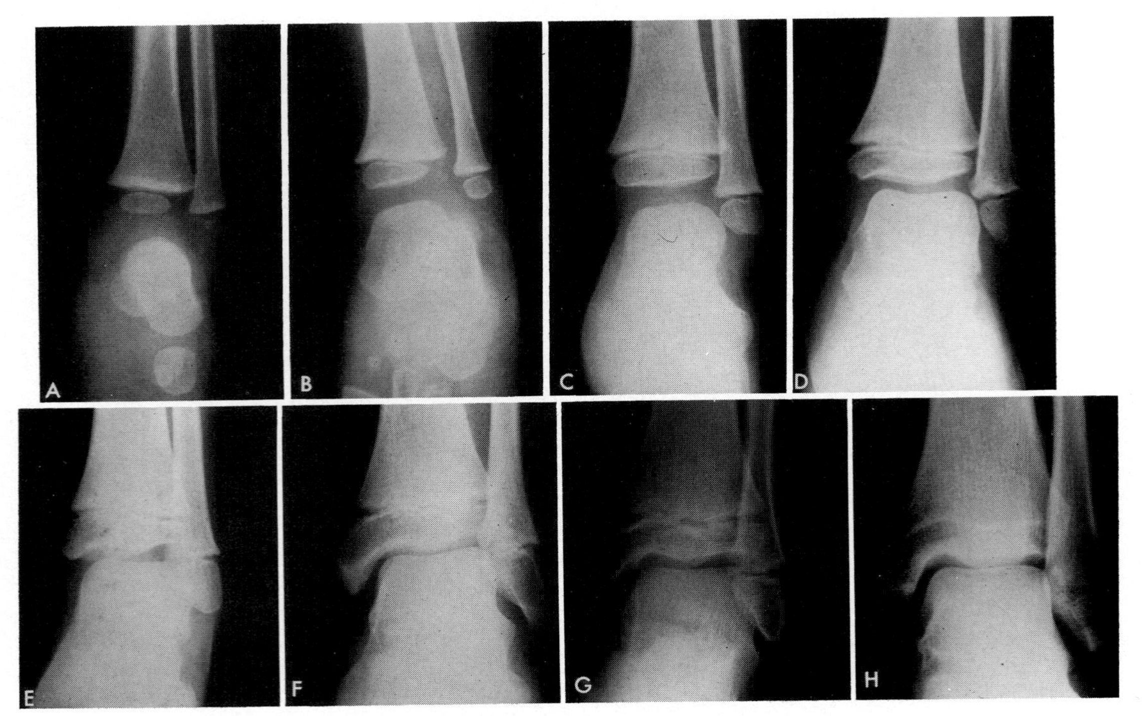

FIGURE 7–6. Ossification of distal epiphyses of tibia and fibula.

A. One year of age. **B.** Two years. **C.** Four years. **D.** Six years. **E.** Seven years. **F.** Ten years. **G.** Twelve years. **H.** Adult.

References

1. Barlow, T. E.: Some observations on the development of the human foot. Thesis, University of Manchester, 1943.
2. Elftman, H., and Manter, J. T.: The evolution of the human foot, with especial reference to the joints. J. Anat., *70*:56, 1935.
3. Gardner, E., Gray, D. J., and O'Rahilly, R.: The prenatal development of the skeleton and joints of the human foot. J. Bone Joint Surg., *41-A*:847, 1959.
4. Harris, B. J.: Observations on the development of the human foot. Thesis, University of California, 1953.
5. O'Rahilly, R., Gardner, E., and Gray, D. J.: The skeletal development of the foot. Clin. Orthop., *16*:7, 1960.
6. Straus, W. L., Jr.: Growth of the human foot and its evolutionary significance. Contrib. Embryol., *19*:93, 1927.

GROWTH OF THE NORMAL FOOT

The pattern of longitudinal growth of the foot is an important consideration in the planning of surgical procedures. Blais, Green, and Anderson have provided normal standards for the length of the growing foot (Fig. 7–7 and Table 7–1). The feet of both boys and girls grow at a sharply decreasing rate from infancy through the age of five years. Then from 5 to 12 years of age in girls and from 5 to 14 years of age in boys, the average increase in the length of the foot is 0.9 cm. per year. This rate of growth decreases markedly after 12 years of age in females and after 14 years of age in males, and the foot attains its mature length at the average age of 14 years in girls and 16 years in boys. Blais, Green, and Anderson also observed that at all times during the growth period, the size of the foot is relatively closer to its adult size than is the total height or the length of the femur and tibia of the same individual. For example, at the age of one year in girls and at one and one half years in boys, the foot has achieved half of its mature length. The femur and tibia, on the other hand, reach half their mature length at three years of age in girls and four years in boys. Thus, the factors that would disturb growth would affect the ultimate length of the foot proportionately less than they would

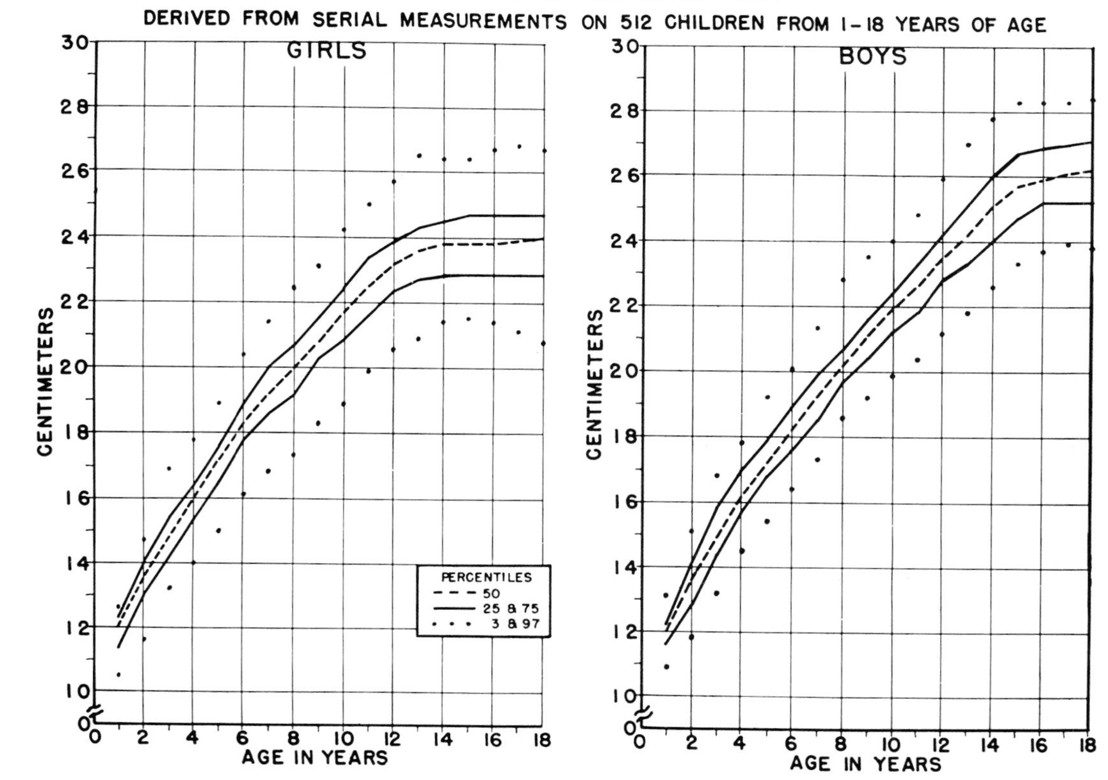

FIGURE 7–7. Length of the growing foot.

Length of normal foot derived from serial measurements of 512 children from 1 to 18 years of age. (From Blais, M. M., Green, W. T., and Anderson, M.: Lengths of the growing foot. J. Bone Joint Surg., *38-A*:998, 1956. Reprinted by permission.)

*Table 7–1. Length of the Normal Foot**

Girls Percentile 3	25	50	75	97	Age	Boys Percentile 3	25	50	75	97
10.5	11.4	12.0	12.3	12.6	1	10.9	11.6	12.0	12.2	13.1
11.6	13.0	13.6	14.0	14.7	2	11.8	12.8	13.6	14.1	15.1
13.2	14.3	14.8	15.4	16.9	3	13.2	14.4	14.9	15.8	16.8
14.0	15.4	16.0	16.4	17.8	4	14.5	15.7	16.2	17.0	17.8
15.0	16.5	17.2	17.6	18.9	5	15.4	16.8	17.2	17.9	19.2
16.1	17.8	18.3	18.9	20.4	6	16.4	17.6	18.2	18.9	20.1
16.8	18.6	19.2	20.0	21.4	7	17.3	18.5	19.2	19.9	21.3
17.3	19.2	20.0	20.7	22.4	8	18.6	19.7	20.2	20.7	22.8
18.3	20.3	20.8	21.5	23.1	9	19.2	20.4	21.1	21.6	23.5
18.9	20.9	21.7	22.4	24.2	10	19.9	21.2	21.9	22.4	24.0
19.9	21.6	22.5	23.4	25.0	11	20.4	21.8	22.6	23.3	24.8
20.6	22.3	23.2	23.9	25.7	12	21.2	22.8	23.5	24.2	25.9
20.9	22.7	23.6	24.3	26.5	13	21.8	23.3	24.2	25.1	27.0
21.4	22.8	23.8	24.5	26.4	14	22.6	24.0	25.1	26.0	27.8
21.5	22.8	23.8	24.7	26.4	15	23.3	24.7	25.7	26.7	28.3
21.4	22.8	23.8	24.7	26.7	16	23.7	25.2	25.9	26.9	28.3
21.1	22.8	23.9	24.7	26.8	17	23.9	25.2	26.1	27.0	28.3
20.8	22.8	24.0	24.7	26.7	18	23.8	25.2	26.2	27.1	28.4

*Caliper measurements in centimeters in weight-bearing position derived from semilongitudinal series of 227 girls and 285 boys.

From Blais, M. M., Green, W. T., and Anderson, M.: Lengths of the growing foot. J. Bone Joint Surg., *38-A*:999, 1956. Reprinted by permission.

the femur or the tibia. If, for example, the linear growth of the foot is completely arrested at the skeletal age of 10 years in girls or at 12 years in boys, the result would be an average reduction in adult length of the foot of only 10 per cent (about 2.5 cm.); or if at the skeletal age of 12 years in girls and 14 years in boys, of only 3 per cent (or about 1 cm.).[1]

Reference

1. Blais, M. M., Green, W. T., and Anderson, M.: Length of the growing foot. J. Bone Joint Surg., *38-A*:998, 1956.

NORMAL VARIATIONS OF THE BONES OF THE FOOT AND ANKLE

The growing tarsal and metatarsal bones are characterized by numerous variations that may simulate pathologic conditions. The orthopedic surgeon should be familiar with these normal anatomic variations in order not to misinterpret them as fractures, osteochondritis, or diseases of bone.

Accessory Bones of the Foot

Numerous accessory bones in the foot have been described. These are shown in the diagrams in Figure 7–8. In the feet of about 22 per cent of children under 16 years of age, one or more accessory bones may be found on radiograms.[49] The accessory navicular and os trigonum are described here in detail because of their clinical importance.

ACCESSORY TARSAL NAVICULAR

The accessory tarsal navicular (also referred to in the literature as *os tibiale externum* or *prehallux*) is present as a separate bone in about 10 per cent of human beings. It has been demonstrated to be a separate center of ossification for the tuberosity of the navicular in the fetus. In adolescence it frequently coalesces with the contiguous navicular; in about 2 per cent of the population, however, it persists as a separate ossicle. It is often bilateral, and may be bifid.

The accessory tarsal navicular is located at the medial end of the navicular. The posterior tibial tendon is attached to it, passing across the medial aspect of the navicular instead of underneath it. Thus, the dynamic support of the longitudinal arch of the foot normally afforded by the posterior tibial muscle is weakened. The result is planovalgus deformity of the foot. Following prolonged walking, the patient will complain of pain in the midfoot. Shoe pressure on the accessory bone may also cause

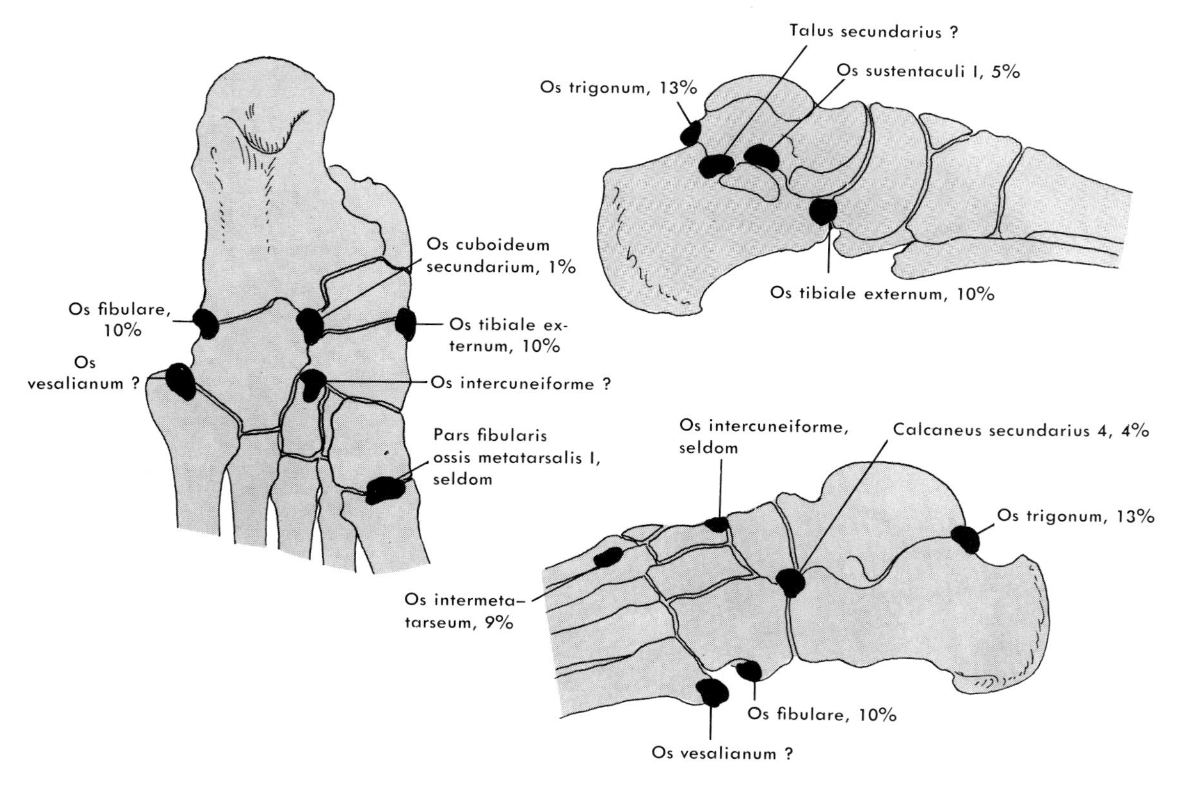

FIGURE 7–8. Accessory bones in the foot.

(Adapted from von Lanz, T., and Wachsmuth, W.: Praktische Anatomie. Berlin, Julius Springer, 1938, p. 359.)

the formation of an inflamed adventitious bursa with local swelling and tenderness (Fig. 7–9 A). There may be associated nonspecific tenosynovitis of the posterior tibial tendon. In the radiograms, the accessory bone will be visible medially and proximal to the navicular bone (Fig. 7–9 B). Its smooth and rounded outline differentiates it from the irregular margin that characterizes a fracture. In later adolescence, the accessory navicular may fuse with the body of the tarsal bone and present as an abnormally prominent and curved medial end of the navicular (Fig. 7–10). This is referred to as a *cornuted navicular* and produces the same symptoms as the accessory navicular.

Initially, treatment should be conservative. A ⅜-inch felt longitudinal arch support is placed in the shoe. When pain is acute, hydrocortisone may be injected into the adventitious bursa and the inflamed posterior tibial tendon sheath, and the foot immobilized in a below-knee walking plaster cast for a period of three weeks.

If symptoms persist and do not respond to these measures, surgical excision of the accessory navicular with rerouting of the posterior tibial tendon to a point well on the plantar aspect of the navicular (Kidner procedure) is performed.[25, 26]

In the Kidner operation the incision is approximately 5 cm. long and begins 1 cm. inferior and 2 cm. distal to the distal tip of the medial malleolus and extends forward to the base of the first metatarsal bone. The subcutaneous tissue and deep fascia are divided, and the wound margins are retracted to expose the posterior tibial tendon and the medial tip of the navicular bone. The posterior tibial tendon inserts into the tuberosity of the navicular bone, into the plantar surfaces of the three cuneiform bones and of the bases of the second, third, and fourth metatarsal bones, and into the cuboid bone. It is detached only from its insertion to the accessory navicular, its other attachments being left intact.

The accessory navicular bone is excised and the medial surface of the navicular is resected until it is flush with the talus and cuneiform. Bleeding cancellous bone is coagulated with electrocautery. The posterior tibial tendon is

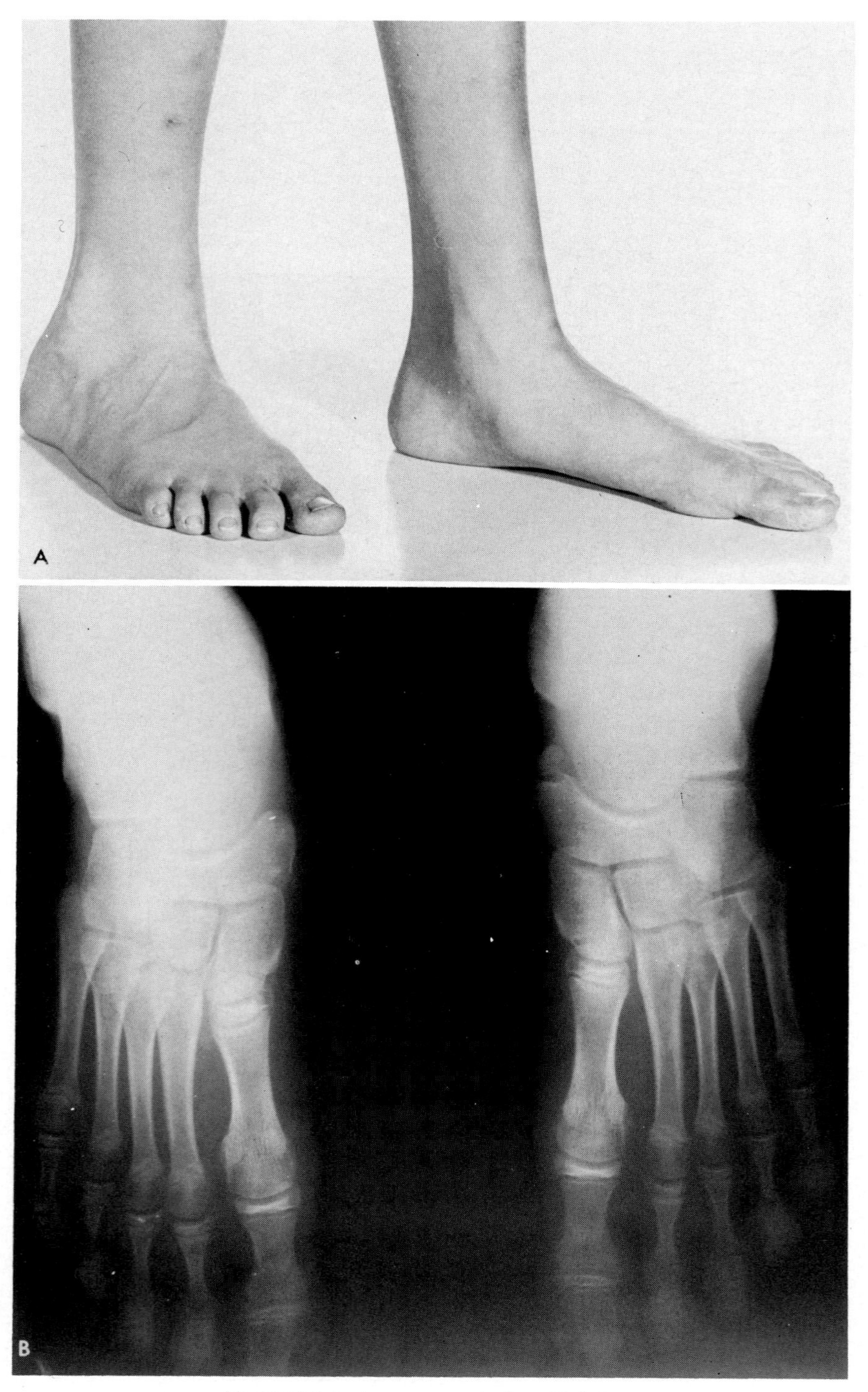

FIGURE 7–9. Accessory navicular of left foot.

A. Clinical appearance—showing the local swelling. **B.** Radiographic appearance. Note the smooth and rounded outline of the accessory ossicle.

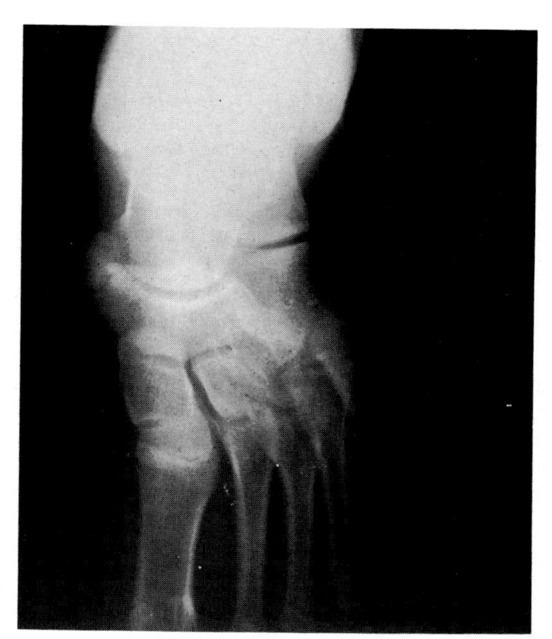

FIGURE 7–10. Accessory navicular fused with the body of the tarsal navicular (cornuted navicular).

transferred laterally and plantarward on the undersurface of the navicular, where it is anchored under tension to the periosteum and plantar ligaments with two or three interrupted sutures. Usually it is not necessary to make drill holes through the navicular. The wound is closed, and a below-knee walking cast is applied.

The cast is removed in three to four weeks, following which a longitudinal arch support is used. The result of the Kidner procedure is good. Pain will subside. One should not, however, expect correction of pes planovalgus deformity in the adolescent.

OS TRIGONUM

On the posterior aspect of the talus there is a groove for the flexor hallucis longus tendon. The bony tubercle lateral to this tendon groove is usually larger than the medial one, and if elongated, it is known as "Stieda's process." Between 8 and 11 years of age, separate centers of ossification appear for the medial and lateral tubercles, and they quickly (usually within a year) fuse with the main body of the talus. The posterior fibers of the lateral ligament of the ankle joint are attached to the lateral tubercle. When the ankle is in full plantar flexion the posterior tubercles of the talus come in full contact with the posterior edge of the distal end of the tibia, serving as a bony block. Repeated minor injury in an active person may cause failure of union of the posterolateral tubercle, which then persists as a separate center of ossification known as *os trigonum* (Fig. 7–11). A fused but large ossicle may be detached by sudden violence, particularly when union of the ossicle to the talus is by synchondrosis (Fig. 7–12). The absence of irregularity between the os trigonum and the main body of the talus distinguishes synchondrosis from a fracture. In doubtful cases, an air arthrogram will settle the diagnosis (Fig. 7–13).[32]

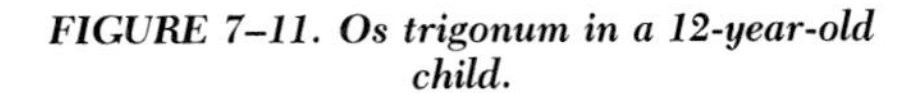

FIGURE 7–11. Os trigonum in a 12-year-old child.

Note also the accessory navicular visible in the lateral projection. The sclerosis of the apophysis of the os calcis is normal.

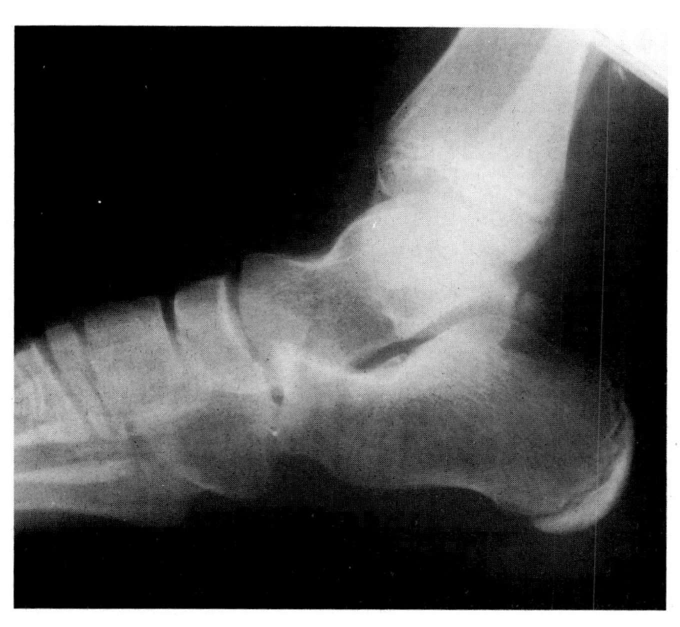

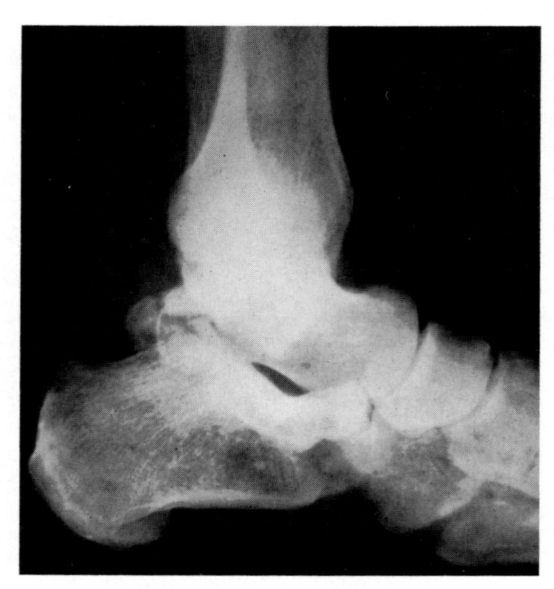

FIGURE 7–12. Fracture of fused os trigonum.

MISCELLANEOUS ACCESSORY BONES

Only a brief listing of the accessory bones and normal anatomic variations of the foot and ankle is given here; for a detailed description the reader should consult the comprehensive reviews of Caffey, O'Rahilly, Trolle, and other cited references.[4, 39, 49, 60]

Medial Malleolus. This may have a separate ossification center (Fig. 7–14). In the literature, the reports of its incidence vary. Selby found it in 47 per cent of girls and 17 per cent of boys, whereas Powell reports 20 per cent.[42, 48] The average age of appearance of a separate center of ossification for the medial malleolus is 7.6 years for girls and 8.7 years for boys; by the twelfth year, the extra center of ossification fuses with the main center.

Distal End of Fibula. The lateral malleolus has a separate center of ossification in 1 per cent of cases. A small accessory ossicle is occasionally present in a notch in the distal fibular metaphysis and should not be mistaken for osteochondritis dissecans; also on oblique views of the lateral malleolus, an area of rarefaction in the medial surface of the distal fibular epiphysis should not be misdiagnosed as a destructive bone lesion.

Talus. In addition to os trigonum, an accessory bone may develop on the dorsal aspect of the head of the talus (os sustentaculare). A separate center of ossification for the head of the talus is a very rare anomaly. *Africoid talus* is a developmental anomaly in which the head and neck of the talus are tilted dorsally (Fig. 7–15).

Os Calcis. A triangular or circular area of radiolucency may appear in the inferior half of the body of the calcaneus, suggesting a pseudocyst (Fig. 7–14 B). It is a normal variation and not a deficiency of spongy bone, occurring in about 10 per cent of children older than seven years.

The enlarged trochlea of the calcaneus may be mistaken for an exostosis.

The apophysis of the os calcis begins to ossify at four to six years of age in the female and at four to nine years in the male. Often a secondary center of ossification in the calcaneal apophysis develops in girls between 10½ and 12 years and in boys between 11½ and 13½ years; it quickly fuses with the body of the calcaneus. A secondary center of ossification may also be present in the tip of the trochlear process on the lateral wall of the calcaneus. Occasionally the body of the calcaneus may ossify from two centers of ossification instead of one, the cartilaginous junction between the two ossific nuclei suggesting a fracture. Sclerosis and fragmentation of the apophysis of the calcaneus are common (see Fig. 7–11).

Cuboid, Navicular, Cuneiforms. Multiple fine ossification centers may be present in the cuboid. In addition to an accessory navicular there may be a small ossicle on the dorsum of the navicular—os supranaviculare. The edges of the cuneiforms may be irregular.

Metatarsals. An accessory ossicle at the base of the fifth metatarsal is quite common (Fig. 7–16); occasionally it may have a fish-scale appearance, simulating a fracture. The distal end of the first metatarsal may have an incomplete synchondrosis.

Phalanges. The skeletal variations of the digits of the foot are numerous. The reader is referred to the statistical study of Venning.[63]

In the hallux the number of phalanges is almost always two, though occasionally a three-phalangeal big toe may be encountered. The lesser toes usually have three phalanges. Not infrequently the fifth toe may have two phalanges, and occasionally the second, third, and fourth toes may have a two-phalangeal form. With the exception of the big toe, toes with two phalanges are nearly always lateral to the toes having three phalanges. The two-phalangeal lesser toes are more preponderant in the female.

The middle phalanx may lack an epiphysis or may be entirely absent. The ossification centers of the epiphyses of the phalanges, particularly the proximal phalanx, may be cone-shaped,

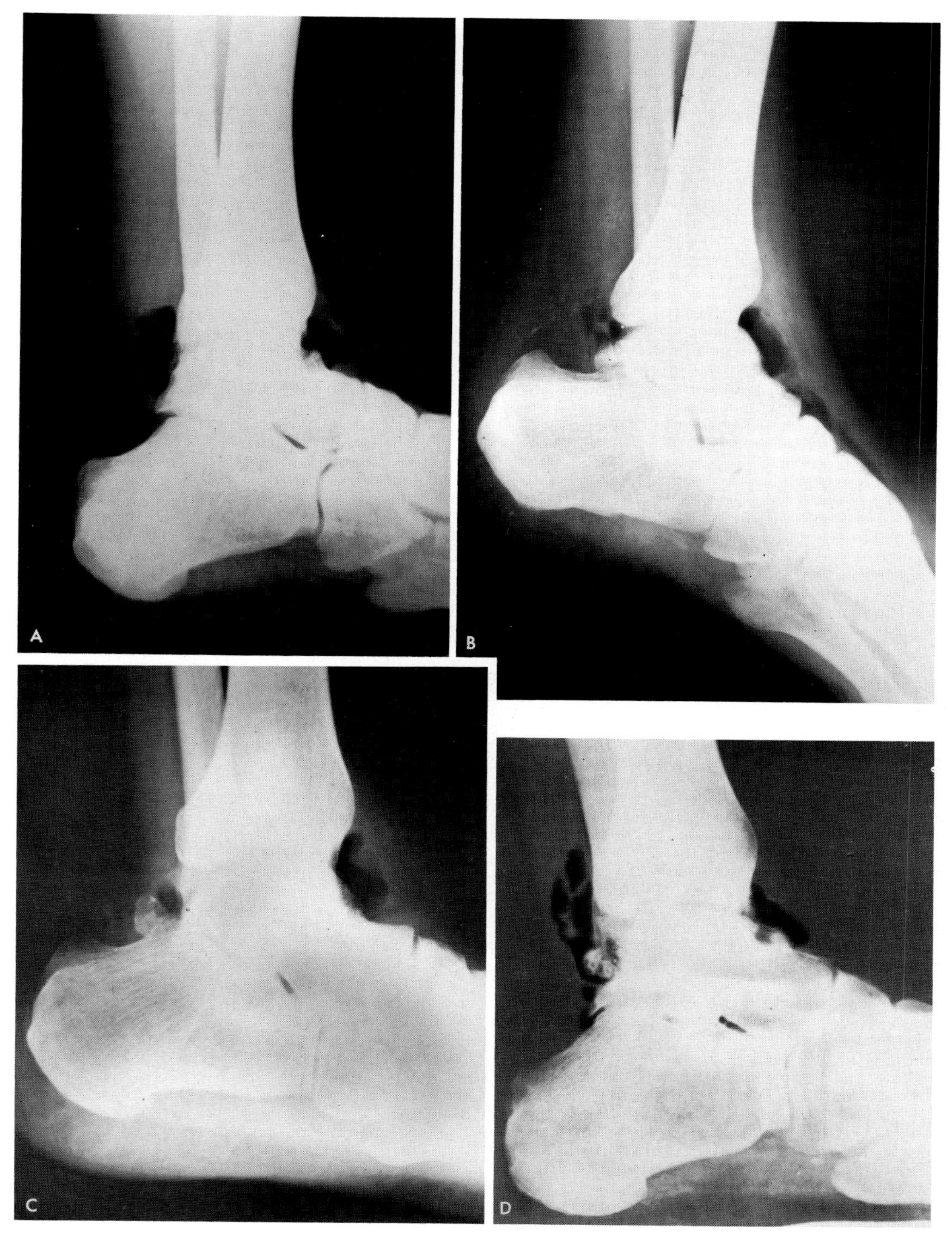

FIGURE 7–13. ***Arthrogram of the ankle.***

A. A normal ankle. **B.** An ankle with os trigonum. Note that the radiolucent shadow cast by the air is located superior to the os trigonum. **C.** In a fracture of a fused os trigonum, the air has sandwiched itself between the detached accessory bone and the main body of the talus. **D.** In an osteocartilaginous loose body of the ankle the air shadow surrounds the loose bone. (Courtesy of Dr. H. Kelikian.)

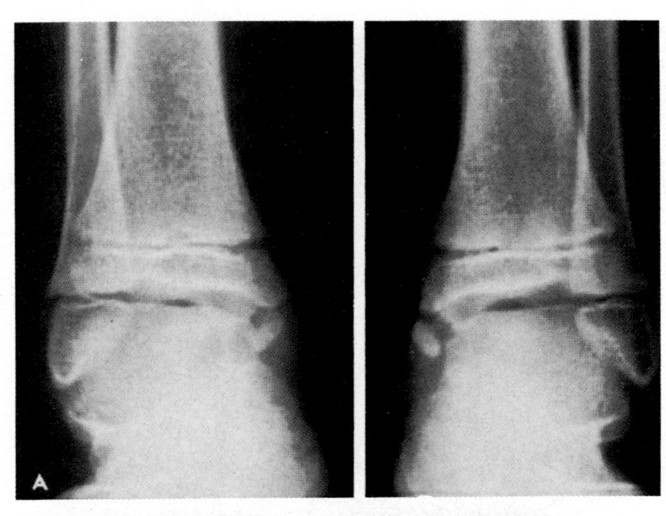

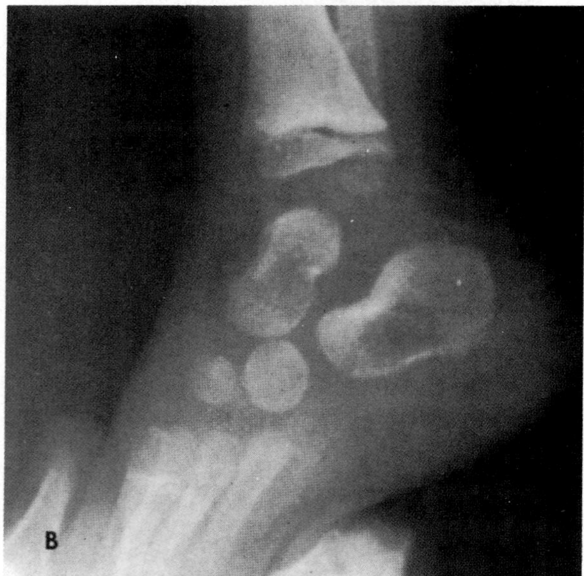

FIGURE 7–14. Normal anatomic variations of the foot and ankle.

A. Accessory ossification center of medial malleolus. **B.** Area of rarefaction in body of os calcis simulating cyst.

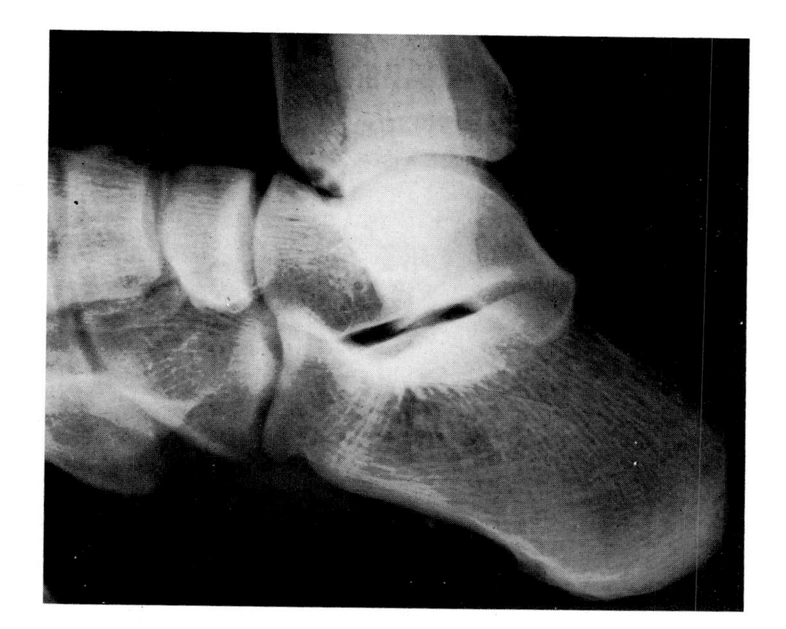

FIGURE 7–15. Africoid talus.

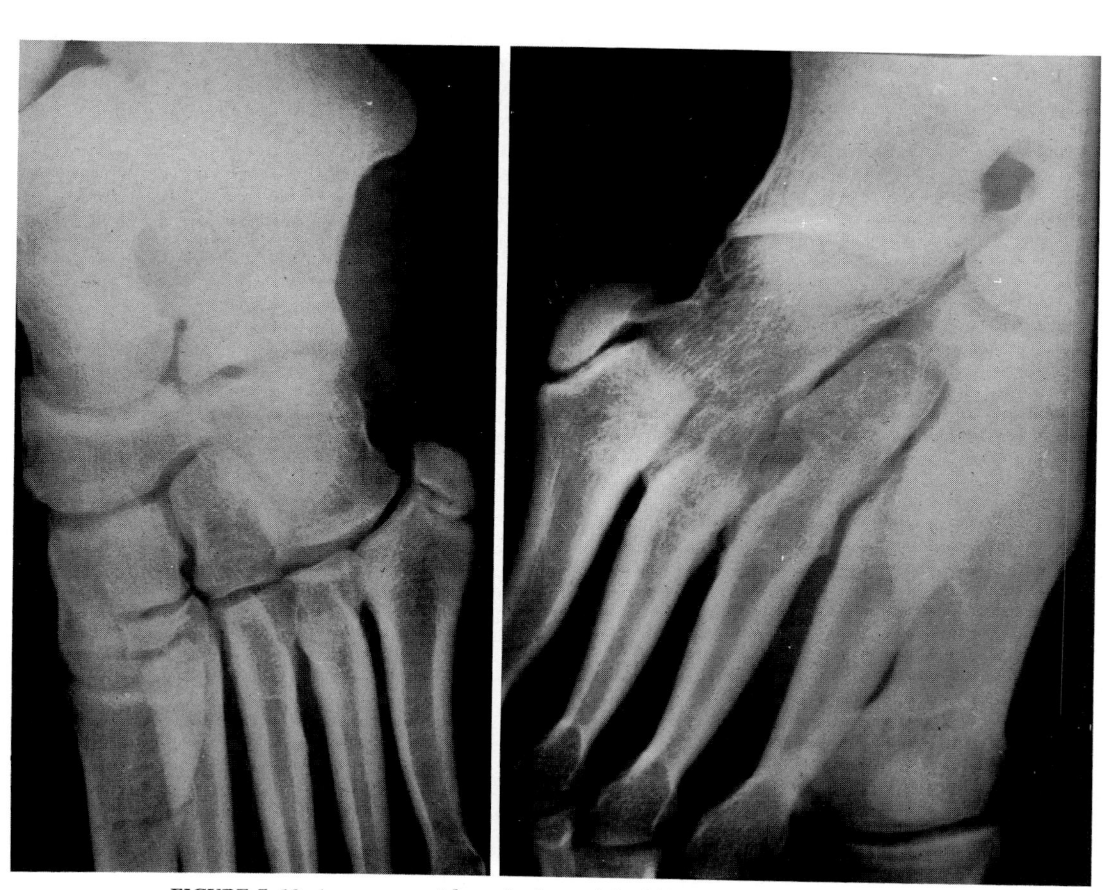

FIGURE 7–16. Accessory ossicle at the base of the fifth metatarsal (os vesalianum).

invaginating into the diaphysis. Fissuring of the epiphyses of the proximal phalanx of the hallux is another variation. The sesamoid may be bipartite and have to be distinguished from fracture.

References

1. Basmajian, J. B., and Stecko, G.: The role of muscles in arch support of the foot. J. Bone Joint Surg., *45-A*:1184, 1963.
2. Bautrier: Cited by Meyer, M., Cuny, J., and Trensz, F.: L'os tibial externe et ses divers aspects radiologiques. Strasbourg Med., *85*:24, 1927.
3. Bjornson, R. G. B.: Developmental anomaly of the lateral malleolus simulating fracture. J. Bone Joint Surg., *38-A*:128, 1956.
4. Caffey, J.: Pediatric X-Ray Diagnosis. 5th Ed. Chicago, Year Book, 1967, p. 744.
5. Chater, E. H.: Foot pain and the accessory navicular bone. Ir. J. Med. Sci., *422*:471, 1962.
6. Dale, G. C., and Harris, W. R.: Prognosis in epiphyseal separation: An experimental study. J. Bone Joint Surg., *40-B*:116, 1958.
7. DuVries, H. L.: *In* Mann, R. A. (ed.): Surgery of the Foot. St. Louis, Mosby, 1978, p. 105.
8. Dwight, T.: Variations of the Bones of the Hands and Feet. Philadelphia, Lippincott, 1907.
9. Faber, A.: Os tibiale externum bein erbgleichen Zwillingen. Erbartz, *4*:83, 1934.
10. Fere, C. H., and Deniker, M.: Note sur des exostosis symetriques des scaphoides tarsiens. Rev. Chir., *29*:544, 1904.
11. Francillon, M. R.: Untersuchungen zur anatomischen und klinischen Bedeutung des Os tibiale externum. Z. Orthop. Chir., *56*:61, 1932.
12. Froelich, R.: Des osselets surnumeraires du tarse et de leur importance pratique. Rev. Med. de l'Est, *41*:433, 1909.
13. Geist, E. S.: Supernumerary bones of the foot: A roentgen study of the feet of 100 normal individuals. Am. J. Orthop. Surg., *12*:403, 1914.
14. Geist, E. S.: The accessory scaphoid bone. J. Bone Joint Surg., *7*:570, 1925.
15. Giannestras, N. J.: Foot Disorders: Medical and Surgical Management. 2nd Ed. Philadelphia, Lea & Febiger, 1973.
16. Gottlieb, C., and Berenbaum, S. L.: Pirie's bone, accessory ossicle on the dorsum of the astragalus—often bilateral. Radiology, *55*:423, 1950.
17. Guntz, E.: Os tibiale und Unfall (Abriss des Os tibiale). Arch. Orthop. Unfallchir., *34*:320, 1933.
18. Haglund, P.: Über Fraktur des Tuberculum ossis navicularis in den Jugendjahren und ihre Bedeutung als Ursache einer typischen Form von Pes valgus. Z. Orthop. Chir., *16*:347, 1906.
19. Harding, V. V.: Time schedule for the appearance and fusion of a secondary center of ossification of the calcaneus. Child Develop., *23*:181, 1952.
20. Harris, R. I., and Beath, T.: Army Foot Survey. Vol. 1. Ottawa, National Research Council of Canada, 1947, p. 52.
21. Hohmann, G.: Fuss und Bein. 5th Auflage Munchen, J. F. Bergmann, 1951.
22. Hubay, C. A.: Sesamoid bones of the hands and feet. A.J.R., *61*:493, 1949.
23. Jones, B. S.: Flat foot: A preliminary report of an operation for severe cases. J. Bone Joint Surg., *57-B*:279, 1975.
24. Jones, R. L.: The human foot. An experimental study of its mechanics and the role of its muscles and ligaments in the support of the arch. Am. J. Anat., *68*:1, 1941.
25. Kidner, F. C.: The prehallux (accessory scaphoid) in its relation to flatfoot. J. Bone Joint Surg., *11*:831, 1929.
26. Kidner, F. C.: The prehallux in relation to flatfoot. J.A.M.A., *101*:1539, 1933.
27. Kienbock, R., and Muller, W.: Os tibiale externum und Verletzung des Fusses. Z. Orthop. Chir., *66*:257, 1937.
28. Langelaan, E. J.: A kinematical analysis of the tarsal joints. An x-ray photogrammetric study. Acta Orthop. Scand. (Suppl.), *204*:1, 1983.
29. Latten, W.: Histologische Beziehungen zwischen Os tibiale und Kahnbein nach Untersuchungen an einem operierten Falle. Dtsch. Z. Chir., *205*:320, 1927.
30. Lawson, J. P., Ogden, J. A., Sella, E., and Barwick, K. W.: The painful accessory navicular. Skeletal Radiol., *12*:250, 1984.
31. Leonard, M. H., Gonzales, S., Breck, L. W., Bason, C., Palafox, M., and Kosicki, Z. W.: Lateral transfer of the posterior tibial tendon in certain selected cases of pes plano valgus (Kidner operation). Clin. Orthop., *40*:139, 1965.
32. McDougall, A.: The os trigonum. J. Bone Joint Surg., *37-B*:257, 1955.
33. Macnicol, M. F., and Voutsinas, S.: Surgical treatment of the systematic accessory navicular. J. Bone Joint Surg., *66-B*:218, 1984.
34. Marti, T.: Kasuistischer Beitrag zum Studium des Os tibiale externum. Praxis, *51*:828, 1962.
35. Meyer, M., Cuny, J., and Trensz, F.: L'os tibial externe et ses divers aspects radiologiques. Strasbourg Med., *85*:24, 1927.
36. Monahan, J. J.: The human pre-hallux. Am. J. Med. Sci., *160*:708, 1920.
37. Mygind, H. B.: The accessory tarsal scaphoid. Acta Orthop. Scand., *23*:142, 1953.
38. Niederecker, K.: Der Plattfuss. Stuttgart, Ferdinand Enke, 1959.
39. O'Rahilly, R.: A survey of carpal and tarsal anomalies. J. Bone Joint Surg., *35-B*:254, 1953.
40. Perry, J.: Anatomy and biomechanics of the hindfoot. Clin. Orthop., *177*:9, 1983.
41. Pfitzner, W.: Beitrage zur Kenntnis des menschlichen Extremitatenskeletts. VII. Die Variationen im Aufbau des Fussskeletts. Schwalbe's Morph. Arb., *6*:245, 1896.
42. Powell, H. D. W.: Extra centre of ossification for the medial malleolus in children. Incidence and significance. J. Bone Joint Surg., *43-B*:107, 1961.
43. Ray, S., and Goldberg, V. M.: Surgical treatment of the accessory navicular. Clin. Orthop., *177*:61, 1983.
44. Roche, A. F., and Sunderland, S.: Multiple ossification centers in the epiphyses of the long bones of the human hand and foot. J. Bone Joint Surg., *41-B*:375, 1959.
45. Ross, S. E., and Caffey, J.: Ossification of the calcaneal apophysis in healthy children: Some normal radiologic features. Stanford Med. Bull., *15*:224, 1957.
46. Salter, R. B., and Harris, W. R.: Injuries involving the epiphyseal plate. J. Bone Joint Surg., *45-A*:587, 1963.
47. Schlüter, K.: Der "Calcaneus bifidus," cine Ossifikationsanomalie des Fersenbeines im Hackenplattfuss. Fortschr. Roentgenstr., *85*:720, 1956.
48. Selby, S.: Separate centers of ossification of the tip of the internal malleolus. A.J.R., *86*:496, 1961.
49. Shands, A. R., Jr.: The accessory bones of the foot. South. Med. Surg., *93*:326, 1931.
50. Shands, A. R., Jr., and Wentz, I. J.: Congenital anomalies, accessory bones, and osteochondritis in the feet of 850 children. Surg. Clin. North Am., *33*:1643, 1953.
51. Shereff, M. J., and Johnson, K. A.: Radiographic anatomy of the hindfoot. Clin. Orthop., *177*:16, 1983.
52. Sirry, A.: The pseudocystic triangle in the normal os calcis. Acta Radiol., *36*:516, 1951.
53. Smith, A. D., Carter, J. R., and Marcus, R. E.: The os vesalianum: An unusual cause of lateral foot pain. Orthopedics, 7:86, 1984.

54. Smith, R. W., and Staple, T. W.: Computerized tomography (CT) scanning technique for the hindfoot. Clin. Orthop., *177*:34, 1983.
55. Specht, E. E.: Minor congenital deformities and anomalies of the foot. *In* Inman, V. T. (ed.): DuVries' Surgery of the Foot. St. Louis, Mosby, 1973, pp. 54–58.
56. Stewart, S. F.: Human gait and the human foot: An ethnological study of the flatfoot. Part I. Clin. Orthop., *70*:111, 1970.
57. Strayhorn, G., and Puhl, J.: The symptomatic accessory navicular bone. J. Fam. Pract., *15*:59, 1982.
58. Sullivan, J. A., and Miller, W. A.: The relationship of the accessory navicular to the development of the flat floot. Clin. Orthop., *144*:233, 1979.
59. Swenson, P. C., and Wilner, D.: Unfused ossification centers associated with pain in the adult. A.J.R., *61*:341, 1949.
60. Trolle, D.: Accessory Bones of the Human Foot. Copenhagen, Munksgaard, 1948.
61. Trott, A. W.: Children's foot problems. Orthop. Clin. North Am., *13*:641, 1982.
62. Veitch, J. M.: Evaluation of the Kidner procedure in the treatment of symptomatic accessory tarsal scaphoid. Clin. Orthop., *131*:210, 1978.
63. Venning, P.: Variation of the digital skeleton of the foot. Clin. Orthop., *16*:26, 1960.
64. Wiley, J. J., and Brown, D. E.: The bipartite tarsal scaphoid. J. Bone Joint Surg., *63-B*:583, 1981.
65. Wood, J. F.: Structure and function as seen in the foot. London, Balliere, Tindall & Cox, 1949.
66. Zadek, I.: The significance of the accessory tarsal scaphoid. J. Bone Joint Surg., *8*:618, 1926.
67. Zadek, I., and Gold, A. M.: The accessory tarsal scaphoid. J. Bone Joint Surg., *30-A*:957, 1948.

Congenital Deformities of the Foot

POSTURAL DEFORMITIES OF THE FOOT AND LEG

Confinement of the human fetus in unnatural positions in the uterus may cause a number of postural deformities of the limbs and trunk. In the foot and leg, intrauterine malpostural deformities are talipes valgus, metarsus adductus, and postural clubfoot. Other common sequelae of intrauterine malposture are: in the knee, extension contracture; in the hip, congenital pelvic obliquity with abduction contracture of one hip and adduction contracture of the contralateral hip; in the spine, infantile scoliosis; and in the head and neck, torticollis and plagiocephaly.

Postural deformities are nonteratologic fetopathies, arising in the postembryonic period after organogenesis; they are the result of deformation of a normally formed part. In contrast, malformations are defects that arise during the period of organogenesis—i.e., they are teratologic embryopathies. The distinguishing features of the two groups are shown in Table 7–2.

Historically Hippocrates proposed a causal relation between postural deformations of the limbs and mechanical forces acting in utero.[12] Browne, Chapple and Davidson, and Dunn have studied the problem in detail.[2, 3, 6–8] Malposition may exist only during a particular phase of development of the limbs, i.e., it may be temporal in addition to being spatial.

The incidence of postural deformations has been investigated by Dunn.[6–8] Of 4,754 infants born in the Birmingham Maternity Hospital, 4,486 (94.4 per cent) were normally formed, 170 (3.6 per cent) were malformed (with or without additional deformities), and 98 (2.0 per cent) had postural deformations. Multiple deformities (two or more) were found in 33 per cent of the cases; there was a total of 151 distinct deformations among the 98 infants. These figures indicate that various postural deformities have a common mechanical origin. Dunn also demonstrated a highly significant clinical association between main groups of postural deformities (Table 7–3).

Normal human fetal posture is dependent upon the sequential development of neuromuscular function. The structural development of the central and peripheral nervous systems proceeds in a craniocaudal direction. Consequently, coordinated muscular contractions appear first in the head and neck, then in the upper limbs, the trunk, and the lower limbs. With activation of different muscle groups the limbs assume different postures. In the human the structural development of the lower limb is usually complete by the end of the eighth week of intrauterine life. With the anatomic level of innervation of muscle groups beginning proximally and proceeding distally, the sequential postures of the lower limbs are as follows: first, hip flexion and medial rotation (L1–L2 level of innervation of iliopsoas muscle); second, hip adduction (L2–L3 level of innervation of hip adductors); and third, knee extension (L3–L4 level of innervation of quadriceps femoris muscle). Therefore, the posture of the lower limbs of the human fetus at the twelfth week of gestation is one of hip flexion–medial rotation–adduction and knee extension (Fig. 7–17 A). This extended breech posture is normal at this stage of development.

The next stage of development of posture in the human fetus is folding of the extended lower limbs as sustained contraction of the short lateral rotators of the hip (level of innervation L4, L5, S1) is activated and the whole lower limb

Table 7–2. Distinguishing Characteristics of Congenital Malformations and Congenital Postural Deformities

	Malformation	*Postural Deformation*
Period of development	Embryonic—during organogenesis (teratologic embryopathy)	Postembryonic—after normal formation of the parts (nonteratologic fetopathy)
Incidence at birth	3.6 per cent*	2.0 per cent*
Structural alterations	Common	Very rare
Response to passive manipulation	Not correctable	Correctable
Spontaneous correction	No	Usual

*Data from Dunn, P. M.: Congenital postural deformities: Perinatal associations. Proc R. Soc. Med., 65:735, 1972.

rotates laterally and the patellae face outward (Fig. 7–17 B). Then the knees flex with activation and sustained contraction of the hamstrings (level of innervation L5, S1, S2). Folding of the lower limbs makes room for trunk flexion to take place, which always precedes cephalic version. The activation of the gluteus maximus (L5, S1, and S2) brings the hips into further lateral rotation. Activity of the peroneals, toe extensors, and anterior tibial muscles (L4, L5, and S1) will make the foot assume a dorsiflexed and everted posture; finally, the foot will be drawn into plantar flexion and inversion with activity of the triceps surae and posterior tibial muscles (L5, S1, and S2). Leg folding takes place between 12 and 26 weeks and vertex posture develops between 26 and 40 weeks of intrauterine life (Fig. 7–17 C).

Arrest of development will cause failure of leg folding, which in turn will prevent spinal flexion and cephalic version from taking place. Arrest of lateral rotation of the hip and flexion of the knee will produce a persistent intrauterine posture in which the hips are flexed and medially rotated and the knees extended (Fig. 7–18). If lateral rotation of the hip takes place but knee flexion is arrested, the hips are locked in flexion and lateral rotation, and the knees in extension (Fig. 7–19). These postures, if present beyond the twenty-eighth week of intrauterine life, constitute breech malposition.

In a survey of 4,000 radiograms of the pelves of pregnant women, Vartan found that breech presentation is common and should be considered normal at the appropriate period of development. The breech posture of about 25 per cent of the fetuses persisted at the thirtieth week. Cephalic version did not take place in those with knees completely extended and hips medially rotated, whereas those with semiflexed

*Table 7–3. Clinical Association Between Certain Postural Deformations: Statistical Analysis**

	Facial Deformities	*Plagiocephaly*	*Mandibular Asymmetry*	*Sternomastoid Contracture*	*Scoliosis (Postural)*	*Congenital Dislocation of Hip*	*Talipes*
Facial deformities	—	S	S+	S	S+	S+	S+
Plagiocephaly	S	—	S+	S+	S+	S+	N
Mandibular asymmetry	S+	S+	—	S+	N	S+	S+
Sternomastoid contracture	S	S+	S+	—	S+	N	S+
Scoliosis (postural)	S+	S+	N	S+	—	S+	S
Congenital dislocation of hip	S+	S+	S+	N	S+	—	S+
Talipes	S+	N	S+	S+	S	S+	—

(N, not significant. S, $P < 0.05$. S+, $P < 0.001$.)

*From Dunn, P. M.: Congenital postural deformities. Perinatal associations. Proc. R. Soc. Med., 65:736, 1972. Reprinted by permission.

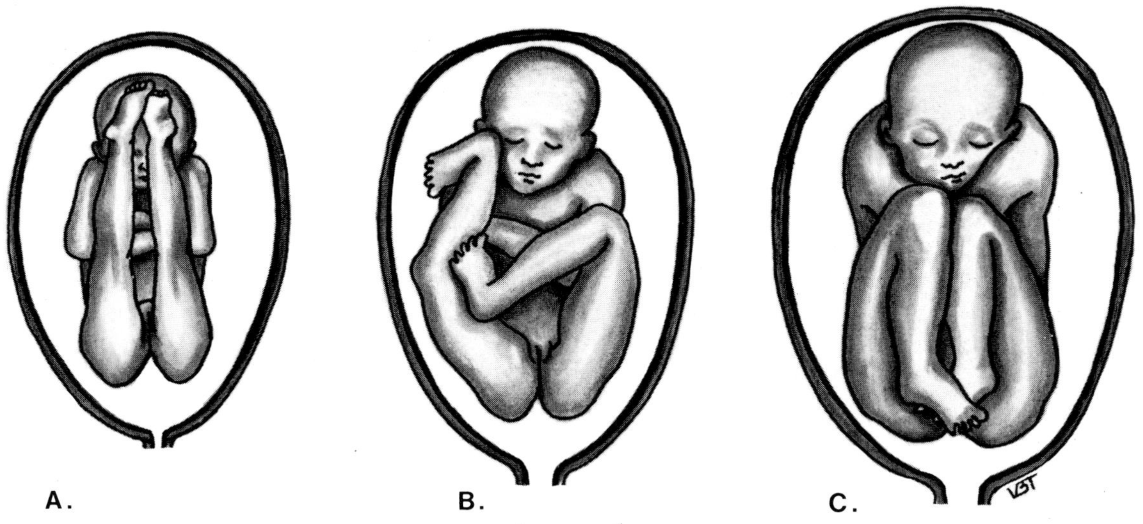

FIGURE 7–17. Development of intrauterine posture.

A. Stage I, extended breech posture. Note the hips are flexed, medially rotated, and adducted, and the knees extended. This is the normal position of the lower limbs in the 8- to 12-week-old human fetus. **B.** Stage II, leg-folding posture. Note the hips are laterally rotated and the knees flexed. Folding of the leg allows trunk flexion to take place, which always precedes cephalic version. The feet are dorsiflexed and everted. This is normal posture for a 12- to 26-week-old fetus. **C.** Stage III, vertex posture. Note the spine is flexed. The ankles and feet are in plantar flexion and inversion. This posture develops between 26 and 40 weeks. (Redrawn from Wilkinson, J. A.: Breech malposition and intrauterine malposition. Proc. R. Soc. Med., 59:1107, 1966.)

knees and laterally rotated hips did undergo cephalic version.[27]

Talipes Calcaneovalgus

This postural deformity is characterized by the dorsiflexion and eversion of the entire foot. The soft tissues on the dorsum and lateral aspect of the foot are contracted and limit plantar flexion and inversion (Fig. 7–20). The degree of severity of deformity varies; in severe cases the foot may touch the anterior aspect of the tibia (Fig. 7–21). Radiograms of the foot and ankle are normal. There is no subluxation or

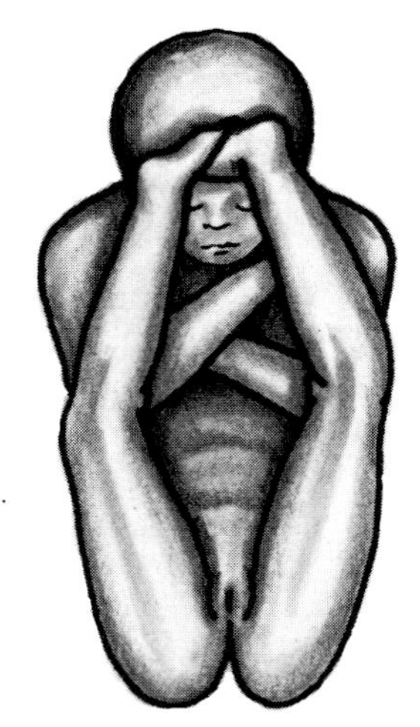

FIGURE 7–18. Neonatal medial rotation breech malposture.

Note the hips are flexed and medially rotated, and the knees are extended. (Redrawn from Wilkinson, J. A.: Breech malposition and intrauterine malposition. Proc. R. Soc. Med., 59:1107, 1966.)

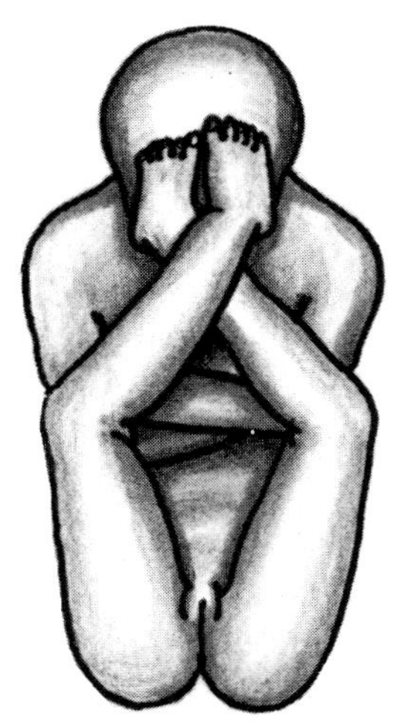

FIGURE 7–19. Neonatal lateral rotation breech malposture.

The hips are flexed and laterally rotated, and the knees are in extension. (Redrawn from Wilkinson, J. A.: Breech malposition and intrauterine malposition. Proc. R. Soc. Med., 59:1107, 1966.)

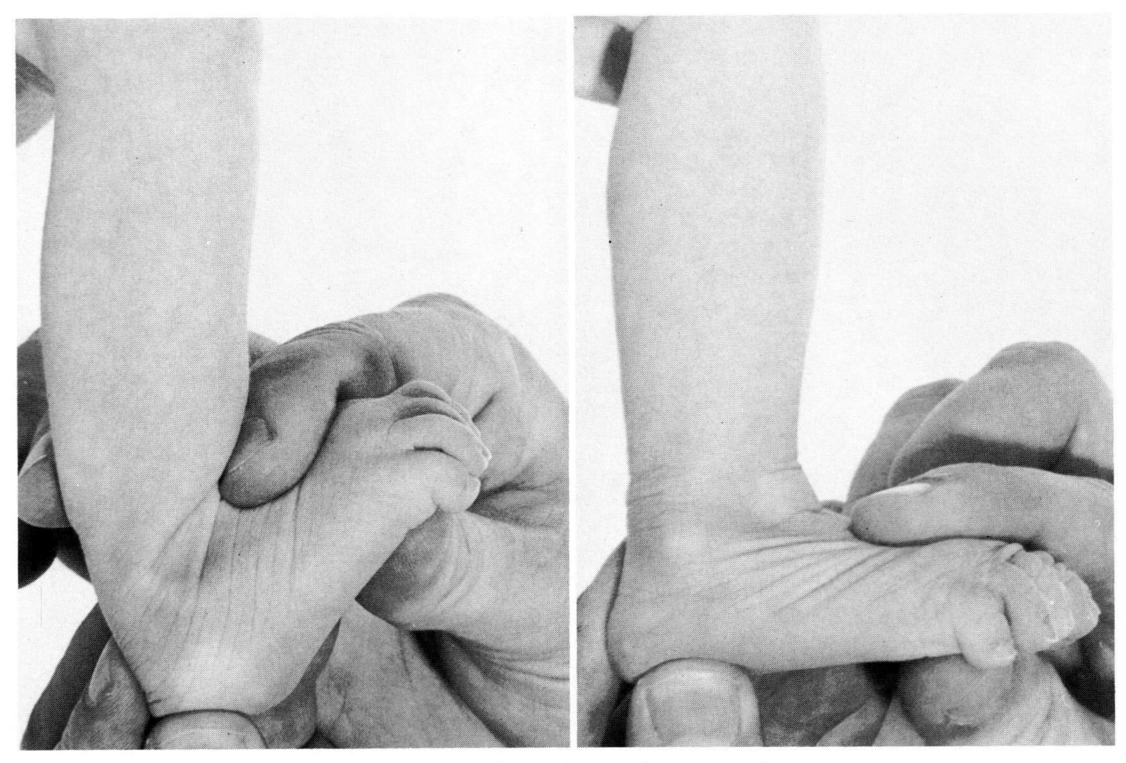

FIGURE 7–20. Talipes calcaneovalgus in an infant.

The foot is dorsiflexed and everted. Note that plantar flexion is limited to neutral position.

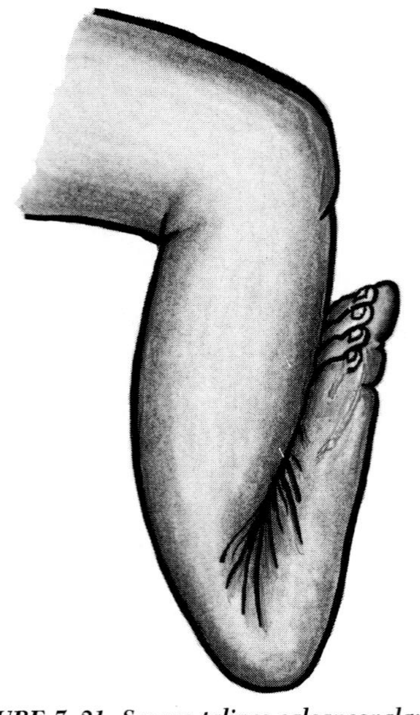

FIGURE 7–21. Severe talipes calcaneovalgus in a newborn.

Note the foot touching the anterior aspect of the tibia. Always examine the hips to rule out congenital dislocations.

dislocation of the tarsal joints and no secondary adaptive bone changes or hypoplasia of the ossification centers.

Talipes calcaneovalgus is the most common deformity of the foot seen at birth. Wetzenstein states that the incidence varies between 30 and 50 per cent.[28] Wynne-Davies, in her family studies, found it to be approximately one per thousand live births. It may be higher, however, as some cases may go unnoticed or ignored.[30] Talipes calcaneovalgus is more common in girls than in boys, with a male-to-female ratio of 0.61:1. Its incidence is significantly greater among first-born children and children of young mothers. The probable cause is intrauterine malposture—the environmental factor being compression acting late in pregnancy, particularly in the primigravida with a small "tight" uterus and strong abdominal muscles.

It is important to distinguish talipes calcaneovalgus from congenital convex pes planovalgus. In the latter, the talocalcaneonavicular joint is dislocated dorsolaterally; the talus is locked in vertical position, the forefoot is in eversion and abduction, and the hindfoot is fixed in equinus position, giving a "rocker-bottom" shape to the sole of the foot. Radiograms of the foot should be taken in doubtful cases. Neuromuscular diseases, particularly spina bifida occulta with neurologic deficit, must be excluded. It is important to demonstrate function in the triceps surae, posterior tibial, and long toe flexor muscles. The hips should be examined to rule out congenital dislocation.

The prognosis is excellent. Mild deformities—if the foot can be plantar-flexed and inverted beyond neutral position—require no treatment. Within three to six months the feet resume normal alignment spontaneously. Moderate deformities—i.e., if it is difficult to plantar-flex the foot and invert it to neutral position by passive manipulation—are treated by daily passive stretching exercises performed by the mother. The shortened dorsolateral muscles and soft tissues are elongated by plantar-flexing and inverting the foot, maintaining the stretched position to the count of 10, and then releasing it. The exercises are performed 20 to 30 times in four sessions daily. Severe and resistant deformities are treated by stretching the soft-tissue contractures by manipulation and retaining the foot in the corrected position with plaster casts or Denis Browne splints, both of which hold the foot in equinovarus posture. Within four to six weeks the deformity will be completely corrected.

Larsen, Reimann, and Becker-Andersen investigated the value of treatment in 125 cases of talipes calcaneovalgus of which 49 per cent were treated with manipulation and elastic bandage and 51 per cent were untreated and observed by regular follow-up examinations. The contractural deformity was marked in 39 per cent of the treated group and 28 per cent of the untreated group. On comparison of the results, there was no significant difference between the two groups. The severity of the contractures found at birth appeared to have no influence on the final results. The follow-up period was 3 to 11 years. At the follow-up examination, the majority of the feet were normal. The only residual finding was pronation of the feet when the infants began to stand and walk. In the series of Larsen, Reimann, and Becker-Andersen, the hindfoot valgus deviation was 0 to 10 degrees in 75 per cent and 10 to 20 degrees in 25 per cent. In 45 per cent of the unilateral cases, the residual valgus deviation of the hindfoot was within the normal range but more exaggerated than on the unaffected side.[15] Giannestras has also noted the high degree of correlation between talipes calcaneovalgus in the newborn and flexible flat foot in the older child.[10] Clinical experience of this author concurs with that of Giannestras; therefore, conservative treatment of moderate and severe cases of talipes calcaneovalgus as just outlined is recommended.

Talipes Varus

In postural talipes varus the forefoot is adducted and inverted, and the hindfoot is inverted, but the range of dorsiflexion of the ankle and foot is normal, a feature that differentiates it from postural clubfoot (Fig. 7–22). Palpation reveals the navicular in normal relation to the head of the talus. One or two fingers can be easily inserted between the medial malleolus and the navicular. The talocalcaneonavicular joint is not subluxated medially. There are no adaptive osseous structural changes. The deformity is flexible, and the foot can be easily manipulated into normal position. The contralateral foot may be in valgus posture. The hips should be examined for congenital pelvic obliquity—with adduction contracture of the hip on the side with talipes varus and abduction contracture of the one on the side with talipes valgus. There is frequent association of these combinations of postural deformities. One should also rule out congenital dislocation of the hip, postural scoliosis, and torticollis.

Treatment consists of manipulative stretching of the foot into valgus position and retention in a below-knee cast. The cast is changed at weekly intervals, the foot being manipulated each time before the application of the new cast. The prognosis is excellent. The deformity will usually be completely corrected within two to four weeks. When this has been achieved, in severe cases the use of a polypropylene or other plastic below-knee splint may be indicated to hold the foot in the corrected position. The infant wears the splint only at night. Passive stretching exercises are performed by the mother several times a day. With this regimen of therapy a normal foot can be expected in three to four months.

Postural Talipes Valgus

In this type of postural deformity, both the forepart of the foot and the hindfoot are everted and abducted; the range of dorsiflexion and plantar flexion of the ankle is normal. Treatment consists of passive stretching exercises and retention of the foot in a below-knee cast. Within three to six weeks full correction of the deformity can be expected.

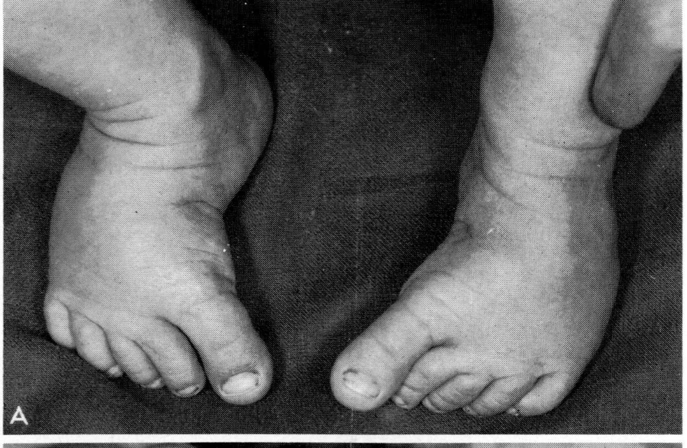

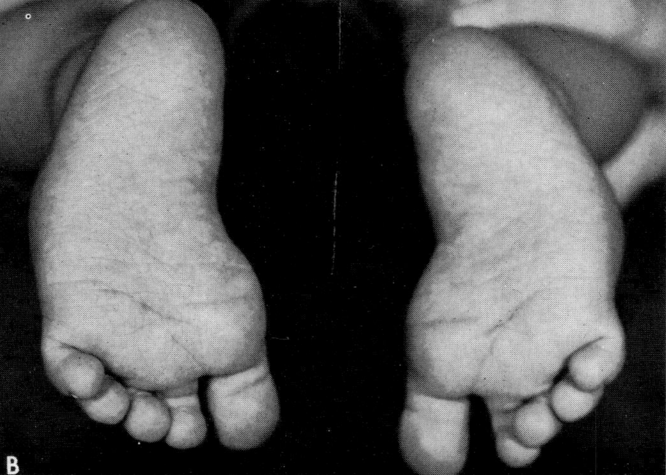

FIGURE 7–22. Bilateral talipes varus.

A. Dorsal view. **B.** Plantar view. The forefoot is inverted and adducted, the hindfoot is inverted, but the range of dorsiflexion of the foot and ankle is normal.

Postural Metatarsus Adductus

In this type of postural deformation of the foot only the forepart of the foot is adducted; the position of the hindfoot is neutral or slightly valgus (Fig. 7–23 A). The articular relations of the tarsometatarsal joints are normal. There is no structural deformity. This condition should be distinguished from congenital metatarsus varus, which is a medial subluxation of the tarsometatarsal joint. In postural metatarsus adductus the forefoot can be brought to neutral position easily, whereas in congenital metatarsus varus the forefoot deformity is rigid, resisting passive manipulation (Fig. 7–23 B and C). Usually no treatment is required. Spontaneous correction within three to four months is the rule. The markedly adducted forefeet can be passively manipulated into abduction several times a day by the mother.

Postural Clubfoot

The forepart of the foot is adducted and inverted, and the hindfoot is inverted in this deformation. The whole foot is plantar-flexed at the ankle so that the toes are carried lower than the heel. The condition is caused by intrauterine malposture. Anatomically the talocalcaneonavicular joint has normal articular relations and shows neither medial nor plantar subluxation. The head and neck of the talus are *not* tilted medially; i.e., the declination angle of the talus is normal. On examination, the skin creases are normal and there are no furrows on the medial and plantar aspects of the midfoot; the navicular does not abut the medial malleolus. The heel is of normal size. There is no calf atrophy. On manipulation the deformity is not rigid. In the literature, postural clubfoot is referred to as extrinsic type of congenital talipes

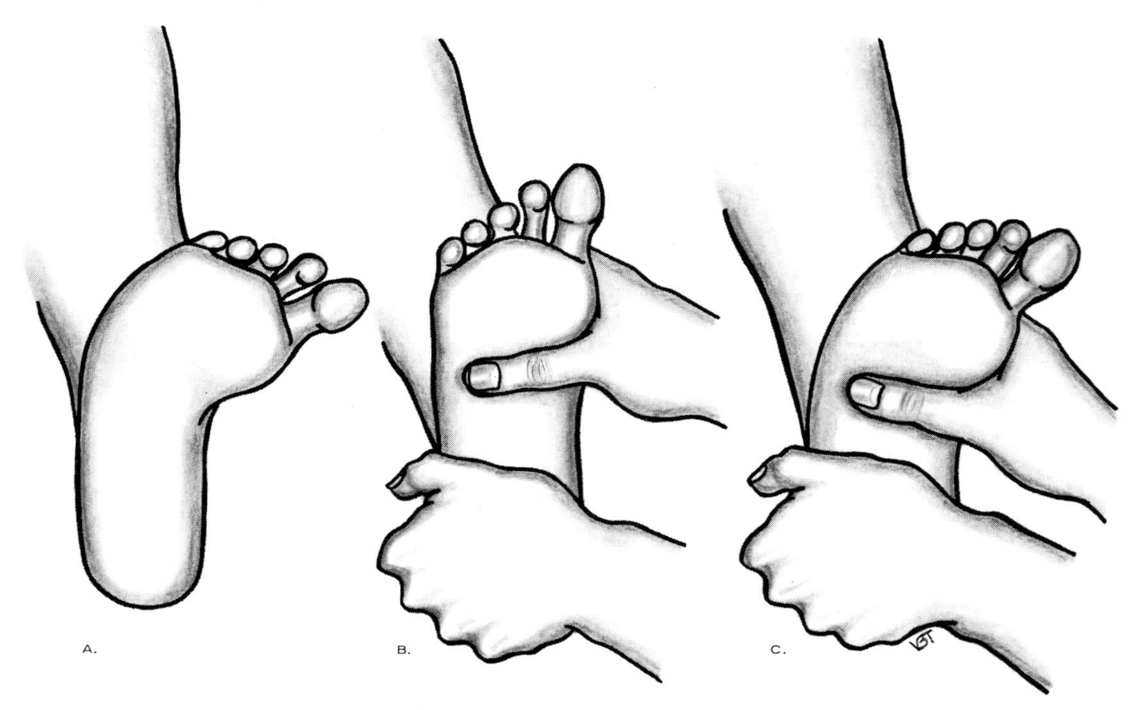

FIGURE 7–23. Postural metatarsus adductus and congenital metatarsus varus.

A. In both conditions the forefoot is adducted. In congenital metatarsus varus the varus deviation of the forefoot is greater and the valgus deviation of the heel is greater. **B.** In postural metatarsus adductus the forefoot can be easily manipulated into neutral position. **C.** In congenital metatarsus varus the forefoot deformity is rigid, resisting passive manipulation.

equinovarus. For the sake of simplicity, however, the author recommends reserving the term *congenital talipes equinovarus* for the true medioplantar displacement of the talocalcaneonavicular joint.

Treatment consists of manipulative stretching of the foot into valgus position and dorsiflexion, and its retention in the corrected position. The choice of retentive apparatus varies with the surgeon's past experience. This author uses a plaster of Paris cast. Others may prefer Robert Jones adhesive strapping or the Denis Browne foot splint. It does not matter which of the aforementioned types of retentive devices is applied.

The prognosis is excellent. With the foregoing regimen of therapy, a normal foot should be obtained within two to three months. The features distinguishing postural clubfoot from congenital talipes equinovarus are given in Table 7–7, page 2451.

References

1. Aronson, J., Nunley, J., and Frankovitch, K.: Lateral talocalcaneal angle in assessment of subtalar valgus: Follow-up of seventy Grice-Green arthrodeses. Foot Ankle, *4*:56, 1983.
2. Browne, D.: Congenital deformities of mechanical origin. Proc. R. Soc. Med., *29*:1409, 1936.
3. Chapple, C. C., and Davidson, D. T.: A study of the relationship between fetal position and certain congenital deformities. J Pediatr., *181*:483, 1941.
4. Citron, N.: Injury of the tibialis posterior tendon: A cause of acquired valgus foot in childhood. Injury, *16*:610, 1985.
5. Damholt, V., and Termansen, N. B.: Asymmetry of plantar flexion strength in the foot. Acta Orthop. Scand., *49*:215, 1978.
6. Dunn, P. M.: The influence of the intrauterine environment in the causation of congenital postural deformities, with special reference to congenital dislocation of the hip. M.D. Thesis, Cambridge University, 1969.
7. Dunn, P. M.: Congenital deformation following premature rupture of the membranes. Teratology, *4*:487, 1971.
8. Dunn, P. M.: Congenital postural deformities: Further perinatal observations. Proc. R. Soc. Med., *67*:1174, 1974.
9. Edwards, E. R., and Menelaus, M. B.: Reverse club foot: Rigid and recalcitrant talipes calcaneovalgus. J. Bone Joint Surg., *69-B*:330, 1987.
10. Giannestras, N. J.: Recognition and treatment of flatfeet in infancy. Clin. Orthop., *70*:10, 1970.
11. Gould, N.: Positional in utero deformities. Am. J. Orthop., *4*:46, 1962.
12. Hippocrates: Vol. 3. Loeb Classical Library. Trans. by E. T. Withington. London, William Heinemann; New York, G. P. Putnam's Sons, 1927.
13. Jahss, M. H., and Kay, B. S.: An anatomic study of the anterior superior process of the os calcis and its clinical application. Foot Ankle, *3*:268, 1983.
14. Krackow, K. A., Hales, D., and Jones, L.: Preoperative

planning and surgical technique for performing a Dwyer calcaneal osteotomy. J. Pediatr. Orthop., 5:214, 1985.
15. Larsen, B., Reimann, I., and Becker-Andersen, H.: Congenital calcaneovalgus. Acta Orthop. Scand., *45*:145, 1974.
16. Letts, R. M., and Sweitzer, R.: A teaching model for instruction in the manipulation of infant foot deformities. J. Bone Joint Surg., *61-A*:791, 1979.
17. McCall, R. E., Lillich, J. S., Harris, J. R., and Johnston, F. A.: The Grice extra-articular subtalar arthrodesis. A clinical review. J. Pediatr. Orthop., 5:442, 1985.
18. Phillips, G. E.: A review of elongation of os calcis for flat feet. J. Bone Joint Surg., *65-B*:15, 1983.
19. Purnell, M. L., Drummond, D. S., Engber, W. D., and Breed, A. L.: Congenital dislocation of the peroneal tendons in the calcaneovalgus foot. J. Bone Joint Surg., *65-B*:316, 1983.
20. Reimann, I. M.: Pathology of congenital metatarsus varus and its relationship to other congenital deformities of the foot. Orthop. Clin. North Am., 9:219, 1978.
21. Shaffer, N. M.: The classic: Non-deforming clubfoot with remarks on its pathology. Clin. Orthop., *125*:2, 1977.
22. Shereff, M. J., and Johnson, K. A.: Radiographic anatomy of the hindfoot. Clin. Orthop., *177*:16, 1983.
23. Simons, G. W.: The diagnosis and treatment of deformity combinations in clubfeet. Clin. Orthop., *150*:229, 1980.
24. Støren, H.: Congenital convex pes valgus with vertical talus. Acta Orthop. Scand. (Suppl.), *94*:21, 1967.
25. Templeton, A. W., McAlister, W. H., and Zim, I. D.: Standardization of terminology and evaluation of osseous relationships in congenitally abnormal feet. A.J.R., *93*:374, 1965.
26. Timmer, H.: Der Zusammenhang des Pes valgus beim Kinder und des Pes calcaneus beim Neugeborenen. Z. Orthop. Chir., *45*:35, 1924.
27. Vartan, C. K.: The behavior of the foetus in utero with special reference to the incidence of breech presentation at term. J. Obstet. Gynaec. Br. Emp., *52*:417, 1945.
28. Wetzenstein, H.: The significance of congenital pes calcaneovalgus in the origin of pes plano-valgus in childhood. Preliminary report. Acta Orthop. Scand., *30*:64, 1960.
29. Wilkinson, J. A.: Breech malposition and intra-uterine dislocations. Proc. R. Soc. Med., *59*:1106, 1966.
30. Wynne-Davies, R.: Family studies of the cause of congenital clubfoot—talipes equinovarus, talipes calcaneovalgus and metatarsus varus. J. Bone Joint Surg., *46-B*:445, 1964.

CONGENITAL TALIPES EQUINOVARUS

Traditionally, the definition of congenital talipes equinovarus has been descriptive: The heel is inverted, the forefoot and midfoot are inverted and adducted *(varus)*, and the ankle is in *equinus* position—the foot is plantar-flexed with the toes at a lower level than the heel. A definition should, however, be specific, be based upon pathologic findings, and offer greater therapeutic insight. Congenital talipes equinovarus is in utero displacement and malalignment of the talocalcaneal navicular and calcaneocuboid joints; the talus is plantar-flexed with its anterior end rotated laterally and its head and neck tilted medially and plantarward; the *calcaneus* is plantar-flexed with its anterior end rotated medially with a medial spin at the subtalar joint and its posterior end tethered to the fibular malleolus; the *navicular* is displaced medially and dorsally, and the cuboid is displaced medially in relation to the calcaneus. These articular malalignments are firmly fixed by capsular, ligamentous, and musculotendinous contractures.

Incidence

Congenital talipes equinovarus is one of the more common congenital deformities of the foot. First described by Hippocrates, it has been known since ancient times.[297]

The incidence of talipes equinovarus varies widely with race and sex. In Caucasians, the birth frequency is 1.2 per thousand, with a male-to-female sex ratio of 2:1, making the rates 1.6 per thousand in boys and 0.8 per thousand in girls.[768, 771, 773]

Stewart, in 1951, noted the incidence of talipes equinovarus to be 4.9 per thousand in part- or full-blooded Hawaiians.[676] This high incidence in Hawaiians was confirmed by Ching and co-workers, who reported it to be 6.81 per thousand in full-blooded Hawaiians, as compared with 1.12 per thousand in Caucasians, and 0.57 per thousand in Orientals of unmixed blood. They also showed that the incidence of talipes equinovarus increased as the proportion of Hawaiian ancestry increased, indicating the racial effects in the risk of talipes equinovarus to be additive.[119] A high frequency of talipes equinovarus in the Maori—another Polynesian group—has been reported by Elliot, by Alldred, and by Veale and associates.[10, 184, 718] On the basis of these data, Beals concluded the birth frequency to be 6.5 to 7.0 per thousand in the Maori.[36]

The incidence of talipes equinovarus in South African blacks (3.5 per thousand) is reported by Pompe van Meerdervoort; and that in Malayans, Indians, and Chinese in Singapore by Pillay, Khong, and Wolfers.[562, 566] The figures for various racial groups are summarized in Table 7–4.

Involvement is bilateral in about 50 per cent of the cases. In unilateral cases the right side is affected slightly more frequently than the left.

Heredity

The pattern of inheritance of talipes equinovarus is polygenic with a threshold effect.[107–109, 772, 773] Single genetic factors or unifactoral dis-

***Table 7–4.** Incidence of Talipes Equinovarus in Various Races**

Race	Cases per Thousand Births
Chinese	.39
Japanese	.53
Malay	.68
Filipino	.76
Caucasian	1.12
Puerto Rican	1.36
Indian	1.51
South African black	3.50
Polynesian	6.81

*From Beals, R. K.: Personal communication; data derived from Ching et al., Chung et al., Pillay et al., and Pompe van Meerdervoort.

orders show discontinuous variation, that is, an all-or-none phenomenon with the malformation being either present or absent. The pattern of inheritance of unifactoral affections is simple, with ratios illustrating dominant, recessive, or sex-linked traits; however, variations may be encountered in malformations caused by single mutant genes. Multiple gene systems or multifactoral disorders show continuous variation and illustrate polygenic patterns of inheritance. The all-or-none nature of talipes equinovarus is explained by the threshold effect, i.e., an underlying gradation of factors related to the deformity that cause it to be present when the level is beyond a certain threshold and absent when the level is under that point.

The polygenic inheritance of talipes equinovarus is supported by the following evidence. (1) The family studies of Wynne-Davies showed a rapid decrease in incidence from first- to second- to third-degree relatives (about 2.9 per cent of siblings, 0.6 per cent of aunts and uncles, and 0.2 per cent of cousins, as listed in Table 7–5). Female index patients are fewer in number than male index patients (the infrequency of talipes equinovarus in the female may be due to some unknown factor that modifies its manifestation) and they have a greater proportion of affected relatives than do the males, indicating a greater deviance from the norm than in the male. (3) The risk of talipes equinovarus developing in subsequent children is increased when both parents are affected or when there is more than one affected individual in the family. In general, talipes equinovarus is less severe in sporadic cases than in familial ones, and the greater the number of talipes equinovarus cases in a family, the greater the probability of having subsequent children with more rigid deformity.*

In the etiology of talipes equinovarus, besides genetic factors, environmental factors must operate. This is shown by the studies of Idelberger, who compared the incidence of talipes equinovarus in identical (monozygotic) twin pairs with that in fraternal (dizygotic) twin pairs. He found that 13 of 40 (32.5 per cent) of the monozygotic co-twins were affected with talipes equinovarus, in contrast to 4 of 134 (2.9 per cent) of the dizygotic co-twins.[319, 320] These data suggest that both genetic and environmental factors play a role in the genesis of deformity. Little is known about the intrauterine environmental factors.[772]

In genetic counseling, one should consider the sex of the index patient, whether or not the parents are affected by talipes equinovarus, and the race of the family. In a Caucasian family, if both parents are normal and the index patient is a male, the risk of a subsequent child being born with talipes equinovarus is about 2 per cent; if the parents are normal and the index patient is a female, the chances are increased to 5 per cent; however, if a parent has talipes equinovarus and already has one child with talipes equinovarus, the odds are much greater—10 to 25 per cent (accurate figures for this group are not yet available).[772, 773]

In a Maori family, if the index patient is a

*See references 107 to 109, 120, 121, 534 to 536, 768, and 770 to 773.

***Table 7–5.** Proportions of First-, Second-, and Third-Degree Relatives Affected with Talipes Equinovarus**

Index Patient		First-Degree Relative: Brother	First-Degree Relative: Sister	Second-Degree Relative: Uncle	Second-Degree Relative: Aunt	Third-Degree Relative: Male Cousins	Third-Degree Relative: Female Cousins
Male	97	4 of 115	0 of 90	0 of 286	2 of 282	2 of 341	0 of 349
Female	47	2 of 33	2 of 34	1 of 138	2 of 117	0 of 166	0 of 136
Total	144	8 of 272		5 of 823		2 of 992	
Per cent		2.9		0.6		0.2	
Appropriate comparison with general population		× 30		× 5		× 1.5	

*Data derived from family studies of Wynne-Davies, 1964 and 1970.

male and the parents are normal, the risk of a subsequent child's having talipes equinovarus is about 9 per cent; if the index patient is a female with normal parents, the chance of a brother's being affected is 9 per cent (there were no sisters affected in the series of Beals). If an index patient has a parent affected with talipes equinovarus, the chance increases to 30 per cent. These differences in incidence of talipes equinovarus in the Caucasian and the Maori are explained by the frequency of the gene in the population rather than by its mode of action. By using the Falconer model for the estimate of heritability, it has been shown that the heritability of talipes equinovarus is simi-ar in the Caucasian and the Maori (i.e., 70 ± 8).[36, 194, 718]

Etiology

The exact cause of talipes equinovarus is unknown. It has, in the past, been the subject of much speculation and theorizing based on a striking paucity of facts.

INTRAUTERINE MECHANICAL FACTORS

The mechanical theory, the oldest, was advocated by Hippocrates. He proposed that the fetal foot was forced into the equinovarus posture by external mechanical forces; that consequent to rapid skeletal growth, the ligaments and muscles developed adaptive shortening; and that the tarsal bones, especially the talus, responded by changes in their contour with subsequent articular malalignment.[297] The theory of intrauterine malposture due to mechanical forces was further elaborated by Parker and Shattock in 1884, Nutt in 1925, and Denis Browne in 1933, 1936, and 1955.[87, 89, 90, 520, 542] This theory is not supported by the observation that the incidence of talipes equinovarus is not increased in prenatal environmental conditions that tend to "overcrowd' the uterus—such as twinning, high birth weight, primiparous uterus, hydramnios, and oligohydramnios.[119, 773] At present, the nature of the intrauterine environmental factors has not yet been determined.

NEUROMUSCULAR DEFECT

In the literature, many theories have been put forward about neuromuscular dysfunction as the cause of talipes equinovarus; to mention a few: a peroneal nerve lesion caused by pressure at the intrauterine stage (White, 1929); maldevelopment of the striated muscle (Middleton, 1934); muscle imbalance due to dysplasia of the peroneals (Flinchum, 1953); and relative shortening of the degenerating muscle fibers during growth (Bechtol and Mossman, 1950).*

Irani and Sherman used fetal material to distinguish primary from adaptive changes. They demonstrated by standard anatomic and routine histologic studies that there are no abnormalities in the muscles, nerves, vessels, or tendinous insertions.[328, 329] The same conclusions have been reached by other investigators.[676, 759] Isaacs and co-workers, however, in 1977, presented a histochemical and electron microscopic study of muscles in talipes equinovarus; there was evidence of neurogenic disease in most instances. They proposed abnormal innervation as the prime factor in the development of the deformity. Minor degrees of muscle imbalance evolving during a period of rapid skeletal growth in early intrauterine periods will produce disproportionately severe deformities.[330]

Ritsila was able to produce equinovarus deformity of the foot in 32 young rabbits (mostly six to seven days old) by soft-tissue alterations; namely a combination of Achilles tenodesis, sectioning of the extensor digitorum longus and both peroneal muscles (longus and brevis), and immobilization of the foot and ankle in an extremely rigid equinovarus posture for three to four weeks. Radiographic examination and analysis of the anatomic deformities by gross dissection and microscopic studies showed the morphologic changes in the experimental animal to be similar to those in the human. Ritsila concluded that primary soft-tissue changes should be considered a factor in provoking skeletal deformities in talipes equinovarus.[593] The primary cause of soft-tissue contractures remains unknown.

In the literature, there are a number of reports on experimental production of talipes equinovarus in animals. Drachman and Coulombre infused chick embryos with curare for periods of up to 48 hours; at the time of hatching, the chicks consistently had limb deformities. The limbs were deformed in the embryonic position, and there was evidence of the external influences of the calcareous shell. The foot deformity was identical to talipes. Active movement of the embryo is required for normal development of joints. The teratogenic effects of curare are due to its paralyzing action. It seems that even relatively brief periods of immobilization will produce ankylosing of

*See references 39, 206, 487, and 748.

joints.[167] Shoro produced clubfoot deformity in rats (38 of 467 fetuses—8.1 per cent) by temporary, brief periods of paralysis and immobilization with tubocurarine injections.[643]

Jackson immobilized the immature and rapidly growing feet of opossums in a deformed position and produced structural adaptations in muscle, tendon, and bone. When structural changes developed, the deformity did not resolve spontaneously. The tendency to resolution was inversely related to the duration of immobilization.[332]

Edwards exposed pregnant guinea pigs to hyperthermia by placing them in an incubator set at 43° Celsius for one hour daily between the eighteenth and twenty-fifth days of gestation. Eleven of the forty newborn guinea pigs showed clubfoot deformity; all of them had associated malformations of the spinal cord.[181] In the human, weak peroneal muscles have been incriminated as the cause of clubfoot. Electromyographic studies, however, have shown no lower motor neuron lesion.[529]

ARREST OF FETAL DEVELOPMENT

Over 100 years ago, Hüter regarded talipes equinovarus as the result of an arrest of development of the foot in one of the physiologic phases of its embryonic life.[318] That there are physiologic positions in the embryonic development of the foot that are similar to clubfoot has been demonstrated by Henke and Reyher, by Schomburg, by Bardeen and Lewis, and by Böhm.[27, 74, 286, 622] The four stages in the evolution of the human foot in the first half of prenatal life were delineated by Böhm.[74]

First Stage (Second Month). The form of the foot is characterized by marked equinus inclination (about 90 degrees of plantar flexion) and by severe adduction of the hindpart and forepart of the foot, with the navicular lying in close proximity to the medial malleolus. The plane of the lower leg and the transverse axis of the knee and the plane of the foot (i.e., the one passing transversely through the long axis of the footplate) are superimposed.

Second Stage (Beginning of Third Month). There is a new development—the foot rotates into a position of marked supination, but remains in 90 degrees of plantar flexion. The first metatarsal is markedly adducted; the lateral four metatarsals are adducted to a lesser extent (Fig. 7–24 A and B).

Third Stage (Middle of Third Month). The equinus inclination decreases to a mild degree, but the marked supination and metatarsus varus persist. In this stage, the long axis of the foot is perpendicular to the plane of the lower leg (Fig. 7–24 C).

Fourth Stage (Beginning at Fourth Month). The foot is in midsupination and there is slight metatarsus varus (Fig. 7–24 D). In this stage, the footplate begins to rotate toward pronation on its long axis, the planes of the foot and lower leg gradually assuming the relative positions seen in the adult human.[74]

It is obvious from the preceding observations that the three clinical deformities of talipes equinovarus, namely plantar flexion, adduction, and supination, are normal in the early stages of physiologic embryonic development of the human foot. This relationship is given in Table 7–6. Studies of the pathologic anatomy of severe talipes equinovarus have shown that in its external appearance it resembles an embryonic foot at the beginning of the second month. Böhm had difficulty explaining his theory of medial and plantar subluxation of the talocalcaneonavicular joint in talipes equinovarus, for this medial displacement of the navicular is not observed in any stage of the development of the normal fetus.[74, 106, 730]

Mau objected to the theory that clubfoot is due to arrested fetal development because the embryonic foot does not show distortion of the bones about the tarsal joints, which is found in clubfoot.[479]

Carroll and associates used a dissecting mi-

Table 7–6. *Stages of Physiologic Development of the Position of the Foot and Ankle in Relation to Origin of Clubfoot*

Stages of Physiologic Embryonic Development	Primary Deformities in Talipes Equinovarus					
	Plantar Flexion		Adduction		Supination	
	Marked	Slight	Tarsus	Metatarsus	Marked	Slight
First stage (second month)	+	–	+	+	–	–
Second stage (beginning of third month)	+	–	–	+	+	–
Third stage (middle of third month)	–	+	–	+	+	–
Fourth stage (beginning of fourth month)	–	–	–	+	–	+

From Böhm, M.: The embryologic origin of clubfoot. J. Bone Joint Surg., *11*:246, 1929. Reproduced by permission of the publisher.

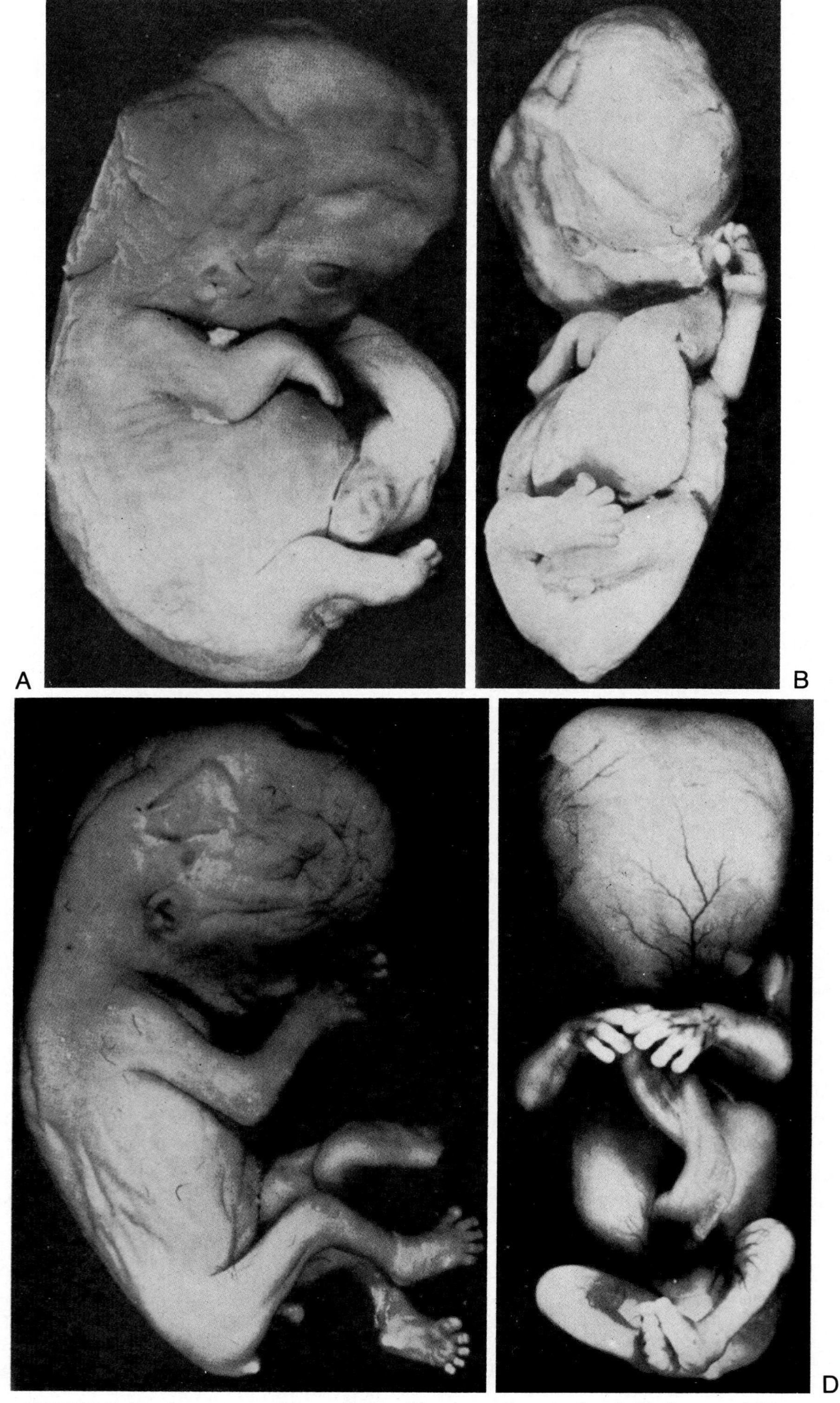

FIGURE 7–24. Appearance of lower limbs of human embryo in first half of prenatal life.

A and **B.** Lateral and anteroposterior views of 23 mm. long (vertex to buttocks) human embryo at nine weeks. Note the 90-degree pes equinus, marked supination of the feet, and the adduction of the metatarsals. **C.** Lateral view of 35-mm. embryo (middle of third month). Note the slight pes equinus, marked supination of the entire foot, and moderate metatarsus varus. **D.** An anteroposterior view of 57 mm. long human embryo (end of third month). Note the midsupination of the feet and the slight metatarsus varus. (From Böhm, M.: The embryologic origin of clubfoot. J. Bone Joint Surg., *11*:246, 1929. Reprinted by permission.)

croscope to examine the normal feet of 17 embryos and fetuses. The youngest embryo studied was eight weeks old; up to that age, the foot was so gelatinous that it could be manipulated into almost any position. In the dissected feet, the mesenchymal condensation or the cartilage model of the navicular had a normal relationship with the head of the talus. The first metatarsal in the younger feet tended to have a varus inclination. These investigators concluded that talipes equinovarus does not reflect persistence of an intrauterine stage of development.[106]

Kaplan studied the comparative anatomy of the talus in relation to talipes equinovarus. He could not find a structure similar to clubfoot in any other species. He concluded that talipes equinovarus does not represent a recapitulation of a pre-existing evolutionary condition.[353]

PRIMARY GERM PLASM DEFECT

The consistent bony deformity in talipes equinovarus is medial and plantar tilting of the head and neck of the talus.[328] Nichols (in 1897) and Elmslie (in 1920) speculated that primary bone dysplasia was the cause of deformation of the talus.[185, 515] The cartilaginous anlage of the tarsal bones is fully formed by six weeks, and that of the tarsal joints by seven weeks, in the embryo.[231] On the basis of this embryologic fact, Irani and Sherman proposed that talipes equinovarus is the result of a defective cartilaginous anlage produced by a primary germ plasm defect, developing in the first trimester of pregnancy.[328, 329]

In the opinion of this author, there is more than one cause of congenital talipes equinovarus. In some cases it is due to a primary germ plasm defect of the talus and decrease of its angle of declination; under the tethering effect of soft-tissue contracture, the talocalcaneonavicular joint progressively subluxates medially and plantarward. In others, there may be a neuromuscular type of congenital talipes equinovarus in which the paralysis, imbalance, and fibrotic contracture of paralyzed muscles are the primary cause of deformity, the changes in the shape of the talus being secondary. There may be a primary ligamentous disorder with excess of myofibroblasts as the cellular cause of soft-tissue contracture. At present the question of the etiology of congenital talipes equinovarus has not been settled.

Pathology

Upon inspection, the gross pathologic changes of talipes equinovarus are characteristic: the foot is plantar-flexed at the ankle and subtalar joints, the hindfoot is inverted, and the mid- and forefoot are adducted, inverted, and in equinus position (Fig. 7–25). These deformities are the result of medial and plantar displacement and medial rotation of the talocalcaneonavicular joint.[612, 613] The navicular and calcaneus are displaced medially and plantarward around the talus, the cuboid is displaced medially on the calcaneus, and the ankle joint assumes the equinus posture because the mechanics of the foot are disturbed. Fixed contractures of the related soft tissue—i.e., the ligaments, capsules, muscles, and tendons—maintain these articular malalignments.

The pathologic changes observed in talipes equinovarus may be either primary (congenital) or secondary (adaptive), the one being distinguished from the other by study of the morbid anatomy in the fetus. Irani and Sherman care-

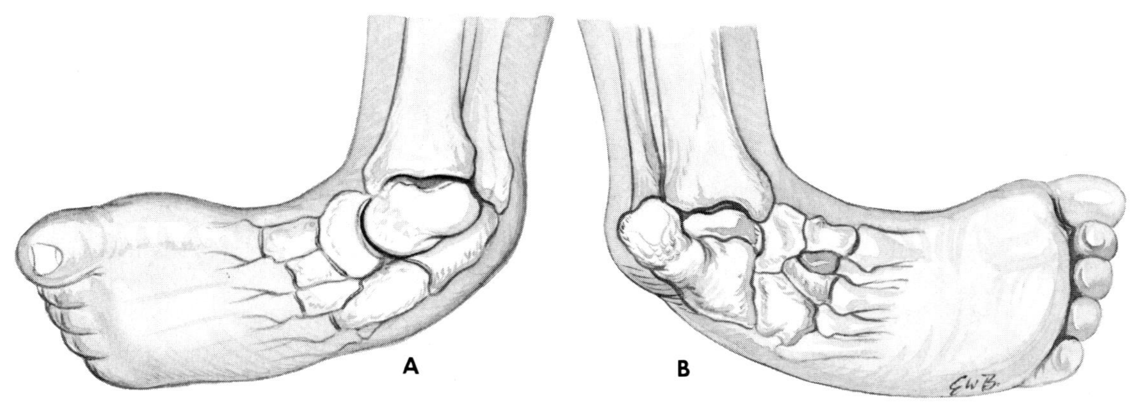

FIGURE 7–25. The deformity of talipes equinovarus (TEV) on gross inspection.

A. Anterior view. **B.** Posterior view.

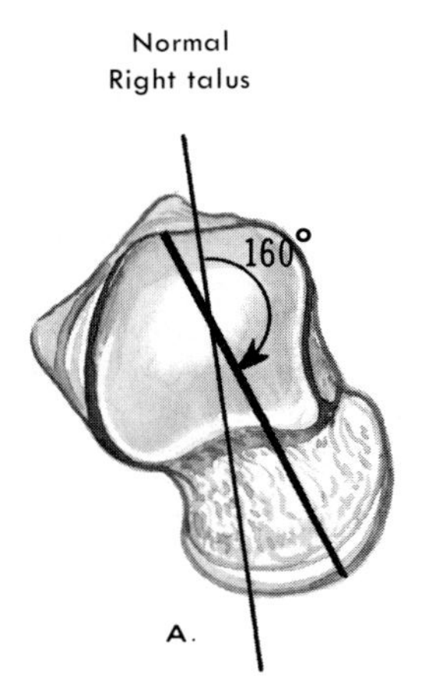

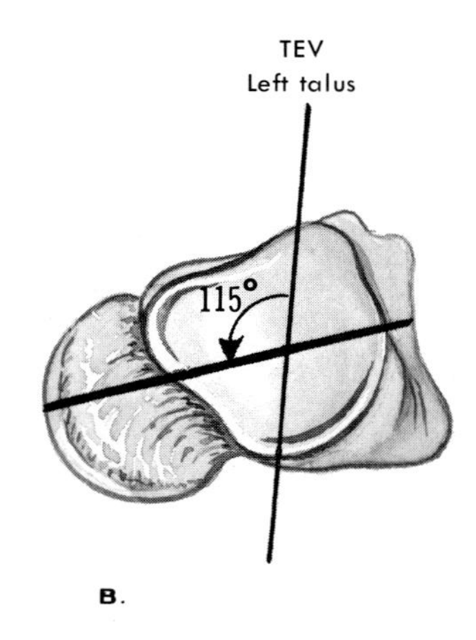

FIGURE 7–26. Declination angle of the talus.

A. Normal foot. Note angle of 150 to 160 degrees. **B.** Talipes equinovarus. The angle is decreased to 115 degrees.

fully dissected 11 fetal limbs with talipes equinovarus deformity, and Settle studied 16 specimens from the late fetal period.[328, 329, 634] In 1970, Müller, reviewing the literature of the past 120 years, found reports of 41 dissections of talipes equinovarus in fetuses.[504] Recently, numerous studies of the morbid anatomy of talipes equinovarus in the different stages of fetal development have been reported.[100, 106, 327, 567, 730] The conclusions reached by these investigators are essentially the same.

BONY DEFORMITIES

The Talus. The primary and basic deformity in talipes equinovarus is medial and plantar deviation of the anterior end of the talus.[328, 329, 634] The angle formed by the long axis of the head and neck of the talus with the long axis of its body is called the "declination angle" of the talus; in the normal adult human foot, it measures between 150 and 160 degrees.[544] In talipes equinovarus, the declination angle of the talus is invariably decreased, measuring 115 to 135 degrees (Fig. 7–26). It is of pathogenetic interest to note that in the young fetus, the head and neck of the talus are tilted toward the medial side of the foot during fetal development; from the sixteenth week onward, the declination angle of the talus increases.[231]

In the literature, medial tilting of the anterior part of the talus is also referred to as obliquity of the neck of the talus.[733] It is measured as follows: the talus is placed with its trochlear articular surface facing superiorly; a horizontal line is drawn across the trochlea between its medial tubercle and lateral process; a longitudinal line is drawn along the center of the trochlear surface, parallel with its inner border

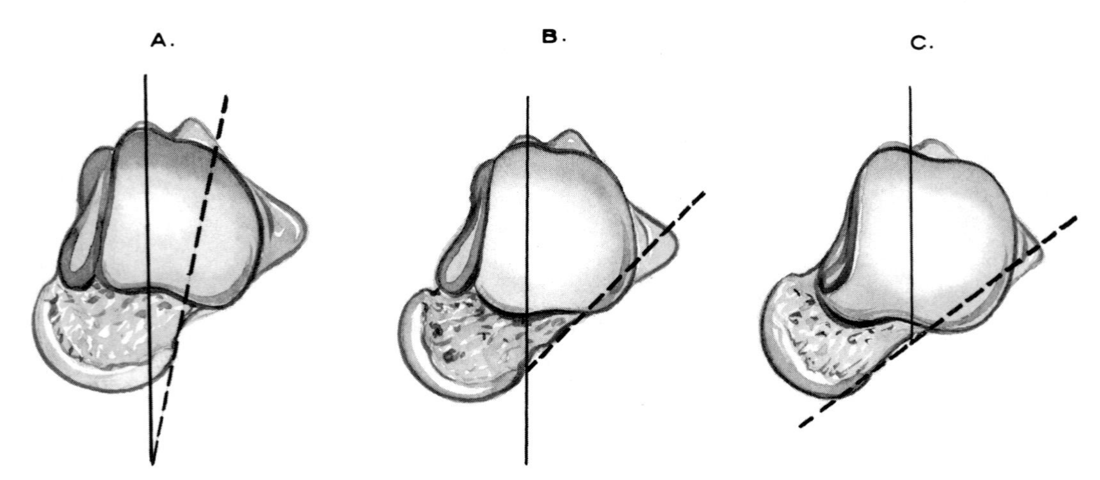

FIGURE 7–27. Obliquity of the neck of the talus.

A. In the normal adult. **B.** In the normal fetus. **C.** In talipes equinovarus. (Redrawn from Walsham, W. J., and Hughes, W. K.: Treatment of talipes equinus. *In* The Deformities of the Human Foot. London, Bailliere, Tindall & Cox, 1895, Chapter VII, pp. 294–320.)

and perpendicular to the horizontal line; then a longitudinal line is drawn parallel to the lateral margin of the neck of the talus. The angle formed between the longitudinal axes of the trochlea and the neck is the measure of the obliquity of the talar neck. Scudder, combining his figures with those of Parker and Shattock, reported the angle of obliquity to be 12 to 32 degrees in the adult, 35 to 75 degrees in the fetus, and 50 to 65 degrees in talipes equinovarus (Fig. 7–27).[542, 627]

The neck of the talus is shortened, sometimes unidentifiable, so that the head appears to be fused with the body. The normal constriction of the talar neck is absent. The anterior articular surface of the talus in the normal foot faces forward and slightly inward and downward in the frontal plane of its body, whereas in talipes equinovarus it is rotated medially and plantarward, facing almost directly inward and markedly downward. The anterior end of the talus is divided by a ridge into two areas; *an inner part,* which is covered by an articular facet and, in the young fetus, in contact with the navicular; and a *lateral part,* which is devoid of articular surface and is covered with a thin layer of fibrous tissue. The lateral part of the anterior end of the talus is unopposed by bone and is palpable as a rounded prominence on the dorsolateral part of the foot. For practical therapeutic purposes, this lateral part is regarded as the "head" of the talus, and the navicular is reduced to articulate with it.

The posterior articular facet on the inferior surface of the talus is relatively normal. The anterior and middle facets, however, are distorted and fused into a single misshapen, articular surface that is tilted medially and downward; inferolaterally, it articulates with the medial surface of the anterior part of the calcaneus. Thus, as seen from above, the anterior portion of the calcaneus is uncovered and the sinus tarsi is widened.

Normally, the ankle mortise is narrower posteriorly than anteriorly, and the corresponding articular surface of the talus is similarly shaped. In talipes equinovarus, however, the talus is plantar-flexed in fixed equinus posture; consequently, the anterior one quarter to one third of its superior articular surface is uncovered (Fig. 7–28). It may be difficult to reposition the wider anterior part of the dome of the talus into the ankle mortise because there is insufficient space; the talus has forfeited its "right of domicile."[445] In general, the trochlear articular surface is normal; but in long-standing untreated talipes equinovarus there may be a distinct ridge separating its anterior uncovered part from the posterior contained parts, as if it had been indented by the anterior ligament of the inferior tibiofibular joint. The medial surface of the talus is grossly deformed and diminished in size. A large part of it is occupied by the deltoid ligament, which seems to have appropriated the articular facet. In the normal foot of the fetus and the neonate, the medial articular facet is pear-shaped, extends farther distally on the medial wall of the talus, and may be continuous with the anterior articular surface for the navicular. In talipes equinovarus, most of the medial facet is obliterated, and only a narrow, posterior stalk remains.

With the rapid growth of the tarsal bones in the fetus, the pull of the contracted calcaneonavicular and tibionavicular ligaments and the posterior tibial tendon will progressively displace the navicular medially and plantarward toward the medial malleolus (Fig. 7–29). The medial surfaces of the calcaneus and the navicular will abut against the medial malleolus and, in severe cases, even be eroded by it. Accessory articulation may develop between the three bones. The lateral surface of the talus appears to be normal, with a relatively well-developed lateral articular facet.

The deformed talus in talipes equinovarus is small in size, and its ossification center may be delayed in appearing and eccentrically situated in a more anterior and lateral location. The vascular channels are scarcer and arranged in a disorganized fashion.[636, 730] The pathologic changes in the talus are more pronounced than those in any of the other tarsal bones.

The Calcaneus. The os calcis is much less deformed than the talus. In general, its contour is relatively normal, with its articular facets normally oriented on its body. Since these facets articulate with those of the talus, the calcaneus, of necessity, is rotated on its long axis inward and downward beneath the talus. The varus position of the heel disappears upon release of its capsular and ligamentous attachments, indicating that the deformity is secondary and postural. There is minimal medial bowing of the calcaneus, its lateral surface being slightly convex and its medial surface concave. The sustentacalum tali is usually underdeveloped and in close proximity to the medial malleolus. The distal calcaneal articular facet for the cuboid bone slants anteriorly, medially, and plantarward; in the normal foot it faces almost forward. This alteration accounts for the medial inclination of the calcaneocuboid joint.

The Forefoot and Tibia. Smaller than normal,

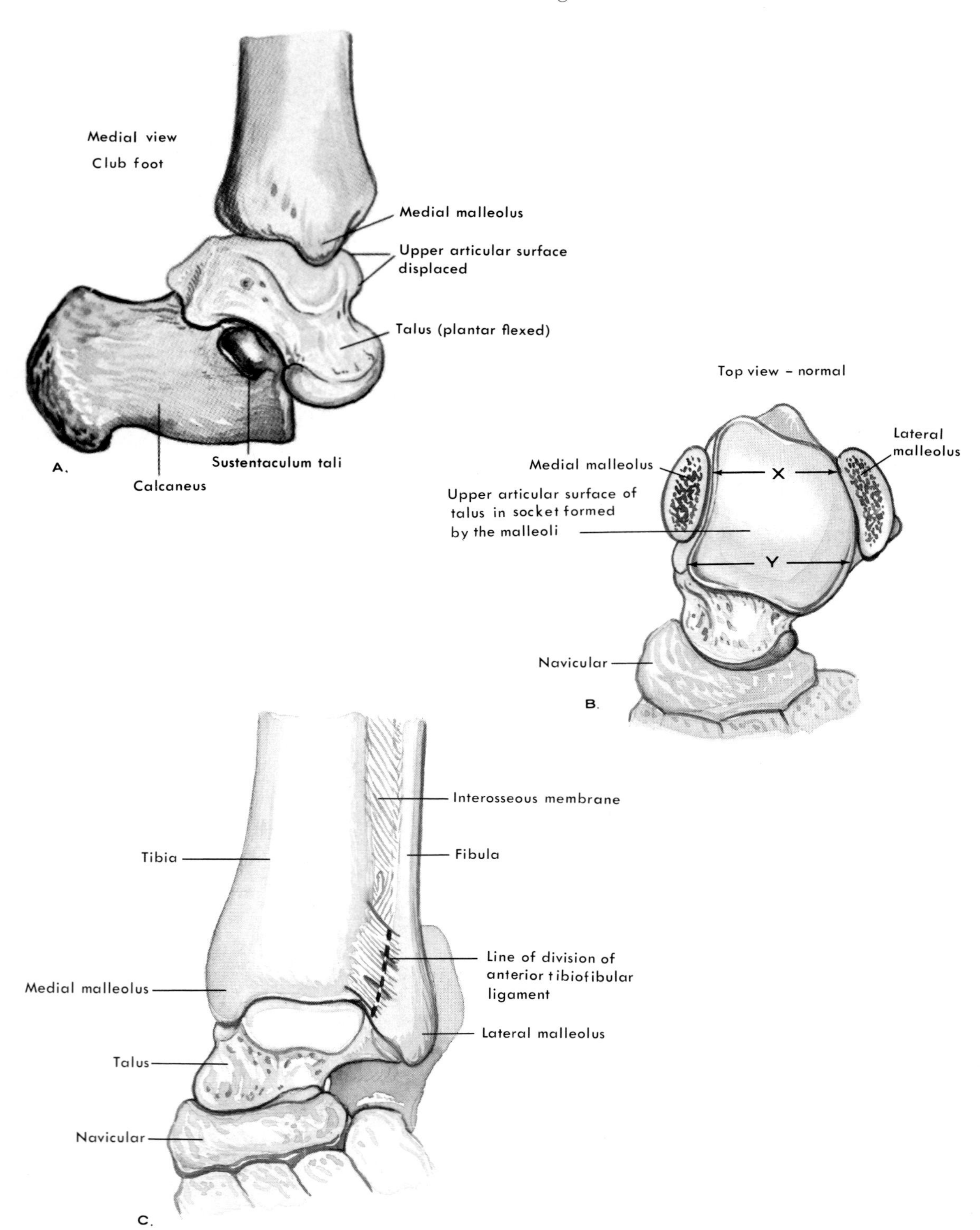

FIGURE 7–28. The anatomic relationships of the talus in the ankle mortise.

A. The talus is plantar-flexed. Note the anterior one fourth to one third of the superior articular surface is uncovered. **B.** The superior articular surface of the talus lying in the mortise formed by the medial and lateral malleoli. Note it is narrower posteriorly than in front. In the older child with talipes equinovarus the plantar-flexed talus may "forfeit its right of domicile," i.e., there may not be room in the ankle mortise to reposition it. **C.** Anterior tibiofibular ligament and lower end of tibiofibular interosseous ligament are sectioned to widen the ankle mortise and make room for the talus.

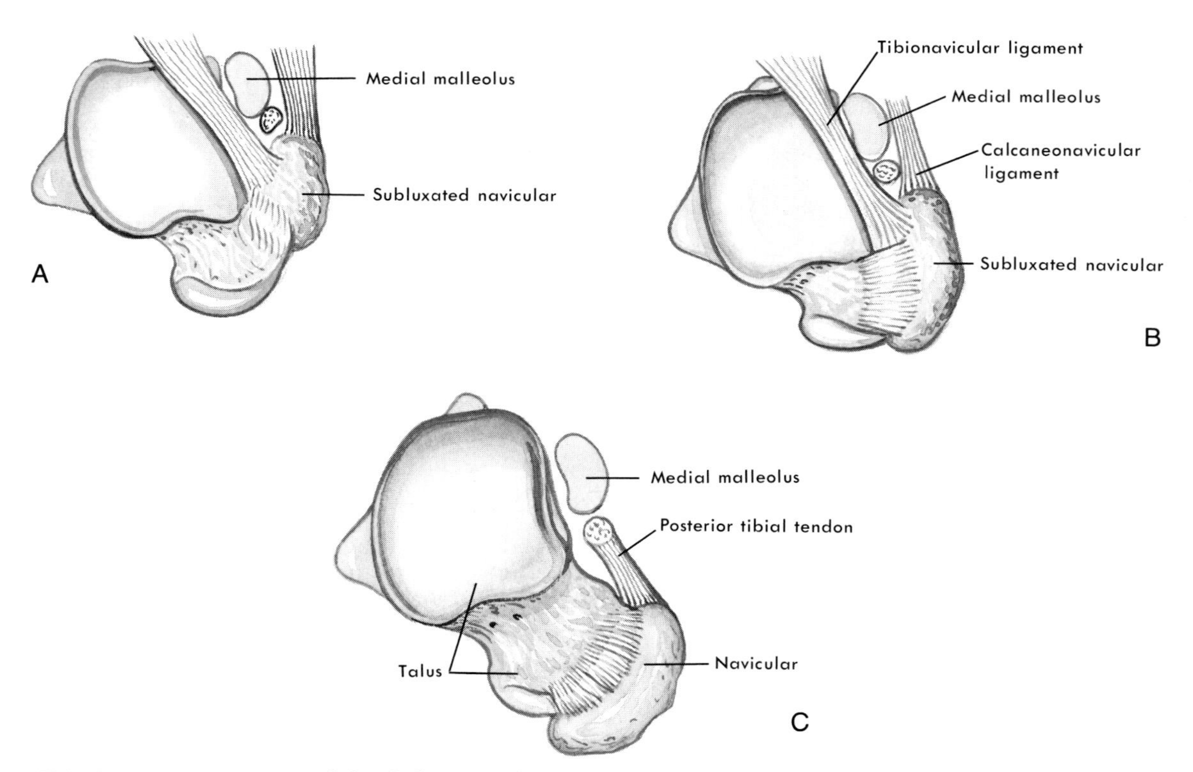

FIGURE 7–29. Progressive medial and plantar displacement of the navicular in relation to the anterior end of the talus.

A. In early fetal life the navicular articulates with the medially tilted head of the talus. **B** and **C.** With rapid growth of the foot of the fetus, the pull of the posterior tibial tendon, the plantar calcaneonavicular ligament, and the tibionavicular ligament, the navicular is displaced medially and plantarward and abuts the medial malleolus.

the navicular is normal in shape. Its medial tuberosity may be hypertrophied. In severe cases, it may have an articular facet for the medial malleolus. The cuboid is essentially normal in shape. The cuneiforms, the metatarsal bones, and the phalanges are normal.

Kite states that exaggerated medial tibial torsion is a commonly associated finding in talipes equinovarus.[363, 375] This is not correct. Tibial torsion is normal. The old concept of exaggerated medial tibial torsion as the fourth element of the complex deformity of talipes equinovarus should be discarded.

ARTICULAR MALALIGNMENTS

Relationship of Talus to Distal Tibia and Fibula. The talus has no muscle attachments; it is stabilized by the ankle mortise. The equinovarus posture of the calcaneus and the medial and plantar displacement of the navicular force the talus to tilt out of the ankle mortise, exposing one fourth to one third of its superior articular surface (see Fig. 7–28 A). In the literature, there is disagreement about whether the talus also rotates in the ankle mortise. There has been a question whether the medial rotation of the foot in talipes equinovarus is due to the medial rotation of the talus in the ankle mortise or to the medial rotation of the foot at the subtalar joint complex. There has also been much controversy as to the etiology of the posterior position of the fibular malleolus. Is it due to the medial or to the lateral rotation of the talus in the ankle mortise? Adams states that he has never observed medial rotation but that, in contrast, there is lateral rotation in the ankle mortise.[3, 4, 139, 244] Walsham and Hughes point out that, because of the greater convexity of the lateral border of the superior articular surface of the talus and the direction of the trochlea, when the ankle joint is plantar-flexed, the talus inclines medially as well as forward and downward. In talipes equinovarus, the talus is in equinus position, and its head therefore inclines medially as well as downward. Hence, on inspection, one finds the lateral malleolar facet of the talus to be displaced anteriorly in front of the lateral malleolus, while the superior and medial surfaces of the talar neck approximate the anterior border of the medial malleolus. In brief, Walsham and Hughes consider the talus to be plantar-flexed and medially rotated at the ankle joint.[733] Goldner believes the talus within the ankle mortise is inverted around a longitudinal (or anteroposterior) axis and slightly medially rotated around a vertical axis. Gould adheres to Goldner's concept of pathoanatomy of talipes equinovarus. In treatment both Goldner and Gould recommend lateral rotation of the talus following surgical release and reconstruction of the deep deltoid ligament.[244, 248–250]

McKay states that in 120 clubfeet he has been unable to observe any medial rotation of the talus in the ankle joint or any abnormal plane of motion of the talus relative to the bimalleolar plane of the talocrural articulation.[447] According to McKay the pathoanatomy of clubfoot is horizontal rotation of the calcaneus at the subtalar joint, the rotation taking place around a vertical axis passing upward through the tibia in the area of the talocalcaneal interosseous ligament.

The computer graphic studies of Herzenberg and Carroll have demonstrated that there is *no medial rotation* of the body of the talus around a vertical axis in the ankle mortise (as proposed by Goldner and Gould), but rather mild lateral rotation of the talar body around a vertical axis. Therefore, Carroll, following surgical release, rotates the body of the talus medially while allowing the calcaneus to rotate in the opposite direction. This author, along with Simons, agrees with the concept of McKay and Carroll.[106, 291, 447–449, 650–652]

Relationship of Navicular to Talus. The navicular is displaced medially and plantarward, leaving the lateral part of the anterior globular end of the talus unopposed (see Fig. 7–29). There is some disagreement about terminology—whether this is true subluxation or dislocation. This author believes that it is imperative to restore normal alignment of the talonavicular joint. Otherwise, the hyaline cartilage on the lateral aspect of the talar anterior end will atrophy and the longitudinal growth of the bone will be retarded.

Relationship of Talus to Calcaneus. The calcaneus is rotated medially and tilted into equinus position beneath the talus. Abnormal movements take place in three dimensions—horizontal, coronal, and sagittal. In the horizontal plane, the calcaneus rotates medially so that, anterior to the ankle joint, it slips underneath the head and neck of the talus, whereas posterior to the ankle joint, the calcaneal tuberosity moves toward the fibular malleolus (Fig. 7–30). The calcaneofibular ligament becomes shortened and thickened. In addition, the calcaneofibular retinaculum (superior peroneal retinaculum, which passes from the posterior aspect of the fibula, encompasses the peroneal tendons, and attaches to the posterolateral aspect of the calcaneus), peroneal tendon sheaths, and posterior talocalcaneal ligament tether the calcaneus to the fibular malleolus.[447]

In talipes equinovarus, the varus appearance of the heel may be difficult to comprehend when, in actuality, the calcaneus is close to the lateral malleolus. This is explained by the rotation of the calcaneus in the coronal plane in addition to the horizontal plane. The heel tips into varus inclination in a fashion very similar

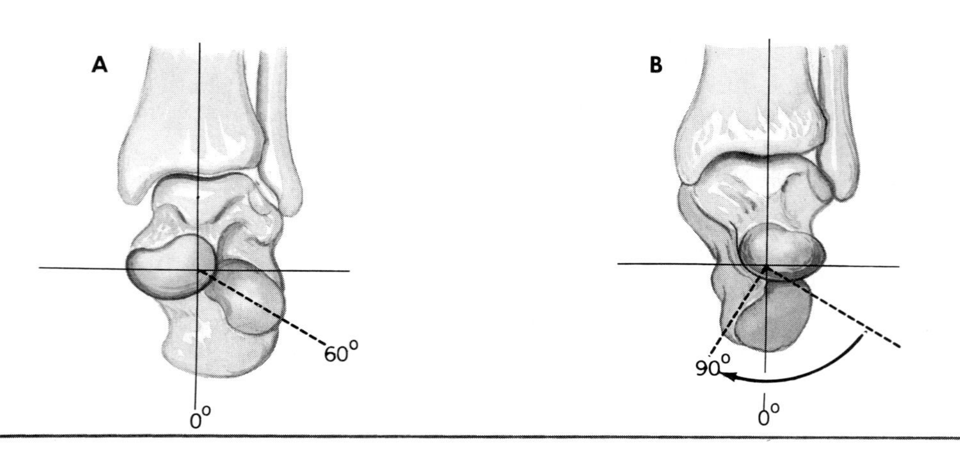

FIGURE 7–30. The articular relationship of the calcaneus to the talus as seen from the front in the left foot.

A. In the normal foot the articular surface of the calcaneus for the cuboid is well to the lateral side of the long axis of the leg. **B.** In talipes equinovarus the medial rotation of the calcaneus in the horizontal plane displaces its posterior tuberosity laterally toward the fibular malleolus and brings the anterior end of the calcaneus beneath the head of the talus instead of lateral to it.

to what happens if one takes a banana and rotates it by one end while looking at the other.[447]

Simons and Sarrafian performed a microsurgical dissection on a seven-month-old stillborn fetus with camptomelic dysplasia. The most important pathologic finding was the marked rotation of the calcaneus beneath the talus around a vertical axis. The anterior half of the calcaneus was rotated medially and downward, whereas the posterior half was rotated laterally and upward. A posterior medial and plantar release failed to realign the hindfoot. The bones of the hindfoot could be repositioned only by a complete subtalar release.[652] The fulcrum upon which the tarsal bones pivot beneath the talus is the interosseous ligament, which is made up of three separate ligaments: the posterior ligament of the talocalcaneal navicular joint, the anterior ligament of the subtalar (posterior talocalcaneal) joint, and the interosseous (cervical) ligament.

Relationship of Calcaneus to Cuboid Bone. The cuboid is displaced medially in relation to the anterior end of the calcaneus, which is inclined inward. With adduction of the cuboid bone on the os calcis, the bifurcated ligament (calcaneocuboid and calcaneonavicular ligaments), long plantar ligament, plantar calcaneocuboid ligament, naviculocuboid ligament, inferior extensor retinaculum, dorsal calcaneocuboid ligament, and cubonavicular oblique ligament become contracted and thereby supinate and adduct the midfoot and forefoot. The cuboid is translated medially in relation to the anterior facet of the calcaneus, which is inclined inward.

With the medial and plantar subluxation of the talocalcaneonavicular joint, the bones in front of the transverse tarsal joint are adducted, medially rotated, and pitched in an equinus inclination.

Carroll and associates dissected feet of stillborn premature and full-term infants with talipes equinovarus, and demonstrated that the lateral malleolus is directed posteriorly, the head of the talus pointed laterally, and the navicular subluxated medially toward the medial malleolus. The anterior part of the calcaneus is pressed downward by the head of the talus, forced into plantar flexion, and rotated medially (Fig. 7–31). The longitudinal axes of the talus and calcaneus become superimposed and parallel. The equinus deformity and inversion of the calcaneus could not be corrected until the talus was derotated medially. Upon medial rotation of the talus and fixation of the head of the talus to the navicular, the foot assumed a normal appearance. By pushing the head of the talus laterally and fixing the navicular in a medially subluxated position, these investigators were able to produce equinus deformity of the ankle, varus deviation of the heel, and adduction of the forefoot in the normal foot of the amputated leg of an eight-year-old boy. They noted the same articular relationships in a one-year-old child with recalcitrant talipes equinovarus. Re-examining patients with residual deformities of talipes equinovarus in the second and third decades of life, they found posterior displacement of the lateral malleolus, lateral direction of the head of the talus, and medial subluxation of the navicular.[106]

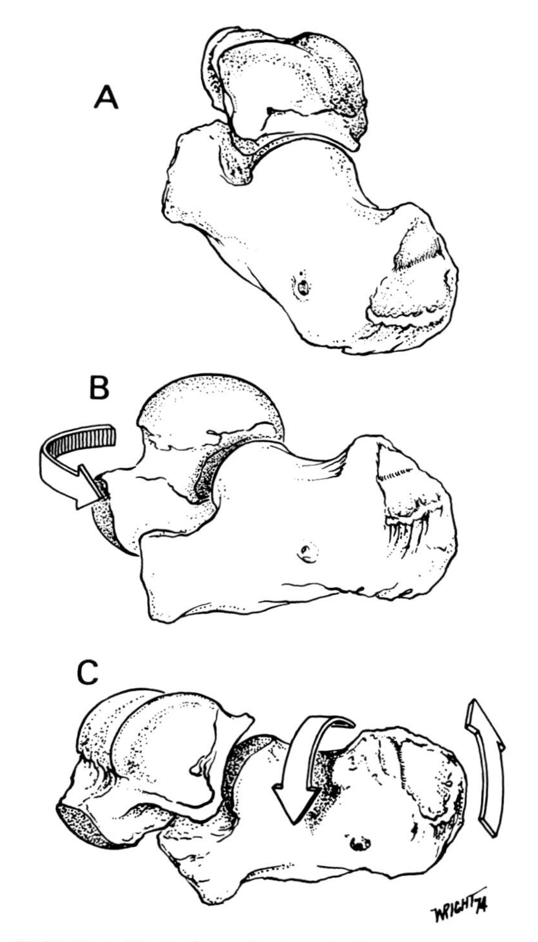

FIGURE 7–31. Pathomechanics of talipes equinovarus.

A. Posterolateral view of the calcaneus and talus of a normal foot. **B.** Lateral rotation of the talus. **C.** The anterior part of the calcaneus is pressed by the head of the talus and forced into plantar flexion, rotation, and varus position. (From Carroll, N., Murphy, R., and Leete, S. F.: The pathoanatomy of congenital clubfoot. Orthop. Clin. North Am., 9:227, 1978. Reprinted by permission.)

SOFT-TISSUE CHANGES

The soft tissues on the medial and posterior aspects of the foot and ankle are shortened. All the components of the tissues participate in the shortening—ligaments and capsules, muscles, tendons, tendon sheaths, vessels, nerves, and skin.

In talipes equinovarus, there are no gross abnormalities of the muscles, tendons, nerves, or vessels. Routine histologic stains have shown no pathologic changes.

Isaacs and co-workers studied the muscles in talipes equinovarus in 60 children, the majority of whom were under the age of five years. The muscle specimens were taken from the posteromedial and peroneal muscle groups, and occasionally from the abductor hallucis. Histologic and histochemical studies were performed in 111 biopsies, of which 53 specimens were examined by electron microscopy. Evidence of neurogenic disease was present in most instances. These abnormalities were found in both the shortened posteromedial (tibialis posterior, soleus, flexor digitorum longus, and flexor hallucis longus) and the lengthened peroneal muscle groups, indicating affection to a varying degree of all of the musculature between the knee and ankle.[330]

The muscle specimens studied by Isaacs and associates were not taken from fetal material; they were obtained at the operating table. There were, therefore, difficulties in distinguishing between congenital and adaptive changes. The neuropathic changes were more obvious in the older children. Isaacs and his coworkers' patients were treated soon after birth by gentle manipulation and stretching casts, which elongate the posteromedial muscles and relax the peronei. The pathologic changes were similar in both muscle groups and therefore not produced by physical trauma from stretching.[330] Scher, Handelsman, and Isaacs have investigated the effects on muscles of immobilization under tension and relaxation. Four young baboons had one foot immobilized in an extreme calcaneovalgus position. The casts were removed after periods of 8 to 25 weeks. Muscle biopsies were then taken from the posteromedial and peroneal muscle groups of both the immobilized and opposite control legs, and were examined histochemically and under the electron microscope. There were no significant changes in any of the muscle groups. The conclusion was that immobilization and the altered muscle tension produced by serial casts in treatment of talipes equinovarus are not the cause of the reported muscle changes.[616]

Repeated forceful manipulations and bruising of the foot or prolonged immobilization of the foot and leg in extreme positions will lead to fibrosis of soft parts.

In the full-term infant, the leg with talipes equinovarus is atrophic and smaller in circumference than the contralateral normal one; in the young fetus, however, the deformed and the opposite normal limb are of the same size. The atrophic changes are generalized and do not involve any one muscle group. The individual muscles have a normal relationship to each other. The insertion of tendons is normal, but the direction of their course is somewhat altered. The *Achilles tendon* inserts more medially and anteriorly on the calcaneus owing to the medial shift of the posterior part of the heel. The *posterior tibial tendon* is displaced anteriorly; passing from its groove behind the medial malleolus, it courses directly downward to insert into the tuberosity of the navicular and other structures on the plantar aspect of the foot. The *anterior tibial tendon* is displaced medially and is prominent as a tense cord crossing over the medial malleolus to its insertion into the base of the first metatarsal and medial cuneiforms. The peroneal tendons appear to be stretched out on the convex lateral border of the foot. The long toe flexors are contracted. On the plantar aspect of the foot, because of the equinus deformity of the forefoot, the plantar fascia, abductor hallucis, short toe flexors, and abductor digiti quinti are shortened.

The soft-tissue contractures, in order of their importance as obstacles to reduction of the talocalcaneonavicular joint, are as follows: (1) the plantar calcaneonavicular ligament; (2) the tibionavicular ligament; (3) the superior, medial, and plantar parts of the talonavicular capsule; and (4) the posterior tibial tendon with its numerous tendinous slips inserting into the navicular and the plantar aspect of the foot. At their attachment to the navicular, these contracted soft-tissue structures are all fused together into a dense mass of fibrous tissue, tethering the navicular and the sustentaculum tali to the medial malleolus (Fig. 7–32). (5) The master knot of Henry is a fibrous slip that envelops the flexor hallucis longus and flexor digitorum longus tendons as they cross each other; it binds them to the undersurface of the navicular. In talipes equinovarus, this fibrous "knot" is very much thickened and prevents anterolateral mobility of the navicular. It must be sectioned during reduction of the talocalcaneonavicular joint. Additional obstacles are (6) the calcaneofibular ligament, (7) the superior

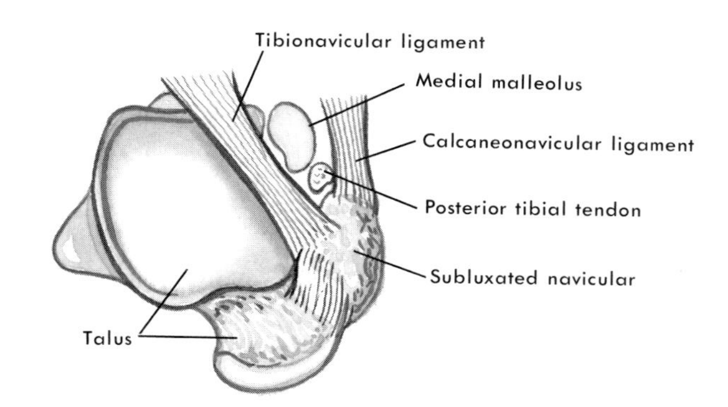

FIGURE 7–32. Primary obstacles to neutral realignment of the navicular on the head of the talus.

(1) The plantar calcaneonavicular ligament: (2) the tibionavicular ligament; (3) the superior, medial, and plantar parts of the capsule of the talonavicular joint; and (4) the posterior tibial tendon with its numerous tendinous slips inserting into the navicular and tethering the navicular to the medial malleolus.

peroneal (calcaneofibular) retinaculum, (8) the posterior talocalcaneal ligament, (9) the posterior capsule of the tibiotalar joint, (10) the tendo Achillis, (11) the interosseous ligament, and (12) the long toe flexors. All these contracted soft tissues are very rigid and prevent concentric reduction of the talocalcaneonavicular joint.

The effect of manipulation on talipes equinovarus in fetal specimens has been reported by Waisbrod. In true talipes equinovarus with deformed tali (decreased angle of declination) the feet could not be manipulated into normal position even by exerting considerable force. When the tali were normal (in postural clubfoot), however, the feet could be manipulated into normal position without difficulty.[730] Irani and Sherman in their study of fetal specimens with talipes equinovarus state that, even after muscles were completely detached from their insertion, the position of the foot could not be corrected by manipulation; it was only after sectioning of all the ligaments between the talonavicular and calcaneonavicular joints together with posterior subtalar joint capsule that the equinovarus deformity could be completely corrected.[328, 329] Repeatedly, the author has observed the same phenomenon; that is, although all the muscles and tendons of the foot and ankle are detached in talipes equinovarus, the deformity of the foot persists; to obtain normal alignment of the talocalcaneonavicular joint, one has to section the ligaments between the talus and navicular, between the talus and calcaneus, and between the navicular and calcaneus, and has to divide the posterior ligaments and capsule of the ankle joint (peritalar release). The talus moves in a plane from anteromedial to posterolateral; therefore, the subtalar joint is always inverted with the talus in plantar flexion. To obtain correction of inversion and to unlock the inverted calcaneus underneath the talus, the equinus deformity must always be corrected.

For better understanding of articular malalignment in talipes equinovarus, the complex mechanism of the talocalcaneonavicular joint is reviewed next. The talocalcaneonavicular joint differs from the ordinary ball-and-socket articulation in that the socket moves around the ball (the head of the talus). The socket is formed anteriorly by the navicular; dorsomedially by the tibionavicular ligament, the capsule of the talonavicular joint, and the posterior tibial tendon; laterally by the calcaneonavicular limb of the bifurcated (Y) ligament; inferiorly by the plantar calcaneonavicular (spring) ligament and the anterior and middle facets on the superior surface of the calcaneus; and posteriorly by the talocalcaneal interosseous ligament. Because of their strong ligamentous connections, the calcaneus and the navicular move as a unit around the talus. The axis of rotation is the interosseous talocalcaneal ligament and the posterior subtalar joint, where minimal motion occurs. Horizontal movements take place at the talonavicular and the anterior and middle subtalar joints. In *eversion*, the navicular and anterior end of the os calcis move *laterally*, whereas in *inversion*, they move medially (Fig. 7–33). Inversion-eversion of the heel cannot take place if the talonavicular joint is internally fixed with a Steinmann pin.[389] Medial rotation of the calcaneus under the talus cannot be corrected unless the navicular is "released" to move distally and laterally on the head of the talus.

Upon plantar flexion and dorsiflexion of the ankle, both the tibiotalar and the talocalcaneonavicular joints move. During plantar flexion, the calcaneus supinates under the talus, with the anterior end moving plantarward and medially, while its posterior tuberosity moves dorsally and laterally. Simultaneously, the navicular moves medially on the head of the talus. During dorsiflexion, the calcaneus pronates under the talus with the anterior end of the calcaneus moving dorsally and laterally, while

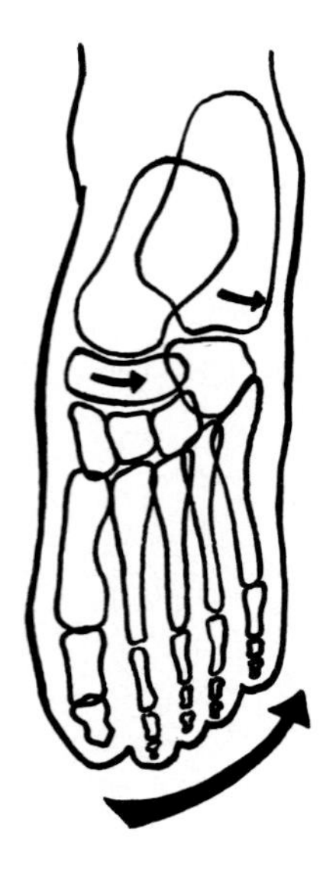

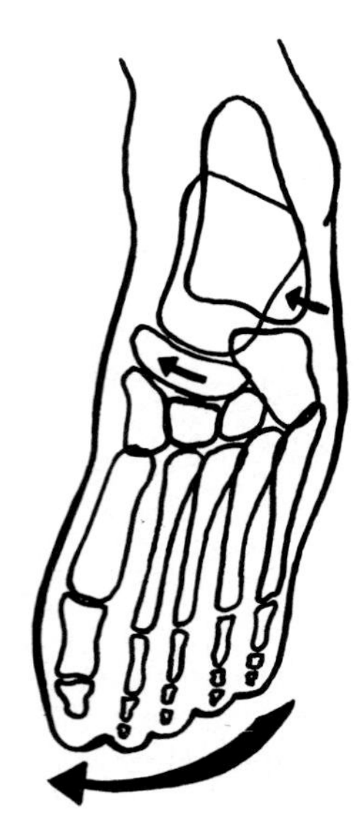

FIGURE 7–33. The calcaneus and navicular move as a unit because of their strong ligamentous connections.

In eversion, the navicular and anterior ends of the os calcis move laterally; in inversion, they move medially.

its posteromedial tubercle moves plantarward. Again simultaneously, the navicular moves laterally as the foot dorsiflexes. The talocalcaneonavicular joint expands and contracts because of its partial ligamentous composition. In dorsiflexion the greater portion of the talar head is covered, and the capacity of the talocalcaneonavicular socket is thereby increased; in plantar flexion, however, more of the talar head is exposed laterally, and the talocalcaneonavicular socket is decreased in volume.[705–707] The calcaneus navigates under the talus like a boat on ocean waves. Its anterior end (the prow of the boat) pitches as its posterior end (the stern of the boat) plunges; and its body turns on itself.[196]

These complex movements of the calcaneus under the talus have been studied experimentally by Campos da Paz, Jr., and De Souza.[100] Indicating the longitudinal axes of the talus and calcaneus by Kirschner wires and marking the axis of the subtalar joint by a Kirschner wire that penetrates the superomedial aspect of the talar neck, crosses the sinus tarsi, and exits at the posteromedial tubercle of the calcaneus, they suspended the connected talus and calcaneus by a specially designed support and analyzed the movements of the calcaneus. Viewed from the lateral side, supination of the calcaneus opened up the sinus tarsi and lowered the anterior end of the calcaneus into plantar flexion (Fig. 7–34 A). Pronation elevated its anterior end into dorsiflexion and depressed the medial tubercle of its posterior tuberosity where the Achilles tendon is inserted (Fig. 7–34 B). Seen from behind when the calcaneus is in maximal supination, the lateral and medial tubercles of its posterior tuberosity are on the same level (Fig. 7–34 C), whereas in pronation, the medial tubercle is depressed plantarward (Fig. 7–34 D). One can best visualize the navigation of the calcaneus under the talus from the front; on transition from supination to pronation, the anterior end is raised superiorly (the pitching of the prow), and the insertion of the Achilles tendon at the medial tubercle of the tuberosity moves inferiorly (plunging of the stern) (Fig. 7–34 E and F). The anteroposterior talocalcaneal angle widens as the calcaneus is shifted from supination to pronation. It is evident, therefore, that to obtain pronation of the calcaneus, the medial tubercle of its posterior tuberosity should move inferiorly into plantar flexion. In talipes equinovarus, this can be accomplished only through lengthening of the triceps surae muscle and sectioning of the posterior contracted soft tissues that restrict dorsiflexion, namely, the posterior capsule of the ankle and subtalar joints, and the posterior talofibular and calcaneofibular ligaments.

With the unified movements of the calcaneus and navicular, the talus and the related joints above the ankle—the knee and hip—move in synchrony. In stance, when the calcaneus of a normal foot is inverted, the anterior part of the calcaneus must first descend plantarward, and then rotate and move medially to lie underneath the head of the talus. Simultaneously, the talar head is elevated into dorsiflexion and moves laterally into lateral rotation; the malleoli rotate, the lateral malleolus moving laterally, and the

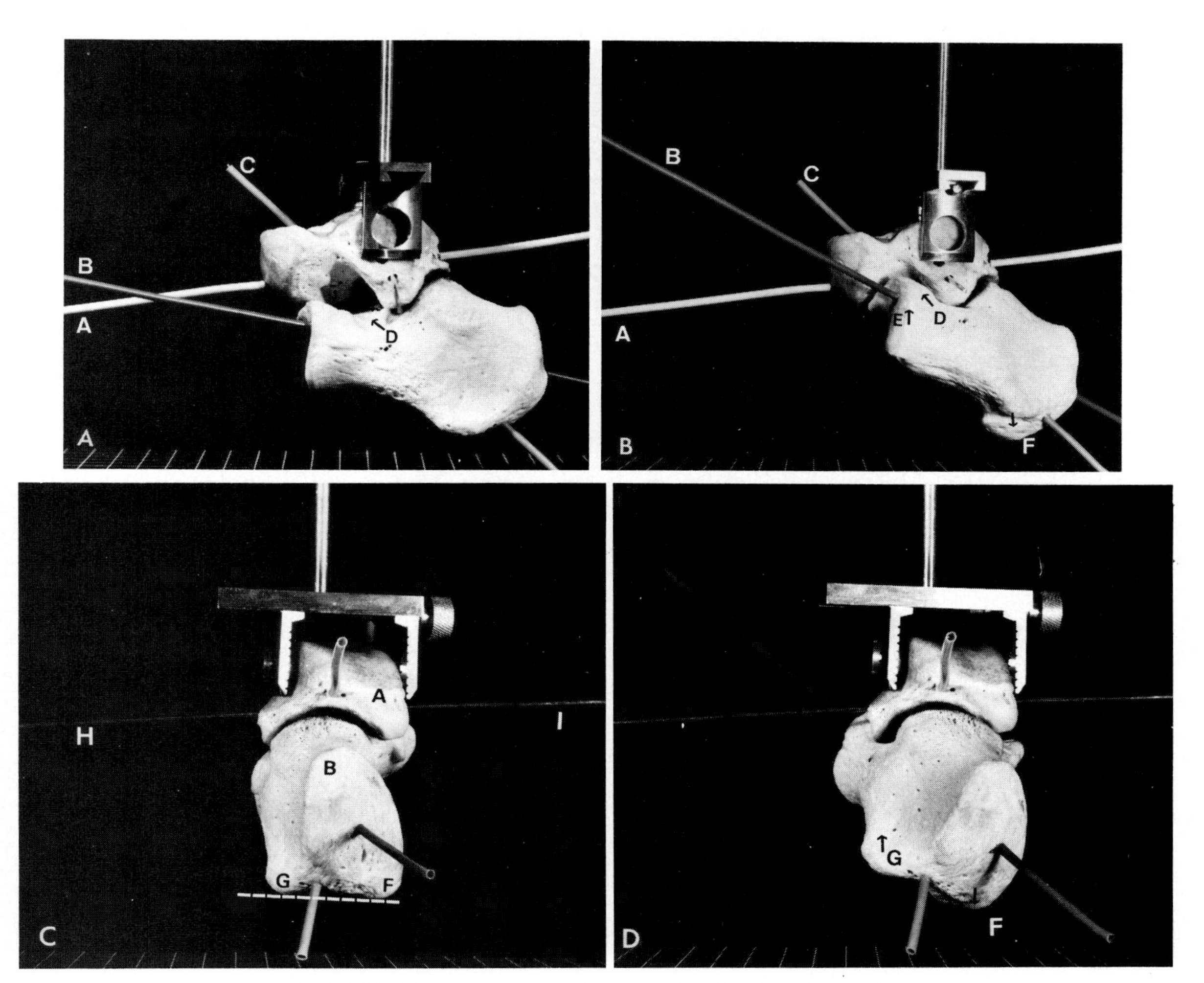

FIGURE 7–34. Movements of the calcaneus under the talus of the left foot.

Kirschner wires mark the longitudinal axes of the talus (A), calcaneus (B), and subtalar joint (C). G is the lateral and F the medial tubercle of the calcaneal tuberosity; E is the anterior end of the calcaneus. D marks the sinus tarsi. **A.** Lateral view in supination. The anterior end of the calcaneus moves in plantar flexion and the sinus tarsi is opened up. **B.** Lateral view in pronation. The sinus tarsi closes, the anterior end of the calcaneus is elevated into dorsiflexion, and the medial tubercle of the posterior tuberosity is displaced into plantar flexion. **C** and **D.** Posterior views of the left foot. In **C,** the calcaneus is in maximal supination—note that the lateral and medial tubercles of the posterior tuberosity of the calcaneus are at the same level. In **D,** the calcaneus is pronated—note the plantar migration of the medial tubercle.

Illustration continued on following page

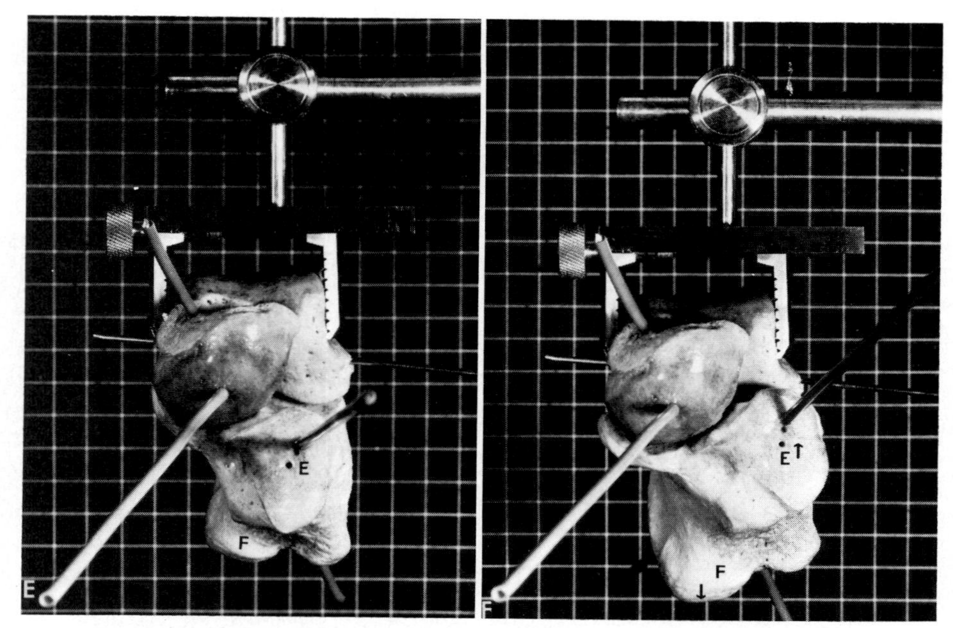

FIGURE 7–34 Continued. Movements of the calcaneus under the talus of the left foot.

E and **F.** Anterior views of the left foot. In **E** the calcaneus is supinated and in **F**, pronated. Note the same movements of the calcaneus under the talus. In transition from supination to pronation, the anterior end of the calcaneus (E) is elevated into dorsiflexion and the medial tubercle of the posterior tuberosity (F) is displaced into plantar flexion. (From Campos da Paz, A., Jr., and De Souza, V.: Talipes equinovarus: Pathomechanical basis of treatment. Orthop. Clin. North Am., 9:172–175, 1978. Reprinted by permission.)

medial malleolus moving anteriorly. Consequently, the whole leg and the hip rotate laterally, with the patellae facing outward (Fig. 7–35 A and B). On eversion of the calcaneus, a reverse chain of movements takes place—the lateral malleolus moves forward, the patellae face inward, and the hips rotate medially (Fig. 7–35 C).

In talipes equinovarus with inversion of the calcaneus, by necessity the malleoli rotate around a vertical axis into lateral rotation. At birth the fibular malleolus is posterior in relation to the medial malleolus. To correct the position of the posteriorly rotated fibular malleolus the anterior end of the talus must be rotated medially (to "unlock" the hindfoot), and the anterior end of the calcaneus must be rotated laterally and elevated dorsally to lie on the lateral side of the head of the talus.

Rotational deformities of the lower limb in talipes equinovarus may be exaggerated during the course of inadequate management. The aggravating and causative factors are improper manipulation and stretching casts, walking on the varus hindfoot, and voluntary compensation at the hip for in-toeing. The levels of lateral rotation are at the ankle, hip, and tibiofibular articulations.

Wynne-Davies and more recently Swann, Lloyd-Roberts, and Catterall have pointed out the effect of improper manipulation and stretching casts on the ankle joint. With fixed contracture of the ligaments (tibionavicular, plantar calcaneonavicular, and talonavicular), correction does not take place at the talocalcaneonavicular joint. The abduction and lateral rotation forces are transmitted to the talus in the ankle mortise. The deformity remains uncorrected in the horizontal plane, and spurious correction takes place at the ankle joint. The talus is rotated laterally in the ankle mortise, carrying the fibular malleolus posteriorly with it (Fig. 7–36). This is called "horizontal breach" by Swann, Lloyd-Roberts, and Catterall.[681, 769]

The already posteriorly positioned lateral malleolus is further displaced posteriorly by premature eversion of the hindfoot. In the lateral radiogram of the foot in a standing position this is easily identified by the posterior location of the fibular malleolus in relation to the medial malleolus and the "flat-topped" appearance of the dome of the talus. The x-ray tube is centered on the hindfoot and ankle, with the foot as nearly as possible at a right angle to the leg. The calcaneus will appear shortened and the forefoot will look relatively

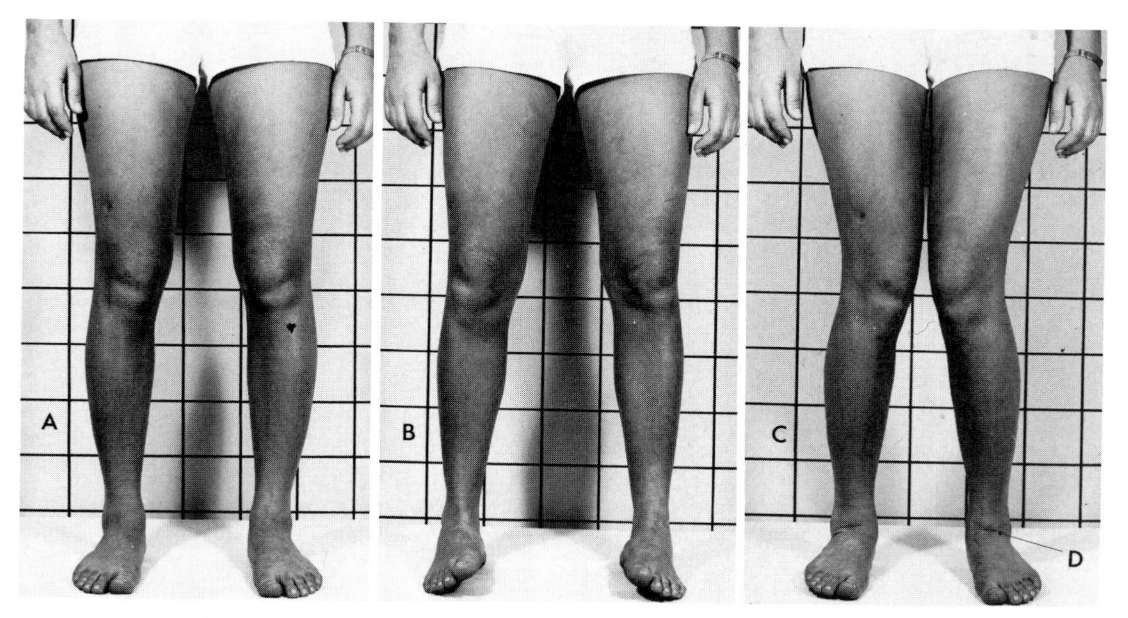

FIGURE 7–35. The relationship of the calcaneus with the ground and the synchronized movements of the subtalar, ankle, knee, and hip joints.

A. Normal. **B.** On inversion of the calcaneus, note the corresponding lateral rotation of the hip joints. **C.** On eversion of the calcaneus, the hip joints rotate medially. (From Campos da Paz, A., Jr., and De Souza, V.: Talipes equinovarus: Pathomechanical basis of treatment. Orthop. Clin. North Am., 9:177, 1978. Reprinted by permission.)

normal. The flat-topped appearance of the talus is spurious, the result of its lateral rotation and projection in a frontal profile in the lateral radiogram. If another radiogram is taken with the leg internally rotated, the summit of the talus will be dome-shaped, and the length and contour of the calcaneus will improve. The forefoot varus inclination will be increased, as shown by the overlap of the cuboid and navicular bones on the calcaneus and talus (Fig. 7–37).

In addition to lateral rotation at the ankle joint, there may be sufficient rotatory force transmitted vertically along the longitudinal axis of the tibia and fibula to the hip joint to cause the entire lower limb to rotate laterally at the hip (Figs. 7–38 and 7–39). In walking, voluntary lateral rotation takes place at the hip to compensate for in-toeing due to the varus foot. With skeletal growth, structural lateral tibiofibular torsion takes place in the older child.[648, 653]

In talipes equinovarus, reduction of medial and plantar subluxation of the talocalcaneonavicular joint is prevented by contracture of soft tissues. It behooves us to remember, when planning surgical division of these soft-tissue contractures, that motions of plantar flexion and inversion at the ankle and talocalcaneonavicular joint take place as synchronized and not as separate isolated movements.

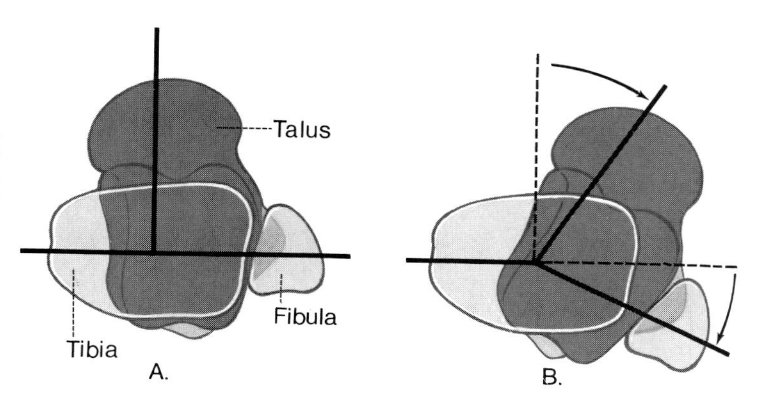

FIGURE 7–36. "Horizontal breach" according to the concept of Swann, Lloyd-Roberts, and Catterall.

A. A cross section through the distal tibia at the level of the ankle shows the normal position of the talus in the ankle mortise. **B.** A cross section through the distal tibia at the level of the ankle shows the position of the talus in the ankle mortise when the "horizontal breach" deformity has occurred. The talus rotates laterally and the fibula moves posteriorly while the tibia remains stationary. (Courtesy of Dr. George Simons.)

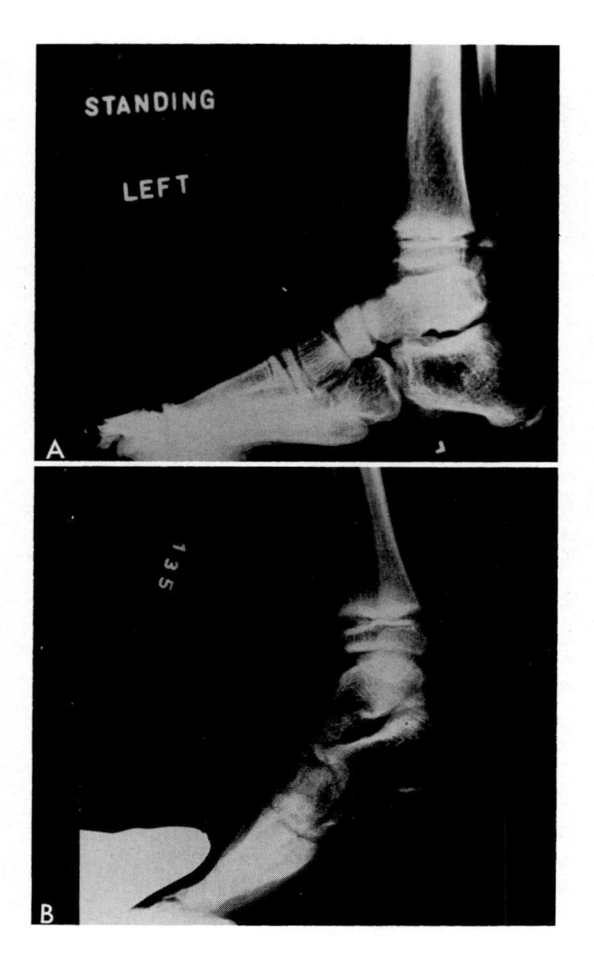

FIGURE 7–37. The radiographic appearance of "horizontal breach" in the lateral projection of the foot and ankle.

A. The fibular malleolus appears to have moved to a posterior position in relation to the medial malleolus. The dome of the body of the talus has assumed a "flat-top" appearance. The anteroposterior diameter of the calcaneus is shortened. **B.** In a lateral projection of the same foot and ankle after the foot has been medially rotated 45 degrees, the fibula has returned to its normal position in relation to the tibia, the shadow of the lateral malleolus overlaps that of the medial malleolus, the dome of the talus has been restored to its normal shape, and the anteroposterior diameter of the calcaneus is of normal length.

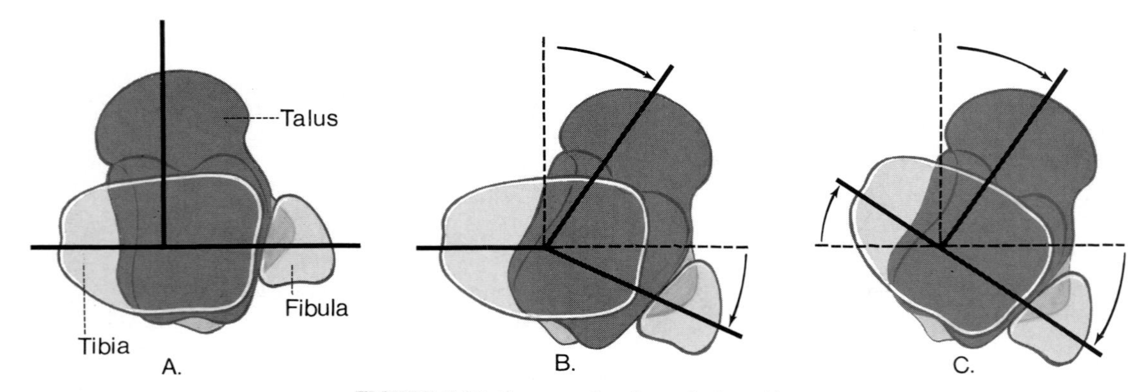

FIGURE 7–38. Cross section through the ankle.

A. The normal relationship of the talus in the ankle mortise *(shaded area)*. **B.** The relationship of the talus in the ankle mortise when "horizontal breach" takes place. Note that the talus rotates laterally, the fibula moves posteriorly, and the tibia remains stationary. **C.** The relationship of the talus in the ankle mortise when compensatory lateral rotation occurs at the hip. Both the tibia and fibula have rotated laterally through the longitudinal axis of the tibia. The talus has maintained its normal relationship to the ankle mortise. (Courtesy of Dr. George Simons.)

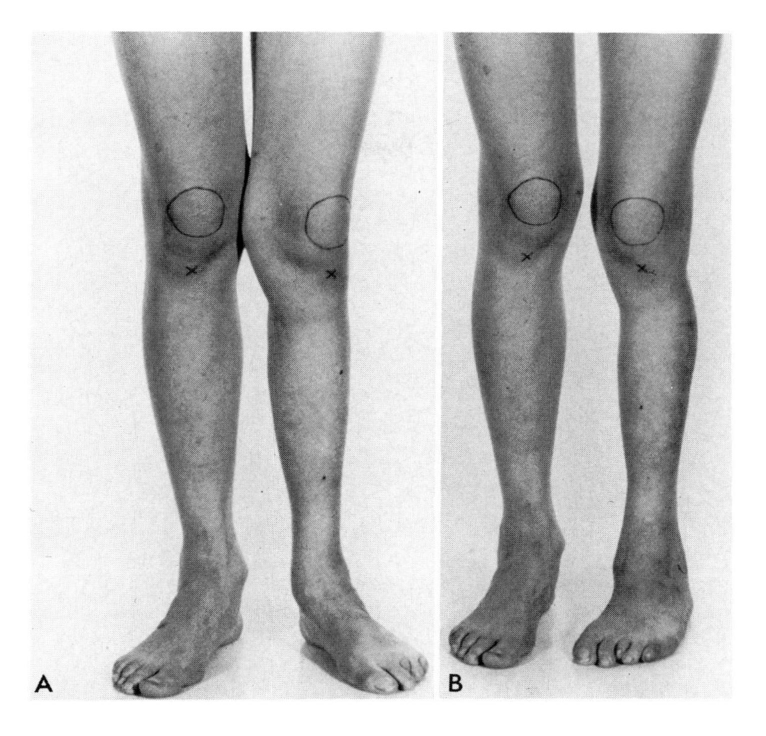

FIGURE 7–39. Clinical and radiographic appearance of the left foot in a seven-year-old child with persistent medial subluxation of the talocalcaneonavicular joint.

A. The medial border of the left foot is parallel to the sagittal plane and the foot is pointing forward. Note the patella of the affected limb is pointing laterally. The right foot is normal. **B.** Note the varus deformity of the left foot when the limb is medially rotated and the patella is facing straight forward.

Illustration continued on following page

The navicular is fixed to the medial malleolus and the sustentaculum tali of the os calcis by the contracted tibionavicular ligament, plantar calcaneonavicular ligament, dorsal medial capsule of the talonavicular joint, and posterior tibial tendon. For the calcaneus to move from supination to pronation and its anterior end to move from plantar flexion to dorsiflexion, the navicular should be released from these soft-tissue checkreins and positioned concentrically in relation to the head of the talus. This cannot be achieved by manipulative stretching in fetal specimens. It is only after the tissues have been sharply divided with a scalpel that one can position the navicular on the head of the talus.

In order to pronate the calcaneus under the talus and obtain normal divergence of the anteroposterior talocalcaneal angle, the posteromedial tubercle of the calcaneal tuberosity should move plantarward. This is prevented by the calcaneofibular ligament, the calcaneofibular retinaculum, the shortened Achilles tendon, and the contracted posterior capsule and ligaments. In fetal specimens with talipes equinovarus, isolated sectioning of the Achilles tendon will not permit dorsiflexion. One has to divide the posterior capsules of the ankle (tibiotalar) and the subtalar (talocalcaneal) joints, and the calcaneofibular ligament.

The interosseous talocalcaneal ligament is relaxed when the foot is in equinovarus posture. In talipes equinovarus, it may become contracted and may bind the inverted calcaneus under the talus. In such an instance, the interosseous talocalcaneal ligament must be sectioned to achieve reduction of the talocalcaneonavicular joint. The calcaneonavicular limb of the bifurcated, or Y, ligament connects the calcaneus to the lateral border of the navicular. When markedly contracted, it will obstruct lateral mobility of the navicular. It is evident, therefore, that to achieve concentric reduction of the talocalcaneonavicular joint, *all soft-tissue obstacles should be sectioned in one stage by complete peritalar release.*

The pathologic changes vary according to the severity of the bony and articular deformity and the degree of the soft-tissue contracture. The age of the patient and the type of prior treatment are also factors to consider.

Diagnosis

The clinical picture of talipes equinovarus is characteristic; the affected foot and leg have a clublike appearance (Fig. 7–40). The foot points plantarward with the small heel drawn up and rolled in under the talus in an inverted position.

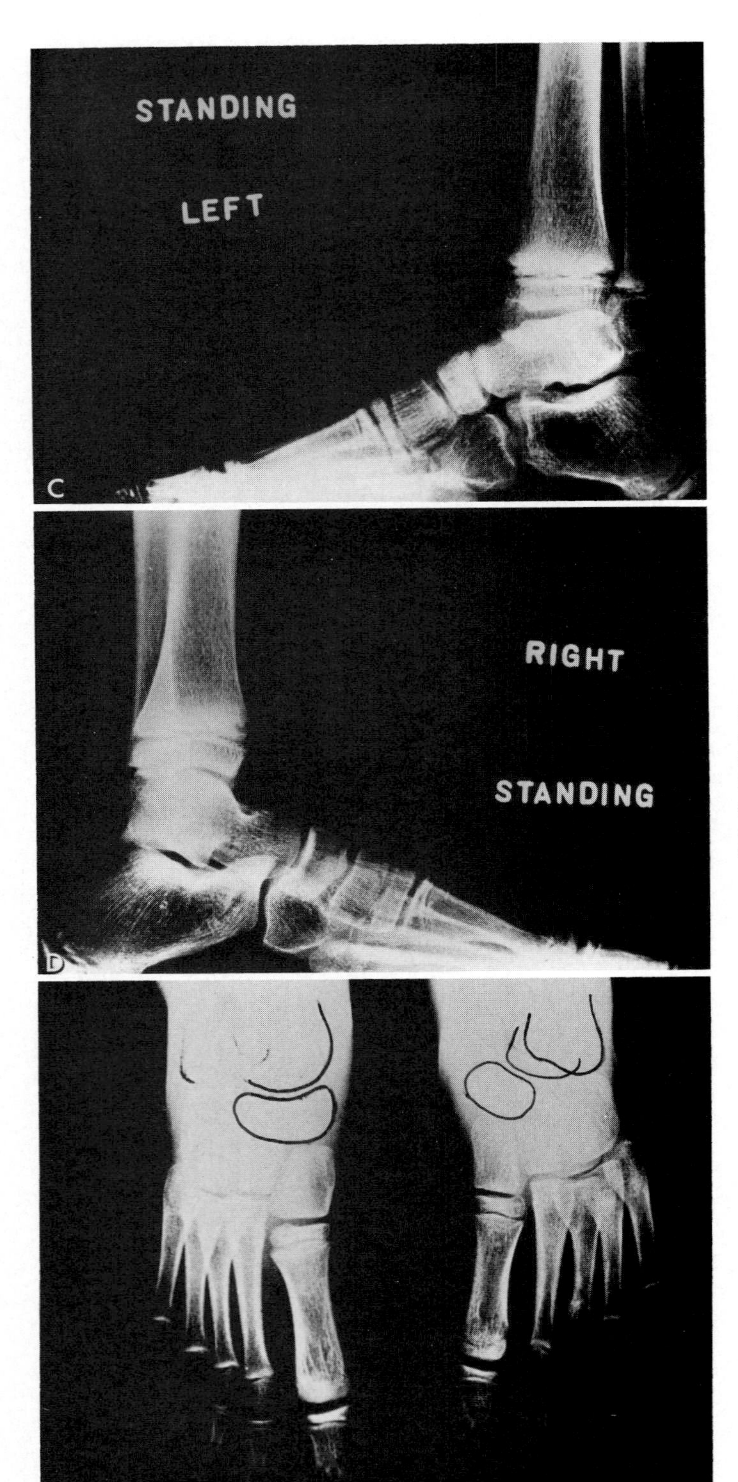

FIGURE 7–39 Continued

C. Lateral radiogram of the left ankle and foot with the toes facing straight forward. Note the posterior position of the fibular malleolus in relation to the medial malleolus and the flattening of the talar dome. **D.** Lateral radiogram of the normal right foot and ankle. **E.** Anteroposterior radiogram of both feet, showing medial subluxation of the navicular.

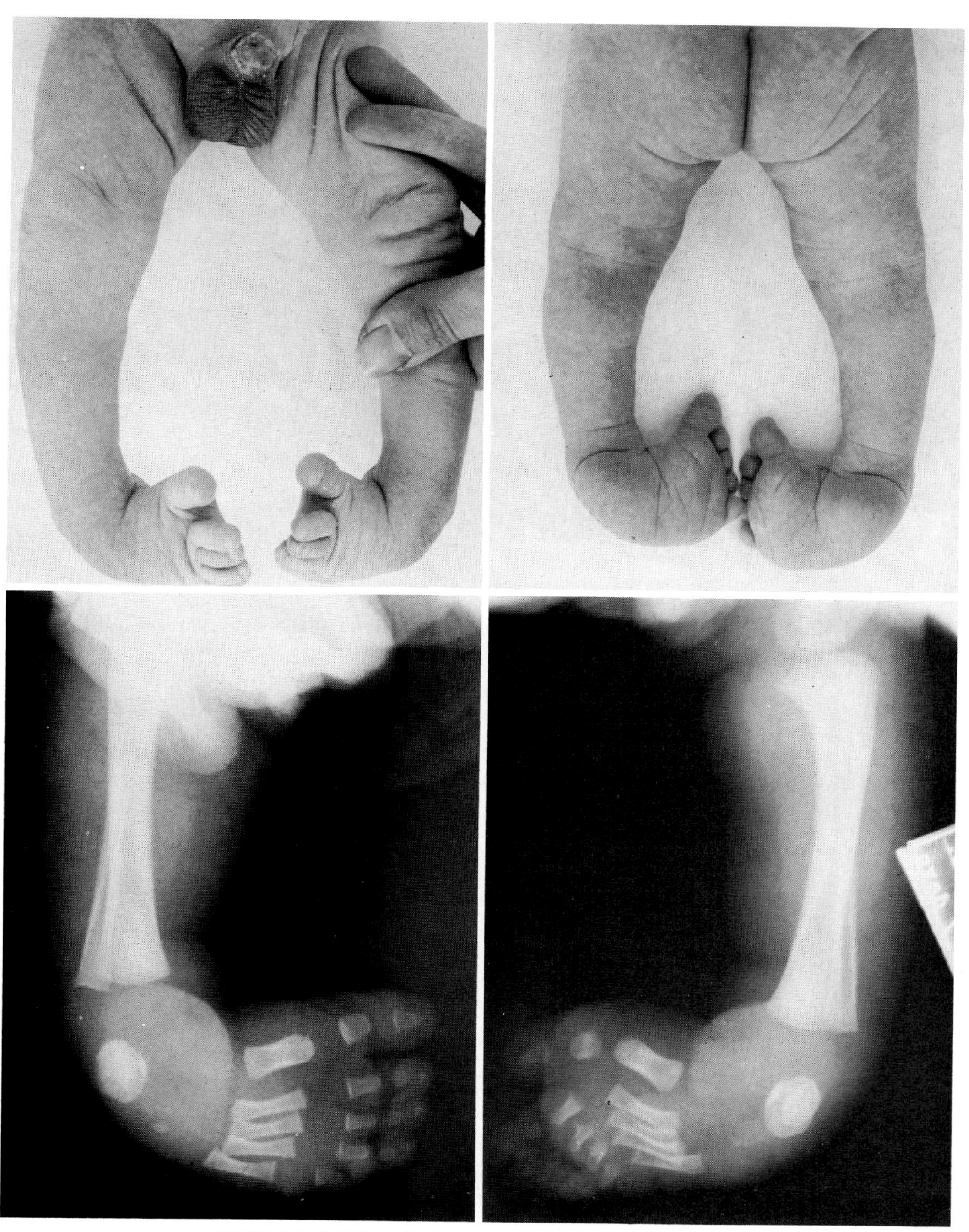

FIGURE 7–40. *Bilateral talipes equinovarus in a newborn infant.*

There are deep creases at the posterior aspect of the ankle joint. The mid- and forefoot are adducted, inverted, and have an equinus pitch. With the inversion of the entire foot and adduction of the forefoot, the anterior end of the talus is the most prominent subcutaneous bone on the lateral side of the dorsum of the foot. The skin in this convex area of the foot is thinned and stretched, and its creases have disappeared. The lateral malleolus is posterior to and more prominent than the medial malleolus. The skin creases are deeply furrowed on the concave medial and plantar aspects of the foot. The navicular bone abuts the anterior and medial margins of the medial malleolus; on palpation, one cannot insert a finger between the two bones. The forefoot is in equinus position, and the soft tissues on the plantar aspect of the foot are contracted.

On passive dorsiflexion and eversion of the foot, the taut triceps surae and posterior tibial tendon can be palpated. One can also feel the thickened and shortened ligaments and joint capsules on the medial aspect of the foot and the posterior aspect of the ankle and subtalar joints. There is usually moderate to severe atrophy of the calf and a varying degree of shortening of the affected leg. The equinovarus deformity is fixed and can be corrected only minimally by passive manipulation. If talipes equinovarus remains untreated, the deformity will progressively increase and the contractures will become more rigid. The child will bear weight on the lateral border of the foot and on the fibular malleolus (Fig. 7–41). Ambulation will be difficult and the gait awkward. Soon painful callosities and bursae will develop over the lateral side of the foot.

It is important to differentiate talipes equinovarus from postural clubfoot (Table 7–7). In the latter, the deformity is mild and can be readily corrected to neutral position by passive manipulation. It most probably is caused by intrauterine malposture. Anatomically, the head and neck of the talus are not tilted medially and there is no subluxation or dislocation of the talocalcaneonavicular joint in postural clubfoot. Clinically, the skin creases on the dorsolateral aspect of the ankle and foot are normal, the heel is of normal size, and the leg is of normal circumference or minimally atrophied. On palpation, there is normal space between the navicular and the medial malleolus. The equinovarus deformity is relatively flexible and can be readily corrected to neutral position by passive manipulation. The opposite foot may be in valgus posture, and there may be associated pelvic obliquity with adduction contracture of the contralateral hip and adduction contracture of the ipsilateral hip.

The foot may have a clubfoot appearance in congenital absence or hypoplasia of the tibia and in congenital dislocation of the ankle. Careful palpation of the anatomic relationship of the hindfoot to the medial and lateral malleoli, and radiograms, will establish the diagnosis.

Talipes equinovarus, a congenital deformity, must also be distinguished from acquired types of clubfoot. In the newborn this is relatively easy, but in the older child it may pose a

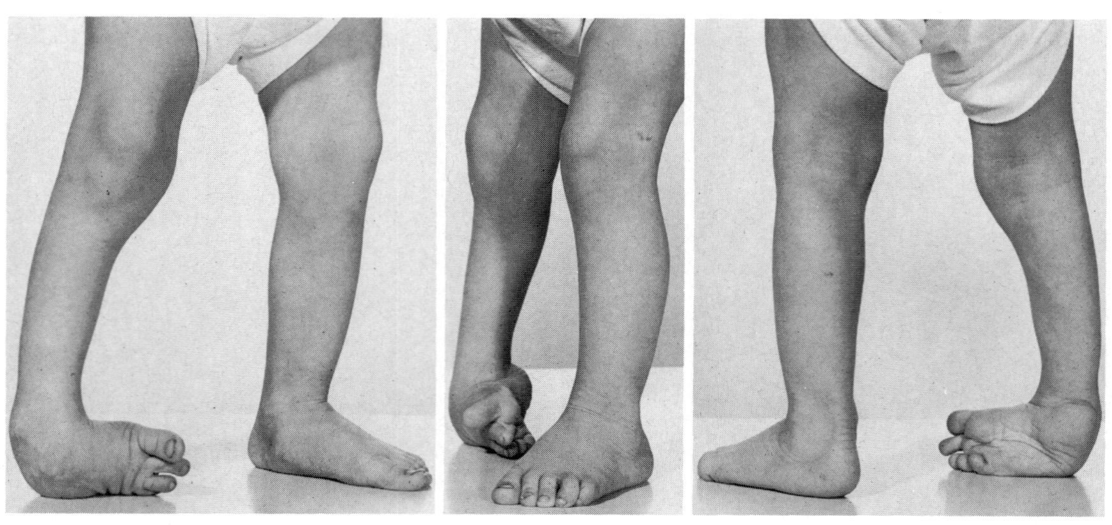

FIGURE 7–41. Untreated severe talipes equinovarus on the right in a three-year-old boy.

The body weight is borne on the lateral border of the foot.

Table 7–7. Differential Diagnosis of Postural Clubfoot and Talipes Equinovarus

	Postural Clubfoot	Talipes Equinovarus
Etiology	Intrauterine malposture	Primary germ plasm defect Defective cartilaginous anlage of the talus
Pathologic Anatomy		
Head and neck of talus	Normal Declination angle of talus normal 150 to 155 degrees	Medial and plantar tilt Declination angle of talus decreased 115 to 135 degrees
Talocalcaneonavicular joint	Normal	Subluxated or dislocated medially and plantarward
Effect of manipulation in fetal specimens	Normal alignment of foot can be restored	Talocalcaneonavicular subluxation cannot be reduced unless ligaments and capsule connecting navicular to calcaneus, talus, and tibia are sectioned and posterior capsule and ligaments divided
Clinical Features		
Severity of deformity	Mild and flexible	Marked and rigid; minimal or no correction on manipulation
Heel	Normal size	Small, drawn up
Relation between navicular and medial malleolus	Normal space between two bones; can insert finger	Navicular abuts medial malleolus: finger cannot be inserted between two bones
Lateral malleolus	Normal position	Posteriorly displaced with anterior part of talus very prominent in front of it
Mobility of lateral malleolus on plantar flexion and dorsiflexion of the ankles	Normal	Fixed to calcaneus with very restricted range of excursion
Lateral border of the foot	Convex; normal relationship of cuboid to calcaneus No step-off	Very convex with cuboid bone displaced medially over anterolateral end of calcaneus Definite step-off; no correction on passive abduction of forefoot
Medial border of foot	Concave with normal skin crease	Concave with furrowed skin No passive manipulation if cannot be straightened
Forefoot	In slight varus, but not in equinus	In fixed equinus and varying degrees of varus
Plantar soft tissues	Not taut	Taut with marked contracture of soft tissues
Skin creases on		
Dorsolateral aspect of foot	Present; normal	Thin or absent
Medial and plantar aspects of foot	No furrowed skin	Furrowed skin
Posterior aspect of ankle	Normal	Deep crease
Calf and leg atrophy	None or very minimal	Moderate to marked
Treatment	Passive manipulation followed by retention by adhesive strapping, splint, or cast	Primary open reduction of talocalcaneonavicular joint often required; surgery is conservative Closed methods of reduction often unsuccessful Prolonged retentive apparatus essential
Prognosis	Excellent; result is normal foot	Poor with closed methods Prolonged cast immobilization results in smaller foot and atrophied leg

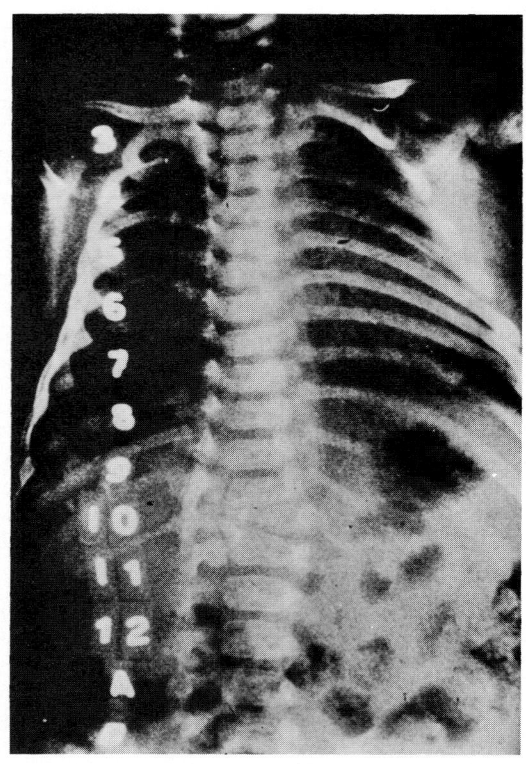

***FIGURE 7–42.** Diastematomyelia of the spine at T_{12}–L_1 level in a newborn infant with bilateral severe talipes equinovarus.*

The spine should be carefully examined for abnormalities.

problem. The spine should be carefully examined for abnormalities, and muscle testing should be performed. Radiograms of the entire vertebral column should be made (Fig. 7–42). The neuromuscular system should be carefully assessed to rule out paralytic disease. Paralytic clubfoot is seen in myelomeningocele, intraspinal tumors, diastematomyelia, poliomyelitis, the distal type of progressive muscular atrophy, cerebral palsy, and Guillain-Barré disease.

Not necessarily an isolated deformity, talipes equinovarus may be associated with multiple congenital malformations or be a part of a generalized developmental syndrome. At the Shriner's Hospital for Crippled Children in Mexico City, 14.15 per cent of the 300 patients with talipes equinovarus had other associated congenital anomalies.[720] It therefore behooves us to examine the whole child.

The deformity is commonly encountered in arthrogryposis multiplex congenita. The hips, knees, elbows, and shoulders must be carefully examined for subluxation or dislocation. What is the range of motion of the peripheral joints? Is there any abnormal extension or flexion contracture? A marked decrease of muscle mass and fibrosis are characteristic of arthrogryposis multiplex congenita (Fig. 7–43).

Bartholini, in 1673, was the first to report association of clubfoot with congenital amputation.[31] Clubfoot is also frequently found along with congenital annular constriction bands (Streeter's dysplasia) (Fig. 7–44). Cowell and Hensinger reviewed 25 cases of congenital annular bands of the limbs and found clubfeet in 56 per cent of them.[134] The frequent association of these two congenital malformations can be explained by early rupture of the amnion with formation of amniotic bands and oligohydramnios.[697, 698] In experiments performed on rats, clubbing of the paws was produced by removal of amniotic fluid during gestation.[156]

"Clubfoot" is frequently encountered in other syndromes. *Diastrophic dwarfism* is manifest at birth and is characterized by small stature; soft cystic masses in the auricle, which later develop into hypertrophic cartilage and give cauliflower deformity of the pinnae; cleft palate; marked shortening of the first metacarpals with proximally set hypermobile thumbs; flexion contracture and varying degrees of webbing of the knees, hips, elbows, shoulders, and interphalangeal joints; and progressive kyphoscoliosis (Fig. 7–45). The equinovarus deformity of the feet is severe and bilateral, and there is increased space between the hallux and second toe. In the radiograms, the metatarsals and

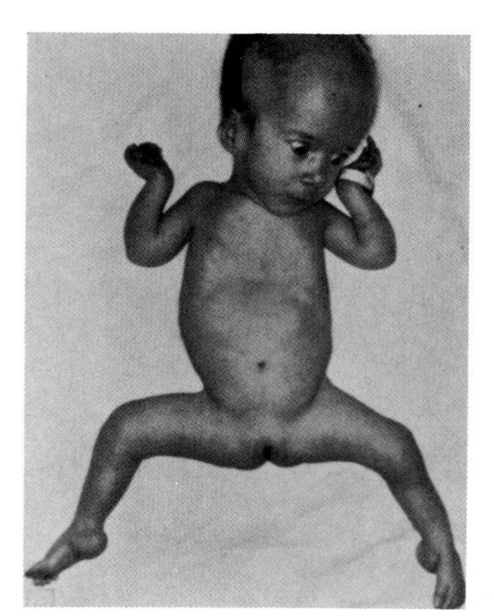

***FIGURE 7–43.** An infant with arthrogryposis multiplex congenita.*

Note the bilateral talipes equinovarus. Both hips are dislocated. The knees are fixed in extension. The radial heads are dislocated. The fingers are clenched in the palm and the thumbs adducted.

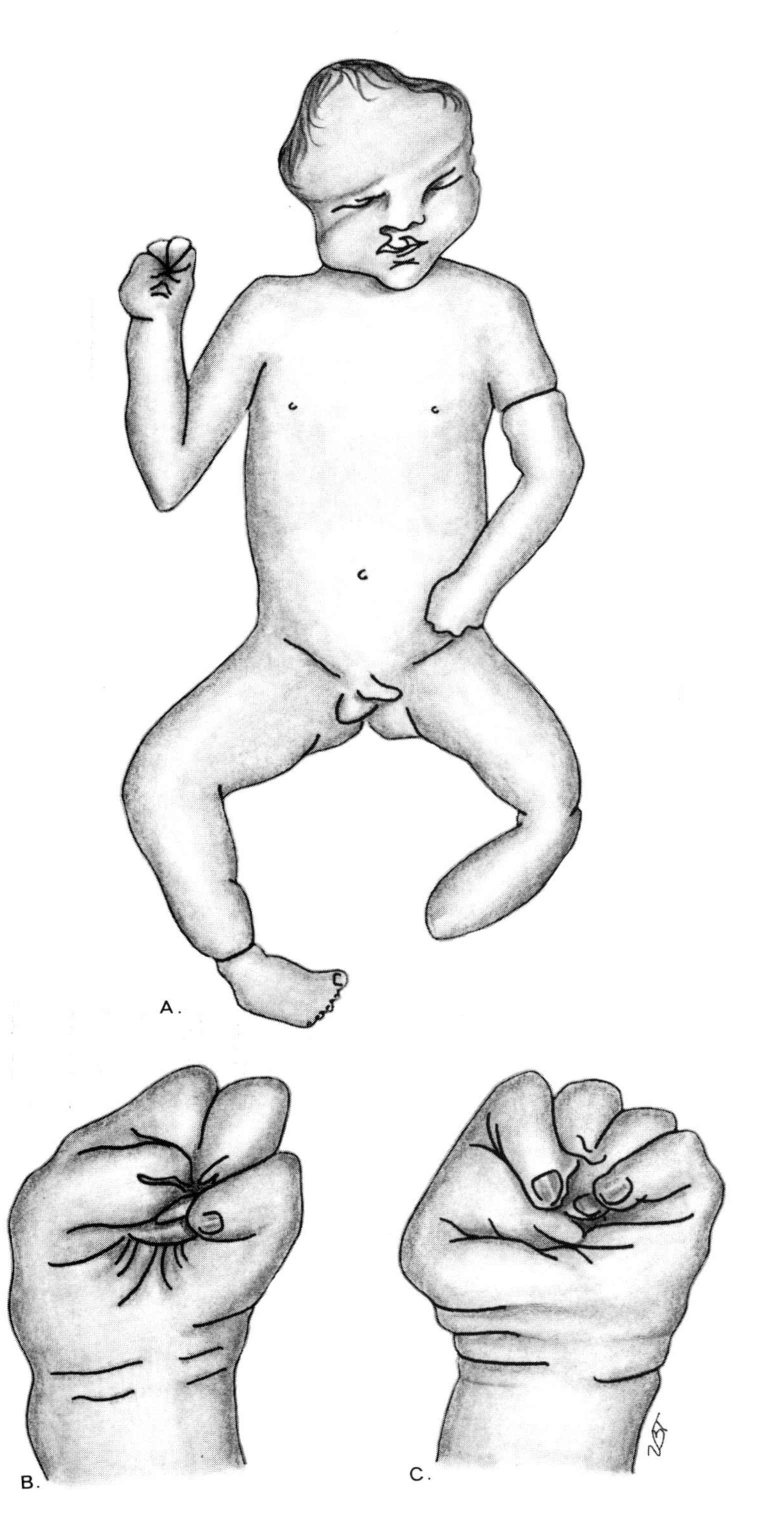

FIGURE 7–44. Talipes equinovarus in an infant with Streeter's dysplasia.

A. Note the constriction band on the lower leg on the right. **B** and **C.** Deformities of the hands.

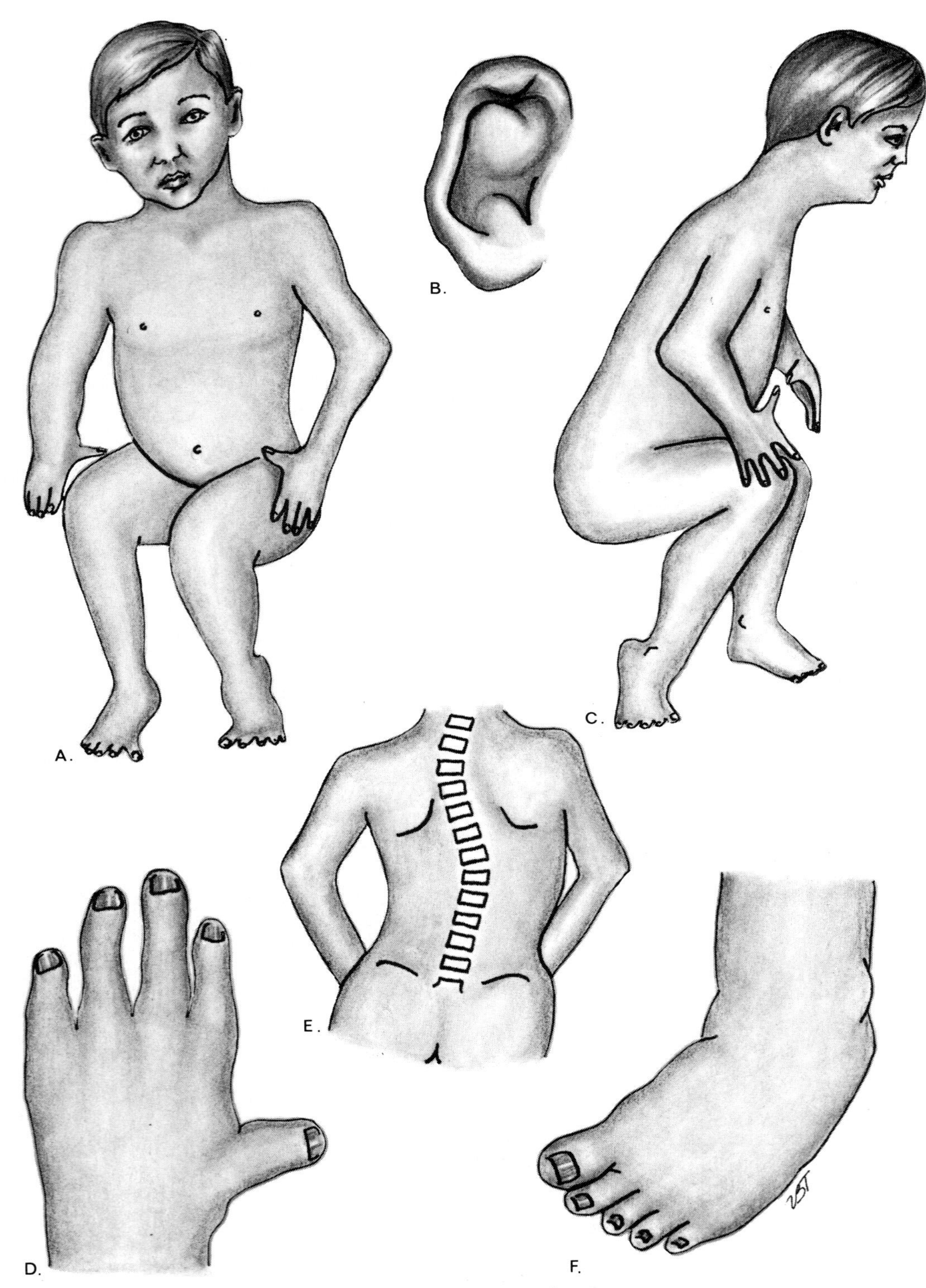

FIGURE 7–45. ***Diastrophic dwarfism.***

Typical physical findings include: **A,** small stature; **B,** auricular masses that give cauliflower deformity of the pinnae; cleft palate; **C,** flexion contracture and varying degrees of webbing of the knees, hips, elbows, shoulders, and interphalangeal joints; **D,** marked shortening of the first metacarpals with proximally set hypermobile thumbs; **E,** progressive kyphoscoliosis; and **F,** severe bilateral equinovarus deformity of the feet.

phalanges appear shortened with widened metaphyses; the first metatarsals are particularly short.[392, 397, 732]

In *Freeman-Sheldon syndrome* (craniocarpotarsal dysplasia), the facies is characteristic. The full forehead, deeply set eyes, flattened midface, and small mouth with protuberant lips give a "whistling" appearance (Fig. 7–46). There may be an H-shaped cutaneous crease pattern on the chin. The palate is high and the speech nasal because motion of the palate is limited. The fingers are deviated upward. Associated with the equinovarus deformity is flexion contracture of the toes.[95, 114, 212, 256, 447, 741]

Larsen's syndrome is characterized by multiple joint dislocations (especially of the knees, hips, and elbows), a flat facies with depressed nasal bridge, prominent forehead, widely spaced eyes, and shortened metacarpals with spatulate thumbs (Fig. 7–47). The ossification centers of the carpus and tarsus may be multiple. Kyphoscoliosis with vertebral malformations is not uncommon.[400, 672]

About one third of the patients with *Möbius syndrome* have talipes equinovarus. The characteristic stigmata of Möbius syndrome are the masklike facies with loss of abduction of the eyes and partial or complete facial nerve paralysis. The affection is usually bilateral and is caused by agenesis or hypoplasia of the sixth and seventh cranial nerve nuclei. Other anomalies of the limbs are syndactyly with bony ankylosis of the proximal interphalangeal joints, absence of the pectoralis major muscle, microdactylia, and failure of development of the three lateral metatarsal rays or absence of all phalanges (Fig. 7–48).[496, 590] *Long arm 18 deletion syndrome* and *aminopterin-induced syndrome* are some other disorders in which multiple malformations, among them talipes equinovarus, are found. (For a complete list, the reader is referred to the textbook of D. W. Smith, *Recognizable Patterns of Human Malformation*.[657]) When clubfoot is associated with other anomalies, or the infant does not look otherwise normal, it is advisable to obtain genetic consultation. The initial management of talipes equinovarus in these syndromes follows the same principles outlined for isolated talipes equinovarus. Generally, however, they have a poorer prognosis, and their early detection will guard against future embarrassment.

Radiographic Assessment

The purpose of radiography is to define precisely the anatomic relationships of talocalcaneonavicular, tibiotalar, midtarsal, and tarsometatarsal joints. Historically, Barwell (in 1896) was the first to propose the value of radiography in the assessment of correction of clubfoot; he used both anteroposterior and lateral views, but did not make angular measurements.[33] In 1932, Wisbrun described the use of the talocalcaneal angle in the anteroposterior (dorsoplantar) projection.[763] Kite and Kandel confirmed the method and stressed the importance of the divergence of the longitudinal axes of the talus and the calcaneus.[351, 362–365] Cabanac and associates, and later Heywood, utilized the talocalcaneal angle in the lateral projection, both in plantar flexion and in dorsiflexion.[97, 295]

In the literature, numerous angle measurements for assessing talipes equinovarus have been described. These are summarized in Table 7–8. Special views such as the suroplantar view described by Kleiger and Mankin and the posterior tangential view are utilized, as are the special techniques of tomography, arthrography, arteriography, and recently, computed tomography (CT scan).[42, 59, 302–304, 378, 527, 570, 671]

Radiograms are indicated in talipes equinovarus to assess the degree of subluxation of the talocalcaneonavicular joint and the severity of the deformity before commencing treatment; to provide an accurate guide to progress during the course of closed nonoperative treatment; to ascertain whether reduction of the talocalcaneonavicular dislocation and normal articular alignment have been achieved; to analyze the composite deformities preoperatively and to plan operative treatment accordingly; to determine intraoperatively whether concentric reduction of the talocalcaneonavicular joint has been obtained; and to ascertain postoperatively whether normal articular alignment is being maintained.

In infancy, the primary centers of ossification of the talus, calcaneus, and cuboid bone are

Table 7–8. *Normal Values of Angular Measurements on Anteroposterior and Lateral Projections of Feet*

	Normal Range (Degrees)
Anteroposterior View	
Talocalcaneal (T-C)	20 to 50
Talo–first metatarsal (T-MT_1)	0 to −20
Talo–fifth metatarsal (T-MT_5)	0
Lateral View	
Talocalcaneal (T-C)	25 to 50
Tibiotalar	70 to 100
Tibiocalcaneal (maximal dorsiflexion	25 to 60
Talocalcaneal Index	
(Sum of T-C angles in anteroposterior and lateral projections)	Greater than 40

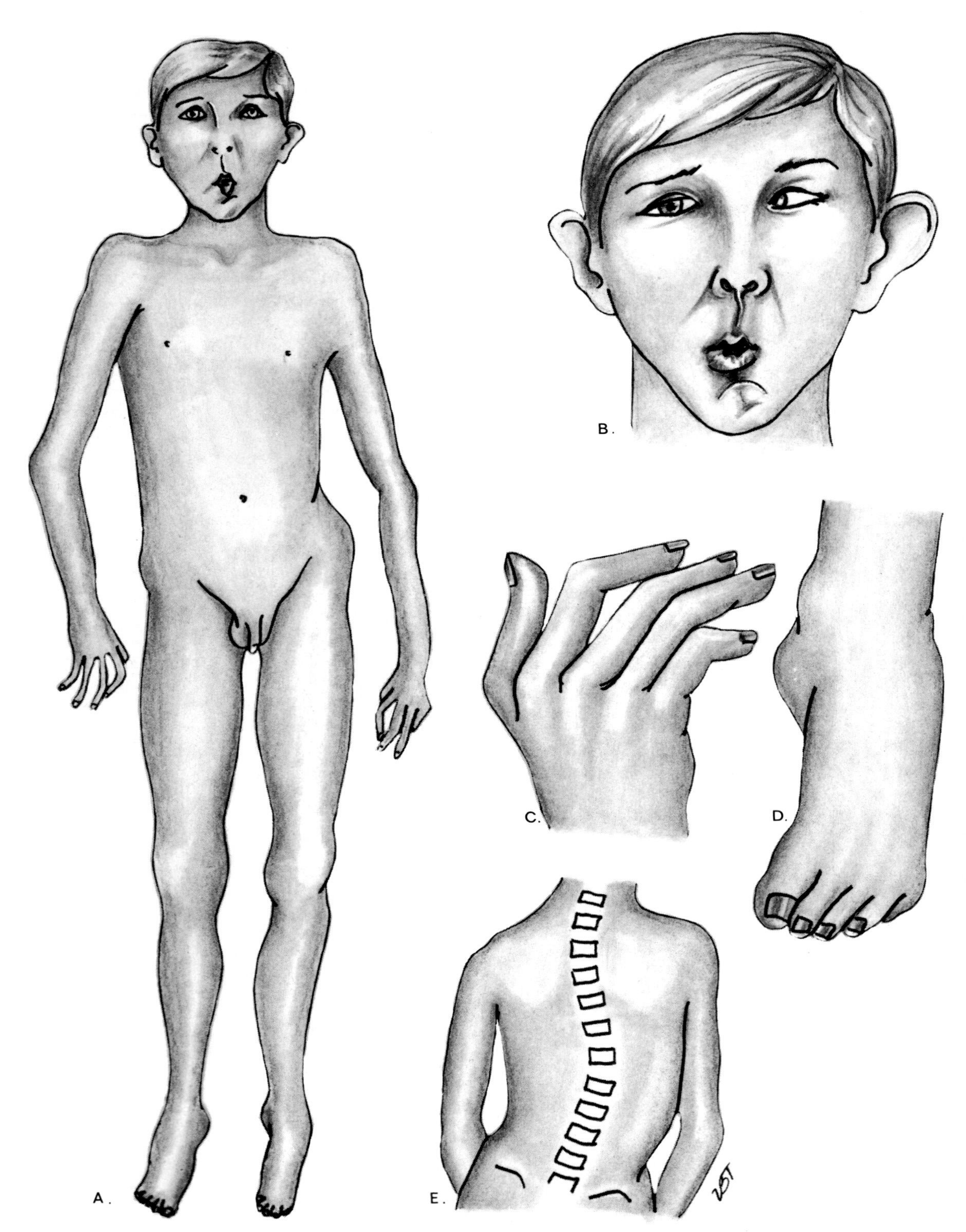

FIGURE 7–46. Freeman-Sheldon syndrome (craniocarpotarsal dysplasia).

A and **B.** Characteristic findings include full forehead, deeply set eyes, flattened midface, and small mouth with protuberant lips that give a "whistling" appearance. **C.** The fingers are deviated ulnarward, and there are equinovarus deformity and flexion contracture of the toes, **D**, and scoliosis, **E.**

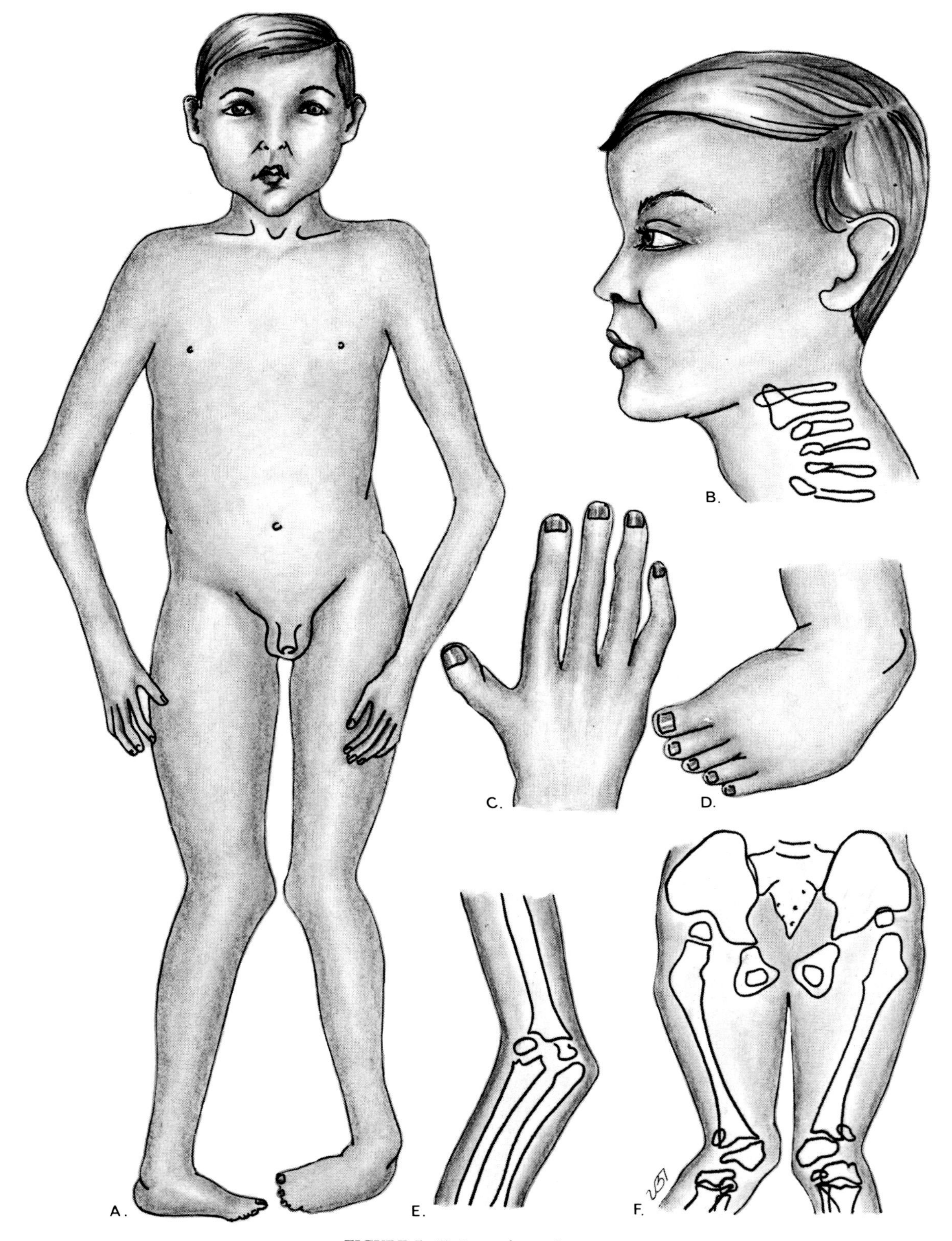

FIGURE 7–47. Larsen's syndrome.

Note the flat facies with depressed nasal bridge and prominent forehead, multiple joint dislocations (knees, hips, and elbows), and vertebral malformations (scoliosis).

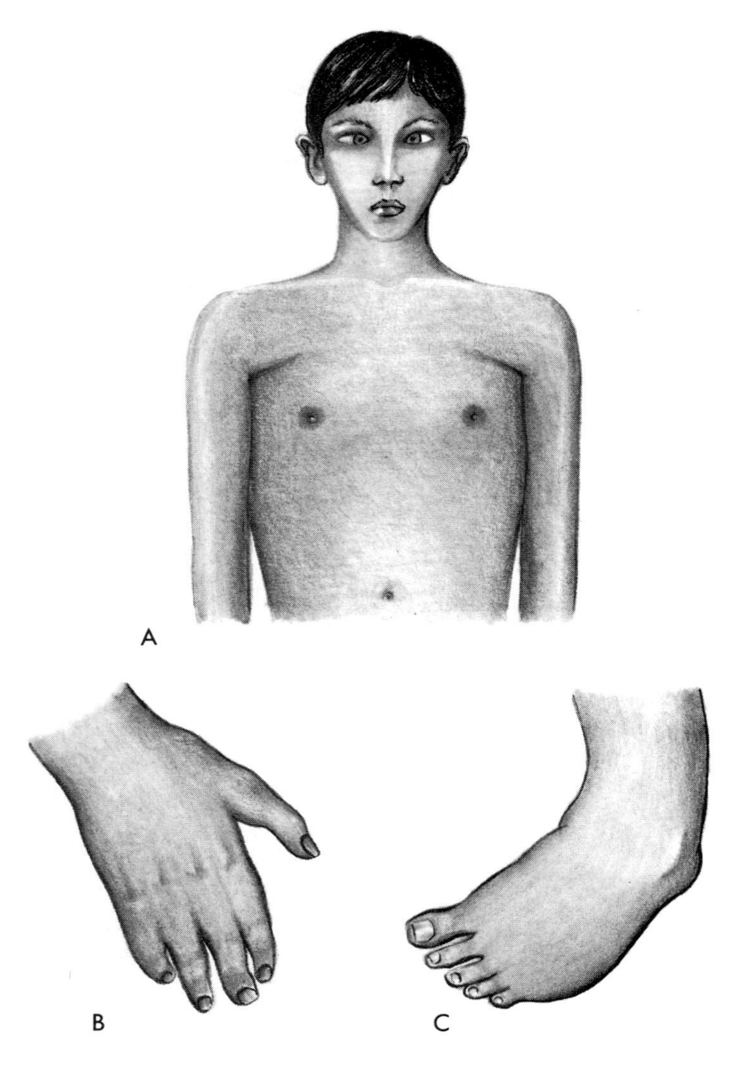

FIGURE 7–48. Möbius syndrome.

Note the masklike facies and loss of abduction of the eyes. There is partial or complete facial nerve paralysis. The pectoralis major muscle is absent, and there is syndactyly with bony ankylosis of the proximal interphalangeal joints. One third of the patients have talipes equinovarus.

well-developed and visible in the plain radiograms; frequently the third cuneiform may be present. The metatarsals and phalanges are also ossified. The navicular is cartilaginous and, like the nonossified femoral head in the first six months of life in congenital dislocation of the hip, is not visualized in the radiograms. The ossification center of the tarsal navicular appears at about three years of age, initially beginning in its lateral quadrant; however, the navicular may not ossify before four years of age or even later.[354] Therefore, lines should be drawn and measurements of angles made to determine the articular relationships in the talocalcaneonavicular joint. It should be remembered that only the small centers of ossification are visualized in the x-ray; the entire bone is not observed, as the surrounding large mass of cartilage has the same density as the soft tissues. An additional difficulty is the delay of skeletal maturation of the tarsus in talipes equinovarus.[411]

TECHNIQUE OF RADIOGRAPHY

In the literature, various methods of radiographic assessment of talipes equinovarus have been described. It is imperative in these studies that the patient's feet be placed in identical positions and that a standard technique be utilized. This author recommends placing the feet in the maximally corrected position, according to the technique described by Simons.[651] Radiograms taken when the feet are not bearing weight or are unstressed do not show the relationship of tarsal bones in the corrected position and are therefore of no value in assessing the correction of deformities.

Positioning. Two persons position the child, preferably a parent and an x-ray technician who is properly instructed by the surgeon. The parent, the child, and the technician should be adequately shielded to minimize the dangers of irradiation. The child is placed in a sitting posture with his knees and hips flexed at right angles; the feet rest on the cassette with their medial borders parallel and touching each other. The forefoot is manually pushed into maximal abduction, and the ankle into maximal dorsiflexion (preferably 15 to 20 degrees), or as close to it as the equinus deformity will allow. If the equinovarus deformity is fixed, or if the child is uncooperative, each foot is held manually in a maximally corrected position; often it is necessary to make a separate exposure of each foot. A translucent splint may be used to hold the foot in the maximally corrected position. An anteroposterior radiogram is made with the x-ray tube directed craniad 30 degrees from the perpendicular toward the dome of the talus and centered on the hindfoot.

For the lateral projection, the cassette is placed on a slotted board or vertical cassette holder for stability. The patient straddles it with the medial border of his *hindfoot* parallel to the edge of the cassette. A maximal dorsiflexion view is made with the leg flexed forward at the ankle without raising the aligned heel off the cassette (the position of the hindfoot is double-checked to assure that it is not elevated). It is essential to have proper alignment of the ankle mortise. It may be necessary to rotate the limb medially 20 to 50 degrees, depending upon the severity of the varus deformity. The x-ray tube is centered on the hindfoot, perpendicular to the cassette.

Films that are not made by the standardized technique should not be accepted. Clues by which improper technique can be recognized are as follows. In the anteroposterior view, the anterior ends of the talus and the calcaneus are at different levels (difference greater than 2 to 3 mm.) This indicates either that the foot was malpositioned in plantar flexion or that the x-ray tube was not tilted craniad at 30 degrees. When the ankle is dorsiflexed inadequately, the shafts of the tibia and the fibula are visualized. In both instances, there will be a spurious decrease in the talocalcaneal angle. On dorsiflexion of the ankle, the anterior end of the calcaneus moves medially, opening the talocalcaneal angle. Marked overlapping of the metatarsals indicates an inverted foot. This appearance may be due to fixed varus deformity or to inverted posture of the foot during x-ray exposure. An inverted posture of the foot diminishes the talocalcaneal angle. The radiographic findings and the clinical appearance of the foot should always be compared and double-checked.

In the lateral view, improper technique is suggested by an extreme posterior position of the fibula and the lateral malleolus in relation to the tibia and medial malleolus, which suggests that the ankle mortise and the hindfoot were in lateral rotation. In the presence of varus deformity of both forefoot and midfoot, the whole foot should not be placed parallel to the cassette, as this will force the hindfoot into external rotation. It is the hindfoot that should be placed parallel to the cassette. If the metatarsals do not overlap and are tiered, it means the foot was inverted when the film was made. The tibiotalar angle in the x-ray should be compared with the clinical range of ankle dorsiflexion.

The accuracy of the preceding technique of two-plane radiography may be affected by two factors: (1) movement of the foot as a unit with no motion between the individual bones, and (2) movement of the foot with motion taking place between the individual bones. Malpositioning of the foot or change in its position by active motion by the patient prior to film exposure will give a difference between the true angle and the angle that is recorded on the radiogram. The experienced technician will see to it that errors in positioning are very minor and will detect and check any significant movement by the patient. Simons has shown mathematically that angle variance (i.e., the difference between the true anatomic angle and the apparent angle on the x-ray) due to minor mistakes of positioning and movement is relatively small and of no practical significance.[651]

During interosseous movement, the true anatomic angle changes; therefore the degree of angle variance due to malposition and the degree due to motion between the individual bones are difficult to determine. Reimann estimated variations in angular measurement from one exposure to another in ten children with talipes equinovarus. Radiograms were made twice, either on the same day or on two consecutive days. The difference between measured values was insignificant.[585] Simons believes the accuracy of the technique described is similar to that of Reimann's method.[651]

Measurement of Angles. In the anteroposterior view, the talocalcaneal angle is measured as follows: in the infant, it is best to trace the outline of the ossific nuclei of the calcaneus and talus with a soft lead pencil. The ossified talus is usually pear-shaped, narrower in front than behind. On its medial and lateral margins, two points are made anteriorly and two points posteriorly. The longitudinal axis of the talus is determined by drawing a line between points made midway between each of the two sets of marginal points. The longitudinal axis of the calcaneus is made by drawing a line parallel to its lateral border. Because its medial border is irregular and somewhat indistinct, this is more accurate than drawing a line between the midpoints of the margins of the calcaneus (Fig. 7–49).

In the normal foot, the long axis of the talus points medially toward the first metatarsal and that of the calcaneus laterally toward the fifth metatarsal, forming a V. This talocalcaneal angle normally measures 20 to 40 degrees, as shown in Figure 7–49.

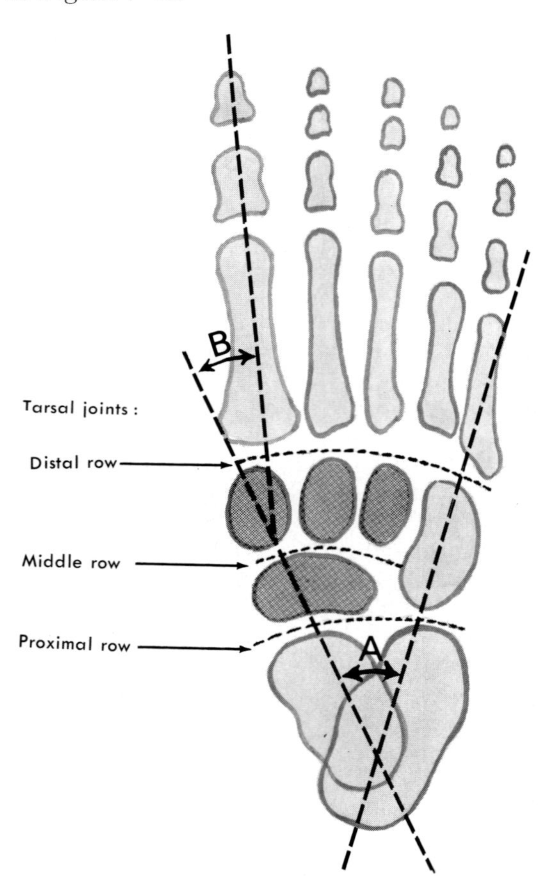

FIGURE 7–49. Measurement of angles in the radiogram of the normal foot.

In the anteroposterior view the long axis of the talus points medially toward the first metatarsal and that of the calcaneus laterally toward the fifth metatarsal, forming the talocalcaneal angle, A, which normally measures 20 to 40 degrees. The angle formed between the longitudinal axis of the talus and that of the first metatarsal is called the talo–first metatarsal (or TMT_1) angle, B. It normally measures zero to minus 15 degrees.

In talipes equinovarus with inversion of the heel, the talocalcaneal angle diminishes and may approach zero. In severe inversion of the hindfoot, the longitudinal axes of the talus and the calcaneus may become superimposed and point laterally to the fourth or fifth metatarsal (Figs. 7–50 to 7–52). As the inversion of the heel is corrected, the head of the talus no longer lies on top of the calcaneus, but projects medially, giving a normal talocalcaneal angle.

The longitudinal axis of the first metatarsal is drawn through the center of the bone. The angle formed between the longitudinal axis of the talus and that of the first metatarsal is called the talo–first metatarsal (or $T\text{-}MT_1$) angle. It normally measures zero to minus 15 degrees (cf. Fig. 7–49). A more negative angle than minus 15 degrees indicates varus deviation of the midfoot or forefoot (Fig. 7–51, angles A and B). In the more skeletally mature foot, one should also note the relationship of the navicular to the cuneiforms and that of the cuneiforms to the metatarsals.[585, 587, 650]

In the normal foot, the lateral margins of the calcaneus and of the cuboid bone form a continuous line. In talipes equinovarus with medial subluxation of the talocalcaneonavicular joint, the cuboid is shifted medially and the calcaneocuboid line is interrupted. On the lateral aspect of the foot, another angle is formed between the longitudinal axis of the calcaneus and that of the fifth metatarsal. Normally the long axis of the calcaneus points toward the fifth metatarsal and the calcaneo–fifth metatarsal angle ($C\text{-}MT_5$) measures zero. In talipes equinovarus the angle is decreased and has a minus value.

In the lateral projection, the talocalcaneal angle is measured as follows: the long axis of the talus is aligned by joining the center points of its head and body, which are determined in the same way as in the anteroposterior view. The long axis of the calcaneus is obtained by drawing a line through its plantar surface, joining the calcaneal tubercles and its anterior plantar convexity. In early infancy, the posterior plantar aspect of the calcaneus is not clearly ossified and is irregular in outline. At this young age, it is best to resort to a tracing technique to determine the midline long axis of the calcaneus as described for the talus (see Fig. 7–52).

The talocalcaneal angle in a lateral radiogram of the normal foot measures between 35 and 50 degrees as shown in Figure 7–52, whereas in talipes equinovarus it is less than 25 degrees and may reach a negative value of minus 10 degrees as shown in Figure 7–52. On forced dorsiflexion, the lateral talocalcaneal angle is

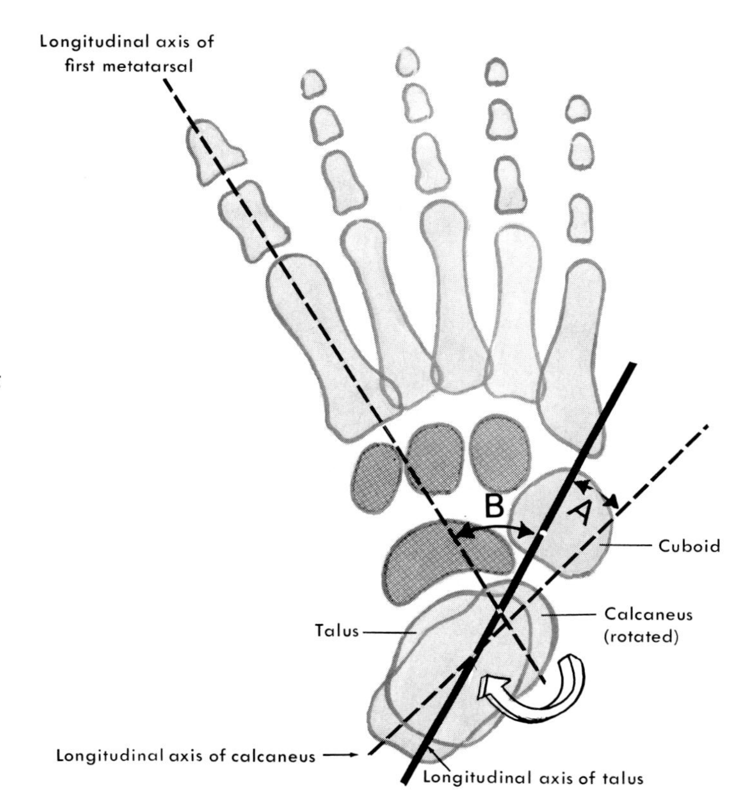

FIGURE 7–50. Line drawing illustrating measurement of angles in talipes equinovarus.

increased in a normal foot because the mobile heel is pulled forward and upward by plantar flexion, but in talipes equinovarus the talocalcaneal angle is decreased further as the calcaneus is tethered in the equinus position by the taut Achilles tendon while the talus moves slightly into dorsiflexion. Therefore, minor differences between a normal and an abnormal foot can be accentuated by the maximal dorsiflexion view.

Talocalcaneonavicular subluxation is present when the talo–first metatarsal angle is greater than 20 degrees and the talocalcaneal angle is less than 15 degrees.

Beatson and Pearson have described the talocalcaneal index—i.e., the sum of the talocalcaneal angles in the anteroposterior and lateral projections. According to them, if the talocalcaneal index is less than 40 degrees in a properly positioned foot, talocalcaneonavicular subluxation has not been reduced.[37]

In the lateral view at birth, the ossific nucleus of the talus in talipes equinovarus appears to be displaced anteriorly and plantarward. The degree of equinus inclination of the ankle can also be measured in the lateral projection of the tibiotalar angle formed between the longitudinal axis of the tibia and the long axis of the talus; this normally measures 70 to 100 degrees. Another method of measuring ankle equinus deviation is the tibiocalcaneal angle, which is formed between the longitudinal axes of the tibia and the calcaneus; its value depends upon the degree of dorsiflexion of the ankle in a normal infant in whom the foot may touch the anterior aspect of the leg. The tibiocalcaneal angle may measure as little as 25 degrees. Normally, with marked dorsiflexion of the ankle, it measures 60 to 90 degrees. Both in the lateral and in the anteroposterior view, the contours of the tarsal bones and the articular surfaces should be inspected. The axial view of the calcaneus is helpful in radiographic assessment of a heel varus deformity in the older child who has started walking. Serial radiograms will demonstrate correction of the heel inversion.

With improper treatment, certain radiographic changes may ensue: "transverse breach," "horizontal or longitudinal breach," and flat-topped talus. A transverse breach in the midtarsal area will give a "rocker-bottom" deformity. This is verified by drawing the longitudinal axis of the sole, which is the line joining the calcaneal tubercle and the head of the third metatarsal. Normally this *sole line* passes below the calcaneocuboid joint; if the line passes through the joint, a "rocker-bottom"

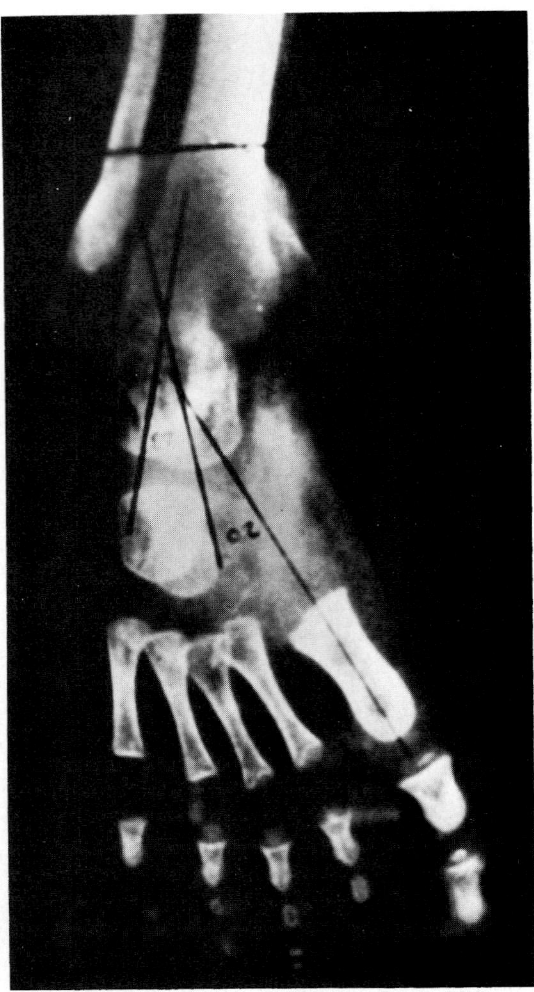

FIGURE 7–51. Measurement of angle between long axes of the talus and the first metatarsal (note it is 20 degrees).

deformity is present. It is an iatrogenic deformity (Fig. 7–53). A longitudinal breach may occur when medial subluxation of the talocalcaneonavicular joint persists in the horizontal plane, as discussed earlier in the section on pathology.

Ono and Hayashi employed frontal tomography perpendicular to the long axis of the foot in 43 cases of treated talipes equinovarus. Tomograms were made with the patient in the supine position initially, but later the weight-bearing posture was employed. Ono and Hayashi found characteristic changes of the hindfoot, namely, increased inclination of the middle subtalar articular surface of the calcaneus (inversion of the calcaneus), hypoplasia of the sustentaculum tali, and narrowing of the talocalcaneal space. They recommended tomography as a simple and easily available method of determining the anatomic status of the foot in talipes equinovarus in children over two years of age.[527] This author recommends computed tomography to determine medial spin of the calcaneus and lateral subluxation of the posterior facet of the subtalar joint.[193]

Arthrography of the ankle joint has been extensively studied by Poulain.[570] Simultaneous arthrography of the ankle and talonavicular joint has been performed by Helmstedt and Sahlstedt. They studied 32 autopsy specimens of feet from 19 children of ages up to three years. Measurements of the size and shape of the talus were made on the films, and the results were compared with corresponding measurements made on the anatomic specimens. With respect to the length of the talus and medial declination of the talonavicular joint, there was a fairly good correlation between the radiographic values and the values obtained on the anatomic specimens. These investigators also studied clinically 24 congenital clubfeet in 18 patients and 6 clubfeet in 5 patients with neurologic disorders. In both groups, there were changes in the talus, consisting of medial deviation of the head with flattening of its dome.[302–304] Experience in arthrography is still limited, however, and computed tomography is replacing it.

Treatment

The objectives of the treatment of talipes equinovarus are: (1) to achieve concentric reduction of the dislocation or subluxation of the talocalcaneonavicular joint; (2) to maintain the reduction; (3) to restore normal articular alignment of the tarsus and the ankle; (4) to establish muscle balance between the evertors and invertors, and the dorsiflexors and plantar flexors; and (5) to provide a mobile foot with normal function and weight-bearing. The principles underlying management of congenital dislocation of the hip should be applied to that of in utero dislocation of the talocalcaneonavicular ball-and-socket joint. Treatment of talipes equinovarus is complex and delicate. Nonoperative reduction of talocalcaneonavicular dislocation in true congenital talipes equinovarus is often impossible, and conservative treatment frequently is open surgical reduction.

Treatment should be started as soon as possible, preferably immediately following birth. A frequently quoted adage is that the prognosis in a breech delivery is better than that in a vertex presentation because exercises and treatment can be begun earlier while awaiting delivery of the head. The first three weeks of life

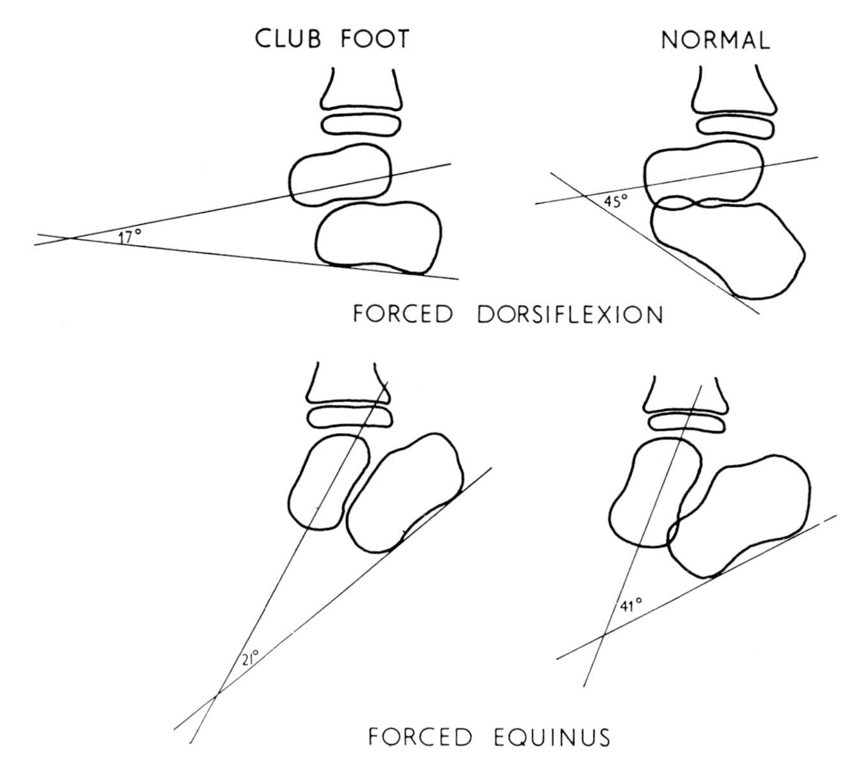

FIGURE 7–52. The talocalcaneal angle in the lateral radiogram in the normal foot and in talipes equinovarus.

The axis of the talus is the line joining the midpoints of the head and body of the talus. The axis of the calcaneus is the line joining the calcaneal tubercles and the anterior plantar convexity of the calcaneus. The normal talocalcaneal angle is between 35 and 50 degrees, and it increases in forced dorsiflexion, whereas in talipes equinovarus, it is less than 35 degrees, and is often decreased further by forced dorsiflexion. (From Heywood, A. W. B.: The mechanics of the hindfoot in clubfoot as demonstrated radiographically. J. Bone Joint Surg., *46B*:105, 1964.)

are the golden period—because the ligamentous tissues of the newborn are still exceedingly lax under the influence of maternal sex hormones. This is the crucial phase in which contracted soft tissues can be elongated by daily repeated manipulations; if the closed method of reduction will ever succeed, this is the time.

Soon after the baby is born, the orthopedic surgeon should explain to the parents the goals, the nature, and the course of treatment. They should understand that management of the child with talipes equinovarus extends over a period of many years until adolescence, when skeletal maturity of the foot is reached, and that uncompromising care and constant vigilance are required through all stages of skeletal growth.

The parents should realize that a foot with talipes equinovarus can never be completely normal. The deformity is the result of a teratologic malformation—a germ plasm defect. There will always be calf atrophy, and the foot will be smaller than the contralateral normal foot. There may be leg length inequality. A realistic approach initially will prevent much disappointment later.

CLOSED NONOPERATIVE METHOD OF MANAGEMENT

The technique of closed manipulative reduction of the medial and plantar subluxation of the talocalcaneonavicular ball-and-socket joint is as follows: The first phase is *elongation of the contracted soft tissues* by passive manipulation. The sacred rule is to be gentle. The soft tissues—ligaments and capsule—are hard; the hard tissues—physis and articular cartilage—are soft and vulnerable to iatrogenic trauma.[157] Forceful manipulation and stretching casts are more radical than surgery.

First the skin of the infant's foot and lower limb is painted or sprayed with a nonirritative adhesive liquid, such as tincture of benzoin or Ace Adherent. The surgeon should use gloves and a 4- by 4-inch sponge, opened up, for a firm grip. The infant is held in the soft lap of the mother or a gentle nurse.

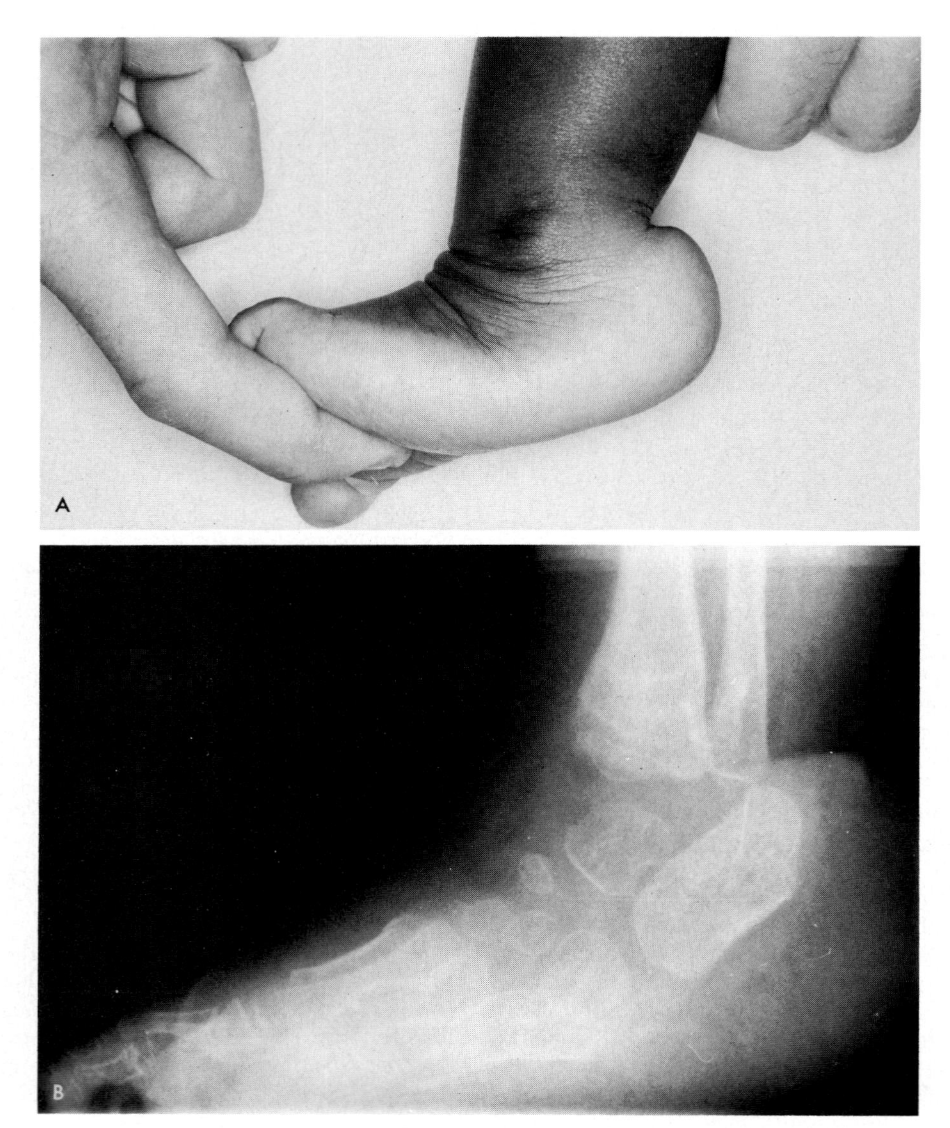

FIGURE 7–53. Rocker-bottom deformity in talipes equinovarus.

Deformity is the result of a transverse breach in the midtarsal area. **A.** Clinical appearance. **B.** Lateral radiogram of the foot and ankle.

Elongation of Triceps Surae Muscle, Posterior Capsule, and Ligaments of Ankle and Subtalar Joints. The manipulative technique is as follows: The os calcis, held between the index finger and thumb of one hand, is pulled *distally*, bringing the heel down, and pushed medially away from the fibular malleolus; with the other hand, the calcaneocuboid area is pushed into dorsiflexion with the whole foot slightly inverted (Fig. 7–54). One should not stretch the midfoot by forced dorsiflexion of the forefoot, or a "rocker-bottom" deformity of the foot will result owing to a transverse breach (see Fig. 7–53). The stretched position is maintained to the count of 10, and then released. Passive stretching of the taut, posterior soft tissues is repeated 20 to 30 times each session.

Elongation of Posterior Tibial Muscle and Tibionavicular Ligament. The navicular is tethered toward the medial malleolus by the contracted posterior tibial muscle and the plantar calcaneonavicular and tibionavicular ligaments. To stretch them, the os calcis is held between the index finger and the thumb of one hand and pulled down distally; with the other hand, the navicular is gripped between the index finger and thumb, and the navicular and the midfoot are pulled distally toward the big toe and then abducted (Fig. 7–54 C). The body of the talus is held steady in the ankle mortise. It is imperative that one does not force the talus into lateral rotation in the ankle mortise and cause horizontal breach (Fig. 7–54 E).

Elongation of Plantar Calcaneonavicular (or Spring) Ligament and Plantar Soft Tissues. Over a hundred years ago, Hugh Owens Thomas stressed the importance of plantar soft tissues as an impediment to correction of talipes equinovarus.[688] It is only recently, however, that we have heeded his advice through the teachings of Wilbur Westin.[641, 747] The plantar calcaneonavicular ligament must be elongated if the navicular bone is to be positioned over the head of the talus. The technique of manipulative stretching is simple. With one hand, the heel is pushed up, and with the other, the midfoot is pushed into dorsiflexion (Fig. 7–54 D). The thumb of one hand is over the medial malleolus, and the thumb of the other hand is over the navicular. Again, care should be taken not to cause lateral rotation of the talus in the ankle mortise (Fig. 7–54 E). The iatrogenic deformity of "horizontal breach" should be avoided. As in elongation of the triceps surae, each stretched position is maintained to the count of 10, then released and repeated 20 to 30 times.

After manipulation and elongation of the contracted soft tissues, the foot and leg are strapped with adhesive tape, a technique described by Sir Robert Jones in 1900. The author prefers an above-knee cast, which is changed every two or three days. The strapping provides a dynamic and nonrigid splint that prevents disuse atrophy and encourages the peroneal and ankle dorsiflexor muscles to function in the first few weeks of life.[341] The technique of its application is shown in Figure 7–55. First, the limb is thoroughly washed with soap and water, and cleansed and dried with alcohol. Tincture of benzoin is applied to the foot, the entire leg (between the knee and the malleoli), and the distal thigh for a distance of 3 to 5 cm. above the knee. The tincture of benzoin protects the skin and improves adherence of the strapping. Next, adhesive orthopedic felt, 3 to 5 cm. wide, is smoothly rolled circumferentially, but not completely, around the foot with the edges about 1 cm. apart in the midline on the dorsum of the foot. The circumferential taping as described by Jones is relatively safe in the first two or three weeks of life. It is imperative that the distal edge of the felt (and the adhesive strapping) end at the base of the toes to support the metatarsal head and dynamically stretch the forefoot out of equinus posture. A longer and wider piece of felt is applied over the dorsum of the 90-degree-flexed knee and the lateral and medial sides of the leg, ending 2 cm. proximal to each malleolus. Adhesive strapping is applied over the felt, rolling it against the varus deformity. With the knee always fully flexed, begin at the lateral edge of the dorsum of the foot and cross it from the lateral to the medial side and around the sole, and then upward on the lateral aspect of the leg. As the strapping is rolled against the deformity, the foot is pulled into eversion and dorsiflexion. To increase correction, an additional layer of adhesive tape may be applied on top of the first. The vertical straps on the leg are secured by two transverse pieces of adhesive tape around the calf, applied one on top of the other. Preferably, the tape should encircle the leg, as it will act as a constrictor and obstruct circulation to the distal part; this is especially true in the older infant and child. The peripheral circulation is checked, and the mother (or nurse, if the child is an inpatient) is properly instructed in how to check it. If the foot is dusky in color, the straps are adjusted to relieve the vascular impediment. If the circulation is still not completely normal after this, the strapping is gently removed and started over again.

Text continued on page 2470

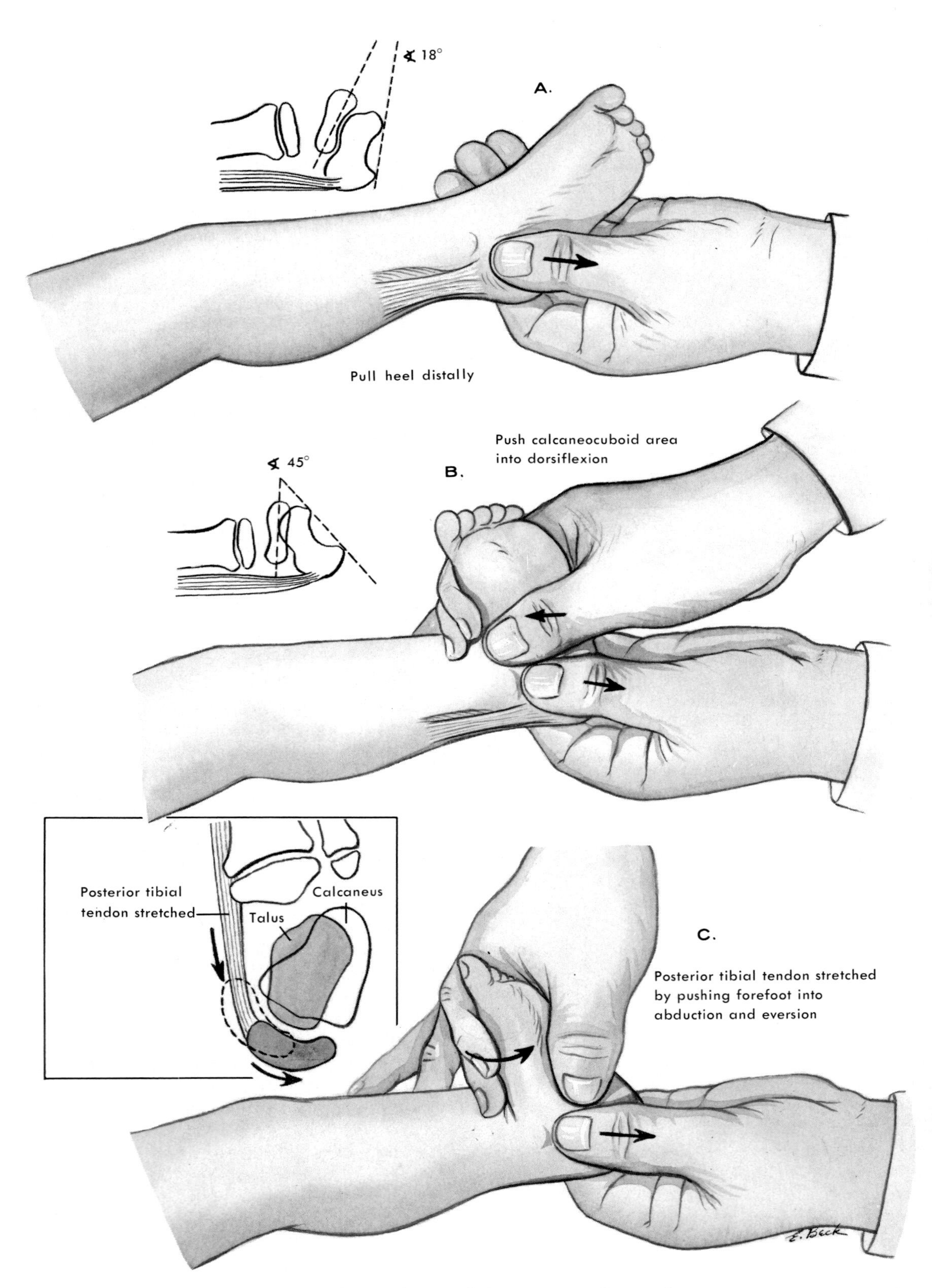

FIGURE 7–54. Technique of manipulation to correct talipes equinovarus.

A and **B.** Elongation of triceps surae muscle and posterior capsule and ligaments of the ankle and subtalar joints. **C.** Elongation of posterior tibial muscle.

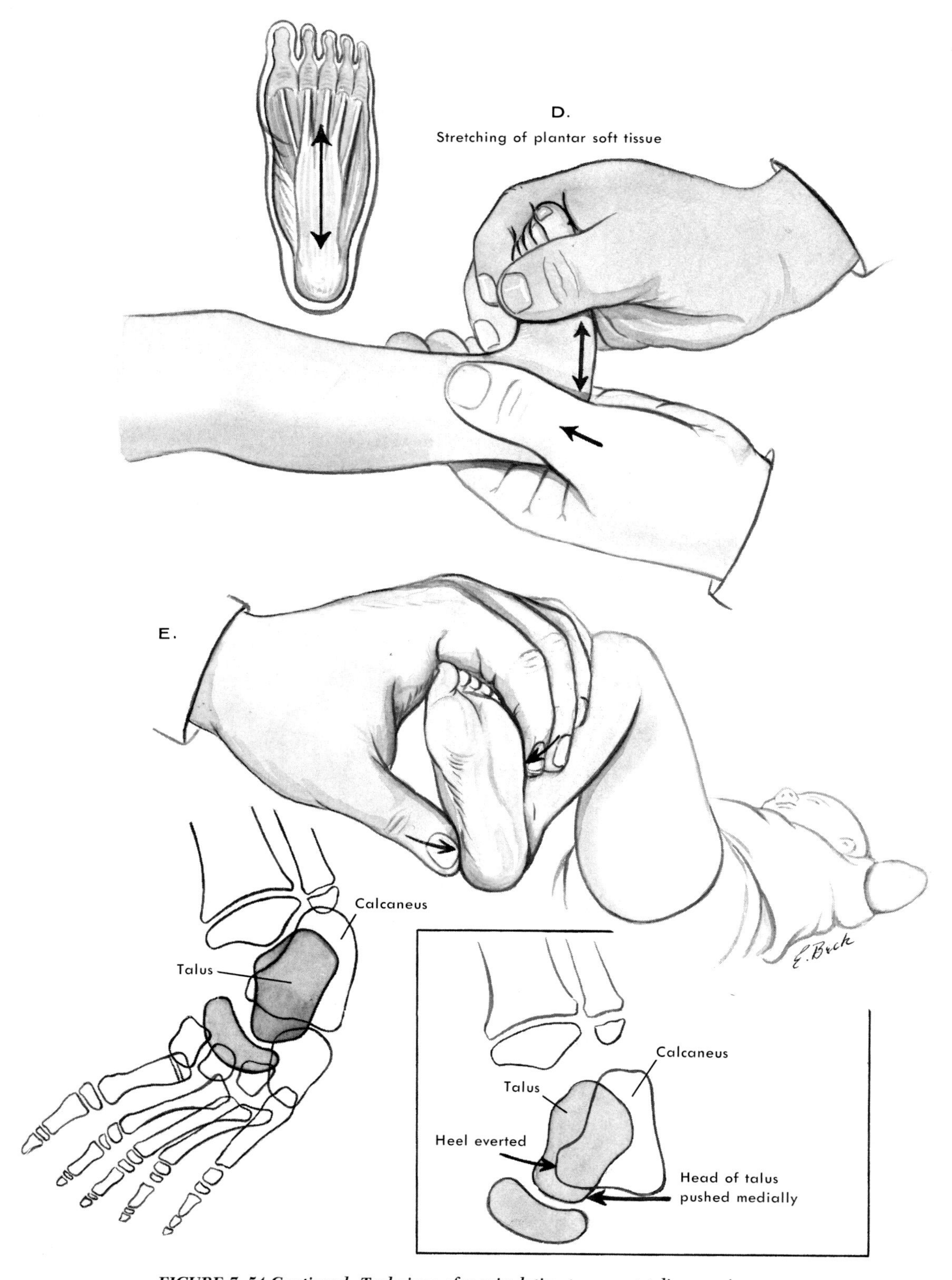

FIGURE 7–54 Continued. Technique of manipulation to correct talipes equinovarus.

D. Elongation of the plantar calcaneonavicular ligament and plantar soft tissue. **E.** Prevention of lateral rotation deformity of the dome of the talus in the ankle mortise. Push the anterior end of the talus medially as the os calcis is everted.

Illustration continued on following page

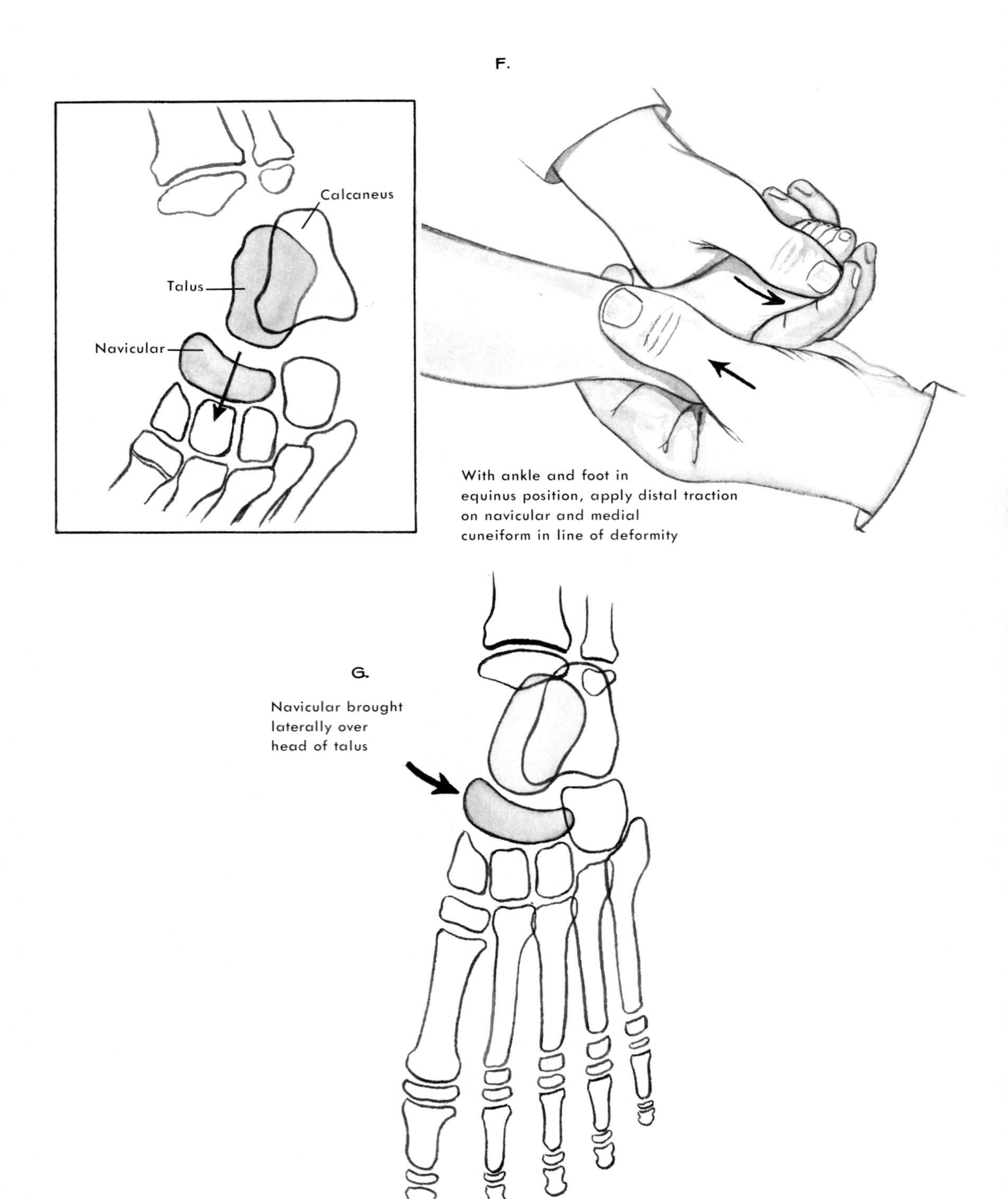

FIGURE 7–54 Continued. Technique of manipulation to correct talipes equinovarus.

F and **G.** Reduction of medial and plantar dislocation of the talocalcaneonavicular joint.

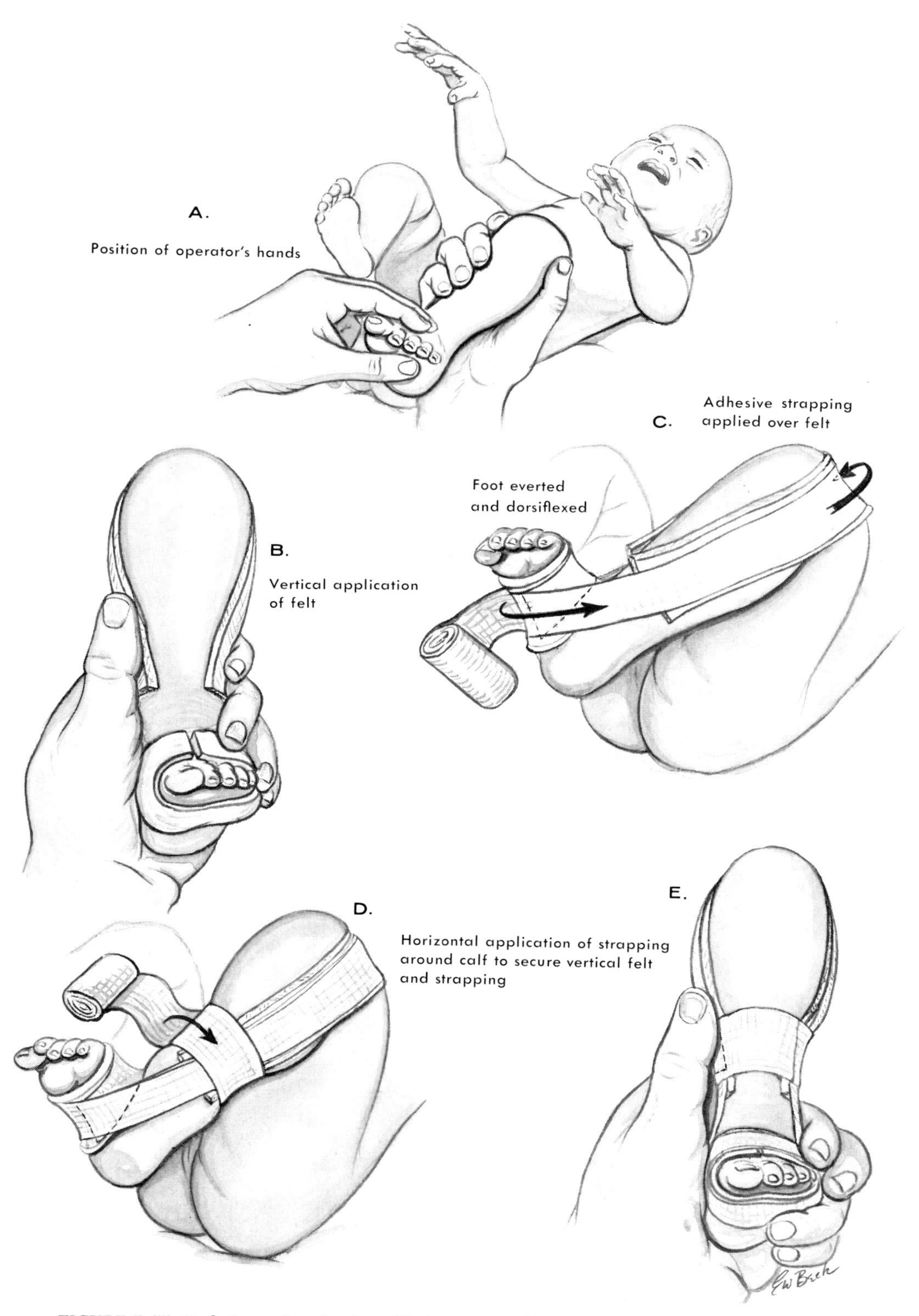

FIGURE 7–55. Technique of application of Robert Jones adhesive strapping for talipes equinovarus.

See text for explanation of the steps of the application.

As the infant kicks the fully flexed knee into extension, a dynamic corrective force is transmitted to the foot. Other advantages of the Robert Jones adhesive strapping are that it is inexpensive and can be applied easily, changed readily, and reapplied at frequent intervals; and it is relatively safe, being least likely to cause pressure sores. The strapping is removed daily and, after manipulation of the foot, is reapplied.

During manipulation, all elements of soft-tissue contracture are elongated. This contrasts with the traditional teaching of Kite, which is that the clubfoot should be corrected in sequence from front to back, and that one should not proceed to the next stage until any distal deformity has been fully corrected. Kite first corrects the varus forefoot, then the inverted hindfoot, and then the equinus ankle and subtalar joints. He has constantly alerted us to the dangers of premature dorsiflexion as a cause of transverse breach at the midtarsal joint, which results in a "rocker-bottom" foot.[362–375] Leaving the hindfoot in the equinus position until the varus deformity is fully corrected, however, allows the contracture of the posterior capsule and ligaments of the ankle and subtalar joints, and the tautness of the triceps surae, to become more rigid. This rigidity is an important factor in the pathogenesis of the "rocker-bottom" foot. Another anatomic factor to consider is that full plantar flexion of the ankle is accompanied by varus posture of the foot, and full dorsiflexion by valgus posture. While the hindfoot is left in the equinus position, the subtalar and midtarsal joints are inverted unless the foot is forcibly breached at the midtarsal joint. It is often stated that it is difficult, if not impossible, to manipulate the small, drawn-up heel of an infant with talipes equinovarus. A common error is to apply the dorsiflexion force on the long anterior lever of the forefoot. The correct approach is to paint the small heel and foot with an adhesive liquid and hold it in an opened-up, 4- by 4-inch surgical gauze and *pull the heel down* (see Fig. 7–54 A and B).

Closed Reduction of Medial and Plantar Dislocation of Talocalcaneonavicular Joint. Once the soft-tissue contractures are sufficiently elongated, the next step is closed reduction of the medial and plantar dislocation of the talocalcaneonavicular joint. A basic principle of reduction of overriding both-bone fractures of the forearm is to apply traction *distally in the line of deformity*. The same principle should be applied to the reduction of the talocalcaneonavicular joint in talipes equinovarus. Grasp the hindfoot with one hand, the index finger over the body of the talus above the sinus tarsi, just anterior and distal to the lateral malleolus, and the thumb of the same hand anterior to the medial malleolus, pushing the navicular distally. With the opposite hand, grasp the fore- and midfoot between the thumb and index finger, and apply *longitudinal* traction distally in the line of deformity—that is, with the foot in equinus posture and inversion. This distracts the forefoot and midfoot from the hindfoot and elongates the foot (Fig. 7–54 F). Next, reduction of the talocalcaneonavicular dislocation is achieved by abducting the midfoot, displacing the navicular laterally, and pushing the anterior end of the talus medially with the opposite thumb (Fig. 7–54 G). The calcaneus is laterally rotated with the cuboid bone as the foot is dorsiflexed at the ankle and subtalar joints. Clinically, reduction is revealed by the normal external contour of the foot in a resting posture. In talipes equinovarus, there is apparent shortening of the hallux; reduction of the dislocation brings the navicular over the distal end of the talus, and the big toe acquires normal length. Digital palpation should disclose a one- or two-fingerbreadth space between the medial malleolus and the navicular.

The success of reduction is confirmed by anteroposterior and lateral radiograms of the foot, made in the standardized positions outlined earlier. In the anteroposterior radiogram, the talocalcaneal angle should be greater than 20 degrees, and the talo–first metatarsal angle less than 15 degrees; in the lateral view, the talocalcaneal angle should be 30 to 45 degrees. Proper positioning of the foot and correct technique of radiography are vital.

Retention of Reduction. Once concentric reduction has been achieved and confirmed by x-ray, an above-knee cast is applied to maintain the reduction. Plaster of Paris cast immobilization is a *static retentive* apparatus. The correct application of a plaster cast to an infant's foot requires considerable skill; it should be applied accurately and with great attention to detail. Three persons working in a harmonious team are necessary: a parent to hold the baby still (the baby may be rebellious, struggling and making every effort to get loose); a trained assistant who will roll the sheet wadding and plaster of Paris cast; and the surgeon, whose responsibility is to hold and mold the cast.

The cast should extend from the toes to the groin with the knee flexed at 60 to 80 degrees to control the heel and prevent the cast from slipping. The infant's lower limb is conical in shape, bulky in the thigh, and tapered distally in the leg and foot. It is best to paint the skin with a nonirritating adhesive liquid, such as tincture of benzoin or Ace Adherent, to protect the skin and prevent slipping of the cast. Narrow sheet wadding should be used: 1 or 1½ inches wide on the foot and lower leg, and 2 inches wide on the upper leg, knee, and thigh. It is rolled snugly against the varus deformity, but not taut and not loose. It should be smooth with no wrinkles. Beginning at the forefoot, the first two turns are applied toward the tips of the toes; then the direction is reversed and the wadding is carried proximally over the rest of the foot, leg, and knee, and up to the upper thigh (Fig. 7–56 A). Each succeeding turn overlaps the preceding turn by one half of its width. Two extra turns are applied at the upper thigh to serve as padding. Because the circumference of the calf and thigh is greater above than below, the sheet wadding is torn slightly at its upper edge as the wrapping proceeds proximally so that the lower part lies flat on the limb, not loose and away from the skin. Small tears are made at varying points in the turns to ensure exact and smooth conformation to the limb. Three layers of sheet wadding are placed over the heel and extending forward to cover both malleoli.

The surgeon then holds the foot and ankle in the desired corrected position, and the assistant rolls the plaster of Paris cast. A 2-inch-wide roll is sufficient for the foot and lower leg; and a 3-inch roll for the upper part of the leg, the knee, and the thigh. In the bigger infant, or if reinforcement is required because the cast cracks on a restless baby, another 3-inch roll may be used. The plaster should be extra-fast setting. Like the sheet wadding, it is rolled against the varus deformity—that is, it begins on the lateral edge of the foot, onto the dorsum, then on the sole, and onto the lateral side again. Each turn covers two thirds of the width of the preceding turn. As the plaster cast is applied, each turn is rubbed to smooth it. The cast should be of uniform thickness. In the uncooperative infant, the plaster is first carried up to the ankle and the lower third of the leg, and then extended up to the upper thigh (Fig. 7–56 B).

Proper and careful molding of the cast is very important. The thenar eminence of one hand is placed over the calcaneocuboid area, pushing the body of the talus medially and also acting as counterpressure. With the other fingers, the back of the heel is molded so that it looks like a normal foot with a prominent, posteriorly displaced heel. The importance of the molding above the heel to give a normal contour to the hindfoot cannot be overemphasized. With the other hand, pressure is applied over the medial and plantar aspects of the mid- and forefoot, not the great toe, pushing it into abduction. The lateral border of the foot should be concave. The midtarsal joint area should be well-molded to prevent a "rocker-bottom" deformity. It should be remembered that the plaster of Paris cast is a retentive, not a corrective, apparatus. Its purpose is to maintain the concentric reduction of the talocalcaneonavicular joint achieved by manipulation. Recently this author has been utilizing a plaster of Paris cast material for the first two layers and then reinforcing it with a synthetic casting tape, which allows a better grip on the infant's foot and firm, rapid setting.

Radiograms are made through the first cast to ensure concentricity of reduction. The cast is changed at two- to three-week intervals in the young infant, whose foot grows rapidly. When solid casts are left on for long periods of time, the soft tissues and the skin become compressed. Soft-tissue fibrosis, pressure sores, and circulatory embarrassment are inherent dangers.

The solid-cast immobilization is continued for an average period of three months. Before discontinuing retention in the solid cast, radiograms are made out of the cast to ensure that concentric reduction is maintained. Then a polypropylene above-knee splint is made to hold the hindfoot in 15 to 20 degrees of eversion, the midfoot and forefoot in 20 degrees of abduction, and the ankle at zero to 5 degrees of dorsiflexion; the knee is flexed 60 degrees. The splint is worn only at night and at nap times. A Reimann dynamic clubfoot splint may be used, if preferred. A prewalker clubfoot shoe is worn during the day (Fig. 7–57). The mother is taught passive stretching exercises to manipulate the mid- and forefoot into abduction and eversion, the heel into eversion, and the foot into dorsiflexion at the ankle joint by pulling the heel down. Again, the parents should be cautioned over and over again not to stretch the midfoot by forced dorsiflexion of the forefoot. Stimulation techniques are used to elicit active exercises promoting inversion and dorsiflexion of the foot. The exercises are performed 15 times slowly in each direction, four to five times a day.

The follow-up care of talipes equinovarus should be continued until skeletal maturity to ensure that there is no recurrence of the deformity. When the child begins to walk, he should wear outflare (tarsal pronator) high-top shoes with 1/8- to 3/16-inch outer lateral side heel

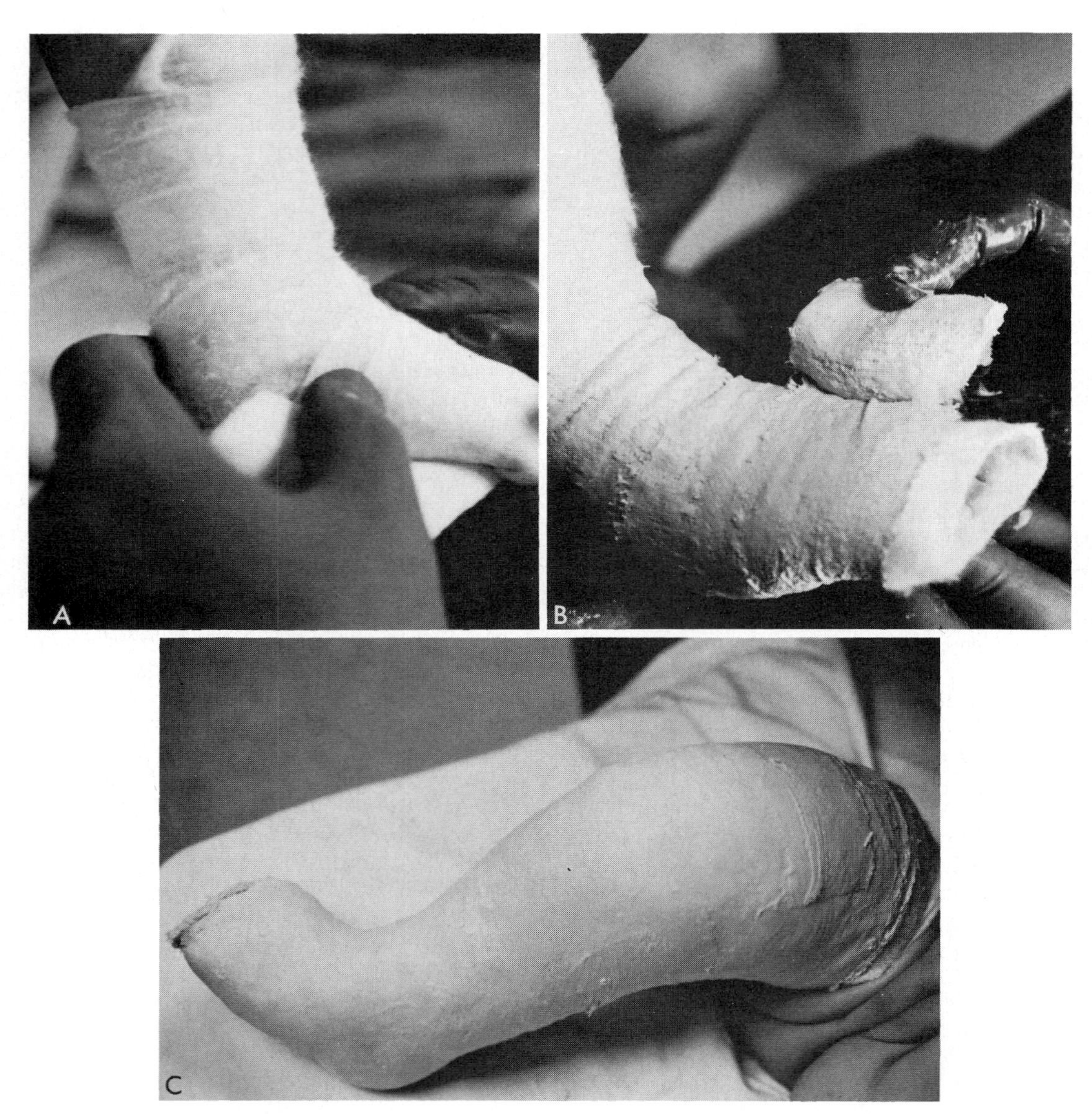

FIGURE 7–56. Technique of plaster of Paris cast application in talipes equinovarus.

A. Rolling of sheet wadding. **B.** Rolling of plaster of Paris cast. **C.** Molding of the cast.

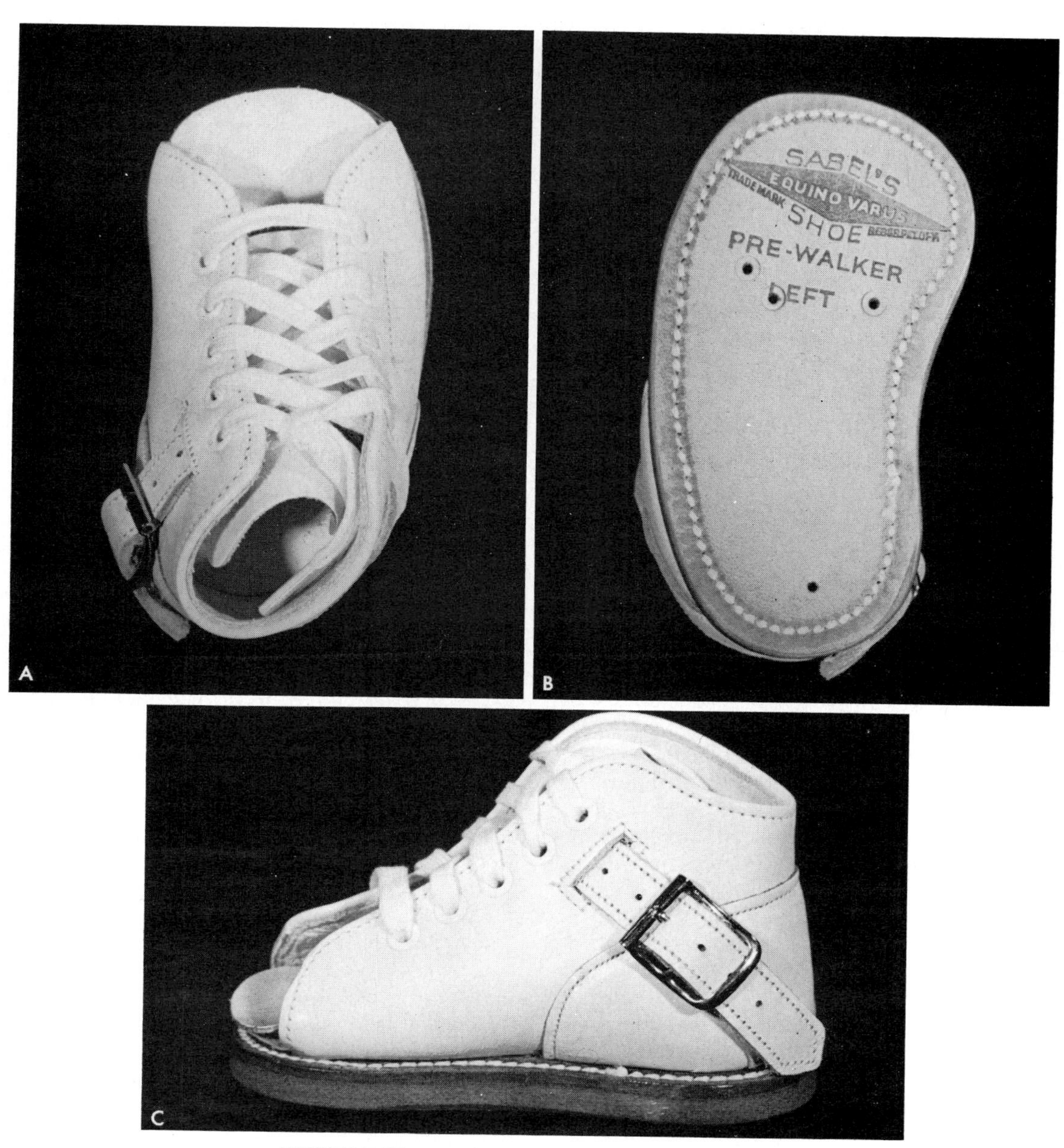

FIGURE 7–57. Prewalker clubfoot shoe with valgus strap.

A. Dorsal view. **B.** Plantar view. **C.** Lateral view.

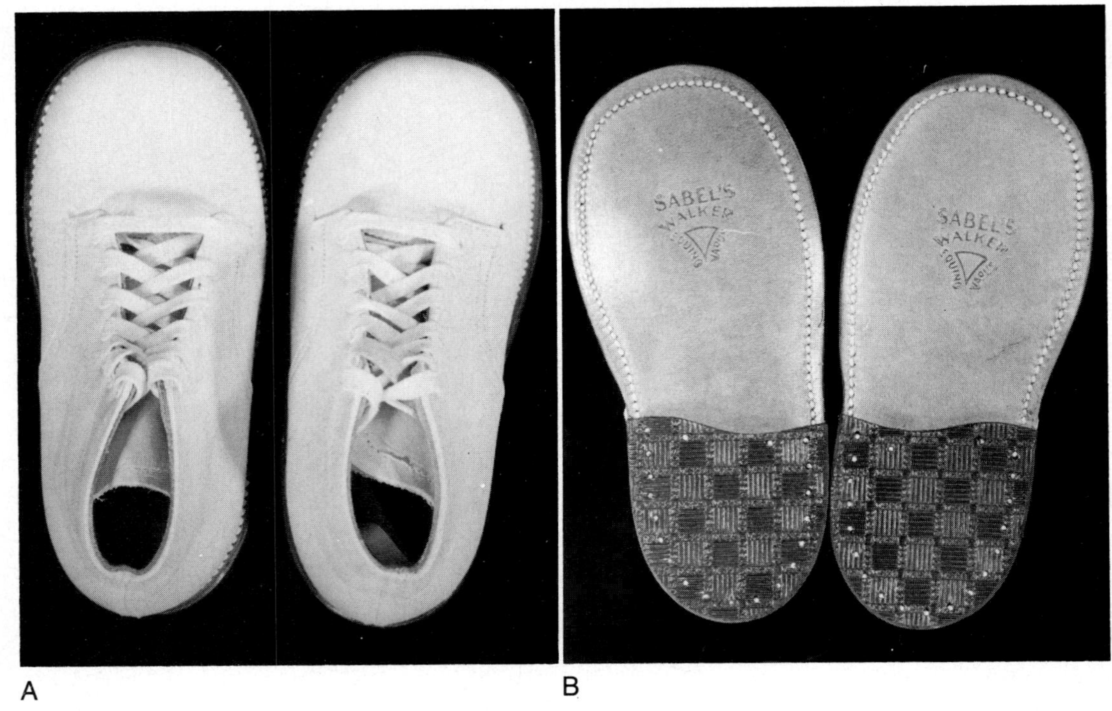

FIGURE 7–58. Outflare (tarsal pronator) shoes.

and sole wedges to encourage walking in eversion and abduction (Fig. 7–58). Radiograms are made periodically. If there is no recurrence of deformity after two years, normal shoes are worn.

Problems and complications of conservative treatment at the ankle joint include failure to correct equinus deformity, growth disturbance of the anterior distal tibial physis, and flat-top talus, which appears as a flattened dome of the talus on the lateral radiogram. This flattening may be due to forceful manipulation, particularly manipulation under anesthesia, or to forceful or prolonged casting with the foot in full dorsiflexion.

Swann, Lloyd-Roberts, and Catterall have reported that the lateral radiogram may show apparent or false talar flattening, which is actually due to improper positioning of the foot during radiography. This lateral oblique radiogram will show the fibula behind the tibia. For an accurate lateral radiogram only the hindfoot should be parallel to the cassette. A lateral arthrogram is required to distinguish between a true flat-top talus and anterior ankle contracture.[681]

Miller and Bernstein observed *flat-top talus* in 83 per cent (20 of 24) of the cases in their study and attributed the complication to forceful conservative treatment.[492] Dunn and Samuelson found some degree of flattening in the tali of all 20 of the patients they studied who were over 30 years of age, most of whom (17 of 20) had been treated initially by manipulation under anesthesia. While these patients had little pain even at 30 years of age, many of them will live to as much as 80 years of age.[172] Therefore, a 30-year follow-up is only an interim evaluation. Prevention of this deformity would appear to be gentle manipulative technique. There is no definitive treatment for this complication.

Anterior ankle contracture develops as a result of prolonged cast treatment with the foot held in maximal dorsiflexion. Clinical examination will show limited range of motion with the ankle relatively immobile and all motion limited to the dorsiflexion part of the arc. Measurement of the lateral talotibial angle on lateral dorsiflexion and plantar-flexion views will show a range of less than 30 degrees. A lateral arthrographic view will differentiate this from flat-top talus, showing a normal or nearly normal arc of the talar dome. Treatment in patients up to six months of age is by plantar-flexion stretching exercises for several weeks or by constant passive motion machine. After the age of six months, anterior ankle capsulotomy is necessary. If an extensive soft-tissue release is anticipated to correct hindfoot varus or equinus, the ankle capsulotomy should be performed first to allow proper repositioning of the foot around the partially plantar-flexed talus. There may be persistent varus and failure to correct medial spin of the calcaneus at the subtalar joint. Rocker-bottom deformity and medial calcaneocuboid joint subluxation are other deformities of the midfoot.

REDUCTION OF TALOCALCANEONAVICULAR JOINT BY OPEN SURGICAL METHODS

What are the chances of success of a closed reduction of the in utero dislocation of the talocalcaneonavicular joint in talipes equinovarus? A review of the literature shows a wide range in the rate of success. Kite reported 90 per cent success in correcting deformity with his method of manipulation and cast.[375] Fripp and Shaw reported 19 per cent success with Denis Browne splints and 71 per cent success with manipulation and stretching casts.[216] Dangelmajer reviewed 200 unselected cases and reported 40 per cent success with nonoperative treatment.[144] Persistence or recurrence of the deformity in 46 per cent was reported by Brockman in 1930, and in 56 per cent by Ponseti and Smoley in 1963.[82, 83, 568] The cause of the confusion and disagreement in the past has been the tendency to group all types of clubfoot into one category. It is imperative that, when discussing the treatment, prognosis, and results of talipes equinovarus, one does not include postural clubfoot. In talipes equinovarus, there is an in utero, rigid dislocation of the talocalcaneonavicular joint that primarily requires open surgical reduction. The likelihood of successful closed manipulative reduction is minimal, probably 5 to 10 per cent, and this is in the mild cases. Closed methods of treatment are performed primarily to elongate the contracted soft tissues. Repeatedly it has been demonstrated in fetal specimens that the talocalcaneonavicular dislocation cannot be reduced by forced manipulation. Again, it is impossible to reduce the dislocation by sectioning of the tendo Achillis and posterior tibial tendons alone. It is only upon the additional division of the plantar calcaneonavicular and tibionavicular ligaments and the capsule of the talonavicular joint, and elongation of contracted posterior and lateral soft tissues of the ankle and subtalar articulations, that one is able to reduce the medial plantar dislocation of the talocalcaneonavicular joint.

Persistent forceful manipulation and prolonged cast immobilization do more harm than good. The articular cartilage, physis, and bone will be damaged before ligaments and capsule will yield to stretching. Rigidity of the joints, fibrosis of soft parts, and disuse atrophy of muscles will develop. The osseous complica-

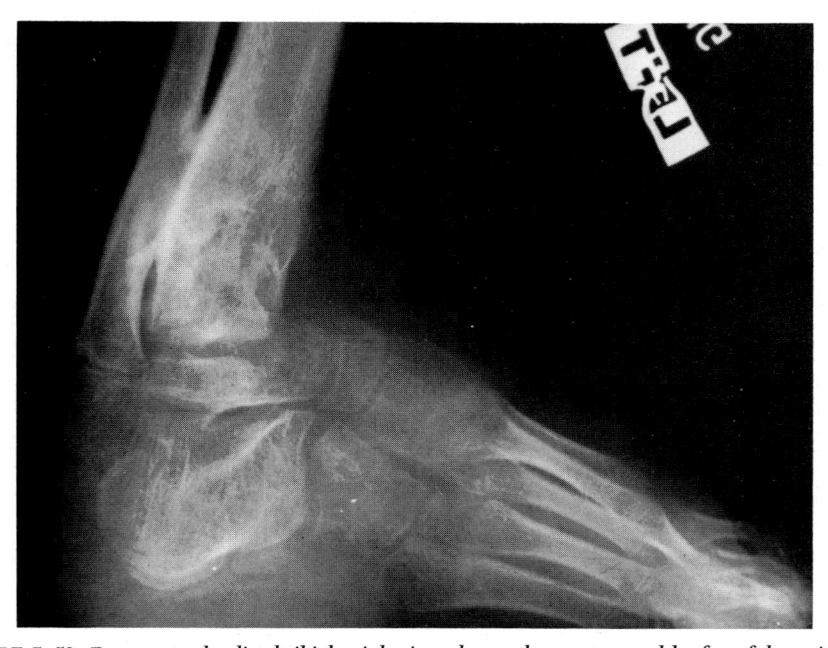

FIGURE 7–59. Damage to the distal tibial epiphysis and growth arrest caused by forceful manipulation to correct talipes equinovarus.

Multiple osteochondral compression fractures have resulted in flat-topped talus. Note the overgrown fibular malleolus.

tions of nonsurgical management—namely, flat-top talus, distal tibial bowing, metaphyseal compression, distal tibial metaphyseal spur, torus fracture of the distal tibial metaphysis, fracture of the distal fibula, and growth injuries to the distal tibial physis as shown in Figure 7–59—vividly support the thesis that the conservative method of treating talipes equinovarus is by open surgery.

Timing of Surgery. The literature on operative management of talipes equinovarus is extensive, and there is considerable difference of opinion as to the indications for surgery, the age at which to operate, and the procedure to be used. This author strongly recommends that if, by six to ten weeks, depending upon the size of the foot, clinical findings and radiograms show that complete correction has not been achieved, open surgical reduction of the talocalcaneonavicular joint be employed. Recently there has been increasing evidence to support this position.* The extremely rapid growth taking place in infancy will quickly restore normal articular alignment and architecture of the foot. It should be pointed out, however, that surgery of the small foot of the infant is very delicate, and the smaller the foot, the greater the risk of iatrogenic trauma. The novice should beware! This operation should be performed only by the knowledgeable and experienced surgeon.

Choice of Operative Procedure. The decision depends on (1) the age of the patient, (2) the degree of rigidity, (3) the deformities present, and (4) the extent of correction obtained by previous treatment.

In general, bony procedures are rarely, if ever, indicated in the infant and young child, as they would disturb the normal growth and development of the foot; if surgery is performed on patients in this age category, it should consist only of soft-tissue procedures.

Under four years of age, open reduction can usually be achieved by complete release of the talocalcaneonavicular and calcaneocuboid joints by sectioning or elongation of the contracted soft tissues on the posterior, medial, plantar, and lateral aspects of the articulation. The calcaneofibular ligament and the posterior capsule of the ankle joint are also divided. If the foot is rigid, to prevent dense scar tissue from retethering contracted soft tissues and causing recurrence of deformity, it is wise to excise ligaments, capsule, and tendon sheaths. In arthrogryposis and myelomeningocele, the tendons of nonfunctioning fibrosed muscles are excised.

In the older child, the tarsal and metatarsal bones become deformed and resist correction; in these patients, various bony procedures are performed. In the five- to eight-year age group, posterior, medial, plantar, and lateral soft-tissue release is performed to reduce the talocalcaneonavicular subluxation. The lateral convex column of the foot is overgrown, however, as compared with the medial column. In addition, the anterior articular surface of the calcaneus faces forward and medially; this medial slant of the calcaneocuboid articulation constitutes a lateral obstacle to eversion and prevents lateral translation of the cuboid, and hence of the navicular. Therefore, between five and eight years of age, the lateral column of the foot is shortened by resection of the distal end of the calcaneus (Lichtblau procedure).[414]

Another alternative method is vertical wedge resection (based laterally) of the anterior part of the calcaneus (as described by Simons).[650, 651] This author prefers Simons' calcaneal osteotomy to the Lichtblau wedge resection because hyaline articular cartilage of the calcaneocuboid joint is preserved.

In the younger child with marked scarring and recurrence of deformity and in the child nine years of age or older with marked incongruity and instability of the talocalcaneonavicular and calcaneocuboid joints, the lateral column of the foot is shortened and stabilized by calcaneocuboid joint resection and fusion (Evans procedure).[188–190] Dynamic imbalance of muscles may cause deformities such as supination of the forefoot or dorsal bunions; in such cases tendon transfers are performed to provide dynamic balance of muscles, such as split anterior tibial tendon transfer for correction of supination deformity of the forefoot.

In the child ten years of age or older, the foot is skeletally mature, and the deformities are fixed; therefore, osteotomy of the os calcis, tarsal reconstruction, or triple arthrodesis is required to provide a plantigrade foot; these are salvage procedures. Metatarsal osteotomy at their bases will correct the varus forefoot. Medial rotation osteotomy of the tibia may be indicated to correct severe lateral rotation malalignment of the tibia and fibula. Occasionally, a talectomy is performed. Table 7–9 gives a brief historic resume of the various operative procedures employed in the surgical treatment of congenital talipes equinovarus. Recent contributions of McKay, Goldner, Simons, Catterall, and Roberts are discussed in the surgical technique in Plate 95.

Procedures on Soft Tissues. The details of open reduction of the talocalcaneonavicular and

*See references 268, 299, 453, 572, 587, 665, and 781.

calcaneocuboid joints for correction of talipes equinovarus are described and illustrated in Plate 95. The procedure advocated by this author is complete subtalar release, as described by Simons and McKay.[447–449, 650] Since the report in 1971 by Turco, posteromedial release has been the operative procedure of choice for most surgeons.[706] In 1977, McKay described his concept of calcaneal rotation, and further reports have shown that simple posteromedial release does not achieve full correction.[447–449] Complete subtalar release is required for full derotation of the calcaneus and concentric alignment of the talocalcaneonavicular and calcaneocuboid joints.

The surgery should be systematic and performed in sequential steps. The progressive approach will ensure correction of all obstacles to reduction. Table 7–10 lists the structures to be sectioned or lengthened. The order of specific surgical steps to obtain correction varies, depending upon the surgical approach and the surgeon's concept of the pathoanatomy of talipes equinovarus.

Tendon Transfers. The equinovarus position of the foot gives a mechanical advantage to the invertors and plantar-flexors of the foot. The evertors and dorsiflexors are in a relatively weak position as they are stretched over the convexity of the dorsolateral aspect of the foot, whereas the anterior and posterior tibial tendons function in a mechanically advantageous position as they run a straight line to their insertions on the concavity of the medial border of the foot.

Muscle imbalance with motor weakness of the peroneals and toe extensor muscles may be a factor in recurrence of equinovarus deformity in the older child. Occasionally tendon transfers may be indicated to balance the dynamic forces acting on the foot and ankle. The muscles available for transfer are the anterior tibial (whole or half), posterior tibial, Achilles tendon, flexor hallucis longus, flexor digitorum longus, and extensor hallucis longus.

Anterior Tibial Tendon Transfer. Lateral transfer of the entire anterior tibial tendon was recommended by Garceau.[223–230] In his last report, Garceau stated that the operation is indicated if there have been multiple recurrences of all components of the deformity, if there is weakness or absence of the peroneus longus and brevis muscles, and if "bowstringing" of the anterior tibial tendon and supination of the forepart of the foot are evident in the swing phase of gait. He stressed the importance of correcting fixed deformity prior to tendon transfer. Radiograms of the foot should be taken, as clinical evaluation of the foot is not necessarily adequate to assess the amount of correction obtained. Garceau also suggested the use of electromyographic studies of the peroneus longus and brevis muscles in order to permit a more accurate assessment of the potential power of these muscles and to minimize the risk of overcorrection.[230] Critchley and Taylor, Ponseti and Campos, Raynal and Judet, and Singer and Fripp have also reported their experience with tibialis anterior transfer in congenital clubfoot.[138, 567, 583, 655] Singer and Fripp found that lateral transfer of the anterior tibial tendon does not increase dorsiflexion power and that relapse occurred in 52 of 76 feet on which the procedure had been performed.[655] Raynal and Judet stated that lateral transfer of all or half of the anterior tibial tendon results in overcorrection, pes cavus, and restriction of plantar flexion. Of the 51 cases they re-examined (with a 9- to 25-year follow-up), only 14 had gained noticeable benefit.[583]

The author does not recommend lateral transfer of the entire anterior tibial tendon in talipes equinovarus for the following reasons: (1) with anterior tibial tendon transfer, a varying degree of loss of power of ankle dorsiflexion occurs and causes recurrence of equinus deformity of the ankle; (2) equinus posture of the first metatarsal and clawing of the great toe result because of the unopposed action of the peroneus longus muscle; and (3) when the varus deformity is corrected, peroneal muscle power returns and provides active eversion of the foot. Even when the anterior tibial tendon is transferred only to the third metatarsal, overcorrection and valgus deformity are potential complications. Lateral transfer of the entire anterior tibial tendon is indicated in calcaneus deformity of the foot (especially in paralytic conditions) when the following requisites are found: (1) the motor strength of the peroneal muscle should be zero or poor minus; (2) the triceps surae muscle is very weak—poor or less in motor strength; (3) the anterior tibial muscle strength is normal or at least good in motor strength; (4) the foot is completely flexible, with no fixed varus, supination, or equinus deformity (a tendon transfer will not correct a fixed deformity); (5) radiograms of the foot should disclose normal alignment of the talocalcaneonavicular and calcaneocuboid joints; and (6) the child is at least four years of age and in a family situation that will provide adequate postoperative training and care. To prevent overcorrection, the tendon should not be transferred farther laterally than the base of the third metatarsal.

Text continued on page 2510

Table 7–9. Operative Correction of Talipes Equinovarus by Soft-Tissue Release and Bony Procedures

	Ober	Brockmann	McCauley	Bost, Schottstaedt, and Larsen
Posterior Release				
Achilles tendon	Subcutaneously Do it at end to assist in driving talus back into mortise	Lengthen by Z-plasty 2 weeks after medial release	Lengthen by Z-plasty 8 weeks after medial release	Lengthen (tri-cut method of Hoke)
Posterior capsule of ankle joint	—	Section 2 weeks after medial release	Section 8 weeks after medial release	Section
Posterior talofibular ligament	—	—	—	—
Posterior capsule of subtalar joint	—	Section 2 weeks after medial release	Section 8 weeks after medial release	Section
Calcaneofibular ligament	—	—	—	—
Posterior insertion of deltoid ligament on calcaneus	Section (whole attachment removed from medial surface of calcaneus subperiosteally)	Section	Section	Section
Flexor digitorum longus	—	—	Excise sheath Lengthen by Z-plasty (if necessary)	—
Flexor hallucis longus	—	—	Excise sheath Lengthen by Z-plasty (if necessary)	—
Kirschner wire in os calcis (to be incorporated in cast)	—	—	—	—
Medial Release				
Posterior tibial tendon	Lengthen	Z-plasty lengthening	Z-plasty lengthening	Detach from insertions (tuberosity of navicular, cuneiform, metatarsals)
Tibionavicular ligament (anterior part of deltoid ligament)	Section	Section	Section	Section
Talonavicular capsule	Section	Section	Section	Section
Calcaneonavicular (spring) ligament	Elevate subperiosteally from calcaneus	—	Section	Section
Deltoid ligament (superficial layer)	Elevate subperiosteally from calcaneus	Section	Section	Section
Deltoid ligament (deep layer)	Elevate subperiosteally from talus	Section	Preserve	Section (sometimes)
Capsule of naviculo-cuneiform joint	—	—	Section (if necessary)	Section
Subtalar Release				
Capsule of medial side of subtalar joint	Lengthen by subperiosteal elevation from calcaneus	Section	Section	Section
Talocalcaneal interosseous ligament	—	—	Section	Section
Bifurcated (Y) ligament (extends from calcaneus to lateral border of navicular and medial border of cuboid)	—	—	—	Section

Gelman	*Turco*	*Evans*	*Dwyer*
Lengthen 2 months after medial release	Z-technique Detach medial half of insertion on os calcis	Lenghten by Z-plasty	Lengthen by Z-plasty
Section 2 months after medial release	Section	Section	—
Section 2 months after medial release	Section	Section	—
Section 2 months after medial release	Section	Section	—
Section 2 months after medial release	Section	Section	—
Section	Section (retract neurovascular bundle posteriorly for exposure)	Section	—
—	—	—	—
—	—	—	—
—	—	—	—
Z-lengthening	Divide above medial malleolus (use distal stump for traction and identification of navicular, then reinsert)	Lengthen by Z-plasty	—
Section	Section	Section	—
Section	Section	Section	—
Preserve—will prevent rocker-bottom deformity	Detach from sustentaculum tali	Section	Subperiosteally elevated from calcaneus
Section	Section	Section	Subperiosteally elevated from calcaneus
Preserve	Preserve	—	—
—	Section (if necessary)	—	—
Section	Section	Section	Elevate subperiosteally and release
Section through medial approach above sustentaculum tali	Section through medial approach above sustentaculum tali	—	—
—	Section	—	—

Table continued on following page

Table 7–9. *Operative Correction of Talipes Equinovarus by Soft-Tissue Release and Bony Procedures* (Continued)

	Ober	*Brockmann*	*McCauley*	*Bost, Schottstaedt, and Larsen*
Plantar Release				
Incision	Subcutaneously	Separate linear incision along anterolateral border of os calcis	—	Medial
Plantar fascia	Section	Excise origin	—	Section
Abductor hallucis Intrinsic toe flexors Abductor digiti quinti	—	Detach all muscles	Superior origin of abductor hallcis detached and displaced downward	Section at origin
Long and short plantar ligaments	—	—	—	Section at the calcaneocuboid joint
Capsule of calcaneocuboid joint	—	—	—	Section
Procedures on Tarsal Bones	No	No	No	No
Internal Fixation	No	No	No	No
Postoperative Care	Change cast at 2 weeks and manipulate foot into overcorrection Change cast monthly, each time manipulating foot into corrected position Total of 4 to 5 months' immobilization Some form of clubfoot brace worn night and day 8 months longer	Posterior release and heel cord lengthening 2 weeks after medial release Change casts to obtain full correction Total of 3 to 5 months' immobilization Below-knee orthosis with medial bar and outside T-strap at night Outside sole and heel wedges on shoe Active exercise to strengthen	Change cast in 2 weeks and manipulate foot into further correction Posterior release and heel cord lengthening at 8 weeks (if necessary) Total of 2 to 4 months' immobilization Cross bar splint attached to shoes at night; ⅛" outer sole and heel wedges on shoes during day Active exercises to strengthen peroneals and dorsiflexors	Foot held in relaxed position until wound healed Repeated changes of casts at 2-week intervals to obtain gradual correction Total of 5 months' immobilization Brace at night to hold foot in corrected position Shoe wedges Periodic cast treatment if necessary
Remarks	Subperiosteal elevation of contracted capsule and ligaments (particularly deltoid) provides stability of ankle joint as they heal and reattach in lengthened position Overcorrect every element of deformity Cure not complete until patient actively can put his foot in a position of overcorrection		Release abductor hallucis to decrease its deforming force More extensive sectioning of capsules and ligaments (particularly of interosseous talocalcaneal ligament, which binds talus and calcaneus in varus position) Following sectioning, marked release of deformity occurs	Thorough plantar dissection and release Section of talocalcaneal interosseous and of bifurcated ligaments stressed

Gelman	*Turco*	*Evans*	*Dwyer*
Medial	Separate (3 cm. long on plantar surface of hindfoot)	Medial	Medial
Section	Excise origin	Section	Section
Section at origin	Strip subperiosteally from os calcis	Section	Section
—	—	—	—
—	—	—	—
No	Excise elongated tuberosity of navicular after reduction (to prevent pressure necrosis of skin)	Shorten lateral column of foot by resection and fusion of calcaneocuboid joint	Osteotomy of calcaneus lever inferior segment inferiorly and laterally (held open by wedge of bone graft)
No	Kirschner wire to transfix talonavicular joint	Two staples across calcaneocuboid joint	—
In long leg cast for 2 to 3 months	Cast change under general anesthesia 3 months after operation	Immobilize in above-knee cast for 5 months Walking in plaster cast permitted in 6 weeks	Immobilize in cast 8 weeks
Posterior release 2 months following medial release if necessary to correct equinus deformity	Remove sutures and Kirschner wire at 6 weeks Total of 4 months' immobilization (last 2½ months can be walking cast in older child) Pronator walking shoes during day Denis Browne splint (25 cm. everting crossbar) at night for 2 years		
Preserve calcaneonavicular ligament to prevent rocker-bottom deformity Preserve deep layer of deltoid ligament (tibiotalar portion)	Preserve deep layer of deltoid ligament (it inserts on the body of the talus) Tilting of the talus and pes valgus will develop if tibiotalar ligament is sectioned Calcaneus must be released at both ends to obtain complete correction Internal fixation of talonavicular joint Note: Ingram divides interosseous talocalcaneal ligament and capsule of calcaneocuboid joint through lateral incision He transfixed calcaneocuboid joint with Kirschner wire in addition to talonavicular joint	Shorten lateral column of foot	Corrects fixed bony varus deformity of hindfoot

Table 7–10. *Structures Divided or Lengthened in the Treatment of Talipes Equinovarus*

A. *Muscles-Tendons*
  1. *Achilles*
     Always; common technique is Z-lengthening with division of distal part medially; McKay lengthens in coronal plane
     Pitfall to avoid—do not overlengthen
  2. *Posterior tibial*
     Always lengthen; supramalleolar level; preserve tendon sheath and canal; maintain function; never section; do not transfer primarily, except in paralytic clubfoot
  3. *Abductor hallucis*
     Always; most surgeons recess at origin; this author recommends excision
  4. *Flexor hallucis longus and flexor digitorum longus*
     Lengthen when toes are flexed and cannot be straightened when the ankle is dorsiflexed to neutral position at the end of surgery
     Recommend musculotendinous recession at two or three sites to obtain desired amount of lengthening; when tendon lengthening, preserve sheath; prevent scarring especially at Henry's knot
  5. *Flexor digitorum brevis,* abductor digiti quinti, and quadratus plantae with plantar aponeurosis and long plantar ligament—from calcaneal origin

B. *Capsule-Ligaments*
  1. *Talonavicular*
     Always: medial, dorsal, plantar, and lateral
  2. *Subtalar*
     Always: medial, anterior, lateral, and posterior
  3. *Calcaneocuboid joint*
     Medial, plantar, and dorsal—always
     Lateral—this author always sections
  4. *Ankle capsule*
     Posterior: always
     Medial: preserve integrity of part of deltoid ligament
     Lateral: divide if necessary, preferably partially
     Anterior: only if contracted, limiting plantar flexion; should be staged
  5. *Contracted ligaments on posterolateral aspect of ankle and subtalar joint*
     Always section:
     a. Calcaneofibular ligament
     b. Posterior talofibular ligament
     c. Superior peroneal retinaculum
  6. *Interosseous talocalcaneal ligament*
     Divide partially or completely when unable to correct medial rotation of calcaneus at the subtalar joint

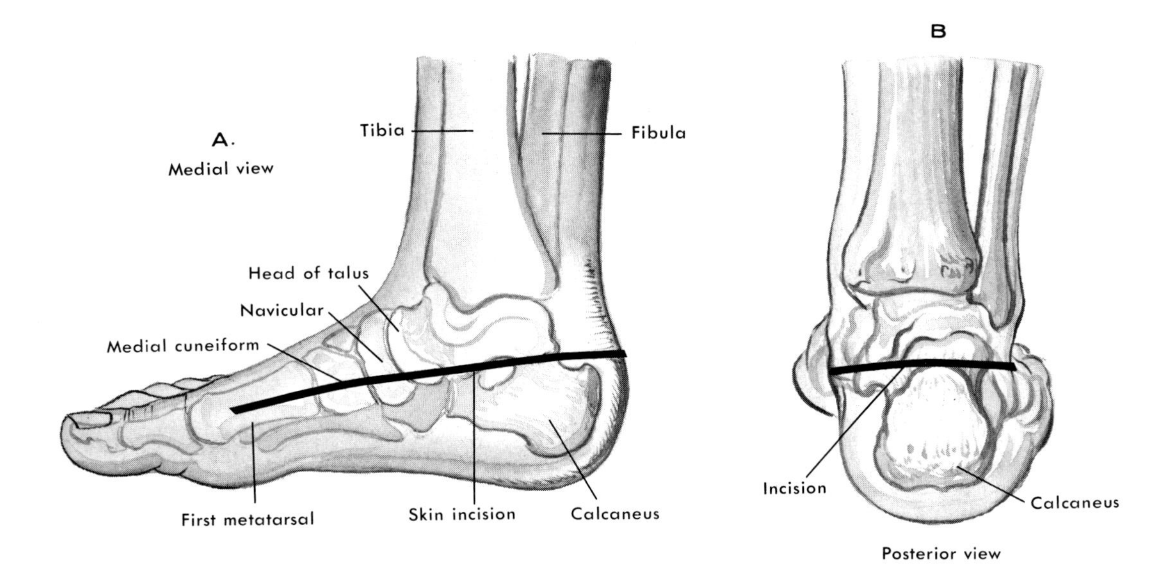

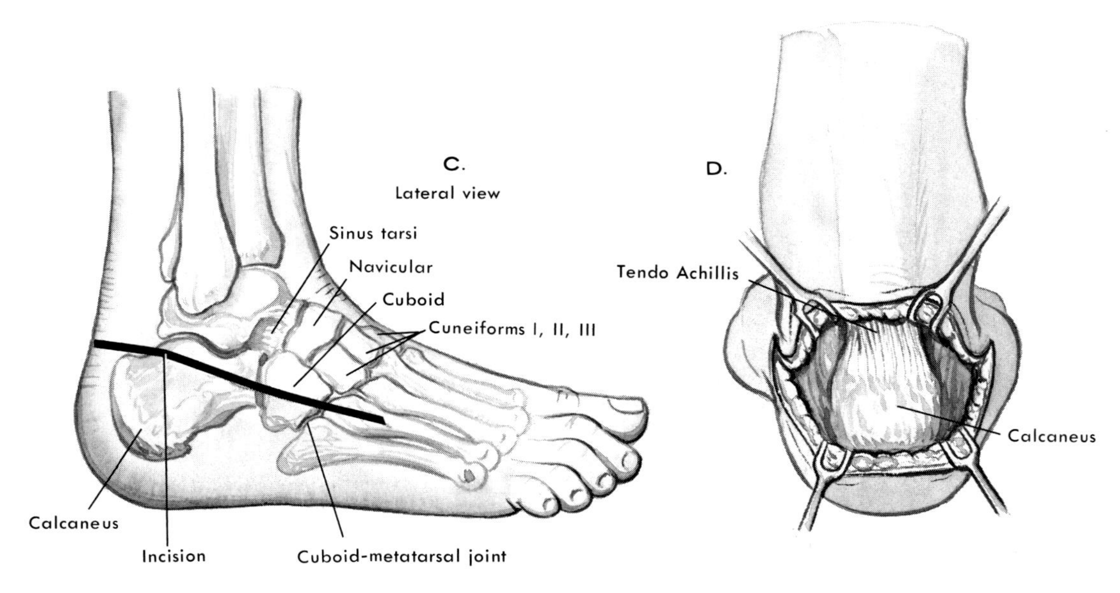

FIGURE 7–60. Cincinnati incision for complete soft-tissue release and open reduction of the talocalcaneonavicular joint in talipes equinovarus.

A to **C.** Transverse incision that starts at the base of the first metatarsal and extends posteriorly 3 mm. superior to the heel crease under the medial malleolus and then posterolaterally to the tip of the lateral malleolus, and distally to the cuboid–fifth metatarsal joint. **D.** Exposure of the Achilles tendon by elevation of subcutaneous tissue proximally and distally. This incision provides an excellent view of the pathologic changes in talipes equinovarus. Its drawbacks are difficulty in dissecting out and exposing the Achilles tendon proximally to permit adequate lengthening of the heel cord, difficulty in supramalleolar lengthening of the posterior tibial tendon, and tautness of the skin posteriorly that does not allow immobilization of the ankle in neutral dorsiflexion.

Open Reduction of Talocalcaneonavicular and Calcaneocuboid Joints by Complete Subtalar Release in Talipes Equinovarus by Posteromedial and Lateral Surgical Approach

OPERATIVE TECHNIQUE

Step I—Surgical Approach: Skin Incisions

The operation is performed in a bloodless field obtained by exsanguinating the limb with an Esmarch bandage and inflating the pneumatic tourniquet to 200 to 250 mm. Hg. The posture of the patient is prone when the Cincinnati or Carroll surgical approach is used, whereas in the posteromedial and lateral surgical approach the patient is supine. The lower limb is washed with Betadine soap, painted with Betadine solution, and draped with the knee free. The patella and proximal tibial tubercle are marked with indelible ink to facilitate determination of appropriate realignment of the foot in relation to the knee.

In the moderately deformed foot the Cincinnati incision is ordinarily used; however, in the severely deformed foot with marked equinus, in which skin necrosis is likely to develop by the transverse Cincinnati incision, this author recommends two incisions: posteromedial and lateral that extends proximally behind the lateral malleolus.

In the *Cincinnati approach* (see Fig. 7–60), the skin incision starts on the medial aspect of the foot at the first metatarsal-cuneiform joint. This author begins the incision at the distal fourth of the first metatarsal. The skin incision extends posteriorly, curving gently beneath the tip of the medial malleolus; then it is carried transversely around the heel over the tendo Achillis in line with the posterior skin crease, approximately at the level of the tibiotalar joint. It then extends forward on the lateral aspect of the foot, gently curving forward over the sinus tarsi and ending on the dorsolateral aspect of the cuboid bone. The anterior ends of the skin incision may be extended further distally on either the medial or lateral side, depending upon the extent of the surgical release. The advantages of the Cincinnati incision are that (1) it provides excellent visualization of the posterior, medial, and lateral aspects of the foot and ankle; and (2) with the patient in prone position, posteromedial release is simple to perform, and the adequacy of correction of calcaneal rotation can be easily determined. Its disadvantages are skin slough and the difficulty of tendo Achillis and supramalleolar posterior tibial lengthening in severe talipes equinovarus.

In the *Carroll technique*, the surgical approach is made by two incisions—a lazy Z medial and a vertical posterior incision. The landmarks for the *medial incision* are (1) the front of the medial malleolus, (2) the center of the medial surface of the os calcis, and (3) the base of the first metatarsal; these three points form a triangle. Bisect this triangle; the *midpoint* of the incision parallels the sole of the foot; the *posterior limb* of the medial incision curves in a plantar direction toward the center of the heel; and the *anterior limb* extends distally around the dorsum of the foot. The posterior part of the incision exposes the plantar structures; the dorsal-anterior part of the incision exposes the talonavicular joint (see Fig. 7–61 A, p. 2510). Behind the medial malleolus there is about one fingerbreadth of intact skin. The *posterior incision* is longitudinal midway between the Achilles tendon and the lateral malleolus; it begins at the heel (2 cm. distal to the tip of the lateral malleolus) and extends proximally to the juncture of the lower one third and the upper two thirds of the calf. The posterior incision exposes the posterolateral structures (see Fig. 7–61 B).

In the Carroll technique the medial-plantar wound is used to release marked plantar soft tissue tethers of the calcaneocuboid joint, but this is technically rather difficult.

A. In the surgical approach illustrated in this plate, two separate incisions are made—a posteromedial and a lateral. The posteromedial incision is curvilinear, beginning 7 to 10 cm. proximal to the medial malleolus, passing 1 cm. behind the posterior margin of the tibia, and extending inferiorly to a point 1.5 cm. distal to the tip of the medial malleolus, where it is gently curved distally and anteriorly along the sustentaculum tali to terminate at the base of the first metatarsal bone. It is important to keep one fingerbreadth of skin intact behind the medial malleolus and not to cross the posterior and plantar skin creases. The lateral skin incision (not illustrated) starts at the base of the fourth metatarsal, 1.5 to 2.0 cm. dorsal to the plantar border of the bone (not the sole, which is quite thick in the infant). Palpate the bone! The skin incision then extends posteriorly 2 to 3 cm. This provides access to the calcaneofibular ligament and superior peroneal retinaculum. Posteriorly there should be adequate width of intact skin between the two incisions.

Plate 95. Open Reduction of Talocalcaneonavicular and Calcaneocuboid Joints by Complete Subtalar Release in Talipes Equinovarus by Posteromedial and Lateral Surgical Approach

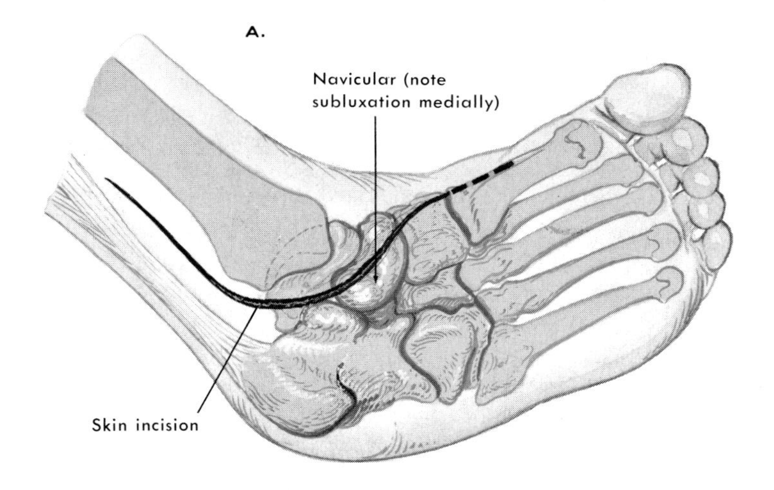

Open Reduction of Talocalcaneonavicular and Calcaneocuboid Joints by Complete Subtalar Release in Talipes Equinovarus by Posteromedial and Lateral Surgical Approach (Continued)

Step I (Continued)

The incised skin margins are elevated with skin hooks, and subcutaneous tissues are divided in line with the skin incision. Superficial blood vessels are clamped and coagulated; if possible, preserve the venous drainage of the foot and leg. Injury to the cutaneous nerves should be avoided. The sural nerve is identified, mobilized, and protected during surgery.

Step II—Dissection and Elongation of the Tendons-Muscles on the Posteromedial Aspect of the Ankle and Foot and Dissection and Mobilization of the Medial Neurovascular Bundle and Its Branches

B and **C**. First, identify the Achilles tendon and dissect it free from the soft tissues on its posterior, medial, and lateral aspects. The paratenon of the triceps surae is divided longitudinally at the medial margin of the tendo Achillis. Inadvertent injury to the neurovascular bundle should be avoided. The tendon is freed of the fibrofatty tissue anterior to it. A tongue-blade is passed deep to the Achilles tendon.

Lengthening of the tendo Achillis by Z-plasty is performed in the anteroposterior (sagittal) plane. With a knife, the Achilles tendon is divided longitudinally into lateral and medial halves for a distance of 5 to 7 cm. The distal end of the medial half is detached from the calcaneus to prevent recurrence of varus deformity of the heel; the lateral half is divided proximally. The medial segment of the divided tendon is reflected proximally, and the lateral segment is reflected distally to its insertion at the calcaneal apophysis. McKay lengthens the tendo Achillis in the coronal plane.[447, 448]

Plate 95. Open Reduction of Talocalcaneonavicular and Calcaneocuboid Joints by Complete Subtalar Release in Talipes Equinovarus by Posteromedial and Lateral Surgical Approach

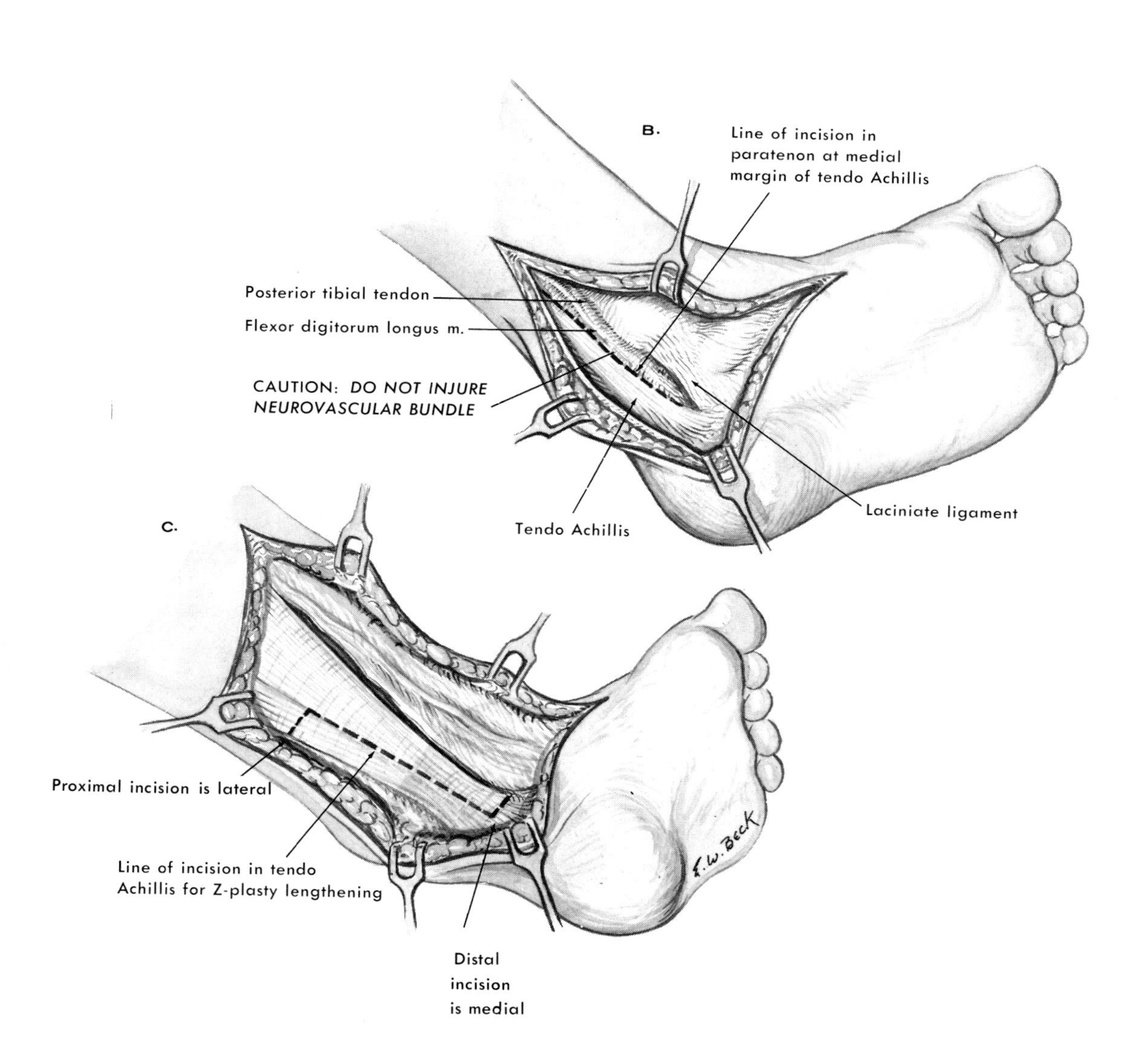

Open Reduction of Talocalcaneonavicular and Calcaneocuboid Joints by Complete Subtalar Release in Talipes Equinovarus by Posteromedial and Lateral Surgical Approach (Continued)

Step II (Continued)

D and **E.** Next, identify and dissect free the *posterior tibial tendon.* In the distal part of the leg, it lies immediately posterior to the tibia; it is deep to the flexor digitorum longus tendon. Pulling on the posterior tibial tendon will invert the midfoot.

Then, identify and dissect free the flexor digitorum longus tendon. It is the most superficial tendon on the posteromedial border of the tibia. Pulling the flexor digitorum tendon will flex the toes. A length of white Silastic tubing is placed around the posterior tibial tendon and another around the flexor digitorum longus tendon for gentle traction.

Then, the medial neurovascular bundle (posterior tibial vessels and tibial nerve) is identified above the medial malleolus; it lies between the flexor digitorum longus and flexor hallucis longus. With a nerve dissector the neurovascular bundle is dissected free and mobilized with its sheath distally to the canal beneath the lacinate ligament (flexor retinaculum). A piece of yellow Silastic tubing is passed around the neurovascular bundle for protection.

Next, with a curved hemostat, locate and identify the *flexor hallucis longus tendon.* It is lateral and deep to the medial neurovascular bundle. Dissect the tendon free from the level of the ankle joint to its canal beneath the talus and pass white Silastic tubing around the tendon.

The *laciniate ligament* is a strong, fibrous band extending from the medial malleolus above to the calcaneus below. It is the "door" to the plantar aspect of the foot, converting a series of bony grooves into four canals for the passage of tendons and the neurovascular bundle. Enumerated anteroposteriorly, these canals transmit (1) the tendon of the tibialis posterior; (2) the tendon of the flexor digitorum longus; (3) the posterior tibial vessels and tibial nerve (neurovascular bundle); and (4) the tendon of the flexor hallucis longus (the last-named canal is partly formed by the talus). The abductor hallucis longus muscle fibers take origin from the lower border of the laciniate ligament. With sharp and dull dissection, the abductor hallucis muscle is freed from its extensive origin—the navicular bone, sustentaculum tali, medial process of the calcaneal tuberosity, first metatarsal, and other structures on the medial aspect of the foot. The abductor hallucis is then elevated and reflected distally and plantarward. The nerve supply to the abductor hallucis muscle (medial plantar nerve) should be preserved.

In the moderately to severely deformed or paralytic or arthrogrypotic type of clubfoot, this author excises the abductor hallucis from its tendinous distal one fourth to its origin. Excision of abductor hallucis facilitates exposure of the medial and plantar aspects of the foot for deep dissection, makes skin closure easier with less tension, and diminishes the likelihood of metatarsus adductus as a postoperative problem. This author has not encountered hallux valgus as a sequela to excision of abductor hallucis. A Freer elevator or a blunt probe is inserted beneath the superior edge of the laciniate ligament to protect the neurovascular bundle. The laciniate ligament is sectioned over the blunt probe near its attachment to the medial malleolus. Do not injure the neurovascular bundle as it enters the plantar aspect of the foot!

The medial neurovascular bundle is traced to the plantar aspect of the foot; its branches (the medial and lateral plantar vessels and nerves and the calcaneal branches) are dissected free, and yellow Silastic tubing is passed around each branch. It is important to be meticulous in freeing and mobilizing the medial neurovascular bundle and all its branches.

Plate 95. Open Reduction of Talocalcaneonavicular and Calcaneocuboid Joints by Complete Subtalar Release in Talipes Equinovarus by Posteromedial and Lateral Surgical Approach

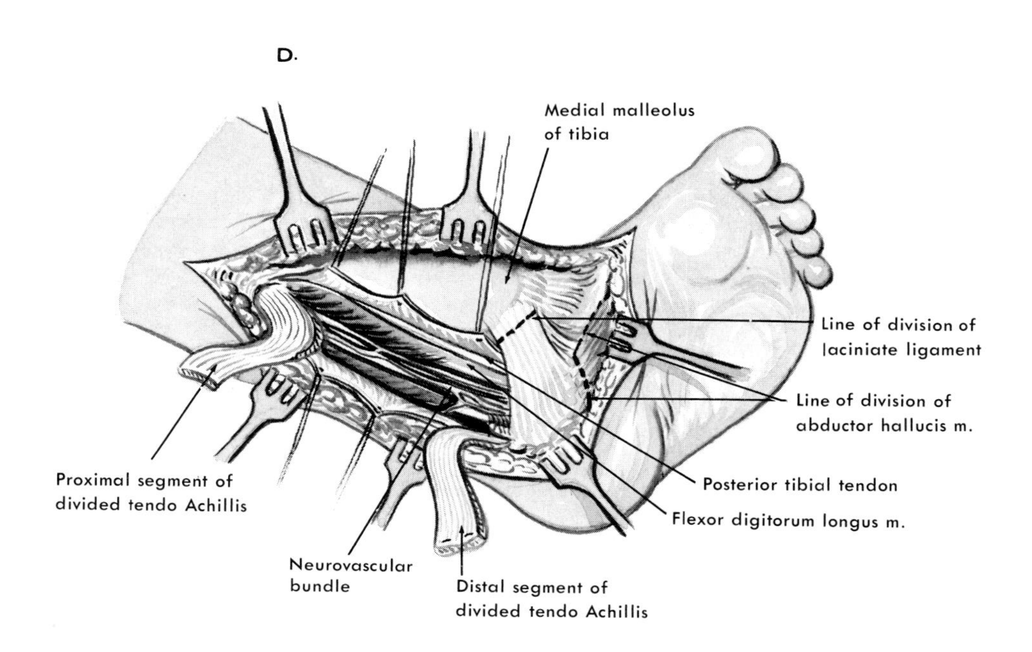

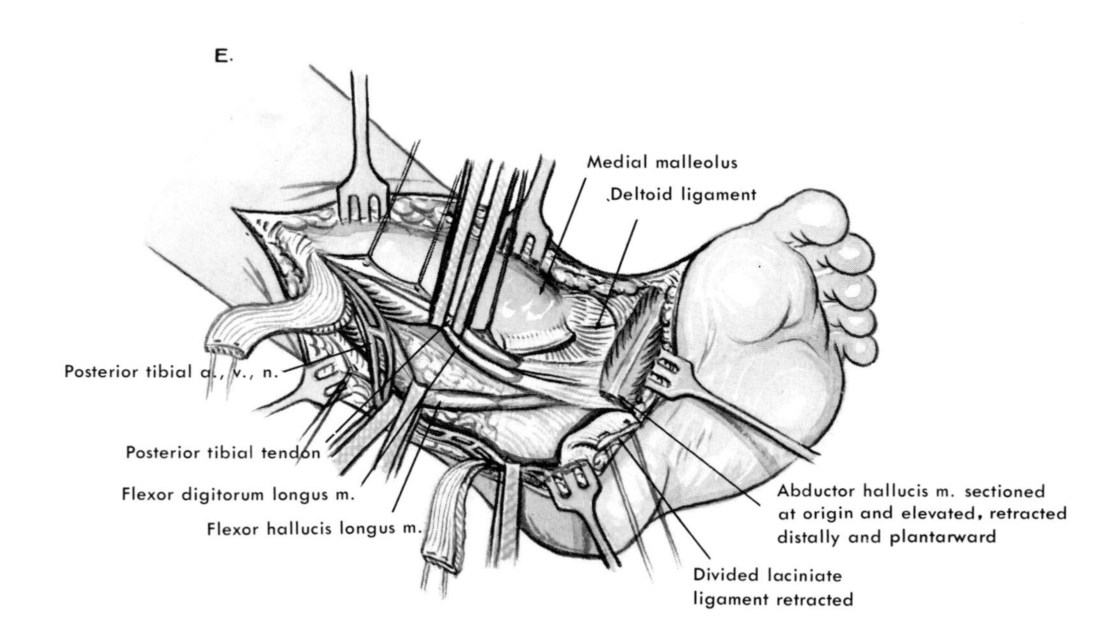

Open Reduction of Talocalcaneonavicular and Calcaneocuboid Joints by Complete Subtalar Release in Talipes Equinovarus by Posteromedial and Lateral Surgical Approach (Continued)

Step II (Continued)

F. The posterior tibial tendon is lengthened by Z-plasty above the medial malleolus. The tendon sheath of the posterior tibial muscle behind the medial malleolus is left intact, because the posterior tibial muscle is an important dynamic force in supporting the medial longitudinal arch of the foot, and its function should be preserved. This author does not section and discard the posterior tibial tendon because overcorrection and pes valgus are definite complications.

Step III—Release of Dorsal and Medial Aspects of the Talonavicular Joint and Dissection of Master Knot of Henry

G and **H.** The proximal segment of the posterior tibial tendon is tagged with 000 Mersilene or Tycron suture. Insert a blunt probe into the canal of the posterior tibial tendon from above the ankle. The tip of the probe is directed toward the navicular, which in severe talipes equinovarus abuts the medial malleolus. Make a small incision (1 to 2 cm.) on the tendon sheath, over the tip of the probe parallel to the course of the tendon and immediately proximal to the tendon's insertion at the navicular. The distal segment of the posterior tibial tendon is pulled out of its sheath distally into the medial part of the foot.

Note: At the end of the surgery, the distal segment of the posterior tibial tendon will be reinserted through its canal and sutured to the proximal segment in elongated position. This technique, in contrast to replacing the tendon in its open sheath, will prevent formation of fibrous adhesions and will allow gliding of the tendon through the pulley and maintain function of the posterior tibial muscle.

The distal segment of the tendon is pulled out of its sheath distally into the medial part of the foot. Traction on the distal posterior tibial stump will serve as a guide in locating the navicular bone and talonavicular joint. The navicular will be found distally medially and plantarward tethered to the medial malleolus and the sustentaculum tali by a dense mass of thick fibrous tissue. The navicular bone lies almost parallel to the long axis of the foot. The joint lines are obscured, making it easy to damage articular cartilage and bone. In order to avoid injury, dissection should proceed distally, not laterally. Sectioning of the neck or head of the talus and the sustentaculum tali should be avoided. Insert a small Chandler retractor on the dorsum of the talus deep to the toe extensor tendons, the anterior tibial tendon, and the dorsalis pedis vessels. With a two-pronged sharp skin hook, pull the navicular distally and section the thick tibionavicular ligament (anterior tibionavicular ligament or anterior part of the deltoid) immediate to the navicular. This is a thickened band that extends from the medial malleolus to the tuberosity of the navicular. By gentle traction on the posterior tibial tendon, the talonavicular joint is identified. With a double skin hook, pull the navicular distally and medially and section the dorsal-medial parts of the talonavicular capsule. It is important to perform an adequate dorsal release in order to get the navicular down from its tethered position. Compromise of dorsal blood supply to the talus (i.e., the leash of vessels that pass from the dorsalis pedis to the talar neck) is avoided by staying distal; section tissues near the navicular. Keep as far distally on the talar head as possible. The capsule of the naviculocuneiform is left intact.

Plate 95. Open Reduction of Talocalcaneonavicular and Calcaneocuboid Joints by Complete Subtalar Release in Talipes Equinovarus by Posteromedial and Lateral Surgical Approach

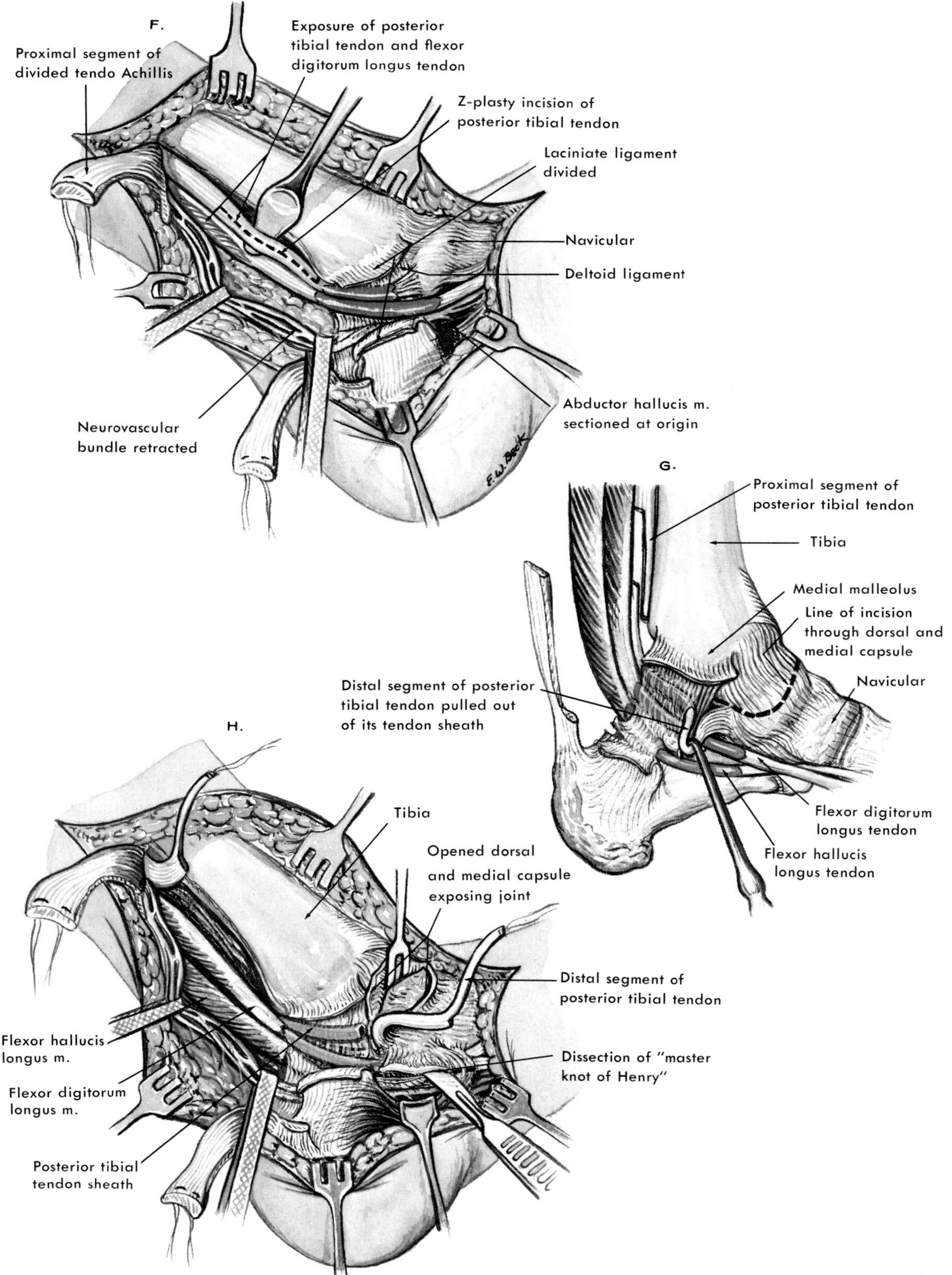

Open Reduction of Talocalcaneonavicular and Calcaneocuboid Joints by Complete Subtalar Release in Talipes Equinovarus by Posteromedial and Lateral Surgical Approach (Continued)

Step III (Continued)

The flexor digitorum and flexor hallucis longus tendons are traced and mobilized from above the ankle to the medial-plantar aspect of the foot.

Distal to the anterior end of the sustentaculum tali, the flexor digitorum longus tendon crosses the flexor hallucis longus tendon from the lateral to the medial side in an oblique course dorsal (i.e., deep) to it. At the crossing point, the flexor hallucis longus and the flexor digitorum longus tendons are bound together by a strong fibrous band—the master knot of Henry—which is attached to the plantar surface of the navicular. With sharp scissors, the master knot of Henry is divided and the long flexor tendons are dissected free, mobilized, and retracted plantarward with the neurovascular bundle. Ordinarily, the long flexor tendons and flexor hallucis longus muscles have a fair amount of excursion and are not markedly contracted; therefore, routine lengthening of the flexor tendons is not indicated. However, when the foot is dorsiflexed to neutral position at the ankle and the toes are still flexed and cannot be passively straightened into full extension, the flexor digitorum longus and flexor hallucis longus are fractionally lengthened at their musculotendinous junction behind the ankle and lower leg. It is best to perform flexor tendon lengthening at the end of the procedure, as traction on the lengthened tendons may cause their discontinuity. It is important not to open the sheaths of the flexor tendons and not to perform Z-lengthening on the medial aspect of the foot, as it may result in adherence of the lengthened tendons to scar tissue. Attention to these details will prevent development of hammertoe and dorsal bunion.

McKay incises the sheaths circumferentially, retaining the tendons within the sheaths. Then he rolls the sheaths proximally to above the level of the ankle joint, whereupon a fractional lengthening of the tendons is performed. The sheaths are left to protect the tendons.[447–449] This author finds the McKay technique of preservation of tendon sheaths and prevention of scar adherence technically difficult.

Plate 95. Open Reduction of Talocalcaneonavicular and Calcaneocuboid Joints by Complete Subtalar Release in Talipes Equinovarus by Posteromedial and Lateral Surgical Approach (Parts F, G, and H repeated)

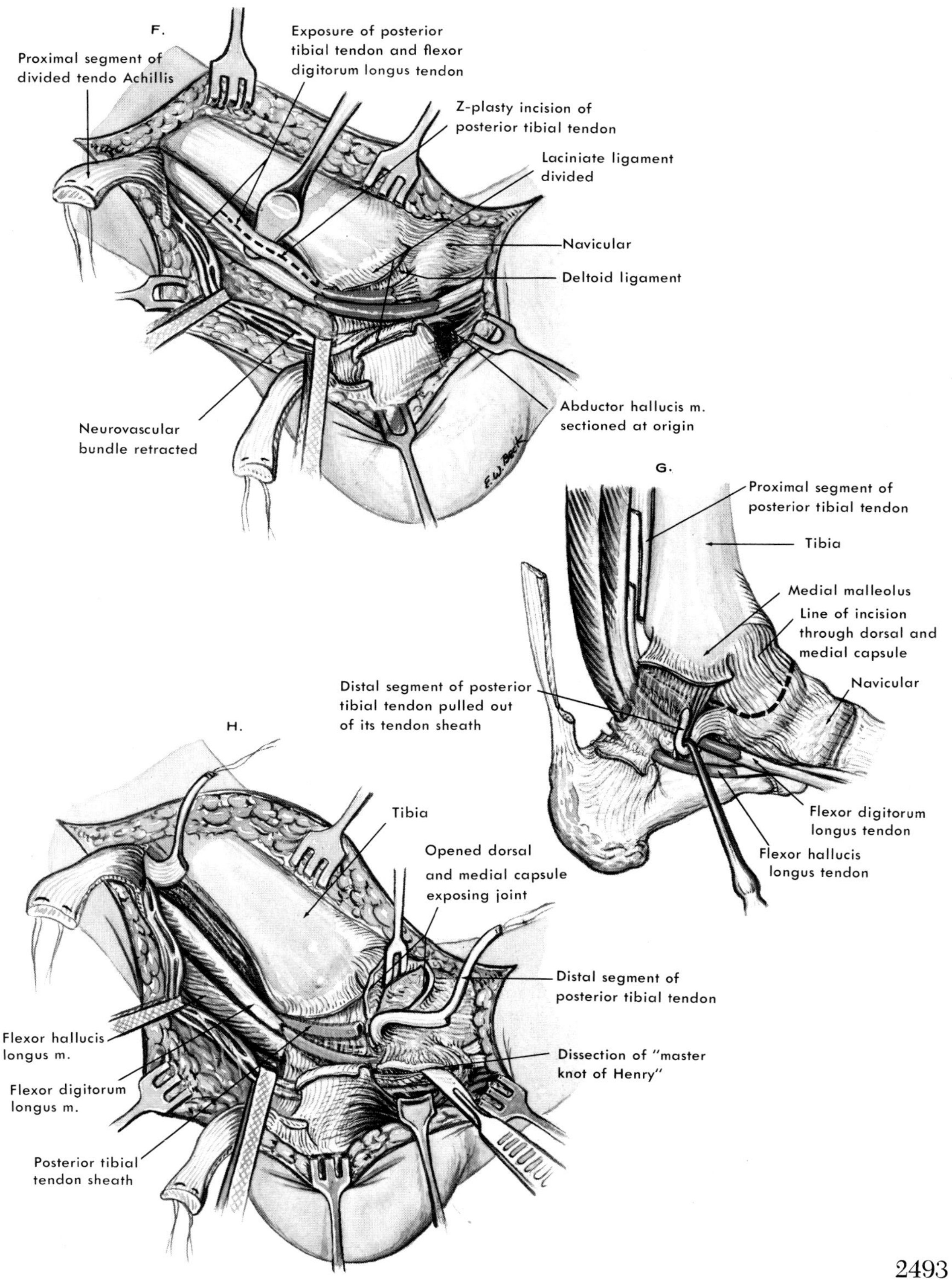

Open Reduction of Talocalcaneonavicular and Calcaneocuboid Joints by Complete Subtalar Release in Talipes Equinovarus by Posteromedial and Lateral Surgical Approach (Continued)

Step IV—Release of the Ligamentous and Capsular Tether and the Plantar and Lateral Sides of the Articulations Between the Talus, Navicular, Calcaneus, and Cuboid

I. This step entails division of (1) plantar and lateral parts of the talonavicular capsule; (2) plantar calcaneonavicular ligament; (3) calcaneonavicular limb of bifurcate ligament; and (4) calcaneocuboid limb of bifurcate ligament.

The goal of release of these structures is to enable lateral translation of the talonavicular and calcaneocuboid joints and also to correct posterior cavus (fixed equinus) at the talonavicular and calcaneocuboid joints.

The plantar aspect of the foot is visualized. The plantar calcaneonavicular ligament (spring ligament) is a thick band connecting the anterior margin of the sustentaculum tali of the calcaneus to the plantar surface of the navicular. It is shortened and is a fixed obstacle to reduction of the talocalcaneonavicular joint; it should be divided after adequate exposure. Normally, the plantar surface of the spring ligament is supported by the posterior tibial tendon medially and the flexor hallucis longus and flexor digitorum longus tendons laterally. (The posterior tibial tendon has already been divided and dissected free to its insertion.)

At this point, the neurovascular bundle and long toe flexors and flexor hallucis longus tendons are retracted inferiorly, and the plantar calcaneonavicular ligament and the plantar and lateral parts of the capsule of the talonavicular joint are sectioned. With medial displacement of the navicular the lateral talonavicular ligament becomes adherent to the anterolateral part of the anterior end of the talus. It is important to release the lateral talonavicular joint capsule for lateral translation of the calcaneocuboid joint.

Next, the calcaneonavicular limb of the bifurcate ligament is sectioned; it attaches the calcaneus to the lateral side of the navicular, and if shortened, will check lateral mobility of the navicular. If on manipulation the cuboid does not translate horizontally, the calcaneocuboid limb of the bifurcate ligament and medial plantar capsule of the calcaneocuboid joint are also sectioned.

Inadvertent division of the peroneus longus tendon should be avoided. Identify the anterior tibial tendon insertion to the base of the first metatarsal; using it as a guide, locate the peroneus longus tendon, which is immediately plantar and lateral to the insertion of the anterior tibial tendon. Divide the sheath of the peroneus longus tendon and retract it out of the way with a long narrow right-angle retractor (an instrument referred to by pediatric surgeons as an infantile rectal retractor).

This author finds it much simpler to release the calcaneocuboid joint through the lateral incision. Should the lateral-dorsal capsule of the calcaneocuboid joint be opened? Yes! It is true that the lateral column of the foot is longer than the medial column of the foot in talipes equinovarus and the lateral capsule of the calcaneocuboid joint is overlengthened; however, it is not loose, and the lateral and dorsal parts of the calcaneocuboid joint become adherent to the anterolateral part of the anterior part of the talus, similar to the lateral talonavicular ligament.

Through the lateral incision, the inferior extensor retinaculum is divided. With scalpel and periosteal elevator the tendinous origin of the extensor digitorum brevis is elevated from the anterolateral part of the calcaneus. The calcaneocuboid joint is exposed. By subperiosteal dissection the peroneus longus tendon is retracted plantarward. The dorsal, lateral, and plantar parts of the capsule of the calcaneocuboid joint are divided. Next, a Freer elevator is inserted into the calcaneocuboid joint lateral to the medial aspect, and all ligamentous tissue on the medial aspect of the calcaneocuboid joint is sectioned. On manipulation the cuboid should translate laterally on the anterior end of the calcaneus.

Plate 95. Open Reduction of Talocalcaneonavicular and Calcaneocuboid Joints by Complete Subtalar Release in Talipes Equinovarus by Posteromedial and Lateral Surgical Approach

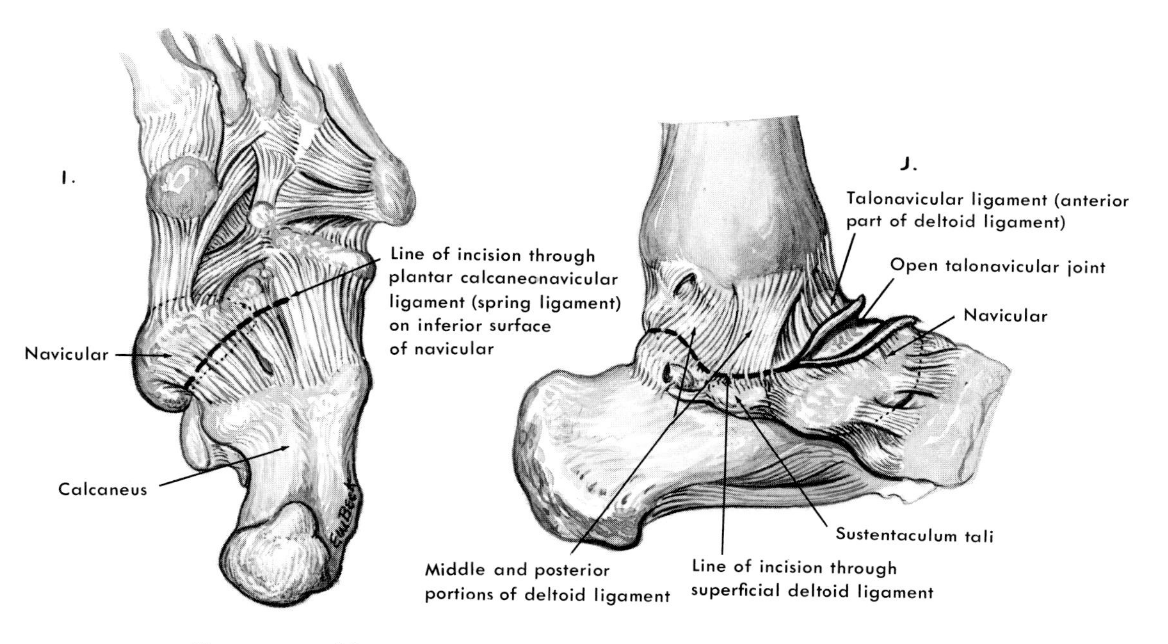

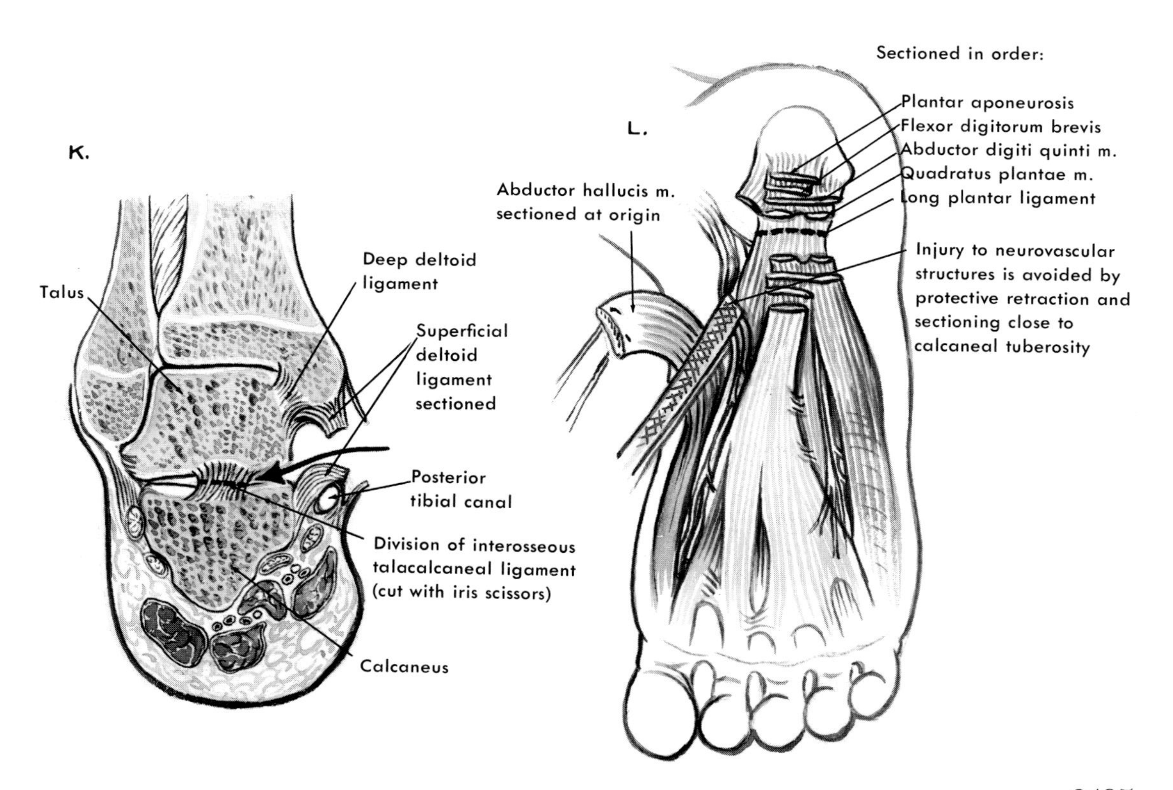

Open Reduction of Talocalcaneonavicular and Calcaneocuboid Joints by Complete Subtalar Release in Talipes Equinovarus by Posteromedial and Lateral Surgical Approach (Continued)

Step IV (Continued)

J. Use the flexor hallucis longus tendon as the guide to the sustentaculum tali. Identify the tibiocalcaneal, or middle, fibers of the superficial deltoid ligament and section them near the calcaneus; they descend almost perpendicularly to the whole length of the sustentaculum tali of the calcaneus. Medially, the subtalar joint runs a sinusoidal course; one should take care not to damage articular cartilage. The posterior fibers of the superficial deltoid ligament (posterior tibiotalar), which passes backward and laterally to the medial side of the talus and its medial tubercle, are divided.

K. The deep portion of the deltoid that inserts to the nonarticular portion of the body of the talus must be left intact, because if it is divided, the body of the talus will tilt laterally and cause valgus deviation of the ankle. If necessary, in the older child or in the infant with very severe rigid deformity, the hindfoot is everted and the interosseous talocalcaneal ligament (located above the sustentaculum tali) is sectioned under direct vision. Release of the talocalcaneal interosseous ligament is a controversial issue. Its indication is failure of correction of subtalar calcaneal rotation. Therefore, it should *not* be performed at this phase of surgery. It should be left toward the end of surgery. If, after complete subtalar release, full correction can be achieved, as documented by intraoperative radiography, the interosseous ligament is retained.

When the interosseous ligament is sectioned, the problem is overcorrection and valgus deformity of the talonavicular and subtalar joints. Therefore, it is important to position the tarsal bones in concentric reduction and internally fix the talocalcaneal joint with one, preferably two, threaded Kirschner wires.

Step V—Plantar Release

L. By blunt dissection develop the space around the medial calcaneal nerve and the lateral plantar vessels and nerve. Insert a blunt instrument or Freer nerve dissector in the axilla and enlarge the aperture. Next insert a long, narrow, right-angle retractor (infantile rectal retractor) in the aperture and dorsally retract the neurovascular bundle with the tendons of flexor digitorum longus and flexor hallucis longus. Place the blades of a Metzenbaum or Mayo scissors over it and release the plantar fascia and plantar soft tissues as they attach to the os calcis. The plantar blade of the scissors is superficial to the plantar fasciae and the dorsal blade next to bone, with the retractor separating it from the neurovascular bundle. Double-check the position of the blades and feel the opposite side on the lateral side of the heel with your fingers. Section from their origin at the tuberosity of the calcaneus: (1) the plantar fascia, (2) flexor digitorum brevis, (3) quadratus plantae, (4) long plantar ligament, (5) abductor digiti quinti, and (6) the remnants of the deep head of abductor hallucis. By staying close to bone, injury to the neurovascular structures is avoided.

Plate 95. Open Reduction of Talocalcaneonavicular and Calcaneocuboid Joints by Complete Subtalar Release in Talipes Equinovarus by Posteromedial and Lateral Surgical Approach (Parts I, J, K, and L repeated)

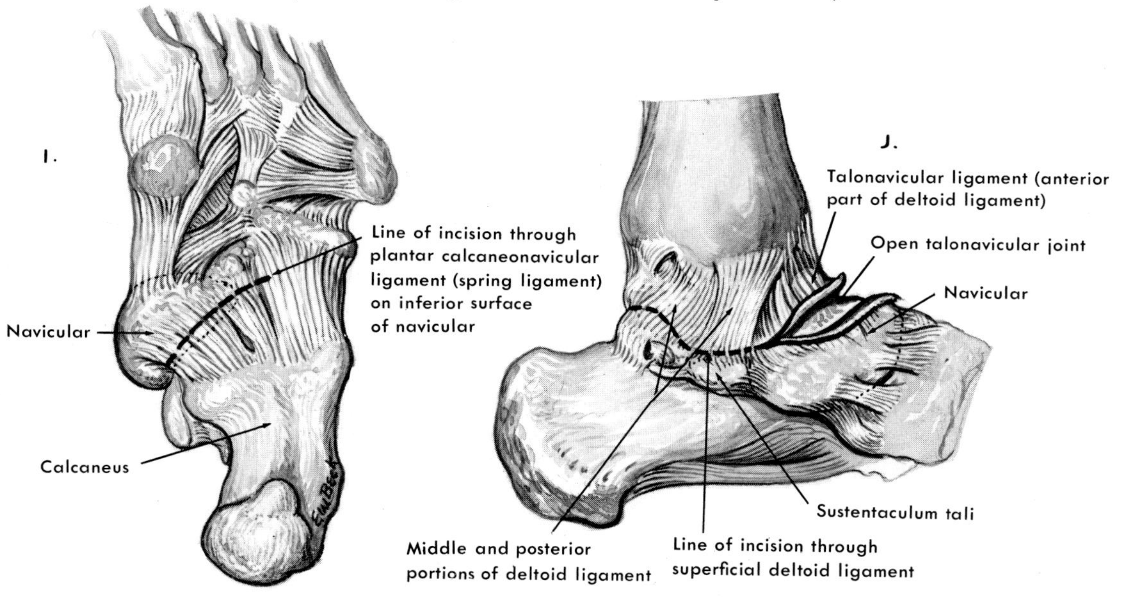

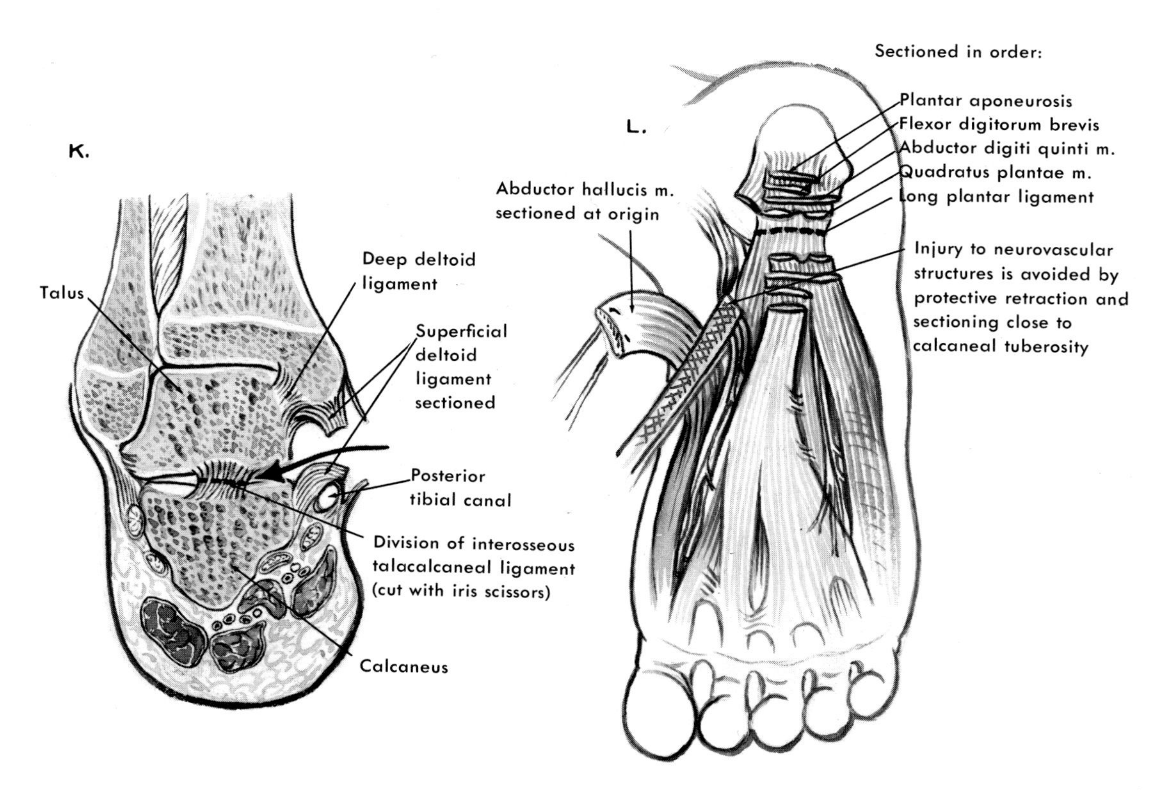

Open Reduction of Talocalcaneonavicular and Calcaneocuboid Joints by Complete Subtalar Release in Talipes Equinovarus by Posteromedial and Lateral Surgical Approach (Continued)

Step VI—Posterior Capsulotomy of the Subtalar and Ankle Joints

M. First incise the superior peroneal retinaculum—this is a ligamentous tissue that runs in the same direction as the calcaneofibular ligament. Identify but do not open the peroneal sheaths at this level. This detail of technique will prevent anterior displacement of the peroneal tendons over the lateral malleolus. Locate the flexor hallucis longus tendon; it lies on the medial side of the subtalar joint and serves as a guide to locating the subtalar joint.

The posterior part of the capsule of the tibiotalar and talocalcaneal joints is exposed by retracting the flexor hallucis longus tendon medially and the peroneal tendons laterally. A Chandler elevator or Davis retractor is used to retract the peroneal tendons and protect them from inadvertent injury. The neurovascular structures behind the medial malleolus are retracted forward. Next, with Mayo or Metzenbaum scissors, completely divide the posterior capsule of the ankle joint by a horizontal incision, and the subtalar joint capsule by a sinusoidal cut. A knife should not be used, as it may damage the articular cartilage. Caution must be exercised so as not to injure the distal tibial physis. If in doubt, radiographic control should be utilized. Posterior capsulotomy of the ankle joint is carried out; it starts laterally at the peroneal tendon sheath and extends medially to the edge of the posterior tibial tendon sheath. There is some controversy as to how far medially the posterior capsulotomy of the ankle should extend. Carroll extends it to the flexor digitorum communis sheath, Catterall to the flexor hallucis longus sheath, and Simons to the posterior tibial tendon sheath; Godner and Gould carry it anteromedially, releasing the deep deltoid ligament, which is reconstructed later.[106, 112, 244, 248–250, 650–652]

This author strongly recommends that the deep deltoid (tibiotalar) ligament not be divided, as the ankle joint will become unstable and valgus ankle deformity may develop. The tibiotalar ligament divided inadvertently or by plan (as in the Goldner technique) should be repaired.

Step VII—Posterolateral Release

N. Dissection of the posterolateral aspect of the foot is carried out, and the following contracted soft-tissue structures between the fibula, os calcis, and talus are released: (1) calcaneofibular ligament, (2) posterolateral talocalcaneal ligament, (3) posterior talofibular ligament, and (4) thickened superior peroneal retinaculum and thick peroneal sheath. These tethers hold the calcaneus close to the lateral malleolus and checkrein rotation of the calcaneus, and they also prevent rotation and posterior movement of the talus in the ankle mortise. The fibula should be free to rotate for the talus to move.

First, divide the sheath of peroneus longus and brevis tendons laterally at the level of the lateral subtalar joint. (As stated, if the peroneal tendon sheaths are divided proximally at the level of the ankle joint, the peroneal tendon may subluxate anteriorly.) Meticulous care is exercised not to section the peroneal tendon inadvertently. Next, the peroneal tendons are mobilized and retracted posteriorly and anteriorly, and the *peroneal tendon sheaths* are completely excised circumferentially. Second, the peroneal tendons and sural nerve are retracted anteriorly, and the thickened short calcaneofibular ligament is exposed. Insert a Freer elevator or a hemostat beneath the calcaneofibular ligament in a posteroanterior direction and divide the ligament close to the calcaneus. McKay cuts the calcaneofibular ligament in an oblique fashion in order to provide a larger surface area and facilitate proper healing and reattachment of the ligament to the calcaneus.[447, 448] Third, retract the peroneal tendon laterally and excise the previously incised thickened fibrous band of *superior peroneal retinaculum.* Fourth, section the posterolateral part of the talocalcaneal capsule. Fifth, identify and vertically section the posterior talofibular ligament, which holds the talus in plantar flexion. McKay prefers to preserve the posterior talofibular ligament; this author finds that in the rigid clubfoot it is difficult to position the talus in the ankle mortise when the posterior talofibular ligament is intact.

Plate 95. Open Reduction of Talocalcaneonavicular and Calcaneocuboid Joints by Complete Subtalar Release in Talipes Equinovarus by Posteromedial and Lateral Surgical Approach

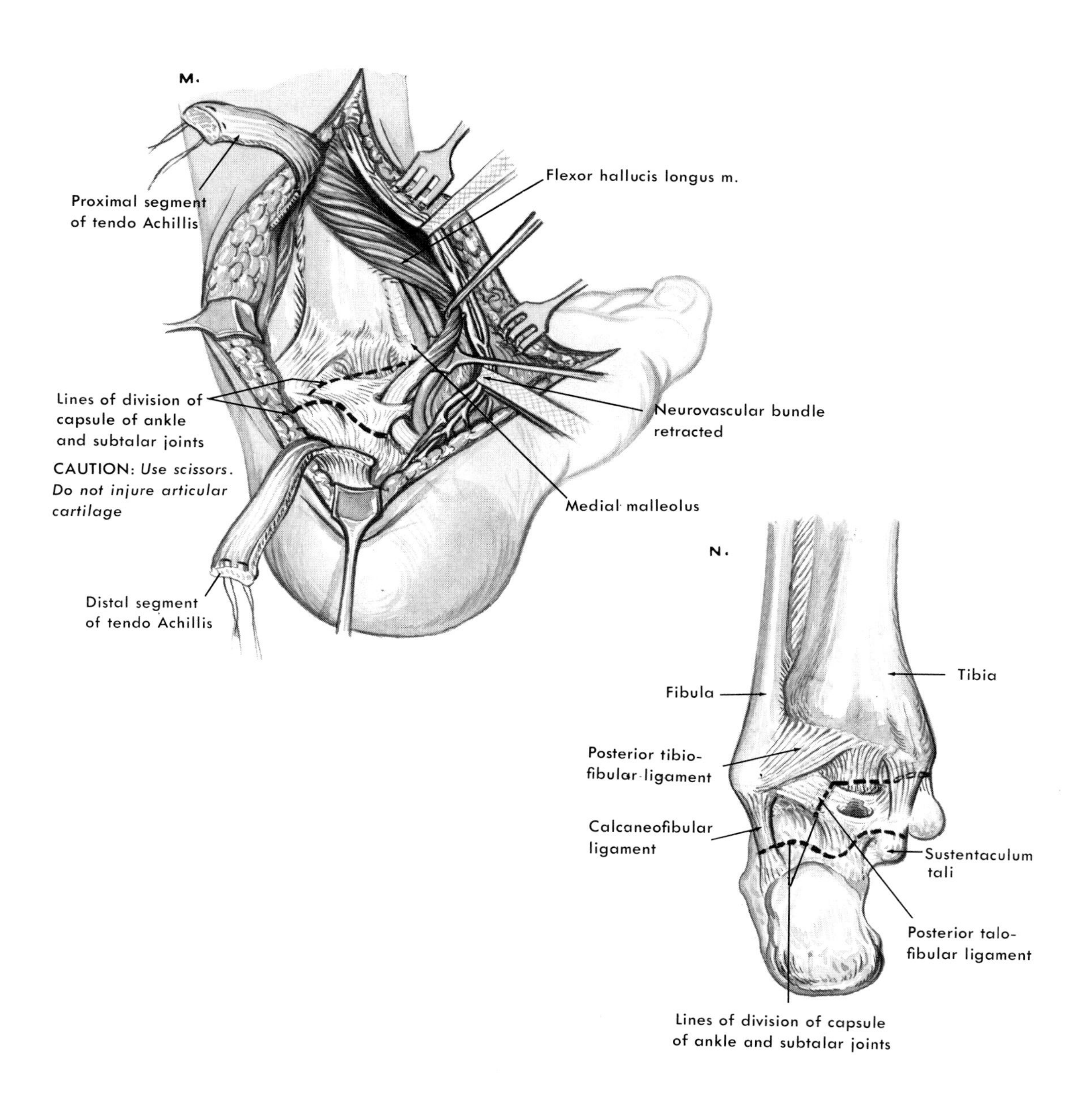

Open Reduction of Talocalcaneonavicular and Calcaneocuboid Joints by Complete Subtalar Release in Talipes Equinovarus by Posteromedial and Lateral Surgical Approach (Continued)

Step VIII—Lateral Subtalar Release

O. With the peroneal tendons retracted posteriorly, the lateral talocalcaneal ligament and joint capsule are completely sectioned. In the Cincinnati approach the capsule and ligaments are divided with scissors from within the joint outward to the level of the lateral part of the talonavicular and calcaneocuboid joints.

Next, by blunt dissection through the lateral part of the wound, the lateral part of the talonavicular joint is exposed and the capsule is divided from its inferior lateral aspect to the dorsum of the foot. Again, meticulous care is exercised in order not to injure blood vessels on the dorsum of the talus. The release of dorsal, medial, lateral, and plantar capsules of the calcaneocuboid joint has already been described in **N.** Next, determine whether the anterior portion of the calcaneus rotates laterally. If subtalar calcaneal rotation cannot be corrected, division of the interosseous ligament is performed.

Plate 95. Open Reduction of Talocalcaneonavicular and Calcaneocuboid Joints by Complete Subtalar Release in Talipes Equinovarus by Posteromedial and Lateral Surgical Approach

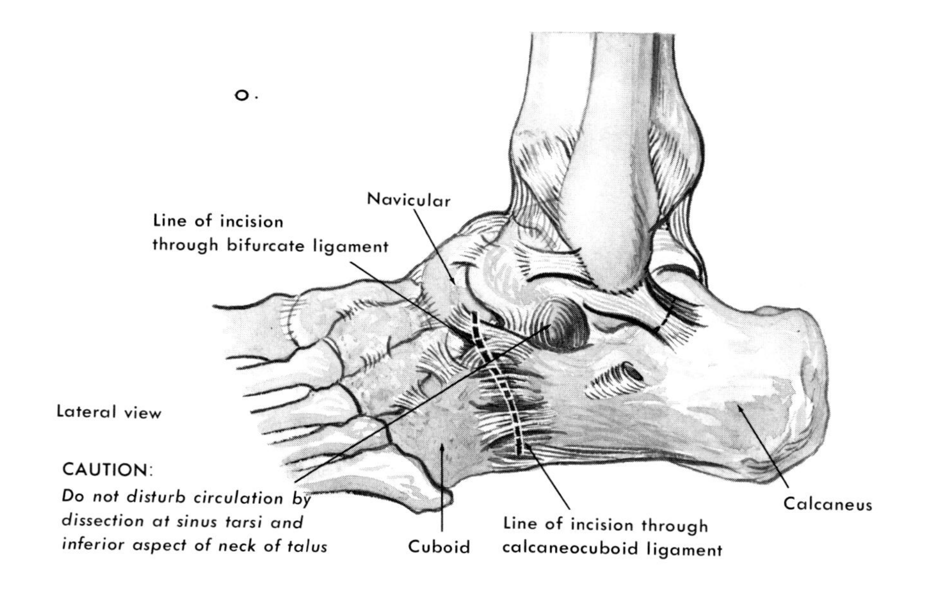

Open Reduction of Talocalcaneonavicular and Calcaneocuboid Joints by Complete Subtalar Release in Talipes Equinovarus by Posteromedial and Lateral Surgical Approach (Continued)

Step IX—Shortening of the Lateral Column of the Foot

P. In the older child, or in very rigid talipes equinovarus, the lateral column of the foot is elongated, acting as an obstacle to reduction of the talocalcaneonavicular joint; the lateral column should therefore be shortened. In the child eight years of age or younger, the anterior end of the calcaneus is resected (see Lichtblau procedure). An alternative method is resection of a vertical wedge from the anterolateral part of the calcaneus—this technique, described by Simons, is preferred by this author in the young child, as it preserves the calcaneocuboid joint.[650, 651] The osteotomy line is 1 cm. posterior to the calcaneocuboid joint; the wedge (0.5 to 1.0 cm. in width) is based laterally. In the child nine years of age or older, and in paralytic clubfoot or in clubfoot associated with extensive medial scarring and recurrent deformity, the calcaneocuboid joint is resected and fused (see Evans operation).[189]

Step X—Concentric Reduction of the Talocalcaneonavicular and Calcaneocuboid Joint by Repositioning of the Bones and Internal Fixation with Threaded Pins

Q and **R.** Next, the foot and ankle are gently manipulated into increasing dorsiflexion. The dome of the talus should be repositioned in the ankle mortise, and on dorsiflexion of the ankle, the posterior surface of the body of the talus should be visualized. In severe fixed equinus deformity, one may have to section the distal tibiofibular syndesmosis. Fractional lengthening of the flexor hallucis longus and flexor digitorum longus muscles at their musculotendinous junction may be required if the toes are acutely flexed upon neutral dorsiflexion of the ankle. In very severe flexion deformity of the hallux, Z-lengthening of the flexor hallucis longus is performed on the plantar aspect of the foot; the problem with Z-lengthening at the level of the master knot of Henry is scarring of the elongated tendon with resultant deformities of clawing of the great toe and dorsal bunion. Whenever possible, it is best to lengthen at the musculotendinous junction by recession; section at two or three sites to obtain the desired length.

Next, through the medial part of the wound, the navicular is displaced laterally, and through the lateral part of the wound, the head of the talus is displaced medially.

Reduction is facilitated by insertion of a threaded Kirschner wire (0.062 or 0.045 cm. in diameter in infants) in the longitudinal axis of the talus from the posterior aspect of its body. The point of entry of the Kirschner wire is immediately lateral to the posterior ridge of the talus; the wire is directed to emerge at the center of the anterior end of the talus. It is vital to use a threaded wire. Smooth pins may migrate, causing loss of alignment and making pin removal very difficult.

The leverage of the pin is used to rotate the anterior end of the talus medially, and that of the calcaneus laterally, obtaining normal talocalcaneal divergence in the anteroposterior plane. Then distal traction is applied on the forefoot, the navicular pushed laterally, and the anterior end of the calcaneus rotated laterally, achieving concentric reduction of the talocalcaneonavicular joint.

Plate 95. Open Reduction of Talocalcaneonavicular and Calcaneocuboid Joints by Complete Subtalar Release in Talipes Equinovarus by Posteromedial and Lateral Surgical Approach

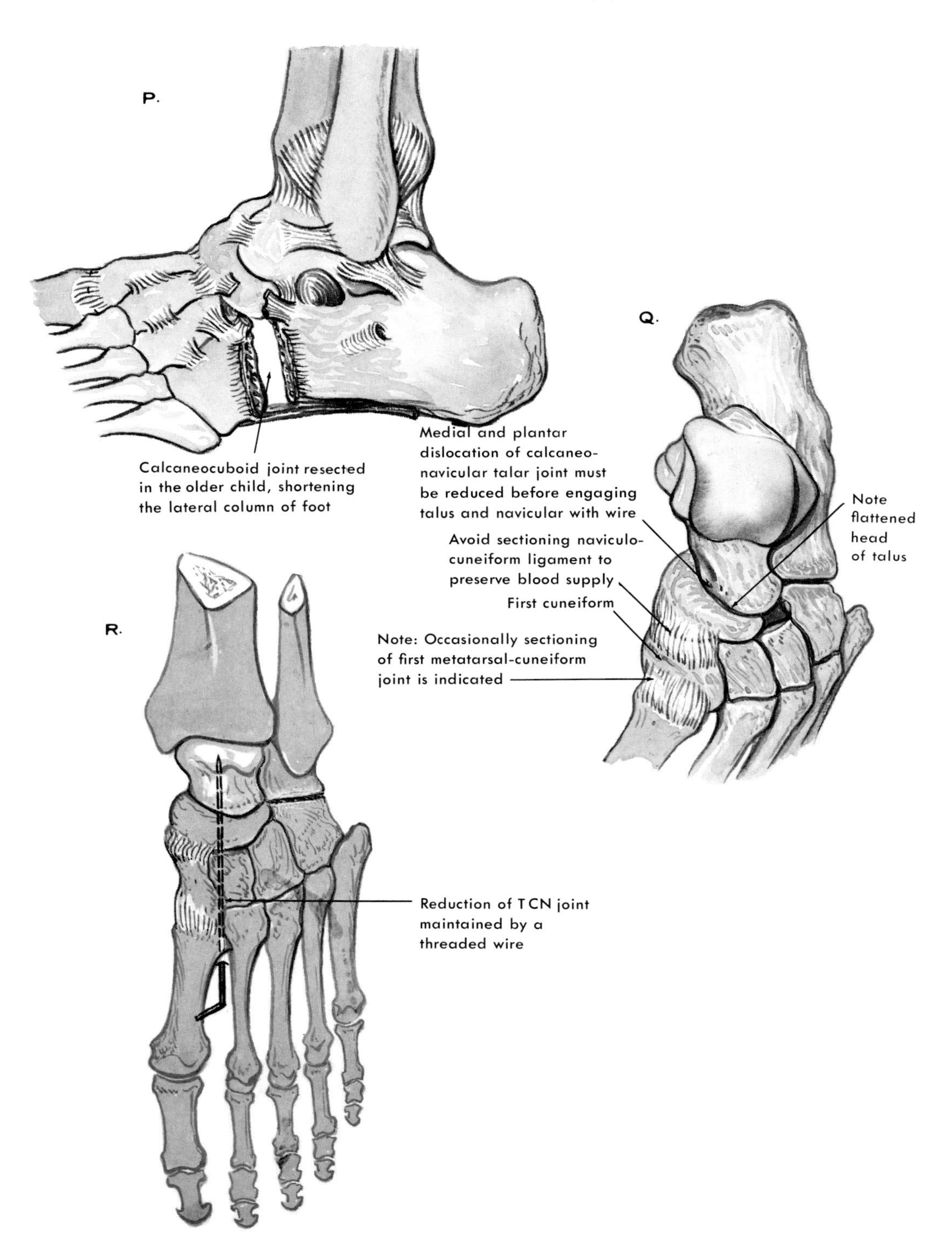

Open Reduction of Talocalcaneonavicular and Calcaneocuboid Joints by Complete Subtalar Release in Talipes Equinovarus by Posteromedial and Lateral Surgical Approach (Continued)

Step X (Continued)

Prior to inserting the pin into the navicular, carefully inspect the relationship of the navicular to the anterior end "head" of the talus. The use of two small Chandler elevator retractors—one dorsal and the other plantar to the talonavicular articulation—will assist proper visualization and palpation of the repositioned bony structures. The medial side of the navicular normally protrudes slightly medially beyond the edge of the talar head and should not be plantar flexed with respect to the navicular; nor should the navicular be displaced superiorly in relationship to the talar head. The lateral side of the talonavicular joint also should be palpated carefully to ensure that there is no lateral step-off at the level of the joint. The relationship of the repositioned bone is determined visually by manual palpation and with an instrument. Overcorrection, a common error after extensive soft-tissue release, should be avoided. The threaded pin is then drilled distally across the talonavicular joint.

Inspection of the position of the foot is necessary before the pin is drilled through the dorsum of the forefoot. The long axis of the foot should be in approximately 10 degrees of lateral rotation with respect to the previously marked tibial tubercle. The foot must not be supinated, and it must not be translated or tilted laterally into a valgus position. If the position is not satisfactory, the talonavicular pin is withdrawn from the navicular, the navicular is repositioned, and the talonavicular pin is reinserted. It is vital that the position of the talonavicular joint and the foot is correct and precise in relation to the leg-knee. The importance of concentric reduction and alignment cannot be overemphasized.

Avoid multiple drilling of the talus and navicular. Fracture of these bones will create a very difficult problem of fixation.

Plate 95. Open Reduction of Talocalcaneonavicular and Calcaneocuboid Joints by Complete Subtalar Release in Talipes Equinovarus by Posteromedial and Lateral Surgical Approach (Parts P, Q, and R repeated)

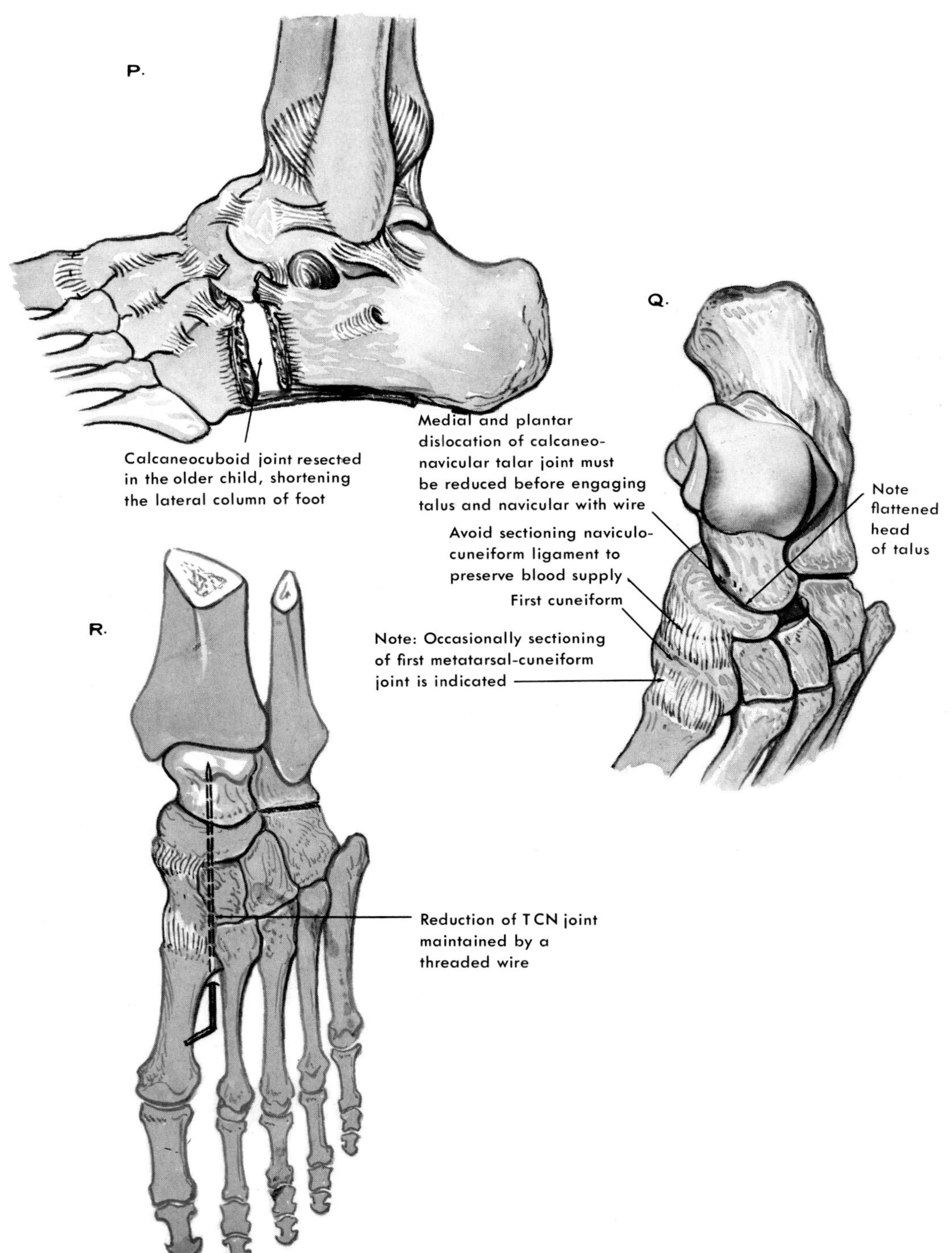

Open Reduction of Talocalcaneonavicular and Calcaneocuboid Joints by Complete Subtalar Release in Talipes Equinovarus by Posteromedial and Lateral Surgical Approach (Continued)

Step XI—Internal Fixation of Talocalcaneal Joint and Repair of Tendons

S and **T.** If the interosseous ligament is sectioned, it is best to fix the calcaneus to the talus with one or two threaded Steinmann pins to maintain corrected horizontal rotation. The pins are inserted from the plantar surface of the calcaneus and up through the talus, but not protruding through the ankle joint. When the talocalcaneal pins are inserted, the subtalar joint should be closed. Anteroposterior and lateral radiograms of the foot and ankle are made in the corrected position to verify concentricity of reduction of the talocalcaneonavicular joint. The value of intraoperative radiograms cannot be overemphasized. If reduction is concentric, the talonavicular pin is drilled out through the dorsum of the forefoot. The drill is changed to the anterior end of the pin, and the pin is withdrawn so that its posterior end is flush with the back of the talus. The protruding anterior end of the pin is cut off subcutaneously or protruding through the skin 1 cm. The talocalcaneal pins are cut protruding 1 cm. out of the sole of the heel.

When vertical closing-wedge osteotomy of the anterolateral part of the calcaneus is performed, the calcaneal osteotomy and calcaneocuboid parts are fixed with a threaded Kirschner wire.

In the severely deformed foot with fixed forefoot varus, capsulotomy of the first metatarsal cuneiform joint and osteotomy of the base of the second metatarsal may be indicated. The wounds are irrigated, a compression bandage is applied, and the tourniquet is released. After a few minutes, the compression bandage is removed and complete hemostasis is obtained.

The distal segment of the posterior tibial tendon is introduced through its canal behind the medial malleolus, delivered into the back of the ankle, and resutured to its proximal segment.

The tendo Achillis is resutured with proper tension with the ankle at only 5 degrees of dorsiflexion. Avoid overlengthening of the triceps surae muscle. The skin margins are observed for adequacy of circulation; they may be blanched from tension when the ankle is maximally dorsiflexed. The foot is plantar flexed 10 degrees farther from the position of the foot at which capillary refill of the skin margin is complete. The subcutaneous tissue is closed with absorbable sutures and the skin with subcuticular or 00 nylon sutures.

A bulky sterile dressing and sheet wadding are applied and reinforced with an above-knee, well-padded plaster of Paris cast. The ankle joint is immobilized in plantar flexion as described above to relax the tension of the skin edges; the knee is in 45 degrees of flexion. If there is any question about circulation to the skin, the cast is omitted and only a Jones compression dressing with a posterior splint is applied.

POSTOPERATIVE CARE

Ten to 14 days after surgery, the patient is taken back to the operating room on an outpatient basis, and under general anesthesia, the dressing is removed and wound healing is assessed. *The sutures and pins are not removed.* The foot is repeatedly manipulated into maximal plantar flexion and neutral dorsiflexion. This manipulation of the foot into plantar flexion is performed in order to prevent contracture of the anterior capsule of the ankle joint. Another above-knee cast is applied with the ankle in neutral or 5 degrees of dorsiflexion. The second cast is removed in two weeks, at which time the pins and sutures are also removed. Again, the ankle joint is manipulated into plantar flexion and dorsiflexion; and another above-knee cast (the third) is applied for an additional period of two weeks. The total period of cast immobilization is about six weeks.

Plate 95. Open Reduction of Talocalcaneonavicular and Calcaneocuboid Joints by Complete Subtalar Release in Talipes Equinovarus by Posteromedial and Lateral Surgical Approach

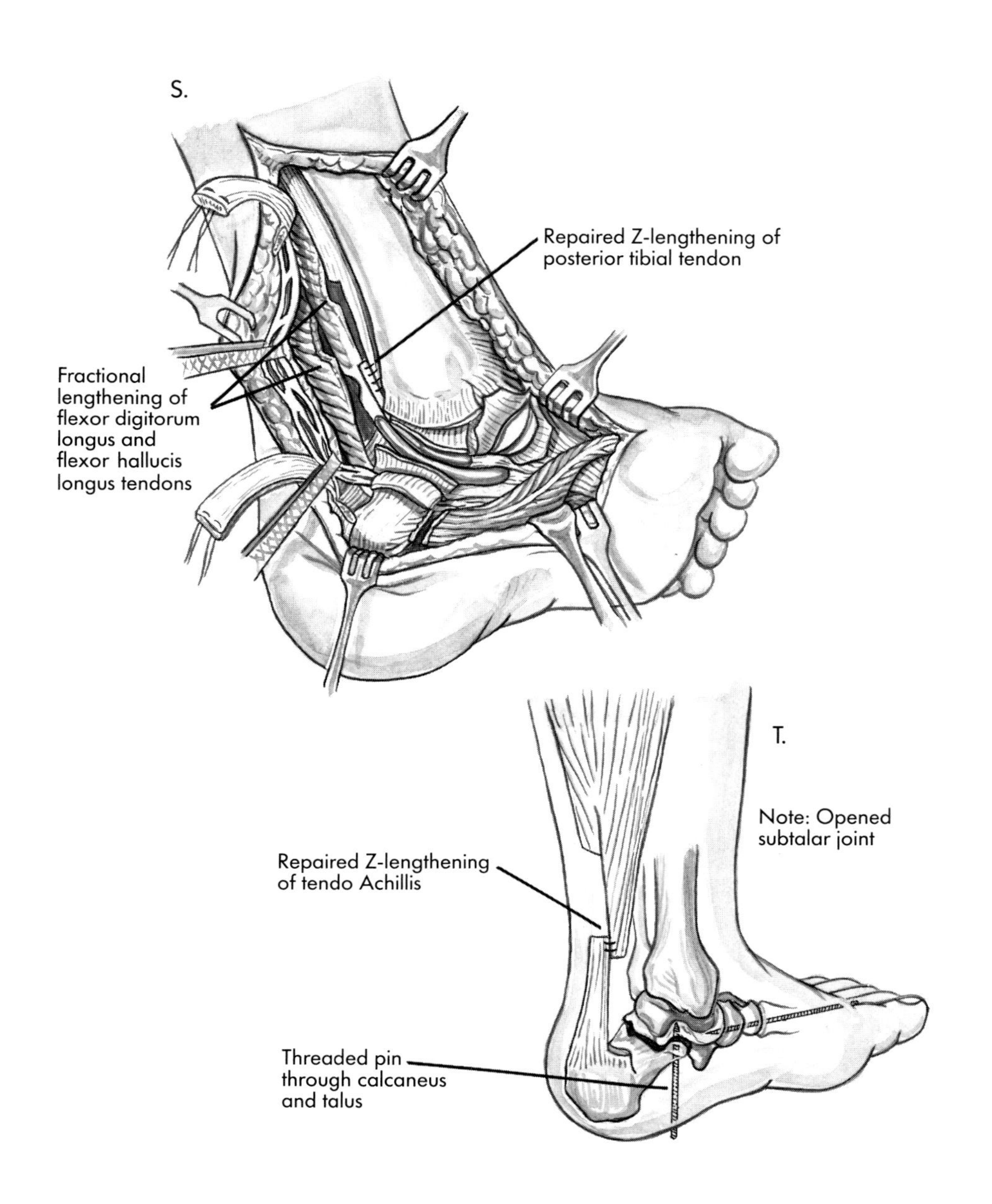

Open Reduction of Talocalcaneonavicular and Calcaneocuboid Joints by Complete Subtalar Release in Talipes Equinovarus by Posteromedial and Lateral Surgical Approach (Continued)

After removal of the cast, the foot and ankle are held at night in a slightly overcorrected position in an above-knee posterior splint made of polypropylene or some other plastic. The purpose of this retentive apparatus is to maintain correction; it is worn only at night and at naptime. It is used for 6 to 12 months until skeletal growth remodels and straightens the medial and plantar tilting of the head and neck of the talus and normal articular relationships are restored. The decreased angle of declination of the talus may be compared with excessive femoral antetorsion in congenital dislocation of the hip; the same principles should be applied.

The Denis Browne splint (with a 10- to 23-cm. everting cross bar between the feet) is not recommended, as it is ineffective in controlling the ankle and hindfoot, and may cause genu valgum and exaggerated lateral tibiofibular torsion.

Passive stretching exercises are performed by the parents on the child's foot and leg two to three times a day, each session consisting of 25 to 40 manipulations of the ankle into dorsiflexion and plantar flexion, heel eversion, forefoot abduction, and stretching of plantar contracted soft tissues. Active exercises are performed by the older child to develop motor function in triceps surae, posterior tibial, and peroneal muscles. In the infant and young child, muscle stimulation techniques are utilized to develop motor power. Children with clubfoot should be followed until the foot is skeletally mature.

Plate 95. Open Reduction of Talocalcaneonavicular and Calcaneocuboid Joints by Complete Subtalar Release in Talipes Equinovarus by Posteromedial and Lateral Surgical Approach (Parts S and T repeated)

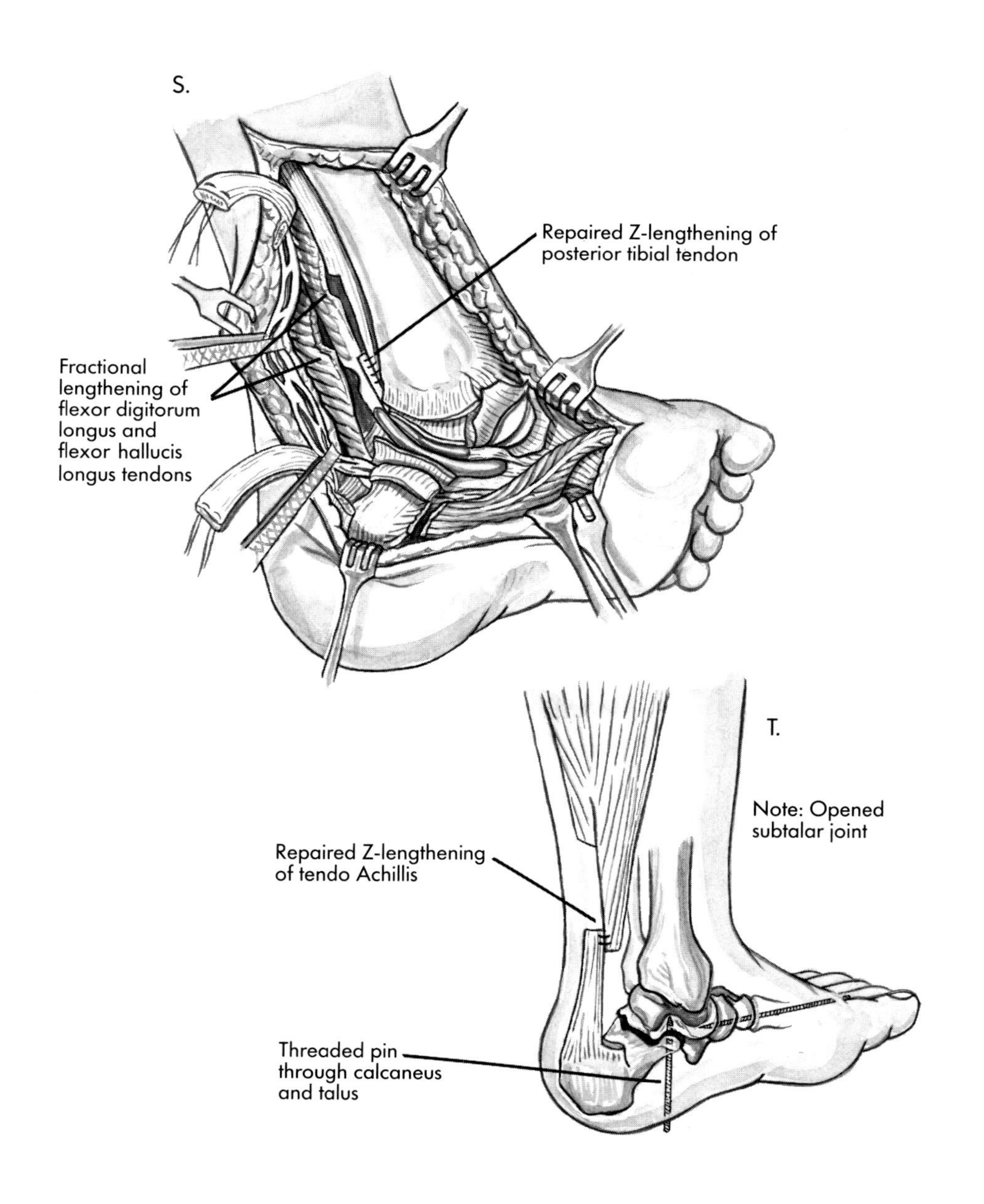

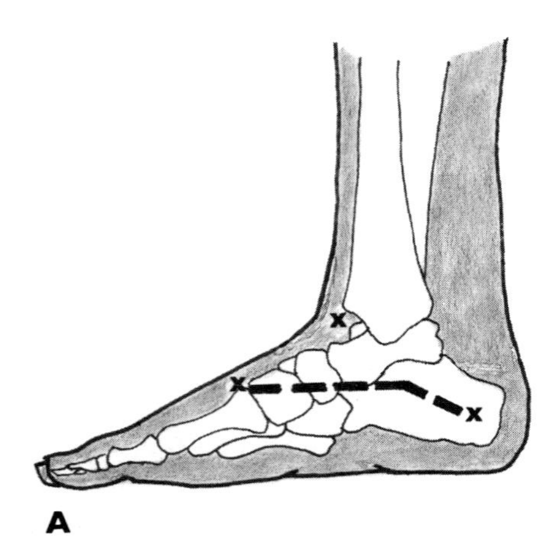

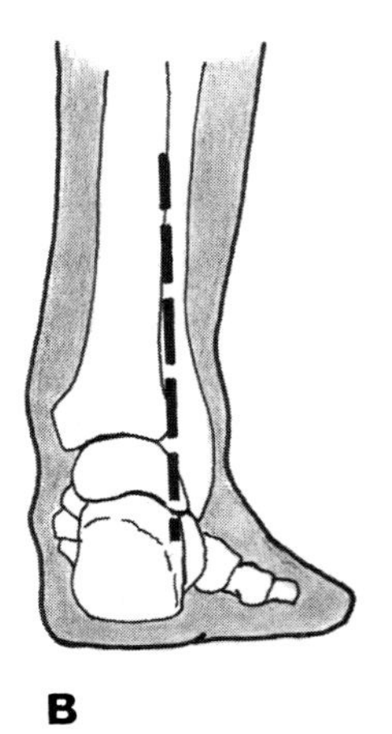

FIGURE 7–61. Skin incisions in the Carroll technique.

A. A lazy Z medial incision. **B.** A vertical posterolateral incision (see text for details).

Split Anterior Tibial Tendon Transfer. This is recommended to correct supination deformity of the forefoot (see section on complications).

Posterior Tibial Tendon Transfer. The posterior tibial tendon is a strong tethering force in talipes equinovarus.[82, 213] A number of ways of treating it have been recorded in the literature: (1) section and discard; (2) Z-lengthening at the insertion; (3) Z-lengthening above the medial malleolus; (4) anterior transfer through the interosseous route simultaneously with open reduction of the talocalcaneonavicular joint, preserving its motor tendon, and transferring it anteriorly through the interosseous route at a later date if necessary; and (5) sectioning and transferring to the lengthened Achilles tendon.

Fried dissected the insertions of the posterior tibial tendon in 54 clubfeet with recurrent deformity and in two clubfeet that had had no previous treatment. The insertions were abnormal in all the cases. Beginning at the level of the medial malleolus, the tendon changed to a thick, hard, fibrous mass that encompassed the entire medial side of the tarsus and inserted with thick strands of fibrous tissue to other parts of the foot, namely, the plantar fascia, deep plantar ligaments, anterior tibial tendon, os calcis, navicular, cuneiforms, and cuboid bone. Fried believed the deforming force of the posterior tibial muscle to be the principal cause of recurrence of clubfoot.[213]

The posterior tibial muscle will function as an active dorsiflexor of the ankle when transferred to the dorsum of the foot through the interosseous membrane. This has been demonstrated by numerous authors in various paralytic conditions such as poliomyelitis, leprosy, Charcot-Marie-Tooth disease, Friedreich's ataxia, and spastic paralysis.[258, 333, 494] Fried recommended transferring the posterior tibial muscle to the dorsum of the foot in talipes equinovarus via the interosseous route and suturing it to the third cuneiform bone. Lengthening of the Achilles tendon and capsulotomy of the posterior parts of the ankle and subtalar joints were performed at the same time to achieve correction of equinus deformity. Capsulotomy of the talonavicular, navicular–first cuneiform, and first cuneiform–first metatarsal joints was also carried out. He reported the results to be good in 12 of the 13 patients who were followed for at least four years. In seven patients, the results were excellent, with full correction of the deformity and satisfactory function. In five patients, minor residual deformity persisted, and walking on tiptoes was still not feasible. In one patient, the result was unsatisfactory because of overcorrection resulting from a too lateral transfer of the tendon to the cuboid rather than only as far as the third cuneiform.[213]

Singer, in 1961, reported that anterior transfer of the posterior tibial tendon in 28 congenital clubfeet stabilized the correction obtained by serial wedging casts. The age range of the patients at surgery was two and one half to eight and one half years. The follow-up period was one to three years. There was no relapse in 27 of the 28 feet. In two thirds of the cases, the tendon was too short and was attached to either the peroneus tertius tendon, if present, or to the lateral two tendons of the extensor digitorum longus. In only one third of the cases was the tendon anchored to the bone, either the lateral or the middle cuneiform. Singer did not recommend the operation when soft-tissue release had been previously performed, because in five such feet, when the posterior tibial tendons were exposed, they proved to be thin, atrophic, adherent to surrounding tissues, and unsatisfactory for transfer.[654]

Gartland suggested that muscle imbalance was the primary cause of relapse in clubfoot, and he recommended anterior transfer of the posterior tibial tendon through the interosseous membrane. He published a preliminary report in 1964. The results in 20 feet in 16 patients were given, and the average follow-up was two years.[232] In 1972, Gartland and Surgent reported the results in 26 feet in 22 children with an average follow-up period of seven years. The results were excellent in 14 feet (54 per cent), satisfactory in 8 feet (31 per cent), and unsatisfactory in 4 feet (15 per cent). The result was graded excellent when the foot was plantigrade and normally aligned, with the transferred posterior tibial muscle functioning as a balancing motor unit and the patient wearing normal shoes. A satisfactory result was a foot with minor residual deformities of heel varus deviation or forefoot adduction that was nevertheless balanced and plantigrade, with a functioning posterior tibial transfer and the ability to wear normal shoes. Unsatisfactory feet were those that could not be evaluated as excellent or satisfactory. Analyses of the failures showed the cause to be inadequate surgical technique rather than any basic fault or breakdown of the procedure. In two feet, severe valgus deformity developed; in both, the tendon had been incorrectly transferred to the cuboid instead of the third cuneiform. In two feet, the posterior tibial muscle failed to function because the tendon adhered in a small opening in the interosseous membrane. Gartland and Surgent emphasized the importance of making an aperture in the interosseous membrane large enough to prevent adherence of the tendon at that site. Upon correlating the result with the age at operation, they found that all seven children operated on at three years of age or younger were in the excellent or satisfactory grade (100 per cent). Of the 19 feet of 15 children who were older than three years of age at surgery, however, the result was excellent or satisfactory in 80 per cent, and unsatisfactory in 20 per cent. Gartland and Surgent believed that, when indicated, the procedure should be performed by the age of two or three years in order to forestall adaptive secondary bony changes.[233]

Turner and Cooper reviewed the experience of posterior tibial transfer at the University Hospitals in Iowa City. The operation was performed in seven cases of very difficult recurrent clubfoot; in five the transfer functioned, in four with good result, and in one with poor result; in two the transfer did not function. In the four feet rated good, the correction of equinovarus deformity was maintained and there was active dorsiflexion of the ankle to neutral or slightly beyond. *In none of the cases, however, did the transferred tendon function as a dorsiflexor during gait.* One patient developed calcaneovalgus deformity. They concluded that in difficult recurrent clubfoot, posterior tibial transfer may be beneficial, provided that: (1) its motor strength is good or better before transfer; (2) deformity is fully corrected by soft-tissue release or bony stabilization; and (3) the tendon is transferred to the midline of the foot, to either the second or third cuneiform.[714]

Del Sel and associates divided the posterior tibial tendon at its insertion to the navicular (which facilitates exposure of the talonavicular and subtalar joints) and dissected it free up to its muscle fibers; then they transferred it posteriorly and sutured it to both segments of the lengthened Achilles tendon. The transfer removes the deforming force of the posterior tibial muscle and reinforces the strength of the triceps surae, which may be weakened because of overlengthening in severe neglected cases of talipes equinovarus.[155]

This author strongly objects to the routine primary anterior transfer of the posterior tibial tendon through the interosseous route to the dorsolateral aspect of the foot. In a two- or three-year-old child, it is very difficult, if not impossible, to train an out-of-phase tendon transfer (e.g., to teach an invertor and plantarflexor to function as an evertor and dorsiflexor). As stated previously, in talipes equinovarus, apart from directional changes, there are no primary abnormalities of the muscles and tendons. The posterior tibial muscle is contracted; this strong deforming force can be weakened by Z-lengthening of its tendon above the medial malleolus. Its action should be preserved, however, to prevent pes planovalgus. Therefore, do not section and discard the posterior tibial tendon.

Anterior transfer of the posterior tibial tendon has an extremely limited place in the treatment of talipes equinovarus. Its sole indication is unquestionable muscle imbalance in which the evertors and dorsiflexors of the ankle and foot are weak and the strong invertors and plantarflexors are pulling the foot into equinovarus position. It is indicated then only when the following prerequisites are met: (1) the deformity of talipes equinovarus and articular malalignment can be corrected with the ankle and foot fully flexible with normal range of passive motion (this basic rule of tendon transfer should not be violated); (2) motor strength of the posterior tibial muscle is good or normal; (3) continuity and length of the tendon are adequate to allow technical feasibility of the transfer; and (4) the age of the child is at least three or four years, i.e., he should be old enough to cooperate in the postoperative re-education program. The tendon should be transferred to the midline of the foot, either to the base of the second metatarsal or to the second or third cuneiform bone, never to the cuboid. The technique of transfer is illustrated in Appendix Plate B. In paralytic equinovarus deformity of the foot, the anterior transfer of the posterior tibial tendon is of definite value in restoring muscle balance.

Other tendon transfers effective in increasing eversion-abduction motor strength of the foot are the extensor hallucis longus to the fifth metatarsal head, and the flexor hallucis longus to the peroneals. This author has had no personal experience with these tendon transfers.

Achilles Tendon Transfers

The Switch Operation on the Tendo Achillis. Stewart proposed that inversion of the heel in talipes equinovarus is caused by malinsertion of the tendo Achillis, which is attached on the calcaneus more medially and farther forward than normal. This acts as a positive deforming force, inverting the heel and twisting the os calcis during its growth period. He recommended sectioning the medial and anterior attachments of the tendo Achillis to the calcaneus, leaving a small lateral attachment. Then the tendon is split longitudinally, and its free tendinous part is transferred to the lateral side of the attached remnant and sutured to the os calcis. Stewart states that he has performed this procedure more than 20 times and has been surprised at the degree of eversion and dorsiflexion of the foot obtained. In only two instances was subsequent lengthening of the tendo Achillis necessary.[676]

Settle, in his dissections, found the fibers of the Achilles tendon to be inserted vertically into the calcaneus, which was rotated into a markedly varus position. When the heel was everted into neutral position, the medial fibers of the Achilles tendon were tighter than the lateral ones.[634] Irani and Sherman noted the tendo Achillis to be inserted slightly on the medial side of the calcaneus as a result of the shift of position of the posterior part of the bone. When the os calcis was placed in neutral position following sectioning of its ligamentous attachments, the apparent medial shift of the insertion of the tendo Achillis disappeared completely.[328]

The author finds that he achieves the same results as Stewart by sectioning the medial half or two thirds of the tendo Achillis insertion to the os calcis during sliding lengthening of the heel cord. Correction of equinus deformity is almost always required at the same time as that of the varus heel.

Lateral Transfer of the Achilles Tendon. Axer and Segal transferred the Achilles tendon to the lateral aspect of the calcaneus for correction of paralytic equinovarus deformity. They based the operation on the following pathomechanical consideration: the rotational movements of the subtalar joint take place along an axis that runs obliquely from the neck of the talus downward, laterally, and posteriorly to the posterolateral surface of the os calcis; the Achilles tendon inserts medially to this axis. Therefore, the triceps surae acts as a powerful invertor of the heel and becomes a major deforming force if its antagonists are paralyzed. Through fascial connections with the forefoot, the triceps surae may increase forefoot varus deviation. Axer and Segal devised the operation to maintain the function of the triceps surae as a plantar-flexor of the ankle and to eliminate its action as a supinator of the hindfoot. An L-shaped incision is made on the posterolateral aspect of the Achilles tendon and the heel. The tendon is sectioned at its insertion together with a piece of the calcaneal apophysis. On the posterolateral aspect of the os calcis (at the estimated site of emergence of the axis of the subtalar joint), a bed is prepared, and the Achilles tendon, with the attached bone, is countersunk and fixed with a screw. It is immobilized in a cast for six weeks. Axer and Segal reported the results in 37 feet. The cause of equinovarus deformity was paralytic in 34 feet, congenital in 2 feet, and spastic cerebral palsy in 1 foot. The results were good in 18 feet, fair in 8 feet, and poor in 11 feet. Complications included growth disturbance of the apophysis of the calcaneus, delayed healing, and tenderness over the screw site.[24] The author has no personal experience with the foregoing procedure and does not recommend lateral transfer of the Achilles tendon in the treatment of talipes equinovarus.

Procedures on Bone. Operative procedures on bone used in the treatment of talipes equinovarus are of three types: osteotomy, arthrodesis, and ostectomy. These procedures are often combined with soft-tissue surgery such as section or excision of the ligamentous and capsular structures, tendon lengthening, or tendon transposition. In general, bony procedures are rarely, if ever, indicated in the infant and young child, as they would disturb the normal growth and development of the foot.

Shortening of Lateral Column of Foot. Evans, in 1961, proposed that the essential deformity in talipes equinovarus was medial displacement and rotation of the navicular on the talus, with all other elements of the deformity being secondary and adaptive. He believed relapse of talipes equinovarus is caused by failure to correct this medial dislocation of the navicular on the head of the talus. The medial column of the foot—consisting of the talus, navicular, medial cuneiform, and first ray—is relatively shortened and is held in varus position by the contracted soft tissues. The lateral column of the foot—composed of the calcaneus, cuboid, and fifth ray—gradually adapts by overgrowth in length and distortion in the shape of the calcaneocuboid joint (primarily medial obliquity of its articular surfaces). These adaptive changes provide a resistant barrier to manipulative correction.[189]

The obstruction by the lateral column of the foot has been noted previously. Ogston, in 1902, advocated enucleation of the cuboid bone, of the anterior part of the calcaneus, and of the head of the talus. His operation, however, was not successful because it weakened rather than restored the medial column of the foot.[525] Johanning, in 1958, proposed enucleating the cuboid bone alone.[339] Another procedure designed to shorten the lateral column of the foot included wedge resection of the midtarsal joint between the cuboid and calcaneus.

Evans described a procedure in which, following medial and posterior release of the contracted soft tissues, a wedge resection of the calcaneocuboid joint was performed. He claimed this resection shortened the lateral column of the foot and permitted the released navicular to be placed on the head of the talus so that the axes of the first metatarsal and the talus are aligned. The varus heel was also corrected. Evans emphasized the importance of carrying out the whole procedure in one stage.[188–190]

In the Evans procedure, nrst an open reduction of the talocalcaneonavicular joint is performed through a posteromedial incision. A lateral incision 4 cm. in length is centered over the calcaneocuboid joint, running parallel to the tendon of the peroneus brevis. The subcutaneous tissue is divided and the skin flaps retracted. The peroneus brevis tendon is retracted plantarward, and the calcaneocuboid joint is fully exposed. A laterally based wedge of the calcaneocuboid joint is resected. If there is associated equinus deformity of the forefoot, the wedge is thicker dorsally; if the foot is rocker-shaped, the wedge is thicker on its plantar surface. With a periosteal elevator, a connection is made between the resected area of the calcaneocuboid joint and the talonavicular joint, ensuring free motion of Chopart's joint as a unit. Next, the foot is manipulated to shift the middle and forepart laterally and align the axes of the first metatarsal and talus. Two staples are inserted to hold the calcaneus and cuboid securely together (one staple is not adequate to prevent rotation). The elongated tendons are then sutured, the incisions are closed, and the limb is immobilized in an above-knee cast, holding the foot in the corrected position. After four to six weeks, a below-knee walking cast is applied. Both Evans and Abrams recommend that immobilization in the cast be continued for about five months.[1, 190]

Initially, Evans routinely transferred the anterior tibial tendon to the lateral side of the foot (26 of 30 feet); this proved unsatisfactory, however, because of the resultant passive dropping of the forefoot. In later cases, he abandoned the tendon transfer as a part of the procedure.[190] Abrams did not transfer the anterior tibial tendon routinely; he found that, with the exception of three cases, there was return of sufficient peroneal power to provide active eversion of the foot.[1]

Evans reported the results of his procedure on 30 feet followed for four to eight years postoperatively. He did not attempt a statistical analysis of the results because the initial factors were too variable and the series was too small. The correction of the deformity obtained at the operation was permanent, and in the experience of Evans, the procedure eliminated all need for aftercare. He also observed that all elements of the deformity, including varus heel, were corrected by the operation.[189]

Abrams reported the results of Evan's operation in 31 feet, with an average follow-up of 44.5 months. The results of his series were roughly comparable to those of Evans; in 74 per cent, good; in 23 per cent, fair; and in 3 per cent, poor. The result was poor when marked scarring and stiffness of the foot were present consequent to extensive or multiple previous surgical procedures. Another important factor determining the outcome of the procedure was the age of the patient. The optimum age, according to both Evans and Abrams, is between four and eight years. They recommended that the operation not be performed before the age of four, as in the immature tarsal bones, wedge resection of the calcaneocuboid joint may remove too much cartilage, and fusion at the site of the joint resection may be difficult to achieve. Abrams also stated that the operation should not be done after the age of nine years. In his experience, the results of this operation were so much

Shortening of the Lateral Column of the Foot

OPERATIVE TECHNIQUE

A. Lateral projection of the foot showing levels of osteotomy. (1) Vertical osteotomy of anterior part of calcaneus. (2) Excision of anterior end of calcaneus (Lichtblau procedure). (3) Excision of calcaneocuboid joint and fusion (Evans operation). (4) Wedge resection and enucleation of cuboid bone.

B. A longitudinal incision about 4 cm. long is made centering over the dorsolateral aspect of the cuboid bone. Subcutaneous tissue and deep fascia are divided in line with the skin incision. The peroneus brevis tendon is identified and retracted plantarward. The extensor digitorum brevis muscle is elevated off the cuboid bone and retracted dorsally and medially. One must be careful not to injure the sural nerve.

C. When the calcaneocuboid joint is tilted medially, a vertical osteotomy with a wedge of bone based laterally is performed. The calcaneocuboid joint is left intact (Simms' procedure).

D. If there is no malalignment of the calcaneocuboid joint, with a sharp osteotome, a ⅜-inch resection of the anterior end of the calcaneus, including the articular cartilage, is carried out (Lichtblau procedure).

E. Evans operation is indicated when there is paralytic clubfoot and stability of the lateral column of the foot is desired. A wedge resection of the calcaneocuboid joint is performed.

F. When there is varus inclination of the midfoot only, a cuboid decancellation is performed. With an osteotome, a wedge of bone based laterally is excised from the cuboid bone, and, with a sharp curet, most of the cancellous bone from the cuboid bone is removed. The foot is then manipulated, bringing the forepart into marked abduction. This author does not recommend the use of staples. The wound is closed and a below-knee cast is applied, holding the forepart of the foot in marked abduction.

POSTOPERATIVE CARE

After two weeks, the cast is changed, the foot is manipulated into corrected position, and a new cast is applied. The foot is immobilized for a total period of six weeks.

Plate 96. Shortening of the Lateral Column of the Foot

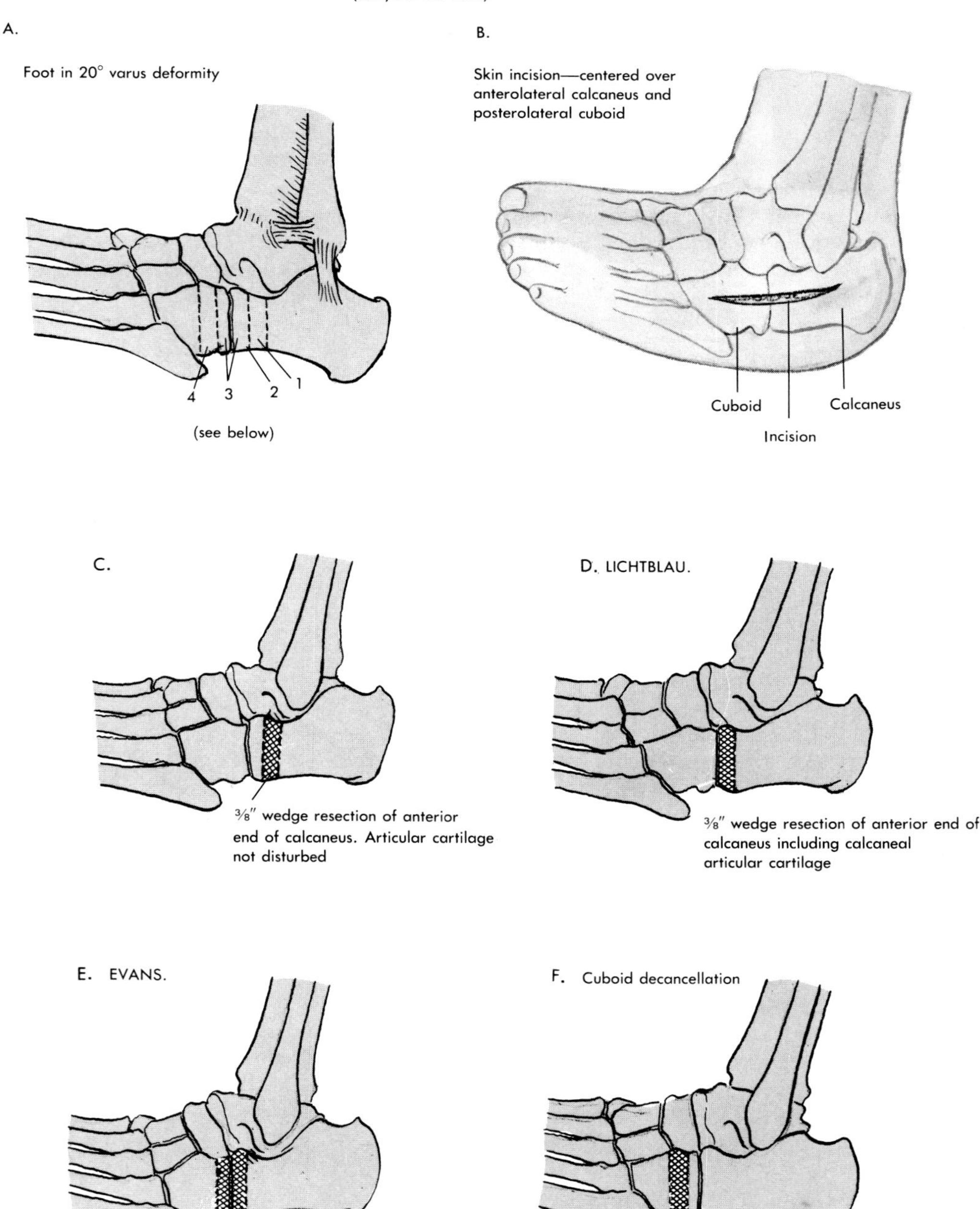

better than those following previous soft-tissue procedures performed after the age of two years that he advised using conservative methods to hold the foot between the ages of two and four years, and then performing the Evans procedure. He also warned that the operation does not correct adduction of the forepart of the foot at the tarsometatarsal joints, and that this should be treated separately.[1]

Evans's principal contribution to this procedure is wedge resection of the calcaneocuboid joint, shortening of the lateral column of the foot, and fusion of the calcaneocuboid joint in order to provide fixed stable correction of the articular malalignment. He noted no ill effects on the mechanics of the foot following calcaneocuboid fusion. A review of the Dillwyn Evans procedure has been given by Addison and colleagues.[5]

After a simplified medial release, Lichtblau recommends resection of the anterior end of the calcaneus instead of a wedge resection and fusion of the calcaneocuboid joint.[414] Through a longitudinal incision, about 4 cm. long and centered over the calcaneocuboid joint, the origin of the extensor digitorum brevis is elevated from the os calcis and reflected distally. The capsule of the calcaneocuboid joint is divided. With a single large osteotome, a wedge-shaped segment of the distal end of the calcaneus at the calcaneocuboid joint is resected. The wedge removed includes about 1 cm. of the distal lateral border of the calcaneus and 2 mm. of the distal medial margin. The foot is manipulated to bring the cuboid into contact with the distal, osteotomized end of the calcaneus. If the gap between the cuboid and calcaneus cannot be closed, it usually is because of insufficient excision of the distal medial portion of the calcaneus. In such an instance, or if the correction of varus deviation is inadequate, more of the distal end of the calcaneus is resected. The origin of the extensor brevis is sutured back to the surrounding soft tissues, and the wound is closed in the usual fashion. An above-knee cast is applied for three weeks, and then is exchanged for a below-knee cast.

Follow-up of Lichtblau's cases disclosed a calcaneocuboid joint space in the radiograms, and none of his patients had pain on walking. In the experimental animal, it has been shown that when a single side of a joint is resected, the excised hyaline cartilage is replaced by fibrocartilage. This permits maintenance of normal joint function.[98]

The author recommends shortening the lateral column of the foot, if necessary, in fixed talipes equinovarus in a child over four years of age. First, open reduction of the talocalcaneonavicular joint is performed by a peritalar release. In a child between four and eight years of age, a resection of the anterior end of the calcaneus (Lichtblau procedure) or vertical osteotomy wedge resection of the anterior part of the calcaneus (Simons' procedure) is performed, with care being taken not to disturb the anterior facet of the subtalar joint (Plate 96). If the calcaneocuboid joint is resected and fused (Evans procedure) with concentric reduction of the talocalcaneonavicular joint is performed in a child under eight years of age, overcorrection into valgus inclination is a definite hazard (Fig. 7–62).

When the child is eight years of age or older, it is relatively safe to fuse the calcaneocuboid joint. Staples are not used for internal fixation at the initial open reduction, however. Initially, the foot and ankle are immobilized in partially corrected position to relax the skin margins and to prevent wound slough. In two weeks, under

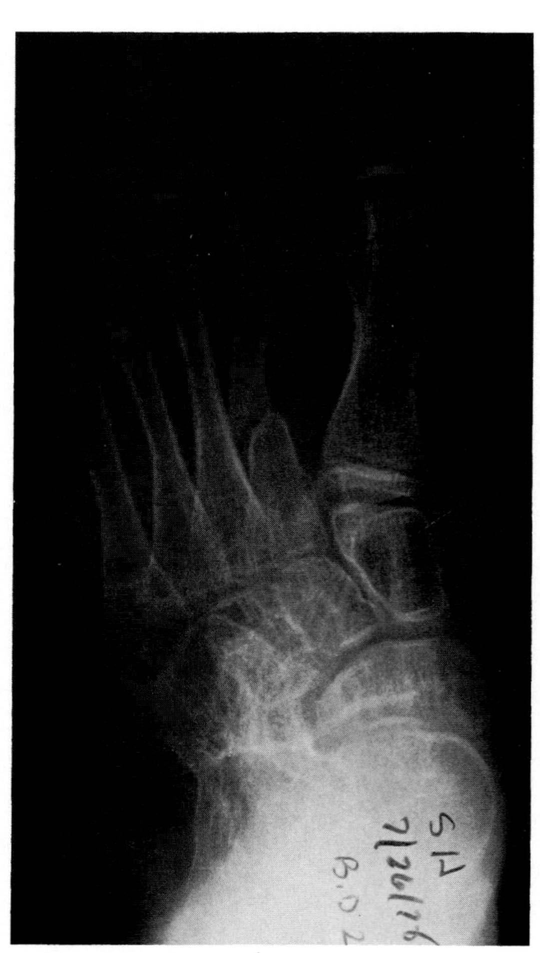

FIGURE 7–62. Valgus deformity of the foot following Evans procedure for correction of talipes equinovarus.

general anesthesia, the foot is manipulated (without removing the sutures) and brought to full correction. At that time, if necessary, one or two large threaded Kirschner wires are inserted to hold the calcaneus, cuboid, and fifth metatarsal firmly together. Often, the author does not utilize internal fixation.

Calcaneal Osteotomy. In 1955, Dwyer first described the lateral close-up calcaneal osteotomy for correction of pes cavus.[174, 175] In 1963, he modified his operation for the treatment of resistant talipes equinovarus by performing an open-up medial osteotomy of the calcaneus, grafting a wedge of tibial bone to correct the hindfoot varus deviation. The procedure was combined with Z-lengthening of the Achilles tendon and medial plantar fasciotomy. The results of the operation on 56 feet in 48 patients were good in 27 and fair in 29 feet.[176, 177]

In recalcitrant talipes equinovarus, the heel is in equinus and varus posture. The fibers of the tendo Achillis sweep more medially and anteriorly in relation to the inverted calcaneus and, with the contracted plantar soft-tissue structures, act as a deforming force. In realigning the heel from the varus into a mild valgus deviation and sectioning the medial half of the calcaneus, the "mechanism of correction of the Dwyer calcaneal osteotomy is dependent upon the flexibility of the subtalar and midtarsal joints." Mobility of these joints is a prerequisite. The Dwyer calcaneal osteotomy shifts the weight-bearing surface of the hindfoot laterally; the center of gravity is shifted into a more medial plane, and the body weight is transmitted through the tibia. In gait, the body weight falls medially onto the axis of the subtalar joint. If the subtalar and midtarsal joints have normal mobility, varus deformity of the midfoot and forefoot tends to improve with each step. If the midfoot and hindfoot are rigid, however, Dwyer's calcaneal osteotomy has no effect on the midfoot and forefoot.

By medial division of the tendo Achillis at the Z-lengthening and by plantar release, inversion forces are removed. The height of the heel is increased. Also, the heel is brought down as low as possible by tilting the posterior calcaneal fragment downward and laterally as the bone graft, a wedge of bone that is wider above than below, is placed in the gap.

An essential prerequisite of the Dwyer calcaneal osteotomy is that there is sufficient ossification of the calcaneus for bone grafting. Dwyer felt that the foot of a three-year-old is large enough for insertion of a medial bony wedge. He stressed that the operation should be performed while the child was still young enough for sufficient further skeletal growth and before gross structural deformity had developed.[177]

Dwyer's osteotomy of the calcaneus does not disturb growth of the foot and preserves mobility of the subtalar and midtarsal joints; these are major advantages over triple arthrodesis. Other positive points for a calcaneal osteotomy are a shorter healing period, lesser magnitude of the surgery, and rapid postoperative recovery. It also does not limit the performance of other surgical procedures in the future if necessary. Dwyer's osteotomy of the calcaneus is, however, ineffective in correcting midfoot and forefoot varus and cavus deformities. It satisfactorily corrects varus heel if the osteotomy is accurately placed and properly executed, and if there is no muscle imbalance. This is well-documented in the reports of Fisher and Shaffer and of Dekel and Weissman.[151, 202] This author disagrees with Dwyer's original claims that, with weight-bearing and walking on a plantigrade hindfoot, there are progressive dynamic correction of forefoot equinus and varus deformities and lateral shift of the navicular, the cuboid, and the anterior end of the calcaneus. Dwyer's osteotomy of the calcaneus does not reduce the medial subluxation of the talocalcaneonavicular joint, does not correct articular malalignment in talipes equinovarus, and has no effect on the forefoot or midfoot. Its sole indication is as a salvage procedure in talipes equinovarus that surgery has failed to improve, that requires bony correction of the heel varus deviation, but in which the foot is skeletally immature for triple arthrodesis. In the older child with a rigid varus deformity of the foot, even if the talus and navicular are normally aligned, residual forefoot adduction cannot be corrected. In such an instance, it is best to stage the operation. First, a plantar release is performed to correct the forefoot equinus and varus deformities. In the postoperative period, it is essential that the child walk on a below-knee cast with an anterior heel. At the second stage, a calcaneal osteotomy is performed.

Should one do a close-up lateral or open-up medial osteotomy? Delayed wound healing, dehiscence, and sloughing are the main problems of a medial open-up osteotomy of the calcaneus. Correction of the varus hindfoot invariably increases the distance between the medial malleolus and the posterior tuberosity of the calcaneus; the insertion of a bone wedge on the medial side of the os calcis further widens the gap, making it impossible to close the wound

Dwyer Open-Up Medial Osteotomy of Calcaneus with Bone Graft Wedge for Correction of Varus Hindfoot

Through a midline plantar incision, the plantar aponeurosis and short plantar muscles are sectioned near their origin from the tuberosity of the calcaneus, as shown in Plate 105.

OPERATIVE TECHNIQUE

A. The skin incision begins at a point in the midline in the posterior prominence of the heel, along the skin creases, and extends distally to the anterior border of the insertion of the tendo Achillis; then it swings obliquely, dorsally and distally, to a point 2 cm. distal to the lower tip of the medial malleolus. This incision differs from that described by Dwyer; as the varus heel is corrected, the skin margins are pulled together rather than apart, thus preventing delayed wound healing and slough. The subcutaneous tissue is divided in line with the skin incision. The elevated wound flaps are retracted and the plexus of veins is coagulated and divided to prevent bleeding later.

B. Next, the medial one third to one half of the insertion of the Achilles tendon to the calcaneus is sectioned. The laciniate ligament is divided near its insertion to the os calcis, at least 2.5 cm. inferior to the flexor hallucis longus tendon and neurovascular bundle. The medial surface of the calcaneus is subperiosteally exposed. The line of incision in the periosteum is 1.5 cm. inferior and in line with the flexor hallucis longus tendon. Injury to neurovascular structures should be avoided. Chandler elevator retractors are used to partially expose the superior and inferior aspects of the calcaneus.

C. With a wide osteotome, the calcaneus is sectioned just inferior to the flexor hallucis longus tendon. The lateral cortex of the calcaneus is left intact; however, its medial, inferior, and superior aspects should be completely divided.

D. Next, a Steinmann pin is inserted transversely into the os calcis. While the pin acts as a lever, with periosteal elevators and a laminectomy spreader, the site of osteotomy is opened. The width of the bone graft wedge is determined by inserting osteotomes of various sizes between the fragments. An appropriate bone graft wedge is taken from the ilium and, with its base medially, is placed in the gap in the calcaneus. The author finds that bone grafts from the upper end of the tibia are usually inadequate and not sturdy enough. The tension of the tissues will firmly hold the bone graft in position; the Steinmann pin is removed, as special fixation is not required. Radiograms are made in the operating room to ensure that the varus deformity of the hindfoot is corrected. The skin is closed with interrupted sutures, and an above-knee cast is applied.

POSTOPERATIVE CARE

The cast and sutures are removed in two to three weeks, and a new above-knee cast is applied. Approximately ten weeks is required for the bone graft to consolidate. Early weight-bearing will result in collapse of the graft and loss of correction. The importance of protecting the foot until the bone graft is fully incorporated cannot be overemphasized.

Plate 97. Dwyer Open-Up Medial Osteotomy of Calcaneus with Bone Graft Wedge for Correction of Varus Hindfoot

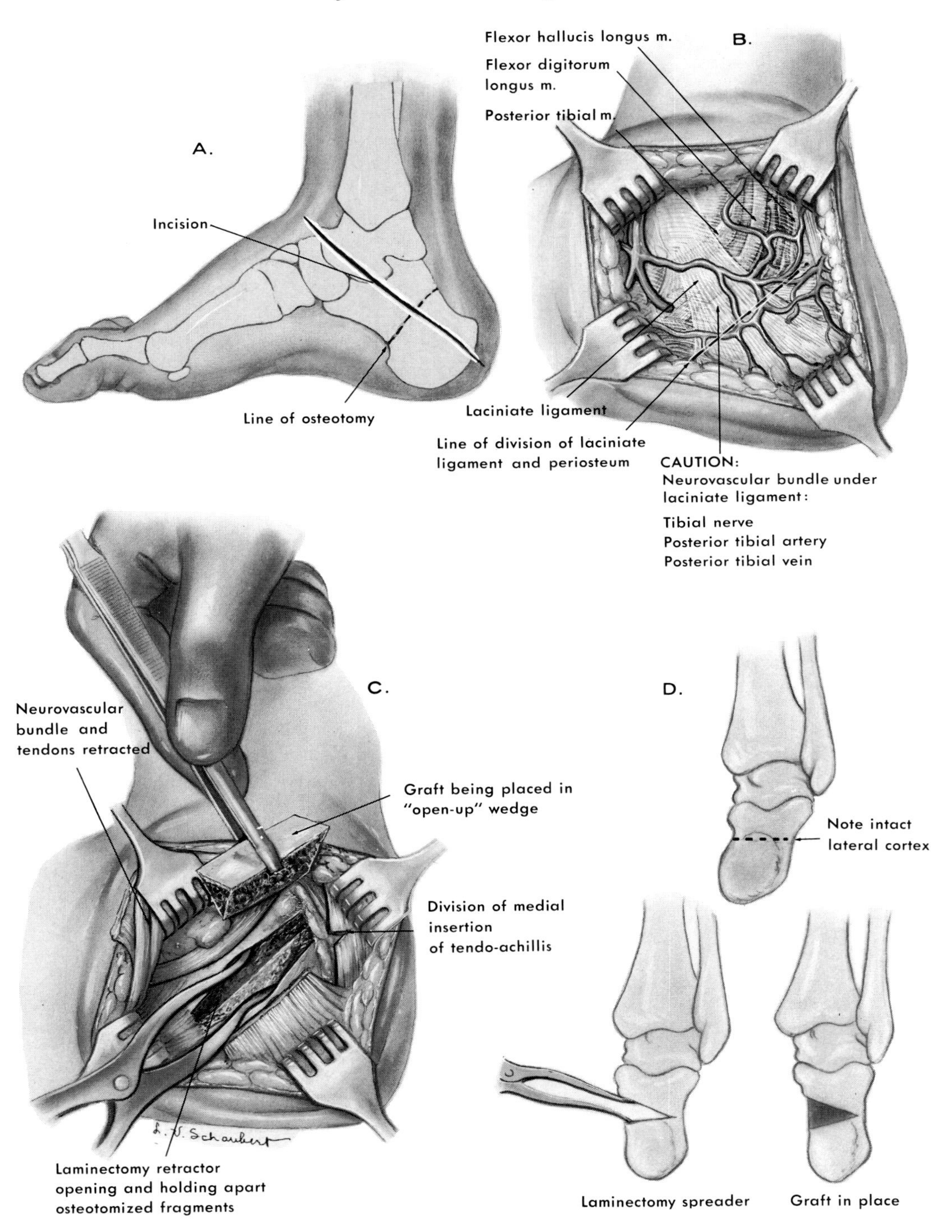

without tension. Originally, Dwyer made a curved incision parallel to the line of osteotomy. This often leaves an oval gap at the apex of the wound whose edges are very difficult to oppose. The wound heals by a hypertrophic scar, which exerts a deforming bowstring effect. Later, Dwyer changed the incision from a single curve to a double curve. The author modified the direction of Dwyer's incision by making it perpendicular to the line of the osteotomy. As the varus heel is corrected, the skin margins are pulled together rather than apart, thus lessening the chances of wound slough (Plate 97).

The problem, however, is complicated by the hypertrophic scar of a previous posteromedial release. In such an instance, one should utilize a Z-plasty incision as advocated by Handelsman and associates (Fig. 7–63). A longitudinal incision is made through the old operative scar along the medial aspect of the tendo Achillis. The proximal part is broken by two oblique limbs at 60 degrees. In the distal part, behind the medial malleolus and over the medial aspect of the midfoot, 60-degree triangles are constructed that allow distal extension of the incision as necessary. The wound is closed by transposing the flaps. This technique provides gain in the vertical length and adequate exposure; previous hypertrophic scars can be readily excised and replaced by the Z-plasty. The bowstring effect is checked by the broken lines of the newly healed scar. In some cases, a full-thickness or split-thickness skin graft may be necessary.[273]

In spite of this Z-plasty technique, when a large varus deviation is corrected, the skin usually does not heal by first intention. Therefore, a lateral close-up osteotomy is preferred by most authors.[103, 151, 202]

Fisher and Shaffer reported the correction of heel varus deformity achieved by the Dwyer calcaneal osteotomy in 26 feet with talipes equi-

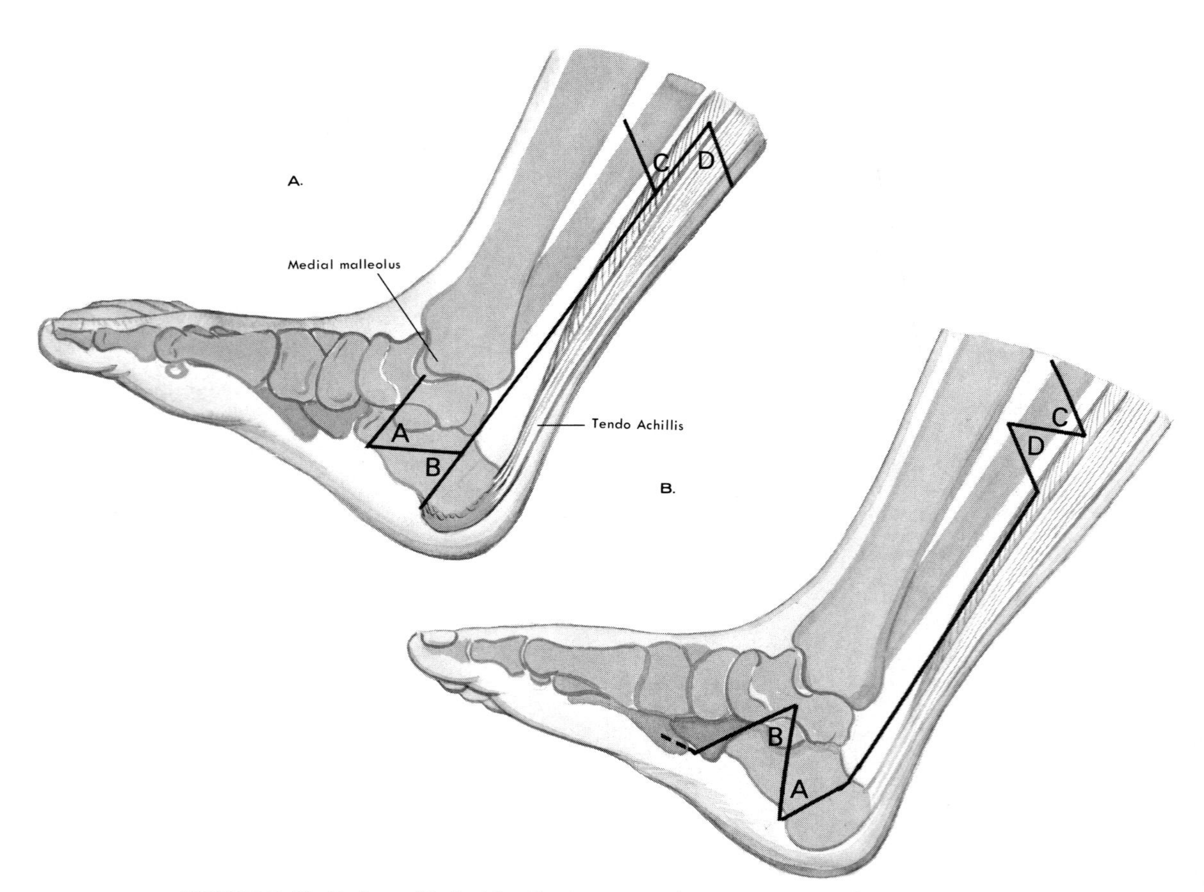

FIGURE 7–63. Z-plasty skin incision for Dwyer os calcis osteotomy in talipes equinovarus.

A. The proximal part of the incision is broken by two oblique limbs at 60 degrees; two 60-degree triangles are constructed in the distal part. **B.** The wound is closed by transposing the flaps.

novarus in 20 patients as good in 13, fair in 7, and poor in 2; 4 were not rated.[202] Dekel and Weissman, using similar methods of rating, reported results in 12 clubfeet as good in 11 and fair in 1.[151] Masse, Taussig, and Bazin presented an excellent study of the value of lateral close-up calcaneal osteotomy in 32 clubfeet. They regarded the operation as a salvage procedure to correct residual fixed heel varus deviation of 5 degrees or more in a child five years old or older. In their experience, previous medial release did not interfere with the lateral calcaneal osteotomy. They recommended the prone position at surgery for better visualization of correction, which must be technically exact. Poor results were due to insufficient correction of the varus inclination during the operation.[473]

Weseley and Barenfeld recommended the open-up osteotomy of the calcaneus in talipes equinovarus. In their experience, wound healing has not been a problem, and they report excellent results. Posterior release is not performed at the same time as the calcaneal osteotomy. The operation is staged: first, an open-up wedge calcaneal osteotomy is performed, combined with Steindler plantar stripping; second, six to eight weeks later, a posterior release is carried out to correct the equinus deformity. Staging the correction avoids stress on the suture line by the increase in the subjacent bony surface due to downward displacement of the calcaneal tuberosity following correction of the equinus deformity.[742–746]

Weseley and Barenfeld utilize a rectangular graft from the proximal tibia. The graft is notched on either side close to one end, and then is inserted into the open osteotomy so that the notches are grasped by the inferomedial cortex of the calcaneus. The remainder of the graft is wedged between the cancellous surfaces of the calcaneus, providing stable fixation.[745] This author strongly feels that an open-up osteotomy should not be performed. Instead, a lateral displacement osteotomy of the calcaneus is recommended. Occasionally, a close-up lateral osteotomy is indicated.

Should one ever perform an open-up osteotomy?

Medial Subtalar Stabilization. Shneider and Smith, in a preliminary report, described a method of medial subtalar stabilization with "posterior medial release" in the treatment of unstable varus hindfoot in children six to ten years of age. First, a "posteromedial release," similar to that described by Turco, is performed. They stress the importance of obtaining complete correction by soft-tissue sectioning. Then, with the foot in corrected position, a smooth pin is inserted from the heel across the subtalar joint and usually up into the tibia. With a 7-mm. dowel plug cutter, a trough is fashioned in the sustentaculum tali of the calcaneus and the plantar aspect of the neck of the talus medially. The fusion is intra-articular, in contrast to the Grice extra-articular arthrodesis. Then a double-cortical graft is taken from the iliac crest with an 8-mm. dowel plug cutter and is placed snugly into the previously cut trough. The authors do not use a pin across the talonavicular joint because they have found that fixation by a single pin across the subtalar joint holds the corrected position firmly. The foot and ankle are immobilized in a below-knee cast for 12 weeks. The pin is removed when weight-bearing is begun at six weeks postoperatively. Short-term results in six patients showed complete correction of the varus deformity in four cases; incomplete correction in two patients was due to the technical failure of inadequate medial release. There were no failures of fusion.[642]

This author has had no experience with medial intra-articular arthrodesis for stabilization of varus hindfoot; it appears, however, to be a sound procedure in a child between six and ten years of age who has marked incongruity and instability of the subtalar joint after open reduction of the talocalcaneonavicular joint.

Triple Arthrodesis. Tarsal reconstruction by wedge resection and fusion of the subtalar and midtarsal joints is an operation of last resort, indicated in the skeletally mature adolescent or adult with persistent rigid equinovarus deformity. It is a salvage procedure. The purpose of triple arthrodesis is to provide stability and prevent future arthritis and pain rather than to improve the cosmetic appearance of the foot. Following triple arthrodesis, the foot is smaller and has, of course, no motion at the subtalar and midtarsal joints. With adequate early treatment of talipes equinovarus, triple arthrodesis should rarely be necessary. Some patients with neglected clubfoot may come from underdeveloped countries; others are occasionally encountered in more developed areas with a high rate of immigration. The primary indication for the procedure should be to provide stability in the paralytic equinovarus deformity of the feet in neuromuscular diseases.

Before starting surgical treatment, it is essential to assess the psychological impact of the disability. An older patient may be accustomed to living with his deformities and managing quite well functionally. It is best to correct the deformities only upon the insistence of the patient and his family. Strong motivation and a genuine desire stimulated by social and cosmetic reasons are imperative prerequisites for a successful overall result. The psychological aspects of the problem are well recorded by Weinberg and Halmosh, and by Herold and Torok.[287, 288, 740] Prolonged walking on a deformed foot causes compensatory rotational deformities at more proximal levels: namely, lateral rotation contracture of the hip, exaggerated lateral tibiofibular torsion and lateral rotation of the talus on the tibia in the ankle mortise, and posterior displacement of the fibular malleolus in relation to the medial malleolus. Prior treatment may have caused flattening of the dome of the talus and distortion of the ankle mortise with narrowing of the joint space.

It should be remembered that triple arthrodesis further compromises the biomechanically stressed ankle joint. In the older patient, the osseous and articular deformities at the ankle joint may be so fixed that, after soft-tissue release and before triple arthrodesis, a medial rotation osteotomy of the tibia may be indicated for proper alignment of the ankle mortise in relation to the leg, as is discussed later. This will accentuate the midfoot and forefoot varus deformity.

Details of surgical treatment should be individualized. In general, it consists of four separate steps: first, a short period of gentle manipulation and cast immobilization to elongate the contracted skin and soft tissues; second, surgical soft-tissue release; third, a period of manipulation and cast retention; and fourth, tarsal bone reconstruction.

Soft-tissue release. The surgical technique of soft-tissue release is described in Plate 95. The following changes are made in the older patient. (1) The skin incision extends distally to the base of the proximal phalanx of the great toe. (2) The posterior tibial tendon is divided at its insertion to the navicular, transferred, and with one or two sutures, attached to the lateral side of the tendo Achillis. (3) The abductor hallucis muscle is detached from its insertion to the base of the proximal phalanx of the hallux and is totally excised. This facilitates exposure of the neurovascular bundle, permits wound closure with less tension, and diminishes the postoperative incidence of forefoot adduction deformity. (4) The joint capsules are resected rather than incised. During division of the deltoid ligament, the deep part, i.e., the tibiotalar band, should not be disturbed. If divided, it should be repaired. There is compensatory valgus deformity at the ankle in the older patient. Division of the tibiotalar ligament medially will result in a severe valgus deformity at the ankle; it will also cause difficulties in further corrections of the foot deformities by manipulation and plaster cast. It is important to close the skin without tension and to apply the immediate postoperative cast in partial correction. Attention to these technical details is vital.

Manipulation and cast retention. Ten to fourteen days after soft-tissue release, the initial cast is removed, and the wound is inspected and re-dressed. It is best not to remove the sutures, as the wound will gape apart at manipulation. Under general anesthesia, the foot and ankle are manipulated to obtain further correction without putting much tension on the skin closure. Manipulation and cast retention are repeated initially at weekly and later at biweekly intervals until maximal correction is achieved. Radiograms are made to assess the anatomic result of the soft-tissue release and the need for further bone reconstruction. Muscle testing is performed; it is imperative to provide a dynamic balance of muscle forces acting on the ankle and foot. Overlengthening of the tendo Achillis and consequent triceps surae insufficiency should be avoided.

Tarsal reconstruction. This stage consists of triple arthrodesis. If there is any question of the vascular supply to the foot, it is studied by arteriography.[42] It is best to perform the operation through two incisions: an anterolateral one extended distally, and a medial one. Prior soft-tissue release and manipulations achieve enough correction so that a triple arthrodesis can be performed with a minimum of bone resection at the articular surfaces. Bone is added rather than resected. The height of the foot is an important consideration, since low-riding malleoli will be irritated by the shoes and walking will be painful and difficult. The midfoot and forefoot are brought into proper alignment with the hindfoot by closing a laterally based wedge through Chopart's joint (the calcaneocuboid and talonavicular), and by shifting the distal segment laterally on the proximal segment to correct the marked medial displacement of the forefoot.

Internal fixation with heavy threaded Kirschner wires or Steinmann pins may be desired by some surgeons; two threaded pins are used—one drilled through the medial cuneiform, through the navicular and into the talus; and the other drilled through the plantar aspect of the foot and up through the calcaneus to the talus.

Correction of the equinus deformity of the

ankle does accentuate that of the forefoot and leads to increased weight-bearing on the metatarsal heads. There may be residual varus deformity of the forefoot. When metatarsalgia and painful pressure keratosis under the prominent metatarsal heads develop, an extension osteotomy of the metatarsals at the base is performed to correct both the equinus and varus deformities of the forefoot.

Talectomy. R. Whitman, in 1901, was the first to advocate excision of the talus for paralytic calcaneus deformity; later on, talectomies were performed for a variety of conditions.[752–754]

A. Whitman, in 1922 and 1931, presented long-term follow-up studies of talectomy and reported varying results. He concluded that the operation is primarily indicated in rigid paralytic deformities of the foot and that best results are obtained in children under four years of age.[750, 751] Young reported a 50-year follow-up in a woman with bilateral talectomy; her feet were most satisfactory.[775]

The operation is a salvage procedure that has a useful place in the management of the severely deformed and rigid foot in some cases of arthrogryposis multiplex congenita, myelomeningocele, and diastrophic dwarfism.[423, 484, 754] Occasionally, it is indicated in a case of surgical failure in talipes equinovarus in which the foot is rigid and deformed, there are multiple scars, and circulation is compromised. Talectomy is unphysiologic and further distorts an already deformed foot; therefore, it is not recommended as a primary operation for rigid talipes equinovarus. When possible, it is best to wait and tide the child over until the age of 10 to 12 years and then to perform a triple arthrodesis to correct the deformity.

The principle of talectomy is that, by excision of the talus, sufficient laxity of soft tissues is provided to correct equinus and varus deformities without tension. It gives a plantigrade foot with a stable and relatively congruous false joint between the calcaneus and the ankle mortise.

The best age for talectomy varies according to the basic disease; in arthrogryposis and myelomeningocele, it is between one and five years; whereas in talipes equinovarus, it is six to nine years. In general, the younger the child, the better the result.

Ablation of the talus does not present any technical problem, but correction of the deformity and internal fixation demand meticulous attention to detail. The incision is curved anterolaterally over the subtalar and talonavicular joints. It begins behind the lateral malleolus and ends over the talonavicular joint. The subcutaneous tissue is divided in line with the skin incision; great care must be taken not to injure the veins. The extensor digitorum brevis muscle is elevated from its origin and reflected distally. The long toe extensors and anterior tibial tendons are retracted medially. The peroneal tendons are divided and tagged with sutures for reattachment. The ligaments and capsule connecting the talus to the distal fibula, tibia, calcaneus, and navicular are divided next. Tenotomy scissors are utilized to avoid damage to hyaline articular cartilage. First, the anterior talofibular ligament is sectioned (it arises from the anterior border of the fibula and runs anteriorly and medially to attach to the neck of the talus). The calcaneofibular ligament is incised proximally at its origin from the lateral malleolus and tagged for resuture later on. Next, the lateral and anterior part of the talocalcaneal ligament is divided. Caution is exercised not to incise the calcaneonavicular and calcaneocuboid limbs of the bifurcate ligament. The dorsal capsule of the talonavicular joint and the interosseous talocalcaneal ligament are sectioned next. At this time, the foot is manipulated into greater equinus and varus inclination, and under direct vision, the medial and posterior ligaments are sectioned. They consist of the medial capsule of the subtalar joint, the tibiotalar (deep part of the deltoid), the posterior tibiotalar and talocalcaneal capsule, and the posterior talofibular ligaments. The talus is grasped with a large towel clip and rotated and displaced in each direction as the dissection proceeds. Usually it can be excised in one piece; if fragments break off, they are removed with bone rongeurs.

The tendo Achillis is sharply divided at its insertion, a small distal segment being left for resuturing later on. Next, the inferior tibiofibular ligament is divided to widen the ankle mortise. Often the lateral malleolus abuts the lateral surface of the calcaneus and prevents a congruous fit of the upper surface of the calcaneus into the ankle mortise. In such an instance, the lower part of the lateral malleolus, distal to its physis, is excised. It is important not to injure the growth plate. With the foot displaced posteriorly, the calcaneus giving a normal contour to the heel, the tip of the medial malleolus should be immediately superoposterior to the navicular, and the lateral malleolus should be just behind the calcaneocuboid joint. It is essential to provide a long lever arm by posterior displacement of the calcaneus to give a mechanical advantage to the triceps surae muscle. If posterior displacement of the hindfoot and correction of the varus inclination are found to be difficult, they are facilitated by partial excision of the cuboid. The foot is laterally rotated 15 to 20 degrees in relation to the leg to stabilize the new articulation. One or two small Steinmann pins are inserted upward through the heel into the tibia for secure fixation. The tendo Achillis is resutured; if it is too lax, a segment is excised. The calcaneofibular ligament is sutured to the lateral malleolus under slight tension. An above-knee plaster of Paris cast is applied with the hindfoot slightly valgus and the ankle in neutral position. The cast and pins are removed after six weeks. Then a below-knee polypropylene orthosis is worn during the day for an additional three to four months. The tendency to rigidity gives stability to the false articulation between the calcaneus and the ankle mortise. It seems that in arthrogryposis, what was an "enemy" working against success turns out to be a "friend."[484]

Osteotomy of the Tibia. Tibial torsion in the newborn with talipes equinovarus is normal, and the old teaching that excessive medial torsion of the tibia is one of the principal deformities in talipes equinovarus should be discarded. The in-toeing one often sees in inadequately treated talipes equinovarus is due to persistence of medial subluxation of the talocalcaneonavicular joint and adduction of the forefoot. Lateral rotation osteotomy of the tibia and fibula should not be performed.

Swann, Lloyd-Roberts, and Catterall have proposed that in improperly treated and uncorrected talipes equinovarus, the talus and the forefoot are laterally rotated in the ankle mortise on the tibia, which has no rotational deformity. The fibular malleolus is displaced posteriorly.[681] Simons has shown that when the child begins to walk with uncorrected talipes equinovarus, compensatory lateral rotation takes place at the hip. In time, structural changes take place with growth, and excessive lateral tibiofibular torsion develops.[644] In the older child, Lloyd-Roberts and associates recommend *medial* rotation osteotomy of the tibia for proper alignment of the ankle mortise in relation to the leg. This will exaggerate the midfoot and forefoot varus deformity, which is corrected at a later stage by open reduction of the talocalcaneonavicular joint, and if necessary, by Evans's procedure.[424]

Metatarsal Osteotomy. Residual forefoot varus deformity in the child over eight years of age may be corrected by valgus osteotomy of the metatarsals at their base. Prior to this age, the Heymann-Herndon soft-tissue procedure described in Plate 101 will give satisfactory results.

*Complications of Surgical Treatment**

Open reduction of the talocalcaneonavicular joint in talipes equinovarus is very delicate surgery, requiring extensive dissection of the small foot of an infant. If meticulous attention to detail is not given, the operative procedure is fraught with hazards and complications, some of which may be disastrous. Clubfoot surgery should be performed by the experienced surgeon—expertise is crucial.

In order to prevent complications it is important to know their cause. Failure to correct deformities results from inadequate surgery; because surgery is required to correct these, they are included here as complications. Deformities also develop from overcorrection and technical errors during surgery. Failure to provide adequate postoperative care may cause recurrence of deformity.

Wound Dehiscence. This can be prevented by the following measures: (1) Preoperative manipulation and stretching of the contracted soft tissues in the medial, posterior, and plantar aspects of the deformed clubfoot. The cast is applied to retain the correction obtained by manipulation. The externally "normal" looking foot provides a better anatomy for placing the skin incisions and also facilitates the handling of soft tissue. Elongation of skin and soft tissues relieves tension on the incised skin margins. (2) Meticulous surgical technique and gentle retraction of skin margins. Sharp hooks are used to retract skin. When using rakes, the pull is on deep soft tissues and not on skin. (3) The tourniquet should be released and complete hemostasis obtained before skin closure. (4) The initial cast is generously padded and applied with the ankle in plantar flexion. The cast is more like a compression dressing. The equinus posture releases tension on the skin margins. The cast is changed 10 to 14 days after the operation, bringing the ankle into dorsiflexion. The sutures are not removed at this time. Paying attention to these details ensures primary wound healing.

Wound dehiscence is still a problem in the rigid clubfoot in arthrogryposis multiplex congenita and myelomeningocele. The previously operated on, scarred foot also presents difficulties with wound healing. When wound slough develops, the foot should be maintained in the

*Written with George W. Simons, M.D., Professor of Orthopedic Surgery, Medical College of Wisconsin; Chief, Department of Orthopedic Surgery, Children's Hospital, Milwaukee.

corrected position in the cast. The wound is allowed to granulate and epithelialize, and Betadine dressings are applied daily through a window in the cast. The cast is changed as necessary. The pin in the talonavicular joint should not be removed. In severe sloughs, consultation with a plastic surgeon may be in order; a split-thickness or full-thickness graft may be indicated.

Wound Infection. If this unfortunate complication develops, the wound is debrided, cleansed, and closed primarily (if possible) with suction drainage. It is best not to leave the wound open to granulate, because this will result in excessive scarring. The talocalcaneonavicular joint is kept in the corrected position in a new cast. If possible, the Steinmann pin is left transfixing the talonavicular joint.

The following complications and problems are discussed according to the joint involved.

COMPLICATIONS INVOLVING THE ANKLE

At this level the complications may include calcaneus deformity, restricted range of plantar flexion of the ankle joint, ankle valgus, equinus of the ankle, and growth arrest of the posterior tibial or distal fibular physis.

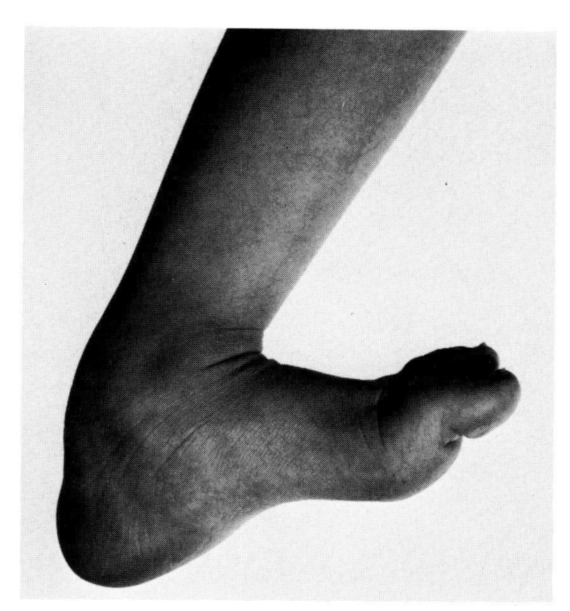

FIGURE 7–64. Calcaneus deformity.

Calcaneus deformity caused by overlengthening of the Achilles tendon and weak triceps surae.

Calcaneus Deformity. This is caused by overcorrection of the equinus deformity (Fig. 7–64). Overlengthening of the Achilles tendon weakens the motor strength of the triceps surae; also, linear growth of the calcaneus is stunted by loss of normal tension of triceps surae on the posterior apophysis of the os calcis. A second pathogenic and aggravating factor in calcaneus deformity is restriction of range of ankle plantar flexion, which further weakens motor function of the triceps surae. A third cause of calcaneus deformity is prolonged immobilization in a cast; the total period of postoperative immobilization should not exceed six weeks. A pitfall in the older child is application of a walking cast with an anterior heel, which will stretch the triceps surae muscle. A walking heel should be applied posteriorly under the midfoot near the longitudinal axis of the tibia. It is preferable to use a cast boot for ambulation.

Calcaneus deformity can be prevented by repairing the Achilles tendon with the ankle in neutral position and definitely in no greater than 10 degrees of dorsiflexion.

Treatment. Conservative measures include plantar-flexion, progressive resistive, and tiptoe rising exercises, and passive stretching of contracted anterior capsule of the ankle joint and ankle dorsiflexor muscles. A continuous passive ankle motion machine may be tried for a period of one to two months to increase range of ankle plantar flexion. When conservative measures fail, operative treatment is indicated; the Achilles tendon is shortened and, if fixed bony calcaneal deformity is present, Achilles tendon shortening is combined with posterior displacement osteotomy of the os calcis. Anterior ankle joint capsular and ligamentous contracture is treated by soft-tissue release.

Restricted Plantar Flexion of the Ankle. Some degree of limitation of ankle motion is present in talipes equinovarus both before and after surgery. Clinical assessment of range of ankle motion in clubfoot is difficult and often inaccurate; motion in the midtarsal and subtalar joints is mistaken for that of the ankle. For accurate determination it is best to make lateral radiograms of the ankle with the foot in maximal dorsiflexion and plantar flexion and to measure the tibiotalar angle (Fig. 7–65). Simons studied passive range of ankle motion in 50 patients with talipes equinovarus who were treated by extensive soft-tissue release; the average range of motion was 31 degrees preoperatively and 29 degrees postoperatively. Following surgery, the range of dorsiflexion increased by an average of 10 degrees, while plantar flexion decreased by an average of 12 degrees.[649] Marked restriction of range of plantar flexion of the ankle in talipes

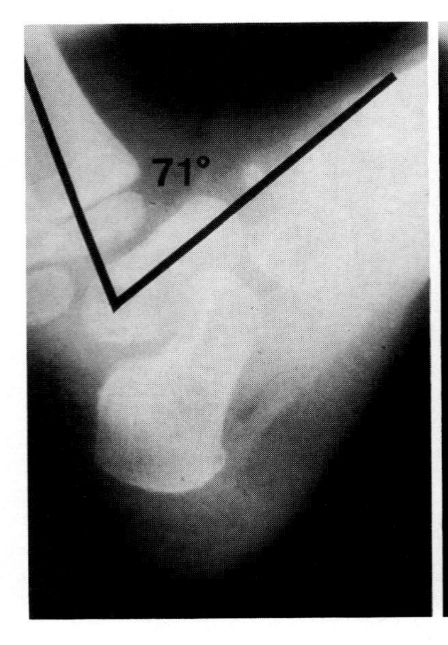

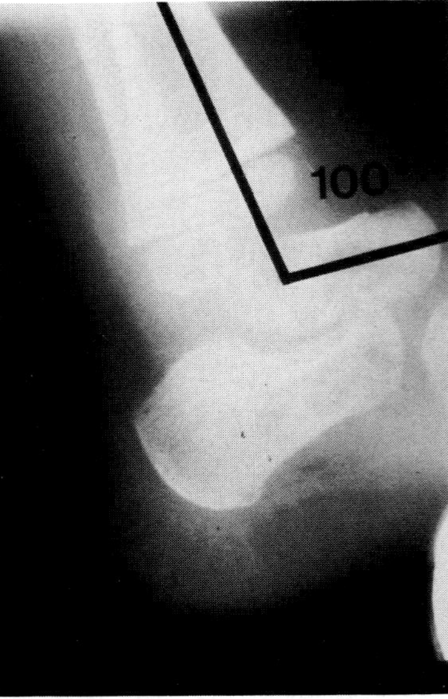

FIGURE 7–65.

Passive range of arc of ankle joint in talipes equinovarus as shown by lateral radiograms of the ankle-foot with the ankle in maximal dorsiflexion and maximal plantar flexion.

equinovarus has also been reported by Nomura and associates and Moreau and Dick.[498, 519]

Etiology. Possible pathogenic factors are contracture of the anterior capsule and ligamentous tissue of the ankle, myostatic contracture of the ankle dorsiflexor nerves, anterior displacement of the peroneal tendons, and incongruity and stiffness of the ankle joint. Ordinarily contracture of the posterior capsule of the ankle is not a causative factor.

Prevention. As mentioned previously, the arc of range of the tibiotalar joint is determined in the neonatal period and during early infancy. During manipulation, in addition to stretching and elongating the contracted posterior soft-tissue structures, the anterior capsule is also stretched by forcing the foot into maximal dorsiflexion and plantar flexion. In nonsurgical management, forceful dorsiflexion manipulation should not be carried out in order to avoid true flat-top talus. Prolonged immobilization of the foot-ankle in maximal dorsiflexion should be avoided, as it will cause contracture of the anterior capsule of the ankle joint. During surgery when posterolateral release is performed, reposition the peroneal tendons behind the lateral malleolus and maintain the tendons in their normal anatomic position by preserving the peroneal sheaths. While performing posterior capsulotomy of the ankle and subtalar joint, do not cause damage to hyaline articular cartilage with the scalpel—use scissors whenever possible! Avoid stiffness of the ankle joint. Following surgery, when changing the cast and bringing the foot into dorsiflexion, repeatedly manipulate the foot into *plantar flexion* and dorsiflexion. Between the second and third postoperative weeks is a critical period to mobilize the ankle joint. This author has not used the hinged cast, as described by McKay, because of its clumsiness and the reluctance of the parents in compliance.

Treatment. Nonsurgical measures are employed initially—they consist of passive exercises, stretching and elongating the contracted anterior capsule and muscles, and temporary use of continuous passive motion ankle machine.

If no improvement is achieved after a conservative trial period of several months, operative correction of the deformity is indicated. Surgery consists of anterior capsulotomy of the ankle joint and lengthening of the shortened anterior tibial and long-toe extensors either fractionally at their musculotendinous junction or in severe calcaneus with rigid contracture of the muscles by Z-plasty. Postoperative cast immobilization should only be used for three weeks. Physical therapy in the form of passive and active muscle strengthening is performed several times a day. At night this author recommends the use of continuous passive motion ankle machine, particularly if there is incongruity of the ankle joint.

Ankle Valgus. This is caused by division of the medial part of the deep deltoid (tibiotalar) ligament. If at surgery the tibiotalar ligament is inadvertently cut, it should be repaired. The child with excessive ligamentous laxity and clubfoot may develop ankle valgus, particularly if the subtalar joint is stiff. Another possible cause is the short fibula with a high-riding lateral malleolus; this is not uncommon when there is marked weakness of triceps surae.

Treatment. Attempts at late repair and tautening of the deep deltoid ligament have been unsuccessful in this author's experience. Best results are obtained by medial displacement horizontal calcaneal osteotomy. Opening-wedge laterally based (Dwyer) osteotomy (see Plate 97) is preferred if the height of the hindfoot is short and a low-riding malleolus is a problem in shoe wear. Postoperatively it is important to support the ankle in a supramalleolar foot-ankle orthosis using the UCBL (University of California Biomechanics Laboratory) principles to elevate the sagging longitudinal arch of the foot. If the ankle valgus is due to a short fibula or high-riding lateral malleolus, varus supramalleolar osteotomy of the distal tibia is indicated, preferably using the Wiltse technique. The varus osteotomy is combined with calcaneofibular tenodesis, using only half of the Achilles tendon; the remaining half of the triceps surae is tautened by shortening. When there is fixed calcaneovalgus deformity of the os calcaneus, posterior and medial displacement osteotomy of the calcaneus is indicated. Often it is best to stage these two procedures.

Equinus of the Ankle

Etiology. This may be *caused* by the following: (1) inadequate release of the posterior ankle and subtalar joint capsules, calcaneofibular ligament, and Achilles tendon; (2) placing the foot in excessive plantar flexion to relieve skin tension during wound closure and maintaining this equinus posture for a long period (the infant becomes ill or noncompliant parents do not keep their follow-up appointment); and (3) failure to provide adequate postoperative care in the form of night-splinting in an ankle-foot orthosis and passive stretching dorsiflexion exercises.

Prevention. At surgery it is vital to section the posterior capsule of the ankle and subtalar joints, posterior talofibular ligament, calcaneofibular ligament, and peroneal retinaculum, and to lengthen the Achilles and posterior tibial tendons. It is also important to untether (unlock) the anterior end of the talus and calcaneus. Intraoperative radiograms should be made to document anatomic repositioning of the talus in the ankle mortise and the establishment of normal tibiotalar and talocalcaneal articular relations. The importance of making appropriate radiograms before closure of the wound cannot be overemphasized. Do not have a false sense of achievement of correction of deformity by external configuration of the foot-ankle!

Treatment. Treatment consists of repeat soft-tissue release and provision of meticulous postoperative care.

Growth Arrest of the Posterior Tibial Physis. This results from injudicious posterior capsulotomy. Locate the ankle joint by palpating with a probe while moving the ankle in maximal plantar flexion and dorsiflexion! In the surgical exploratory approach, move distal to proximal, i.e., subtalar to ankle joint. If in doubt, make intraoperative radiograms.

Treatment. The osseous bridge is resected after appropriate tomographic determination of its extent and location. Fat is interposed as a spacer to prevent recurrence of bony bridge formation across the physis. If physeal bar excision fails, repeat posteriorly based opening-wedge osteotomy of the distal tibial metaphysis may be required. Distraction-lengthening of the distal tibial physis (either Ilizarov or DeBastiani's chondrodiatasis technique) is another alternative method of management; its drawbacks are stiffness of the ankle due to hyaline cartilage compression, risk of sepsis, and arrest of the remainder of the open growth plate of the distal tibia.

Growth Arrest of the Distal Fibular Physis. Inadvertent trauma to the growth plate may result when the calcaneofibular ligament or the peroneal retinaculum is sectioned. It is important to make adequate surgical exposure; do not operate through a small aperture! With disturbance of growth of the distal fibula, high-riding lateral malleolus and ankle valgus may develop.

Treatment. Options are (1) physeal bar excision, (2) lengthening of the fibula, and (3) varization supramalleolar osteotomy of the tibia. Factors to consider in decision-making are the extent of the bony bridge as determined by computed tomography, age of the patient, and severity of the deformity. Lengthening of the fibula is technically difficult because of the rigidity of the distal tibiofibular syndesmosis.

COMPLICATIONS INVOLVING THE SUBTALAR JOINT

At this level the following complications may occur: valgus deformity (hinged or rotatory), varus deformity, and stiffness with marked limitation of subtalar joint motion.

Valgus Deformity at the Subtalar Joint. This deformity may be either of two types: (1) *hinge valgus*, in which the talocalcaneal joint opens up in the *horizontal* axis in the anteroposterior plane; or (2) *rotatory valgus*, in which lateral deviation of the subtalar joint takes place in the *vertical* axis.

Etiology. Hinged valgus at the subtalar joint occurs when complete posteromedial release and division of talocalcaneal interosseous ligament are performed but the lateral subtalar capsule is left intact; the result is the calcaneus hinges beneath the talus. *Rotatory valgus* results from overcorrection of the horizontal rotation of the calcaneus beneath the talus around a vertical axis that passes in the area of the talocalcaneal interosseous ligament upward through the tibia. Other possible causes of rotatory valgus are (1) lateral displacement of the navicular on the head of the talus due to excessive soft-tissue release and (2) failure to correct calcaneocuboid medial subluxation with consequent compensatory valgus at the subtalar joint. Occasionally rotatory valgus at the subtalar joint develops gradually following surgery in children with excessive ligamentous hyperlaxity.

Prevention. Hinged valgus is prevented by completely or partially leaving the talocalcaneal interosseous ligament intact when only posteromedial release is performed. The lateral talocalcaneal capsule should be divided during posteromedial plantar release; i.e., perform a complete subtalar release. *Rotatory valgus* at the subtalar joint is prevented by pinning the subtalar joint, with one or two threaded Steinmann pins, in normal anatomic position when complete peritalar release is performed with sectioning of the talocalcaneal interosseous ligament. An additional preventive measure is anatomic concentric reduction of the calcaneocuboid and talonavicular joints. Also, when performing clubfoot surgery in children with ligamentous hyperlaxity or in infants whose siblings or one or both parents have marked ligamentous laxity, correct the deformities to only the lower limits of the normal radiographic range!

Treatment. Hinged valgus is treated by complete subtalar release and internal fixation of the subtalar joint by one or preferably two threaded Steinmann pins. Rotatory valgus is corrected by open reduction of the subtalar joint in anatomic position and internal fixation with pins. The rigid valgus deformity at the subtalar joint is best treated by horizontal medial displacement osteotomy of the calcaneus. The stiff painful valgus foot in the adolescent is best treated by triple arthrodesis.

Varus Deformity at the Subtalar Joint

Etiology. This deformity results from incomplete release of (1) the medial capsule of the subtalar joint (superficial deltoid ligament), (2) the capsule of the talonavicular joint, and (3) the interosseous ligament. This was a common deformity in the past when surgical correction of talipes equinovarus consisted of only posterior or extended posterior release and serial casts were employed to correct medial-plantar contracted soft tissues. At present the inadequacy of such posterior release is obvious.

Prevention and Treatment. A complete subtalar soft-tissue release should be performed for concentric reduction of the talocalcaneal navicular and calcaneocuboid joints. In the older patient with rigid subtalar varus, lateral displacement closing-wedge osteotomy of the os calcis is performed to correct the deformity. Triple arthrodesis is indicated in the adolescent when the subtalar inversion is associated with rigid midfoot varus and incongruity of the talocalcaneonavicular and calcaneocuboid joints.

Restricted Range of Subtalar Motion. Factors in pathogenesis of the deformity are iatrogenic damage to the hyaline articular cartilage when performing subtalar capsular release, failure to release cartilaginous subtalar coalition, postsurgical osseous bridge formation in the region of the sustentaculum tali, and incongruity of the subtalar joint due to failure of normal development of the talocalcaneal articular facets in the inadequately treated cases.

Prevention and Treatment. Some degree of limitation of subtalar joint motion is inherent in talipes equinovarus; this persists when the deformity is corrected. Prolonged immobilization in a cast should be avoided. Motion should be restored early in the postoperative period. It is important to remove the internal fixation pins at three weeks and the cast at six weeks following surgery. Active and passive exercises are employed to improve and maintain mobility.

COMPLICATIONS INVOLVING THE PROXIMAL TARSAL JOINT (TALONAVICULAR AND CALCANEOCUBOID)

At this level the following deformities may develop or persist following surgery: (1) talonavicular subluxation, which may be medial, dorsal, or lateral; (2) calcaneocuboid subluxation, which may be medial or lateral; (3) posterior cavus with plantar subluxation of the talonavicular and calcaneocuboid joints; the posterior cavus may be simple (i.e., neutral ankle joint) or associated with varying degrees of ankle equinus (i.e., equinocavus) or calcaneus (i.e., calcaneocavus); (4) sagging and collapse of the medial longitudinal arch; and (5) supination deformity taking place at the talonavicular joint with varying degrees of involvement of the calcaneocuboid joint.

Medial Talonavicular Subluxation

Etiology. This complication is caused by inadequate release of the navicular from its tethering contracted soft tissues, namely (1) medial, plantar, dorsal, and lateral capsule of the talonavicular articulation; (2) plantar calcaneonavicular ligament; and (3) tibionavicular ligament (anterior part of deltoid ligament).

Prevention. This complication can be prevented by complete subtalar release.

Treatment. Minimal medial subluxation of the talonavicular joint requires no treatment as it is adequately compensated by lateral rotation of the hip. Moderate to severe subluxations require complex subtalar release. In the older child with varus hindfoot a lateral closing and horizontal displacement osteotomy of the calcaneus is indicated. The painful varus hindfoot in the skeletally mature foot is best treated by triple arthrodesis.

Dorsal Talonavicular Subluxation

Etiology. This complication is quite common following Turco's posteromedial release. It occurred in 43 per cent of the cases in the series of Schlafly and associates and in 54 per cent (13 of 24 feet) of the cases in the report of Miller and Bernstein.[492, 618, 708, 709] It is caused by failure to release tibionavicular ligaments and the dorsal capsule of the talonavicular joint and improper positioning and fixation at the time of surgery. Dorsal subluxation of the navicular may be associated with dorsal displacement of the calcaneocuboid joint and by wedging of the navicular (Fig. 7–66).

Prevention. During surgery the navicular should be placed in normal anatomic position in relation to the anterior end of the talus; this should be verified clinically by inspection and palpation (i.e., the dorsum of the navicular and talus are at the same level) and also by intraoperative true lateral radiograms of the foot. In infancy the navicular is not ossified; therefore, the relationship of the talus to the first metatarsal is determined. When the alignment of the talonavicular joint is normal, the longitudinal axis of the talus bisects that of the first metatarsal. When the longitudinal axis of the talus passes plantar to that of the first metatarsal, the navicular is subluxated dorsally. By paying meticulous attention to these clinical and radiographic guidelines and by internal fixation of the talonavicular joint by *threaded* pin, dorsal talonavicular subluxation can be prevented.

Treatment. Dorsal subluxation of the talonavicular joint is divided into three grades: *Grade 1*—less than one third; *Grade 2*—one third to two thirds; and *Grade 3*—two thirds to complete dislocation. Grade 1 dorsal subluxations require no treatment, since functionally the foot is very satisfactory. Grade 2 and particularly Grade 3 dorsal subluxation of the talonavicular joint, however, may cause functional impairment of the foot and pain in the dorsum of the midfoot over the bony prominence; treatment is therefore recommended. In order to correct the deformity, often an extensive soft-tissue release and realignment of the entire midfoot and hindfoot are necessary. Dorsal subluxation of the midfoot is often associated with midfoot varus; therefore, in addition to the dorsal and medial release, a radical plantar release is also required. A simple open reduction of the talo-

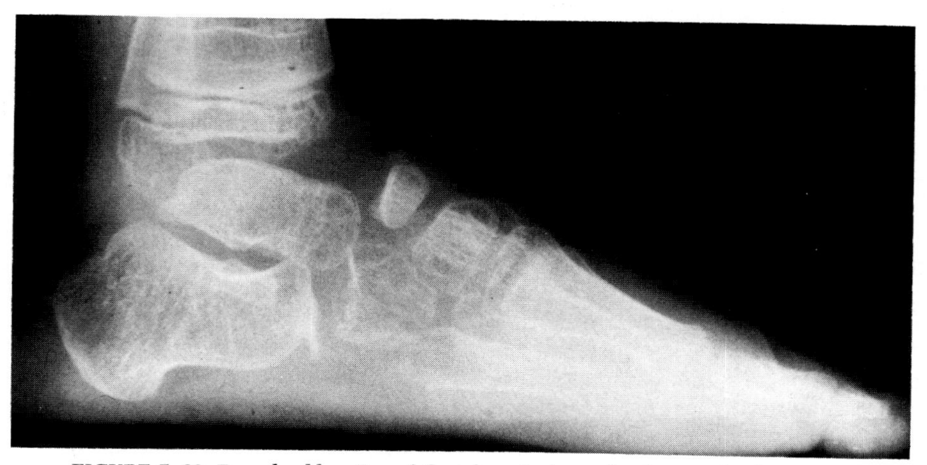

FIGURE 7–66. Dorsal subluxation of the talonavicular and calcaneocuboid joints.

navicular joint is inadequate. In the patient 12 years of age and older, triple arthrodesis may be necessary.

Lateral Talonavicular Subluxation

Etiology. This almost always results from overcorrection. Occasionally, in children with marked ligamentous hyperlaxity it develops later due to gradual lateral drift of the navicular on the head of the talus. In these rare cases due to ligamentous hyperlaxity, there is often associated rotatory valgus of the calcaneus.

Prevention. During open reduction and internal fixation of the talocalcaneonavicular joint the medial side of the navicular should *not* be flush with the medial side of the talus; instead, the navicular must be allowed to protrude medially to a slight degree—2 to 3 mm. in the infant to 5 to 7 mm. in the older child. There should be no step-off on the lateral side of the talonavicular joint. Paying attention and adhering to these anatomic criteria at surgery will greatly diminish the incidence of lateral talonavicular subluxation.

Treatment. Minimal lateral talonavicular subluxation does not require treatment, as there is no functional disability; this is in contrast to medial talonavicular subluxation, which is usually associated with poor results. Severe lateral talonavicular subluxation causes valgus at the midfoot. It is treated by repeat open reduction with extensive soft-tissue surgery. The rigid valgus foot in the older child is treated by medial displacement osteotomy: in the adolescent or adult triple arthrodesis may be required in order to provide a painless asymptomatic plantigrade foot.

Posterior Pes Cavus (Equinus Deformity of the Fore- and Midpart of the Foot at the Proximal Tarsal Joints). This is often associated with varying degrees of anterior cavus. It is caused by failure to adequately release the contracted plantar soft tissues.

Treatment. This is by thorough plantar release in the young child. The fixed deformity in the older child may require dorsal wedge resection of the tarsus.

Sagging of the Medial Longitudinal Arch (Pes Planus)

Etiology. Following the Turco procedure most clubfeet are flat; this is due to sectioning of the posterior tibial and not reattaching it. Collapse of the medial longitudinal arch also develops following anterolateral transfer of the posterior tibial tendon. Another cause of severe pes planus in clubfoot is radical plantar release in the presence of rocker-bottom foot or excessive ligamentous hyperlaxity.

Prevention. Posterior tibial release or primary transfer is contraindicated in clubfoot. Instead, the posterior tibial muscle function should be preserved by lengthening the tendon, preferably at the supramalleolar level; the Z-lengthened tendon should be repaired meticulously. Also, do not perform plantar release when there is rocker-bottom deformity. In children with clubfoot and excessive ligamentous hyperlaxity, preserve function of the plantar calcaneonavicular ligament.

Treatment. In the experience of Turco most of his clubfoot cases with resultant flat foot improved with growth and required no treatment.[706, 709] In the experience of this author, however, severe pes planovalgus due to sectioning of the posterior tibial tendon and plantar calcaneonavicular ligament persists; it does not improve with growth and can cause problems with abnormal shoe wear. In adult life the foot may become symptomatic. In childhood, support to the medial longitudinal arch by UCBL foot orthosis is indicated. Attempts at repair and reattachment of the posterior tibial tendon have been futile. In the skeletally mature foot with marked rigid planovalgum deformity and pain, bony procedures in the form of reverse Evans procedure with medial displacement osteotomy of the calcaneus or triple arthrodesis may be indicated.

Supination at the Midfoot. This deformity is due to incomplete correction at the talonavicular joint. Often, however, supination occurs at the forefoot due to dynamic muscle imbalance between an anterior tibial muscle of normal motor strength and a weak peroneus longus muscle.

Prevention. Supination at the midfoot can be prevented by careful concentric reduction and internal fixation of the talonavicular joint. Muscle imbalance between the anterior tibial and peroneus longus is not preventable—it is inherent in talipes equinovarus. Active progressive resistive exercises are performed to strengthen the weak peroneus longus muscle, and passive stretching exercises are carried out to elongate the shortened anterior tibial muscle. Dorsal bunion may develop in conjunction with supination deformity of the forefoot because the anterior tibial muscle dorsiflexes the first metatarsal, whereas the peroneus longus muscle plantar-flexes the first metatarsal.

Treatment. One may try a period of nonsurgical treatment in the form of an ankle-foot orthosis that pronates and plantar-flexes the forefoot; the orthosis is worn at night. Active and passive exercises are performed several times a day as outlined above. Often, however, when supination deformity becomes fixed, surgical treatment is indicated. A medial and dorsal release of the talonavicular, naviculocuneiform, and cuneiform–first metatarsal joints is performed. The bases of the second and third metatarsals are osteotomized if necessary. The mid- and forepart of the foot should passively pronate 20 to 30 degrees. Dynamic muscle balance is provided by split anterior tibial tendon transfer—the split lateral half of the anterior tibial tendon is transferred to the base of the cuboid bone, leaving its medial half intact and attached to its insertion. This preserves some function of the anterior tibial tendon as a dorsiflexor of the first metatarsal to balance its antagonist, the peroneus longus muscle, as a plantar-flexor of the first metatarsal. The operative technique is described and illustrated in Plate 98. In the experience of this author the results of split anterior tibial tendon transfer have been very satisfactory.

Medial Calcaneocuboid Subluxation. This is due to failure to reduce it at the time of open reduction of talipes equinovarus, due to inadequate release of the medial, plantar, and dorsal capsules and contracted ligaments of the calcaneocuboid joint. If a complete subtalar release is then performed, including an interosseous talocalcaneal ligament, and the lateral capsule of the calcaneocuboid joint is left intact, the calcaneus may rotate laterally to a markedly abnormal degree.

When calcaneocuboid medial subluxation is mild, i.e., *Grade 1,* which is equivalent to half the transverse distance of the calcaneus on the anteroposterior view, no treatment is indicated. When it is subluxated more than this, i.e., *Grade 2 or 3,* the calcaneocuboid joint should be opened completely on all four sides and reduced and pinned. If left untreated, it may cause hindfoot valgus when the navicular is reduced on the talar head. In *Grade 4* calcaneocuboid subluxation, the cuboid slips off the medial anterior end of the calcaneus and migrates proximally, and the whole midfoot seems to shift proximally. When the midfoot is then reduced on the hindfoot, the skin is under considerable tension and may not close. In treatment of *Grade 4* the distal end of the calcaneus is resected to reduce the cuboid.

COMPLICATIONS AT THE METATARSOTARSAL JOINTS

Complications that can occur at this level are metatarsus varus, metatarsus valgus, anterior pes cavus, and growth arrest of the physis of the first metatarsal.

Metatarsus Varus

Etiology. Metatarsus varus is due to inadequate release of or failure to release the contracted soft tissues on the medial aspect of the foot, namely, abductor hallucis, capsules of the first metatarsal–cuneiform and medial cuneiform–navicular joints, plantar fascia, and ligaments and muscles on the medial plantar aspect of the foot. Lowe and Hannon reviewed 73 clubfeet in 51 children between the ages of 4 and 14 years to determine the presence or absence of forefoot adduction as a residual deformity. The alignment of the feet was assessed clinically and by weight-bearing anteroposterior radiograms. The authors measured the degree of metatarsus varus by relating the position of the first metatarsal to the navicular bone. First, a line is drawn to join the extremities of the proximal articular surface of the navicular; then a central line is drawn through the longitudinal axis of the first metatarsal. The lateral angle formed by the junction of these two lines is the "naviculometatarsal angle" (Fig. 7–67). The authors admit the contribution of the naviculocuneiform and cuneiform-metatarsal joints to this measurement, but state that such distinction is of no practical value. The average naviculometatarsal angle of a normal foot is 93.5 degrees. A value in excess of 100 degrees repre-

Text continued on page 2538

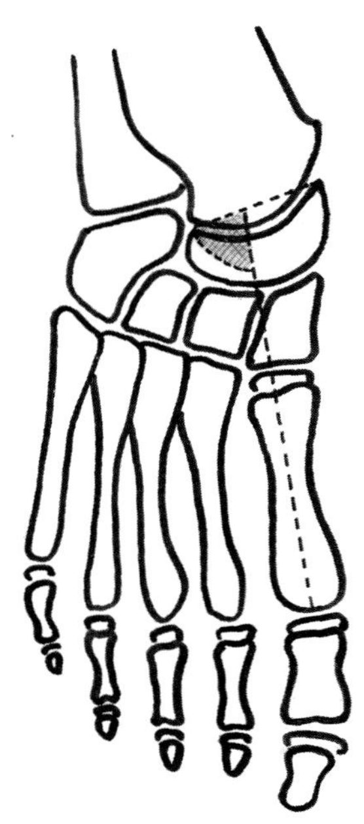

FIGURE 7–67. The naviculometatarsal angle.

The method of measurement is described in the text. (Redrawn after Lowe, L. W., and Hannon, M. A.: Residual adduction of the forefoot in treated congenital clubfoot. J. Bone Joint Surg., 55-*B*:810, 1973.)

Split Anterior Tibial Tendon Transfer

Operative Technique

A. A 5 cm. long incision is made over the dorsomedial aspect of the foot centered over the medial cuneiform. The subcutaneous tissue is divided in line with the skin incision. The skin margins are retracted. A second longitudinal incision, 5 to 7 cm. long, is made over the anterior aspect of the distal one third of the leg lateral to the crest of the tibia. The subcutaneous tissue is divided, and the anterior tibial tendon is identified at the musculotendinous juncture.

B. The anterior tibial tendon is identified with its sheath and carefully dissected to its insertion into the medial plantar aspect of the base of the first metatarsal.

Plate 98. Split Anterior Tibial Tendon Transfer

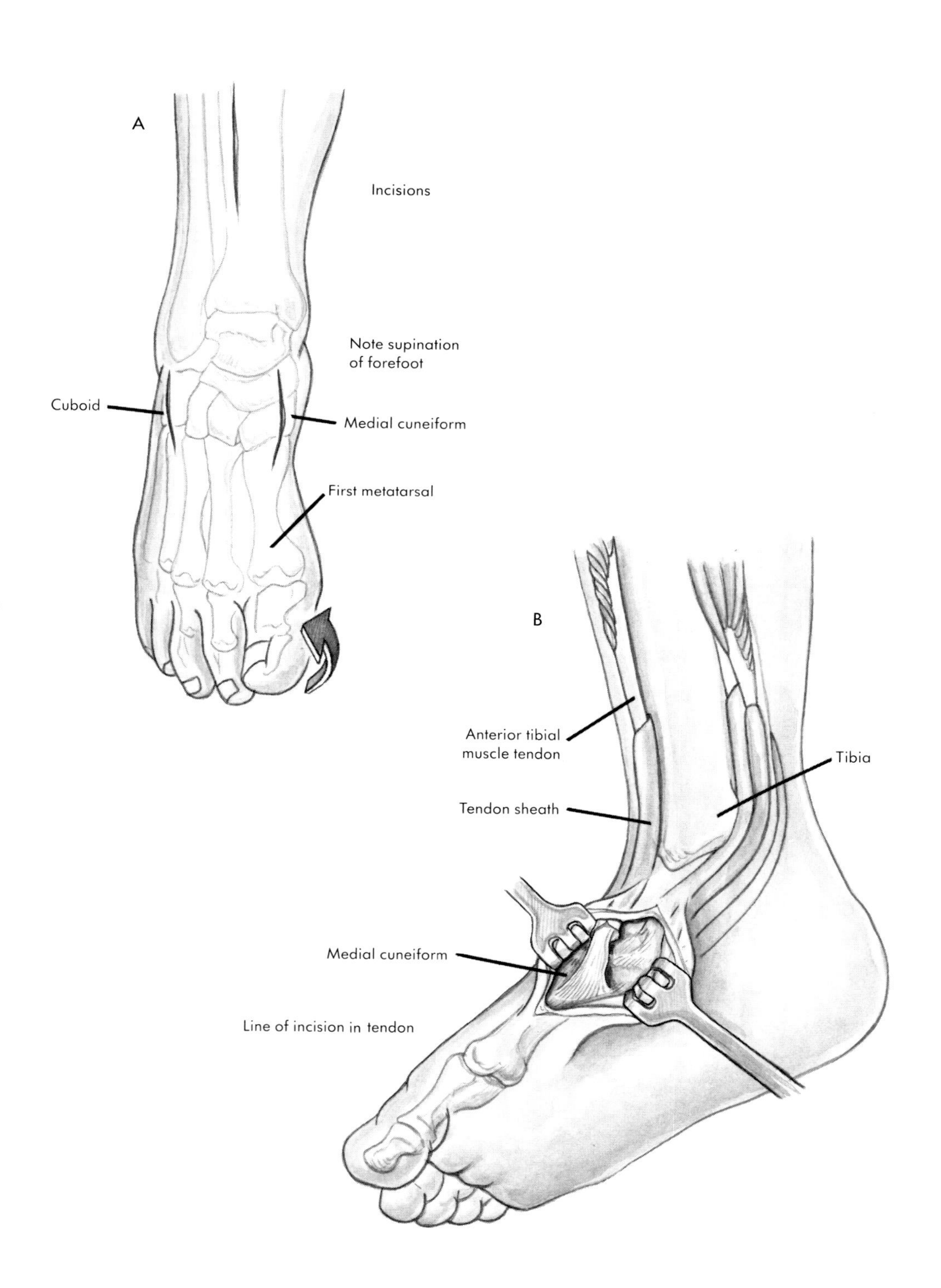

Split Anterior Tibial Tendon Transfer (*Continued*)

C. The anterior tibial tendon is split into two halves. The lateral half of the tendon is sectioned near its insertion to the base of the first metatarsal, taking meticulous attention not in injure the growth plate of the first metatarsal. The lateral half of the tendon is tagged with 00 Tycron suture.

D and E. An Ober tendon passer is inserted in the tendon shaft of the anterior tibial tendon, and the split lateral half of the tendon is delivered into the proximal wound.

Plate 98. Split Anterior Tibial Tendon Transfer

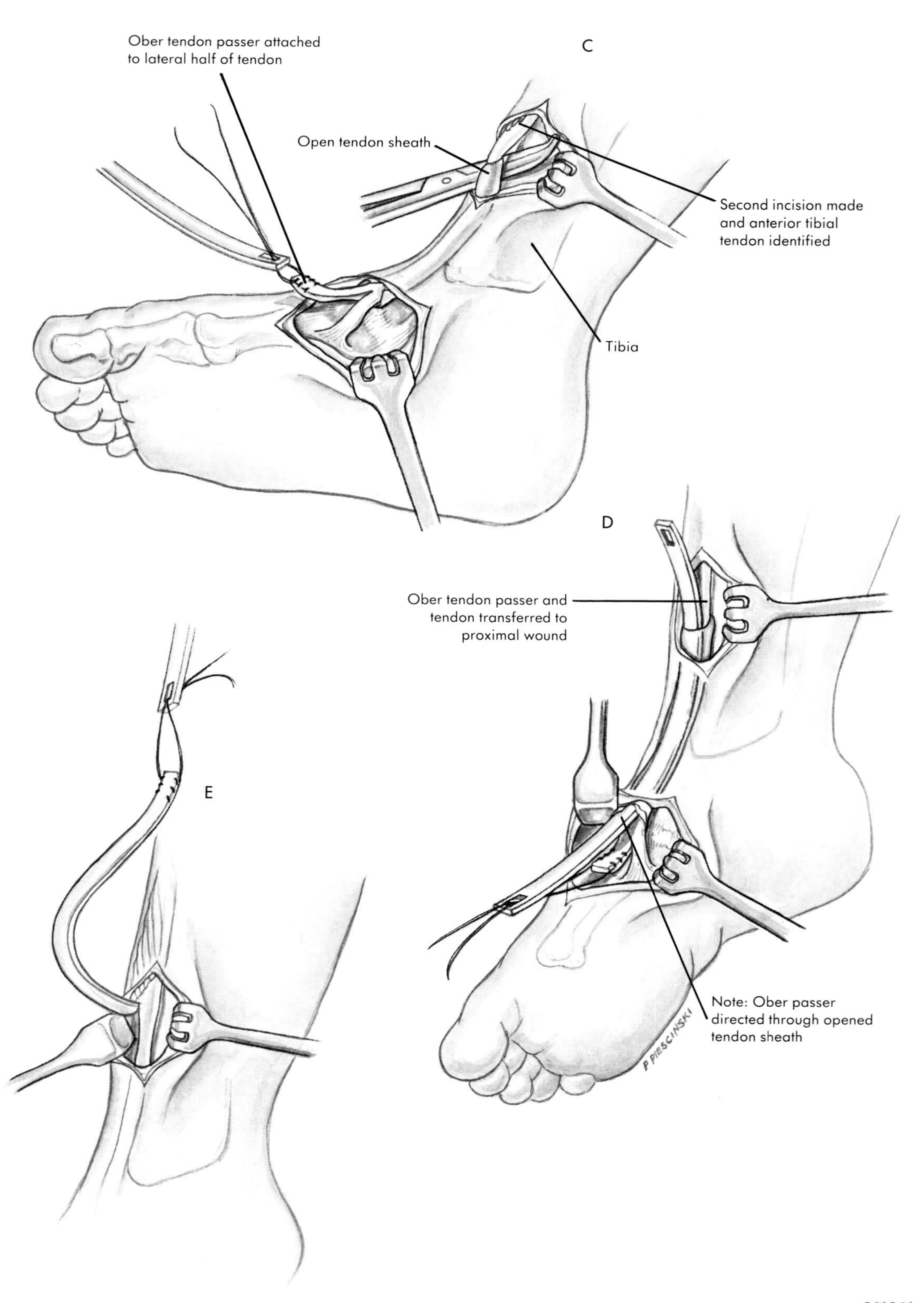

Split Anterior Tibial Tendon Transfer (Continued)

F and G. A third longitudinal incision is made over the dorsolateral aspect of the foot, 5 cm. longitudinal and centered over the cuboid. The lateral half of the anterior tibial tendon is delivered into a third wound subcutaneously deep to the extensor retinaculum with an Ober tendon passer. With an electric drill, two holes are made on the cuboid at converging angles.

H and I. The holes are joined at their depth with a small curet. Preserve the dorsal roof of the cuboid! Do not fracture it! The lateral half of the split anterior tibial tendon is passed into the holes and sutured to itself with the ankle in 5 to 10 degrees of dorsiflexion.

If the child's foot is small or the cuboid bone is osteoporotic, a drill hole is made in the cuboid bone, and with two Keith needles, the whip suture at the distal end of the split tendon is delivered into the plantar aspect of the foot. The tendon is firmly anchored in the hole in the cuboid bone, and the sutures are tied down firmly over a piece of sterile felt and a button with the foot in 5 degrees of dorsiflexion. (This technique is not illustrated in this drawing.) The tourniquet is released, and after complete hemostasis the wounds are closed in the usual fashion and a below-knee cast is applied.

Postoperative Care

Four weeks postoperatively, the cast is removed and active and passive exercises are performed to develop motor function over the anterior tibial muscle. A plastic splint is made to be worn at night, holding the ankle in 5 degrees of dorsiflexion or neutral position and the forefoot in 10 to 15 degrees of pronation.

Plate 98. Split Anterior Tibial Tendon Transfer

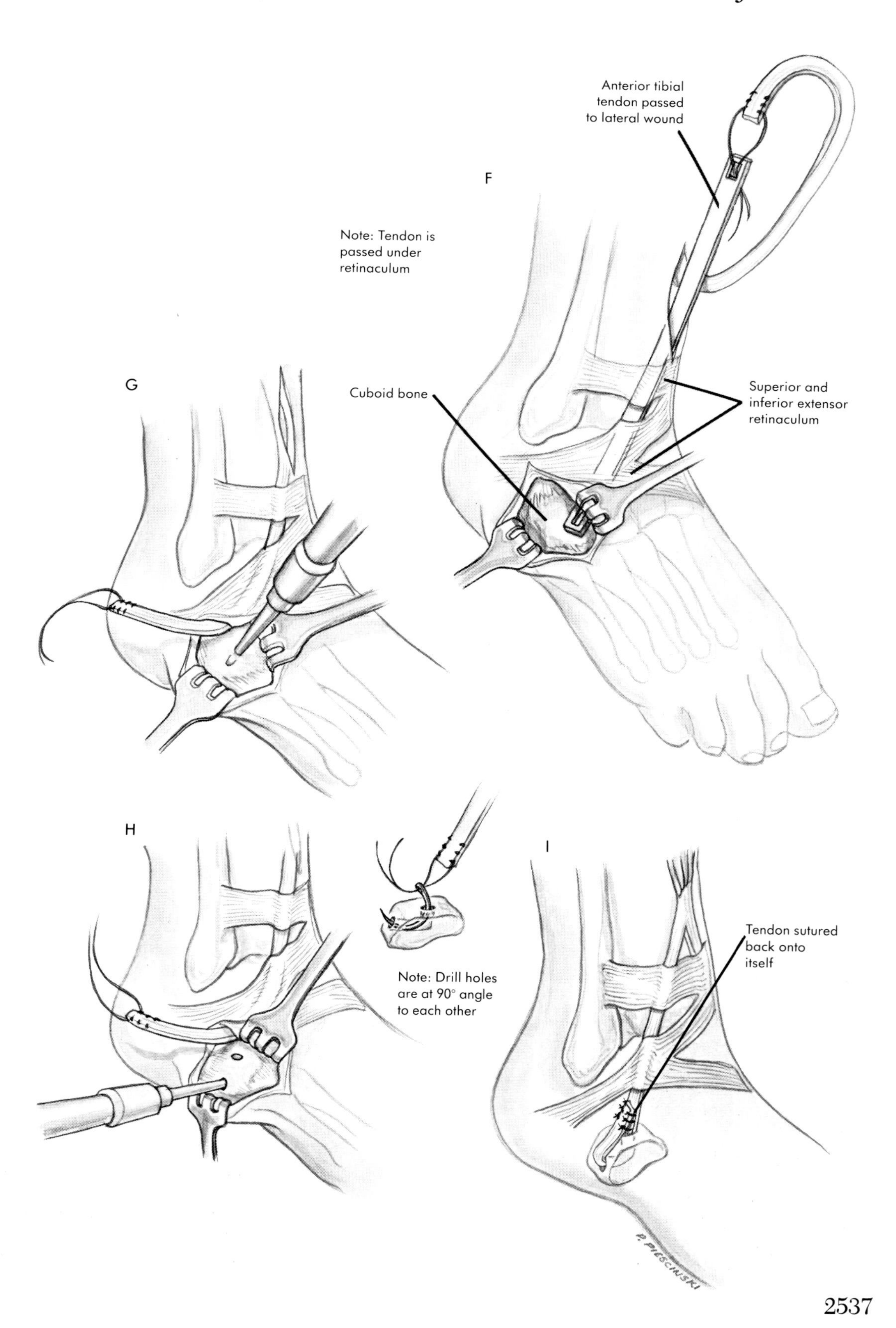

sents some degree of metatarsus varus. On clinical examination, they found forefoot adduction in 38 of 73 treated clubfeet (52 per cent). Radiographic study of the group with adduction showed metatarsus varus alone in 45 per cent and medial subluxation of the talonavicular joint alone in 26 per cent. Therefore, meticulous radiographic assessment and measurement showed that 74 per cent of the group with forefoot adduction had metatarsus varus. In the 35 feet with no residual forefoot adduction, only 45 per cent had normal radiographic features; in the remainder, i.e., 55 per cent, there were various forms of spurious correction—metatarsus varus with valgus overcorrection of the talonavicular joint, talonavicular medial subluxation with metatarsus valgus, and talonavicular medial subluxation with outward rotation of the ankle joint. Lowe and Hannon recommended detachment of the origin of the abductor hallucis muscle at the time of extended posterior release, with tenotomy of the tendon of insertion through a separate incision as an additional measure.[427]

Metatarsus varus may be associated with overcorrection of the hindfoot (hinged valgus), resulting in skew or serpentine foot.[709]

Prevention. The problem of forefoot varus can be obviated by performing a meticulous medial and plantar release. This author recommends excision of the abductor hallucis muscle; other surgeons may prefer to section or recess the origin of the abductor hallucis. Capsulotomy of the first metatarsal cuneiform joint may be indicated. In the severe clubfoot it can be combined with osteotomy of the base of the second metatarsal.

Treatment. Wynne-Davies has stated that metatarsus varus corrects spontaneously with time.[769] In the experience of this author, spontaneous correction generally does not occur, and in the cases when there is some improvement, it is incomplete. The *mild* deformities are treated by stretching exercises, cast, and night splinting. The moderate cases require surgical treatment in the form of medial release—abductor hallucis resection and capsulotomy of the first metatarsal-tarsal joint and osteotomy of the bases of the second metatarsal or second and third metatarsals at their base. The severe metatarsus varus deformity is corrected by Heymann-Herndon-Strong tarsometatarsal capsulotomies and intermetatarsal ligamentous release if the child is less than six years of age; in a child seven years age or older, valgus osteotomy at the bases of the second to fourth metatarsals with capsulotomy of the first metatarsal-tarsal joint is performed. If there is associated midfoot varus the procedure can be combined with closing-wedge osteotomy of the cuboid and opening-wedge osteotomy of the medial cuneiform.

Forefoot Abduction

Etiology. This rare complication is a late consequence of calcaneocuboid joint resection and fusion (Evans procedure), especially when performed at a young age; valgus of the mid- and forefoot develops with subsequent overgrowth of the medial column and tethering of the lateral column of the foot. Overcorrection into valgus during metatarsal osteotomy and capsulotomy ligamentous release of the tarsometatarsal joints (Heymann-Herndon-Strong procedure) are other occasional causes of forefoot abduction.

Prevention. Evans procedure should not be performed for shortening of the lateral column of the foot in children under eight years of age. Instead, for correction of midfoot or forefoot varus this author recommends anterolateral vertical closing-wedge osteotomy of the calcaneus or resection of the anterior end of the calcaneus. Overcorrection into valgus when performing metatarsal osteotomy should be avoided.

Treatment. Reverse Evans procedure, i.e., opening-wedge osteotomy of the fused calcaneocuboid joint or anterior calcaneus, will correct the deformity if the cause of the deformity was the Evans procedure. When the forefoot valgus is due to overcorrection by previous metatarsal-tarsal soft-tissue release or metatarsal osteotomy, medial angulation osteotomy of the metatarsals or repeat soft-tissue release may be indicated. This author recommends a trial period of stretching cast initially, prior to surgical intervention.

Anterior Pes Cavus. In this form of pes cavus the forefoot is in fixed equinus at the metatarsal-tarsal joint. It is due to failure to perform adequate plantar release. Prevention and treatment are by thorough plantar release. In the older child with fixed bony deformity, dorsal wedge osteotomy is indicated, either of the first ray alone or at the metatarsal (cuneiform-cuboid) area if all the metatarsals are fixed in equinus.

Growth Arrest of the Physis of the First Metatarsal. This is caused inadvertently when performing capsulotomy of the first metatarsal-tarsal joint or osteotomy at the base of the first metatarsal. It results in a short first metatarsal with abnormal stresses of weight-bearing on the second or third metatarsal heads. The deformity can be quite disabling. If the physeal arrest is asymmetrical, i.e., medial part fused and lateral part open, the short first metatarsal will deviate into varus.

Prevention. During capsulotomy use the anterior tibial tendon insertion as a guide to the first metatarsal-cuneiform joint and dissect distally from the medial cuneiform to the articulation. If in doubt, radiograms should be made to determine the level of the metatarsophalangeal joint.

Treatment. Physeal bar excision may be attempted if less than 50 per cent of the growth plate is closed by the osseous bridge. Angular deformity may be corrected by a single or multiple open-up wedge osteotomy. The first ray can be lengthened instantaneously and bone grafted; or it may be lengthened gradually using Ilizarov or DeBastiani technique.

COMPLICATIONS AT THE METATARSOPHALANGEAL JOINT LEVEL

Complications include dorsal bunion, hammer toe, and hallux varus.

Dorsal Bunion. This is caused by dynamic imbalance of motor strength between a strong anterior tibial muscle (dorsiflexor of the first metatarsal) and a weak peroneus longus muscle (plantar-flexor of the first metatarsal). The peroneus longus may be inherently weak due to stretched-out muscle or occasionally it may have been inadvertently transected at surgery. In the young child electromyographic studies may be employed to ascertain motor status of the peroneal muscles. Other causes of dorsal bunion are conditions that markedly sag the medial longitudinal arch of the foot. The dorsal bunion is produced by the following mechanism: decrease of the medial longitudinal arch increases tension on the flexor hallucis brevis, which in turn places tension on the proximal interphalangeal joint and gradually elevates the fixed metatarsal head. Various factors that may cause loss of the longitudinal arch are pre-existing flat foot, rocker-bottom deformity of the foot, excessive plantar release, ligamentous laxity, release or transfer of the posterior tibial tendon, and overlengthening of the Achilles tendon. Other etiologic factors are a short flexor hallucis longus or an adhesed flexor hallucis longus following previous lengthening, contracted flexor hallucis brevis, and pin fixation of the talonavicular joint with the forefoot in supination.

Prevention. Plantar release is contraindicated in the presence of either flat foot or rocker-bottom deformity, as it will only enhance these deformities, which may then lead to dorsal bunion formation.

Split anterior tibial tendon transfer, with the lateral half transferred to the peroneus longus tendon as it passes underneath the cuboid bone, will balance muscle forces acting on the first metatarsal.

Treatment. McKay's procedure—transferring the flexor hallucis brevis and the adductor and abductor tendons to the dorsum of the first metatarsal—often corrects dorsal bunion. In the older patient, volar wedge osteotomy of the proximal first metatarsal and transfer of the flexor hallucis longus to the neck of the first metatarsal may be required.

Hammer Toe. This rare complication develops when the long toe flexors are taut and not lengthened during extensive soft-tissue surgery. When at the time of open reduction of the talocalcaneonavicular and calcaneocuboid joint the toes cannot be extended passively to neutral position, the long-toe flexors and the flexor hallucis longus tendons should be lengthened at their musculotendinous junction at several levels. It is best not to perform Z-plasty of the long-toe flexors and flexor hallucis longus on the plantar aspect of the foot because of risk of scar formation and adherence and contracture.

Treatment. Interphalangeal joint fusion will correct the rigid hammer toe.

Hallux Varus. This is often associated with flexion deformity in the first ray, due to contracture of the flexor hallucis brevis. The deformity is corrected by Z-lengthening of the tendon just proximal to its insertion. Occasionally, the lateral toes tend to follow the great toe into varus derotation; this is treated by lengthening the common flexor tendon.

BONE COMPLICATIONS

These include transection of the sustentaculum tali, sectioning of the head of the talus, aseptic necrosis of the talus, and aseptic necrosis of the navicular.

Transection of the Sustentaculum Tali. This can occur inadvertently in the hands of the inexperienced surgeon when performing medial subtalar release. It is important to be cognizant of the sinusoidal S-shaped configuration of the subtalar joint medially. Use the flexor hallucis longus tendon as a guide to medial subtalar joint for release—the tendon traverses beneath the sustentaculum tali. Occasionally there may be cartilaginous coalition medially between the talus and calcaneus; when excising this cartilaginous bar it should be done very cautiously in order not to transect the sustentaculum tali. Treatment consists of repositioning of the detached sustentaculum tali and fixing it with two threaded Kirschner wires.

Transection of the Talar Head. This occurs when the inexperienced surgeon attempts to open the talonavicular joint, not recognizing that the talar head often lies deep within the joint. When it is difficult to visualize the head of the talus, this author recommends continuing dissection from both the lateral and medial aspects. The navicular is displaced medially and proximally on the talus; it is important to free the navicular in the proximal to distal (heel to toe) direction and not in a medial to lateral direction. If the talar head is transected it should be replaced and fixed with one or two threaded Kirschner wires. Occasionally, the talar head will have been flattened by cast treatment, leading the surgeon to suspect that the head has been amputated.

Aseptic Necrosis of Talus. The blood supply of the talus is derived principally from the artery of the tarsal sinus entering from the anterolateral side of the talus, from the artery of the tarsal canal on its posteromedial aspect, and from a rich source from the medial surface distal to the articular facet of the medial malleolus. The major blood supply to the body of the talus enters through the neck of the talus.[264] There is a definite hazard of interruption of the blood supply to the body of the talus when extensive peritalar release is performed. Vascular injury to the three major blood sources proximal to their anastomoses may occur, or one may interrupt circulation at the entrance of the vascular network into the anteroinferior portion of the talar neck. Aplington and Riddle studied 321 congenital clubfeet in 203 patients retrospectively. Thirty-five of these patients had extensive combined medial and lateral release; five of them, or 14.3 per cent, developed aseptic necrosis of the body of the talus. No aseptic necrosis of the talus was found when the medial release was done alone or combined with posterior release, even when the subtalar joint was released from the medial side. In all cases with aseptic necrosis, however, the medial release was combined with extensive lateral dissection, including the sinus tarsi and the subtalar joint, which was released both medially and laterally. Aplington and Riddle strongly urged the surgeon to refrain from lateral dissection of the subtalar joint, particularly of the sinus tarsi, in conjunction with medial release.[15]

Schlafly and associates reported one instance of avascular necrosis of the talus in 51 cases of clubfeet.[618]

This author has avoided aseptic necrosis of the talus by not disturbing the circulation of the superolateral aspect of the neck of the talus and by not entering the sinus tarsi.

Treatment. Treatment consists of supporting the talus by a patellar tendon bearing (PTB) ankle-foot orthosis. Cancellous and cortical autogenous bone grafting may be tried; this author has had satisfactory results with bone grafting in post-traumatic avascular necrosis of the talus, but has had no personal experience in aseptic necrosis of the talus in clubfoot.

Aseptic Necrosis of the Navicular. This complication is especially likely to occur if the naviculocuneiform capsule is released. Schlafly and co-workers reported two cases of aseptic necrosis of the navicular in their 81 surgical cases; an additional five patients experienced fragmentation of the navicular. All of these were associated with either delayed ossification or multiple ossification centers.[618] Miller and Bernstein observed wedging and truncation of the navicular in 20 of their 24 feet (86 per cent), but did not comment on the long-term effect.[492] These changes, however, may be related to excessive pressure rather than to avascular changes.

Treatment. Treatment consists of support to the longitudinal arch of the foot. There is no functional impairment. Revascularization of the navicular bone will take place without difficulty and the bone will reossify.

Rigidity of the Foot. Rigidity is prevented by carrying out very gentle manipulations and avoiding hyaline cartilage compression and cartilage necrosis. During surgery, injury to joint cartilage should be avoided.

NEUROVASCULAR COMPLICATIONS

Spasm of the posterior tibial artery may occur occasionally following dissection around the neurovascular bundle. The tourniquet should be released and the blood supply checked; if no transection is located, bathing the vessels in a papavarine-soaked sponge relieves the spasm.

Transection of the neurovascular bundle is extremely rare and usually is associated with badly scarred, previously operated feet or an anomalous position of the neurovascular bundle. When dissecting a previously operated foot, it is helpful to dissect the neurovascular bundle "en bloc" along with the encasing fibrous tissue off the medial surface of the talus to the level of the branching vessels in the subtalar region. If the bundle is transected, the assistance of a microsurgeon or vascular surgeon should be obtained immediately.

The transfixation pins may puncture or spear the neurovascular bundle or its branches. It is important to release the tourniquet and achieve complete hemostasis before wound closure.

LOSS OF REDUCTION AND RECURRENCE OF DEFORMITY

Recurrence of deformity may result from the following: (1) failure to achieve concentric reduction initially—this is a spurious recurrence; (2) loss of reduction in the immediate postoperative period due to inadequate internal fixation; (3) persistence of primary deformity of the talus, i.e., decreased angle of declination of the head-neck of the talus; (4) scar tissue formation; and (5) dynamic imbalance of muscles acting on the foot-ankle.

So-called recurrence of deformity is often due to failure to achieve concentric reduction at the time of initial surgery. To ensure restoration of normal articular relations, it is imperative that intraoperative radiograms of the foot and ankle be made in two planes—true anteroposterior and true lateral. Is there a normal angle of talocalcaneal divergence in the anteroposterior and lateral projections? This author uses a threaded Steinmann pin to transfix the talonavicular joint. If the talocalcaneal interosseous ligament is divided, the talocalcaneal joint should be internally fixed with one or two threaded Steinmann pins. A smooth pin may slip out. It is vital to provide secure internal fixation to maintain reduction for a period of three to four weeks; the soft tissues should heal.

A retentive apparatus, such as an ankle-foot orthosis (AFO) holding the foot-ankle in slightly overcorrected position, should be utilized at night and at naptime for an adequate period. The decreased angle of declination of the talus should straighten to normal, and all articular malalignments should be corrected with skeletal growth and remodeling.

In some cases talocalcaneal navicular subluxation recurs because of persistent medial and plantar tilting of the head and neck of the talus. Hjelmstedt and Sahlstedt performed a chevron osteotomy of the neck of the talus to correct the deformity and realign the declination angle of the talus to normal.[301, 305, 306] Roberts described an open-up osteotomy of the neck of the talus with bone graft from the ilium.[594] This author concurs with Roberts and recommends his technique; it should not, however, be a primary procedure and should not be performed on a child under three years of age.

It is essential to pay meticulous attention to postoperative care; passive exercises are performed to maintain a normal range of joint motion, and active exercises are carried out to establish a dynamic balance of muscles acting on the foot and ankle. Scarring on the medial and plantar aspects of the foot should be avoided; the tethering pull of scar tissue will cause recurrence of deformity.

References

1. Abrams, R. C.: Relapsed club foot. The early results of an evaluation of Dillwyn Evans' operation. J. Bone Joint Surg., *51-A*:270, 1969.
2. Adam, A.: Tibialis posterior transfer in relapsed clubfoot. J. Bone Joint Surg., *45-B*:804, 1963.
3. Adams, W.: A series of four specimens illustrating the morbid anatomy of congenital club-foot (talipes varus). Trans. Pathol. Soc. London, *6*:348, 1854–1855.
4. Adams, W.: Club Foot, Its Causes, Pathology and Treatment. London, J. & A. Churchill, 1866.
5. Addison, A., Fixsen, J. A., and Lloyd-Roberts, G. C.: A review of the Dillwyn Evans-type collateral operation in severe club feet. J. Bone Joint Surg., *65-B*:12, 1983.
6. Adelaar, R. S., and Kyles, M. K.: Surgical correction of resistant talipes equinovarus: Observations and analysis—preliminary report. Foot Ankle, *2*:126, 1981.
7. Agerholm-Christensen, J.: On Denis Browne's treatment of club-foot. Acta Orthop. Scand., *19*:134, 1949.
8. Albanese, M., Basile, N., and Carbone, C.: Rilievi clinici statistici sul piede torto congenito. Orriz. Ortop. Odierna. Riabilit., *5*:443, 1960.
9. Alberman, E. D.: The causes of congenital club foot. Arch. Dis. Child., *40*:548, 1965.
10. Alldred, A. J.: Early surgery for the correction of congenital clubfoot. N. Z. Med. J., *65*:665, 1966.
11. Altchek, M.: Molding the talus. A method of treating clubfoot. Clin. Orthop., *84*:44, 1972.
12. Altchek, M., and Bleck, E. E.: Congenital club feet. Clin. Orthop., *130*:303, 1978.
13. Amor, R., Pener, E., and Yannez, P. R.: The treatment of congenital clubfoot. *In* Delchef, J. (ed.): Orthopaedic Surgery and Traumatology. Congenital clubfoot. d. Neglected and inveterate cases. New York, American Elsevier, 1973.
14. Apley, A. G.: Talipes (clubfoot). *In* A System of Orthopaedics and Fractures. 3rd Ed. New York, Appleton-Century-Crofts, 1968, pp. 194–220.
15. Aplington, J. P., and Riddle, C. D.: Avascular necrosis of the body of the talus after combined medial and lateral release of congenital clubfoot. South. Med. J., *69*:1037, 1976.
16. Aranes, A., and Villadot, P.: Clinica y tratamiento de las enfermedades del pie. Pie equino varo congenito. Barcelona, Editorial Cientifico Medica, 1956, p. 201.
17. Aritamur, A.: Une malformation congénitale rare de pied. Rev. Chir. Orthop., *57*:151, 1971.
18. Ashby, M. E.: Roentgenographic assessment of soft tissue medial release operations in clubfoot deformity. Clin. Orthop., *90*:146, 1973.
19. Asher, M.: Plantar release in the correction of deformities of the foot in childhood (letter). J. Bone Joint Surg., *64-A*:790, 1982.
20. Assum, H. W.: Untersuchungen über die Erblichkeit des angeborenen Klumpfussleidens. Z. Orthop., *65*:1, 1936.
21. Atlas, S.: The morbid anatomy of clubfoot in the embryo and fetus. *In* Delchef, J. (ed.): Orthopaedic Surgery and Traumatology. Congenital clubfoot. a. Anatomy and pathology of the disease. New York, American Elsevier, 1973, pp. 753–754.
22. Attenborough, C. G.: Severe congenital talipes equinovarus. J. Bone Joint Surg., *48-B*:31, 1966.
23. Attenborough, C. G.: Early posterior soft-tissue re-

lease in severe congenital talipes equinovarus. Clin. Orthop., *84*:71, 1972.
24. Axer, A., and Segal, D.: Transfer of Achilles tendon to the lateral aspect of the calcaneus in the treatment of clubfeet. *In* Delchef, J. (ed.): Orthopaedic Surgery and Traumatology. Congenital clubfoot. c. Surgical treatment in later childhood. New York, American Elsevier, 1973, pp. 769–771.
25. Bachmann, R.: Klinisches und röntgenologisches Behandlungsergebnis angeborener Klumpfüsse nach 5 Jahren. Zentralbl. Chir., *78*:1738, 1953.
26. Barcat, J., and Preyssas, J.: Le rôle des transplantations tendineuses dans le pied bot varus équin congenital. J. Chir., *79*:29, 1960.
27. Bardeen, C. R., and Lewis, W. H.: Development of limbs, body-wall and back in man. Am. J. Anat., *1*:1, 1901.
28. Barenfeld, P. A., and Weseley, M. S.: Surgical treatment of congenital clubfoot. Clin. Orthop., *84*:79, 1972.
29. Barenfeld, P. A., and Weseley, M. S.: Talipes equinovarus: "Hard" versus "soft" tissues. Clin. Orthop., *123*:109, 1977.
30. Barenfeld, P. A., Weseley, M. S., and Munter, M.: Dwyer calcaneal osteotomy. Clin. Orthop., *84*:79, 1972.
31. Bartholini, T.: De Observationibus Raris Medicorum. Acta Med. et Phil. Hafn., *2*:1, 1673.
32. Bartsolas, C. S.: Hephaestus and clubfoot. J. Hist. Med. Allied Sci., *27*:450, 1972.
33. Barwell, R.: On various forms of talipes as depicted by x-ray. Lancet, *2*:160, 234, 1521, 1896.
34. Batchelor, J. S.: Treatment of the uncorrected clubfoot in childhood. Proc. R. Soc. Med., *39*:713, 1946.
35. Batory, I.: Contribution to the etiology of congenital torticollis and congenital clubfoot. Z. Orthop., *120*:742, 1982.
36. Beals, R. K.: Club foot in the Maori: A genetic study of 50 kindreds. N. Z. Med. J., *88*:144, 1978.
37. Beatson, R. R., and Pearson, J. R.: A method assessing correction in club feet. J. Bone Joint Surg., *48-B*:40, 1966.
38. Beau, A., Prevot, J., and Mathieu, P.: Resultats de l'allongement des parties molles internes et postérieures dans le traitement du pied bot varus équin congénital. Ann. Chir. Infant., *1*:91, 1960.
39. Bechtol, C. O., and Mossman, H. W.: Club-foot; embryological study of associated muscle abnormalities. J. Bone Joint Surg., *32-A*:827, 1950.
40. Bell, J. F., and Grice, D. S.: Treatment of congenital talipes equinovarus with the modified Denis Browne splint. J. Bone Joint Surg., *26*:799, 1944.
41. Belloc, J.: Congenital talipes equinovarus. Bol. Med. Hosp. Infant. Mex., *22*:13, 1965.
42. Ben-Menachem, Y., and Butler, J. E.: Arteriography of the foot in congenital deformities. J. Bone Joint Surg., *56-A*:1625, 1974.
43. Bennet, G. A., and Bauer, W.: Further studies concerning the repair of articular cartilage in dog joints. J. Bone Joint Surg., *17*:141, 1935.
44. Bensahel, H.: Bilan de vingt années de traitement fonctionnel du pied-bot dans le premier âge. *In* Delchef, J. (ed.): Orthopaedic Surgery and Traumatology. Congenital clubfoot. b. Early childhood conservative and surgical treatment. New York, American Elsevier, 1973, p. 759.
45. Bensahel, H., Degrippes, Y., and Billot, C.: Comments about 600 club feet. Chir. Pediatr., *21*:335, 1980.
46. Bensahel, H., Huguenin, P., and Themar-Noel, C.: The functional anatomy of clubfoot. J. Pediatr. Orthop., *3*:191, 1983.
47. Bensahel, H., Csukonyi, Z., Desgrippes, Y., and Chaumien, J. P.: Surgery in residual clubfoot: One-stage medioposterior release "a la carte." J. Pediatr. Orthop., *7*:145, 1987.
48. Bentzon, P. G. K., and Thomasen, E.: On treatment of congenital clubfoot. Acta Orthop. Scand., *11*:129, 1940.
49. Berenstein, S. S.: Classification of congenital clubfoot. Ortop. Travmatol. Protez., *5*:32, 1983.
50. Berg, H. W.: Club-foot. Arch. Med., *8*:226, 1882.
51. Bergonzoli, E.: Contributo alla cura del piede torto congenito. Risultati delgi interventi cruenti sulle parti molli del piede torto recidivo. Arch. Ital. Ortop., *56*:378, 1940.
52. Berman, A., and Gartland, J. J.: Metatarsal osteotomy for the correction of adduction of the forepart of the foot in children. J. Bone Joint Surg., *53-A*:498, 1971.
53. Bernardczyk, K., Marciniak, W., and Lempicki, A.: Dwyer's operation in the treatment of equino-varus talipes. Chir. Narzadow Ruchu Ortop. Pol., *43*:179, 1978.
54. Bernbeck, R.: Zur Pathologie des angeborenen Klumpfusses. Das Klumpfussproblem im Lichte der pathologischen Anatomie und Histologie. Z. Orthop., *79*:521, 1950.
55. Bertelsen, A.: Treatment of congenital club foot. J. Bone Joint Surg., *39-B*:599, 1957.
56. Bertelsen, A., and Jansen, K.: Treatment of congenital clubfoot. J. Bone Joint Surg., *39-B*:599, 1957.
57. Bertini, S., Guerra, A., and Romano, B.: L'intervento di Codivilla nella cura del piede torto congenito. Chir. Organi Mov., *59*:460, 1970.
58. Bertola, L.: Sindesmocapsulotomia tibio-astragalica posteriore ei allungamento plastico del tendine di Achille nella cura precoce del piede torto congenito. Arch. Ortop., *62*:229, 1949.
59. Bertrand, P.: L'arthrographie dans le pied bot congénital. Rev. Orthop., *33*:548, 1947.
60. Bessel-Hagen, F. C.: Die Pathologie und Therapie des Klumpfusses. Heidelberg, O. Peters, 1889.
61. Bethem, D., and Weiner, D.: Radical one-stage postero-medial release for the resistant clubfoot. Clin. Orthop., *131*:214, 1978.
62. Bick, E. M.: Morphology and genetics. *In* Source Book of Orthopaedics. 2nd Ed. Baltimore, Williams & Wilkins, 1948, pp. 140–153.
63. Biezin, A. P.: Modification of the operation of soft tissues in children with congenital clubfoot. Khirurgiia (Mosk.), *41*:115, 1965.
64. Bissell, J. B.: The morbid anatomy of congenital talipes equinovarus. Arch. Pediatr., *5*:406, 1888.
65. Bjonnes, T.: Congenital clubfoot. A follow-up of 95 persons treated in Sweden from 1940–1945 with special reference to their social adaptation and subjective symptoms from the foot. Acta Orthop. Scand., *46*:848, 1975.
66. Bleck, E. E.: Congenital clubfoot. Pathomechanics, radiographic analysis, and results of surgical treatment. Clin. Orthop., *125*:119, 1977.
67. Blockey, N. J., and Smith, M. G. H.: The treatment of congenital club foot. J. Bone Joint Surg., *48-B*:660, 1966.
68. Blokhin, V. N.: Plastic splints for therapy of congenital clubfoot. Vestn. Khir., *70*:55, 1950.
69. Bluhm, M.: Modification of the Denis Browne splint. J. Bone Joint Surg., *29*:248, 1947.
70. Blumenfeld, I.: The treatment of clubfoot in the newborn by the Denis Browne splint. *In* Delchef, J. (ed.): Orthopaedic Surgery and Traumatology. Congenital clubfoot. b. Early childhood—conservative and surgical treatment. New York, American Elsevier, 1973, pp. 756–758.
71. Blumenfeld, I., Kaplan, N., and Hicks, E. O.: The conservative treatment of congenital talipes equinovarus. J. Bone Joint Surg., *28*:765, 1946.
72. Bogdanov, F. R., and Melikdzhanian, Z. G.: Congen-

ital clubfoot and its surgical treatment. Ortop. Travmatol. Protez., *35:*33, 1974.
73. Böhm, M.: Zur Pathologie und Röntgenologie des angeborenen Klumfusses. Munchen Med. Wochenschr., *55:*1492, 1928.
74. Böhm, M.: The embryologic origin of clubfoot. J. Bone Joint Surg., *11:*229, 1929.
75. Book, M.: A contribution to the genetics of clubfoot. Hereditas (Lund), *34:*289, 1948.
76. Boppe and Estève: Le traitement du pied bot varus équin congénital de la deuxieme ou moyenne. Rev. Chir. Orthop., *34:*403, 1948.
77. Bornbeck, R.: Zur Pathologie des angeborenen Klumpfusses. Z. Orthop., *79:*521, 1950.
78. Bösch, I.: Zur Technik der Klumpfussbehandlung. Z. Orthop., *94:*159, 1961.
79. Bost, F. C., Schottstaedt, E. R., and Larsen, L. J.: Plantar dissection. An operation to release the soft tissues in recurrent or recalcitrant talipes equinovarus. J. Bone Joint Surg., *42-A:*151, 1960.
80. Bostos-Mora, F.: On the surgical treatment of congenital talipes equinovarus. Cir. Ginec. Urol. (Madrid), *19:*265, 1965.
81. Bouvier, H.: Leçons cliniques sur les maladies chroniques de l'appareil locomoteur. Paris, J. B. Ballière, 1858.
82. Brockman, E. P.: Congenital Clubfoot (Talipes Equinovarus). Bristol, John Wright & Sons; New York, William Wood & Co., 1930.
83. Brockman, E. P.: Modern methods of treatment of clubfoot. Br. Med. J., *2:*572, 1937.
84. Brockway, A.: Surgical correction of talipes cavus deformities. J. Bone Joint Surg., *22:*81, 1940.
85. Brodell, J. D., Axon, D. L., and McCollister Evarts, C.: The Robert Jones bandage. J. Bone Joint Surg., *69-B:*776, 1987.
86. Brown, L. T.: The treatment of club feet. J. Bone Joint Surg., *18:*173, 1936.
87. Browne, D.: Congenital malformations. Practitioner, *131:*20, 1933.
88. Browne, D.: Talipes equinovarus. Lancet, *2:*909, 1934.
89. Browne, D.: Congenital deformities of mechanical origin. Proc. R. Soc. Med., *29:*1409, 1936.
90. Browne, D.: Congenital deformities of mechanical origin. Arch. Dis. Child., *30:*37, 1955.
91. Browne, D.: Splinting for controlled movement. Clin. Orthop., *8:*91, 1956.
92. Browne, D.: The pathology and classification of talipes. Aust. N. Z. J. Surg., *29:*85, 1959.
93. Browne, D.: Talipes equinovarus (letter to the editor). Lancet, *1:*863, 1962.
94. Burgess, E. M.: Dynamic restoration of muscle imbalance in recurrent club foot. *In* Proceedings. Annual Meeting of the Association of Bone and Joint Surgeons. J. Bone Joint Surg., *38-A:*947, 1956.
95. Burian, F.: The "whistling face" characteristic in a compound cranio-facio-corporal syndrome. Br. J. Plast. Surg., *46:*140, 1963.
96. Burrell, H. L.: A contribution to the anatomy of congenital equinovarus. Ann. Surg., *17:*293, 1893.
97. Cabanac, J., Petit, P., and Maschas, A.: Le traitement du pied bot varus équin congénital. Reports XXVII Réunion Annuelle de la Société Française D'Orthopédie et de Traumatologie. Rev. Chir. Orthop., *38:*314, 1952.
98. Calandruccio, R. A., and Gilmer, W. S.: Proliferation, regeneration and repair of articular cartilage of immature animals. J. Bone Joint Surg., *44-A:*314, 1952.
99. Camera, U.: Mon expérience dans le traitement de pied bot congénital. Rev. Chir. Orthop., *38:*525, 1952.
100. Campos da Paz, A., Jr., and DeSouza, V.: Talipes equinovarus: Pathomechanical basis of treatment. Orthop. Clin. North Am., *9:*171, 1978.
101. Capecchi, V., and Casini, E.: Sul trattamento chirurgico del piede torto congenito inveterato. Arch. Putti Chir. Organi Mov., *3:*121, 1953.
102. Capener, N.: Congenital clubfoot. J. Bone Joint Surg., *44-B:*956, 1962.
103. Carlioz, H.: Les ostéotomies calcanéennes et tibiales dans le traitement du pied bot varus. *In* Le pied bot varus équin congénital. Cahiers d'enseignement de la S.O.F.C.O.T. Paris, Expansion Scientifique Française, 1976.
104. Carmack, J. C., and Hallock, H.: Tibiotarsal arthrodesis after astragalectomy. A report of eight cases. J. Bone Joint Surg., *29:*476, 1947.
105. Carpenter, E. B., and Huff, S. H.: Selective tendon transfers for recurrent club foot. South. Med. J., *46:*220, 1953.
106a. Carroll, N. C.: Pathoanatomy and treatment of talipes equinovarus. *In* Symposium: Current Practices in the Treatment of Idiopathic Club Foot in the Child Between Birth and Five Years of Age. Parts I and II. Contemp. Orthop., *1* and *2,* 1988.
106. Carroll, N. C., McMurtry, R., and Leete, S. F.: The pathoanatomy of congenital clubfoot. Orthop. Clin. North Am., *9:*225, 1978.
107. Carter, C. O.: Genetics of common disorders. Br. Med. Bull., *25:*52, 1969.
108. Carter, C. O.: Talipes equinovarus. *In* Sorsby, A. (ed.): Clinical Genetics: The Skeletal System. 2nd Ed. London, Butterworths, 1973, pp. 200–201.
109. Carter, C. O., and Fairbank, J. J.: Talipes equinovarus. *In* The Genetics of Locomotor Disorder. London, Oxford University Press, 1974, pp. 100–102.
110. Castellana, A.: Lengthening of Achilles tendon and posterior capsulotomy of tibiotarsal joint in therapy of congenital twisted foot. Minerva Ortop., *3:*139, 1952.
111. Cattaneo, R.: Development and therapy of tibial torsion in congenital clubfoot. Arch. Ortop. (Milano), *72:*1045, 1955.
112. Catterall, A.: Symposium: Current Practices in the Treatment of Idiopathic Club Foot in the Child Between Birth and Five Years of Age. Parts I and II. Contemp. Orthop., *1* and *2,* 1988.
113. Cavanaugh, C. J.: Clubfoot and congenital hand anomalies. J. Hered., *44:*53, 1953.
114. Cervenka, J., Figalova, P., and Gorlin, R. J.: Craniocarpo-tarsal dysplasia or the whistling face syndrome. Am. J. Dis. Child., *117:*434, 1969.
115. Cervenka, J., Gorlin, R. J., Figalova, P., and Farkasova, J.: Cranio-carpo-tarsal dysplasia or whistling face syndrome. Arch. Otolaryngol. (Chicago), *91:*183, 1970.
116. Chaiz, O., Masse, P., and Taussig, G.: Double arthrodesis in the treatment of congenital talipes equinovarus. Rev. Chir. Orthop., *2:*Suppl.:141, 1983.
117. Chapchal, G.: Operative treatment of congenital clubfoot. *In* Delchef, J. (ed.): Orthopaedic Surgery and Traumatology. Congenital clubfoot. c. Surgical treatment in later childhood. New York, American Elsevier, 1973, pp. 764–765.
118. Chiappara, P.: La funzione delle articolazioni astragalo-calcaneari. Minerva Ortop., *24:*6, 1973.
119. Ching, G. H. S., Chung, C. S., and Nemechek, R. W.: Genetic and epidemiological studies of clubfoot in Hawaii: Ascertainment and incidence. Am. J. Hum. Genet., *21:*566, 1969.
120. Chung, C. S., and Myrianthopoulos, N. C.: Racial and prenatal factors in major congenital malformations. Am. J. Hum. Genet., *20:*40, 1968.
121. Chung, C. S., Nemechek, R. W., Larsen, I. J., and Ching, G. H. S.: Genetic and epidemiological studies

of clubfoot in Hawaii: General and medical considerations. Hum. Hered., *19*:321, 1969.

122. Clark, J. M. P.: Treatment of clubfoot. Early detection and management of the unreduced clubfoot. Proc. R. Soc. Med., *61*:779, 1968.
123. Clark, J. M. P., and Silk, F. F.: Congenital talipes. *In* Clark, J. M. P.: Tether Contracture and Deformity. London, Heinemann, 1976, pp. 119–155.
124. Claus, D., and Lang, H.: Differential diagnosis of acquired clubfoot. Z. Orthop., *119*:416, 1981.
125. Codivilla, A.: New procedure for surgical treatment of the congenital pes equinus varus. Arch. Soc. Ital. Chir., *18*:1906.
126. Codivilla, A.: Sulla cura del piede equino varo congenito. Nuovo metodo di cura cruenta. Arch. Chir. Ortop., *23*:245, 1906.
127. Coleman, S. S.: Complex Foot Deformities in Children. Philadelphia, Lea & Febiger, 1983, p. 26.
128. Collburn, R. C.: Flat-top talus in recurrent clubfoot. J. Bone Joint Surg., *44-A*:1018, 1962.
129. Commerell, J.: New approach to the untreated or relapsed clubfoot in adults. J. Bone Joint Surg., *45-B*:430, 1963.
130. Compere, E. L.: Congenital talipes equinovarus. Surg. Clin. North Am., *15*:767, 1935.
131. Condon, V. R.: Radiology of practical orthopedic problems. Radiol. Clin. North Am., *10*:203, 1972.
132. Conrad, J. A., and Frost, H. M.: Evaluation of subcutaneous heel cord lengthening. Clin. Orthop., *64*:121, 1969.
133. Contargyris, A.: Le traitement operatoire précoce du pied bot congénital chez les nouveau-nés. Rev. Orthop. (3e Série), *18*:719, 1931.
134. Cowell, H. R., and Hensinger, R. N.: The relationship of clubfoot to congenital annular bands. *In* Bateman, J. E. (ed.): Foot Science. Philadelphia, Saunders, 1976, pp. 41–46.
135. Cowell, H. R., and Wein, L. K.: Genetic aspects of clubfoot. J. Bone Joint Surg., *62-B*:1381, 1980.
136. Crabbe, W. A.: Aetiology of congenital talipes. Br. Med. J., *2*:1060, 1960.
137. Crawford, A. H., Marxsen, J. L., and Osterfeld, D. L.: The Cincinnati incision: A comprehensive approach for surgical procedures for the foot and ankle in childhood. J. Bone Joint Surg., *64-A*:1355, 1982.
138. Critchley, J. E., and Taylor, R. G.: Transfer of the tibialis anterior tendon for relapsed clubfoot. J. Bone Joint Surg., *34-B*:49, 1952.
139. Curtis, B. H., and Butterfield, W. L.: Surgical treatment of congenital clubfoot. *In* Delchef, J. (ed.): Dixième Congrès International de Chirurgie Orthopédique et de Traumatologie, Paris, 4–9 Septembre, 1966. Bruxelles, Les Publications "Acta Medica Belgica," 1967, p. 1150.
140. Curtis, F. E., and Muro, F.: Decancellation of the os calcis, astragalus, and cuboid in correction of congenital talipes equinovarus. J. Bone Joint Surg., *16*:220, 1934.
141. Czernihowski, M.: Tibial torsion in children with congenital talipes equinovarus. Chir. Narzadow Ruchu Ortop. Pol., *44*:71, 1979.
142. Dabadie, J.: Intérêt de l'allongement précoce du tendon d'Achille dans le traitement des pieds bots varus équins congénitaux, sévères. Ann. Chir. Infant. (Paris), *12*:77, 1971.
143. Dahmen, G.: Principles for the treatment of the juvenile club-foot. Ther. Ggw., *117*:378, 1978.
144. Dangelmajer, R. C.: A review of 200 clubfeet. Bull. Hosp. Spec. Surg., *4*:73, 1961.
145. Davis, L. A., and Hatt, W. S.: Congenital abnormalities of the feet. Radiology, *64*:818, 1955.
146. Debeugny, P.: Treatment of congenital clubfoot in the newborn and infants. Lille Med., *10*:Suppl.:1103, 1965.
147. Debrunner, H.: Der angeboren Klumpfuss. Stuttgart, Ferdinand Enke Verlag, 1936.
148. Debrunner, H.: De Klumpfuss und andere orthopädische Missbildungen als Erbleiden. Schweiz. Med. Wochenschr., *75*:981, 1945.
149. Debrunner, H.: Die Therapie des angeborenen Klumpfusses. Stuttgart, Ferdinand Enke Verlag, 1957.
150. Declercq, F.: Talipes equino varus. Etiology patogenése. Behandelung en resultaten. Acta Orthop. Belg., *33*:799, 1967.
151. Dekel, S., and Weissman, S. L.: Osteotomy of the calcaneus and concomitant plantar stripping in children with talipes cavo-varus. J. Bone Joint Surg., *55-A*:802, 1973.
152. Dekelver, L., Fabry, G., and Mulier, J. C.: Triple arthrodesis and Lambrinudi arthrodesis. Literature review and follow-up study. Arch. Orthop. Trauma. Surg., *96*:23, 1980.
153. DeLangh, R., Mulier, J. C., Fabry, G., and Martens, M.: Treatment of clubfoot by posterior capsulectomy. Clin. Orthop., *106*:248, 1975.
154. Dellapiccola, B., and Capra, L.: Dermatoglyphics in Larsen's syndrome. Lancet, *1*:493, 1973.
155. Del Sel, J. M., DePaoli, J. M., Calvo, A., and Espagnol, R. O.: Clubfoot—neglected and resistant cases. *In* Delchef, J. (ed.): Orthopaedic Surgery and Traumatology. Congenital clubfoot. d. Neglected and inveterate cases. New York, American Elsevier, 1973, pp. 774–776.
156. DeMeyer, W., and Baird, I.: Mortality and skeletal malformations from amniocentesis and oligohydramnios in rats: Cleft palate, clubfoot, microstomia and adactyly. Teratology, *2*:33, 1969.
157. Denham, R. A.: Congenital talipes equinovarus. J. Bone Joint Surg., *49-B*:583, 1967.
158. Denham, R. A.: Early operation for severe congenital talipes equinovarus. J. Bone Joint Surg., *59-B*:116, 1977.
159. Depinski, K.: Correction of the varus positioning of the first bone of the metatarsus by means of "geometric" osteotomy. Chir. Narzadow Ruchu Ortop. Pol., *46*:581, 1981.
160. Dessaint, J. J.: Tomographie de pied bots. Presse Med., *62*:188, 1954.
161. DeWet, I. S.: Postero-medial release in clubfoot (abstract). 20th Congress of South African Orthopedic Association, 1975. J. Bone Joint Surg., *57-B*:257, 1975.
162. Dietz, F. R., Ponseti, I. V., and Buckwalter, J. A.: Morphometric study of clubfoot tendon sheaths. J. Pediatr. Orthop., *3*:311, 1983.
163. Dimeglio, A., and Pous, J. G.: Le pied bot varus équin: Un conflict autour de l'articulation mediotarsien. Du traitement orthopédique au traitement chirurgicale. *In* Cahiers d'enseignement de la S.O.F.C.O.T. Paris, Expansion Scientifique Française, 1977, p. 73.
164. Dittrich, R. J.: Pathogenesis of congenital club foot. J. Bone Joint Surg., *12*:373, 1930.
165. Domeniconi, S., and Perricone, F.: L'operazione di Codivilla nel trattamento precoce del piedo torto congenito. Minerva Ortop., *3*:176, 1952.
166. Van Domselaar, F.: Application de las gotieras de Denis Browne para el pie-bot. Bol. Trab. Soc. Argent. Cir. Ortop., *8*:95, 1943.
167. Drachman, D. B., and Coulombre, A. J.: Experimental clubfoot and arthrogryposis multiplex congenita. Lancet, *2*:523, 1962.
168. Dubowitz, V., and Sharrard, J.: Congenital clubfoot with central core disease of muscle. Proc. R. Soc. Med., *61*:1258, 1968.
169. Ducci, L., and Grilli, E. P.: Studio clinico-statistico sul piede torto congenito. Arch. Putti Chir. Organi Mov., *5*:517, 1954.

170. Dumeau, C. L.: L'astragalectomie temporaire subtotale dans le traitement des pieds bots. Thèse Médecine, Bordeaux, 1942.
171. Dunaj, W.: Microscopic examination of muscles in congenital clubfoot. Chir. Narzadow Ruchu Ortop. Pol., *36*:197, 1971.
172. Dunn, H. K., and Samuelson, K. M.: Flat-top talus. A long-term report of twenty club feet. J. Bone Joint Surg., *56-A*:57, 1974.
173. Dunn, N.: The treatment of congenital talipes equinovarus. Br. Med. J., *2*:216, 1923.
174. Dwyer, F. C.: A new approach to the treatment of pes cavus. Société Internationale de Chirurgie Orthopédique. Sixiéme Congrès International de Chirurgie Orthopédique. Brussels, M. A. Bailleux, 1955, pp. 551–558.
175. Dwyer, F. C.: Osteotomy of the calcaneum for pes cavus. J. Bone Joint Surg., *41-B*:80, 1959.
176. Dwyer, F. C.: The treatment of relapsed clubfoot by the insertion of a wedge into the calcaneum. J. Bone Joint Surg., *45-B*:67, 1963.
177. Dwyer, F. C.: Treatment of the relapsed clubfoot. Proc. R. Soc. Med., *61*:783, 1968.
178. Edelson, J. G., and Husseini, N.: The pulseless club foot. J. Bone Joint Surg., *66-B*:700, 1984.
179. Editorial: Club foot. Br. Med. J., *2*:593, 1962.
180. Edwards, E. R., and Menelaus, M. B.: Reverse club foot: Rigid and recalcitrant talipes calcaneovalgus. J. Bone Joint Surg., *69-B*:330, 1987.
181. Edwards, M. J.: The experimental production of clubfoot in guinea-pigs by maternal hyperthermia during gestation. J. Pathol., *103*:49, 1971.
182. Ehrenfried, A.: The occurrence and etiology of clubfoot. J.A.M.A., *59*:1940, 1912.
183. Eikenbary, C. F.: Congenital equinovarus, report of 114 cases. Surg. Gynecol. Obstet., *30*:555, 1920.
184. Elliot, J. K.: Club foot in the Polynesian. J. Bone Joint Surg., *43-B*:190, 1961.
185. Elmslie, R. C.: The principles of treatment of congenital talipes equino-varus. J. Orthop. Surg., *2*:669, 1920.
186. Elsner, H.: Die Osteotomie und zeitweilige Nagelung des Calcaneus bei blutiger Klumpfuss operation. Zentralbl. Chir., *51*:429, 1924.
187. Erlacher: Totale Tibialisvereisung bei der Behandlung hartnackiger Klumpfusse. Verh. Dtsch. Orthop., *21*:495, 1927.
188. Evans, D.: Treatment of cavo-varus foot and clubfoot. J. Bone Joint Surg., *39-B*:789, 1957.
189. Evans, D.: Relapsed club foot. J. Bone Joint Surg., *43-B*:722, 1961.
190. Evans, D.: Treatment of unreduced or lapsed clubfoot in older children. Proc. R. Soc. Med., *61*:782, 1968.
191. Evans, D.: Calcaneo-valgus deformity. J. Bone Joint Surg., *57-B*:270, 1975.
192. Eyre-Brook, A. L.: Talipes equino cavo varus. J. Bone Joint Surg., *45-B*:428, 1963.
193. Fahrenbach, G., Kuehn, D., and Tachdjian, M. O.: The use of computerized tomography in assessing residual deformities in talipes equinovarus. J. Pediatr. Orthop., *6*:334, 1986.
194. Falconer, D. S.: The inheritance of liability to certain diseases estimated from the incidence among relatives. Ann. Hum. Genet., *29*:51, 1965.
195. Fang, H. S. Y., and Yu, F. Y. K.: Foot binding in Chinese women. Can. J. Surg., *3*:195, 1960.
196. Farabeuf: Cited by Kapandji, I. A.: The physiology of the joints. *In* Annotated Diagrams of the Mechanics of Human Joints. 2nd Ed. Edinburgh, E. & S. Livingstone, 1970, Vol. 2, pp. 138–195.
197. Farill, J.: Elongación del tendon de Aquiles. Gac. Med. Mex., *72*:69, 1942.
198. Farill, J.: Splints in talipes equinovarus. Orthopedic Correspondence. Club Letter, Dec. 10, 1945.
199. Farill, J.: Tratamiento del pie varus equino-congénito en los niños pequeños. Bol. Med. Hosp. Infant., *2*:252, 1946.
200. Farrill, J.: Tibioperoneal tenoplasty for congenital clubfoot with peroneal insufficiency. J. Bone Joint Surg., *38-A*:329, 1956.
201. Feoksistov, G. F.: Functional splint for correction of pes equinus and its retention in the position of correction in congenital clubfoot. Ortop. Travmatol. Protez., *34*:74, 1973.
202. Fisher, R. L., and Shaffer, S. R.: An evaluation of calcaneal osteotomy in congenital clubfoot and other disorders. Clin. Orthop., *70*:141, 1970.
203. Fisk, J. R., House, J. H., and Bradford, D. S.: Congenital ulnar deviation of the fingers with clubfoot deformities. Clin. Orthop., *104*:200, 1974.
204. Fiske, E. W.: The prognosis of congenital clubfoot and its relation to nonoperative treatment. J.A.M.A., *65*:375, 1915.
205. Fjeldborg, O. C.: Medfødt Klumpfod. En biomeckanisk analyse af el Klinisk materiale. Arhus, Universitetsforlaget i Arhus, 1971.
206. Flinchum, D.: Pathologic anatomy in talipes equinovarus. J. Bone Joint Surg., *35-A*:111, 1953.
207. Forrester-Brown, M.: The treatment of congenital equinovarus (clubfoot). J. Bone Joint Surg., *17*:661, 1935.
208. Forrester-Brown, M.: A clamp for stretching congenital club-feet. Lancet, *1*:897, 1936.
209. Fraser, F. C., Pashayan, H., and Kadish, M. E.: Cranio-carpo-tarsal dysplasia. Report of a case in father and son. J.A.M.A., *211*:1374, 1979.
210. Frassi, G. A.: Lateral transplant of the tibialis anterior in the treatment of congenital clubfoot and its recurrences. Arch. Ortop., *76*:93, 1963.
211. Fredenhagen, H.: Der Klumpfuss, Vorkommen, Anatomie, Behandlung und Spätresultate. Z. Orthop., *85*:305, 1955.
212. Freeman, E. A., and Sheldon, J. H.: Cranio-carpaltarsal dystrophy. An undescribed congenital malformation. Arch. Dis. Child., *13*:277, 1938.
213. Fried, A.: Recurrent congenital club-foot. The role of the m. tibialis posterior in etiology and treatment. J. Bone Joint Surg., *41-A*:243, 1959.
214. Fripp, A. T.: The relapsed clubfoot. Proc. R. Soc. Med., *44*:873, 1951.
215. Fripp, A. T.: Editorial: The problem of the relapsed clubfoot. J. Bone Joint Surg., *43-B*:626, 1961.
216. Fripp, A. T., and Shaw, N. E.: Club-foot. Edinburgh and London, E. & S. Livingstone, 1967.
217. Fujii, H.: Early treatment and surgical indication in congenital clubfoot. Shujutsu, *26*:368, 1972.
218. Furmento, A., Silberman, F., and Khoury, S. C.: Pie varo equino congénito evolución y pronostico de acuerdo el estudio radiografico. Presna Med. Argent., *48*:1617, 1961.
219. Fusari, A.: Sul trattamento precoce del piede torto congenito. Arch. Ortop., *62*:208, 1949.
220. Gafarov, KhZ.: Apparatus for functional treatment of congenital clubfoot. Ortop. Travmatol. Protez., *5*:46, 1978.
221. Gafarov, KhZ.: Results of the conservative treatment of congenital clubfoot in children. Ortop. Travmatol. Protez., *2*:45, 1978.
222. Gambier, N.: Les résultats éloignés de l'opération de Codivilla dans le traitement du pied bot congénital. Rev. Chir. Orthop., *38*:531, 1952.
223. Garceau, G. J.: Anterior tibial transposition in recurrent congenital club-foot. J. Bone Joint Surg., *22*:932, 1940.
224. Garceau, G. J.: Talipes equinovarus. A.A.O.S. Instr. Course Lect., *7*:119, 1950.
225. Garceau, G. J.: Recurrent clubfoot. Bull. Hosp. Jt. Dis., *15*:143, 1954.

226. Garceau, G. J.: Talipes equinovarus. A.A.O.S. Instr. Course Lect., *12*:90, 1955.
227. Garceau, G. J.: Congenital talipes equinovarus. A.A.O.S. Instr. Course Lect., *18*:178, 1961.
228. Garceau, G. J.: Anterior tibial tendon transfer for recurrent clubfoot. Clin. Orthop., *84*:61, 1972.
229. Garceau, G. J., and Manning, K. R.: Transposition of the anterior tibial tendon in the treatment of recurrent congenital club-foot. J. Bone Joint Surg., *29*:1044, 1947.
230. Garceau, G. J., and Palmer, R. M.: Transfer of the anterior tibial tendon for recurrent clubfoot. A long-term follow-up. J. Bone Joint Surg., *49-A*:207, 1967.
231. Gardner, E.: Prenatal development of the skeleton and joints of the human foot. J. Bone Joint Surg., *44-A*:847, 1959.
232. Gartland, J. J.: Posterior tibial transplant in the surgical treatment of recurrent club foot. A preliminary report. J. Bone Joint Surg., *46-A*:1217, 1964.
233. Gartland, J. J., and Surgent, R. E.: Posterior tibial transplant in the surgical treatment of recurrent club foot. Clin. Orthop., *84*:66, 1972.
234. Gaston, S. R.: Management of club foot deformities. Bull. N.Y. Orthop. Hosp., *2*:12, 1958.
235. Gaul, J. S., Jr.: The evolution of biomechanical analysis in the management of congenital clubfoot. Clin. Orthop., *76*:141, 1971.
236. Geist, E. S.: An operation for the after treatment of some cases of congenital club-foot. J. Bone Joint Surg., *22*:50, 1924.
237. Gelman, W. B.: Soft-tissue releasing procedure for persisting heel varus in the uncorrected clubfoot. Clin. Orthop., *15*:177, 1960.
238. Ghali, N. N., Smith, R. B., Clayden, A. D., and Silk, F. F.: The results of pantalar reduction in the management of congenital talipes equinovarus. J. Bone Joint Surg., *65-B*:1, 1983.
239. Ghinst, Van De H. M., and Claessens, H.: Talipes equinovarus. Verslag by M. Van De Ghinst en H. Claessens. Acta Orthop. Belg., *33*:797, 1967.
240. Gibson, A.: A universal joint clubfoot splint. J. Bone Joint Surg., *36-A*:658, 1954.
241. Gibson, D. A., and Urs, N. D. K.: Arthrogryposis multiplex congenita. J. Bone Joint Surg., *52-B*:483, 1970.
242. Glicenstein, J., and Bensahel, H.: Surgical treatment of severe club foot: Cutaneous plasty. Nouv. Presse Med., *7*:2469, 1978.
243. Gluckman, L. K.: Club foot in the Maori (letter). N.Z. Med. J., *88*:298, 1978.
244. Goldner, J. L.: Congenital talipes equinovarus—fifteen years of surgical treatment. Curr. Pract. Orthop. Surg., *4*:61, 1969.
245. Goldwny, R. M.: Z-plasty skin closure after lengthening the Achilles tendon. Plast. Reconstr. Surg., *52*:431, 1973.
246. Gordon, H., Davies, D., and Bermen, M.: Camptodactyly, cleft palate and club foot. A syndrome showing the autosomal-dominant pattern of inheritance. J. Med. Genet., *6*:266, 1969.
247. Gordon, S. L., and Dunn, E. J.: Peroneal nerve palsy as a complication of clubfoot treatment. Clin. Orthop., *101*:229, 1974.
248. Gould, J. S.: Surgical reconstruction of the talipes equinovarus deformity. *In* Bateman, J. E., and Trott, A. W. (eds.): The Foot and Ankle. New York, Brian C. Decker, 1980, pp. 207–214.
249. Gould, J. S.: Reconstructive surgery for club foot. *In* Kiene, R. H., and Johnson, K. A. (eds.): A.A.O.S. Symposium on the Foot and Ankle. St. Louis, C. V. Mosby, 1983, pp. 237–252.
250. Gould, J. S.: Clubfoot. *In* Gould, J. S. (ed.): The Foot. Baltimore, Williams & Wilkins, 1988, pp. 159–160.
251. Gray, D. H., and Katz, J. M.: A histochemical study of muscle in clubfoot. J. Bone Joint Surg., *63-B*:417, 1981.
252. Green, A. D. L., Fixsen, J. A., and Lloyd-Roberts, G. C.: Talectomy for arthrogryposis multiplex congenita. J. Bone Joint Surg., *66-B*:697, 1984.
253. Green, A. D. L., and Lloyd-Roberts, G. C.: The results of early posterior release in resistant club feet. A long-term review. J. Bone Joint Surg., *67-B*:588, 1985.
254. Greider, T. D., Siff, S. J., Gerson, P., and Donovan, M. M.: Arteriography in club foot. J. Bone Joint Surg., *64-A*:837, 1982.
255. Grill, F., and Franke, J.: The Ilizarov distractor for the correction of relapsed or neglected clubfoot. J. Bone Joint Surg., *69-B*:593, 1987.
256. Gross-Kieselstein, E., Abrahamov, A., and Ben-Hur, N.: Familial occurrence of the Freeman-Sheldon syndrome: Craniocarpotarsal dysplasia. Pediatrics, *47*:1064, 1971.
257. Gulledge, W. C.: Skintight casts for the treatment of clubfoot, a follow-up report. Pacif. Med. Surg., *74*:28, 1966.
258. Gunn, D. R., and Molesworth, B. D.: The use of tibialis posterior as a dorsiflexor. J. Bone Joint Surg., *39-B*:674, 1957.
259. Hadidi, H.: Management of congenital talipes equinovarus. Orthop. Clin. North Am., *5*:53, 1974.
260. Van Haelst, A.: Traitment du pied bot congénital après deux ans. Rev. Orthop. (3ᵉ Série), *18*:712, 1931.
261. Hahn, F.: Über der Ätiologie des kongenitalen Klumpfusses. Z. Orthop. Chir., *42*:151, 1922.
262. Haicl, A.: Empirical hazards in talipes equinovarus. Acta Chir. Orthop. Traumatol. Cech., *38*:205, 1971.
263. Haicl, Z., and Frydl, J.: Personal experience with surgery of congenital pes equinovarus using Turco's technic. Acta Chir. Orthop. Traumatol. Cech., *50*:530, 1983.
264. Haliburton, R. A., Sullivan, C. R., Kelly, P. J., and Peterson, L. F.: Extra-osseous and intra-osseous blood supply of the talus. J. Bone Joint Surg., *40-A*:1115, 1958.
265. Hall, C. B.: Congenital skeletal deficiencies of the extremities. J.A.M.A., *181*:590, 1962.
266. Hamada, G.: Orthopaedics and orthopaedic diseases in ancient and modern Egypt. Clin. Orthop., *89*:253, 1972.
267. Hamsa, W. R., and Burney, D. W., Jr.: Open correction of recurrent talipes equinovarus. A study of end-result. Clin. Orthop., *26*:104, 1963.
268. Handelsman, J. E.: The surgical treatment of clubfoot in later childhood. *In* Delchef, J. (ed.): Orthopaedic Surgery and Traumatology. Congenital clubfoot. c. Surgical treatment in later childhood. New York, American Elsevier, 1973, pp. 766–768.
269. Handelsman, J. E., and Badalamente, M. A.: Neuromuscular studies in clubfoot. J. Pediatr. Orthop., *1*:23, 1973.
270. Handelsman, J. E., and Badalamente, M. A.: Club foot: A neuromuscular disease. Dev. Med. Child Neurol., *24*:3, 1982.
271. Handelsman, J. E., and Isaacs, H.: Aetiology of club foot. Proceedings: 20th Congress of S. Afr. Orthop. Assoc. (abstract). J. Bone Joint Surg., *57-B*:262, 1975.
272. Handelsman, J. E., and Solomon, L.: The assessment of correction in club foot. S. Afr. Med. J., *47*:1909, 1973.
273. Handelsman, J. E., Youngleson, J., and Malkin, C.: A modified approach to the Dwyer os calcis osteotomy in club foot. S. Afr. Med. J., *39*:989, 1965.
274. Hansteen, I. L., Schirmer, L., and Hestetun, S.: Trisomy 12p syndrome. Clin. Genet., *13*:339, 1978.
275. Harrold, A. J., and Walker, C. J.: Treatment and

prognosis in congenital club foot. J. Bone Joint Surg., *65-B:*8, 1983.

276. Harry, N. M.: Denis Browne splints in the treatment of talipes equinovarus. Aust. N.Z. J. Surg., *10:*117, 1940.
277. Haudek, M.: Zur Behandlung des angeborenen Klumpfusses beim Neugeborenen und Saugling. Z. Orthop., *25:*761, 1910.
278. Hauser, E. D. W.: A manipulative method of treatment for recalcitrant and neglected clubfoot. J.A.M.A., *93:*688, 1929.
279. Hauser, E. D. W.: Cohesive bandage for clubfoot in newborn infants. J.A.M.A., *138:*19, 1948.
280. Hauser, E. D. W.: Origin and etiology of clubfoot. Q. Bull. Northwest. Med. Sch., *28:*274, 1954.
281. Hauser, E. D. W.: Congenital clubfoot. Springfield, Ill., Charles C Thomas, 1966.
282. Hayashi, H.: Structural deformity and dynamic deformity in congenital club foot. J. Jpn. Orthop. Assoc., *46:*939, 1972.
283. Hehne, H. J., and Baumann, J. U.: Dwyer's calcaneal osteotomy for varus deformity of the foot. (A follow-up study including gait analysis). Z. Orthop., *117:*202, 1979.
284. Hendel, H. L., Wood, G. G., and Arnold, M.: Die Muskulatur beim angeborenen Klumpfuss. Z. Orthop., *108:*604, 1971.
285. Hendrix, G., and Marneffe, R. de: Pied bot congénital: Étude radiologique complementaire. Acta Orthop. Belg., *26:*341, 1960.
286. Henke, W., and Reyher, C.: Studien über die Entwicklung der Extremitäten des Menschen insbesondere der Gelenkflächen. Sitzungsberichte d.k. Akademie d. Wissenschaften Wiener Math. Naturwissenschäftliche Klasse, Ed. 3, *50:*217, 1874.
287. Herold, H. Z.: Surgical correction of previously untreated clubfeet in older children and adults. *In* Delchef, J. (ed.): Orthopaedic Surgery and Traumatology. Congenital clubfoot. c. Neglected and inveterate cases. New York, American Elsevier, 1973, p. 777.
288. Herold, H. Z., and Torok, G.: Surgical correction of neglected club foot in the older child and adults. J. Bone Joint Surg., *55-A:*1385, 1973.
289. Hersh, A.: The role of surgery in the treatment of club feet. J. Bone Joint Surg., *49-A:*1684, 1967.
290. Hersh, A., and Fuchs, L. A.: Treatment of the uncorrected clubfoot by triple arthrodesis. Orthop. Clin. North Am., *4:*103, 1973.
291. Herzenberg, J., Carroll, N., and Christofferson, M.: Clubfoot analysis with three-dimensional computer modelling. A.A.O.S. Instr. Course Lect., *36:*117, 1987.
292. Heyman, C. H.: Ober operation for congenital clubfoot. End-results in fifteen cases. Surg. Gynecol. Obstet., *49:*706, 1929.
293. Heyman, C. H.: The surgical release of fibrous tissue structures resisting correction of congenital clubfoot and metatarsus varus. A.A.O.S. Instr. Course Lect., *16:*100, 1959.
294. Heyman, C. H., Herndon, C. H., and Strong, J. M.: Mobilization of the tarsometatarsal and intermetatarsal joints for the correction of resistant adduction of the forepart of the foot in congenital clubfoot or congenital metatarsus varus. J. Bone Joint Surg., *40-A:*299, 1958.
295. Heywood, A. W. B.: The mechanics of the hindfoot in clubfoot as demonstrated radiographically. J. Bone Joint Surg., *46-B:*102, 1964.
296. Hicks, J. H.: Mechanics of foot; joints. J. Anat., *87:*345, 1953.
297. Hippocrates: Vol. 3. Loeb Classical Library. Trans. by E. T. Withington. London, William Heinemann; New York: G. P. Putnam's Sons, 1927.
298. Hirsch, C.: Modfödd Klumpfot och höftledsluxation. Nord. Med., *62:*1138, 1959.
299. Hirsch, C.: Observations on early operative treatment of congenital club-foot. Bull. Hosp. Jt. Dis., *21:*173, 1960.
300. Hjelmstedt, A.: The importance of analysis of skeletal deformities in congenital clubfeet for adequate surgical treatment. Proceedings of the Scandinavian Orthopaedic Society, 37th Assembly, 1974 (abstract). Acta Orthop. Scand., *45:*953, 1974.
301. Hjelmstedt, A.: Correction osteotomy of the talus and calcaneus in relapsing or incorrigible clubfeet. Principles and technique. Proceedings of the Scandinavian Orthopaedic Society, 37th Assembly, 1974 (abstract). Acta Orthop. Scand., *45:*978, 1974.
302. Hjelmstedt, A., and Sahlstedt, B.: The anatomy of the talus in clubfeet. Results of an arthrographic study. Proceedings of the Scandinavian Orthopaedic Society, 36th Assembly, 1972 (abstract). Acta Orthop. Scand., *44:*128, 1973.
303. Hjelmstedt, A., and Sahlstedt, B.: Talar deformity in congenital clubfeet. Acta Orthop. Scand., *45:*628, 1974.
304. Hjelmstedt, A., and Sahlstedt, B.: Simultaneous arthrography of the talocrural and talonavicular joints in children. II. Comparison between anatomic and arthrographic measurements. Acta Radiol. [Diagn.] (Stockh.), *17:*557, 1976.
305. Hjelmstedt, A., and Sahlstedt, B.: Arthrography as a guide in the treatment of congenital clubfoot. Findings and treatment results in a consecutive series. Acta Orthop. Scand., *52:*321, 1980.
306. Hjelmstedt, A., and Sahlstedt, B.: Talo-calcaneal osteotomy and soft-tissue procedures in the treatment of clubfeet. I. Indications, principles and technique. Acta Orthop. Scand., *51:*335, 1980.
307. Hjelmstedt, A., and Sahlstedt, B.: Talo-calcaneal osteotomy and soft-tissue procedures in the treatment of clubfeet. II. Results in 36 surgically treated feet. Acta Orthop. Scand., *51:*349, 1980.
308. Hoeer, N. L., Pyle, S. E., and Krancis, C. C.: Radiographic Atlas of Skeletal Development of the Foot and Ankle, a Standard of Reference. Springfield, Ill., Charles C Thomas, 1962.
309. Hoffa, A.: Lehrbuch der Orthopädischen Chirurgie. 5th Ed. Stuttgart, Ferdinand Enke Verlag, 1905, pp. 734–782.
310. Hofmann, A. A., Constine, R. M., McBride, G. G., and Coleman, S. S.: Osteotomy of the first cuneiform as treatment of residual adduction of the fore part of the foot in club foot. J. Bone Joint Surg., *66-A:*985, 1984.
311. Hoke, M.: An operative plan for the correction of relapsed and untreated talipes equinovarus. Am. J. Orthop. Surg., *9:*379, 1911.
312. Holmadhl, H. C.: Astragalectomy as a stabilizing operation for foot paralysis following poliomyelitis: Results of a follow-up investigation of 153 cases. Acta Orthop. Scand., *25:*207, 1956.
313. Hootnick, D. R., Levinsohn, E. M., Crider, R. J., and Packard, D. S., Jr.: Congenital arterial malformations associated with clubfoot. A report of two cases. Clin. Orthop., *167:*160, 1982.
314. Hopf, A.: Die operative Klumpfussbehandlung im späten Kindesalter und beim Erwachsenen. Verh. Dtsch. Orthop. Ges. 42 Kongress Beil, Z. Orthop., *86:*162, 1954.
315. Howorth, M. B.: Textbook of Orthopaedics. Collingdale, Pa., Dorman Printers, 1959, pp. 426–428.
316. Hsu, L. C. S., Jaffray, D., and Leong, J. C. Y.: Talectomy for club foot in arthrogryposis. J. Bone Joint Surg., *66-B:*694, 1984.
317. Huguenin, P., Themar-Noel, C., and Bensahel, H.:

Study of the foot ground pressure pattern in children. Rev. Chir. Orthop., *67*:765, 1981.
318. Hüter, C.: Zur der Frage über das Wesen des angeborenen Klumpfusses. Dtsch. Klinik, *15*:487, 1863.
319. Idelberger, K.: Die Ergebnisse der Zwillingsforschung beim angeborenen Klumpfuss. Verh. Dtsch. Orthop. Ges., *33*:272, 1939.
320. Idelberger, K.: Die Zwillingspathologie der angeborenen Klumpfuss. Z. Orthop., Suppl. 69, 1939.
321. Imhäuser, G.: Die Frühbehandlung des angeborenen, muskulären Klumpfusses. Monatsschr. Kinderheilkd., *117*:645, 1969.
322. Inclán, A.: Anomalies of the tendinous insertions in the pathogenesis of club foot. J. Bone Joint Surg., *40-B*:159, 1958.
323. Inclán, A.: Las anomalias de las inserciones tendinosas en la pathogenia del pié bot varo equino congénito. Rev. Ortop. Trauma., *5*:173, 1960.
324. Ingelrans, P.: Report. Rev. Chir. Orthop., *38*:535, 1952.
325. Ingelrans, P.: Results of treatment of congenital inturned clubfoot before one year of age by Denis Browne splint. Acta Orthop. Belg., *34*:19, 1969.
326. Ingram, A. J., and Sprague, B.: Congenital clubfeet with associated absence of the anterior compartment musculature. *In* Delchef, J. (ed.): Orthopaedic Surgery and Traumatology. Congenital clubfoot. a. Anatomy and pathology of the disease. New York, American Elsevier, 1973, pp. 744–745.
327. Ippolito, E., and Ponseti, I. V.: Congenital club foot in the human fetus. J. Bone Joint Surg., *62-A*:8, 1980.
328. Irani, R. N., and Sherman, M. S.: The pathological anatomy of clubfoot. J. Bone Joint Surg., *45-A*:45, 1963.
329. Irani, R. N., and Sherman, M. S.: The pathological anatomy of idiopathic clubfoot. Clin. Orthop., *84*:14, 1972.
330. Isaacs, H., Handelsman, J. E., Badenhorst, M., and Pickering, A.: The muscles in club foot—a histological, histochemical and electron microscopic study. J. Bone Joint Surg., *59-B*:465, 1977.
331. Ivy, R. H.: Congenital anomalies; as recorded on birth certificates in the Division of Vital Statistics of the Pennsylvania Department of Health, for the period of 1951–1955, inclusive. Plast. Reconstr. Surg., *20*:400, 1957.
332. Jackson, R. K.: Experimental talipes in the Virginia opossum. Clin. Orthop., *81*:152, 1971.
333. Jacobs, J. E., and Carr, C. R.: Progressive muscular atrophy of the peroneal type (Charcot-Marie-Tooth disease), orthopedic management and end-result study. J. Bone Joint Surg., *32-A*:27, 1950.
334. Jacquemain, B.: Der angeborenen Klumpfuss in therapeutischer Insicht. Z. Kinderchir., *6*:80, 1968.
335. Jahss, M. H.: Tarsometatarsal truncated-wedge arthrodesis for pes cavus and equinovarus deformity of the fore part of the foot. J. Bone Joint Surg., *62-A*:713, 1980.
336. Janacek, M., and Liphardt, H. P.: Beitrage zur Therapie des equinovarus congenitus. Beitr. Orthop. Trauma., *12*:408, 1965.
337. Jansen, K.: Treatment of congenital club foot. J. Bone Joint Surg., *39-B*:599, 1957.
338. Jergesen, F. H.: The treatment of unilateral congenital talipes equinovarus with the Denis Browne splint. J. Bone Joint Surg., *25*:185, 1943.
339. Johanning, K.: Excochleatio ossis cuboidei in the treatment of pes equinovarus. Acta Orthop. Scand., *27*:310, 1958.
340. Johanson, J. E., Horak, R. D., and Winter, R. B.: Gillette Children's Hospital experience with the Turco procedure for clubfeet (talipes equinovarus). Minn. Med., *64*:745, 1981.
341. Jones, R., and Lovett, R. W.: Club-foot. *In* Orthopaedic Surgery. New York, William Wood & Co., 1926, pp. 578–598.
342. Jorring, K., and Christiansen, L.: Congenital clubfoot. A follow-up of 58 children treated during 1964–1969. Acta Orthop. Scand., *46*:152, 1975.
343. Judet, H., and Judet, J.: La réorientation de l'articulation tibio-tarsienne. Chirurgie, *97*:638, 1971.
344. Judet, J.: A propos du traitement des pieds bots. Rev. Chir. Orthop., *28*:538, 1952.
345. Judet, J.: Principes et technique de la réposition des os du pied dans le traitement des pieds bots rebelles ou récidivés. Acta Orthop. Belg., *33*:876, 1967.
346. Judet, J.: New concepts in the corrective surgery of congenital talipes equinovarus and congenital and neurologic flatfeet. Clin. Orthop., *70*:56, 1970.
347. Judet, J.: Le pied bot varus équin de l'adulte. *In* Cahiers d'enseignement des la S.O.F.C.O.T. Paris, Expansion Scientifique Française, 1977, p. 113.
348. Judet, J., Raynal, L., and Rigault, P.: Traitment des piedes bots varus équin rebelles ou récidivés chez des enfants âgés de 18 mois à 6 ans (préambule). Acta Orthop. Belg., *33*:866, 1967.
349. Kalamchi, A.: Operative management of the resistant clubfoot. A.A.O.S. Instr. Course Lect., *31*:256, 1982.
350. Kalman, E.: Einige Bemerkungen zur operativen Therapie des Klumpfusses. Beitr. Orthop. Trauma., *15*:597, 1968.
351. Kandel, B.: The suroplantar projection in the congenital clubfoot of the infant. Acta Orthop. Scand., *22*:161, 1952.
352. Kaneda, K.: Posteromedial release operation in congenital clubfoot. Shujutsu, *26*:391, 1972.
353. Kaplan, E. B.: Comparative anatomy of the talus in relation to idiopathic clubfoot. Clin. Orthop., *85*:32, 1972.
354. Karp, M.: Kohler's disease of the tarsal scaphoid. J. Bone Joint Surg., *19*:84, 1937.
355. Keim, H. A., and Ritchie, G. W.: "Nutcracker" treatment of clubfoot. J.A.M.A., *189*:613, 1964.
356. Keith, A.: Concerning the origin and nature of certain malformations of the face, head and foot. Br. J. Surg., *28*:173, 1940.
357. Kelly, J. P.: Clubfoot. J. Bone Joint Surg., *44-B*:748, 1962.
358. Kendrick, R. E., Sharma, N. K., Hassler, W. L., and Herndon, C. H.: Tarsometatarsal mobilization for resistant adduction of the forepart of the foot. A follow-up study. J. Bone Joint Surg., *52-A*:61, 1970.
359. Kerkiacharian, A.: Considérations techniques dans les capsulotomies du coup-de-pied. Presse Med., *76*:1192, 1968.
360. Kilfoyle, R. M., Broome, J. S., Hardy, J. H., and Curtis, B. H.: Talectomy. *In* Bateman, J. E. (ed.): Foot Science. Philadelphia, Saunders, 1976, p. 162.
361. Kinder, F. C.: Clubfoot. J.A.M.A., *98*:1736, 1932.
362. Kite, J. H.: Non-operative treatment of congenital clubfeet. South. Med. J., *23*:337, 1930.
363. Kite, J. H.: The treatment of congenital clubfeet. A study of the results in two hundred cases. J.A.M.A., *99*:1156, 1932.
364. Kite, J. H.: The surgical treatment of congenital clubfeet. Surg. Gynecol. Obstet., *61*:100, 1935.
365. Kite, J. H.: Principles involved in the treatment of congenital club-foot. The results of treatment. J. Bone Joint Surg., *21*:595, 1939.
366. Kite, J. H.: Treatment of congenital clubfoot. A.A.O.S. Instr. Course Lect., *7*:117, 1950.
367. Kite, J. H.: Treatment of congenital clubfoot. A.A.O.S. Instr. Course Lect., *8*:181, 1951.
368. Kite, J. H.: Treatment of resistant clubfeet. Discussion of tendon transference. A.A.O.S. Instr. Course Lect., *10*:171, 1953.

369. Kite, J. H.: The operative treatment of congenital clubfeet. A.A.O.S. Instr. Course Lect., *12*:100, 1955.
370. Kite, J. H.: Congenital clubfeet: Facts designed to aid in providing answers for anxious parents. Am. J. Orthopsychiatry, *1*:58, 1959.
371. Kite, J. H.: Some suggestions on treatment of clubfoot by casts. J. Bone Joint Surg., *45-A*:406, 1963.
372. Kite, J. H.: The Clubfoot. New York, Grune & Stratton, 1964.
373. Kite, J. H.: Errors and complications in treating foot conditions in children. Clin. Orthop., *53*:31, 1967.
374. Kite, J. H.: Conservative treatment of the resistant recurrent clubfoot. Clin. Orthop., *70*:93, 1970.
375. Kite, J. H.: Nonoperative treatment of congenital clubfoot. Clin. Orthop., *84*:29, 1972.
376. Kleiger, B.: Significance of tibiotalar navicular complex in congenital clubfoot. Bull. Hosp. Jt. Dis., *23*:158, 1962.
377. Kleiger, B.: Anomalies of the posterior tibial tendon observed during medial release operation. Bull. Hosp. Jt. Dis., *27*:9, 1966.
378. Kleiger, B., and Mankin, H. J.: A roentgenographic study of the development of the calcaneus by means of the posterior tangential view. J. Bone Joint Surg., *43-A*:961, 1961.
379. Kocher: Zur Aetiologie und Therapie des pes varus congenitus. Dtsch. Z. Chir., *9*:329, 1879.
380. Kovalevich, M. D., and Stavskaia, E. A.: Early surgical treatment of congenital clubfoot. Khirurgiia (Mosk.), *47*:111, 1971.
381. Kranicz, J., Barta, O., and Bellyei, A.: Early surgery of the soft tissues in congenital clubfoot. Magy. Traumatol. Orthop., *20*:143, 1977.
382. Kranicz, J., Barta, O., and Bellyei, A.: A method for the evaluation of treatment results in congenital clubfoot. Magy. Traumatol. Orthop., *20*:287, 1977.
383. Kranicz, J., Barta, O., and Bellyei, A.: The effect of operations on soft tissues in the development of tarsal bones in patients with clubfoot. Magy. Traumatol. Orthop. Helyreallito Sebesz., *23*:14, 1980.
384. Kranicz, J., Barta, O., and Bellyei, A.: Results of soft tissue operations in the management of congenital club foot. Magy. Traumatol. Orthop. Helyreallito Sebesz., *23*:191, 1980.
385. Kreuz, L., and Stope, H.: Pes equino-varus congenitus. *In* Hohmann, G. (ed.): Handbuch der Orthopadie. Stuttgart, George Thiem Verlag, 1961, Vol. IV, Part II, pp. 788–821.
386. Kuhlmann, R. F.: Conservative management of congenital clubfoot deformity. Am. J. Dis. Child., *87*:440, 1954.
387. Kuhlmann, R. F.: A survey and clinical evaluation of the operative treatment for congenital talipes equinovarus. Clin. Orthop., *84*:88, 1972.
388. Kuhlmann, R. F., and Bell, J. F.: A clinical evaluation of operative procedures for congenital talipes equinovarus. J. Bone Joint Surg., *39-A*:265, 1957.
389. Kumar, K.: The role of footprints in the management of clubfeet. Clin. Orthop., *140*:32, 1979.
390. Laaveg, S. J., and Ponseti, I. V.: Long term results of treatment of congenital clubfoot. J. Bone Joint Surg., *62-A*:23, 1980.
391. Lamy, M., and Maroteaux, P.: Le nanisme diastrophique. Presse Med., *68*:1977, 1960.
392. Lamy, M., and Maroteaux, P.: The genetic study of limb malformations. *In* Swinyard, C. A. (ed.): Limb Development and Deformity. Springfield, Ill., Charles C Thomas, 1969, pp. 170–175.
393. Landi, F.: L'ereditarieta del piede torto-congenito. Chir. Organi Mov., *34*:234, 1950.
394. Lanfranchi, R., and Sabetta, F.: Risultati del trattamento ortopedico e fisiochinesiterapico del P.T.C. nei primi giorni di vita. Chir. Organi Mov., *59*:523, 1970.
395. Lange, M.: Orthopädische-Chirurgische. Operationslehre. München, J. Bergman, 1951.
396. Langenskiöld, A., and Ritsalä, V.: Supination deformity of the forefoot. Acta Orthop. Scand., *48*:325, 1977.
397. Langer, L. O.: Diastrophic dwarfism in early infancy. A.J.R., *93*:399, 1965.
398. Lapidus, P. W.: Congenital bilateral talipes equinus in twins. J. Bone Joint Surg., *21*:792, 1939.
399. Larsen, E. H.: Congenital clubfoot. J. Bone Joint Surg., *45-B*:620, 1963.
400. Larsen, L. J., Schottstaedt, E. R., and Bost, F. C.: Multiple congenital dislocations associated with characteristic facial abnormality. J. Pediatr., *37*:574, 1950.
401. Latta, R. J., Graham, B., Aase, J., Scham, S. M., and Smith, D. W.: Larsen's syndrome: A skeletal dysplasia with multiple joint dislocation and unusual facies. J. Pediatr., *78*:291, 1971.
402. Lauterburg, W.: Zur Behandlung des angeborenen Klumpfusses in Säuglingsalter. Schweiz. Med. Wochenschr., *75*:954, 1945.
403. Lazzareschi, M., Bruschili, S., Verniera, J., and Laredo, J.: Early surgery for resistant congenital talipes equino-varus. *In* Delchef, J. (ed.): Orthopaedic Surgery and Traumatology. Congenital clubfoot. b. Early childhood—conservative and surgical treatment. New York, American Elsevier, 1973, pp. 761–762.
404. Leck, J.: Incidence of malformations. In Davis, J. A. (ed.): Scientific Foundations of Paediatrics. Paediatric Aspect of Epidemiology. Philadelphia, Saunders, 1974, pp. 705–726.
405. Leclerc, G. C.: Etude sur les résultats thérapeutiques dans les pieds bots varus équins. Rev. Chir. Orthop., *47*:578, 1961.
406. Lehman, W. B.: The Clubfoot. Philadelphia, Lippincott, 1980.
407. Lelievre, J.: Pied varus équin congénital. *In* Pathologie du Pied. 2nd Ed. rev. Paris, Masson & Cie, 1961, pp. 154–175.
408. Lemperg, R.: Subastragalar triarticular arthrodesis for congenital clubfoot in children aged 2½–15 years. Acta Orthop. Scand., *36*:203, 1965.
409. LeNoir, J. L.: Congenital Idiopathic Talipes. Springfield, Ill., Charles C Thomas, 1966.
410. LeNoir, J. L.: A perspective focus on the indicated surgical treatment of resistant clubfoot in the infant. South. Med. J., *69*:837, 1976.
411. Leonard, D. W.: The significance of delayed ossification in the treatment of congenital clubfoot. J. Pediatr., *26*:379, 1945.
412. Leun, W.: Nachtschiene gegen Klumpfuss. Z. Orthop., *72*:250, 1941.
413. Leveuf, J., and Bertrand, P.: La réduction sanglante du pied bot chez le jeune enfant. Rev. Orthop., *34*:97, 1948.
414. Lichtblau, S.: A medial and lateral release operation for clubfoot. A preliminary report. J. Bone Joint Surg., *55-A*:1377, 1973.
415. Lichtblau, S.: External rotation tibial osteotomy in clubfoot: Adverse late effects. Clin. Orthop., *136*:225, 1978.
416. Liebermann, B.: Über eine Merkwurdige Exostosenbildung bei Klumpfuss. Arch. Orthop. Chir., *32*:16, 1952.
417. Lipmann Kessel, A. W.: The Kite method in the treatment of clubfoot. J. Bone Joint Surg., *33-B*:463, 1951.
418. Little, W. J.: A Treatise on the Nature of Club-Foot and Analogous Distortions: Including Their Treatment Both With or Without Surgical Operation. London, W. Jeffs, 1839.
419. Lloyd-Roberts, G. C.: Editorial: "Congenital club foot." J. Bone Joint Surg., *46-B*:369, 1964.
420. Lloyd-Roberts, G. C.: Clubfoot. Dev. Med. Child Neurol., *6*:507, 1965.
421. Lloyd-Roberts, G. C.: The treatment of clubfoot. Manitoba Med. Rev., *48*:198, 1968.

422. Lloyd-Roberts, G. C.: Orthopaedic abnormalities, the foot and ankle. *In* Norman, A. P. (ed.): Congenital Abnormalities in Infancy. 2nd Ed. Oxford, Blackwell, 1971, pp. 282–287.
423. Lloyd-Roberts, G. C., and Lettin, A. W. R.: Arthrogryposis multiplex congenita. J. Bone Joint Surg., *52-B*:494, 1970.
424. Lloyd-Roberts, G. C., Swann, M., and Catterall, A.: Medial rotational osteotomy for severe residual deformity in club foot. A preliminary report on a new method of treatment. J. Bone Joint Surg., *56-B*:37, 1974.
425. Lombard, P.: Les bases du traitement dans le pied bot varus équin congénital. Rev. Orthop., *36*:46, 1950.
426. Lombard, P.: Note sur la pathogénie et le traitement du pied bot varus équin congénital. Rev. Chir. Orthop., *38*:542, 1952.
427. Lowe, L. W., and Hannon, M. A.: Residual adduction of the forefoot in treated congenital clubfoot. J. Bone Joint Surg., *55-B*:809, 1973.
428. Lowell, W. W., and Hancock, C. I.: Treatment of congenital talipes equinovarus. Clin. Orthop., *70*:79, 1970.
429. Lozano, E., and Padilla, F.: Pié equino varo congénito. Rev. Mex. Pediat., *28*:481, 1959.
430. Lubrano di Diego, J. G., Noyer, D., Daudet, M., Kohler, R., Dodat, H., Vidal, P., Louis, D., and Chappius, J. P.: A new orthopedic apparatus for the treatment of congenital equinovarus clubfoot. The active-passive articulated splint. Critical study apropos of 72 cases treated in our department. Chir. Pediatr., *20*:371, 1979.
431. Lucas, L. S.: Surgical procedures in treatment of chronic clubfoot. West. J. Surg., *56*:542, 1948.
432. Lucas, L. S., and Cottrell, G. W.: Notched rotation osteotomy. A method employed in the corrections of torsion of the tibia and other conditions. West. J. Surg., *57*:5, 1949.
433. Lundberg, B. J.: Early Dwyer operation in talipes equinovarus. Clin. Orthop., *154*:223, 1981.
434. Lusskin, H.: Nonrigid method of treatment for early clubfoot. J. Int. Coll. Surg., *14*:444, 1950.
435. McBride, E. D.: Congenital and hereditary anomalies. *In* Crippled Children. Their Treatment and Orthopedic Nursing. St. Louis, Mosby, 1937, pp. 278–316.
436. McCauley, J. C., Jr.: Operative treatment of clubfeet. N.Y. J. Med., *47*:255, 1947.
437. McCauley, J. C., Jr.: Surgical treatment of clubfoot. Surg. Clin. North Am., *31*:561, 1951.
438. McCauley, J. C., Jr.: A release operation for problem clubfoot. N.Y. J. Med., *52*:2997, 1952.
439. McCauley, J. C., Jr.: Triple arthrodesis for congenital talipes equinovarus deformities. Clin. Orthop., *34*:25, 1964.
440. McCauley, J. C., Jr.: Clubfoot. History of the development and the concepts of pathogenesis and treatment. Clin. Orthop., *44*:51, 1966.
441. McCauley, J. C., Jr.: The history of conservative and surgical methods of clubfoot treatment. Clin. Orthop., *84*:25, 1972.
442. McCauley, J. C., Jr., and Krida, A.: The early treatment of equinus in congenital clubfoot. Am. J. Surg., *22*:491, 1933.
443. McCollum, R. G.: A functional brace for congenital clubfoot. A preliminary report. Clin. Orthop., *89*:197, 1972.
444. MacEwen, G. D., Scott, D. J., Jr., and Shands, A. R., Jr.: Follow-up survey of clubfoot treated at Alfred I. duPont Institute. With special reference to the value of plaster therapy, instituted during earliest signs of recurrence, and the use of night splints to prevent or minimize the manifestations. J.A.M.A., *175*:427, 1961.
445. McGregor, A. L.: Congenital clubfoot: An analysis of the deformity and the principles of its treatment. Lancet, *2*:20, 1933.
446. McIntosh, R., Merritt, K. K., Richards, M. R., Samuels, M. H., and Bellows, M. T.: The incidence of congenital malformations: A study of 5,964 pregnancies. Pediatrics, *14*:505, 1954.
447. McKay, D. W.: New concept of and approach to clubfoot treatment: Section I—Principles and morbid anatomy. J. Pediatr. Orthop., *2*:347, 1982.
448. McKay, D. W.: New concept of and approach to clubfoot treatment: Section II—Correction of the clubfoot. J. Pediatr. Orthop., *3*:10, 1983.
449. McKay, D. W.: New concept of and approach to clubfoot treatment: Section III—Evaluation and results. J. Pediatr. Orthop., *3*:141, 1983.
450. Mackenney, R. P., and Oni, O. O.: The Cincinnati incision: A comprehensive approach for surgical procedures of the foot and ankle in childhood (letter). J. Bone Joint Surg., *66-A*:313, 1984.
451. Magnusson, R.: Rotation osteotomy—a method employed in case of congenital club-foot. J. Bone Joint Surg., *28*:262, 1946.
452. Main, B. J., and Crider, R. J.: An analysis of residual deformity in club feet submitted to early operation. J. Bone Joint Surg., *60-B*:536, 1978.
453. Main, B. J., Crider, R. J., Polk, M., Lloyd-Roberts, G. C., Swann, M., and Kamdar, B. A.: The results of early operation in talipes equinovarus. J. Bone Joint Surg., *59-B*:337, 1977.
454. Malagon Castro, V.: Pié varus equino congénito (factores etiológicos). Rev. Fac. Med. (Bogotá), *22*:427, 1955.
455. Marciniak, W.: Guidelines for the evaluation of treatment of congenital clubfoot. Chir. Narzadow Ruchu Ortop. Pol., *36*:213, 1971.
456. Marciniak, W.: Results of conservative management of congenital clubfoot in infants in the light of 5-year follow-up. Chir. Narzadow Ruchu Ortop. Pol., *36*:507, 1971.
457. Marciniak, W.: Single-stage peritalar reposition of congenital club foot in children. Chir. Narzadow Ruchu Ortop. Pol., *37*:589, 1972.
458. Marciniak, W.: Reasons for and description of pseudocorrections in conservative treatment of congenital clubfoot. Chir. Narzadow Ruchu Ortop. Pol., *37*:679, 1972.
459. Marciniak, W.: Anatomical analysis of deformities in congenital clubfoot and its pseudo-corrections. Selection of surgical method. Chir. Narzadow Ruchu Ortop. Pol., *38*:45, 1973.
460. Marciniak, W.: Die anatomische Analyse der Veränderungen beim angeborenen Klumpfuss and bei seinen Pseudokorrektionen als Beitrag zur Auswahl der Methode einer operativen Behandlung. Beitr. Orthop. Traumatol., *22*:163, 1975.
461. Marciniak, W.: Modification of the Kite's method of conservative treatment of congenital talipes equinovarus (preliminary report). Chir. Narzadow Ruchu Ortop. Pol., *43*:471, 1978.
462. Marciniak, W., and Koczocik-Prezedpelska, J.: Occurrence of action potentials in the calf muscles of children with clubfoot during walking. Chir. Narzadow Ruchu Ortop. Pol., *46*:295, 1981.
463. Marciniak, W., and Koczocik-Przedpelska, J.: Electrogoniometric studies of the knee and foot movements in children during walking after surgical treatment of clubfoot. Chir. Narzadow Ruchu Ortop. Pol., *46*:453, 1981.
464. Marciniak, W., and Koczocik-Prezedpelska, J.: Relations between the action of the leg muscles and the knee and foot movements in children during walking after treatment of congenital equino-varus talipes. Chir. Narzadow Ruchu Ortop. Pol., *47*:71, 1982.

465. Maresca, A.: Considerazioni sulla lussazione congenital astragalo scafoidea nel quadro del cosidetto piede a dondolo. Orriz. Ortop. Odierna Riabilit., *4*:187, 1959.
466. Marique, P.: La réintegration non sanglante de l'astragale. Méthode nouvelle pour la réduction du pied bot varus équin. Rev. Orthop., *27*:37, 1942.
467. Marique, P.: La subluxation du pied bot. Presse Med., *54*:411, 1946.
468. Marique, P., and De Meuter, W.: Le controle radiographique au cours du traitement du pied bot par la méthode de Denis Browne. Rev. Chir. Orthop., *37*:250, 1951.
469. Marique, P., and Steebenruggen, C. A.: Le traitement du pied bot varus équin congénital. Acta Orthop. Belg., *13*:90, 1947.
470. Marquez Gubern, A.: Some aspects in the treatment of congenital talipes equinovarus (TEV). An. Med. Espec., *51*:49, 1965.
471. Martini, G., and Tos, L.: Corrective manual treatment of the congenital talus valgus foot. Gazz. Med. Ital., *124*:108, 1965.
472. Massart, R.: Le traitement chirurgical précoce au pied bot congénital. Bull. Mem. Soc. Chir. Paris, June:382, 1931.
473. Masse, P., Taussig, G., and Bazin, G.: External wedge-shaped osteotomy of the calcaneus in the treatment of talipes equinovarus. Rev. Chir. Orthop., *60*:Suppl. 2:135, 1974.
474. Masse, P., Taussig, G., and Jacob, P.: Osteotomy of the calcaneus in the treatment of congenital varus equinus clubfoot. Rev. Chir. Orthop., *66*:51, 1980.
475. Masse, P., Benichou, J., Dimeglio, A., Morel, J. M., Onimus, M., Padovani, J., and Seringe, R.: Pied bot varus équin congénital. S.O.F.C.O.T., Réunion annuelle, Nov., 1975. Rev. Chir. Orthop., *62*:Suppl. 2:37, 1976.
476. Masse, R.: Le traitement du pied bot par la méthode fonctionelle. *In* Cahiers d'enseignement de la S.O.F.C.O.T. Paris, Expansion Scientifique Française, 1977, p. 51.
477. Match, R. M.: Onycho-osteo-arthrodysplasia with equinovarus. Study of affected family. N.Y. J. Med., *73*:1105, 1973.
478. Matheis, H.: Die Sofortbehandlung des angeborenen Klumpfusses. Wien. Klin. Wochenschr., *59*:55, 1947.
479. Mau, C.: Der Klumpfuss. Ergeb. Chir. Orthop., *20*:361, 1927.
480. Mau, C.: Muskelbefunde und ihre Bedeutung beim angeborenen Klumpfussleiden. Arch. Orthop. Unfallchir., *28*:292, 1930.
481. Mau, H.: Klumpfuss. Dtsch. Med. Wochenschr., *98*:1782, 1973.
482. Melville, R. S.: Utilization of the body weight in treatment of the residual deformity in clubfeet. J. Bone Joint Surg., *21*:456, 1939.
483. Memmi, G.: Lo svilippo embriologico del piede e i suoi riflessi sulla patogenesi del piede torto congenito. Minerva Ginec., *15*:508, 1963.
484. Menelaus, M. B.: Talectomy in equinovarus deformity in arthrogryposis and spina bifida. J. Bone Joint Surg., *53-B*:468, 1971.
485. Mezzari, A.: La capsultomia posteriore nella cura del piede torto congenito. Atti Soc. Ital. Ortop. Trauma., *32*:354, 1947.
486. Michel, L.: Le pied bot varus équin congénital et son traitement actuel. Rev. Orthop., *35*:167, 1949.
487. Middleton, D. S.: Studies on prenatal lesions of striated muscle as a cause of congenital deformity. Edinburgh Med. J., N.S., *41*:401, 1934.
488. Migeon, B. R.: Short arm deletions in group E and chromosomal "deletion" syndromes. J. Pediatr., *69*:432, 1966.
489. Mikyska, V., and Stehlik, V.: Corrective splint with horizontal rotation for follow-up treatment of congenital clubfoot. Beitr. Orthop. Traumatol., *14*:403, 1967.
490. Miller, E. A.: Congenital clubfoot. Surg. Clin. North Am., *45*:231, 1965.
491. Miller, G. M., Hsu, J. D., Hoffer, M. M., and Rentfro, R.: Posterior tibial tendon transfer: A review of the literature and analysis of 74 procedures. J. Pediatr. Orthop., *2*:363, 1982.
492. Miller, J. H., and Bernstein, S.: The roentgenographic appearance of the corrected clubfoot. Foot Ankle, *6*:177, 1986.
493. Miller, W. E.: Congenital clubfeet. Bull. Univ. Miami Sch. Med. & Jackson Mem. Hosp., *13*:1, 1959.
494. Mimran, R.: Transplantation du jambier postérieur sur le dos du pied. Rev. Chir. Orthop., *52*:681, 1966.
495. Mitroszewska, H., and Jaworski, W.: Congenital hypoplasia of the fibula associated with talipes equinovarus. Chir. Narzadow Ruchu Ortop. Pol., *43*:283, 1978.
496. Möbius, P. J.: Ueber angeborene doppelseitige Abducens-Facialis-Lähmung. Munchen Med. Wochenschr., *35*:91, 1888.
497. Moore, J. R.: Clubfoot braces. *In* Orthopaedic Appliances Atlas. Ann Arbor, J. W. Edwards, 1952, Vol. 1, pp. 479–495.
498. Moreau, M., and Dick, D.: Ankle motion in the surgically corrected club foot. Presented at the annual meeting of the Pediatric Orthopedic Society of North America, Toronto, May 1987.
499. Morel, G.: La correction chirurgicale du pied bot chez le grand enfant. *In* Cahiers d'enseignement de la S.O.F.C.O.T. Paris, Expansion Scientifique Française, 1977, p. 91.
500. Morita, S.: A method for the treatment of resistant congenital clubfoot in infants by gradual correction with leverage-wire correction and wire-traction cast. J. Bone Joint Surg., *44-A*:149, 1962.
501. Moroz, P. F.: The method of operative treatment of congenital talipes in children. Ortop. Travmatol. Protez., *27*:47, 1966.
502. Morris, R. H.: Skeletal traction as a method of treatment for certain foot deformities. Arch. Surg. (Chicago), *46*:737, 1943.
503. Mulfinger, G. L., and Trueta, J.: The blood supply of talus. J. Bone Joint Surg., *52-B*:160, 1970.
504. Müller, G.: Die morphologischen Ergebnisse der Klumpfussbehandlung aus klinischer und röntgenologischer Sicht. Beitr. Orthop. Traumatol., *17*:594, 1970.
505. Müller, G.: Clubfoot therapy. Kinderarztl. Prax., *41*:7, 1973.
506. Müller, R.: Über das Geschlechtsverhältnis beim angeborenen Klumpfussleiden. Z. Orthop., *72*:237, 1941.
507. Murray, W. R.: Treatment of clubfoot. Postgrad. Med., *37*:105, 1965.
508. Musial, W. W.: Results of surgical treatment of pes equinovarus. Folia Med. Cracov., *7*:559, 1965.
509. Myers-Ralfs, M.: Seltene Muskelanomalie bei angeborenen Klumpfuss. Z. Orthop., *111*:801, 1973.
510. Nagura, S.: Zur Ätiologie des angeborenen Klumpfusses. Zentralbl. Chir., *81*:187, 1956.
511. Nagura, S.: Zur Frage der Vererbung des angeborenen Klumpfusses. Arch. Orthop. Unfallchir., *52*:48, 1960.
512. Neel, J. V., Falls, H. T., and Test, A. R.: Pedigree of club-foot. Am. J. Dis. Child., *79*:442, 1950.
513. Negron, A. J.: Un concepto fundamental en el tratamiento precoz del pié bot congénito. Rev. Hosp. Niño (Lima), *54*:119, 1953.
514. Nemechek, R. W.: Long-term follow-up and family study in congenital talipes equinovarus. J. Bone Joint Surg., *50-A*:1064, 1968.
515. Nichols, E. H.: Anatomy of congenital equinovarus. Boston Med. Surg. J., *36*:150, 1897.

516. Nicoladoni, C.: The classic. On the treatment of pes equinus paralyticus. Clin. Orthop., *135*:2, 1978.
517. Niedzwiecki, T., Lejman, T., and Marchewczyk, J.: Radiological picture of the Chopart's joint in talipes equinovarus. Chir. Narzadow Ruchu Ortop. Pol., *44*:265, 1979.
518. Nilsonne, H.: Eine statistische Studie über den kongenitalen Klumpfuss. Z. Orthop. Chir., *48*:219, 1927.
519. Nomura, S., Kondo, M., Maekawa, M., Himeno, S., and Matsui, T.: Limited plantar flexion of the ankle in the surgically treated congenital club foot. Fukuoka Acta Med., *73*:476, 1982.
520. Nutt, J. J.: Congenital club-foot. *In* Diseases and Deformities of the Foot. New York, E.B. Treat & Co., 1925, pp. 113–173.
521. Nyga, W.: Results of relocating the anterior tibial muscle in treating congenital clubfoot. Beitr. Orthop. Traumatol., *26*:44, 1979.
522. Ober, F. R.: An operation for the relief of congenital equinovarus deformity. Preliminary report. J.A.M.A., *65*:621, 1915.
523. Ober, F. R.: An operation for the relief of congenital equinovarus deformities. J. Orthop. Surg., *2*:558, 1920.
524. Ode, A.: Zur histologischen Pathologie des kongenitalen Spitz-Klumpfüsses mit Nachuntersuchungsergebnissen operierter Spitz-Klumpfüsses. Z. Orthop., *82*:102, 1952.
525. Ogston, A.: A new principle of curing club-foot in severe cases in children a few years old. Br. Med. J., *1*:1524, 1902.
526. Oliver, G.: Formation du sequelette des membres. Paris, Vigot Frères, 1962.
527. Ono, K., and Hayashi, H.: Residual deformity of treated congenital club foot. A clinical study employing frontal tomography of the hind part of the foot. J. Bone Joint Surg., *56-A*:1577, 1974.
528. O'Rahilly, R.: Morphological patterns in limb deficiencies and duplications. Am. J. Anat., *89*:135, 1951.
529. Orofino, C. F.: The etiology of congenital club foot. Acta Orthop. Scand., *29*:59, 1960.
530. Otremski, I., Salama, R., Khermosh, O., and Wientroub, S.: An analysis of the results of a modified one-stage posteromedial release (Turco operation) for the treatment of clubfoot. J. Pediatr. Orthop., *7*:149, 1987.
531. Otto, F. M. G.: Die "Cranio-carpo-tarsal Dystrophie" (Freeman-Sheldon); ein kasuistischer Beitrag. Z. Kinderheilkd., *73*:240, 1953.
532. Padovani, J. P., Rigault, P., Pouliquen, J. C., Guyonvarch, G., and Durand, Y.: L'astragalectomie chez l'enfant. Rev. Chir. Orthop., *62*:475, 1976.
533. Pages, R.: Treatment of congenital talipes equinovarus. Bull. Soc. Chir. Paris, *59*:252, 1969.
534. Palmer, R. M.: Hereditary club foot. Clin. Orthop., *33*:138, 1964.
535. Palmer, R. M.: The genetics of talipes equinovarus. J. Bone Joint Surg., *46-A*:542, 1964.
536. Palmer, R. M., Conneally, P. M., and Yu, P. L.: Studies of the inheritance of idiopathic talipes equinovarus. Orthop. Clin. North Am., *5*:99, 1974.
537. Pandey, S., Jha, S. S., and Pandey, A. K.: "T" osteotomy of the calcaneum. Int. Orthop., *4*:219, 1980.
538. Pansini, A.: Indicazioni e risultati dell'operazione di Codivilla nel trattamento del piede torto congenito. Minerva Ortop., *16*:158, 1965.
539. Papin, E.: Le Phelps-Kirmisson dans le traitment du pied bot congénital après deux ans. Rev. Orthop., *18*:698, 1931.
540. Parker, R. W.: Congenital clubfoot. The part played by the tarsal ligaments in maintaining the deformity and the value of the subcutaneous section in the cure. Br. Med. J., *2*:10, 1886.
541. Parker, R. W.: Congenital Club-foot: Its Nature and Treatment. London, Lewis & Co., 1887.
542. Parker, R. W., and Shattock, S. G.: The pathology and etiology of congenital club-foot. Trans. Pathol. Soc. Lond., *35*:423, 1884.
543. Pasila, M., and Sulamaa, M.: Early operation on severe club foot. Nord. Med., *66*:1274, 1961.
544. Paturet, G.: Traite d'Anatomie Humaine. Tome II. Paris, Masson & Cie, 1951.
545. Paulos, L., Coleman, S. S., and Samuelson, K. M.: Pes cavovarus. Review of a surgical approach using selective soft-tissue procedures. J. Bone Joint Surg., *62A*:942, 1980.
546. da Paz, A. C., Jr., and de Souza, V.: Talipes equinovarus: pathomechanical basis of treatment. Orthop. Clin. North Am., *9*:171, 1978.
547. Pearocca, A.: Contribution of the therapy of congenital clubfoot. Minerva Orthop., *11*:180, 1960.
548. Peleska, L.: Surgical treatment of talipes equino-varus deformity: A commentary. Acta Chir. Orthop. Traumatol. Cech., *45*:483, 1978.
549. Penners, R.: Muskelanomalien bei angeborenen Klumpfüssen. Z. Orthop., *83*:103, 1954.
550. Pennino, C.: Late therapy of congenital twisted foot. Arch. Chir. Ortop., *19*:47, 1954.
551. Peretti, G., and Surace, A.: Club foot, classification, etiology and pathogenesis. Ital. J. Orthop. Traumatol., *2*:Suppl.:11, 1976.
552. Pérez Lorié, J.: Pié varo equino congénito. Cir. Ortop. Trauma., *3*:39, 1935.
553. Perkins, G.: Orthopaedics. London, Athlone Press, 1961, p. 585.
554. Perugia, L., and Maffucci, M.: Valutazione elettrodiagnostica dell squilibrio muscolare nel piede torto congenito. Orriz. Ortop. Odierna Riabilit., *4*:219, 1959.
555. Petri, C.: Congenital club-foot. Ther. Umsch., *28*:309, 1971.
556. Petri, C.: The results of the early treatment of congenital clubfoot. Orthopaede, *8*:159, 1979.
557. Pfeiffer, R. A., Ammermann, M., Baisch, C., and Bolhoff, G.: Das Syndrom von Freeman und Sheldon. 3 neue Beobachtung. Z. Kinderheilkd., *112*:43, 1973.
558. Phelps, A. M.: The present status of the open incision method for talipes equinovarus. Med. Res., *38*:22, 1890.
559. Picazo, G.: Pié varus equino congenito. IV Cong. Nacl. Soc. Mex. Ortop. Trauma, 1956, p. 59.
560. Picazo, G.: Algunas consideraciones sobre pié equinovaro congenito o pié bot. Primeras jornadas Nc. de Ortop. y Trauma., 1961, p. 70.
561. Pierre, M.: Subluxation of clubfoot. Presse Med., *54*:411, 1946.
562. Pillay, V. K., Khong, B. T., and Wolfers, D.: The inheritance of club foot in Singapore. Proc. Third Malaysian Cong. Med., *3*:102, 1967.
563. Piskorski, Z.: Failures of conservative management of congenital clubfoot. Chir. Narzadow Ruchu Ortop. Pol., *36*:221, 1971.
564. Pizio, Z.: Internal torsion of the tibia and foot as a component of clubfoot. Chir. Narzadow Ruchu Ortop. Pol., *33*:215, 1967.
565. Pokrassa, M. A., and Rodgveller, B.: Talipes equinovarus: Current concepts. J. Am. Podiatry Assoc., *71*:472, 1981.
566. Pompe van Meerdervoort, H. P.: Congenital muscular-skeletal disorders in the South African Negro. J. Bone Joint Surg., *59-B*:257, 1977.
567. Ponseti, I. V., and Campos, J.: Observations on pathogenesis and treatment of congenital clubfoot. Clin. Orthop., *84*:50, 1972.
568. Ponseti, I. V., and Smoley, E. N.: Congenital club foot: The results of treatment. J. Bone Joint Surg., *45-A*:261, 1963.

569. Porat, S., Milgrom, C., and Bentley, G.: The history of treatment of congenital clubfoot at the Royal Liverpool Children's Hospital: Improvement of results by early extensive posteromedial release. J. Pediatr. Orthop., *4*:331, 1984.
570. Poulain, J.: L'arthrographie tibio-tarsienne dans le pied bot varus équin congénital du premier âge. Thèse pour le Doctorat en Médicine. Paris, Libraire Arnette, 1949.
571. Pous, J. G.: La chirurgie de transplantation tendineuse dans le pied bot varus équin. *In* Cahiers d'enseignement de la S.O.F.C.O.T. Paris, Expansion Scientifique Française, 1977, p. 87.
572. Pous, J. G., and Dimeglio, A.: La chirurgie néonatale du pied bot varus équin: Pourquoi pas? *In* Cahiers d'enseignement de la S.O.F.C.O.T. Paris, Expansion Scientifique Française, 1977, p. 65.
573. Preston, E. T., and Fett, T. W., Jr.: Congenital idiopathic clubfoot. Clin. Orthop., *122*:102, 1977.
574. Pridie, K. H.: Complications of the treatment of club foot. Proc. South-West Orth. Club (abstract). J. Bone Joint Surg., *35-B*:53, 1952.
575. Primrose, D. A.: Talipes equinovarus in mental defectives. J. Bone Joint Surg., *51-B*:60, 1969.
576. Prochiantz, A.: La fonction et la forme, double préoccupation du traitement du pied bot varus équin. Ann. Chir. Infant. (Paris), *16*:211, 1975.
577. Proppe, P.: Häufigkeit des angeborenen Klumpfusses und der angeborenen Hüftluxation. Z. Orthop., *42*:308, 1922.
578. Pyka, R. A., and Coventry, M. B.: Avascular necrosis of the skin after operation on the foot. J. Bone Joint Surg., *43-A*:955, 1961.
579. Rabl, C. R. H.: Herunterholen der Klumpfuss-Ferse ohne Tenotomie. Z. Orthop., *82*:599, 1952.
580. Rabl, C. R. H.: Zur Methode der Klumpfussbehandlung. Beitr. Orthop. Traumatol., *15*:125, 1968.
581. Radke, J., and Janssen, R.: Clinical aspects and therapy of congenital clubfoot. Med. Monatsschr., *28*:293, 1974.
582. Ranieri, L.: Patogenesi e terapia del piede torto congenito. Chir. Organi Mov., *52*:64, 1963.
583. Raynal, L., and Judet, J.: Traitement du pied bot varus équin congénital de l'âge de deux à cinq ans. Acta Orthop. Belg., *33*:867, 1967.
584. Raynal, L., Judet, J., and Judet, R.: Traitement du pied bot varus équin congénital de l'âge de deux à cinq ans. Acta Orthop. Belg., *25*:479, 1959.
585. Reimann, I.: Congenital idiopathic club foot. Thesis. Copenhagen, Munsgaard, 1967.
586. Reimann, I., and Lyquist, E.: Dynamic splint used in the treatment of clubfoot. Acta Orthop. Scand., *40*:817, 1970.
587. Reimann, I., and Becker-Andersen, H.: Early surgical treatment of congenital clubfoot. Clin. Orthop., *102*:200, 1974.
588. Repetto, P.: Early surgery of congenital clubfoot in the first two years of life. Minerva Nipiol., *6*:72, 1956.
589. Resnick, D.: Radiology of the talocalcaneal articulations. Radiology, *111*:581, 1974.
590. Richards, R. M.: The Möbius syndrome. J. Bone Joint Surg., *41-A*:473, 1953.
591. Rigault, P.: Résultats du traitement des pieds bots varus équins congénitaux rebelles ou récidives per allongement ou section des parties molles avec correction de la malposition osseuse. Acta Orthop. Belg., *33*:883, 1967.
592. Rintala, A.: Freeman-Sheldon's syndrome. Craniocarpo-tarsal dystrophy. Acta Paediatr. Scand., *57*:553, 1968.
593. Ritsila, V. A.: Talipes equinovarus and vertical talus produced experimentally in newborn rabbits. Acta Orthop. Scand., Suppl. 121, 1969.
594. Roberts, J. M.: Paper presented at the Pediatric Orthopedic International Seminar, San Francisco, May 1988.
595. Rogala, E. J., Wynne-Davies, R., Littlejon, A., and Gormley, J.: Congenital limb anomalies: Frequency and aetiological factors. Data from the Edinburgh Register of the Newborn (1964–68). J. Med. Genet., *11*:221, 1974.
596. Romanini, L., and Mollica, Q.: I trattamento del piede torto congenito nella storia della medicina. Orriz. Ortop. Odierna Riabilit., *5*:183, 1960.
597. Roper, A.: A simple and effective method of treatment of congenital clubfoot. Cent. Afr. J. Med., *13*:226, 1967.
598. Rosa, G.: Deformita del piede da esostosi solitaria dell'astragalo. Orriz. Ortop. Odierna Riabilit., *8*:103, 1963.
599. Rubin, A., and Friedenberg, Z. B.: Clubfoot (talipes). *In* Rubin, A. (ed.): Handbook of Congenital Malformations. Philadelphia, Saunders, 1969, Chapter 5.
600. Rydell, N. W., and Magnusson, A.: A new brace for the treatment of congenital clubfoot. Acta Orthop. Scand., *41*:501, 1970.
601. Ryoppy, S., and Sarinen, H.: Neonatal operative treatment of club foot. A preliminary report. J. Bone Joint Surg., *65-B*:320, 1983.
602. Sahlstedt, B.: Simultaneous arthrography of the talocrural and talonavicular joints in children. I. Technique. (Part II. see Hjelmstedt, A.). Acta Radiol. [Diagn.] (Stockh.), *17*:545, 1976.
603. Salle, B., Picot, C., Vauzelle, J. L., Deffrenne, P., Mounet, P., Francois, R., and Robert, J. M.: Le nanisme diastrophique. A propos de trois observations chez le nouveau-né. Pediatrie, *21*:311, 1966.
604. Salter, R. B.: Present trends in treatment of club feet. A.A.O.S. Instr. Course Lect. Sound-Slide Program, 1965, No. 7.
605. Salter, R. B., and Field, P.: The effects of continuous compression on living articular cartilage. J. Bone Joint Surg., *42-A*:31, 1960.
606. Salzer, M., and Schwagerl, W.: Die operative Klumpfussbehandlung mit Transfixation des Ruckfusses. Z. Orthop., *106*:368, 1969.
607. Savini, R., and Gualdrini, G.: Report on two cases of Freeman-Sheldon syndrome ("whistling face"). Ital. J. Orthop. Trauma., *6*:105, 1980.
608. Sayre, L. E.: Practical Manual of the Treatment of Clubfoot. New York, Appleton & Co., 1869.
609. Scaglietti, O.: Studio clinico statistico sui casi piede torto congenito oservati all'Instituto Orthopedico Rizzoli dal 1899 al 1933. Chir. Organi Mov., *19*:225, 1934.
610. Scaglietti, O.: Considerazioni sulla patogenesi del piede torto congenito. Chir. Organi Mov., *20*:25, 1935.
611. Scarlini, G.: Sulla cura del piede torto congenito. Arch. Ital. Chir., *13*:726, 1925.
612. Scarpa, A.: Memoria chirurgica sui piedi torti congeniti dei fanciulli e sulla maniera di corregger questa deformita. 2nd Ed. Pavia, B. Comino, 1806.
613. Scarpa, A.: A Memoir on the Congenital Club Foot in Children. Translated from Italian by J. W. Wishart. Edinburgh, Constable & Co., 1818.
614. Scheel, P. F.: Beobachtungen bei der Behandlung des kongenitalen Klumpfusses. Z. Orthop., *79*:546, 1950.
615. Scheel, P. F.: Fehlerquellen in der operativen Behandlung des Säuglingsklumpfusses. Z. Orthop., *90*:343, 1958.
616. Scher, M. A., Handelsman, J. E., and Isaacs, H.: The effect on muscle of immobilization under tension and relaxation. J. Bone Joint Surg., *59-B*:257, 1977.
617. Scherb, R.: Zur Ätiologie kongenitaler und Kongeni-

talbedingter. Fussdeformitäten mit besonderer Berucksichtingung des Pes equino-varus congenitus. Acta Chir. Scand., *67*:717, 1930.
618. Schlafly, B., Butler, J. E., Siff, S. J., Criswell, A., and Cain, T.: The appearance of the tarsal navicular after postero-medial release for club foot. Foot Ankle, *5*:222, 1985.
619. Schlicht, D.: The pathologic anatomy of talipes equinovarus. Aust. N.Z. J. Surg., *33*:2, 1963.
620. Schmid, W., D'Apuzzo, V., and Rossi, E.: Trisomy 6q25 to 6qter in a severely retarded 7-year-old boy with turricephaly, bow-shaped mouth, hypogenitalism and club feet. Hum. Genet., *46*:279, 1979.
621. Scholder, P.: Surgical treatment of congenital clubfoot. Ther. Umsch., *28*:315, 1971.
622. Schomburg, H.: Untersuchung der Entwicklung der Muskeln und Knochen des menschlichen Fusses an Serienschnitten und Rekonstruktionen und unter Zuhulfenahme Makrosko-pischer Präparation. Gottingen, Kaestner, 1900.
623. Schultze, C.: A plastic splint for the treatment of clubfoot in newborn infants. Beitr. Orthop. Traumatol., *19*:55, 1972.
624. Schulze, H.: Korrekturschiene zur Behandlung eines veralteten angeborenen Klumpfusses und der Innenrotation eines Hüftgelenkes. Beitr. Orthop. Traumatol., *18*:479, 1971.
625. Scolari, F.: Considerzioni sulla cura del piede torto congenito. Arch. Ortop., *62*:235, 1949.
626. Scott, W. A., Hosking, S. W., and Catterall, A.: Clubfoot. Observations on the surgical anatomy of dorsiflexion. J. Bone Joint Surg., *66-B*:71, 1984.
627. Scudder, C. L.: Congenital talipes equinovarus. Boston Med. Surg. J., *117*:397, 1887.
628. Sell, L. S.: The conservative treatment of congenital clubfeet in infants. South. Med. J., *32*:1199, 1939.
629. Sell, L. S.: Tibial torsion accompanying congenital clubfoot. J. Bone Joint Surg., *23*:561, 1941.
630. Semb, H. T.: The treatment of club-foot and its results. Acta Orthop. Scand., *34*:271, 1964.
631. Seringe, R.: Anatomie pathologique et physiopathologie du pied bot varus équin congénital. *In* Cahiers d'enseignement de la S.O.F.C.O.T. Paris, Expansion Scientifique Française, 1977, p. 11.
632. Seringe, R.: Etude clinique et radiologique de pied bot varus équin congénital. *In* Cahiers d'enseignement de la S.O.F.C.O.T. Paris, Expansion Scientifique Française, 1977, p. 25.
633. Seringe, R.: Traitement du pied bot varus équin congénital chez l'enfant. *In* Cahiers d'enseignement de la S.O.F.C.O.T. Paris, Expansion Scientifique Française, 1977, p. 57.
634. Settle, G. W.: The anatomy of congenital talipes equinovarus: Sixteen dissected specimens. J. Bone Joint Surg., *45-A*:1341, 1963.
635. Shaffer, N. M.: The classic non-deforming club-foot. With remarks on its pathology. Med. Rec., *27*:561, 1885.
636. Shapiro, F., and Glimcher, J. J.: Gross and histological abnormalities of the talus in congenital clubfoot. J. Bone Joint Surg., *61-A*:522, 1979.
637. Sharrard, W. J. W., and Grosfield, I.: The management of deformity and paralysis of the foot in myelomeningocele. J. Bone Joint Surg., *50-B*:456, 1968.
638. Shaw, N. E.: The primary treatment of congenital talipes equinovarus. Proc. 11th Annual Meeting Br. Assoc. Paediatr. Surg., 1964 (abstract). Arch. Dis. Child., *40*:230, 1965.
639. Shaw, N. E.: Comparison of three methods for treatment of congenital clubfoot. Br. Med. J., *1*:1084, 1966.
640. Shaw, N. E.: The early management of clubfoot. Clin. Orthop., *84*:39, 1972.
641. Sherman, F. C., and Westin, G. W.: Plantar release in the correction of deformities of the foot in childhood. J. Bone Joint Surg., *63-A*:1382, 1981.
642. Shneider, D. A., and Smith, C. F.: Medial subtalar stabilization with posterior medial release in the treatment of varus feet: A preliminary report. Orthop. Clin. North Am., *7*:949, 1976.
643. Siegel, M. I.: Letters: Reply to "comparative anatomy of the talus in relation to idiopathic club foot." Clin. Orthop., *102*:268, 1974.
644. Simons, G. W.: External rotational deformities in club feet. Clin. Orthop., *126*:239, 1977.
645. Simons, G. W.: Analytical radiography of clubfeet. J. Bone Joint Surg., *59-B*:485, 1977.
646. Simons, G. W.: Analytical radiography and the progressive approach in talipes equinovarus. Orthop. Clin. North Am., *9*:187, 1978.
647. Simons, G. W.: A standardized method for the radiographic evaluation of clubfeet. Clin. Orthop., *135*:107–118, 1978.
648. Simons, G. W.: Lateral talo-navicular subluxation—A complication of extensive soft tissue release for club feet. Orthop. Trans., *8*:448, 1984.
649. Simons, G. W.: Ankle range of motion in club feet. Presented at the Annual Meeting of the Pediatric Orthopedic Society of North America, San Antonio, Texas, May 1985.
650. Simons, G. W.: Complete subtalar release in club feet: Part I—A preliminary report. J. Bone Joint Surg., *67A*:1044, 1985.
651. Simons, G. W.: Complete subtalar release in club feet: Part II—Comparison with less extensive procedures. J. Bone Joint Surg., *67A*:1056, 1985.
652. Simons, G. W.: Symposium: Current practices in the treatment of idiopathic club foot in the child between birth and five years of age. Parts I and II. Contemp. Orthop., *1* and *2*, 1988.
653. Simons, G. W., and Sarrafian, S.: The microsurgical dissection of a stillborn fetal clubfoot. Clin. Orthop., *173*:275, 1983.
654. Singer, M.: Tibialis posterior transfer in congenital club foot. J. Bone Joint Surg., *43-B*:717, 1961.
655. Singer, M., and Fripp, A. T.: Tibialis anterior transfer in congenital club foot. J. Bone Joint Surg., *40-B*:252, 1958.
656. Slavik, J.: The clubfoot and its occurrence. Acta Chir. Orthop. Traumatol. Cech., *34*:74, 1967.
657. Smith, D. W.: Recognizable Patterns of Human Malformation. 2nd Ed. Philadelphia, Saunders, 1976.
658. Smith, R. B.: Dysplasia and the effects of soft tissue release in congenital talipes equinovarus. Clin. Orthop., *174*:303, 1983.
659. Smith, W. A., Jr., Campbell, P., and Bonnett, C.: Early posterior ankle release in the treatment of congenital clubfoot. Orthop. Clin. North Am., *7*:889, 1976.
660. Smoczynski, A., and Grabowski, M.: Tibialis anterior tendon transfer in the treatment of clubfoot and flatfoot in adolescents. Chir. Narzadow Ruchu Ortop. Pol., *44*:595, 1979.
661. Sofield, H. A.: Elastic traction assisting correction of club feet. J. Bone Joint Surg., *13*:283, 1931.
662. Soifer, H., and Palew, P.: Proper use of the Denis Browne splint. J. Pediatr., *61*:648, 1962.
663. Solomon, L., and Handelsman, J. E.: The treatment of club-foot. S. Afr. J. Surg., *5*:31, 1967.
664. Solonen, K. A., and Parkkulainen, K. V.: Congenital clubfoot, results of treatment. Ann. Chir. Gynaecol. Fenn. (Helsinki), *48*:130, 1958.
665. Somppi, E., and Sulamaa, M.: Early operative treatment of congenital club foot. Acta Orthop. Scand., *42*:513, 1971.
666. Sonnenschein, A.: Blutige oder unblutige Klumpfuss Behandlung? Acta Orthop. Scand., *18*:266, 1949.
667. Sostegni, A., and Paleari, L.: Il trattamento precoce

chirurgico del piede torto congenito e i suoi risultati a distanza. Arch. Ortop., *62*:225, 1949.
668. Sotirow, B.: Congenital club foot. Pathomechanism and treatment. Chir. Narzadow Ruchu Ortop. Pol., *38*:337, 1973.
669. Spires, T. D., Gross, R. H., Low, W., and Barringer, W.: Management of the resistant myelodysplastic or arthrogrypotic clubfoot with the Verebelyi-Ogston procedure. J. Pediatr. Orthop., *4*:705, 1984.
670. Spotorno, A.: Stabilization of congenital equinovarus following surgical and non-surgical therapy by means of transplantation of anterior tibial onto fifth metatarsal. Arch. Ortop., *63*:98, 1950.
671. Steel, H. H.: Computerized axial tomography (C-T scan) in assessment of correction of talipes equinovarus. Personal communication; paper read at Sixth Pediatric Orthopedic International Seminar, San Francisco, 1978.
672. Steel, H. H., and Kohl, J.: Multiple congenital dislocations associated with other skeletal anomalies (Larsen's syndrome) in three siblings. J. Bone Joint Surg., *54-A*:75, 1972.
673. Stein, V., and Weickert, H.: Treatment results of congenital clubfoot with special reference to recurrence. Beitr. Orthop. Traumatol., *30*:475, 1983.
674. Steindler, A.: Stripping of the os calcis. J. Orthop. Surg., *2*:8, 1920.
675. Steindler, A.: Orthopedic Operations, Indications, Techniques and End Results. Springfield, Ill., Charles C Thomas, 1950, Vol. I, pp. 178–196.
676. Stewart, S. F.: Club-foot: Its incidence, cause and treatment. Anatomical-physiological study. J. Bone Joint Surg., *33-A*:577, 1951.
677. Steyler, J. C. A., and Van Der Walt, I. D.: Correction of resistant adduction of the forefoot in congenital clubfoot and congenital metatarsus varus by metatarsal osteotomy. Br. J. Surg., *53*:558, 1966.
678. Storen, H.: Operative treatment of club foot in older children and adults. Acta Orthop. Scand., *18*:233, 1949.
679. Stover, C. N., Hayes, J. T., and Holt, J. F.: Diastrophic dwarfism. A. J. R., *89*:914, 1963.
680. Sudman, E., Hald, J. K., Jr., and Skandfer, B.: Features resisting primary treatment of congenital club foot. Acta Orthop. Scand., *54*:850, 1983.
681. Swann, M., Lloyd-Roberts, G. C., and Catterall, A.: The anatomy of uncorrected clubfeet. A study of rotation deformity. J. Bone Joint Surg., *51-B*:263, 1969.
682. Taylor, H. L.: Treatment of club foot by leverage. Trans. Am. Orthop. Assoc., *5*:178, 1892.
683. Taylor, J. F., Oyemade, G. A. A., Shaw, E., Ankers, P., Davies, C., and Jenkins, A. C.: Primary treatment of rigid congenital talipes equinovarus. Physiotherapy, *62*:89, 1976.
684. Tayton, K., and Thompson, P.: Relapsing club feet. Late results of delayed operation. J. Bone Joint Surg., *61-B*:474, 1979.
685. Templeton, A. W., McAlister, W. H., and Zim, I. D.: Standardization of terminology and evaluation of osseous relationships in congenitally abnormal feet. A. J. R., *93*:374, 1965.
686. Terry, R. J.: Sprengel's deformity and clubfoot: An anthropological interpretation. Am. J. Phys. Anthropol., *17*:251, 1959.
687. Thomas, W.: On translocation surgery of the tendon of the musculus peroneus brevis (M. fibularis brevis) in clubfoot. Z. Orthop., *116*:379, 1978.
688. Thompson, G. H., Richardson, A. B., and Westin, G. W.: Surgical management of resistant congenital talipes equinovarus deformities. J. Bone Joint Surg., *64-A*:652, 1982.
689. Thomson, S. A.: Treatment of congenital talipes equinovarus with a modification of the Denis Browne method and splint. J. Bone Joint Surg., *24*:291, 1942.
690. Thomson, S. A.: A splint treatment of recurrent clubfoot. J. Bone Joint Surg., *28*:778, 1946.
691. Thomson, S. A.: The treatment of congenital clubfoot. Nine years' experience with a modification of the Denis Browne method and splint. J. Bone Joint Surg., *31-A*:431, 1949.
692. Thomson, S. A.: Modified Denis Browne splint for unilateral club-foot to protect the normal foot. J. Bone Joint Surg., *37-A*:1286, 1955.
693. Thyes, A.: Le traitement du pied bot varus équin congénital par la méthode de Scheib. Acta Orthop. Belg., *13*:299, 1947.
694. Tokarowski, A.: Osteotomoclasis for tibial detorsion in the treatment of congenital club-foot. Chir. Narzadow Ruchu Ortop. Pol., *38*:173, 1977.
695. Tompkins, S. F., Millers, R. J., and O'Donoghue, D. H.: An evolution of astragalectomy. South. Med. J., *49*:1128, 1956.
696. Tönnis, D., and Bikadorov, V.: Untersuchungen über die Ergebnisse verschiedener Behandlungsmethoden bei angeborenen Klumpfuss. Z. Orthop., *104*:218, 1968.
697. Torpin, R.: Fetal Malformations: Caused by Amnion Rupture During Gestation. Springfield, Ill., Charles C Thomas, 1968.
698. Torpin, R., Miller, G. T., Jr., and Culpepper, B. W.: Amniogenic fetal amputations associated with clubfoot. Obstet. Gynecol., *24*:379, 1964.
699. del Torto, V.: Arthrodesis for verticalization of astragalus in pes equinus. Rif. Med., *66*:1128, 1952.
700. de la Tourette, G.: Pathogénie et traitement des pieds bots. Sem. Med., *16*:517, 1897.
701. Treves, A.: Traitement du pied bot varus équin congénital. Rev. Orthop., *18*:393, 1931.
702. Treves, A.: Traitement du pied bot varus équin congénital après deux ans. Rev. Orthop., *18*:695, 1931.
703. Trias, A.: Effect of persistent pressure on articular cartilage. J. Bone Joint Surg., *43-B*:376, 1961.
704. Tripathi, R. P., and Chaturvedi, S. N.: Treatment of clubfoot by one stage medial soft tissue release operation. J. Indian Med. Assoc., *16*:73, 1979.
705. Turco, V. J.: Surgical corrections of the resistant congenital club-foot—one-stage release with internal fixation. A.A.O.S. Film Library, Chicago, Illinois, 1980.
706. Turco, V. J.: Surgical correction of the resistant club foot. One-stage posteromedial release with internal fixation: A preliminary report. J. Bone Joint Surg., *53-A*:477, 1971.
707. Turco, V. J.: Resistant congenital clubfoot. A.A.O.S. Instr. Course Lect., *24*:104, 1975.
708. Turco, V. J.: Resistant congenital club foot—one-stage posteromedial release with internal fixation. A follow-up report of a fifteen-year experience. J. Bone Joint Surg., *61-A*:805, 1979.
709. Turco, V. J.: Clubfoot. *In* Current Problems in Orthopaedics. New York, Churchill-Livingstone, 1981.
710. Turco, V. J., and Spinella, A. J.: Current management of clubfoot. A.A.O.S. Instr. Course Lect., *31*:218, 1982.
711. Turcu, G.: Congenital talipes equinovarus in infants less than 1 year of age. Clinical and laboratory studies. Rev. Med. Chir. Soc. Med. Nat. ISI, *78*:25, 1974.
712. Turcu, G.: Role and value of the footprint in evaluation of development of congenital talipes equinovarus. Rev. Chir., *24*:65, 1975.
713. Turek, S. L.: Orthopedics—Principles and Their Application. 2nd Ed. Philadelphia, Lippincott, 1967.
714. Turner, J. W., and Cooper, R. R.: Anterior transfer of the tibialis posterior through the interosseous membrane. Clin. Orthop., *83*:241, 1972.
715. Turra, S., Pavanini, G., and Volpe, A.: Surgical treatment of congenital club foot. (Comparison of the results of Codivilla's operation with those of Turco's modification). Ital. J. Orthop. Traumatol., *4*:155, 1978.

716. Valentin, Z. N.: La immovilización enyesada, su tecnica y sus apliaciones. La immovilizacion del pié equino varo congenita. Buenos Aires, Editorial El Ateneo, 1945, pp. 443–462.
717. Veale, A. M. O.: Polygenic inheritance. N.Z. Med. J., *67*:344, 1968.
718. Veale, A. M. O., Tapsel, P. W., and Tyler, K. R.: Club foot in Maoris. *In* Proceedings, Third International Congress of Human Genetics, 1966, p. 102.
719. Velasco, A., and Diaz, E.: Pié bot (estudio de 50 casos). An. Orthop. Trauma., *2*:115, 1952.
720. Velasco Polo, G. de, and Ponchener-Lechtman, C.: Surgical treatment of congenital talipes equinovarus adductus. Clin. Orthop., *70*:87, 1970.
721. Vereanu, D., Socolesco, M., and Georgesco, P.: Le traitement chirurgical du pied bot congénital varus-équin par libération des voutes plantaires. *In* Delchef, J. (ed.): Orthopaedic Surgery and Traumatology. Congenital clubfoot. a. Anatomy and pathology of the disease. New York, American Elsevier, 1973, pp. 751–752.
722. Vesely, D. G.: A method of application of a clubfoot cast. Clin. Orthop., *84*:47, 1972.
723. Vesely, J., Kordos, J., and Sijka, P.: Surgical treatment of severe recidivating deformities in pes equinovarus (clubfoot). Acta Chir. Orthop. Traumatol. Cech., *49*:63, 1982.
724. Vigliani, F.: Codivilla's operation after seventy years. Ital. J. Orthop. Trauma., *1*:297, 1975.
725. Vilenskii, V. I.: Polymeric devices in early conservative treatment of congenital clubfoot (modification of method of therapy). Ortop. Travmatol. Protez., *34*:24, 1973.
726. Vladimirova, N. A.: Physical therapeutic factors in the complex treatment of congenital clubfoot in radical reconstructive surgery. Ortop. Travmatol. Protez., *34*:72, 1973.
727. Wagner, E. J., and Haney, P. J.: Case report 230: Camptomelic syndrome. Skeletal Radiol., *9*:283, 1983.
728. Wagner, L. C., and Butterfield, W. L.: Surgical release of contracted tissues for resistant congenital clubfoot. Am. J. Surg., *84*:82, 1952.
729. Wahren, H.: Über die Korrektur der Tibiatorsion bei kongenitalen Klumpfuss. Acta Chir. Scand., *67*:928, 1930.
730. Waisbrod, H.: Congenital club foot. An anatomical study. J. Bone Joint Surg., *55-B*:796, 1973.
731. Waisbrod, H.: High medial release operation for resistant clubfoot. Isr. J. Med. Sci., *16*:444, 1980.
732. Walker, B. A., Scott, C. I., Hall, J. G., Murdoch, J. L., and McKusick, V. A.: Diastrophic dwarfism. Medicine (Baltimore), *51*:41, 1972.
733. Walsham, W. J., and Hughes, W. K.: Treatment of talipes equinus. *In* The Deformities of the Human Foot. London, Bailliere, Tindall & Cox, 1895, pp. 294–320.
734. Warkany, J.: Clubfoot (talipes equinovarus). *In* Congenital Malformations. Chicago, Year Book, 1971, pp. 1004–1010.
735. Watkins, M., Jones, J. B., Ryder, C. T., and Brown, T. H.: Transplantation of the posterior tibial tendon. J. Bone Joint Surg., *36-A*:1181, 1964.
736. Watts, A. W.: Anterior transplantation of tibialis posterior tendon. Aust. N.Z. J. Surg., *34*:284, 1965.
737. Weickert, H.: Ergebnisse konservativer und operativer Klumpfussbehandlung. Beitr. Orthop. Traumatol., *15*:753, 1968.
738. Weickert, H., and Stein, V.: Principles of treatment of congenital clubfoot and analysis of results. Beitr. Orthop. Traumatol., *26*:409, 1979.
739. Weinberg, H.: Congenital clubfoot. J. Bone Joint Surg., *45-B*:807, 1963.
740. Weinberg, H., and Halmosh, A. F.: Emotional maladjustment in the surgical correction of long-standing deformity. J. Bone Joint Surg., *41-A*:1310, 1959.
741. Weinstein, S., and Gorlin, R. J.: Cranio-carpo-tarsal dysplasia or the whistling face syndrome. Am. J. Dis. Child., *117*:427, 1969.
742. Weseley, M. S., and Barenfeld, P. A.: Operative treatment of congenital clubfoot. Clin. Orthop., *59*:161, 1968.
743. Weseley, M. S., and Barenfeld, P. A.: Calcaneal osteotomy for the treatment of cavus deformity. Bull. Hosp. Jt. Dis., *31*:93, 1970.
744. Weseley, M. S., and Barenfeld, P. A.: Mechanism of the Dwyer calcaneal osteotomy. Clin. Orthop., *70*:137, 1970.
745. Weseley, M. S., and Barenfeld, P. A.: Hard tissue correction of congenital clubfoot. Orthop. Rev., *5*:19, 1976.
746. Weseley, M. S., Barenfeld, P. A., and Barrett, N.: Complications of the treatment of clubfoot. Clin. Orthop., *84*:93, 1972.
747. Westin, G. W.: Plantar release in talipes equinovarus. Personal communication, 1975.
748. White, J. W.: The importance of the tibialis in the production and recurrence of clubfoot. South. Med. J., *22*:675, 1929.
749. White, J. W., and Gulledge, W. H.: Skin-tight casts for treatment of club-foot. J. Bone Joint Surg., *33-A*:475, 1951.
750. Whitman, A.: The Whitman operation as applied to various types of paralytic deformities of the foot. Results in the average cases. Med. Rec., *4*:266, 1922.
751. Whitman, A.: Astragalectomy. Ultimate results. Am. J. Surg., *11*:357, 1931.
752. Whitman, R.: The operative treatment of paralytic talipes of the calcaneus type. Am. J. Med. Sci., *192*:593, 1901.
753. Whitman, R.: Further observation on the treatment of paralytic talipes of the calcaneus by astragalectomy and backward displacement of the foot. Ann. Surg., *47*:264, 1908.
754. Whitman, R.: Further observation on the treatment of paralytic talipes, calcaneus and allied distortions. Med. Rec., *81*:47, 1914.
755. Wiberg, G.: Tiding behandling av den kongenitala Klumfoten. Nord. Med., *8*:2660, 1940.
756. Wickstrom, J., and Williams, R. A.: Shoe corrections and orthopaedic foot supports. Clin. Orthop., *70*:30, 1970.
757. Widolf, G. A.: Congenital clubfoot—a better splint for conservative treatment. Med. J. Aust., *1*:846, 1973.
758. Wiedemann, H. R., and Dibbern, H.: Larsen's syndrome. Med. Welt, *24*:1548, 1980.
759. Wiley, A. M.: Club foot. An anatomical and experimental study of muscle growth. J. Bone Joint Surg., *41-B*:821, 1959.
760. Wilhelm, R.: Mangelhafte Entwicklung des os naviculare beim angeborenen Klumpfuss. Fortschr. Rontgenstr., *35*:735, 1927.
761. Williams, P.: Principles in treatment of talipes equinovarus. Personal communication: Paper presented at Sixth Pediatric Orthopedic Seminar, San Francisco, 1978.
762. Wiltse, L. L., and Bateman, J. G.: Removing plaster from clubfeet. Clin. Orthop., *103*:63, 1974.
763. Wisbrun, W.: Neue Gesichtspunkte zum Redressement des angeborenen Klumpfusses und daraus sich ergebende Schlussfolgerungen dezuglich der Atiologie. Arch. Orthop. Unfallchir., *31*:451, 1932.
764. Wolff, J.: Ueber die Ursachen, das Wesen und die Behandlung das Klumpfusses. Berlin, August Hirschwald, 1903.
765. Wolff, J. R., and Tönnis, D.: Elektronenmikroskopische Untersuchungen der Muskulatur bei angeborenen Klumpfuss und angeborener Huftluxation. Arch. Orthop. Unfallchir., *68*:95, 1970.
766. Wolff, L. V.: The development of the human foot as

an organ of locomotion. Am. J. Dis. Child., *37*:1212, 1929.
767. Wood-Jones, F.: Structure and Function as Seen in the Foot. Baltimore, Williams & Wilkins, 1944, pp. 133–135.
768. Wynne-Davies, R.: Family studies and cause of congenital clubfoot. J. Bone Joint Surg., *46-B*:445, 1964.
769. Wynne-Davies, R.: Talipes equinovarus. A review of eighty-four cases after completion of treatment. J. Bone Joint Surg., *46-B*:464, 1964.
770. Wynne-Davies, R.: Family studies and aetiology of clubfoot. J. Med. Genet., *2*:227, 1965.
771. Wynne-Davies, R.: The genetics of some common congenital malformations. *In* Emery, A. (ed.): Modern Trends in Human Genetics. London, Butterworths, 1970, Chapter 11.
772. Wynne-Davies, R.: Genetic and environmental factors in the etiology of talipes equinovarus. Clin. Orthop., *84*:9, 1972.
773. Wynne-Davies, R.: Heritable Disorders in Orthopaedic Practice. Oxford, Blackwell, 1973, p. 206.
774. Wynne-Davies, R.: A review of genetics in orthopaedics. Acta Orthop. Scand., *46*:338, 1975.
775. Young, A. B.: Club foot treated by astragalectomy. 50-year follow-up of a case. Lancet, *1*:670, 1962.
776. Zadek, I., and Barnett, E. I.: The importance of the ligaments of the ankle in correction of congenital clubfoot. J.A.M.A., *69*:1057, 1917.
777. Zatsepin, T. S.: Operation on tendinoligamentous apparatus in congenital clubfoot in children. Mosk, Khirurgiia, No. *11*:59, 1944.
778. Zavialov, P. V., and Stavskaia, E. A.: Treatment of congenital clubfoot by a distraction-compression method. Ortop. Travmatol. Protez., *2*:41, 1978.
779. Zenker, H.: Ossare Klumpfussbehandlung beim Kleinkind. Arch. Orthop. Unfallchir., *68*:255, 1970.
780. Zerbi, E.: Sulla cura del piede torto congenito. Minerva Ortop., *9*:1, 1958.
781. Zergollern, J.: Biochemical basis for the need of surgical treatment of pes equinovarus congenitus in resistant cases. Acta Med. Iugosl., *25*:91, 1971.
782. Zergollern, J.: Importance of early treatment of pes equinovarus congenitus. Lijec. Vjesn., *93*:543, 1971.
783. Zimbler, S.: Practical considerations in the early treatment of congenital talipes equinovarus. Orthop. Clin. North Am., *3*:257, 1972.
784. Zimmer, J.: Das Geschlechtsverhaltnis beim angeborenen Klumpfuss. Z. Orthop. Chir., *69*:126, 1939.
785. Zwierzchowski, H.: Growth disorders of the distal epiphysis of the tibia in patients treated for clubfoot. Chir. Narzadow Ruchu Ortop. Pol., *42*:425, 1977.

CONGENITAL CONVEX PES VALGUS

Congenital convex pes valgus is a primary dorsal and lateral dislocation of the talocalcaneonavicular joint, developing in utero at some time during the first trimester of pregnancy. The navicular bone articulates with the dorsal aspect of the talus, locking it in a plantar-flexed vertical position. The deformity is commonly referred to as congenital vertical talus or simply vertical talus—a usage to be discouraged, as it focuses attention upon only one facet of this severe deformity.[58]

The condition was first described by Henken in 1914.[37] Its characteristic features were reviewed by Lamy and Weissman, who also presented a comprehensive study of the literature up to 1939.[48]

The entity is known by various synonyms. Originally, it was called congenital flatfoot due to vertical talus (pied plat congénital par subluxation sous-astragalienne congénitale et orientation vertical de l'astragale) by Rocher and Pouyanne.[66] "Congenital rocker-bottom flatfoot"; "rocker-foot due to congenital subluxation of the talus"; and "rocker-foot, or congenital flatfoot, due to talonavicular dislocation" are other names given the condition. The term *congenital convex pes valgus* was initially proposed by Lamy and Weissman, and later adopted in preference to others by Heyman and Herndon.[39, 48]

Teratologic dorsolateral dislocation of the talocalcaneonavicular joint is a more accurate name because it directs attention to the pathogenesis and therapeutic implications.

The condition may occur as an isolated primary deformity or in association with abnormalities of the central nervous and musculoskeletal systems. Sharrard and Grosfield found the incidence of congenital convex pes valgus to be 10 per cent in a large series of patients with myelomeningocele who had foot deformities.[69] Drennan and Sharrard proposed that a neuromuscular imbalance, i.e., a weak posterior tibial muscle and strong evertors of the foot, is responsible for the development of congenital convex pes valgus in myelomeningocele. They also noted the high incidence of abnormalities of the central nervous system in the reported cases of congenital vertical talus, and emphasized the importance of ruling out such associated anomalies prior to accepting the condition as an isolated primary deformity.[20] Arthrogryposis multiplex congenita, talipes equinovarus, pollex varus, dislocation of the hip, and neurofibromatosis are some of the neuromusculoskeletal abnormalities associated with it, and it may also be one of the numerous anomalies associated with autosomal trisomy, occurring with both trisomy 13–15 and trisomy 18.[78, 79] It is common with ischiocalcaneal bands.

The cause of the primary isolated form is unknown. Campos da Paz, Jr., and his associates proposed that congenital convex pes valgus probably is the result of an arrest of prenatal development of the foot.[11] At the seventh week of pregnancy the foot is in dorsiflexion, and the calcaneus is in close proximity to the lateral malleolus; in the twelfth week of pregnancy it moves away from the fibula to lie under the talus (Fig. 7–68).[83] The posture of the foot and

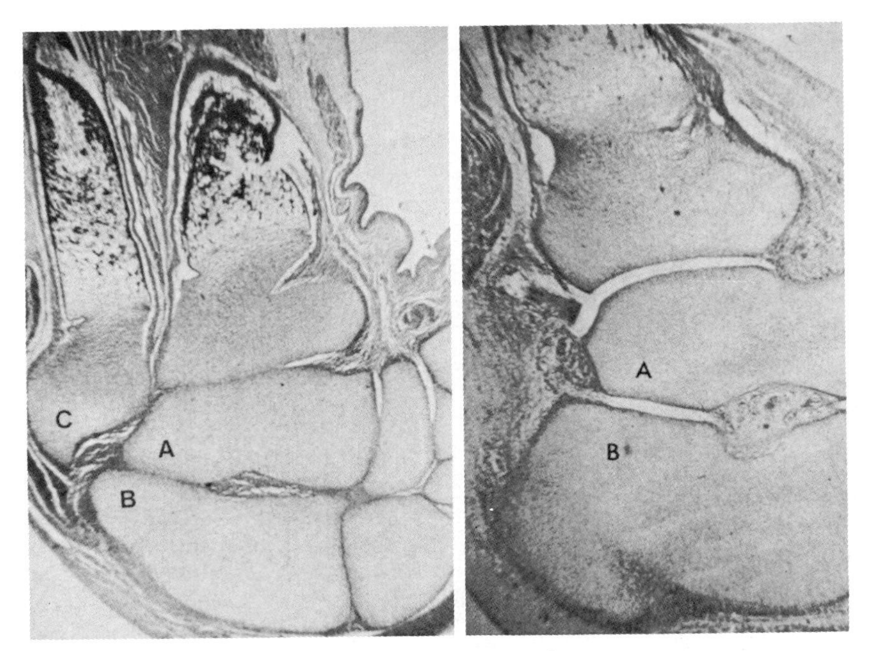

FIGURE 7–68. The relationship of the tarsal bones during development of a normal fetus.

A. At the seventh week of pregnancy, the ossification of the tarsal bones and distal fibula and tibia has commenced. Note the dorsiflexed posture of the foot and the close proximity of the calcaneus (B) to the distal end of the fibula (C). **B.** At the twelfth week of pregnancy, the calcaneus (B) has moved to lie under the talus (A) and away from the fibular malleolus. (From Campos da Paz, A., Jr., de Souza, V., and Conceicao de Souza, D.: Congenital convex pes valgus. Orthop. Clin. North Am., 9:207, 1978. Reprinted by permission.)

leg is dependent upon consecutive development of muscle function and muscular dominance.[84] The structural development of the central and peripheral nervous systems proceeds in a craniocaudal direction, and coordinated muscle contractions appear in the different muscle groups in a sequence corresponding to their anatomic level of innervation. Therefore, as the fourth and fifth lumbar and first sacral levels are innervated, the foot is in dorsiflexion and eversion; and as the fifth lumbar and first and second sacral levels are innervated, the foot changes its posture to plantar flexion and inversion.

Ritsilä produced vertical talus in rabbits by causing simultaneous shortening of the triceps surae muscle and dorsiflexor muscles of the foot, and sectioning the extensor digitorum longus, the tibialis anterior, and the ligamentum transversum cruris. (The divided tendons of the extensor digitorum longus and tibialis anterior adhered to the dorsum of the foot and acted as the deforming force.) Vertical talus also developed when either the extensor digitorum longus or the anterior tibial muscles were resected in addition to sectioning of the ligamentum transversum cruris and fixation of the Achilles tendon. Two types of vertical talus were produced, an anterior tibial type and an extensor digitorum type. In the *anterior tibial type* the tibialis anterior is taut and is the shortened element on the front of the ankle, whereas in the *extensor digitorum type* the long toe extensor and peroneal tendons are tightened and shortened. In both types as seen in the lateral projection, the sole has the rocker-bottom shape with the forepart of the foot dorsiflexed and the hindfoot in equinus posture, the talus is vertical, pointing to the plantar aspect of the foot, and the navicular articulates with the dorsal surface of the talar neck and not with the head of the talus. The anteroposterior projection shows the forefoot slightly supinated in the anterior tibial type (Fig. 7–69) and definitely pronated in the extensor digitorum type (Fig. 7–70). Ritsilä concluded that primary soft-tissue changes should be considered in the pathogenesis of congenital convex pes valgus.[64]

Heredity may be a factor. Familial incidence in parent and child has been observed by Aschner and Engelmann, by Robbins, and by Lamy and Weissman.[2, 48, 65] Armknecht found congenital convex pes valgus in identical twins.[1]

The incidence of teratologic dislocation of the

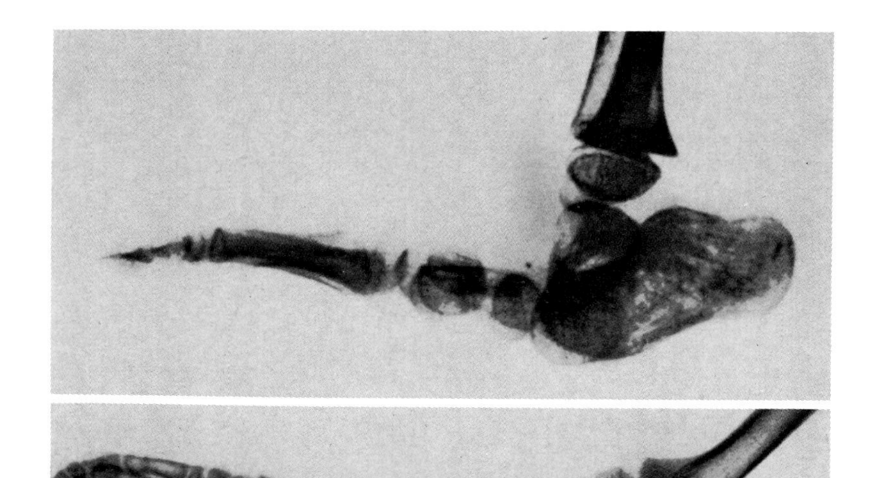

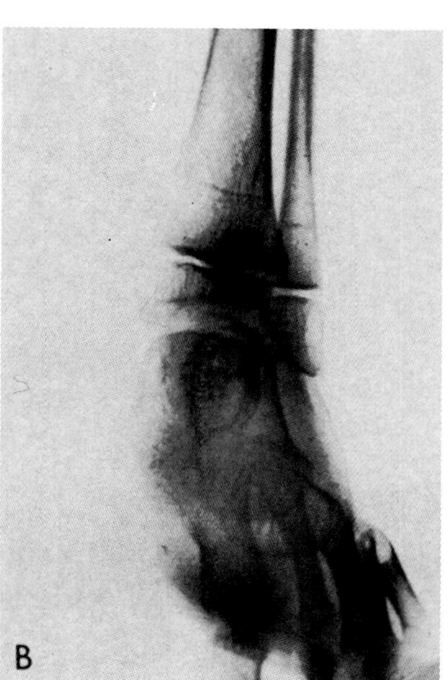

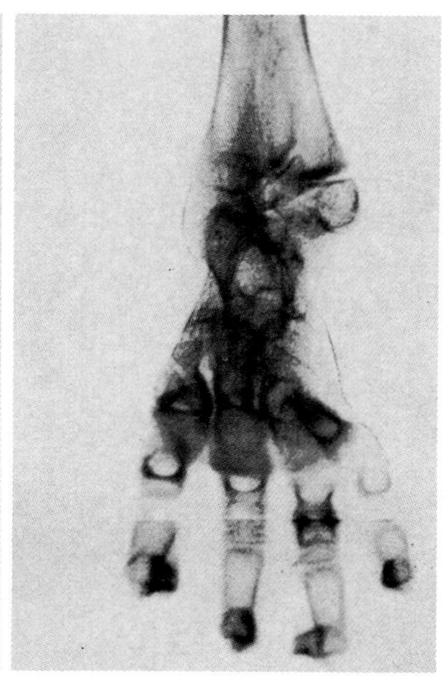

FIGURE 7–69. Congenital convex pes valgus of the "anterior tibial" type.

A. The deformity as seen in lateral radiograms in a child *(top)* and in a rabbit *(bottom)*. **B.** Anteroposterior radiograms of the deformity in a child *(left)* and in a rabbit *(right)*. From Ritsila, V. A.: Talipes equinovarus and vertical talus produced experimentally in newborn rabbits. Acta Orthop. Scand., Suppl. 121, 1969, p. 54. Reprinted by permission.)

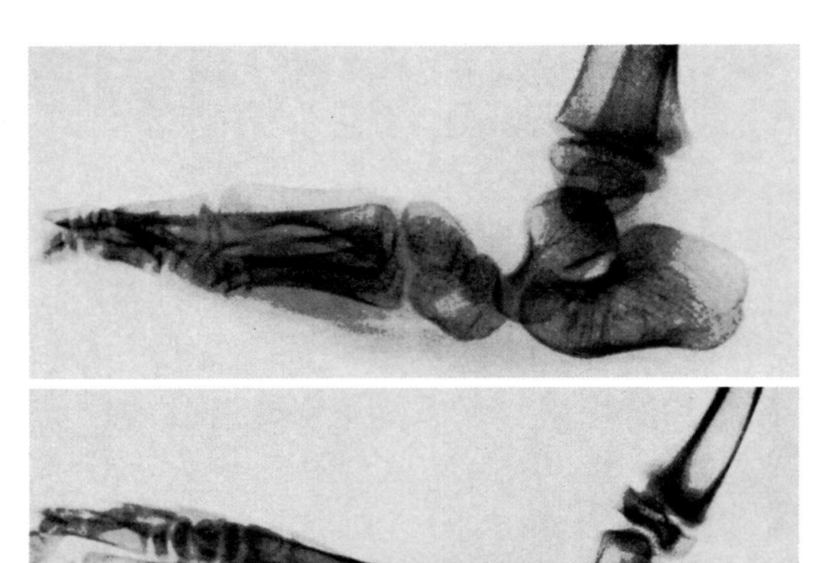

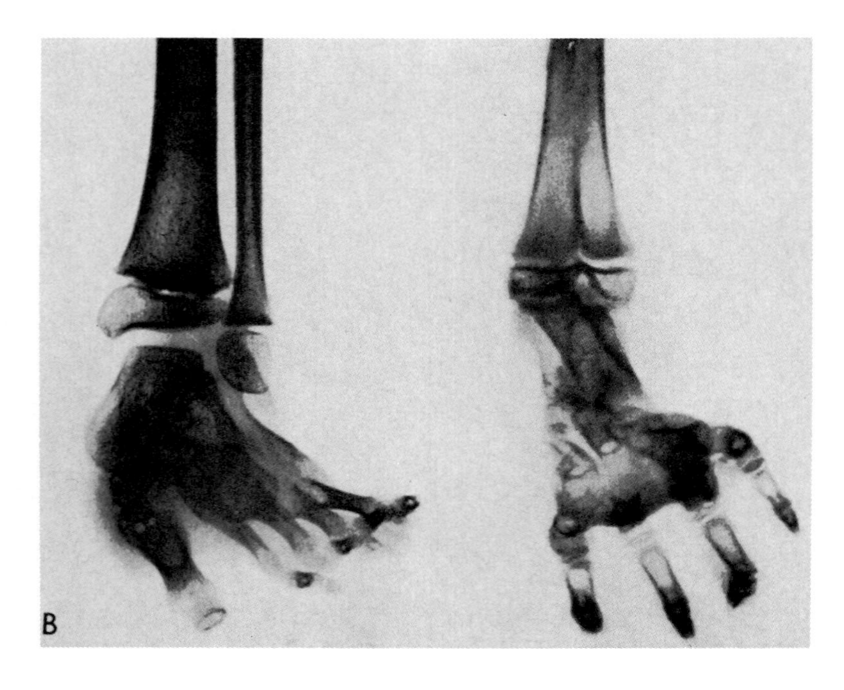

FIGURE 7–70. Congenital convex pes valgus of the "extensor digitorum" type.

A. The deformity as seen in lateral radiograms in a child *(top)* and in a rabbit *(bottom)*. **B.** Anteroposterior radiograms of the deformity in a child *(left)* and in a rabbit *(right)*. Note abduction and eversion of the forefoot. (From Ritsila, V. A.: Talipes equinovarus and vertical talus produced experimentally in newborn rabbits. Acta Orthop. Scand., Suppl. 121, 1969, p. 54. Reprinted by permission.)

talonavicular joint is unknown. The deformity is very rare, as judged by the small number of case reports from major children's hospitals. It is more common in boys than in girls. Involvement may be bilateral or unilateral; in the latter, the opposite foot may have a calcaneovalgus, equinovarus, or metatarsus varus deformity.

Pathologic Anatomy

The gross anatomic and histologic features of congenital convex pes valgus have been described in several investigators: by Güntz in a stillborn with bilateral involvement; by Patterson, Fitz, and Smith in a six-week-old girl who succumbed to congenital heart disease; by Drennan and Sharrard, who reported the findings in an 11-hour-old-girl with myelomeningocele who died of cardiac arrest following spinal osteotomy; and by Campos da Paz, Jr., and his colleagues in an eight-hour-old infant with myelomeningocele who died of atelectasis and hemorrhage.[11, 20, 29, 61] In Patterson and associates' case, the spinal cord was not examined. Observations at operation have also contributed to our knowledge of the deformity's pathologic anatomy. The anatomic abnormalities may be subdivided into those of the bones and joints, those of the ligaments, and those of the muscles and tendons.

BONE AND JOINT CHANGES

The navicular will be found articulating with the dorsal aspect of the neck of the talus, locking it in a vertical position (Fig. 7–71). The proximal articular surface of the navicular is tilted plantarward. The head of the talus develops an abnormal shape and is flattened superiorly, somewhat pointed, and oval rather than spherical. The neck of the talus is hypoplastic and may have an abnormal facet on its dorsal surface that articulates with the navicular. The calcaneus is displaced posterolaterally in relation to the talus, is in close contact with the distal end of the fibula, and is tilted into equinus posture. The anterior part of the calcaneus is deviated laterally, and the talocalcaneal angle (formed by the longitudinal axes of the talus and the calcaneus) is abnormally increased. The sustentaculum tali is hypoplastic and blunted, offering no support to the head of the talus. The calcaneus may be convex on its plantar aspect. There are abnormalities in the facets of the subtalar joint; the anterior articular facet is absent, the

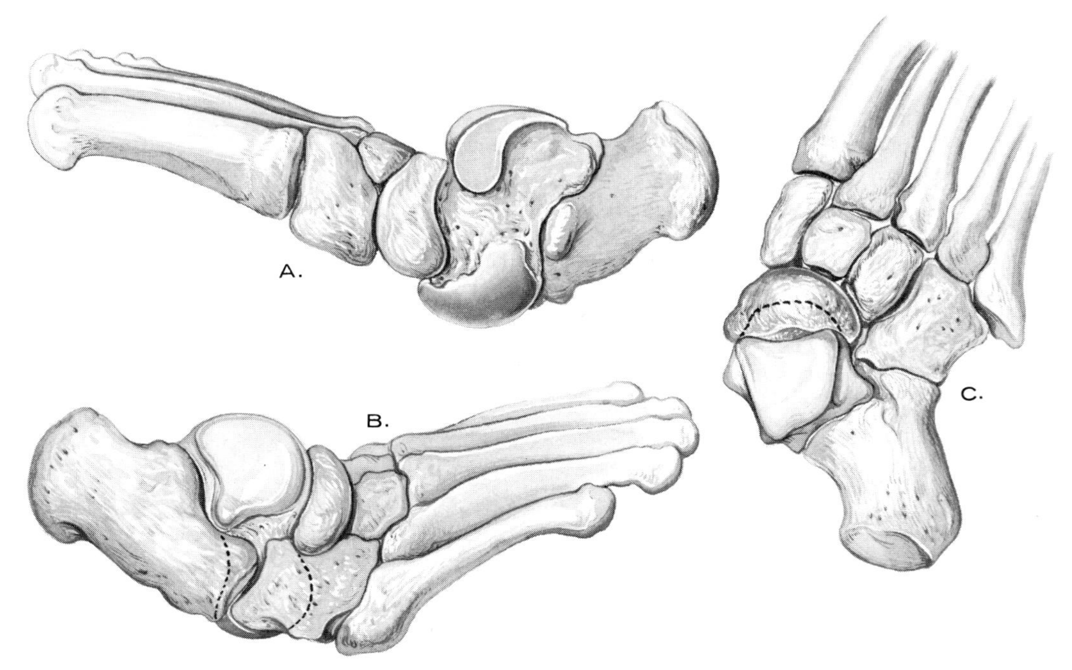

FIGURE 7–71. Bone and joint changes in congenital convex pes valgus.

A. Medial aspect of right foot showing dorsiflexion of forefoot at midtarsal joint; vertical talus producing a rocker-bottom convexity; subluxation of the navicular upon the neck of the talus, locking talus vertically; calcaneus 20 to 25 degrees equinus. **B.** Lateral aspect of right foot. Dotted lines indicate displaced head of talus. **C.** Dorsal aspect showing abducted forefoot beginning at midtarsus. Dotted lines indicate head of talus subluxated below navicular bone. (From Tachdjian, M. O.: Congenital convex pes valgus. Orthop. Clin. North Am., *3*:133, 1972. Reprinted by permission.)

middle one is hypoplastic, and the posterior one is misshapen and has an increased lateral tilt. These changes are most probably produced by the lack of contact between the normally congruent surfaces of the talus and calcaneus. The lateral column of the foot is concave, and the articular facet of the calcaneus for the cuboid is inclined dorsally and laterally. There is a variable degree of dorsolateral subluxation of the calcaneocuboid joint. The medial column of the foot is elongated, obstructing normal alignment of the navicular over the head of the talus. The anatomic relations of the navicular and cuboid with the cuneiforms and the metatarsals are normal and not disturbed.

LIGAMENTOUS CHANGES

As shown in Figures 7–72, 7–73, and 7–74, the tibionavicular ligament (which is a part of the anterior portion of the deltoid ligament) and the lateral parts of the dorsal medial talonavicular ligament are markedly contracted and present a major obstacle to successful reduction. The bifurcated, or Y, ligament, located between the upper lateral part of the calcaneus and the navicular and cuboid bones, is shortened, causing the forefoot to be held in abduction. Contracture of the interosseous talocalcaneal and calcaneofibular ligaments takes place, preventing reduction of the posterolaterally subluxated os calcis. In untreated cases, the posterior capsule of the ankle and subtalar joints is also shortened.

The plantar calcaneonavicular ligament, or spring ligament, is stretched and moderately attenuated. The capsule of the talonavicular joint is elongated on its medial and plantar aspects.

MUSCLE AND TENDON ABNORMALITIES

The anterior tibial, extensor hallucis longus, extensor digitorum longus, peroneus brevis,

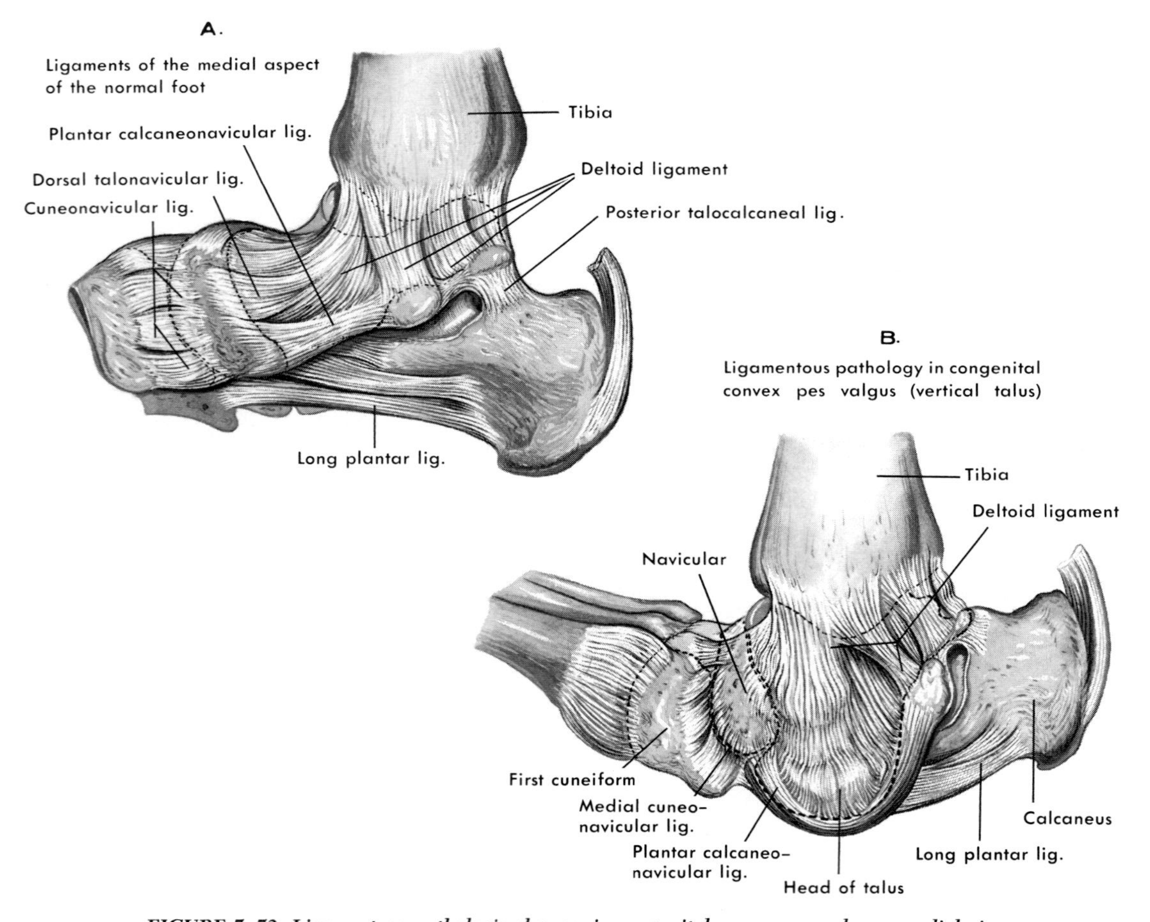

FIGURE 7–72. Ligamentous pathologic changes in congenital convex pes valgus—medial view.

A. Normal foot. **B.** Malformed foot with congenital convex pes valgus.

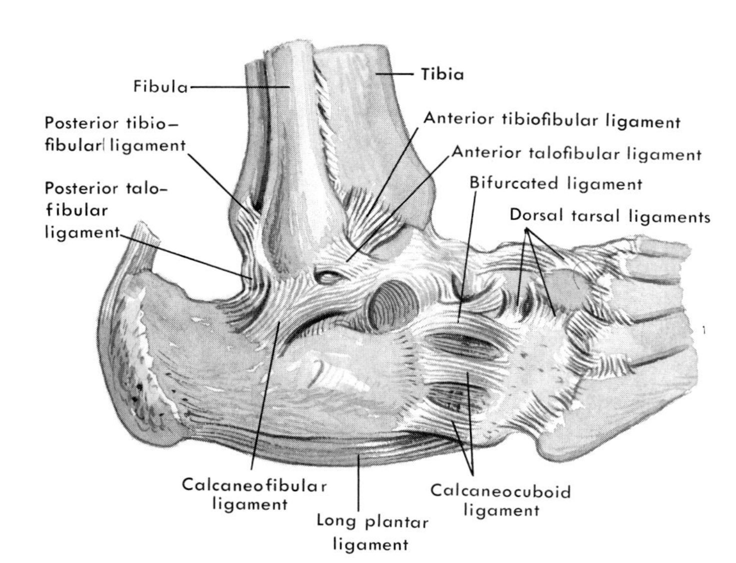

FIGURE 7–73. Ligamentous pathologic changes in congenital convex pes valgus—lateral view.

and triceps surae muscles are contracted. The posterior tibial and peroneal tendons are usually anteriorly displaced, lying in grooves on the malleoli and acting as dorsiflexors rather than plantar flexors. In severe cases, they may "bowstring" across the ankle joint (Figs. 7–75 and 7–76). Patterson and co-workers found these muscles to be grossly and histologically normal, and proposed that their contracture is secondary to length deficit.[61] Drennan and Sharrard reported moderate atrophy of the posterior tibial and quadratus plantae muscles and hypertrophy of the extensor digitorum longus muscle; it should be remembered, however, that their anatomic specimen was from a child with myelomeningocele.[20] In an arthrogrypotic child with congenital convex pes valgus, the author has observed fibrosis of the anterior tibial, long toe extensor, and peroneal muscles.

The effect of manipulation in stillborn and fetal specimens with congenital convex pes valgus has been studied by Güntz and by Campos da Paz, Jr., and associates.[11, 29] Talocalcaneonavicular dislocation was not reduced by forceful manipulation; only after division of the aforementioned contracted ligaments and tendons could normal articular alignment be restored.

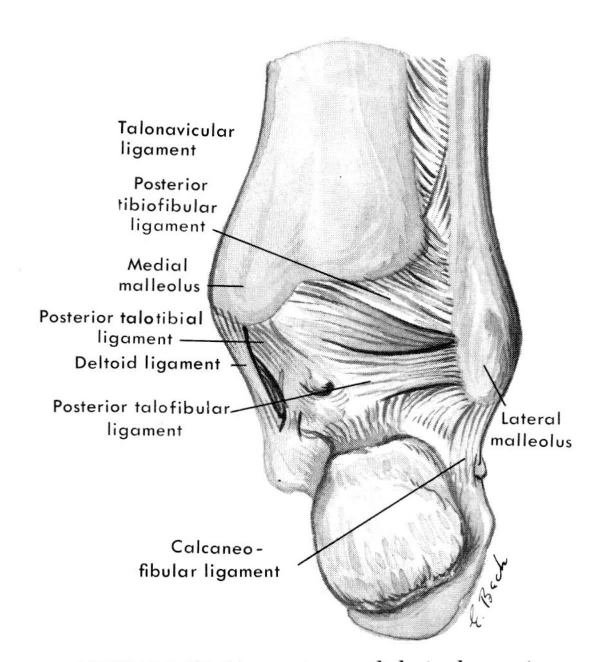

FIGURE 7–74. Ligamentous pathologic changes in congenital convex pes valgus—posterior view.

Clinical Features

The rigid deformity of the foot is present at birth and is so distinct that the condition can be diagnosed at that time. The sole of the foot is convex and has a rocker-bottom appearance (Fig. 7–77). The head of the talus is markedly prominent on the medial and plantar aspects of the foot. The forefoot is abducted and dorsiflexed at the midtarsal joint. The long toe extensor, anterior tibial, and peroneal muscles are markedly shortened. The calcaneovalgus deformity of the forefoot is fixed; the taut muscles and the contracted tibionavicular and talonavicular ligaments resist plantar flexion and inversion of the forefoot. The hindfoot posture is equinovalgus; the triceps surae muscle is

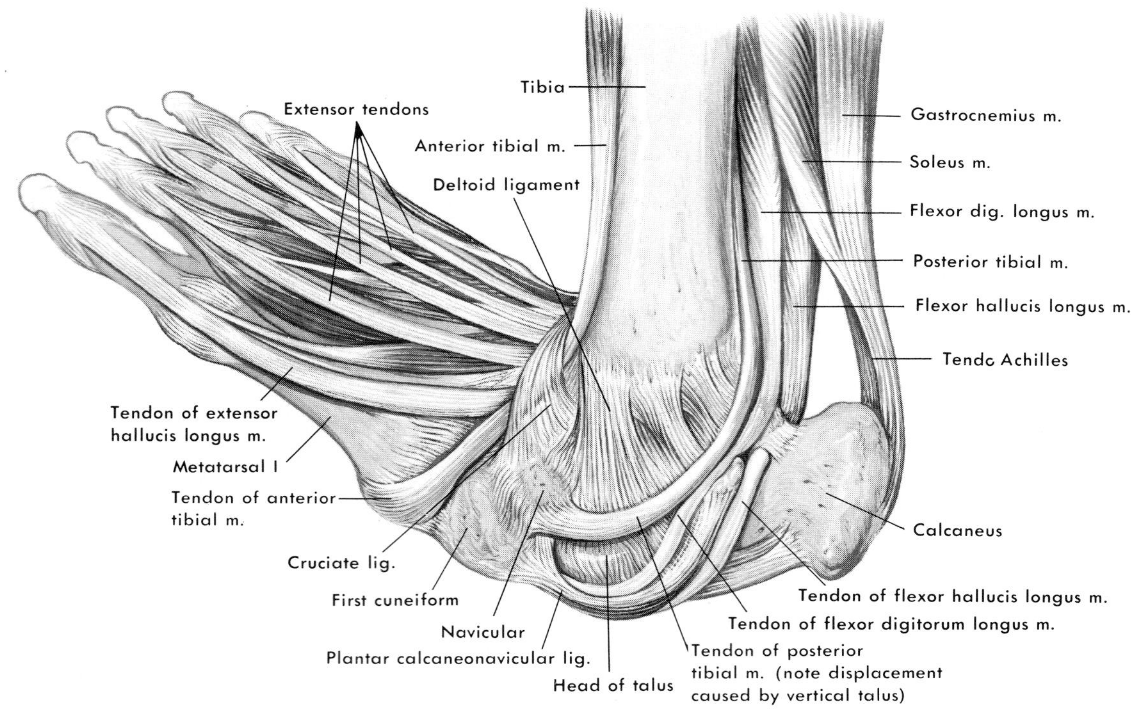

FIGURE 7–75. Abnormalities of muscles and tendons in congenital convex pes valgus.

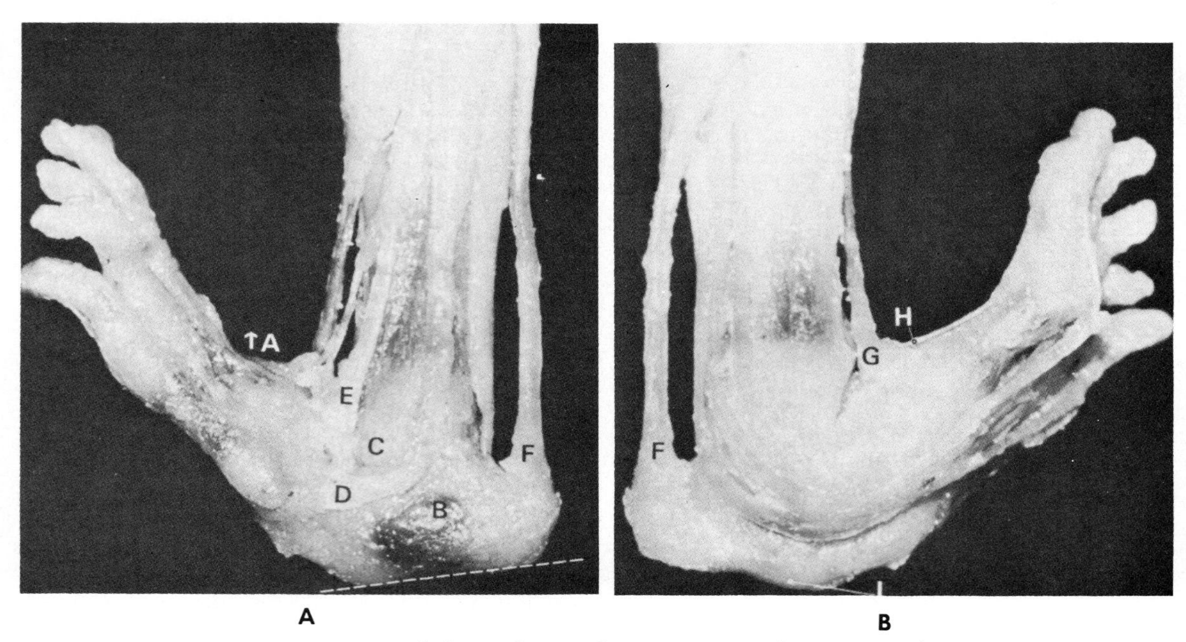

FIGURE 7–76. Pathologic soft-tissue changes in congenital convex pes valgus.

Anatomic findings in an infant who died eight hours after birth. **A.** Lateral view. Note the rocker-bottom foot with dorsiflexion of the forefoot (A) and equinus deformity of the heel. The apex of the angulation of the lateral column is at the calcaneonavicular joint. The calcaneus (B) is displaced laterally under the talus, lying in close proximity to the distal end of the fibula (C). The triceps surae (F) is contracted, holding the calcaneus in plantar flexion. The peroneus longus (D) and peroneus tertius (E) are shortened. **B.** Medial view. The anterior tibial (G) and extensor hallucis longus (H) muscles are shortened. (The extensor digitorum longus is also contracted, but it does not show in this photograph.) The triceps surae muscle (F) is shortened. These musculotendinous contractures are secondary obstacles to anatomic alignment of the talocalcaneonavicular joint. (From Campos da Paz, A., Jr., De Souza, V., and Conceicao de Souza, D.: Congenital convex pes valgus. Orthop. Clin. North Am., *9*:207, 1978, p. 210. Reprinted by permission.)

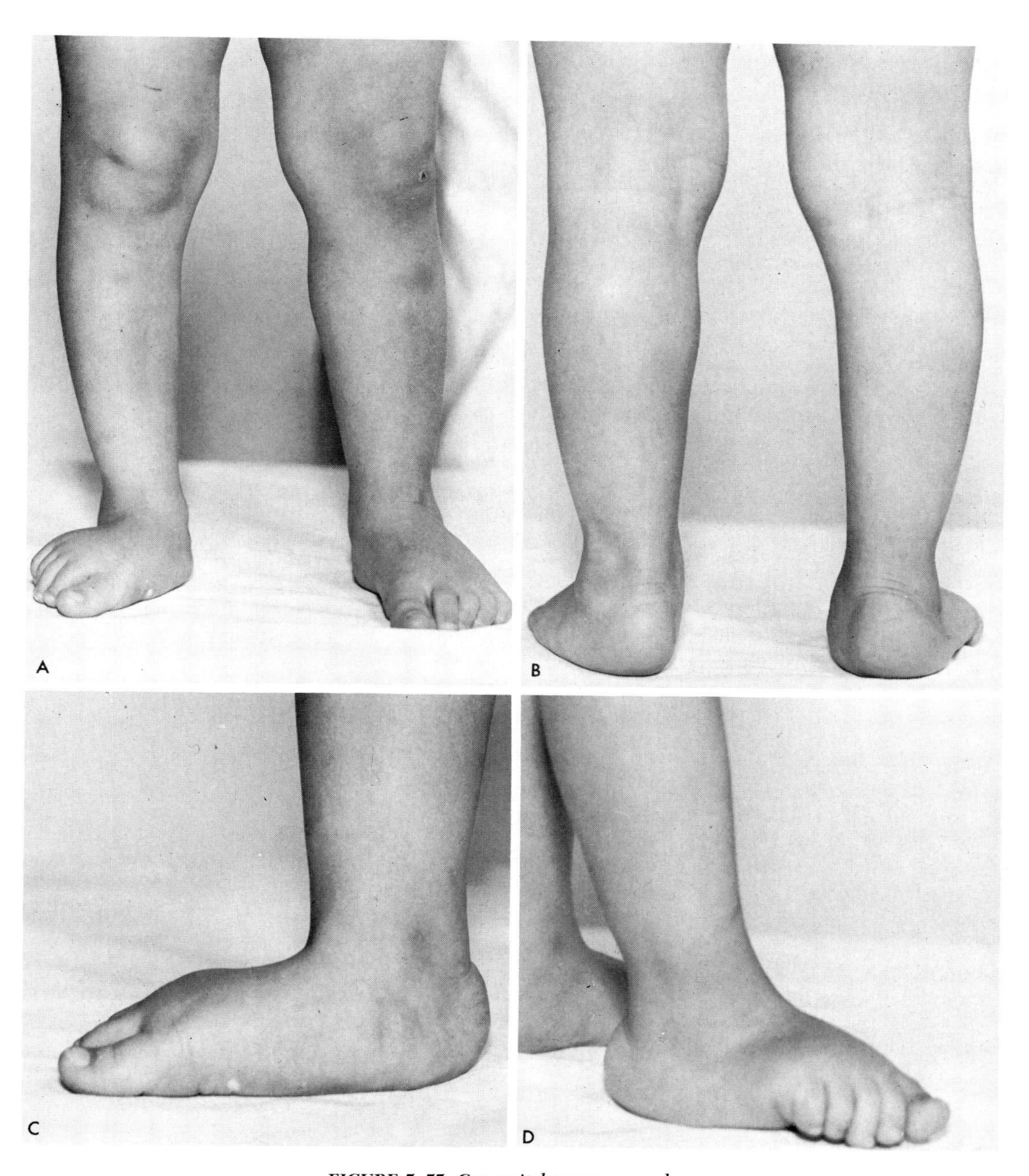

FIGURE 7–77. Congenital convex pes valgus.

A to **D.** Clinical appearance of the deformity in a child.

contracted, and the calcaneus is everted and tilted downward in plantar flexion. The dislocated navicular may be palpable on the dorsum of the neck of the talus. Deep creases appear on the dorsolateral aspect of the foot near the ankle joint. The deformity is so rigid that on plantar flexion without weight-bearing the fixed convex planovalgus appearance of the foot persists; the longitudinal arch cannot be restored.

Walking is usually not delayed. The older child stands with the involved hindfoot in markedly valgus position with the posterior part of the heel not touching the floor. The forefoot is abducted, and most of the body weight is borne on the head of the talus. The gait is awkward, clumsy, almost peglike, the feet toeing out and rolling into a valgus posture. The balance is poor. Shoes rapidly become distorted, the medial part of the heel and the upper over the longitudinal arch wearing down within a few weeks. Pain is not a symptom in childhood, but it usually becomes a complaint in later adolescence.

Radiographic Findings

There is considerable variation in the time for radiographic appearance of the ossification centers of the tarsal bones. At birth those of the talus, calcaneus, and metatarsals are clearly visible; however, the ossific nucleus of the cuboid bone may be present or delayed in its appearance until the third to the twentieth day after birth. The cuneiform bones become visible later than the cuboid. The ossification center of the navicular usually appears at three years of age (one and one half to four years); hence it cannot be seen in the radiograms at birth. To define their relationships one has to draw lines through the longitudinal axes of the talus, the calcaneus, and the first metatarsal bones as described in the section on radiographic investigation of talipes equinovarus.

The radiographic findings in congenital convex pes valgus are characteristic, even in the newborn. The talus is vertical, lying parallel with the longitudinal axis of the tibia, and the calcaneus is in equinus position, whereas the forepart of the foot is dorsiflexed and deviated laterally at the midtarsal level. The outline of the soft tissues of the sole is convex. The anteroposterior talocalcaneal angle is abnormally increased. To make the definitive diagnosis, it is imperative to demonstrate that the navicular is dislocated dorsally on the neck of the talus when the foot is maintained in extreme plantar flexion.[23]

The location of the cartilaginous navicular can be determined by drawing the longitudinal axis of the first metatarsal and noting its relation to the head of the talus. In congenital convex pes valgus, on forced plantar flexion, the long axis of the first metatarsal will point dorsally to the head of the talus. In a normal foot it bisects the head of the talus.

The relationship of the long axes of the talus and calcaneus should be noted. In a normal foot the long axis of the talus passes through the lower half of the cuboid, and that of the calcaneus cuts through the upper half of the cuboid (Fig. 7–78). In congenital convex pes valgus the long axis of the talus passes below and posterior to the cuboid and often cuts through the anterior part of the calcaneus or passes very close to its anterior end (Figs. 7–79 and 7–80); and the long axis of the calcaneus passes plantar to the cuboid. By the age of three years, the navicular ossifies and its complete dislocation over the dorsal surface of the neck of the talus is clearly visible (Fig. 7–81).

In paralytic pes valgus in which the feet are severely pronated, the talus may be tilted into vertical position (particularly if there is contracture of the triceps surae), and the navicular will sag on the head of the talus, suggesting subluxation of the talonavicular joint. On close scrutiny, however, it is evident that there is definite contact between the articular surfaces of the navicular and the head of the talus. On forced

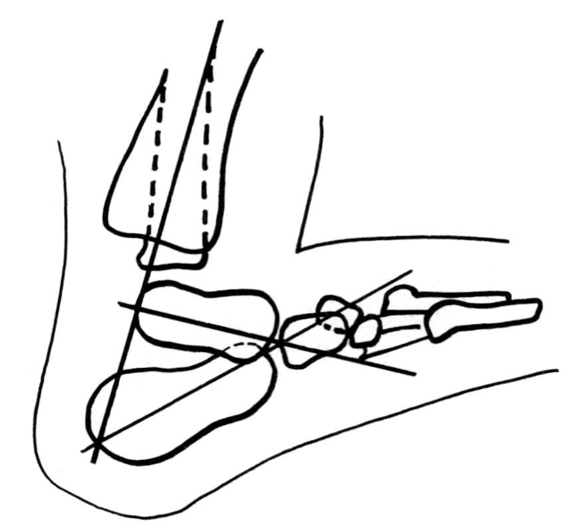

FIGURE 7–78. Line drawing of the lateral radiogram of a normal foot.

The long axis of the talus cuts the lower half of the cuboid, whereas the long axis of the calcaneus passes through the upper half of the cuboid.

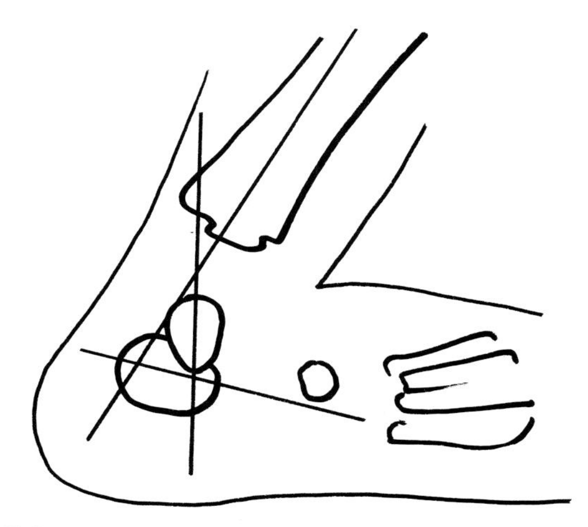

FIGURE 7–79. Line drawing of the lateral radiogram of a foot with congenital convex pes valgus.

The long axis of the talus passes below and behind the cuboid bone and cuts through the anterior part of the calcaneus, and the long axis of the calcaneus passes plantar to the cuboid.

plantar flexion of the foot one can restore normal talonavicular relations.

The navicular bone, in congenital convex pes valgus, may be irregularly ossified, suggesting Köhler's disease. With increasing age, it becomes wedge-shaped toward its plantar aspect, and upward tilting of its anterior end gives it a beak-shaped appearance. With dorsal and lateral displacement of the forepart of the foot, dorsolateral subluxation of the calcaneocuboid joint is evident. The first metatarsal is dorsiflexed and the hallux is plantar-flexed at the metatarsophalangeal joint, compensating for the elevated first metatarsal bone.

The talus is underdeveloped, particularly at its waist, resembling an hourglass. In the lateral projection it will be seen that only the posterior portion of the superior surface of the talus is contained in the tibiofibular mortise.

Differential Diagnosis

In early infancy, congenital convex pes valgus is commonly mistaken for talipes calcaneovalgus. In both conditions, the forepart of the foot is dorsiflexed and everted, and there is limitation of plantar flexion and inversion. The heel in congenital convex pes valgus is in equinus position, the sole of the foot convex, and the deformity very rigid, whereas in talipes calcaneovalgus, the os calcis and talus are in dorsiflexion, and the deformity is quite flexible and responds rapidly to stretching exercises and treatment with corrective casts.

The presence of pes valgus with myostatic contracture of the triceps surae muscle may present a problem in differential diagnosis. In stance, the heel position is equinovalgus, and the talus is plantar-flexed with its head prominent on the medial and plantar aspects of the midfoot; the deformity is not rigid, however, and when not bearing weight, the heel can be manipulated into neutral position and the head of the talus into dorsiflexion, giving a normal longitudinal arch to the foot. In congenital convex pes valgus, the deformity is fixed and does not improve when not bearing weight. Radiograms made with the foot in plantar flexion will establish the diagnosis.

Paralytic pes valgus due to cerebral palsy, myelomeningocele, or poliomyelitis should not be difficult to distinguish from congenital convex pes valgus. Although the clinical appearance of peroneal spastic flatfoot due to tarsal coalition may resemble congenital vertical talus, the radiographic findings are distinctive. An accessory navicular produces a prominence on the medial aspect of the foot, which is in a valgus position. Again, radiograms should settle the diagnosis.

Treatment

The objectives of therapy are to place the navicular and calcaneus in a normal anatomic relationship to the talus and to maintain the reduction.

The method of treatment depends upon the age of the patient and the degree and severity of the deformity. A number of methods and

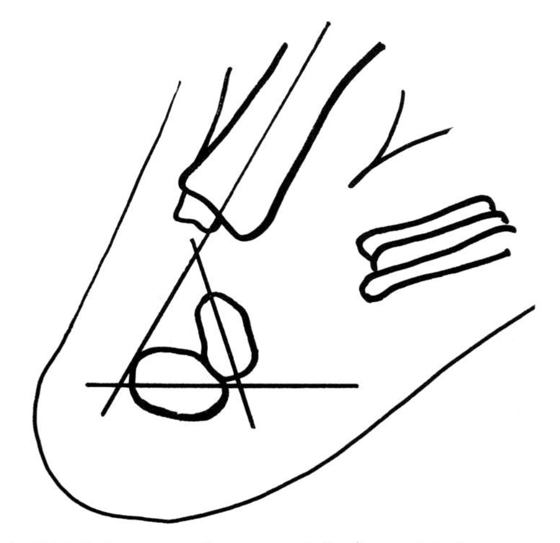

FIGURE 7–80. Line drawing of the lateral radiogram of a foot with congenital convex pes valgus.

The long axis of the talus passes very close to the anterior end of the calcaneus.

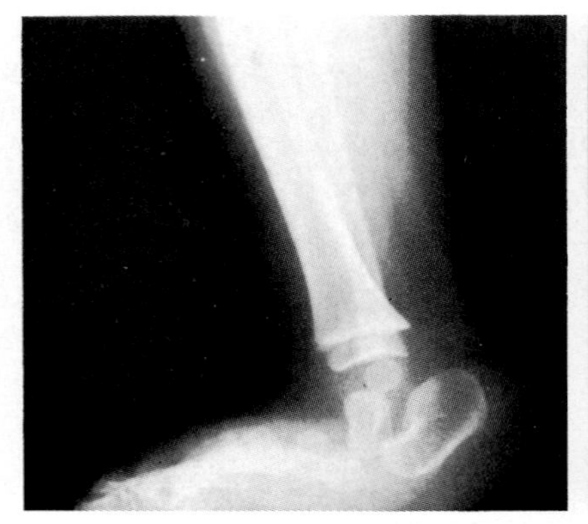

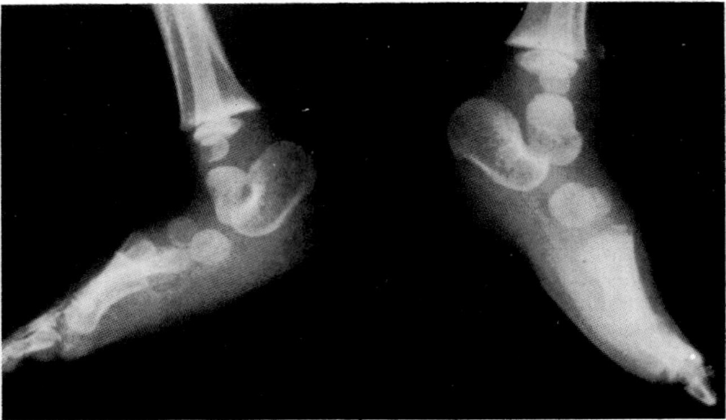

FIGURE 7–81. Radiographic appearance of congenital convex pes valgus in a two-year-old child.

Lateral projection of the foot and ankle. The navicular is ossified, and its complete dislocation over the head of the talus is clearly visualized.

techniques of treatment that have been proposed by various authors in the literature are summarized in Table 7–11.

The condition may be diagnosed at birth by the characteristic rocker-bottom convex shape of the foot, the rigidity of the deformity, and its distinctive radiographic features. Treatment should begin at birth. The first three weeks of life is the golden period when there may be a chance to achieve and retain reduction of the dorsolateral dislocation of the talocalcaneonavicular joint by the closed method. In general, however, this is extremely difficult, and often one has to employ open surgery to obtain and maintain reduction. Any delay in diagnosis will lead to a crippling deformity of the foot. The older the patient at the time treatment is initiated, the more rigid will be the ligamentous, capsular, and soft-tissue contractures, and the greater the structural osseous changes.

ELONGATION OF CONTRACTED SOFT TISSUES BY MANIPULATIVE STRETCHING

In the neonate and young infant a preliminary period of stretching of the shortened ligaments and muscles by passive manipulation is indicated. As in talipes equinovarus, one should remember that soft tissues are hard and hard tissues are soft. Gentleness is the basic principle. The technique of manipulation is as follows: first, the triceps surae and calcaneofibular ligament are stretched by pulling them distally and medially with one hand and pushing the anterior end of the os calcis (not the cuboid) with the other hand. The stretched position is maintained to the count of 10, then released. The ankle dorsiflexor and evertor muscles are stretched by pulling the forefoot into plantar flexion, inversion, and adduction. Then the tibionavicular and talonavicular ligaments are elongated by applying *distal traction* on the forefoot and navicular bone and gradually bringing them into adduction and inversion. Each time the corrected positions are maintained to the count of 10 and then released. The manipulations are performed for 15 minutes. The skin is then painted with a nonirritating adhesive liquid such as tincture of benzoin to prevent slipping of the cast, and the limb is immobilized in a long leg cast with the foot and ankle in the corrected position—the forepart of the foot in equinus position and inversion, and the heel well molded in the degree of dorsiflexion obtained by passive manipulation. During application of the cast on the foot, thumb pressure is applied on the anterior end of the os calcis. The successive plaster casts are changed twice a week; each time the foot is gently manipulated for 15 minutes to further stretch the soft-tissue contracture.

Following manipulative elongation of the contracted ligaments and muscles over a period of four to six weeks, closed reduction of the talocalcaneonavicular dislocation is attempted. This is performed by applying distal traction on the forefoot and navicular, first in the line of deformity, i.e., into dorsiflexion and eversion. After bringing the navicular over the talar head and the calcaneus under the talus, the forefoot and midfoot are brought into plantar flexion as the head of the talus is pushed into dorsiflexion and the heel is pulled distally and into inversion. Restoration of the normal articular relationship of the navicular with the head of the talus should be verified by radiographic examination. As previously stated, because the navicular is not ossified in infancy, the anatomic relationship of

Table 7–11. *Methods of Treatment of Congenital Convex Pes Valgus*

Procedures on Talus
- Excision of head and neck of talus (Lange, 1912; Nové-Josserand, 1923)
- Curettage of talus with excision of its cuneiform portion (Camera, 1926)
- Complete astragalectomy (Lamy and Weissman, 1939)
- Open-up wedge osteotomy of neck of talus with insertion of bone graft on its plantar aspect (Hughes, 1957)

Procedures on Navicular
- Excision of navicular (Stone, 1963)
- Excision of dorsal wedge from navicular and placement of the wedge under elevated head of talus combined with open reduction, reefing of spring ligament, and shortening of posterior tibial tendon (Eyre-Brook, 1967)

Procedures on Talonavicular Joint
- Open reduction with or without lengthening of Achilles tendon and release of shortened musculotendinous units, ligaments, and capsules on dorsolateral aspect of foot
- Reduction maintained with plaster cast (Rocher and Pouyanne, 1934)
- Reduction maintained with Kirschner wire across talonavicular joint (Hark, 1950; Heyman, 1959; Herndon and Heyman, 1963)
- Reduction maintained with transfer of peroneus brevis tendon to neck of talus (Osmond-Clarke, 1956)
- Reduction maintained with scarification of talonavicular joint with or without Kirschner wire through navicular into head of talus (Hughes, 1957)
- Reduction maintained with reefing of capsule and rerouting of anterior tibial tendon under neck of talus and fixing to navicular (Grice, 1959)
- Reduction maintained with subtalar arthrodesis (Grice, 1959; Coleman et al., 1966)
- Reduction maintained with plication of calcaneonavicular ligament and reattaching of posterior tibial tendon with shortening (Eyre-Brook, 1967; Harrold, 1967; Storen, 1967)
- Release of capsule of calcaneocuboid joint on its dorsolateral aspect (Coleman et al., 1966)
- Closed reduction in young infant (under 3 months of age) following elongation of shortened soft tissues by serial stretching casts (Harrold, 1967; Støren, 1967)

Reconstructive or Stabilization Procedures on Tarsus
- Triple arthrodesis (Hark, 1950; Lloyd-Roberts, 1958; and others)
- Wedge tarsectomy (Lloyd-Roberts, 1958)

the talonavicular articulation is difficult to establish. The exact location of the cartilaginous navicular between the ossified medial cuneiform and the head of the talus is determined. Arthrography of the articulation may be attempted in borderline or doubtful cases.

Occasionally, closed reduction of teratologic dislocation of the talonavicular joint is successful.[34, 74, 75, 81] In such an instance, the author recommends maintenance of reduction by "blind" pinning of the talonavicular joint. Image-intensifier radiographic control will make the procedure a simple one. A heavy threaded Kirschner wire is inserted in the web interspace between the great and second toes, and is then drilled proximally across the talonavicular joint, holding the forefoot in marked plantar flexion and inversion. Initially, the hindfoot and ankle joint are immobilized in plantar flexion. After two to three weeks, the cast is changed and the foot is brought into increasing dorsiflexion. Immobilization should be continued for at least two months.

OPEN REDUCTION

If closed reduction proves unsuccessful, open reduction should be performed at three months of age (Plate 99).

The reduction of the talonaviculocuneiform joint in congenital convex pes valgus is obstructed by the following structures (in order of priority). *Ligaments:* (1) the dorsal and lateral part of the talonavicular ligament; (2) the tibionavicular ligament; (3) the bifurcated, or Y, ligament (both the calcaneonavicular and the calcaneocuboid limbs); (4) the dorsal and lateral parts of the calcaneocuboid capsule; (5) the calcaneofibular ligament; and (6) the interosseous talocalcaneal ligament. *Musculotendinous tissues:* (1) the triceps surae, (2) the anterior tibial, (3) the long toe extensors, and (4) the peroneals. These permanently shortened muscles serve as secondary obstacles to reduction. In a systematic step-by-step approach these contracted soft tissues should be lengthened by open surgical division under direct vision. In the older child or in the one with very severe rigid deformity, the medial skeletal column of the foot is too long and prevents normal restoration of articular alignment of the talus and navicular; therefore, it is shortened by excision of the dorsally dislocated navicular.

During open reduction it is essential to take measures to maintain the correction. Capsular plication and tightening of the calcaneonavicular (spring) ligament and posterior tibial tendon under the head of the talus by distal transfer should be performed in all cases. Muscle and tendon transfers may be performed to suspend the head of the talus in dorsiflexion: transferring the peroneus brevis as recommended by Osmond-Clarke; splitting the anterior tibial tendon and transferring half of it to the head of the talus as recommended by Grice; or transferring the entire anterior tibial tendon to the head and neck of the talus as recommended by Lloyd-Roberts. In the older child the Grice extra-articular arthrodesis is performed to maintain the reduction and give stability to the subtalar joint.

Text continued on page 2576

Open Reduction of Dorsolateral Dislocation of Talocalcaneonavicular Joint (Congenital Convex Pes Valgus)

OPERATIVE TECHNIQUE

A. A longitudinal incision is made lateral to the tendo calcaneus, beginning at the heel and extending proximally for a distance of 7 to 10 cm. The subcutaneous tissue and tendon sheath are divided in line with the skin incision, and the wound flaps are retracted, exposing the Achilles tendon.

B. Z-plastic lengthening is performed in the anteroposterior plane. With a knife the Achilles tendon is divided longitudinally into lateral and medial halves for a distance of 5 to 7 cm. The distal end of the lateral half is detached from the calcaneus to prevent recurrence of valgus deformity of the heel; the medial half is divided proximally. When the equinus deformity is not marked, sliding lengthening of the heel cord is performed.

C and **D.** A posterior capsulotomy of the ankle and subtalar joint is performed if necessary. The calcaneofibular ligament is sectioned. The thickened capsule of the calcaneocuboid joint and the bifurcated ligament are divided through a separate lateral incision. The Cincinnati transverse incision shown in Figure 7–60 is an alternative surgical approach; it is preferred by this author.

Plate 99. Open Reduction of Dorsolateral Dislocation of Talocalcaneonavicular Joint (Congenital Convex Pes Valgus)

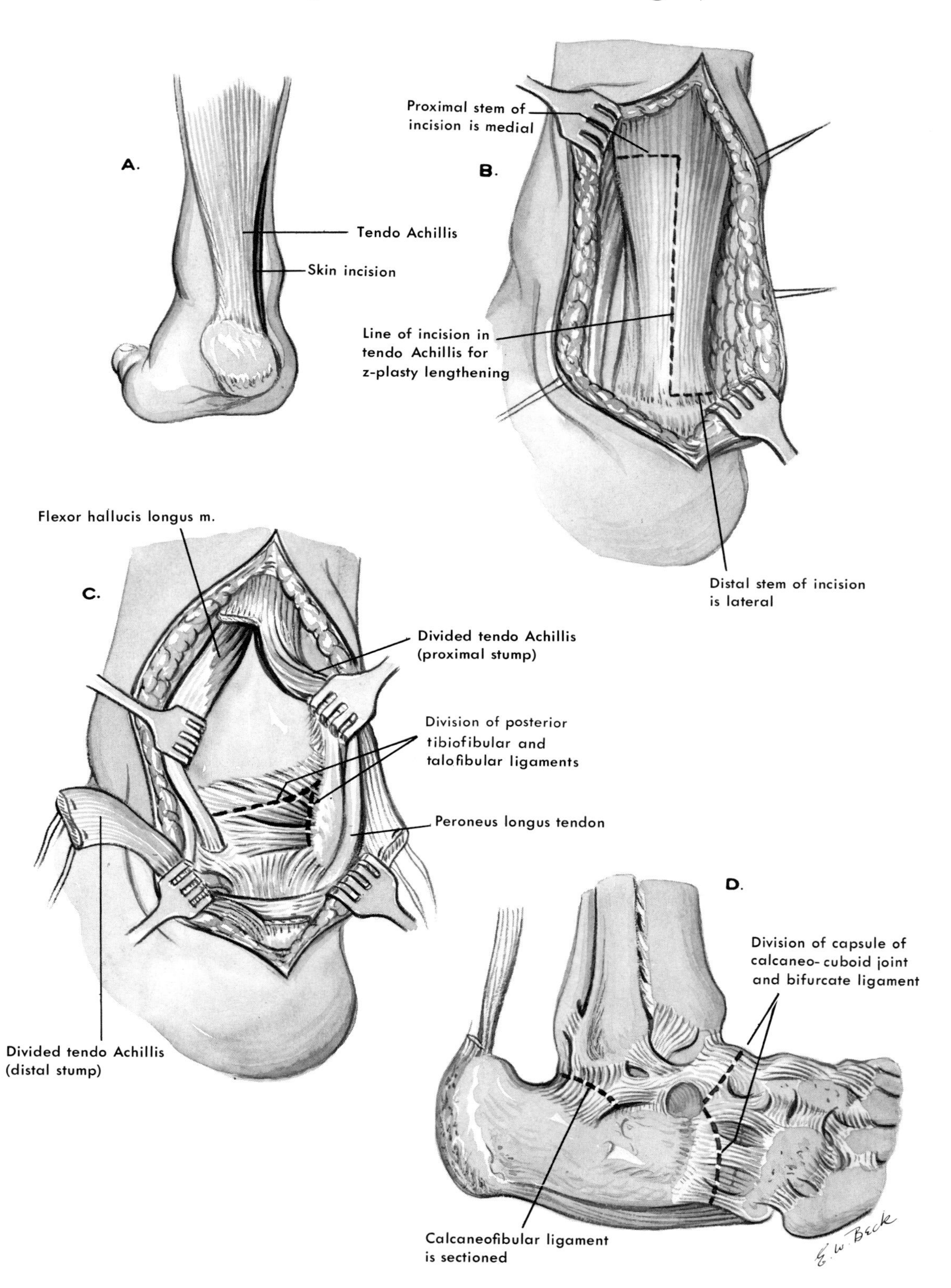

Open Reduction of Dorsolateral Dislocation of Talocalcaneonavicular Joint (Congenital Convex Pes Valgus)(Continued)

E. The medial skin incision begins at a point 2 cm. posterior and 1 cm. distal to the tip of the medial malleolus and extends distally to the base of the first metatarsal. The subcutaneous tissue is divided. The skin margins are mobilized and retracted to expose the dorsal, medial, and plantar aspects of the tarsus.

F and **G.** The posterior tibial tendon is identified, dissected, and divided at its insertion to the tuberosity of the navicular. The end of the tendon is marked with 0 Mersilene suture for later reattachment. The articular surface of the head of the talus points steeply downward and medially to the sole of the foot and is covered by the capsule and ligament. The navicular will be found against the dorsal aspect of the neck of the talus, locking it in vertical position. The pathologic anatomy of the ligaments and capsule is noted and the incisions planned so that a secure capsuloplasty can be performed and the talus maintained in its normal anatomic position. Circulation to the talus is another important consideration; it should be disturbed as little as possible by exercising great care and gentleness during dissection. Avascular necrosis of the talus is always a potential serious complication of open reduction. The plantar calcaneonavicular ligament is identified and divided distally from its attachment to the sustentaculum tali, and a 00 Mersilene suture is inserted in its end for later reattachment. The talonavicular articulation is exposed by a T-incision. The transverse limb of the T is made distally over the tibionavicular ligament (the anterior portion of the deltoid ligament) and over the dorsal and medial portions of the talonavicular ligament. A cuff of capsule is left attached to the navicular for plication on completion of surgery. The longitudinal limb of the incision is made over the head and neck of the talus inferiorly.

The articular surface of the head of the talus is identified, and a large threaded Kirschner wire is inserted in its center. With a skid and the leverage of the Kirschner wire, the head and neck of the talus are lifted dorsally and the forefoot is manipulated into plantar flexion and inversion, bringing the articular surfaces of the navicular and head of the talus into normal anatomic position.

Plate 99. Open Reduction of Dorsolateral Dislocation of Talocalcaneonavicular Joint (Congenital Convex Pes Valgus)

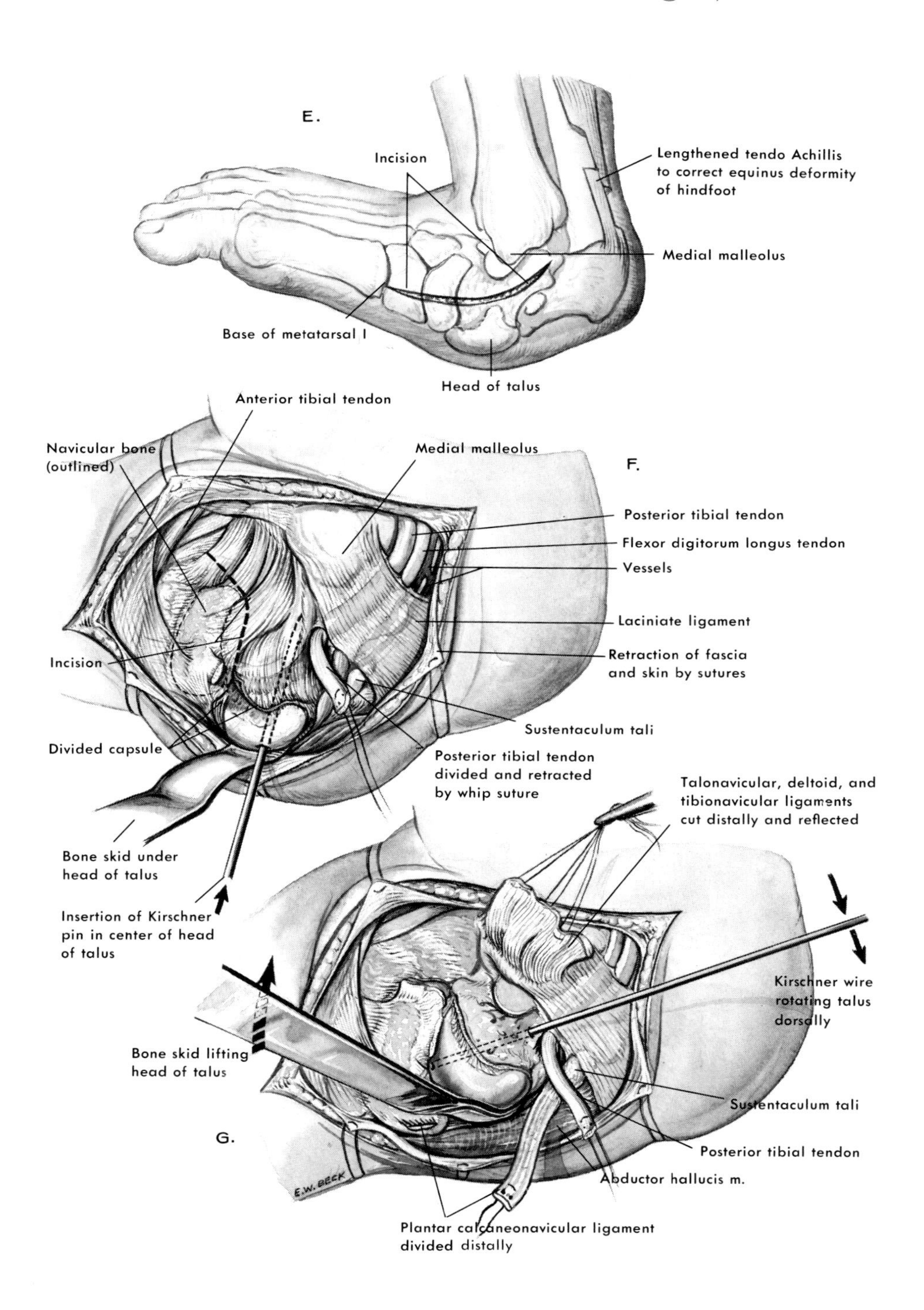

Open Reduction of Dorsolateral Dislocation of Talocalcaneonavicular Joint (Congenital Convex Pes Valgus)(Continued)

H. The Kirschner wire is drilled retrograde into the navicular, cuneiform, and first metatarsal bones, maintaining the reduction. Radiograms of the foot are taken at this time to verify the reduction.

In the older child the calcaneocuboid and talocalcaneal interosseous ligaments may prevent reduction of the laterally subluxated Chopart's and subtalar joints. If necessary, they are divided through a separate anterolateral incision. The anterior tibial, extensor hallucis longus, extensor digitorum longus, and peroneal muscles may also be so shortened that they prevent reduction; if so, they are lengthened. The author prefers fractional lengthening of these muscles through a separate longitudinal incision over the anterior tibial compartment. Others prefer to lengthen them by a Z-plasty over the dorsum of the foot.[15, 16]

I and **J.** A careful capsuloplasty is very important for maintaining the reduction and the normal anatomic relationship of the talus and navicular. The redundant inferior part of the capsule should be tightened by plication and overlapping of its free edges. First, the plantar-proximal segment of the T of the capsule is pulled dorsally and distally and sutured to the dorsal corner of the inner surface of the distal capsule. Next, the dorsoproximal segment of the T is brought plantarward and distally over the plantar-proximal segment of the capsule and sutured to the plantar corner on the inner surface of the distal capsule. Then, interrupted sutures are used to tighten the capsule on its plantar and medial aspects by bringing the distal segment over the proximal segments.

The plantar calcaneonavicular ligament is sutured under tension to the base of the first metatarsal. To tighten the posterior tibial tendon under the head of the talus, it is advanced distally and sutured to the inferior surface of the first cuneiform.

The anterior tibial may be transferred to provide additional dynamic force for maintaining the navicular in correct relationship to the talus. The tendon is detached from its insertion to the medial cuneiform and first metatarsal bone, and dissected free proximally and medially for a distance of 5 cm. Then it is redirected to pass along the medial aspect of the neck of the talus and beneath the head of the talus, where it is fixed to the inferior aspects of the talus and navicular with 00 Mersilene sutures. Normally the lower end of the anterior tibial tendon may be split near its insertion. Often the author leaves intact the attachment to the first metatarsal, dividing only the insertion to the medial cuneiform. The tendon is split (if not normally bifurcated), and the portion to the medial cuneiform bone is transferred to the head of the talus and the navicular. Sometimes, following adequate capsuloplasty, the reduction of the talonavicular joint is so stable that anterior tibial transfer is not necessary to restore support to the head of the talus.

K. The wounds are then closed in routine fashion. The Kirschner wire across the talonavicular joint is cut subcutaneously. To maintain the normal anatomic relationship of the os calcis to the talus, a Kirschner wire is inserted transversely in the os calcis and incorporated into the cast. An alternate method is to pass the wire from the sole of the foot upward through the calcaneus into the talus. The author prefers the former, as it controls the heel in the cast and prevents recurrence of both equinus deformity and eversion of the hindfoot. An above-knee cast is applied, with the knee in 45 degrees of flexion, the ankle in 10 to 15 degrees of dorsiflexion, the heel in 10 degrees of inversion, and the forefoot in plantar flexion and inversion. The longitudinal arch and the heel in the cast are well molded.

POSTOPERATIVE CARE

The Kirschner wires are removed in six weeks, but the foot and ankle are immobilized in a solid above-knee cast for an additional two to three weeks. After removal of the cast, an above-knee polypropylene splint is worn at night for one to two years. In the splint, the knee is held in 50 to 60 degrees of flexion, the ankle in neutral dorsiflexion, the heel inverted, and the forefoot plantar-flexed and inverted. Passive exercises to develop and maintain range of joint motion and active exercises to develop muscle function are performed several times a day.

Plate 99. Open Reduction of Dorsolateral Dislocation of Talocalcaneonavicular Joint (Congenital Convex Pes Valgus)

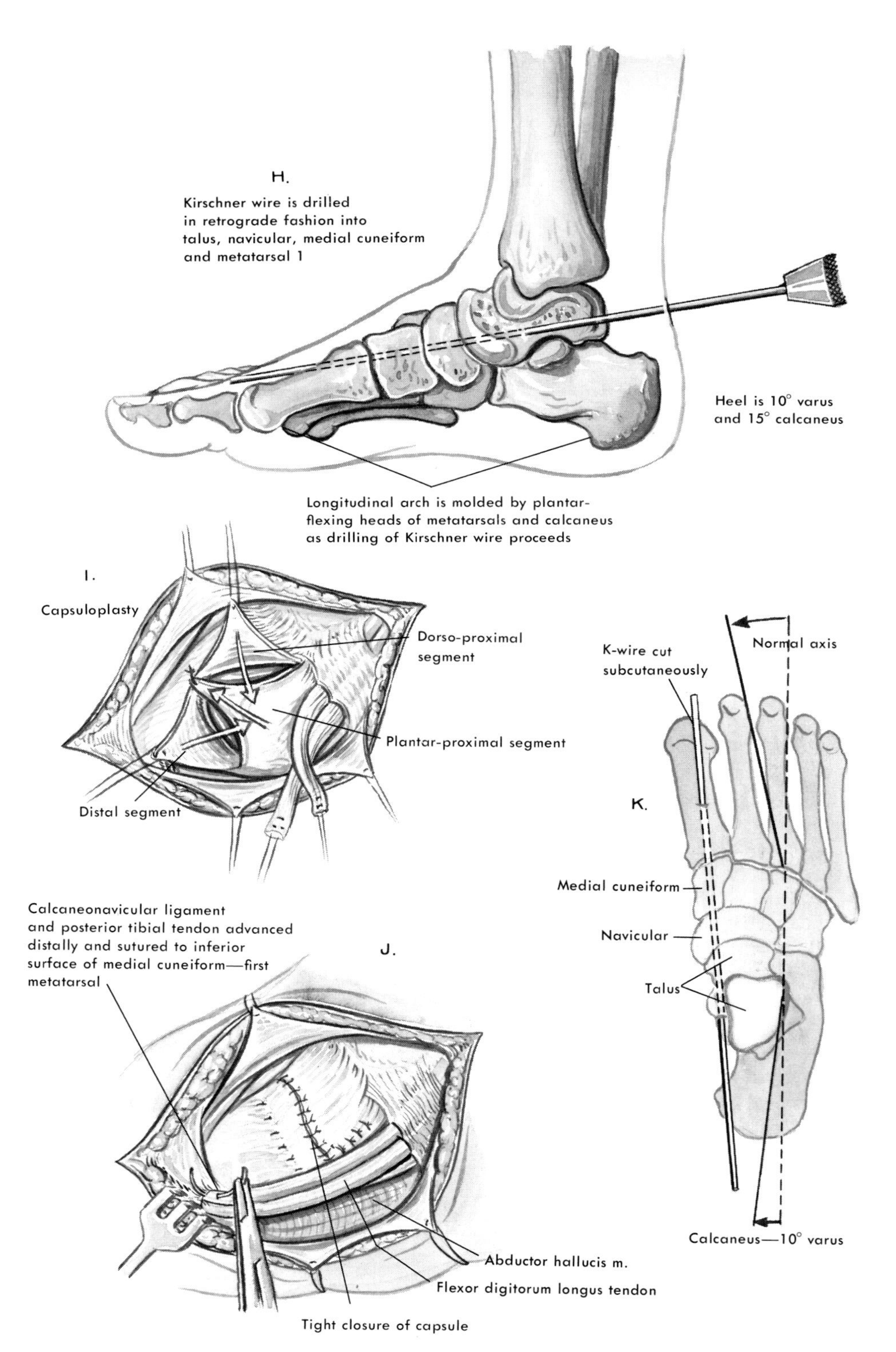

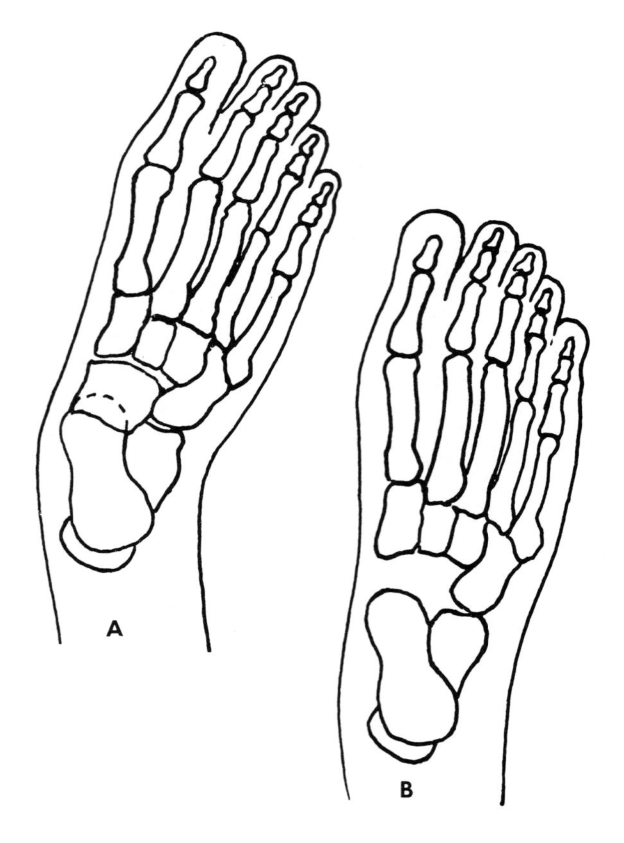

FIGURE 7–82. Principle of excision of navicular in treatment of rigid congenital convex pes valgus.

A. The deformed foot. Note the excessive length of the medial skeletal column. **B.** By excision of the navicular, a vacant space is provided to allow alignment of the forepart of the foot with the hindfoot. The medial cuneiform is brought into line with the talus. With growth and remodeling of the tarsus, the vacant area is filled with the head of the talus. (From Clark, M. W., D'Ambrosia, R. D., and Ferguson, A. B.: Congenital vertical talus. J. Bone Joint Surg., 59-A:816, 1977, p. 822. Reprinted by permission.)

In the age range of three to six years, and in the rigid dislocation of arthrogryposis or myelomeningocele, the author recommends excision of the navicular. It will effectively reduce the length of the medial skeletal column of the foot and facilitate reduction (Fig. 7–82). The medial cuneiform is aligned with the head of the talus, and with growth and remodeling of the tarsus, the vacant space is gradually filled with the head of the talus.

Eyre-Brook excised a wedge of the navicular and used it to prop up the head of the talus and maintain reduction. He reported the results in four cases; five to ten years after operation, stable reduction was maintained. Eyre-Brook suggested that the entire navicular be excised, at least in the more severe deformities.[23] Earlier, Stone, reporting for Lloyd-Roberts, had described excision of the entire navicular combined with posterior capsulotomy of the ankle, lengthening of the Achilles tendon, and transfer of the anterior tibial tendon through the neck of the talus.[73] Colton followed the technique of Lloyd-Roberts and reported good results in six feet.[17] Clark, D'Ambrosia, and Ferguson performed open reduction and excision of the navicular in 16 feet (12 patients) with true congenital vertical talus. The follow-up was for 2 to 15 years. The anatomic results in 15 of the feet were excellent in 3, good in 7, fair in 4, and poor in 1. Anatomic reduction was best achieved and maintained when the operation was performed in patients less than 18 months of age. Incomplete reductions, however, appeared to be compatible with satisfactory asymptomatic function. In this age group the sustentaculum tali is very hypoplastic and does not support the talar head. Tightening of the calcaneonavicular ligament and dynamic support by the anterior tibial and posterior tibial muscles usually are not sufficient to prevent recurrence of dislocation. The author recommends stabilization of the subtalar joint by the Grice extra-articular subtalar arthrodesis.

In the child over six years of age the deformity is very rigid, and attempts at open reduction are usually unsuccessful. Avascular necrosis of the talus is a definite complication. It is best to wait until the patient is 10 or 12 years old, at which time a reconstructive stabilization procedure on the foot is carried out. Following a preliminary period of corrective casts and soft-tissue lengthening, a triple arthrodesis is performed. The head and neck of the talus and part of the navicular are excised, and appropriate wedges (their bases plantar and medial) are resected at the calcaneocuboid joint to restore the longitudinal arch of the foot. The valgus deformity of the hindfoot is corrected by inserting a bone graft in the sinus tarsi, as in the Grice extra-articular arthrodesis. The excised head of the talus is used as a bone graft. It is not necessary to disturb the posterior subtalar joint.

References

1. Armknecht, P.: Orthopadische Leiden bei Zwillingen. Verh. Dtsch. Orthop. Ges., *26*:62, 1931.
2. Aschner, B., and Engelmann, G.: Konstitutionspathologie in der Orthopädie. Erbbiologie des peripheren Bewegungsapparates. Vienna, Julius Springer, 1928.
3. Becker-Andersen, H., and Reimann, I.: Congenital vertical talus. Reevaluation of early manipulative treatment. Acta Orthop. Scand., *45*:130, 1974.
4. Bender, G., and Horvath, F.: Über eine seltene Entwicklungsanomalie des Talus und des Os naviculare pedis. Fortschr. Rontgenstr., *94*:281, 1961.
5. Berman, J. L., Rankin, J. K., Harrison, P. A., Donovan, D. J., Hogan, W. J., and Bearn, A. O.: Autosomal trisomy of a group 16–18 chromosome. J. Pediatr., *60*:503, 1962.
6. Böhm, M.: Der Kongenitale Plattfuss. Zentralbl. Chir., p. 2987, 1932.
7. Bratberg, J. J., and Scheer, G. E.: Extra-articular arthrodesis of the subtalar joint: A clinical study and review. Clin. Orthop., *126*:220, 1977.
8. Browne, D.: Congenital vertical talus in infancy. J. Bone Joint Surg., *48-B*:588, 1966.
9. Caffey, J.: Congenital spastic flat feet. *In* Pediatric X-ray Diagnosis, the Extremities. Diseases of Bones, Congenital Malformations. 4th Ed. Chicago, Year Book, 1961, Section V, pp. 866–867.
10. Camera, V.: A proposito del piede piatto valgo congenito. Arch. Ortop., *42*:432, 1926.
11. Campos da Paz, A., Jr., De Souza, V., and De Souza, D. C.: Congenital convex pes valgus. Orthop. Clin. North Am., *9*:207, 1978.
12. Canale, G., and Bagliani, G. P.: Considerazioni sull' intervento di Grice per la correzione del piede piatto valgo. Minerva Ortop., *19*:442, 1968.
13. Chiappara, P.: Le valgus du talon. Podologie, *4*:139, 1965.
14. Clark, M. W., D'Ambrosia, R. D., and Ferguson, A. B., Jr.: Congenital vertical talus. J. Bone Joint Surg., *59-A*:816, 1977.
15. Coleman, S. S., Martin, A. F., and Jarrett, J.: Congenital vertical talus: Pathogenesis and treatment. J. Bone Joint Surg., *48-A*:1442, 1966.
16. Coleman, S., Stelling, F. H., and Jarrett, J.: Pathomechanics and treatment of congenital vertical talus. Clin. Orthop., *70*:62, 1970.
17. Colton, C. L.: The surgical management of congenital vertical talus. J. Bone Joint Surg., *55-B*:566, 1973.
18. Connolly, J. F., Dornenburg, P., and Holmes, C. D.: Congenital convex pes valgus deformities. *In* Bateman, J. E. (ed.): Foot Science. A selection of papers from the proceedings of the American Orthopaedic Foot Society, Inc., 1974 and 1975. Philadelphia, Saunders, 1976, pp. 47–66.
19. Dommisse, F. G.: Flat foot. II. S. Afr. Med. J., *45*:726, 1971.
20. Drennan, J. C., and Sharrard, W. J. W.: The pathological anatomy of convex pes valgus. J. Bone Joint Surg., *53-B*:455, 1971.
21. Duckworth, T., and Smith, T. W.: The treatment of paralytic convex pes valgus. J. Bone Joint Surg., *56-B*:305, 1974.
22. Ellis, J. N., and Scheer, G. E.: Congenital convex pes valgus. Clin. Orthop., *99*:168, 1974.
23. Eyre-Brook, A.: Congenital vertical talus. J. Bone Joint Surg., *49-B*:618, 1967.
24. Ghisellini, F., and Manaresi, C.: Il piede piatto reflesso congenito. Chir. Organi Mov., *50*:37, 1961.
25. Giannestras, N. J.: The congenital rigid flatfoot. Its recognition and treatment in infants. *In* Proceedings of the American Orthopaedic Foot Society. Orthop. Clin. North Am., *4*:49, 1973.
26. Gray, E. R.: The role of leg muscles in variations of the arches in normal and flat feet. Phys. Ther., *49*:1084, 1969.
27. Gregersen, H. N.: Malformatio congenita articuli talocruralis. Acta Orthop. Scand., *45*:462, 1974.
28. Grice, D. S.: The role of subtalar fusion in the treatment of valgus deformities of the feet. A.A.O.S. Instr. Course Lect., *16*:127, 1959.
29. Güntz, E.: Die pathologische Anatomie der angeborenen Plattfusses. Z. Orthop., *69*:219, 1939.
30. Haliburton, R. A., Sullivan, C. R., Kelly, P., and Peterson, L. F. A.: The extra-osseous and intra-osseous blood supply of the talus. J. Bone Joint Surg., *40-A*:1115, 1958.
31. Handelsman, J. E.: Treatment of congenital vertical talus. J. Bone Joint Surg., *50-B*:439, 1968.
32. Hansteen, I. L., Schirmer, L., and Hestetun, S.: Trisomy 12p syndrome. Clin. Genet., *13*:339, 1978.
33. Hark, F. W.: Rocker-foot due to congenital subluxation of the talus. J. Bone Joint Surg., *32-A*:344, 1950.
34. Harrold, A. J.: Congenital vertical talus in infancy. J. Bone Joint Surg., *49-B*:634, 1967.
35. Harrold, A. J.: The problem of congenital vertical talus. Clin. Orthop., *97*:133, 1973.
36. Haveson, S. B.: Congenital flatfoot due to talonavicular dislocation (vertical talus). Radiology, *72*:19, 1959.
37. Henken, R.: Contribution a l'étude des formes osseuses du pied valgus congénital. These de Lyon, 1914.
38. Henssge, J., and Allmeling, W.: Therapeutic experiences in congenital flatfoot with vertical talus. Arch. Orthop. Unfallchir., *59*:74, 1966.
39. Herndon, C. H., and Heyman, C. H.: Problems in the recognition and treatment of congenital convex pes valgus. J. Bone Joint Surg., *45-A*:413, 1963.
40. Heyman, C. H.: The diagnosis and treatment of congenital convex pes valgus or vertical talus. A.A.O.S. Instr. Course Lect., *16*:117, 1959.
41. Hohmann, G.: Fuss und Bein. Munchen, I. F. Bergann, 1934, pp. 26–33.
42. Hohmann, G.: Pes plano-valgus congenitus. *In* Hohmann, G. (ed.): Handbuch der Orthopadie. Stuttgart, Georg Thieme Verlag, 1961, Vol. IV, Part II, pp. 832–840.
43. Hughes, J. R.: Congenital vertical talus. J. Bone Joint Surg., *39-B*:580, 1957.
44. Hughes, J. R.: Pathologic anatomy and pathogenesis of congenital vertical talus and its practical significance. J. Bone Joint Surg., *52-B*:777, 1970.
45. Joachimsthal: Ueber pes valgus congenitus. Dtsch. Med. Wochensschr., *29*:(Vereins-Beilage):123, 1903.
46. Judet, J., Estève, P., Masse, P., and Rigault, P.: Congenital convex foot. Rev. Chir. Orthop., *60*:Suppl. 2:370, 1974.
47. Laburthe-Tolra, Y., and Bensahel, H.: Congenital convex talipes valgus (apropos of 19 cases). Ann. Chir., *26*:203, 1972.
48. Lamy, L., and Weissman, L.: Congenital convex pes valgus. J. Bone Joint Surg., *21*:79, 1939.

49. Lange, F.: Plattfussbeschwerben und Plattfussbehandlung. Munchen Med. Wochensschr., *59*:300, 1912.
50. Leveuf, J.: Le traitement du pied convexe valgus congénital. Rev. Orthop., *27*:129, 1941.
51. Lloyd-Roberts, G. C., and Spence, A. J.: Congenital vertical talus. J. Bone Joint Surg., *40-B*:33, 1958.
52. McFarland, B.: Congenital vertical talus. J. Bone Joint Surg., *39-B*:480, 1957.
53. Maresca, A.: Considerazioni sulla lussazione congenita astragalo scafoidea nel quadro del cosidetto piede a dondolo. Orriz. Ortop. Odierna Riabilit., *4*:187, 1959.
54. Mau, C.: Muskelbefunde und ihre Bedeutung beim angeborenen Klumpfussleiden. Arch. Orthop. Unfallchir., *28*:292, 1930.
55. Mead, N. C., and Anast, G.: Vertical talus. Clin. Orthop., *21*:198, 1961.
56. Nové-Josserand: Formes anatomiques du pied plat. Rev. Orthop., *10*:117, 1923.
57. Ogata, K., Schoenecker, P. S., and Sheridan, J.: Congenital vertical talus and its familial occurrence. Clin. Orthop., *139*:128, 1979.
58. Osmond-Clarke, H.: Congenital vertical talus. J. Bone Joint Surg., *38-B*:334, 1956.
59. Outland, T., and Sherk, H. H.: Congenital vertical talus. A.A.O.S. Instr. Course Lect., *16*:214, 1959.
60. Parrish, T. F.: Congenital convex pes valgus accompanied by previously undescribed anatomic derangements. South. Med. J., *60*:983, 1967.
61. Patterson, W. R., Fitz, D. A., and Smith, W. S.: The pathologic anatomy of congenital convex pes valgus. J. Bone Joint Surg., *50-A*:458, 1968.
62. Pouliquen, J. C.: Pied convexe congénital. Rev. Chir. Orthop., Suppl. 2:370, 1974.
63. Rigault, P., and Pouliquen, J. C.: Le pied convexe congénital. Ann. Chir. Infant., Paris, *11*:261, 1970.
64. Ritsilä, V. A.: Talipes equinovarus and vertical talus produced experimentally in newborn rabbits. Acta Orthop. Scand., Suppl. 121, 1969.
65. Robbins, H.: Naviculectomy for congenital vertical talus. Bull. Hosp. Jt. Dis., *37*:77, 1976.
66. Rocher, H. L., and Pouyanne, L.: Pied plat congénital par subluxation sous-astragalienne congénitale et orientation verticale de l'astragale. Bordeaux Chir., *5*:249, 1934.
67. Schulitz, K. P., Schumacher, G., and Parsch, K.: Der angeborene Schaukelfuss. Z. Orthop., *115*:55, 1977.
68. Searfoss, R., Bendana, A., King, G., and Miller, G.: Vertical talus of unusual etiology. Case report. J. Bone Joint Surg., *57-A*:409, 1975.
69. Sharrard, W. J. W., and Grosfield, I.: The management of deformity and paralysis of the foot in myelomeningocele. J. Bone Joint Surg., *50-B*:456, 1968.
70. Silk, F. F., and Wainwright, D.: The recognition and treatment of congenital flat foot in infancy. J. Bone Joint Surg., *49-B*:628, 1967.
71. Slavik, M., and Stryhal, F.: Congenital steep talus. (Congenital convex pes valgus, congenital vertical talus.) Acta Chir. Orthop. Traumatol. Cech., *37*:367, 1970.
72. Specht, E. E.: Congenital paralytic vertical talus. J. Bone Joint Surg., *57-A*:842, 1975.
73. Stone, K. H., and Lloyd-Roberts, G. C.: Congenital vertical talus: A new operation. Proc. R. Soc. Med., *56*:12, 1963.
74. Støren, H.: On the closed and open correction of congenital convex pes valgus with a vertical astragalus. Acta Orthop. Scand., *36*:352, 1965.
75. Støren, H.: Congenital convex pes valgus with vertical talus. Acta Orthop. Scand., Suppl. 94:1, 1967.
76. Syntheses Bibliographiques: Pied convexe valgus congénital. Rev. Chir. Orthop., *67*:27, 1970.
77. Tachdjian, M. O.: Congenital convex pes valgus. Orthop. Clin. North Am., *3*:131, 1972.
78. Towns, P. L., Dettart, G. K., Hecht, F., and Manning, J. A.: Trisomy 13–15 in a male infant. J. Pediatr., *60*:528, 1962.
79. Uchida, I. A., Lewis, A. J., Bowman, J. M., and Wang, H. C.: A case of double trisomy: No. 18 and triple-X. J. Pediatr., *60*:498, 1962.
80. Wainwright, D.: The recognition and cure of congenital flat foot. Proc. R. Soc. Med., *57*:357, 1964.
81. Wainwright, D.: Congenital vertical talus in infancy. J. Bone Joint Surg., *48-B*:588, 1966.
82. Weiss, P.: Principles of development. New York, Henry Holt & Co., 1939.
83. Wertheimer, L. G.: Personal communication to Campos da Paz, Jr. (see ref. 11).
84. Wilkinson, J. A.: Breech malposition and intra-uterine dislocations. Proc. R. Soc. Med., *59*:1106, 1966.

TARSAL COALITION

In this congenital abnormality, varying degrees of union occur between two or more tarsal bones, producing a rigid planovalgus foot. Buffon, in 1769, was probably the first to recognize tarsal coalition.[21] Since then, Cruveilhier, in 1829, reported the first recorded example of calcaneonavicular coalition; Zuckerkandl is credited with the first anatomic description, in 1877, of talocalcaneal coalition; and Anderson, in 1880, with that of talonavicular synostosis.[4, 38, 194] Heiple and Lovejoy described bilateral talocalcaneal bridges, one complete and one incomplete, in a pre-Columbian Indian skeleton found in Ohio and dating from approximately A.D. 1000.[79] Their report documents the existence of this anomaly in man in ancient times.

The clinical significance of these intertarsal bridges was not appreciated until 1880, when Holl proposed a possible relationship between flatfoot and intertarsal bar.[83] Sir Robert Jones gave the first clinical description of peroneal spastic flatfoot in 1897; but it remained for Slomann and later Badgley to show that at least some cases of rigid pes planovalgus with peroneal spasm are caused by calcaneonavicular bar.[8, 94, 162, 163] In 1948, Harris and Beath reported the correlation between medial talocalcaneal bridge and peroneal spastic flatfoot.[74]

Table 7–12. *Incidence of Tarsal Coalition*

Author	*Material*	*Incidence (Per Cent)*
Pfitzner[142]	Autopsy	0.38 (2 of 524)
Harris and Beath[73]	Army recruits	0.03 (1 of 3,619)*
Vaughan and Segal[179]	Army personnel	1 (21 of 2,000)
Shands and Wentz[157]	Children's clinic	0.9 (11 of 1,232)

*Of 3,619, 72 (2 per cent) had peroneal spastic flat foot.

Table 7–13. Classification of Types of Tarsal Condition

Isolated anomaly
Dual between two tarsal bones
Talocalcaneal
Medial
Complete
Incomplete
Rudimentary
Posterior
Anterior
Calcaneonavicular
Talonavicular
Calcaneocuboid
Naviculocuneiform
Multiple—various combinations of the preceding, e.g., talocalcaneal and calcaneocuboid
Massive—all major tarsal bones fused into a single block of bone
Part of complex malformation
In association with other synostoses
Carpal coalition
Symphalangism
As one of manifestations of a syndrome
Nievergelt-Pearlman
Apert's
In association with major limb anomalies
Absence of toes or rays
"Ball-and-socket" ankle joint
Fibular hemimelia
Phocomelia
Proximal focal femoral deficiency

Incidence and Classification

The exact incidence of tarsal coalition in the general population is unknown because the reported studies have been based on selected materials (Table 7–12).[73, 142, 157, 179] Probably it is 1 per cent or less, as in none of the series is it above this figure.

Intertarsal coalition may be of many types. It may occur as an isolated anomaly or sometimes be associated with fusions between other bones (such as those of the carpus or the phalanges). Occasionally tarsal coalitions are part of a generalized syndrome. A classification of the various forms is given in Table 7–13. The coalition may be completely osseous (synostosis), or the bones may be divided by a fissure of varying depth consisting of cartilage (synchondrosis) or fibrous tissue (syndesmosis).

The most common coalitions in the tarsus are between the calcaneus and the navicular, and between the talus and the calcaneus. Harris reported the following distribution of the various types of intertarsal bridges found in 102 patients: medial talocalcaneal bridge in 62, calcaneonavicular bar in 29, posterior talocalcaneal bridge in 4, multiple intertarsal fusions in 4, talonavicular fusion in 1, calcaneocuboid fusion in 1, and cubonavicular fusion in 1.[69–75] In this author's clinical practice, calcaneonavicular coalition is the most common type.

Of the intertarsal coalitions, medial talocalcaneal bridge and calcaneonavicular bar are the more significant clinically, as they are responsible for the majority of cases of peroneal spastic flatfoot and cause the greater disability.

Medial talocalcaneal bridge may take a variety of forms: complete, in which a bony bridge connects the talus and calcaneus, as illustrated in Figures 7–83 A and 7–84; incomplete, in which a mass of bone projecting from the talus is united to a mass of bone projecting from the sustentaculum tali by a thin plate of fibrous tissue or cartilage, as shown in Figure 7–83 B; or rudimentary, in which only one element of the bridge is present, i.e., the bony mass projects either upward from the posterior margin of the sustentaculum tali or downward from the medial surface of the body of the talus posterior to the sustentaculum tali, in either instance blocking inversion of the os calcis (Fig. 7–83 C and D).[72] The complete and incomplete forms are readily recognizable, but in the rudimentary form the radiographic changes are equivocal.

Talonavicular coalition is very rare. The total number of cases reported in the world literature is less than 40; Schreiber has suggested, however, that it may be more common than the literature indicates.[154] Involvement may be unilateral or bilateral, with a definite hereditary factor in the latter.[81, 150]

Calcaneocuboid synostosis was first described by Wagoner in 1928, and isolated case reports have since appeared in the literature.[20, 119, 182] The condition is of anatomic interest only, as it is asymptomatic and does not require any orthopedic care.

Cubonavicular synostosis is rare. Waugh reported a case of peroneal spastic flatfoot caused by cubonavicular coalition.[183] Naviculocuneiform synostosis was first described by Lusby; Gregersen reported a bilateral case of symptomatic flatfoot.[64, 118]

Tarsal and carpal coalitions may coexist. Leonard, on clinical and radiographic examination, however, did not find any abnormality of the carpus in 69 patients with tarsal coalition. Despite the developmental similarity of the carpus and tarsus, the two conditions seem to be unrelated.[114, 115] Symphalangism (congenital fusion of the proximal or distal interphalangeal joints) may be present in tarsal and carpal coalitions.[7, 24, 48, 67] Tarsal synostoses may occur in phocomelia, fibular hemimelia, or proximal focal femoral deficiency; other anomalies associated with tarsal coalition are "ball-and-socket" ankle joint and absence of toes.[53, 109, 136]

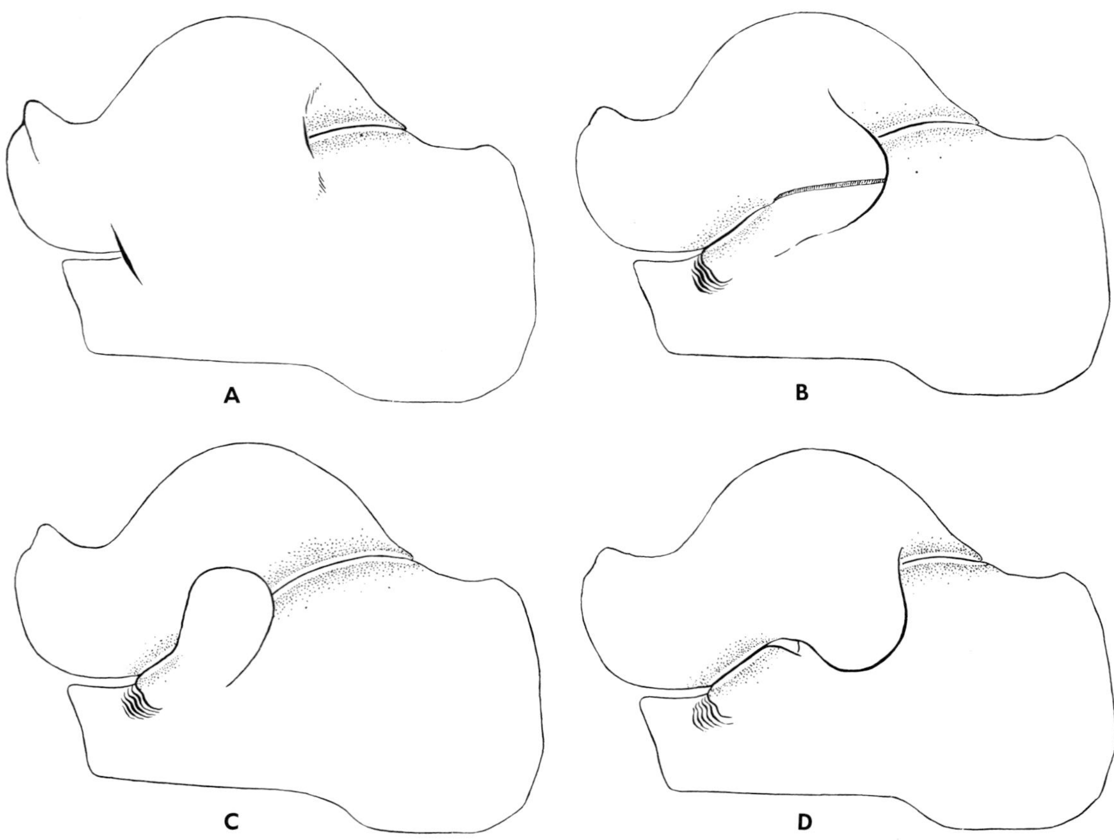

FIGURE 7–83. Diagrams of variations in medial talocalcaneal coalition (bridge).

A. Complete medial talocalcaneal coalition. **B.** Incomplete medial talocalcaneal coalition—syndesmosis and synchondrosis. **C.** Rudimentary medial talocalcaneal coalition—sustentacular element. (The bony mass projects upward from the posterior margin of the sustentaculum tali and impinges on the medial side of the body of the talus.) **D.** Rudimentary medial talocalcaneal coalition—talar element. (Bony mass projects downward from the medial surface of the body of the talus posterior to the sustentaculum tali. It impinges on the calcaneus on inversion, though not attached to it.) (From Harris, R. I.: Retrospect—peroneal spastic flat foot (rigid valgus foot). J. Bone Joint Surg., *47-A*:1661, 1965. Reprinted by permission.)

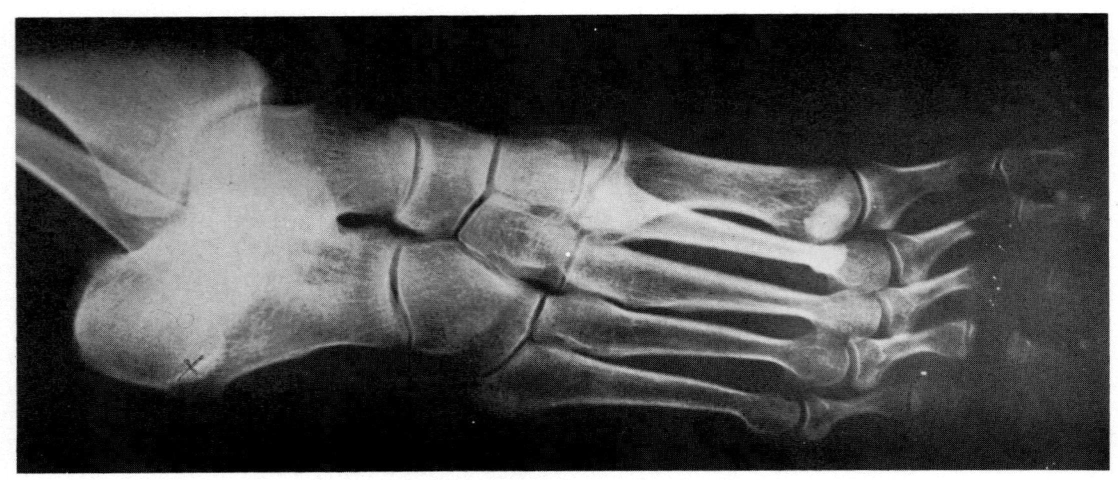

FIGURE 7–84. Complete medial talocalcaneal coalition.

Multiple or massive tarsal coalitions may be part of a more complex syndrome. Nievergelt, in 1944, described a syndrome consisting of tarsal synostosis with clubfeet, bilateral elbow dysplasia with radioulnar synostosis and subluxation of the radial head, and dysplasia of the tibia and fibula with the fibula relatively long because of lesser involvement.[134] Twenty years later, Pearlman, Edkin, and Warren reported a similar combination of deformities in a mother and her daughter; their patients did not have dysplasia of the tibia. The case of Pearlman and associates also presented carpal synostosis, symphalangism, brachydactylia, and clinocamptodactylia. They proposed the name *Nievergelt syndrome*.[141] Dubois reported a case, confirming the descriptions by Nievergelt and Pearlman; the x-rays, in addition, showed a typical ball-and-socket ankle (Fig. 7–85). Dubois suggested that *Nievergelt-Pearlman syndrome* would be more correct.[49] Clinically, when there is dysplasia of the tibia and fibula, the lower legs are short and the deformity is apparent at birth. Radiograms will disclose the thick and markedly shortened tibiae, which are triangular in shape. Pronation and supination of the forearms are restricted because of radioulnar synostosis. The syndrome is transmitted as an autosomal dominant trait; it is of interest that Nievergelt's original patient was one of the principal figures in a legal case of disputed paternity—the genetic trait was transmitted to three illegitimate children from three different mothers. Murakami reported three cases of Nievergelt-Pearlman syndrome in a family with impairment of hearing due to bony fusion of the ossicles of the middle ear.[132]

In Apert's syndrome there may be massive synostosis of the tarsal bones (Fig. 7–86). The condition is characterized by craniosynostosis, midfacial hypoplasia, osseous or cutaneous syndactyly of all digits (or commonly, of the second, third, and fourth fingers and toes), and a broad distal phalanx of the thumb and hallux.

Etiology

The exact cause of tarsal coalition is unknown. It seems to arise from failure of differentiation and segmentation of the primitive mesenchyme with resultant lack of joint formation. This theory is supported and confirmed by the finding of intertarsal bridges in fetal feet (Fig. 7–87).

In the past, anatomists such as Pfitzner proposed that tarsal coalition was caused by incorporation of the accessory intertarsal ossicles into the adjacent major tarsal bones.[142] Thus calcaneonavicular coalition was believed to result from the union of the os calcaneus secundarius with the adjacent calcaneus and navicular bones, and incorporation of the os sustentaculare with its neighboring os calcis and talus was believed to cause medial talocaneal coalition. Similarly, one might implicate the os trigonum in posterior talocalcaneal fusion, the os tibiale externum in talonavicular synostosis, the os peroneum in calcaneocuboid fusion, and multiple accessory ossicles in massive tarsal coalition. This hypothesis of incorporation of accessory ossicles is not acceptable, however, as it fails to explain the presence of tarsal coalition in the fetus.

Heredity

In the literature there are several reports of the occurrence of tarsal coalition in several members of the same family. For example, Webster and Roberts described talocalcaneal coalition in two sisters; Boyd reported a family with bilateral talonavicular bars in three generations; Rothberg, Feldman, and Schuster reported familial incidence of bilateral talonavicular synostosis; and Bersani and Samilson reported similar cases involving several tarsal bones.[15, 17, 150, 185] Wray and Herndon, describing the occurrence of calcaneonavicular coalition in three generations of one family, proposed that at least some, perhaps all, cases of calcaneonavicular bar are caused by a specific gene mutation that is autosomally dominant, probably with reduced penetrance.[190] Harris noted calcaneonavicular bars in identical twins and also in a father and son.[72] Glessner and Davis reported monozygotic twins with peroneal spastic flatfoot and tarsal coalition.[61]

Leonard conducted a family survey of 31 patients known to have had treatment for peroneal spastic flatfoot and tarsal coalition (27 calcaneonavicular and 4 talocalcaneal). The pattern of inheritance was studied by clinical and radiographic examination of the hands and feet of the 31 index patients and their 98 first-degree relatives—parents, siblings, and children. Some type of tarsal coalition was found in 39 per cent of the first-degree relatives (33 per cent of the parents and 46.5 per cent of the siblings). Of the first-degree relatives of the 27 index patients with calcaneonavicular coalition, 25 per cent had calcaneonavicular fusion, but 14 per cent had talocalcaneal or some other type of tarsal synostosis. In all 11 of the affected first-degree relatives of the four index patients with talocalcaneal coalitions, however, a similar type of

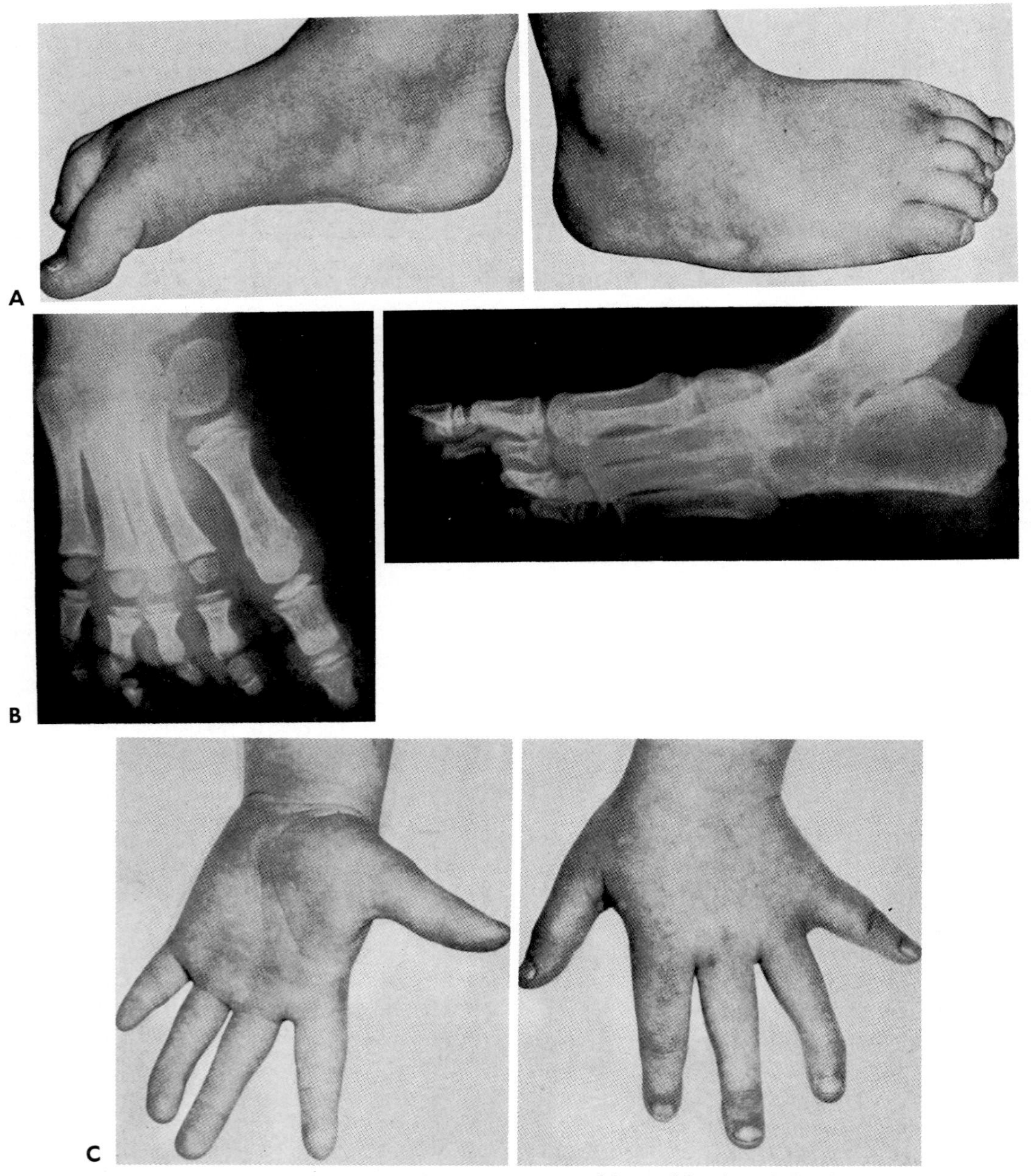

FIGURE 7–85. Nievergelt-Pearlman syndrome—synostoses of feet and hands with dysplasia of the elbows.

A. and **B.** Photographs and radiograms of feet. There is varus deformity of both feet and massive synostosis of the talus, calcaneus, cuboid, and cuneiform bones. The second, third, and fourth metatarsal bases are fused, with a bony bridge between them and the one tarsal bone. **C.** Photographs of the hands.

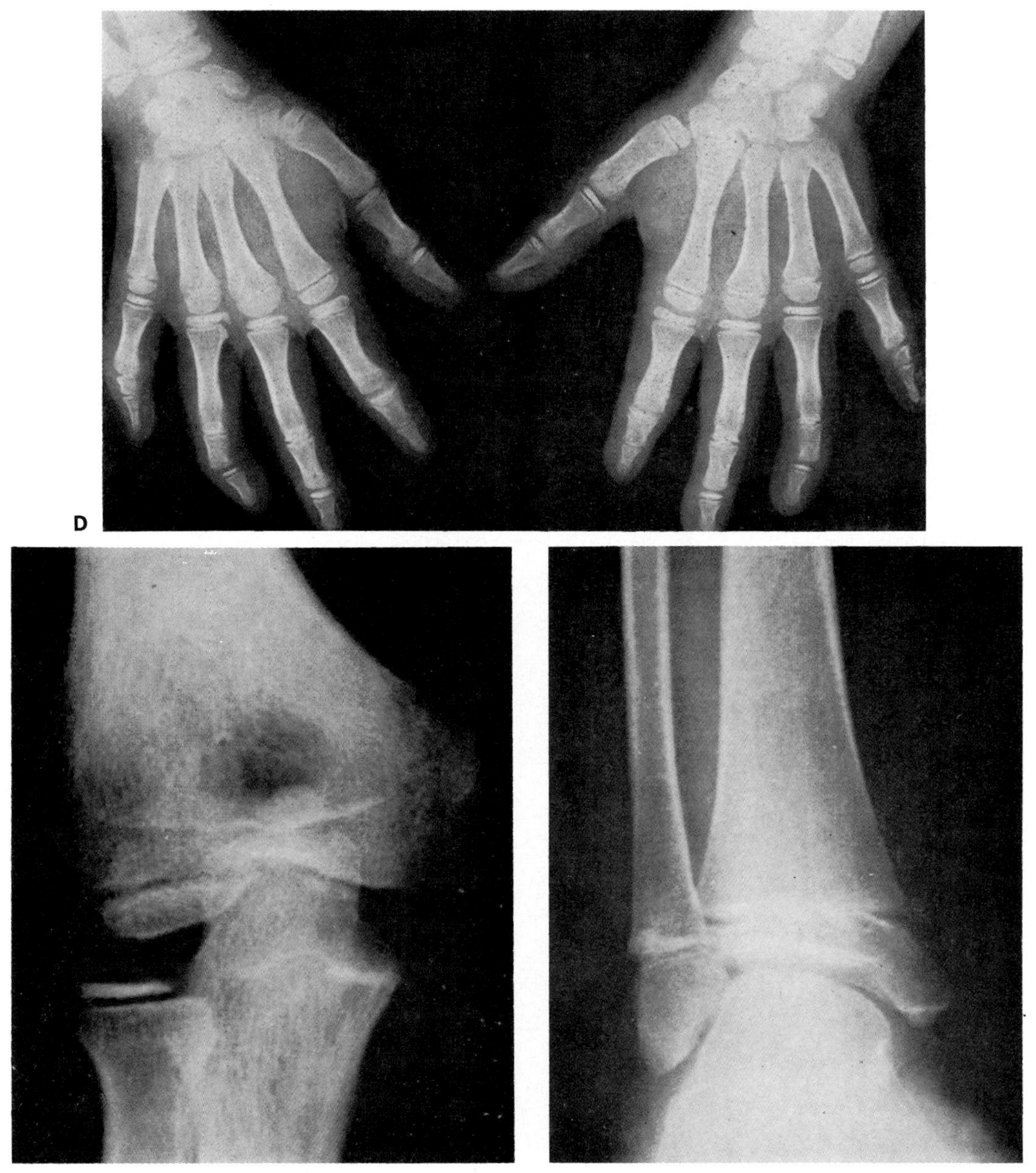

FIGURE 7–85 Continued. Nievergelt-Pearlman syndrome—synostoses of feet and hands with dysplasia of the elbows.

D. Radiograms of the hands. The capitate and trapezoid, and the triquetrum and hamate are fused. Note the symphalangism of the proximal interphalangeal joints of the middle and ring fingers and the distal interphalangeal joints of the index and little fingers. **E.** Anteroposterior projections of the elbow and ankle showing dysplasia of the elbow and the typical "ball-and-socket" deformity of the ankle. (From Dubois, H. J.: Nievergelt-Pearlman syndrome. J. Bone Joint Surg., *52-B*:325, 1970. Reprinted by permission.)

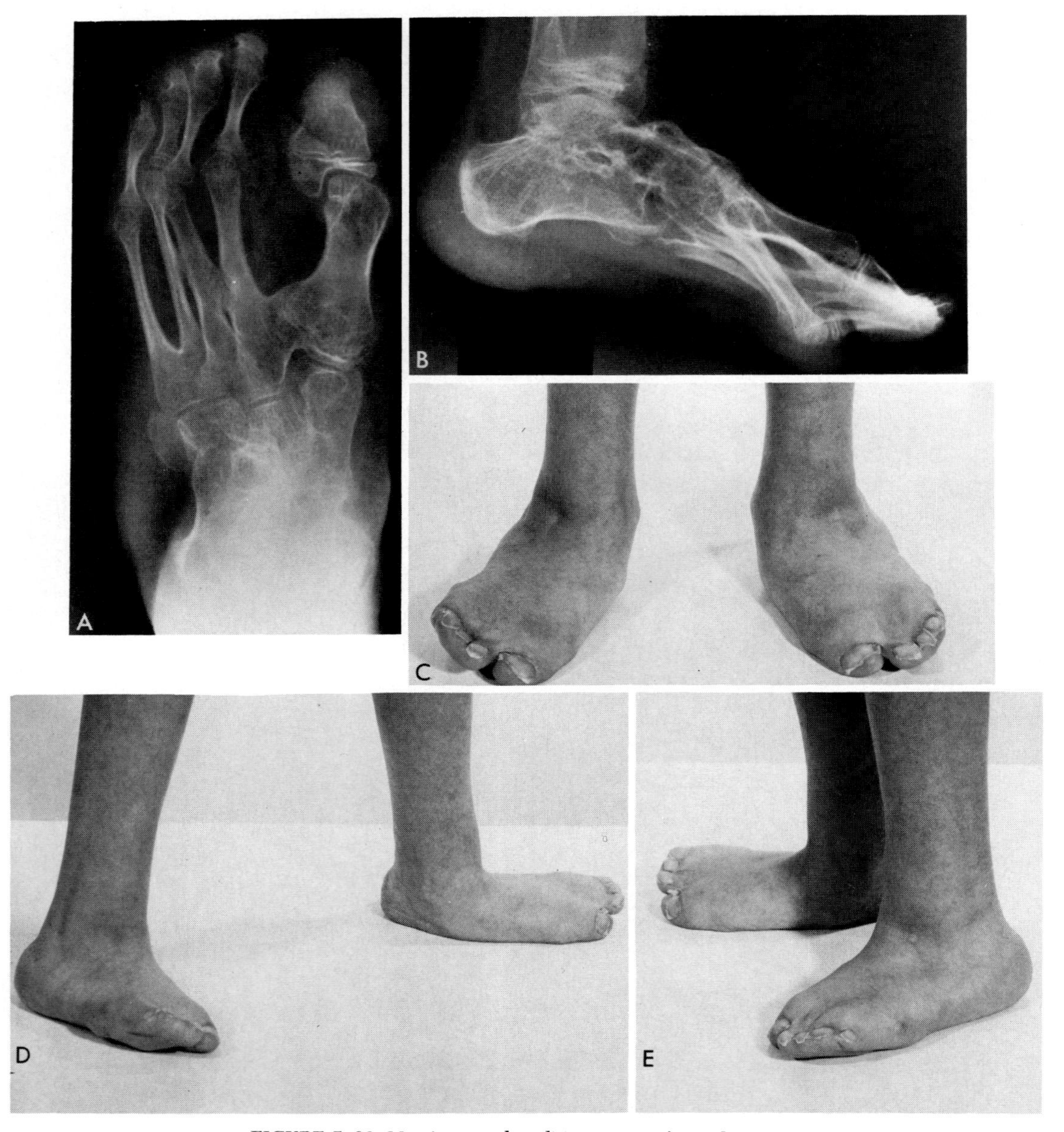

FIGURE 7–86. Massive tarsal coalition in Apert's syndrome.

A and **B**. Radiograms of feet. **C**, **D**, and **E**. Characteristic clinical appearance.

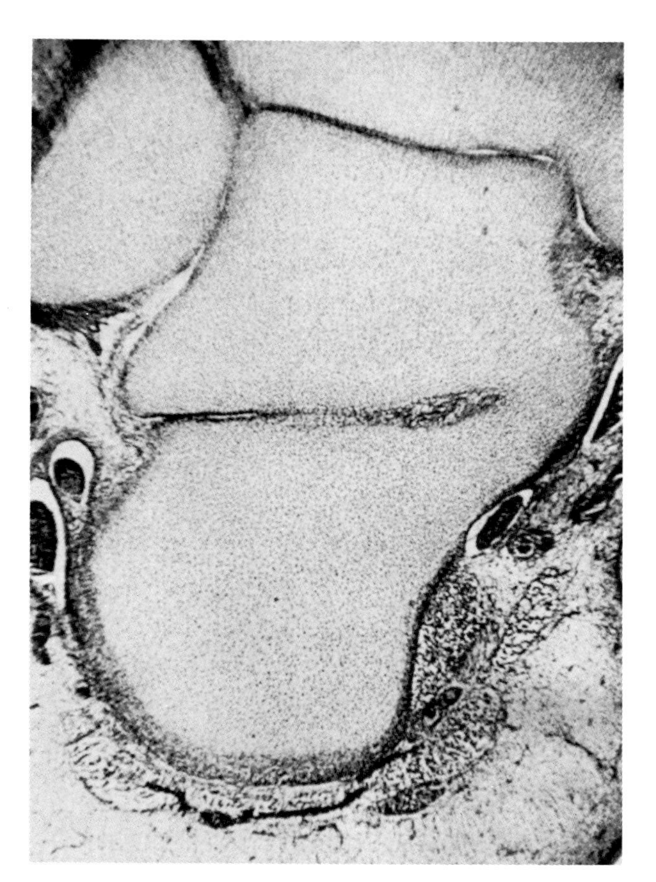

FIGURE 7–87. Complete medial talocalcaneal bridge in the foot of a 72.3-mm. fetus (coronal section).

(Courtesy of Barbara Anne Harris Monie; from Harris, R. I.: Retrospect—peroneal spastic flat foot. J. Bone Joint Surg., *47-A*:1658, 1965. Reprinted by permission.)

fusion was discovered. The findings of Leonard indicate that tarsal coalitions are most probably an inherited autosomal dominant disorder with almost full penetrance. The presence of a different type of tarsal coalition in 14 per cent of the relatives shows that there is no genetic difference in the inheritance of the various coalitions.[114, 115]

Clinical Features

Tarsal coalitions may occur bilaterally or unilaterally. As a rule talonavicular fusions are present in both feet; calcaneonavicular coalition is bilateral in 60 per cent of patients, and talocalcaneal coalition, in 50 per cent.

In infancy and early childhood the condition is usually asymptomatic and is seldom recognized. When the child begins to walk, varying degrees of restriction of motion between the involved tarsal bones may become apparent; during this period, however, the condition is not likely to be suspected, as pain is not a clinical feature, the bar is fibrous or cartilaginous, and the radiograms are normal.

Tarsal coalition may be totally asymptomatic and an accidental finding in the radiogram. For example, in studying 23 patients with tarsal coalition, Jack found that 5 (22 per cent) were free of symptoms.[87] Leonard was surprised to find that not one of the 38 affected first-degree relatives of the index patients with tarsal coalition had ever had symptoms referable to their feet.[115]

The occurrence of symptoms and the age of their onset are dependent upon the period at which ossification of the coalition takes place. All coalitions are cartilaginous at birth and may allow motion, whereas a bony union between two or more tarsal bones restricts motion, causing symptoms. According to Cowell, clinical complaints related to talonavicular coalition may develop as early as two years of age, whereas symptoms of calcaneonavicular coalition usually appear between 8 and 12 years of age, and those of talocalcaneal coalition occur during adolescence.[35, 36]

Another factor to consider is the increasing stress and strain exerted on the foot with greater body weight and strenuous physical activity as in sports.

The biomechanics of the foot is disturbed in tarsal coalition. During normal gait the tibia rotates medially 18 degrees during swing phase and the first 15 per cent of stance phase; then lateral rotation of the tibia takes place, reaching its maximum immediately after toe-off, when medial rotation begins again. In the ankle mortise these rotatory motions are transmitted to the talus. The axis of rotation of the subtalar joint is oblique, similar to that of an oblique hinge. Medial rotation of the tibia results in eversion of the calcaneus; conversely lateral rotation of the tibia produces inversion of the calcaneus. With progressive restriction of motion in the subtalar joint, compensatory movement must take place at levels either proximal or distal to it. In the ankle joint the increasing laxity of ligaments predisposes to recurrent ankle sprain; in the transverse tarsal joints the navicular bone gradually becomes displaced dorsolaterally over the head of the talus, causing progressive eversion and valgus deviation of the calcaneus. The peroneal muscles gradually shorten with no true spasticity. When inversion of the hindfoot is attempted, the peroneal muscles are stretched, they contract, and the tautened tendons pull the forefoot into abduction. In medial talocalcaneal coalition, there is progressive restriction of motion on the medial aspect of the joint but not on the lateral aspect, which forces the calcaneus into valgus position, and the longitudinal arch becomes flattened.

The degree of pes valgus varies greatly; it may be very marked or so minimal that it may be overlooked. In general, medial talocalcaneal bridges cause more valgus deformity than do calcaneonavicular coalitions.

Restriction of motion at the subtalar and midtarsal joints is the characteristic physical finding. When the medial talocalcaneal coalition is complete, the hindfoot will be rigidly fixed in some degree of valgus deformity; midtarsal motion may also be restricted. In calcaneonavicular coalitions, motion at the subtalar and midtarsal joints is moderately limited, but usually not completely obliterated.

The most common symptom of tarsal coalition is pain in the subtalar or midtarsal area of the involved foot. It often develops in adolescence, though not in all patients. It is usually noted after some unusual activity or minor trauma, and is aggravated by walking over rough terrain, prolonged standing, jumping, or participating in athletics. Rest relieves the pain. In severe cases the gait may be antalgic.

"Spasm" of the peroneal tendons may develop during the course of the disease. The characteristic findings of peroneal "spastic" flatfoot are restricted subtalar motion, hindfoot valgus deformity, abduction of the forefoot, and tautness of the peroneal tendon. Forced passive inversion of the calcaneus is painful and stretches the peroneal muscles, which contract, increasing the valgus deformity of the foot (Fig. 7–88). In severe cases, the extensor digitorum longus may also be involved. Muscle spasm may occur intermittently or be present continuously in varying severity; overactivity increases it, and rest relieves it.

Occasionally in tarsal coalition, the anterior tibial and posterior tibial muscles are in spasm and cause a varus deformity of the foot (Fig. 7–89).

Peroneal spastic flatfoot may be caused by any condition that restricts the motion and normal biomechanics of the talocalcaneonavicular joint. For example, rheumatoid arthritis may involve the subtalar joint, and it is not uncommon in pauciarticular arthritis for painful peroneal spastic flatfoot to be the presenting complaint. Other conditions include osteochondral fractures involving the anterior or middle facets of the talocalcaneal joint and lesions such as osteoid osteoma or fibrosarcoma.[36]

In talonavicular coalition, the presenting complaint is usually a hard prominence on the medial side of the foot rather than pain. Some cases are discovered accidentally. The longitudinal arch is well maintained. Immobility of the talonavicular joint, however, increases the strain of body weight on the joints adjacent to the fused bones and the cuneiforms. This excess stress may predispose the patient to arthritic changes in adult life. Sanghi and Roby have reported a case of bilateral peroneal spastic flatfoot associated with talonavicular coalition.[152]

Radiographic Findings

The radiographic appearance of tarsal coalition depends upon its site and whether it is bony or fibrocartilaginous. The radiologic examination of the foot should proceed in an orderly manner from the routine and simple to more sophisticated studies. Initial radiograms include anteroposterior, lateral, and oblique projections; these will clearly show coalitions between the talus and the navicular and between the calcaneus and the cuboid.

Calcaneonavicular coalitions are best demonstrated in a 45-degree oblique view of the foot made with the patient standing on the film and the x-ray beam projected through the middle of the foot from the lateral to the medial

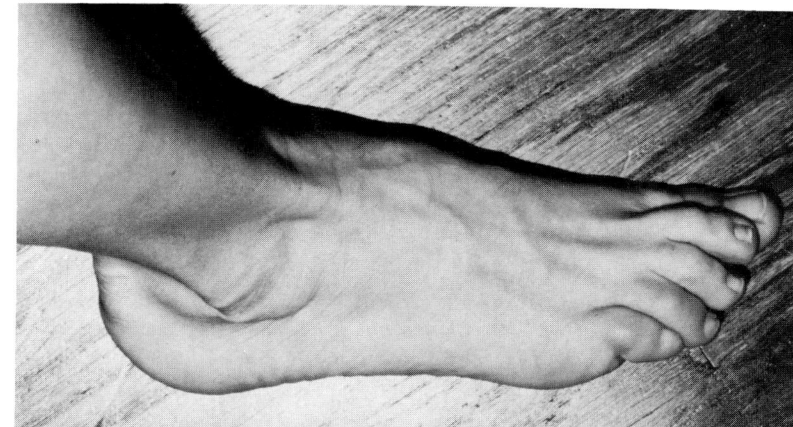

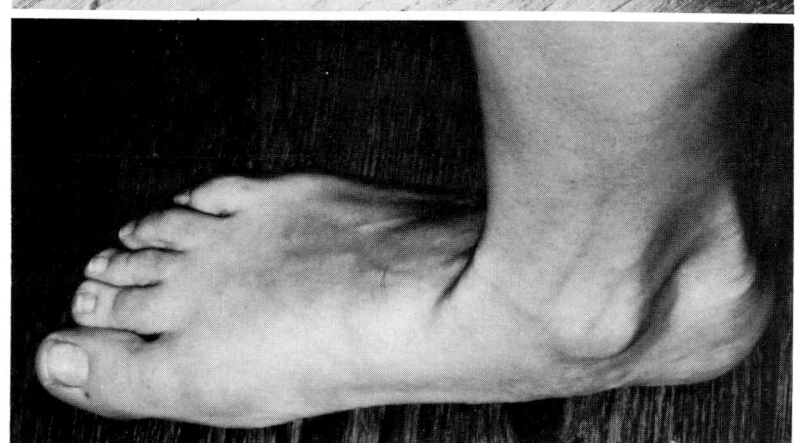

FIGURE 7–88. The clinical findings in peroneal "spastic" flatfoot.

Note the severe pes planovalgus with abduction of the forefoot. The peroneal tendons are taut, and there is marked restriction of subtalar motion.

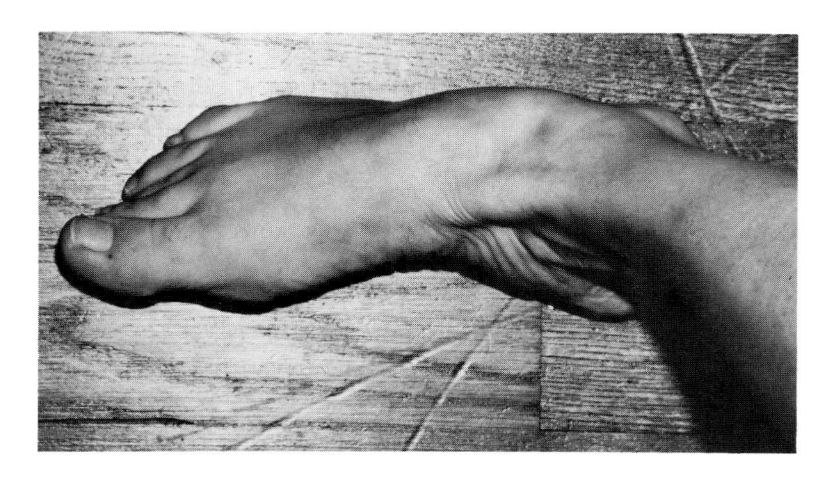

FIGURE 7–89. Pes varus due to tautness of the anterior tibial muscle in calcaneonavicular coalition.

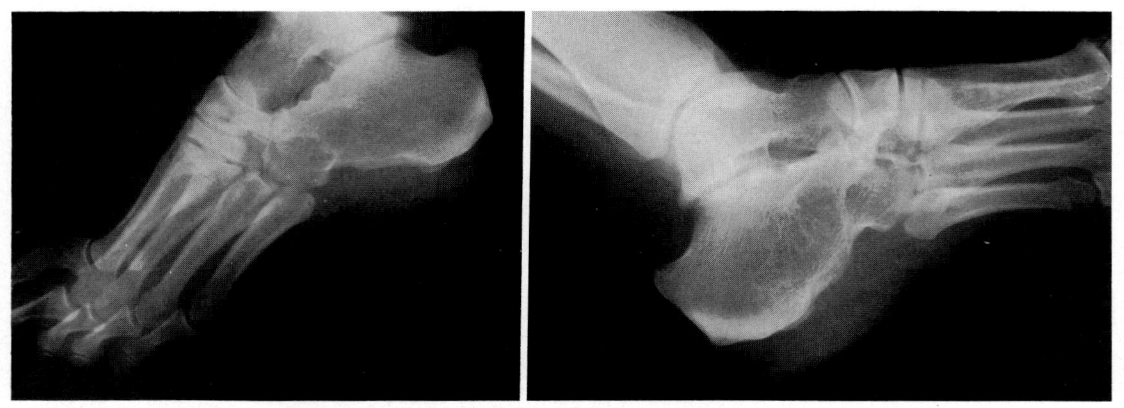

FIGURE 7–90. Calcaneonavicular synostosis is best visualized in the oblique view.

Note the bony bridge obliterating the space between the anterior process of the calcaneus and the navicular of both feet.

side (Fig. 7–90). Overlap of the tarsal bones may be mistaken for synostosis; in such instances, oblique projections at various angles are necessary for a definitive diagnosis. The importance of these oblique views cannot be overemphasized, as often in the regular anteroposterior and lateral views of the foot, a calcaneonavicular bar may be entirely overlooked.

The connecting bar between the calcaneus and the navicular may be either bony or cartilaginous. When bony, the bridge is at least 1 cm. wide, completely obliterates the space between the calcaneus and the navicular, and is clearly visible in the oblique radiogram. When the union is cartilaginous or fibrous, however, diagnosis is not that simple. Such a possibility should be suspected when the anterior medial end of the calcaneus and the navicular are in close proximity and their contiguous cortical surfaces are flattened, having the appearance of a pseudarthritic joint (Fig. 7–91). Hypoplasia of the head of the talus is another associated finding. Fracture of the anterior process of the calcaneus and the presence of an os calcaneus secundarius should be considered in the differential diagnosis (Fig. 7–92). In chip fracture the bone fragment has a well-delineated trabecular structure, and its surfaces are smooth and clearly demarcated.

Occasionally, the oblique radiograms of the foot may show a slender prolongation of the anterior process of the calcaneus; this may contain a cartilaginous bar and be pathologic (Fig. 7–93). To determine whether it is, one may have to resort to arthrography, as described later, or wait until further ossification takes place.

Special projections are necessary to demonstrate talocalcaneal coalitions. Korvin, in 1934, was the first to describe use of the axial view of the calcaneus to reveal talocalcaneal coalition.[105] Harris and Beath, in 1948, emphasized the relation of peroneal spastic flatfoot to talocalcaneal bridge and recommended a 45-degree-angle axial view of the calcaneus for its demonstration.[74]

The subtalar joint is complex, consisting of anterior, middle, and posterior joints that are formed by three separate pairs of facets on the superior surface of the calcaneus and the inferior surface of the talus. The middle and anterior facets are located in the anterior compartment, and the posterior facet is in the posterior compartment (Fig. 7–94). The two compartments are separated by the interosseous talocalcaneal ligament. All three parts of the subtalar joint should be studied to rule out the presence of talocalcaneal coalition. The middle and posterior facet joints usually lie in approximately parallel planes and within the same plane as the sustentaculum (Fig. 7–95). The angle of the sustentaculum (an angle of 30 to 45 degrees to the longitudinal axis of the calcaneus) is determined in the standing lateral radiogram, and the axial view of the calcaneus is made at that angle (usually 30, 35, 40, or 45 degrees) (Fig. 7–96). The anterior facet joint is a variable structure; it may be separate and distinct, or it may extend from the middle facet; on occasion it may be absent. When the calcaneus is viewed from above and posteriorly (as in the axial radiographic projection) the posterior and middle facets lie in a horizontal plane, but the anterior facet is inclined downward and

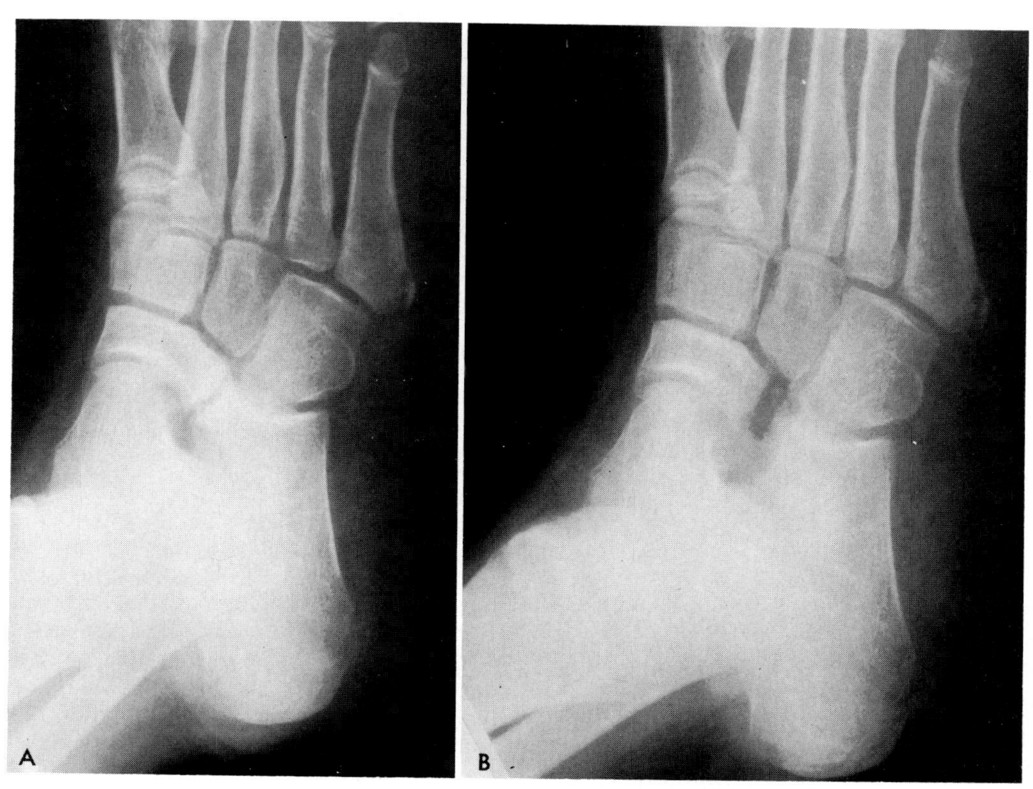

FIGURE 7–91. Calcaneonavicular coalition.

A. Oblique projection of the foot shows a cartilaginous bar; note the flattened ends of the two bones on either side of the cartilaginous bridge. **B.** Postoperative radiogram after the bar was excised. Following surgery peroneal spasm disappeared and full range of motion of the subtalar joint was achieved.

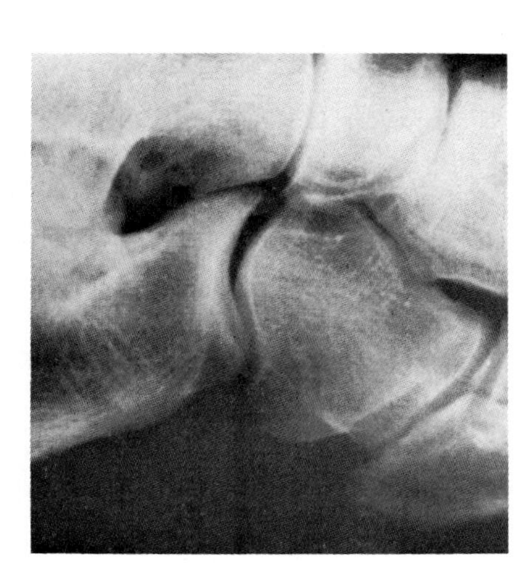

FIGURE 7–92. Oblique radiogram of the foot shows os calcaneus secundarius in the calcaneonavicular interspace.

(From Leonard, M. A.: The inheritance of tarsal coalition and its relation to spastic flatfoot. J. Bone Joint Surg., *56-B*:522, 1974. Reprinted by permission.)

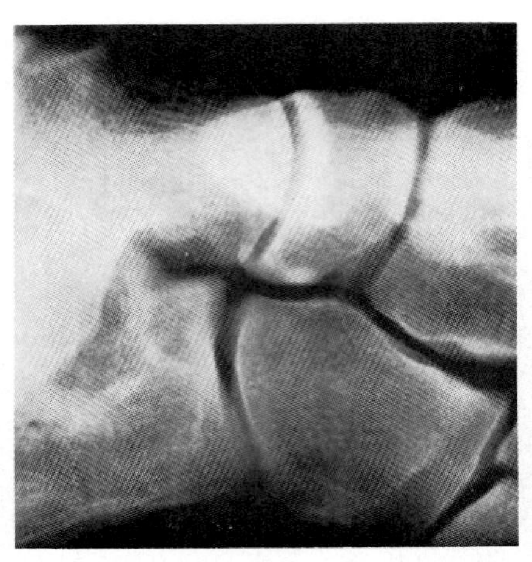
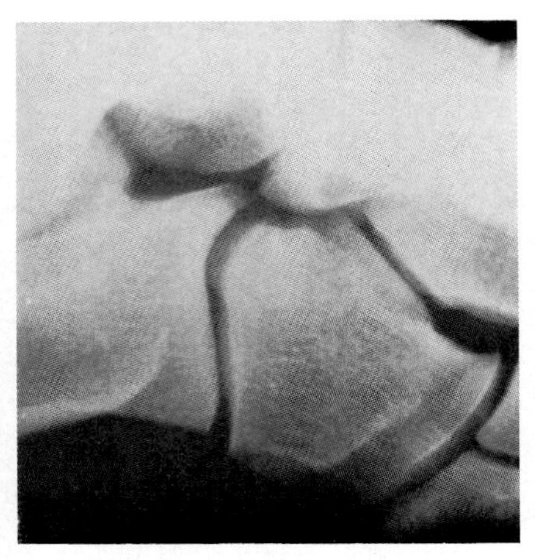

FIGURE 7–93. Slender prolongation of the anterior process of the calcaneus.

A. An oblique radiogram of a normal foot. **B.** An oblique radiogram of the foot showing a slender prolongation of the anterior process of the calcaneus; there may be a cartilaginous bar. (From Leonard, M. A.: The inheritance of tarsal coalition and its relation to spastic flatfoot. J. Bone Joint Surg., *56-B*:521, 1974. Reprinted by permission.)

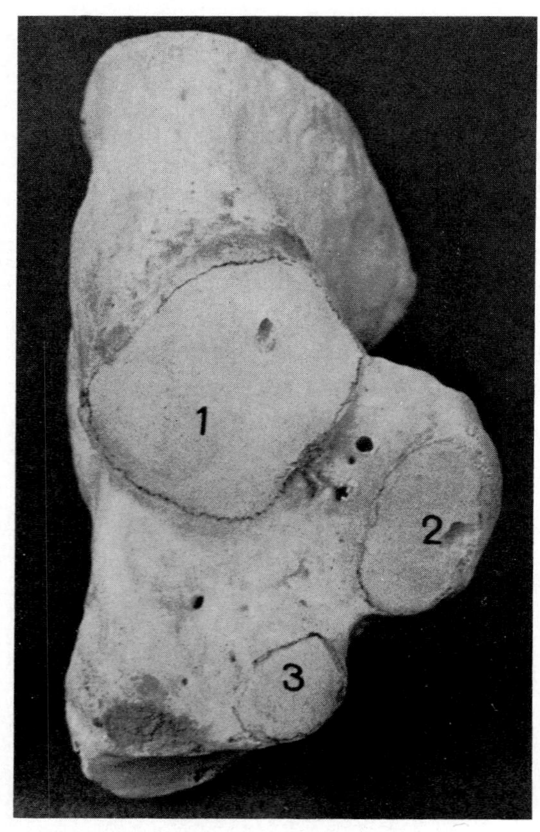

FIGURE 7–94. The dorsal surface of the calcaneus.

Note the three facets of the talocalcaneal joint. The posterior facet (1) is in the posterior compartment. The middle facet (2) and the anterior facet (3) are in the anterior compartment. (Courtesy of Dr. H. Cowell.)

medially. In the standard lateral radiogram of the foot, the middle and posterior facets are clearly visible; the anterior facet, however, is obscured because of its downward and medial inclination. When the foot is rotated so that the projection is not truly lateral, or the x-ray tube is not centered correctly, the middle joint may not be visualized because it is superimposed on the body of the calcaneus. In pes planovalgus, penetrated axial views should be utilized.

A bony coalition across the middle subtalar joint will show continuity of osseous trabeculae between the sustentaculum tali and the talus, obliterating the cartilage space in the axial view (Fig. 7–97). When the coalition is fibrous or cartilaginous a radiolucent line separates the sustentaculum tali from the talus; the margins of this radiolucent line are irregular and lack cortication. In addition, the plane of the radiolucent line in medial talocalcaneal coalition is inclined medially and downward, in contrast to the more horizontal position of the normal middle facet joint (Fig. 7–98).

Isherwood recommends the following projections for the radiographic study of the talocalcaneonavicular joint. The *oblique lateral dorsoplantar view* will often demonstrate the anterior facet joint (Fig. 7–99). The medial border of the foot is placed on the film, with the sole tilted at 45 degrees to the cassette. The tube is centered 2.5 cm. distal and 2.5 cm. anterior to the lateral malleolus.[86]

The *medial oblique axial view* will show the middle joint, and a tangential projection of the

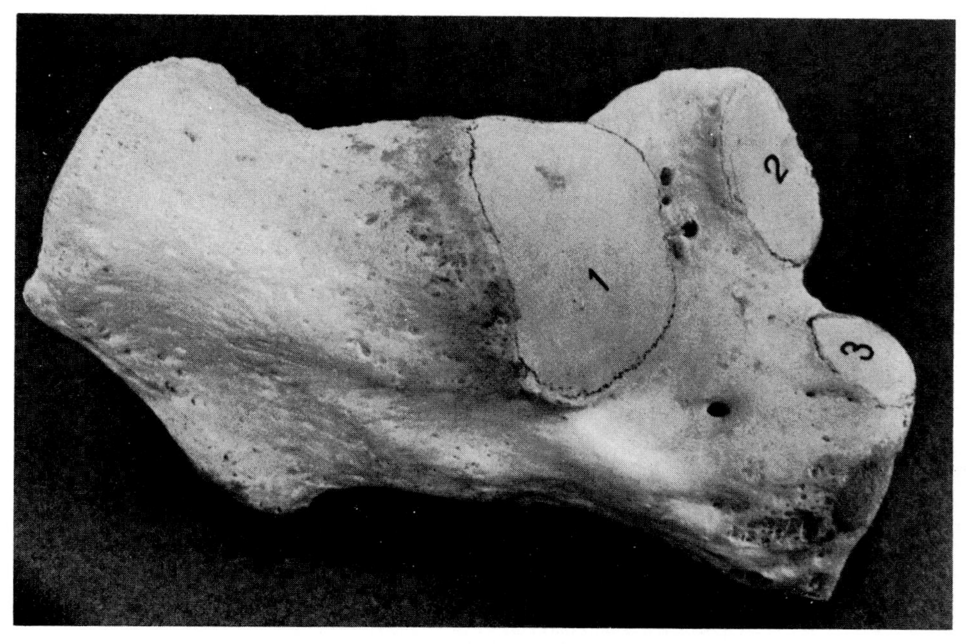

FIGURE 7–95. Facets of the subtalar joint.

In this anatomic specimen the posterior and middle facets (1 and 2) are in the same plane and can be easily visualized in the proper axial projection, whereas the anterior facet (3) is in a different plane and usually is obscured by the head of the talus in the axial view. (Courtesy of Dr. H. Cowell.)

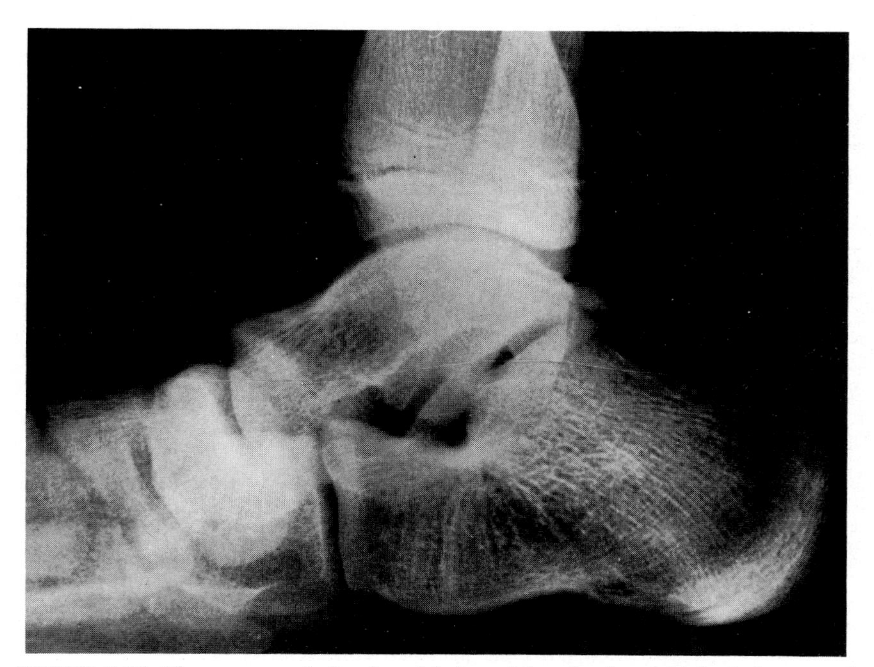

FIGURE 7–96. The proper angle for the axial view of the talocalcaneal joint is determined in the standing lateral radiogram.

Note in this extreme example the variation in the plane of the posterior and middle facets; an angle of 40 degrees is necessary to visualize the posterior facet, and an angle of 55 degrees is required for the middle facet. (Ordinarily the middle and posterior facet joints lie within the same plane as the sustentaculum.) (Courtesy of Dr. H. Cowell.)

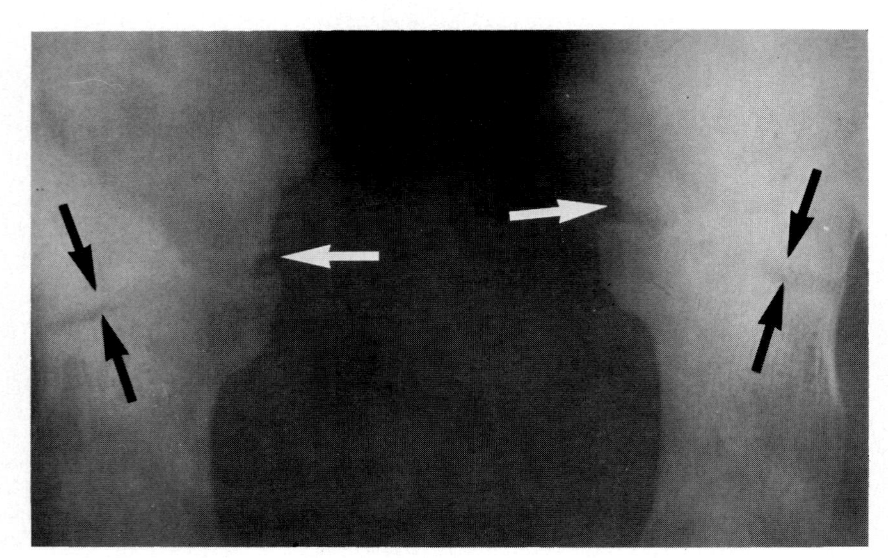

FIGURE 7–97. ***Penetrated axial view showing a complete bony coalition of the middle facet joint (right) with continuous bony trabeculae between the talus and the sustentaculum.***

On the left, there is cartilaginous coalition; note that the radiolucent line lacks normal cortication and is narrowed and inclined downward and medially.

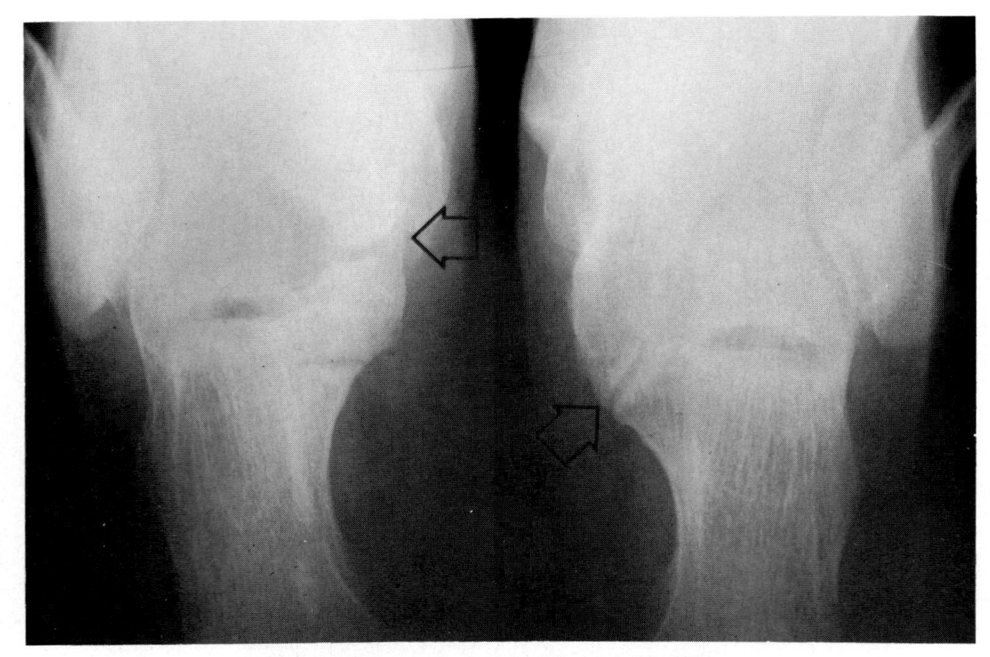

FIGURE 7–98. ***Penetrated axial view of both feet.***

On the left the middle facet joint is normal; note the radiolucent articular cartilage space lies horizontally. On the right there is fibrocartilaginous coalition of the middle facet joint—its radiolucent line is tilted medially and downward with irregular margins that lack cortication.

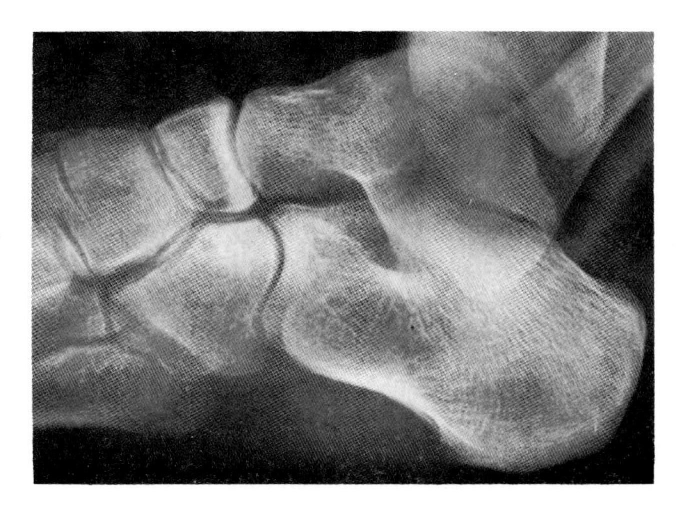

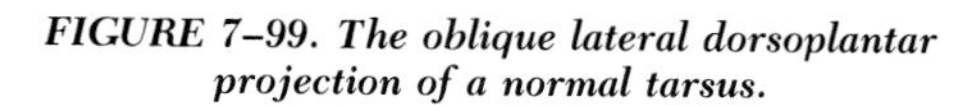

FIGURE 7–99. The oblique lateral dorsoplantar projection of a normal tarsus.

Note the clear visualization of the anterior part of the talocalcaneonavicular joint. (From Isherwood, I.: A radiological approach to the subtalar joint. J. Bone Joint Surg., *43-B*:566–574, 1961. Reprinted by permission.)

convexity of the posterior joint will be depicted (Figs. 7–100 and 7–101). The film is made with the foot dorsiflexed and, when possible, inverted. The position is maintained by strapping with a wide bandage. The limb is rotated 60 degrees medially, and the foot is placed on a 30-degree wedge. The tube is directed axially, tilted 10 degrees cephalad, and centered 2.5 cm. below and 2.5 cm. anterior to the lateral malleolus. The asymmetrical pull of the strapping will maintain inverted posture. The sustentaculum tali is close to the film for bone detail, and an "end-on" view of the tarsal canal is given.[86]

The *lateral oblique axial view* will demonstrate the posterior joint in profile (Fig. 7–102). The foot is dorsiflexed and, when possible, everted, the position being maintained by the asymmetrical pull of the strapping. The limb is rotated laterally 60 degrees, the knee flexed when necessary, and the foot placed on a 30-degree wedge. The tube is directed axially, tilted 10 degrees cephalad, and centered 2.5 cm. below the medial malleolus. Tube direction and tilt may be fixed for both oblique axial views.[86]

When the middle facet joints are more nearly horizontal than usual in the axial view, the articular cartilage space may be obscured and misinterpreted as coalition. Even multiple axial views may fail to demonstrate the middle facet joint, but normal joint spaces will be seen in the oblique, axial and lateral projections (Fig. 7–103).[11] Occult coalitions of the anterior and middle joints are best demonstrated by tomography (Figs. 7–104 and 7–105). Conway and Cowell have described the tomographic technique for demonstrating the talocalcaneal

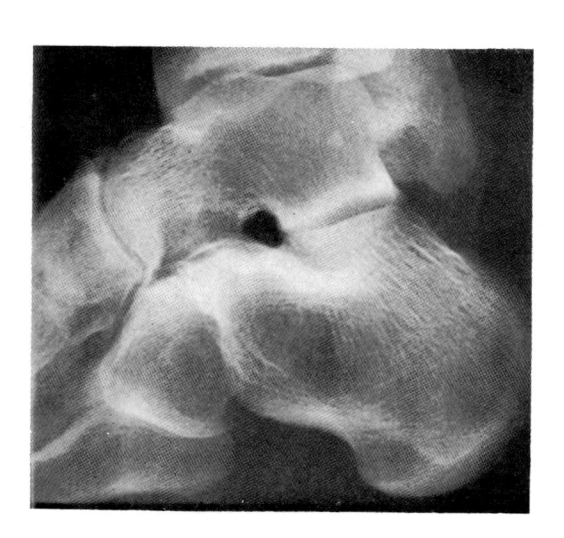

FIGURE 7–100. Medial oblique axial projection of a normal foot.

The middle facet joint is well seen. Also depicted is a tangential view of the convexity of the posterior facet joint. (From Isherwood, I.: A radiological approach to the subtalar joint. J. Bone Joint Surg., *43-B*:566–574, 1961. Reprinted by permission.)

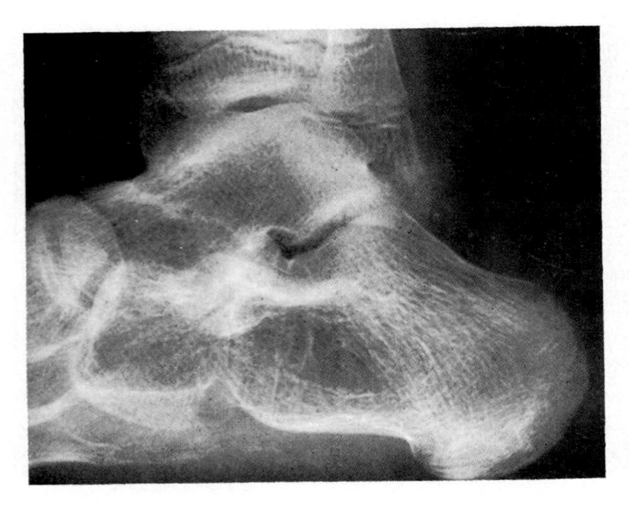

FIGURE 7–101. Medial oblique axial projection of a foot with talocalcaneal coalition.

Note the bony union in the posterior aspect of the middle facet joint. (From Isherwood, I.: A radiological approach to the subtalar joint. J. Bone Joint Surg., *43-B*:566–574, 1961. Reprinted by permission.)

joint.[32] Computed tomography will clearly visualize the coalition of the talocalcaneal joint (Fig. 7–105).

One should be cautious in interpreting lateral plain tomograms, as obliquity of the anterior joint may give a false appearance of coalition. The anterior facet joint is clearly demonstrated in plain films made in the lateral oblique position; therefore in dubious cases when tomography is indicated, the lateral oblique or the coronal plane should be used.[11]

Restriction of movement between the talus above and the calcaneus, cuboid, and navicular below results in certain secondary changes visible in the plain radiogram. These vary in intensity, depending upon the type of coalition, whether the intertarsal bridge is complete or incomplete, and the age of the patient. They are best seen in standing lateral radiograms of the foot (i.e., the patient standing, the film vertical on the medial side of the foot, and the x-ray beam projected from the lateral side with the rays parallel to the ground).

The most striking secondary change is beaking on the dorsal and lateral aspect of the head of the talus adjacent to the talonavicular joint (Fig. 7–106). There is obvious absence of other signs of degenerative arthritis. There are no hypertrophic changes on the navicular, the articular cartilage space is not narrowed, and there is no associated subchondral sclerosis nor any cystic bony changes. The cause of talar beak is the repeated minute elevation of the talus in response to abnormal mechanics of the subtalar joint; it is not a true degenerative arthritic process, though that may develop later in untreated cases of long standing.

Outland and Murphy proposed that talar beak is produced by impingement of the dorsal part of the navicular on the head of the talus during

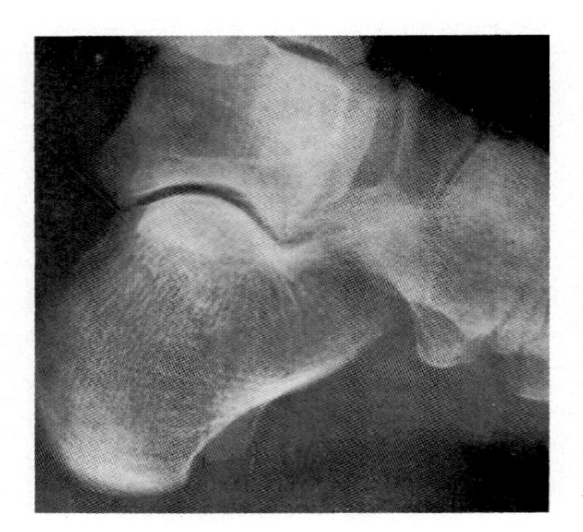

FIGURE 7–102. Lateral oblique axial projection of a normal foot.

The posterior facet joint is clearly depicted. (From Isherwood, I.: A radiological approach to the subtalar joint. J. Bone Joint Surg., *43-B*:566–574, 1961. Reprinted by permission.)

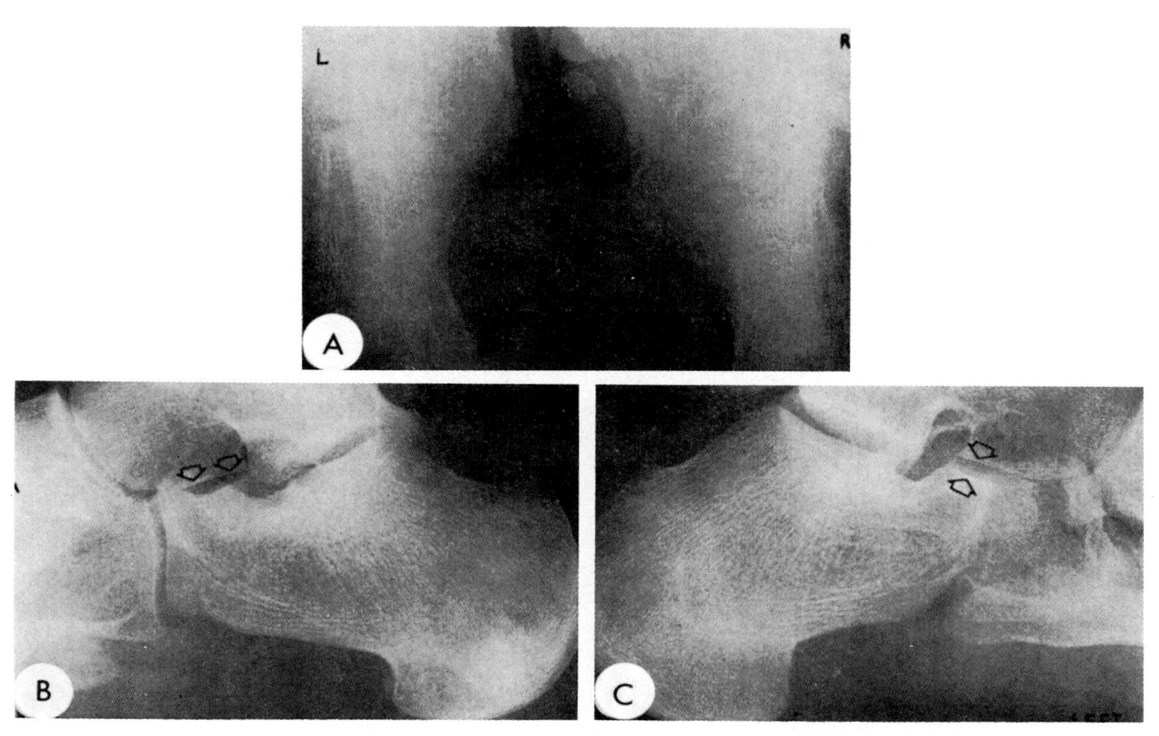

FIGURE 7–103. Apparent bony coalition between the talus and the sustentaculum.

A. Penetrated axial projection. Note the absence of the middle joint space. Multiple axial views using different tube angulations failed to show any middle joint cartilage space. **B.** Lateral view of the same foot shows the middle facet joint space. Note the axis of the middle facet joint is more nearly horizontal than usual; it is not in the same oblique plane as the posterior facet joint. **C.** Medial oblique axial view of the same foot clearly demonstrates the middle facet joint space. (From Beckly, D. E., Anderson, P. W., and Pedegana, L. R.: The radiology of the subtalar joint with special reference to talo-calcaneal coalition. Clin. Radiol., *26*:340, 1975. Reprinted by permission.)

dorsiflexion. The navicular is rigidly held to the calcaneus by the plantar and lateral calcaneonavicular ligaments. When motion of the subtalar joint is limited, the dorsal aspect of the navicular will impinge on the head of the talus.[139, 140]

Other secondary changes in talocalcaneal coalition are narrowing of the posterior talocalcaneal facet joint space and broadening of the lateral process of the talus, which has a rounded appearance. This may be associated with flattening and even concavity on the undersurface of the neck of the talus on the side with coalition (Fig. 7–106).[29] A ball-and-socket ankle joint may be present.[109]

Talonavicular coalition is readily diagnosed by the evident absence of the talonavicular joint space as seen on the lateral radiogram.

Arthrography of the talocalcaneonavicular joint with tangential views of the subtalar articulation (Harris views) provides another way to detect talocalcaneal coalition. It is indicated when the routine radiograms are normal in painful rigid flatfoot. This author, however, recommends computed tomography of the hindfoot because it is noninvasive and accurate.

The technique of arthrography of the talocalcaneonavicular joint is as follows: the foot and leg are prepared, and sterile drapes are applied. Following local skin anesthesia, 3 to 4 ml. of positive contrast material is instilled through a 22-gauge needle into the talonavicular joint from its dorsal aspect. The site of injection is located 1 cm. lateral to the pulsation of the dorsalis pedis artery. Brief visualization of the lateral projection with image intensification will facilitate correct placement of the needle. Upon entrance into the joint cavity, the contrast material is introduced; it should flow easily, outlining the talocalcaneonavicular joint space. The films taken are the anteroposterior, lateral, and oblique projections of the foot, and tangential Harris views at 35-, 45-, and 55-degree angles from the horizontal.[146]

In the normal foot the talocalcaneonavicular joint space is filled with the contrast material.

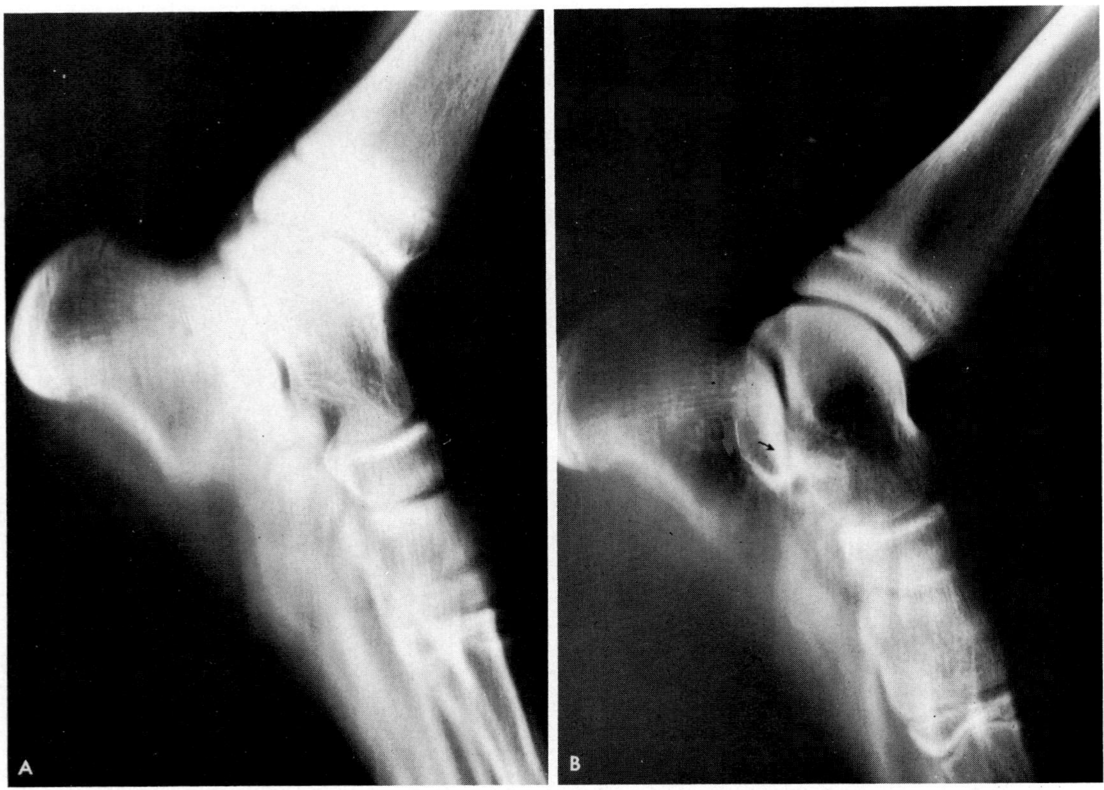

FIGURE 7–104. Coalitions of the middle facet of the talocalcaneal joint.

A and **B.** Simple tomograms. **A.** Normal foot. **B.** Foot with a middle facet coalition.

Therefore, in the lateral view the contrast material can be seen extending above the sustentaculum tali (Fig. 7–107). In the Harris tangential views the thin medial joint space filled by the contrast material can be clearly visualized. These findings exclude a fibrous, cartilaginous, or bony coalition. In the presence of talocalcaneal coalition the arthrogram will fail to show contrast material in the talocalcaneonavicular joint area.

The posterior compartment does not communicate with the anterior compartment, and the posterior joint is clearly visible in standard radiograms. Its arthrography is rarely warranted. The injection may, however, be made through a medial approach. The site of insertion of the needle is 1 cm. inferior to the medial malleolus and 1 cm. posterior to the pulsation of the posterior to the pulsation of the posterior tibial vessels. Under image-intensifier control, the needle is advanced distally (toward the toes) and dorsally into the space between the posterior facets of the talus and calcaneus. Care is taken to stay away from the interosseous talocalcaneal ligament and the anterior compartment. Contrast material (1.5 to 2.5 ml.) is instilled, and radiograms in the anteroposterior, lateral, and oblique projections are made (Fig. 7–108).[146]

Treatment

The treatment varies according to the type of coalition, the age of the patient, the severity of deformity, and the degree of disability caused by pain and muscle spasm.

Many patients with tarsal coalition have little discomfort and will not require treatment. During the growing years ⅛- to 3⁄16 inch inner heel wedges on the shoes, Thomas heel, extended medial heel counter, and longitudinal arch support may be used. If the valgus deformity is of significant degree, however, a well-fitted UCBL (University of California Biomechanical Laboratory) foot orthosis will prove more effective in diminishing stress on the rigid hindfoot.

If peroneal muscle spasm and pain do develop, more aggressive measures are indicated; initially these should be conservative. Acute symptoms following trauma or unusual stress may be relieved by immobilizing the foot and

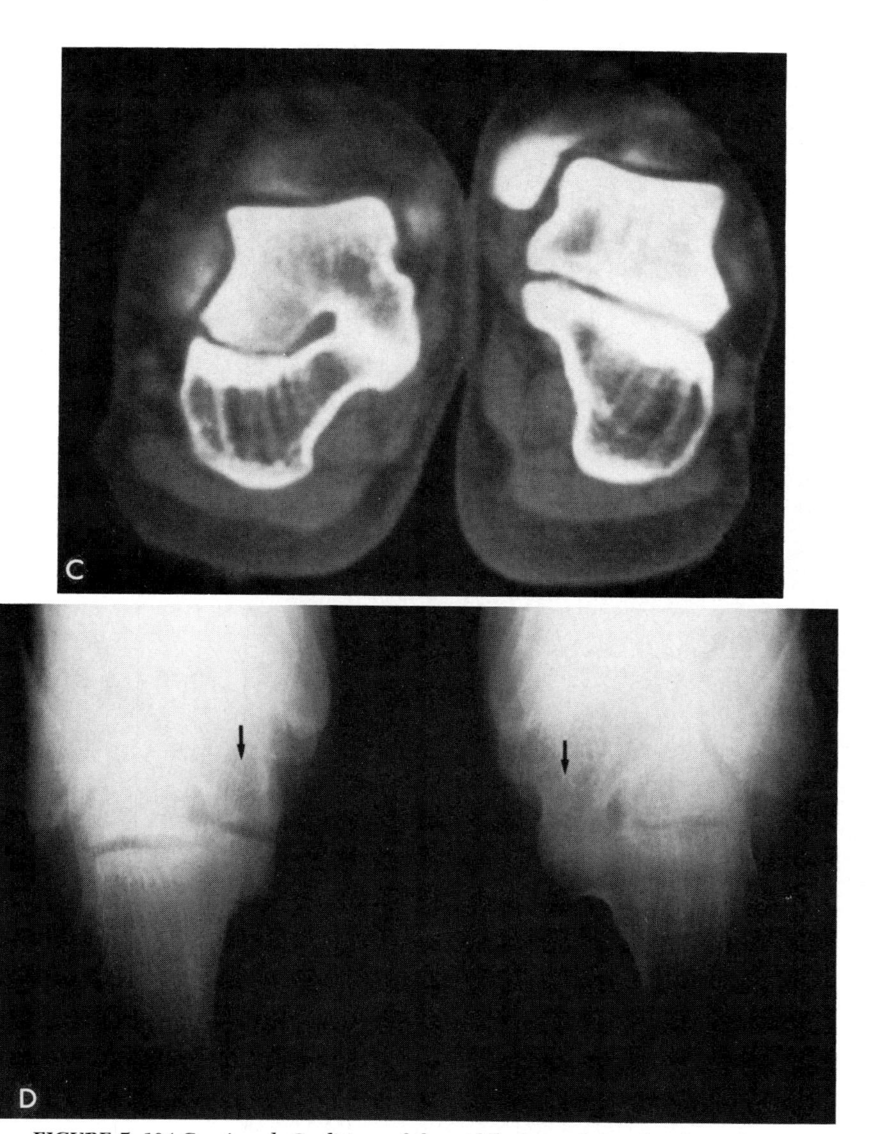

FIGURE 7–104 Continued. Coalitions of the middle facet of the talocalcaneal joint.

C. CT scan of both feet showing medial talocalcaneal coalition of right foot. **D.** Harris axial views of both feet of same patient showing medial talocalcaneal coalition of the right foot. (Courtesy of Dr. H. Cowell.)

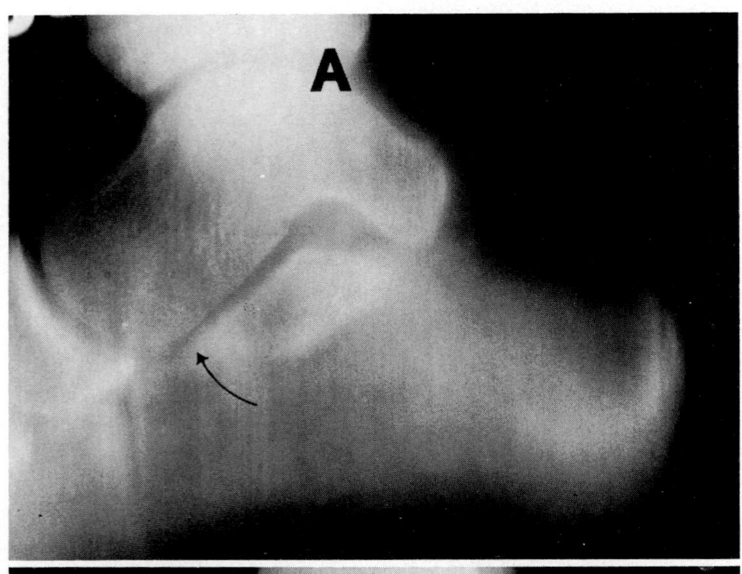

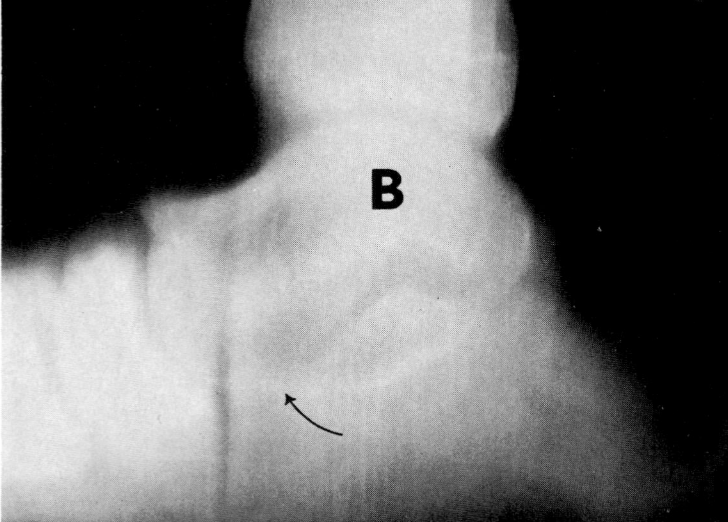

FIGURE 7–105. Tomograms of anterior facet of talocalcaneal joint.

A. Normal foot. **B.** Foot with talocalcaneal coalition. Note the talar beak and the irregularity and haziness of anterior facet, indicating coalition. (Courtesy of Dr. H. Cowell.)

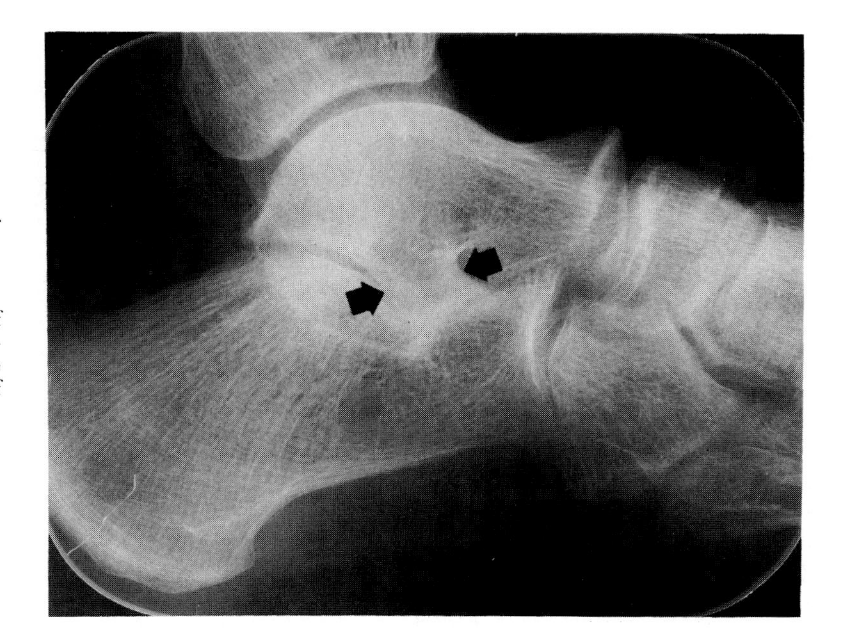

FIGURE 7–106. Secondary signs of calcaneonavicular coalition as seen in the lateral radiogram of the foot.

Note the beaking of the head of the talus, the broadening of the lateral process of the talus, and the narrowing of the cartilage space of the posterior subtalar joint.

ankle in a below-knee walking cast for a period of three to four weeks.

It is doubtful whether manipulation of the foot under anesthesia is of any value. The hindfoot should not be forced into inversion while the cast is being applied, as it will be uncomfortable and the result will be more spasm. Following removal of the cast the foot is supported in a foot-ankle orthosis made of polypropylene or another plastic for an additional three months. Injection of corticosteroids into the subtalar joint is not recommended.

Braddock studied the natural history of peroneal spastic flatfoot in 28 patients (24 males and 4 females; 15 with bilateral involvement, making a total of 43 feet). The first symptoms

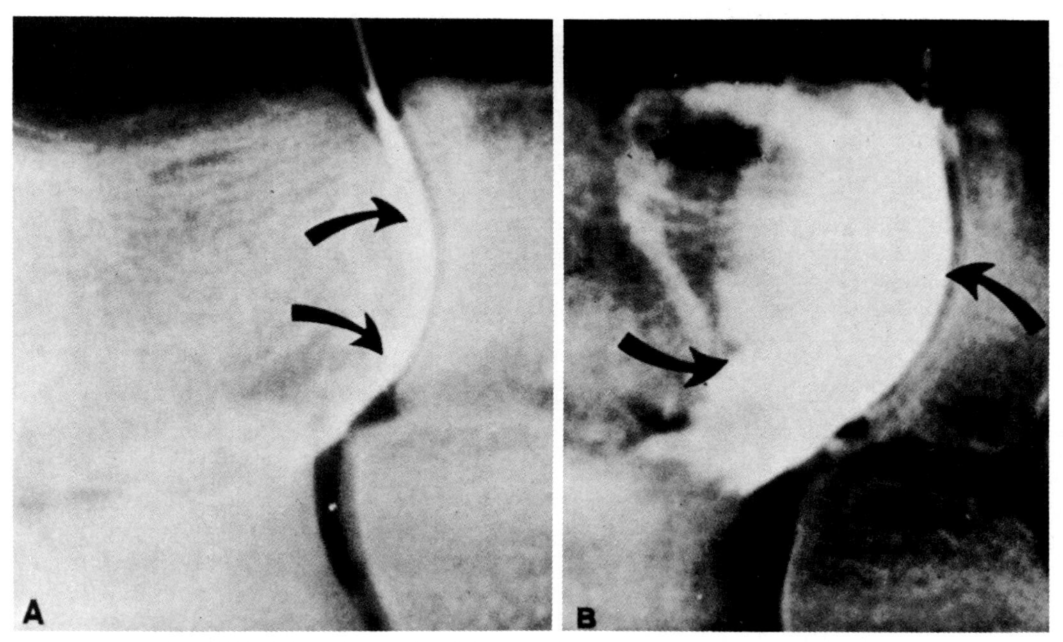

FIGURE 7–107. Arthrography of the talocalcaneonavicular joint of a normal foot.

The contrast material is introduced through the dorsal capsule of the talonavicular joint. Oblique projections show, **A**, partial filling and, **B**, complete filling of the synovial cavity *(curved arrows)*. (From Resnick, D.: Radiology of the talocalcaneal articulation. Radiology, *111*:586, 1974. Reprinted by permission.)

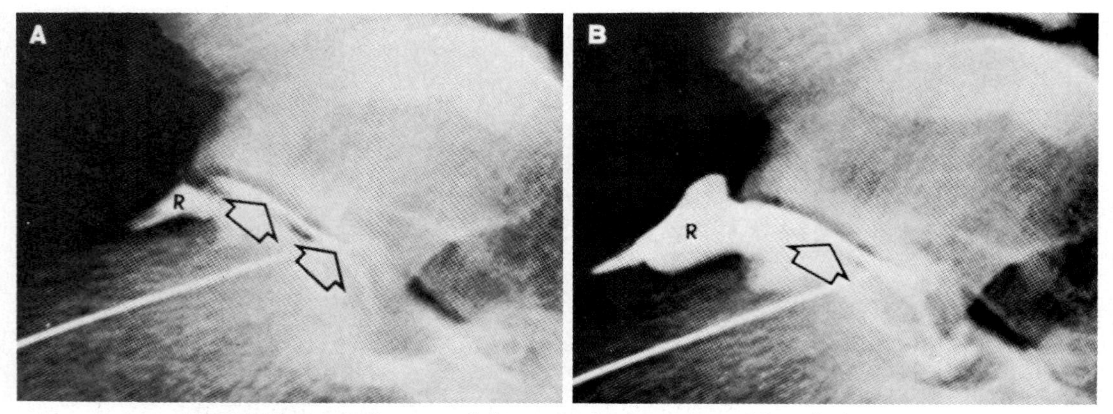

FIGURE 7–108. Arthrogram of the posterior compartment of the subtalar joint.

A and **B**. Lateral radiograms showing partial and complete filling. (From Resnick, D.: Radiology of the talocalcaneal articulation. Radiology, *111*:586, 1974. Reprinted by permission.)

appeared during adolescence. In 22 of the feet, tarsal coalition was disclosed in the radiograms. These patients were treated with manipulation under anesthesia, a below-knee walking plaster cast, or an orthosis with valgus T-strap. The average period of follow-up was 21 years, the longest being 34 years and the shortest 13 years. About half these patients continued to have minor symptoms for many years, but only 10 per cent were disabled with persistent pain and required operative treatment.[18] An interesting finding in this report was that severe symptoms were more persistent in those patients without apparent tarsal anomalies than in those with obvious bars. Probably more thorough radiographic examination including computed tomography (particularly of the anterior and middle facets of the talocalcaneal joint) would have disclosed partial or occult coalitions.

When pain and muscle spasm recur and become chronic or when the deformity is severe, surgical treatment is indicated. The operative procedure employed depends upon the type of coalition and the presence or absence of secondary changes in the talonavicular joint.

MEDIAL TALOCALCANEAL COALITION

For medial talocalcaneal coalition, a medial curvilinear incision is made, beginning at the base of the first cuneiform bone and terminating 2 cm. inferior and posterior to the tip of the medial malleolus. This medial approach, recommended by Harris, provides adequate exposure of the talonavicular joint and the medial aspect of the subtalar joint (Fig. 7–109). It also permits the surgeon to assess the pathologic anatomy of the talocalcaneal coalition, the degree and rigidity of pes valgus, and the changes in the talonavicular joint.[70]

If there is complete union of the medial talocalcaneal articulation, and the fixed valgus deformity of the hindfoot is functionally acceptable (i.e., not exceeding 15 degrees), only the talonavicular joint is fused. It is not necessary to osteotomize and mobilize the synostosis of the subtalar joints, nor is stabilization of the calcaneoocuboid joint required. Occasionally the large bony mass of the medial talocalcaneal coalition is partially resected, which diminishes its prominence and prevents irritation from the shoe.

If the talocalcaneal coalition is incomplete, the subtalar joint should be stabilized. Harris recommends fusion of only the talocalcaneal and talonavicular joints; the author, however, prefers to include the calcaneocuboid joint in the fusion (i.e., triple arthrodesis). If the pes valgus exceeds 15 degrees, the intertarsal bony bridge is osteotomized and appropriate wedges are resected, while triple arthrodesis is performed to give the foot a normal configuration. The peroneal muscles usually do not require lengthening, except in an occasional severe long-standing case with marked myostatic contracture. In such an instance, sliding lengthening of the peroneals is performed; i.e., through a separate incision on the lateral aspect of the middle third of the leg, the tendinous fibers are divided at two levels 3 to 4 cm. apart, and the sectioned fibers are slid over the underlying muscles by applying traction distally on the peroneal tendons. Excision of incomplete or rudimentary medial talocalcaneal coalition may be tried. In the experience of this author it was successful in restoring painless subtalar motion in two cases.

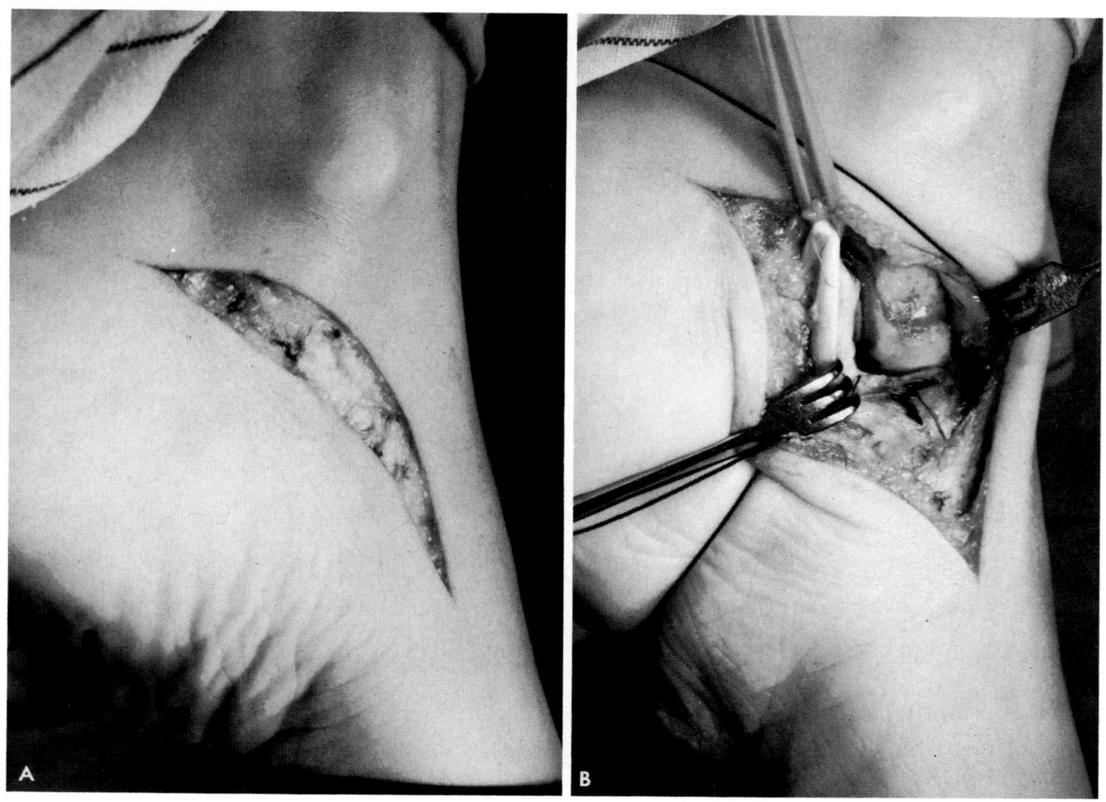

FIGURE 7–109. Medial approach to subtalar joint.

A. Skin incision begins at the base of the first cuneiform bone and ends 2 cm. inferior and posterior to the tip of the medial malleolus (the bony prominence in the photograph). **B.** Posterior tibial tendon is elevated and retracted inferiorly and posteriorly, exposing the subtalar joint.

The surgical treatment of the rare anterior and posterior talocalcaneal coalitions follows the same principles as those outlined for the medial one.

CALCANEONAVICULAR COALITION

Surgical treatment is indicated when there is persistent pain, muscle spasm, and deformity. Resection of the calcaneonavicular bar was suggested by Badgley and Bentzon more than 50 years ago; their results were disappointing, however, because the operations were carried out in older individuals who had developed degenerative changes in the tarsus.[8, 13]

Mitchell and Gibson recommended excision of the calcaneonavicular bar in children under 14 years of age who showed no radiographic evidence of adaptive changes. In their experience, the procedure had an excellent chance of abolishing symptoms and restoring mobility to the foot without any restriction of future activity.[129] In Mitchell's personal series of 13 consecutive selected cases, excision of the bar restored mobility and abolished symptoms in all the cases.[128] In their original communication, Mitchell and Gibson reported their results in unselected series of 41 feet; there were eight failures following excision of the bar—these occurred in feet with long-standing deformity or with adaptive changes in the tarsal joints. They recommended triple arthrodesis in these late cases.[129]

Cowell resected the calcaneonavicular bar, but in addition interposed the extensor digitorum brevis to obliterate the dead space and prevent re-formation of bone. According to Cowell, resection of the bar and extensor brevis arthroplasty are indicated in a patient under 14 years of age who has pain in the foot, limited subtalar motion, and a cartilaginous bar. These procedures should not be performed in the presence of degenerative changes in the talonavicular joint with accompanying talar beak or when there is an additional coalition between the talus and the calcaneus. Cowell reported the results of the procedure on 26 bars in 15 patients. Twenty-three of the twenty-six feet demonstrated no symptoms following surgery,

Text continued on page 2608

Resection of Calcaneonavicular Coalition with Interposition of Extensor Digitorum Brevis Muscle or Adipose Tissue

OPERATIVE TECHNIQUE

A. A lateral Ollier approach is made. The incision starts immediately below the lateral malleolus and curves upward to end on the lateral aspect of the talonavicular joint.

B. The peroneal tendons are retracted posteriorly and the long toe extensors are retracted dorsally. The origin of the extensor digitorum brevis muscle is detached and elevated in one piece, and reflected distally.

Plate 100. Resection of Calcaneonavicular Coalition with Interposition of Extensor Digitorum Brevis Muscle or Adipose Tissue

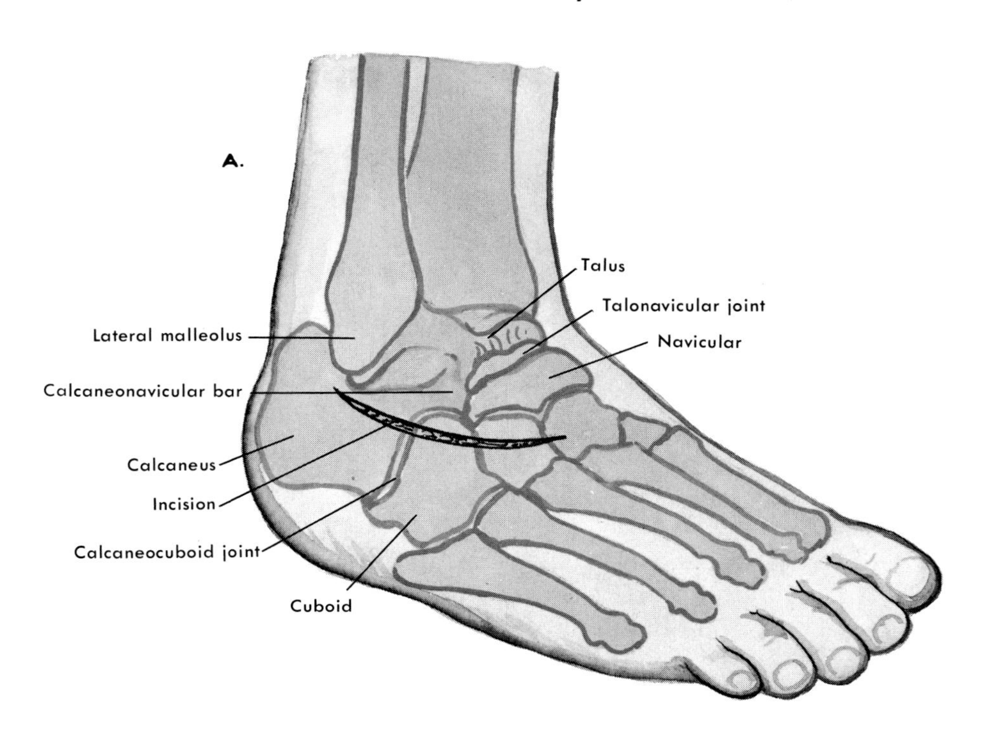

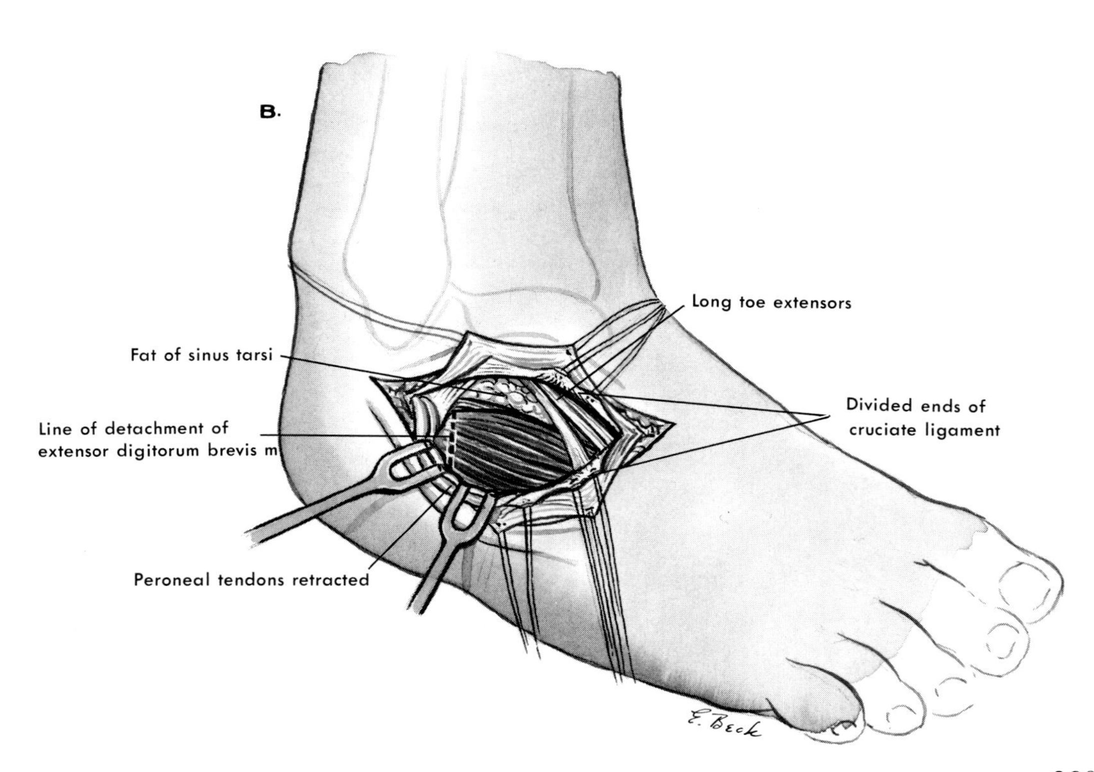

Resection of Calcaneonavicular Coalition with Interposition of Extensor Digitorum Brevis Muscle or Adipose Tissue (Continued)

C. The calcaneus, cuboid, and navicular bones are identified. The capsule of the calcaneocuboid joint is incised to facilitate exposure of the calcaneonavicular bar. Do not divide the talonavicular capsule, or dorsal subluxation of the navicular on the head of the talus may result. Next, the entire bar is resected as a rectangle, not a wedge, with two straight osteotomes. The osteotome for the calcaneal portion of the bar is directed almost horizontally, whereas the one for the navicular portion is angled plantarward. An oscillating electric saw may be used if preferred.

D. It is imperative to remove the bar adequately, with generous portions of the calcaneal and navicular components. The plantar aspects of the navicular and the talar head should be level. The raw cancellous bleeding bases of the excised bar are coagulated. Caution! Do not disturb the circulation between the talus and the navicular.

Plate 100. Resection of Calcaneonavicular Coalition with Interposition of Extensor Digitorum Brevis Muscle or Adipose Tissue

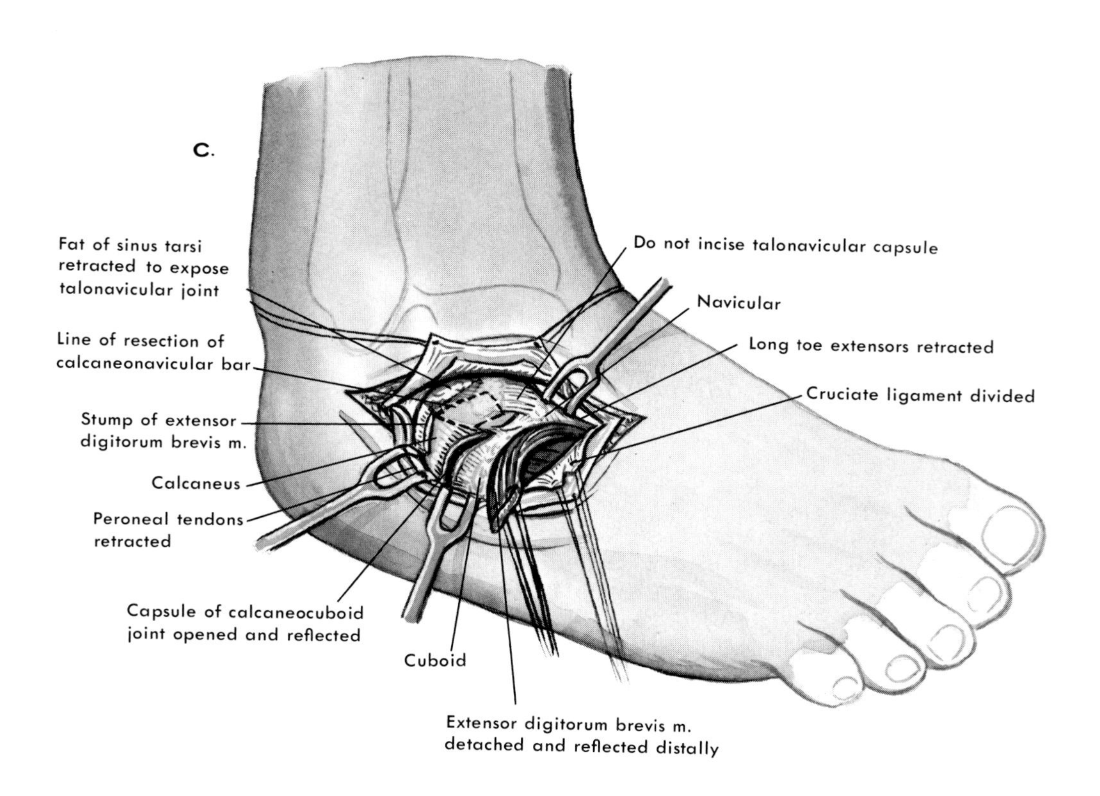

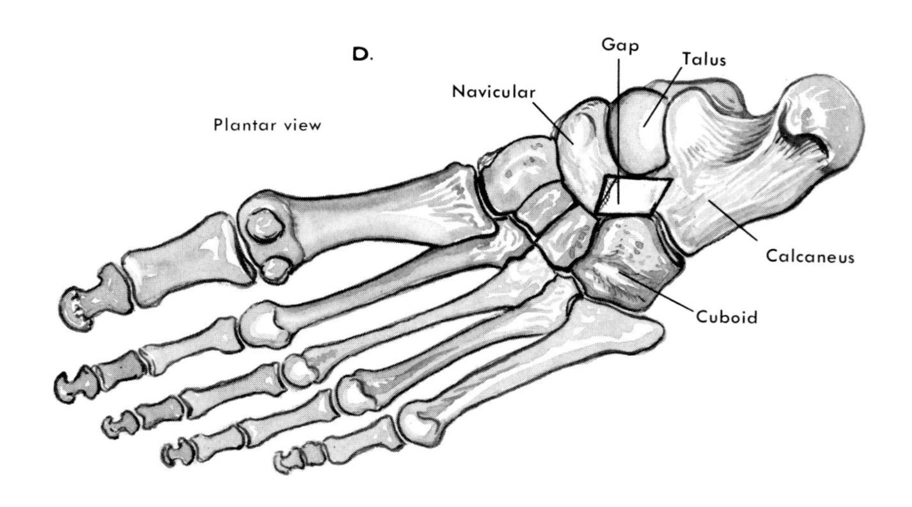

Resection of Calcaneonavicular Coalition with Interposition of Extensor Digitorum Brevis Muscle or Adipose Tissue (Continued)

E. In Cowell's technique the entire origin of the extensor digitorum brevis muscle is placed in the defect and secured with a chromic suture. Two Keith needles are used, one on each end of the suture; they are pulled out on the medial side of the foot, where the suture is tied over a well-padded button or over a rectangular piece of sterile felt.

F. The author prefers to place adipose tissue from the gluteal area in the gap created by excision of the bar to obliterate dead space and prevent new bone formation. The extensor digitorum brevis is sutured back to its origin. The wound is closed, and the foot and ankle are immobilized in a below-knee cast.

POSTOPERATIVE CARE

In about ten days the cast is bivalved, and passive and active exercises are performed to develop inversion and eversion of the hindfoot. The foot and ankle are supported in neutral position in a posterior splint made of polypropylene or other plastic material. Full weight-bearing is not permitted; the splint support is continued until the patient obtains full active subtalar motion. This will usually require eight to ten weeks.

Plate 100. Resection of Calcaneonavicular Coalition with Interposition of Extensor Digitorum Brevis Muscle or Adipose Tissue

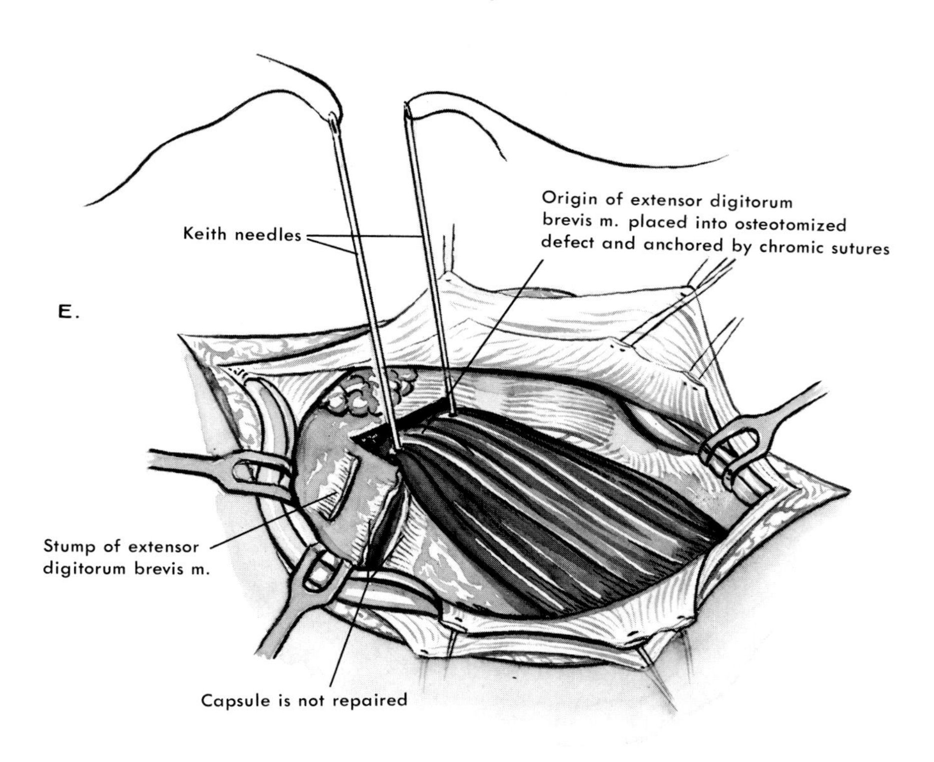

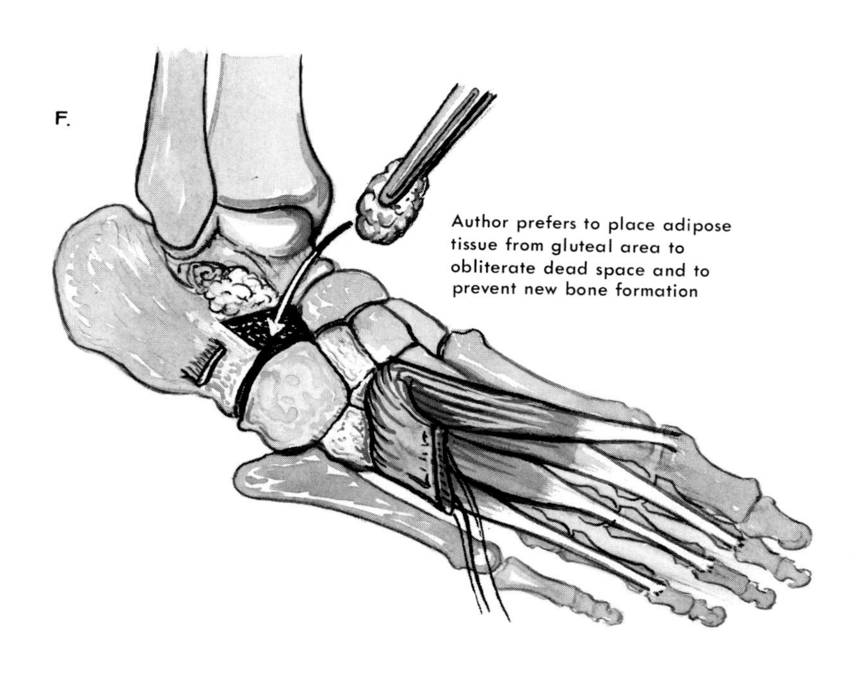

and the patients were able to resume full activity, including participation in sports. According to Cowell, when proper indications are observed, satisfactory results may be expected in 90 per cent of the patients.[34]

This author concurs with Cowell, but he also excises the calcaneonavicular bar when it is ossified in a patient over 14 years of age, provided there are no talonavicular degenerative changes. Instead of interposing the extensor digitorum brevis, he uses adipose tissue from the gluteal region and places it between the resected ends of the calcaneus and navicular as a spacer and to prevent reossification.

The technique of resection of the calcaneonavicular bar with the extensor digitorum brevis arthroplasty or gluteal fat interposition is illustrated in Plate 100.

A triple arthrodesis is performed when there are degenerative changes in the talonavicular joint or when excision of the bar fails to relieve the symptoms.

Talonavicular coalition usually does not require treatment, as the condition is asymptomatic. In adult life, naviculocuneiform fusion may be indicated if hypertrophic changes and pain develop. Subtalar and calcaneocuboid fusion is performed in the occasional case associated with painful and persistent peroneal spastic flatfoot.

Treatment of the other rare tarsal coalitions should be individualized.

References

1. Achterman, C., and Kalamchi, A.: Congenital deficiency of the fibula. J. Bone Joint Surg., *61–B:*133, 1979.
2. Adler, J. B.: Radiologic notes: Case No. 358: Tarsal coalition—calcaneo-naviculo-cuboid. Mt. Sinai J. Med. (N.Y.), *39:*321, 1972.
3. Amr, F., and El-Hadidi, H.: Spasmodic valgus foot: A contribution to its aetiology and treatment. Egypt. Orthop. J., *7:*175, 1972.
4. Anderson, R. J.: The presence of an astragalo-scaphoid bone in man. J. Anat. Physiol., *14:*452, 1880.
5. Anthonsen, W.: An oblique projection for roentgen examination of the talocalcaneal joint, particularly regarding intra-articular fracture of the calcaneus. Acta Radiol., *24:*306, 1943.
6. Asher, M., and Mosier, K.: Coalition of the talocalcaneal middle facet: Treatment by surgical excision and fat graft interposition. Orthop. Trans., *7:*149, 1983.
7. Austin, F. H.: Symphalangism and related fusions of tarsal bones. Radiology, *56:*882, 1951.
8. Badgley, C. E.: Coalition of the calcaneus and the navicular. Arch. Surg. (Chicago), *15:*75, 1927.
9. Bargellini, D.: Fusione calcenao-cuboidea e piede piatto. Arch. Ital. Chir., *21:*386, 1928.
10. Basu, S. S.: Naviculo-cuneo-metatarso-phalangeal synostoses. Indian J. Surg., *27:*750, 1963.
11. Beckly, D. E., Anderson, P. W., and Pedegana, L. R.: The radiology of the subtalar joint with special reference to talo-calcaneal coalition. Clin. Radiol., *26:*333, 1975.
12. Behr, F.: Ueber eine sym. Synostose der Hand und Fusswurzel Knochen. Arch. Orthop. Chir., *32:*12, 1932.
13. Bentzon, P. G. K.: Coalitio calcaneo-navicularis, mit besondere Bezugnahme auf die operative Behandlung des durch diese Anomalie bedingten Plattfusses. Verh. Dtsch. Orthop. Ges., *23:*269, 1929.
14. Bentzon, P. G. K.: Bilateral congenital deformity of the astragalo-calcaneal joint—bony coalescence between os trigonum and the calcaneus? Acta Orthop. Scand., *1:*359, 1930.
15. Bersani, F. A., and Samilson, R. L.: Massive familial tarsal synostosis. J. Bone Joint Surg., *39-A:*1187, 1957.
16. Blockey, N. J.: Peroneal spastic flat foot. J. Bone Joint Surg., *37-B:*191, 1955.
17. Boyd, H. B.: Congenital talonavicular synostosis. J. Bone Joint Surg., *26:*682, 1944.
18. Braddock, G. T. F.: A prolonged follow-up of peroneal spastic flat foot. J. Bone Joint Surg., *43-B:*734, 1961.
19. Brand, C.: Über die Bedeutung und spec. Diagnostik der Coalitio calcaneonavicularis. Arch. Orthop. Unfallchir., *48:*202, 1956.
20. Brobeck, O.: Congenital bilateral synostosis of the calcaneus and cuboid and the triquetral and hamate bones. Report of a case. Acta Orthop. Scand., *26:*217, 1957.
21. Buffon, G. L. L.: Histoire Naturelle, Génerale et Particuliere. Tome 3, p. 47. Paris, Panekoucke, 1769.
22. Bullitt, J. B.: Variations of the bones of the foot. Fusion of the talus and navicular, bilateral and congenital. A. J. R., *20:*548, 1928.
23. Cain, T. J., and Hyman, S.: Peroneal spastic flat foot. Its treatment by osteotomy of the os calcis. J. Bone Joint Surg., *60-B:*527, 1978.
24. Calvert, J. P.: A case of symphalangism, with associated carpal and tarsal fusions. Hand, *6:*291, 1974.
25. Cavallaro, D. C., and Hadden, H. R.: An unusual case of tarsal coalition: A cuboid navicular synostosis. J. Am. Podiatry Assoc., *68:*71, 1978.
26. Challis, J.: Hereditary transmission of talonavicular coalition in association with anomaly of the little finger. J. Bone Joint Surg., *56-A:*1273, 1974.
27. Chambers, C. H.: Congenital anomalies of the tarsal navicular with particular reference to calcaneonavicular coalition. Br. J. Radiol., *23:*580, 1974.
28. Chambers, R. B., Cook, T. M., and Cowell, H. R.: Surgical reconstruction for calcaneonavicular coalition. Evaluation of function and gait. J. Bone Joint Surg., *64-A:*829, 1982.
29. Christian, J. C., Franken, E. A., Jr., Lindemann, J. P., Lindseth, R. E., Reed, T., and Scott, C. I., Jr.: A dominant syndrome of metacarpal and metatarsal asymmetry with tarsal and carpal fusions, syndactyly, articular dysplasia and platyspondyly. Clin. Genet., *8:*75, 1975.
30. Close, J. R., Inman, V. T., Poor, P. M., and Todd, F. N.: The function of the subtalar joint. Clin. Orthop., *50:*159, 1967.
31. Cobey, J. C.: Posterior roentgenogram of the foot. Clin. Orthop., *118:*202, 1976.
32. Conway, J. J., and Cowell, H. R.: Tarsal coalition: Clinical significance and roentgenographic demonstration. Radiology, *92:*799, 1969.
33. Coventry, M. B.: Flatfoot, with special consideration of tarsal coalition. Minn. Med., *33:*1091, 1950.
34. Cowell, H. R.: Extensor brevis arthroplasty. J. Bone Joint Surg., *52-A:*820, 1970.
35. Cowell, H. R.: Talocalcaneal coalition and new causes of peroneal spastic flatfoot. Clin. Orthop., *85:*16, 1972.
36. Cowell, H. R.: Diagnosis and management of peroneal spastic flatfoot. A.A.O.S. Instr. Course Lect., *24:*94, 1975.

37. Cowell, H. R., and Elener, V.: Rigid painful flatfoot secondary to tarsal coalition. Clin. Orthop., *177*:54, 1983.
38. Cruveilhier, J.: Anatomie Pathologique du Corps Humain. Tome I, 1829.
39. Del Sel, J. M., and Grand, N. E.: Cubonavicular synostosis: A rare tarsal synostosis. J. Bone Joint Surg., *41-B*:149, 1959.
40. De Marchi, E., Gambier, R., and Vespignani, L.: Les synostoses tarsiennes dans le pied plat valgus douloureux. J. Radiol. Electr., *36*:665, 1955.
41. Deutsch, A. L., Resnick, D., and Campbell, G.: Computed tomography and bone scintigraphy in the evaluation of tarsal coalition. Radiology, *144*:137, 1982.
42. Devoldere, J.: A case of familial congenital synostosis in the carpal and tarsal bones. Arch. Chir. Neerl., *12*:185, 1960.
43. Diamond, L. S.: A possible new syndrome—clinodactyly, voluntary shoulder dislocation and massive tarsal coalition. Birth Defects, *10*:527, 1974.
44. Domenella, G.: Dimonstrazione ed analisi delle sinostosi calcaneo-scafoidee nel piede piatto-valgo contratto, atraverso una nuova technica proiettiva radiografica. Chir. Organi Mov., *52*:501, 1963.
45. Dommisse, G. F.: Flat foot. S. Afr. Med. J., *45*:726, 1971.
46. Drawbert, J. P., Stevens, D. B., Cadle, R. G., and Hall, B. D.: Tarsal and carpal coalition and symphalangism of the Fuhrmann type. Report of a family. J. Bone Joint Surg., *67-A*:884, 1985.
47. Drewes, J.: Die angeborenen Synostosen der Fusswurzelknochen. *In* Kremer, K. (ed.): Die chirurgische Behandlung der angeborenen Fehlbildungen. Stuttgart, Georg Thieme Verlag, 1961, pp. 517–524.
48. Drinkwater, H.: Phalangeal anarthrosis (synostosis, ankylosis) transmitted through fourteen generations. Proc. R. Soc. Med. (Section of Pathology), *10*:60, 1917.
49. Dubois, H. J.: Nievergelt-Pearlman syndrome. Synostosis in feet and hands with dysplasia of elbows. Report of a case. J. Bone Joint Surg., *52-B*:325, 1970.
50. Dwight, T.: A Clinical Atlas. Variations of the Bones of the Hands and Feet. Philadelphia, Lippincott, 1907.
51. Ernsting, G.: Zur klinischen Bedeutung der Coalito calcaneo-navicularis. Arch. Orthop. Unfallchir., *48*:433, 1956.
52. Ertel, A. N., and O'Connell, F. D.: Talonavicular coalition following avascular necrosis of the tarsal navicular. J. Pediatr. Orthop., *4*:482, 1984.
53. Esau, P.: Angeborene Missbildungen der Fuss (Randdefekt). Dtsch. Z. Chir., *194*:236, 1926.
54. Esau, P.: Angeborene Synostosen im Bereich des Carpus and Tarsus. Roentgenpraxis, *5*:235, 1933.
55. Feist, J. H., and Mankin, H. J.: The tarsus. Radiology, *79*:250, 1962.
56. Galinski, A. W., Crovo, R. T., and Ditmars, J. J., Jr.: Os trigonum as a cause of tarsal coalition. J. Am. Podiatry Assoc., *69*:191, 1979.
57. Garelli, R.: Piede valghi e piatti infantili. Minerva Pediatr., *26*:506, 1974.
58. Gaynor, S. S.: Congenital astragalocalcaneal fusion. J. Bone Joint Surg., *18*:479, 1936.
59. Geelhoed, G. W., Neel, J. V., and Davidson, R. T.: Symphalangism and tarsal coalitions: A hereditary syndrome. J. Bone Joint Surg., *51-B*:278, 1969.
60. Geyer, E.: Beitrag zu den Synostosenbildungen der Hand und Fusswerzel. Z. Orthop., *90*:395, 1958.
61. Glessner, J. R., Jr., and Davis, G. L.: Bilateral calcaneo-navicular coalition occurring in twin boys. A case report. Clin. Orthop., *47*:173, 1966.
62. Goldman, A. B., Pavlov, H., and Schneider, R.: Radionuclide bone scanning in subtalar coalitions: Differential considerations. A. J. R., *138*:427, 1982.
63. Grashey, R.: Articulatio talo-calcanea (os sustentaculi). Roentgenpraxis, *14*:139, 1942.
64. Gregersen, H. N.: Naviculocuneiform coalition. J. Bone Joint Surg., *59-A*:128, 1977.
65. Hall, M. C.: The normal movement of the sub-talar joint. Can. J. Surg., *2*:287, 1959.
66. Hark, F. W.: Congenital anomalies of the tarsal bones. Clin. Orthop., *16*:21, 1960.
67. Harle, T. S., and Stevenson, J. R.: Hereditary symphalangism associated with carpal and tarsal fusions. Radiology, *89*:91, 1967.
68. Harold, A. J.: Rigid valgus foot from fibrous contracture of the peronei. J. Bone Joint Surg., *47-B*:743, 1965.
69. Harris, B. J.: Anomalous structures in the developing human foot (abstract). Anat. Rec., *121*:399, 1955. (Original thesis in University of California library).
70. Harris, R. I.: Rigid valgus foot due to talocalcaneal bridge. J. Bone Joint Surg., *37-A*:169, 1955.
71. Harris, R. I.: Peroneal spastic flat foot. A.A.O.S. Instr. Course Lect., *15*:116, 1958.
72. Harris, R. I.: Retrospect: Peroneal spastic flat foot (rigid valgus foot). J. Bone Joint Surg., *47-A*:1657, 1965.
73. Harris, R. I., and Beath, T.: Army Foot Survey. Ottawa, National Research Council of Canada, 1947, p. 44.
74. Harris, R. I., and Beath, T.: Etiology of peroneal spastic flat foot. J. Bone Joint Surg., *30-B*:624, 1948.
75. Harris, R. I., and Beath, T.: John Hunter's specimen of talocalcaneal bridge. J. Bone Joint Surg., *32-B*:203, 1950.
76. Hayd, F. W.: Die Coalitio calcaneo-navicularis und ihre Klinische Bedeutung. Z. Orthop., *78*:292, 1949.
77. Hayek, W.: Synostosis talonavicularis. Z. Orthop. Chir., *69*:231, 1934.
78. Heikel, H. V. A.: Coalition calcaneo-navicularis and calcaneus secundarius. A clinical and radiographic study of twenty-three patients. Acta Orthop. Scand., *32*:72, 1962.
79. Heiple, K. G., and Lovejoy, C. O.: The antiquity of tarsal coalition. Bilateral deformity in a pre-Columbian Indian skeleton. J. Bone Joint Surg., *51-A*:979, 1969.
80. Herschel, H., and Von Ronnen, J. R.: The occurrence of calcaneonavicular synostosis in pes valgus contractus. J. Bone Joint Surg., *32-A*:280, 1950.
81. Hodgson, F. G.: Talonavicular synostosis. South. Med. J., *39*:940, 1946.
82. Hohmann, G.: Angeborene Synostosen zwischen Fusswurzelknochen. Pes planovalgus congenitus. *In* Hohmann, G. (ed.): Handbuch der Orthopadie. Stuttgart, Georg Thieme Verlag, 1961, Part II, Vol. 4, pp. 840–842.
83. Holl, M.: Beitrage zur chirurgischen Osteologie des Fusses. Arch. Klin. Chir., *25*:211, 1880.
84. Holland, C. T.: Two cases of rare deformity of feet and hands. Arch. Radiol. Electrother., *22*:234, 1918.
85. Illievitz, A. B.: Congenital malformation of the feet. Report of the case of congenital fusion of the scaphoid with astragalus and complete absence of one toe. Am. J. Surg., *4*:550, 1928.
86. Isherwood, I.: A radiological approach to the subtalar joint. J. Bone Joint Surg., *43-B*:566, 1961.
87. Jack, E. A.: Bone anomalies of the tarsus in relation to "peroneal spastic flat foot." J. Bone Joint Surg., *36-B*:530, 1954.
88. Jacobs, A. M., Sollecito, V., Oloff, L., and Klein, N.: Tarsal coalitions: An instructional review. J. Foot Surg., *20*:214, 1981.
89. James, A. E., Jr.: Tarsal coalitions and peroneal spastic flat foot. Australas. Radiol., *14*:80, 1970.
90. Jaubert De Beaujeu, A., and Benmussa: Synostose astragalo-scaphoidienne congenitale, bilaterale et isolee. J. Radiol. Electr., *23*:348, 1939.

91. Jayakumar, S., and Cowell, H. R.: Rigid flatfoot. Clin. Orthop., *122*:77, 1977.
92. Johansson, S.: A case of congenital ankylosis of the ankle joints and other malformations. Acta Orthop. Scand., *5*:231, 1934.
93. Johnson, J. C.: Peroneal spastic flatfoot syndrome. South. Med. J., *69*:807, 1976.
94. Jones, R.: Peroneal spasm and its treatment. Report of meeting of Liverpool Medical Institution held 22nd April, 1897. Liverpool Med. Chir. J., *17*:442, 1897.
95. Jones, R.: The soldier's foot and the treatment of common deformities of the foot. Br. Med. J., *1*:709, 1916.
96. Judet, R., Judet, J., and Rigault, P.: Possibilités de correction chirurgical des malformations des os du pied. Presse Med., *74*:157, 1966.
97. Kadelbach, G.: Ein Beitrag zur den Fusswurzelsynostosen. Arch. Orthop. Unfallchir., *40*:363, 1949.
98. Kaplan, E. G., Kaplan, G. W., and Vaccari, O. A.: Tarsal coalition: Review and preliminary conclusions. J. Foot Surg., *16*:136, 1977.
99. Kaye, J. J., Ghelman, B., and Schneider, R.: Talocalcaneonavicular joint arthrography for sustentacular-talar tarsal coalitions. Radiology, *115*:730, 1975.
100. Kendrick, J. I.: Treatment of calcaneonavicular bar. J.A.M.A., *172*:1242, 1960.
101. Kendrick, J. I.: Tarsal coalition. Clin. Orthop., *85*:62, 1972.
102. Kewesh, E. L.: Über hereditäre Verschmelzung der Hand-und Fusswurzelknochen. Fortschr. Rongenstr., *50*:550, 1934.
103. Kirmisson, E.: Double pied bot varus par malformation osseuse primitive associée à des ankyloses congénitales des doigts et des orteils chez quatre membres d'une même famille. Rev. Orthop., *9*:392, 1898.
104. Kolbel, R., and Hermann, H. J.: Ball and socket ankle joint and tarsal synostosis. Z. Orthop. Chir., *60*:105, 1934.
105. Korvin, H.: Coalition talocalcanea. Z. Orthop. Chir., *60*:105, 1934.
106. Kozlowski, K.: Hypoplasie bilatérale congénitale du cubitus et synostose bilatérale calcaneo-cuboïde chez une fillette. Ann. Radiol. (Paris), *8*:389, 1965.
107. Kyne, P. J., and Mankin, H. J.: Changes in intra-articular pressure with subtalar joint motion with special reference to the etiology of peroneal spastic flat foot. Bull. Hosp. J. Dis., *26*:181, 1965.
108. LaGrange, M.: Anomalie du pied. Soudure des os du tarse et du metatarse. Prog. Med. (Paris), *10*:367, 1882.
109. Lamb, D.: The ball-and-socket ankle joint. J. Bone Joint Surg., *40-B*:240, 1958.
110. Lapidus, P. W.: Congenital fusion of the bones of the foot; with a report of a case of congenital tragaloscaphoid fusion. J. Bone Joint Surg., *14*:888, 1932.
111. Lapidus, P. W.: Bilateral congenital talonavicular fusion. Report of a case. J. Bone Joint Surg., *20*:775, 1938.
112. Lapidus, P. W.: Spastic flat foot. J. Bone Joint Surg., *28*:126, 1946.
113. Lawson, J. P.: Symptomatic radiographic variants in extremities. Radiology, *157*:625, 1985.
114. Leonard, M. A.: Inheritance of tarsal coalition and its relationship to spastic flat foot. Proceedings, British Orthopaedic Association, 1973 (abstract). J. Bone Joint Surg., *55-B*:881, 1973.
115. Leonard, M. A.: The inheritance of tarsal coalition and its relationship to spastic flat foot. J. Bone Joint Surg., *56-B*:520, 1974.
116. Levens, A. S., Inman, V. T., and Blosser, J. A.: Transverse rotation of the segments of the lower extremity in locomotion. J. Bone Joint Surg., *30-A*:859, 1948.
117. Lissoos, I., and Soussi, J.: Tarsal synostosis with partial adactylia. Med. Proc., *11*:224, 1965.
118. Lusby, H. L. J.: Naviculo-cuneiform synostosis. J. Bone Joint Surg., *41-B*:150, 1959.
119. Mahaffey, H. W.: Bilateral congenital calcaneocuboid synostosis. Case report. J. Bone Joint Surg., *27*:164, 1945.
120. Manley, M. T.: Biomechanics of the foot. *In* Helfet, A. J., and Lee, D. M. G. (eds.): Disorders of the Foot. Philadelphia, Lippincott, 1980.
121. Manter, J. T.: Movements of the subtalar and transverse tarsal joints. Anat. Rec., *80*:397, 1941.
122. Martinez, S., Herzenberg, J. E., and Apple, J. S.: Computed tomography of the hindfoot. Orthop. Clin. North Am., *16*:481, 1985.
123. Maudsley, R. S.: Spastic pes varus. Proc. R. Soc. Med., *49*:181, 1956.
124. Merryweather, R.: Spastic valgus of the foot. Proc. R. Soc. Med., *48*:103, 1955.
125. Michailow, S.: Über eine angeborene Synostosis zwischen Talus and Kalkaneus. Beitr. Orthop. Traumatol., *19*:278, 1972.
126. Miki, T., Yamamuro, T., Iida, H., Ohta, S., and Oka, M.: Naviculo-cuneiform coalition. A report of two cases. Clin. Orthop., *196*:256, 1985.
127. Miller, E. M.: Congenital ankylosis of joints of hands and feet. J. Bone Joint Surg., *4*:560, 1922.
128. Mitchell, G. P.: Spasmodic flat foot. Clin. Orthop., *70*:73, 1970.
129. Mitchell, G. P., and Gibson, J. M. C.: Excision of calcaneonavicular bar for painful spasmodic flat foot. J. Bone Joint Surg., *49-B*:281, 1967.
130. Mommsen, F.: Das klinische Bild und die klinische Analyse der Varusdeformitaet des Fusses und ihre unblutige Korrektur. Z. Orthop. Chir., *50*:173, 1929.
131. Mosier, K. M., and Asher, M.: Tarsal coalitions and peroneal spastic flatfoot. A review. J. Bone Joint Surg., *66-A*:976, 1984.
132. Murakami, Y.: Nievergelt-Pearlman syndrome with impairment of hearing. Report of three cases in a family. J. Bone Joint Surg., *57-B*:367, 1975.
133. Nierderecker, K.: Der Plattfuss, Klinik, Pathologie, Konservative und Operative Behandlung. Stuttgart. Ferdinand Enke Verlag, 1959, pp. 53–109.
134. Nievergelt, K.: Positiver Vaterschaftsnachweis auf Grand erblicher Missbildungen der Extremitäten. Arch. Klaus Stift Vererbungforsch., *19*:157, 1944.
135. O'Donoghue, D. H., and Sell, L. S.: Congenital talonavicular synostosis. J. Bone Joint Surg., *25*:925, 1943.
136. O'Rahilly, R.: A survey of carpal and tarsal anomalies. J. Bone Joint Surg., *35-A*:626, 1953.
137. O'Rahilly, R.: Developmental deviations in carpus and tarsus. Clin. Orthop., *10*:9, 1957.
138. O'Rahilly, R., Gardner, E., and Gray, D. J.: The skeletal development of the foot. Clin. Orthop., *16*:7, 1960.
139. Outland, T., and Murphy, I. D.: Relation of tarsal anomalies to spastic and rigid flat feet. Clin. Orthop., *1*:217, 1953.
140. Outland, T., and Murphy, I.: The pathomechanics of peroneal spastic flat foot. Clin. Orthop., *16*:64, 1960.
141. Pearlman, H. S., Edkin, R. E., and Warren, R. F.: Familial tarsal and carpal synostosis with radial head subluxation. J. Bone Joint Surg., *46-A*:585, 1964.
142. Pfitzner, W.: Die Variationen im Aufbar des Fusskelts Beitrage zur Kenntniss des menschlichen Extremitäten-skelets. VII. Morphol. Arbeit., *6*:245, 1896.
143. Poznanski, A. K.: Foot manifestations of the congenital malformation syndromes. Semin. Roentgenol., *5*:354, 1970.
144. Poznanski, A. K., Stern, A. M., and Gall, J. C., Jr.: Radiographic findings in the hand-foot-uterus syndrome (H.F.U.S.). Radiology, *95*:129, 1970.

145. Rankin, E. A., and Baker, G. I.: Rigid flat foot in the young adult. Clin. Orthop., *104*:244, 1974.
146. Resnick, D.: Radiology of the talocalcaneal articulation. Radiology, *111*:581, 1974.
147. Richards, R. R., Evans, J. G., and McGoey, P. F.: Fracture of the calcaneonavicular bar: A complication of tarsal coalition. A case report. Clin. Orthop., *185*:220, 1984.
148. Roger, A., and Meary, R.: Les synostoses congénitales des os du tarse. A propos de 41 cas. Rev. Chir. Orthop., *55*:721, 1969.
149. Rompe, G.: Ankylosen des unteren Sprunggelenkes nach offenem Unterschenkelbruch. Arch. Orthop. Unfallchir., *54*:339, 1962.
150. Rothberg, A. S., Feldman, J. W., and Schuster, O. F.: Congenital fusion of astragalus and scaphoid: Bilateral inherited. N.Y. J. Med., *35*:29, 1935.
151. Rutt, A.: Zur Genese der Coalitio calcaneo naviculare. Z. Orthop., *96*:96, 1962.
152. Sanghi, J. K., and Roby, H. R.: Bilateral peroneal spastic flat feet associated with congenital fusion of the navicular and talus. A case report. J. Bone Joint Surg., *43-A*:1237, 1961.
153. Sartorius, D. J., et al.: Tarsal coalition. Arthritis Rheum., *28*:331, 1985.
154. Schreiber, R. R.: Talonavicular synostosis. J. Bone Joint Surg., *45-A*:170, 1963.
155. Seddon, H. J.: Calcaneo-scaphoid coalition. Proc. R. Soc. Med. (Section of Orthopedics), *26*:419, 1932.
156. Shaffer, H. A., Jr., and Harrison, R. B.: Tarsal pseudocoalition—positional artifact. J. Can. Assoc. Radiol., *31*:236, 1980.
157. Shands, A. R., and Wentz, I. J.: Congenital anomalies, accessory bones, and osteochondritis in the feet of 850 children. Surg. Clin. North Am., *33*:1643, 1953.
158. Sicard, A., and Moreau, R.: Synostose astragalocalcanéenne bilateral. Rev. Chir. Orthop., *50*:233, 1964.
159. Simmons, E. H.: Spastic tibialis varus with tarsal coalition. J. Bone Joint Surg., *47-B*:533, 1965.
160. Slater, P., and Rubinstein, H.: Aplasia of interphalangeal joints associated with synostosis of carpal and tarsal bones. Q. Bull. Sea View Hosp., *7*:429, 1942.
161. Sloane, M. W. M.: A case of anomalous development in the foot. Anat. Rec., *96*:23, 1946.
162. Slomann, H. C.: On coalitio calcaneo-navicularis. J. Orthop. Surg., *3*:586, 1921.
163. Slomann, H. C.: On demonstration and analysis of calcaneo-navicular coalition by roentgen examination. Acta Radiol., *5*:304, 1926.
164. Smith, R. W., and Staple, T. W.: Computerized tomography (CT) scanning technique for the hindfoot. Clin. Orthop., *177*:34, 1983.
165. Snyder, R. B., Lipscomb, A. B., and Johnston, R. K.: The relationship of tarsal coalition to ankle sprains in athletes. Am. J. Sports Med., *9*:313, 1981.
166. Soeur, R.: Le Pied plat contracture. Rev. Chir. Orthop., *45*:817, 1959.
167. Solger, B.: Ueber abnorme Verschmelzung knorpeliger Skelettheile beim Fotus. Zentralbl. Allg. Pathol., *1*:124, 1890.
168. Solonen, K. A., and Sulamma, M.: Nievergelt syndrome and its treatment. Ann. Chir. Gynaecol. Fenn., *47*:142, 1958.
169. Spoendlin, H.: Congenital stapes ankylosis and fusion of tarsal and carpal bones as a dominant hereditary syndrome. Arch. Otorhinolaryngol. (Chicago), *206*: 173, 1974.
170. Steinhauser, J.: Further ball-type ankle-joints observed in cases of congenital tarsosynostoses. Z. Orthop., *112*:433, 1974.
171. Stormont, D. M., and Peterson, H. A.: The relative incidence of tarsal coalition. Clin. Orthop., *181*:28, 1983.
172. Stoskopf, C. A., Hernandez, R. J., Kelikian, A., Tachdjian, M. O., and Dias, L. S.: Evaluation of tarsal coalition by computed tomography. J. Pediatr. Orthop., *4*:365, 1984.
173. Sutro, G.: Anomalous talocalcaneal articulation. Cause for limited subtalar movements. Am. J. Surg., *74*:64, 1947.
174. Swiontkowski, M. F., Scranton, P. E., and Hansen, S.: Tarsal coalitions: Long-term results of surgical treatment. J. Pediatr. Orthop., *3*:287, 1983.
175. Templeton, A. W., McAlister, W. H., and Zim, I. D.: Standardization of terminology and evaluation of osseous relationships in congenitally abnormal feet. A. J. R., *93*:374, 1965.
176. Tomeno, B.: Flatfoot caused by congenital synostosis of the tarsus. Rev. Chir. Orthop., *63*:783, 1977.
177. Trolle, D.: Accessory Bones of the Human Foot. (Transl. by E. Aagesen.) Copenhagen, Munksgaard, 1949.
178. Umidon, M.: Architettura, topografia e morfogenesi dei retinacoli perioniery e del legamento anulare laterale del tarso, nell'uomo. Chir. Organi Mov., *52*:305, 1963.
179. Vaughan, W. H., and Segal, G.: Tarsal coalition with special reference to roentgenographic interpretation. Radiology, *60*:855, 1953.
180. Veneruso, L. C.: Unilateral congenital calcaneocuboid synostosis with complete absence of a metatarsal and toe. Case report. J. Bone Joint Surg., *27*:718, 1945.
181. Voutey, H.: Traitement chirurgical du pied plat de l'enfant. Rev. Chir. Orthop., *58*:489, 1972.
182. Wagoner, G. W.: A case of bilateral congenital fusion of the calcanei and cuboids. J. Bone Joint Surg., *10*:220, 1928.
183. Waugh, H.: Partial cubo-navicular coalition as a cause of peroneal spastic flat foot. J. Bone Joint Surg., *39-B*:520, 1957.
184. Weber, V.: Multiple symmetrische Synostosen an Hand und Fuss. Arch. Orthop. Unfallchir., *46*:277, 1954.
185. Webster, F. C., and Roberts, W. M.: Tarsal anomalies and peroneal spastic flat foot. J.A.M.A., *146*:1099, 1951.
186. Weitzner, I.: Congenital talonavicular synostosis associated with hereditary multiple ankylosis arthropathies. A. J. R., *56*:185, 1946.
187. Wheeler, R., Guevara, A., and Bleck, E. E.: Tarsal coalitions: Review of the literature and case report of bilateral dual calcaneonavicular and talocalcaneal coalitions. Clin. Orthop., *156*:175, 1981.
188. Widervank, L. S., Goedhard, G., and Meijer, S.: Proximal symphalangism of fingers associated with fusion of os naviculare and talus and occurrence of two accessory bones in the feet (os paranaviculare and os tibiale externum) in a European-Indonesian-Chinese family. Acta Genet. (Basel), *17*:166, 1967.
189. Wisbrun, W.: Zur Morphologie und Funktion der articulatio talocalcanea. Arch. Orthop. Unfallchir., *44*:606, 1951.
190. Wray, J. B., and Herndon, C. N.: Hereditary transmission of congenital coalition of the calcaneus to the navicular. J. Bone Joint Surg., *45-A*:365, 1963.
191. Wright, D. G., Desai, S. M., and Henderson, W. H.: Action of the subtalar and ankle-joint complex during the stance phase of walking. J. Bone Joint Surg., *46-A*:361, 1964.
192. Zeidel, M. S., Wiessel, S. W., and Terry, R. L.: Talonavicular coalition. Clin. Orthop., *126*:225, 1977.
193. Zock, E.: Ein Beitrag zu den Synostosen der Fusswurzel. Zentralbl. Chir., *78*:845, 1953.
194. Zuckerkandl, E.: Ueber eine Fall von Synostose zwischen Talus und Calcaneus. Allg. Wein. Med. Zeit., *22*:293, 1877.

CONGENITAL METATARSUS VARUS

Congenital metatarsus varus is medial subluxation of the tarsometatarsal joints with adduction and inversion deformity of all five metatarsals; the hindfoot is in a slightly valgus or neutral position. The commonly used term *a third of a clubfoot* is a misnomer, as the navicular articulates normally with the head of the talus or is displaced laterally to compensate for the varus deviation of the forefoot; the talonavicular joint is not subluxated medially as seen in talipes equinovarus. The term *congenital metatarsus adductus* is used by the author when the forepart of the foot is adducted as a result of intrauterine malposition. Metatarsus adductus is a postural deformation of the forefoot with an excellent prognosis, correcting itself spontaneously without treatment within a few months, whereas congenital metatarsus varus is an in utero subluxation that will increase in severity without treatment. It is vital to distinguish the two conditions. The terms *skewfoot* and *serpentine foot* were suggested by McCormick and Blount to describe the complex deformity of the varus forefoot and valgus hindfoot. The condition may result from delayed and improper treatment of congenital metatarsus varus.[33]

Congenital metatarsus varus was first described by Henke.[19] Its incidence is about one per thousand live births, according to Wynne-Davies, and it occurs more frequently in the female, with a female-to-male ratio of 100:76. Approximately 4.5 per cent of first-degree relatives of a person with metatarsus varus are similarly affected. Thus, if one child is affected, the risk of a second occurrence in a family is about 1 in 20. There is no clear pattern of inheritance, the cause being partly genetic and partly environmental.[55]

Reimann and Werner investigated the pathogenesis of metatarsus varus by means of a series of dissections of 14 normal feet of infants who were stillborn or died during the perinatal period. A slight valgus deformity of the hindfoot was produced by maximal dorsiflexion of the ankle. On dissection, the navicular bone was found to be displaced laterally in relation to the head of the talus. The anterior tibial tendon was sectioned. The hindfoot was then fixed in dorsiflexion and experiments were carried out to obtain adduction and inversion of the forefoot—with the following results: (1) traction on the anterior tibial tendon, even with extreme force, could not produce metatarsus varus; (2) capsulotomy of the first metatarsal—medial cuneiform joint and traction on the anterior tibial tendon did not result in the deformity; but (3) only after extensive capsulotomies of all tarsometatarsal joints could the bones be displaced into a position similar to metatarsus varus (Fig. 7–110). Reimann and Werner suggest that congenital metatarsus varus is a primary medial subluxation of the tarsometatarsal joints, taking place in utero when the foot is dorsiflexed. Contracture of the soft tissues and adaptive bony changes are secondary deformities.[43]

Clinical Features

The deformity is present at birth, but may often go unnoticed for as long as several months. Involvement may be unilateral or bilateral.

On inspection of the dorsal and plantar aspects of the foot, all the metatarsals are seen to be adducted and inverted, but the heel is in either valgus or neutral position. The great toe is usually widely separated from the second toe. The base of the fifth metatarsal is prominent. The medial border of the foot is concave, and the lateral border convex. The medial longitudinal arch is high (normally, an infant's foot appears flat because of the presence of a large fat pad under the arch).

There is usually a deep skin crease on the medial aspect of the foot at the tarsometatarsal joint area. Decreased plantar flexion of the ankle and contracture of the anterior tibial muscle are commonly present at birth. On stimulation and contraction of the peroneal muscles, the foot fails to abduct actively, and it cannot be passively abducted to neutral position. The abductor hallucis muscle is taut, pulling the forefoot into varus position. A simple way to demonstrate the tight abductor hallucis tendon is to hold the hindfoot with one hand, with the index finger of the same hand applying counterpressure at the cuboid–fifth metatarsal area, and with the thumb of the opposite hand to push the medial aspect of the first metatarsal head into abduction. The taut tendon of the abductor hallucis is stretched like a bowstring near its insertion and can be seen and palpated with the index finger (Fig. 7–111).[29] Exaggerated medial tibial torsion is often present in metatarsus varus.

When the older child starts to walk, he toes in, his weight being borne on the lateral side of the sole. It is difficult to fit shoes, and shoe wear is noticeably abnormal, with early breakdown of the inner side of the upper of the shoe and the lateral side of the sole.

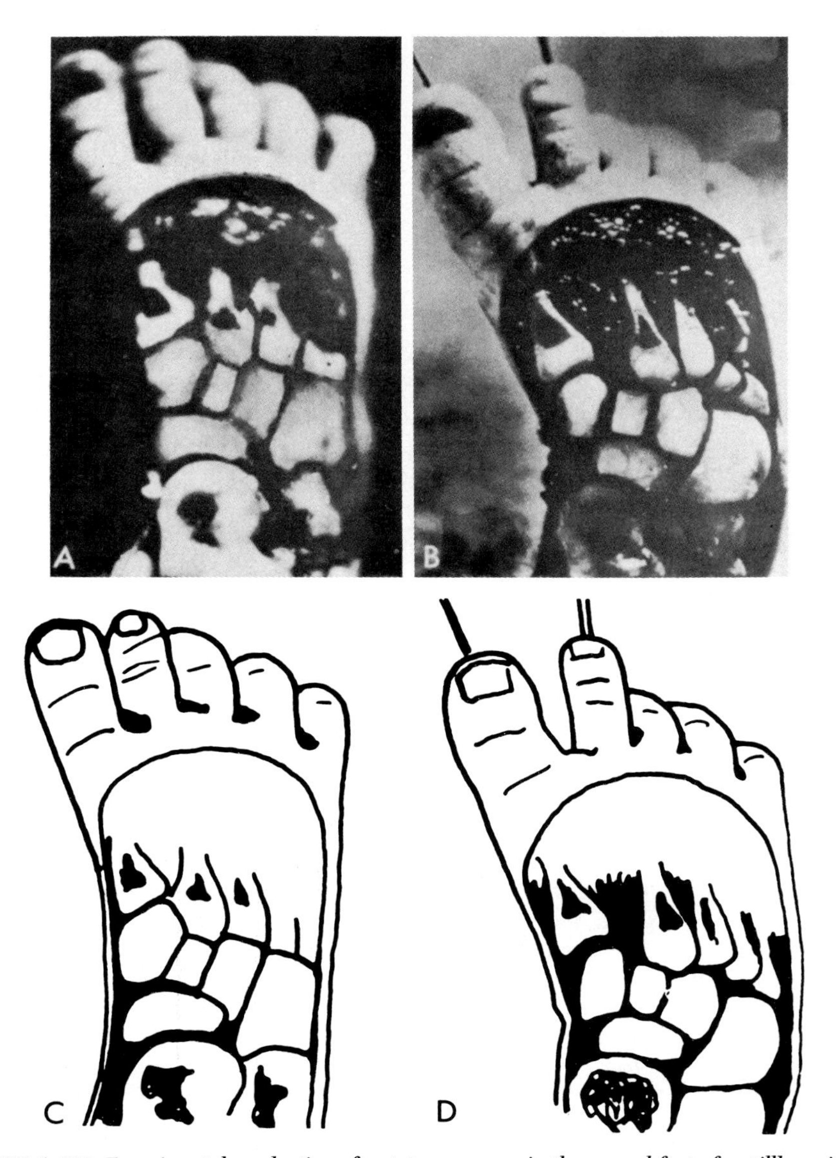

FIGURE 7–110. Experimental production of metatarsus varus in the normal foot of a stillborn infant.

A and **C.** Photograph and diagram of the normal foot. They show the normal articular relations of the bones in neutral position. **B** and **D.** Photograph and diagram of the same foot demonstrating the findings after the hindfoot is fixed in dorsiflexion and the forepart of the foot is adducted and inverted after capsulotomies of all the tarsometatarsal joints and sectioning of all the intermetatarsal interosseous ligaments. Note the medial subluxation of the tarsometatarsal joint; it is most marked between the first metatarsal and medial cuneiform, and there is increased space between the first and second rays. The second to the fifth metatarsals are slightly adducted and inverted. The lateral border of the foot is convex. The navicular is displaced laterally in relation to the head of the talus, and the hindfoot is in valgus position. (From Reimann, I., and Werner, H. H.: Congenital metatarsus varus. A suggestion for a possible mechanism and relation to other foot deformities. Clin. Orthop., *110*:224, 1975. Reprinted by permission.)

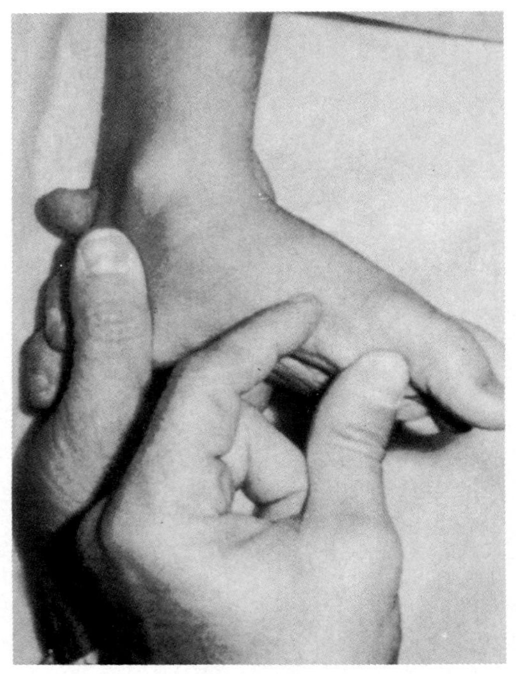

FIGURE 7–111. Lichtblau's test to demonstrate tautness of the abductor hallucis muscle in congenital metatarsus varus.

(From Lichtblau, S.: Section of the abductor hallucis tendon for correction of metatarsus varus deformity. Clin. Orthop., *110*:228, 1975. Reprinted by permission.)

Diagnosis

Functional metatarsus varus may be confused with congenital metatarsus varus. The former is caused by hyperactivity of the abductor hallucis and short toe flexors. All infants have an active plantar grasp reflex and on stimulation will actively hold the forefoot in adduction and the toes in flexion. When the infant is placed at rest in a comfortable prone position, however, the foot has normal contours and range of abduction.

Postural metatarsus adductus is a postural deformation of the forepart of the foot; there is no subluxation of the tarsometatarsal joints. Actively and passively, the forefoot can be brought to neutral position. The varus posture is flexible and not fixed. In addition, in postural metatarsus adductus the foot can be plantar-flexed fully, the anterior tibial is not taut, and the skin creases of the instep are normal.

Congenital metatarsus varus is occasionally misdiagnosed as talipes equinovarus. Clinically, in both conditions the foot is adducted and inverted, but in congenital metatarsus varus the hindfoot is slightly valgus without equinus deformity; in talipes equinovarus the hindfoot is in severe equinovarus position.

Radiograms, although they should not be required to establish the diagnosis, will depict the adducted and inverted position of all the metatarsals at the tarsometatarsal joints. The medial angular deformity is greatest at the medial cuneiform–first metatarsal joint area, with a progressive decrease from the first to the fifth tarsometatarsal joints. The talocalcaneal angle in the anteroposterior view is normal or increased (in talipes equinovarus, the talocalcaneal angle is decreased). When the child is over the age of three years and the bone is ossified, the navicular may be either in normal relationship to the head of the talus or lateral to it (in talipes equinovarus, it is displaced medially on the head). On the lateral radiogram, the talocalcaneal angle is normal.

Treatment

When a pediatrician makes the diagnosis of congenital metatarsus varus, the infant should be referred to an orthopedic surgeon for immediate treatment. It is very unfortunate that mild deformities are often kept under observation by the pediatrician to see whether they will correct themselves spontaneously. During this period of procrastination the deformity increases and becomes more rigid and progressively more resistant to correction. The importance of treatment of true congenital metatarsus varus within the first week of life cannot be overemphasized.

Certain pitfalls of management should be avoided. (1) Stretching exercises are often poorly and improperly executed by the parents, the entire foot being abducted and pronated. The valgus inclination of the hindfoot is exaggerated, the navicular is displaced dorsolaterally on the head of the talus, which is plantar-flexed, and the metatarsals are fixed in varus position. The resultant "Z" deformity of the foot (fixed varus forefoot and valgus hindfoot) is then much more difficult to treat than the original metatarsus varus. (2) Reversing shoes—putting the left shoe on the right foot—will not correct the deformity. (3) "Swung-out" or tarsal pronator shoes or prewalker clubfoot shoes should not be used, as they accentuate the hindfoot valgus deformity by forcing the heel into eversion. (4) An abduction bar on the shoes (the usual Denis Browne splint or any of its modifications such as the Fillauer bar) should not be used as a corrective device, as the valgus force of the splint is exerted on the hindpart as well as on the forepart of the foot.

NONOPERATIVE MANAGEMENT

The only effective way to correct the fixed deformity of congenital metatarsus varus is by manipulative stretching exercises and retention of the foot in the corrected position in an above-knee cast.

The technique of gentle manipulative exercises to stretch the soft-tissue contracture and application of the corrective plaster cast is well described by Kite, by McCormick and Blount, and by Ponseti and Becker.[25–28, 33, 42] It is imperative that the details of technique be followed meticulously (Fig. 7–112).

The tendency is to abduct and evert the whole foot during manipulation and application of the cast. This will increase the valgus deformity of the heel and provide only minimal corrective force at the tarsometatarsal joints (Fig. 7–112 A and B). The correct method of manipulation is as follows: (1) The hindfoot is placed in slight plantar flexion and the anterior process of the calcaneus is pushed medially beneath the head of the talus. (2) The metatarsals are forced into abduction while counterpressure is applied over the cuboid, immediately proximal to the base of the fifth metatarsal. The forepart of the foot is everted (Fig. 7–112 C and D). It is important not to produce an iatrogenic valgus deformity of the hindfoot. The corrected position is maintained to the count of 10 and then released. The exercises are performed for five to ten minutes. The manipulations should be gentle. Then an above-knee corrective cast is applied in two sections (Fig. 7–112 E to G). First the plaster is wrapped over the foot and ankle, and is rolled against the deformity. Again, the hindfoot is maintained in inversion and slight plantar flexion, correcting the valgus deformity of the heel. With pressure over the cuboid bone, the metatarsals are pushed into maximal abduction, but not eversion. Pressure is exerted on the head and neck of the first metatarsal, not on the great toe. After the plaster sets, the cast is extended proximally to include the knee and thigh. Ponseti and Becker laterally rotate the leg when applying the proximal part of the cast to correct the associated medial torsion of the tibia. There is, however, no evidence that immobilizing the leg of an infant in lateral rotation for six to ten weeks will correct exaggerated medial tibial torsion; all it will accomplish is stretching of the soft tissues. If there is associated contracture of the invertors of the foot, the author laterally rotates the leg. In children under the age of one year, below-knee casts are ineffective for controlling the heel in correct position. This author recommends the combined use of the plaster of Paris cast and plastic tape, as it permits better grip and molding. An above-knee cast that holds the knee in 60 to 70 degrees of flexion will provide much better control of the heel and will prevent the cast from slipping. Casts are changed at 10- to 14-day intervals, the total duration of cast treatment varying from four to ten weeks, depending upon the rigidity of the deformity and its resistance to correction.

According to Kite, the following three criteria must be met before cast treatment is discontinued: (1) Complete correction of the convexity of the lateral border of the foot must be achieved (in fact, it is preferable to obtain slight overcorrection so that the convexity is reversed to slight concavity). (2) The prominence at the base of the fifth metatarsal must be no longer palpable. (3) Muscular balance must be restored so that active abduction of the forefoot is just as strong as active adduction.[25–28] In children over one year of age, overcorrection is almost impossible, and in the small infant, it should be avoided, as it will produce a valgus foot. Following cast removal, corrective shoes usually are not required. When the deformity was severe initially or definitive cast treatment was delayed, it is best that the forepart of the foot be held in slight overcorrection in plastic splints during sleep. Again attention should be paid to seeing that the heel is in slight inversion but without valgus distortion. A Denis Browne splint with reversed shoes should *not* be used for this purpose.

SURGICAL TREATMENT

When a patient with metatarsus varus is seen late, i.e., at over one or two years of age, the deformity may have become so fixed that it does not respond to conservative measures. Forceful manipulation in an attempt to correct the deformity of the forepart of the foot may force the heel into valgus position, producing a skewfoot. In such an instance, surgical measures are indicated.

In children under two years of age, the deformity can be satisfactorily corrected by capsulotomy of the first metatarsocuneiform joint and soft-tissue release of the abductor hallucis followed by a stretching plaster of Paris cast for six to eight weeks.

Tarsometatarsal and intermetatarsal soft-tissue release is performed in children between the ages of three and seven years. This procedure is described and illustrated in Plate 101.

Osteotomies at the base of the metatarsals are performed in children over eight years of

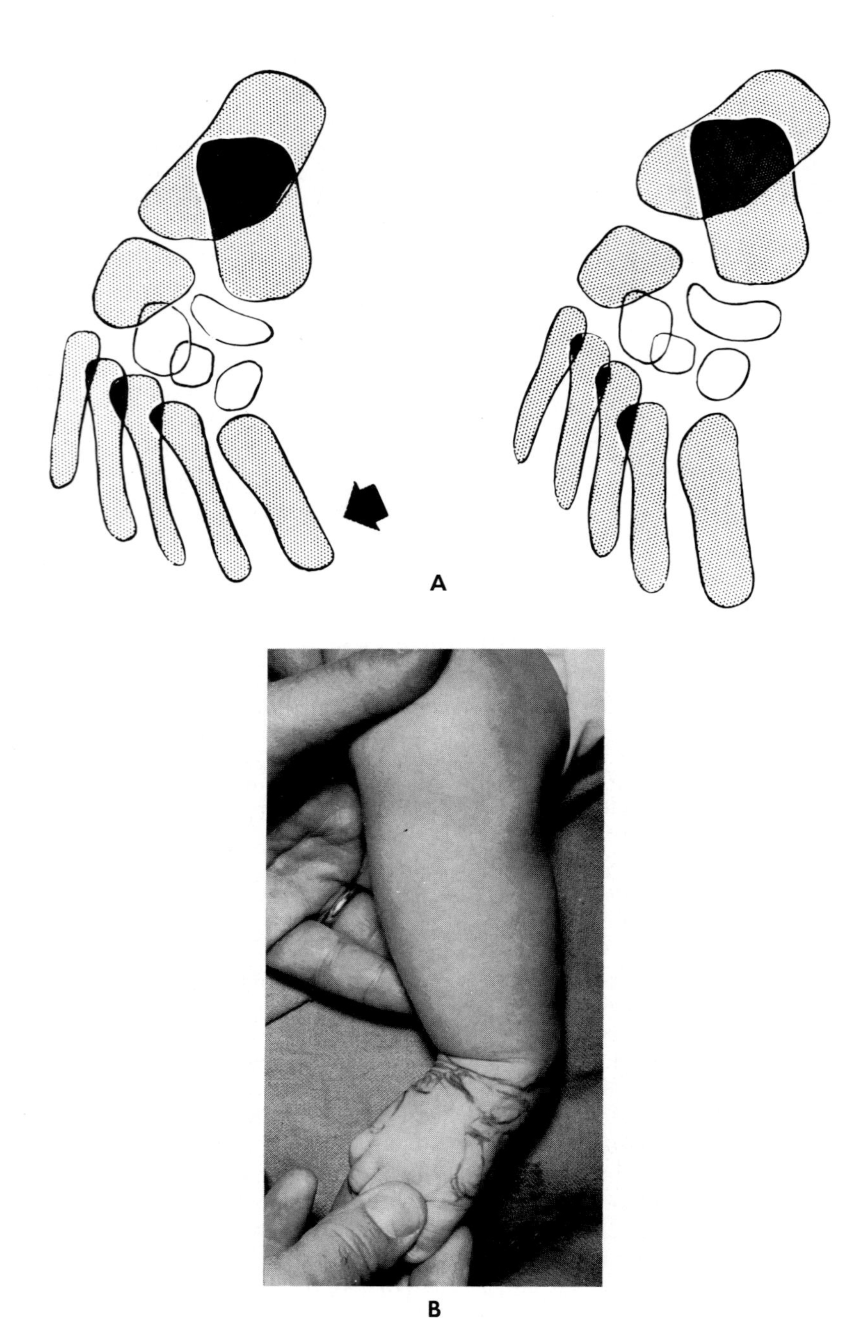

FIGURE 7–112. Correction of congenital metatarsus varus by passive stretching and retention in above-knee cast.

A and **B.** *The incorrect method of manipulation.* The entire foot is abducted and everted by forcefully abducting and everting the forefoot without counterpressure on the hindfoot. The foot is simply being twisted at the ankle, with little corrective force being exerted at the metatarsotarsal joints. The diagram illustrates how the valgus deformity of the heel is increased and shows that the improved appearance of the varus deformity of the forepart of the foot is spurious and not real correction.

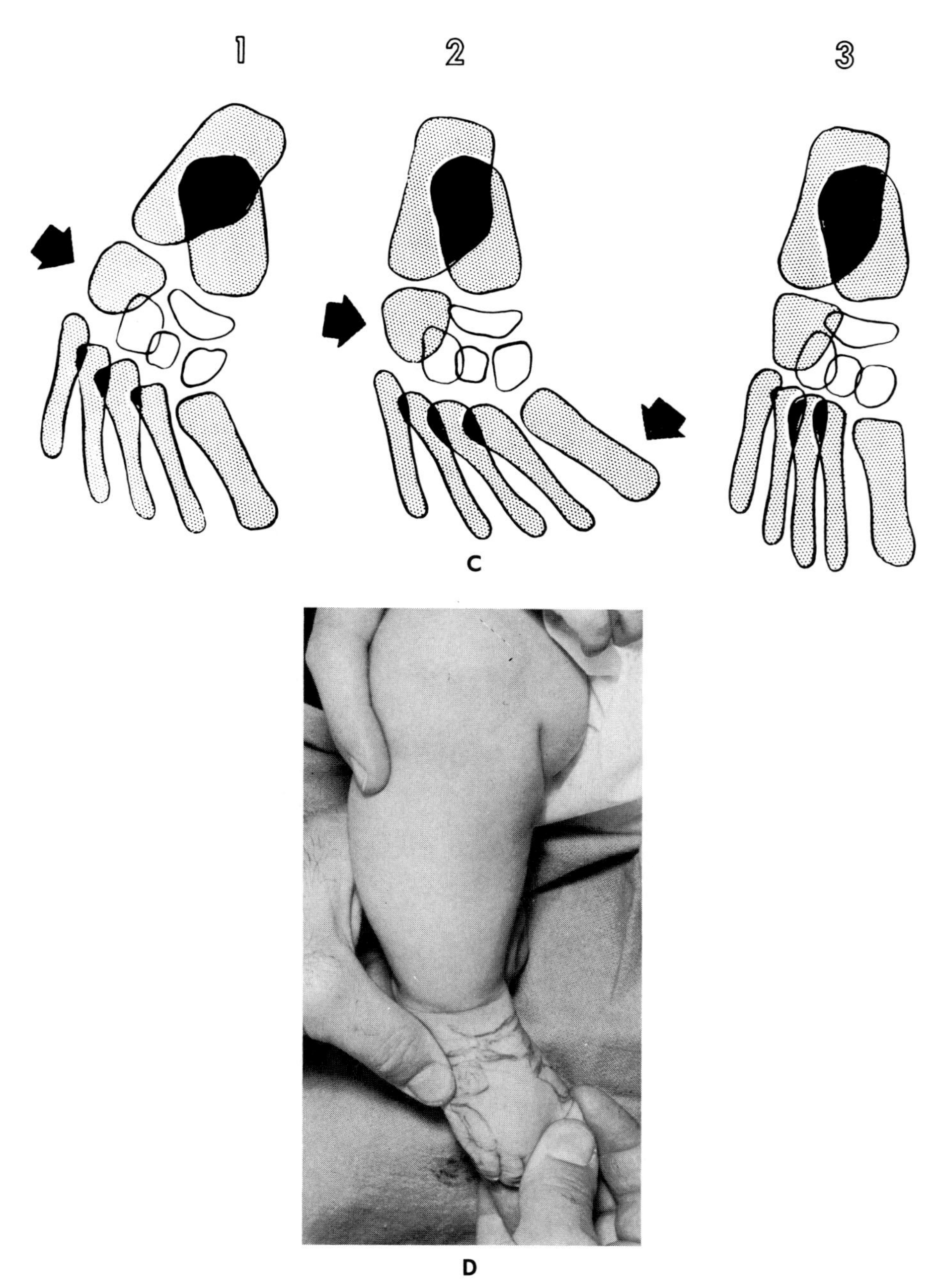

FIGURE 7–112 Continued. Correction of congenital metatarsus varus by passive stretching and retention in above-knee cast.

C and **D.** *The correct method of manipulation.* The hindfoot is slightly plantar-flexed, and the anterior process of the talus is displaced medially underneath the head of the talus; the metatarsals are pushed into abduction while counterpressure is applied over the cuboid. The diagram illustrates the proper method.

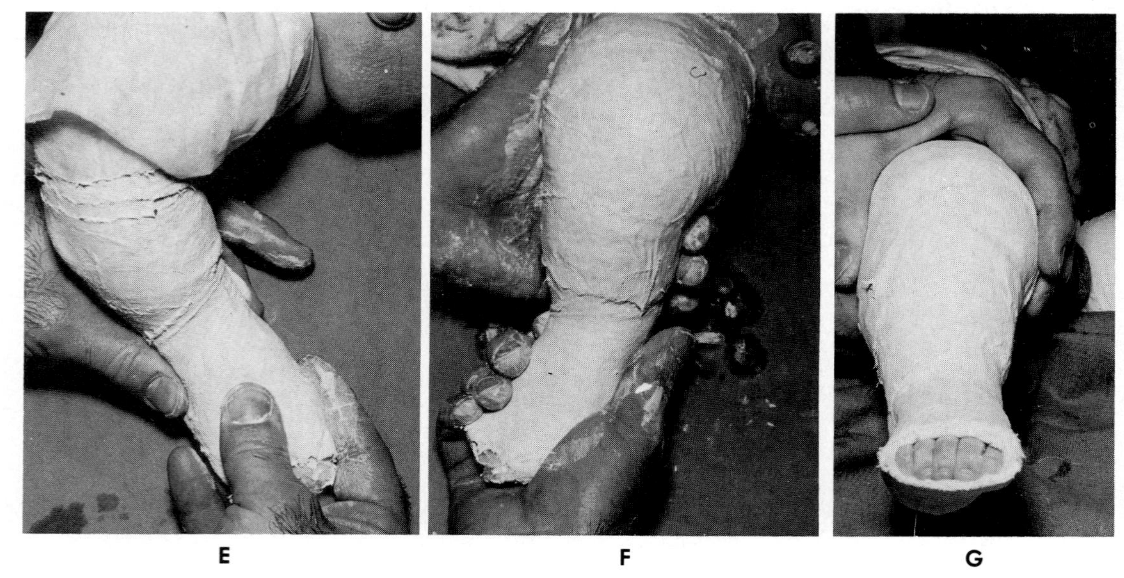

FIGURE 7–112 Continued. Correction of congenital metatarsus varus by passive stretching and retention in above-knee cast.

E. The foot points somewhat medialward while the first section of the plaster cast is applied. **F.** The foot and leg are in slight external rotation while the second section of the plaster cast is applied. **G.** Completed plaster cast. The heel and anterior part of the foot are immobilized in a position as near normal as possible. (From Ponseti, I. V., and Becker, J. R.: Congenital metatarsus adductus: The results of treatment. J. Bone Joint Surg., *48-A*:706–707, 1966. Reprinted by permission.)

age. The operative technique is described and illustrated in Plate 102.

Walking on a foot with rigid metatarsus varus forces the hindfoot into valgus position, producing a skewfoot. In such an instance, when only the varus deformity of the forepart of the foot is corrected, a severe pes valgus more disabling than the original skewfoot may be produced. If surgical correction is warranted, a two-stage procedure should be performed: first, a Grice extra-articular arthrodesis to correct the hindfoot valgus deformity; then soft-tissue release or metatarsal osteotomies, depending upon the age of the patient, to correct the forefoot varus deformity.

References

1. Bankart, A. S.: Metatarsus varus. Br. Med. J., *2*:685, 1921.
2. Berg, E. F.: A reappraisal of metatarsus adductus and skewfoot. J. Bone Joint Surg., *68-A*:1185, 1986.
3. Berman, A., and Gartland, J. J.: Metatarsal osteotomy for the correction of adduction of the forepart of the foot in children. J. Bone Joint Surg., *53-A*:498, 1971.
4. Bleck, E. E.: Metatarsus adductus: Classification and relationship to outcomes of treatment. J. Pediatr. Orthop., *3*:2, 1983.
5. Bleck, E. E., and Minaire, P.: Persistent medial deviation of the neck of the talus: A common cause of intoeing in children. J. Pediatr. Orthop., *3*:149, 1983.
6. Bonnat, H., Bensahel, H., and Themar-Noel, C.: Congenital metatarsus varus. Anatomic and therapeutic considerations. Chir. Pediatr., *22*:405, 1981.
7. Browne, R. S., and Paton, D. F.: Anomalous insertion of the tibialis posterior tendon in congenital metatarsus varus. J. Bone Joint Surg., *61-B*:74, 1979.
8. Coleman, S. S.: Complex Foot Deformities in Children. Philadelphia, Lea & Febiger, 1983, pp. 267–290.
9. Cramer, K.: Metatarsus varus congenitus. Arch. Orthop. Unfallchir., *2*:370, 1904.
10. Cramer, K.: Metatarsus adductus congenitus. Z. Chir. Mechanische Orthop., *3*:329, 1909.
11. DalMonte, A., Manes, E., Soncini, G., Bandini, E., and Andrisano, A.: Surgical treatment of metatarsus varus during the growth period. Ital. J. Orthop. Traumatol., *8*:390, 1982.
12. Diamond, L. S., Lynne, D., and Sigman, B.: Orthopedic disorders in patients with Down's syndrome. Orthop. Clin. North Am., *12*:57, 1981.
13. Duckworth, T.: The hindfoot and its relation to rotational deformities of the forefoot. Clin. Orthop., *177*:39, 1983.
14. Ettore, E.: Metatarso varo congenito. Arch. Ortop., *37*:185, 1921.
15. Ferguson, A. B.: Orthopedic Surgery in Infancy and Childhood. 2nd. Ed. Baltimore, Williams & Wilkins, 1963.
16. Ghali, N. N., Abberton, M. J., and Silk, F. F.: The management of metatarsus adductus et supinatus. J. Bone Joint Surg., *66-B*:376, 1984.
17. Grace, D. L., and Cracchiolo, A., III: A method of evaluating the results of forefoot surgery. Clin. Orthop., *198*:208, 1985.
18. Helbing, C.: Ueber den Metatarsus Varus. Dtsch. Med. Wochenschr., *2*:1312, 1905.
19. Henke, W.: Contracteur des metatarsus. Z. Rat. Med., *17*:188, 1863.
20. Herndon, C. H.: Discussion of paper by Berman, A., and Gartland, J. J.: J. Bone Joint Surg., *53-A*:505, 1971.
21. Heyman, C. H., Herndon, C. H., and Strong, J. M.: Mobilization of the tarsometatarsal and intermetatarsal joints for the correction of resistant adduction of the forepart of the foot in congenital clubfoot or congenital metatarsus varus. J. Bone Joint Surg., *40-A*:299, 1958.
22. Holden, D., Siff, S., Butler, J., and Cain, T.: Shortening of the first metatarsal as a complication of metatarsal osteotomies. J. Bone Joint Surg., *66-B*:582, 1984.
23. Jacobs, J. E.: Metatarsus varus and hip dysplasia. Clin. Orthop., *16*:19, 203, 1960.
24. Kendrick, R. E., Sharman, N. K., Hassler, W. L., and Herndon, C. H.: Tarsometatarsal mobilization for resistant adduction of the forepart of the foot. J. Bone Joint Surg., *52-A*:61, 1970.
25. Kite, J. H.: Congenital metatarsus varus. Report of 300 cases. J. Bone Joint Surg., *32-A*:500, 1950.
26. Kite, J. H.: Congenital metatarsus varus. A.A.O.S. Instr. Course Lect., *7*:126, 1950.
27. Kite, J. H.: Congenital metatarsus varus. J. Bone Joint Surg., *46-A*:525, 1964.
28. Kite, J. H.: Congenital metatarsus varus. J. Bone Joint Surg., *49-A*:388, 1967.
29. Lichtblau, S.: Section of the abductor hallucis tendon for correction of metatarsus varus deformity. Clin. Orthop., *110*:227, 1975.
30. Lloyd-Roberts, G. C., and Clark, R. C.: Ball and socket ankle joint in metatarsus adductus varus (S-shaped or serpentine foot). J. Bone Joint Surg., *55-B*:193, 1973.
31. Lusskin, R., and Lusskin, H.: A metatarsus varus splint for the prewalker. J. Bone Joint Surg., *41-A*:363, 1959.
32. McCauley, J., Jr., Lusskin, R., and Bromley, J.: Recurrence in congenital metatarsus varus. J. Bone Joint Surg., *46-A*:525, 1964.
33. McCormick, D. W., and Blount, W. P.: Metatarsus adductovarus. "Skewfoot." J.A.M.A., *141*:449, 1949.
34. Mau, H., and Ling, W.: The pathogenesis and treatment of metatarsus adductus. Z. Orthop., *122*:841, 1985.
35. Meier, P. J., and Kenzora, J. E.: The risks and benefits of distal first metatarsal osteotomies. Foot Ankle, *6*:7, 1985.
36. Mitchell, G.: Personal communication, 1978.
37. Mitchell, G. P.: Abductor hallucis release in congenital metatarsus varus. Int. Orthop., *3*:299, 1980.
38. Peabody, C. W., and Muro, F.: Congenital metatarsus varus. J. Bone Joint Surg., *15*:171, 1933.
39. Peterson, H. A.: Congenital anomalies of the lower extremities. *In* Goldsmith, H. S. (ed.): Practice of Surgery. Orthopaedics. Philadelphia, Harper & Row, 1980, pp. 1–9.
40. Peterson, H. A.: Skewfoot (forefoot adduction and heel valgus) (abstract). Orthop. Trans., *6*:134, 1982.
41. Peterson, H. A.: Skewfoot (forefoot adduction and heel valgus). J. Pediatr. Orthop., *6*:24, 1986.
42. Ponseti, I. V., and Becker, J. R.: Congenital metatarsus adductus: The results of treatment. J. Bone Joint Surg., *48-A*:702, 1966.
43. Reimann, I., and Werner, H. H.: Congenital metatarsus varus. A suggestion for possible mechanism and relation to other foot deformities. Clin. Orthop., *110*:223, 1975.
44. Reimann, I., and Werner, H. H.: Congenital metatarsus varus. On the advantages of early treatment. Acta Orthop. Scand., *46*:857, 1975.
45. Reimann, I., and Werner, H. H.: The pathology of congenital metatarsus varus. A post-mortem study of a newborn infant. Acta Orthop. Scand., *54*:847, 1983.
46. Rushforth, G. F.: The natural history of hooked foot. J. Bone Joint Surg., *60-B*:530, 1978.
47. Sharrard, W. J. W.: Paediatric Orthopaedics and Fractures. Oxford, Blackwell, 1971.

Text continued on page 2626

Mobilization of Tarsometatarsal and Intermetatarsal Joints by Capsulotomy and Ligamentous Release for Resistant Varus Deformity of the Forefoot (Heyman, Herndon, and Strong)

OPERATIVE TECHNIQUE

A. A curved transverse skin incision is made, extending from the base of the first metatarsal to the lateral border of the cuboid bone. It runs obliquely across the dorsum of the forepart of the foot just distal to the tarsometatarsal joints.

An alternative method of exposure of the tarsometatarsal joints is to make three longitudinal incisions on the dorsum of the foot—the first overlies the first ray, the second is between the second and third rays, and the third overlies the fourth ray. In the young child, two instead of three linear skin incisions may be made—one between the first and second rays and the other overlying the fourth ray.

B. The subcutaneous tissue and deep fascia are divided. The skin flaps are mobilized and retracted with 00 silk sutures. By meticulous linear dissection the tendons of the extensor digitorum longus, extensor hallucis longus, anterior tibial, and peroneus brevis are exposed and freed. The dorsalis pedis vessels are identified. Meticulous care is taken not to injure the neurovascular structures.

C. The anterior tibial tendon is retracted medially, and the extensor hallucis longus tendon with the dorsalis pedis vessels is retracted laterally. The intermetatarsal space between the first and second metatarsals is identified with a small hemostat and the intermetatarsal ligament is divided, beginning distally and progressing proximally. By this method the first metatarsocuneiform joint is located. The epiphyseal plate of the first metatarsal is proximally located; it should not be damaged. The medial and dorsal capsules are divided. The plantar capsule is not sectioned at this time. The anterior tibial tendon should be carefully protected in order to prevent its inadvertent sectioning. The articular cartilage should not be injured.

Plate 101. Mobilization of Tarsometatarsal and Intermetatarsal Joints by Capsulotomy and Ligamentous Release for Resistant Varus Deformity of the Forefoot (Heyman, Herndon, and Strong)

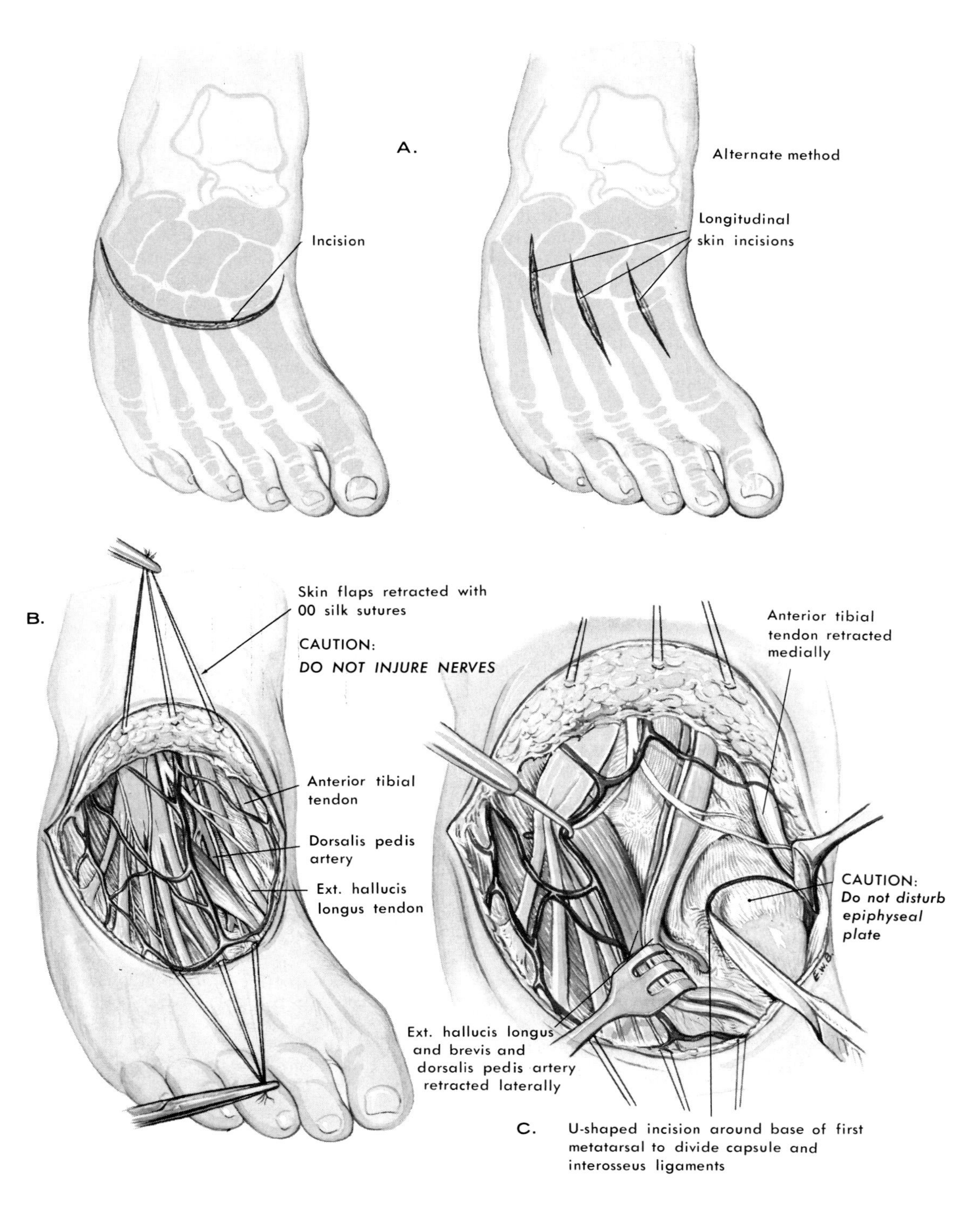

Mobilization of Tarsometatarsal and Intermetatarsal Joints by Capsulotomy and Ligamentous Release for Resistant Varus Deformity of the Forefoot (Heyman, Herndon, and Strong) (Continued)

D. Next, the second metatarsocuneiform joint is exposed; it is located slightly proximal to the first metatarsocuneiform joint. The intermetatarsal ligaments and dorsal capsule are divided. Then longitudinal dissection is carried out in a plane overlying the third ray, taking care to protect the neurovascular structures and the extensor tendons. Again, with a small hemostat, the intermetatarsal space between the second and third metatarsals is identified, and the intermetatarsal ligaments are sectioned. Dorsal capsulotomy of the second and third metatarsocuneiform joints is completed. The fourth metatarsotarsal joint is essentially at the same level as the second and third; the articulation is readily identified after division of the intermetatarsal ligaments. Dorsal capsulotomy is similarly carried out.

At the fifth metatarsocuboid joint the attachment of the peroneus brevis is protected and the lateral capsule is not disturbed; the latter will serve as a hinge that prevents lateral displacement of the fifth metatarsal as the foot is manipulated.

E. Attention is then directed to the plantar capsule and the plantar ligaments. The metatarsotarsal joints are opened by plantar flexion of the forefoot and distal traction on the individual metatarsals. The medial two thirds of the plantar capsule and ligaments at each joint are divided, leaving the lateral one third intact. This will provide sufficient stability to prevent displacement of the metatarsals while the forefoot is manipulated out of adduction. The intermetatarsal ligaments must be divided completely to permit gliding of the metatarsals as the deformity is corrected.

F and **G.** The forefoot is manipulated into abduction and eversion. After correction is achieved there will be considerable incongruity of the articular surfaces. If there is marked instability of the tarsometatarsal joints, Kirschner wires may be inserted to fix the first metatarsal to the first cuneiform and the fifth to the cuboid. The author, however, has not found routine use of Kirschner wires to be necessary.

The tourniquet is released and complete hemostasis is secured. The wound is closed with *interrupted* sutures, and a well-molded above-knee cast is applied, holding the foot in the corrected position.

POSTOPERATIVE CARE

For the first few days after surgery, the leg should be elevated to prevent excessive swelling. In 10 to 14 days, when the reactive swelling has subsided, the cast is changed and a new snug, well-molded one is applied. It is best to carry this out with the patient under general anesthesia and his foot manipulated into the corrected position prior to application of the cast. The skin sutures should not be removed at this time, as the wound edges will separate.

Three weeks later (about four to five weeks after surgery) the cast and sutures are removed, and a carefully molded below-knee walking cast is applied. Immobilization in the cast is continued for a minimum of three to four months; this is important to allow adequate time for remodeling of articular surfaces. The casts are changed every three to four weeks (depending on how robust the child is, as walking is encouraged). Each time the foot is manipulated into the corrected position.

Plate 101. Mobilization of Tarsometatarsal and Intermetatarsal Joints by Capsulotomy and Ligamentous Release for Resistant Varus Deformity of the Forefoot (Heyman, Herndon, and Strong)

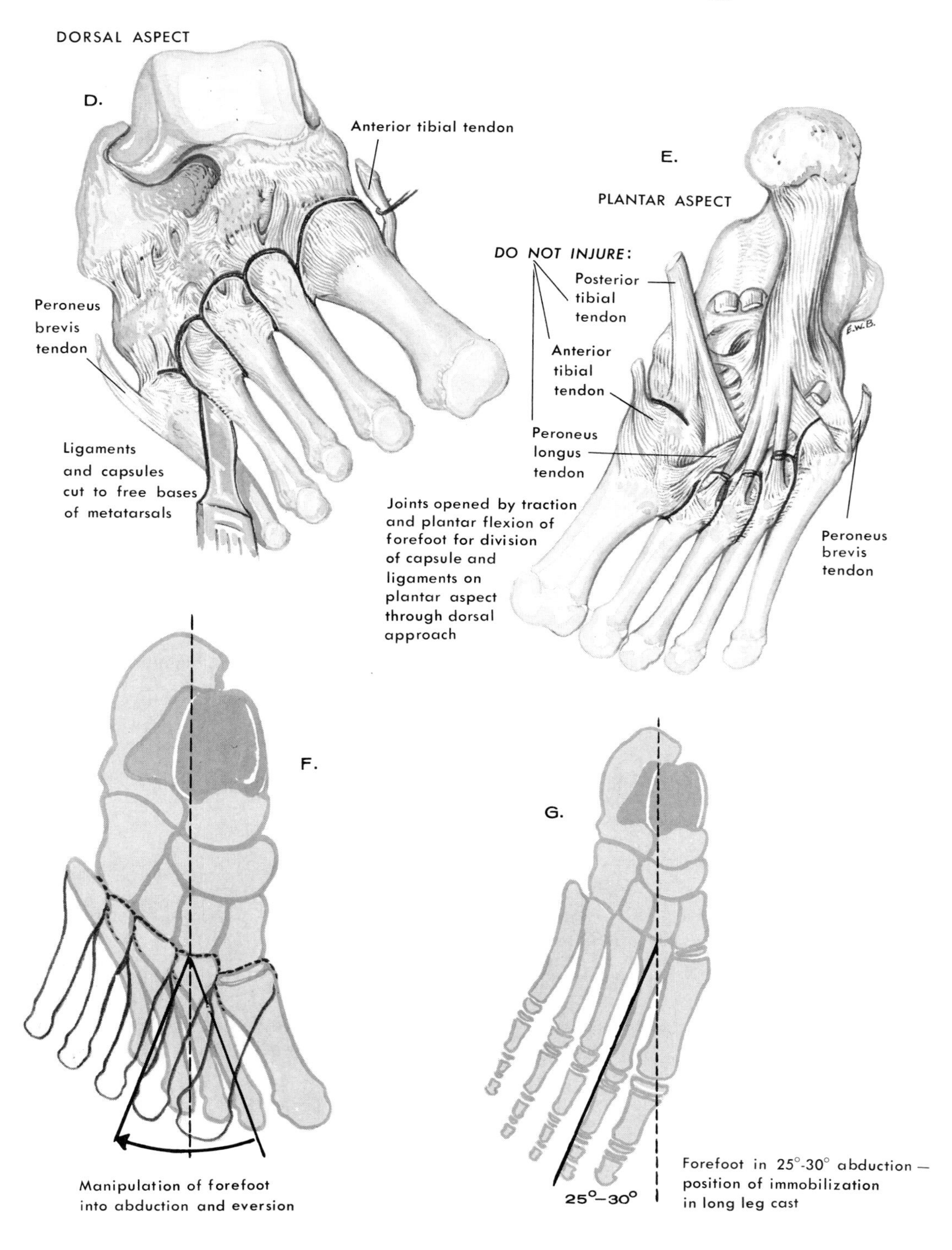

Osteotomy of Bases of Metatarsals for Correction of Varus Deformity of Forepart of Foot

OPERATIVE TECHNIQUE

A. The bases of all five metatarsals are exposed by three longitudinal skin incisions, all approximately 5 cm. long—the first on the medial side of the first metatarsal; the second, in the interval between the second and third rays; and the third, between the fourth and fifth rays. The subcutaneous tissue and fascia are divided in line with the skin incisions. The dorsal cutaneous nerves and the dorsalis pedis and metatarsal vessels should be protected from injury. The epiphyseal plate of the first metatarsal, in contrast to the lateral four metatarsals, is proximal in location and should not be damaged. By appropriate retraction of the extensor tendons and the anterior tibial tendon, the bases of all metatarsals are exposed.

B. The lines of osteotomy may be marked with a small starter and drill holes. The osteotomies are dome-shaped, with their apices directed posteriorly. In the first four metatarsals the medial limb is longer than the lateral limb, whereas in the fifth metatarsal the lateral (fibular) limb is longer than the medial one in order to prevent lateral displacement of the distal fragment when the forefoot is manipulated into abduction. In moderate varus deformity, osteotomy of the fifth metatarsal is not necessary. Often a laterally based wedge is excised from the lateral half of the base of the first metatarsal. The osteotomy is completed with a sharp dental osteotome or a small oscillating electric saw.

C. A heavy threaded Kirschner wire is inserted across the distal one fourth of the metatarsal shafts. The wound is closed and the foot is manipulated, swinging the forepart into abduction. An alternate method is internal fixation of the osteotomized fragments with two Kirschner wires—one inserted across the first metatarsal to the medial cuneiform and the other across the fifth metatarsal to the cuboid. A well-molded above- or below-knee cast is applied, holding the forepart of the foot in 5 to 10 degrees of abduction. The heel should be in neutral position. Weight-bearing is not allowed.

Radiograms are made in the operating room with the patient under anesthesia to ensure that the desired degree of correction is achieved and that the osteotomized bone fragments are in satisfactory apposition.

POSTOPERATIVE CARE

At three to four weeks, the cast, Kirschner wires, and sutures are removed. A below-knee walking cast is applied while the foot is held in the corrected position. Immobilization in the cast is continued for an additional two to three weeks.

Plate 102. Osteotomy of Bases of Metatarsals for Correction of Varus Deformity of Forepart of Foot

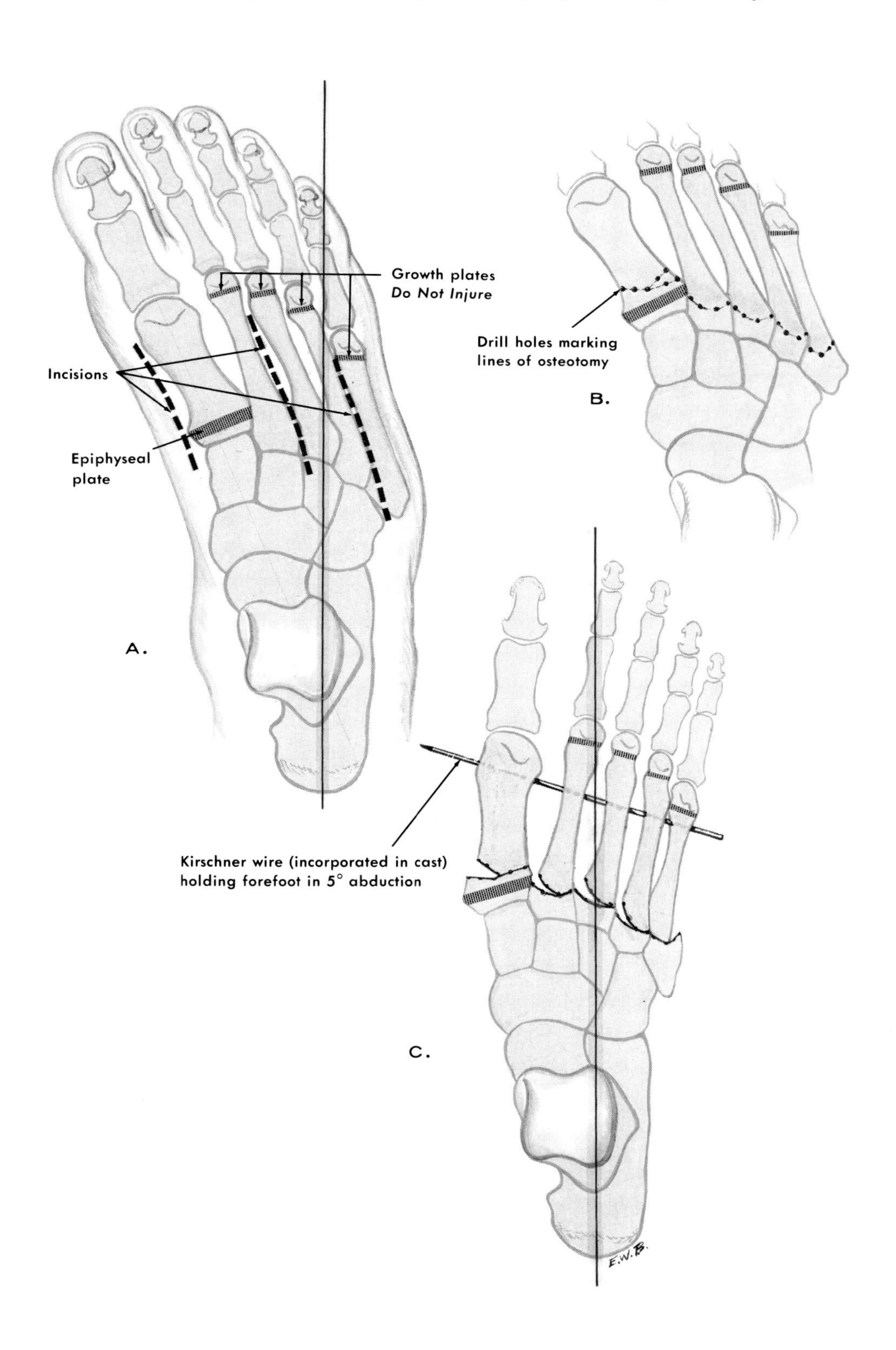

48. Staheli, L. T.: In-toeing and out-toeing in children. J. Fam. Pract., *16*:1005, 1983.
49. Stark, J. G., Johanson, J. E., and Winter, R. B.: The Heyman-Herndon tarsometatarsal capsulotomy for metatarsus adductus: Results in 48 feet. J. Pediatr. Orthop., *7*:305, 1987.
50. Taussig, G., and Pilliard, D.: Congenital metatarsus varus. Value of orthopedic treatment and role of surgery. Apropos of 200 cases. Rev. Chir. Orthop., *69*:29, 1983.
51. Thomson, S. A.: Hallux varus and metatarsus varus. Clin. Orthop., *16*:109, 1960.
52. Tonnis, D.: Congenital metatarsus adductus ("Sichel-Fuss"). (Abstract Oestreich, A. E.) Orthopade, *15*:174, 1986.
53. Turek, S. L.: Orthopaedics: Principles and Their Application. 4th Ed. Philadelphia, Lippincott, 1984, pp. 325–326.
54. Weseley, M. S., Barenfeld, P. A., and Eisenstein, A. L.: Thoughts on in-toeing and out-toeing: Twenty years' experience with over 5,000 cases and a review of the literature. Foot Ankle, *2*:49, 1981.
55. Wynne-Davies, R.: Family studies and the cause of congenital club-foot—talipes equinovarus, talipes calcaneovalgus and metatarsus varus. J. Bone Joint Surg., *46-B*:455, 1964.

CONGENITAL METATARSUS PRIMUS VARUS AND HALLUX VALGUS

Metatarsus Primus Varus

This is a congenital deformity in which the first metatarsal is deviated medially to an abnormal degree. The lateral four metatarsals have normal alignment (Fig. 7–113). In the standing anteroposterior radiogram of the foot, the angle between the first and second metatarsals measures about 7 degrees in the normal foot; an angle greater than 10 degrees is considered pathologic.

The condition is hereditary, with a marked preponderance in girls. Because of the trivial nature of this anomaly, it is often not recognized in infancy and early childhood. This is unfortunate because, in adolescence, the great toe will be gradually pushed into abduction, and the secondary deformities of hallux valgus and bunion will develop (Fig. 7–114). When detected in infancy, metatarsus primus varus is treated by passive stretching and a corrective cast.

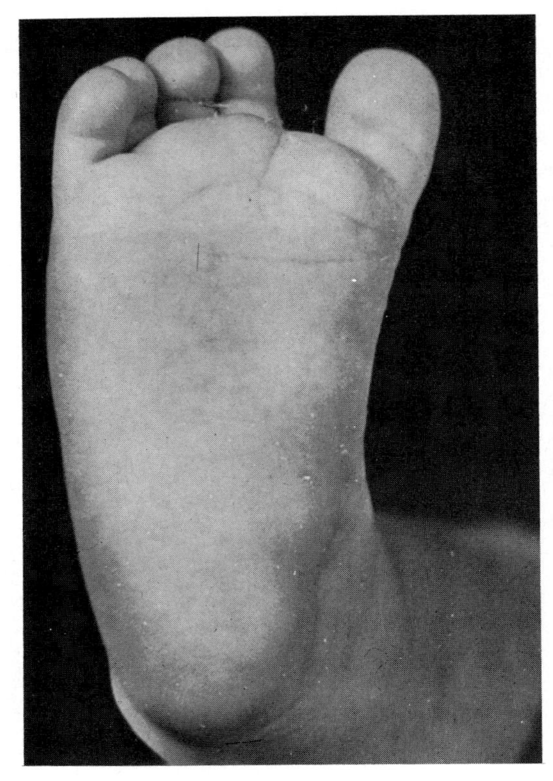

FIGURE 7–113. Metatarsus primus varus.

Note that only the first metatarsal is deviated medially to an abnormal degree. The lateral four metatarsals have normal alignment.

Hallux Valgus and Bunion

These two terms, commonly used synonymously, refer to separate elements of the same syndrome, namely, the lateral deviation of the great toe at the metatarsophalangeal joint and the prominence on the medial aspect of the forefoot produced by the bony deformity together with its acquired bursa. Since the deformity usually causes disability in patients at or past middle age, the pathologic changes are not discussed here, and the presentation of the treatment of hallux valgus is very brief. The literature on the subject is voluminous; one excellent treatise is the monograph by Kelikian.[47]

The symptoms comprise those due to the bunion and those due to the secondary deformities and metatarsalgia. The initial presenting complaint is tenderness over the bunion from pressure and friction against the shoe. The adventitious bursa becomes inflamed and may also be secondarily infected and may suppurate. Metatarsalgia and secondary deformities such as hammertoe and callosities are other causes of discomfort.

Treatment

Conservative measures will provide symptomatic relief, but they will not correct the primary deformity. Shoes of adequate width in the forefoot are provided, the bunion is protected with pads of felt, and a rubber wedge

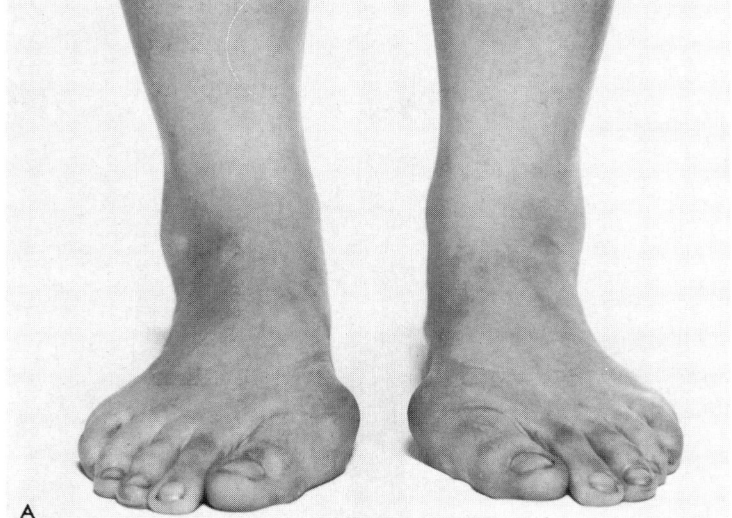

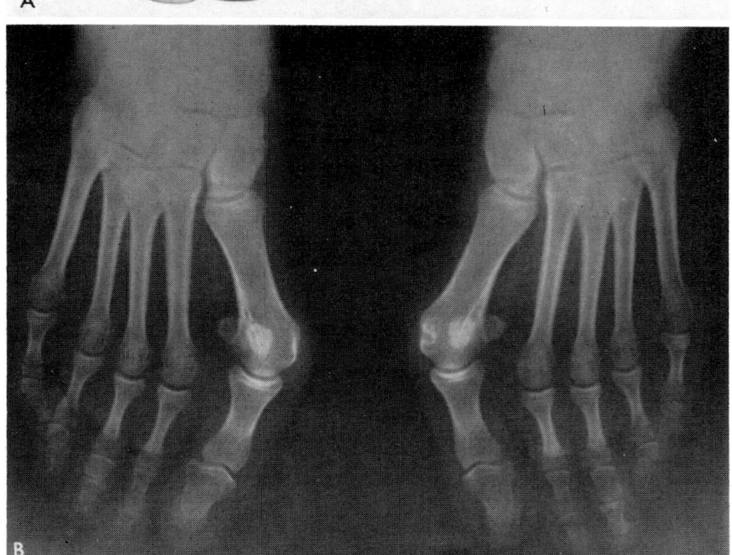

FIGURE 7–114. ***Severe bilateral metatarsus primus varus, hallux valgus, and bunion in an adolescent girl.***

A. Clinical appearance. **B.** Standing anteroposterior radiogram.

between the great and second toes or special bunion splints to hold the hallux straight are given to be worn at night. Metatarsal arch support in the form of appropriate insole pads is provided to treat metatarsalgia.

Operative treatment is indicated when conservative measures fail to give symptomatic relief and when the deformity is very severe. Surgical methods that have been described are many and include the following general technical features: (1) osteotomy of the first metatarsal at its base or neck to correct the metatarsus primus varus deformity; (2) soft-tissue procedures to correct the hallux valgus deformity at the metatarsophalangeal joint; (3) section and transfer of the adductor hallucis to the first metatarsal head; (4) partial excision of the medial prominence of the first metatarsal head; and (5) resection of the proximal two thirds of the proximal phalanx of the great toe.

In adolescents, degenerative changes in the first metatarsophalangeal joint are usually absent and arthroplasty by the Keller procedure is not indicated. If there is associated hallux rigidus with restriction of dorsiflexion of the great toe, osteotomy of the first metatarsal near its neck, displacing the metatarsal head plantarward as well as laterally, is advisable. One or two Kirschner wires are inserted to maintain alignment of the osteotomy. Otherwise, the

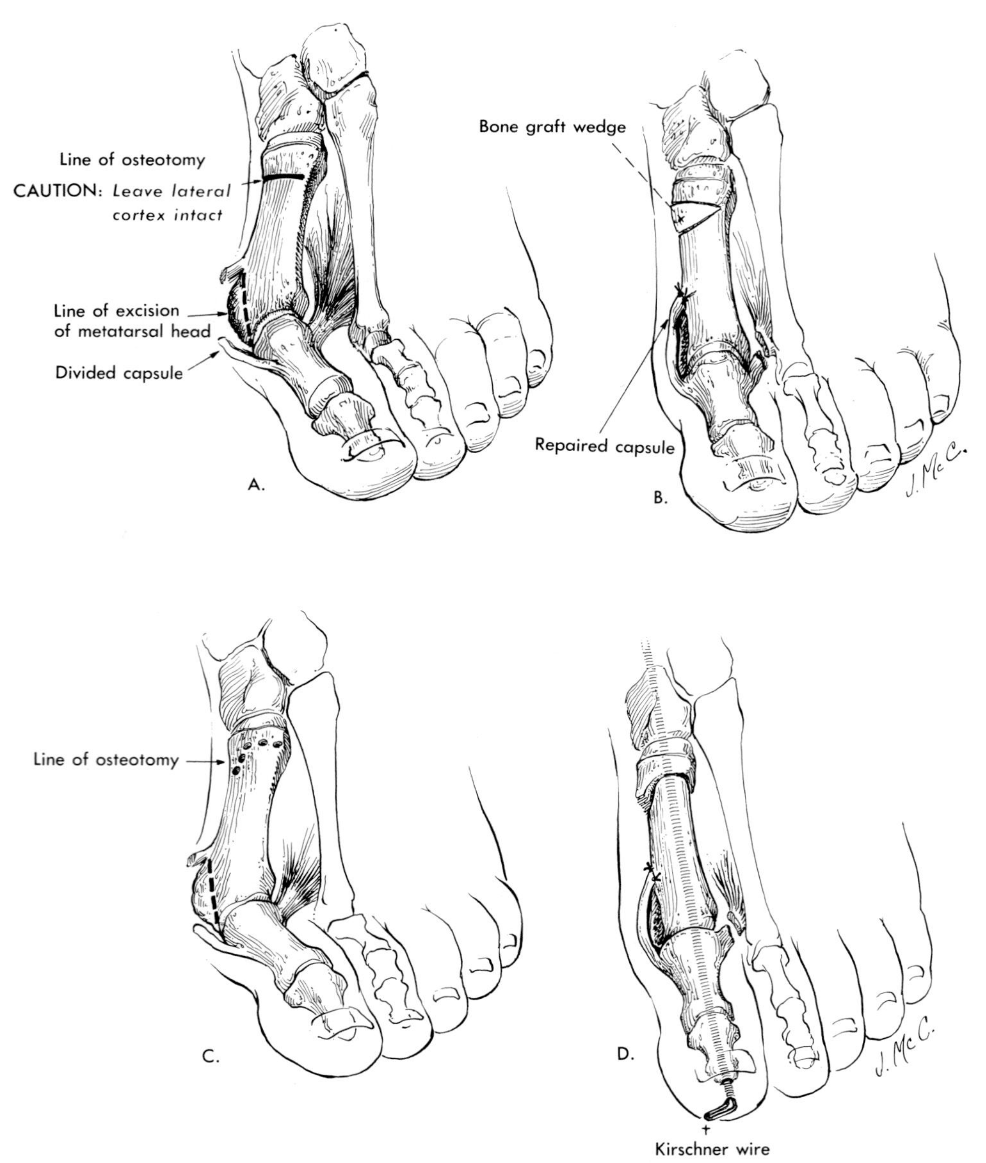

FIGURE 7–115. Correction of hallux valgus and metatarsus primus varus.

Diagrams showing the deformity (**A**) and the postoperative correction (**B**). The hallux valgus is corrected by medial capsular tightening and sectioning of the adductor hallucis longus tendon and lateral capsule. The medial prominence of the first metatarsal head is excised and is used for bone graft. Metatarsus primus varus deformity is corrected by an open-up transverse osteotomy at the base of the metatarsal. The lateral cortex is left intact. **C** and **D.** Correction of metatarsus primus varus and hallux valgus by modified dome osteotomy of the first metatarsal at its base (note the medial buttress) and internal fixation with Kirschner wire. The author, however, recommends that the distal part of the first metatarsal shaft be fixed to the lateral metatarsals with a threaded Steinmann pin.

author prefers the following technique for correcting metatarsus primus varus and hallux valgus (Fig. 7–115).

A dorsomedial incision is made, extending from the middle of the proximal phalanx of the great toe to the base of the first metatarsal. The subcutaneous tissue is divided in line with the skin incision; the digital nerves are identified, care being taken not to injure them inadvertently. Three sets of silk sutures are placed on the skin edges for retraction; the loops are passed distal to the toes, and the ends of the sutures are tied on the lateral side of the forefoot. A U-shaped incision is made on the medial aspect of the capsule of the first metatarsophalangeal joint; the width of the U should be at least 2 cm. The capsule is divided as close to its metatarsal attachment as possible and is reflected distally, leaving its base attached to the proximal phalanx. With an osteotome, the prominent nonarticular portion of the metatarsal head is resected in one piece and kept sterile in a moist sterile sponge. The big toe is laterally displaced, and with Mayo or tenotomy scissors, the lateral part of the capsule of the metatarsophalangeal joint and the adductor hallucis tendon are sectioned. (The author has not found it necessary to transfer the adductor hallucis to the head of the first metatarsal, the only exception to this being in hallux valgus in a spastic foot—in which instance a separate short dorsolateral incision is made and the adductor hallucis longus tendon is divided under direct vision and transferred to the first metatarsal head.) Then a 00 Mersilene whip suture is inserted on the proximal end of the capsule, which is attached firmly to the distal shaft of the first metatarsal through two drill holes. If the abductor hallucis tendon is displaced plantarward, it is detached at its insertion and transferred to a more dorsal site on the medial aspect of the base of the proximal phalanx. Next, *without stripping the periosteum*, the site of osteotomy is marked with a sharp starter and drill holes at the base of the first metatarsal. The lateral cortex is left intact. The bone is divided transversely with a thin osteotome, and the bone previously removed from the metatarsal head is shaped into a wedge and driven in between the osteotomized bone fragments—with care that the lateral cortex is not broken. Precautions should be taken to avoid elevating or depressing the first metatarsal unless this is indicated. This open-up osteotomy will correct only moderate medial divergence of the first metatarsal. If the metatarsus primus varus is severe, a modified dome-shaped osteotomy with a medial buttress in the proximal segment will more effectively correct the deformity. In such an instance, the alignment of the osteotomized fragments is maintained by fixation with a heavy threaded Steinmann pin that fixes the shaft of the first metatarsal to the lateral metatarsals. The pin protrudes on the lateral aspect of the foot for ease of removal when the osteotomy is healed. The wound is closed in the usual manner, and a below-knee walking cast with a toe cap is applied. Ordinarily the osteotomy will heal in six weeks, at which time the cast and pin are removed and a new below-knee walking cast is applied for 10 to 14 days, and then weight-bearing is permitted without restriction. Passive exercises of the first metatarsophalangeal joint are performed several times a day until full range of motion is obtained.

References

1. Alvarez, R., Haddad, R. J., Gould, N., and Trevino, S.: The simple bunion: Anatomy at the metatarsophalangeal joint of the great toe. Foot Ankle, *4*:229, 1984.
2. Antrobus, J. N.: The primary deformity in hallux valgus and metatarsus primus varus. Clin. Orthop., *184*:251, 1984.
3. Aseyo, D., and Nathan, H.: Hallux sesamoid bones. Anatomical observations with special reference to osteoarthritis and hallux valgus. Int. Orthop., *8*:67, 1984.
4. Austin, D. W., and Leventen, E. O.: A new osteotomy for hallux valgus: A horizontally directed "V" displacement osteotomy of the metatarsal head for hallux valgus and primus varus. Clin. Orthop., *157*:25, 1981.
5. Beverly, M. C., Horan, F. T., and Hutton, W. C.: Load cell analysis following Silastic arthroplasty of the hallux. Int. Orthop., *9*:101, 1985.
6. Bishop, J., Kahn, A., and Turba, J.: Surgical correction of the splay-foot: The Giannestras procedure. Clin. Orthop., *146*:234, 1980.
7. Bonney, G., and Macnab, I.: Hallux valgus and hallux rigidus. A critical survey of operative results. J. Bone Joint Surg., *34-B*:366, 1952.
8. Brahms, M. A.: Hallux valgus—the Akin procedure. Clin. Orthop., *157*:47, 1981.
9. Carr, C. R., and Boyd, B. M.: Correctional osteotomy for metatarsus primus varus and hallux valgus. J. Bone Joint Surg., *50-A*:1353, 1968.
10. Cedell, C. A., and Astrom, M.: Proximal metatarsal osteotomy in hallux valgus. Acta Orthop. Scand., *53*:1013, 1982.
11. Chana, G. S., Andrew, T. A., and Cotterill, C. P.: A simple method of arthrodesis of the first metatarsophalangeal joint. J. Bone Joint Surg., *66-B*:703, 1984.
12. Chang, J. W., Griffiths, H., and Chan, D. P.: A new radiological technique for the forefoot. Foot Ankle, *5*:77, 1984.
13. Chiappara, P.: Treatment of symptomatic first metatarsal shortened by surgery. Foot Ankle, *6*:39, 1985.
14. Cholmeley, J. A.: Hallux valgus in adolescents. Proc. R. Soc. Med. (Section of Orthopaedics), *51*:903, 1958.
15. Colloff, B., and Weitz, E.: Proximal phalangeal osteotomy in hallux valgus. Clin. Orthop., *54*:105, 1976.
16. Coughlin, M. J., and Mann, R. A.: Arthrodesis of the first metatarsophalangeal joint as salvage for the failed Keller procedure. J. Bone Joint Surg., *69-A*:68, 1987.

17. Das, De S.: Comparative review of distal first metatarsal osteotomy for hallux valgus (Thesis for the M. Ch. Orth.). Liverpool, University of Liverpool, 1980.
18. Das De, S.: Distal metatarsal osteotomy for adolescent hallux valgus. J. Pediatr. Orthop., *4*:32, 1984.
19. Dhanendran, M., Pollard, J. P., and Hutton, W. C.: Mechanics of the hallux valgus foot and the effect of Keller's operation. Acta Orthop. Scand., *51*:1007, 1980.
20. Ellis, V. H.: A method of correcting metatarsus primus varus. Preliminary report. J. Bone Joint Surg., *33-B*:415, 1951.
21. Fenton, C. F., III, and McGlamry, E. D.: Reverse buckling to reduce metatarsus primus varus: A preliminary investigation. J. Am. Podiatry Assoc., *72*:342, 1982.
22. Fitzgerald, J. A., and Wilkenson, J. M.: Arthrodesis of the metatarsophalangeal joint of the big toe. Clin. Orthop., *157*:70, 1981.
23. Ghali, N. N., Abberton, M. J., and Silk, F. F.: The management of metatarsus adductus et supinatus. J. Bone Joint Surg., *66-B*:376, 1984.
24. Glynn, M. K., Dunlop, J. B., and Fitzpatrick, D.: The Mitchell distal metatarsal osteotomy for hallux valgus. J. Bone Joint Surg., *62-B*:188, 1980.
25. Goldberg, I., Bahar, A., and Yosipovitch, Z.: Late results after correction of hallux valgus deformity by basilar phalangeal osteotomy. J. Bone Joint Surg., *69-A*:58, 1987.
26. Goldner, J. L.: Hallux valgus and hallux flexus associated with cerebral palsy: Analysis and treatment. Clin. Orthop., *157*:98, 1981.
27. Goldner, J. L., and Gaines, R. W.: Adult and juvenile hallux valgus: Analysis and treatment. Orthop. Clin. North Am., *7*:863, 1976.
28. Haines, R. W., and McDougall, A.: The anatomy of hallux valgus. J. Bone Joint Surg., *36-B*:272, 1954.
29. Halebian, J. D., and Gaines, S. S.: Juvenile hallux valgus. J. Foot Surg., *22*:290, 1983.
30. Hardy, R. H., and Clapham, J. C. R.: Observations on hallux valgus. Based on controlled series. J. Bone Joint Surg., *33-B*:376, 1951.
31. Hart, J. A. L., and Bentley, G.: Metatarsal osteotomy in the treatment of hallux valgus. J. Bone Joint Surg., *58-B*:261, 1976.
32. Hattrup, S. J., and Johnson, K. A.: Chevron osteotomy: Analysis of factors in patients' dissatisfaction. Foot Ankle, *5*:327, 1985.
33. Helal, B.: Metatarsal osteotomy for metatarsalgia. J. Bone Joint Surg., *57-B*:187, 1975.
34. Helal, B.: Surgery for adolescent hallux valgus. Clin. Orthop., *157*:50, 1981.
35. Helal, B., Gupta, S. K., and Gojeseni, P.: Surgery for adolescent hallux valgus. Acta Orthop. Scand., *45*:271, 1974.
36. Henry, A. P. J., and Waugh, W.: The use of footprints in assessing the results of operations for hallux valgus. A comparison of Keller's operation and arthrodesis. J. Bone Joint Surg., *57-B*:478, 1975.
37. Hodstein, A.: Hallux valgus—an acquired deformity in the foot in cerebral palsy. Foot Ankle, *1*:33, 1980.
38. Horne, G., Tanzer, T., and Ford, M.: Chevron osteotomy for the treatment of hallux valgus. Clin. Orthop., *183*:32, 1984.
39. Houghton, G. R., and Dickson, R. A.: Hallux valgus in the younger patient: The structural abnormality. J. Bone Joint Surg., *61-B*:176, 1979.
40. Hutton, W. C., and Dhanendian, M.: The mechanics of normal and hallux valgus feet—a quantitative study. Clin. Orthop., *157*:7, 1981.
41. Jahss, M. H.: Hallux valgus: Further considerations—the first metatarsal head. Foot Ankle, *2*:1, 1981.
42. Jahss, M. H., Troy, A. I., and Kummer, F.: Roentgenographic and mathematical analysis of first metatarsal osteotomies for metatarsus primus varus: A comparative study. Foot Ankle, *5*:280, 1985.
43. Johansson, J. E., and Barrington, T. W.: Cone arthrodesis of the first metatarsophalangeal joint. Foot Ankle, *4*:244, 1984.
44. Johnson, K. A., Cofield, R. H., and Morrey, B. F.: Chevron osteotomy for hallux valgus. Clin. Orthop., *142*:44, 1979.
45. Jones, A. R.: Hallux valgus in the adolescent. Proc. R. Soc. Med. (Section of Orthopaedics), *41*:392, 1948.
46. Kato, T., and Watanabe, S.: The etiology of hallux valgus in Japan. Clin. Orthop., *157*:78, 1981.
47. Kelikian, H.: Hallux Valgus, Allied Deformities of the Forefoot and Metatarsalgia. Philadelphia, Saunders, 1965.
48. Keller, W. L.: Surgical treatment of bunion and hallux valgus. N.Y. Med. J., *80*:741, 1904.
49. Keller, W. L.: Further observations on the surgical treatment of hallux valgus and bunions. N.Y. Med. J., *95*:696, 1912.
50. Kinnard, P., and Gordon, D.: A comparison between Chevron and Mitchell osteotomies for hallux valgus. Foot Ankle, *4*:241, 1984.
51. Lapidus, P. W.: Operative correction of the metatarsus varus primus in hallux valgus. Surg. Gynecol. Obstet., *58*:183, 1934.
52. Lemon, R. A., Engber, W. D., and McBeath, A. A.: A complication of Silastic hemiarthroplasty in bunion surgery. Foot Ankle, *4*:262, 1984.
53. Lewis, R. J., and Feffer, H. L.: Modified chevron osteotomy of the first metatarsal. Clin. Orthop., *157*:105, 1981.
54. Lindgren, U., and Turan, I.: A new operation for hallux valgus. Clin. Orthop., *175*:179, 1981.
55. Luba, R., and Rosman, M.: Bunions in children: Treatment with a modified Mitchell osteotomy. J. Pediatr. Orthop., *4*:44, 1984.
56. McBride, E. D.: A conservative operation for bunions. J. Bone Joint Surg., *10*:735, 1928.
57. McBride, E. D.: Hallux valgus, bunion deformity; its treatment in mild, moderate and severe stages. J. Int. Coll. Surg., *21*:99, 1954.
58. McBride, E. D.: The McBride bunion hallux valgus operation. Refinements in the successive surgical steps of the operation. J. Bone Joint Surg., *42-A*:965, 1960.
59. McKay, D. W.: Dorsal bunions in children. J. Bone Joint Surg., *65-A*:975, 1983.
60. Magerl, F.: Stable osteotomies for treatment of hallux valgus and metatarsus primus varus. Foot Ankle, *11*:170, 1982.
61. Mann, R. A., and Coughlin, M. J.: Hallux valgus—etiology, anatomy, treatment and surgical considerations. Clin. Orthop., *157*:31, 1981.
62. Mann, R. A., and Thompson, F. M.: Arthrodesis of the first metatarsophalangeal joint for hallux valgus in rheumatoid arthritis. J. Bone Joint Surg., *66-A*:687, 1984.
63. Martorell, J. M.: Hallux disorder and metatarsal alignment. Clin. Orthop., *157*:14, 1981.
64. May, C.: The surgical treatment of bunions. Am. Surg., *48*:300, 1980.
65. Meier, P. J., and Kenzora, J. E.: The risks and benefits of distal first metatarsal osteotomies. Foot Ankle, *6*:7, 1985.
66. Merkel, K. D., Katoh, Y., Johnson, E. W., Jr., and Chao, E. Y.: Mitchell osteotomy for hallux valgus: Long-term follow-up and gait analysis. Foot Ankle, *3*:189, 1983.
67. Miller, J. W.: Distal first metatarsal displacement osteotomy. J. Bone Joint Surg., *56-A*:923, 1974.
68. Miller, R. J., Rattan, N., and Sorto, L.: The geriatric bunion: Correction of metatarsus primus varus and hallux valgus with the Swanson total joint implant. J. Foot Surg., *22*:263, 1983.
69. Mitchell, C. L., Fleming, J. L., Allen, R., Glenney, C., and Sanford, G. A.: Osteotomy-bunionectomy for hallux valgus. J. Bone Joint Surg., *40-A*:41, 1958.

70. Panacos, N.: A new surgical technique for metatarsus primus varus correction with radical bunionectomy: A preliminary report. J. Foot Surg., *16*:98, 1977.
71. Pelet, D.: Osteotomy and fixation for hallux valgus. Clin. Orthop., *157*:42, 1981.
72. Piggott, H.: The natural history of hallux valgus in adolescence and early adult life. J. Bone Joint Surg., *42-B*:749, 1960.
73. Price, G. F.: Metatarsus primus varus: Including various clinicoradiologic features of the female foot. Clin. Orthop., *145*:217, 1979.
74. Renshaw, J., Sirkin, R., and Drennan, J.: The management of hallux valgus in cerebral palsy. Dev. Med. Child Neurol., *21*:202, 1979.
75. Riggs, S. A., Jr., and Johnson, E. W., Jr.: McKeever arthrodesis for the painful hallux. Foot Ankle, *3*:248, 1983.
76. Robbins, H. M.: The unified forefoot. II. The relationship between hallux valgus and metatarsus primus adductus. J. Foot Surg., *22*:320, 1983.
77. Rokkanen, P., Isolauri, J., Avikainen, V., Tervo, T., and Vaherto, H.: Basal osteotomy of the first metatarsal bone in hallux valgus: Experiences with the use of AO plate. Arch. Orthop. Trauma. Surg., *92*:233, 1978.
78. Rowe, P. H., Coutinho, J., and Fearn, B. D.: Fixation of Hohmann's osteotomy for hallux valgus. Acta Orthop. Scand., *56*:419, 1985.
79. Sarrafian, S. K.: A method of predicting the degree of functional correction of the metatarsus primus varus with a distal lateral displacement osteotomy in hallux valgus. Foot Ankle, *5*:322, 1985.
80. Scheck, M.: Etiology of acquired hammertoe deformity. Clin. Orthop., *123*:63, 1977.
81. Schnepp, J., Carret, J. P., Courcelles, P., Revel, J. J., Texier, A., and Vallat, M. P.: Treatment of hallux valgus with irreducible metatarsus varus of the first metatarsus. Bipolar metatarsal osteotomy. Rev. Chir. Orthop., Suppl. 2:113, 1983.
82. Scranton, P. E., Jr.: Adolescent bunions: Diagnosis and management. Pediatr. Annu., *11*:518, 1982.
83. Scranton, P. E., Jr.: Principles in bunion surgery. J. Bone Joint Surg., *65-A*:1026, 1983.
84. Scranton, P. E., Jr., and Rutkowski, R.: Anatomic variations in the first ray: Part I. Anatomic aspects related to bunion surgery. Clin. Orthop., *151*:244, 1980.
85. Scranton, P. E., Jr., and Zuckerman, J. D.: Bunion surgery in adolescents: Results of surgical treatment. J. Pediatr. Orthop., *4*:39, 1984.
86. Sherman, K. P., Douglas, D. L., and Benson, M. K.: Keller's arthroplasty: Is distraction useful? A prospective trial. J. Bone Joint Surg., *66-B*:765, 1984.
87. Silver, D.: The operative treatment of hallux valgus. J. Bone Joint Surg., *5*:225, 1923.
88. Simmonds, F. A., and Menelaus, M. B.: Hallux valgus in adolescents. J. Bone Joint Surg., *42-B*:761, 1960.
89. Smith, R. W., Reynolds, J. C., and Stewart, M. J.: Hallux valgus assessment: Report of research committee of American Orthopaedic Foot and Ankle Society. Foot Ankle, *5*:92, 1984.
90. Wagner, F. W., Jr.: Technique and rationale: Bunion surgery. Contemp. Orthop., *3*:1040, 1981.
91. Zhuber, K., and Salzer, M.: Operative treatment of hallux valgus with varus of the first metatarsal. Z. Orthop., *115*:916, 1977.

CONGENITAL BALL-AND-SOCKET ANKLE JOINT

In this rare malformation, the contour of the ankle joint is abnormal. The proximal articular surface of the normal talus is dome-shaped in the lateral, but not in the anteroposterior, view. In the ball-and-socket ankle joint the upper end of the talus is dome-shaped in both the anteroposterior and lateral projections, and articulates in a reciprocal manner with the concave distal end of the tibia (Fig. 7–116). The fibular malleolus may or may not participate in the ball-and-socket ankle.

Lamb, in 1958, described five cases of this rare entity; four of his patients had associated coalition of the tarsal bones; the fifth patient had congenital shortening of the lower limb without tarsal fusion.[12] Brahme reported another case with bilateral involvement and used the term *upper talar enarthrosis.*[1] Congenital ball-and-socket joint may also be seen in association with congenital hypoplasia or absence of the fibula and failure of segmentation of the vertebrae. Lloyd-Roberts and Clark reported three children with ball-and-socket ankle joints who also had metatarsus adductus varus (S-shaped or serpentine foot).[13] Schreiber reported 27 congenital ball-and-socket ankle joints in 21 patients; the abnormality was found in 10 of 26 cases of congenital shortening of the leg (38 per cent), in 11 of 64 cases of tarsal coalition (17 per cent), and in 4 of 18 cases of congenital hypoplasia or absence of the fibula (22 per cent). No associated deformity of the lower limb could be found with 6 of the 27 congenital ball-and-socket joints (22 per cent).[18]

The condition is twice as common in the male as in the female. Jacobs has reported a familial occurrence in a father and daughter, each of whom had bilateral involvement.[10] The exact cause is unknown.

The basic underlying pathogenic factor appears to be loss of subtalar joint motion and resultant increased motion and stress at the ankle joint.[11] By means of serial radiograms taken from the first month of life to puberty, Imhauser studied three feet with congenital synostosis of the tarsal bones. He demonstrated that the transformation of the ankle joints to spherical shape is a secondary process taking place between the second and fourth years of life. It is a morphologic response to altered function caused by restriction of motion in the tarsus. He also showed that shortening of the fibular malleolus, a radiographic finding associated with ball-and-socket ankle joint, is not of pathogenic significance.[8]

Congenital ball-and-socket ankle joint is usually asymptomatic. The abnormal lateral mobility at the ankle may cause repeated sprains of the joint, and patients often complain of weak-

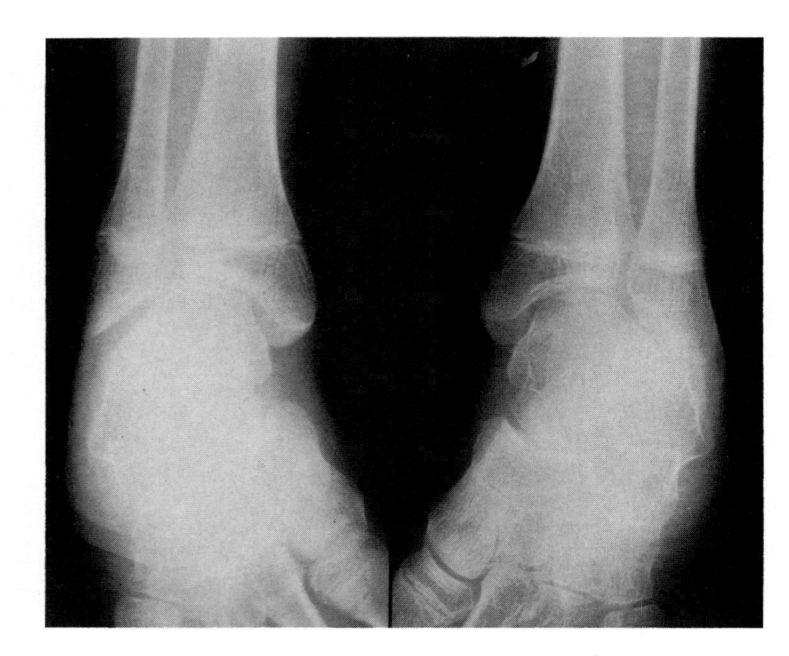

FIGURE 7–116. Radiogram of ankle showing ball-and-socket joint.

ness of the ankle. When there is associated loss of subtalar motion, degenerative arthritis of the ankle may develop in adult life because of excessive stress and repeated minor trauma to the joint.

The radiographic appearance is characteristic. The trochlear surface of the talus, which is normally convex in the anteroposterior plane and gently concave from side to side, loses its concavity in this deformity and becomes spheroid in shape. The lower end of the tibia is correspondingly molded into a cuplike cavity, forming the socket of a ball-and-socket joint. In infancy and late childhood, it is difficult to determine the exact shape of the ankle joint because of the great amount of cartilage in the unossified tibia, talus, and fibula.

Treatment is not indicated, as the condition is asymptomatic. Ankle fusion is performed if degenerative arthritic changes in late adult life cause the deformity to become very disabling.

An acquired form of ball-and-socket ankle joint is sometimes seen in which the rounding of the talus is not as smooth as in the congenital variety. It is reported to follow subtalar arthrodesis (Grice procedure) performed at an early age and probably represents an attempt to compensate for loss of subtalar motion. It is also found in congenital insensitivity to pain. It seems to be associated with marked abnormal laxity of the ligaments about the ankle joint. Robins studied the ankle joints of 52 patients with poliomyelitis who had had arthrodesis of their feet: triple arthrodesis (42 cases), subtalar arthrodesis (4 cases), Lambrinudi arthrodesis (4 cases), and Campbell's bone block (2 cases). Eight feet (15 per cent) disclosed some compensatory increase in lateral movement of the talus within the tibiofibular mortise, and radiograms showed some rounding of the margins of the talus.[17]

References

1. Brahme, F.: Upper talar enarthrosis. Acta Radiol., *55*:221, 1961.
2. Channon, G. M., and Brotherton, B. J.: The ball and socket ankle joint. J. Bone Joint Surg., *61-B*:85, 1979.
3. Dwyer, F. C.: Cause, significance and treatment of stiffness of the subtaloid joint. Proc. R. Soc. Med., *69*:97, 1976.
4. Fischer, V., and Refior, H. J.: Talo-crurales Kugelgelenk bei Ruckfusssynostosen. Arch. Orthop. Unfallchir., *73*:278, 1972.
5. Henssge, J., and Engelke, B.: Die fibulo-ulnare Hypoplasie mit kugelformigem Knochelgelenk, Strahlendefekten und Synostosen. Z. Orthop., *107*:502, 1970.
6. Hiroshima, K., Kurata, Y., Nakamura, M., and Ono, K.: Ball-and-socket ankle joint: Anatomical and kinematic analysis of the hindfoot. J. Pediatr. Orthop., *4*:564, 1984.
7. Hohmann, D., and Eckhoff, P. U.: Kompensationsbewegungen des Tarsus bei Versteifung des Talokruralgelenkes. Z. Orthop., *111*:444, 1973.
8. Imhauser, G.: Veranderungen des oberen Sprunggelenkes bei Fusswurzelsynostosen. Verh. Dtsch. Orthop. Ges., *48*:299, 1960.
9. Imhauser, G.: Kugelformige Knochelgelenke bei angeborenen Fusswurzelsynostosen. Beitrag zur Form-Funktions-Beziehung. Z. Orthop., *108*:247, 1970.
10. Jacobs, P.: Some uncommon deformities of the ankle and foot. Br. J. Radiol., *35*:776, 1962.

11. Jensen, J. K.: Ball and socket ankle joint. Clin. Orthop., *85*:28, 1972.
12. Lamb, D.: The ball-and-socket ankle joint. J. Bone Joint Surg., *40-B*:240, 1958.
13. Lloyd-Roberts, G. C., and Clark, R. C.: Ball and socket joint in metatarsus adductus varus. S-shaped or serpentine foot in poliomyelitis. J. Bone Joint Surg., *41-B*:337, 1959.
14. Murakami, Y.: Nievergelt-Pearlman syndrome with impairment of hearing. Report of three cases in a family. J. Bone Joint Surg., *57-B*:367, 1975.
15. Pappas, A. M., and Miller, J. T.: Congenital ball-and-socket ankle joints and related lower-extremity malformations. J. Bone Joint Surg., *64-A*:672, 1982.
16. Penrose, J. H.: Tarsal synostosis and the ball and socket ankle joint. *In* Proceedings of the British Orthopaedic Association. J. Bone Joint Surg., *56-B*:202, 1974.
17. Robins, R. H. G.: The ankle joint in relation to arthrodesis of the foot in poliomyelitis. J. Bone Joint Surg., *41-B*:337, 1959.
18. Schreiber, R. R.: Congenital and acquired ball-and-socket ankle joint. Radiology, *84*:940, 1963.
19. Steinhauser, J.: Beitrage zur Umformung des Knochelgelenkes zum Kugelgelenk bei angeborenen Fusswurzelsynostosen. Z. Orthop, *112*:433, 1974.
20. Takakura, Y., Tamai, S., and Mashuhara, K.: Genesis of the ball and socket ankle. J. Bone Joint Surg., *68-B*:834, 1986.
21. Vichard, P., Pinon, P., and Peltre, G.: Ball and socket ankle associated with congenital synostosis of the tarsus. Report of a case (author's transl.). Rev. Chir. Orthop., *66*:387, 1980.
22. Weston, W. J.: Congenital ball and socket ankle joint. Br. J. Radiol., *35*:871, 1962.
23. Wroble, R. R.: Congenital ball and socket ankle joints and related lower extremity malformations (letter). J. Bone Joint Surg., *65-A*:121, 1983.

BRACHYMETATARSIA (CONGENITAL SHORT METATARSAL)

Congenital shortening of one or more metatarsals is not uncommon. Frequently the first metatarsal is shortened, a condition known as metatarsus primus atavicus. The length of the first metatarsal in relation to that of the second metatarsal may vary considerably in the normal foot. This was determined by Harris and Beath on standardized dorsoplantar radiograms that showed all the bones of the foot with equal clarity from the posterior end of the calcaneus to the tips of the distal phalanges. They measured the distance from the posterior end of the calcaneus to the head of the second metatarsal in 7,167 individual feet. In 2,878 feet (40 per cent), the first metatarsal was *shorter* than the second by 1 mm. or more; in 2,693 feet (38 per cent), the first metatarsal was *longer* than the second by 1 mm. or more; and in 1,596 feet (22 per cent), the first and second metatarsals were of equal length (within 1 mm.).[3]

Morton, in 1935, in his monograph *The Human Foot*, proposed that shortness of the first metatarsal can cause disability by disturbing the transmission of weight and thrust forces through the forepart of the foot. According to his thesis, the head of the short first metatarsal does not reach the ground as readily as that of the longer second metatarsal. Hence, the greater part of the body weight that is borne through the forepart of the foot is shifted from the first metatarsal to the second or to the second and third metatarsals. The forefoot pronates in an attempt to put the head of the first metatarsal into a weight-bearing position on the ground. This compensatory mechanism lowers the longitudinal arch, which is then subjected to undue strain. In response to this increased stress, callosities develop beneath the heads of the second and third metatarsals, and the shaft of the second metatarsal may thicken. Morton, however, emphasized that shortness of the first metatarsal is but *occasionally* the cause of foot disability, and then only in adult life.[4] Despite his observations, however, the presence of this anomaly was commonly believed to be the cause of symptomatic flat foot.

The fallacy of this assumption was proved by Harris and Beath, who found in the Canadian Army Foot Survey that the short first metatarsal is seldom if ever the cause of foot disability.[2] They stressed that callus under the heads of the central metatarsals is not specifically related to the short first metatarsal, as it occurred almost as frequently in those feet in which the first metatarsal was longer than the second. That the first metatarsal is short does not necessarily indicate that it cannot reach the ground as readily or that less weight will be transmitted through this bone. The obliquity of the metatarsals in relation to the ground demonstrates that all can share equally in weight-bearing, provided the longer metatarsals are on a higher plane than the shorter. Depression of the central metatarsals and marked pressure under their prominent heads cause the callosity. Limitation of plantar flexion of the toes and fixation of the toes in dorsiflexed position will further exaggerate the depression of the metatarsal heads.

Primary marked shortening of the first metatarsal may be encountered as a rare isolated anomaly. It may also occur in association with metatarsus varus and talipes equinovarus. These may lead to abnormal stress and cause painful callosities under the remaining metatarsal heads. Treatment consists of fitting a metatarsal pad that is elongated medially under the first metatarsal to redistribute the body weight.

The next most common shortened metatarsal is the fourth. Figures 7–117 through 7–121 illustrate other types of shortening of the meta-

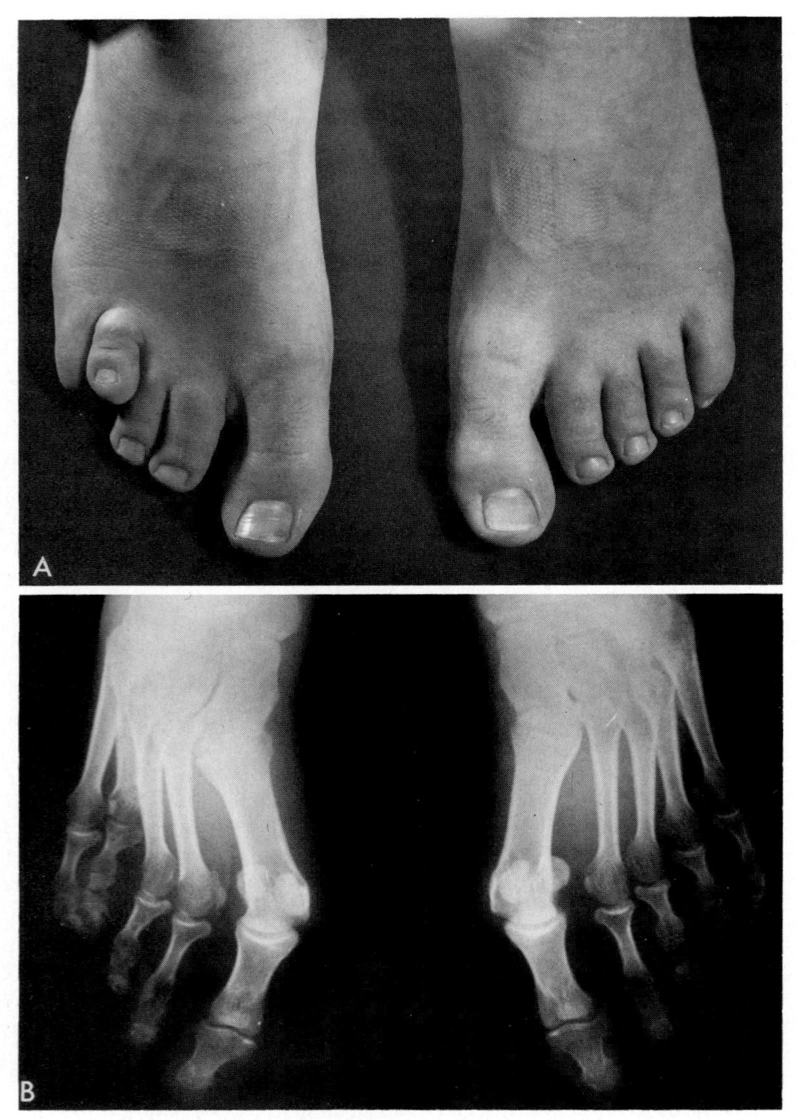

FIGURE 7–117. Congenital shortening of the right fourth metatarsal.

A. Clinical appearance. Note the "apparent" shortening of the right fourth toe. Left foot is normal. **B.** Anteroposterior radiogram of both feet, showing the short fourth metatarsal of the right foot.

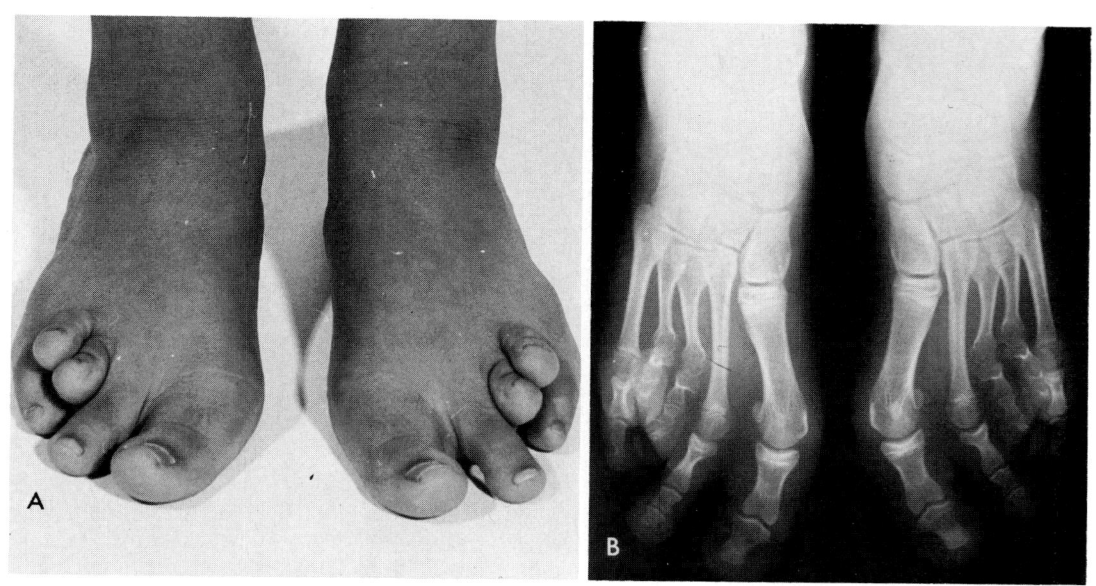

FIGURE 7–118. Congenital shortening of third and fourth metatarsals.

A. Clinical appearance. **B.** Anteroposterior radiogram of both feet.

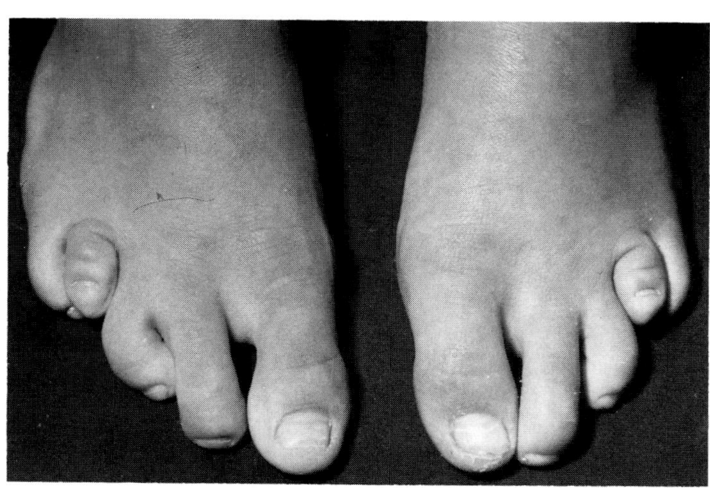

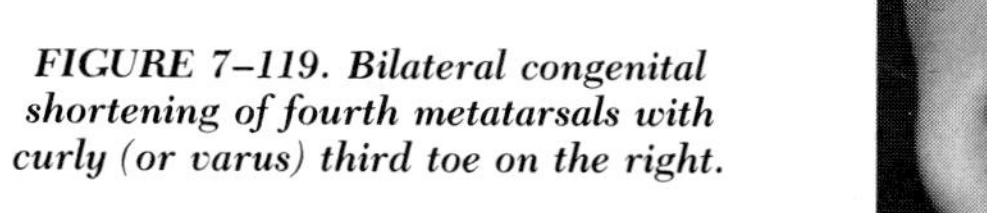

FIGURE 7–119. Bilateral congenital shortening of fourth metatarsals with curly (or varus) third toe on the right.

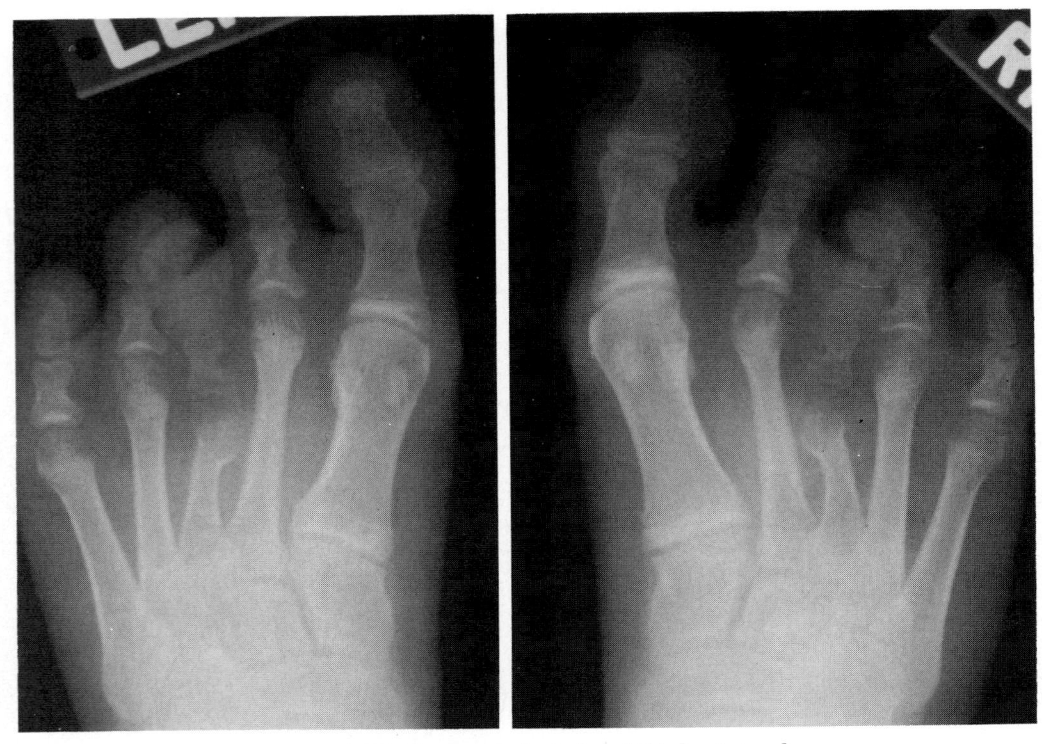

FIGURE 7–120. Congenital shortening of third metatarsal.

Anteroposterior radiograms of both feet show congenital shortening of the third metatarsal.

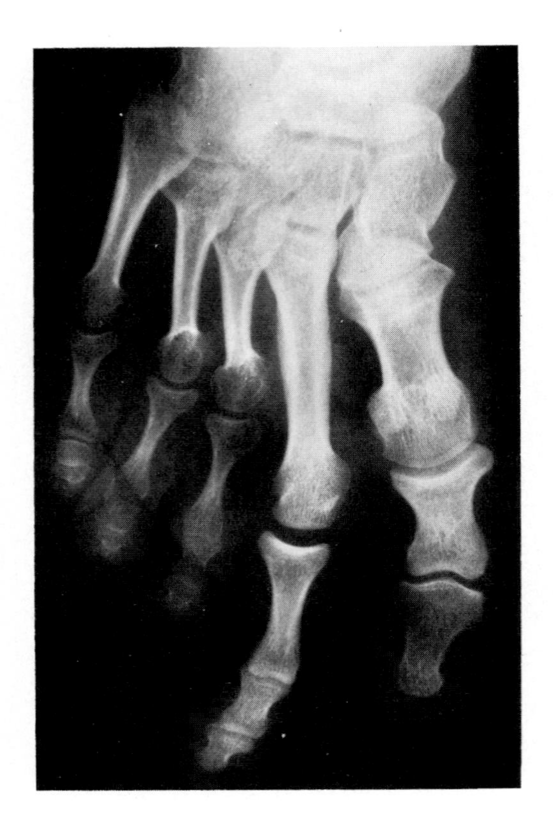

FIGURE 7–121. Anteroposterior radiogram of foot showing congenital shortening of the first, third, fourth, and fifth metatarsals.

tarsals. Usually no treatment is required unless there is difficulty with pressure from the shoe on the upriding toes. Lengthening of the metatarsals has been performed successfully by using the technique for shortened metacarpals.

References

1. Fischer, F. J., and Vandemark, R. E.: Bilateral symmetrical brachymetacarpalia and brachymetatarsalia. Report of a case. J. Bone Joint Surg., *27*:145, 1945.
2. Harris, R. I., and Beath, T.: Report 1574, Army Foot Survey. Ottawa, National Research Council of Canada, 1947.
3. Harris, R. I., and Beath, T.: The short first metatarsal. J. Bone Joint Surg., *31-A*:553, 1949.
4. Morton, D.: The Human Foot. New York, Columbia University Press, 1935.
5. Tashiro, Y., and Takagi, K.: Asthelische Verlanger des Knochens. Mitt. Med. Ges. Tokio, *35*:262, 1921.
6. Urano, Y., and Kobayashi, A.: Bone-lengthening for shortness of the fourth toe. J. Bone Joint Surg., *60-A*:91, 1978.
7. Urbaniak, J. R., and Richardson, W. J.: Diaphyseal lengthening for shortness of the toe. Foot Ankle, *5*:251, 1985.

CONGENITAL SPLIT OR CLEFT FOOT (LOBSTER CLAW)

Congenital split foot is a form of ectrodactyly characterized by the absence of two or three central digital rays of the foot. The cone-shaped cleft in the forefoot tapers proximally. The first metatarsal may be of normal size, or it may be broad and connected with the intermediate cuneiform at its base, representing fusion of the first and second metatarsals. Valgus deformity of the great toe is common. The lateral digital ray may consist of only the fifth metatarsal or the fifth and fourth metatarsals. The phalanges of the lateral ray usually deviate toward the midline. The hindfoot is normal (Figs. 7–122 to 7–125).

Split foot (lobster claw) is a very rare malformation; it exists in two forms. In the typical form, the deformity is always bilateral and is inherited as an autosomal dominant trait with incomplete penetrance.[2, 11] In the less common atypical form, the deformity is unilateral and there is no evidence of familial inheritance.

Although bilateral split foot may be an isolated deformity, it usually occurs in conjunction with lobster clawing of the hand.[2, 19] Other associated abnormalities are cleft lip and palate, reduction in number and size of phalanges, syndactyly and polydactyly, triphalangeal thumb, and deafness.[10, 14, 15, 23]

Surgical correction of split foot is indicated to facilitate the fitting of shoes and to improve the objectionable appearance. Surgery is performed between one and two years of age. The divergent metatarsals are approximated by osteotomy at their bases, the deformed toes are normally aligned, and the split forefoot and toes are surgically syndactylized to maintain correction.

References

1. Ayer, A. A., and Rao, V. S.: Split hand and split foot. J. Indian Med. Assoc., *24*:108, 1954.
2. Barsky, A. J.: Cleft hand: Classification, incidence and treatment. J. Bone Joint Surg., *46-A*:1707, 1964.
3. Berndorfer, A.: Gesichtsspalten gemeinsam mit Hand- und Fusspalten. Z. Orthop., *107*:344, 1970.
4. Blankenburg, H.: Spalthand- und Spaltfussbildungen in typischen and atypischen Formen. Beitr. Orthop. Traumatol., *14*:209, 1967.
5. Cockayne, E. A.: Cleft palate, hare lip, dacryocystitis, and cleft hand and feet. Biometrika, *28*:60, 1936.
6. Cowan, R. J.: Surgical problems associated with congenital malformations of the forefoot. Can. J. Surg., *8*:29, 1965.
7. Eder, H., and Port, J.: Familial cleft foot—a clinical study over 4 generations (author's transl.). Z. Orthop., *116*:189, 1978.
8. Grand, M. J. H., and Dolan, D. J.: Heredofamilial cleft foot. Am. J. Dis. Child., *51*:338, 1936.
9. Lange, M.: Grundsätzliches über die Beurteilung der Entstehung und Bewertung atypischer Hand- und Fussmissbildung. Z. Orthop., *66*:8, 1937.
10. Lewis, T., and Embleton, D.: Split-hand and split-foot deformities, their types, origin and transmission. Biometrika, *6*:26, 1908.
11. McMullen, G., and Pearson, K.: On the inheritance of the deformity known as split foot or lobster claw. Biometrika, *9*:381, 1913.
12. Meyerding, H. W., and Upshaw, J. E.: Heredofamilial cleft foot deformity (lobster-claw or split foot). Am. J. Surg., *74*:889, 1947.
13. Pfeiffer, R. A., and Verbeck, C.: Spalthand und Spaltfuss. Ektodermale Dysplasie und Lippen-Kiefer-Gaumen-Spalte: Ein autosomal-dominant vererbtes Syndrom. Z. Kinderheilkd., *115*:235, 1973.
14. Phillips, R. S.: Congenital split foot (lobster claw) and triphalangeal thumb. J. Bone Joint Surg., *53-B*:247, 1971.
15. Potter, E. L., and Nadelhoffer, L.: A familial lobster claw. J. Hered., *38*:331, 1947.
16. Ray, A. K.: Another case of split foot mutation in two sibs. J. Hered., *61*:169, 1970.
17. Robinson, G. C., Wildervanck, L. S., Chiang, T. P., and Hyg, S. M.: Ectrodactyly, ectodermal dysplasia, and cleft lip-palate syndrome. J. Pediatr. *82*:107, 1973.
18. Rudiger, R. A., Haase, W., and Passarge, E.: Association of ectrodactyly, ectodermal dysplasia, and cleft lip-palate. Am. J. Dis. Child., *120*:160, 1970.
19. Stiles, K. A., and Pickard, I. S.: Hereditary malformations of the hands and feet. J. Hered., *34*:341, 1943.
20. Sumiya, N., and Onizuka, T.: Seven years' survey of our new cleft foot repair. Plast. Reconstr. Surg., *65*:447, 1980.
21. Van Den Berghe, H., Dequeker, J., Fryns, J. P., and David, G.: Familial occurrence of severe ulnar aplasia and lobster claw feet: A new syndrome. Hum. Genet., *42*:109, 1978.
22. Vogel, F.: Verzögerte Mutation beim Menschen; einige

Text continued on page 2642

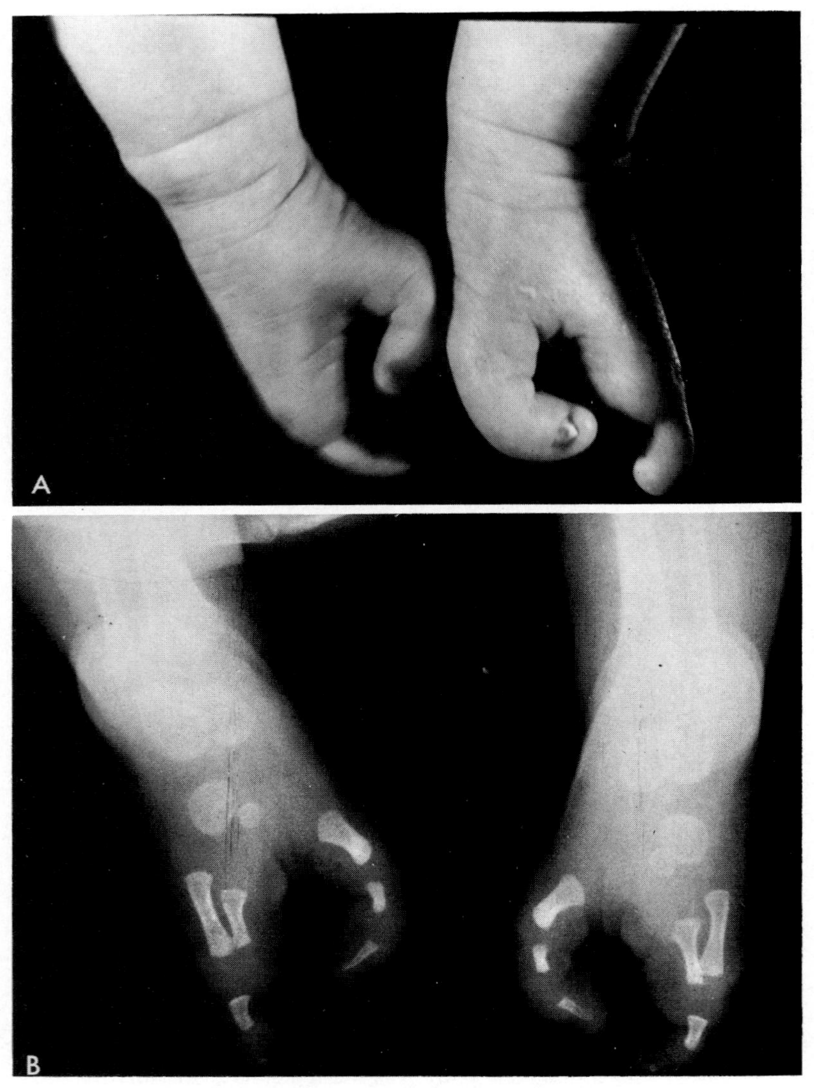

FIGURE 7–122. Congenital split or cleft foot.

A and **B.** Clinical appearance and radiogram of both feet in an 18-month-old child.

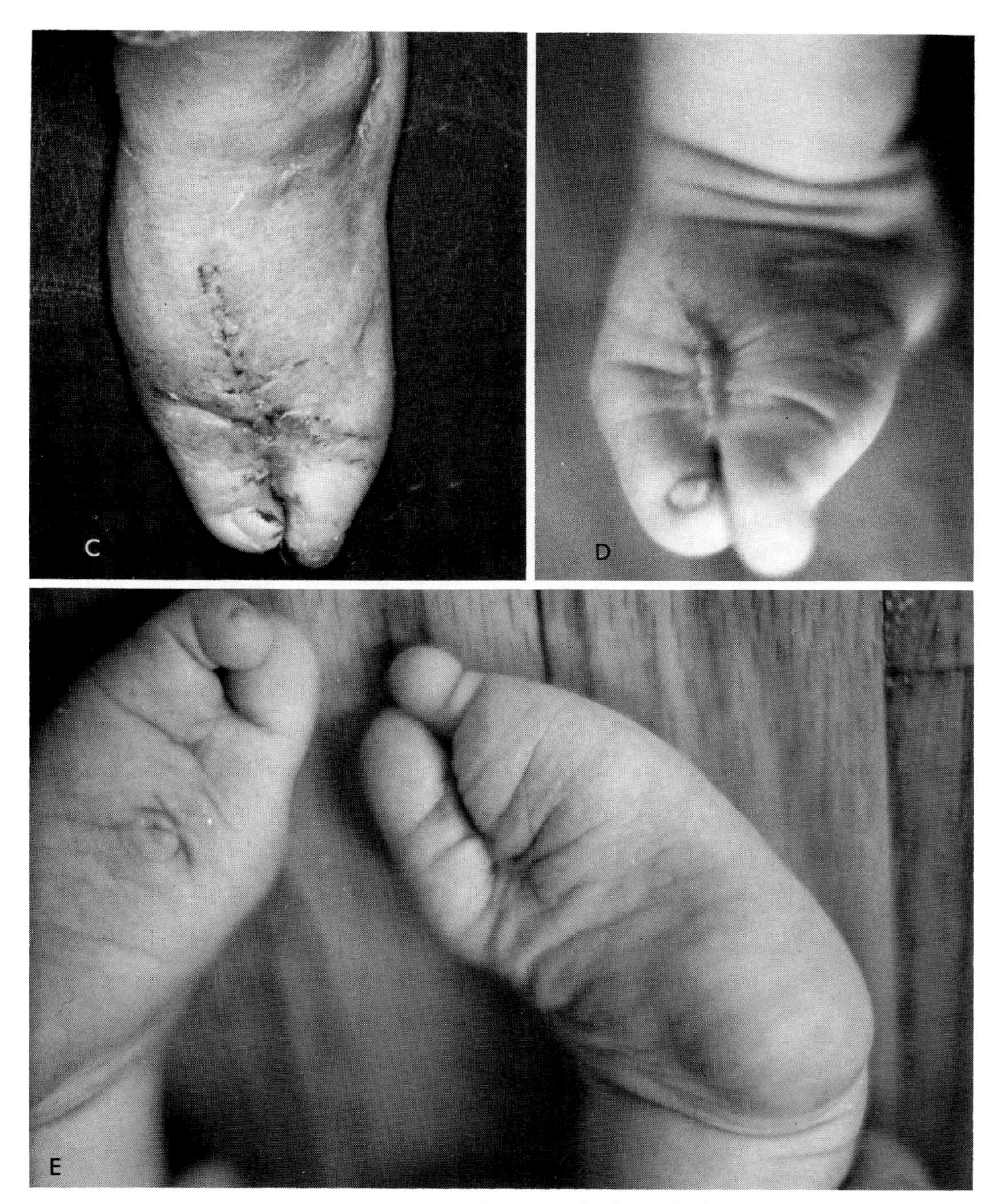

FIGURE 7–122 Continued. Congenital split or cleft foot.

C. Immediate postoperative photograph of left foot. The divergent metatarsals were brought together by osteotomy at their bases, the toes were normally aligned, and the split forefoot was surgically syndactylized to maintain correction. **D.** Dorsal photograph of the left foot six months later. **E.** Plantar photograph of both feet six months postoperatively.

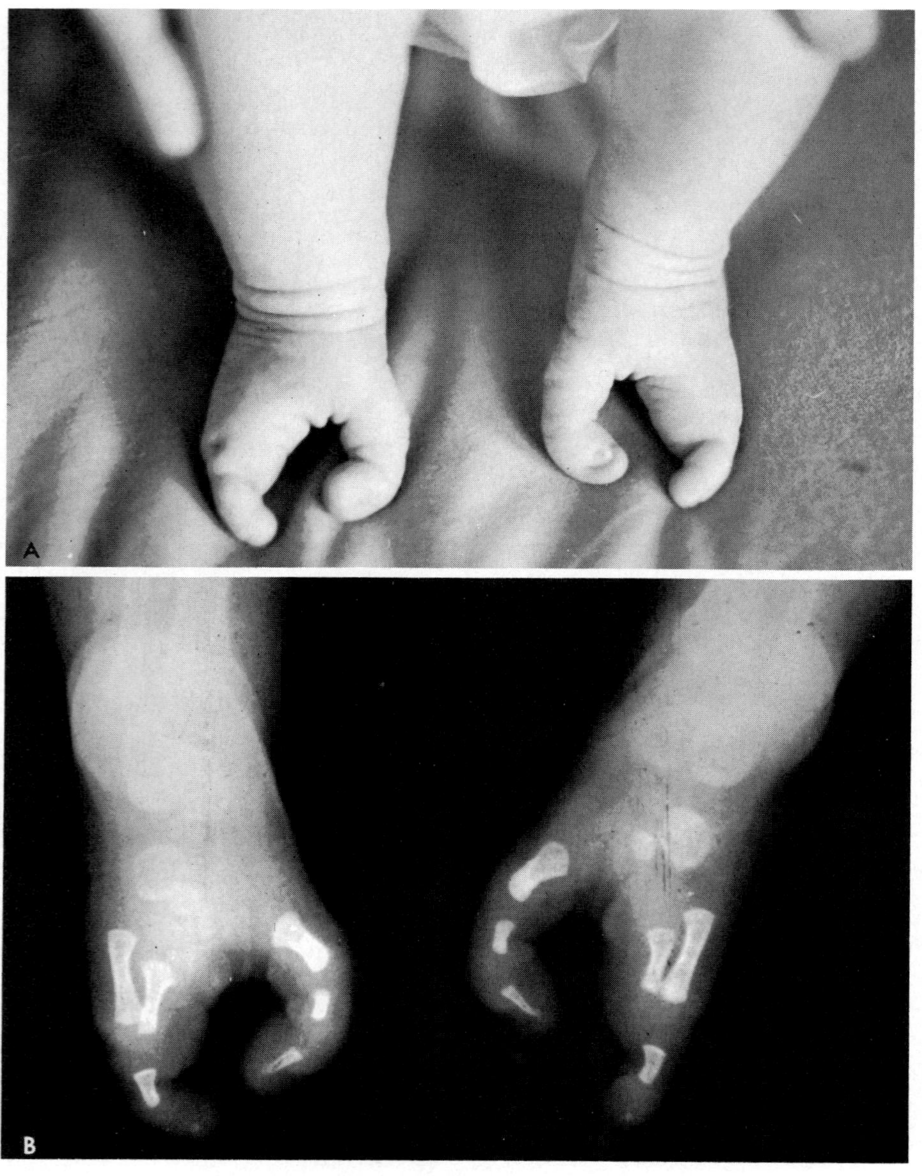

FIGURE 7–123. Congenital split or cleft foot (lobster claw).

A. Clinical appearance in a six-month-old infant. **B.** Radiogram of both feet.

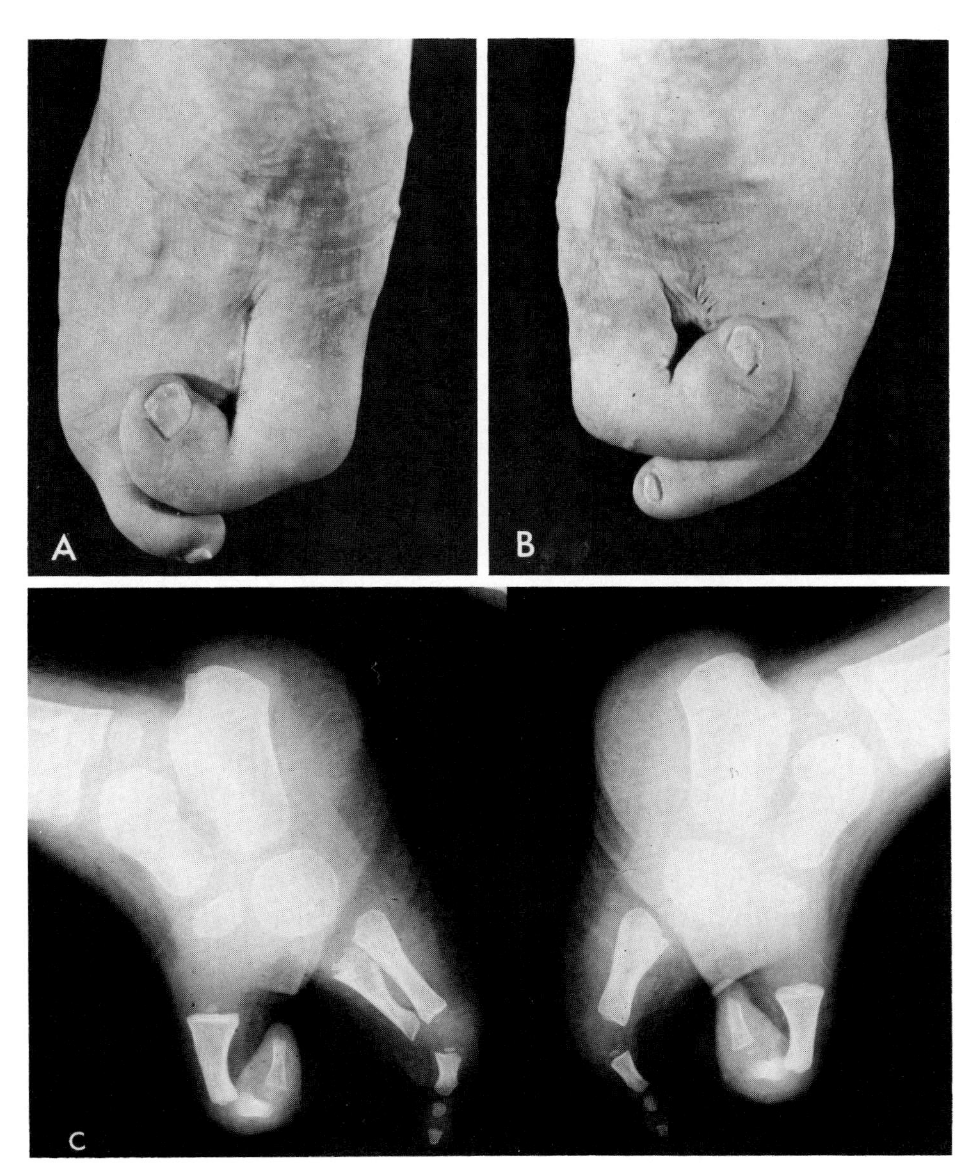

FIGURE 7–124. Lobster claw or split foot in 12-year-old child.

A and **B.** Clinical appearance of both feet. **C.** Radiogram. To facilitate shoe wear, deformity is usually corrected by walking age. Note the adaptation of the toes to the external pressure of the shoes.

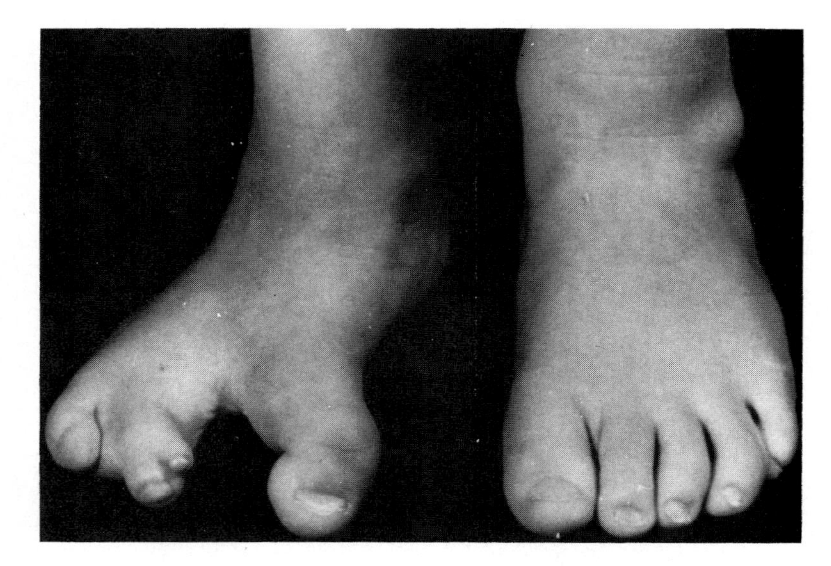

FIGURE 7–125. Atypical form of split foot.

Only the right foot was malformed. The left foot and both hands were normal. (Courtesy of Dr. H. Kelikian.)

kritische Bemerkungen zu Ch. Auberbachs Arbeit (1956). Ann. Hum. Genet., *22*:132, 1958.
23. Walker, J. C., and Clodius, L.: The syndromes of cleft lip, cleft palate and lobster-claw deformities of hands and feet. Plast. Reconstr. Surg., *32*:627, 1963.

POLYDACTYLISM

Supernumerary digits are common in the foot; they occur more frequently in the black and in the female. Polydactyly is usually transmitted as an autosomal dominant trait, but sporadic cases are caused by mutant genes. The supernumerary toe may be associated with polydactyly in the hand or other major congenital malformations such as absence or hypoplasia of the tibia. The whole child should be examined to rule out association with syndromes such as Ellis–van Creveld chondroectodermal dysplasia or Jeunes's infantile thoracic dystrophy.

Morphologically the extra digit may be preaxial, on the medial (big toe) side; postaxial, on the lateral (little toe) side; or it may be a duplication of one of the middle toes (central). The various forms of digital duplications of the foot are illustrated in Figures 7–126 to 7–133.

Surgical removal of the supernumerary toes is indicated for cosmetic reasons as well as for the sake of comfort in wearing shoes. The optimum age for surgery is between 9 and 12 months, when the infant begins to stand and walk. In deciding which toe is to be excised, the important consideration is the general contour of the foot. Usually the most peripheral toe is amputated, despite the fact that it may be more normal than the one adjacent to it. Radiograms of the foot should also be considered in the decision. The extra toe is amputated through a racquet-shaped incision at its base, and the tendons are divided near their insertion and sutured to the adjacent tendon to preserve function. A transverse incision is made in the capsule of the metatarsophalangeal joint, and the toe is disarticulated. Injury to the growth centers of the adjacent digits should be avoided. Any bony protrusion of the common metatarsal is sharply excised; if there is a corresponding supernumerary metatarsal, it is ablated through a proximal extension of the skin incision on the dorsolateral aspect of the foot. The capsule and ligaments are reconstructed to prevent malalignment of the neighboring toes.

References

1. Crawford, M. D., and Saldana-Garcia, P.: Brachydactyly and polydactyly with dermal ridge dissociation and ridge hypoplasia. J. Med. Genet., *16*:402, 1979.
2. Funderbunk, S. J., Sparkes, R. S., and Klisak, I.: The 9P syndrome. J. Med. Genet., *16*:75, 1979.
3. Mollica, F., Volti, S. L., and Sorge, G.: Autosomal recessive postaxial polydactyly type A in a Sicilian family. J. Med. Genet., *15*:212, 1978.
4. Pfeiffer, R. A., and Santelmann, R.: Limb anomalies in chromosomal aberrations. Birth Defects, *13*:319, 1977.
5. Schinzel, A.: Postaxial polydactyly, hallux duplication, absence of the corpus callosum, macrencephaly and severe mental retardation: A new syndrome? Helv. Paediatr. Acta, *34*:141, 1979.
6. Venn-Watson, E. A.: Problems in polydactyly of the foot. Orthop. Clin. North Am., *7*:909, 1976.
7. Waldrigues, A., Grohmann, L. C., Takahashi, T., and Reis, H. M.: Ellis–van Creveld syndrome. An inbred kindred with five cases. Rev. Bras. Pesqui. Med. Biol., *10*:193, 1977.

Text continued on page 2649

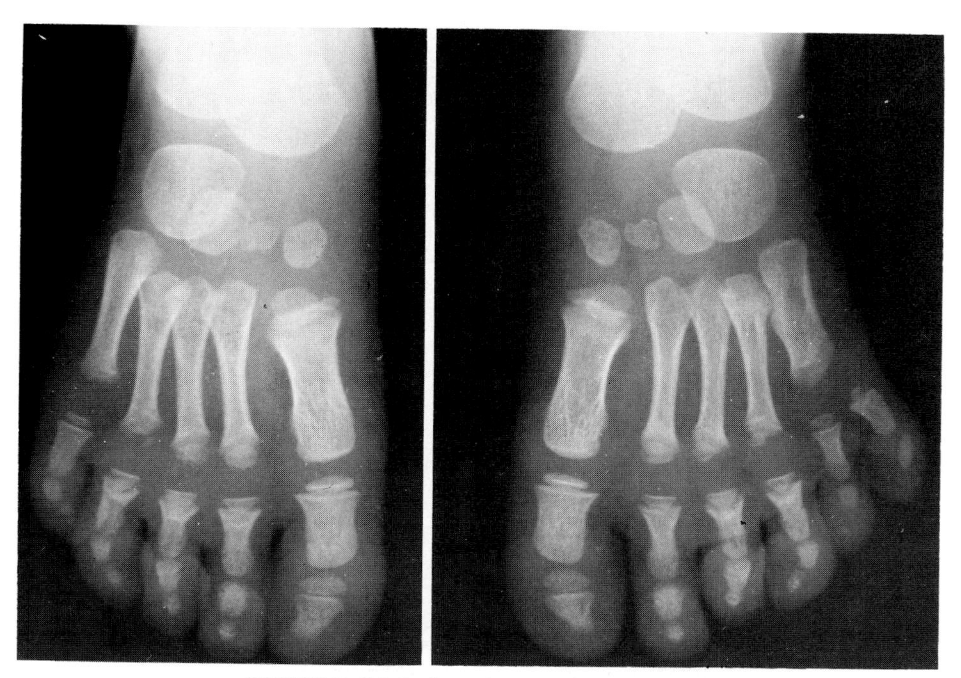

FIGURE 7–126. Unilateral postaxial polydactyly.

The fifth and sixth toes share a common fifth metatarsal.

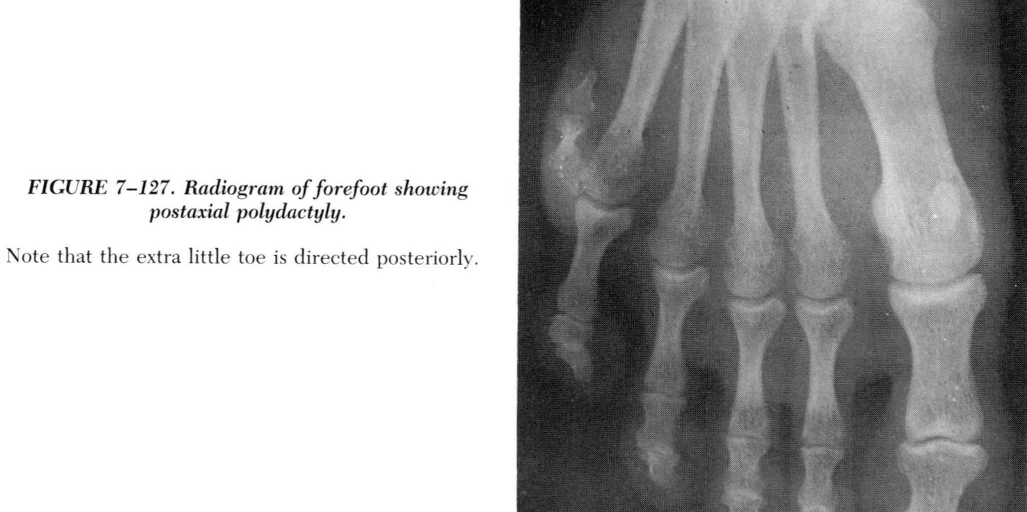

FIGURE 7–127. Radiogram of forefoot showing postaxial polydactyly.

Note that the extra little toe is directed posteriorly.

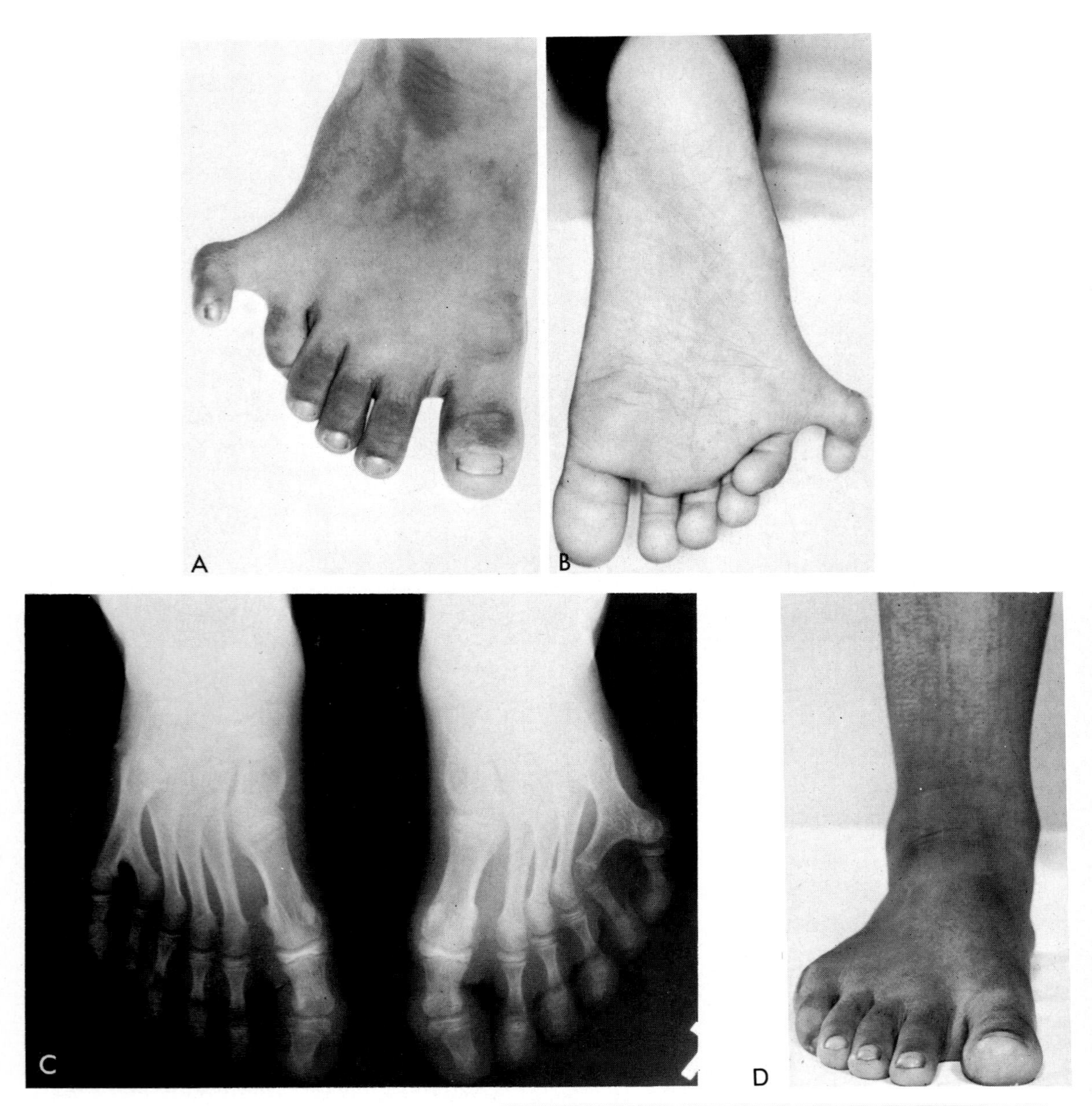

FIGURE 7–128. Postaxial polydactyly.

A and **B.** Clinical appearance of right foot. **C.** Anteroposterior radiogram of both feet. Note the bilateral involvement and fusion of the supernumerary metatarsals at their distal third. **D** and **E.** Postoperative photographs of the right foot showing result.

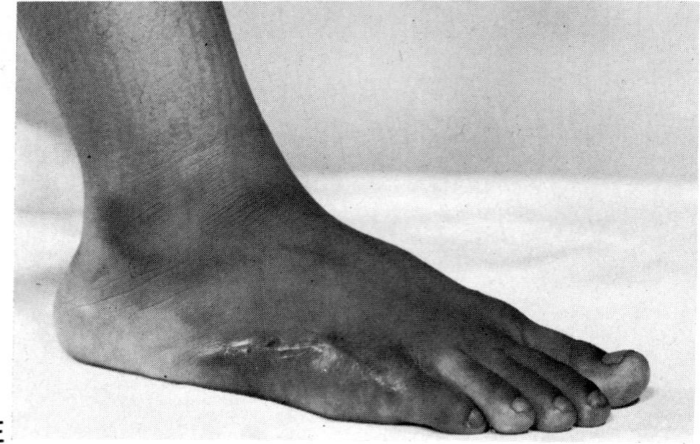

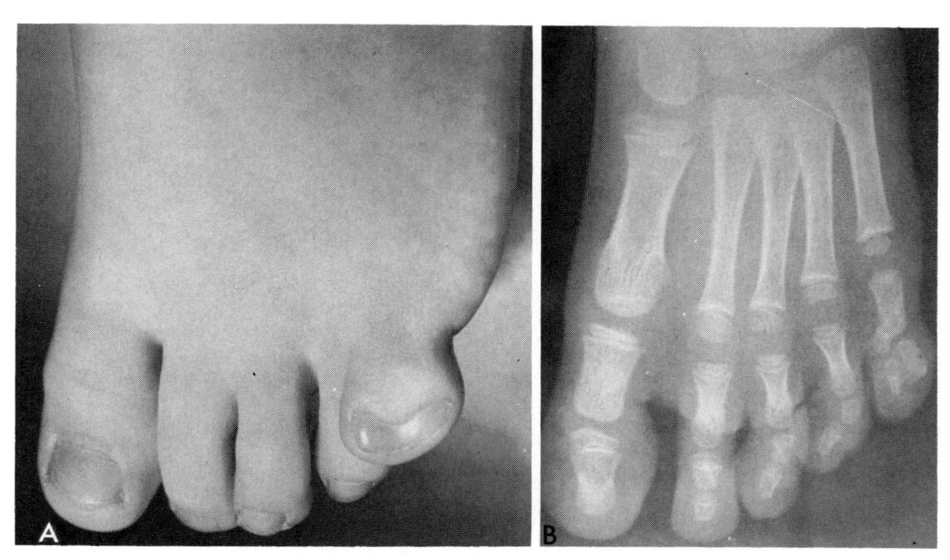

FIGURE 7–129. Postaxial polydactyly with syndactyly of little toe.

A. Clinical appearance. **B.** Radiogram showing that only the distal and middle phalanges are duplicated. This is best treated by excision of the distal and middle phalanges of the extra digit on the tibial side and surgical syndactyly of the sixth toe to the fourth toe.

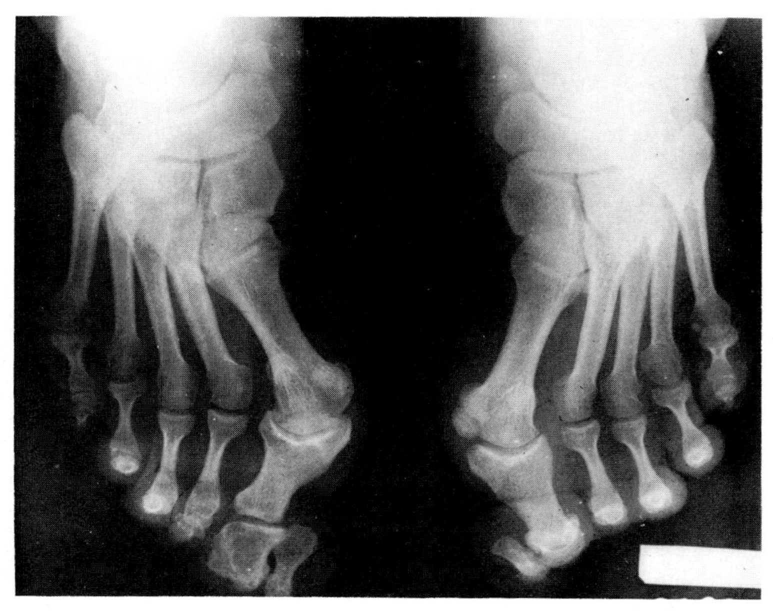

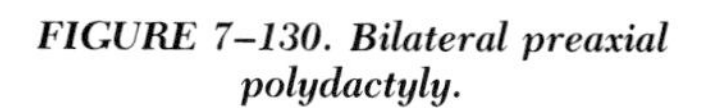

FIGURE 7–130. Bilateral preaxial polydactyly.

The radiogram shows that only the distal phalanx of the great toe is duplicated. There is associated hallux valgus and metatarsus primus varus.

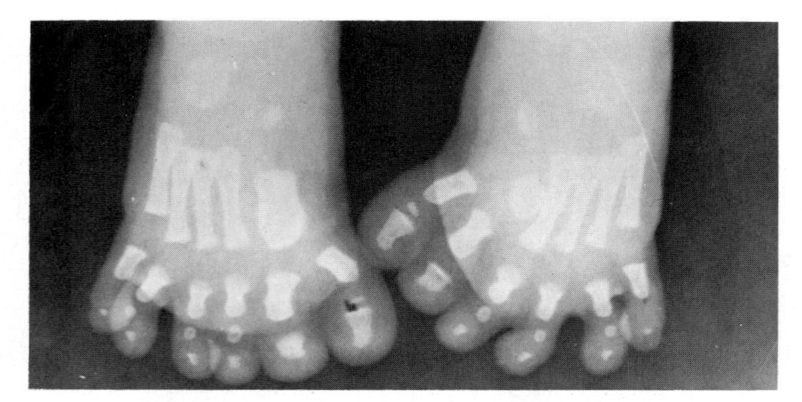

FIGURE 7–131. *Bilateral preaxial polydactyly.*

Both phalanges of the great toe are duplicated.

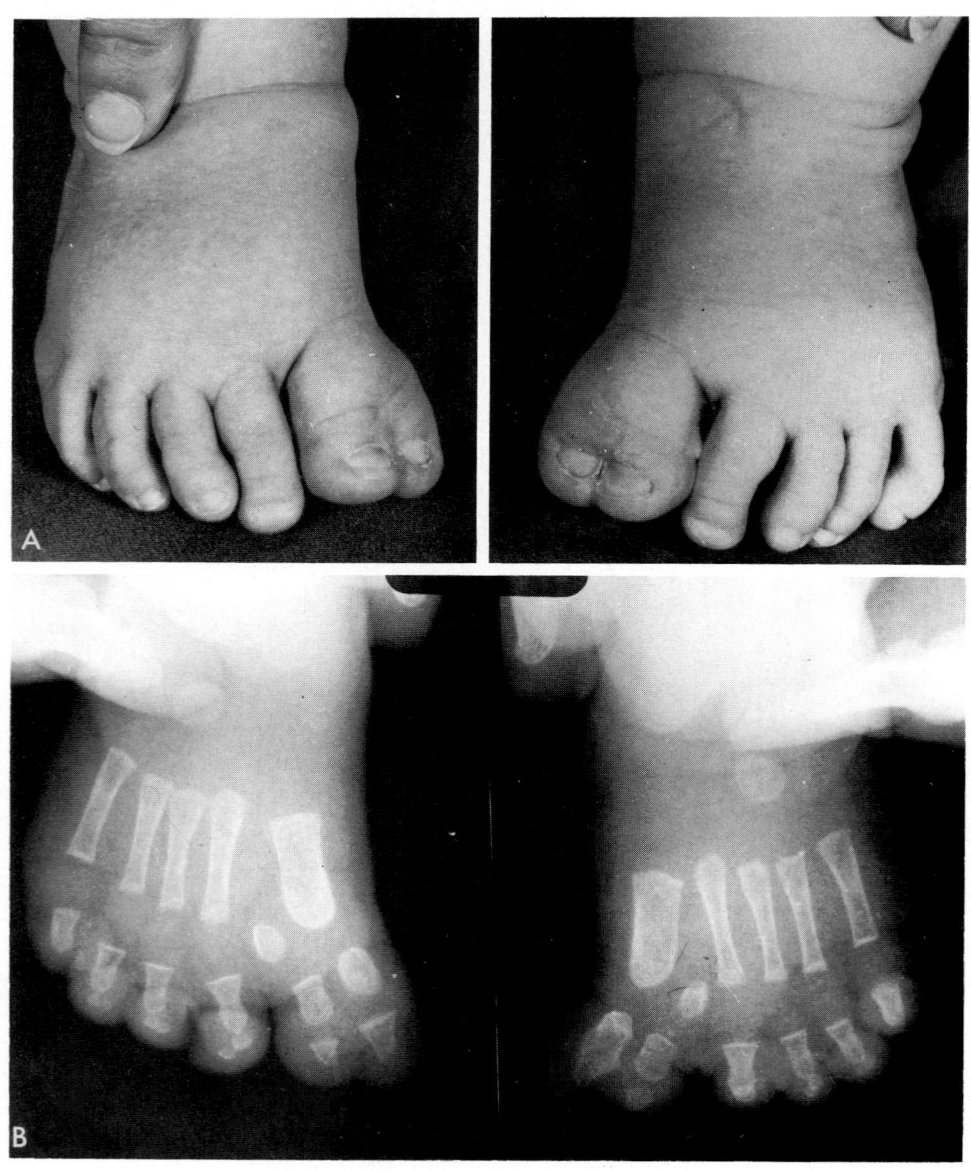

FIGURE 7–132. *Bilateral preaxial polydactyly.*

Both distal and proximal phalanges of the great toes and the distal end of the metatarsals are duplicated. **A.** Clinical appearance. **B.** Anteroposterior radiograms of the feet.

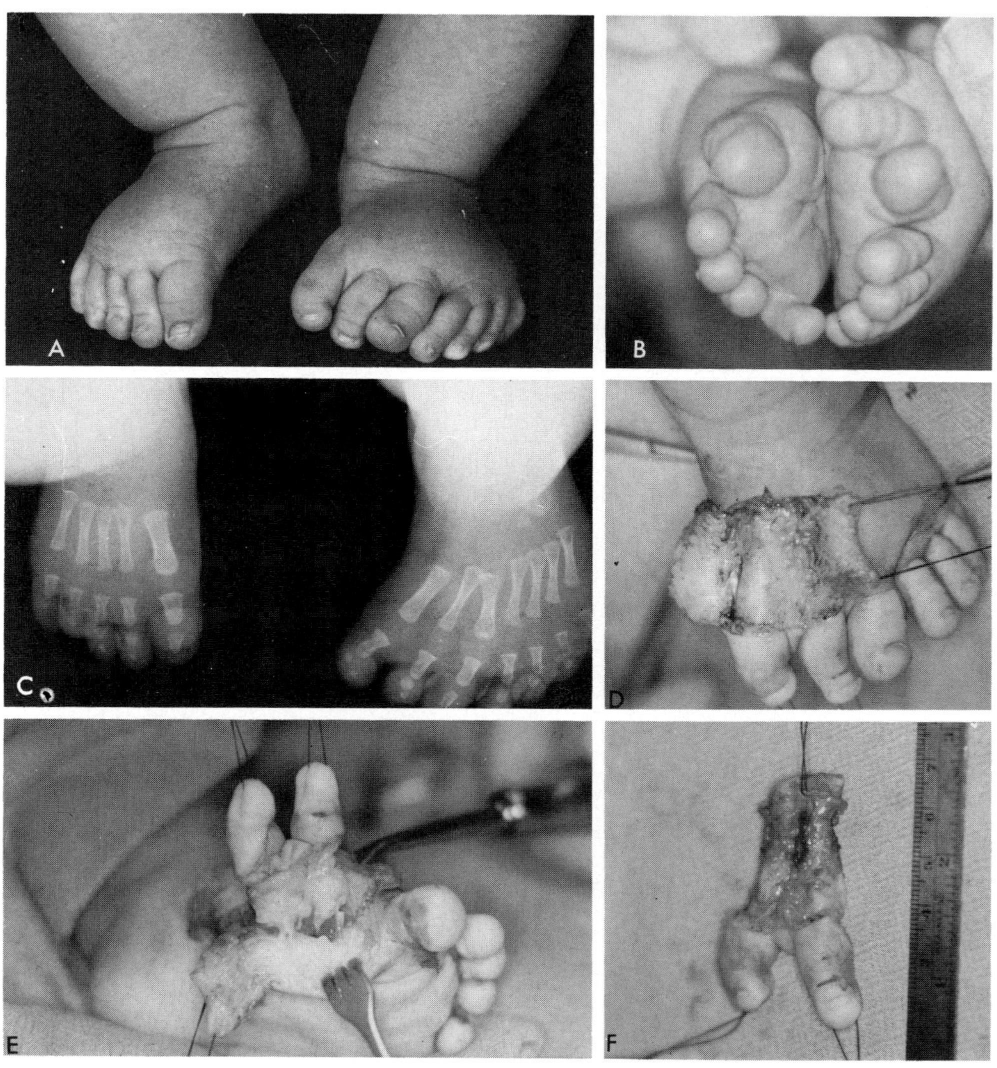

FIGURE 7–133. Polydactyly of left foot.

A and **B.** Clinical appearance. Note the swan toes on the left foot. **C.** Radiogram showing that both the phalanges and metatarsals of the supernumerary digital rays are present. **D.** The skin incision and the raising of the wound flaps. **E** and **F.** The medial two digital rays are dissected and excised.

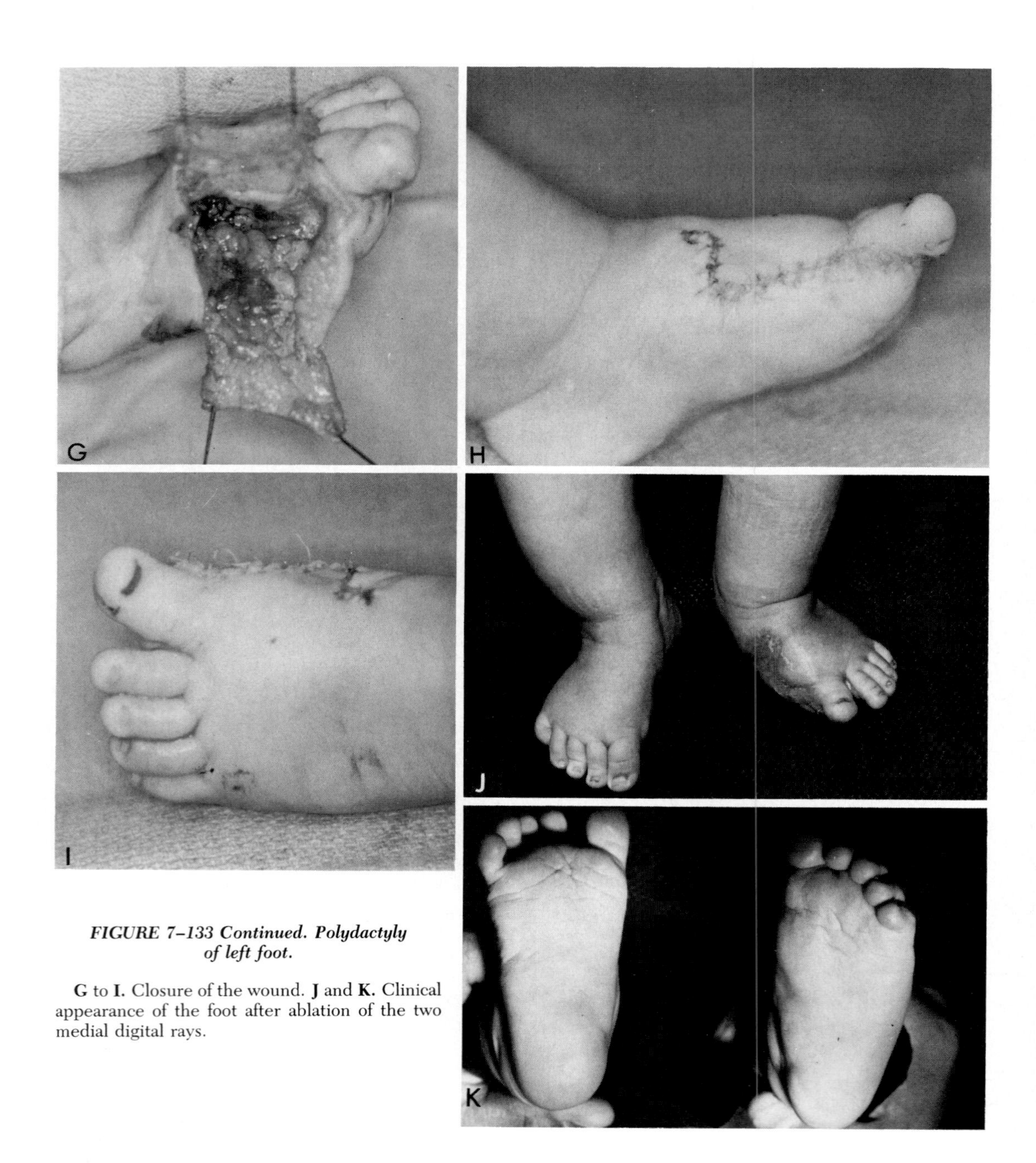

FIGURE 7–133 Continued. Polydactyly of left foot.

G to **I.** Closure of the wound. **J** and **K.** Clinical appearance of the foot after ablation of the two medial digital rays.

CONGENITAL HALLUX VARUS

In this deformity there is congenital medial angulation of the great toe at the metatarsophalangeal joint. There are several types of congenital hallux varus: (1) a primary type, not associated with any other congenital anomaly, in which a taut fibrous band extends from the medial side of the great toe to the base of the first metatarsal and progressively pulls the great toe toward the midline; (2) a type associated with congenital deformities of the forepart of the foot, namely hallux varus with metatarsus varus, hallux varus with isolated congenital marked shortening of the first metatarsal, and hallux varus with accessory bones or toes, as shown in Figures 7–134 and 7–135; and (3) hallux varus associated with extensive developmental affections of the skeleton, as in diastrophic dwarfism.

The method of treatment depends upon the type of hallux varus. The deformity is satisfactorily corrected by any one of the surgical methods of McElvenny, Farmer, or Kelikian and associates.[2, 10, 13] The contracted fibrous band on the medial aspect of the great toe, the taut abductor hallucis, and the shortened medial capsule of the metatarsophalangeal joint of the big toe are released. Any accessory phalanx or bone is excised, and surgical syndactylism between the great and second toes is carried out to maintain correction. Capsuloplasty on the lateral side of the metatarsophalangeal joint and extensor hallucis tendon rerouting will assist in holding the hallux in proper anatomic alignment. A Kirschner wire is inserted into

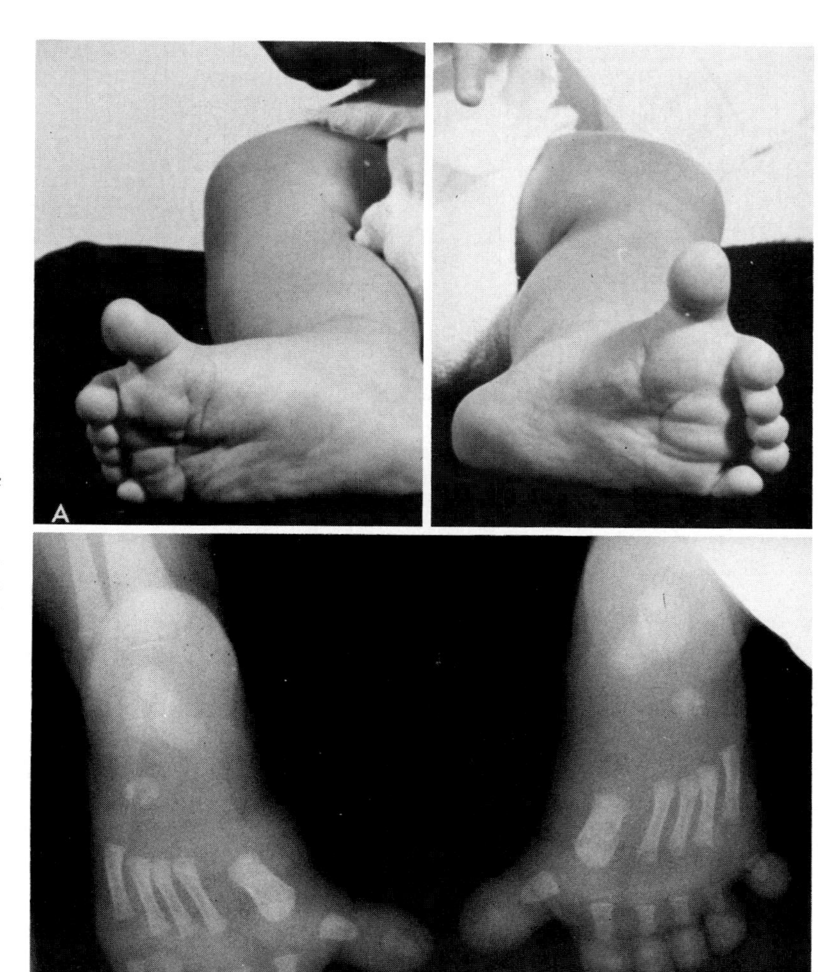

FIGURE 7–134. Congenital hallux varus due to preaxial polydactyly of great toe.

A. Clinical appearance. **B.** Radiogram. Only the phalanges of the hallux are duplicated; note also the stout first metatarsal.

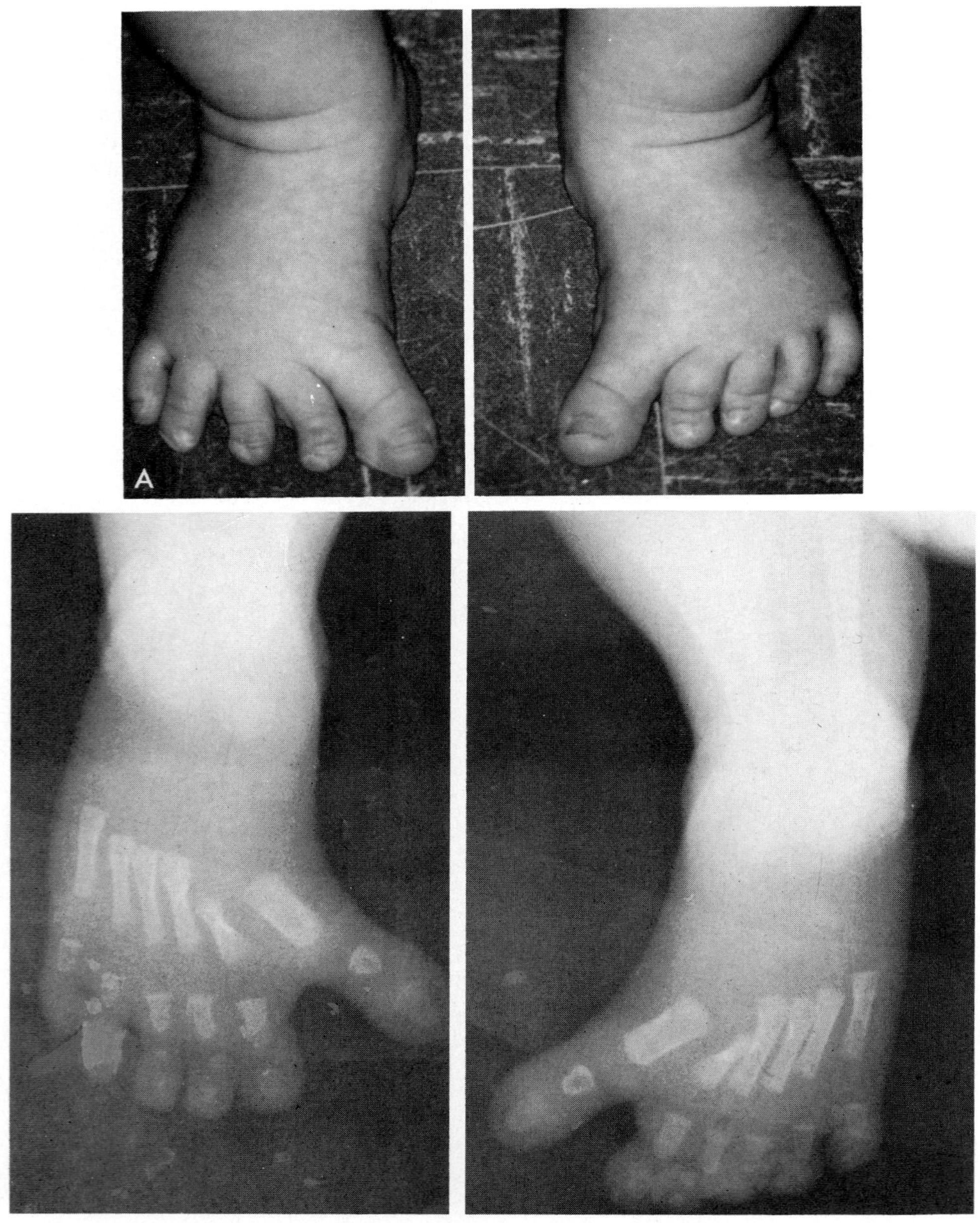

FIGURE 7–135. Bilateral congenital hallux varus due to preaxial polydactyly of great toe.

A. Clinical appearance. **B.** Radiograms of the feet.

the great toe, across the metatarsophalangeal joint, and into the first metatarsal for three weeks to maintain correction.

References

1. Bishop, J., Kahn, A. D., and Turba, J. E.: Surgical correction of the splayfoot. The Giannestras procedure. Clin. Orthop., *146*:234, 1980.
2. Farmer, A. W.: Congenital hallux varus. Am. J. Surg., *95*:274, 1958.
3. Haas, S. L.: An operation for correction of hallux varus. J. Bone Joint Surg., *20*:705, 1938.
4. Hawkins, F. B.: Acquired hallux varus: Cause, prevention and correction. Clin. Orthop., *76*:169, 1971.
5. Horwitz, M. T.: An unusual hallux varus deformity and its surgical correction. J. Bone Joint Surg., *19*:828, 1937.
6. Huurman, W. W.: Congenital foot deformities. *In* Mann, R. A. (ed.): Surgery of the Foot. St. Louis, Mosby, 1986, p. 555.
7. Jahss, M. H.: Spontaneous hallux varus: Relation to poliomyelitis and congenital absence of fibular sesamoid. Foot Ankle, *3*:224, 1983.
8. Johnson, K. A., and Spiegl, P. V.: Extensor hallucis longus transfer for hallux varus deformity. J. Bone Joint Surg., *66-A*:681, 1984.
9. Kelikian, H.: The hallux. *In* Jahss, M. H. (ed.): Disorders of the Foot. Philadelphia, Saunders, 1982, pp. 616–618.
10. Kelikian, H., Clayton, L., and Loseff, H.: Surgical syndactylism of the toes. Clin. Orthop., *19*:208, 1961.
11. Kimizuka, M., and Miyanaga, Y.: The treatment of acquired hallux varus after the McBride procedure. J. Foot Surg., *19*:135, 1980.
12. Kleiner, B. C., and Holmes, L. B.: Brief clinical report: Hallux varus and preaxial polysyndactyly in brothers. Am. J. Med. Genet., *6*:113, 1980.
13. McElvenny, R. T.: Hallux varus. Q. Bull. Northwest. Med. Sch., *15*:277, 1941.
14. Miller, J. W.: Acquired hallux varus: A preventable and correctable disorder. J. Bone Joint Surg., *57-A*:183, 1975.
15. Myginal, H. B.: Surgical correction of congenital hallux varus. Nord. Med., *49*:914, 1953.
16. Poehling, G. G., and DeTorre, J.: Hallux varus and hammertoe deformity. Orthop. Trans., *6*:186, 1982.
17. Sloane, D.: Congenital hallux varus. Operative correction. J. Bone Joint Surg., *17*:209, 1935.
18. Thomson, S. A.: Hallux varus and metatarsus varus. Clin. Orthop., *16*:109, 1960.
19. Turner, R. S.: Dynamic post-surgical hallux varus after lateral sesamoidectomy: Treatment and prevention. Orthopedics, *9*:963, 1986.
20. Wood, W. A.: Acquired hallux varus: A new corrective procedure. J. Foot Surg., *20*:194, 1981.

MACRODACTYLISM

Gigantism of one or more toes is a rare deformity. The hypertrophy is frequently caused either by neurofibromatosis or by congenital hyperplasia of lymphatic and adipose tissue (Figs. 7–136 and 7–137). A grotesque appearance, difficulty in shoe-fitting, and interference with weight-bearing are indications for surgical treatment.

The operation is performed in two or three steps. First, the proximal phalanx is resected, and the toe is partially defatted on one side. The growth plate of the middle phalanx is arrested. Alignment is maintained by syndactyly of the affected toe with its neighboring toe. Several months later, hypertrophied tissue is resected on the opposite side (Fig. 7–138). If the corresponding metatarsal is enlarged, its growth is arrested by epiphyseodesis at the appropriate age. Amputation of a gigantic second toe should not be performed, as its removal will lead to hallux valgus deformity. Severe macrodactyly of the third toe, however, may be treated by amputation of the affected toe, partial resection of the corresponding metatarsal, and surgical syndactyly of the second toe to the fourth toe.

References

1. Ackland, M. K., and Uhthoff, H. K.: Idiopathic localized gigantism: 26 year follow-up. J. Pediatr. Orthop., *6*:618, 1986.
2. Barsky, A. J.: Macrodactyly. J. Bone Joint Surg., *49-A*:1255, 1967.
3. Bouvet, J. P., Huc de Bat, J. M., Benoit, J., and Ramadier, J. O.: Bilateral symmetrical macrodactyly of the toes (author's transl.). Rev. Chir. Orthop., *66*:331, 1980.
4. Charters, A. D.: Local gigantism. J. Bone Joint Surg., *39-B*:542, 1957.
5. Dennyson, W. G., Bear, J. N., and Bhoola, K. D.: Macrodactyly in the foot. J. Bone Joint Surg., *59-B*:355, 1977.
6. Devalentine, S., Scurran, B. L., Tuerk, D., and Karlin, J. M.: Macrodactyly of the lower extremity: A review with two case reports. J. Am. Podiatry Assoc., *71*:175, 1981.
7. El-Shami, I. N.: Congenital partial gigantism. Surgery, *65*:683, 1969.
8. Gonzalez-Crussi, F.: The pathology of congenital localized gigantism. Plast. Reconstr. Surg., *59*:411, 1977.
9. Herring, J. A., and Tolo, V. T.: Macrodactyly. J. Pediatr. Orthop., *4*:503, 1984.
10. Kumar, K., Kumar, D., Gadegone, W. M., and Kapahtia, N. K.: Macrodactyly of the hand and foot. Int. Orthop., *9*:259, 1985.
11. Ofodile, F. A., and Oluwasanmi, J.: Pedal macrodactyly—report of seven cases. East Afr. Med. J., *56*:283, 1979.
12. Perdive, R. L., Mason, W. H., and Bernard, T. M.: Macrodactyly: A rare malformation. Review of the literature and case report. J. Am. Podiatry Assoc., *69*:657, 1979.
13. Tsuge, K.: Treatment of macrodactyly. Plast. Reconstr. Surg., *41*:232, 1968.
14. Tuli, S. M., Khanna, N. N., and Sinha, G. P.: Congenital macrodactyly. Br. J. Plast. Surg., *22*:237, 1969.

MISCELLANEOUS DEFORMITIES OF TOES

Microdactylism

Small toes may be an isolated deformity, with or without hypoplasia of the corresponding metatarsals, or may be associated with Streeter's

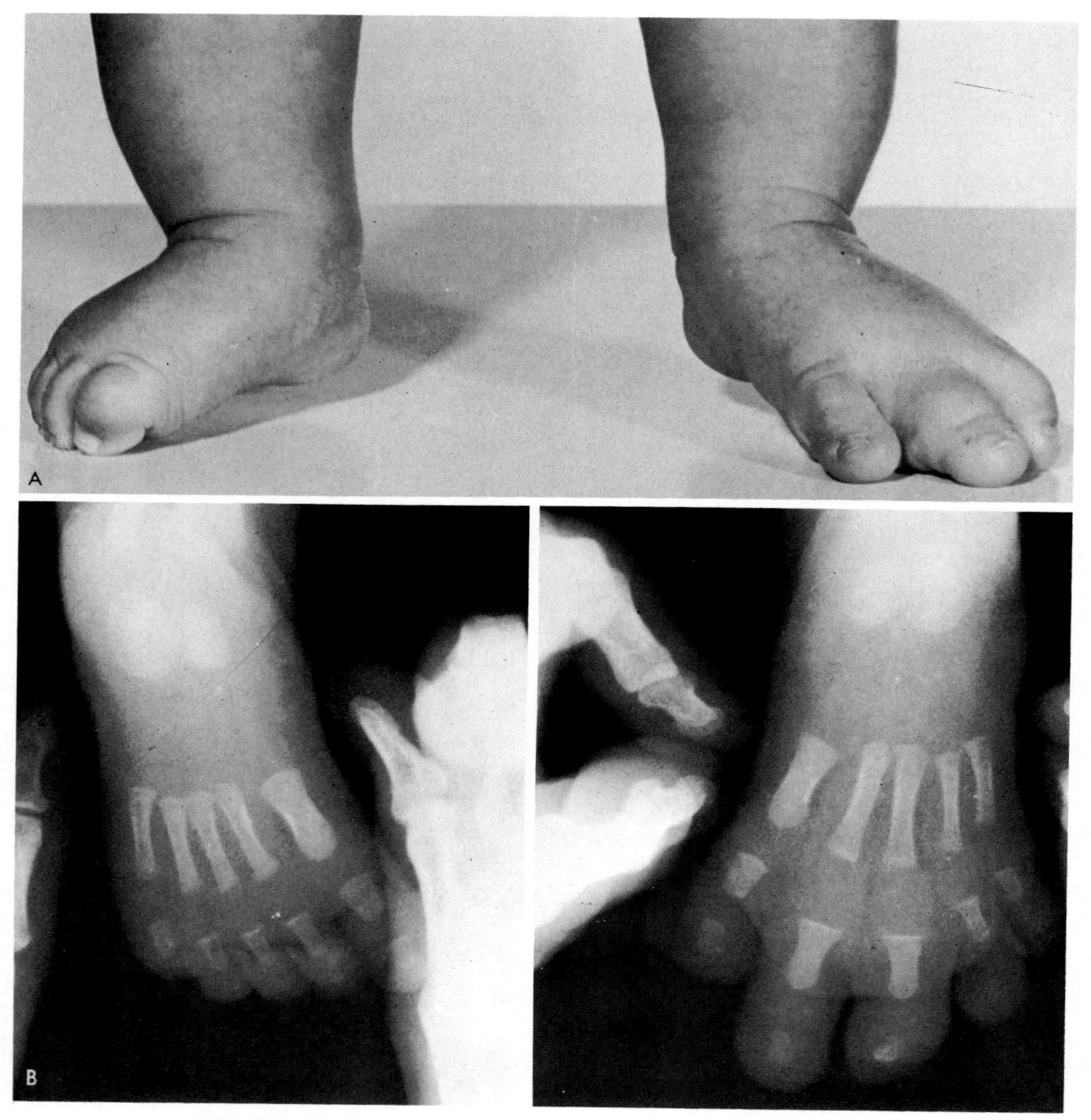

FIGURE 7–136. Macrodactyly of the second and third digits of the left foot.

A. Clinical appearance. **B.** Radiograms of the feet.

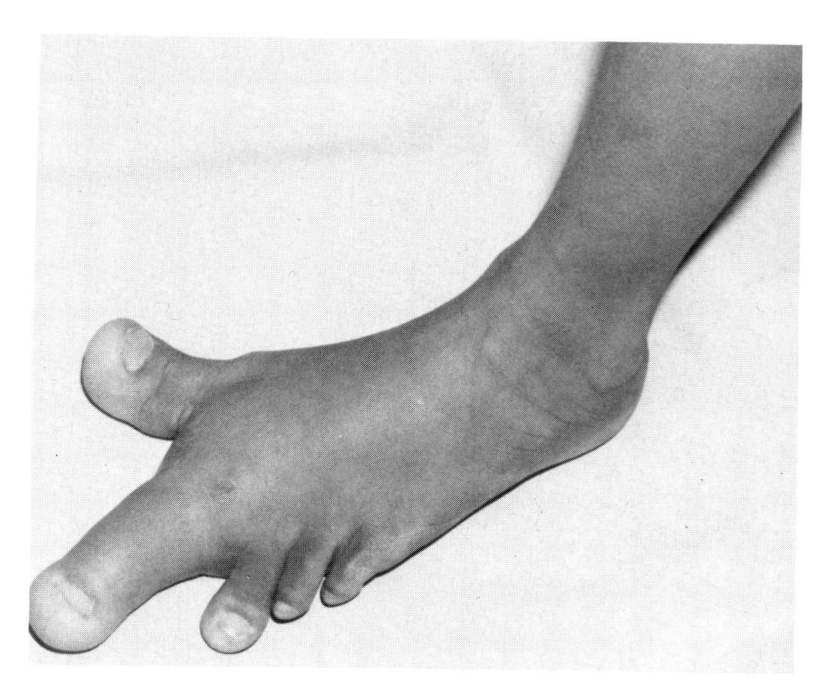

FIGURE 7–137. Macrodactyly of the second toe in an adolescent.

dysplasia. Because they do not usually cause disability, treatment is not required.

Syndactylism

Congenital webbing of the toes neither causes disability nor interferes with function. Cosmetically it is usually not objectionable, and no treatment is necessary (Figs. 7–139 to 7–141). If webbing is associated with polydactylism, the most peripheral digit is excised to facilitate shoe wear (Fig. 7–142).

Divergent or Convergent Toes

These may occur as an isolated angular deformity, without flexion contracture of the distal interphalangeal joint (Fig. 7–143). In minimal deformity, treatment is not necessary. In severe cases, when the angulated toe underrides or overrides the adjacent toe, surgical syndactylism of the affected toes is indicated; in adolescents, it is combined with proximal phalangectomy.

Congenital Digitus Minimus Varus

Congenital dorsal overriding of the fifth toe is a common familial deformity in which the fifth metatarsophalangeal joint is subluxated dorsomedially. The fifth toe is hyperextended and adducted, lying across the base of the fourth toe (Fig. 7–144). The capsule of the metatarsophalangeal joint is contracted on its dorsomedial aspect. The extensor tendon is shortened, and the skin on the dorsum of the fifth and between the fourth and fifth toes is taut. In severe deformity, the fifth toe becomes rotated on its longitudinal axis with its nail pointing laterally. There is no flexion deformity of the interphalangeal joints. A hard callus often develops over the dorsum of the fifth toe because of irritation caused by the shoe. The condition is usually bilateral. It causes disability in about half the affected patients.

TREATMENT

In the infant and the young child, conservative measures are indicated: passive stretching of the little toe in plantar flexion and abduction, and strapping of the little toe in normal alignment with adhesive tape. Usually, however, these methods do not correct the deformity and, in the adolescent, if symptoms warrant it, operative correction is necessary.

Numerous surgical procedures have been proposed in the literature: (1) transfer of the extensor tendon of the fifth toe to the neck of the fifth metatarsal (Lantzounis); (2) division of the extensor tendon of the fifth toe over the dorsum of the midfoot and transfer of its distal

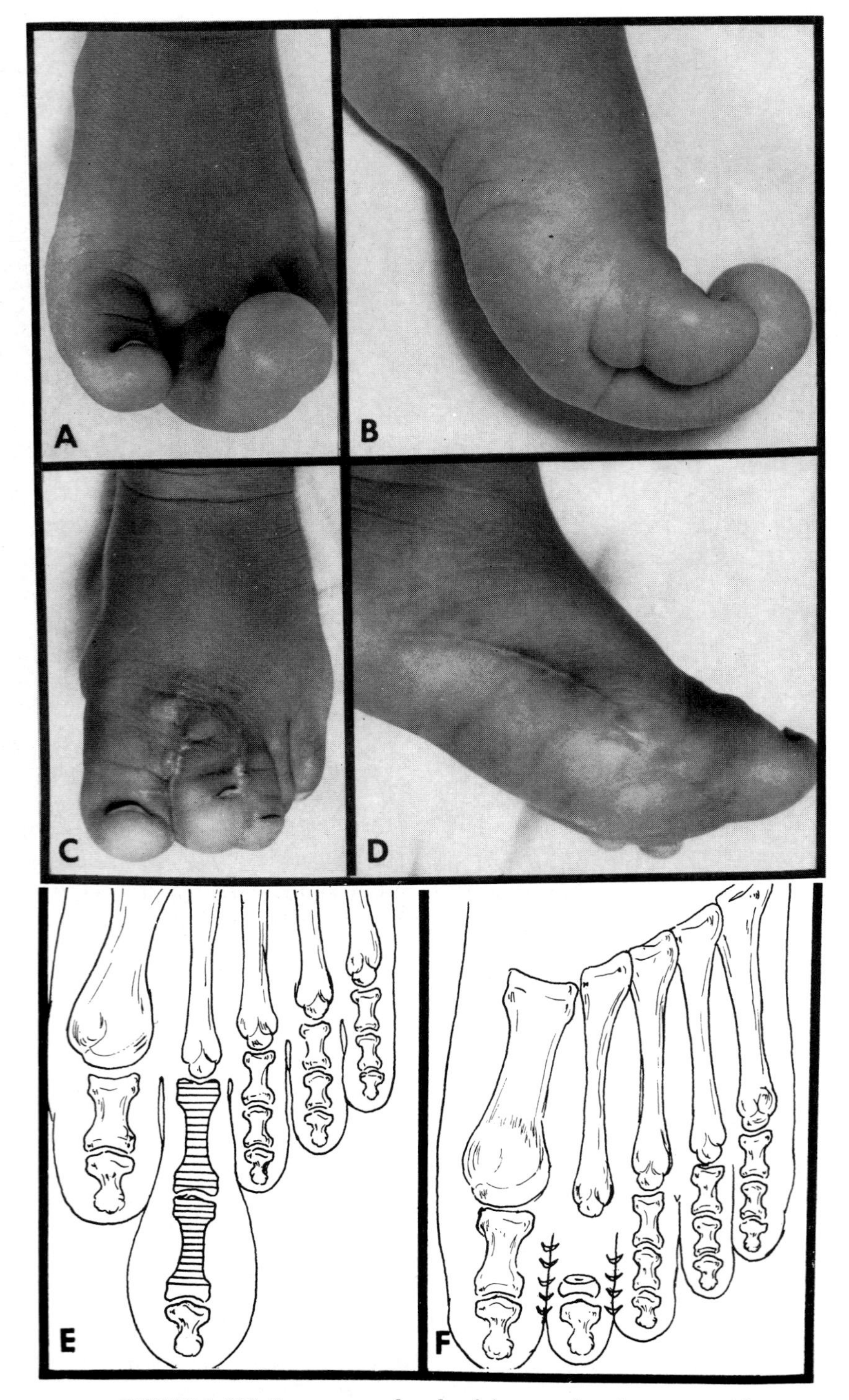

FIGURE 7–138. Severe macrodactyly of the second toe in a young girl.

A and **B.** Preoperative photographs. The deformity was treated in two stages: first the proximal phalanx of the second toe was excised, and the toe was defatted from its medial side and syndactylized to the big toe; three months later, the middle phalanx of the second toe was excised, and the toe was defatted from its lateral side and syndactylized with the third digit. The medial plantar nerve was normal on exploration. **C** and **D.** Postoperative photographs. **E** and **F.** Interpretive diagrams show the amount of bone resected. Amputation of the second toe should not be performed, as it will lead to hallux valgus. (From Kelikian, H.: Hallux Valgus, Allied Deformities of the Forefoot and Metatarsalgia. Philadelphia, Saunders, 1965, p. 332. Reprinted by permission.)

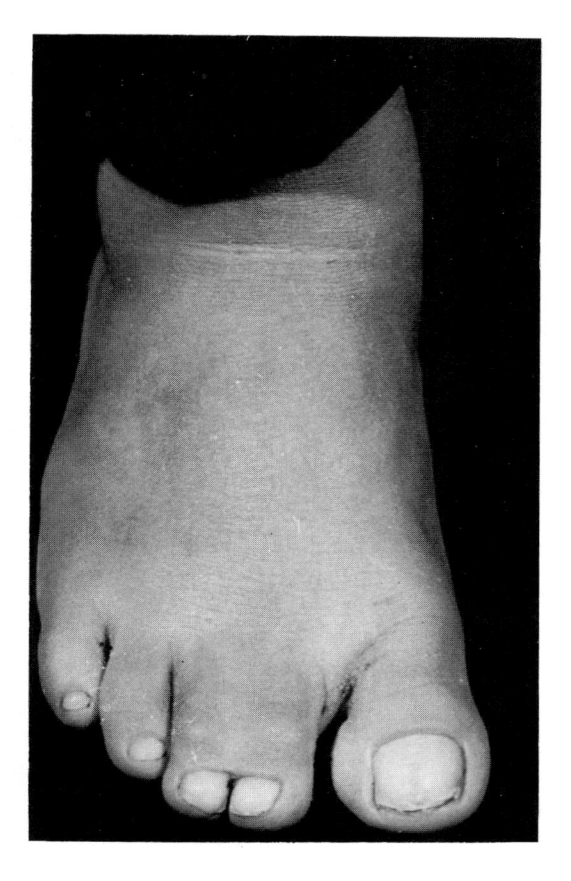

FIGURE 7–139. Syndactyly of the second and third toes.

segment to the abductor digiti quinti by rerouting the tendon from the medial to the lateral side of the proximal phalanx (Lapidus); (3) Z-plastic lengthening of the extensor tendon, dorsal and medial capsulotomy of the metatarsophalangeal joint, and plastic lengthening of the contracted skin fold (Goodwin and Swisher Y-plasty, Wilson and DuVries V and Y–plasty, Thompson Z-plasty); (4) excision of the proximal phalanx through a lateral incision (Gocht and DeBrunner); (5) excision of the proximal phalanx and surgical syndactyly of the fourth and fifth toes; and (6) amputation of the fifth toe.[12–14, 19–23, 31, 32]

The author recommends tenotomy of the extensor tendon, dorsal and medial capsulotomy of the fifth metatarsophalangeal joint, excision of the proximal phalanx, and fusion of the skin (surgical syndactylism) of the fourth and fifth toes as shown in Figure 7–145. The operative technique is described and illustrated in Plate 103 (see p. 2662). In children the proximal phalanx is partially excised, leaving the growth plate at its base intact. The results of the McFarland operation are very satisfactory.[23]

Plastic procedures involving V-Y elongation of the skin and soft tissues are not recommended by the author because they often result in an ugly scar that is cosmetically undesirable. Sometimes a keloid may form, which may be irritated by the shoe.

Cockin recommends the Butler operation, as it is safe and simple, and full correction of the deformity is obtained without tension.[10] He reported the results of 70 operations performed on 19 male and 36 female patients; the result was good in 91 per cent, fair in 6 per cent, and poor in 3 per cent. In the failures, the deformity recurred rapidly (within a year) and was then treated by amputation. Circulatory embarrassment to the little toe is prevented by avoiding traction on the neurovascular bundles. In the experience of Cockin, there has been no circulatory damage to the toe, and wound healing has not been a problem. The operative technique of the Butler operation is as follows:

A dorsal racquet incision is made on the skin; then a second handle is added to the racquet on the plantar aspect (the plantar handle inclined laterally and a little longer than the dorsal handle) (Fig. 7–145 A and B). The wound flaps are undermined and elevated, exposing the

Text continued on page 2661

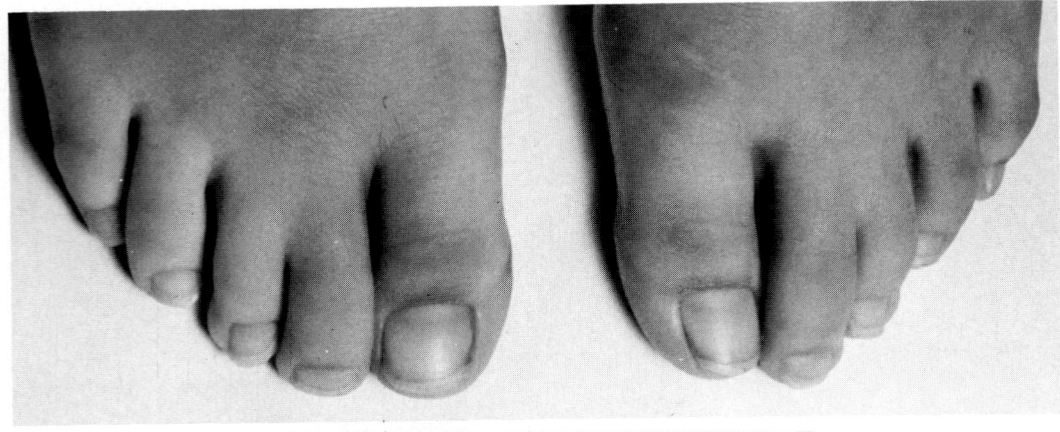

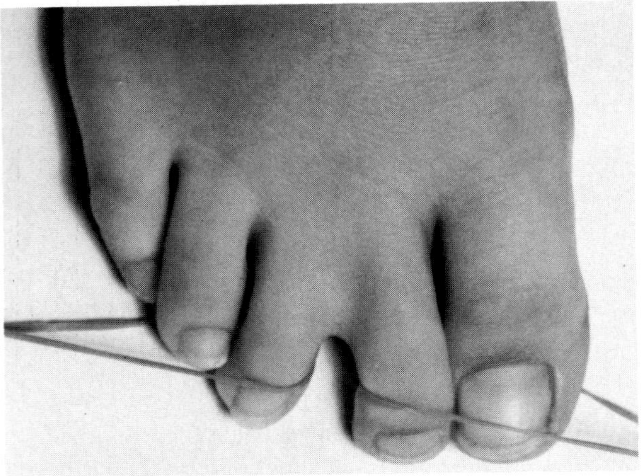

FIGURE 7–140. Congenital webbing of toes.

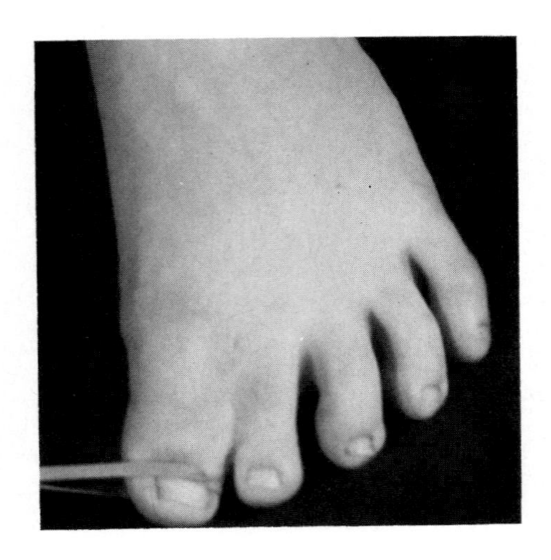

FIGURE 7–141. Congenital syndactyly between the great and second toes.

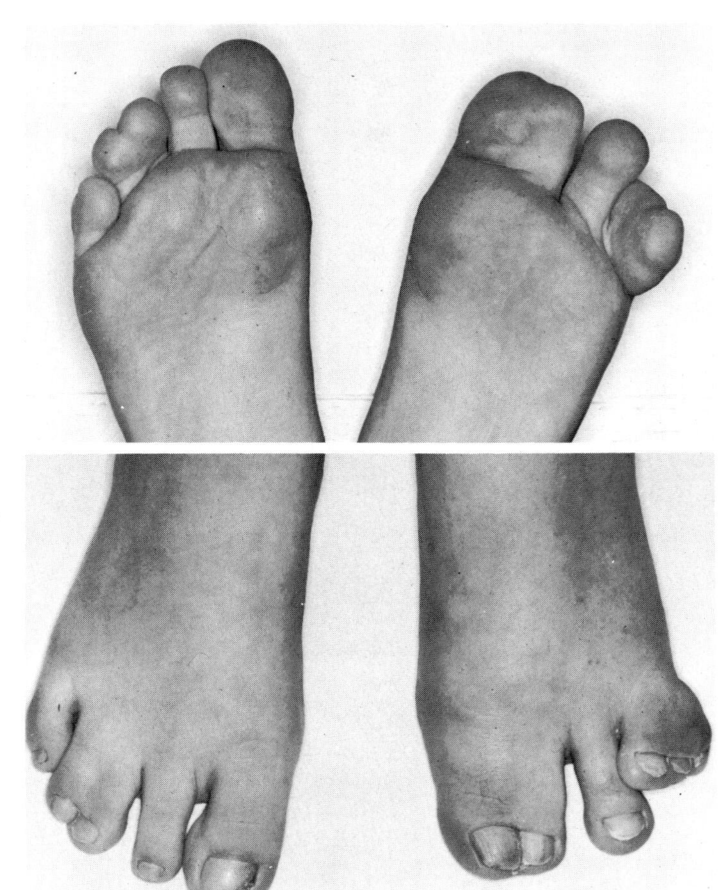

FIGURE 7–142. Congenital syndactylism of the fourth and fifth toes and the first and second toes on the right foot and the third and fourth toes on the left foot.

In the right foot, there is a supernumerary digit. It was surgically excised.

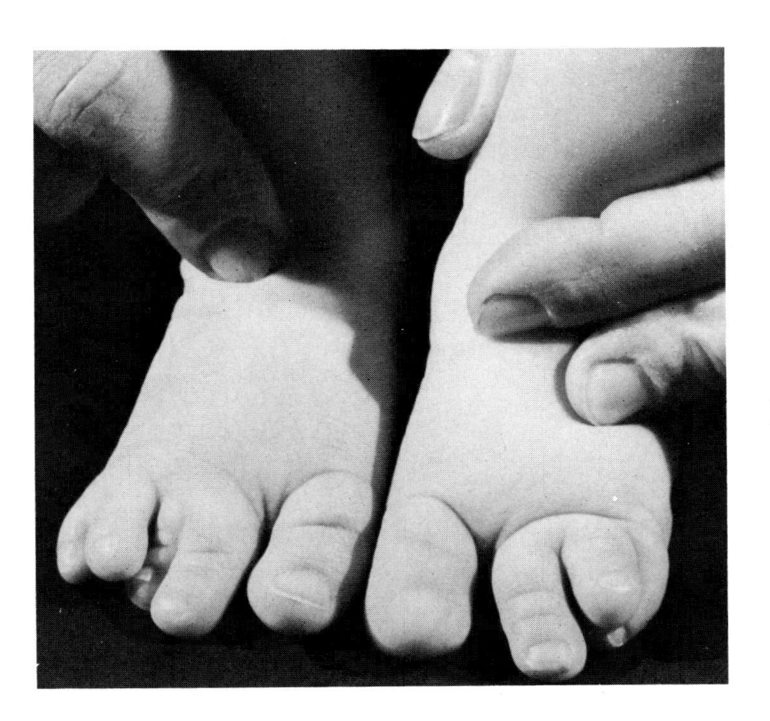

FIGURE 7–143. Angular deformity of toes.

Fourth toe on the right foot overrides the third toe. In the left foot, there are only three lesser toes and metatarsals.

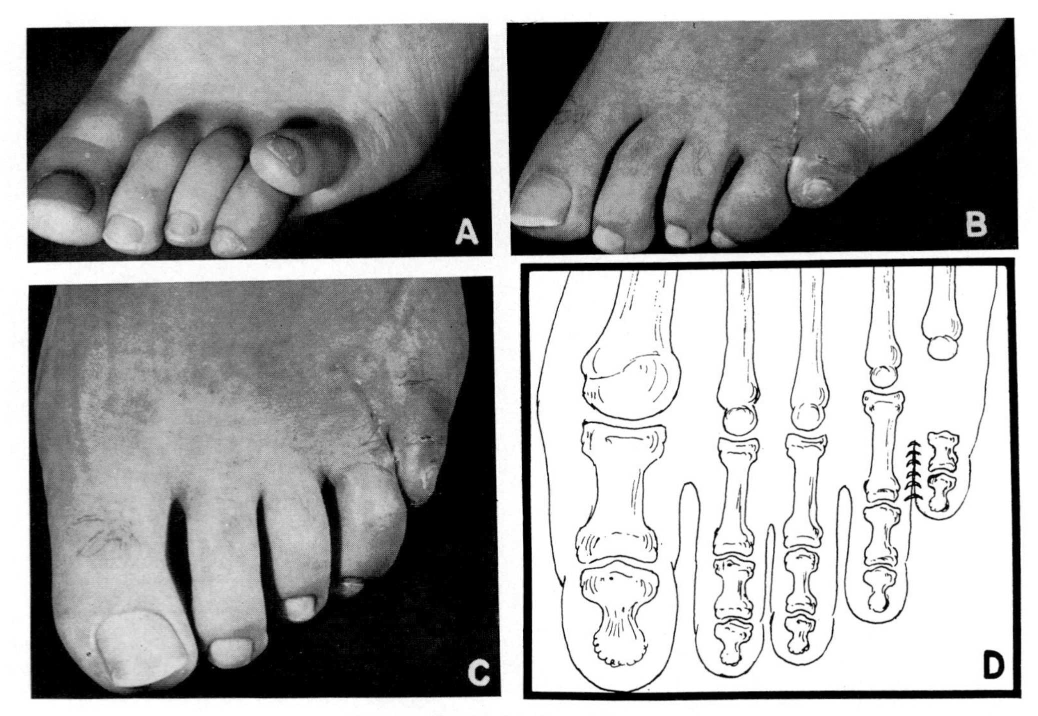

FIGURE 7–144. Digitus minimus varus.

Deformity was treated by excision of the proximal phalanx of the little toe, extensor tenotomy, dorsal capsulotomy of the fifth metatarsophalangeal joint, and surgical syndactyly of the fifth and fourth toes. **A.** Preoperative photograph. **B** and **C.** Postoperative photographs. **D.** Interpretive diagram. (From Kelikian H.: Hallux Valgus, Allied Deformities of the Forefoot and Metatarsalgia. Philadelphia, Saunders, 1965, p. 328. Reprinted by permission.)

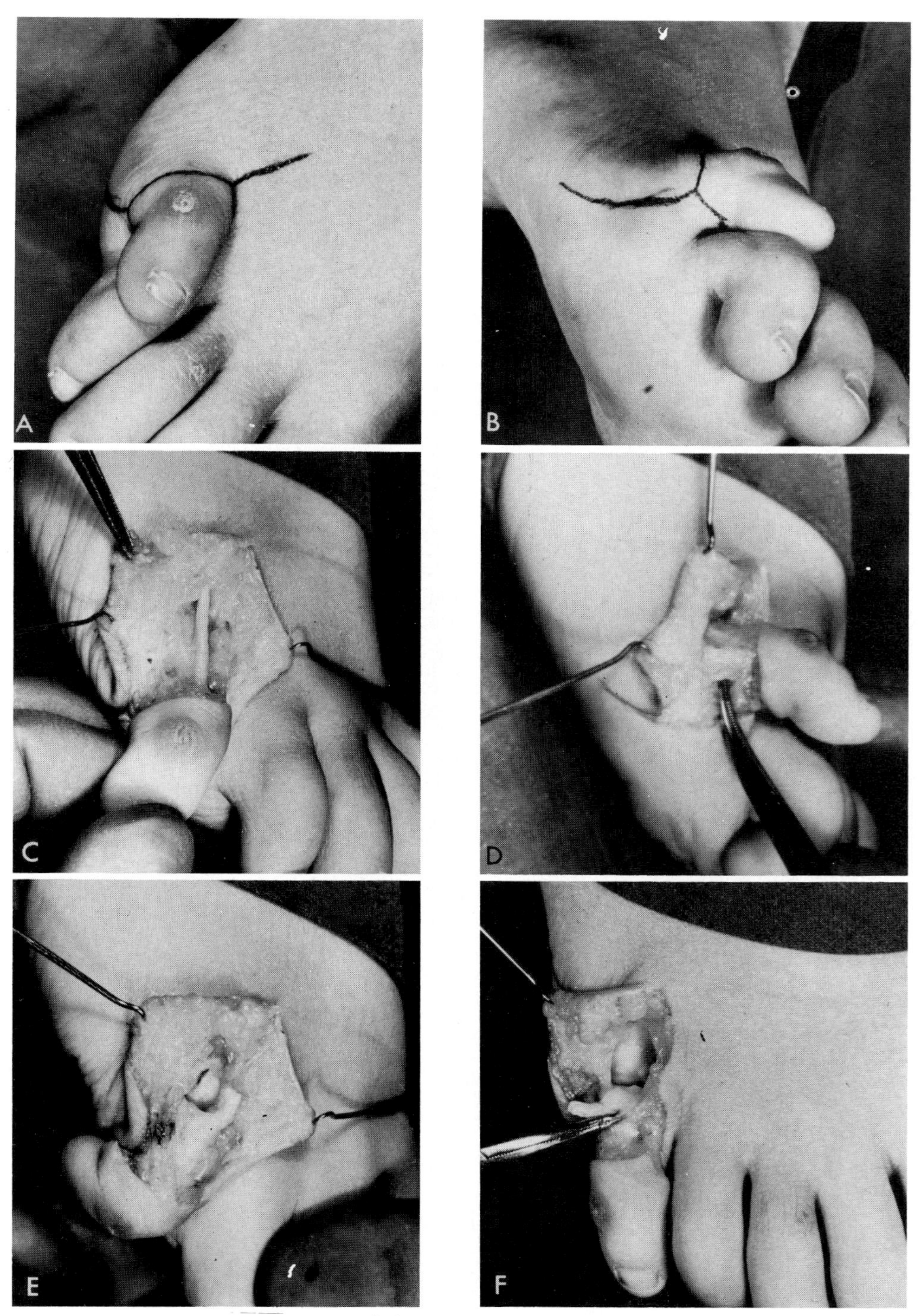

FIGURE 7–145. Butler's operation for an overriding fifth toe.

A and **B.** A dorsal racquet incision is made with a second handle added on the plantar aspect. The plantar handle is inclined laterally and is a little longer than the dorsal handle. **C** and **D.** The contracted extensor tendon to the fifth toe is exposed by elevating the skin flaps. The neurovascular bundles should be identified and carefully preserved. **E.** Sectioning of the extensor tendon and the dorsomedial part of the capsule of the metatarsophalangeal joint. **F.** In severe deformity, the articular surfaces of the metatarsophalangeal joints may be incongruous. This is due to plantar capsular adhesions.

Illustration continued on following page

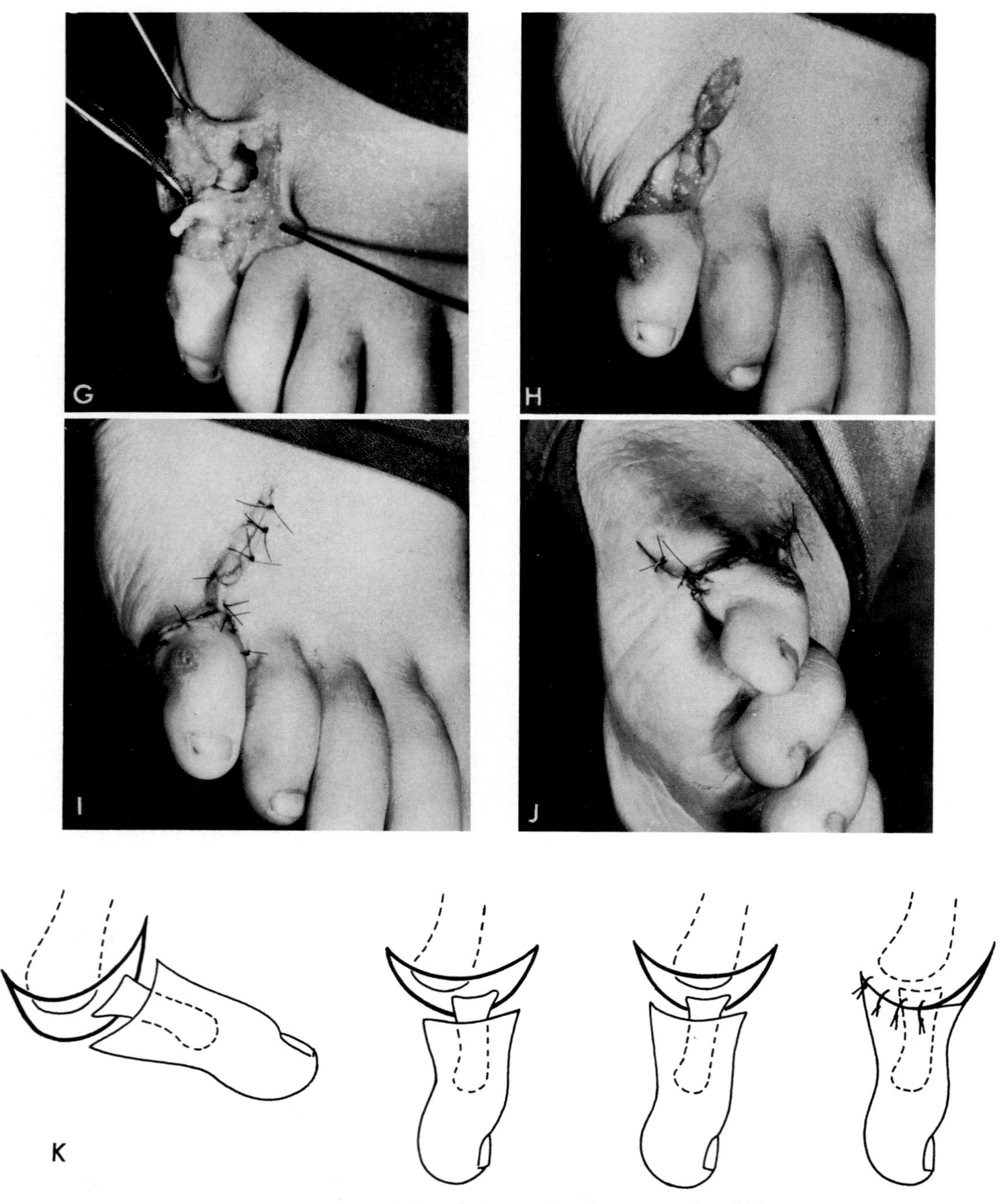

FIGURE 7–145 Continued. Butler's operation for an overriding fifth toe.

G. Adhesions on the plantar part of the capsule are freed by blunt dissection. Note the little toe now lies in the fully corrected position. **H.** Appearance of the toe before skin closure. It lies freely in normal alignment without tension. **I** and **J.** Closure of the wound. Skin sutures securely hold the toe in the correct position. **K.** Diagrammatic illustration of the mechanics of the operation. (From Cockin, J.: Butler's operation for an overriding fifth toe. J. Bone Joint Surg., *50-B*:78–80, 1968. Reprinted by permission.)

shortened extensor tendon of the fifth toe (Fig. 7–145 C). The neurovascular bundle is identified and carefully protected from injury (Fig. 7–145 D). The extensor tendon and the dorsomedial part of the capsule of the metatarsophalangeal joint are sectioned (Fig. 7–145 E). The toe can now be manipulated freely downward and laterally into correct alignment. Occasionally, in severe long-standing cases, adhesions on the plantar aspect of the capsule are separated from the metatarsal head by blunt dissection (Fig. 7–145 F and G). Now the toe moves into the plantar handle of the incision and dangles in normal alignment without any tension (Fig. 7–145 H). The wound is closed so the surrounding skin sutures hold the toe in the corrected position (Fig. 7–145 I and J). Figure 7–145 K is a diagrammatic illustration of the mechanics of the operation.

Skin dressing is applied. Splints to immobilize the toe in the corrected position are not required. The sutures are removed in 10 to 14 days, and normal activity is then allowed.

The author has utilized the Butler operation in children and has found it to be very satisfactory. In adolescents and adults, however, the potential embarrassment to circulation of the little toe is a definite drawback to the procedure.

Hallux Valgus Interphalangeus

In this congenital deformity the distal phalanx of the great toe is deviated laterally toward the second toe at the interphalangeal joint. The degree of valgus deviation varies from mild to marked (Figs. 7–146 and 7–147). In moderately severe cases the shoe pressure irritates the skin over the interphalangeal joint of the hallux, and gradually adventitious bursae and blisters develop.

In childhood treatment consists of cuneiform osteotomy through the shaft of the proximal phalanx of the hallux. The resected wedge of bone is based medially, and the bone fragments are aligned and fixed internally with a Kirschner wire (Fig. 7–148). In the skeletally mature foot, the interphalangeal joint of the great toe is fused in correct alignment following partial excision of the hypertrophied medial portion of the epiphysis.

Congenital Curly (or Varus) Toe

In this common congenital deformity one or more toes are bent plantarward, deviated medially, and rotated laterally at the distal interphalangeal joint (Fig. 7–149). The twisted terminal pulp then gradually begins to impinge upon and curl under the adjacent toe.

This affection is usually bilateral and symmetrical, and has a high familial incidence. It is most probably caused by hypoplasia of the intrinsic muscles of the affected toe. Trethowan regarded the anomaly as a congenital form of hammer toe.[43] Sweetnam coined the term *congenital curly toe*, and also observed that the

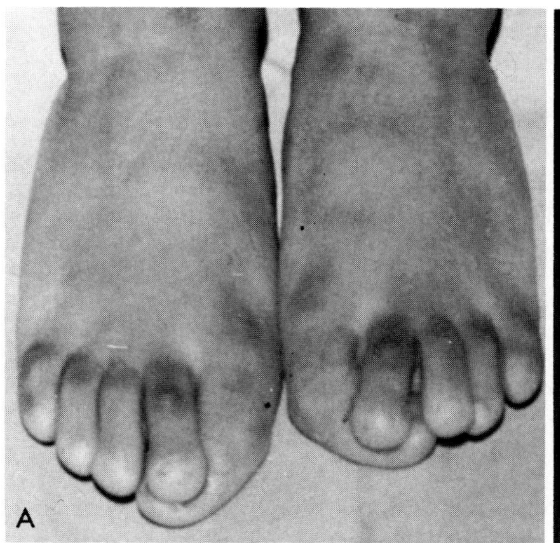

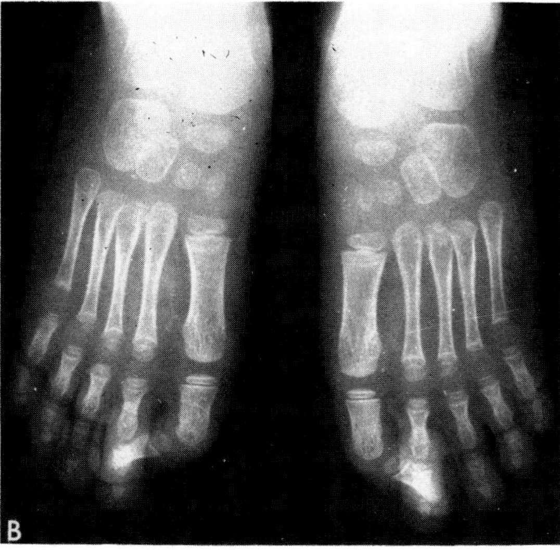

FIGURE 7–146. Bilateral hallux valgus interphalangeus.

A. Clinical appearance. Note the lateral deviation of the distal phalanx of the great toe. **B.** Anteroposterior radiogram of both feet showing lateral subluxation of the interphalangeal joint of the hallux.

Correction of Digitus Minimus Varus (McFarland, Kelikian)

OPERATIVE TECHNIQUE

A. First, a 00 silk whip suture is passed through the pulps of the fourth and fifth toes. The suture ends are clamped with hemostats and the toes are pulled apart, bringing the web space into full view.

B. Three sets of incisions are made: (1) a web-bisecting incision that starts on the dorsum of the forefoot in the groove between the metatarsal heads and extends distally to bisect the web, and then passes plantarward to terminate at about the same point posteriorly on the plantar aspect of the forefoot as it does on the dorsum; (2) two *paradigital incisions,* one for each toe, which begin at the point where the web-bisecting incision begins to dip plantarward and extend lengthwise along the adjacent side of each toe. The paradigital incision for the little toe ends on the side of the distal phalanx at a point plantar and just proximal to the base of the nail, whereas the incision for the fourth toe is the same length as that for the fifth. The paradigital incisions are placed slightly toward the plantar border of the toe to give a semblance of an interdigital groove after surgical syndactylism. (3) Two connecting oblique incisions extend from the terminal point of the paradigital incision on each side to the proximal end of the web-bisecting incision on the plantar aspect.

C. The triangular patches of skin between the paradigital and oblique connecting incisions are excised. In dissection of subcutaneous tissue in this area, care is taken not to injure the plexus of veins. The skin flaps are mobilized and retracted to their respective sides. The digital nerves and vessels should be identified and protected from injury.

D and **E.** The long extensor tendon of the fifth toe is divided at its insertion; a 00 silk whip suture is applied to its distal end. (This end is later transferred to the fifth metatarsal head according to the technique for the Jones procedure described in Plate 106.) Next, the long flexor of the fifth toe is dissected free of the proximal phalanx. Small retractors are placed on the dorsal and plantar aspects of the bone to protect the soft tissues. The capsules of the metatarsophalangeal and proximal interphalangeal joints of the little toe are divided, and the proximal phalanx is excised. The long fifth toe extensor is transferred to the fifth metatarsal head. The wound is packed with moist gauze, the pneumatic tourniquet is deflated, and bleeding vessels are clamped and coagulated.

F. The terminal points of the paradigital incisions are sutured together with 0000 nylon, bringing the toes together. The alignment of the toes is inspected. Care is taken to avoid eversion or inversion of the toes; if necessary, the terminal suture is removed and reapplied. The dorsal wound is closed with 0000 nylon and the plantar skin edges with 0000 plain catgut.

POSTOPERATIVE CARE

A below-knee walking cast is applied. Three to four weeks following surgery, the cast and sutures are removed. The patient is allowed to bear weight and resume normal activities.

Plate 103. Correction of Digitus Minimus Varus (McFarland, Kelikian)

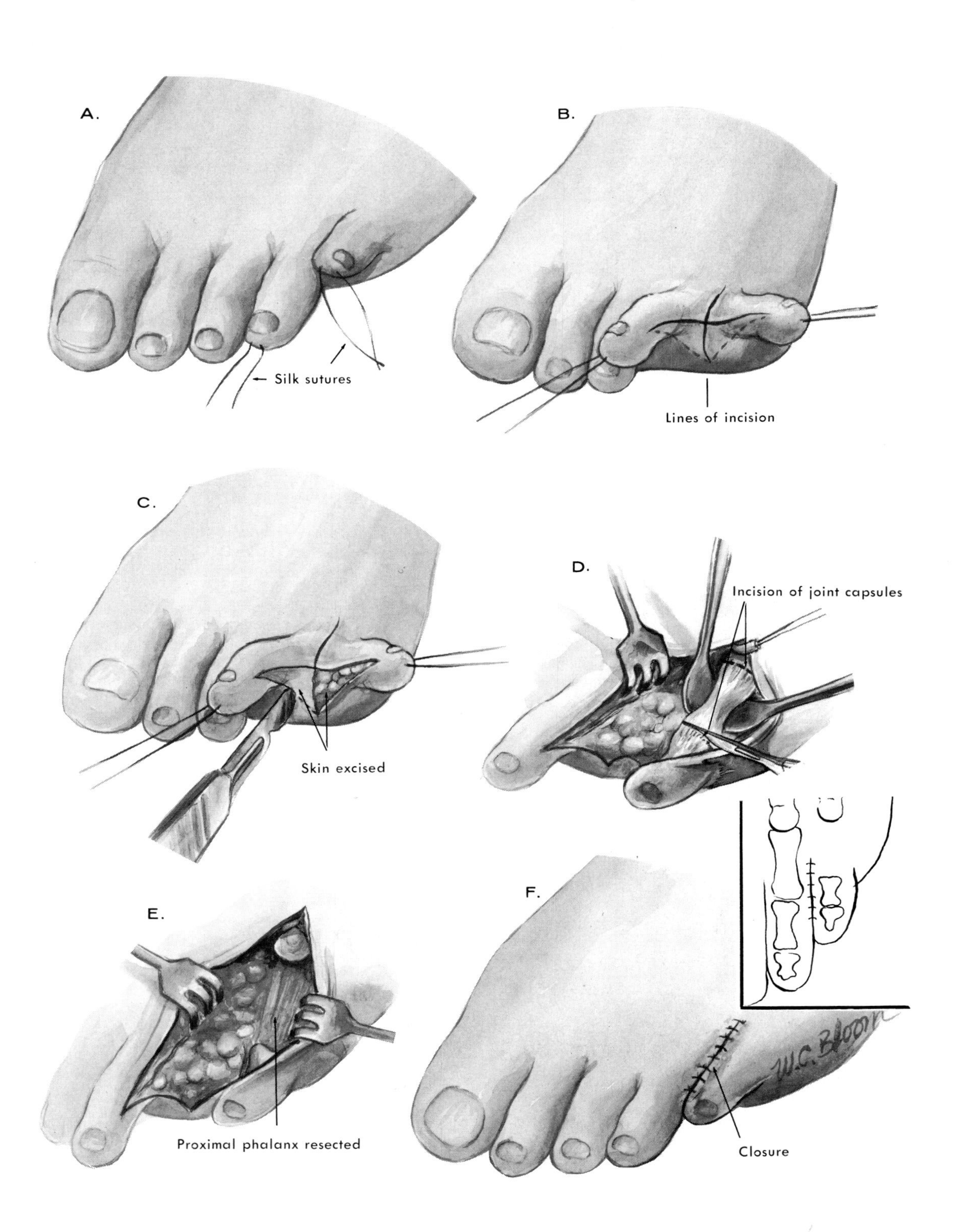

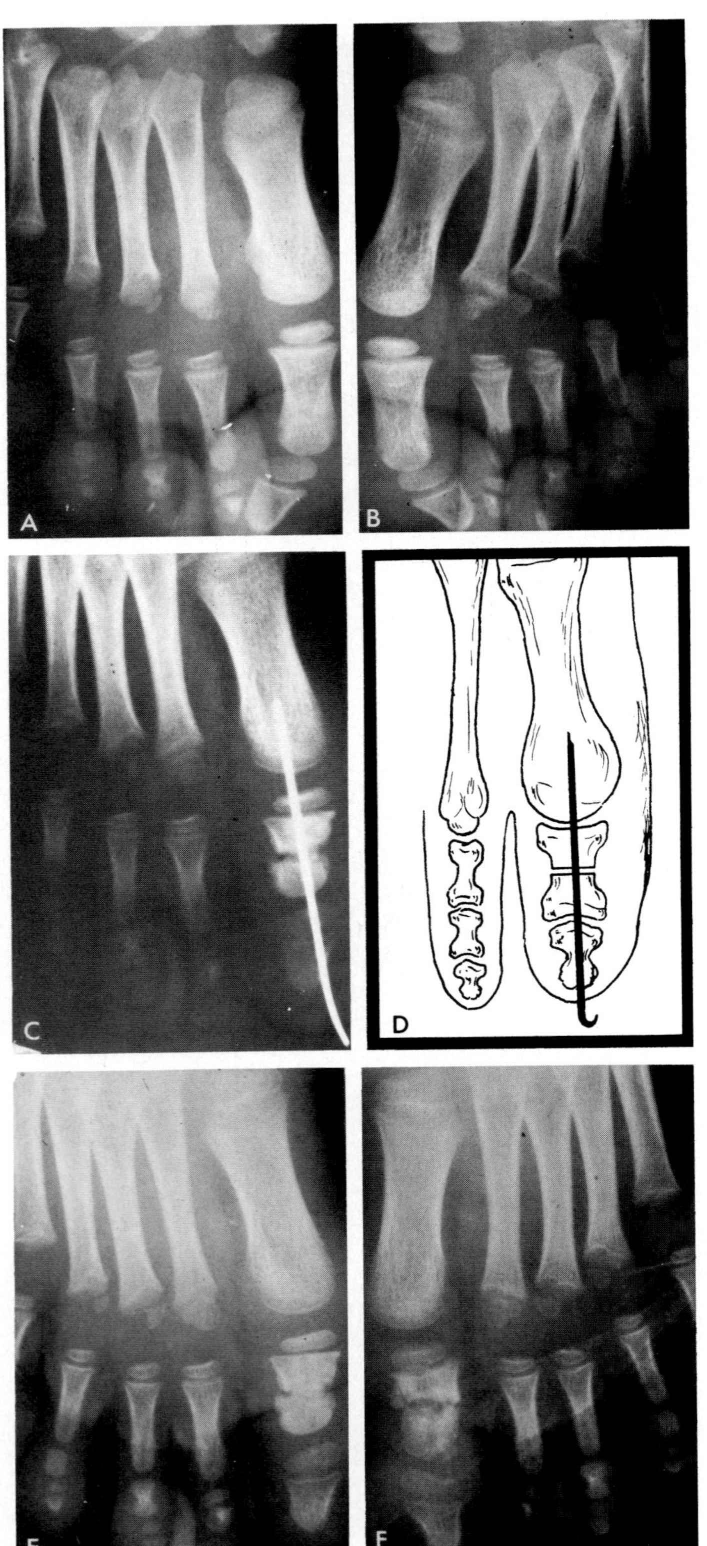

FIGURE 7–147. Congenital hallux valgus interphalangeus in a two-year-old child.

Treatment consisted of cuneiform osteotomy of the shaft of the proximal phalanx with the base of the resected wedge of bone passing medially, and internal fixation of the bone fragments with Kirschner wire. **A** and **B.** Preoperative radiograms. **C.** Radiogram showing correction maintained by Kirschner wire. **D.** Interpretive diagram. **E** and **F.** Postoperative radiograms of the forefeet showing excellent correction. (From Kelikian, H.: Hallux Valgus, Allied Deformities of the Forefoot and Metatarsalgia. Philadelphia, Saunders, 1965, p. 461. Reprinted by permission.)

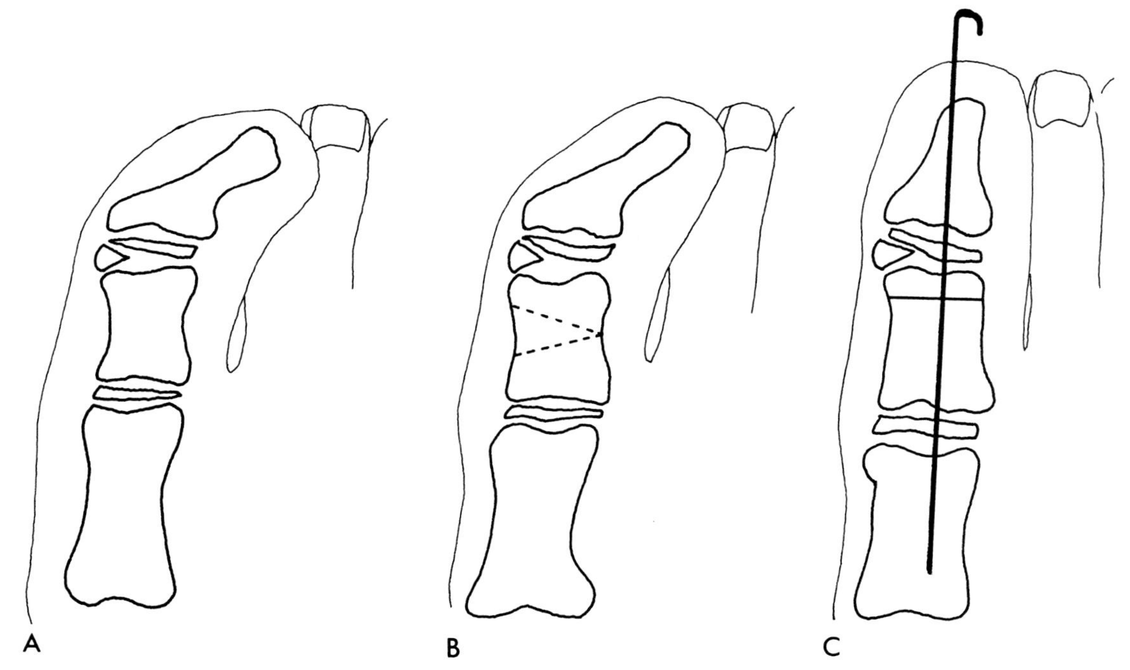

FIGURE 7–148. Hallux valgus interphalangeus—diagram showing method of correction in childhood.

A. Deformity. **B.** Cuneiform osteotomy of the diaphysis of the proximal phalanx of the great toe. The base of the resected bone wedge lies medially. **C.** The bone fragments are aligned and fixed internally with Kirschner wire.

deformity does not correct itself spontaneously and usually becomes exaggerated with growth.[41]

TREATMENT

If the deformity is mild and the curly toe does not impinge upon its adjacent toe, the condition can be ignored and no treatment is necessary. Over-and-under strapping is useless and has no permanent effect.

If the affected toe curls under the neighboring one, disabling symptoms are most likely to ensue later in life, particularly in women, in whom discomfort results from the pressure of tight shoes. Pain under the adjacent medial metatarsal head develops as the underlying toe does not permit its neighboring medial toe to touch the floor; thus more body weight is transmitted to the metatarsal head. In children, Kelikian recommends surgical syndactyly of the curly toe with its normal neighbor on the medial side.[36] Another alternative is to transfer the flexor digitorum longus tendon of the affected toe to the dorsal and lateral aspect of the extensor hood.[39, 42] This is especially indicated in children in whom the deformity is not very severe or rigid. The operative technique is as follows:

A 3-cm. longitudinal incision is made on the dorsolateral aspect of the deformed toe. The subcutaneous tissue is divided, and the digital nerve and long toe extensor tendon are pulled medially with a blunt retractor. The affected toe is acutely flexed, and on its plantar aspect the long toe flexor tendon is identified. A longitudinal incision is made in the flexor tendon sheath, and the tendon is pulled dorsally with a small hook and sectioned near its insertion. After manipulation of the distal interphalangeal joint into normal alignment, the long flexor tendon is sutured to the extensor expansion with the interphalangeal joints of the toe in full extension and with the metatarsophalangeal joint in flexion. The tourniquet is released, and the wound closed in the usual manner. Alignment of the affected toe is maintained by a smooth Kirschner wire drilled from the distal end of the toe into the base of the proximal phalanx. Adhesive strapping or a below-knee walking cast is applied. The cast and wire are removed three to four weeks after surgery. In

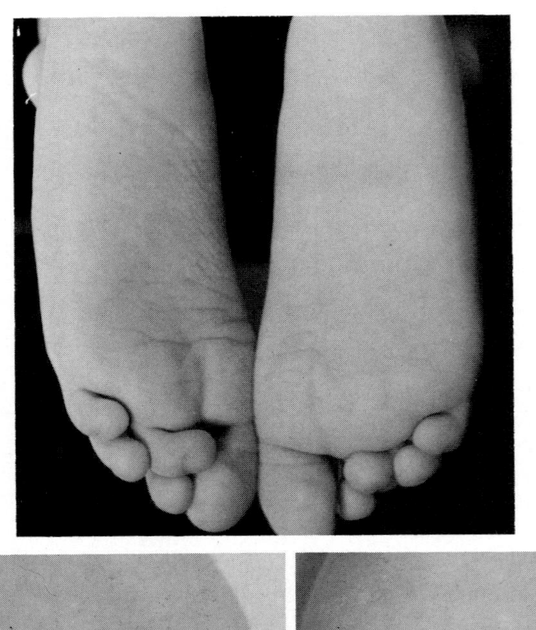

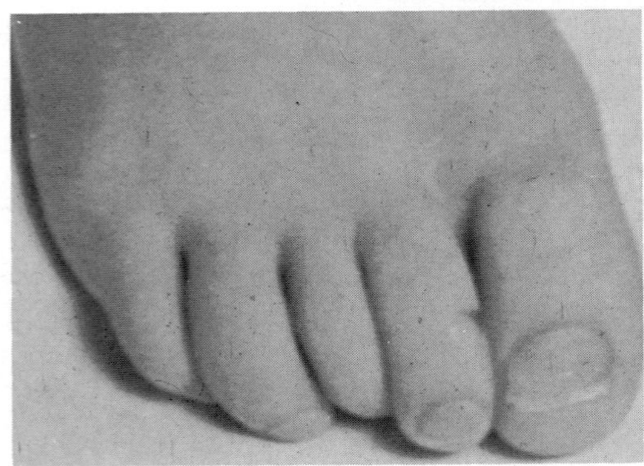

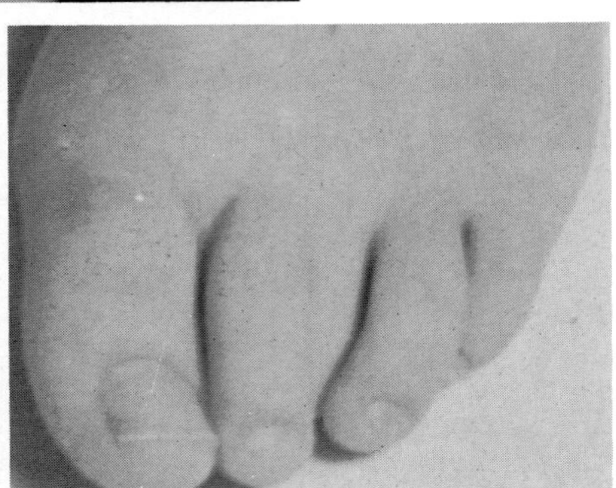

FIGURE 7–149. *Curly toes.*

adults, Kelikian recommends partial proximal phalangectomy with surgical syndactyly of the toes.[36]

References

SYNDACTYLISM

1. Blauth, W.: Congenital digital syndactylia. (Author's transl.) Z. Kinderchir. Grenzgeb., *30*:42, 1980.
2. Blauth, W., and Helbig, B.: Syndactylia recurrences and their treatment (author's transl.). Z. Kinderchir. Grenzgeb., *30*:53, 1980.
3. Kleiner, B. C., and Holmes, L. B.: Brief clinical report: Hallux varus and preaxial polysyndactyly in brothers. Am. J. Med. Genet., *6*:113, 1980.
4. Losch, G. M., Schrader, M., and Eckert, P.: Malformation syndrome with constriction rings, pseudoligaments, acral defects and syndactylism: Diagnosis and treatment. (Author's transl.) Z. Kinderchir. Grenzgeb., *30*:85, 1980.
5. Piza, H., and Meissl, G.: Long term results following surgical correction of syndactylia. (Author's transl.) Z. Kinderchir. Grenzgeb., *30*:57, 1980.
6. Reuter, G.: Pitfalls in surgery of syndactylism. (Author's transl.) Z. Kinderchir. Grenzgeb., *30*:61, 1980.
7. Teot, L., and Gilbert, A.: Measure of the web-space in children. (Author's transl.) Chir. Pediatr. *22*:31, 1981.

CONGENITAL DIGITUS MINIMUS VARUS (CONGENITAL DORSAL OVERRIDING OF FIFTH TOE)

8. Black, G. B., Grogan, D. P., and Bobechko, W. P.: Butler arthroplasty for correction of the adducted fifth toe: A retrospective study of 36 operations between 1968 and 1982. J. Pediatr. Orthop., *5*:439, 1985.
9. Brahms, M. A.: The small toes. *In* Jahss, M. H. (ed.): Disorders of the Foot. Philadelphia, Saunders, 1982, pp. 646–647.
10. Cockin, J.: Butler's operation for an overriding fifth toe. J. Bone Joint Surg., *50-B*:78, 1968.
11. Coughlin, M. J., and Mann, R. A.: Lesser toe deformities. *In* Mann, R. A. (ed.): Surgery of the Foot. St. Louis, Mosby, 1986, pp. 152–157.
12. DuVries, H. L.: Surgery of the Foot. St. Louis, Mosby, 1959, p. 347.
13. Gocht, H., and DeBrunner, H.: Orthopaedische Therapie. Leipzig, F. C. W. Vogel, 1925, p. 238.
14. Goodwin, F. C., and Swisher, F. M.: The treatment of congenital hyperextension of the great toe. J. Bone Joint Surg., *25*:193, 1943.
15. Hulman, S.: Simple operation for the overlapping fifth toe. Br. Med. J., *11*:1506, 1964.
16. Jones, R., and Lovett, R. W.: Orthopaedic Surgery. London, Oxford University Press, 1929, p. 666.
17. Jordan, R. P., and Caselli, M. A.: Overlapping deformity of the digits in the pediatric patient: A conservative approach to treatment. J. Am. Podiatry Assoc., *68*:503, 1978.
18. Karchinov, K.: Varusnyi V palets stopy. Ortop. Travmatol. Protez., *6*:84, 1978.
19. Kelikian, H.: Hallux Valgus, Allied Deformities of the Forefoot, and Metatarsalgia. Philadelphia, Saunders, 1965.
20. Kelikian, H., Clayton, L., and Loseff, H.: Surgical syndactylia of the toes. Clin. Orthop., *19*:208, 1961.
21. Lantzounis, L. A.: Congenital subluxation of the fifth toe and its correction by a periosteocapsuloplasty and tendon transplantation. J. Bone Joint Surg., *22*:147, 1940.
22. Lapidus, P. C.: Transplantation of the extensor tendon for correction of the overlapping fifth toe. J. Bone Joint Surg., *24*:555, 1942.
23. McFarland, B.: Congenital deformities of the spine and limbs. *In* Platt, H. (ed.): Modern Trends in Orthopedics. New York, P. B. Hoeber, 1950, p. 107.
24. Morris, E. W., Scullion, J. E., and Mann, T. S.: Varus fifth toe. J. Bone Joint Surg., *64-B*:99, 1982.
25. Ruiz-Mora, J.: Orthopaedic surgery. *In* Cecil, R. (ed.): The Specialties in General Practice. Philadelphia, Saunders, 1951, p. 60.
26. Ruiz-Mora, J.: Personal communication to L. R. Straub, 1954.
27. Scrase, W. H.: The treatment of dorsal adduction deformities of the fifth toe. J. Bone Joint Surg., *36-B*:146, 1954.
28. Stamm, T. T.: Minor surgery of the foot—elevated fifth toe. *In* Carling, E. R., and Ross, J. P. (eds.): British Surgical Practice. London, Butterworth & Co., 1948, pp. 161–162.
29. Stamm, T. T.: Surgery of the foot. *In* British Surgical Practice. Vol. IV. St. Louis, Mosby, 1948, p. 160.
30. Straub, L. R.: Orthopedic surgery. *In* Cecil, R. (ed.): The Specialties in General Practice. Philadelphia, Saunders, 1951, p. 60.
31. Thompson, C. T.: Surgical treatment of disorders of the forepart of the foot. J. Bone Joint Surg., *46-A*:1117, 1964.
32. Wilson, J. N.: V-Y correction for varus deformity of the fifth toe. Br. J. Surg., *41*:133, 1953.

CONGENITAL CURLY (OR VARUS) TOES

33. Giannestras, N. J.: Foot Disorders. Philadelphia, Lea & Febiger, 1978, pp. 102–107.
34. Huurman, W. W.: Congenital foot deformities. *In* Mann, R. A. (ed.): Surgery of the Foot. 5th Ed. St. Louis, Mosby, 1986, p. 559.
35. Jahss, M. H.: Disorders of the Foot. Philadelphia, Saunders, 1982, pp. 214–215.
36. Kelikian, H.: Hallux Valgus, Allied Deformities of the Forefoot, and Metatarsalgia. Philadelphia, Saunders, 1965, p. 330.
37. Pollard, J. P., and Morrison, P. J. M.: Flexor tenotomy in the treatment of curly toes. Proc. R. Soc. Med., *68*:480, 1975.
38. Ross, E. R., and Menelaus, M. B.: Open flexor tenotomy for hammer toes and curly toes in childhood. J. Bone Joint Surg., *66-B*:770, 1984.
39. Sharrard, W. J. W.: The surgery of deformed toes in children. Br. J. Clin. Pract., *17*:263, 1963.
40. Sharrard, W. J. W.: Congenital varus (curly) toes. *In* Paediatric Orthopaedics and Fractures and Developmental Abnormalities of the Foot and Toes. Oxford, Blackwell, 1971, pp. 295–299.
41. Sweetnam, R.: Congenital curly toes. An investigation into the value of treatment. Lancet, *2*:398, 1958.
42. Taylor, R. G.: The treatment of claw toes by multiple transfers of flexor with extensor tendons. J. Bone Joint Surg., *33-B*:539, 1951.
43. Trethowan, W. H.: The treatment of hammertoe. Lancet, *1*:1257, 1312, 1925.
44. Watson, H. K., and Boyes, J. H.: Congenital angular deformities of the digits. J. Bone Joint Surg., *49-A*:333, 1967.

HAMMER TOE

Hammer toe is a deformity characterized by flexion contracture of the proximal interphalangeal joint. The distal interphalangeal joint may be in flexion, in neutral extension, or in slight

Correction of Hammer Toe by Resection and Arthrodesis of Proximal Interphalangeal Joint

OPERATIVE TECHNIQUE

A. A 3- to 4-cm. longitudinal incision is made over the dorsal aspect of the proximal interphalangeal joint parallel to and at the lateral border of the extensor digitorum longus tendon. The subcutaneous tissue is divided and the skin flaps are retracted.

B. The long extensor tendon is split and retracted to expose the capsule of the proximal interphalangeal joint. The digital vessels and nerves are protected from injury. A transverse incision is made in the capsule and the joint surfaces are widely exposed.

C and **D.** With a rongeur, wedges of bone based dorsally are resected from the head of the proximal phalanx and the base of the middle phalanx. Enough bone should be removed to allow correction of deformity.

E and **F.** The proximal and middle phalanges are held together by internal fixation with a Kirschner wire that is inserted retrograde. The Kirschner wire should not cross the metatarsophalangeal joint. The cancellous bony surfaces of the middle and proximal phalanges should be apposed, and the rotational alignment should be correct. The capsule is resutured tightly by reefing. The wound is closed in routine manner. With a pair of nose pliers, the end of the Kirschner wire is bent 90 degrees and cut, leaving 0.5 cm. protruding through the skin.

POSTOPERATIVE CARE

A below-knee walking cast is applied with a band of plaster of Paris protecting the toe. The wire and cast are removed in six weeks, when the radiograms show fusion of the interphalangeal joint.

Plate 104. Correction of Hammer Toe by Resection and Arthrodesis of Proximal Interphalangeal Joint

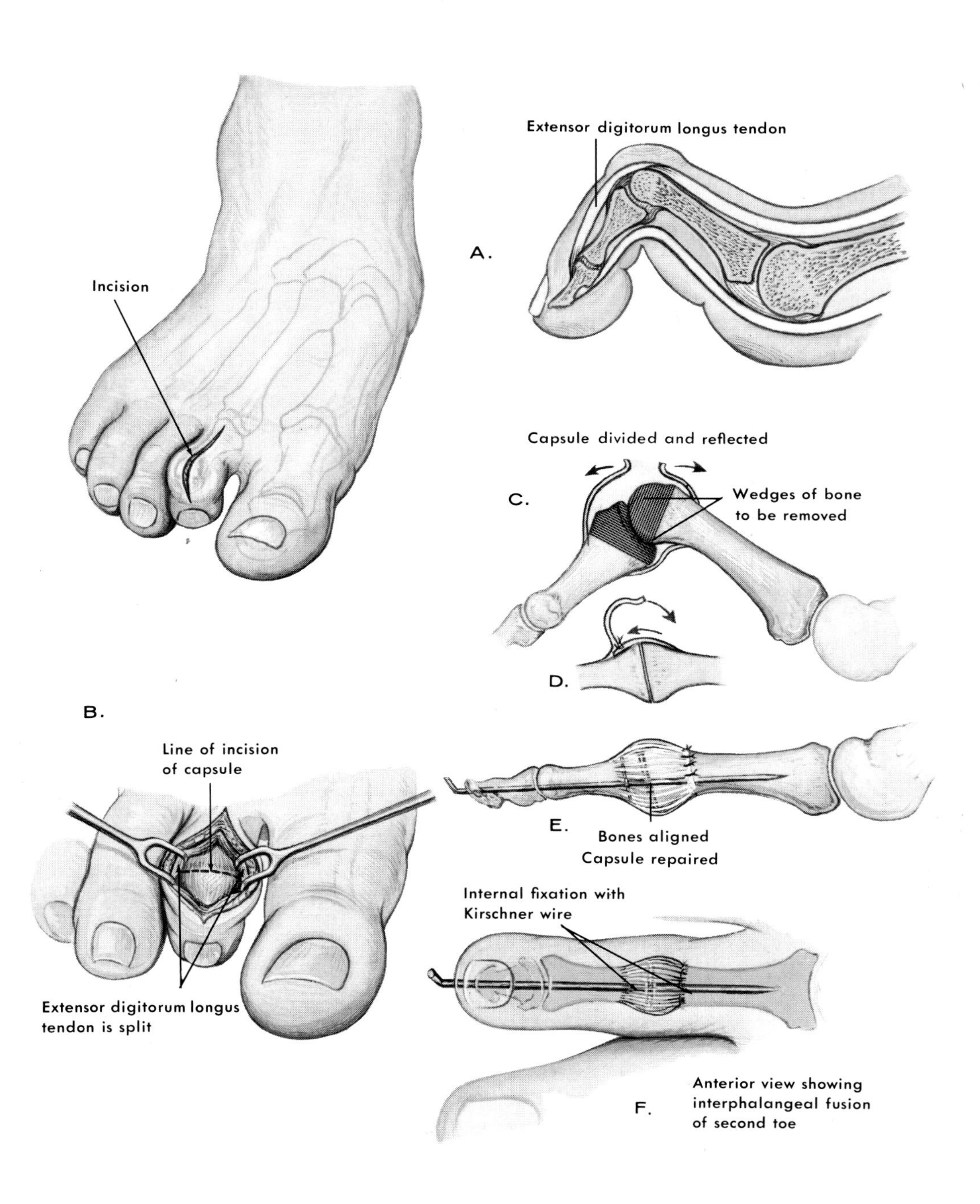

hyperextension. Eventually, with depression of the metatarsal head, the metatarsophalangeal joint becomes hyperextended. Painful calluses develop under the metatarsal heads. The capsules and ligaments on the plantar aspect of the flexed joints and on the dorsal aspect of the hyperextended joints become contracted. The interosseous tendons become shifted dorsally. Constant irritation caused by shoe pressure may cause calluses to develop over the dorsum of the flexed interphalangeal joint and on the end of the toe. An adventitious bursa may also appear between the indurated skin and subjacent bone.

Hammer toe is often bilateral and symmetrical. There is a very high familial incidence. The second toe is most frequently affected, and less often the third and fourth toes. The deformity is usually congenital; acquired cases are ordinarily caused by mechanical pressure of a too-small shoe on an abnormally long toe that is forced to flex at its interphalangeal joints. Hammer toe may occur in association with hallux valgus.

Treatment

In infants and children, the deformity should be treated conservatively. Passive stretching exercises are performed by the parents. The deformity is usually not fixed; if it is marked, the interphalangeal joint is manipulated into extension and strapped with adhesive tape in the corrected position. When the child begins to walk, it is important to provide him with shoes that have adequate room. Pain from inflamed calluses over the dorsum of the flexed interphalangeal joint is alleviated by protective pads.

In the adolescent, if the deformity is severe and disabling, surgical correction is indicated. Various operative procedures are available. A simple and very satisfactory method is resection of the proximal interphalangeal joint and arthrodesis of the joint in neutral position. This was first reported by Soule, in 1910, and later was popularized by Sir Robert Jones.[6, 17] The operative correction of hammer toe by resection and fusion of the proximal interphalangeal joint is described and illustrated in Plate 104. The procedure is combined with dorsal capsulotomy of the metatarsophalangeal joint if the latter has developed fixed hyperextension contracture. In the presence of marked depression of the metatarsal head, the long toe extensor is transferred to the metatarsal head.

When the hammer toe deformity is severe with *irreducible* dorsal subluxation of the metatarsophalangeal joints, partial proximal phalangectomy is preferred and the adjacent digits are syndactylized surgically.

The Girdlestone operation was designed to provide active plantar flexion of the proximal phalanx by transfer of the toe flexor to the extensor hood. The author is dissatisfied with the procedure and does not recommend it because lateral deformities of the toes frequently develop following the transfer and also because it does not always correct the deformity.

References

1. Blum, A.: De l'orteil en marteau. Bull. Mem. Soc. Chir. Paris, *9:*738, 1883.
2. Brahms, M. A.: Common foot problems. J. Bone Joint Surg., *49-A:*1653, 1967.
3. Cahill, B. R., and Connor, D. E.: A long-term follow-up on proximal phalangectomy for hammer toes. Clin. Orthop., *86:*91, 1972.
4. Ely, L. W.: Hammertoe. Surg. Clin. North Am., *6:*433, 1926.
5. Glassman, F., Wallin, L., and Sideman, S.: Phalangectomy for toe deformities. Surg. Clin. North Am., *29:*275, 1949.
6. Jones, R.: Notes on Military Orthopaedics. New York, P. B. Hoeber, 1917, pp. 38–57.
7. Krenz, L.: Die Hammerzehen und ihre Operation nacht Bocht. Arch. Orthop. Unfallchir., *21:*459, 1923.
8. Lapidus, P. W.: Operation for correction of hammertoe. J. Bone Joint Surg., *21:*977, 1939.
9. McConnell, B. E.: Hammer toe surgery. South. Med. J., *68:*595, 1975.
10. Margo, M. K.: Surgical treatment of conditions of the fore part of the foot. J. Bone Joint Surg., *49-A:*1665, 1976.
11. Merrill, W. J.: Conservative operative treatment of hammertoe. Am. J. Orthop. Surg., *10:*262, 1912.
12. Michele, A. A., and Krueger, F. J.: Operative correction for hammertoe. Milit. Surg., *103:*52, 1948.
13. Milgram, J. E.: Office measures for relief of painful foot. J. Bone Joint Surg., *46-A:*1095, 1964.
14. O'Neil, J.: An arthroplastic operation for hammertoe. J.A.M.A., *57:*1207, 1911.
15. Ross, E. R. S., and Menelaus, M. B.: Open flexor tenotomy for hammer toes and curly toes in childhood. J. Bone Joint Surg., *66-B:*770, 1984.
16. Sehig, S.: Hammertoe: A new procedure for its correction. Surg. Gynecol. Obstet., *72:*101, 1941.
17. Soule, R. E.: Operation for the cure of hammertoe. N.Y. Med. J., *91:*649, March 26, 1910.
18. Taylor, R. G.: An operative procedure for the treatment of hammer toe and claw toe. J. Bone Joint Surg., *22:*608, 1940.
19. Trethowan, W. H.: The treatment of hammertoe. Lancet, *1:*1257–1312, 1925.
20. Young, C. S.: An operation for correction of hammertoe and claw toe. J. Bone Joint Surg., *20:*715, 1938.

MALLET TOE

This deformity is characterized by flexion deformity at the distal interphalangeal joint of any of the lesser toes (Fig. 7–150). Usually a single toe or two neighboring ones are affected.

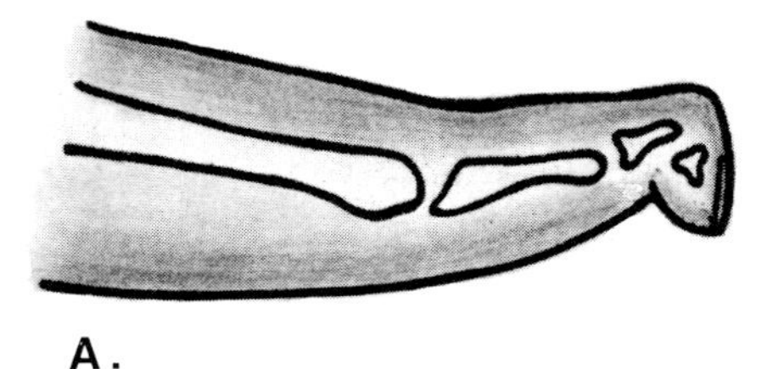

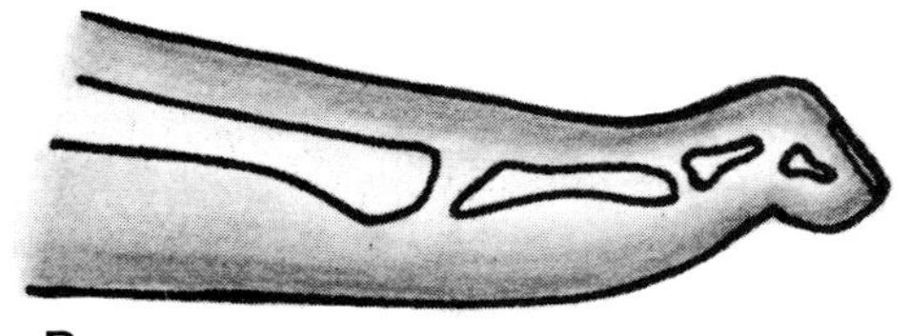

FIGURE 7–150. Mallet toe.

A. Severe. **B.** Mild.

The condition is less common than hammer toe, in which the flexion deformity is at the proximal interphalangeal joint. Mallet toes are asymptomatic in childhood, but in adolescence or early adult life, the development of a painful corn on the tip of the toe close to the nail may be very disabling.

Conservative measures such as adhesive strapping and passive stretching exercises do not correct the deformity. Shaving the corn and padding the toe will give symptomatic relief, but surgery is often preferred. Fusion of the distal interphalangeal joint in normal alignment and section of the long toe flexor corrects the deformity. A simpler method that provides immediate relief of symptoms is amputation of the distal phalanx, but this is esthetically undesirable.

Pes Cavus and Claw Toes

PES CAVUS

Pes cavus is a fixed equinus deformity of the forefoot on the hindfoot (Fig. 7–151). When associated with clawing of the toes, the term *clawfoot* is sometimes used to describe the condition.

Etiology and Pathogenesis

Cavus deformity of the foot is usually a manifestation of some underlying neuromuscular disease. The lesion may be in muscle (myopathic pes cavus), peripheral nerves or lumbosacral spinal nerve roots, anterior horn cells of the spinal cord, spinocerebellar tracts, pyramidal or extrapyramidal systems of the brain, or cerebral cortex. Examples are: at the *muscular level*, muscular dystrophy (particularly the distal type); at the *peripheral nerve or spinal nerve root level*, Déjérine-Sottas interstitial hypertrophic neuritis, Charcot-Marie-Tooth disease, polyneuritis, and traumatic lesions of the sciatic nerve; at the *spinal cord level*, poliomyelitis, myelomeningocele, diastematomyelia, and cord tumors; as heredofamilial affections of spinocerebellar tracts, Friedreich's ataxia and Roussy-Lévy syndrome; at the *pyramidal and extrapyramidal levels*, cerebral palsy (spastic hemiplegia or athetosis) and dystonia musculorum deformans; and at the *cerebral level*, hysteria in which, when the position of pes cavus is maintained constantly for prolonged periods, permanent contracture and fixed deformity may develop. Some cases of pes cavus are congenital; in others no specific cause or neurologic deficit can be demonstrated, in which case the term *idiopathic pes cavus* is used.

In the pathogenesis of pes cavus, several factors should be considered:

Muscle Imbalance Between Weak Anterior Tibial and Strong Peroneus Longus Muscles. The medial cuneiform and the base of the first metatarsal are elevated by the action of the anterior tibial muscle and depressed by the peroneus longus muscle. Bentzon advanced the theory that when the anterior tibial muscle is weak, the first metatarsal is plantar-flexed by a strong peroneus longus muscle. The forefoot is pronated by the action of the peroneus longus muscle, and the valgus deviation is further aggravated by the pull of the long toe extensors. Varying degrees of equinus deformity due to contracture of the triceps surae muscle and posterior soft tissues of the ankle are usually found. In attempting to substitute for the dorsiflexing action of the weakened anterior tibial muscle, the long toe extensors pull the proximal phalanges of the toes into hyperextension; and the tension on the long toe flexor muscle brings the distal two phalanges of the toes into plantar flexion.[11] The "windlass" mechanism pulls the metatarsals, especially the first, into plantar

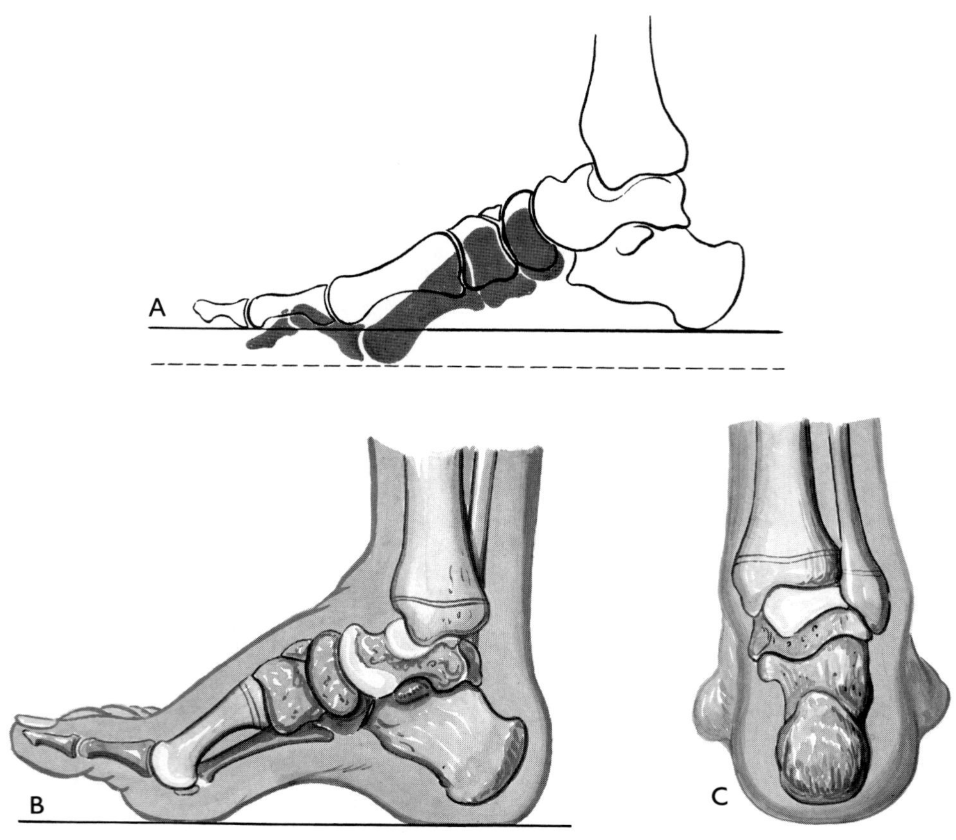

FIGURE 7–151. Cavus deformity of the foot.

A. Pes cavus. There is fixed equinus deformity of the forefoot on the hindfoot. **B** and **C.** Simple pes cavus. The plantar flexion deformity of the forefoot is equal in its medial and lateral columns and the heel is in neutral position.

flexion and elevates the medial longitudinal arch. The plantar soft tissues become shortened. This hypothesis of dynamic imbalance between a weak anterior muscle and a strong peroneus longus muscle sounds very plausible and is of definite value in planning treatment. It is supported by the studies of Missirian and Mann.[104] It fails, however, to explain the actual clinical findings. In poliomyelitis, when the anterior tibial muscle is weak and the peroneal muscles are strong, a valgus deformity results. The os calcis is everted, the head of the talus is plantar-flexed, the medial longitudinal arch is flattened, and the toes are flat on the ground. In walking, however, although the toe extensors do pull the toes into extension, a fixed claw toe deformity does not develop. Also in contradiction to the theory of Bentzon is the absence of definite anterior tibial muscle weakness in most cases of pes cavus.

Isolated Weakness of the Peroneus Brevis Muscle. Another theory is that, in an attempt to compensate for the paralysis of the peroneus brevis muscle, the peroneus longus hypertrophies and overpowers the action of the anterior tibial muscle. The first metatarsal and medial cuneiform are pulled into plantar flexion, and the forefoot is pronated. The long toe extensors are hyperactive to compensate for dorsiflexion insufficiency caused by peroneus brevis muscle weakness; consequently, the proximal phalanges of the toes are pulled into hyperextension and their distal phalanges into flexion by the tension on the long toe flexors. The hindfoot inverts to compensate for eversion of the forefoot, enabling the first and fifth metatarsals to rest evenly on the ground. The dynamic imbalance between a weak peroneus brevis and a strong posterior tibial muscle may also be a factor in producing a varus heel. In support of this attractive theory, one finds an occasional patient with poliomyelitis who has isolated paralysis of the peroneus brevis muscle and a deformity of the foot quite similar to pes cavus.

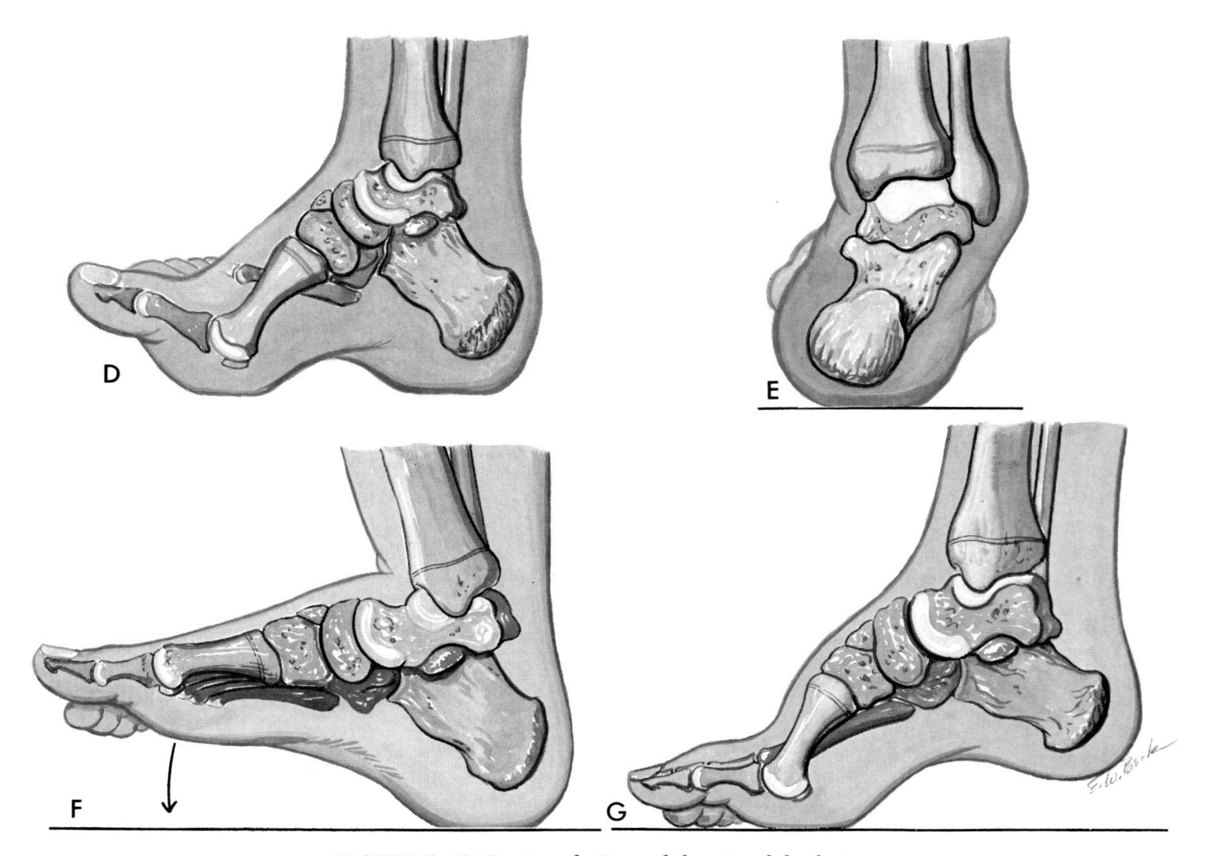

FIGURE 7–151 Continued. Cavus deformity of the foot.

D and **E.** Pes cavovarus. Note the plantar flexion of the medial column of the forefoot and the inversion of the heel. **F.** Calcaneocavus deformity. Note the calcaneus position of the hindfoot. The forefoot drops into equinus position, developing calcaneocavus deformity. **G.** Pes equinocavus. In addition to the forefoot, the hindfoot and ankle are in equinus position.

Paralysis of Intrinsic Muscles of Foot. Duchenne described a cavus clawfoot with atrophy of the muscles that insert into the sesamoids of the great toe and the interossei of the foot. The proximal phalanges are hyperextended so that they are subluxated on the metatarsal heads, and the middle and distal phalanges are flexed. The result is clawing of the toes and a considerable increase in the curvature of the plantar arch. Duchenne proposed the following theory of the pathogenesis of cavus clawfoot:

> When the interossei are paralyzed or weakened, the force of the muscles which extend the proximal phalanges and the muscles which flex the middle and distal phalanges lose the moderating action of the interossei. The clawing of the toes sets in and gradually increases. The bases of the proximal phalanges progressively depress the heads of the metatarsals with increase of the degree of subluxation of the proximal phalanges; the curvature of the plantar arch increases considerably and the plantar aponeurosis contracts in time. Following this, all the joints, especially the mediotarsal joints and their ligaments, become deformed in a manner characteristic of all cavus feet.[38]

Duchenne believed the mechanism of the clawing of the foot to be similar to that of the clawhand seen following paralysis of the intrinsic muscles of the hand, i.e.,

> . . . the heads of the medial four metacarpals are equally pushed by the proximal phalanges of the fingers, resulting in a form of cavus of the palm and of the hand.[38]

It should be noted, however, that the interossei in the foot insert mainly into the bases of the proximal phalanges, an anatomic fact that contradicts the theory of Duchenne of the "moderating action of the interossei" on the middle and distal phalanges in preventing flexion at the interphalangeal joints.[85]

Paralysis of the intrinsic muscles of the foot produces pes planovalgus, not pes cavus. Coonrad, Irwin, Gucker, and Wray observed that persistent function of the short toe flexors and other intrinsic muscles of the foot in an otherwise flail foot resulted in the development of cavovarus deformity of the foot.[31] Garceau and Brahms demonstrated the importance of functioning intrinsic muscles in the production of pes cavus and pes cavovarus; they recommended resection of the motor branches of both the medial and lateral plantar nerves. In their experience the results of 47 operations in 40 patients were encouraging.[53]

Electromyographic studies of the intrinsic muscles of the foot and the extrinsic muscles of the foot and leg in patients with pes cavus have been performed by Bertrand and Ingelrans. Both authors have documented definite abnormality in the short toe flexors and other intrinsic muscles of the foot. Ingelrans also observed abnormal activity in the long toe extensor and peroneus longus muscles.[12, 78] The author has repeatedly observed such changes, but has found it difficult to correlate electromyographic findings in pes cavus with dynamic muscle imbalance and abnormal forces causing the cavus deformity.

Lambrinudi supported Duchenne's theory of interosseus insufficiency as the cause of clawfoot and devised an operation consisting of arthrodeses of both interphalangeal joints and sectioning of the long toe extensors. Stiffening the interphalangeal joints brings the entire action of the long toe flexor to bear on the metatarsophalangeal joint; thus, during locomotion, the toes are pressed on the ground and the metatarsal heads are supported.[89]

Triceps Surae Muscle. The triceps surae muscle has been blamed as a factor in the pathogenesis of pes cavus. When the gastrocnemius-soleus muscles are paralyzed, the normal long toe flexor muscles substitute for the lost action of the triceps surae during the push-off phase of gait, with resultant clawing of the toes. The forefoot becomes plantar-flexed because of the depressing action of the claw toes. In paralytic neuromuscular disease, calcaneocavus deformity may result from such a mechanism.

Hyperactivity of Intrinsic Muscles of Foot. This is considered by Coonrad and associates and by Garceau and Brahms to be a cause of pes cavovarus.[31, 53] This theory fails, however, to explain the hyperextension deformity of the proximal phalanges of the toes.

Muscle Fibrosis and Contracture. Fibrosis and permanent contracture of the short toe flexors and other intrinsic muscles of the foot and plantar aponeurosis have been repeatedly demonstrated at surgery in pes cavus. As stated previously, the intrinsic muscles of the foot insert into the bases of the proximal phalanges, not into the metatarsal heads. The proximal phalanx of the toes in pes cavus is hyperextended, not flexed.

Genetic Factors. In idiopathic pes cavus there is a high rate of familial incidence; an exact method of hereditary transmission has not, however, been delineated. The genetic aspects of degenerative diseases of the spinocerebellar tracts and spina bifida are discussed in Chapter 5.

In summary, the exact pathogenesis of pes cavus is not known. Diverse factors may be operative in it. In some cases, equinus forefoot may be the primary deformity; in others, clawing of the toes; and occasionally, inversion of the hindfoot. Pes cavus is a manifestation of neuromuscular disease unless proved otherwise. It is imperative, therefore, that the following studies be performed to determine various possible etiologic factors: (1) a thorough family history (which should include foot examinations and neurologic assessments of the siblings and parents); (2) a muscle examination to rule out paralytic disease; (3) a thorough neurologic evaluation (often it is best to obtain consultation with a pediatric neurologist); (4) radiography of the *entire* spine; (5) nerve conduction and electromyographic studies; and (6) in selected cases when indicated, lumbar puncture, myelography, and computed tomography of the spine.

Clinical Features

There are various types of pes cavus that should be distinguished: In *simple pes cavus*, the plantar flexion deformity of the forefoot is equal in its medial and lateral columns, with even distribution of weight on the first and fifth metatarsal heads. The heel is in neutral position or a few degrees valgus, which is normal (see Fig. 7–151 B and C). In *pes cavovarus* only the medial column of the forefoot is dropped in plantar flexion; consequently, the longitudinal axes of the first metatarsal and, to a lesser degree, of the second metatarsal are at a marked equinus angle, while that of the fifth metatarsal is in normal horizontal position (Figs. 7–151 D and E and 7–152 A to C). Examination of the non-weight-bearing foot (with the patient sitting and his leg hanging at the edge of the table) will reveal that the fifth metatarsal can easily be dorsiflexed into neutral position, whereas the first metatarsal is fixed in equinus position and cannot be passively manipulated into neu-

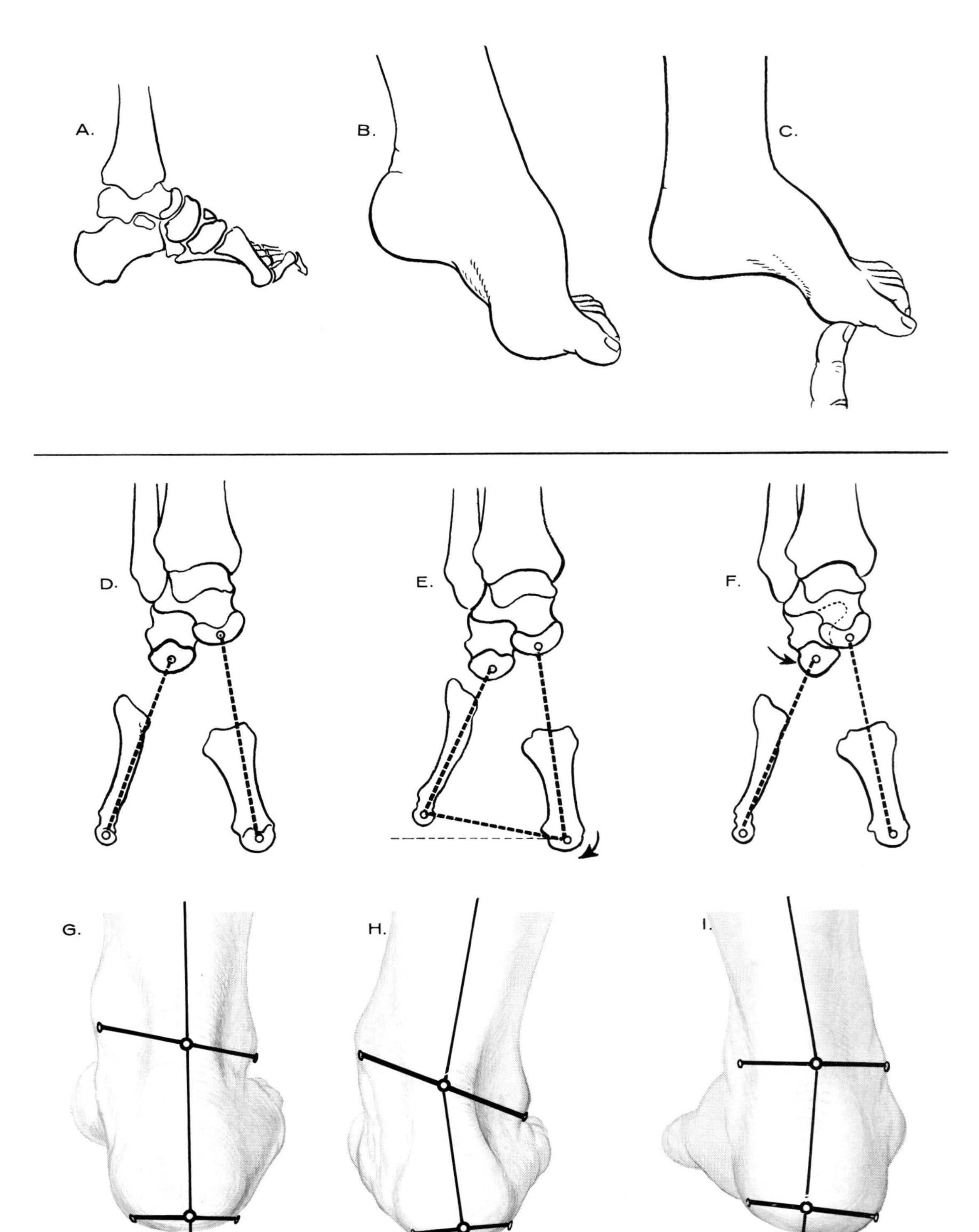

FIGURE 7–152. Pes cavovarus.

A to **C.** Diagrams of mediolateral view of the foot demonstrating that only the medial column of the forefoot is dropped in plantar flexion. Note the longitudinal axis of the first metatarsal is markedly equinus, whereas that of the fifth metatarsal is in normal alignment. On push-up test, the first metatarsal cannot be passively manipulated into neutral extension. **D** to **F.** Diagrams of the mechanism of inversion of the hindfoot in pes cavovarus. In the normal foot, the weight-bearing forces are equally distributed on the first and fifth metatarsal heads (**D**). In pes cavovarus the first metatarsal is fixed in equinus position and the forefoot is in 20 to 30 degrees of pronation. In stance and locomotion, there is excessive pressure on the pronated first metatarsal head (**E**). Excessive pressure on the first metatarsal head is relieved by inverting the whole foot (both forefoot and hindfoot) (**F**). **G** to **I.** Posterior views of the ankle and foot, showing the normal, pronated, and inverted hindfoot. The hindfoot assumes a varus inclination as the forefoot is inverted.

tral extension. Closer scrutiny and analysis will disclose that the forefoot, particularly the first metatarsal, is in 20 to 30 degrees of pronation. The longitudinal arch is elevated. In the early stages the hindfoot is in neutral position, and in stance and locomotion there is excessive pressure on the pronated first metatarsal head; in order to relieve this pressure the whole foot (forefoot and hindfoot) is inverted (Fig. 7–152 D to I). Initially, the varus deformity of the hindfoot is reducible and can be expected to disappear when the fixed equinus deformity and pronation of the first metatarsal are corrected. With time, however, the hindfoot deformity becomes fixed and cannot be corrected by aligning the forefoot (Fig. 7–153). *Calcaneocavus deformity* of the foot usually occurs in flaccid paralysis, such as that seen in poliomyelitis or myelomeningocele. The triceps surae muscle is paralyzed. The hindfoot is in calcaneus position and the forefoot is fixed in equinus position (cf. Fig. 7–151 F). *Pes equinocavus* is usually secondary to talipes equinovarus; in addition to the forefoot, the hindfoot and ankle are in equinus posture (cf. Fig. 7–151 G). Occasionally cavus deformity of the feet is present at birth. The terms *talipes cavus* and *congenital cavus foot* are used to describe the condition.

On examination, the forefoot of the cavovarus foot (especially the first metatarsal) is plantarflexed and pronated, whereas the hindfoot is in varus supination. The hindfoot and forefoot are interdependent; i.e., the forefoot pronation supinates the flexible hindfoot owing to the "tripod" effect. The medial longitudinal arch is elevated and the soft tissues in the plantar aspect of the foot are taut, fixing the forefoot in plantar flexion. The contracted structures are the plantar aponeurosis, the abductor hallucis, the flexor hallucis brevis, the flexor digitorum brevis, the abductor digiti quinti, the interossei, the tendinous insertions of the posterior tibial tendon on the plantar aspect of the cuneiform and the base of the metatarsals, the Y-ligament (calcaneocuboid and calcaneonavicular), and the capsule on the plantar aspect of the naviculocuneiform and the cuneiform-metatarsal joints. Bony and articular deformities gradually follow the soft-tissue contracture. The head of the first metatarsal is prominent beneath the sole of the foot.

In pes cavus the toes may be normal, but usually they become progressively retracted and clawed, with hyperextension of the metatarsophalangeal joints and flexion of the interphalangeal joints. The great toe and the fifth toe are ordinarily the most severely deformed (Fig. 7–153 D). A painful adventitious bursa may develop over the dorsum of the interphalangeal joint as a result of irritation by the shoe; with dorsal subluxation of the metatarsophalangeal joints, the bases of the proximal phalanges press against the metatarsal heads and exaggerate the forefoot equinus deformity. In severe claw toe deformity, the toes do not touch the ground at all and lose their function of propulsion in gait; consequently, most of the body weight is transmitted to the metatarsal heads, and plantar keratosis develops.

Depending upon the type of pes cavus, the position of the hindfoot may be neutral, inverted, equinus, or calcaneus. In pes cavovarus, the heel is inverted and the talocalcaneal angle is decreased on the radiogram. In pes equinocavus, contracture of the triceps surae muscle causes the hindfoot to be fixed in plantar flexion, and in stance the heel does not touch the floor (Fig. 7–153 C). Most of the body weight is borne on the metatarsal heads. If the equinus deformity is not corrected, painful callosities develop on the plantar aspect of the metatarsal heads. The keratotic skin eventually ulcerates and secondary infection sets in.

Radiographic Findings

Weight-bearing anteroposterior and lateral radiograms of the feet are made. Lateral projections of the foot in maximal dorsiflexion demonstrate the apex of the cavus deformity. In the normal foot, the distal and proximal articular surfaces of the first cuneiform bone are almost parallel to each other. In pes cavus the forefoot equinus inclination is usually maximal at the first cuneiform bone, and the articular surfaces of the bone converge in the plantar aspect of the foot. Less often the tarsal navicular is at the apex of the cavus deformity. Occasionally the forefoot will drop into equinus posture more distally at the tarsometatarsal joints.

Different methods may be used to gauge the degree of pes cavus. Hibbs measures the angle formed between two lines drawn through the centers of the longitudinal axes of the calcaneus and the first metatarsal (Fig. 7–154 C).[71] Méary measures the angle formed between two lines drawn through the centers of the longitudinal axes of the talus and the first metatarsal (Fig. 7–154 B).[100]

The talocalcaneal angle is measured on the anteroposterior radiogram; in pes cavovarus it will be decreased. Routine standing radiograms of the ankle should be made also to detect any

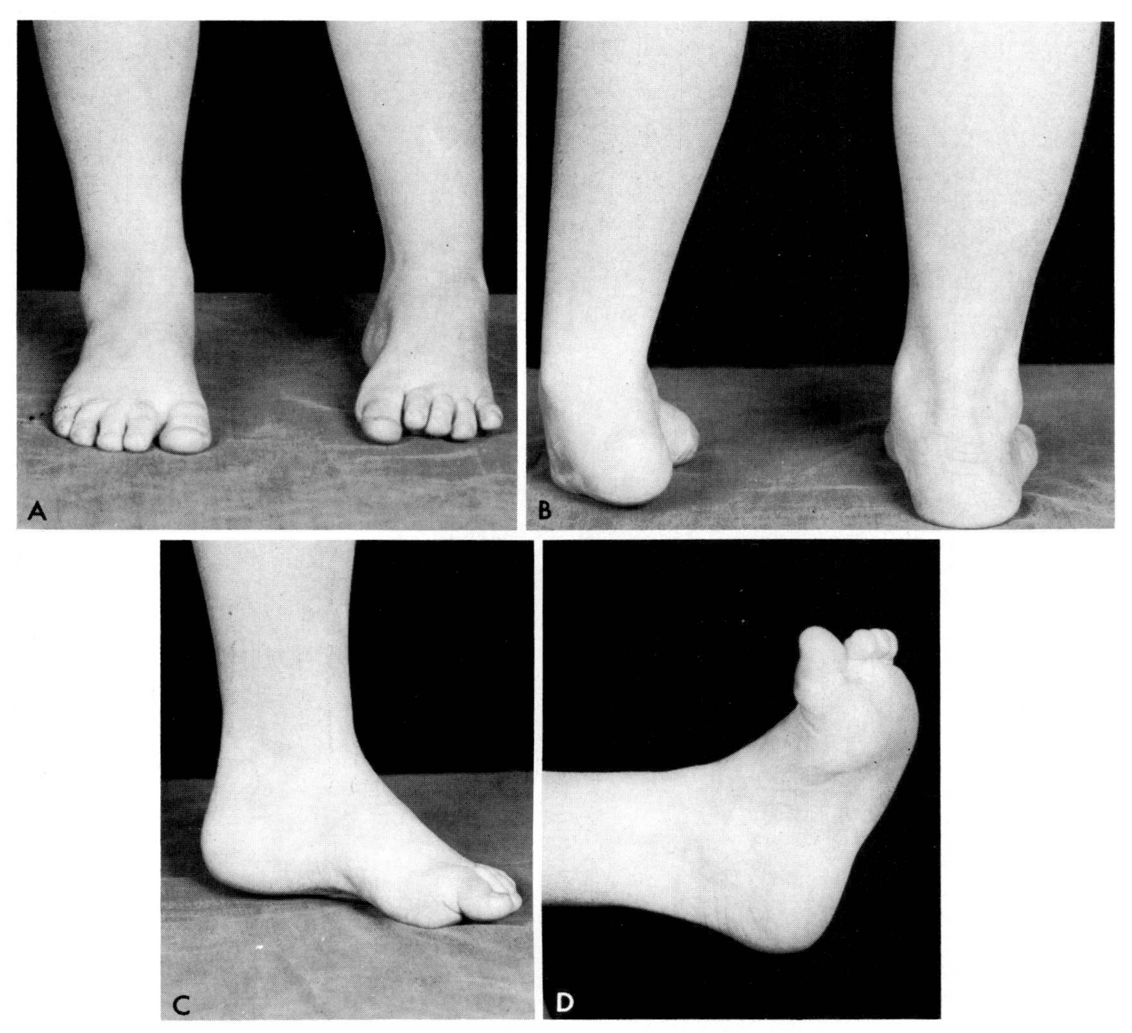

FIGURE 7–153. Cavovarus deformity of left foot.

A and **B.** Anterior and posterior views showing varus deformity of both forefoot and hindfoot. **C.** Medial view of left foot showing the equinus forefoot. Note also that the heel is not touching the floor, indicating associated contracture of the triceps surae muscle. **D.** Range of active dorsiflexion of ankle and foot. Note the clawing of the great toe.

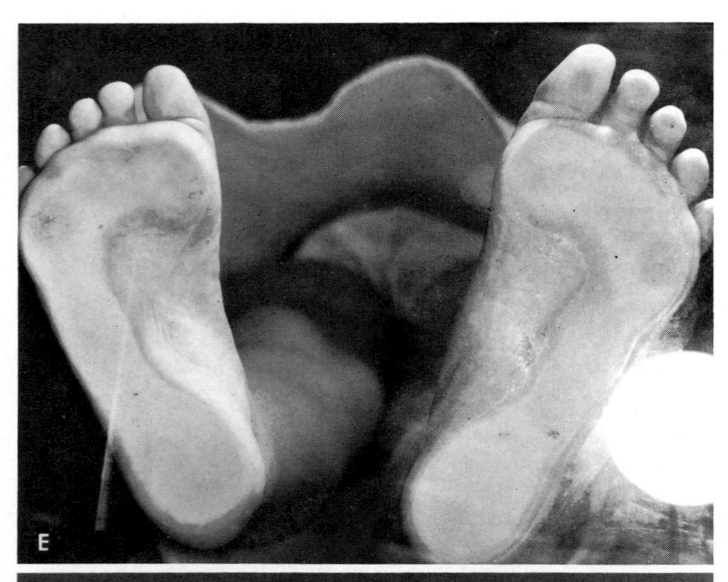

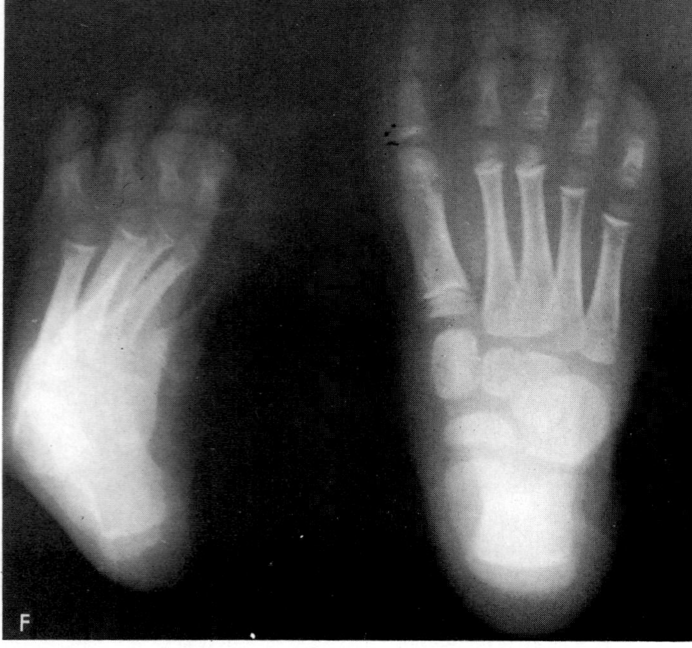

FIGURE 7–153 Continued Cavovarus deformity of left foot.

E. Plantar standing view. **F.** Weight-bearing anteroposterior radiogram of both feet, depicting the varus deformity of forefoot and hindfoot on the left.

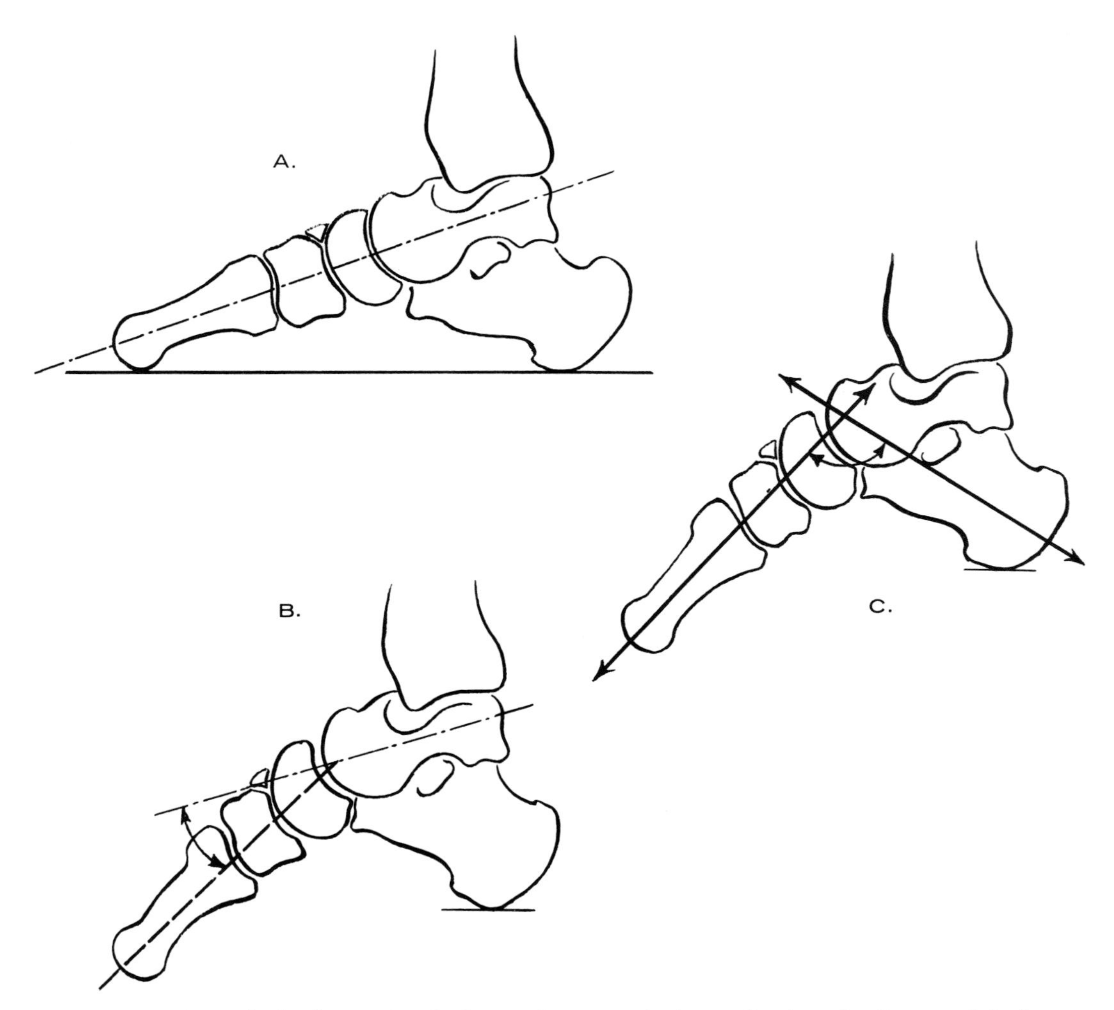

FIGURE 7–154. Methods of measuring the degree of pes cavus in the standing lateral radiogram of the foot.

A. In the normal foot, the longitudinal axis of the talus is parallel with that of the first metatarsal. **B.** *Méary* measures the angle formed between lines drawn through the centers of the longitudinal axes of the talus and the first metatarsal. **C.** *Hibbs* measures the angle formed between two lines drawn through the centers of the longitudinal axes of the calcaneus and the first metatarsal.

medial tilting of the ankle mortise, which may be the cause of varus deformity of the hindfoot.

Treatment

Conservative measures are indicated in early and mild cases. Passive stretching exercises of the contracted plantar fascia and the short plantar muscles are performed several times a day. For comfort, a supportive insole with a 1-cm. pad just behind the metatarsals is placed in the shoe to relieve pressure from the metatarsal heads and redistribute the weight (Fig. 7–155). A Plastizote shoe insert of medium density is usually used. The toe portion of the shoes should be wide enough not to press on the toes. A ⅛- to 3/16-inch wedge on the lateral side of the heel is given if the hindfoot tends to go into inversion. Thin padding on the tongue of the shoe will relieve pressure on the dorsum of the foot. The objective of these measures is to provide symptomatic relief. Special shoes, shoe inserts, and ankle-foot orthoses neither correct cavovarus deformity of the foot nor prevent it from increasing in severity.

Surgical measures are indicated when the deformity is severe and disabling. Preoperative assessment should be thorough. The factors that determine the type of operation are as follows: (1) The *location of the apex of cavus deformity.* Is it anterior at the naviculocuneiform or tarsometatarsal joints or more posterior at the talonavicular and calcaneocuboid articulations? (2) The *type of pes cavus.* Is it a simple cavus or a cavovarus deformity? Is there pronation of the forefoot, particularly of the first metatarsal? (3) The *position of the hindfoot.* Is it inverted, neutral, or everted? Is there calcaneus or equinus deformity of the heel? (4) The *deformity of the toes.* Are they clawed? Do the tips of the toes touch the ground? Is there painful adventitious bursitis over the dorsum of the interphalangeal joints? How flexible is the deformity of the toes? On passive dorsiflexion of the metatarsal heads do the metatarsophalangeal joints flex from hyperextension to neutral position and do the flexed toes extend fully (Fig. 7–156)? The passive range of motion of the proximal and distal interphalangeal joints is noted. On weight-bearing, do the tips of the

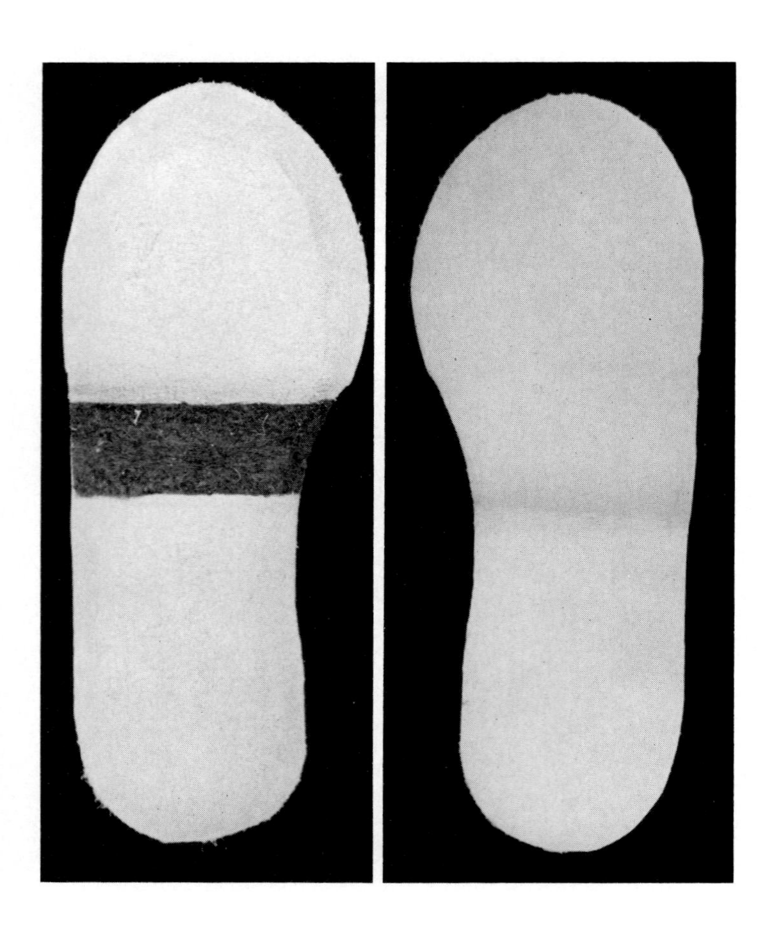

FIGURE 7–155. Insole with a ⅜-inch pad placed just behind metatarsal heads.

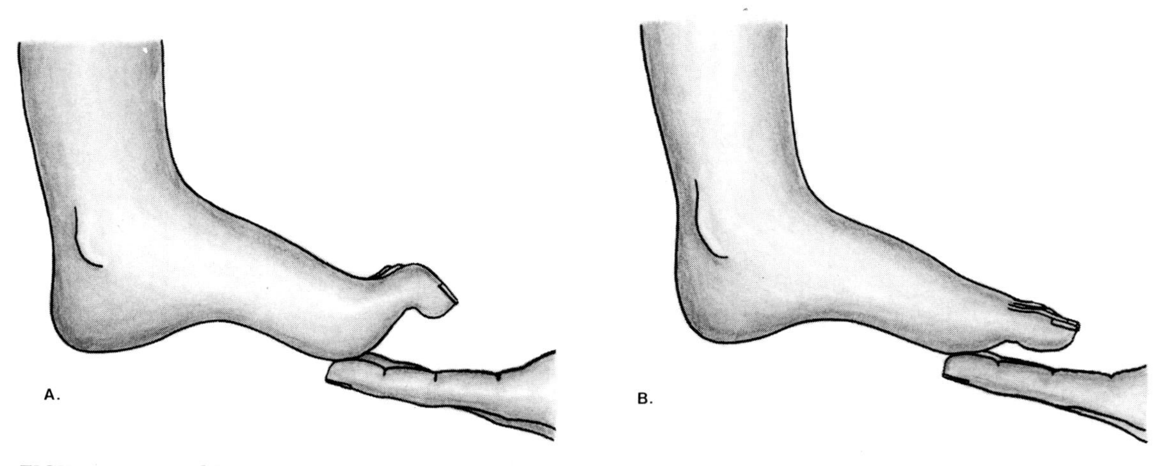

FIGURE 7–156. Kelikian's "push-up" test for flexibility of the metatarsophalangeal and interphalangeal joints in clawfoot.

On passive dorsiflexion of the metatarsal heads the hyperextended metatarsophalangeal joints extend to neutral position and the interphalangeal joints extend fully.

toes touch the floor? (5) The *condition of the sole* on the plantar aspect of the metatarsal heads. Are there painful callosities? Is the skin ulcerated? (6) The *shoe wear.* Is it abnormal? (7) The *rigidity of the deformities* and their severity. How taut are the plantar soft tissues? How far can the forefoot be dorsiflexed out of equinus posture? Is there contracture of the triceps surae muscle? Does the hindfoot evert beyond neutral on passive manipulation?

Coleman and Chestnut have described a simple test for hindfoot flexibility in the cavovarus foot (Fig. 7–157). The "cavovarus test," or standing lateral block test, is performed as follows: Place the patient's foot on a 2.5- to 4-cm.-thick wooden block with the heel and the lateral border of the foot on the block and bearing full weight while the first through third metatarsals are allowed to hang freely into plantar flexion and full pronation; this maneuver neutralizes the tripod mechanism and negates any effect that the forefoot may have on the hindfoot in stance (Fig. 7–157 A to C). A flexible hindfoot will assume a normal valgus position. The degree of correction of hindfoot varus deviation is recorded by photographs and radiograms. An anteroposterior radiogram is made of the foot with the tube directed 30 degrees cephalad toward the dome of the talus; then, with the patient still standing on the block (but without increasing the height of the block), normal weight-bearing and lateral anteroposterior radiograms of the foot are also made. The talocalcaneal angle is measured. If the decreased talocalcaneal angle is restored to normal value by this maneuver, the hindfoot is flexible and therapeutic efforts should be directed toward the forefoot. If, however, the talocalcaneal angle remains decreased it means the varus deformity of the hindfoot is fixed and surgical measures should be employed to correct both the forefoot and hindfoot deformations (Fig. 7–157 D to F).[29] This author finds the test to be reliable in assessing and documenting whether or not the hindfoot is flexible during stance phase. (8) *Strength of muscles* controlling foot and ankle. Is there any dynamic imbalance between the anterior tibial (dorsiflexor of the first metatarsal bone) and the peroneus longus (plantar flexor of the first metatarsal bone) and between the evertors and invertors of the foot and dorsiflexors and plantar flexors of the ankle? Is it necessary to provide stability to the foot by arthodesis? (9) *Stability of the neurologic picture.* Is there any progressive neuromuscular deficit? Can the primary neurologic affection be corrected by appropriate neurosurgical treatment? Determination of the nature of the disease process is vital. What is the rate and pattern of progression of paralysis? For example, in Charcot-Marie-Tooth disease, the posterior tibial muscle may be the only muscle left functioning for effective anterior transfer. (10) The *age of the patient* and the skeletal maturity of the foot.

In general, operative measures should be delayed until several periodic examinations have ruled out progressive neuromuscular deficit. As a rule surgical correction of pes cavus should be executed in stages in a systematic, progressive approach. First, a plantar release is always carried out. Sectioning of the taut plantar

Text continued on page 2686

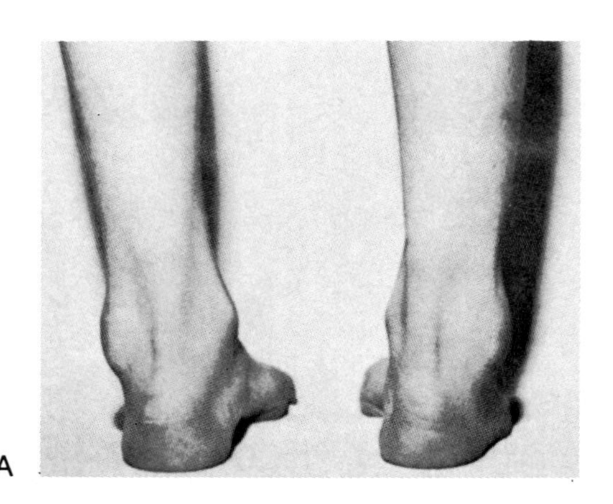

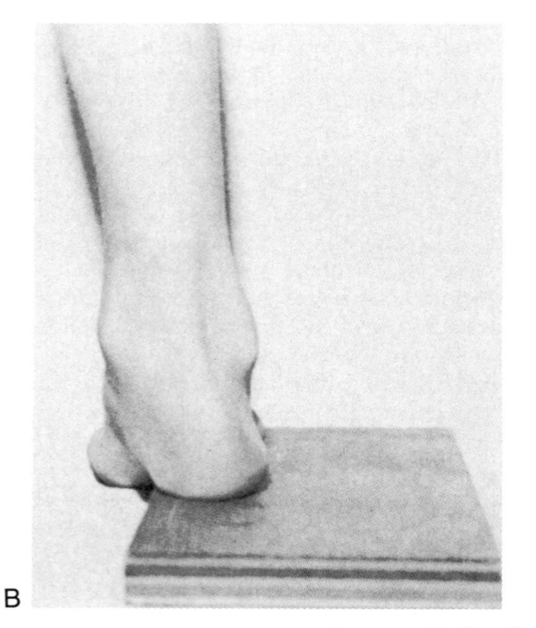

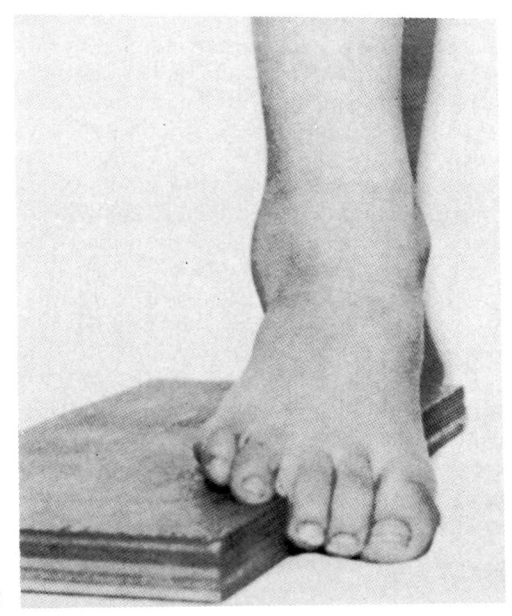

FIGURE 7–157. Test to determine hindfoot flexibility in cavovarus foot (Coleman's cavovarus test).

A. Posterior view of both feet, standing. Note the varus deformity of the right heel. **B** and **C.** Posterior and anterior views of the right foot, standing. The heel and the lateral border of the foot are bearing full weight on a block 2.5 cm. thick, whereas the first through third metatarsals are plantar-flexed into pronation.

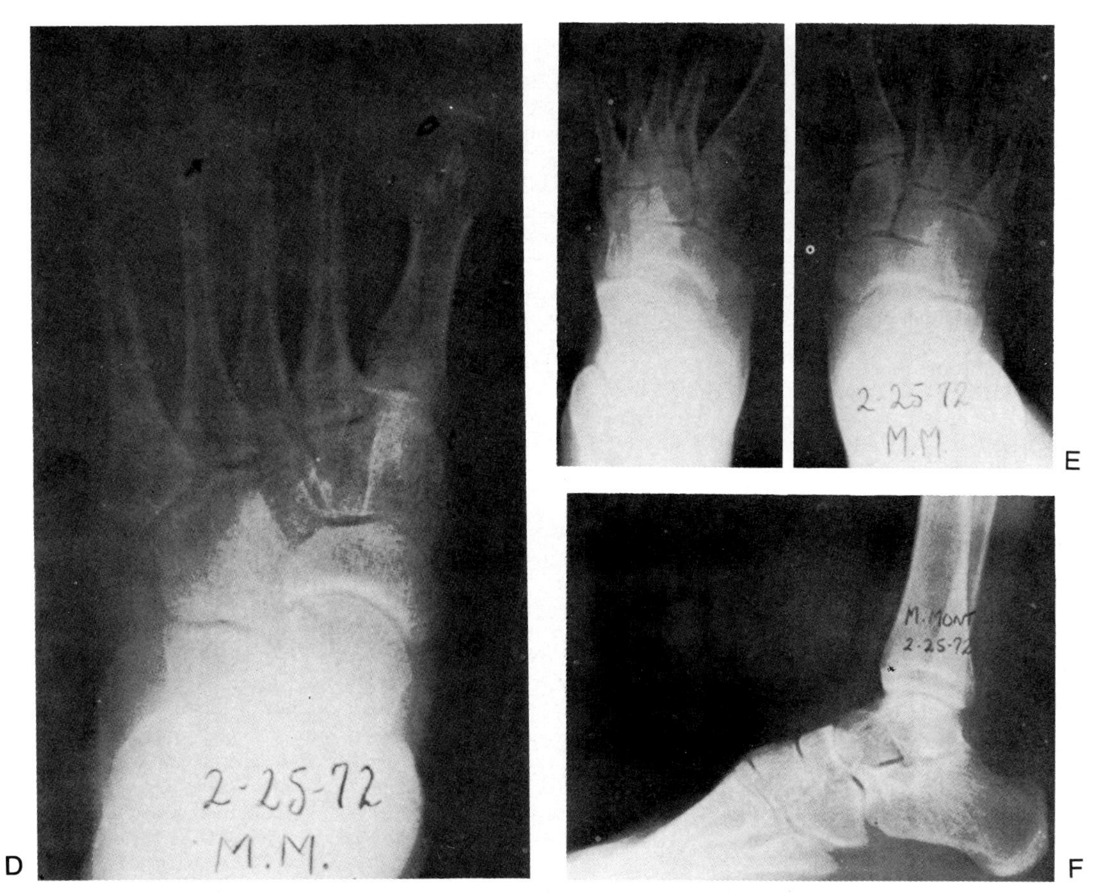

FIGURE 7–157 Continued. Test to determine flexibility in cavovarus foot (Coleman's cavovarus test).

D. Anteroposterior radiogram of the right foot with the patient standing on the block. Note the restoration of normal articulation between the talus and calcaneus; the talocalcaneal angle is normal. **E.** Standing anteroposterior radiograms of the feet. Note the decreased talocalcaneal angle of the cavovarus foot (on the left of the photograph). **F.** Standing lateral radiogram of the same right foot. Note the forefoot equinus deformity, the high arch, and the "through-and-through" visualization of the subtalar joint. (From Coleman, S. S., and Chesnut, W. J.: A simple test for hindfoot flexibility in the cavovarus foot. Clin. Orthop., *123*:60, 1977. Reprinted by permission.)

Plantar Fasciotomy and Release of Contracted Soft Tissues on Plantar Aspect of Cavus Foot

SUBCUTANEOUS SECTION OF PLANTAR APONEUROSIS

A. This procedure is performed when contracture of the plantar fascia is moderate and that of the short plantar muscles is minimal. It is not recommended by this author.

A sharp Ryerson knife is inserted deep to the plantar fascia with the blade flat to the skin. Then the sharp edge of the blade is rotated 90 degrees, bringing its sharp edge toward the plantar fascia. By pushing it against the knife with the index finger of the opposite hand, the plantar fascia is completely divided. It is sectioned at two levels about 2.5 cm. apart, and stretched by holding the heel steady and bringing the forefoot into dorsiflexion. A below-knee walking cast is applied. The cast is changed every two to three weeks, and each time the forefoot is manipulated into further dorsiflexion. The metatarsal heads and the heel should be adequately padded and the cast well molded to prevent pressure sores.

The total period for which stretching casts should be used is about eight weeks, depending upon the severity and fixity of deformity. At night, following removal of the solid cast, the forefoot is held out of equinus and in neutral position in a posterior ankle-foot polypropylene splint; the metatarsal heads can be elevated into further dorsiflexion by a Plastizote metatarsal insert glued to the insole of the splint. The night splints are worn for several years, depending upon the cause of pes cavus and the severity of deformity. Metatarsal pads are worn in the shoes during the day. Passive stretching exercises of the plantar fascia are performed several times a day.

SECTION OF PLANTAR APONEUROSIS AND SHORT PLANTAR MUSCLES THROUGH MIDLINE INCISION

B. The Steindler stripping operation for pes cavus should not be performed because of its possible inherent complications of contracture of the scar in the instep, injury to neurovascular structures, and inadequate correction of equinus forefoot. The author recommends the following technique when contracture of plantar soft tissues is moderate.

A midline incision is made on the sole of the foot, extending from 1 cm. distal to the tuberosity of the calcaneus to the base of the metatarsals. The subcutaneous tissue is divided and the wound flaps are undermined and elevated. The central, medial, and lateral portions of the plantar aponeurosis are widely excised. The abductor hallucis is sectioned at its origin from the medial process of the tuberosity of the calcaneus and the laciniate ligament. The flexor digitorum brevis, abductor digiti quinti, and quadratus plantae muscles and the long plantar ligaments are detached from their origin on the tuberosity of the calcaneus. By keeping the dissection immediately adjacent to bone, injury to neurovascular structures is avoided. The pneumatic tourniquet is released and after complete hemostasis the skin is approximated by interrupted sutures. A below-knee walking cast is applied with the heel held in valgus posture and the forefoot in some degree of supination. This position of the foot in the cast tends to correct the cavovarus deformity by flattening the longitudinal arch. Weight-bearing is not allowed during the first postoperative week. Ten to fourteen days after surgery the cast is removed; the wound is inspected for healing, but the sutures are not removed. A new below-knee walking cast is applied. This author uses plaster of Paris cast for the first two layers and then reinforces it with several layers of plastic adhesive tape. This allows better molding of the cast and makes it much stronger. An anterior heel is applied to the cast. If the wound edges are healthy the heel is manipulated and held into a greater valgus inclination and the forefoot into further supination, obtaining additional correction of the cavovarus deformity. The patient is allowed and encouraged to walk on the cast. The casts are changed biweekly, for a total period of cast immobilization of eight weeks.

Plate 105. Plantar Fasciotomy and Release of Contracted Soft Tissues on Plantar Aspect of Cavus Foot

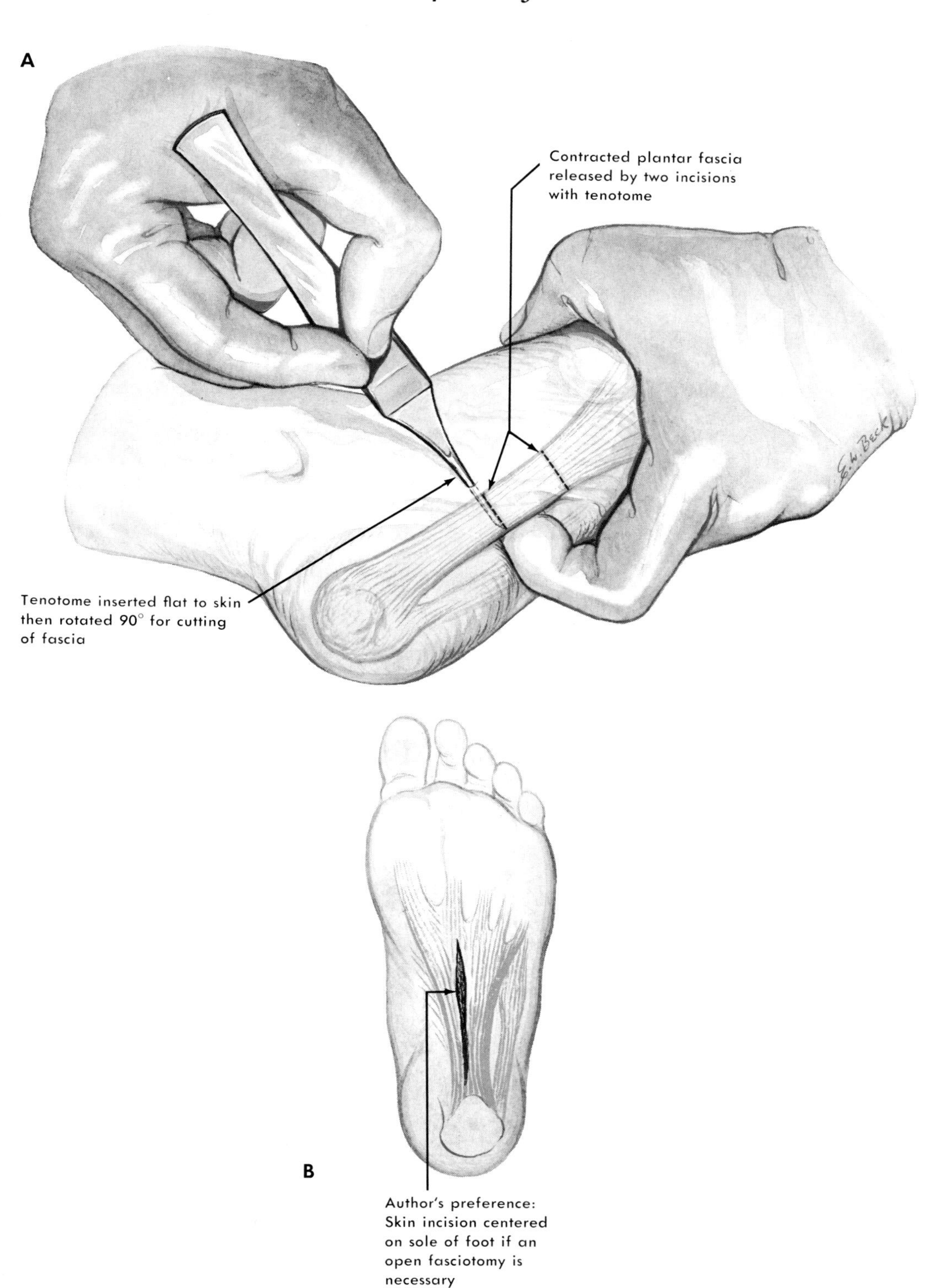

fascia, short plantar muscles, and plantar ligaments will allow the forefoot to be elevated from equinus posture into neutral dorsiflexion. This basic dictum should never be violated. Second, the correction obtained is assessed clinically and radiologically to determine the degree of rigidity of the osseous changes. If the hindfoot varus deformity is flexible, the long toe extensor tendons are transferred to the metatarsal heads, and any invertor-evertor dynamic muscle imbalance is corrected by appropriate muscle and tendon transfers. If the varus hindfoot is rigid on the lateral block test and the forefoot cannot be elevated to neutral position, the fixed osseous changes are corrected by appropriate bony procedures prior to tendon transfers. Pes cavus is a dynamic deformity during the period of skeletal growth. Success or failure in correcting it is often determined by the diligence of detailed postoperative care.

SOFT-TISSUE PROCEDURES

Release of Contractures on Plantar Aspect of Foot

Subcutaneous Section of Plantar Aponeurosis. In the past, in paralytic pes cavus due to poliomyelitis, this procedure was performed when the contracture of the plantar fascia was moderate and that of the short plantar muscles was minimal. It was followed by a series of stretching casts to obtain full correction. The technique is illustrated in Plate 105. Fibrositis of the plantar fascia is an occasional but bothersome complication of this simple procedure. This author recommends that the contracted plantar fascia be excised by open surgery rather than released by percutaneous section.

Section of Plantar Aponeurosis and Short Plantar Muscles Near Their Origin from Tuberosity of Calcaneus. In 1920, Steindler described a stripping operation for pes cavus in which a longitudinal incision was made on the medial side of the calcaneus, and the long plantar ligament was transversely sectioned. The flexor digitorum brevis, abductor digiti quinti, and abductor hallucis brevis were also subperiosteally stripped and released from the calcaneus.[138–140] The Steindler procedure should not be performed because the operative scar in the instep contracts, hypertrophies because of irritation from the shoe, and acts as a deforming force. Other drawbacks of the Steindler plantar fascial stripping are the potential injury to neurovascular structures and the inadequate correction of forefoot equinus deformity.

The author prefers a midline incision on the sole of the foot when contracture of plantar soft tissues is moderate and not very rigid. The resultant scar is minimal and not bothersome, and the exposure is adequate for the complete release of moderately contracted plantar soft tissues. The operative technique is described in Plate 105.[130, 152] Westin, after Lucas, performs the plantar release through a lateral incision.[152] Inadvertent injury to neurovascular structures should be avoided. It is imperative postoperatively to apply a series of stretching casts with an anterior heel for a total period of at least eight weeks.

If more extensive soft-tissue release is indicated, the procedure described by Bost, Schottstaedt, and Larsen is carried out:[16]

A curvilinear incision is made over the medial aspect of the foot; it begins over the posterior tuberosity of the calcaneus in line with skin creases, extends dorsally and anteriorly to a point 1 cm. inferior to the medial malleolus, and then extends distally to terminate at the base of the first metatarsal. Subcutaneous tissues are elevated in line with the skin incision. The wound edges are undermined, elevated, and retracted. The abductor hallucis muscle is released entirely at its origin and retracted distally. In severe cavovarus deformity this author excises the abductor hallucis muscle; it facilitates surgical exposure and closure of the wound.

Next, the neurovascular bundle is identified, isolated, and traced to its bifurcation into medial and lateral plantar branches. The flexor digitorum longus and flexor hallucis longus tendons are identified, and the master knot of Henry is sectioned. A generous portion of the plantar aponeurosis is excised. Next, the short flexors and plantar muscles are sectioned extraperiosteally from their calcaneal origin and dissected distally up to the talonavicular and calcaneocuboid joints. The contracted tendinous expansions of the posterior tibial tendon should be sectioned at their metatarsal and cuneiform attachments because they fix the first metatarsal in equinus posture. The Y-ligament (the calcaneocuboid and calcaneonavicular ligaments) and the plantar portion of the capsules of the cuneiforms and the first three metatarsals are sectioned. The tourniquet is released, and after complete hemostasis the wound is closed with closed suction Hemovac tubes. A below-knee cast is applied. The postoperative care is similar to that after plantar release through a midline incision.

Transfer of Long Toe Extensors to Heads of Metatarsals.[25, 50, 83, 131] This procedure is indicated when, on active dorsiflexion of the foot, the toes hyperextend but the metatarsal heads do not elevate and remain in equinus posture. The tendon transfer will increase the power of dorsiflexion of the foot and elevate the metatarsal heads, providing a dynamic force against forefoot equinus deformity. By routing the tendons from the medial to the lateral side, the transfer will also be given some inversion power, which acts against the pronation deformity of the forefoot in pes cavovarus.

For the tendon transfers to function effectively, the foot should be flexible. First, a release of contracted soft tissues on the plantar aspect of the foot is carried out. In cases of mild deformity the two procedures can be combined at the same operation; however, in moderate and severe deformities, the use of stretching casts for a period of two to three months is essential to correct the position of the forefoot. Tendon transfers are performed only when fixed cavus deformity has been fully corrected—the importance of this prerequisite cannot be overemphasized.

In 1919, Hibbs described an operation for correction of clawing of the lesser toes. The tendons of the extensor digitorum longus were divided as far distally as possible and anchored en masse into the third cuneiform bone.[71] The Hibbs operation should not be performed for pes cavus, as it fails to provide a dynamic force to elevate the metatarsal heads.

The operative technique of transfer of the long toe extensors to the metatarsal heads is described and illustrated in Plate 106. When there is associated clawing of the toes, it is combined with fusion of the proximal interphalangeal joints.

Transfer of Anterior Tibial Tendon to Dorsum of Base of First Metatarsal. This procedure, described by Fowler and associates, is combined with an opening-wedge vertical extension osteotomy of the medial cuneiform.[49] The osteotomy site is opened up on its plantar aspect and held by a triangular wedge of autogenous bone based plantarward. The osteotomized fragments are transfixed by a threaded Steinmann pin. Plantar release is always performed first. The transferred anterior tibial tendon acts as a dorsiflexor of the first metatarsal. The opening-wedge dorsiflexion osteotomy of the medial cuneiform bone elevates and elongates the medial ray of the foot. In Fowler's experience, when the hindfoot is flexible and there is satisfactory extrinsic muscle balance, the procedure will correct the cavovarus deformity. When there is fixed plantar-flexion deformity of the first ray, this author recommends combination of Fowler's procedure with transfer of the extensor hallucis longus to the first metatarsal head, as shown in Figure 7–158; and of the long toe extensors to the second, third, and fourth metatarsal necks.

The anterior tibial tendon should not be transferred laterally to decrease the inversion deformity in pes cavovarus because it will enhance the action of the peroneus longus as plantar flexor of the first metatarsal, nor should the posterior tibial tendons be lengthened in an attempt to correct hindfoot varus deformity. In paralytic pes cavovarus, as in Charcot-Marie-Tooth disease, function of the posterior tibial muscle must be preserved because it will have to be transferred anteriorly to provide dorsiflexion of the ankle and foot (see Chapter 5).

In idiopathic flexible pes cavovarus, fractional lengthening at the musculotendinous junction of the peroneus longus may be indicated to weaken its action as plantar flexor and pronator of the first metatarsal when the anterior tibial tendon is transferred to the dorsum of the base of the first metatarsal.

Selective neurectomy of the motor nerves to plantar muscles in pes cavus is not recommended by the author, as, in his experience, the results have been poor. The procedure was described by Garceau and Brahms for the treatment of paralytic cavovarus deformity of the feet following poliomyelitis; they reported encouraging results.[53] Coonrad and co-workers recommend neurectomy of the motor branches of the lateral plantar nerve and partial excision of the short toe flexors and plantar fascia in paralytic pes cavovarus.[31] Such a procedure is indicated only when the short toe flexors and other intrinsic muscles of the foot are functioning in an otherwise flail foot.

PROCEDURES ON BONE

In the adolescent or adult patient with a skeletally mature foot, osseous structural changes may fix the forefoot in marked equinus position and pronation and the hindfoot in rigid varus position. Such rigid cavovarus feet require bony procedures to correct the deformity. A number of operations have been described in the literature. In general they can be subdivided into those to correct the equinus deformity of the forefoot and those to correct the varus deformity of the hindfoot. As mentioned previously, prior to performing operations on bone, one should release the contracted soft tissues on the plantar aspect of the foot. These two procedures should be performed in separate stages.

Transfer of Long Toe Extensors to Heads of Metatarsals

A. A longitudinal incision is made on the dorsomedial aspect of the first metatarsal, extending from the base of the proximal phalanx to the proximal one fourth of the metatarsal shaft. The incision should be placed medial to the extensor hallucis longus tendon, toward the second metatarsal. The subcutaneous tissue is divided and the wound flaps are retracted with 0 silk sutures. The digital nerves and vessels should not be injured.

B. The extensor hallucis longus and brevis tendons are identified and sectioned at the base of the proximal phalanx. An alternate technique is to leave the insertion of the extensor hallucis brevis tendon intact; the stump of the extensor hallucis longus tendon is sutured to the intact brevis tendon. (This latter method is faster and is utilized by the author when the long toe extensors of all five toes are to be transferred to the heads of the metatarsals.)

C. Silk whip sutures (00) are inserted in the ends of the long and short toe extensors. The long toe extensor is dissected free, and with a sharp scalpel its sheath is thoroughly excised as far proximally as possible.

D. The epiphyseal plate of the first metatarsal is proximal, whereas that of the lateral four metatarsals is distal in location. The extensor hallucis longus tendon is transferred to the head of the first metatarsal. The long toe extensors of the lesser toes are transferred to the distal one third of the metatarsal shafts, with care taken not to disturb the growth plate. When the patient is over the age of 10 to 12 years, the tendons are transferred to the heads of the metatarsals, as, by then, growth of the foot is almost complete.

With small Chandler elevator retractors, the soft tissues are retracted. The periosteum is not stripped. Through a stab wound in the periosteum, a hole is drilled in the center of the first metatarsal head and is enlarged to receive the tendon. The extensor hallucis longus tendon is passed through the hole in the first metatarsal in a medial to lateral direction and sutured to itself, with the forefoot in maximal dorsiflexion.

E. The extensor hallucis brevis tendon is then sutured to the stump of the long toe extensor, holding the toe in neutral extension or in 10 degrees of dorsiflexion.

A similar technique is employed to transfer the long extensor tendons of the lesser toes. Longitudinal incisions are made between the second and third metatarsals, and between the fourth and fifth metatarsals. The extensor brevis tendon of the little toe is either absent or not of adequate size to transfer to the stump of the longus.

The tourniquet is released and complete hemostasis is obtained. The wounds are closed with interrupted sutures. A below-knee walking cast is applied, to be worn for four to six weeks. A sturdy, well-padded toe plate is made in the cast. The plantar aspect of the metatarsals should be well padded.

Special muscle training for the transferred tendons is not required, as the transfer is in phase.

Plate 106. Transfer of Long Toe Extensors to Heads of Metatarsals

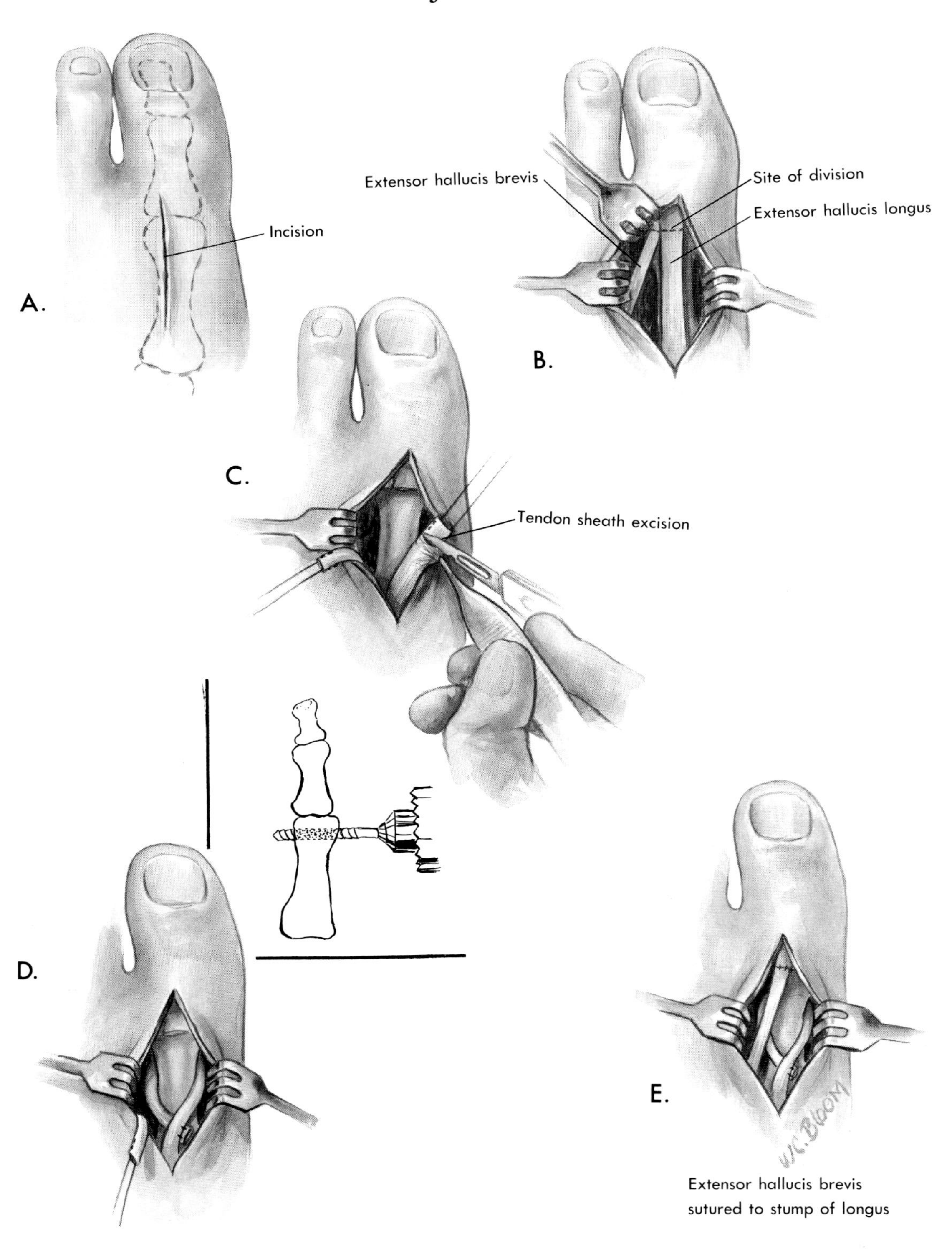

Extensor hallucis longus passed through hole in metatarsal head and sutured to itself

Extensor hallucis brevis sutured to stump of longus

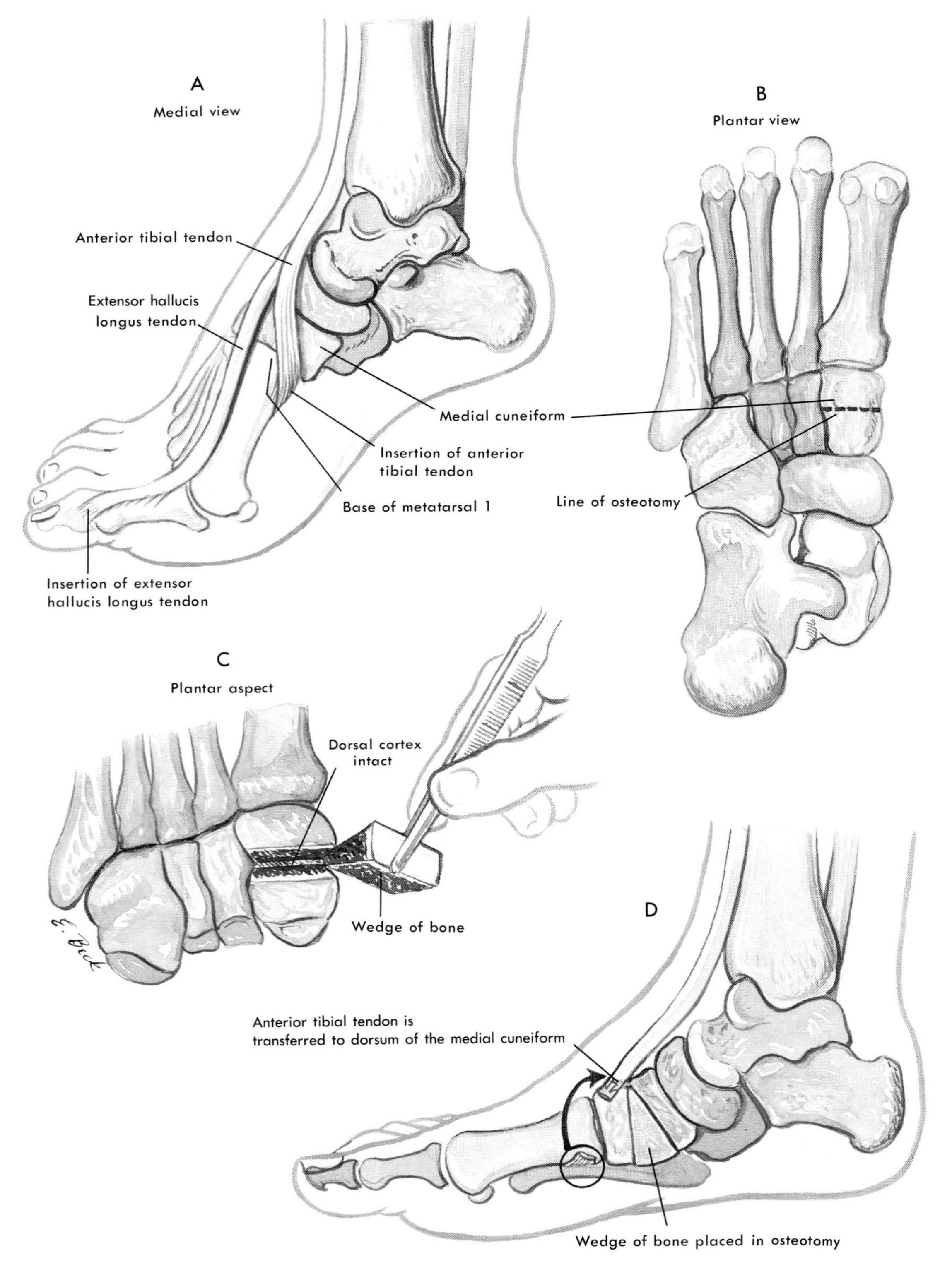

FIGURE 7–158. Vertical osteotomy of the medial cuneiform with a wedge of bone graft based on the plantar aspect.

This is usually combined with transfer of the anterior tibial tendon to increase action as a dorsiflexor of the first metatarsal. The extensor hallucis longus is transferred to the head of the first metatarsal.

Bony Procedures to Correct Forefoot Equinus Deformity

Dorsal Tarsal Wedge Osteotomy. Dorsal wedge resection at the level of the cuneiform and cuboid bones was devised by Saunders and popularized by Cole.[27, 122] It is described and illustrated in Plate 107. While preserving motion at the metatarsotarsal, midtarsal, and subtalar joints, the operation corrects the cavus deformity, provided the apex of the arch is at the midfoot. It should always be preceded by release of the contracted plantar soft tissues. Often equinus deformity of the first metatarsal will persist, necessitating a dorsiflexion osteotomy of the first metatarsal at its base or first metatarsocuneiform fusion for correction at a later stage. Wedge resection of the tarsus will shorten the foot—it should therefore never be performed in a skeletally immature foot. Circulatory insufficiency of the toes is a definite hazard. The procedure should not be combined with Dwyer osteotomy of the os calcis for correction of varus heel, since gangrene of the toes is a probable complication.

V-Osteotomy of the Tarsus. This procedure for pes cavus, originally described by Japas, is shown in Plate 108.[82] The foot is not shortened by resection of a bone wedge. The forefoot is elevated by depressing the base of the distal fragment plantarward. The procedure lengthens the concave plantar surface of the foot. Japas recommends the operation in children over six years of age. The author's personal experience with the procedure is limited; at present it is utilized in the skeletally mature foot in cases of unilateral involvement when length of the foot and shoe size are important considerations.

First Metatarsotarsal Dorsal Wedge Resection with Fusion and Dorsal Wedge Osteotomy of Lateral Four Metatarsals at Their Bases. This procedure is indicated in the skeletally immature foot when the apex of the cavus deformity is located anteriorly in the metatarsotarsal area, especially when painful keratoses develop on the plantar aspect of the foot under the metatarsal heads. The physes of the lateral four metatarsals are distal, and osteotomy at their bases will not disturb growth. The growth plate of the first metatarsal is proximal; therefore, to prevent physeal injury, dorsal wedge resection and fusion of the first metatarsocuneiform joint is performed (Fig. 7–159). The lateral four tarsometatarsal joints are left intact. The base of the wedge is dorsal, measuring 8 to 15 mm. The osteotomy is performed with an oscillating saw and finished with an osteotome. Care is exercised to avoid rotational malalignment. The joint of the first metatarsal and the cuneiform is fixed internally with a Steinmann pin.

In the skeletally mature foot in which previous dorsal tarsal wedge resection has failed to correct fixed equinus deformity of the metatarsals, and when the apex of the deformity is at the tarsometatarsal joints, dorsal wedge osteotomy of all five metatarsals is performed at their bases, leaving the tarsometatarsal articulation intact (Fig. 7–160). The slight remaining mobility of the Lisfranc joint will be of definite functional help. The bases of all five metatarsals and the tarsometatarsal joints are exposed through a transverse or longitudinal incision. The shape of the osteotomy is cuneiform, with a buttress based plantarward. In order to avoid sloughing of the skin edges, the wound flaps should be retracted gently and the cast should be padded on the dorsum of the foot. Excessive correction will result in painful bony prominences at the bases of the metatarsals. Rotational malalignment or adduction or abduction of the distal fragments will produce deformities of the forefoot.

Fusion of the First Metatarsocuneiform Joint. McElvenny and Caldwell proposed that varus distortion of the hindfoot in pes cavovarus is caused by pronation of the first metatarsal. They recommended elevation and supination of the first metatarsal and fusion of the first metatarsocuneiform joint in this position. If the forefoot dropped into equinus position in this area, they also fused the naviculocuneiform joint. They stressed that only the first metatarsal should be supinated, not the entire forefoot. If the cavovarus deformity was fixed, they recommended plantar fasciotomy and a series of stretching casts to correct the hindfoot varus deformity and to provide flexibility to the forefoot.[95]

Vertical Opening-Wedge Osteotomy of Medial Cuneiform. The vertical osteotomy with a wedge of bone graft based on the plantar aspect was recommended by Fowler and associates to elevate the first metatarsal into dorsiflexion as described earlier.[49]

Dorsal Wedge Resection and Fusion of Talonavicular and Calcaneocuboid Joints. This is carried out when the apex of pes cavus is more posterior in the midtarsal area. It is usually combined with subtalar fusion to correct any hindfoot varus distortion that is present. In paralytic pes cavovarus, triple arthrodesis will provide stability and at the same time correct the deformity.

"Beak" Triple Arthrodesis. In this technique, described by Siffert, correction of severe pes cavus and flattening of the arch is obtained by

Text continued on page 2700

Dorsal Wedge Resection for Pes Cavus

The dorsal aspect of the tarsal bones may be exposed by several means. Cole and Japas make a single dorsal longitudinal incision approximately 6 to 8 cm. long in the midline of the foot, centering over the midtarsal arch (naviculocuneiform junction). Subcutaneous tissue is divided, and the long toe extensors are identified and separated. The plane between the long extensor tendons of the second and third toes is developed, and the extensor digitorum brevis muscle is identified, elevated, and retracted laterally with the peroneus brevis tendon. The anterior tibial tendon and the long extensor tendons of the second and big toes are retracted medially. The periosteum is incised, longitudinally elevated, and retracted medially and laterally.[27, 82]

Méary makes two longitudinal incisions, each about 5 to 6 cm. in length, on the dorsum of the foot. The medial incision is parallel to the longitudinal axis of the second metatarsal and is centered over the intermediate cuneiform bone. The extensor hallucis longus tendon, dorsalis pedis vessels, and the anterior tibial tendon are identified, dissected free, and retracted medially. The lateral incision is about 3 cm. long and is centered over the cuboid bone. The peroneus brevis is identified and retracted laterally.

This author uses two longitudinal incisions, one dorsolateral and the other medial.

OPERATIVE TECHNIQUE

A and **B.** Two longitudinal skin incisions are made. The medial incision, about 5 cm. long, is over the medial aspect of the navicular and first cuneiform bones in the interval between the anterior tibial and posterior tibial tendons. The subcutaneous tissue is divided. The anterior tibial tendon is retracted dorsally; the posterior tibial tendon is partially detached from the tuberosity of the navicular and is retracted plantarward to expose the medial and dorsal aspects of the navicular and first cuneiform bones. The dorsolateral incision, about 4 cm. long, is centered over the cuboid bone. The extensor brevis muscle is identified, elevated, and retracted distally and laterally with the peroneus brevis tendon. The long toe extensors are retracted medially.

C. Next, through the medial wound, the capsule and periosteum of the navicular and first cuneiform bones are incised and elevated. The soft tissues are retracted dorsally and plantarward with Chandler elevator retractors. The capsule of the talonavicular joint should not be disturbed. If in doubt, one should take radiograms to identify the tarsal bones with certainty.

D and **E.** With osteotomes, a wedge of bone is excised, including the naviculocuneiform articulation. The base of the wedge is dorsal, its width depending upon the severity of the forefoot equinus deformity to be corrected. Through the dorsolateral incision, the wedge osteotomy of the cuboid is completed.

F. The forefoot is then manipulated into dorsiflexion. If the plantar fascia is contracted, a plantar fasciotomy is performed. In severe cases the short plantar muscles are also sectioned. The first cuneiform bone should be dorsally displaced over the navicular bone. Two Steinmann pins are inserted to transfix the tarsal osteotomy. The medial pin is inserted into the shaft of the first metatarsal, directed posteriorly through the first cuneiform, across the osteotomy site into the navicular and the head of the talus. The lateral pin is started posteriorly along the longitudinal axis of the calcaneus, across the calcaneocuboid joint, into the cuboid and the base of the fifth metatarsal. (Méary uses staples to maintain position of the osteotomy.) Radiograms are taken to verify the position of the pins and the maintenance of correction of forefoot equinus deformity. The tourniquet is released and complete hemostasis is obtained. The incisions are closed. The pins are cut subcutaneously and a below-knee cast is applied.

POSTOPERATIVE CARE

The foot and leg are immobilized for six weeks, at which time the cast, pins, and sutures are removed. A new below-knee walking cast is given—to be worn for another two to four weeks.

Plate 107. Dorsal Wedge Resection for Pes Cavus

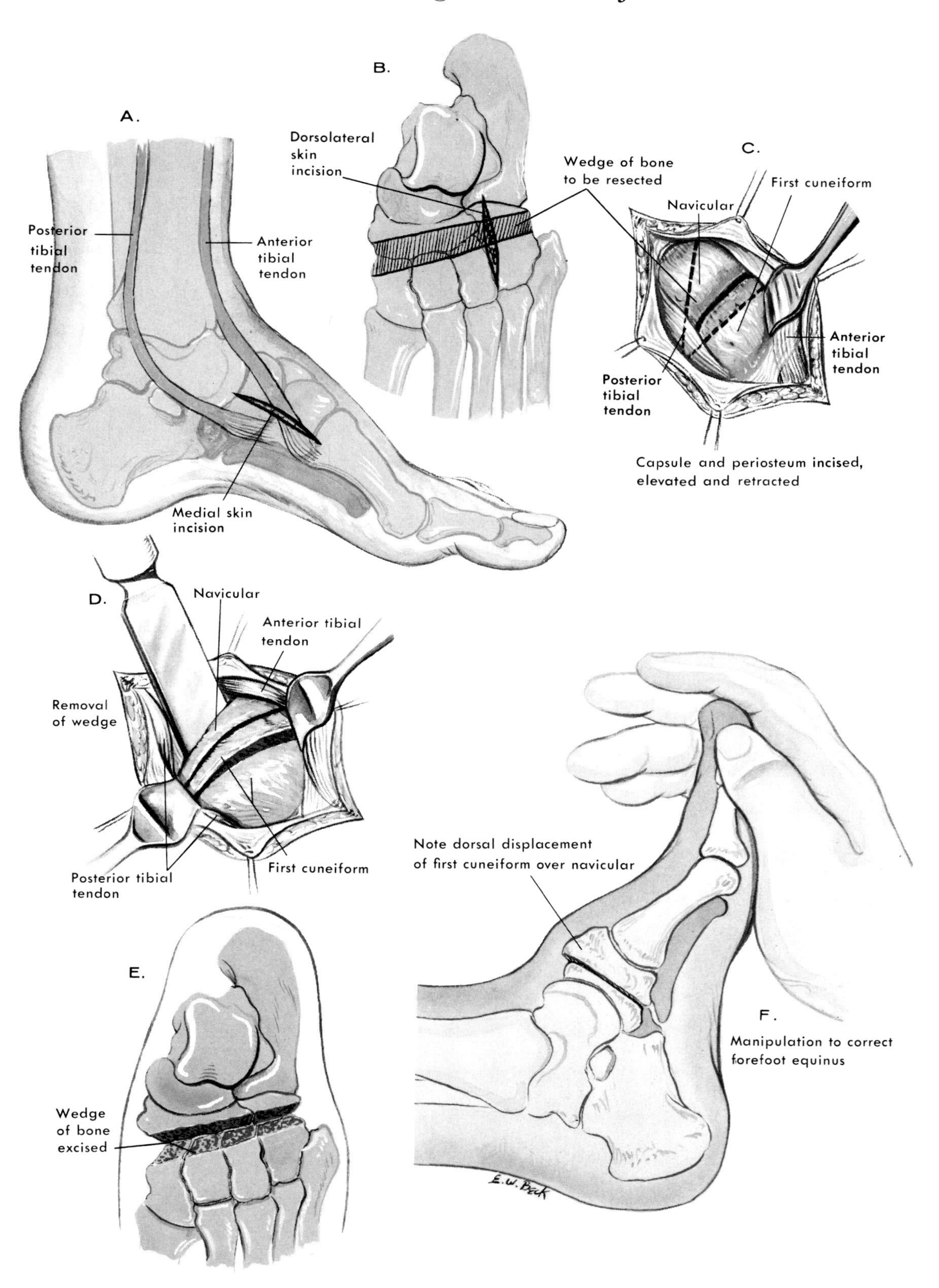

Japas V-Osteotomy of the Tarsus

OPERATIVE TECHNIQUE

A. The dorsal aspect of the tarsal bones is exposed by a longitudinal incision 6 to 8 cm. long in the midline of the foot, i.e., between the second and third rays; it is centered over the midtarsal area at the naviculocuneiform junction.

B and **C.** The subcutaneous tissue is divided. The superficial nerves are isolated and protected. The long toe extensor tendons are identified and separated, and the plane between those of the second and third toes is developed. The extensor digitorum brevis muscle is identified, extraperiosteally elevated, and retracted laterally with the peroneal tendons. The extensor hallucis longus tendon, dorsalis pedis vessels, and anterior tibial tendon are identified, dissected free, and retracted medially. The osteotomy site is exposed extraperiosteally.

The talonavicular joint is identified next. Caution! Do not injure the midtarsal joint and compromise its function. If bony landmarks are distorted, radiograms are made for proper orientation. Inadvertent partial ostectomy of the head of the talus will result in aseptic necrosis and traumatic arthritis. The V line of the osteotomy is marked; its apex is located in the midline of the foot at the height of the arch of the cavus deformity; its medial limb extends to the middle of the medial cuneiform, exiting proximal to the cuneiform–first metatarsal joint, and its lateral limb extends to the middle of the cuboid, emerging proximal to the cuboid–fifth metatarsal joint. Often the V is shallow, shaped more like a dome.

Plate 108. Japas V-Osteotomy of the Tarsus

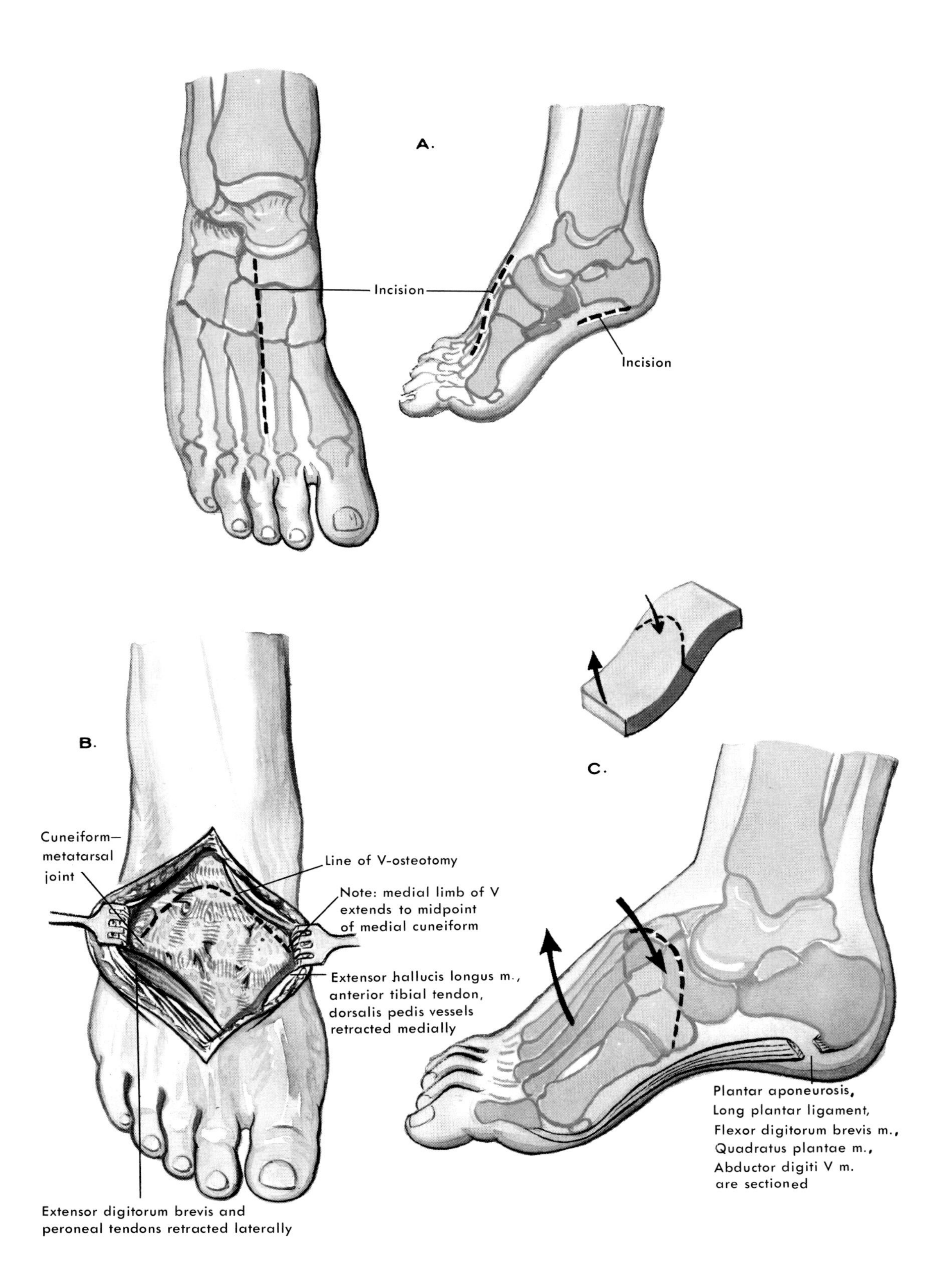

Japas V-Osteotomy of the Tarsus *(Continued)*

D and **E.** The osteotomy is begun with an oscillating bone saw and completed with an osteotome. Splintering of the ends of the medial and lateral limbs should be avoided. Next, a curved periosteal elevator is inserted into the osteotomy site, manual traction is applied on the forefoot, and with the elevator used as a lever, the base of the distal fragment is depressed plantarward. This maneuver corrects the cavus deformity and lengthens the concave plantar surface of the foot. The foot is not shortened, as it would be by resection of a bone wedge, and any abduction or adduction deformity can be corrected if necessary.

F. Once desired alignment is achieved, a single Steinmann pin is inserted through the distal part of the first metatarsal and directed posteriorly and laterally to terminate in the lateral part of the calcaneus or the cuboid. Radiograms are made to verify the completeness of correction. Then the tourniquet is removed, hemostasis obtained, and the wound closed with interrupted sutures. The pin is cut subcutaneously, and a below-knee cast is applied.

POSTOPERATIVE CARE

Two weeks after surgery, a walking heel is placed posteriorly—under the long axis of the tibia—and gradual partial weight-bearing is permitted with crutches. In six weeks the cast, sutures, and Steinmann pin are removed. Radiograms are made. If healing is not adequate, another below-knee cast is applied for an additional two to four weeks.

Plate 108. Japas V-Osteotomy of the Tarsus

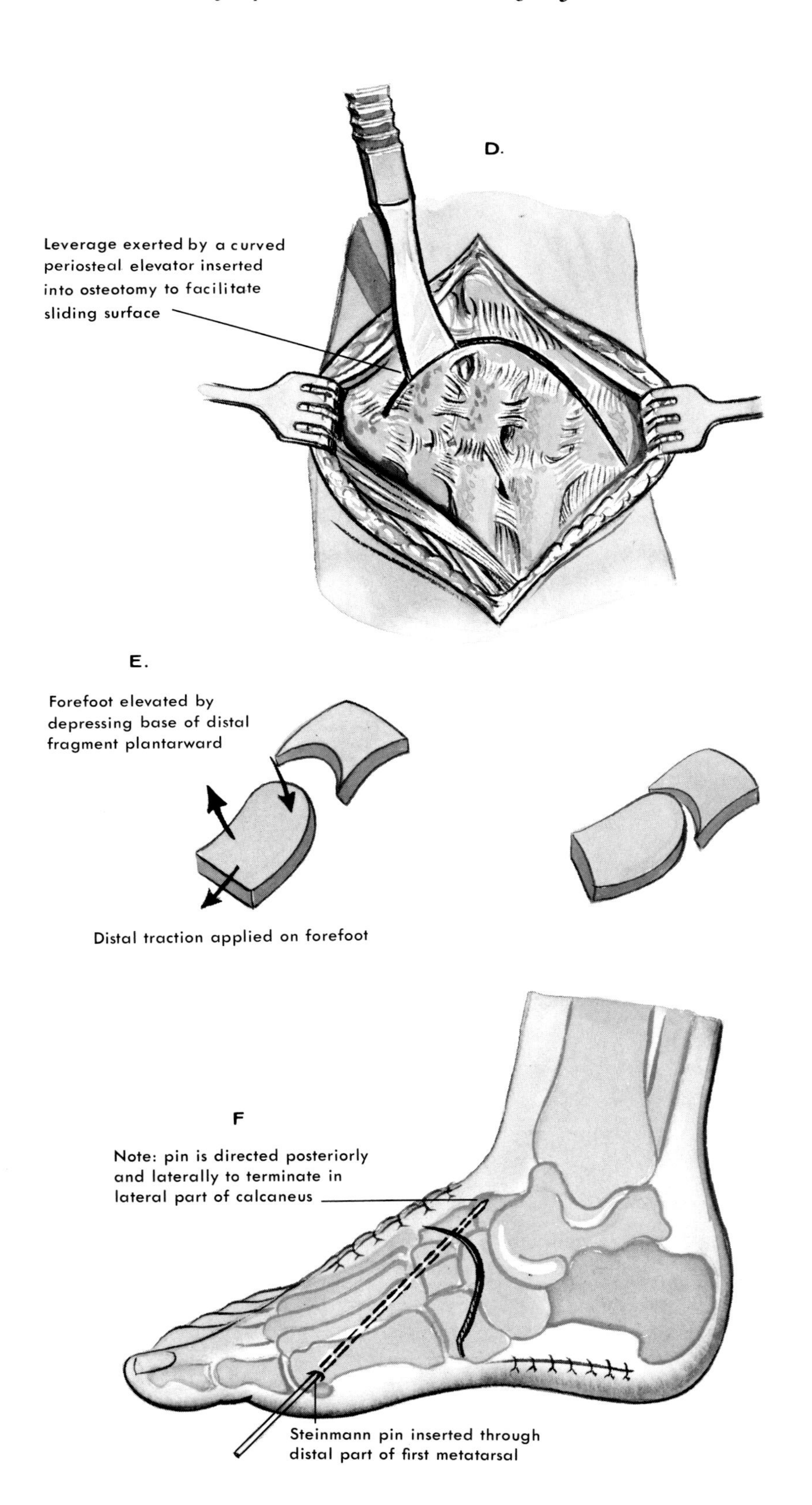

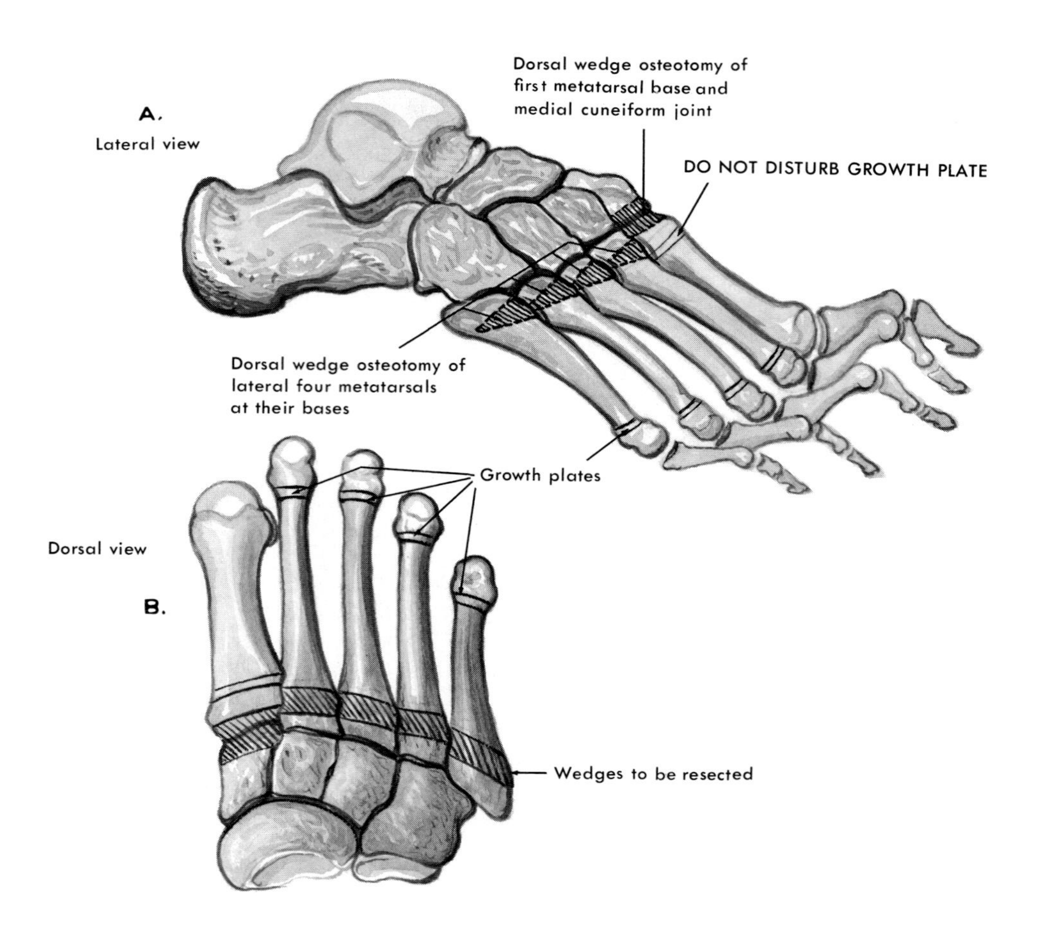

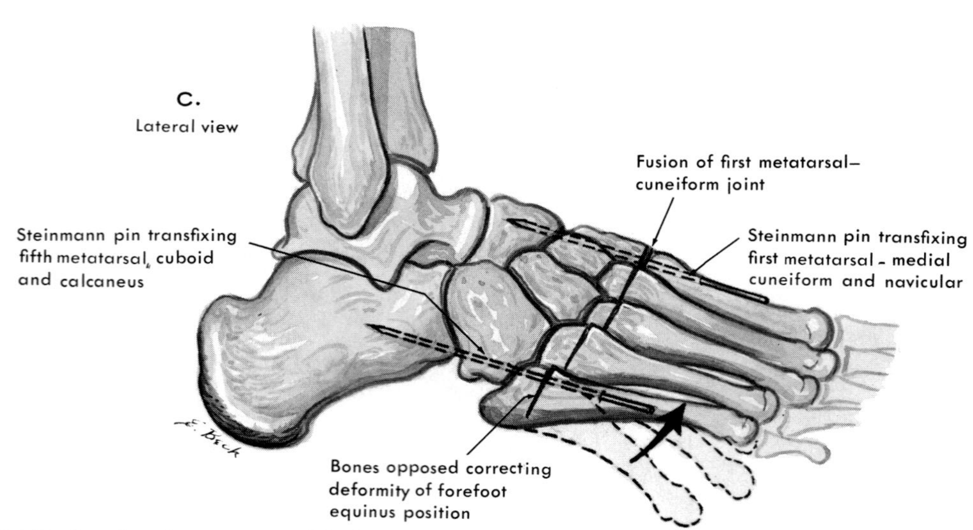

FIGURE 7–159. Dorsal wedge osteotomy of the lateral four metatarsals at their bases with dorsal wedge osteotomy and fusion of the first metatarsal–cuneiform joint.

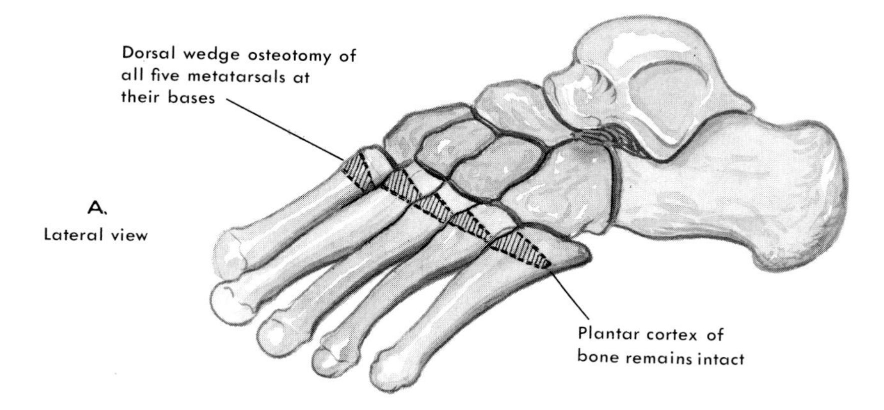

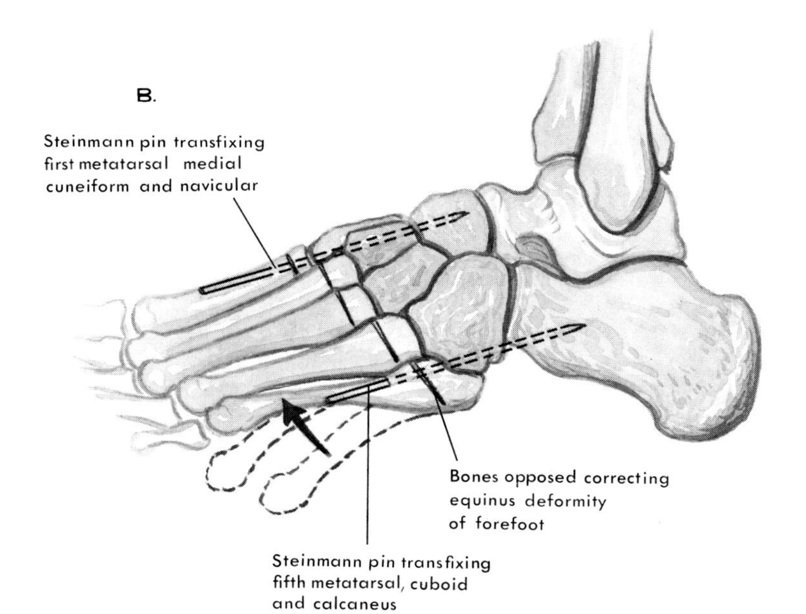

FIGURE 7–160. Dorsal wedge osteotomy of all five metatarsals at their base.

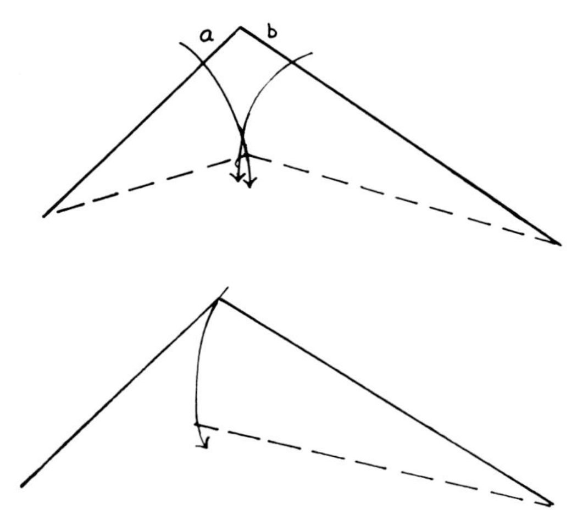

FIGURE 7–161. The principle of "beak" triple arthrodesis for correction of severe posterior cavus deformity.

Top. In order to obtain adequate flattening of the arch, an extensive amount of bone has to be resected from the talar head (a) and the navicular and cuneiform bones (b). This may compromise circulation to the talus. *Bottom.* The same degree of flattening of the arch is achieved by plantar displacement and depression of the proximal end of the forefoot segment under the head and neck of the talus. (From Siffert, R. S., Forster, R. I., and Nachamie, B.: "Beak" triple arthrodesis for correction of severe cavus deformity. Clin. Orthop., *45*:102, 1966. Reprinted by permission.)

downward displacement and depression of the proximal end of the forefoot segment under the head and neck of the talus (Figs. 7–161, 7–162, and 7–163). The operation is performed through medial and lateral incisions. The subtalar and calcaneocuboid joints are denuded of hyaline articular cartilage as in an ordinary triple arthrodesis. The cartilage on the proximal surface and the cortex on the dorsal surface of the navicular bone are resected. Appropriate wedges are resected from the calcaneocuboid joint. The soft tissues on the dorsum of the talus and anterior part of the talus should not be disturbed. In severe deformity the navicular may have to be excised; in such an instance the proximal and dorsal surfaces of the medial cuneiform are denuded. Then the inferior one half or one third of the talar head and neck are undercut to form a "beak" (a dorsal buttress). Next, the proximal end of the forefoot is pushed downward, and the navicular is locked under the talar beak. The bone segments are usually stable in their corrected position, and a plaster cast is adequate to maintain it. Occasionally one or two staples or threaded Steinmann pins (across the talocalcaneal and calcaneocuboid joints) are inserted for secure internal fixation.[132] This author finds the procedure effective in correcting posterior cavus deformity. It has the definite advantages of preserving circulation to the neck of the talus and maintaining the integrity of the anterior capsular and ligamentous structures of the ankle joint.

Close-Up Lateral Wedge Osteotomy of Calcaneus (Dwyer). This procedure is combined

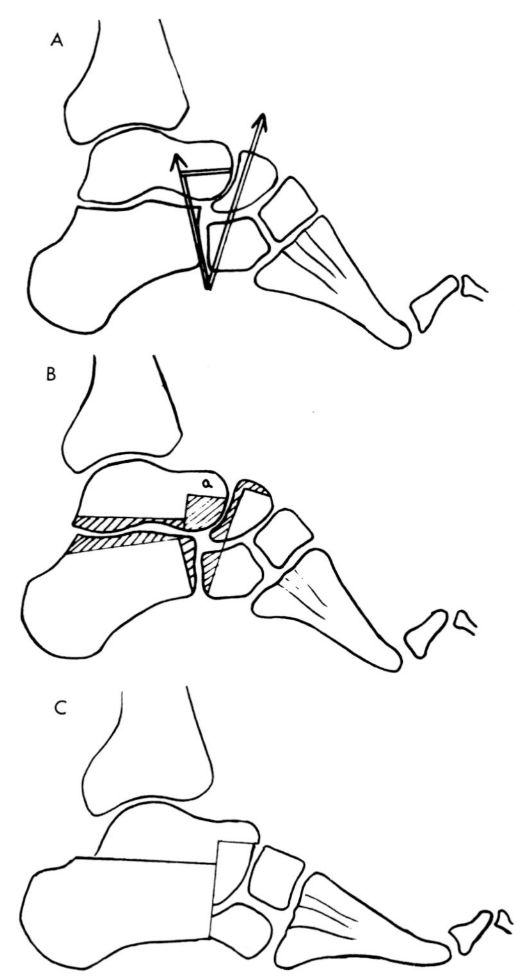

FIGURE 7–162. Technique of "beak" triple arthrodesis for correction of severe pes cavus deformity.

Medial and lateral incisions are employed for exposure of the subtalar, talonavicular, and calcaneocuboid joints. With the exception of the head of the talus, all joint surfaces are denuded of hyaline cartilage as in an ordinary triple arthrodesis. A dorsal-based wedge is removed from the calcaneocuboid joint and navicular bone. The plantar half or one third of the talar head-neck is resected to form a beak. Care is taken not to disturb the soft tissues in the superior aspect of the talus and anterior part of the ankle joint. **A.** The lines of osteotomy are indicated. **B.** The area of bone resected is shown by hatched areas. **C.** The final result demonstrating correction of the cavus deformity. Note that the forefoot is displaced plantarward and locked under the talar beak. (From Siffert, R. S., Forster, R. I., and Nachamie, B.: "Beak" triple arthrodesis for correction of severe cavus deformity. Clin. Orthop., *45*:102, 1966. Reprinted by permission.)

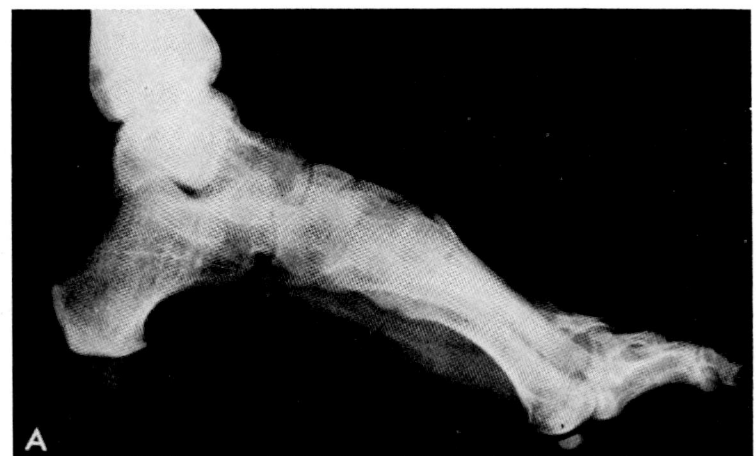

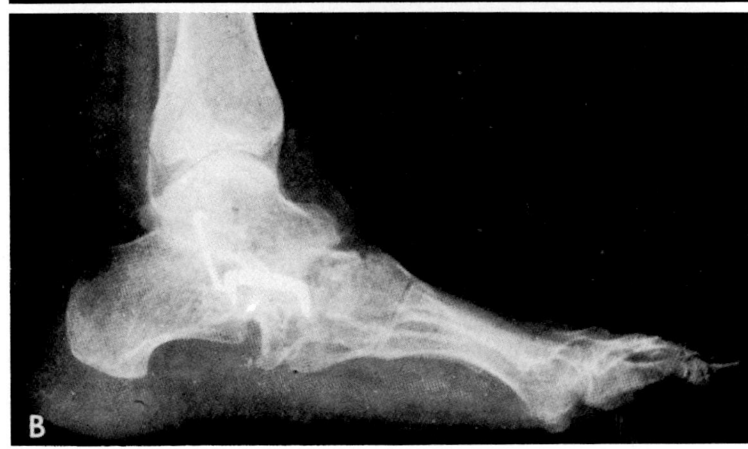

FIGURE 7–163. Radiograms of the left foot showing the correction obtained by "beak" triple arthrodesis in a postpoliomyelitic cavus foot.

A. Preoperative radiogram. **B.** Postoperative radiogram. Note the displacement of the forefoot under the talar beak and the excellent degree of correction obtained. (From Siffert, R. S., Forster, R. I., and Nachamie, B.: "Beak" triple arthrodesis for correction of severe cavus deformity. Clin. Orthop., *45*:104, 1966. Reprinted by permission.)

with a release of contracted soft tissues on the plantar aspect of the foot for correction of varus hindfoot.[39] The operation should be performed only in children over eight years of age; the operative technique is described and illustrated in Plate 109.

Bony Procedures to Correct Hindfoot Varus Deformity. In the skeletally mature foot the varus deformity of the hindfoot may be so rigid that soft-tissue releases alone are ineffective and bony procedures are required for correction. In the orthopedic arsenal, procedures available are Dwyer's osteotomy of the calcaneus (either medial opening- or lateral closing-wedge), lateral displacement osteotomy of the calcaneus, and triple arthrodesis. An axial (or Harris) view of the calcaneus is made. If there is true varus deformity of the calcaneus, Dwyer's close-up lateral wedge osteotomy of the calcaneus is indicated.[39] This author does not recommend opening-wedge osteotomy of the calcaneus, as the vertical height of the hindfoot is not a consideration in pes cavus and wound healing problems are greater in opening-wedge than in closing-wedge osteotomy. The operation should be performed only in children over eight years of age and it should be preceded by or combined with a plantar release.

Lateral displacement osteotomy of the calcaneus is indicated when the hindfoot varus deformity is fixed but the calcaneus is not derotated medially. Triple arthrodesis is indicated in paralytic pes cavovarus when provision of stability is desirable or when the fixed varus deformity is at the subtalar or talocalcaneonavicular joint. This author recommends that in general it is best not to combine forefoot and hindfoot operations in one stage.

Osteotomy of the Calcaneus for Correction of Pes Calcaneocavus. In the past pes calcaneus was corrected by an Elmsie type of triple arthrodesis in which a posteriorly based wedge was resected from the subtalar joint. The operation is difficult and complicated.

Dwyer, in 1964, reported on dorsal wedge osteotomy of the calcaneus for correction of

Dwyer Lateral Wedge Resection of Calcaneus for Pes Cavus

Forefoot equinus deformity is corrected first, either by plantar soft-tissue release or by dorsal wedge tarsal resection, depending upon the age of the patient and the severity of the deformity. Close-up lateral wedge resection of the os calcis is designed to correct the varus deformity of the hindfoot in which the heel is of adequate height and size.

OPERATIVE TECHNIQUE

A. A 5-cm.-long oblique incision is made on the lateral aspect of the calcaneus parallel to, but 1.5 cm. posterior and inferior to, the peroneus longus tendon. The subcutaneous tissue is divided and the wound flaps are retracted.

B and **C.** The peroneal tendons are identified and retracted dorsally and distally. The calcaneofibular ligament is sectioned, and the periosteum is incised. The lateral surface of the calcaneus is subperiosteally exposed; with Chandler elevator retractors, the superior and inferior aspects of the calcaneus are partially exposed. With a pair of osteotomes of adequate width, a wedge of the os calcis with its base directed laterally is excised. The site of osteotomy is immediately inferior and posterior to the peroneus longus tendon. The medial cortex should be left intact. The width of the base of the wedge depends upon the severity of the varus deformity of the heel.

D. Next, a Steinmann pin is inserted transversely across the posterior segment of the calcaneus. The forefoot is dorsiflexed, putting tension on the Achilles tendon, and, the Steinmann pin serving as a lever, the bone gap is closed. The heel should be in 5 degrees of valgus. The wound is closed and an above-knee cast is applied, the pin being incorporated in the cast. The knee is in 45 degrees of flexion.

POSTOPERATIVE CARE

The cast, pin, and sutures are removed in four weeks. Then a below-knee walking cast is applied for an additional two weeks, by which time the osteotomy should be healed.

Plate 109. Dwyer Lateral Wedge Resection of Calcaneus for Pes Cavus

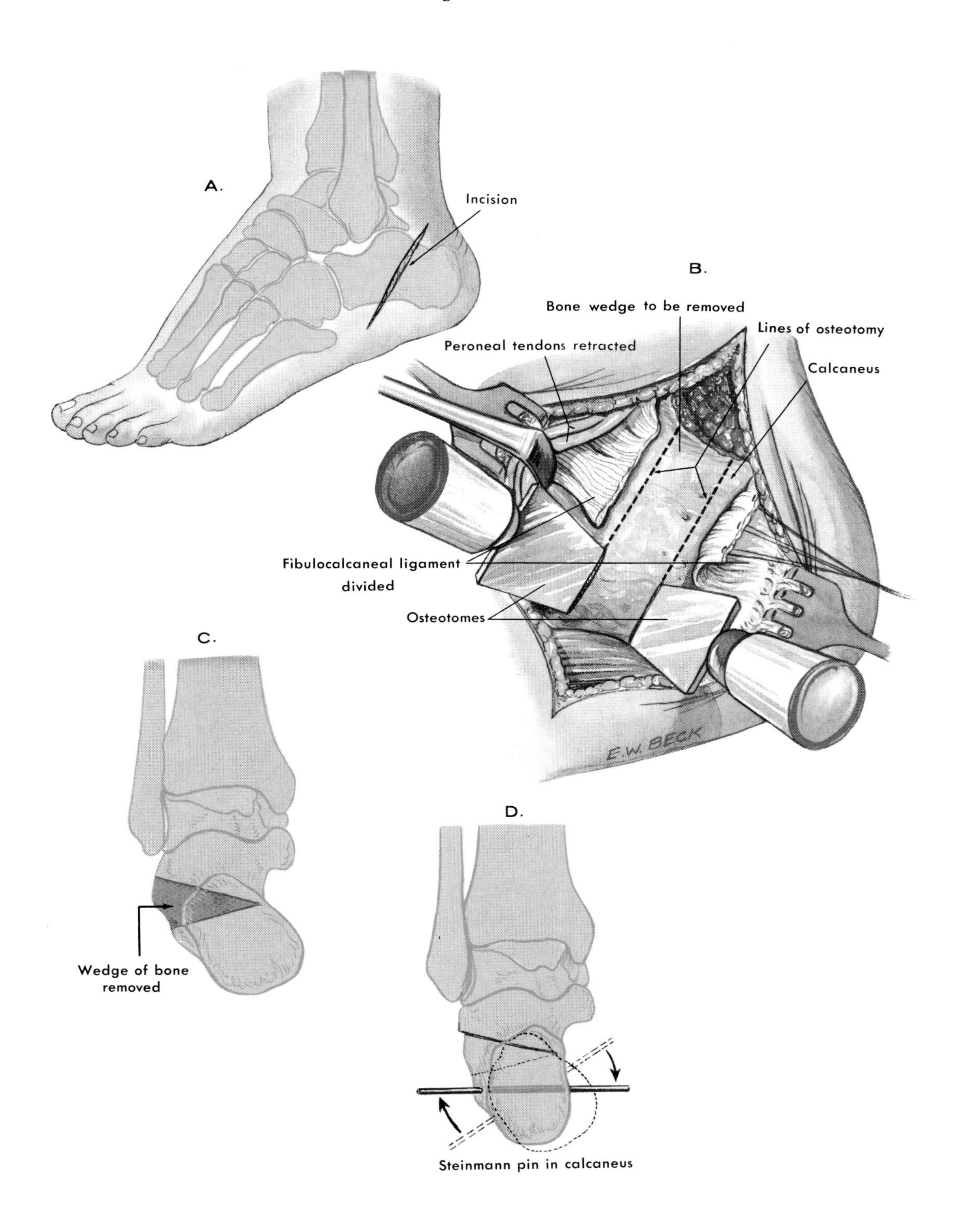

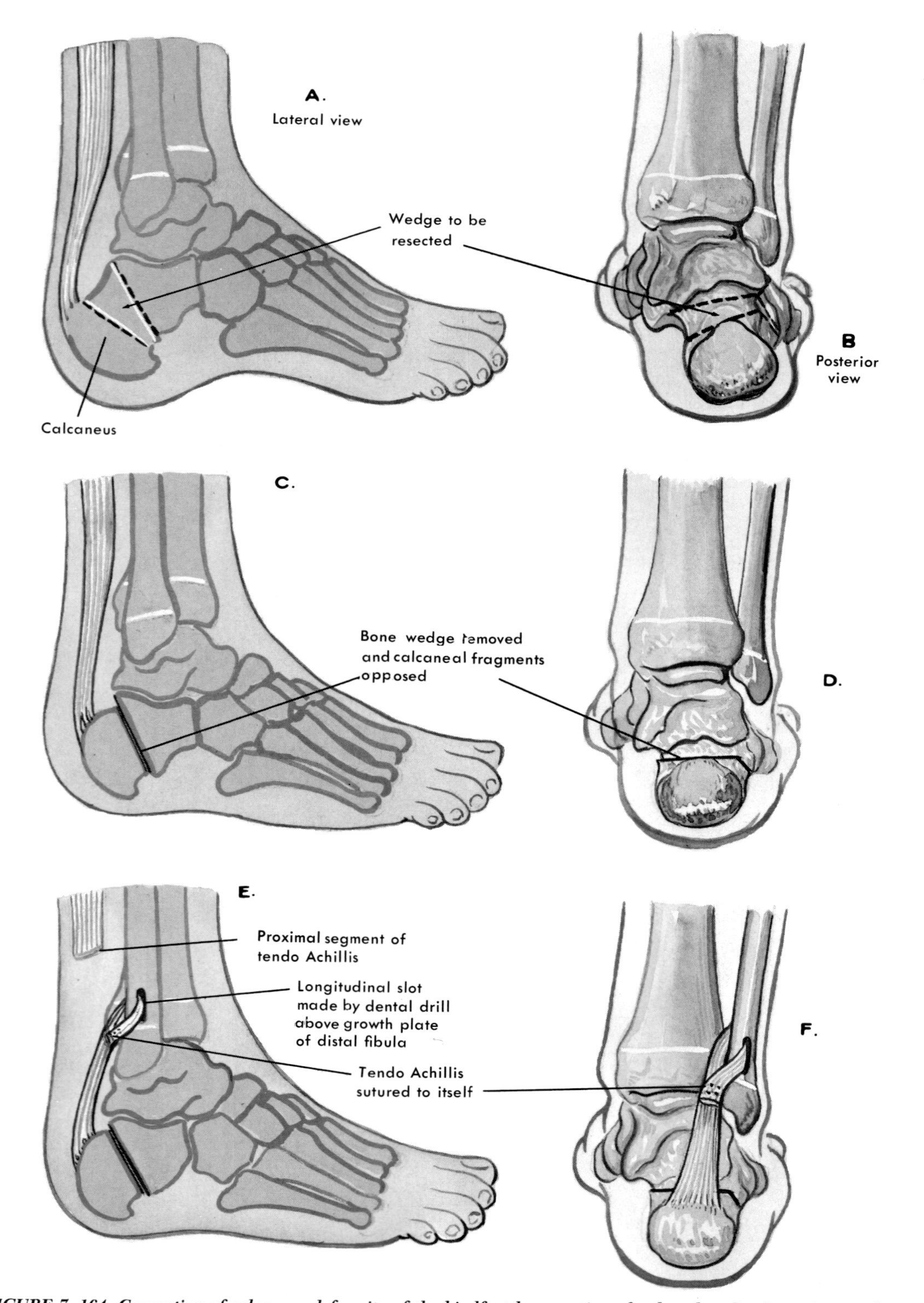

FIGURE 7–164. Correction of calcaneus deformity of the hindfoot by resection of a dorsal wedge from the os calcis.

A and **C.** A wedge, based superiorly and as wide as possible, is excised from the dorsal surface of the calcaneus. The height of the os calcis is reduced and the heel is brought closer to the plane of the forefoot. **B** and **D.** By taking the bone wedge wider on its medial or lateral side, valgus or varus deformity of the hindfoot can be corrected. In this drawing the base of the wedge is medial to correct the valgus heel. **E** and **F.** Tenodesis of the Achilles tendon to the distal fibular metaphysis is performed when the triceps surae is zero in motor strength and there is associated valgus deformity of the ankle.

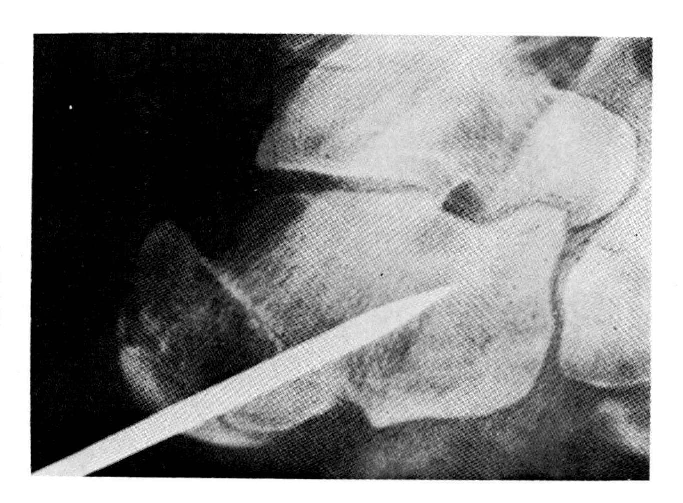

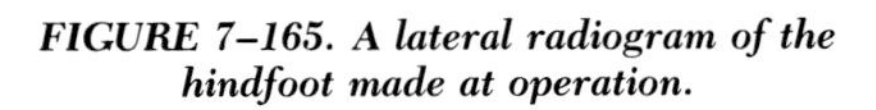

FIGURE 7–165. A lateral radiogram of the hindfoot made at operation.

Note the typical displacement of the osteotomy transfixed by a Steinmann pin. (From Mitchell, G. P.: Posterior displacement osteotomy of the calcaneus. J. Bone Joint Surg., 59-*B*:233, 1977. Reprinted by permission.)

calcaneus deformity.[40] The objective of surgery was to reduce the height of the calcaneus so that the heel would be brought closer to the plane of the forefoot. By taking the wedge wider on its medial or lateral aspect any valgus or varus deformity of the hindfoot could be corrected at the same time. In addition, leveling of the forefoot with the hindfoot allowed weight-bearing on the metatarsal heads (Fig. 7–164). Dwyer recommended preserving the wedge taken from the calcaneus; it was trimmed and inserted into a V-shaped cut in the neck of the talus to act as a permanent bone block, preventing excessive dorsiflexion of the ankle. Dwyer gave credit to Professor Bryan McFarland as the originator of the operation. This author does not recommend bone block; a more functional result is achieved with a tenodesis of the Achilles tendon to the distal fibular metaphysis (see Fig. 7–164 E and F). The McFarland-Dwyer dorsal wedge resection of the calcaneus has the definite drawback of shortening the os calcis.

Since 1956, Mr. George P. Mitchell of Edinburgh, Scotland, has performed a posterior and upward displacement osteotomy of the calcaneus; it is combined with an extensive plantar release. The calcaneocavus deformity is corrected without resection of bone (Fig. 7–165). The procedure is simple and has the advantage of lengthening the posterior lever arm of the calcaneus.[105] The technique of the Mitchell operation is depicted in Plate 110 L and M).

It is imperative to perform an extensive plantar release. Mr. Mitchell carries it out through a short horizontal medial incision. This author is concerned with the potential contracture and hypertrophy of the operative scar in the instep, because it may act as a deforming force in the calcaneocavovarus foot. In pes calcaneocavovalgus, however, it does not cause any difficulty. In moderate cases this author performs plantar release through a lateral or a midline incision; in severe contractures the surgical approach advocated by Bost, Schottstaedt, and Larsen is carried out.

Mr. Mitchell reviewed the long-term results in 15 feet. In five patients the triceps surae was weak and was reinforced by posterior tendon transfers. Eight feet required triple arthrodesis at a later stage.[105]

Samilson described a crescentic osteotomy of the os calcis for calcaneocavus feet.[119] The operative technique is described in Plate 110. Samilson uses staples or Kirschner wires for internal fixation. The results in 11 feet were excellent at follow-up between 5 and 12 years later. The indications for surgery were symptoms related to the calcaneocavus deformity of the feet; seven of the patients were spastics and four had idiopathic pes calcaneocavus. Before surgery the calcaneal pitch was 41 degrees, and postoperatively it was 19.5 degrees (Fig. 7–166). There were no infections, and all osteotomies healed. The motor strength of the triceps surae muscle did not change after surgery. Samilson found the procedure to be simple and effective in correcting calcaneocavus deformity; it does not, however, correct cavus deformity when the apex is located at the midtarsal or tarsometatarsal area.[119]

Sesamoidectomy. In the adult patient, irritation of the sesamoids under the first metatarsal head causes them to hypertrophy and become inflamed. Axial views demonstrate enlargement of the sesamoids and irregularity on their plan-

Text continued on page 2713

Posterior and Superior Displacement Osteotomy of Os Calcis for Correction of Pes Calcaneocavus

OPERATIVE TECHNIQUE

A. The entire lower limb is prepared and draped in the usual manner, and the operation is performed under tourniquet ischemia. An oblique lateral incision is made over the body of the calcaneus, behind the peroneal tendons and the subtalar joint. The upper end of the incision is 3 cm. posterior to its plantar end.

B. The subcutaneous tissue is divided in line with the skin incision. First, an extensive plantar release is performed. This is vital; otherwise an adequate backward and upward displacement of the posterior segment of the calcaneus is not feasible. Mitchell uses a medial horizontal incision, as described in the text. This author carries out the plantar release as follows: the plantar fascia, abductor digiti quinti, and lateral part of the short plantar muscles are divided with scissors through the lateral incision. If one stays close to bone, this maneuver is safe and neurovascular injury is avoided.

C. An alternative approach for plantar release is through a midline plantar incision. Next, a longitudinal incision, 5 cm. long, is made on the plantar aspect of the foot, in line with the second ray.

D and **E.** With a periosteal elevator the plantar fascia and short plantar muscles are stripped from the tuberosity of the calcaneus and elevated forward.

The short and long plantar ligaments, the plantar calcaneonavicular ligament, and the capsule of the calcaneocuboid joint are divided. The foot is manipulated to correct the cavus deformity as much as possible.

At this time the lateral and plantar wounds are packed with hot moist sponges and the tourniquet is released. In a few minutes the packing is removed and the wounds are thoroughly inspected for bleeding. After complete hemostasis the tourniquet is reinflated.

Plate 110. Posterior and Superior Displacement Osteotomy of Os Calcis for Correction of Pes Calcaneocavus

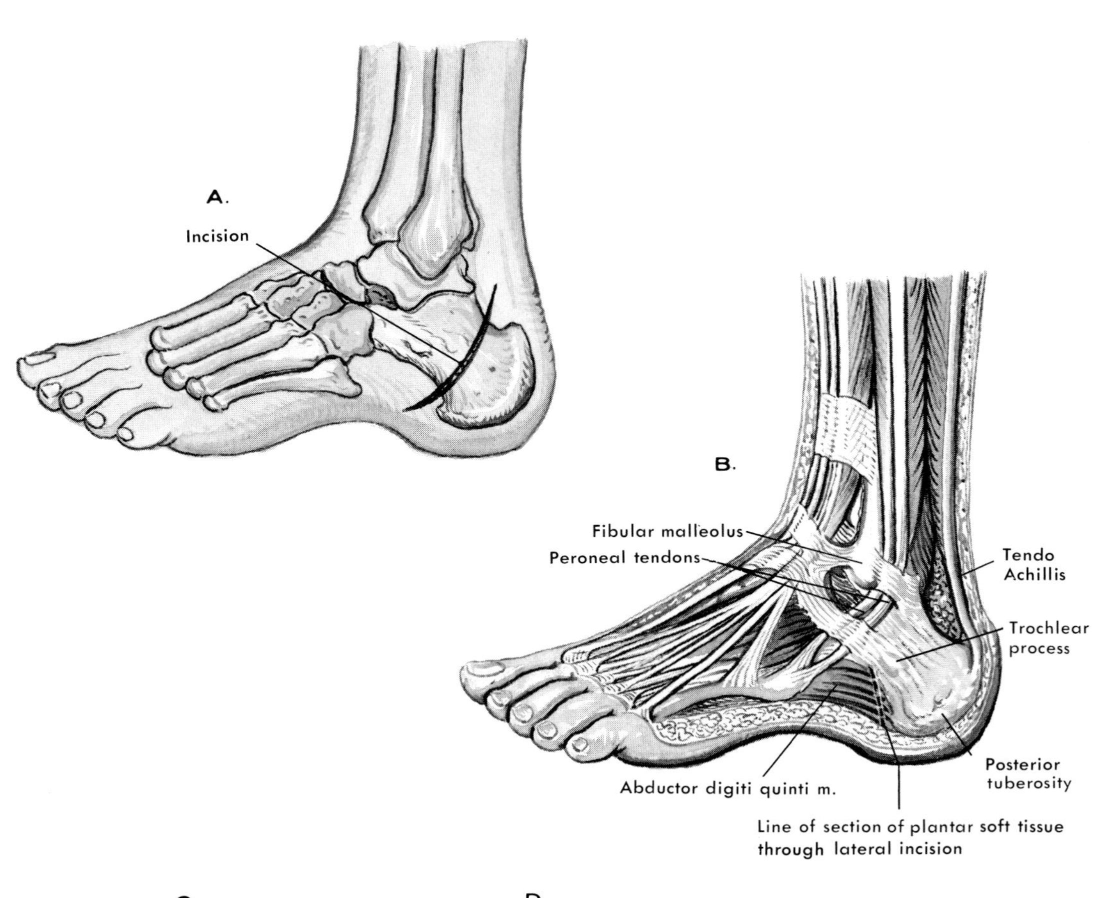

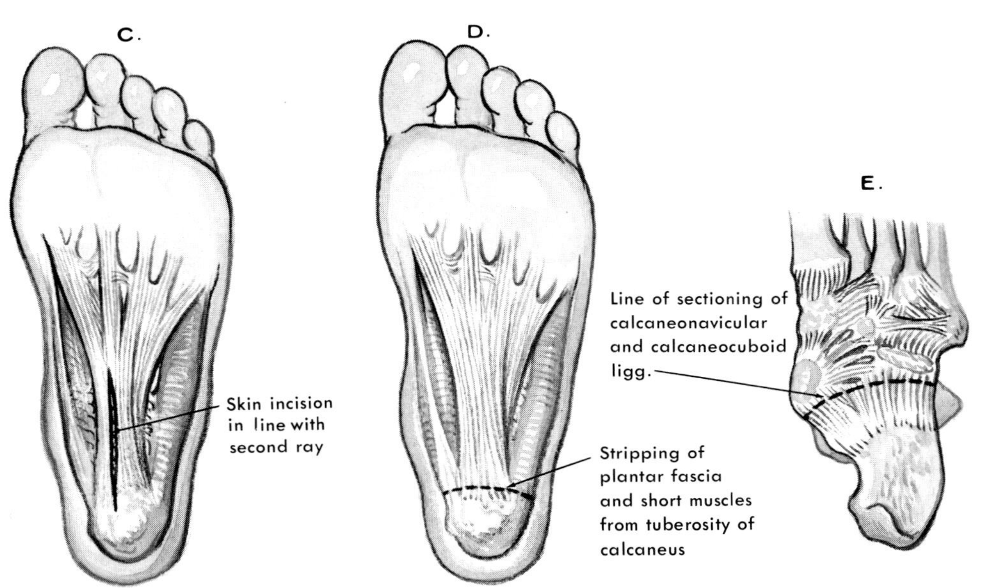

Posterior and Superior Displacement Osteotomy of Os Calcis for Correction of Pes Calcaneocavus (Continued)

F to **J.** Then, the lateral surface of the body of the calcaneus is exposed. The calcaneofibular ligament is sectioned and retracted. The peroneal tendons are pulled forward as far as possible, but there is no need to elevate them from their groove. Chandler elevators are placed on the superior and plantar surfaces of the calcaneus. The line of osteotomy is marked with multiple drill holes. Samilson makes a crescentic osteotomy (**I, J,** and **K**), whereas Mitchell's osteotomy is oblique transverse, inclining forward and plantarward (see **L** and **M**).

With an electric bone saw or a large curved sharp osteotome, the osteotomy is made.

K. A threaded Steinmann pin is inserted through the skin into the center of the apophysis of the calcaneus and the posterior bone segment. By manipulation and by using the Steinmann pin as a lever, the posterior fragment is displaced backward and upward, reducing the calcaneocavus deformity. The degree of correction obtained is checked on stress-lateral radiograms of the foot. The calcaneal pitch should be 10 to 20 degrees. (The calcaneal pitch is the angle formed between the sole line—joining the plantar aspects of the metatarsal heads and the calcaneal tuberosity—and the plantar calcaneal line—drawn between the posterior and anterior calcaneal tuberosities [see Fig. 7–177].) If correction is satisfactory the Steinmann pin is drilled into the anterior part of the os calcis, transfixing the osteotomized bones securely. This author prefers that the threaded Steinmann pin exit through the skin over the dorsolateral aspect of the midfoot and remain subcutaneous or flush with the calcaneus posteriorly.

Plate 110. Posterior and Superior Displacement Osteotomy of Os Calcis for Correction of Pes Calcaneocavus

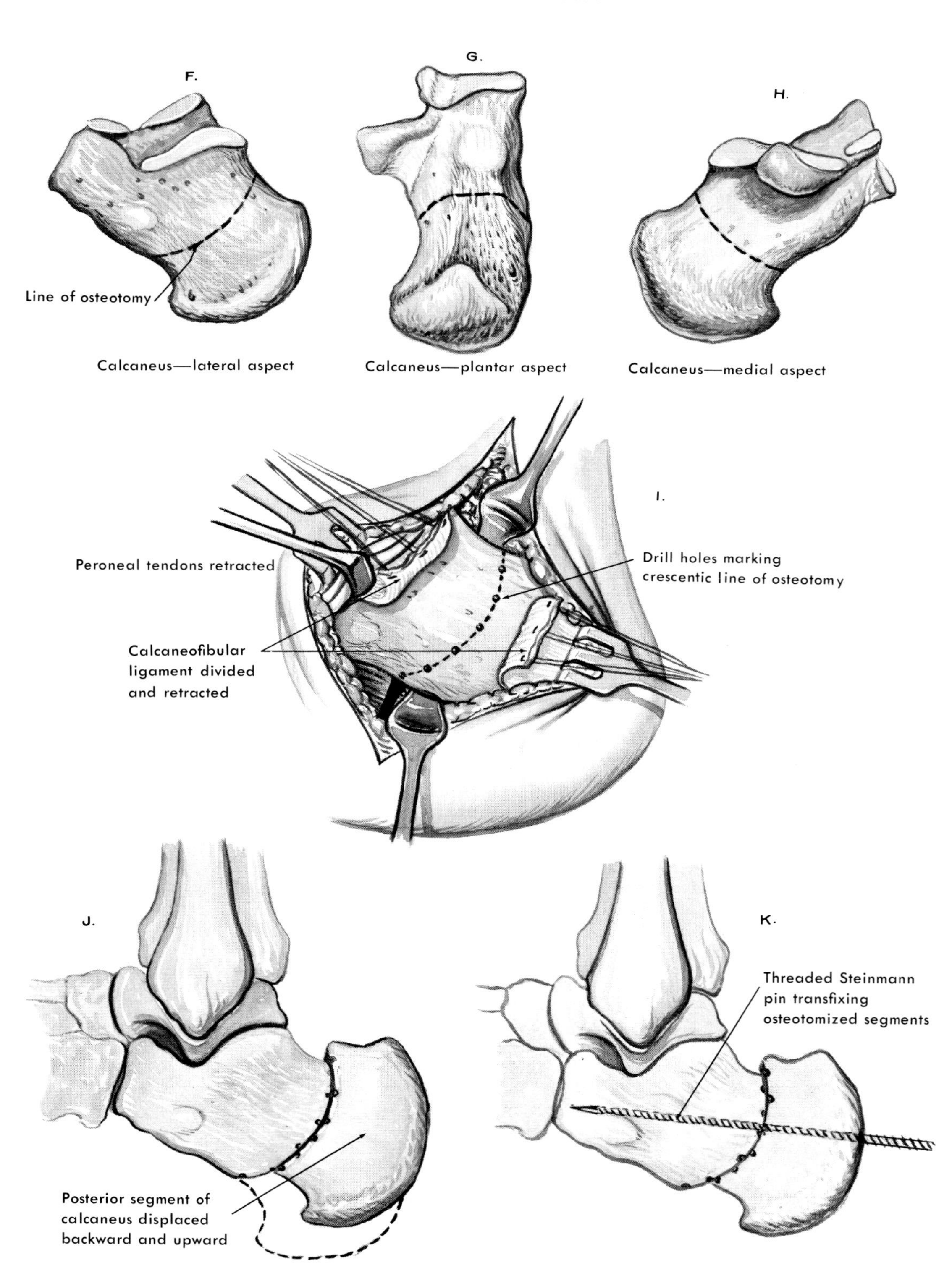

Posterior and Superior Displacement Osteotomy of Os Calcis for Correction of Pes Calcaneocavus (Continued)

L, M, and **N.** Oblique transverse osteotomy according to the technique of Mitchell. The line of osteotomy from the superior part inclines downward and forward. Drill holes are not made in the soft cancellous bone. The osteotomy is performed with a wide straight osteotome. The foot is manipulated, and with the leverage of the Steinmann pin, the posterior fragment is displaced backward and upward. This is easily done if all plantar soft tissues attached to the posterior tuberosity of the calcaneus are divided.

The wound is closed in the usual manner. A below-knee plaster of Paris cast is applied, incorporating the pin in the cast. This author prefers an above-knee cast with the knee flexed 45 degrees.

POSTOPERATIVE CARE

Weight-bearing is not allowed for three to four weeks, at which time the first cast and pin are removed. A new below-knee walking cast is applied for another two to three weeks. Then weight-bearing is permitted.

Plate 110. Posterior and Superior Displacement Osteotomy of Os Calcis for Correction of Pes Calcaneocavus

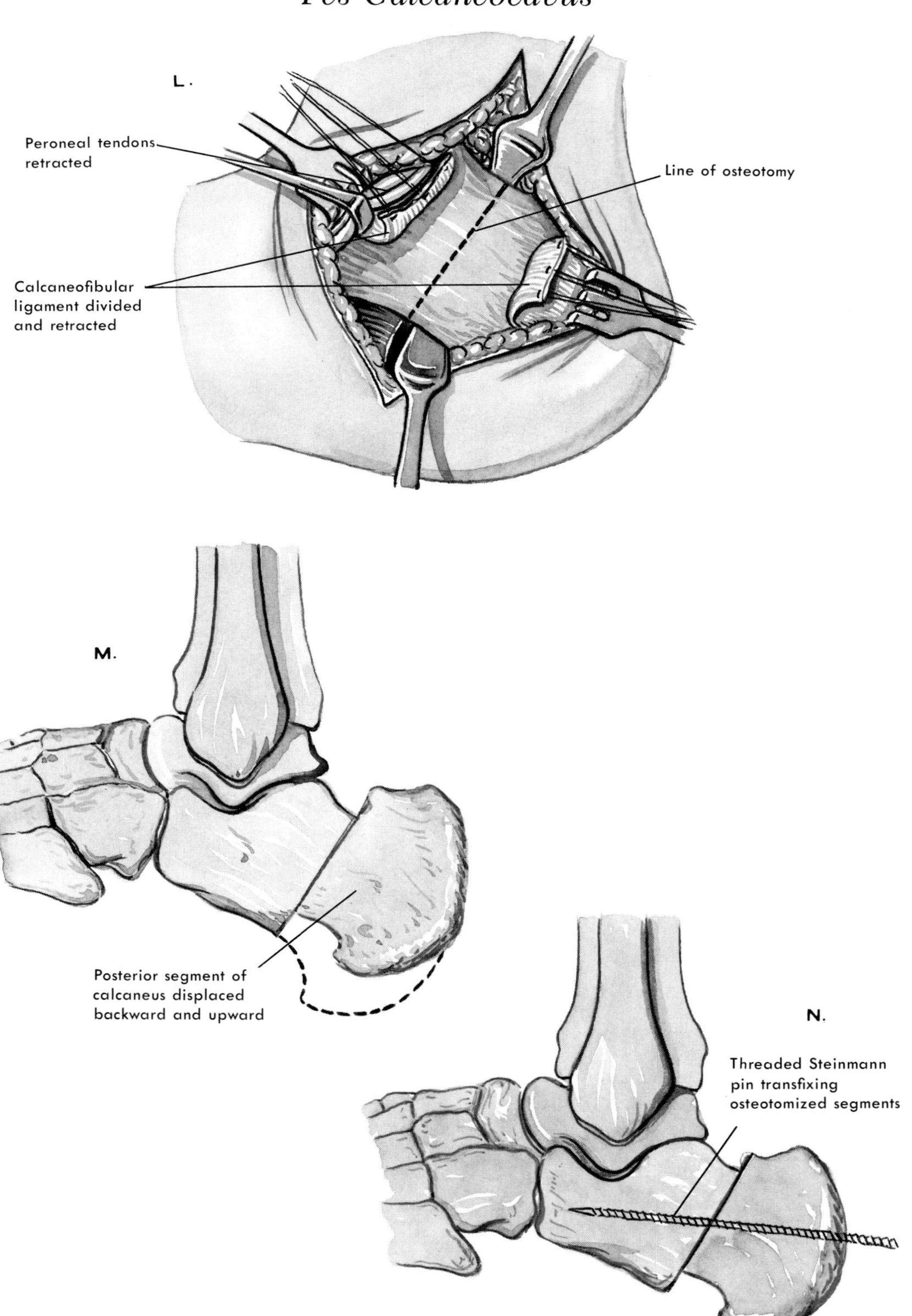

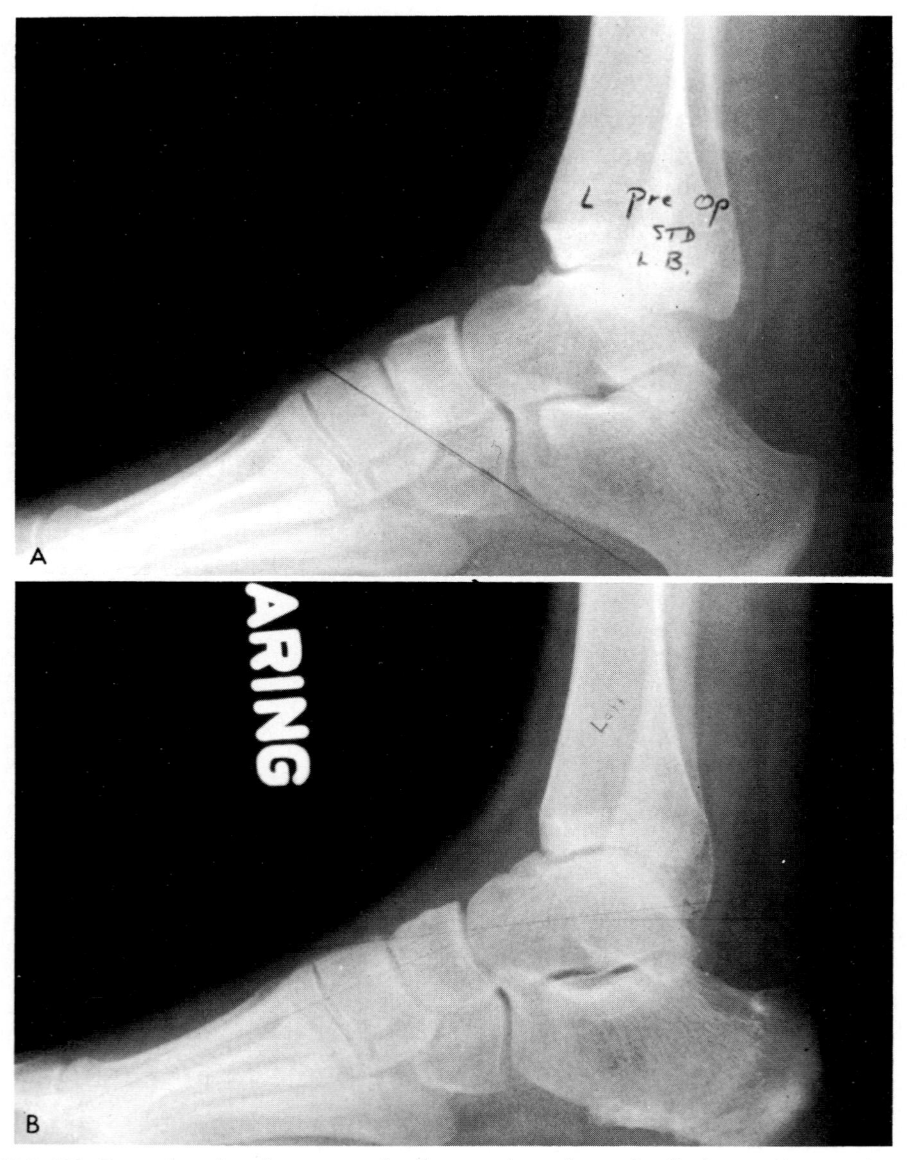

FIGURE 7–166. Correction of a calcaneocavus foot by posterior and superior displacement crescentic osteotomy of the os calcis.

Standing lateral radiograms of the foot. **A.** Preoperatively. **B.** Five years postoperatively. (From Samilson, R. L.: Crescentic osteotomy of the os calcis for calcaneocavus feet. *In* Bateman, J. E. (ed.): Foot Science. Philadelphia, Saunders, 1976, pp. 18–25. Reprinted by permission.)

tar surfaces. In such an instance, excision of one or both sesamoid bones affords complete symptomatic relief.

Subtotal Excision of the Talus. This may be indicated in a paralyzed cavovarus foot. Occasionally amputation of the toes is carried out if they are so deformed and inflamed that fitting shoes poses a formidable problem.

References

1. Adelaar, R. S., Dannelly, E. A., and Meunier, P. A.: A long term study of triple arthrodesis in children. Orthop. Clin. North Am., *7*:895, 1976.
2. Alvik, I.: Operative treatment of pes cavus. Acta Orthop. Scand., *23*:137, 1953.
3. Anzoletti, A.: Annotazioni intorno al peide equino cavo acquisito ed all'equinocavismo quale sintomo di affenzione nervosa non ancora descritta. Arch. Ortop., *22*:356–377, 1905.
4. Arandes Adan, R., Viladot Perice, A., and Vilanova Montiu, X.: Pie cavo. *In* Clinica y tratamiento de las enfermedades del pie (podologia). Barcelona, Editorial Cientifico Medical, 1956, pp. 149–159.
5. Barenfeld, P. A., Weseley, M. S., and Munter, M.: Dwyer calcaneal osteotomy. Clin. Orthop., *53*:147, 1967.
6. Barenfeld, P. A., Weseley, M. S., and Shea, J. M.: The congenital cavus foot. Clin. Orthop., *79*:119, 1971.
7. Bargellini, D.: Sul piede cavo con spina bifida occulta. Arch. Ortop., *32*:65, 1915.
8. Bartolini, G.: Il trattamento chirurgico del piede cavo anteriore: La metatarsectomia (Note di tecnica). Arch. Ortop., *73*:650, 1960.
9. Barwell, R.: Pes planus and pes cavus: An anatomical and clinical study. Edinburgh Med. J., *3*:113, 1898.
10. Benages, A.: Chirurgie du pied creux. Revista espanola orthopedia et traumatologia. Rev. Esp. Cir. Osteoart., *1*:115, 1966.
11. Bentzon, P. G. K.: Pes cavus and the m. peroneus longus. Acta Orthop. Scand., *4*:50, 1933.
12. Bertrand, P.: Discussion. Symposium—le pied creux essentiel. Rev. Chir. Orthop., *53*:423, 1967.
13. Beykirch, A.: Ein Beitrag zur Ätiologie und Therapie des Klanenhohlfusses. Z. Orthop. Chir., *52*:41, 1929.
14. Boppe, M., and Janvier: A propos du pied creux essentiel de la second enfance. Rev. Med. Franc., *19*:519, 1938.
15. Bosch, J.: Die Osteotomie nach Dwyer beim Ballenhohlfuss. Z. Orthop., *94*:325, 1961.
16. Bost, F. C., Schottstaedt, E. R., and Larsen, L. J.: Plantar dissection. An operation to release the soft tissues in recurrent or recalcitrant talipes equinovarus. J. Bone Joint Surg., *42-A*:151, 1960.
17. Bradley, G. W., and Coleman, S. S.: Treatment of the calcaneo-cavus foot deformity. J. Bone Joint Surg., *63-A*:1159, 1981.
18. Brewerton, D. A., Sandifer, P. H., and Sweetman, D. R.: "Idiopathic" pes cavus, an investigation of its etiology. Br. Med. J., *358*:659, 1963.
19. Brewster, S. H., and Larson, C. B.: Cavus feet. J. Bone Joint Surg., *22*:361, 1940.
20. Brockway, A.: Surgical correction of talipes cavus deformities. J. Bone Joint Surg., *22*:81, 1940.
21. Busatti, R.: Cura del piede cavo. Atti del XVI Congr. Soc. Ital. di Ortop., 1925.
22. Camera, U.: Il mio indirizzo sul trattamento delle deformita neurogene sul piede in equinismo e cavismo con particolare riguardo al piede cavo anteriore dell'adolescenza. Boll. Mem. Soc. Piemontese Chir., *9*:216, 1939.
23. Catalano, V.: Sul trattamento chirurgico del piede cavo. Arch. Putti, *5*:431, 1954.
24. Chawap, A. R.: Rôle et chirurgie de l'aponévrose plantaire dans la déformation en pied creux. Thèse médecine, Paris, 1956.
25. Chuinard, E. G., and Baskin, M.: Claw-foot deformity. Treatment by transferring the long extensors into the metatarsals and fusion of the interphalangeal joints. J. Bone Joint Surg., *55-A*:351, 1973.
26. Ciaccia, S.: Sul trattamento del piede cavo. Chir. Organi Mov., *11*:483, 1926.
27. Cole, W. H.: The treatment of claw-foot. J. Bone Joint Surg., *22*:895, 1940.
28. Coleman, S. S.: Complex Foot Deformities in Children. Philadelphia, Lea & Febiger, 1983.
29. Coleman, S. S., and Chesnut, W. J.: A simple test for hindfoot flexibility in the cavovarus foot. Clin. Orthop., *123*:60, 1977.
30. Colon, M. J., Whitton, K. E., and Schwartz, N.: Treatment of pes cavus in a patient with Charcot-Marie-Tooth disease. J. Foot Surg., *19*:41, 1980.
31. Coonrad, R. W., Irwin, C. E., Gucker, T., III, and Wray, J. B.: The importance of plantar muscles in paralytic varus feet: Results of treatment by neurectomy and myoneurectomy. J. Bone Joint Surg., *38-A*:563, 1956.
32. Cralley, J., Fitch, K., and McGonagle, W.: Lumbrical muscles and contracted toes. Anat. Anz., *138*:348, 1975.
33. Davis, G. G.: The treatment of hollow foot (pes cavus). Am. J. Orthop. Surg., *11*:231, 1913.
34. Daw, S. W.: Claw-foot. Clin. J., *61*:13, 1932.
35. Debrunner, W.: Ueber die Wirkung einiger Fussmuskeln insbesondere im Hinblick auf den Hohlfuss. Z. Orthop., *45*:111, 1924.
36. Dekel, S., and Weissman, S. L.: Osteotomy of the calcaneus and concomitant plantar stripping in children with talipes cavo-varus. J. Bone Joint Surg., *55-B*:802, 1973.
37. DeLuca, P. A., et al.: Pes cavovarus as a late consequence of peroneus longus tendon laceration. J. Pediatr. Orthop., *5*:582, 1985.
38. Duchenne, B. G.: Physiology of Motion. (Translated and edited by E. B. Kaplan.) Philadelphia, Saunders, 1959, p. 384.
39. Dwyer, F. C.: Osteotomy of the calcaneum for pes cavus. J. Bone Joint Surg., *41-B*:80, 1959.
40. Dwyer, F. C.: Relationship of variations in the size and inclination of the calcaneum to the shape and function of the whole foot. Ann. R. Coll. Surg. Engl., *34*:120, 1964.
41. Dwyer, F. C.: The present status of the problem of pes cavus. Clin. Orthop., *106*:254, 1975.
42. Farill, J.: A tendon transfer for the treatment of certain cases of cavus deformity of the foot. J. Bone Joint Surg., *45-A*:1779, 1963.
43. Faye, C. L.: A propos de 50 observations de pied creux. Étude étiologique et thérapeutique (Traitement chirurgical). Thèse médecine, Paris, 1961.
44. Fenton, C. F., III, McGlamry, E. D., and Perrone, M.: Severe pes cavus deformity secondary to Charcot-Marie-Tooth disease: A case report. J. Am. Podiatry Assoc., *72*:171, 1982.
45. Filipe, G., and Queneau, P.: Osteotomy of the calcaneus for pes cavus in childhood. Rev. Chir. Orthop., *63*:563, 1977.
46. Fixsen, J. A.: Pes cavus. *In* Klenerman, L. (ed.): The Foot and Its Disorders. The Foot in Childhood. Oxford, Blackwell, 1976, pp. 69–72.
47. Flint, M., and Sweetnam, R.: Amputation of all toes. A review of forty-seven amputations. J. Bone Joint Surg., *42-B*:90, 1960.

48. Forrester-Brown, M. F.: Tendon transplantation for clawing of great toe. J. Bone Joint Surg., *20*:57, 1938.
49. Fowler, B., Brooks, A. L., and Parrish, T. F.: The cavo-varus foot. J. Bone Joint Surg., *41-A*:757, 1959.
50. Frank, G. R., and Johnson, W. M.: The extensor shift procedure in the correction of clawtoe deformities in children. South. Med. J., *59*:889, 1966.
51. Galeazzi, R.: Pes cavus and principles for effectual treatment. Arch. Ital. Chir., *13*:697, 1925.
52. Garceau, G. J.: Pes cavus. A.A.O.S. Instr. Course Lect., *18*:184, 1961.
53. Garceau, G. J., and Brahms, M. A.: A preliminary study of selective plantar-muscle denervation for pes cavus. J. Bone Joint Surg., *38-A*:553, 1956.
54. Gaunel, C., Louyot, P., and Tréheux, A.: Étude radiologique des desaxation en pronation ou supination du pied. Rev. Rhum., *28*:591, 1971.
55. Geiges, F.: Ein Beitrag zur Aetiologie des Klauenhohlfusses. Bruns Beitr. Klin. Chir., *1*:78, 1912.
56. Giaccai, L., and Simonetti, E.: Caratteristiche patogenetiche del peide cavo cosidetto essenziale e suo trattamento conla resezione-artrodesimodellante della medio-tarsica. Arch. Putti Chir. Organi Mov., *25*:303, 1970.
57. Giannini, S., et al.: Modified Jones operation in the treatment of pes cavovarus. Ital. J. Orthop. Traumatol., *11*:165, 1985.
58. Gilroy, E.: Pes cavus: A clinical study with special reference to its etiology. Edinburgh Med. J., *36*:749, 1929.
59. Girardi, V. C.: Pie cavo. Semana Med., *2*:776, 851, 1942.
60. Giriat, A., Taussig, G., and Masse, P.: Plantar release in the treatment of pes cavus in childhood. Technique and indications. (Author's transl.) Rev. Chir. Orthop., *65*:77, 1979.
61. Giuntini, L.: Modalita e risultati della cura chirurgica nel piede cavo. Arch. Ortop., *54*:459, 1938.
62. Goff, C. W.: The pes cavus of congenital syphilis. J.A.M.A., *86*:392, 1926.
63. Grevtsov, V. V.: Military medical expertise on recruits with flatfoot and pes cavus. Ortop. Travmatol. Protez., *10*:50, 1980.
64. Gudas, C. J.: Mechanism and reconstruction of pes cavus. J. Foot Surg., *16*:1, 1977.
65. Guradze: Operative Behandlung des Klauenhohlfusses mit Exstirpation des Os naviculare. Verh. Dtsch. Orthop. Ges., *15*:348, 1921.
66. Hackenbrock, M.: Der Hohlfuss. Ergeb. Chir. Orthop., *17*:457, 1924.
67. Halgrimssen, S.: Pes cavus, seine Behandlung und einige Bemerkungen "über seine" Ätiologie. Acta Orthop. Scand., *10*:73, 1939.
68. Hammond, G.: Elevation of the first metatarsal bone with hallux equinus. Surgery, *13*:240, 1943.
69. Heron, J. R.: Neurological syndromes associated with pes cavus. Proc. R. Soc. Med., *62*:270, 1969.
70. Heyman, C. H.: The operative treatment of clawfoot. J. Bone Joint Surg., *14*:335, 1932.
71. Hibbs, R. A.: An operation for "claw-foot." J.A.M.A., *73*:1583, 1919.
72. Hoffmann-Kuhnt, H.: Der Tibialis Auticus beim Plattfuss und beim Hohlfuss. Z. Orthop., *79*:519, 1950.
73. Horne, G.: Pes cavovarus following ankle fractures. Clin. Orthop., *184*:249, 1984.
74. Howard, R. J.: Operative treatment of early cavus feet. South. Med. J., *4*:558, 1971.
75. Hsu, J. D., and Inbus, C. E.: Pes cavus. *In* Jahss, M. H. (ed.): Disorders of the Foot. Philadelphia, Saunders, 1982, pp. 463–485.
76. Hughes, W. K.: Talipes cavus. Br. Med. J., *2*:902, 1940.
77. Imhauser, G.: Surgical treatment of pes cavus with or without claw toes. Z. Orthop., *106*:488, 1969.
78. Ingelrans, P.: Discussion. Symposium—le pied creux essential (Méary, R., ed.). Rev. Chir. Orthop., *53*:422, 1967.
79. Jahss, M. H.: Tarsometatarsal truncated-wedge arthrodesis for pes cavus and equinovarus deformity of the forepart of the foot. J. Bone Joint Surg., *62-A*:713, 1980.
80. Jahss, M. H.: Evaluation of the cavus foot for orthopedic treatment. Clin. Orthop., *181*:52, 1983.
81. James, H. E., McLaurin, R. L., and Watkins, W. T.: Remission of pes cavus in surgically treated spinal dysraphism. Report of a case. J. Bone Joint Surg., *61-A*:1096, 1979.
82. Japas, L. M.: Surgical treatment of pes cavus by tarsal V-osteotomy. Preliminary report. J. Bone Joint Surg., *50-A*:927, 1968.
83. Jones, R.: The soldier's foot and the treatment of common deformities of the foot. Part II: Claw-foot. Br. Med. J., *1*:749, 1968.
84. Karlstrom, G., Lonnerholm, T., and Olerud, S.: Cavus deformity of the foot after fracture of the tibial shaft. J. Bone Joint Surg., *57-A*:893, 1975.
85. Kelikian, H.: Hallux Valgus, Allied Deformities of the Forefoot, and Metatarsalgia. Philadelphia, Saunders, 1965, p. 305.
86. Kleinberg, S., Horwitz, T., and Sobel, R.: Pes cavus. Bull. Hosp. J. Dis., *10*:252, 1949.
87. Kollicker: Der Hohlfuss. Z. Orthop., *45*:106, 1924.
88. Lake, N. C.: Pes cavus. *In* The Foot. 3rd Ed. Baltimore, Williams & Wilkins, 1948, p. 284–287.
89. Lambrinudi, C.: An operation for claw-toes. Proc. R. Soc. Med., *21*:239, 1927.
90. Lelievre, J.: Le pied creux anterieur. *In* Pathologie du Pied. Paris, Masson & Cie, 1970, p. 405.
91. Lenzi, L., and Manzoni, A.: Piede cavo essenziale e piede cavo mielodisplasico. Chir. Organi Mov., *54*:123, 1965.
92. Little, N. J.: Claw foot. Med. J. Aust., *2*:495, 1938.
93. Lorenz, A.: Zum Redressement des Hohlfuss. Z. Orthop., *62*:149, 1934.
94. Lumsden, R. M., Schottstaedt, E. F., and Tsou, P. M.: Pes cavus. *In* Samilson, R. L. (ed.): Children's Foot, Ankle and Leg Problems. Course Syllabus, September, 1971. San Francisco, American Academy of Orthopedic Surgeons, 1971, pp. 197–214.
95. McElvenny, R. T., and Caldwell, G. D.: A new operation for correction of cavus foot. Fusion of first metatarso-cuneiform-navicular joints. Clin. Orthop., *11*:85, 1958.
96. Mann, R., and Inman, V. T.: Phasic activity of intrinsic muscles of the foot. J. Bone Joint Surg., *46-A*:469, 1964.
97. Mattéi, C. R.: La tarsectomie antérieure dans la correction du pied creux. Thèse médecine, Paris, 1974.
98. Mau, C.: Die Calcaneusosteotomie beim Hohlfuss. Verh. Dtsch. Orthop. Ges., *21*:488, 1927.
99. Mayer, P. J.: Pes cavus: A diagnostic and therapeutic challenge. Orthop. Rev., *7*:105, 1978.
100. Méary, R.: Le pied creux essentiel. Symposium. Rev. Chir. Orthop., *53*:389, 1967.
101. Méary, R., Mattei, C. R., and Tomeno, B.: Tarsectomie antérieure pour pied creux. Indications et résults lointains. Rev. Chir. Orthop., *62*:231, 1976.
102. Milano, C., Sessa, G., and Amicone, A.: Tarso-metatarsal arthrodesis in therapy of anterior pes cavus. Long-term results. Chir. Organi Mov., *66*:715, 1980.
103. Mills, G. P.: The etiology and treatment of claw foot. J. Bone Joint Surg., *6*:142, 1924.
104. Missirian, J., and Mann, R. A.: Pathophysiology of Charcot-Marie-Tooth disease. Presented at Foot Society, Anaheim, California, March, 1983.
105. Mitchell, G. P.: Posterior displacement osteotomy of the calcaneus. J. Bone Joint Surg., *59-B*:233, 1977.

106. Mitroszewska, H., and Szulc, W.: Idiopathic pes cavus and its surgical treatment. Chir. Narzadow Ruchu Ortop. Pol., *42*:543, 1977.
107. Ollerenshaw, R.: The treatment of pes cavus. Proc. R. Soc. Med. (Section of Orthopaedics), *20*:1126, 1927.
108. Parkin, A.: Causation and mode of production of pes cavus. Br. Med. J., *1*:1285, 1891.
109. Paulos, C. E., Coleman, S. S., and Samuelson, K. M.: Pes cavovarus: Review of a surgical approach using soft tissue procedures. J. Bone Joint Surg., *62-A*:942, 1980.
110. Pitzen, P.: Development of medial arch in newborn. Z. Orthop., *84*:44, 1953.
111. Pizziolo, I.: Sul trattamento del piede cavo. Arch. Ortop., *56*:157, 1940.
112. Rivera-Dominguez, M., DiBenedetto, M., Frisbie, J. H., and Rossier, A. B.: Pes cavus and claw toes deformity in patients with spinal cord injury and multiple sclerosis. Paraplegia, *16*:375, 1979.
113. Rocher, H. L., and Dupin, J.: Aplasie musculaire jambière presque totale dans un double pied bot "varus cavus" congenital. Tarsectomie. Guérison, J. Med. Bordeaux, *130*:920, 1953.
114. Rosati, G., Graniere, E., Aiello, I., Pinna, L., De-Bastiani, P., and Tola, R.: Ataxia telangiectasia: Apropos of a case with pes cavus and distal neural amyotrophy. Acta Neurol. (Napoli), *32*:764, 1977.
115. Rosenzweig, A.: Die operative Behandlung des Hohlfusses. Zentrolbl. Chir., *61*:2037, 1934.
116. Rugh, J. T.: An operation for the correction of plantar and adduction contraction of the foot arch. J. Bone Joint Surg., *6*:664, 1924.
117. Rutt, A.: Der Hohlfuss (Pes cavus). *In* Hohmann, G. (ed.): Handbuch der Orthopädie. Stuttgart, Georg Thieme Verlag, 1961, Vol. IV, Part II, pp. 1068–1095.
118. Sabir, M., and Lyttie, D.: Pathogenesis of pes cavus in Charcot-Marie-Tooth disease. Clin. Orthop., *175*:173, 1983.
119. Samilson, R. L.: Crescentic osteotomy of the os calcis for calcaneocavus feet. *In* Bateman, J. E. (ed.): Foot Science. Philadelphia, Saunders, 1976, pp. 18–25.
120. Samilson, R. L.: Calcaneocavus feet—a plan of management in children. Orthop. Rev., *10*:121, 1981.
121. Samilson, R. L., and Dillin, W.: Cavus, cavovarus and calcaneocavus. An update. Clin. Orthop., *177*:125, 1983.
122. Saunders, J. T.: Etiology and treatment of clawfoot. Arch. Surg. (Chicago), *30*:179, 1935.
123. Scalone, I.: Sul trattamento operativo del piede cavo. Chir. Organi Mov., *6*:83, 1922.
124. Scheer, G. E., and Crego, C. H., Jr.: A two-stage stabilization procedure for correction of calcaneocavus. J. Bone Joint Surg., *38-A*:1247, 1956.
125. Scherb, R.: Bemerkungen zur Aetiologie des Klauenhohlfusses. Z. Orthop., *44*:564, 1924.
126. Schlegel, K. F.: Spina bifida occulta and pes cavus with marked hammertoes. On the pathogenesis and causal treatment of so-called idiopathic talipes cavus. Ergeb. Chir. Orthop., *45*:268, 1964.
127. Schnepp, K. H.: Hammer-toe and claw-foot. Am. J. Surg., *36*:351, 1937.
128. Sell, L. S.: Pes cavus. Spectator Correspondence Club Letter, December 11, 1961.
129. Sharrard, W. J. W.: Congenital pes cavus (arcuatus). *In* Paediatric Orthopaedics and Fractures. Oxford, Blackwell, 1979, pp. 547–549.
130. Sherman, F. C., and Westin, G. W.: Plantar release in the correction of deformities of the foot in childhood. J. Bone Joint Surg., *63-A*:1382, 1981.
131. Sherman, H. M.: The operative treatment of pes cavus. Am. J. Orthop. Surg., *2*:374, 1904–1905.
132. Siffert, R. S., and del Torto, U.: "Beak" triple arthrodesis for severe cavus deformity. Clin. Orthop., *181*:64, 1983.
133. Siffert, R. S., Forster, R. I., and Nachamie, B.: "Beak" triple arthrodesis for correction of severe cavus deformity. Clin. Orthop., *45*:101, 1966.
134. Spillane, J. D.: Familial pes cavus and absent tendon-jerks: Its relationship with Friedreich's disease and peroneal muscular atrophy. Brain, *63*:275, 1940.
135. Spitzy, H.: Operative correction of claw foot. Surg. Gynecol. Obstet., *45*:813, 1927.
136. Staheli, L. T., Chew, D. E., and Corbett, M.: The longitudinal arch. A survey of eight hundred eighty-two feet in normal children and adults. J. Bone Joint Surg., *69-A*:426, 1987.
137. Stauffer, R. N., Nelson, G. E., and Bianco, A. J.: Calcaneal osteotomy in treatment of cavovarus foot. Mayo Clin. Proc., *45*:624, 1970.
138. Steindler, A.: Operative treatment of pes cavus. Surg. Gynecol. Obstet., *24*:612, 1917.
139. Steindler, A.: Stripping of the os calcis. J. Orthop. Surg., *2*:8, 1920.
140. Steindler, A.: The treatment of pes cavus. Arch. Surg. (Chicago), *2*:325, 1921.
141. Stuart, W.: Claw-foot—its treatment. J. Bone Joint Surg., *6*:360, 1924.
142. Swanson, A. B., Browne, H. S., and Coleman, J. D.: The cavus foot concept of protection and treatment by metatarsal osteotomy. J. Bone Joint Surg., *48-A*:1019, 1966.
143. Taylor, T. G.: The treatment of claw toes by multiple transfer of flexors into extensor tendons. J. Bone Joint Surg., *33-B*:539, 1951.
144. Thomas, W.: Treatment of talipes cavus. Birmingham Med. Rev., *34*:1, 1893.
145. Todd, A.: Treatment of pes cavus. Lancet, *2*:758, 1934.
146. Tomeno, B.: Essential pes cavus. Rev. Prat., *31*:1019, 1981.
147. Turner, M.: Pathogenesis of pes cavus, chronaximetric study. Arch. Argent. Pediat., *38*:38, 1952.
148. Walsham, W. J., and Hughes, W. K.: Talipes cavus. *In* The Deformities of the Human Foot. London, Bailliere, Tindall & Co., 1895, Chap. XIII, pp. 490–495.
149. Wang, G., and Shaffer, L. W.: Osteotomy of the metatarsals for pes cavus. South. Med. J., *79*:77, 1977.
150. Weseley, M. S.: Calcaneal osteotomy for the treatment of the cavus deformity. Bull. Hosp. Joint Dis., *31*:93, 1970.
151. Weseley, M. S., and Barenfield, P. A.: Mechanism of the Dwyer calcaneal osteotomy. Clin. Orthop., *70*:137, 1970.
152. Westin, G. W.: Personal communication, 1978.
153. Whitman, R.: Orthopaedic Surgery. Philadelphia, Lea & Febiger, 1930, pp. 853, 896.
154. Wilcox, P. G., and Weiner, D. S.: The Akron midtarsal dome osteotomy in the treatment of rigid pes cavus: A preliminary review. J. Pediatr. Orthop., *5*:333, 1985.
155. Williams, M., and Lissner, H. R.: Parallel forces in one plane. *In* Biomechanics of Human Motion. Philadelphia, Saunders, 1962, pp. 34–68.
156. Williams, P. F., and Menelaus, M. B.: Triple arthrodesis by inlay grafting—a method suitable for the undeformed or valgus foot. J. Bone Joint Surg., *59-B*:333, 1977.
157. Yale, A. C., and Hugar, D. W.: Pes cavus: The deformity and its etiology. J. Foot Surg., *20*:159, 1981.

CLAW TOES

Clawing of the toes is characterized by hyperextension of the metatarsophalangeal joint

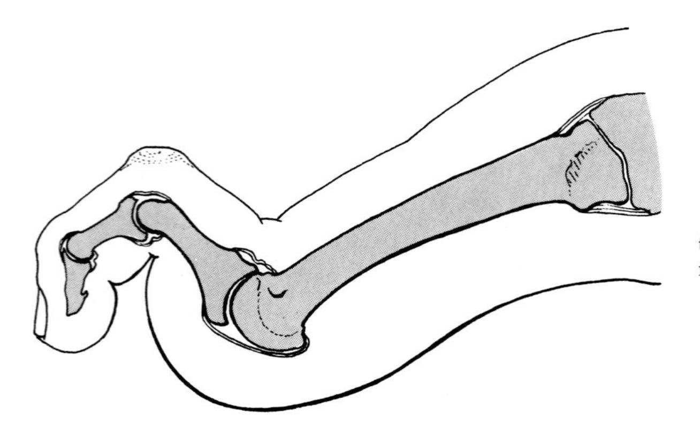

FIGURE 7–167. Claw toe.

The deformity is characterized by hyperextension of the metatarsophalangeal joint and flexion of both proximal and distal interphalangeal joints.

and flexion of both the proximal and distal interphalangeal joints (Figs. 7–167 and 7–168). The deformity may be secondary to pes cavus, or it may be paralytic in its pathogenesis. During the push-off phase of gait, when the long toe flexors contract to substitute for the paralyzed triceps surae muscle, the interphalangeal joints of the toes are flexed, and the metatarsophalangeal joints are hyperextended. A reverse mechanism by which clawing of the toes may also occur acts when the anterior tibialis muscle is weakened or zero in motor strength, and the extensor hallucis longus and extensor digitorum longus muscles are used to substitute for its action. In this latter type, clawing of the toes is produced during the swing phase of the gait. The great toe is usually more severely affected than the lesser toes. Painful callosities gradually develop over the dorsum of the interphalangeal joints, which become fixed in flexion. Pressure keratoses under the metatarsal heads aggravate the disability.

Treatment

Treatment is dependent upon the type of claw toes, the degree of flexibility of the interphalangeal and metatarsophalangeal joints, and the age of the patient. The Girdlestone-Taylor operation (in which the long toe flexor is transferred to the dorsal expansion of the long toe extensors) should *not* be performed for clawing of the toes, as it causes rotational malalignment of the toes.[6, 14] The experience of Taylor, who obtained good results in 27 of 38 patients, is not shared by others. Pyper, reviewing the results of the Girdlestone-Taylor operation in 45 feet with clawing of the toes, found that in approximately 20 per cent of cases, the extensor tendons regenerated and the deformity recurred. The interphalangeal joints were stiff in 60 per cent, and in no case was there significant improvement in metatarsal pain and callosities. Worthwhile improvement was achieved in about 50 per cent of the cases, with the best results in those with only the mildest symptoms. The advantages observed by Pyper were: improvement in the shape of the toes with consequent easier fitting of shoes, disappearance of corns over the interphalangeal joints, and general improvement in walking.[11]

For clawing of the great toe, Dickson and Dively advise transfer of the extensor hallucis longus tendon to the flexor hallucis longus tendon, and resection and arthrodesis of the interphalangeal joint in normal alignment.[3] This author has had no experience with this operation.

In paralytic claw toes, the dynamic imbalance causing the deformity should be corrected whenever feasible. In the presence of anterior tibial muscle weakness, the motor power of ankle dorsiflexion should be restored by appropriate tendon transfer. First, associated equinus

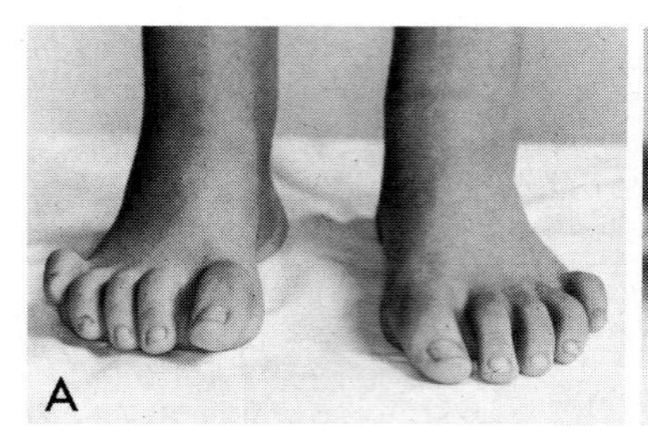

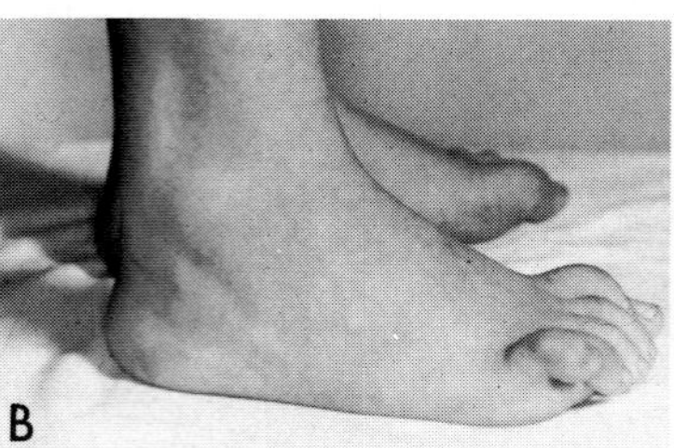

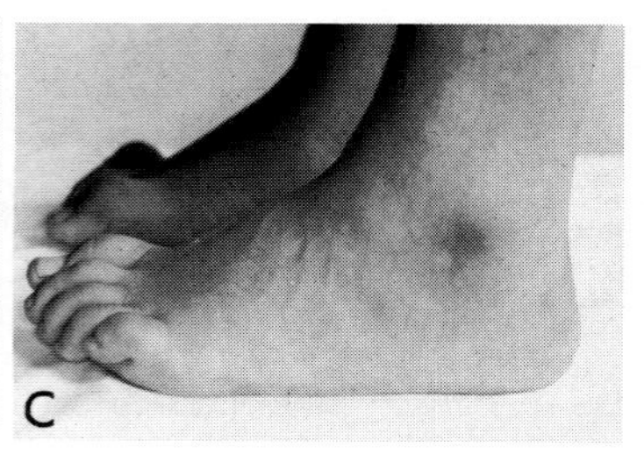

FIGURE 7–168. Bilateral clawing of the toes.

deformity is corrected by stretching casts; then the peroneal muscles are transferred to the base of the second metatarsal, or in the presence of peroneal muscle weakness, the long toe extensors are transferred to the metatarsal heads. The fixed flexion deformity of the interphalangeal joints is corrected by wedge resections and arthrodesis. If the primary cause of claw toes is triceps surae muscle weakness and hyperactive long toe flexors, posterior transfer of the appropriate muscles to the os calcis is performed to restore active power of plantar flexion. If the claw toes represent triceps surae muscle weakness and hyperactive long toe flexors, posterior transfer of the appropriate muscles to the os calcis is performed to restore active power of plantar flexion. If the claw toes are secondary to pes cavus, equinus deformity of the forefoot is corrected. Fixed claw toes are treated by dorsal capsulotomy of the metatarsophalangeal joints and transfer of the long toe extensors to the metatarsal heads and fusion of the interphalangeal joints as described in Plates 104 and 106 for correction of hammer toes.

References

1. Barbari, S. G., and Brevig, K.: Correction of clawtoes by the Girdlestone-Taylor flexor-extensor transfer procedure. Foot Ankle, *5*:67, 1984.
2. Coughlin, M. J., and Mann, R. A.: Lesser toe deformities. *In* Mann, R. A. (ed.): Surgery of the Foot. St. Louis, Mosby, 1986, pp. 132–148.
3. Dickson, F. D., and Dively, R. L.: Operation for correction of mild claw foot, the result of infantile paralysis. J.A.M.A., *87*:1275, 1926.
4. Forrester-Brown, M. F.: Tendon transplantation for clawing of the great toe. J. Bone Joint Surg., *20*:57, 1938.
5. Frank, G. R., and Johnson, W. M.: The extensor shift procedure in the correction of clawtoe deformities in children. South. Med. J., *59*:889, 1966.
6. Girdlestone, G. R.: Physiotherapy for hand and foot. Journal of Chartered Society of Physiotherapy, *32*:176, 1947.
7. Heyman, C. H.: Operative treatment of claw foot. J. Bone Joint Surg., *14*:335, 1932.
8. Hibbs, R. A.: An operation for "claw foot." J.A.M.A., *73*:1583, 1919.
9. Lambrinudi, C.: An operation for claw-toes. Proc. R. Soc. Med., *21*:239, 1927.
10. Parrish, T. F.: Dynamic correction of clawtoes. Orthop. Clin. North Am., *4*:97, 1973.
11. Pyper, J. B.: The flexor-extensor transplant operation for claw toes. J. Bone Joint Surg., *40-B*:528, 1958.
12. Sharrard, W. J. W., and Smith, T. W. D.: Tenodesis of the flexor hallucis longus for paralytic clawing of the hallux in childhood. J. Bone Joint Surg., *58-B*:224, 1976.
13. Taylor, T. G.: An operative procedure for the treatment of hammer toe and claw toe. J. Bone Joint Surg., *22*:608, 1940.
14. Taylor, T. G.: The treatment of claw toes by multiple transfers of flexor into extensor tendons. J. Bone Joint Surg., *33-B*:539, 1951.
15. Young, C. S.: An operation for correction of hammertoe and claw toe. J. Bone Joint Surg., *20*:715, 1938.

Flexible Pes Planovalgus (Flat Foot)

Flat foot is a loose generic term used to describe any condition of the foot in which the longitudinal arch is abnormally low or absent. It covers a multitude of conditions that differ in their etiology, pathology, degree of severity, prognosis, and treatment. The term *pes planus* is more esoteric. In the literature *pes planus* is often modified by adjectives such as *rigid* or *flexible, static* or *paralytic, congenital* or *acquired* and is sometimes denoted by more complex combinations of terms such as *congenital rigid pes planus with vertical talus* or *congenital convex pes valgus.*

The simplicity of the term *flat foot,* or *pes planus,* is deceptive, resulting in faulty diagnosis in a large number of children with normal feet that appear flat. It is vital to avoid vagaries and to be more exact in terminology. A classification of flat foot is given in Table 7–14. The disorder includes both congenital and acquired forms, with the deformity either rigid or flexible. In the acquired type the defect may be ligamentous, muscular, articular, bony, or contractural. This section deals with flat foot due to excessive ligamentous laxity; the other entities are described in other sections of this book.

The integrity of the longitudinal and transverse arches of the foot is dependent upon the configuration of tarsal bones and joints and the strength of the ligaments that bind them together. The longitudinal arch of the foot is *not* maintained by the active contraction of muscles. Electromyographic studies by Basmajian and associates demonstrated minimal or no electrical activity in the intrinsic and extrinsic muscles of the foot and leg of the person standing at rest. The main concerns of the primary muscles of the lower limb are to maintain balance, to propel the body forward, and to protect the ligaments from abnormal stress such as in walking on rough terrain.[7, 8]

The exact cause of hyperlaxity of ligaments in flexible pes planovalgus is unknown; the condition is, however, familial.

Analysis of Deformity and Radiographic Features

In flat foot the basic deformity is depression of the longitudinal arch. The sag in the arch may result from plantar deviation of any one or all three of the components that constitute the

Table 7–14. Classification of Flat Foot

Congenital
Rigid
Congenital convex pes valgus
Tarsal coalition
Flexible
Talipes calcaneovalgus
Talipes valgus due to contracture of triceps surae muscle (calcaneal equinus deformity)
Hypoplasia of sustentaculum tali
Acquired
Due to *ligamentous hyperlaxity*
Familial
Part of a generalized syndrome (e.g., Ehlers-Danlos, Marfan's, Down's, osteogenesis imperfecta)
Due to *muscle weakness and imbalance*
Accessory tarsal navicular with insufficiency of tibialis posterior muscle
Myopathic (e.g., muscular dystrophy)
Peripheral nerve injuries
Spinal cord affections (e.g., poliomyelitis, myelodysplasia)
Cerebral palsy (spastic or hypotonic)
Arthritic
Inflammatory conditions involving subtalar and midtarsal joints (e.g., rheumatoid arthritis)
Traumatic arthritis (in children usually in rare conditions such as congenital insensitivity to pain)
Contractural
Due to myostatic contracture of peroneal muscles
Due to acquired contracture of triceps surae

arch—namely, the talocalcaneal, talonavicular, and naviculocuneiform joints. The cuneiform-metatarsal articulation does not sag because it is a stable joint with very limited range of motion.

When the hypermobile foot is loaded under the static force of body weight the calcaneus pronates under the talus. The anterior end of the calcaneus moves laterally and dorsally, whereas the head of the talus moves medially and plantarward (Fig. 7–169). The plantar calcaneonavicular ligament is elongated because of ligamentous hyperlaxity and does not support the head of the talus. The talocalcaneal interosseous ligament is lax, allowing the heel to evert. Horizontal movement takes place at the talonavicular joint; the navicular abducts in relation to the talar head, moving in unison with the anterior end of the calcaneus. The forepart of the foot follows the navicular, and the center of gravity of the body is shifted over or medial to the first metatarsal bone (Fig. 7–170 A). Normally the weight falls between the second and third rays, which is the center of the foot. A foot that on weight-bearing assumes a valgus posture because of extreme laxity of the ligaments with medial displacement of the static load of body weight produces excessive stress and strain on the foot. It is not the flatness of the longitudinal arch but rather the medial shift in weight-bearing that makes the pronated foot mechanically weak. Nature makes the child toe-in actively so that the center of gravity of the body is shifted laterally toward the center of the foot (Fig. 7–170 B). With toeing-in the forepart of the foot is adducted. In the literature there is some controversy over whether the active supination and adduction of the forefoot are part of the complex deformity of flexible pes planovalgus. This author proposes that toeing-in in gait and supination of the medial rays of the forefoot in stance are secondary

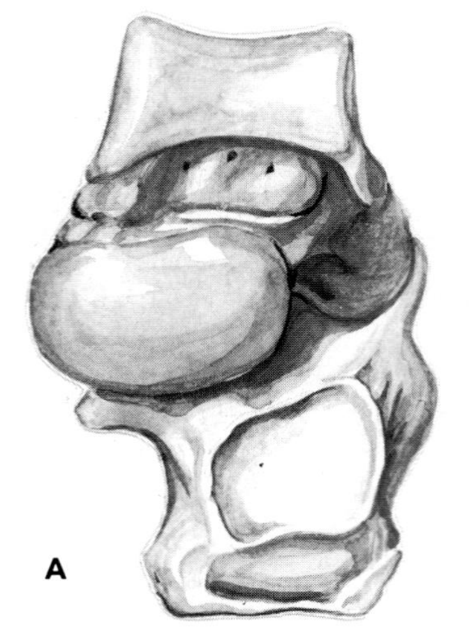

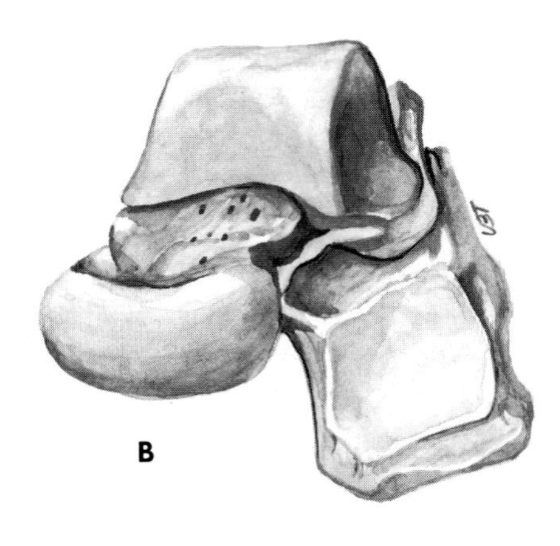

FIGURE 7–169. Hypermobile flat foot.

A. Non-weight-bearing. **B.** Weight-bearing. Note that the anterior end of the calcaneus moves laterally and dorsally, whereas the head of the talus moves medially and plantarward.

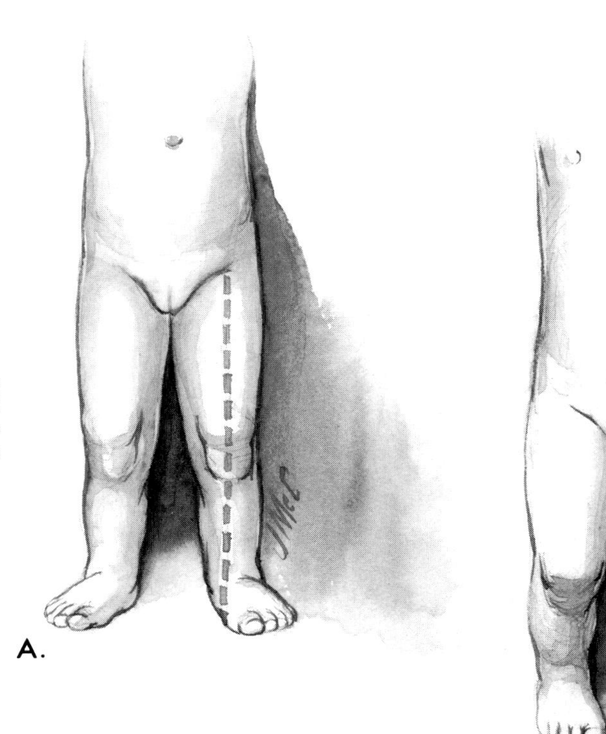

FIGURE 7–170. Flexible flat foot.

A. In stance, the center of gravity of the body is over or medial to the first metatarsal bone. **B.** Protective toeing-in so that the body weight is shifted laterally toward the center of the foot.

compensatory mechanisms and not the primary deformity.

In the flexible flat foot caused by excessive ligamentous laxity there is no fixed deformity—in stance the foot assumes valgus posture, but when not bearing weight it has a normal contour and longitudinal arch (Fig. 7–171).

When there is associated myostatic contracture of the triceps surae muscle, the calcaneus is tilted into plantar flexion, losing its normal pitch, the valgus posture of the foot in stance is exaggerated, and the child is unable to protect his feet by compensatory toeing-in.

Radiographic examination of the feet will demonstrate the malalignment of the joints and the anatomic site of the break in the longitudinal arch, whether at the talonavicular joint, the

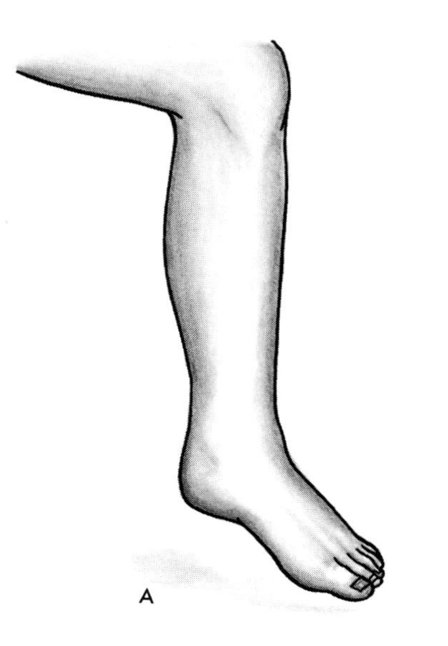

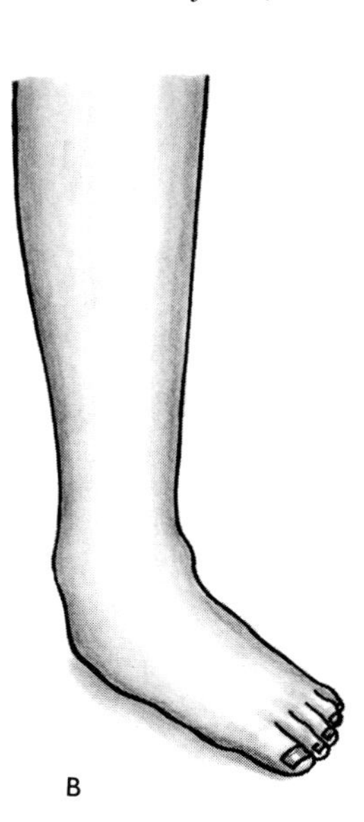

FIGURE 7–171. Flexible flat foot.

A. When not weight-bearing, the suspended foot has normal contour and longitudinal arch. **B.** On weight-bearing the longitudinal arch is flattened.

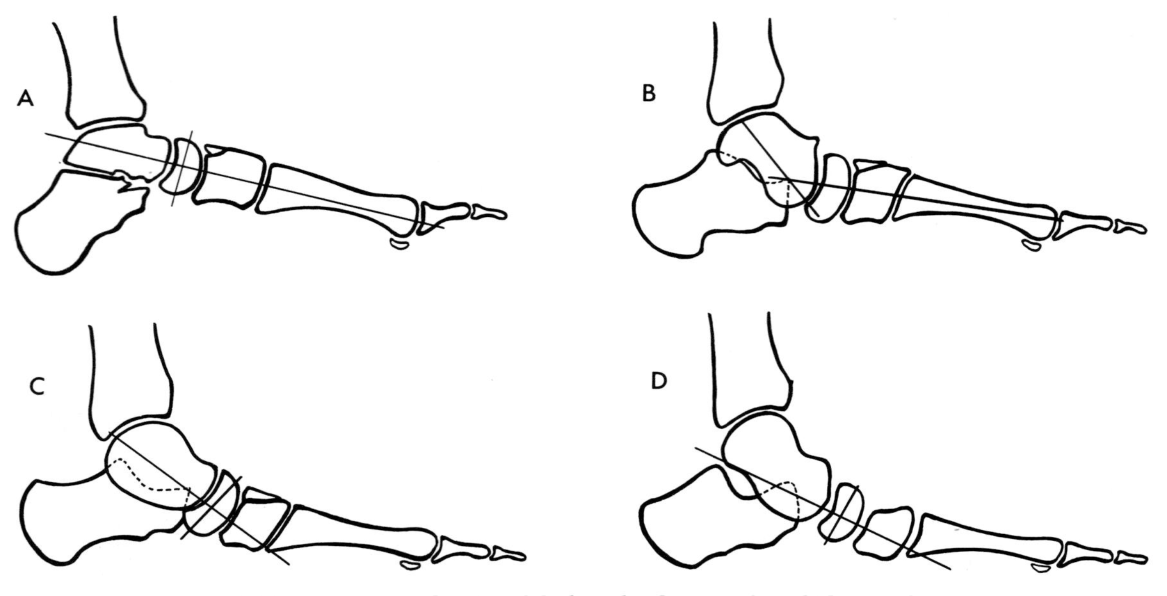

FIGURE 7–172. Line drawing of the lateral radiogram of weight-bearing feet.

Lines are drawn through the center of the longitudinal axes of the talus, navicular, medial cuneiform, and first metatarsal. A vertical line is drawn through the center of the navicular parallel to its proximal articular surface. **A.** *Normal foot.* The longitudinal axes of the talus, navicular, medial cuneiform, and first metatarsal form a straight line; the longitudinal axis of the talus crosses the navicular vertical line at a right angle. **B.** Flexible flat foot due to *talonavicular sag.* The longitudinal axis of the talus points plantarward, exiting on the inferior quadrant of the navicular, behind the medial cuneiform. The long axes of the first metatarsal, medial cuneiform, and navicular are in a straight line and cross the long axis of the talus at an angle. **C.** Flexible flat foot due to *naviculocuneiform sag.* The longitudinal axes of the talus and navicular make a straight line and bisect the navicular vertical line at right angles, but they exit on the plantar aspect of the medial cuneiform proximal to the base of the first metatarsal. **D.** Flexible flat foot due to sag at both the talonavicular and naviculocuneiform joints. The line drawn through the longitudinal axis of the navicular when extended proximally and distally lies plantar to the center of the talar and first metatarsal segments.

naviculocuneiform joint, or both joints. The radiograms should be made with the patient standing with the muscles relaxed. If the feet are flexible clinically, non-weight-bearing radiograms are not usually required.

In the lateral projection of a normal weight-bearing foot, lines drawn through the center of the longitudinal axes of the talus, navicular, medial cuneiform, and first metatarsal form a straight line (Fig. 7–172 A). A vertical line is drawn through the center of the navicular parallel to its proximal articular surface. In the normal foot the longitudinal axis of the talus crosses the navicular vertical line at a right angle (Figs. 7–172 A and 7–173).

When the break occurs *at the talonavicular joint alone,* the long axis of the talus points plantarward, exiting on the lower quarter of the navicular, posterior to the medial cuneiform. The long axes of the first metatarsal, medial cuneiform, and navicular, however, remain in a straight line and intersect the long axis of the talus at an angle (Fig. 7–172 B).

The *plantar-flexion angle of the talus* is defined as the angle formed between the horizontal plantar line and a line drawn through the center of the longitudinal axis of the talus (bisecting the talar neck and head) on a weight-bearing lateral projection. The normal plantar-flexion angle of the talus measures 26.5 degrees (S.D., 5.3 degrees).[14]

The talus, in addition to being plantar-flexed, deviates medially. In the anteroposterior radiogram, with the medial deviation of the talus and the lateral tilting of the anterior end of the calcaneus, the anteroposterior talocalcaneal angle is widened, usually to more than 35 degrees. The navicular is displaced laterally in relation to the head of the talus. Giannestras assesses the degree of medial deviation of the talar head in relation to the navicular by the dorsoplantar talonavicular angle. One line is drawn parallel to the distal articular surface of the navicular; another line is drawn through the longitudinal axis of the talus (bisecting the talar head-neck). The two lines form an angle of between 60 and 80 degrees. An angle of less than 60 degrees is abnormal and indicates medial deviation of the talus (Figs. 7–173 and 7–174).[48]

When the break takes place *at the naviculo-*

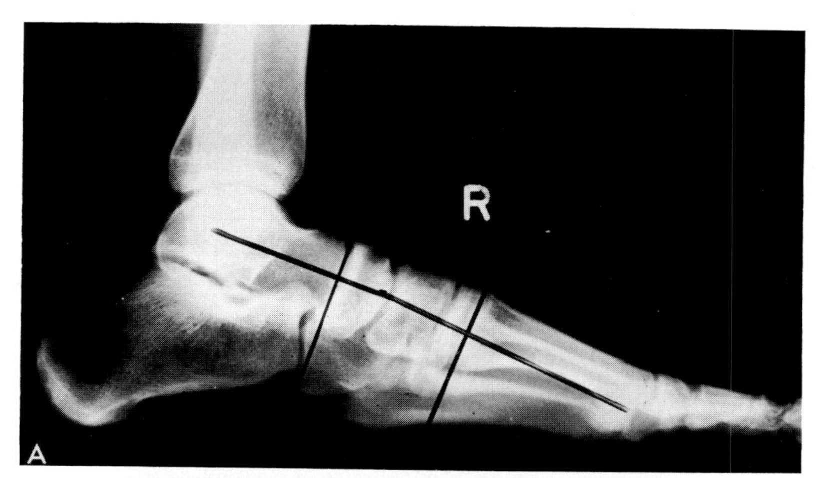

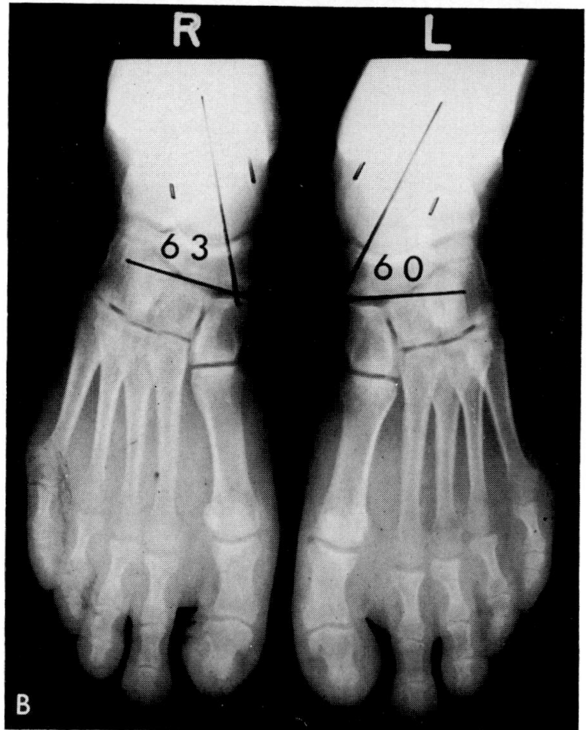

FIGURE 7–173. Radiograms of a normal foot, weight-bearing in stance.

A. Lateral view. Lines are drawn parallel to the proximal articular surface of the navicular and the distal articular surface of the medial cuneiform. The line drawn through the center of the longitudinal axis of the talus bisects the navicular line at a right angle. On forward projection the long axis of the talus crosses the medial cuneiform line at a right angle and extends to the plantar aspect of the first metatarsal head. Note the line is slightly angulated dorsally at the naviculocuneiform joint. A straight line is considered the lower limit of normal. **B.** Anteroposterior view. The dorsoplantar talonavicular angle is that formed between the longitudinal axis of the talus (bisecting the talar head-neck) and a line drawn parallel to the distal articular surface of the navicular. The normal value is between 60 and 80 degrees. Note that in the right foot it is 63 degrees and in the left foot 60 degrees. An angle less than 60 degrees is considered abnormal. (From Giannestras, N.: Flexible valgus flatfoot resulting from naviculocuneiform and talonavicular sag. Surgical correction in the adolescent. *In* Bateman, J. E. (ed.): Foot Science. Philadelphia, Saunders, 1976, pp. 67–105. Reprinted by permission.)

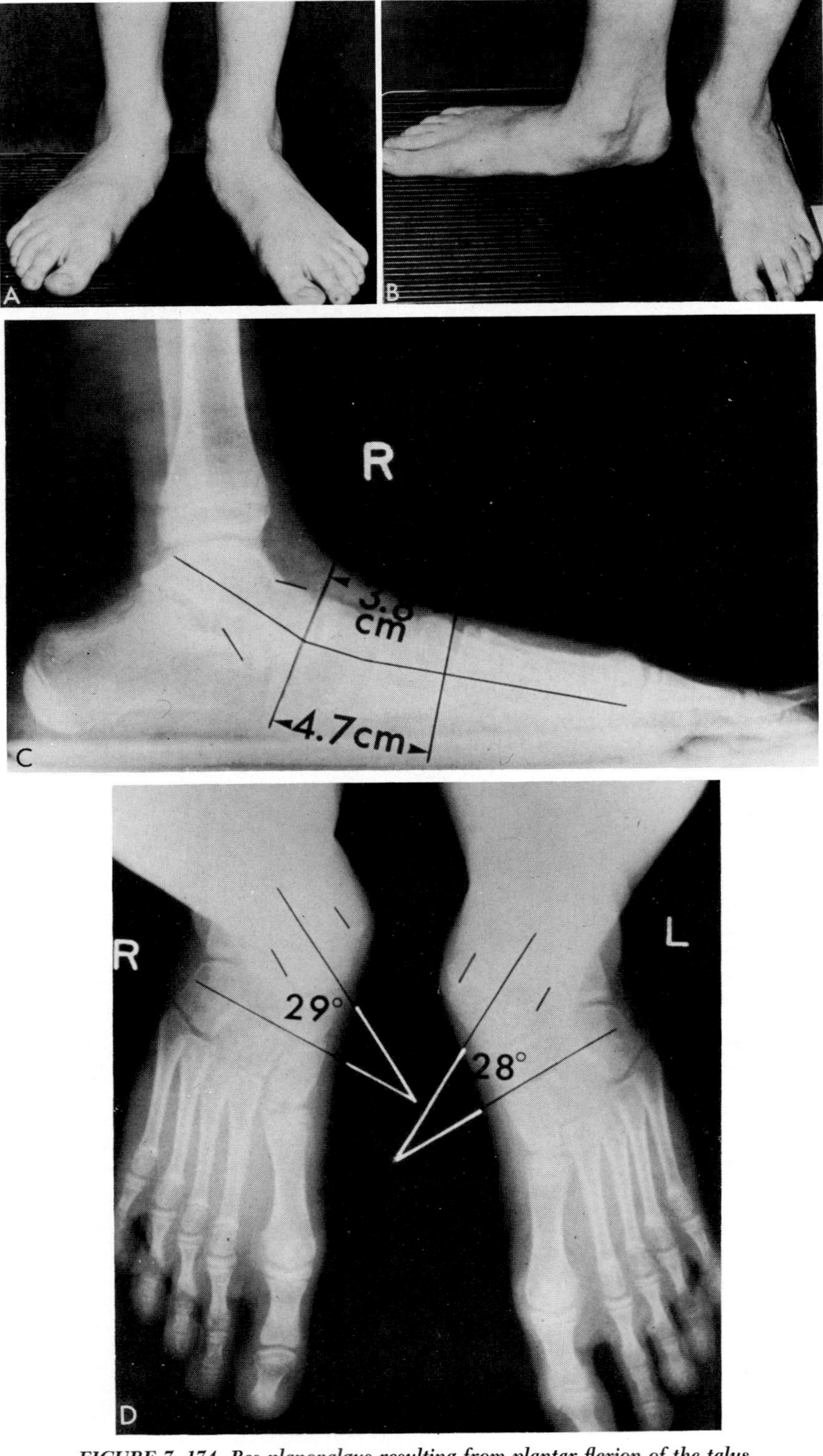

FIGURE 7–174. Pes planovalgus resulting from plantar flexion of the talus.

A and **B.** Clinical appearance showing complete absence of the longitudinal arch and the prominent plantar-flexed head of the talus just below the medial malleolus. The heels are in valgus position. **C.** Standing lateral radiogram of the right foot. The talus is plantar-flexed. The sag at the naviculocuneiform joint is minimal. **D.** Anteroposterior standing radiogram of both feet. The head of the talus is deviated medially, and the dorsoplantar talonavicular angle is markedly diminished. (From Giannestras, N.: Flexible valgus flatfoot resulting from naviculocuneiform and talonavicular sag. Surgical correction in the adolescent. *In* Bateman, J. E. (ed.): Foot Science. Philadelphia, Saunders, 1976, pp. 67–105. Reprinted by permission.)

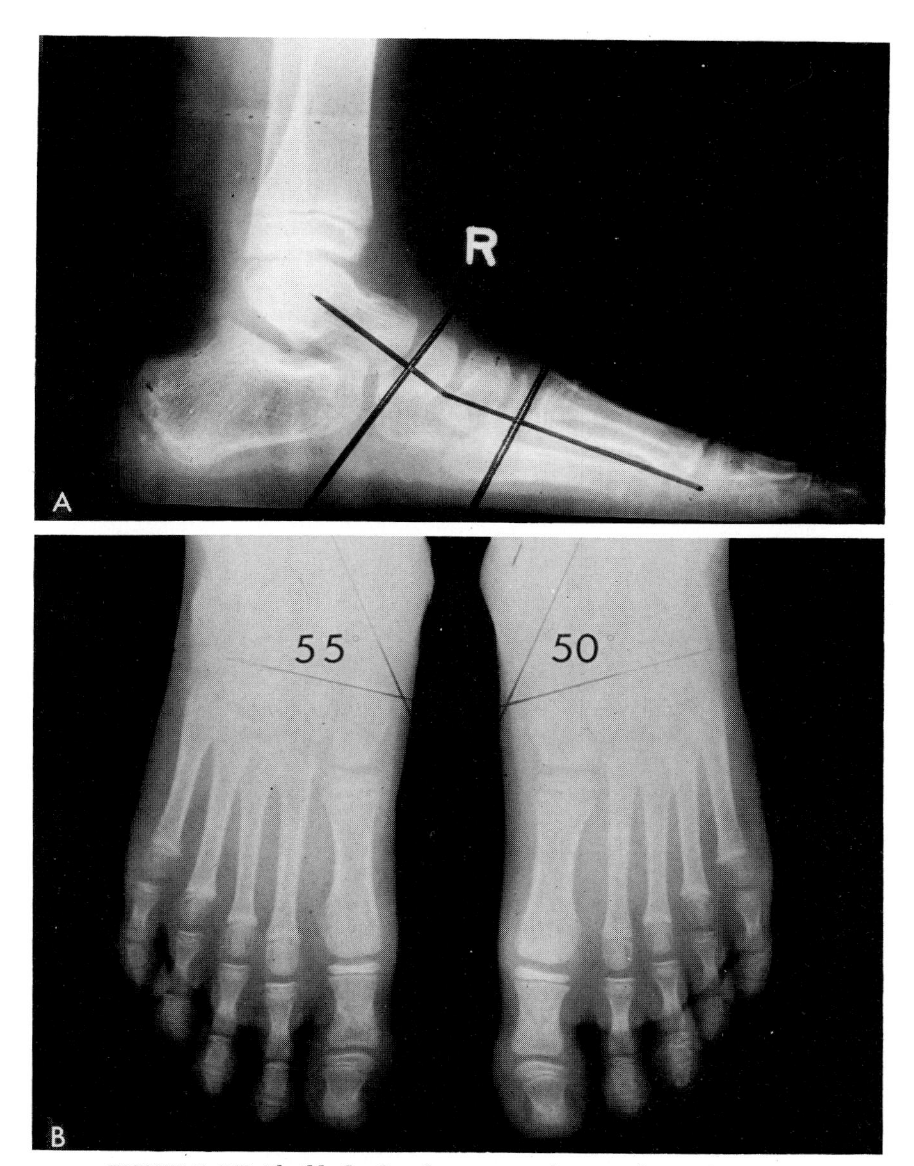

FIGURE 7–175. Flexible flat foot due to sag at the naviculocuneiform joint.

A. In the standing lateral radiogram the lines drawn through the long axes of the talus and the first metatarsal are angulated plantarward at the naviculocuneiform joint. **B.** The standing anteroposterior radiogram of both feet shows the decrease in the dorsoplantar talonavicular angles (the lower limit of normal is 60 degrees). (From Giannestras, N.: Flexible valgus flatfoot resulting from naviculocuneiform and talonavicular sag. Surgical correction in the adolescent. *In* Bateman, J. E. (ed.): Foot Science. Philadelphia, Saunders, 1976, pp. 67–105. Reprinted by permission.)

cuneiform joint alone, in the lateral radiogram of the foot the longitudinal axes of the talus and the navicular make a straight line and bisect the navicular vertical line perpendicularly, but they exit on the plantar aspect of the medial cuneiform proximal to the base of the first metatarsal (see Fig. 7–172 C). In the lateral view of the standing radiogram of the foot, Giannestras draws lines over the proximal articular surface of the navicular and over the distal articular surface of the medial cuneiform. In a normal foot the longitudinal axis of the talus (bisecting the talar head) crosses the navicular articular line at a right angle. A line drawn from the plantar aspect of the first metatarsal head is perpendicular to the medial cuneiform articular line. The line running through the long axis of the talus to the plantar aspect of the first metatarsal head in the normal foot is slightly angulated dorsally at the naviculocuneiform joint as shown in Figure 7–173 A; when the line is straight it is considered to be the lower limit of the normal. When there is a sag at the naviculocuneiform joint the line is angulated plantarward (Fig. 7–175).[48]

When the break occurs *at both the talonavicular and naviculocuneiform joints*, Jack recommends drawing a line through the longitudinal axis of the navicular, which, when extended proximally and distally, lies plantar to the talar and first metatarsal segments (see Fig. 7–172 D).[76]

An example of severe flexible flat foot due to breaks in all three components that make up the longitudinal arch—talocalcaneal, talonavicular, and naviculocuneiform joints—is illustrated in Figure 7–176.

The angle formed between the horizontal and a line drawn along the plantar border of the calcaneus extending between its posterior and anterior tuberosities on the lateral projection of the weight-bearing radiogram of the foot is called the calcaneal pitch; its normal value is 15 to 20 degrees. In flat foot with contracture of the triceps surae muscle, the calcaneal pitch is low (less than 15 degrees); in pes calcaneus it is high (30 degrees or more) (Fig. 7–177).

Clinical Features

In children, flexible flat foot is asymptomatic. It is the parents who are concerned about the appearance of the feet; or it may be a problem of abnormal shoe wear. In the obese older child or the adolescent, prolonged standing may give rise to foot strain, with pain in the longitudinal arch, abnormal fatigue, and discomfort extending upward on the legs. If there is associated myostatic contracture of the triceps surae muscle, the presenting complaint may be pain in the calf. The permanent shortening of the gastrocnemius-soleus muscle is demonstrated by testing the range of passive dorsiflexion of the ankle with the hindfoot in slight inversion or neutral (never valgus) position and the knee in neutral extension. The angle that the plantar aspect of the foot makes with the longitudinal axis of the leg is observed from the fibular side. During this test, the dorsiflexors of the ankle should not contract actively, as their contraction will cause reciprocal relaxation of the triceps surae muscles.

Faulty shoes or abusive use of the feet will aggravate the symptoms. Prolonged bed rest due to ill health will increase the ligamentous laxity and consequently exaggerate pronation of the feet.

Flexible flat foot is divided into three categories of severity: *mild* or *first degree*—in which on weight-bearing the longitudinal arch is depressed but still visible; *moderate* or *second degree*—in which the longitudinal arch is not visible in stance; and *severe* or *third degree*—in which the longitudinal arch is absent and the medial border of the foot is convex with the head of the talus presenting on the plantar aspect of the foot immediately below and anterior to the medial malleolus (Fig. 7–178).

When not bearing weight, as when the patient is sitting on the examining table with the legs dangling, the feet have normal longitudinal arch and contour; under the weight of the body, however, the longitudinal arch becomes obliterated and the foot appears flat. There may be varying degrees of valgus deviation of the hindfoot and plantar flexion and medial deviation of the talus.

On clinical examination it is difficult to detect the site of the sag, whether it is at the naviculocuneiform joint, at the talonavicular joint, or combined in both joints. The "toe-raising test" described by Jack will give an indication but is not infallible.[76] The patient stands bearing weight on both feet. On passive hyperextension of the big toe the longitudinal arch is elevated in all cases of naviculocuneiform sag and in most cases of combined (naviculocuneiform and talonavicular) breaks; this maneuver, however, does not restore the arch when the talus is plantar-flexed and the sag is at only the talonavicular joint (Fig. 7–179). It seems the flexor hallucis longus does not have sufficient leverage to force the navicular under the head of the talus. When the triceps surae is contracted, the toe-raising test cannot be performed because the flexor hallucis is inefficient.

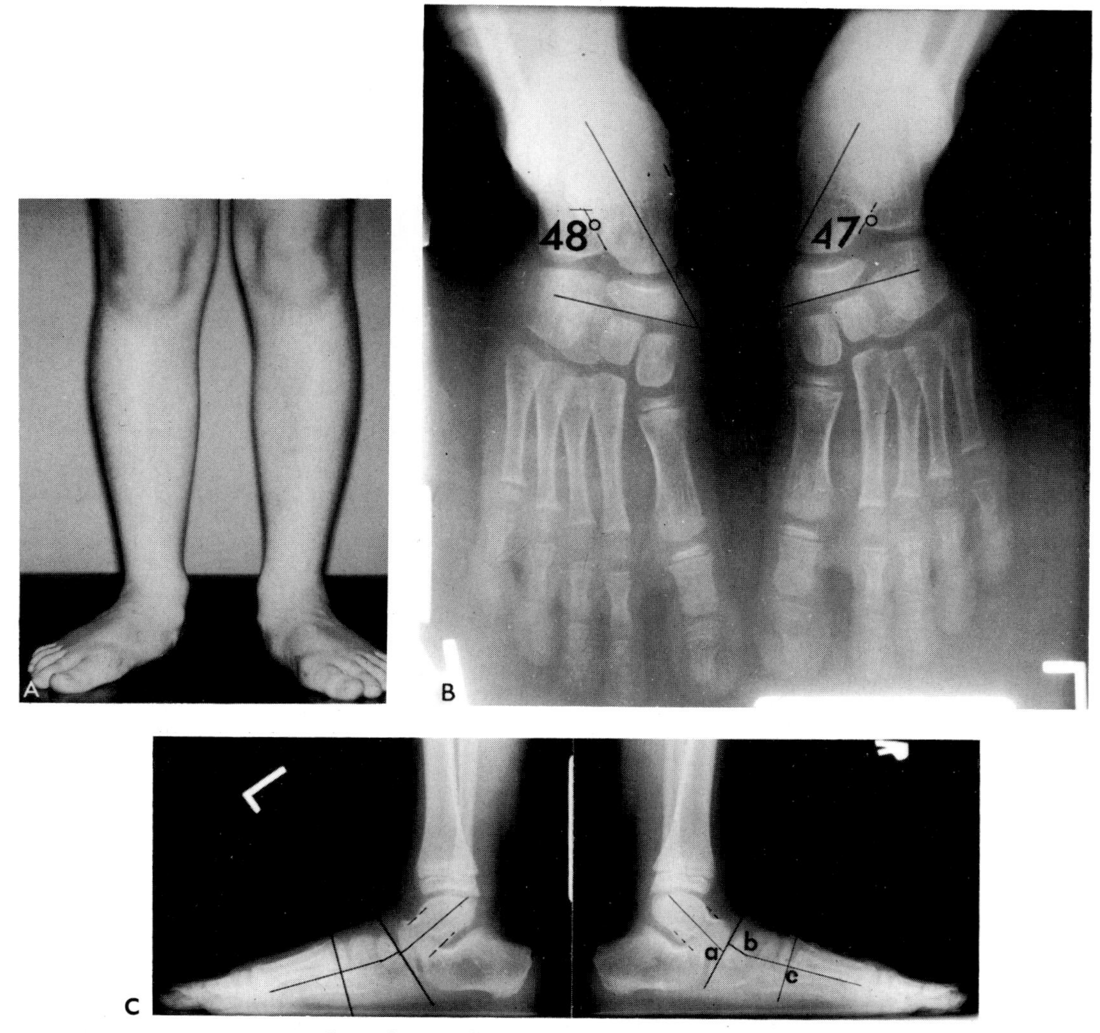

FIGURE 7–176. Severe pes planovalgus resulting from malalignment of the talocalcaneal, talonavicular, and naviculocuneiform joints.

A. Clinical appearance. **B.** Anteroposterior standing radiograms of both feet show decrease in the dorsoplantar talonavicular angle, 48 degrees on the right and 47 degrees on the left. **C.** In the lateral view note that the talus is plantar-flexed (a) with a plantar sag at the talonavicular joint (b). The longitudinal line drawn perpendicular to the distal articular surface of the cuneiform extends to the plantar aspect of the first metatarsal head, indicating a normal tarsometatarsal joint (c). (From Giannestras, N.: Flexible valgus flatfoot resulting from naviculocuneiform and talonavicular sag. Surgical correction in the adolescent. *In* Bateman, J. E. (ed.): Foot Science. Philadelphia, Saunders, 1976, pp. 67–105. Reprinted by permission.)

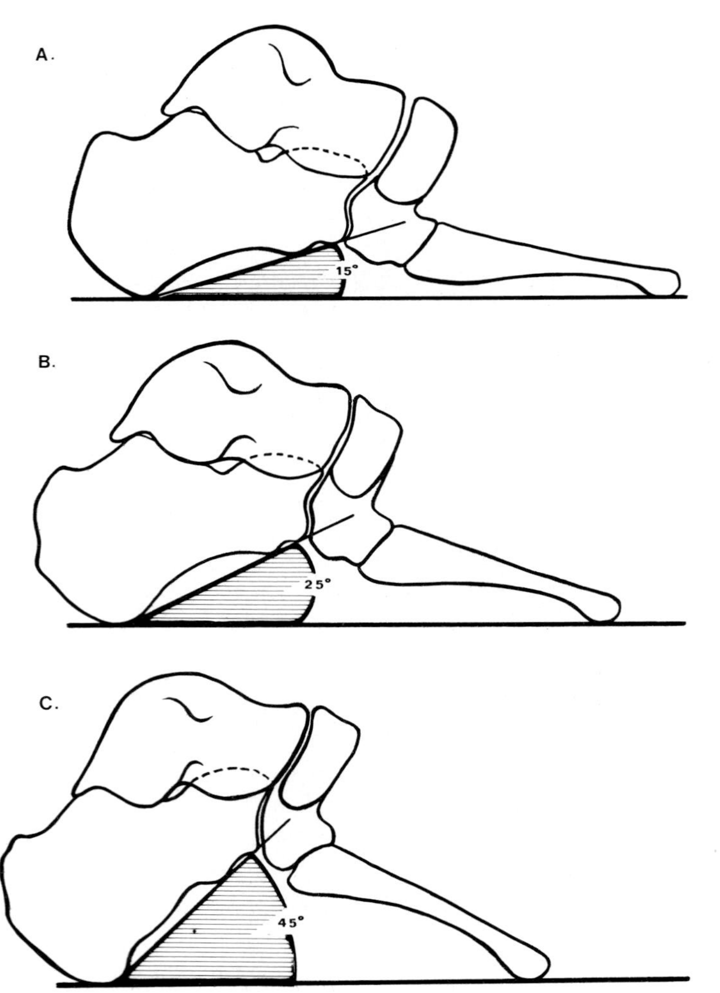

FIGURE 7–177. Calcaneal pitch.

Calcaneal pitch is determined on the standing lateral radiogram of the foot. It is the angle formed between the horizontal and a line drawn along the plantar border of the calcaneus extending between its posterior and anterior tuberosities. **A.** In flat foot it is decreased to less than 15 degrees. **B.** Its normal value is 20 to 25 degrees. **C.** In calcaneus feet the calcaneal pitch is high—over 30 degrees. (Redrawn from Gamble, F. O., and Yale, I.: Clinical Foot Roentgenology. 2nd Ed. New York, Robert E. Krieger, 1975, p. 194.)

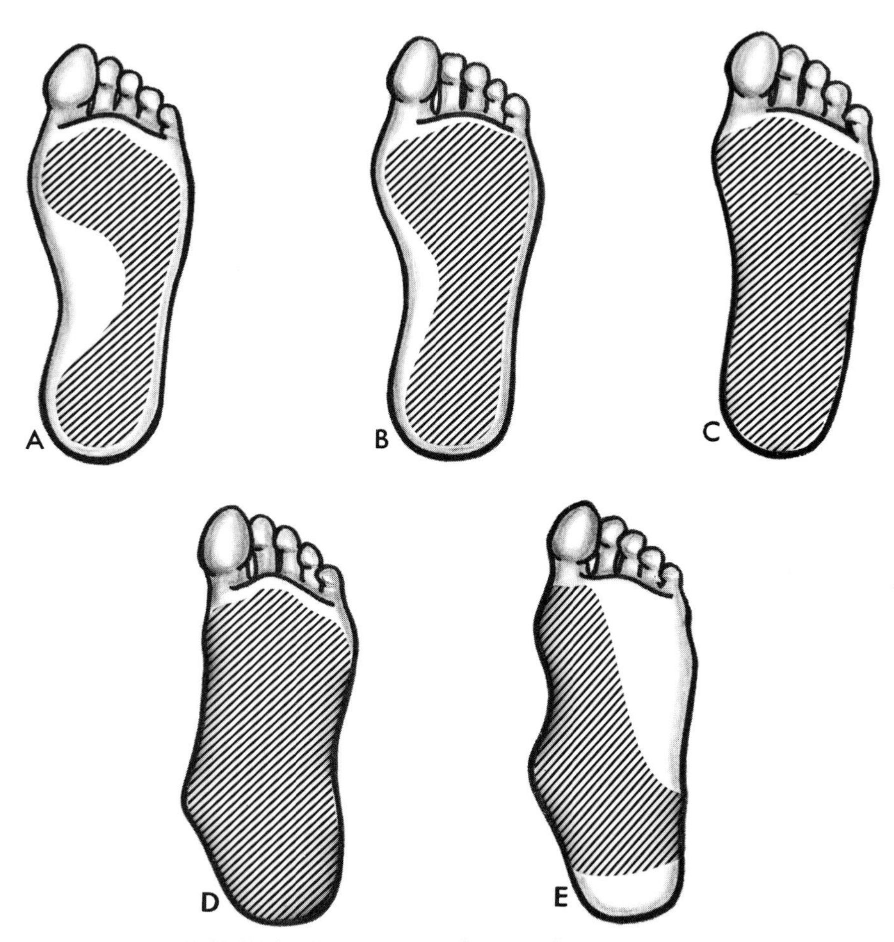

FIGURE 7–178. Foot prints of varying degrees of flat foot.

A. Normal. **B.** Mild or first-degree. The longitudinal arch is low but still visible. **C.** Moderate or second degree—the longitudinal arch is absent. **D.** Severe or third degree—the longitudinal arch is absent and the medial border of the foot is convex with the head of the talus pressing on the plantar aspect of the foot. **E.** Rocker-bottom deformity in congenital convex pes valgus. The heel is in equinus position, the forefoot is dorsiflexed and everted, and the head of the talus is prominent on the sole. The deformity is rigid; it does not disappear when not weight-bearing.

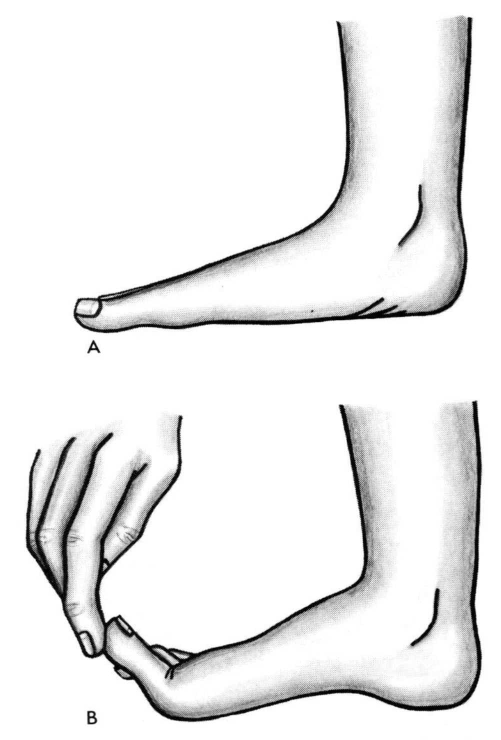

FIGURE 7–179. The "toe-raising test" of Jack.

A. Pes planus due to sag at the naviculocuneiform joint. **B.** On passive dorsiflexion of the great toe the longitudinal arch is elevated. When the talus is plantar-flexed and the sag is only at the talonavicular joint, hyperextension of the big toe does not restore the longitudinal arch. The test is not reliable in the presence of triceps surae contracture.

Examination of the child often reveals that the excessive ligamentous laxity is generalized, as shown by the hyperextensibility of the elbows, wrists, thumbs, and knees. Muscle testing is performed to rule out muscle weakness and imbalance. A neurologic examination is carried out to detect neurologic defect.

In adult life, structural changes may gradually develop in the tarsal bones, and the planovalgus deformity may become progressively rigid. Eventually foot strain may cause disabling pain. Adult women tend to have more discomfort in the forepart of the foot (the so-called anterior or transverse arch) because of wearing shoes with high heels, which causes the weight to be transmitted to the metatarsal heads.

Treatment

In the infant and the young child up to three years of age the plantar surface of the foot appears to be flat. The portion of the foot that subsequently becomes the longitudinal arch is filled with a pad of fat. These feet are normal. As the child gets older this fat pad shrinks, the ligaments become taut, and a normal longitudinal arch develops. These normal feet should be left alone.

The mild or first-degree flat foot requires no treatment. A proportion of the human race has low longitudinal arches; such "flat feet" are normal provided they are flexible and have good muscle control, the hindfoot is not pronated more than 10 to 15 degrees, and there is no associated myostatic contracture of the triceps surae muscle. They will stand as much hard usage without producing pain or disability as do feet with so-called "normal arches." As stated earlier, the child with moderately flat feet toes-in actively so that the center of gravity of the body is shifted laterally toward the center of the foot (see Fig. 7–170 B). That such toeing-in is Nature's way of protecting a child's foot and is therefore good for him should be explained to the parents, who may find it difficult to comprehend, especially when they have sought medical advice because their child is toeing-in. The toeing-in calls into action the tibialis anterior and posterior muscles, the long and short toe flexors, and the adductors of the foot; using them gives additional muscular support to the longitudinal arch. Toeing-in should *not* be discouraged nor should any effort be made to prevent it by reversing shoes, putting lateral wedges on the soles of the shoes, or using Denis Browne splints or other orthoses. The more the child toes-in and shifts the center of the body weight to the center of the foot, the sooner he will correct the associated physiologic genu valgum. The parents are assured of satisfactory foot function later on in life. Nature should be left alone.

Flexible flat foot in children does not cause pain. Pain is indicative of the presence of some other pathologic condition. Commonly it is the result of contracture of the triceps surae muscle, and occasionally it is due to tarsal coalition or an inflammatory process such as rheumatoid arthritis involving the subtalar and midtarsal joints. Radiograms of the foot are made and, if indicated, bone imaging with technetium-99m is performed to rule out rare lesions such as osteoid osteoma or stress fracture. If there is restriction of motion of the tarsal joints, a CT scan of the foot may be indicated to detect obscure tarsal coalition.

Foot strain may occur in children with normal arches as well as in those with flat feet. It is not the flatness of the longitudinal arch, but rather the medial shift in weight-bearing that is the important factor in producing foot strain. It occurs more commonly in children who are overweight and physically sluggish. A foot with a high arch is more susceptible to pain and disability than is the flexible flat foot.

CONSERVATIVE MANAGEMENT

Children with mild or moderate flexible flat foot should be allowed to go without shoes on sand at the beach, on grass in a yard or park, or on a thick rug at home. The bare foot will respond to contact with natural terrain by dynamic action of all the muscles controlling the foot and normal motion of the joints. There is absolutely no scientific evidence that encasing the foot in stiff leather above-ankle shoes and shoe modifications such as built-in longitudinal arch supports, scaphoid pads, Thomas heels, medial heel wedges, or extended medial heel counters are of any therapeutic value for correcting flexible flat foot.[13, 136, 137] Unfortunately, in urban living, a child may have to spend hours walking on hard floors and pavements. Nature did not plan the human foot for such hard terrain. In such circumstances the feet are supported in a pair of good Oxford shoes.

Various exercise programs to strengthen the muscles of the foot and leg have been advocated in the literature.[10, 24, 73, 154] This author does not, however, believe that muscle weakness causes flexible pes planovalgus. Active exercises such as toe curling or picking up objects with the toes or tip-toe walking or walking with the feet inverted have no therapeutic value. It is archaic to force these children to perform exercises for 15 to 30 minutes each day. Such "toe twiddling" should be abandoned. Instead of being forced to stay in his room and pick up marbles with his toes, the poor child should be allowed to go out in the yard and play with his friends. The overanxious parents should be soothed through some other outlet, such as jogging or swimming and exercising themselves. Often the parents require more reassurance than the children with flat feet need treatment.

The only exercise recommended is elongation of the contracted triceps surae muscle by passive stretching exercises performed manually or against the wall (Fig. 7–180).

In growing children over three or four years of age, the third-degree or severe flexible flat foot is treated by supporting the hindfoot and providing adequate room for the forepart of the foot. An attempt is made to shift weight-bearing laterally over the center of the foot to prevent foot strain. A common practice is to apply a wedged raise (⅛ to ³⁄₁₆ inch) on the medial side of the heel and a Thomas heel to the shoe. A longitudinal arch support in the form of a ⅜-inch-thick flexible felt, leather, or rubber pad is glued to the insole; and, often, additional support is provided by extending the medial counter of the heel forward. The purpose is to tilt the hindfoot into inversion. This will not be accomplished, because the uprights of the heel of the shoe do not grip the heel snugly, and the hindfoot simply twists into eversion. Numerous heel inserts (cups) are available commercially. Such devices satisfy the anxious parents and the shoe salesmen, but do little, if anything, to correct the deformity. In symptomatic flexible flat foot, however, they may relieve pain in a certain percentage of the cases.

Basta and Mital and their associates presented a clinical and radiographic study of 50 children with symptomatic flexible flat feet treated over a period of four years with varying combinations of shoes, custom-made arch supports, and pads. They concluded that conservative treatment of symptomatic flat feet in children can be successful in relieving subjective discomfort. They realized pain is a subjective patient response, but the success could be correlated with objective radiographic measurements. They recommended that children with symptomatic flexible flat foot be fitted initially with laced high-top shoes containing a steel shank and firm counter. A custom-made navicular pad is added if the recommended shoe does not afford adequate symptomatic relief. Navicular "cookies" were found to be less effective than navicular pads.[9]

Bleck and Berzins performed a prospective study of 71 cases of flexible pes valgus with plantar-flexed talus followed up for periods of more than one year. The UCBL (University of California Biomechanics Laboratory) foot orthosis, shown in Figure 7–181, and Helfet heel seat improved the clinical and radiographic appearance of the feet in 79 per cent of the patients. These authors recommended the use of the Helfet heel seat when the plantar-flexion angle of the talus is 35 to 45 degrees, and the UCBL foot orthosis in those cases in which the plantar-flexion angle of the talus is greater than 45 degrees.[14]

Mereday, Dolan, and Lusskin reported the results of treatment of flexible pes planus by UCBL foot orthoses worn by 12 children over a two-year period. The study was documented by photographic and radiographic measurements, gait analysis, and a subjective questionnaire. It was concluded (1) that protracted wearing of the UCBL foot orthosis relieved local

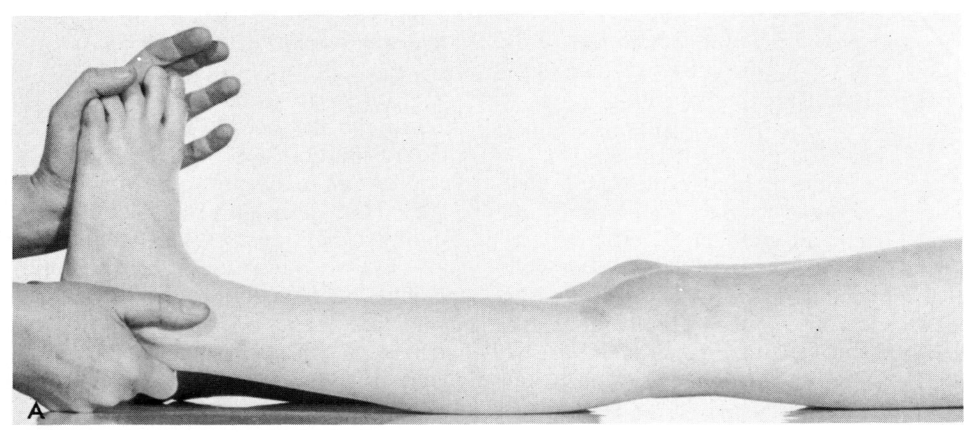

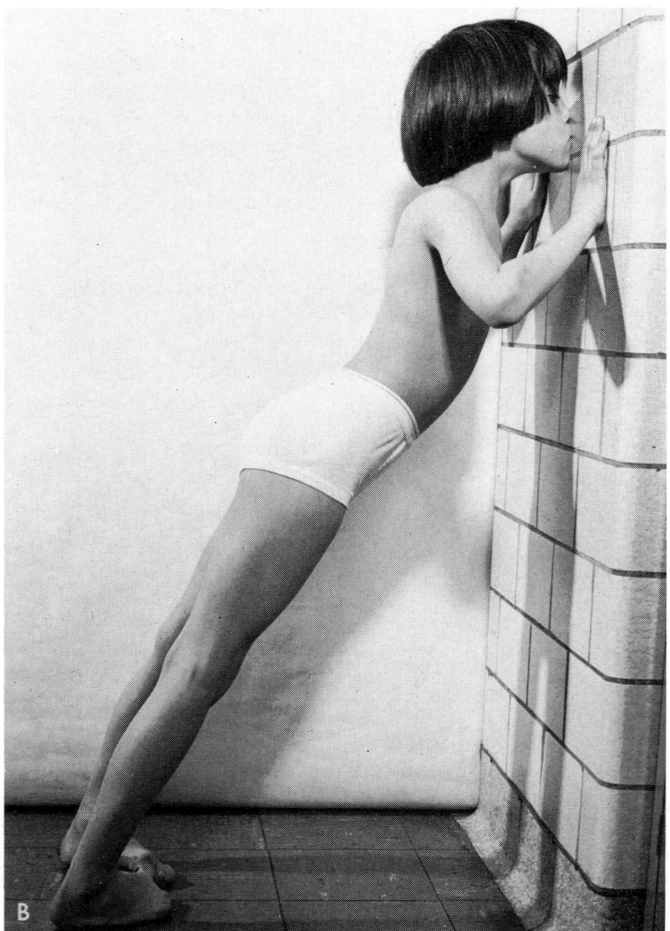

FIGURE 7–180. Passive stretching of contracted triceps surae muscle.

A. Manual stretching by the parents. Note the knee should be in extended position and the hindfoot slightly inverted. The child should not actively dorsiflex the ankle, as contraction of the anterior tibial muscle will relax the gastrocnemius-soleus muscles—its reciprocal antagonists. The maximally dorsiflexed position is maintained to the count of 10 and then relaxed. Exercises are performed 20 times each at three sessions a day. **B.** Passive stretching of triceps surae muscles against the wall is indicated in the older cooperative child. Note the feet are in inversion. The knees should not be hyperextended.

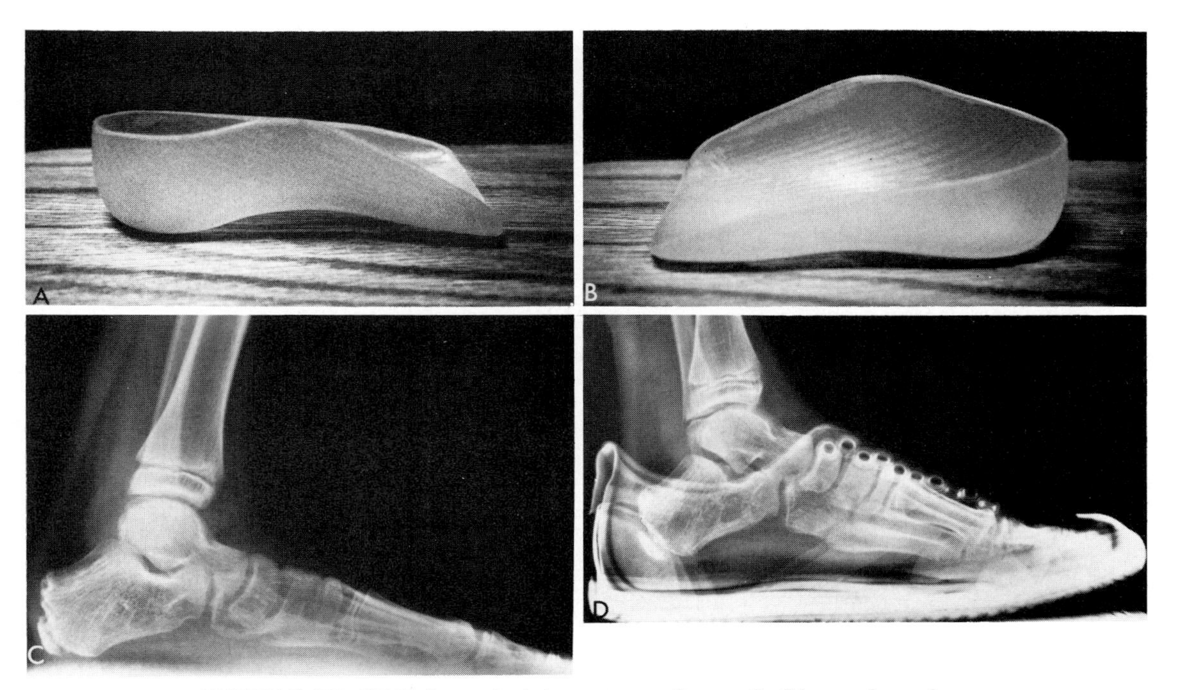

FIGURE 7–181. UCBL foot orthosis in treatment of severe flexible pes planovalgus.

A. Medial view of foot orthosis. **B.** Lateral view of foot orthosis. **C.** Standing lateral radiogram of left foot. Note the sag at the naviculocuneiform and talonavicular joints. **D.** Standing lateral radiogram with UCBL orthosis. The normal articular relations between the naviculocuneiform and talonavicular joints are restored, and the calcaneal pitch has improved to normal.

pain in the anterior tibial muscles and diffuse pain in six children; (2) that there was some improvement in gait in eight patients, and that shoe wear was more even while the inserts were worn; and (3) that in the presence of relatively fixed foot deformity, the inserts failed to achieve lasting structural changes.[103]

In summary, factors to consider in treatment are (1) the age of the patient; (2) the severity of deformity; (3) the shoe wear; and (4) the symptoms. Mild and moderate degrees of flexible flat foot require no treatment in any age group. A well-fitted pair of good Oxford shoes is all that is needed. The symptomatic moderate flat foot in the older child is usually associated with contracture of the triceps surae; passive stretching exercises are performed to elongate the shortened calf muscles. A shoe prescription may be given for the symptomatic flat foot. It consists of a Thomas heel, a ⅛- to 3/16-inch medial heel wedge, an extended medial counter, and a ⅜-inch-high longitudinal arch support glued to the insole. The objective of such a shoe prescription is to relieve mild local discomfort of foot strain and not to correct flat foot. Older children with flat feet wear down the lateral part of the heels; raising the medial side of the shoe in such cases will increase the excessive wear of the lateral side of the heel. In these children the heel of the shoe is not altered; instead a Helfet plastic heel seat or, preferably, a UCBL foot orthosis is prescribed if the symptoms warrant it.

When a child presents with severe flexible flat foot one should rule out an underlying neuromuscular disorder such as benign congenital hypotonia, muscular dystrophy, Down's syndrome, Marfan's syndrome, osteogenesis imperfecta, or Ehlers-Danlos syndrome. These feet are symptomatic and cause rapid abnormal shoe wear. They should be supported by UCBL foot orthoses during the period of rapid skeletal growth of the foot (up to 8 to 10 years in girls and 10 to 12 years in boys). With the UCBL foot orthoses these children can wear any type of shoe and appear normal to their peers. The UCBL foot orthosis is also given to the juvenile or adolescent with severe flat foot to alleviate pain prior to consideration for surgery.

SURGICAL MANAGEMENT

Operative correction of pes planovalgus is indicated when the deformity is so marked that it causes rapid abnormal wear of the shoes as shown in Figure 7–182, or the discomfort in the foot persists despite proper conservative

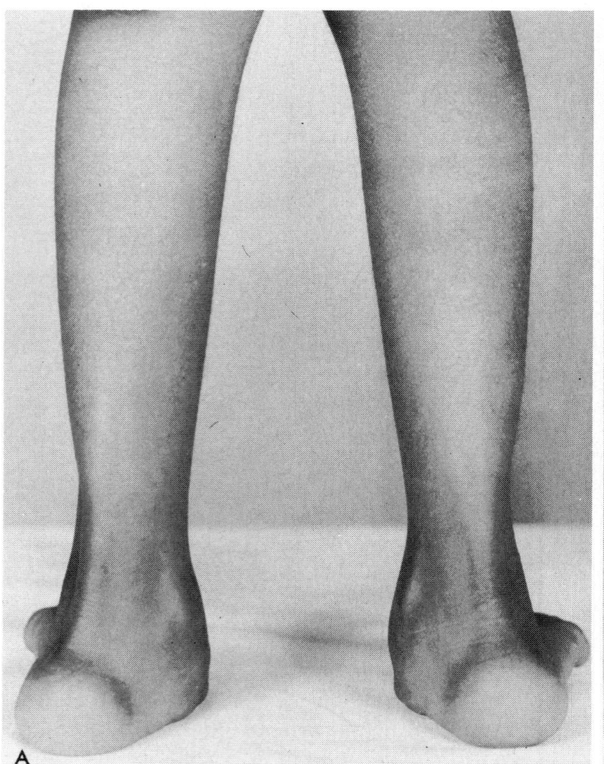

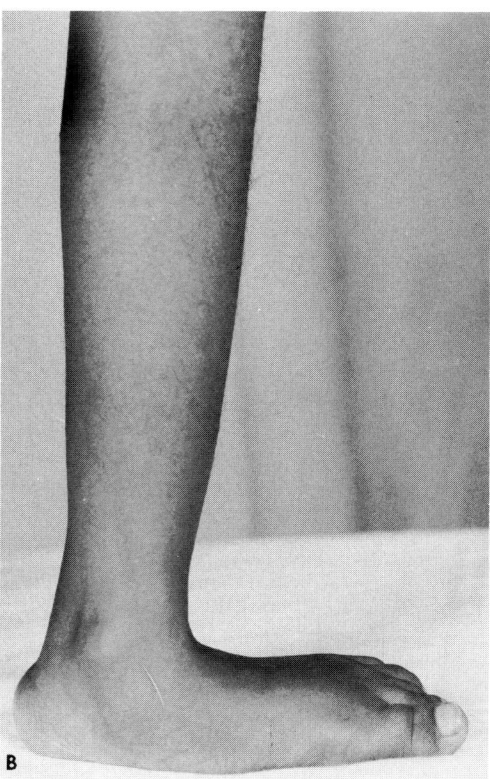

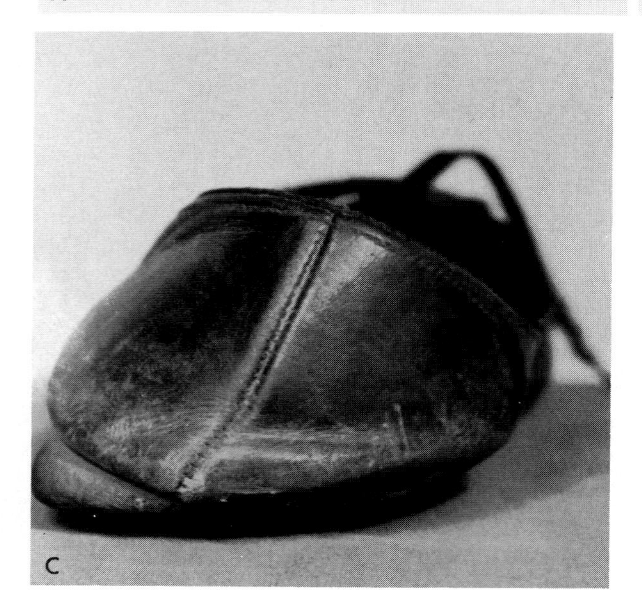

FIGURE 7–182. Severe flexible flat foot in an eight-year-old girl.

Surgical correction of deformity is indicated in such a case. **A.** Posterior view of both feet and legs. **B.** Medial view of left foot. **C.** Abnormal wear of left shoe.

measures and prevents the patient from taking part in normal activities. Only a small percentage of patients with symptomatic flat foot fail to respond to conservative measures. Surgery should not be considered before the age of ten years.

Ideally surgical correction of flexible flat foot should provide a foot with a normal longitudinal arch that is free of pain and has normal range of motion and function. This is not always possible.

In the literature numerous operative procedures have been described for correction of flexible pes planovalgus. In general they can be divided into four groups: (1) soft-tissue procedures alone—ligamentous tightening, release of contracted soft tissue, and muscle-tendon transfer; (2) arthrodesis of tarsal joints; (3) osteotomy of tarsal bones with or without bone grafts (calcaneus, cuboid, or medial cuneiform); and (4) bone and joint operations combined with soft-tissue procedures (Table 7–15). Some of the operations have been discarded and are of historical interest only; they are therefore not considered in this text.

In the choice of operative procedure to correct flexible pes planovalgus the following factors should be considered: (1) the anatomic *site of the sag* in the longitudinal arch (Is it at the naviculocuneiform joint, at the talonavicular joint, or at both joints?); (2) the *plantar-flexion angle of the talus* (Is it normal or is the talus tilted into an excessively equinus posture? Does the lateral radiogram of the foot indicate that the anatomic relationship between the talus and calcaneus and between the navicular and talar head can be restored to normal by full plantar flexion of the ankle and forefoot?); (3) the *degree of medial deviation of the talar axis* (What is the dorsoplantar talonavicular angle? Is the navicular displaced laterally in relation to the head of the talus?); (4) the *degree of hindfoot valgus deviation* (Is the anteroposterior talocalcaneal angle widened? Is there any valgus deformity of the ankle?). It is imperative to have standing anteroposterior radiograms of the ankle and to note the relationship of the distal fibular physis to the level of the ankle. Is there abnormal lateral tilting of the dome contracture of the talus?); (5) the *calcaneal pitch* (Is it low or flat

Table 7–15. *Surgical Procedures for Correction of Flexible Flat Foot*

Operation	Objective	Indication	Comment
Operations on Soft Tissues			
Distal advancement of plantar calcaneonavicular ligament and posterior tibial tendon (Miller)	Tauten "sling" that supports medial longitudinal arch	Naviculocuneiform sag	Effective if combined with arthrodesis of naviculocuneiform joint
Transfer of anterior tibial tendon dorsally to the navicular bone (Lowman, Young)	Alter direction of pull of anterior tibial tendon from dorsiflexion of first metatarsal to dorsal elevation of navicular bone and apex of medial longitudinal arch	Naviculocuneiform sag	Effective if combined with stabilization of naviculocuneiform or talonavicular joint and distal advancement of posterior tibial tendon and plantar calcaneonavicular ligament
Transfer of medial half of Achilles tendon to first metatarsal neck (Jones)	Reinforce incompetent plantar fascia	Talonavicular and naviculocuneiform sag	No experience with this procedure
Proximal transfer of deltoid ligament (Schoolfield)	Maintain calcaneus in neutral position	Valgus hindfoot	Ineffective—will stretch out
Lengthening of Achilles tendon	Correct eversion pull on os calcis by contracted triceps surae	Taut triceps surae not responding to passive stretching exercises	Perform sliding lengthening. Section lateral half of heel cord insertion distally
Stabilization of Joints by Arthrodesis			
Naviculocuneiform fusion (Hoke)	Provide longer and more stable lever arm on which muscles act and maintain longitudinal arch	Naviculocuneiform sag	Effective if combined with distal transfer of plantar calcaneonavicular ligament and posterior tibial tendon. Caution—added stress on adjacent joints
Talonavicular fusion (Lowman)	Give stability of lever arm and correct plantar deviation of talus	Talonavicular sag	Lowman combined with transfer of anterior tibial tendon to navicular. Caution—causes stiffness of hindfoot. Grice or triple arthrodesis better

Table continued on following page

Table 7–15. *Surgical Procedures for Correction of Flexible Flat Foot* (Continued)

Operation	*Objective*	*Indication*	*Comment*
Extra-articular subtalar arthrodesis (Grice)	Stabilize subtalar joint in neutral position	Valgus malalignment at talocalcaneal and talonavicular joints	Does not correct midfoot valgus deformity. Transfer distally plantar calcaneonavicular and posterior tibial tendon if talonavicular and naviculocuneiform sag
Triple arthrodesis	Stabilize talocalcaneonavicular and calcaneocuboid joints	Valgus malalignment of all three components of longitudinal arch	Stiff hindfoot. Rule out ankle valgus deviation prior to surgery. Recommended lateral inlay graft technique of Williams/Menelaus
Osteotomies of Calcaneus			
Anterolateral part of calcaneus, beneath anterolateral facet of calcaneus and immediately posterior to calcaneocuboid joint (Chambers)	Provide bony buttress to maintain normal alignment of talocalcaneal joint	Plantar flexion and valgus malalignment of talocalcaneal joint	Preserves some subtalar motion. Causes incongruity of talocalcaneal joint—stiffness a postoperative problem. Not recommended by author
Horizontal osteotomy through base of posterior articular process of calcaneus with lateral wedge graft (Baker)	Invert os calcis without disturbing subtalar joint motion	Valgus malalignment of talocalcaneal joint	Good but technically difficult operation. Use iliac double cortical wedge graft. Do not break medial cortex of calcaneus!
Lateral open-up osteotomy of calcaneus with bone graft wedge (Dwyer)	Invert os calcis without disturbing subtalar joint motion	Valgus malalignment of talocalcaneal joint	Technically easier but not as effective as Baker operation. Not recommended in flexible pes planovalgus
Medical displacement osteotomy of calcaneus (Pridie, Koutsogiannis)	Restore normal weight-bearing on calcaneus	Valgus heel	Correct triceps surae contracture by heel cord lengthening. Medial displacement should be adequate
Elongation of lateral column of foot by osteotomy of os calcis and insertion of bone graft immediately behind calcaneocuboid joint (reverse Evans)	To elongate lateral column of foot	Valgus midfoot with lateral subluxation of navicular over head of talus and lateral tilting of calcaneocuboid joint	Effective in correcting midfoot valgus deformity

or at an equinus angle owing to contracture of the triceps surae muscle?); (6) the presence of *soft-tissue contracture* (Is it ligamentous or myostatic? Is there any muscle imbalance?); (7) the *age* of the patient; (8) the *rigidity* of flat foot (Can the foot be passively corrected to normal? Are there arthritic changes in the tarsal joints?).

Treatment of Flexible Pes Planovalgus Due to Sag at Naviculocuneiform Joint

Naviculocuneiform Fusion. Hoke, in 1931, introduced naviculocuneiform fusion for correction of flexible pes planus; he believed fusion gives a longer and more stable level on which the muscles act to maintain the longitudinal arch.[73] Butte, in 1937, reported unsatisfactory results in 50 per cent of the naviculocuneiform fusions for flat foot.[21] Crego and Ford, in 1952, criticized the operation as being insufficient to support the flattened longitudinal arch.[32] Jack, in 1953, reported the results of naviculocuneiform fusion in 46 feet in 25 patients, aged 11 to 14 years, with flexible flat foot with a break at the naviculocuneiform joint; 15 months to five years after operation, the results were excellent in 54 per cent, good in 28 per cent, and unsatisfactory in 18 per cent. Jack stressed that proper selection of patients was most important and that the procedure reconstructed the longitudinal arch only if radiographically verified collapse was restricted to the naviculocuneiform joint.[76] In 1967, 16 to 19 years after the surgery, Seymour reassessed 17 of the 25 patients on whom Jack had operated. The results were excellent in 31 per cent, good in 19 per cent, and unsatisfactory in 50 per cent. Seymour pointed out that it is unlikely that only naviculocuneiform ligaments are affected and solely responsible for the flattening of the medial longitudinal arch, and the stabilization of only one segment of the complex cannot be expected to prevent collapse of the entire arch. He also cautioned that the procedure will cause degenerative arthritis in the adjacent joints, which are subjected to additional load and stress following naviculocuneiform arthrodesis.[129] This author agrees with Seymour and does not recommend arthrodesis of the naviculocuneiform joint alone.

Tendon Transfers and Ligamentous Tautening Procedures. In the literature a number of tendon transfers have been proposed to provide a dynamic force to elevate the apex of the medial longitudinal arch. Transfer of the anterior tibial tendon to the dorsum of the navicular bone (without arthrodesis of the tarsal joints) was first performed by Müller, modified by Legg, and popularized by Young.[89, 107, 153] Both peroneal tendons were transferred dorsally into the medial cuneiform by Ryerson.[122] Osmond-Clarke transferred the peroneus brevis to the head of the talus.[111]

Transfer of the medial half of the Achilles tendon to the first metatarsal neck was described by Jones.[78] He emphasized the importance of the medial plantar fascia in maintaining the structural integrity of the longitudinal arch of the foot. He designed an operation by which the incompetent plantar fascia is reinforced by transferring the medial half of the Achilles tendon to the first metatarsal neck. A longitudinal incision is made on the medial side of the tendo Achillis. The subcutaneous tissue and paratenon are divided in line with the skin incision. The Achilles tendon is split sagittally into halves. The medial half with its fascial prolongations over the muscle belly is divided at its proximal end but is left attached at its insertion to the calcaneus. The plantar and medial aspects of the calcaneus are exposed by undermining and elevating subcutaneous tissues. Next, a second incision is made over the medial aspect of the first metatarsal neck. With an Ober tendon passer or Kocher forceps a subcutaneous tunnel is made from the metatarsal incision to the back of the heel. The free separated upper end of the medial strip of the Achilles tendon is pulled out and delivered into the second wound. A drill hole of appropriate diameter is made in the neck of the first metatarsal; the rolled-up fascial prolongation of the calcaneal tendon is passed through the hole and tautly sutured to itself, holding the longitudinal arch of the foot in the corrected position. After closure of the wounds, a below-knee cast is applied and worn for three months. During the last six weeks, a walking heel is added and weight-bearing is allowed. Jones reported satisfactory results in three patients, two, six, and seven years after surgery (Fig. 7–183).[78] This author has had no personal experience with this operation.

Ogston tautened the soft tissues on the medial aspect of the foot by division and shortening or by plication.[110] Schoolfield transferred the deltoid ligament proximally; he believed pes planovalgus is caused by insufficiency of the deltoid ligament, which is unable to hold the calcaneus in erect attitude during weight-bearing. He therefore shortened the deltoid ligament by transferring it proximally with a periosteal flap. He claimed the advantage of the procedure was that mobility of the joints was preserved and not destroyed by arthrodesis.[126]

Ligamentous tightening and tendon advancement operations alone are not recommended by this author, as they generally do not stand the stresses of body weight and the deformity recurs.

Combination of Naviculocuneiform Fusion and Soft-Tissue Tautening with Tendon Transfer. In the properly selected patient, this combination of procedures is effective in correcting flat foot due to sag at the naviculocuneiform joint.

Miller described an operation in which the articulations between the navicular and medial cuneiform, and between the medial cuneiform and first metatarsal, are fused in corrected position, and in which the plantar calcaneonavicular ligament and posterior tibial tendon are transferred distally, thus tightening the "sling" that supports the medial longitudinal arch and holding up the head of the talus in normal relationship with the anterior end of the calcaneus.[105] Fusion of the first metatarsal and medial cuneiform articulation is not recommended by this author because this joint is stable anatomically and does not sag.

The Durham operation differs from that of Miller in two aspects: first, the cuneiform–first metatarsal joint is not fused; second, a ligamentous-periosteal flap is raised from the medial and plantar aspect of the navicular and medial cuneiform with its base left attached distally at the base of the first metatarsal. After navicular cuneiform fusion the flap is pulled taut and attached to the sustentaculum tali, thereby reinforcing the plantar calcaneonavicular (spring) ligament and supporting the medial longitudinal arch.[22]

The Scottish-Rite operation, described by Lovell, differs from the Miller procedure in two ways: a dorsally based wedge osteotomy of the

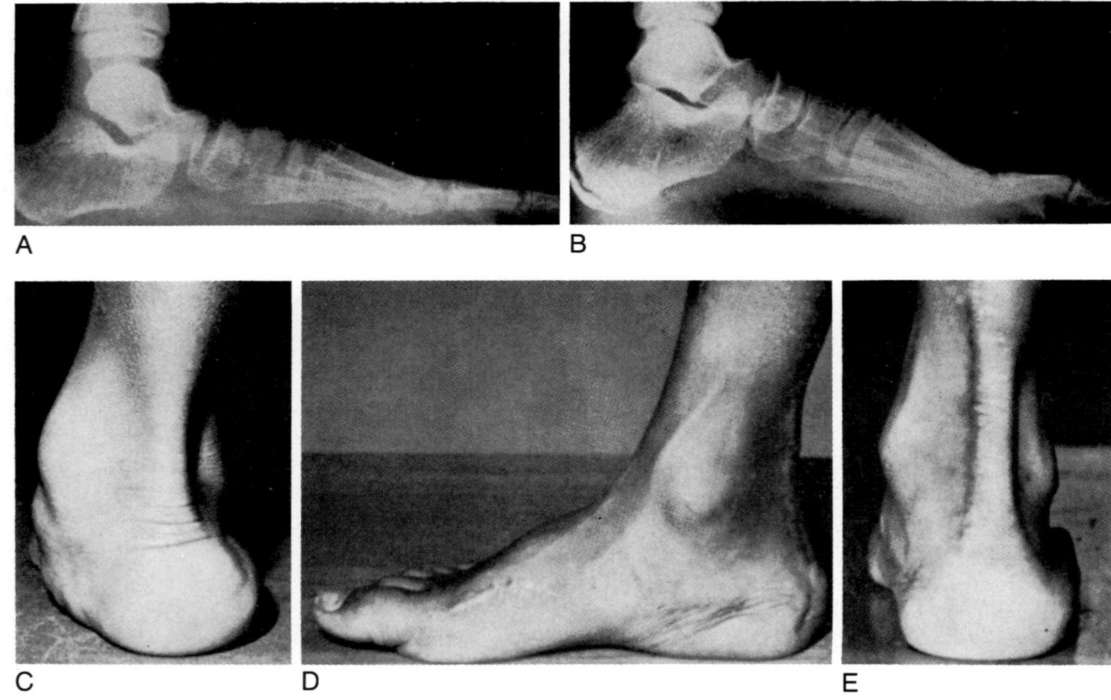

FIGURE 7–183. Jones's operation for severe flat foot.

The medial half of the tendo Achillis is transferred to the first metatarsal neck to reinforce the incompetent plantar fascia. **A.** Radiogram of the foot before operation. **B.** Postoperative radiogram. **C.** Clinical appearance of the foot before surgery. **D** and **E.** Weight-bearing photographs of the foot three years after surgery. (From Jones, B. S.: Flat foot. A preliminary report of an operation for severe cases. J. Bone Joint Surg., *57-B*:281, 1975. Reprinted by permission.)

medial cuneiform is performed to elevate the longitudinal arch, and the cuneiform–first metatarsal joint is left intact.[98]

Giannestras described an operation that is similar to that of Miller with the exceptions that the cuneiform–first metatarsal joint is not fused and that the tendons of the anterior tibial and posterior tibial muscles are transferred to the plantar surface of the navicular.[50] The Giannestras operation corrects the plantar sag of the naviculocuneiform joint and to a certain degree the medial sag of the talonavicular joint. This author finds it to be very effective. It is described in Plate 111. Giannestras strongly recommends that a suture be used to stabilize the medial cuneiform and navicular bones. He states that K-wires should not be used for internal fixation. This author, however, finds a small-fragment cancellous screw or two threaded K-wires are much more effective in transfixing the naviculocuneiform joint.

Treatment of Flexible Pes Planovalgus Due to Plantar Sag at Talonavicular Joint. In this type of flat foot the talus is tilted at an excessive equinus slant and the calcaneal pitch is low or flat owing to contracture of the triceps surae muscle. Often the talar axis is deviated medially and the dorsoplantar-talonavicular angle is markedly diminished (see Fig. 7–174). The navicular may be displaced laterally in relation to the head of the talus. The first step in treatment of this type of flat foot is correction of the contracture of the triceps surae muscle by passive stretching exercises and, if necessary, by a below-knee walking cast with an anteriorly placed heel. In the rigid equinus deformity that does not respond to a stretching cast, sliding lengthening of the heel cord is performed. The distal cut is made laterally. Excessive lengthening of the heel cord must be avoided.

Lowman advocated *fusion of the talonavicular joint* and transfer of the anterior tibial tendon dorsally to the navicular bone.[99] Fusion between the talus and navicular results in almost complete loss of motion of the talocalcaneonavicular joint. Because patients will have difficulty in walking on irregular terrain, this author does not recommend the Lowman operation.

Fogel and associates reported clinical, radiographic, and gait analysis of 11 patients in whom talonavicular fusion had been performed to relieve pain from isolated arthrosis. At a mean follow-up of 9.5 years (range 2.5 to 21 years) 3 of the 11 patients had radiographic evidence of arthrosis of adjacent tarsal joints that previously were unaffected. This late development of intertarsal arthrosis, however, did not cause symptoms. Isolated talonavicular arthrodesis did give relief of pain, and the patients were satisfied.[47] This author recommends talonavicular arthrodesis primarily for traumatic arthritis to provide relief of pain.

The patients who require surgical correction of flexible flat foot usually have disability and rapid abnormal wear of shoes because of valgus malalignment at the talocalcaneal and talonavicular joints. It is the pronated hindfoot that causes problems. *Extra-articular subtalar arthrodesis (Grice procedure)* corrects the hindfoot valgus deformity and restores the plantar-flexion angle of the talus to normal; however, fusion eliminates motion of the subtalar joint. In paralytic pes planovalgus, stability provided by a talocalcaneal arthrodesis is desirable; for flexible pes planovalgus, however, the Grice extra-articular arthrodesis is not recommended by this author. The only indication is severe flexible pes planovalgus in syndromes with marked ligamentous hyperlaxity such as Marfan's syndrome. In such feet, valgus deformity is in the hindfoot as well as in the midfoot, and in the skeletally mature foot, triple arthrodesis is the most effective procedure (see section on triple arthrodesis). In the growing foot, a Grice extra-articular subtalar arthrodesis is recommended because it does not disturb the growth of the foot. The technique is described in Plate 65.

Dennyson and Fulford have described a technique of subtalar arthrodesis by means of metallic internal fixation and autogeneous cancellous bone grafting (Fig. 7–184). It is a modification of the Batchelor operation, but uses a metal screw instead of a bone peg to maintain the corrected position, and cancellous graft instead of cortical bone to stimulate union. The authors claim that it obviates technical problems of obtaining a satisfactory position of the hindfoot. Results of treatment of 48 feet with flexible pes planus by this method were

Text continued on page 2748

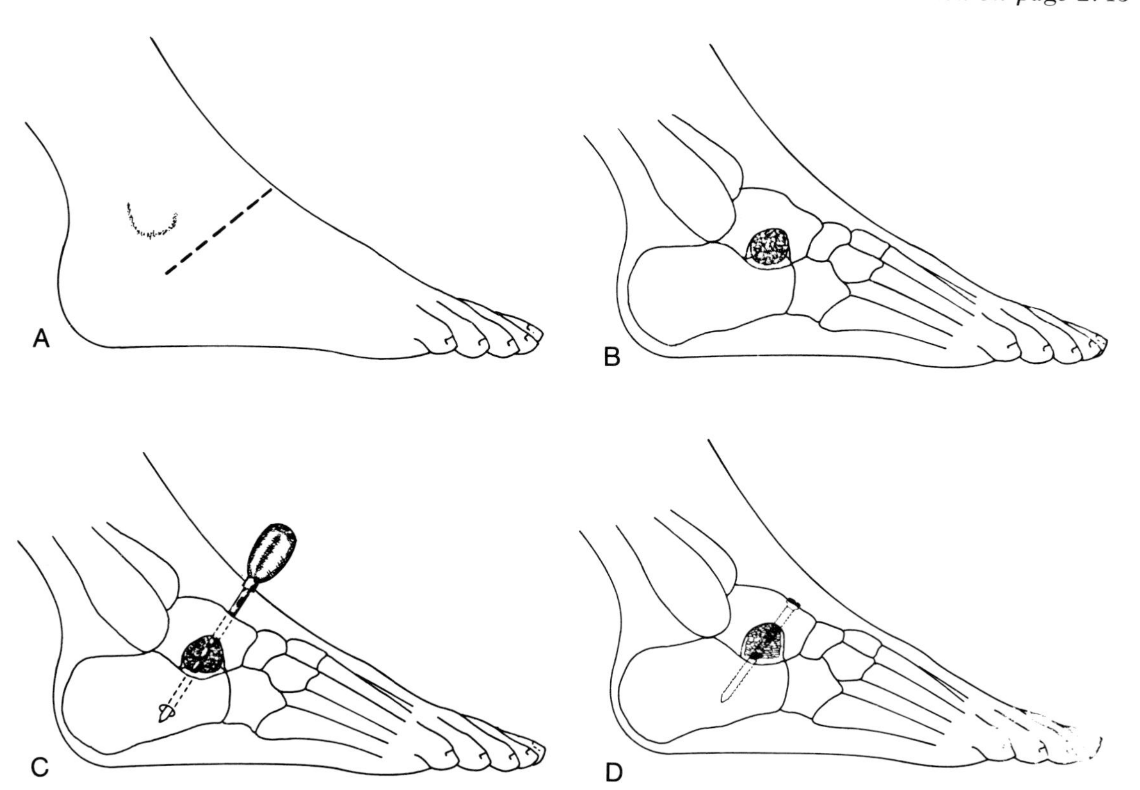

FIGURE 7–184. Subtalar arthrodesis by cancellous grafts and metallic internal fixation.

A. The incision. **B.** Area of cortical bone removed from sinus tarsi. **C.** Note the position of the bone awl. **D.** Internal fixation screw and packing of the sinus tarsi with cancellous bone chips. (From Dennyson, W. G., and Fulford, G. E.: Subtalar arthrodesis by cancellous grafts and metallic internal fixation. J. Bone Joint Surg., *58-B*:507, 1976. Reprinted by permission.)

Correction of Flexible Pes Planovalgus Due to Plantar Sag of Naviculocuneiform Joint and Medial Sag of Talonavicular Joint (Giannestras)

OPERATIVE TECHNIQUE

A. A slightly dorsally curved incision is made on the medial aspect of the foot; it begins immediately posterior to the medial malleolus, extends anteriorly to the navicular tubercle, and ends at the middle of the midshaft of the first metatarsal. The subcutaneous tissue is divided in line with the skin incision; and the wound margins are undermined, elevated, and gently retracted. Avoid a short and inadequate incision.

B. The abductor hallucis muscle is detached and elevated from the medial and plantar surfaces of the medial cuneiform, navicular, plantar calcaneonavicular (spring), and laciniate ligaments. Care is taken not to injure the muscle's nerve supply.

C. Next, the posterior tibial tendon is identified. In the posterior part of the wound immediately behind the posterior tibial tendon are the flexor digitorum longus tendon and medial plantar branch of the tibial nerve; they are retracted posteriorly and plantarward. Over a blunt elevator the sheath of the posterior tibial tendon is split longitudinally from the medial malleolus to its insertion at the tuberosity of the navicular.

Plate 111. Correction of Flexible Pes Planovalgus Due to Plantar Sag of Naviculocuneiform Joint and Medial Sag of Talonavicular Joint (Giannestras)

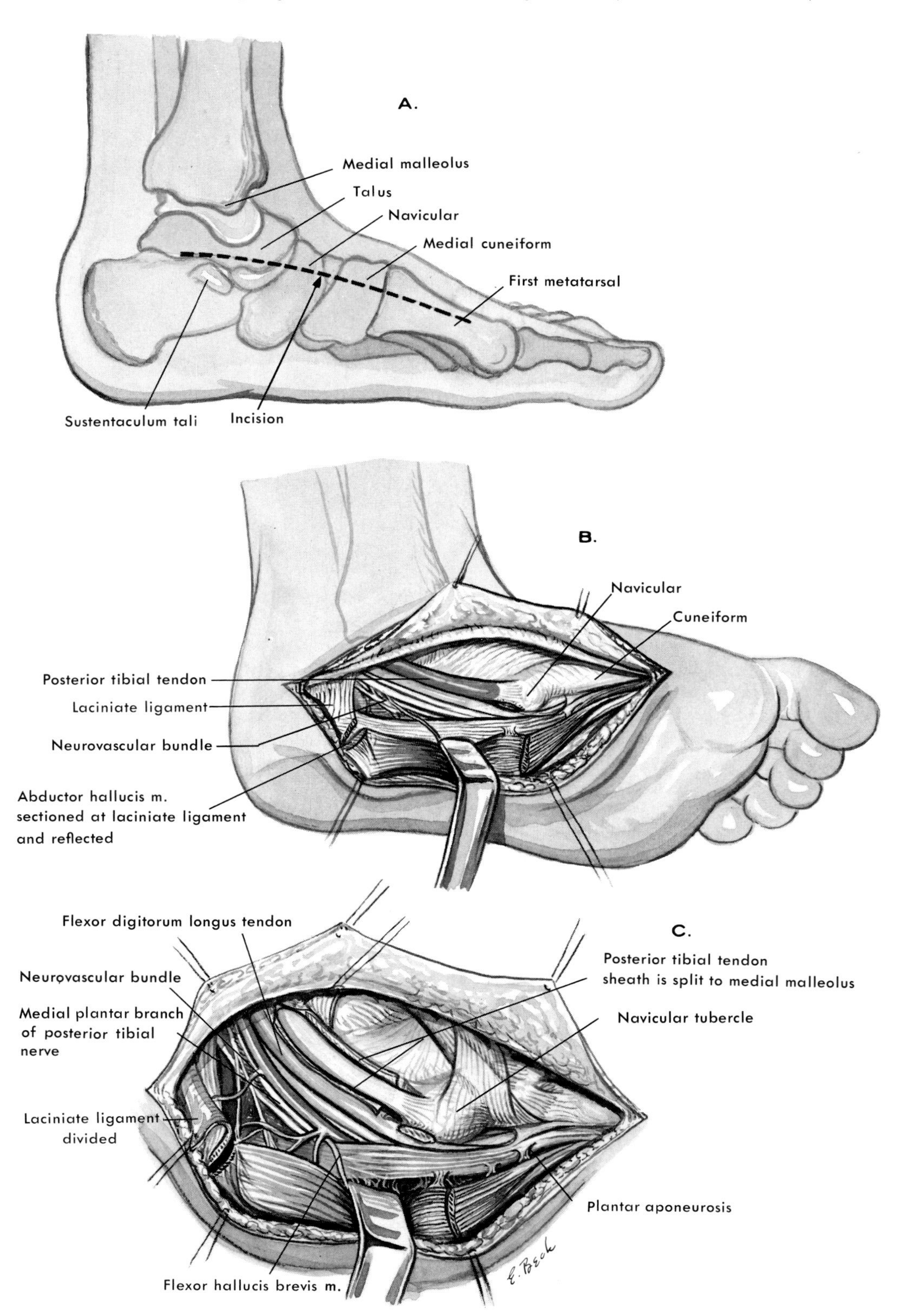

Correction of Flexible Pes Planovalgus Due to Plantar Sag of Naviculocuneiform Joint and Medial Sag of Talonavicular Joint (Giannestras) (Continued)

D. The posterior tibial tendon is sectioned from its insertion to the navicular tubercle, and a 00 Mersilene "whip" suture is passed through the distal end of the tendon for traction and later reattachment. Caution! It is imperative to leave a moderate amount of stump of posterior tibial tendon covering the navicular tuberosity.

E. The anterior tibial tendon is identified in the dorsal and anterior part of the wound. The inferior extensor retinaculum is sectioned, and the sheath of the anterior tibial tendon is split longitudinally. The tendon is divided at its insertion to the base of the first metatarsal, and a 00 Mersilene suture is passed through its distal end.

F. The talonavicular, naviculocuneiform, and cuneiform–first metatarsal joints are identified; this should not be difficult, but, if in doubt, can be verified by making a radiogram with a Keith needle marking the first metatarsocuneiform joint. Next, on the medial aspect of the foot, 1.5 cm. apart, two parallel incisions are made down to underlying bone, dividing the capsule and ligamentous tissues; the two incisions extend from the distal end of the medial cuneiform to the neck of the talus adjacent to the sustentaculum tali. Do not divide the flexor digitorum longus tendon or the neurovascular bundle in the posterior part of the wound. The capsule of the first metatarsocuneiform joint is sectioned between the two parallel incisions, and, with a sharp, thin osteotome, an osteocartilaginous flap is elevated. The flap begins at the distal end of the medial cuneiform and extends proximally to include a thin cortical layer of the medial cuneiform and the navicular.

Plate 111. Correction of Flexible Pes Planovalgus Due to Plantar Sag of Naviculocuneiform Joint and Medial Sag of Talonavicular Joint (Giannestras)

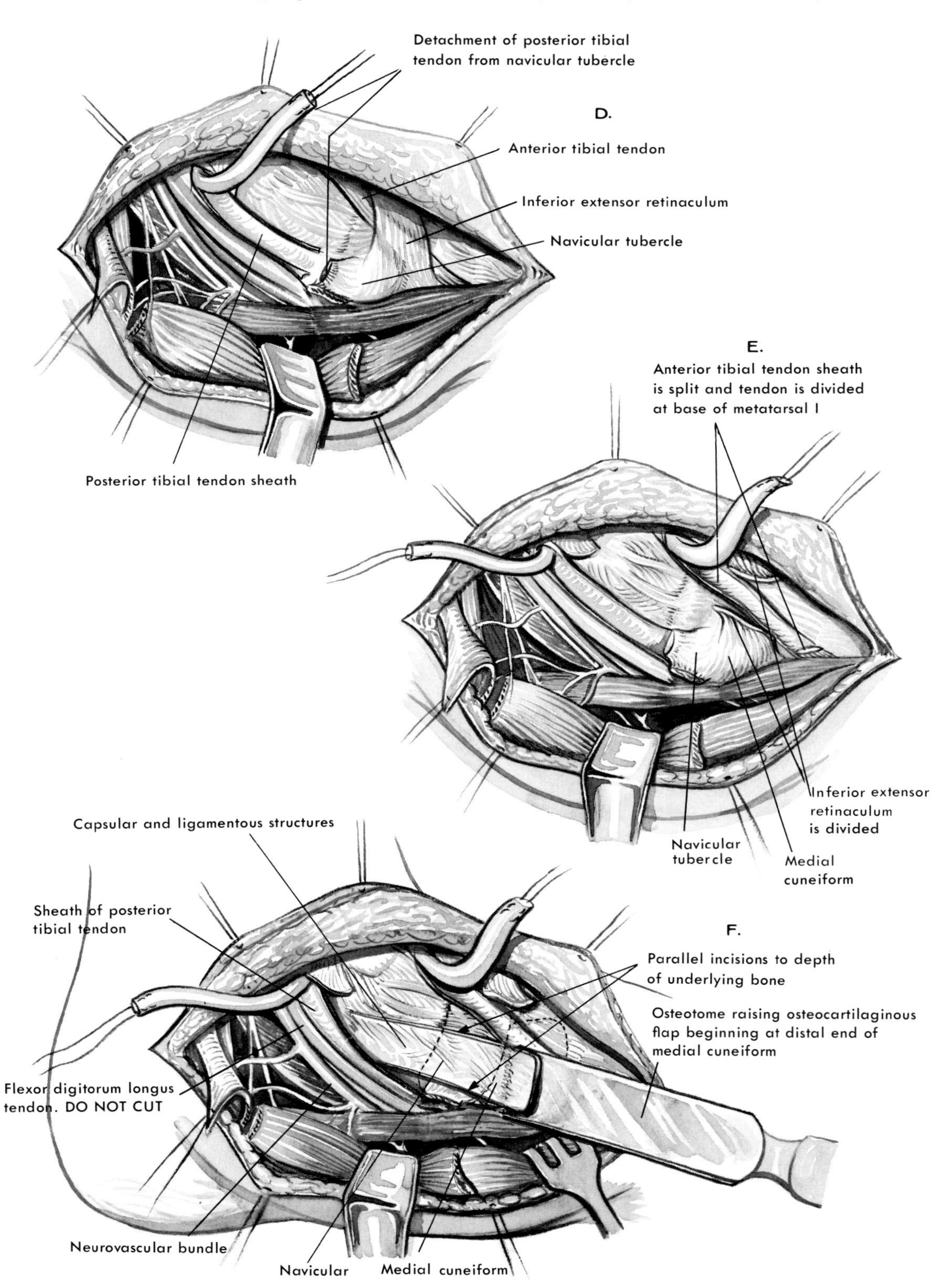

Correction of Flexible Pes Planovalgus Due to Plantar Sag of Naviculocuneiform Joint and Medial Sag of Talonavicular Joint (Giannestras) (Continued)

G. The osteocartilaginous flap and the capsular and ligamentous tissues are reflected. Care is taken not to tear the thin ligamentous structure between the navicular and cuneiform. The hyaline articular cartilage of the talonavicular joint should not be disturbed.

H. The plantar calcaneonavicular (or spring) ligament is identified and divided from its attachment to the navicular. It is dissected free and lifted back to its origin from the sustentaculum tali.

I. The ligamentous and capsular structures are gently dissected and elevated to expose the dorsal, medial, and plantar surfaces of the navicular and medial cuneiform bones.

Plate 111. Correction of Flexible Pes Planovalgus Due to Plantar Sag of Naviculocuneiform Joint and Medial Sag of Talonavicular Joint (Giannestras)

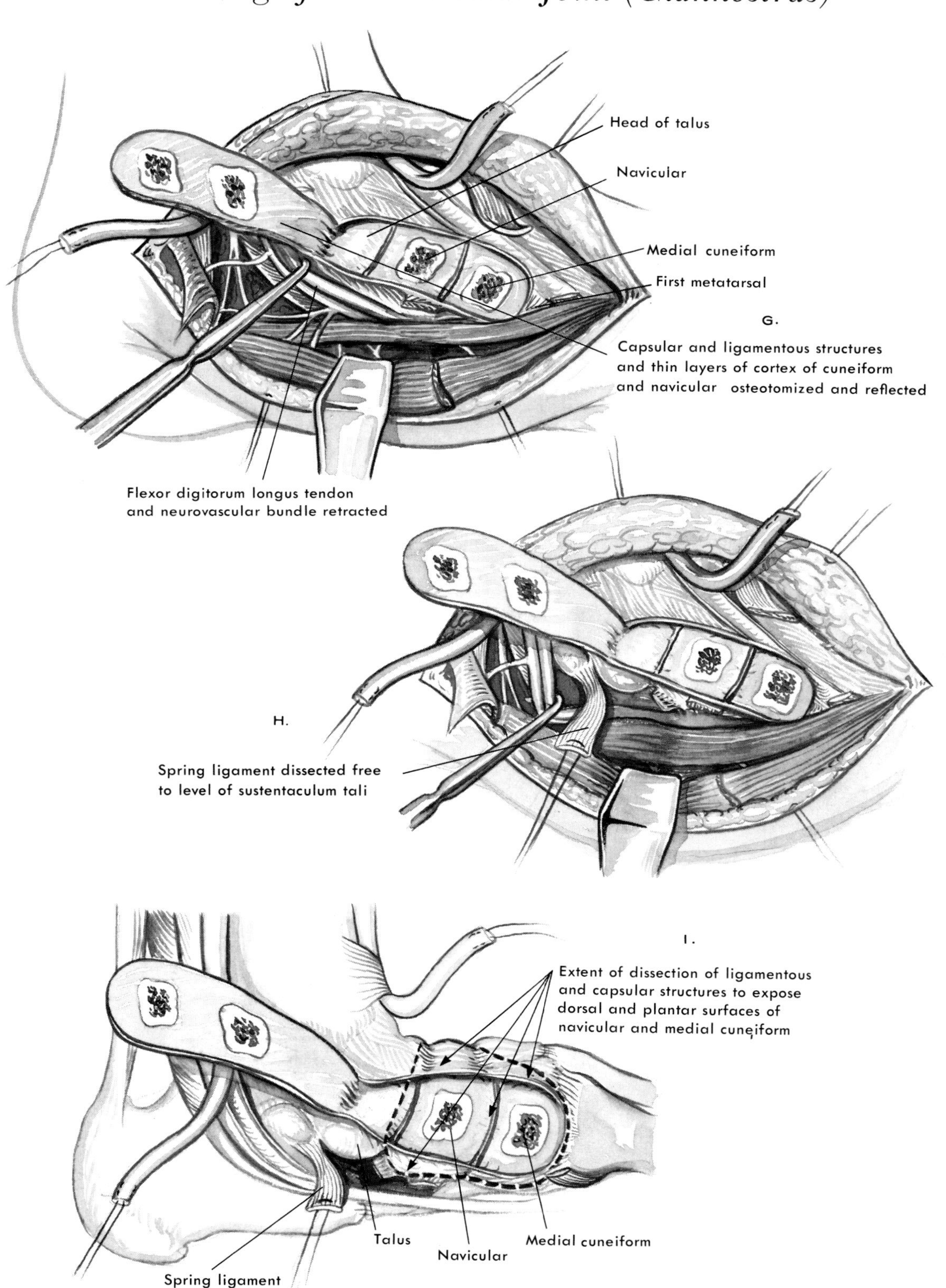

Correction of Flexible Pes Planovalgus Due to Plantar Sag of Naviculocuneiform Joint and Medial Sag of Talonavicular Joint (Giannestras) (Continued)

J. Next, the plantar aspect of the navicular is denuded of soft tissue, and the cortex is roughened with a sharp curet or rasp.

K. With a thin, sharp osteotome, a wedge of bone is excised from the proximal surface of the medial cuneiform. The base of the wedge, directed plantarward, is about 2 to 3 mm. in width. The opposing distal articular cartilage of the navicular is excised, exposing the subjacent cortical bone.

L. Next, the adequacy of correction of the plantar sag of the naviculocuneiform joint is checked by pronation and plantar flexion of the forepart of the foot. There should be close apposition of the bone surfaces between the medial cuneiform and navicular. Then a drill hole 5/16 inch in diameter is made in the navicular, beginning on its plantar surface; it is directed dorsally and distally to exit at the center of the denuded distal articular surface of the navicular. A second drill hole, 5/16 inch in diameter, is made in the medial cuneiform; it begins on the plantar surface, extends dorsally and proximally, and exits on the proximal denuded joint surface immediately below the dorsal cortex. An adequate amount of cortex should be left in both bones so that the suture does not tear out of the cancellous bone.

M. Giannestras does not recommend the use of staples or Kirschner wires across the naviculocuneiform joint for internal fixation. A double No. 2 chromic suture is passed through the holes from the plantar surface of the navicular into the dorsal holes in the navicular and medial cuneiform, exiting on the plantar aspect of the cuneiform. The forefoot is held in plantar flexion and pronation, and the suture is tied. This author recommends the use of a small-fragment cancellous screw or two threaded Kirschner wires for transfixing the naviculocuneiform joint.

Plate 111. Correction of Flexible Pes Planovalgus Due to Plantar Sag of Naviculocuneiform Joint and Medial Sag of Talonavicular Joint (Giannestras)

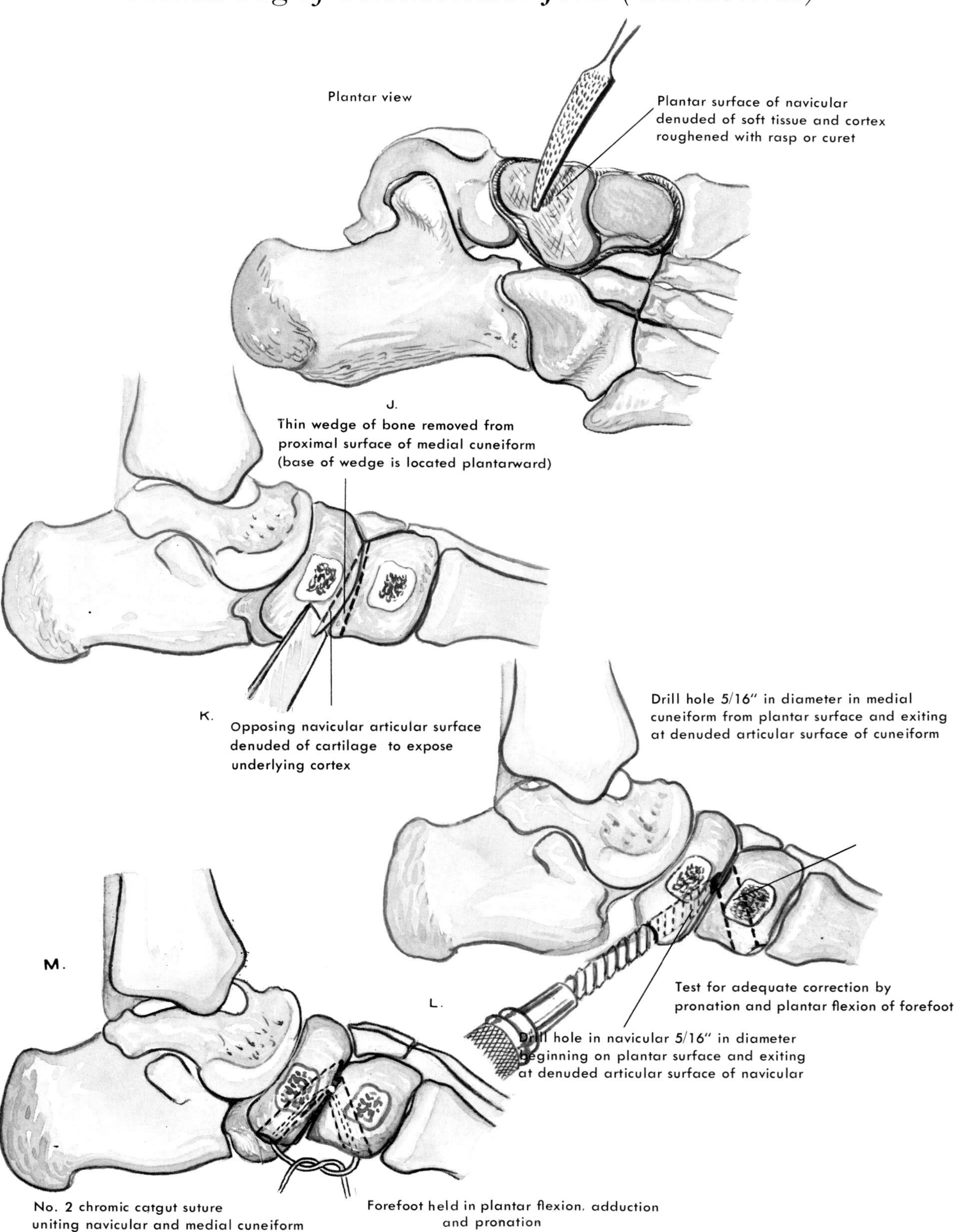

Correction of Flexible Pes Planovalgus Due to Plantar Sag of Naviculocuneiform Joint and Medial Sag of Talonavicular Joint (Giannestras) (Continued)

N. With the foot held in maximally corrected position—i.e., the forepart of the foot plantar-flexed and adducted—the osteocartilaginous flap is pulled distally with a Kocher clamp to cover the denuded surfaces of the navicular and cuneiform bones. The distal end is anchored securely to the base of the first metatarsal with 00 Mersilene suture. The flap should be taut, forming a bowstring on the medial and plantar aspects of the foot. With a fine small cutting needle, the dorsal and plantar margins of the flap are anchored to adjacent capsular structures with interrupted sutures. Any distal redundant portion of the flap is excised. The spring ligament is tautly resutured to the navicular. The security of fixation and degree of correction are checked with the foot released.

O. A drill hole 7/64 inch in diameter is made in the navicular from the dorsal to the plantar surface, approximately 1.5 to 2.0 cm. lateral to the medial edge of the navicular tubercle. The plantar surface of the navicular is denuded of all fibrous tissue and roughened with a sharp curet exposing raw cancellous bone.

P. The ends of the tibialis anterior and tibialis posterior tendons are sutured together with 00 Mersilene suture, which is passed in a figure of eight fashion. The two ends of the suture are loose, one coming out of the end of the tibialis anterior and the other through the end of the tibialis posterior, similar to Bunnell's suture but without the pull-out wire. Then the two suture ends are threaded through a large, slightly curved needle and passed through the plantar drill hole and up through the dorsal drill hole. The suture ends are then separated, and each one is threaded through a sharp cutting needle and passed separately through the overlying capsular and ligamentous soft tissues. Next, with a forceps the two tendons are pulled and held down snugly under the plantar aspect of the navicular and the sutures are tied. The tendons are against the plantar aspect of the navicular, but are not pulled up through the drill hole; only the sutures pass up through the drill hole. Additional sutures are applied through the two tendons to the overlying spring ligament.

The tourniquet is deflated and complete hemostasis obtained. It is best to insert a closed-suction Hemovac unit. The subcutaneous tissues are closed with interrupted sutures and the skin with a subcuticular suture.

A below-knee cast is applied for immobilization. An overcorrected position should be avoided. The purpose of the cast is to retain the correction achieved surgically. Giannestras recommends that the cast be applied in two sections. The heel should be slightly varus, the plaster under the newly formed longitudinal arch well-molded, and the forefoot in maximal pronation.[50]

Before the patient leaves the operating room, anteroposterior and lateral radiograms of the foot are made to determine the position of the talonavicular and naviculocuneiform joints.

POSTOPERATIVE CARE

Immobilization in the cast is maintained for eight weeks. The cast is changed as necessary. Radiograms of the foot are made to ascertain the fusion of the naviculocuneiform joint. If union is delayed or does not take place, a below-knee walking cast is applied for another four weeks. Persistence of non-union is ignored, however, as it usually does not cause any symptoms.

Upon removal of the cast the foot may appear overcorrected; parents should be reassured that it will return to normal position after two to three weeks of walking. In the beginning a three- or four-point crutch gait is used to protect the limb. Active exercises are performed to strengthen the triceps surae, toe extensor, tibialis posterior, and tibialis anterior muscles.

Initially the tendency is to walk on the lateral aspect of the foot. Proper heel-toe gait should be taught by the physical therapist. The child is fitted with simple Oxford shoes with a rigid shank. No arch supports of any type in the shoe are required.

Plate 111. Correction of Flexible Pes Planovalgus Due to Plantar Sag of Naviculocuneiform Joint and Medial Sag of Talonavicular Joint (Giannestras)

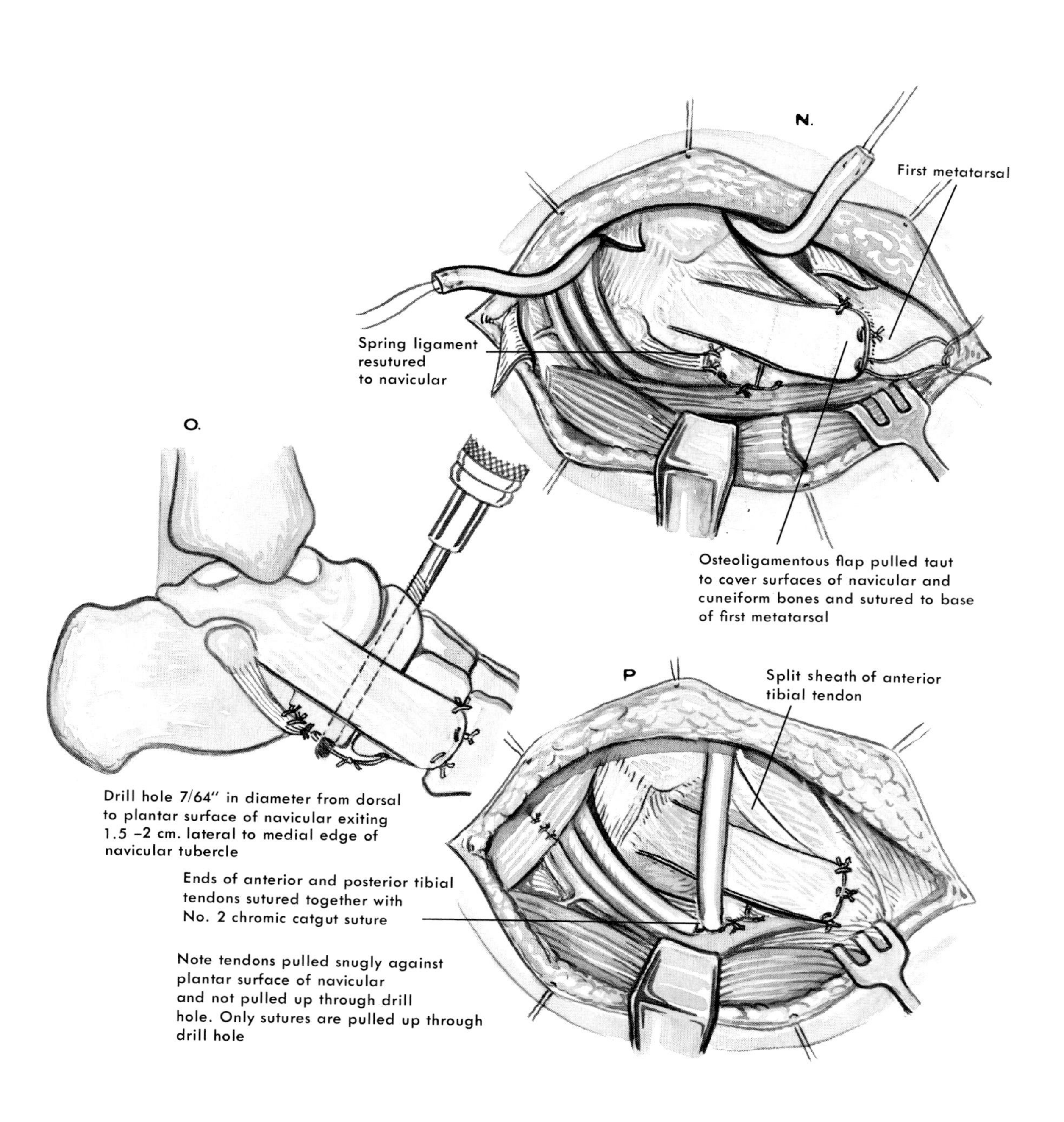

satisfactory in 45 feet. Union occurred after an average of seven and a half weeks in a below-knee weight-bearing plaster cast. An example is shown in Figure 7–185.[35]

In the experience of this author the technique described by Grice is very adequate, and he has found it unnecessary to use internal fixation by screw or transfixation by fibular bone graft.

In flexible pes planovalgus, relief of pain is the primary indication for *triple arthrodesis*. This author has performed it in adolescents with symptomatic flat feet caused by excessive ligamentous laxity associated with such generalized syndromes as Marfan's or Down's. Equinus deformity, if present, is corrected by elongating the tendo Achillis.

Arthrodesis by excision of articular cartilage and variable amounts of subjacent bone is not desirable in stabilization of the valgus foot. The base of the bone wedge to be removed must face medially. Following resection of bone, the foot becomes floppy and shorter than its mate. It is much better to leave the joints undisturbed and to insert a lateral inlay graft to achieve stabilization. According to Williams and Menelaus, the operation was first elaborated by Littlejohn in 1930 (unpublished) and later popularized by Price.[152] The technique of the operation is described in Plate 112.

Williams and Menelaus reported the results of 88 triple arthrodeses by inlay grafting in 70 patients. The only significant complication was failure of fusion of the midtarsal joint; it occurred in 3 of 85 feet (3.5 per cent). In these three feet repeat inlay grafting of the midtarsal joint resulted in complete fusion. There were no failures of fusion of the subtalar joint.[152]

Osteotomies of Os Calcis to Correct Hindfoot Valgus Deformity

The Chambers Procedure. The operation is illustrated in Figure 7–186 and is performed as follows: first a lengthening of the tendo Achillis is carried out. Next the lateral part of the calcaneus is exposed through an oblique incision over the sinus tarsi, beginning 2 cm. inferior to the tip of the lateral malleolus and extending dorsally and distally to the talonavicular joint. The subcutaneous tissues are incised in line with the skin incision. Superficial fat is left intact. The deep fat in the sinus tarsi is excised. The talocalcaneal, calcaneocuboid, and talonavicular joints are identified. The capsule of the talonavicular joint is completely sectioned inferiorly, laterally, dorsally, and medially, to permit upward and backward shifting of the talus. With dorsal elevation of the head of the talus the calcaneus shifts medially and the sustentaculum tali rotates to lie underneath the talar head. The calcaneus becomes anteriorly displaced in relation to the talus. The soft-tissue release permits restoration of normal articular relations of the foot. Next, an osteotomy of the anterolateral part of the calcaneus is performed, beneath the anterolateral facet and immediately posterior to the calcaneocuboid joint. The osteotomized segment of the calcaneus is elevated dorsally and medially against the talus—cautiously, so as not to enter the subtalar joint. The position of the elevated calcaneal segment is maintained by a triangular autogenous bone graft. The wounds are closed, and an above-knee cast is applied and worn for four weeks, after which a below-knee walking cast is used for an additional eight weeks. By the end of this period there is usually solid bone healing and adequate remodeling of the anterior subtalar joint.[23]

Miller reported the results of the Chambers osteotomy of the anterolateral aspect of the calcaneus in 81 hypermobile flat feet with an average follow-up of six and one half years (range—1 to 22 years). In 70 feet tendo Achillis lengthening was performed with the calcaneal osteotomy, and in 95 per cent of them an excellent or good clinical result was obtained. Radiograms disclosed normal foot alignment and normal articular cartilage spaces in only 72.8 per cent of the feet, however; in 22.2 per cent the talonavicular joint was narrowed, and in 5 per cent the subtalar joint was narrow. Postoperatively, in nine feet there was minimal loss of motion, in two feet moderate loss of motion, and in three feet marked restriction of joint motion. It seems the technique of complete release of the talonavicular joint disturbs circulation to the talus and damages articular cartilage. Miller states that should disabling pain develop later on, the feet are in good position for talonavicular or triple arthrodesis.[104] Because it causes incongruity and stiffness of the talocalcaneal joint, the Chambers procedure is not recommended by this author.

Dwyer's Osteotomy. Dwyer's calcaneal osteotomy to correct valgus hindfoot may be either the lateral open-up or the medial close-up type. It is discussed in the section on cerebral palsy in Chapter 5. This author does not recommend this procedure for treatment of flexible pes planovalgus. The medial displacement osteotomy is simpler and as effective.

Medial Displacement Osteotomy. Koutsogiannis described medial displacement osteotomy of the calcaneus; he credited Mr. Pridie with having been the first to perform the operation.[82]

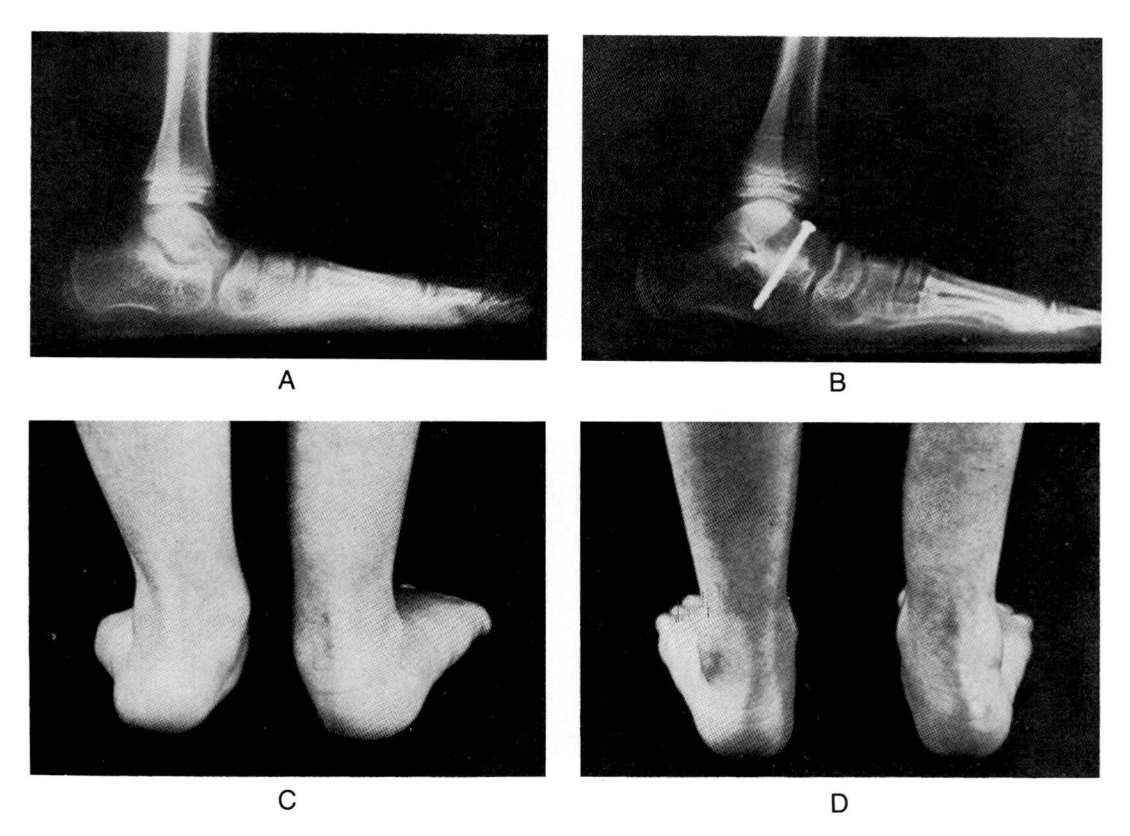

FIGURE 7–185. Subtalar arthrodesis by cancellous grafts and internal fixation with a screw.

A. Preoperative lateral radiogram of the foot. **B.** Lateral radiogram three years after operation. **C** and **D.** Preoperative and postoperative appearance of the foot. (From Dennyson, W. G., and Fulford, G. E.: Subtalar arthrodesis by cancellous grafts and metallic internal fixation. J. Bone Joint Surg., *58-B*:507, 1976. Reprinted by permission.)

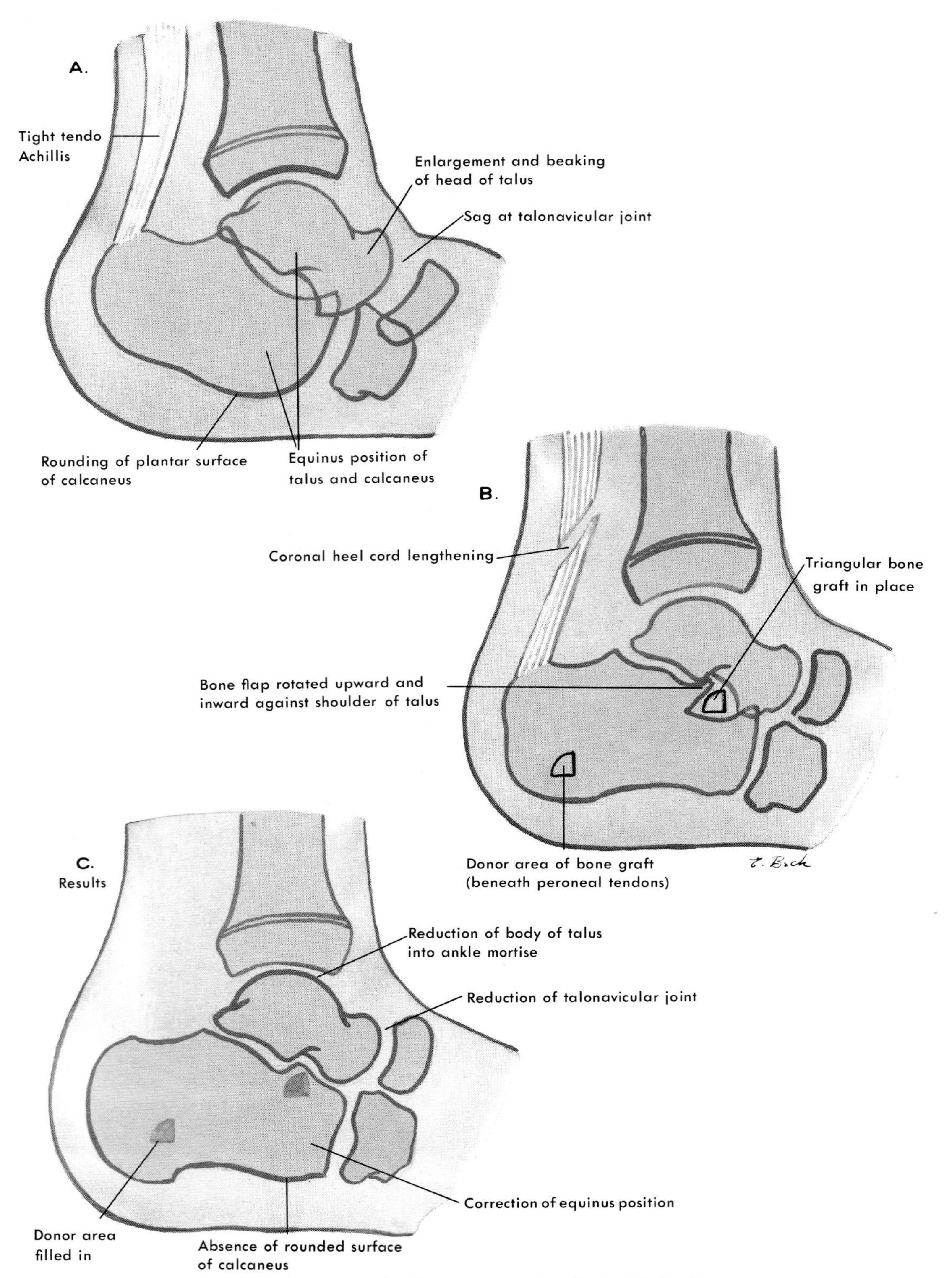

FIGURE 7–186. The Chambers procedure for flexible flat foot.

A. Diagram illustrating preoperative abnormality. The talus and calcaneus are in equinus position owing to the taut triceps surae and the plantar sag at the talonavicular joint, with forward and downward displacement of the talus and posterolateral displacement of the calcaneus. **B.** Diagram of the operative correction showing the coronal lengthening of the heel cord and the osteotomy of the anterolateral part of the calcaneus beneath the anterolateral facet and immediately posterior to the calcaneocuboid joint. Note the triangular bone graft holding the osteotomized segment of the calcaneus dorsally and medially against the talus. **C.** Diagram showing remodeling of the calcaneal bone flap. It acts as a buttress to maintain normal alignment of the talocalcaneal joint. (Redrawn after Miller, G. R.: The operative treatment of hypermobile flatfeet in the young child. Clin. Orthop., *122*:95, 1977.)

In flexible pes planovalgus the line along which body weight is transmitted through the talus passes medial to the calcaneus (Fig. 7–187 B). The objective of the operation is to displace the posterior part of the calcaneus medially, thereby restoring normal weight-bearing (Fig. 7–187 C). The patient is placed in prone position with the knee flexed 30 to 45 degrees by a sandbag under the lower leg. An incision is made on the lateral aspect of the body of the calcaneus, parallel and immediately posterior to the peroneal tendons. It extends proximally from the lateral margin of the tendo Achillis to the plantar aspect of the heel. Damage to the sural nerve should be avoided. The wound margins are undermined, elevated, and held apart by self-retaining retractors. Two Chandler elevator retractors are inserted, one on the superior and the other on the inferior surface of the os calcis, exposing its dorsal, lateral, and plantar surfaces. The periosteum is incised and elevated in line with the skin incision. With an

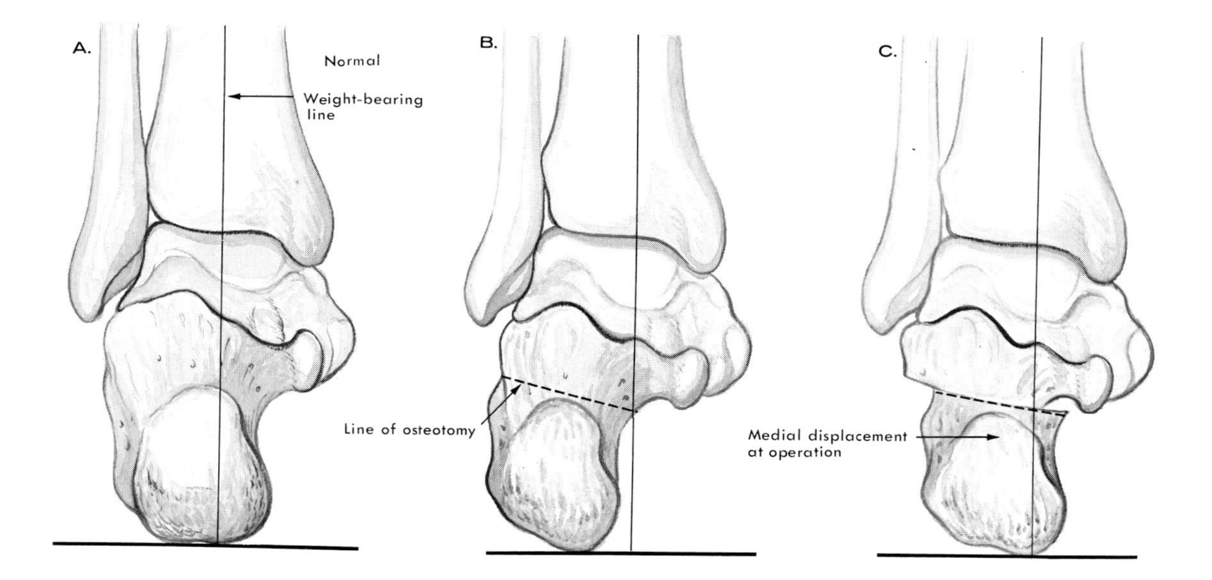

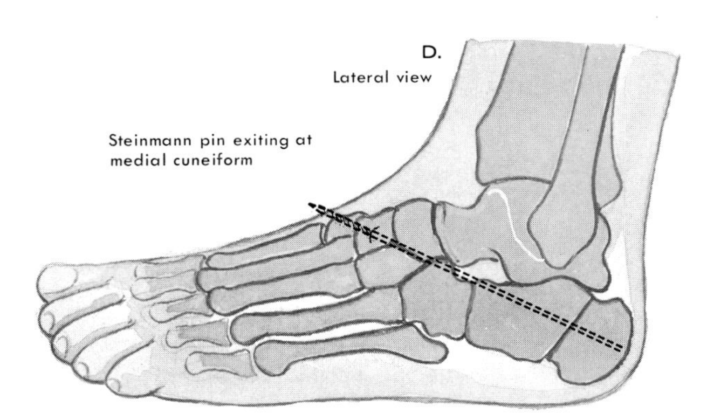

FIGURE 7–187. Medial displacement osteotomy of the calcaneus in severe pes planovalgus.

The weight-bearing line and relation of the talus to the calcaneus are visualized from the posterosuperior aspect. **A.** In normal foot. **B.** In pes planovalgus. Note that the weight transmitted through the talus passes medial to the calcaneus. The line of osteotomy of the calcaneus is shown. **C.** After medial displacement osteotomy of the calcaneus. The medial margin of the posterior calcaneal fragment is placed in line with the sustentaculum tali, and normal weight-bearing is restored. **D.** Threaded Steinmann pin transfixing the osteotomized calcaneus.

Triple Arthrodesis by Inlay Grafting (Williams and Menelaus)

OPERATIVE TECHNIQUE

A. A curved longitudinal incision is made on the anterolateral aspect of the dorsum of the foot. It extends from immediately distal to the tip of the lateral malleolus to the second cuneiform. The subcutaneous tissue and deep fascia are divided in line with the skin incision.

B. The extensor digitorum brevis is elevated from its origin and reflected distally. The extensor digitorum longus tendons are retracted medially. The contents of the sinus tarsi and the capsules of the talonavicular, calcaneocuboid, and subtalar joints are excised.

C. Next, the foot is manipulated and securely held in the desired plantigrade position, with the valgus deviation corrected and a normal longitudinal arch. In the very flaccid foot it is best to stabilize the tarsus by drilling two stout Kirschner wires longitudinally, one across the talonavicular and the other across the calcaneocuboid joint. A square or oblong trough is cut across the midfoot—extending across the talonavicular, anterior subtalar, calcaneocuboid, and naviculocuboid joints.

D and **E.** A bone graft, slightly larger than the resected block, is taken from the upper third of the same tibia and is then hammered snugly into the trough in the tarsus.

With a gauge, the articular cartilage from the adjacent subtalar joint is removed and the defect is filled with the bone previously removed from the trough. The tourniquet is released, and after complete hemostasis the leg and foot wounds are closed in the usual fashion. Absorbable sutures are put in the skin. An above-knee cast is applied.

POSTOPERATIVE CARE

The foot and leg are immobilized in a plaster cast for a total period of three months. Then bone healing is assessed clinically and radiologically. The cortical bone graft may appear dense initially, but in time it will become revascularized.

Plate 112. Triple Arthrodesis by Inlay Grafting (Williams and Menelaus)

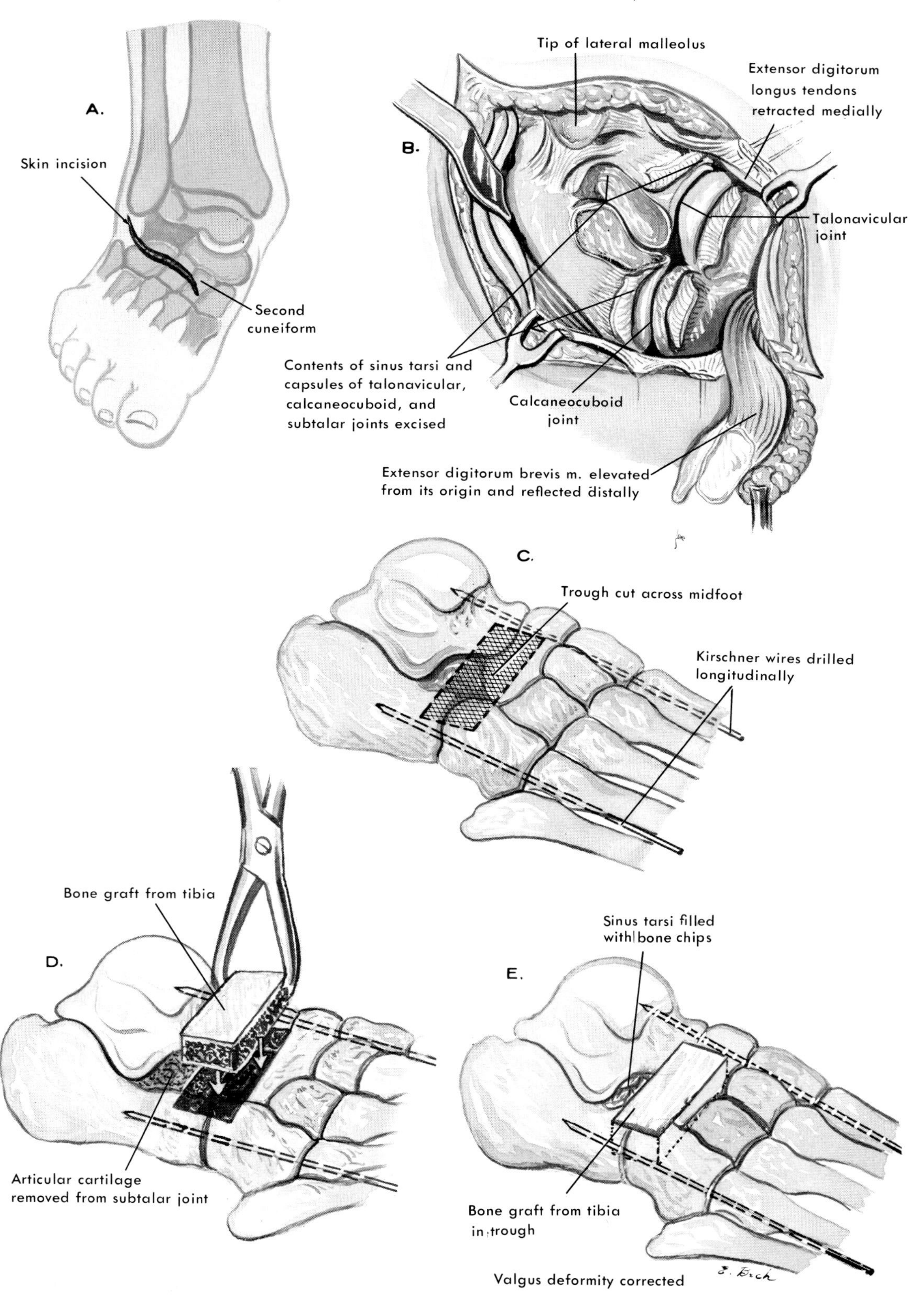

electric oscillating saw or a wide osteotome the calcaneus is sectioned. If necessary, the segments are spread open with a laminectomy spreader to allow the periosteum on the medial aspect of the calcaneus to be divided; sometimes the taut plantar ligament is sectioned to achieve sufficient medial displacement. Next the posterior fragment of the calcaneus is displaced medially until its medial margin is in line with the sustentaculum tali. It is usually necessary to displace a third to a half of the width of the calcaneus. The calcaneal fragments are transfixed by one large threaded Steinmann pin, inserted obliquely from the posteroplantar aspect of the os calcis. The pin exits through the skin over the medial or intermediate cuneiform and should be subcutaneous or flush with the calcaneus posteriorly. The wound is closed in the usual fashion, and a well-padded above-knee cast is applied with the ankle in neutral position and the knee in 45 degrees of flexion.[82]

Four weeks after the operation the cast is changed. The threaded Steinmann pin and the sutures are removed. By then bony union usually has taken place. A below-knee walking cast is applied for an additional two weeks.

The operation was performed by Koutsogiannis in 34 feet in 19 patients. Two patients were over 17 years of age at the time of surgery; on exclusion of these two older patients, the mean age was 12 years. The follow-up ranged from six years to a few months. In 17 of the 19 patients, function was markedly improved. According to Koutsogiannis the two failures were probably due to a taut Achilles tendon or to inadequate medial displacement of the posterior calcaneal fragment.[82] This author highly recommends medial displacement osteotomy of the calcaneus to correct hindfoot valgus deformity in severe symptomatic flexible pes planovalgus.

Evans Operations. Evans operation for lengthening the lateral column of the foot for correction of calcaneovalgus deformity is performed as follows:

A 7-cm.-long incision is made over the lateral aspect of the calcaneus and cuboid bone, parallel with and immediately dorsal to the peroneal tendon. Subcutaneous tissue is divided in line with the skin incision. Avoid inadvertent division of the sural nerve. The calcaneocuboid joint is identified and the calcaneus is exposed. With a straight sharp osteotome the anterior end of the calcaneus is sectioned in front of the peroneal tubercle. The line of osteotomy is parallel with and 1.5 cm. behind the calcaneocuboid joint. The osteotomized segments are prised apart with a spreader. Broad straight osteotomes of various sizes (1.25 to 3.0 cm. or more) are inserted into the osteotomy site to determine the optimum width of the bone graft to be used. The foot is inspected clinically, and radiograms are made to ensure that the desired degree of correction is obtained. Next, a cortical bone graft is taken from the tibia. (This author prefers iliac bone with both cortices intact.) The graft is inserted between the calcaneal fragments. The spreader is removed, and the degree of correction is ascertained again by radiograms. The forepart of the foot should be adducted and the heel slightly inverted. The tourniquet is deflated, and after complete hemostasis, the wound is closed in the usual fashion. A below-knee cast is applied for immobilization.[42]

The cast is changed in four weeks. Radiograms are made to assess bone healing. A new below-knee cast with an anterior heel is applied, and weight-bearing is allowed. The total period of cast immobilization is two months for solid consolidation of the graft. (Mr. Evans recommended the plaster cast be retained for about four months; this author finds two months to be adequate.) No special corrective shoes or shoe inserts are needed when the plaster is removed.[42] This author recommends the reverse Evans procedure for midfoot valgus deformity with lateral subluxation of the navicular on the head of the talus and lateral tilting of the calcaneocuboid joint. If the calcaneocuboid joint is not tilted, he finds open-wedge osteotomy of the cuboid with iliac bone graft effective in correcting lateral subluxation of the navicular on the head of the talus. He combines it with tautening of the posterior tibial tendon and plantar calcaneonavicular ligament.

In summary, surgical treatment of pes planovalgus is rarely indicated and should not be performed in patients under the age of ten years. Contracture of the triceps surae muscles should be corrected in all cases; if it does not respond to passive stretching exercises or a below-knee walking cast with an anterior heel, a sliding lengthening of the heel cord is performed. The distal cut of the Achilles tendon should be lateral. When flexible pes planovalgus is due to sag at the naviculocuneiform joint, the recommended procedure is naviculocuneiform fusion and tautening of the posterior tibial tendon and plantar calcaneonavicular ligament. Proximal transfer of the anterior tibial tendon to the navicular will provide a dynamic force to elevate the medial longitudinal arch of the foot, and this author highly recommends the Giannestras modification. When the problem is severe hindfoot valgus deformity, medial displacement osteotomy of the calcaneus is the procedure of choice. This may be combined with naviculocuneiform fusion and tautening of the plantar calcaneonavicular ligament and distal transfer of the posterior tibial tendon. It is best to stage these two procedures. When the navicular is displaced laterally on the head of the talus and the medial column of the foot is elongated, elongation of the lateral column of the foot is recommended. If the calcaneocuboid joint is tilted laterally, the reverse Evans operation is performed with a wedge of bone graft placed in the anterior part of the calcaneus. If the calcaneocuboid joint orientation is normal, an open-up osteotomy of the cuboid bone is performed with the base of the wedge lateral; the plantar calcaneonavicular ligament and the posterior tibial tendon are tautened, but they should not be detached from the navicular or advanced distally. In severe flexible pes planovalgus due to excessive ligamentous laxity and in syndromes such as Down's or Marfan's, the inlay graft triple arthrodesis of Williams and Menelaus is recommended. When pes planovalgus is rigid and painful, a triple arthrodesis is performed with a subtalar bone block as in the Grice procedure and talonavicular and calcaneocuboid joint fusion with the wedges based plantarward.

References

1. Anderson, A. F., and Fowler, S. B.: Anterior calcaneal osteotomy for symptomatic juvenile pes planus. Foot Ankle, *4*:274, 1984.
2. Armstrong, G.: Evans elongation of lateral column of the foot for valgus deformity. J. Bone Joint Surg., *57-B*:530, 1975.
3. Asher, C.: Flat foot and valgus heel. *In* Postural Variations in Childhood. London, Butterworth & Co., 1975, pp. 76–101.
4. Baker, L. D., and Hill, L. M.: Foot alignment in the cerebral palsy patient. J. Bone Joint Surg., *46-A*:1, 1964.
5. Barrasso, J. A., Wile, P. B., and Gage, J. R.: Extraarticular subtalar arthrodesis with internal fixation. J. Pediatr. Orthop., *4*:555, 1984.
6. Barry, R. J., and Scranton, P. E., Jr.: Flat feet in children. Clin. Orthop., *181*:68, 1983.
7. Basmajian, J. R., and Bentzon, J. W.: An electromyographic study of certain muscles of the leg and foot in the standing position. Surg. Gynecol. Obstet., *98*:662, 1954.
8. Basmajian, J. R., and Stecko, G.: The role of muscles in arch support of the foot. An electromyographic study. J. Bone Joint Surg., *45-A*:1184, 1963.
9. Basta, N. W., Mital, M. A., Bonadio, O., Johnson, A., Kang, S. Y., and O'Connor, J.: A comparative study of the role of shoe, arch supports, and navicular cookies in the management of symptomatic mobile flat feet in children. Int. Orthop., *1*:143, 1977.
10. Bettmann, E.: The treatment of flat-foot by means of exercise. J. Bone Joint Surg., *19*:821, 1937.
11. Bick, E. M.: Static deformities of the foot. *In* Source Book of Orthopaedics. Baltimore, Williams & Wilkins, 1948, pp. 449–458.
12. Bivings, L.: Heel printing in flat feet. Am. J. Dis. Child., *46*:1050, 1933.
13. Bleck, E. E.: The shoeing of children: Sham or science? Dev. Med. Child Neurol., *13*:188, 1971.
14. Bleck, E. E., and Berzins, U. J.: Conservative management of pes valgus with plantar flexed, talus flexible. Clin. Orthop., *22*:85, 1977.
15. Bohm, M.: Der Foetal Fuss. Beitrage zur Entstehung des Pes planus, des Pes valgus und des Pes planovalgus. Z. Orthop. Chir., p. 57, 1932.
16. Bordelon, R. L.: Correction of hypermobile flatfoot in children by molded insert. Foot Ankle, *1*:132, 1980.
17. Bordelon, R. L.: Hypermobile flatfoot in children. Comprehension, evaluation and treatment. Clin. Orthop., *181*:7, 1983.
18. Brahdy, B. M.: Flat-foot in children. Arch. Pediatr., *44*:86, 1927.
19. Brown, L. T.: The end results of stabilizing operations on the foot. J. Bone Joint Surg., *6*:839, 1924.
20. Bruce, J. M., and Walmsley, R.: Some observations on the arches of the foot and flatfoot. Lancet, *2*:656, 1938.
21. Butte, F. L.: Navicular-cuneiform arthrodesis for flatfoot. J. Bone Joint Surg., *19*:496, 1937.
22. Caldwell, G. D.: Surgical correction of relaxed flatfoot by the Durham flatfootplasty. Clin. Orthop., *2*:221, 1953.
23. Chambers, E. F. S.: An operation for correction of flexible flat feet of adolescents. West. J. Surg., *54*:77, 1946.
24. Chandler, F. A.: Children's feet, normal and presenting common abnormalities. Am. J. Dis. Child., *63*:1136, 1942.
25. Chiappara, R., Vaerrina, F., Dagnino, G., and Pedroni Menconi, F.: The surgical treatment of mobile valgus flat foot in children. Ital. J. Orthop. Traumatol., *10*:469, 1984.
26. Chigot, P. L., and Sananes, P.: Arthrodese de Grice. Rev. Chir. Orthop., *51*:53, 1965.
27. Clark, W. A.: A rebalancing operation for pronated feet. J. Bone Joint Surg., *13*:867, 1931.
28. Compere, E. L.: Flat feet in children. Med. Clin. North Am., *30*:147, 1946.
29. Connolly, J., Regen, E., and Hillman, J. W.: Pigeontoes and flatfeet. Pediatr. Clin. North Am., *17*:291, 1970.
30. Cowell, H. R., and Elener, V.: Rigid painful flatfoot secondary to tarsal coalition. Clin. Orthop., *177*:54, 1983.
31. Craxford, A. D., Minna, R. J., and Park, C.: Plantar pressures and gait parameters: A study of foot shape and limb rotations in children. J. Pediatr. Orthop., *4*:477, 1984.
32. Crego, C. H., Jr., and Ford, L. T.: An end-result study of various operative procedures for correcting flat feet in children. J. Bone Joint Surg., *34-A*:183, 1952.
33. Debrunner, H. U.: Fussdeformitaten. Ther. Umsch., *29*:447, 1972.
34. DeDoncker, E.: Le traitement du pied valgus souple. Acta Orthop. Belg., *28*:709, 1962.
35. Dennyson, W. G., and Fulford, G. E.: Subtalar arthrodesis by cancellous grafts and metallic internal fixation. J. Bone Joint Surg., *58-B*:507, 1976.
36. Dickson, F. D., and Dively, R. L.: Functional Disorders of the Foot. Philadelphia, Lippincott, 1944.
37. Dommisse, G. F.: Flat foot. II. S. Afr. Med. J., *45*:726, July, 1971.
38. Duncan, J. W., and Lovell, W. W.: Modified Hoke-Miller flatfoot procedure. Clin. Orthop., *181*:24, 1983.
39. Dwyer, F. C.: Osteotomy of the calcaneum in the

treatment of grossly everted feet with special reference to cerebral palsy. *In* Huitième Congrès de la Société Internationale de Chirurgie Orthopédique et de Traumatologie. New York, 4–9 September, 1960. Brussels, Imprimerie des Sciences, 1961, pp. 892–897.

40. Dwyer, F. C.: The relationship of variations in the size and inclination of the calcaneus to the shape and function of the whole foot. Ann. R. Coll. Surg., *34*:120, 1964.
41. Engel, G. M., and Staheli, L. T.: The natural history of torsion and other factors influencing gait in childhood. A study of the angle of gait, tibial torsion, knee angle, hip rotation, and development of the arch in normal children. Clin. Orthop., *99*:12, 1974.
42. Evans, D. C.: Calcaneovalgus deformity. J. Bone Joint Surg., *57-B*:270, 1975.
43. Ewald, P.: Ueber den Knick und Plattfuss. Z. Orthop. Chir., *25*:229, 1910.
44. Faggiana, F.: Il piede piatto. Acta Orthop. Ital., *1*:141, 1955.
45. Ferciot, C. F.: The etiology of developmental flat foot. Clin. Orthop., *85*:7, 1972.
46. Ferguson, A. B.: Flat feet in childhood. Penn. Med. J., *57*:330, 1954.
47. Fogel, G. R., Katoh, Y., Rand, J. A., and Chao, E. Y. S.: Talonavicular arthrodesis for isolated arthrosis: 9.5-year results and gait analysis. Foot Ankle, *3*:105, 1982.
48. Giannestras, N. J.: Static foot problems in the preadolescent and adolescent stages. *In* Foot Disorders. Medical and Surgical Management. Philadelphia, Lea & Febiger, 1967, pp. 119–155.
49. Giannestras, N. J.: Static deformities of the foot. Editorial comment. Clin. Orthop., *70*:2, 1970.
50. Giannestras, N. J.: Flexible valgus flatfoot resulting from naviculocuneiform and talonavicular sag. Surgical correction in the adolescent. *In* Bateman, J. E. (ed.): Foot Science. Philadelphia, Saunders, 1976, pp. 67–105.
51. Giannestras, N. J.: Long term results of surgical treatment of flexible pes planovalgum. Paper presented at Pediatric International Orthopedic Seminars, Chicago, 1978.
52. Giannini, S., Girolami, M., and Ceccarelli, F.: The surgical treatment of infantile flat foot. A new expanding endo-orthotic implant. Ital. J. Orthop. Traumatol., *11*:315, 1985.
53. Gleich, A.: Beitrag zur operativen Plattfussbehandlung. Arch. Klin. Chir., *46*:358, 1893.
54. Golding-Bird, C. H.: Pes valgus acquisitus. Pes pronatus acquisitus. Pes cavus. Guy's Hosp. Rep., *41*:439, 1883.
55. Gomez, A. J.: Consideraciones Generales Acerca del Pie valgo Plano en el Nino. Conceptos Modernos de su Tratamiento Ortopedico y Quirurgico. Monograph. Caracas, Venezuela, 1965.
56. Gottlieb, A.: The acquired pes valgus in childhood. Arch. Pediatr., *55*:166, 1938.
57. Gresham, J. L.: Correction of flat feet in children. Grice-Green subastragalar arthrodesis. South. Med. J., *61*:177, 1968.
58. Grice, D. S.: An extra-articular arthrodesis of the subastragalar joint for correction of paralytic flat-feet in children. J. Bone Joint Surg., *34-A*:929, 1952.
59. Grice, D. S.: Further experience with extra-articular arthrodesis of the subtalar joint. J. Bone Joint Surg., *37-A*:246, 1955.
60. Grice, D. S.: The role of subtalar fusion in the treatment of valgus deformities of the foot. A.A.O.S. Instr. Course Lect., *16*:127, 1959.
61. Hackenbroch, M.: Der Plattfus. *In* Hohmann, G. (ed.): Handbuch der Orthopaedie. Stuttgart, Georg Thieme Verlag, 1961 IV(II), p. 998.
62. Haraldsson, S.: Pes plano-valgus staticus juvenilis and its operative treatment. Acta Orthop. Scand., *35*:234, 1965.
63. Harris, R. I., and Beath, T.: Hypermobile flat-foot with short tendo-Achillis. J. Bone Joint Surg., *30-A*:116, 1948.
64. Hatt, W. S., and Davis, L. A.: Analysis of the foot in infant, radiographic criteria and clinical aspects. South. Med. J., *50*:720, 1954.
65. Hazlett, J. W.: Pes planus. Bull Hosp. Spec. Surg., *3*:23, February, 1960.
66. Helfet, A. J.: A new way of treating flat feet in children. Lancet, *1*:262, 1956.
67. Henderson, W. H., and Campbell, J. W.: UCBL shoe insert: Casting and fabrication. The Biomechanics Laboratory. University of California at San Francisco and Berkeley. Technical Report 53, August 1967.
68. Herzmark, M. H.: Floor pad for foot-exercising. J. Bone Joint Surg., *29*:1098, 1947.
69. Hicks, J. H.: The function of the plantar aponeurosis. J. Anat., *85*:414, 1951.
70. Hicks, J. H.: The mechanics of the foot. I. The joints. J. Anat., *87*:343, 1953.
71. Hicks, J. H.: The mechanics of the foot. II. The joints. J. Anat., *88*:25, 1954.
72. Hohmann, G.: Zur operativen Plattfussbehandlung. Chirurg, *3*:593, 1931.
73. Hoke, M.: An operation for the correction of extremely relaxed flat feet. J. Bone Joint Surg., *13*:773, 1931.
74. Imhauser, G., and Schoberlein, J.: What does Schede flatfoot operation accomplish? Assessment based on follow-up examinations after two decades. Z. Orthop., *112*:139, 1974.
75. Inman, V. T.: UCBL dual axis control system and UCBL shoe insert. Bull. Prosthet. Res., *10*:11, 1969.
76. Jack, E. A.: Naviculocuneiform fusion in the treatment of flat foot. J. Bone Joint Surg., *35-B*:279, 1953.
77. Jayakumar, S., and Cowell, H. R.: Rigid flatfoot. Clin. Orthop., *122*:77, 1977.
78. Jones, B. S.: Flat foot. A preliminary report of an operation for severe cases. J. Bone Joint Surg., *57-B*:279, 1975.
79. Jones, R. L.: The human foot. An experimental study of the mechanics and role of its muscles and ligaments in the support of the arch. Am. J. Anat., *68*:1, 1941.
80. Keith, A.: The history of the human foot and its bearing on orthopaedic practice. J. Bone Joint Surg., *11*:10, 1929.
81. Kite, J. H.: The treatment of flatfeet in small children. Postgrad. Med., *15*:75, 1954.
82. Koutsogiannis, E.: Treatment of mobile flat foot by displacement osteotomy of a calcaneus. J. Bone Joint Surg., *53-B*:96, 1971.
83. Krause, W.: The operative treatment of juvenile flat and abducted feet. Ortopädische Klinik Kassel-Wilhelmshöne, West Germany, 1971.
84. Lake, N. C.: Flat foot. *In* The Foot. 3rd Ed. Baltimore, Williams & Wilkins, 1948, pp. 165–198.
85. Lang, G., Kehr, P., Sejourne, P., Paternotte, H., Mathevon, H., and Pointu, J.: Reflections concerning the radiological assessment of static flat foot in the child. J. Radiol. Electrol. Med. Nucl., *59*:497, 1978.
86. Lange, F.: Neue Plattfusseneinlagen aus Celluloid-Stahldraht. Munchen Med. Wochenschr., 7, 1903.
87. Lanfranchi, R., and Zinghi, G. F.: L'Artrodesi estraarticolare della sotta-astragalica associata alla transposizione del tibialae posteriore nel trattamento del piede plato dell'adulto. Chir. Organi Mov., *57*:395, 1968.
88. Leavitt, D. G.: Subastragaloid arthrodesis for the os calcis type of flat foot. Am. J. Surg., *59*:501, 1943.
89. Legg, A. T.: The treatment of congenital flatfoot by

tendon transplantation. Am. J. Orthop. Surg., *10*:584, 1912–1913.
90. Lelièvre, J.: Le pied plat valgus statique. *In* Pathologie du Pied. 2nd Ed. Paris, Masson & Cie, 1961, pp. 387–399.
91. Lelièvre, J.: Current concepts and corrections in the valgus foot. Clin. Orthop., *70*:43, 1970.
92. Leonard, M. H., Gonzalez, S., Beck, L. W., Basom, C., Palafox, M., and Kosick, Z. W.: Lateral transfer of posterior tibial tendon in certain selected cases of pes planovalgus (Kidner operation). Clin. Orthop., *40*:139, 1965.
93. L'Episcopo, J. B., and Sabatelle, P. E.: The Hoke operation for flat feet. J. Bone Joint Surg., *21*:92, 1939.
94. Lewin, P.: Flat foot in infants and children. Am. J. Dis. Child., *31*:704, 1926.
95. Lignac, F., and Rigault, P.: Essential flat foot in the child. Definition, diagnosis and therapeutic indications. Nouv. Presse, *6*:3321, 1977.
96. Lonergan, R. C.: Surgical treatment of flat feet: Indication and technic. Surg. Clin. North Am., *19*:21, 1934.
97. Lord, J. P.: Correction of extreme flatfoot. Value of osteotomy of os calcis (Gleich operation). J.A.M.A., *81*:1502, 1923.
98. Lovell, W. W., Price, C. T., and Meehan, P. L.: *In* Winter, R. B., and Lovell, W. W. (eds.): Pediatric Orthopedics. Philadelphia, Lippincott, 1978.
99. Lowman, C. L.: An operative method for correction of certain forms of flat foot. J.A.M.A., *81*:1500, 1923.
100. Lowman, C. L.: The treatment of flat foot. Orthopedic Correspondence Club Letter, 1941.
101. Lund, S. H.: Arthrodesis for flat foot. Acta Orthop. Scand., *33*:234, 1965.
102. Mann, R. A., and Thompson, F. M.: Rupture of the posterior tibial tendon causing flat foot. Surgical treatment. J. Bone Joint Surg., *67-A*:556, 1985.
103. Mereday, C., Dolan, C. M. E., and Lusskin, R.: Evaluation of the University of California Biomechanics Laboratory shoe insert in "flexible" pes planus. Clin. Orthop., *82*:45, 1972.
104. Miller, G. R.: The operative treatment of hypermobile flatfeet in the young child. Clin. Orthop., *122*:95, 1977.
105. Miller, O. L.: A plastic flat foot operation. J. Bone Joint Surg., *9*:84, 1927.
106. Mitch, H.: Reinforcement of the deltoid ligament for pronated foot. Surg. Gynecol. Obstet., *74*:876, 1942.
107. Müller, E.: Ueber die Resultate der Ernst Muller'schen Plattfussoperation. Beitr. Klin. Chir., *75*:424, 1913.
108. Niederecker, K.: Der Plattfuss. Stuttgart, F. Enke, 1959.
109. Ogilvy, C.: An operation for the permanent correction of weak feet in children. J. Orthop. Surg., *1*:343, 1919.
110. Ogston, A.: On flatfoot and its cure by operation. Br. Med. J., *9*:110, 1884.
111. Osmond-Clarke, H.: Congenital vertical talus. J. Bone Joint Surg., *38-B*:334, 1956.
112. Penneau, K., Lutter, L. D., and Winter, R. B.: Pes planus: Radiographic changes with foot orthoses and shoes. Foot Ankle, *2*:299, 1982.
113. Penners, W., and Penners, R.: Surgical treatment of acquired flat foot. Fortschr. Med., *96*:1973, 1978.
114. Phillips, G. E.: A review of elongation of os calcis for flat feet. J. Bone Joint Surg., *65-B*:15, 1983.
115. Powell, H. D.: Pes planovalgus in children. Clin. Orthop., *177*:133, 1983.
116. Purvis, G. D.: Surgery of the relaxed flat foot. Clin. Orthop., *57*:221, 1968.
117. Romanini, L., Carfagni, A., and Amorese, V.: Grice's operation for spastic flat foot. Ital. J. Orthop. Traumatol., *9*:439, 1983.
118. Rose, G. K.: Correction of the pronated foot. J. Bone Joint Surg., *40-B*:674, 1958.
119. Rose, G. K., Welton, E. A., and Marshall, T.: The diagnosis of flat foot in the child. J. Bone Joint Surg., *67-B*:71, 1985.
120. Rugtveit, A.: Extra-articular subtalar arthrodesis according to Green-Grice in flat feet. Acta Orthop. Scand., *34*:367, 1964.
121. Rupture of the posterior tibial tendon causing flat foot. Surgical treatment (letter). J. Bone Joint Surg., *67-A*:1448, 1985.
122. Ryerson, E. W.: Tendon transplantation in flatfoot. Am. J. Orthop. Surg., *34*:367, 1964.
123. Schede, F.: Die Operation des Platfusses. Z. Orthop. Chir., *50*:528, 1929.
124. Schellenberg, K.: Extra-artikulare subtalar arthrodese nach Grice. Arch. Orthop. Unfallchir., *56*:604, 1964.
125. Schmied, H. R.: Late results of translocation of the anterior tibial tendon around the navicular bone in plano-valgus feet. Z. Orthop., *104*:309, 1968.
126. Schoolfield, B. L.: An operation for the cure of flatfoot. Ann. Surg., *110*:437, 1939.
127. Schwartz, R. P., and Heath, A. L.: Conservative treatment of functional disorders of feet in adolescents and adults. J. Bone Joint Surg., *31-A*:501, 1969.
128. Seitz, D. G., and Carpenter, E. B.: Triple arthrodesis in children. A ten-year review. South. Med. J., *67*:1420, 1974.
129. Seymour, N.: The late results of naviculo-cuneiform fusion. J. Bone Joint Surg., *49-B*:558, 1967.
130. Seymour, N., and Evans, D. K.: A modification of the Grice subtalar arthrodesis. J. Bone Joint Surg., *50-B*:372, 1968.
131. Sharrard, W. J. W.: Minor orthopedic disabilities in childhood. Practitioner, *180*:415, 1958.
132. Silver, C. M., Simon, S. D., Spindell, E., Litchman, H. M., and Scala, M.: Calcaneal osteotomy for valgus and varus deformities of the feet in cerebral palsy. J. Bone Joint Surg., *49-A*:232, 1967.
133. Smith, J. B., and Westin, G. W.: Follow-up notes on articles previously published, subtalar extra-articular arthrodesis. J. Bone Joint Surg., *50-A*:1027, 1968.
134. Smith, J. W.: Muscular control of the arches of the foot in standing, an electromyographic assessment. J. Anat., *88*:152, 1954.
135. Smith, S. D., and Millar, E. A.: Arthrosis by means of a subtalar polyethylene peg implant for correction of hindfoot pronation in children. Clin. Orthop., *181*:15, 1983.
136. Staheli, L. T.: Corrective shoes for children. Pediatr. Digest, *20*:22, 1978.
137. Staheli, L. T., and Griffin, L.: Corrective shoes for children: A survey of current practice. Pediatrics, *65*:13, 1980.
138. Staheli, L. T., Chew, D. E., and Corbett, M.: The longitudinal arch. A survey of 882 feet in normal children and adults. J. Bone Joint Surg., *69-A*:426, 1987.
139. Steindler, A.: The pathomechanics of the static deformities of foot and ankle. *In* Kinesiology of the Human Body Under Normal and Pathological Conditions. 2nd Ed. Springfield, Ill., Charles C Thomas, 1970, p. 339.
140. Tanz, S. S.: The so-called tight heel cord. Clin. Orthop., *16*:184, 1960.
141. Tax, H. R.: Flexible flatfoot in children. J. Am. Podiatry Assoc., *67*:616, 1977.
142. Thomson, J. E. M.: Treatment of congenital flat foot. J. Bone Joint Surg., *28*:787, 1946.
143. Trendelenburg, F.: Über Plattsfussoperationen. Arch. Klin. Chir., *39*:751, 1889.
144. Vanden Brink, K. D.: Childhood foot and leg problems. Pediatr. Annu., *5*:61, 1976.
145. Vigliani, F., Maranzano, G., and Novati, G.: Grice-Green extra-articular subtalar arthrodesis in the treat-

ment of infantile valgus pronated flat foot. Ital. J. Orthop. Traumatol., 9:411, 1983.
146. Voutey, H.: Traitment chirurgical du pied plat de l'enfant. Rev. Chir. Orthop., 58:489, 1972.
147. Walsham, W. J., and Hughes, W. K.: Treatment of acquired flat foot. *In* The Deformities of the Human Foot. London, Bailliere, Tindall & Cox, 1895, pp. 412–489.
148. Weissman, S. L., Torok, G., and Kharmosh, O.: L'arthrodèse extraarticulaire avec transplantation tendineuse concomitante dans le traitment du pied plat valgus paralytique du jeune enfant. Rev. Chir. Orthop., 43:79, 1957.
149. Wenger, D. R., Mauldin, D., Morgan, D., Sobol, M. G., Pennebaker, M., and Thaler, R.: Foot growth rate in children age one to six years. Foot Ankle, 3:207, 1983.
150. Wetzenstein, H.: Prognosis of pes calcaneovalgus congenita. Acta Orthop. Scand., 41:122, 1970.
151. Westin, G. W., and Hall, C. B.: Subtalar extra-articular arthrodesis. J. Bone Joint Surg., 39-A:501, 1957.
152. Williams, P. F., and Menelaus, M. B.: Triple arthrodesis by inlay grafting—a method suitable for the undeformed or valgus foot. J. Bone Joint Surg., 59-B:333, 1977.
153. Young, C. S.: Operative treatment of pes planus. Surg. Gynecol. Obstet., 68:1099, 1939.
154. Zadek, I.: Transverse wedge arthrodesis for the relief of pain in rigid flatfoot. J. Bone Joint Surg., 17:453, 1935.

Acquired Affections of the Toes

HALLUX RIGIDUS

Pain and stiffness in the metatarsophalangeal joint of the great toe are quite common in adults but occur in children only very occasionally. The condition is referred to by a variety of terms—as *hallux rigidus* by Cotterill, as *hallux flexus* by Davies-Colley, as *hallux dolorosus* by Walsham and Hughes, and as *metatarsus primus elevatus* by Lambrinudi.[6, 7, 24, 40]

Etiology

In adolescent patients, hallux rigidus is often a familial affliction. Bonney and Macnab report that 50 per cent of patients whose symptoms began prior to the age of 20 had a positive family history.[2]

More preponderant in females in adolescence, the condition shows equal sex incidence in the adult.

Hallux rigidus may be caused either by intrinsic disorders of the metatarsophalangeal joint or by extrinsic mechanical abnormalities acting on the joint.

Elevation of First Metatarsal. Lambrinudi observed that hallux rigidus is associated with dorsal hyperextension of the first metatarsal.[24] In about two thirds of the cases of Jack and of Bonney and Macnab, metatarsus primus elevatus was found in hallux rigidus.[2, 17] Kessel and Bonney reported two adult patients with acquired metatarsus primus elevatus (resulting from an osteotomy of the first metatarsal done for hallux valgus in one and following triple arthrodesis in the other) who developed typical hallux rigidus later. Thus evidence was presented that in some patients, hyperextension of the first metatarsal is the primary deformity and hallux rigidus is secondary.[22] One must, however, add that cases have been observed in which metatarsus primus elevatus developed because of marked flexor spasm following the operative production of a stiff and painful first metatarsophalangeal joint. The question of which is the cause and which the effect in adolescent hallux rigidus has not, as yet, been answered. Bingold and Collins believe that in the majority of cases metatarsus primus elevatus is secondary to flexor spasm of the first metatarsophalangeal joint.[1]

Relative Length of First and Second Metatarsals. Nilsonne observed that most of his adolescent patients with hallux rigidus had long narrow feet with a first metatarsal that was longer than the second.[36] This finding was also noted by Bonney and Macnab in 22 of the 53 feet examined, the discrepancy in length being 0.5 cm. or more.[2] The common association of a long great toe with hallux rigidus was also noted by McMurray.[29] It seems the pathomechanical factor is the increased pressure transmitted from the hallux to the first metatarsal head.

Stress on First Metatarsophalangeal Joint. A number of other conditions predispose to excessive pressure on the base of the proximal phalanx of the great toe. In hallux rigidus, the feet are frequently pronated and the center of gravity of body weight is shifted toward the first metatarsal head. Bingold and Collins proposed that the cause of hallux rigidus is an abnormal gait developed either to protect an injured or inflamed metatarsophalangeal joint from the pressure of weight-bearing or to stabilize a hypermobile first metatarsal. As a result, excessive pressure is transmitted from the flexor hallucis brevis tendon and the two sesamoids to the base of the first phalanx and the great toe. They found evidence of this abnormal gait in the peculiarities of wear seen in old shoes and observed a high degree of correlation between unilateral hallux rigidus and the patient's foot dominance.[1]

Local Inflammation of the Joint. In some cases, there is a definite history of injury precipitating these symptoms, and traumatic arthritis may be a factor. In other patients, hallux rigidus may be a local manifestation of generalized rheumatoid arthritis.

Osteochondritis Dissecans of First Metatarsal Head. This may be an occasional cause of hallux rigidus (Fig. 7–188). Increased density and fragmentation of the epiphysis of the proximal phalanx of the great toe was considered by Glissan to represent aseptic necrosis of bone, a condition similar to Legg-Perthes disease of the femoral head.[10] Pathologic studies by Bingold and Collins have, however, demonstrated that the increased density of the epiphysis of the proximal phalanx is caused by close packing of live trabeculae, and that fragmentation of the epiphysis represents irregular ossification, not aseptic necrosis.[1] Similar changes are observed in normal feet of adolescents; they are of no etiologic significance in hallux rigidus.

Clinical Features

The presenting complaint is pain in and around the metatarsophalangeal joint of the great toe. Usually the symptoms are of gradual onset, developing in adolescence. Occasionally pain occurs suddenly, precipitated by acute trauma. It is aggravated by walking or rising on the toes and is relieved by rest.

Abnormal patterns of wear in the shoes are suggestive of hallux rigidus. The shoes are often too narrow and short, and show excessive wear on the outer side of the heel, on the posterior half of the sole, and under the terminal phalanx of the great toe. The uppers are bulged outward over the outer side of the heel and the posterior half of the sole. Their toe spring is shortened, and there are furrows over the medial side of the toe cap caused by the hypermobile interphalangeal joint of the great toe. In gait the foot is inverted on push-off.

The feet of these patients are long and narrow and are usually pronated. The base of the first metatarsal is pushed plantarward, and its head is tilted dorsally. The first metatarsophalangeal

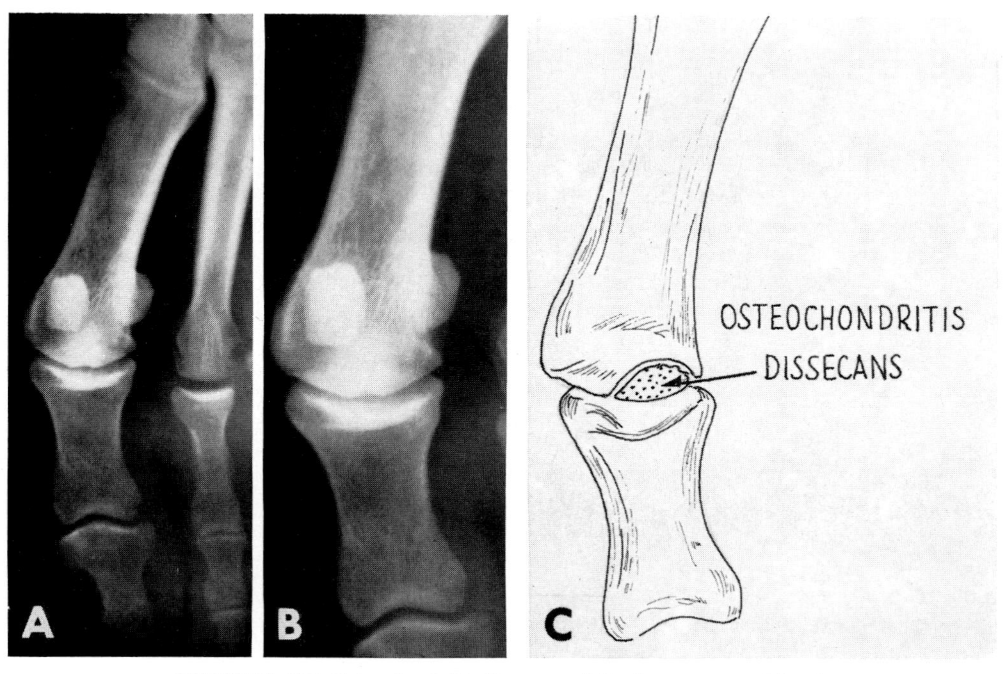

FIGURE 7–188. Osteochondritis dissecans of the first metatarsal head.

This condition is an occasional cause of hallux rigidus. (From Kelikian, H.: Hallux Valgus, Allied Deformities of the Forefoot and Metatarsalgia. Philadelphia, Saunders, 1965, p. 273. Reprinted by permission.)

joint is enlarged, and the great toe is held in a varying degree of flexion (hallux flexus). There is a callosity underneath the base of the proximal phalanx of the great toe, but the skin on the plantar aspect of the first metatarsal head is smooth (lacking its normal thickness). On palpation the metatarsophalangeal joint of the great toe is found to be tender and thickened. In severe cases one may palpate osteophytes at the articular margins. Active extension of the metatarsophalangeal joint is markedly restricted, but in the early stages of the disease, flexion is within normal range. Passive dorsiflexion of the great toe is limited and very painful (Fig. 7–189). Passive motions of the joint may be accompanied by crepitus. A taut flexor hallucis brevis may be palpated on the plantar aspect. The interphalangeal joint of the great toe is hypermobile in adolescents; in adults, its motion may be restricted and somewhat painful.

There is a rare variety of hallux rigidus referred to as hallux extensus in which the first metatarsal is plantar-flexed and the great toe is fixed in hyperextension at the metatarsophalangeal joint (Fig. 7–190).

Radiographic Features

Early in the course of the disease, the x-rays may be normal or show thickening of the soft tissues around the affected joint. The standing lateral radiogram of the foot shows the first metatarsal hyperextended with its head tilting dorsally. Later on, the articular cartilage space becomes narrowed and the metatarsal head flattened. Soon osteophytes form at the joint margins (Fig. 7–191).

In hallux rigidus due to rheumatoid arthritis there will be local osteoporosis and erosion at the articular margins. Gout is very rare in the adolescent, but in the adult a punched-out erosion due to a tophus on the articular surface is characteristic.

Treatment

Initially conservative treatment should always be tried. The sole of the shoe between the shank and toe portions medially under the first metatarsal head is stiffened. A slightly larger shoe with its leather softened dorsally over the first metatarsophalangeal joint will give symptomatic relief. Passive manipulative exercises are performed several times a day to increase the range of dorsiflexion of the great toe. In most cases, with conservative management, the symptoms will regress if the joint is protected for a few weeks or months. If the symptoms persist and disability remains moderately severe, operative correction of the deformity is required.

In these resistant cases, Kessel and Bonney (following an earlier suggestion of Bonney and Macnab) perform an extension osteotomy at the base of the proximal phalanx of the great toe, converting the normal range of plantar flexion at the metatarsophalangeal joint to a functional range of dorsiflexion and plantar flexion (Fig. 7–192).[2, 22]

The operative technique is as follows:

A curved dorsal incision about 4 cm. long is made, centering over the base of the proximal phalanx. The subcutaneous tissue is divided. The extensor hallucis longus tendon and digital nerves are retracted to one side to expose the proximal phalanx and metatarsophalangeal joint of the great toe. With small osteotomes, a wedge of bone with a dorsal base of predetermined width is resected from the phalanx as far proximally as possible. The cortex and periosteum on the plantar aspect are left intact. It is best to use drill holes to mark and control the extent of osteotomy. The phalanx is angulated dorsally to close the gap. One or two Kirschner wires are placed obliquely to keep the osteotomized fragments firmly together. The wound is closed, and a below-knee walking cast with a sturdy toe plate is applied. The great toe should be held in extension by appropriate padding underneath. In four to six weeks the osteotomy will heal.

Kessel and Bonney report satisfactory results following their procedure, with a mean improvement of dorsiflexion from 5 degrees before operation to 44 degrees afterward (Fig. 7–192).[22]

Watermann, in 1927, recommended a cuneiform osteotomy of the head of the first metatarsal with the base of the wedge directed dorsally and including the hypertrophic spurs (cf. Fig. 7–193).[41] Kelikian recommends the Watermann osteotomy in growing children in order to avoid injury to the growth plate of the proximal phalanx.[20]

A plantar capsulotomy of the first metatarsophalangeal joint is performed if the capsule is contracted and limits extension. One may have to release the flexor hallucis brevis from the proximal phalanx.

Whether extension osteotomy of the base of the proximal phalanx or the first metatarsal head will prevent the development of hallux rigidus in adult life has not been determined, as long-

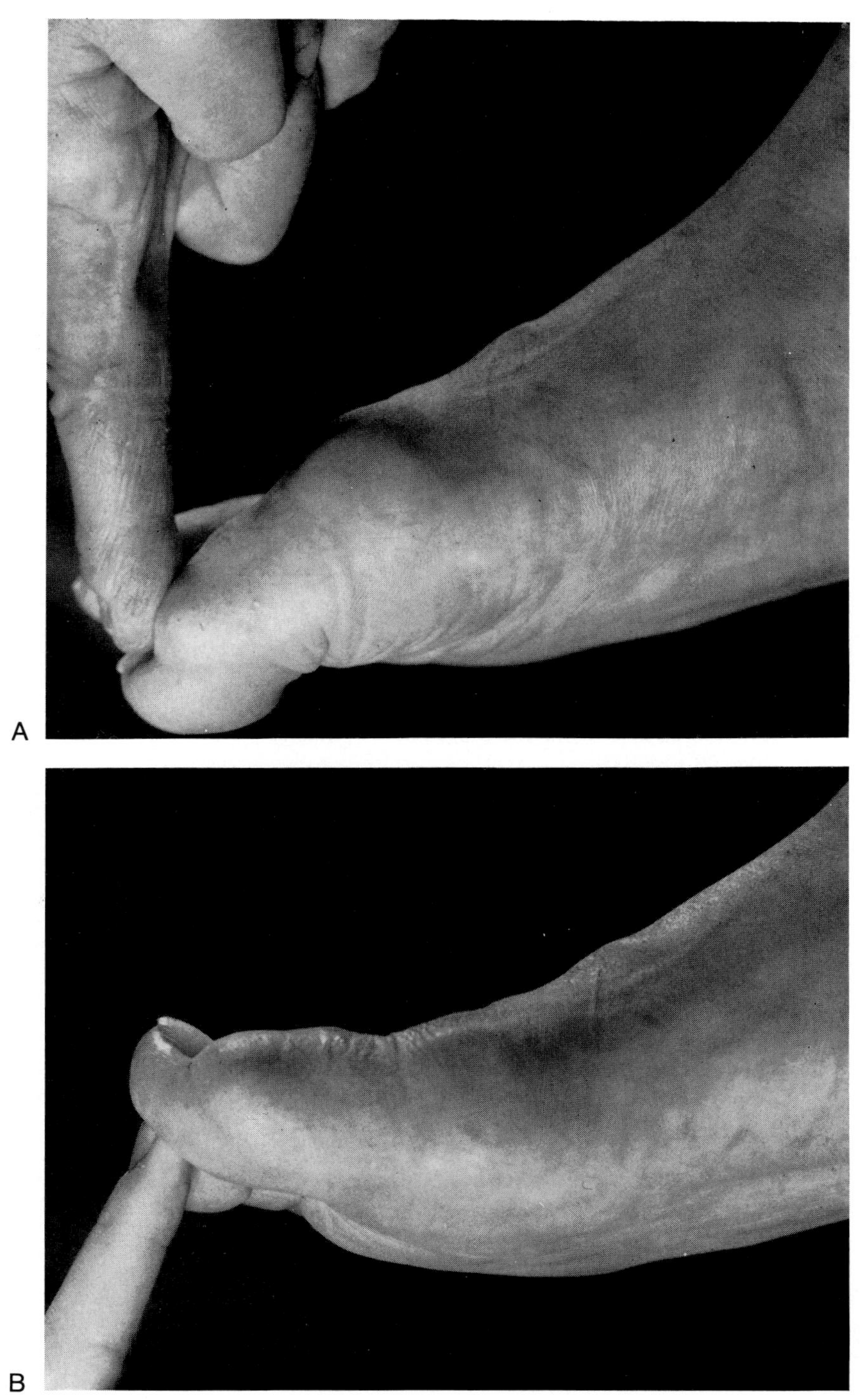

FIGURE 7–189. Hallux rigidus.

The metatarsophalangeal joint is enlarged, and dorsiflexion of the great toe is markedly limited. (From Kelikian, H.: Hallux Valgus, Allied Deformities of the Forefoot and Metatarsalgia. Philadelphia, Saunders, 1965, p. 268. Reprinted by permission.)

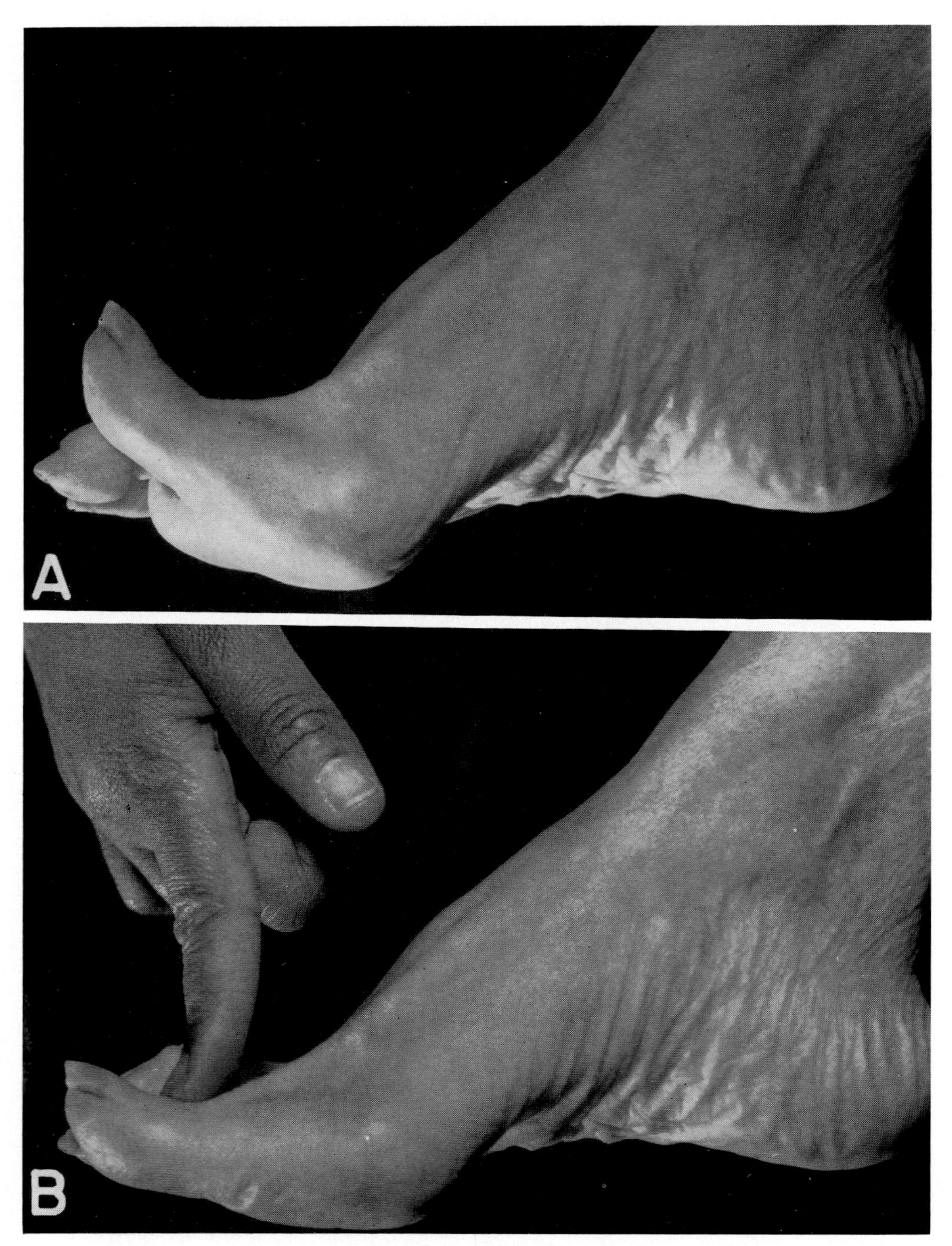

FIGURE 7–190. Hallux extensus.

A rare variety of hallux rigidus in which the first metatarsal is plantar-flexed and the great toe is held in hyperextension at the metatarsophalangeal joint. Note the hallux cannot be pushed plantarward. (From Kelikian, H.: Hallux Valgus, Allied Deformities of the Forefoot and Metatarsalgia. Philadelphia, Saunders, 1965, p. 269. Reprinted by permission.)

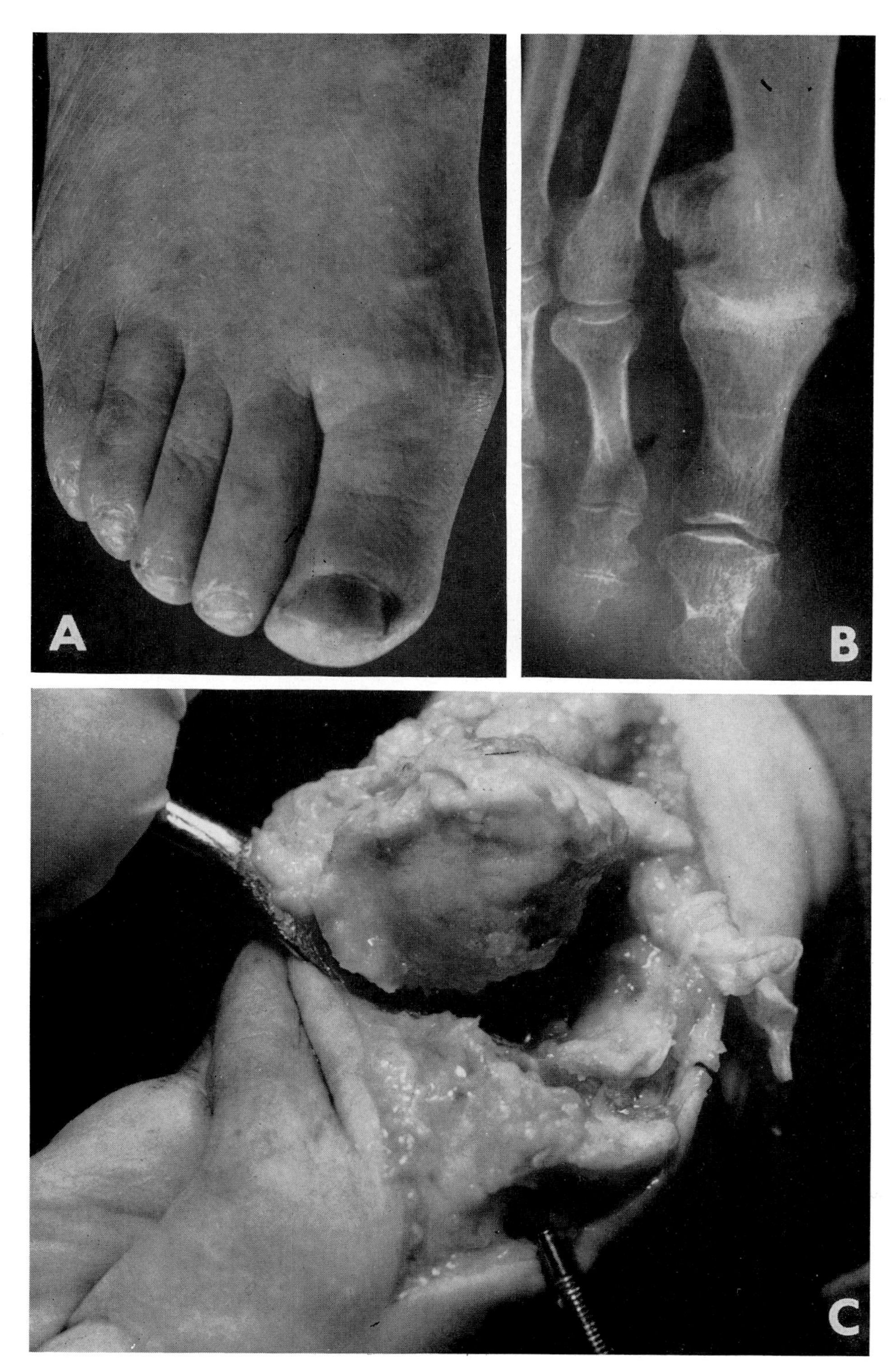

FIGURE 7–191. Hallux rigidus.

A. Photograph of the forefoot, showing enlargement of the first metatarsophalangeal joint. **B.** Radiograms. Note the degenerative changes—the articular cartilage space is obliterated and osteophytes have formed at the joint margins. **C.** Findings at operation. The hyaline articular cartilage is eroded, the synovium is thickened, and there is marked proliferation of new bone. (From Kelikian, H.: Hallux Valgus, Allied Deformities of the Forefoot and Metatarsalgia. Philadelphia, Saunders, 1965, p. 271. Reprinted by permission.)

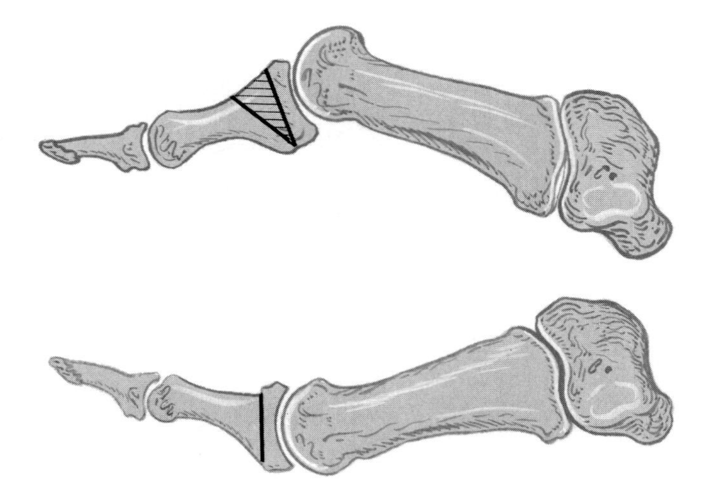

FIGURE 7–192. Kessel and Bonney osteotomy.

term follow-ups are not available. If metatarsus primus elevatus is the primary cause of hallux rigidus, the symptoms being due to restriction of dorsiflexion of the first metatarsophalangeal joint, extension osteotomy of the base of the first phalanx is worth a trial.

Depression of the first metatarsal head by a wedge osteotomy (with its base on the plantar aspect) was recommended by Jack.[17] This may prevent the development of hallux rigidus; however, experience with this procedure is limited.

In the adult in whom hallux rigidus is symptomatic and disabling, resection of the proximal half of the first phalanx of the great toe is recommended. If the sesamoid bones are involved in the arthritic process, they are also excised.

When hallux valgus is accompanied by metatarsalgia, Kelikian recommends fusion of the metatarsophalangeal joint of the great toe; in such an instance, the distal third of the second metatarsal is resected and its digit is syndactylized with the first or third toe. The optimum position of arthrodesis is 20 to 30 degrees valgus and 10 to 15 degrees of dorsiflexion in the male, 15 to 20 degrees of dorsiflexion in the female.

The operation is performed through a dorsomedial longitudinal incision. The joint cartilage is excised, and the denuded bony surfaces of the first metatarsal head and base of the proximal phalanx are snugly held in the desired position and internally fixed with a screw. The drill is directed proximally through the base of the proximal phalanx into the metatarsal, emerging on the side of the metatarsal. The screw head is countersunk and lies against the flare of the base of the proximal phalanx (Fig. 7–194). The foot is immobilized in a below-knee walking cast for six weeks.

Other methods are compression arthrodesis

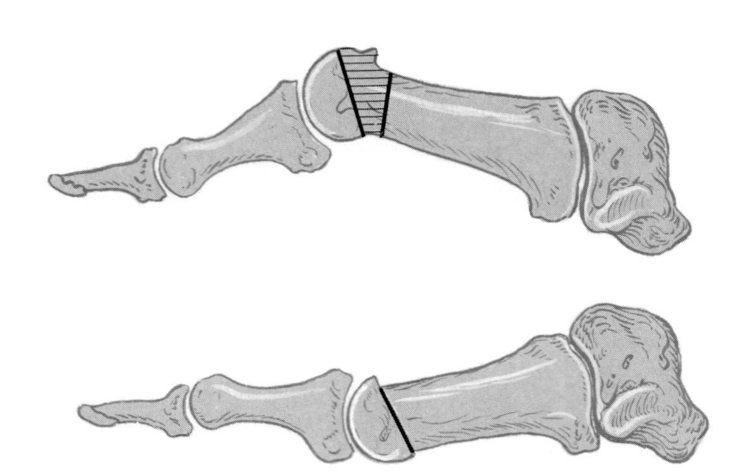

FIGURE 7–193. Watermann's cuneiform osteotomy of the first metatarsal bone.

Base of the wedge is directed dorsally and includes the hypertrophic spurs.

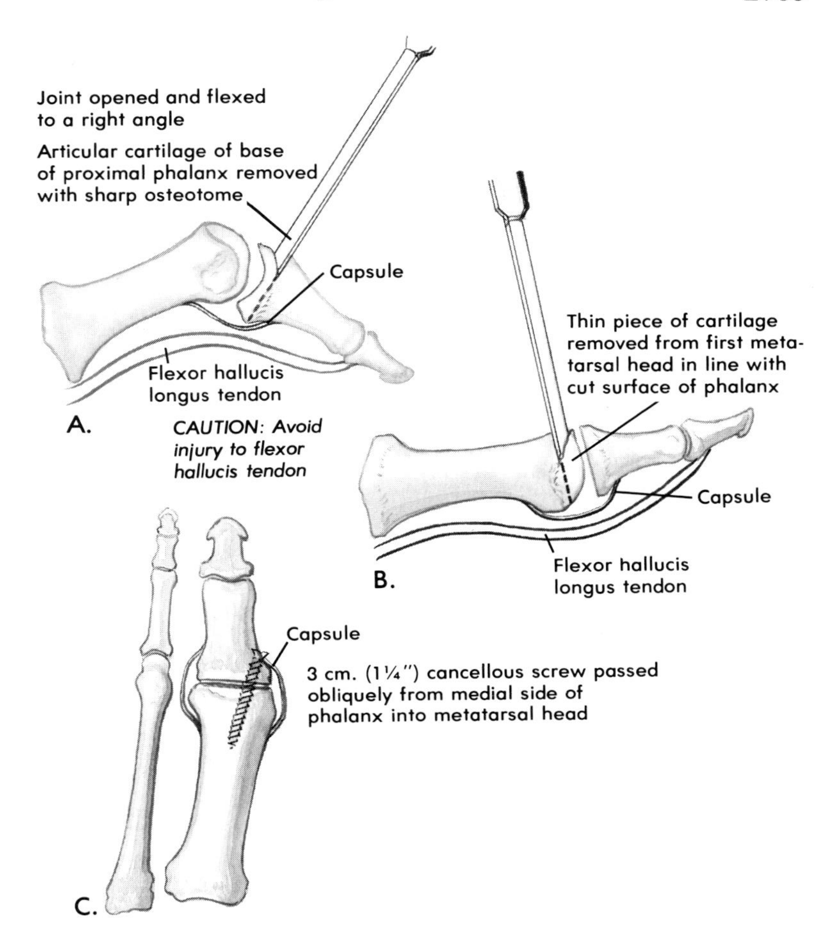

***FIGURE 7–194.** Arthrodesis of metatarsophalangeal joint of great toe and internal fixation with screw.*

(used by Harrison and Harvey) and cone fusion (used by Wilson).[15, 43] Long-term results of metatarsophalangeal joint fusion of the great toe reported by Fitzgerald are excellent.[8]

References

1. Bingold, A. C., and Collins, D. H.: Hallux rigidus. J. Bone Joint Surg., *32-B:*214, 1950.
2. Bonney, G., and Macnab, I.: Hallux valgus and hallux rigidus. A critical survey of operative results. J. Bone Joint Surg., *34-B:*366, 1952.
3. Breitenfelder, G.: Hallux rigidus Jugendlicher. Verh. Dtsch. Orthop. Ges., *80:*313, 1951.
4. Citron, N., and Neil, M.: Dorsal wedge osteotomy of the proximal phalanx for hallux rigidus. J. Bone Joint Surg., *69-B:*835, 1987.
5. Cochrane, W. A.: An operation for hallux rigidus. Br. Med. J., *1:*1095, 1927.
6. Cotterill, J. M.: On the condition of stiff great toe in adolescents. Edinburgh, Trans. Med. Chir. Soc., 1886–1887, p. 277.
7. Davies-Colley, N.: On contraction of the metatarso-phalangeal joint of the great toe (hallux flexus). Trans. Clin. Soc. Lond., *20:*165, 1887.
8. Fitzgerald, J. A. W.: Review of long-term results in arthrodesis of the first metatarsophalangeal joint. J. Bone Joint Surg., *51-B:*488, 1969.
9. Fixsen, J. A.: Hallux valgus and hallux rigidus. *In* Harris, N. H. (ed.): Postgraduate Textbook of Clinical Orthopaedics. Bristol, Wright PSG, 1983, pp. 166–167.
10. Glissan, D. J.: Hallux valgus and hallux rigidus. Med. J. Aust., *2:*585, 1946.
11. Goodfellow, J.: Aetiology of hallux rigidus. Proc. R. Soc. Med., *59:*821, 1966.
12. Gould, N.: Hallux rigidus: Cheilotomy or implant? Foot Ankle, *1:*315, 1981.
13. Harris, N. H.: Hallux rigidus. *In* Harris, N. H. (ed.): Postgraduate Textbook of Clinical Orthopaedics. Bristol, Wright PSG, 1983, pp. 859–860.
14. Harrison, M.: Hallux limitus. J. Bone Joint Surg., *53-B:*772, 1971.
15. Harrison, M. H. M., and Harvey, F. J.: Arthrodesis of the first metatarsophalangeal joint for hallux valgus and rigidus. J. Bone Joint Surg., *45-A:*471, 1963.
16. Heany, S. H.: Phalangeal osteotomy for hallux rigidus. J. Bone Joint Surg., *52-B:*799, 1970.
17. Jack, E. A.: The aetiology of hallus rigidus. Br. J. Surg., *27:*492, 1940.
18. Jansen, M.: Hallux valgus, rigidus and malleus. J. Orthop. Surg., *3:*27, 1921.
19. Judas, G. J.: An etiology of hallux rigidus. J. Foot Surg., *10:*113, 1971.
20. Kelikian, H.: Hallux Valgus, Allied Deformities of the Forefoot, and Metatarsalgia. Philadelphia, Saunders, 1965, p. 273.

21. Kelikian, H.: The hallux. *In* Jahss, M. H. (ed.): Disorders of the Foot. Philadelphia, Saunders, 1983, pp. 608–613.
22. Kessel, L., and Bonney, G.: Hallux rigidus in the adolescent. J. Bone Joint Surg., *40-B*:668, 1958.
23. Kingreen, O.: Zur Aetiologie des Hallux flexus. Zentralbl. Chir., *60*:2116, 1933.
24. Lambrinudi, C.: Metartarsus primus elevatus. Proc. R. Soc. Med. (Section of Orthopaedics), *31*:1273, 1938.
25. Lapidus, P. W.: "Dorsal bunion": Its mechanics and operative correction. J. Bone Joint Surg., *22*:627, 1940.
26. Lipscomb, P. R.: Arthrodesis of the first metatarsophalangeal joint for severe bunions and hallux rigidus. Clin. Orthop., *142*:48, 1979.
27. McKeever, D. C.: Arthrodesis of the first metatarsophalangeal joint for hallux valgus, hallux rigidus and metatarsus primus varus. J. Bone Joint Surg., *34-A*:129, 1952.
28. McMaster, M. J.: The pathogenesis of hallux rigidus. J. Bone Joint Surg., *60-B*:82, 1978.
29. McMurray, T. P.: The treatment of hallux valgus and rigidus. Br. Med. J., *2*:218, 1936.
30. Mann, R. A., Coughlin, M. J., and DuVries, H. L.: Hallux rigidus. A review of the literature and a method of treatment. Clin. Orthop., *142*:57, 1979.
31. Mau, C.: Das Krankheitsbild des Hallux rigidus. Munchen Med. Wochenschr., *75*:1193, 1928.
32. Miller, L. F., and Arendt, J.: Deformity of first metatarsal head due to faulty foot mechanics. J. Bone Joint Surg., *22*:349, 1940.
33. Moberg, E.: A simple operation for hallux rigidus. Clin. Orthop., *142*:55, 1979.
34. Molster, A. O., Lunde, O. D., and Rait, M.: Hallux rigidus treated with the Swanson Silastic hemi-joint prosthesis. Acta Orthop. Scand., *51*:853, 1980.
35. Moynihan, F. J.: Arthrodesis of the metatarsophalangeal joint of the great toe. J. Bone Joint Surg., *49-B*:544, 1967.
36. Nilsonne, H.: Hallux rigidus and its treatment. Acta Orthop. Scand., *1*:295, 1930.
37. Severin, E.: Removal of the base of the proximal phalanx in hallus rigidus. Acta Orthop. Scand., *17*:77, 1947.
38. Steinhauser, W.: Osteochondrose der basalen Epiphyse der Grandphalanx, Grosszehe und Hallux rigidus. Beitr. Ges. Orthop., *6*:177, 1959.
39. Thompson, F. M., and Mann, R. A.: Arthritides. *In* Mann, R. A. (ed.): Surgery of the Foot. St. Louis, Mosby, 1986, pp. 159–164.
40. Walsham, W. J., and Hughes, W. K.: The Deformities of the Human Foot. London, Bailliere, Tindall & Cox, 1895, pp. 512–514.
41. Watermann, H.: Die Arthritis deformans Grosszehengrundgelenkes. Z. Orthop. Chir., *48*:346, 1927.
42. Watson-Jones, R.: Treatment of hallux rigidus. Br. Med. J., *1*:1165, 1927.
43. Wilson, J. N.: Oblique displacement osteotomy of hallux valgus. J. Bone Joint Surg., *45-B*:552, 1963.

Tumors of the Foot

Tumors of the foot are uncommon in children. If they do occur, they may originate in either the soft tissues or bone, and may be either benign or malignant. Metastatic tumors distal to the knee are extremely rare.

The usual presenting complaints are a swelling or mass, difficulty in fitting shoes, and local pain or a limp. To detect minimal findings, it is essential to examine both feet, comparing the suspected pathologic limb with the contralateral normal limb. The exact site of the problem should be determined, whether it is in the soft tissues (subcutaneous tissue, fascia, muscle, tendon, or nerve), the joint, or the bone. Is the consistency of the swelling cystic, firm, or bony? Is the mass fixed to subjacent bone or is it freely movable? Are its boundaries well-delineated or ill-defined and does it infiltrate adjacent tissues? Can it be transilluminated? What is the color of the overlying skin? Are the superficial veins dilated? Is there increased local heat? Does the mass pulsate? Upon tourniquet ischemia, does it decrease in size? The regional lymph nodes of the entire lower limb are also palpated for enlargement and tenderness. Radiograms of the foot are made to determine bony and soft-tissue alterations. The more common tumors causing problems in the foot are briefly described here.

SOFT-TISSUE TUMORS

Lipoma

Lipoma, one of the more common tumors in the foot, is seen in infants as well as in older children. It is usually located in the subcutaneous tissue of the instep of the foot, or deep to the plantar fascia (Figs. 7–195 and 7–196). Occasionally it may be found on the dorsum of the foot involving tendon sheaths or digital nerves. The mass is soft, generally lobulated, and surrounded by a definite capsule. The histologic picture varies, depending upon the amount of fibrous and myxomatous tissue associated with the fat.

On palpation, the mass has a soft flabby feeling, suggesting fluctuation. Its boundaries are usually not distinct. On the radiograms, the lipoma casts a soft-tissue shadow of "fatty density."

Treatment consists of surgical excision of the tumor. If the lesion is not completely removed, it may recur. It is best to perform the procedure with tourniquet ischemia with the child under general anesthesia.

Ganglion

The usual locations of this common tumorous lesion are on the dorsum of the foot in the

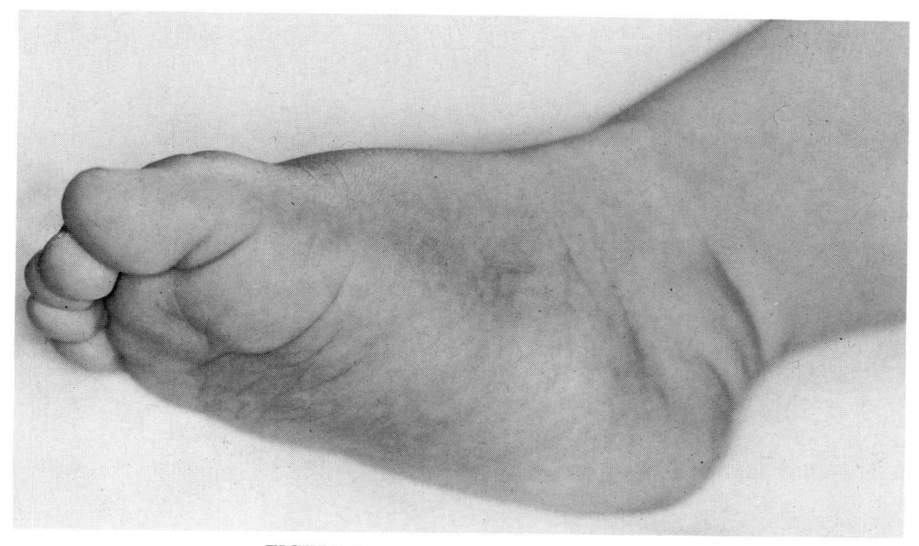

FIGURE 7–195. Lipoma of the right foot.

The mass was encapsulated and located deep to the plantar fascia.

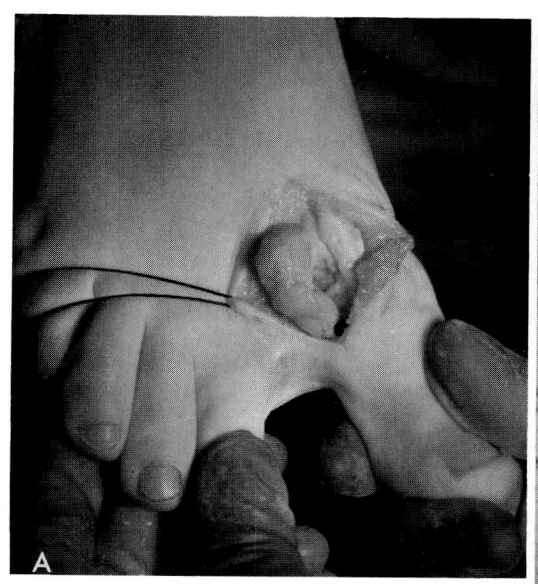

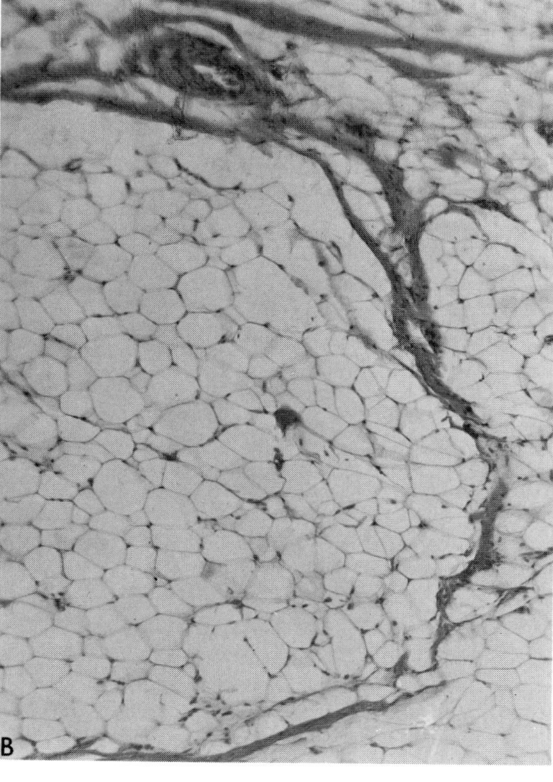

FIGURE 7–196. Lipoma on dorsum of the foot between the first and second metatarsal heads.

A. Appearance at surgery. **B.** Photomicrograph showing the fat cells (× 100).

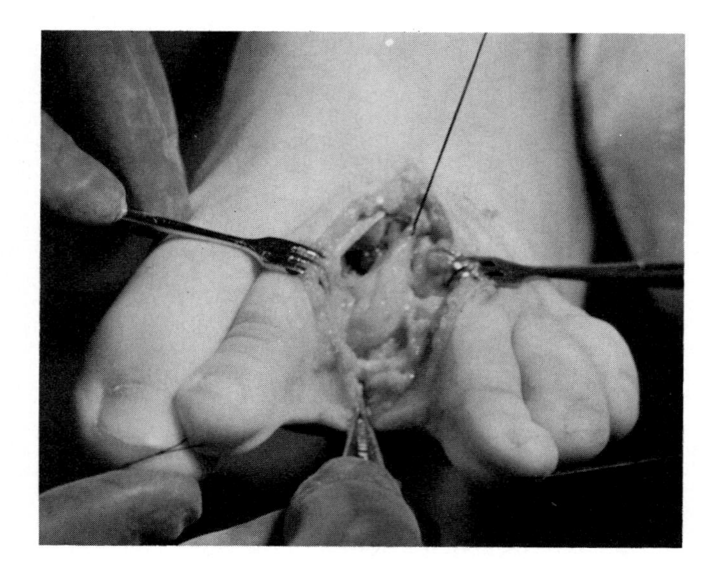

FIGURE 7–197. Ganglion between the second and third toes.

Gross appearance of the cyst at operation.

midtarsal area, in between the toes, and in the region of the ankle adjacent to the lateral or medial malleolus (Figs. 7–197 and 7–198). The thin-walled cyst contains clear colorless gelatinous fluid and seems to arise from tendon sheaths or from within the connective tissue of the subjacent joint capsule. Surgical excision of ganglia is usually indicated if they interfere with the normal fit of the shoe or if they are painful on weight-bearing (Fig. 7–199). Rupture of the cyst by external force or aspiration of its contents and injection of hydrocortisone are, as a rule, inadequate, and the ganglion eventually recurs. The best treatment is complete excision, which should be performed in the operating room with the child under general anesthesia and tourniquet ischemia. The ligamentous tissue at the base of the stalk of the ganglion should be removed or scarified to prevent recurrence.

Hemangioma

Angiomata may be of congenital origin, presenting at birth, or they may develop in childhood or adolescence. The cavernous type is more common. In the foot, hemangioma may involve the skin and subcutaneous tissue, or it may involve the muscle and tendon (Figs. 7–200, 7–201, and 7–202). The tarsal bones may be invaded. The instep and plantar aspect of the foot are favored locations. Occasionally the lesion affecting the foot may be part of diffuse hemangiomatosis affecting the entire lower limb (Fig. 7–203).

The presenting complaint is of a compressible mass, which may be irritated by the shoe. When one obstructs the venous return, the mass enlarges. Occasionally the lesion may be painful when it invades nervous tissue or when it is located in bone and expansion is taking place. When hemangioma involves the skin, its external appearance is characteristic and diagnosis is not difficult.

Treatment consists of meticulous and complete excision of the lesion. Large tumors may require surgical resection in two or three stages. Tourniquet ischemia controls hemorrhage, but it is disadvantageous because part of the lesion may be overlooked. Because the tissues often heal poorly, careful handling and hemostasis of the wound are required. Radiation therapy should not be employed in the treatment of hemangioma in children, but cryotherapy may occasionally be indicated.

Aneurysm in the foot and ankle may result from blunt trauma, which weakens the vessel walls, or from penetrating wounds. During triple arthrodesis, aneurysm of the posterior tibial vessels may be caused by injury with an osteotome (Fig. 7–204).

Lymphangiectasis

In this condition the foot and often the entire lower limb are edematous and enlarged owing to replacement of normal subcutaneous tissue by dilated lymphatics (Fig. 7–205). In later life, fibrous changes take place in the lesion. When the abnormality is familial, it is known as "Mil-

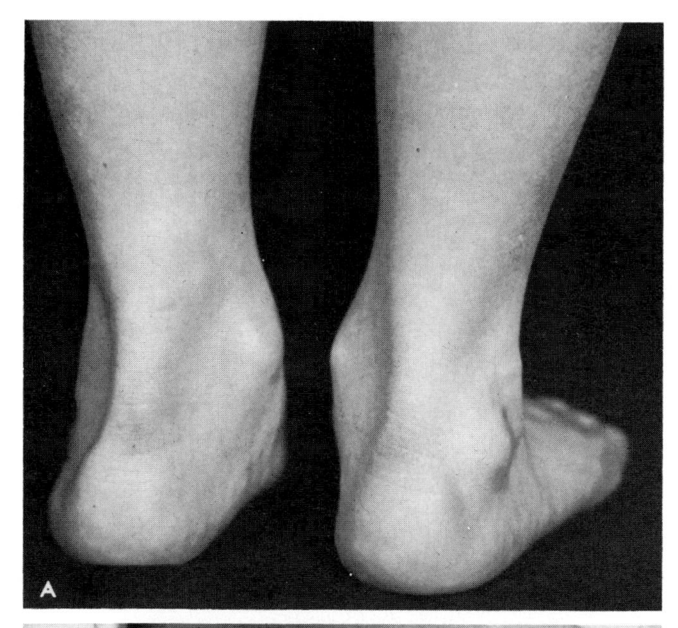

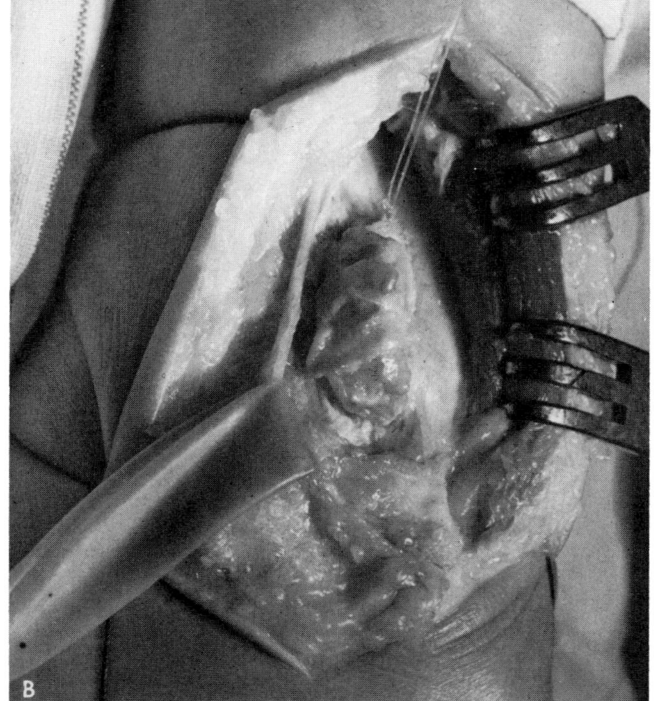

FIGURE 7–198. Ganglion in the region of the right ankle behind the lateral malleolus.

A. Photograph shows the mass behind the lateral malleolus. **B.** Gross appearance of the cyst at surgery.

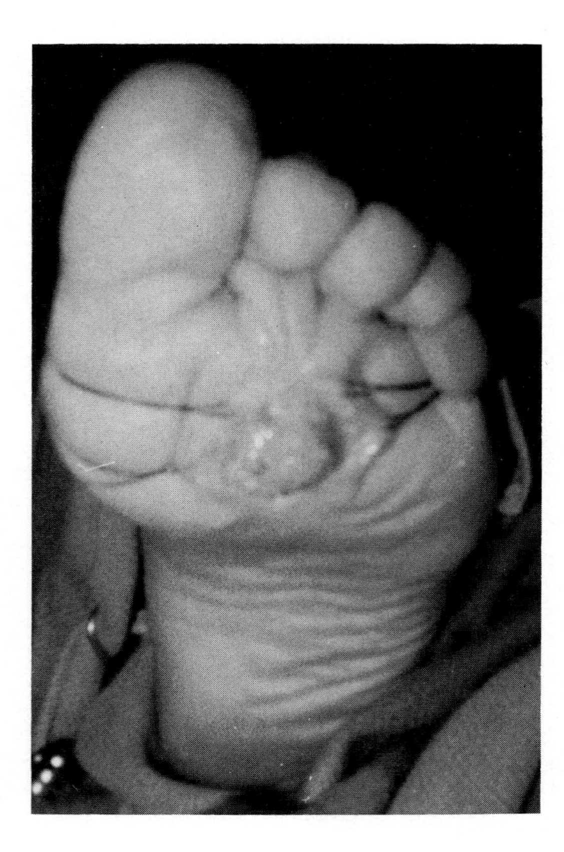

FIGURE 7–199. Ganglion on the sole of the foot, presenting as a painful mass.

roy's disease." The condition should not be mistaken for a tumor; in doubtful cases, lymphangiography will establish the diagnosis.

Treatment consists of application of elastic bandages or stockings at night to shrink the dilated lymphatics. Excision of abnormal tissue is difficult but possible. The resulting defects are covered by salvaged skin and skin grafts.

Recurrent Digital Fibroma in Childhood

Digital fibrous tumors in infancy and childhood are rare.* They are limited to the fingers and toes and have a marked tendency to recur. There is no sex predilection. The lesions are multiple in about 50 per cent of cases. The tumors either are present at birth or, with few exceptions, develop in the first few months of infancy.

The tumors appear as small nodules on the lateral surfaces of the distal parts of the fingers and toes; occasionally they may be on the dorsal aspect of a digit. In multicentric cases the opposing surfaces of the toes are affected. The color of the overlying skin is normal or slightly red. The mass is firm in consistency, nontender, and fixed to the skin and underlying deep tissues. The tumor may grow either slowly or rapidly, reaching enormous size and encircling the digit. It is grayish white in color, fibrous, and not encapsulated.

On histologic examination of the lesion the epidermis is normal. The tumor is located in the dermis and consists of interlacing bands of fibrous connective tissue with abundant collagen. The size of nuclei varies; mitosis is infrequent.

Two forms of fibroblasts can be visualized on electron microscopy: in Type I the nucleus is large and lobulated with scanty endoplasmic reticulum; and in Type II the nucleus is small and flattened with a greater amount of endoplasmic reticulum. Some authors have demonstrated the presence of cytoplasmic inclusion bodies; others were unable to find them despite a thorough search.[4]

*See references 1, 2, 4, 7, 8, 30, 33, 42.

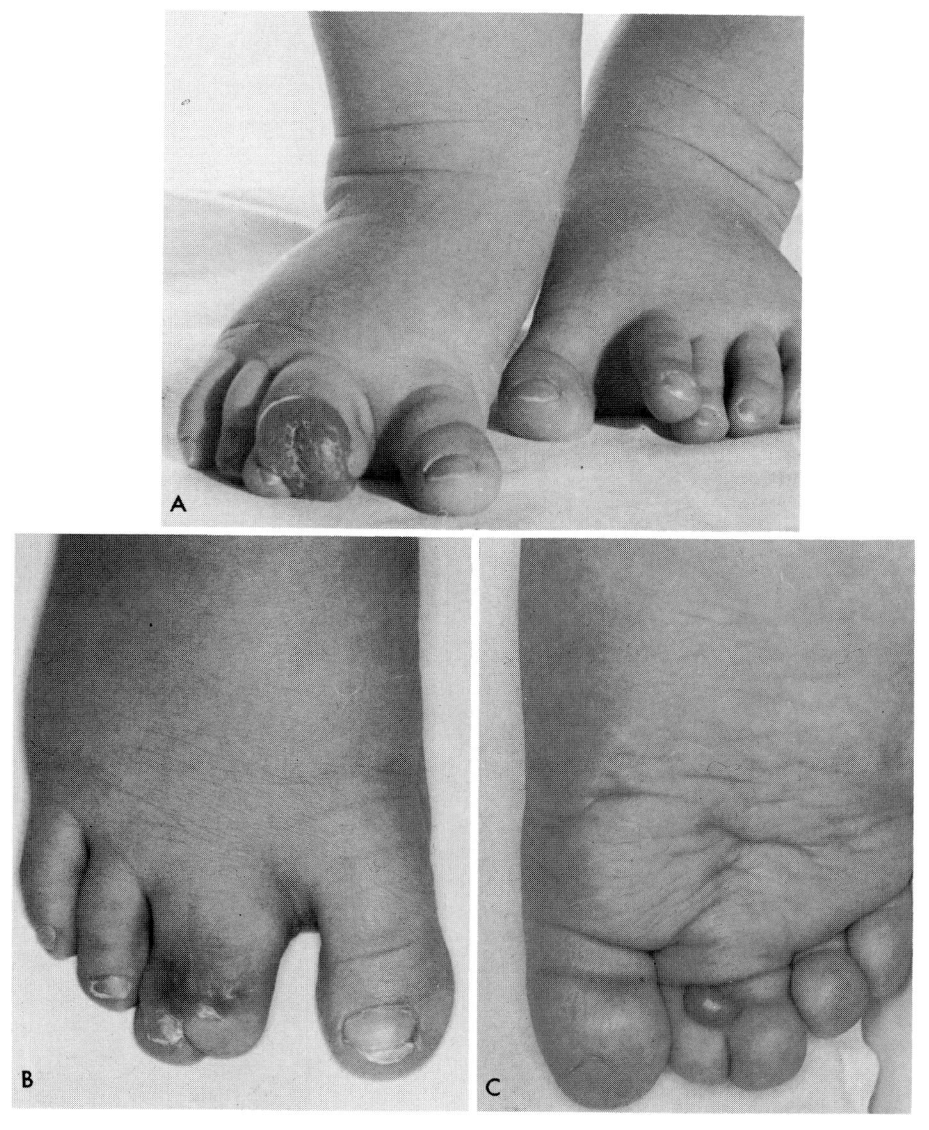

FIGURE 7–200. Hemangioma involving skin and subcutaneous tissue of the second and third toes.

A. Preoperative appearance. **B** and **C.** The lesion recurred one year following surgical removal. Again it was totally excised and the second and third toes were surgically syndactylized. Five-year follow-up showed no recurrence of the tumor.

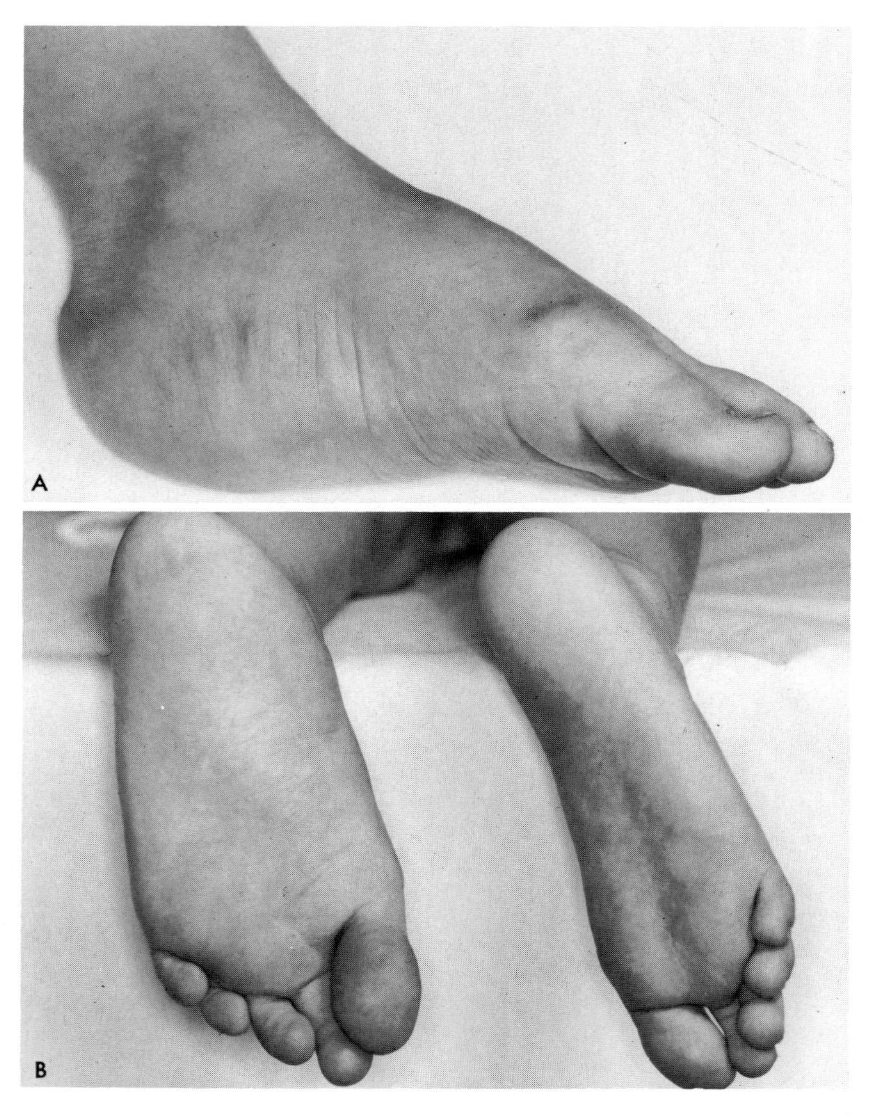

FIGURE 7–201. Cavernous hemangioma involving the subcutaneous tissue of the instep and the short plantar muscles.

A and **B.** Clinical appearance.

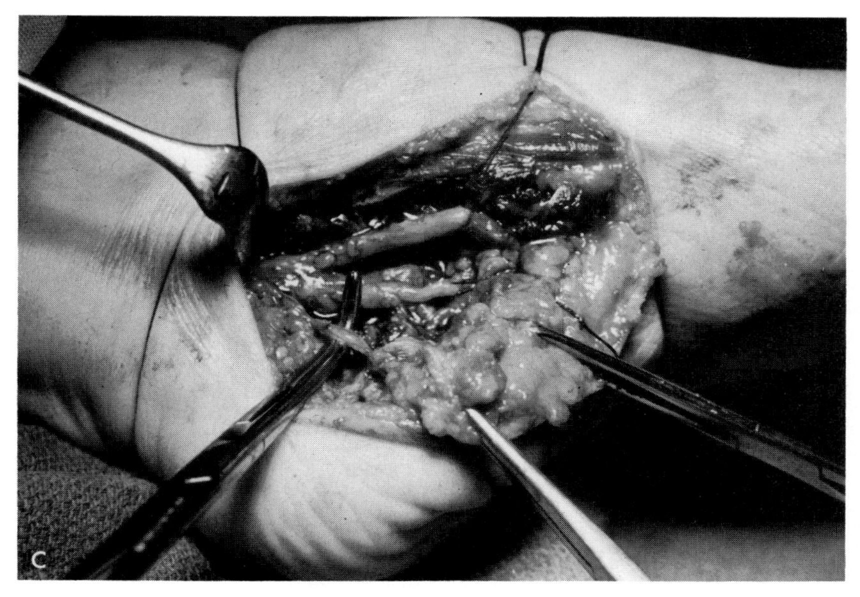

FIGURE 7–201 Continued. Cavernous hemangioma involving the subcutaneous tissue of the instep and the short plantar muscles.

C. Gross appearance at surgery.

A virus is believed to be the cause of the tumor, but its presence has not been demonstrated by tissue culture.

The natural history of the tumor is local recurrence after excision, followed by slow spontaneous regression. There is no recorded case of metastasis and no reported case of persistence into adult life. Therefore, a conservative approach in management is recommended. Treatment consists of local excision with skin grafting, if necessary. The surgeon is strongly urged to refrain from amputation and impairment of the function of the part. In certain cases, this calls for the establishment of a high level of confidence between parent and surgeon.

Nerve Sheath Tumors

The *benign encapsulated neurilemoma* is the most common type. In the past there has been some controversy as to its origin, but tissue culture studies favor development from the Schwann cells.[28] The tumor presents as a round or fusiform white mass within the sheath of the medial or lateral plantar nerve or in the smaller digital branches (Fig. 7–206). On palpation the tumor is firm in consistency, although occasionally it may be cystic. When located in weight-bearing areas of the foot it is painful and tender on pressure. It is usually solitary, but may be multiple.

On surgical exploration the tumor is usually well encapsulated. When the capsule is opened by a longitudinal incision it can be easily enucleated. Histologically the lesion is classified by Thorsrud into three types: in *Type I* there are a loose reticulum of cells with small nuclei and radiating fibrils with areas of cystic degeneration (Antoni B areas); in *Type II* the lesion predominantly consists of long slender cells with the nuclei arranged in a palisade fashion (Antoni A areas); *Type III* is a combination of Type I and Type II.[42]

Treatment is surgical excision; the encapsulated tumors are easy to shell out without damaging continuity of the nerve. The lesion is benign and the prognosis excellent.

Malignant neurilemomas are extremely rare in children; often they are associated with von Recklinghausen's disease.

Miscellaneous Tumors

Solitary fibroma is rare but may occur at any site in the foot and ankle; treatment is by surgical excision. Fibromatosis of plantar fascia does occur in adolescents, causing pain and disability; it is treated by excision of the plantar fascia.

Text continued on page 2780

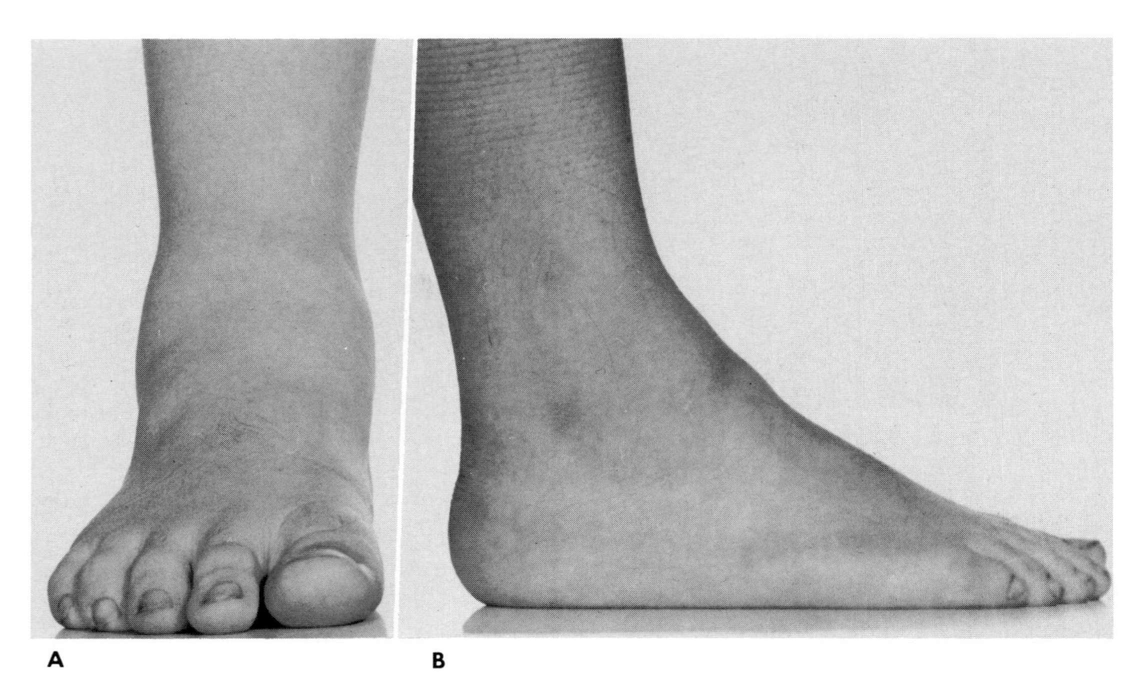

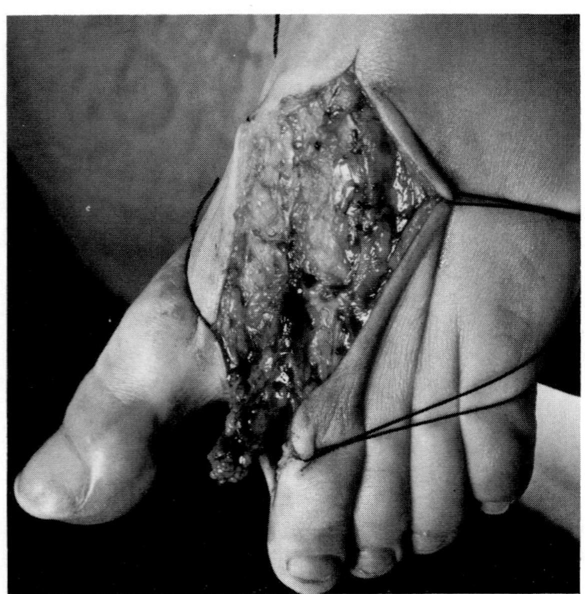

FIGURE 7–202. Cavernous hemangioma involving tendon sheaths on the dorsum of the foot.

A and **B.** Preoperative appearance. The condition was misdiagnosed, and the patient was treated for rheumatoid arthritis of the ankle and subtalar joints. Note the soft-tissue swelling. **C.** Gross appearance at surgery.

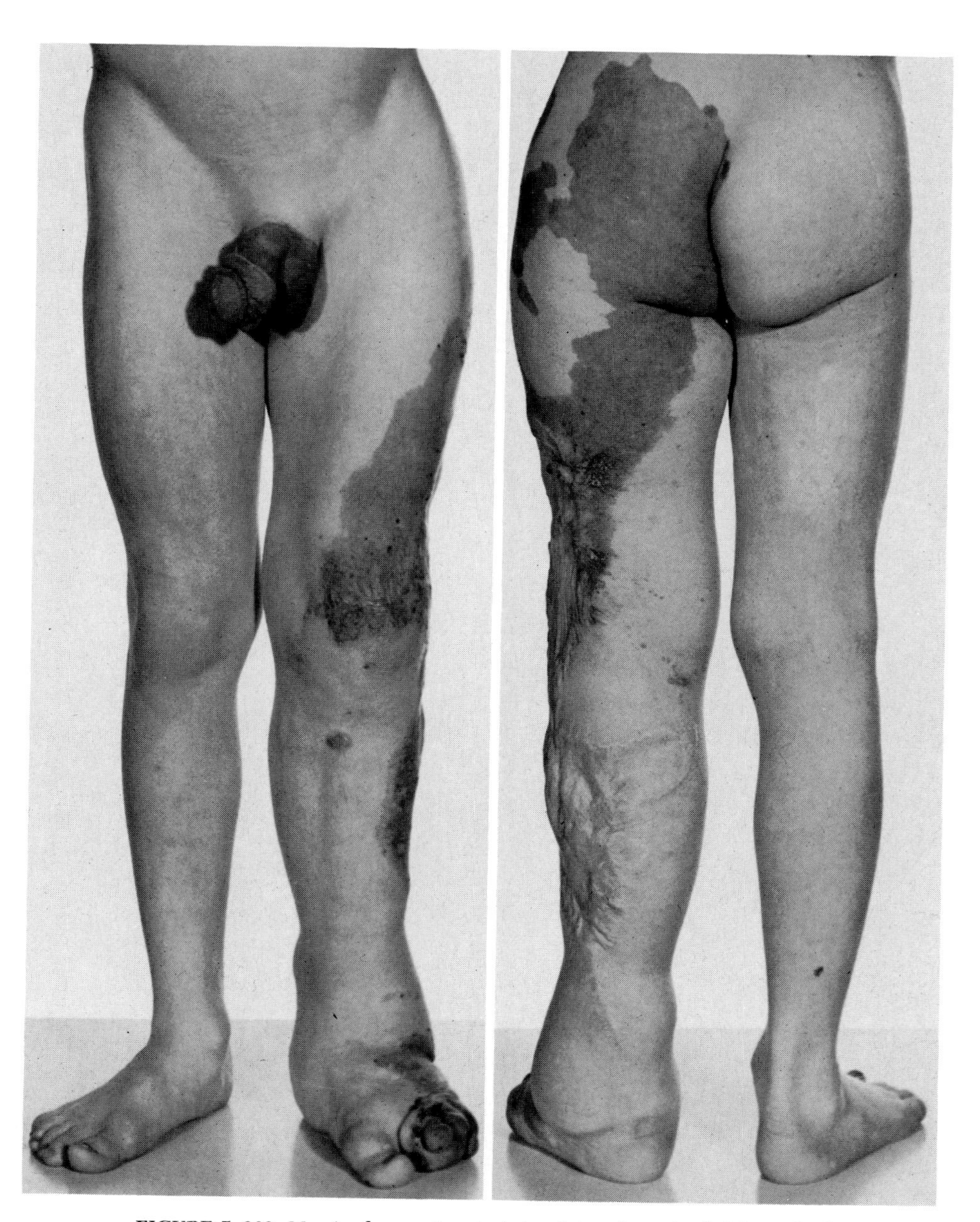

FIGURE 7–203. Massive hemangiomatosis involving the entire left lower limb.

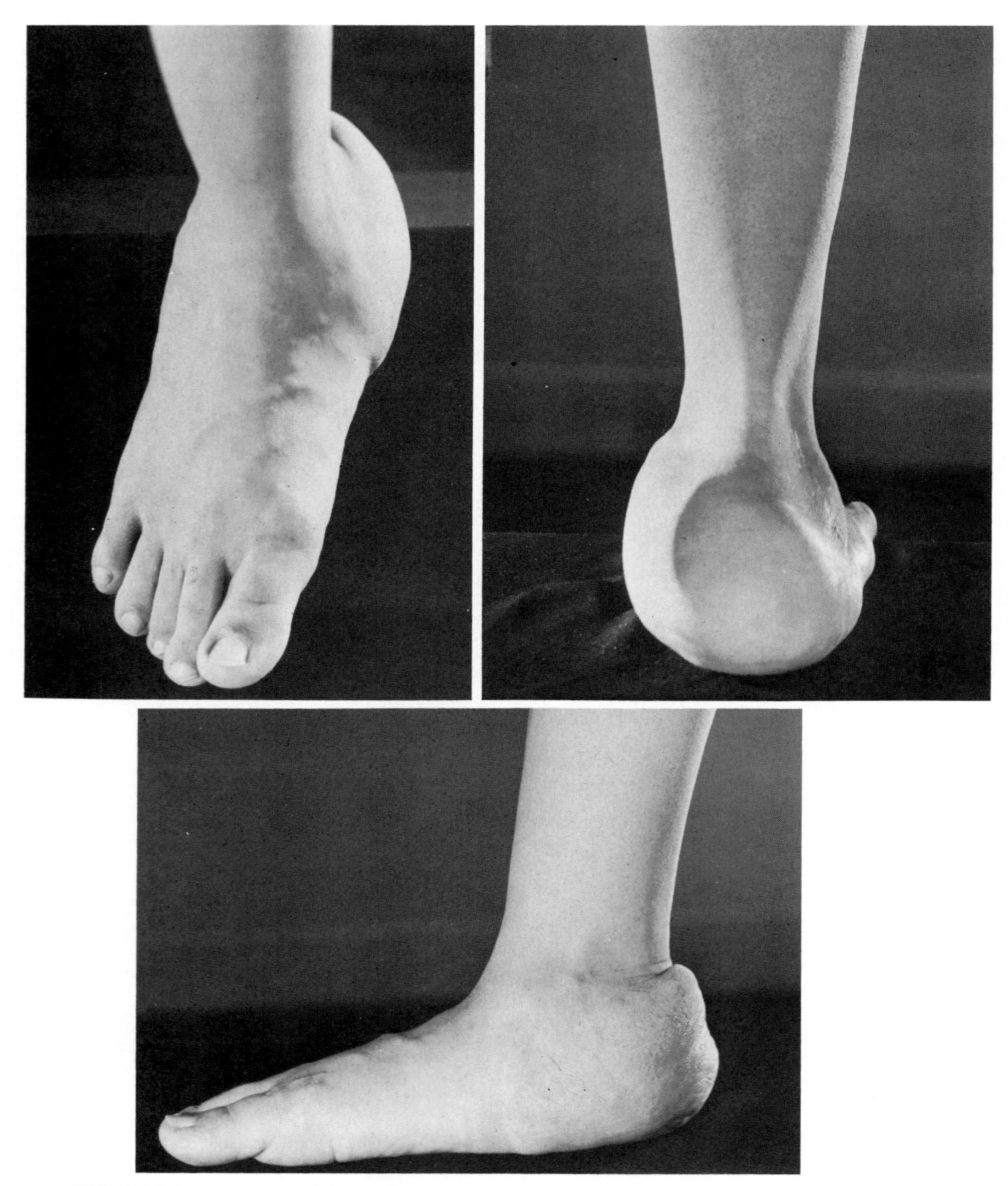

FIGURE 7–204. Aneurysm of the posterior tibial artery caused by injury during triple arthrodesis.

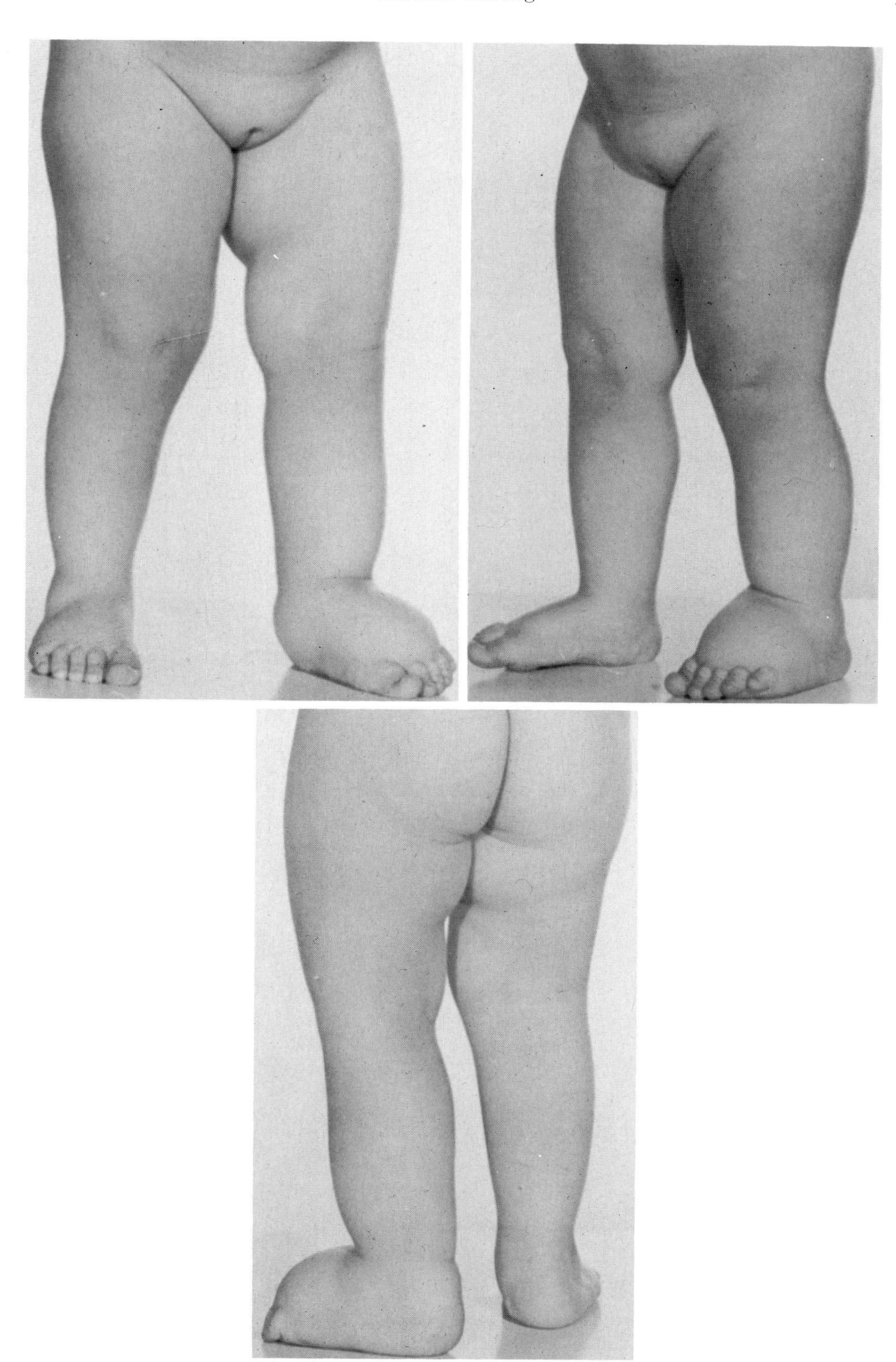

FIGURE 7–205. Lymphangiectasis of the left foot and leg.

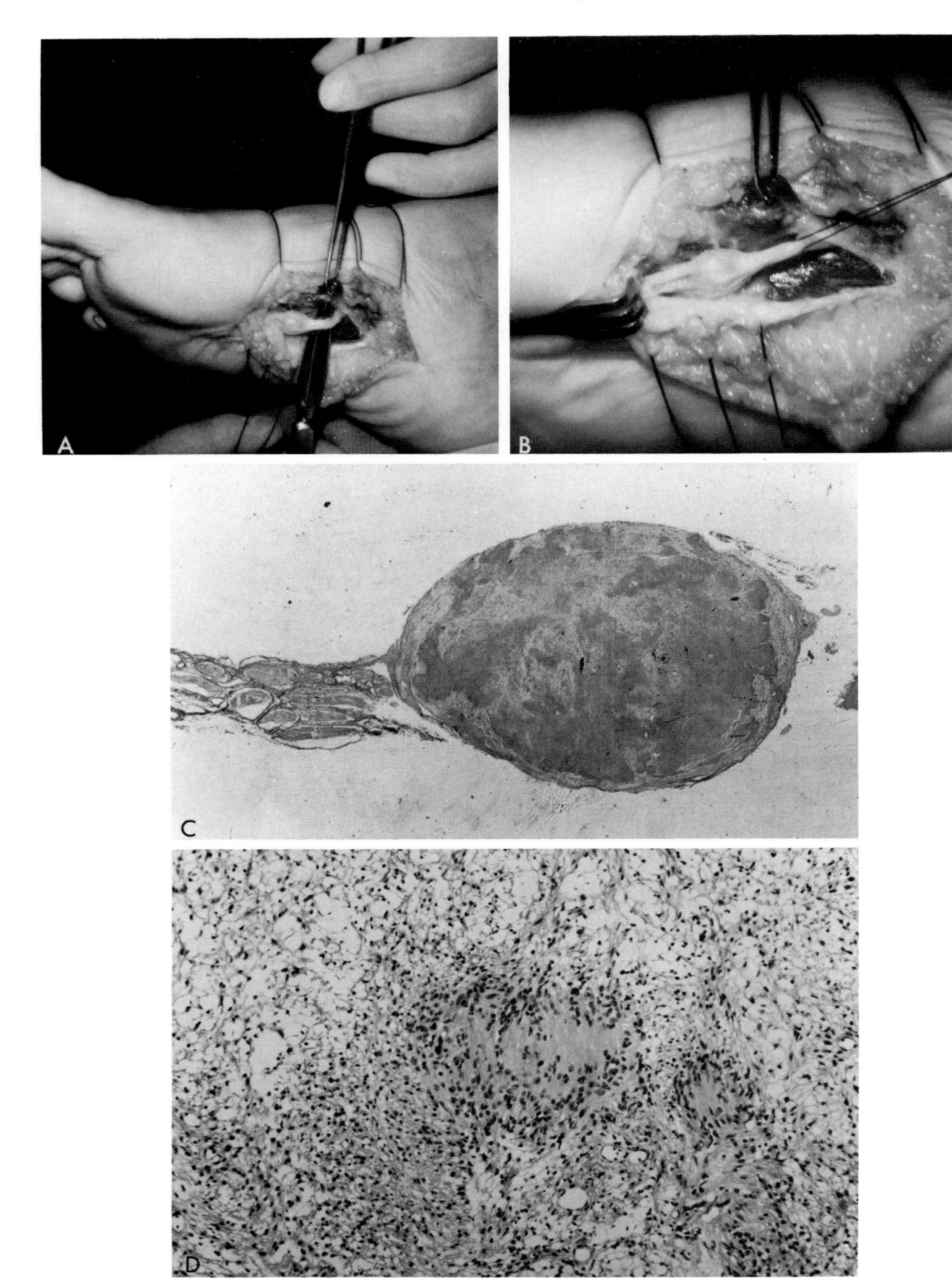

FIGURE 7–206. Solitary benign encapsulated neurilemoma of the medial plantar nerve.

A. Gross appearance in the wound. **B.** Close-up view showing the fusiform encapsulated mass. **C.** Photomicrograph of tumor (× 10). **D.** Photomicrograph showing palisading of long slender cells mixed with areas of loose reticulum cells with small nuclei (× 100). Note areas of cystic degeneration.

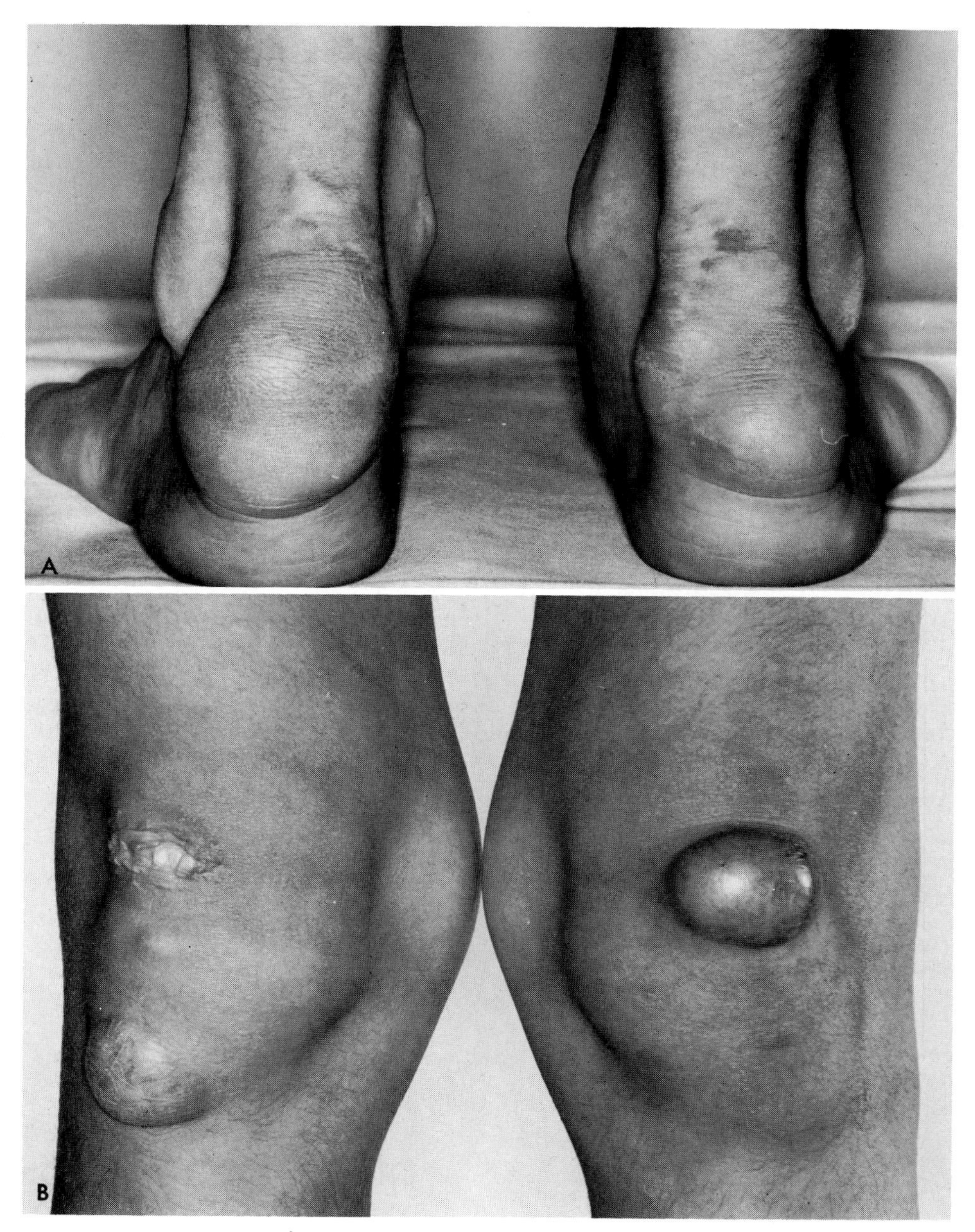

FIGURE 7–207. Multiple xanthomatosis involving both heels (A) and the extensor surfaces of knees (B).

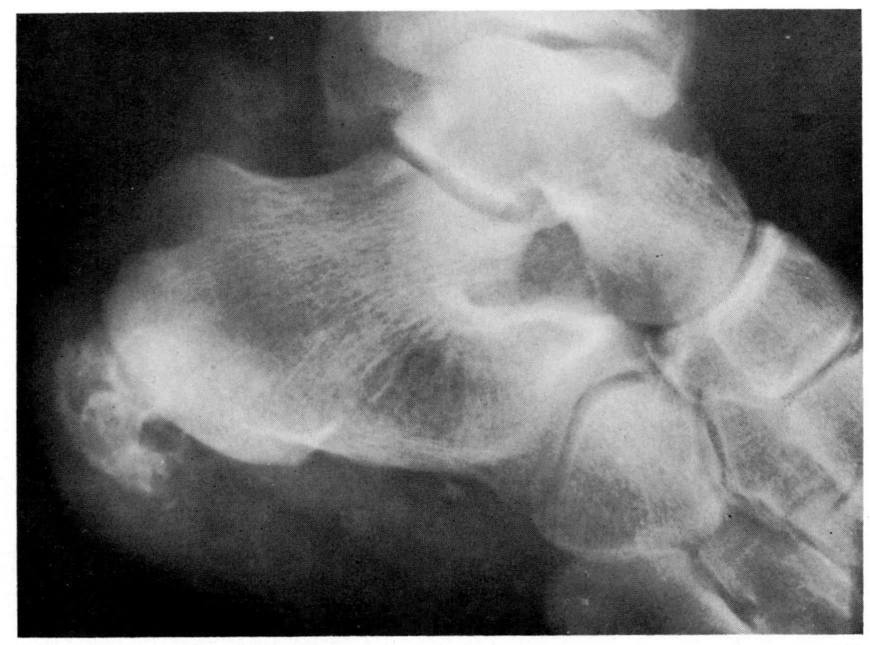

FIGURE 7–208. Tumoral calcinosis presenting as firm calcified mass in the posterior aspect of the heel.

Other soft-tissue tumors that may affect the foot are multiple xanthomatosis, tumoral calcinosis, and pigmented villonodular synovitis (Figs. 7–207 to 7–209). Glomus tumor is rarely found in children. Foreign body granuloma may present as a mass in the feet (Fig. 7–210).

Synovioma is very rare in childhood and adolescence but can occur (Fig. 7–211). Fibrosarcoma is extremely rare (Fig. 7–212).

TUMORS OF BONE

Tumors of bone occasionally occur in the foot, involving the tarsal and metatarsal bones. Osteoid osteoma (shown in Fig. 7–213), enchondroma, aneurysmal bone cyst (shown in Fig. 7–214), unicameral bone cyst (shown in Figs. 7–215 and 7–216), intraosseous lipoma (Fig. 7–217), and multiple hereditary exostoses are some of the lesions encountered; the reader is referred to the excellent textbooks of Dahlin, Jaffe, and Lichtenstein.[9, 18, 23]

A bony tumor characteristically found in the foot is subungual exostosis. It presents as a bony growth from the dorsal surface of the distal part of the terminal phalanx of a toe, usually the great toe. A history of previous injury may be obtained in some cases; its cause, however, is unknown. The condition is usually encountered in adolescents or young adults and is preponderant in females. The tumor projects upward and forward between the tip of the nail and the terminal pulp. The nail is deformed, becomes elevated, and eventually undergoes degenerative changes. The tumor is very painful, especially when pressure is applied over the nail. Diagnosis is made by demonstration of the exostosis on the radiogram (Fig. 7–218). It is treated by excision through a transverse incision at the distal end of the nail.

Malignant tumors of the bone in the region of the foot and ankle are very rare in childhood (Fig. 7–219).

References

1. Ahlqvist, J., Pohjanpelto, P., Hjelt, L., and Hurme, K.: Recurring digital fibrous tumor of childhood. 1. Clinical and morphological aspects of a case. Acta Pathol. Microbiol. Scand., *70*:291, 1967.
2. Battifora, H., and Hines, J. R.: Recurrent digital fibromas of childhood. Cancer, *27*:1530, 1971.
3. Bergstrand, H.: Über eine eigenartige wahrscheinlich bisher nicht beschriebene osteoblastische Krankheit in den longen Knochen der Hand und der Fusses. Acta Radiol., *11*:597, 1930.
4. Bloem, J. J., Vuzevski, V. D., and Huffstadt, A. J. C.: Recurring digital fibroma of infancy. J. Bone Joint Surg., *56-B*:746, 1974.
5. Boyle, W. J.: Cystic angiomatosis of bone. A report of three cases and review of the literature. J. Bone Joint Surg., *54-B*:626, 1972.
6. Brown, R. C., and Ghormley, R. K.: Solitary eccentric (cortical) abscess in bone. Surgery, *14*:541, 1943.
7. Burry, A. F., Kerr, J. F. R., and Pope, J. H.: Recurring digital fibrous tumour of childhood: An electron microscopic and virological study. Pathology, *2*:287, 1970.

Text continued on page 2785

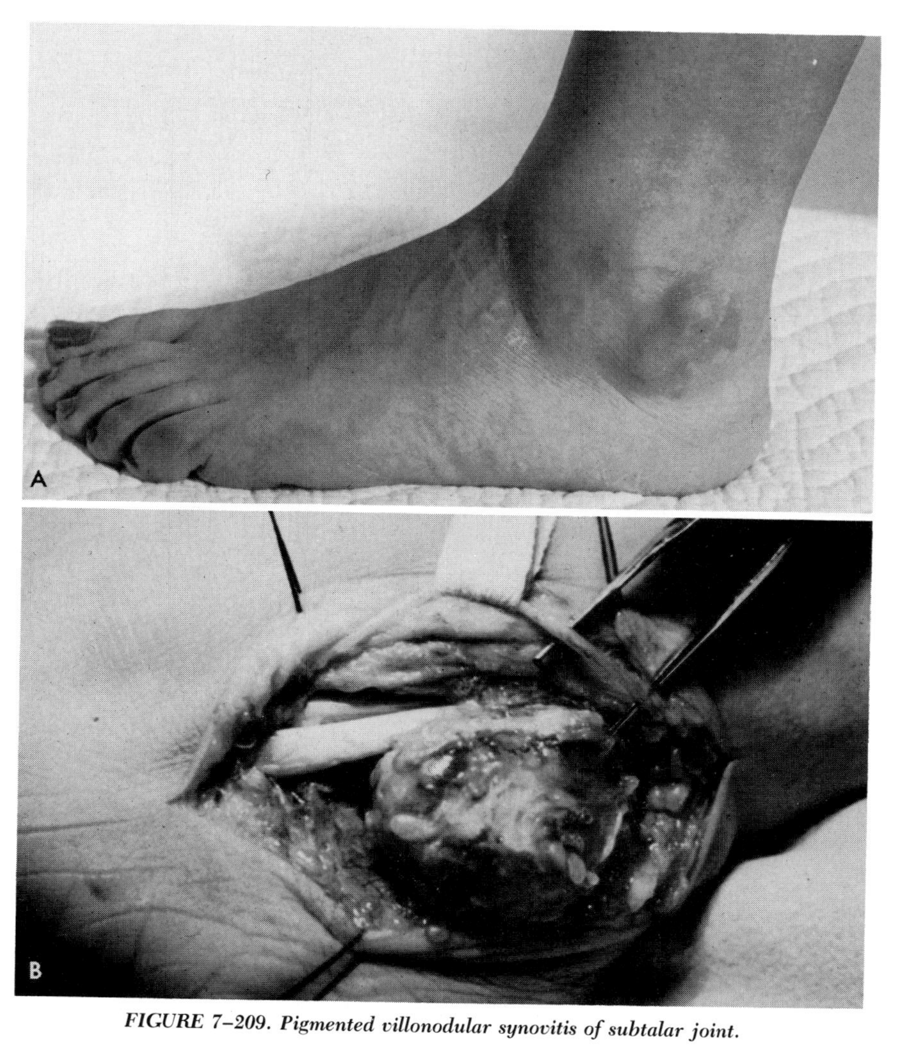

FIGURE 7–209. Pigmented villonodular synovitis of subtalar joint.

A. Photograph showing soft-tissue mass below the lateral malleolus. **B.** Gross appearance at surgery.

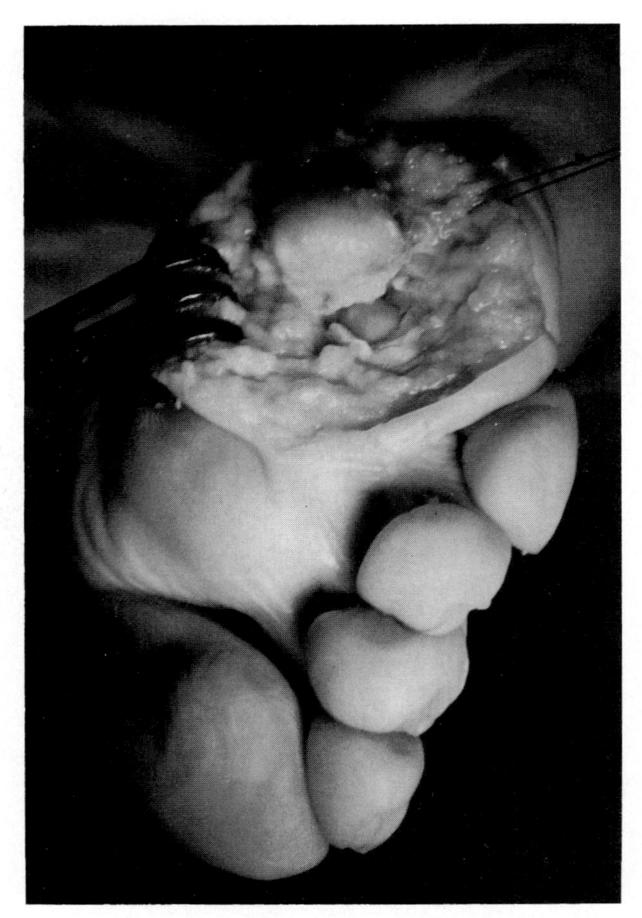

FIGURE 7–210. Foreign body granuloma in sole of foot—caused by a piece of broken glass.

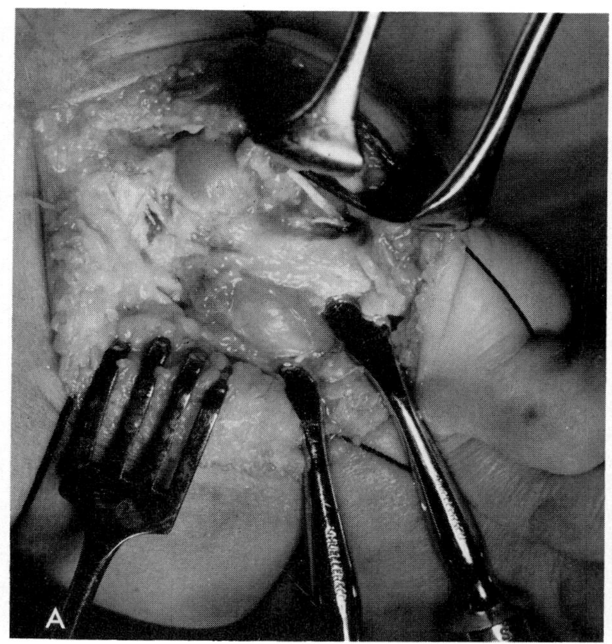

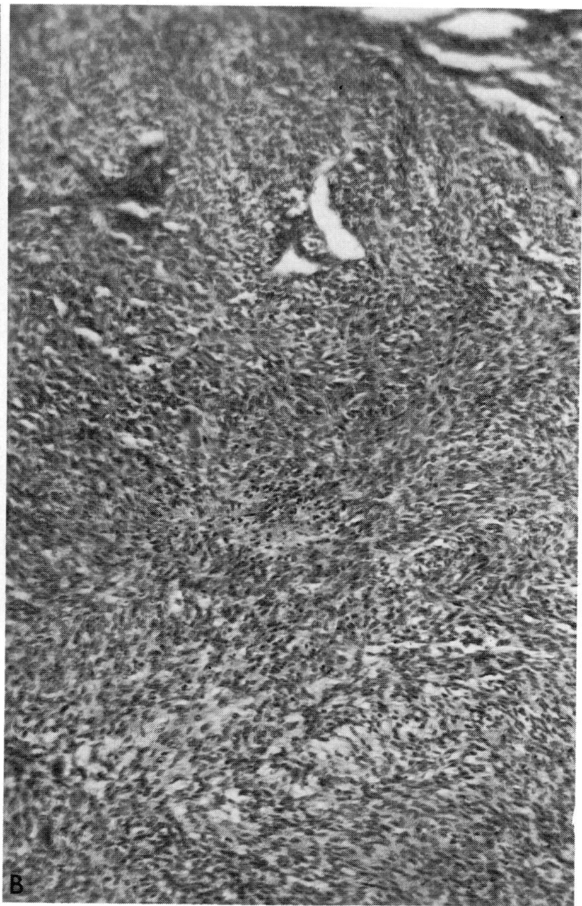

FIGURE 7–211. Synovioma in the plantar aspect of the foot.

A. Gross appearance at surgery. **B.** Photomicrograph (× 130)

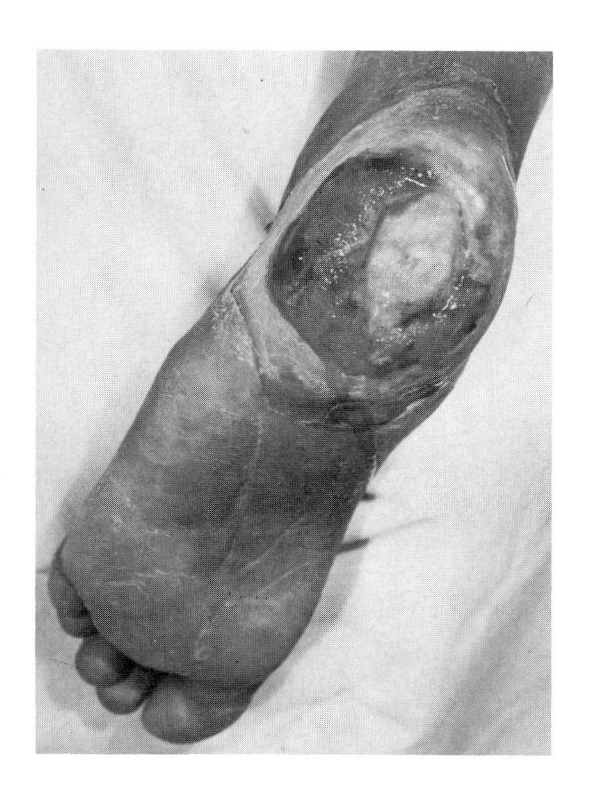

FIGURE 7–212. Fibrosarcoma of the heel.

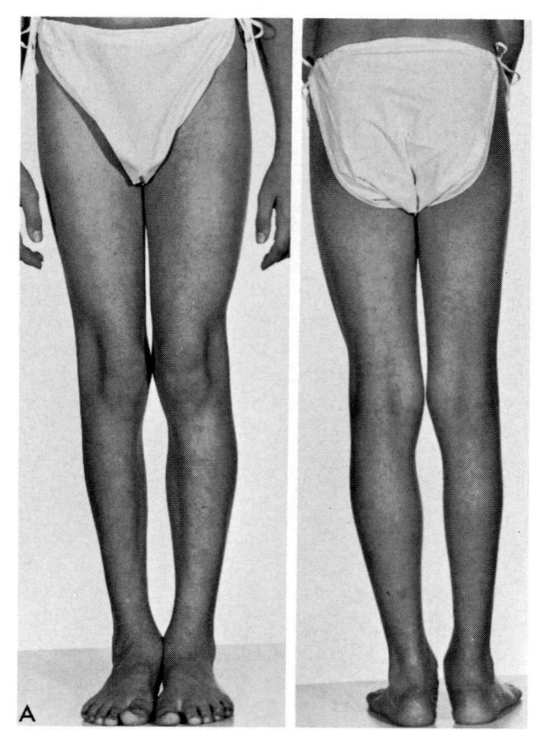

FIGURE 7–213. Osteoid osteoma of the talus.

A 12-year-old girl presented with a right antalgic limp of one year's duration. **A.** Photographs of the patient show disuse atrophy of the right leg. **B** and **C.** Radiograms of ankle. Note the radiolucent lesion in the superomedial area of the talus. Clinically, there was excruciating local tenderness on palpation.

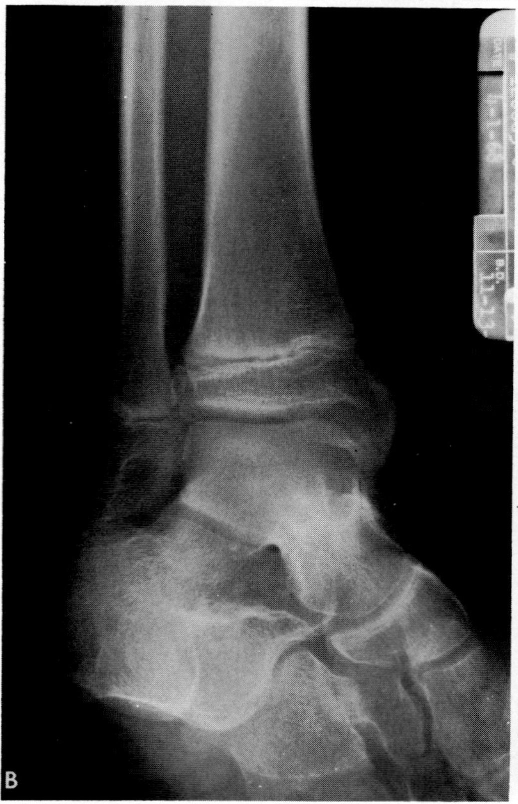

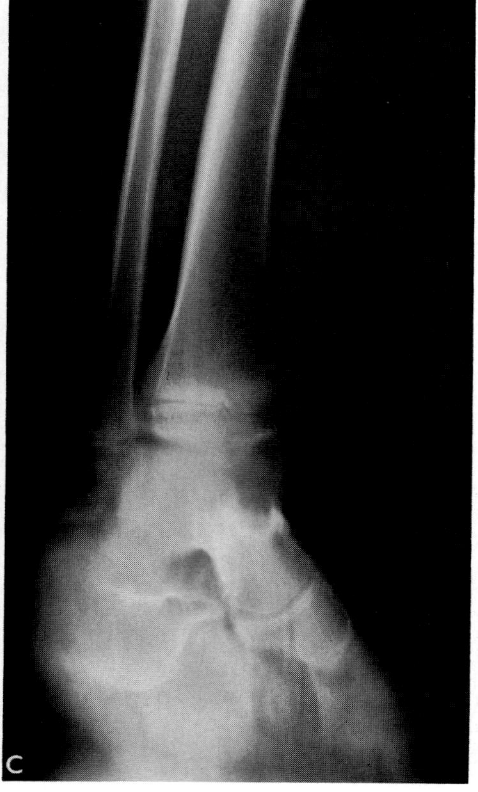

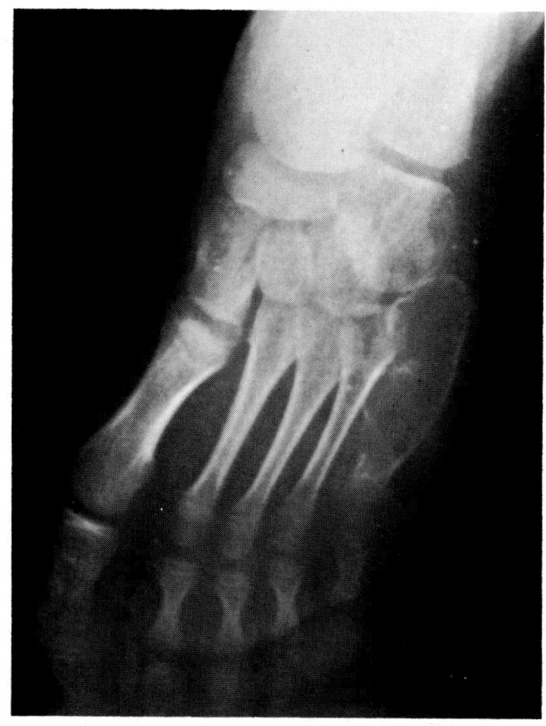

FIGURE 7–214. Aneurysmal bone cyst of the fifth metatarsal.

8. Cutler, E. C., and Gross, R. E.: The surgical treatment of tumors of peripheral nerves. Ann. Surg., *104*:436, 1936.
9. Dahlin, D. C.: Bone Tumors. 3rd Ed. Springfield, Ill., Charles C Thomas, 1978.
10. Enneking, W. F.: Clinical Musculoskeletal Pathology. Gainesville, Fla., Storter Printing, 1977.
11. Glynn, J. J., and Lichtenstein, L.: Osteoid-osteoma with multicentric nidus. A report of two cases. J. Bone Joint Surg., *55-A*:855, 1973.
12. Golding, J. S. R.: The natural history of osteoid osteoma. J. Bone Joint Surg., *36-B*:218, 1954.
13. Gould, N.: Articular osteoid osteoma of the talus: A case report. Foot Ankle, *1*:284, 1981.
14. Grunnet, N., Genner, J., Mogensen, B., and Myhre-Jensen, O.: Recurring digital fibrous tumour of childhood. Acta Pathol. Microbiol. Scand., Section A, *81*:167, 1973.
15. Heiple, K., Perrin, E., and Aikawa, M.: Congenital generalized fibromatosis. A case limited to osseous lesions. J. Bone Joint Surg., *54-A*:663, 1972.
16. Huvos, A. G.: Bone Tumors: Diagnosis, Treatment, Prognosis. Philadelphia, Saunders, 1979.
17. Jaffe, H. L.: Osteoid osteoma. A benign osteoblastic tumor composed of osteoid and atypical bone. Arch. Surg. (Chicago), *31*:709, 1935.
18. Jaffe, H. L.: Tumors and Tumorous Conditions of the Bones and Joints. Philadelphia, Lea & Febiger, 1958.
19. Jaffe, H. L., and Lichtenstein, L.: Osteoid-osteoma: Further experience with this benign tumour of bone. J. Bone Joint Surg., *22*:645, 1940.
20. Jensen, A. R., Martin, L. W., and Longino, L. A.: Digital neurofibrosarcoma in infancy. J. Pediatr., *51*:566, 1957.
21. Kauffman, S. L., and Stout, A. P.: Histiocytic tumors (fibrous xanthoma and histiocytoma) in children. Cancer, *14*:469, 1961.
22. Keller, R. B., and Baez-Giangreco, A.: Juvenile aponeurotic fibroma. Report of three cases and review of the literature. Clin. Orthop., *106*:198, 1975.
23. Lichtenstein, L.: Bone Tumors. 5th Ed. St. Louis, Mosby, 1977.
24. Lichtenstein, L., and Goldman, R. L.: Cartilage tumors in soft tissues, particularly in the hand and foot. Cancer, *17*:1203, 1964.
25. Lichtenstein, L., and Goldman, R. L.: The cartilage analogue of fibromatosis. A reinterpretation of the condition called "juvenile aponeurotic fibroma." Cancer, *17*:810, 1964.
26. Lindbom, A., Lindvall, N., Soderberg, G., and Spjut, H.: Angiography in osteoid osteoma. Acta Radiol., *54*:327, 1960.
27. Moberg, E.: The natural course of osteoid osteoma. J. Bone Joint Surg., *33-A*:166, 1951.
28. Murray, M. R., and Stout, A. P.: Schwann cell versus fibroblast as the origin of the specific nerve sheath tumor. Am. J. Pathol., *16*:41, 1940.
29. Norman, A., and Dorfman, H. D.: Osteoid-osteoma inducing pronounced overgrowth and deformity of bone. Clin. Orthop., *110*:233, 1975.
30. Pohjanpelto, P., Ahlqvist, J., Hurme, K., and Hjelt, L.: Recurring digital fibrous tumor of childhood. 2. Isolation of a cell transforming agent. Acta Pathol. Microbiol. Scand., *70*:297, 1967.
31. Posch, J. L.: Tumors of the hand. J. Bone Joint Surg., *38-A*:517, 1956.
32. Quick, D., and Cutler, M.: Neurogenic sarcoma. Ann. Surg., *86*:810, 1927.

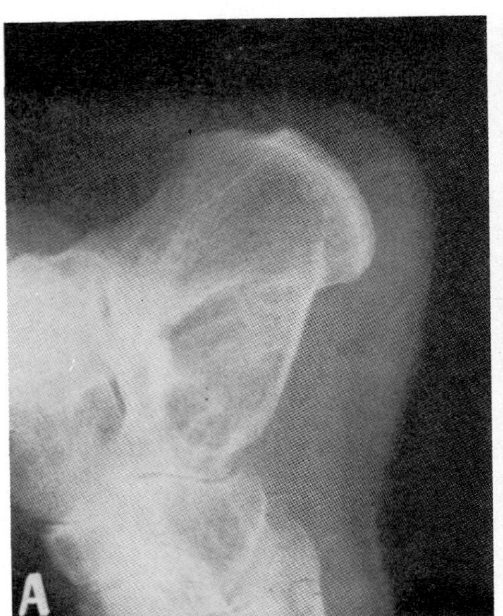

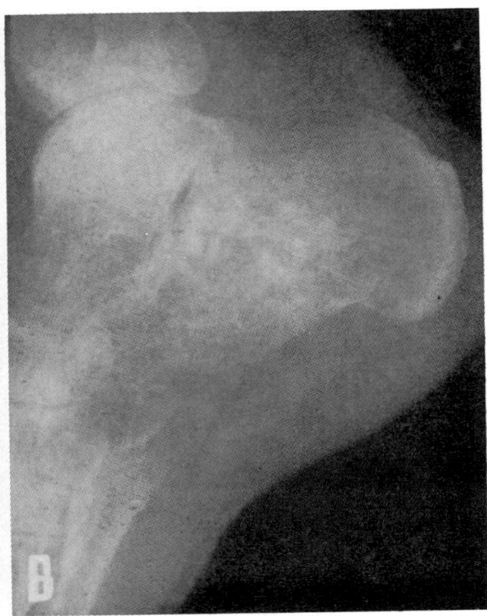

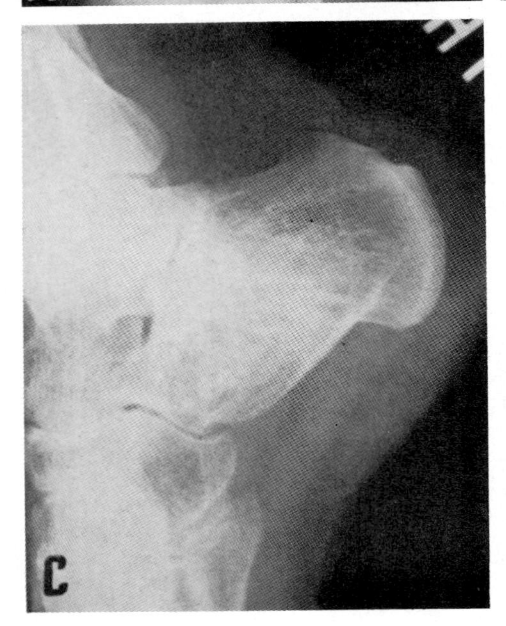

FIGURE 7–215. Radiograms of hindfoot showing solitary unicameral bone cyst in the calcaneus.

A. Preoperative. Note the radiolucency of the cyst. **B.** After curettage and implantation of bone chips. **C.** Five years after operation. (From Garceau, G. J., and Gregory, C. F.: Solitary unicameral bone cyst. J. Bone Joint Surg., *36-A*:267, 1954. Reprinted by permission.)

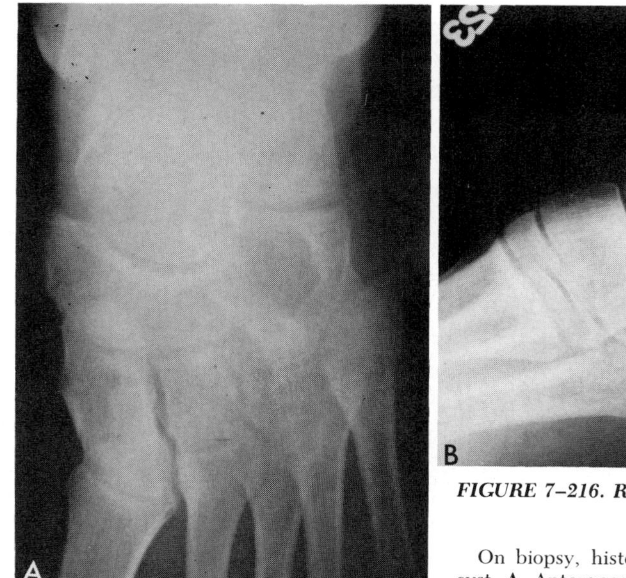

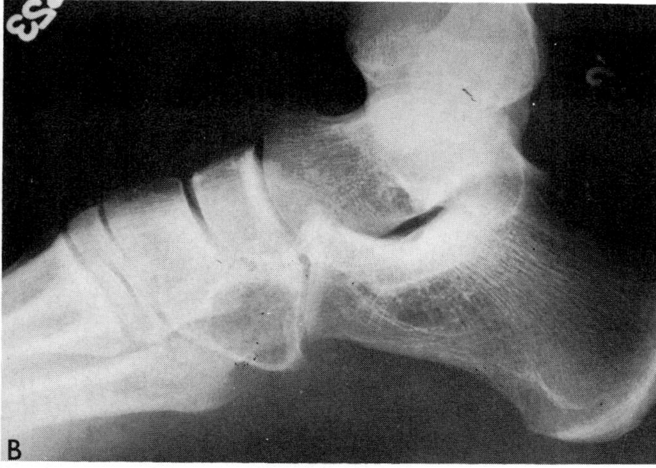

FIGURE 7–216. Radiograms of the foot showing a radiolucent lesion in the cuboid.

On biopsy, histologic findings were consistent with solitary bone cyst. **A.** Anteroposterior view. **B.** Lateral view.

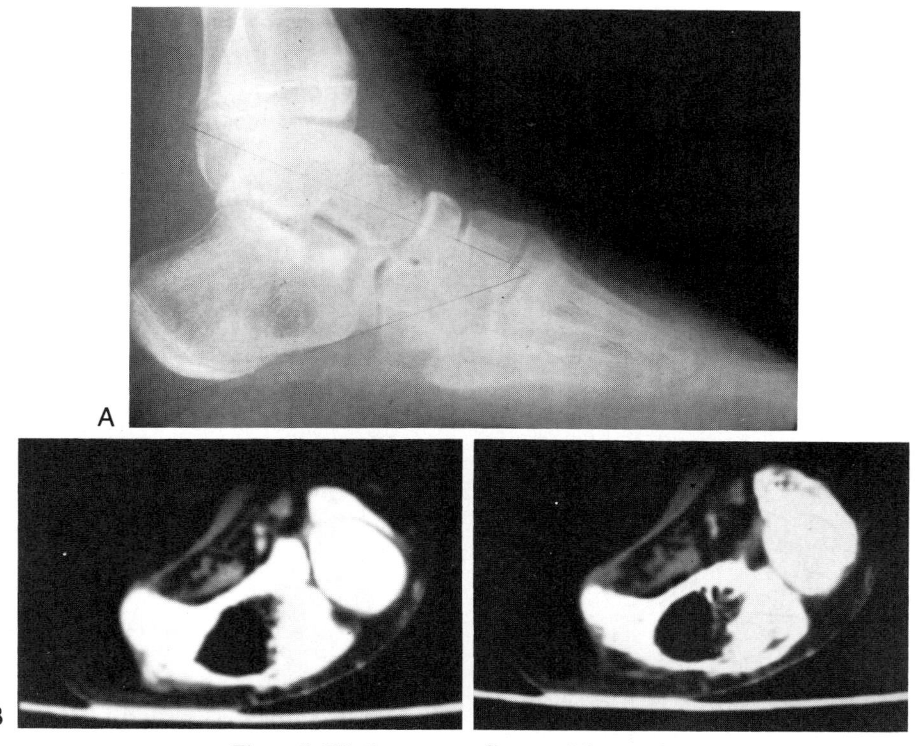

Figure 7–217. Intraosseous lipoma of the os calcis.

A. Lateral radiogram of the foot showing the radiolucent lesion in the body of the calcaneus. **B.** CT scan of the hindfoot showing the radidolucent lesion. On excisional biopsy the pathologic diagnosis was intraosseous lipoma.

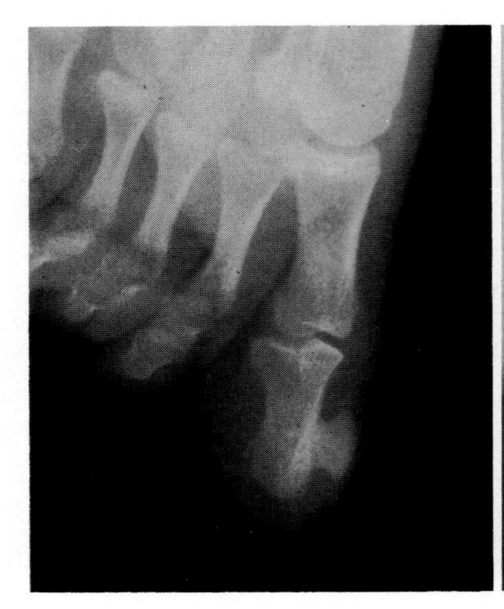
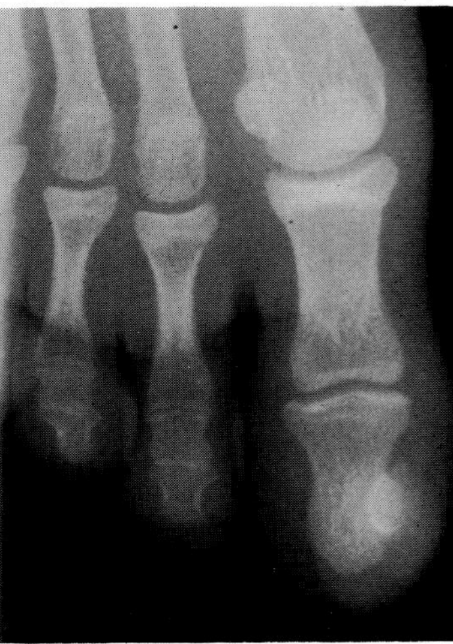

FIGURE 7–218. Subungual exostosis of the distal phalanx of the great toe.

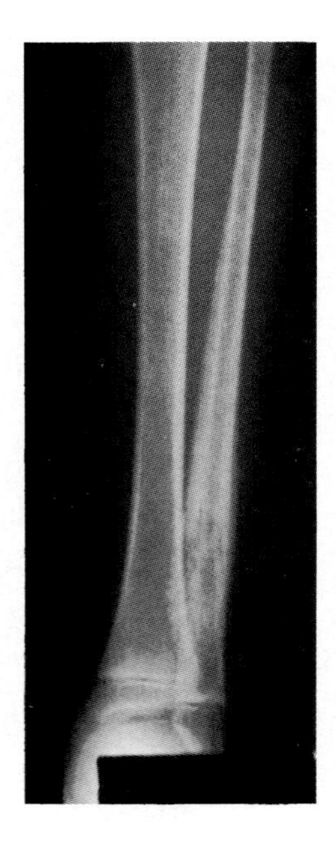

FIGURE 7–219. Osteogenic sarcoma in distal fibula of a five-and-a-half-year-old girl.

33. Reye, R. D. K.: Recurring digital fibrous tumors of childhood. Arch. Pathol. (Chicago), *80*:228, 1965.
34. Schaffzin, E. A., Chung, S. M. K., and Kaye, R.: Congenital generalized fibromatosis with complete spontaneous regression. A case report. J. Bone Joint Surg., *54-A*:657, 1973.
35. Schajowicz, F., Aiello, C. L., Francone, M. V., and Giannini, R. E.: Cystic angiomatosis (hamartous haemolymphangiomatoisis) of bone. A clinicopathological study of three cases. J. Bone Joint Surg., *60-B*:100, 1978.
36. Shapiro, L.: Infantile digital fibromatosis and aponeurotic fibroma. Arch. Dermatol. (Chicago), *99*:37, 1969.
37. Sim, F. J., Dahlin, D. C., and Beabout, J. W.: Osteoid-osteoma: Diagnostic problems. J. Bone Joint Surg., *57-A*:154, 1975.
38. Soren, A.: Pathogenesis and treatment of ganglion. Clin. Orthop., *48*:173, 1966.
39. Spjut, H. J., Dorfman, H. D., Fechner, R. E., and Ackerman, L. V.: Tumors of Bone and Cartilage. Washington, D. C., Armed Forces Institute of Pathology, 1971.
40. Stout, A. P.: Juvenile fibromatoses. Cancer, *7*:953, 1954.
41. Stout, A. P., and Lattes, R.: Tumors of the Soft Tissues. Washington, D. C., Armed Forces Institute of Pathology, 1967.
42. Thorsrud, G.: Neurinoma. Acta Chir. Scand. (Suppl.), *252*:3–38, 1960.

Skin and Nail Lesions

The skin of the foot responds to the stress of body weight and to external pressure from the shoes. The *epidermis,* the outermost layer of the skin, is an epithelial tissue derived from ectoderm; the *dermis,* the subjacent deeper layer, is of mesodermal origin and consists of dense connective tissue. In the sole of the foot, the epidermis is very thick. In the embryo, the nails first appear in the third lunar month as invasions of epidermis into the subjacent dermis over the distal ends of the toes. This epidermal plate forms the matrix of the nail from which the epidermal cells proliferate and gradually become transformed into hard keratinous nail tissue that is pushed distally over the nail bed. The matrix of the nail, extending from its root to the crescentic whitish lunula, is the only site where longitudinal growth of the nail takes place, normal growth being about 1 mm. per week. If the matrix of the nail is destroyed, longitudinal growth of the nail will be arrested, and instead of a hard smooth nail appendage, the nail bed will be covered with irregular, corrugated, horny tissue.

The skin and nails are affected by a great variety of lesions; only the common ones are briefly discussed here. More extensive details are given in general textbooks of dermatology and the cited references.

HARD CORN (CLAVUS DURUS)

A hard corn is a localized cornification of the skin resulting from shoe pressure on a bony prominence. It is most commonly seen over the dorsolateral aspect of the proximal interphalangeal joint of the fifth toe and over the tip of a flexed toe close to its nail. In the central area of the corn there is a deeply penetrating nucleus of hyperkeratosis that is partly degenerated. Beneath this hyperkeratotic central nucleus, there may be a sac containing fluid; irritation and inflammation of this sac and consequent pressure on the nerve endings in the papillary layer of the dermis are the cause of pain.

The immediate cause of the corn must be corrected to eliminate the possibility of recurrence; it may be a badly fitted shoe, deformed toes, or excessive use of the feet. The keratinized skin is softened with preparations containing salicylic acid; the horny layer and central nucleus will then eventually separate and fall away. Occasionally surgical excision of deep-rooted corns is required; this should be done under strict aseptic conditions to prevent infection.

SOFT CORN (CLAVUS MOLLIS)

Soft corns are rare in children. They usually occur between the toes, the most frequent sites being the fourth and fifth toes, where they are caused by bony pressure from a small exostosis on the lateral aspect of the base of the proximal phalanx of the fourth toe. They are soft and of whitish appearance and have a depressed central area (Fig. 7–220).

The condition is painful and disabling. Treatment consists of excision of the interdigital clavus, resection of the exostosis or the proximal half of the proximal phalanx of the fourth toe, or surgical syndactylism of the fourth and fifth toes.

PLANTAR WART (VERRUCA PLANTARIS)

These are very common in children and may be found on any part of the plantar aspect of the foot, on either weight-bearing or non-

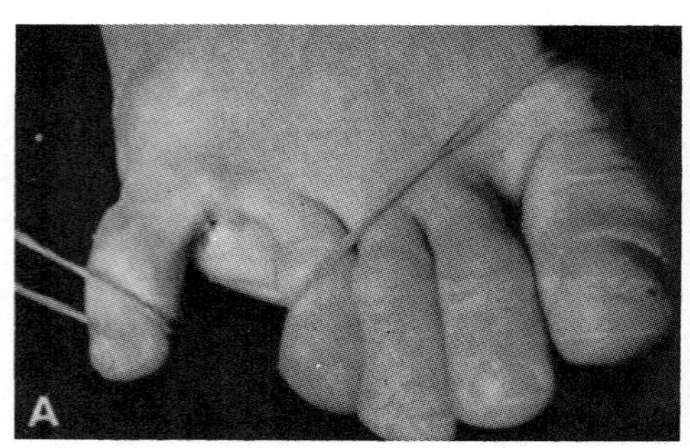

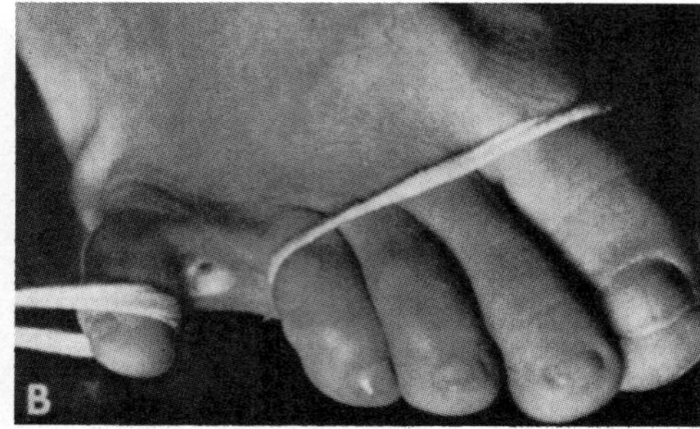

FIGURE 7–220. Two cases of interdigital soft corn.

(From Kelikian, H.: Hallux Valgus, Allied Deformities of the Forefoot and Metatarsalgia. Philadelphia, Saunders, 1965, p. 290. Reprinted by permission.)

weight-bearing surfaces. Frequent sites are the heel, under the metatarsal heads, and the big toe. They may be single or surrounded by a whole crop of daughter warts, their size ranging from a few millimeters to 2 or 3 cm. A multitude of tiny warts may conglomerate into a large "mosaic wart." Plantar warts are infectious and may be transferred from one child to another by direct contact or indirectly by agents such as bath mats. Epidemics have been known to occur in schools.

Anatomically, a plantar wart is a papillomatous growth, but instead of projecting beyond the skin surface (like warts elsewhere), they are buried under the stratum corneum of the skin, with only the ends of the papillae showing through. They are extremely vascular and bleed profusely when trimmed. Plantar warts have a dark, punctate surface and are clearly demarcated from the surrounding skin. On direct pressure and lateral compression of the skin, the lesion is markedly tender.

Treatment

In children, a conservative approach is advised. Small lesions can be ignored, but if they are especially painful, the area is padded to relieve pressure of body weight on the wart. Larger or persistent lesions are destroyed by a caustic or keratolytic agent. Lapidus recommends applying 50 per cent salicylic acid ointment, covering the entire area of the wart with 40 per cent salicylic acid plaster (manufactured by Duke Laboratories, Inc.), and strapping it with adhesive tape. In three or four days, the dressing is removed and the foot is re-examined. The keratolytic medication may not be tolerated by some children and may produce irritation and aggravate the pain, in which case the dressing is removed and the foot is soaked in pHisoHex solution and zinc oxide ointment is applied. Most patients do tolerate the salicylic acid ointment. At weekly intervals the macerated skin is debrided, bleeding vessels are cauterized with silver nitrate stick, and again salicylic acid ointment and plaster are applied. Intractable plantar warts, particularly the mosaic warts, may require several weeks of treatment before being cured. Parents should be advised of the stubborn nature of the condition.[1]

Electrocoagulation of the plantar wart under local infiltration anesthesia may result in an intractable ulcer; it should be performed in only a few selected cases. Excision of the lesion may result in a disabling postoperative scar and is not recommended. Irradiation is contraindicated, as it may cause chronic indolent ulceration.

Reference

1. Lapidus, P. W.: Orthopedic skin lesions of the soles and the toes. Clin. Orthop., *45*:87, 1966.

INGROWING TOENAIL

Ingrowing toenail most commonly involves the great toe. It is caused by external pressure from tight shoes or hose on an improperly trimmed nail that has been cut too short so that its corners dig into the pulp. The edges of the nail become thickened and press into the neighboring soft tissues, which respond by hypertrophy. Soon the overgrown soft tissues obliterate the medial or lateral nail groove. This mechanical irritation is followed by infection of the skin fold. Pus then spreads around the edge of the nail and between the nail and the matrix, the great toe becoming red, swollen, locally tender, and painful.

Conservative treatment is indicated in mild and early cases. A pledget of cotton or gauze soaked in an antiseptic (such as aqueous Zephiran) is tucked beneath the corner of the nail so that it does not dig into the skin. This is done once or twice a day; then the nail is allowed to grow until its edges project beyond the skin folds. Local hot soaks may be used three or four times a day or continuously, depending upon the severity of infection. The toenails should subsequently be cut with square corners and the child should be fitted with proper shoes and socks to prevent recurrence.

Surgery is indicated in long-standing cases or when conservative measures have failed, the simplest method being excision of a wedge of nail bed together with the margin of skin fold. In very severe or recurrent cases, permanent ablation of the nail by excision of the nail bed is indicated.

Torsional (or Rotational) Deformities of the Lower Limbs

Torsion is defined as the twisting of a long bone on its longitudinal axis. In *tibial torsion* the distal segment of the tibia may be rotated toward the medial malleolus (medial tibial torsion) or toward the lateral malleolus (lateral tibial torsion). As the tibia twists, the relative planes of the transverse axes of the knee and ankle joints are altered in the axial plane. In *femoral torsion* the lower or condylar portion is the fixed end upon which the proximal part rotates on its longitudinal axis. In *antetorsion* the femoral neck axis is twisted forward or anteriorly in relation to the frontal or coronal plane of the femoral condyles, whereas in *retrotorsion* the plane of the femoral neck axis is rotated posteriorly or directed backward with reference to the coronal condylar plane.

In the past, the term "angle of declination" was used interchangeably with "femoral torsion." Such usage is misleading and should be discontinued, as the "angle of declination" is often confused with the "angle of inclination," which is that angle formed by the femoral neck axis with the femoral shaft axis (the so-called shaft-neck angle).

Pathophysiologic Considerations

The shape of a bone is determined by both intrinsic and extrinsic factors. In order to clarify the pathogenesis and rationale of therapy of torsional deformities of the lower limb, certain basic facts and experimental work are reviewed here.

Deformation of growing bones by abnormal pressure has been known for centuries, as attested by the Chinese bound-foot deformities and the elongated skull of the Egyptians. This quality of bone was well portrayed by Nicholas André in his familiar picture of the crooked tree bound to the straight rod as a symbol of the plasticity of the skeleton of the growing child.

Abnormal pressure can alter the shape of the growing skeleton only when applied more or less continuously over a period of time. Osseous tissue, being a crystalline structure, is elastic rather than plastic in the true sense. The "plasticity" of the skeleton is biologic, apparent only after the passage of time and existing only during periods of growth.[136] According to Wolff, "Every change in the form and function of bones or their function alone is followed by certain definite changes in their external configuration in accordance with mathematical laws."[140]

The rate of physeal growth is affected by pressures applied to its axes; i.e., increased pressure inhibits growth and decreased pressure accelerates it, a relationship that was originally noted by Delpech in 1829 and later recognized by Hueter and Volkmann in 1862; it is often referred to as the Hueter-Volkmann law.[26, 48, 132]

There have been a number of experimental studies on the effects of pressure on physeal growth:

Appleton, in 1934, demonstrated that minor degrees of pressure can slow growth without stopping it entirely. He applied abnormal pressures to the growing bones of young rabbits by creating postural abnormalities by surgical section of certain muscle groups; for example, by division of the lateral rotators of the hip, he could produce medial deformation of the femur. He also found that the opposite limb was held in lateral rotation and the femur became retroverted.[2] Haas caused total arrest of physeal growth by means of compression with a wire loop.[44]

Arkin and Katz applied pressure over the growing epiphyses of young rabbits by means of plaster casts that immobilized the limbs in deformed positions. They demonstrated that when a growing epiphysis is subjected to a stress, the rate or direction of growth (or both) of that epiphysis is modified by that stress. Physeal growth is inhibited by pressure applied parallel to its direction of growth. Cartilaginous growth is completely arrested by considerable pressure, but pressure does not inhibit it by an all-or-none law. Rather, growth is retarded by slight or intermittent pressures, such as those from a plaster cast, postural stress, or gravitational and muscular forces. In vertical weight-bearing bones, the gravitational force of normal weight-bearing seems to slow cartilaginous growth, whereas lack of normal weight-bearing stresses results in overgrowth. Pressures applied perpendicularly to the direction of physeal growth deflect such growth, resulting in lateral or spiral (torsional) displacement of the newly laid-down bone. The diameter of a bone is a determining factor in the ease with which angular or torsional deformities are produced—the narrower the bone, the greater its "plasticity."[4]

The effect of splinting the hind limbs of immature animals in different positions, with particular reference to rotation, has been studied by a number of investigators. Bernbeck produced increased femoral antetorsion by immobilizing the hind legs of kittens in medial rotation.[11]

Wilkinson used six- to eight-week-old rabbits for his experiments, rabbits being chosen because of the similarity of the normal posture of their hind limbs in flexion, abduction, and lateral rotation to the human prenatal and neonatal postures. He showed that (1) prolonged medial rotation of the femur produces antetorsion, whether the hip is in flexion or extension, abduction or adduction; (2) prolonged lateral rotation of the femur, with the hip flexed and abducted, increases retroversion; and (3) prolonged fixation of the femur in the Lorenz position corrects or prevents the development of retrotorsion. The deformity occurred mostly in the metaphyseal region and was twice as great in the distal metaphysis as in the proximal metaphysis, reflecting the relative growth in these areas.[138] Salter performed similar experiments and demonstrated that antetorsion is produced by the strain of medial rotation on the femoral epiphyses, and that retrotorsion is produced by the strain of lateral rotation.[107] The bone displacement in a rotational deformity is always in the direction opposite to that of the deforming force.

Salter, in a series of experiments in newborn pigs, also studied the effect on the acetabulum of maintained extension and flexion of the hip. A position of forced extension of the hip for a period of six to eight weeks resulted in dysplasia and maldirection of the acetabulum, whereas maintained flexion was associated with normal acetabular development. The restricting bandages were removed from one group of animals that were then allowed to run free; the acetabular dysplasia was reversed and the maldirection of the entire acetabulum reverted to normal.[107]

Brookes and Wardle studied the effect of muscle action on the shape of decalcified femora. They showed that an iliopsoas force acting at the lesser trochanter causes an immediate valgus deformity, posterior deflection of the neck, and lateral rotation of the shaft with an increase in its anterior convexity. Conversely, the effect of gluteal action at the greater trochanter produced by the iliopsoas force was abolished by a gluteal force acting on the greater trochanter when these were in a ratio of 5:3. Adductor action causes medial deflection and torsion of the diaphysis with some varus deformity of the neck of the femur.[18]

Rotation of the Limb Bud

In humans, the evolution of upright posture requires the limb buds to rotate during embryonic development. The lower limbs originate in a laterally abducted and flexed position relative to the pelvis and acetabular anlage. Around the third month of intrauterine life, the femoral neck and shaft become adducted (almost 90 degrees) to a position parallel with the longitudinal axis of the trunk and rotate medially to allow the patella and leg to face forward.[8]

This rotation phenomenon of the lower limb necessitates certain adaptive changes in the direction in which the acetabulum faces. Dega studied 100 fetal skeletons and found the angle of forward inclination of the acetabulum to be 29.5 degrees and its angle of downward inclination in relation to the transverse plane to be 62.8 degrees.[25] With the change in the position of the hip from the intrauterine posture of flexion and abduction to that of erect posture of hip extension and neutral adduction, the forward inclination of the acetabulum decreases. Some degree of retention of fetal position of the lower limbs is common and normal in early infancy.

Etiologic Considerations

The exact cause of torsional deformities of the lower limb is not known. A number of possible factors should be considered.

PERSISTENT FETAL ALIGNMENT

Böhm observed that human beings have an inherent predisposition to certain infantile deformities of the ankles, knees, and hips, and he proposed that these are caused by an arrest of skeletal development. The proximal tibial epiphysis of the adult gorilla was noted by Böhm to have marked asymmetry—the lateral condyle is overdeveloped, whereas the medial condyle is underdeveloped. In the human fetus, the *proximal tibial epiphysis* has certain anthropoid characteristics—the lateral condyle is high and convex, the medial condyle is low and concave, and the tibial diaphysis is deviated medially, producing a genu varum.[15]

In the newborn child the fetal configuration of the tibia with a high lateral condyle, a low medial condyle, and varus inclination of the shaft is still present. This tibia vara deformity will gradually correct itself with growth. If the tibia retains its fetal shape, a genu varum deformity results. Böhm calls attention to the difference in the volume and height of the *femoral condyles* in the anthropoid knee; the medial femoral condyle is much larger and higher than the lateral condyle. In his studies of the human knee in different age groups, Böhm has observed underdevelopment of the *lateral femoral condyle* in the fetus, and believes that genu valgum results from persistence of underdevelopment of the lateral condyles.[15]

Somerville proposed that abnormal femoral antetorsion represented a persistent fetal alignment of the hip due to failure of normal derotation of the femur in utero.[114] Embryologic evidence supports his theory.

HEREDITY

Abnormal femoral antetorsion and medial tibial torsion are familial afflictions. Blumel, Eggers, and Evans reported eight cases of bilateral medial tibial torsion in four generations. In their pedigree they demonstrated a mendelian autosomal dominant type of inheritance.[14] That a genetic factor is partly responsible in the causation of abnormal femoral torsion is supported by the report of Crane—in 21 of his 72 patients (29 per cent), siblings or a parent were similarly affected. An exact clear pattern of inheritance could not be demonstrated, however.[24]

PERSISTENT MALPOSTURE IN POSTNATAL LIFE

Intrauterine posture and molding affect the rotational alignment of the lower limbs. In the fetus the hips are flexed and laterally rotated; as a result, the hips have a greater degree of lateral than of medial rotation. The legs and feet are medially rotated and adducted. In the neonate this fetal posture is present to a varying degree. With longitudinal growth, ligamentous and muscular forces, and static forces of body weight across the physes, the gradual spontaneous resolution of the fetal posture takes place: The femoral antetorsion decreases and the tibia rotates laterally.

That the sleeping, sitting, and play habits of the infant and child may disturb the normal developmental pattern of the lower limbs and even cause deformities has been much emphasized in the literature.[39, 50, 63–66, 68] Fitzhugh reviewed the sleeping positions of children, and found that of 100 infants who slept in the knee-chest position, 84 per cent had a deviation of their lower limbs, either inward or outward, of more than 10 degrees.[39] The importance of intrauterine malposture as a factor in the causation of deformities of the newborn is well known. A logical corollary is that sleeping and sitting habits may well influence the persistence of these positional deformities as well as increase their severity.

The following outline, given by Knight, shows the deformities of the lower limbs that are associated with certain habitual sleeping or sitting positions:[68]

SLEEPING HABITS

I. Prone knee-chest position with:
   a. Extremities internally rotated, results in:
      (1) internal rotation deformity of the hips,
      (2) medial tibial torsion,
      (3) bow-leg,
      (4) ankle equinus,
      (5) adduction and varus of the fore part of the foot (may appear to be a metatarsus varus).
   b. Extremities externally rotated, results in:
      (1) external rotational deformity in the knees,
      (2) knock-knee,
      (3) ankle equinus,
      (4) valgus of the feet.
   c. Extremities neutral, results in:
      (1) ankle equinus (toe-walking of early childhood).
II. Frog-leg position, most frequently prone but occasionally supine, resulting in:
      (1) external rotation deformity of the hips,
      (2) external rotation deformity in the knee joints, in conjunction with

shortening of the iliotibial band and of the biceps femoris,
(3) knock-knee,
(4) valgus and abduction of the feet.

III. Prone, with hips extended and:
  a. Internally rotated, may result in:
    (1) internal rotation contracture of the hips,
    (2) medial tibial torsion (to a lesser degree than that which results from the knee-chest position),
    (3) ankle equinus,
    (4) varus of the metatarsus, with or without adduction.
  b. Externally rotated, may result in:
    (1) external rotation contracture of the hips,
    (2) external rotation deformity in the knee joints,
    (3) ankle equinus,
    (4) valgus of the feet.

SITTING HABITS

I. Reversed tailor position with:
  a. Feet internally rotated beneath the buttocks (sitting on the feet), results in:
    (1) internal rotation contracture of the hips,
    (2) medial tibial torsion,
    (3) adduction of the fore part of the foot.
  b. Feet externally rotated, results in:
    (1) internal rotation contracture of the hips,
    (2) external rotation deformity in the knees,
    (3) knock-knee, with relaxation or stretching of medial collateral ligaments,
    (4) valgus deformity of the feet.
  c. One foot internally rotated and the other externally rotated.*

Crane cites two examples to support the postnatal malposition theory. Both these patients had cerebral atrophy, were unable to talk or walk, and were confined to mental institutions. The first patient was a seven-year-old boy who constantly sat in the reverse tailor's position with the feet laterally rotated, a position that provided a broader base and greater stability. With the hips in extension, medial rotation of the hips was 75 degrees and lateral rotation only 5 to 10 degrees. The angle of antetorsion was 50 degrees on the right and 53 degrees on the left (Fig. 7–221 A to C). The second patient, in the next bed, sat continually in the tailor's position. Upon straightening his lower limbs, he reverted to this position. With the hips extended, medial rotation of the hip was 10 degrees and lateral rotation 80 degrees. Femoral antetorsion was less than 10 degrees (Fig. 7–221 D to F).[24]

There is no evidence that, in *normal* infants and children, static forces of malposition are of etiologic significance. Normal children constantly move around and do not remain in one position long enough for the force of gravity to be a factor in the causation of torsional or angular deformities of the lower limbs. Often they assume the tailor's or reverse tailor's position because it is more comfortable for them.

Torsional (or Rotational) Profile

In order to accurately assess lower limb rotational problems in the transverse plane, Staheli has proposed the use of the torsional profile. The goal is to provide an accurate record of measurements for future comparison and reproduceable results by the same surgeon or another physician. The torsional profile consists of measurement of six parameters of each lower limb: (1) the foot-progression angle; (2) the medial hip rotation in extension; (3) the lateral hip rotation in extension; (4) the thigh-foot angle; (5) the angle of the transmalleolar axis; and (6) the configuration of the foot. Staheli et al. studied 1000 normal lower limbs in children and adults (279 females and 221 males) and established normal values for torsional and rotational profiles in various age groups.[121] *Normal* is that which occurs within two standard deviations (SD) of the mean. *Rotational variation* is a torsional problem with values within the normal range. *Torsional deformity* is a rotational problem outside the normal range.

Foot-Progression Angle. This is the angular difference between the long axis of the foot and the line of progression (Fig. 7–222). Clinically this is determined by observing the patient's gait and estimating in degrees the amount of in- or out-toeing. A plus sign denotes an out-toeing angle, whereas an in-toeing angle is designated by a minus sign. In the study by Staheli et al. the mean foot-progression angle was approximately plus 10 degrees with a normal range between minus 3 and plus 20 degrees.[121] Young children toe-out more than older children owing to a greater range of lateral rotation of the hip. The foot-progression angle data of Staheli et al. are consistent with those of Scrutton and Robson, who studied the gait

*From Knight, R. A.: Developmental deformities of the lower extremities. J. Bone Joint Surg., *36-A*:521, 1954. Reprinted with permission.

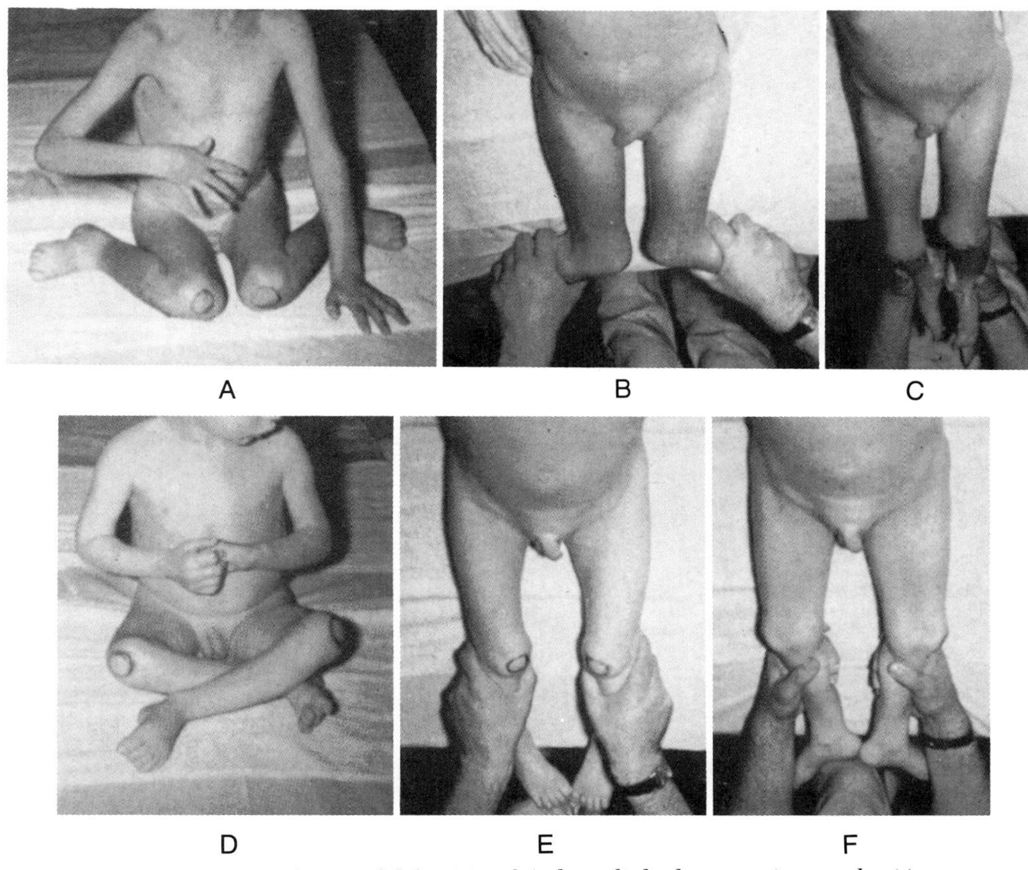

FIGURE 7–221. Developmental deformities of the lower limbs due to persistent malposition.

Both patients had cerebral atrophy, were confined to mental institutions, and could not talk or walk. **A** to **C**. A seven-year-old boy who sat constantly in the reverse tailor's position with the feet externally rotated (**A**). Maximum internal rotation of the hips (**B**)—75 degrees; maximum external rotation of the hips (**C**)—5 to 10 degrees; femoral antetorsion was exaggerated bilaterally—right, 50 degrees; left, 53 degrees. **D** to **F**. A five-year-old boy who persistently sat in the tailor's position. He always reverted to this posture after his legs were straightened (**D**). Maximum internal rotation of the hips (**E**) is 10 degrees and maximum external rotation is 80 degrees (**F**). Femoral anteversion was less than 10 degrees. (From Crane, L.: Femoral torsion and its relation to toeing-in and toeing-out. J. Bone Joint Surg., *41-A*:427, 1959.)

of 50 normal children. In the latter report in the one- to three-year age group the mean foot-progression angle was plus (+) 6 degrees with a range from minus (−) 5 to plus (+) 15 degrees; in children older than four years of age, the mean foot-progression angle was plus (+) 4 degrees with a range from minus (−) 2 to plus (+) 12 degrees.[110] Schwartz et al., in a study of walking patterns of normal adults, found the foot-progression angle to be between plus (+) 5 and 9 degrees—the greater out-toeing was found in the older age group.[109]

In excessive femoral antetorsion (medial torsion) the foot-progression angle may be normal owing to compensatory lateral tibial torsion.[36, 37] In the anatomic study of dry bones, Kobyliansky et al. reported a high incidence of compensatory lateral tibial torsion with excessive femoral antetorsion of the same limb.[70]

Medial and Lateral Hip Rotation. Hip rotation is measured with the patient prone and the knees flexed to 90 degrees. It is important for the patient to be relaxed and for the pelvis to be level. The thighs are rotated to the angle that would be maintained by gravity alone (Figs. 7–223 and 7–224). If necessary, hip rotation can be measured also with the patient supine with the hips in full extension, the pelvis flat on the examining table, and the knees in 90 degrees of flexion with the legs hanging free at the edge of the table. The range of medial rotation of the hip declines with increasing age.

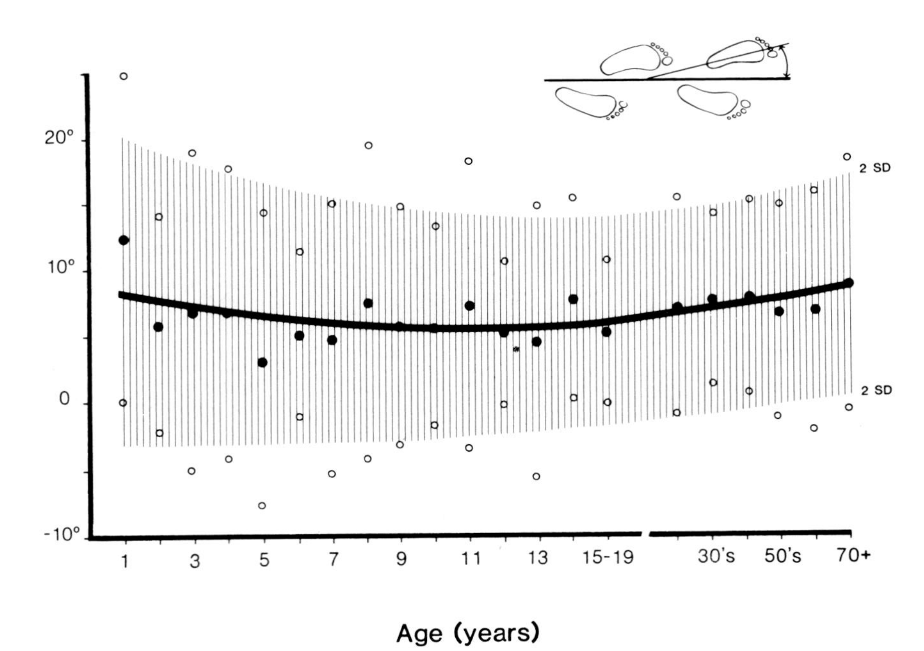

FIGURE 7–222. Foot-progression angle.

(From Staheli, L. T., Corbett, M., Wyss, C., and King, H.: Lower extremity rotational problems in children. Normal values to guide management. J. Bone Joint Surg., *67-A*:39, 1985.)

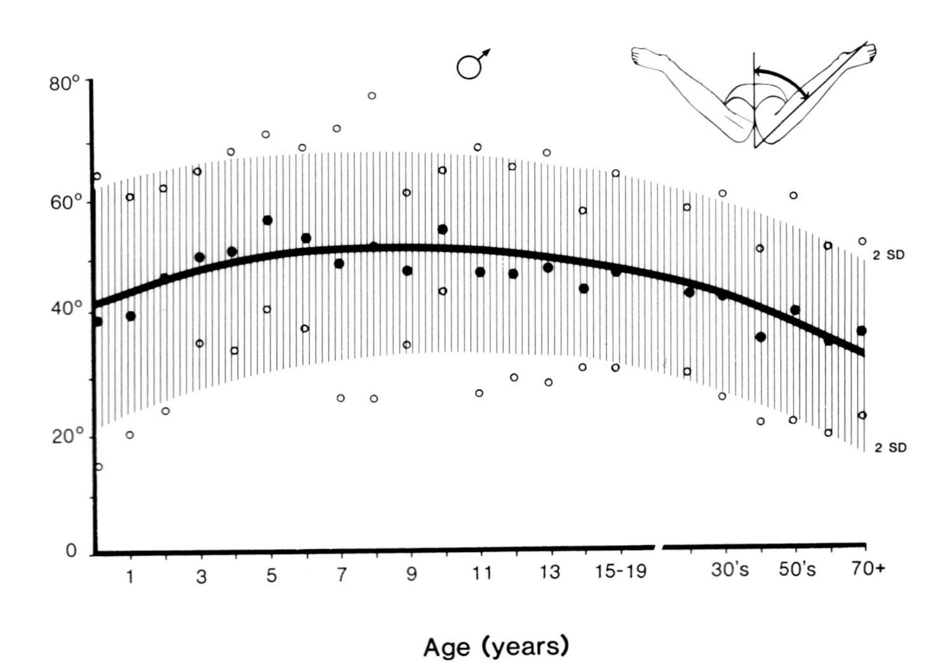

FIGURE 7–223. Medial rotation of the hip in the male.

(From Staheli, L. T., Corbett, M., Wyss, C., and King, H.: Lower extremity rotational problems in children. Normal values to guide management. J. Bone Joint Surg., *67-A*:39, 1985.)

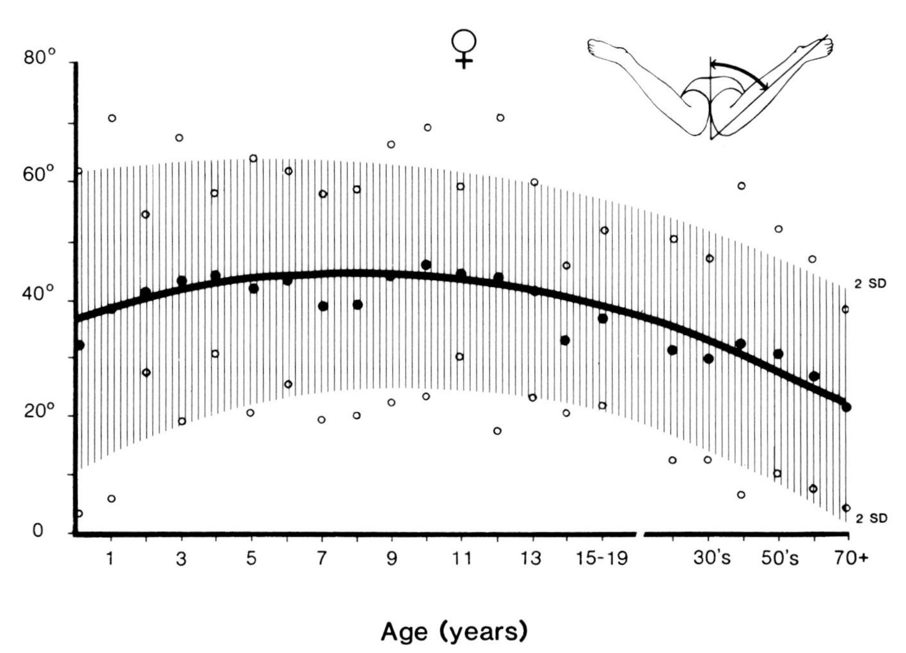

FIGURE 7–224. Medial rotation of the hip in the female.

(From Staheli, L. T., Corbett, M., Wyss, C., and King, H.: Lower extremity rotational problems in children. Normal values to guide management. J. Bone Joint Surg., *67-A*:39, 1985.)

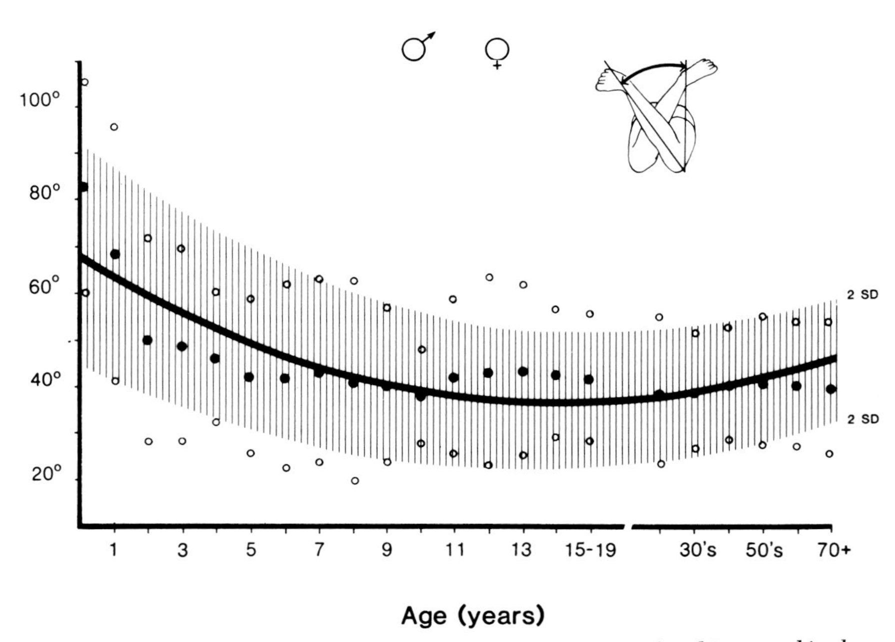

FIGURE 7–225. Lateral rotation of the hip in the male and female subjects combined.

(From Staheli, L. T., Corbett, M., Wyss, C., and King, H.: Lower extremity rotational problems in children. Normal values to guide management. J. Bone Joint Surg., *67-A*:39, 1985.)

In early infancy, lateral rotation of the hip is greater than medial rotation; as the child gets older the range of lateral rotation decreases. The upper limit of medial rotation is 65 degrees in boys and 60 degrees in girls. The lower limit of lateral rotation is about 25 degrees for males and females.[121]

According to Staheli et al., the degree of hip rotation correlates with the degree of femoral antetorsion as measured radiographically.[120, 121] The severity of femoral torsion is graded *severe* if medial rotation is greater than 90 degrees and lateral rotation is less than 0 degrees; *moderate* if medial rotation is 80 to 90 degrees and lateral rotation 0 to 10 degrees; and *mild* if medial rotation is 70 to 80 degrees and lateral rotation is 10 to 20 degrees.[121] It should be noted that acetabular inclination affects range of hip rotation, and joint laxity increases both medial and lateral rotation of the hip. The mean *medial rotation* of the hip for girls is 40 degrees, with a normal range of 15 to 60 degrees; for boys the mean is 50 degrees, with a normal range of 25 to 65 degrees (Figs. 7–223 and 7–224). The mean *lateral rotation* of the hip is 45 degrees (with a normal range from 25 to 65 degrees) (Fig. 7–225). There is no sex difference in the range of lateral rotation of the hip.

Thigh-Foot Angle (Fig. 7–226). This parameter assesses tibial torsion. It is measured with the patient in prone position, the knees flexed 90 degrees and the ankles in neutral position. The angular difference between the longitudinal axis of the foot and the longitudinal axis of the thigh is the thigh-foot angle. A negative value is given for in-toeing angle and a positive value for out-toeing angle. The thigh-foot angle is negative in infancy; with increasing age it becomes progressively lateral. In the study by Staheli et al., from the middle of childhood on the mean thigh-foot angle remained about plus (+) 10 degrees, with a range of normal values from minus (−) 5 to plus (+) 30 degrees. It should be noted that the thigh-foot angle is a composite measurement, depicting rotation of the tibia and the hindfoot.

Angle of the Transmalleolar Axis. This is also determined with the patient prone, knees flexed to 90 degrees and ankles in neutral position. The center points of medial and lateral malleolus are marked and joined by a line across the sole of the foot. This represents the transmalleolar axis. Next, a line is projected toward the heel perpendicular to the transmalleolar axis. The angle of the transmalleolar axis is the angular difference between this projected line (toward the heel and the axis of the thigh) (Fig. 7–227). The angle of transmalleolar axis increases with age; its approximate mean value from the middle of childhood on is plus (+) 20 degrees, with ranges of normal from 0 to plus (+) 45 degrees.

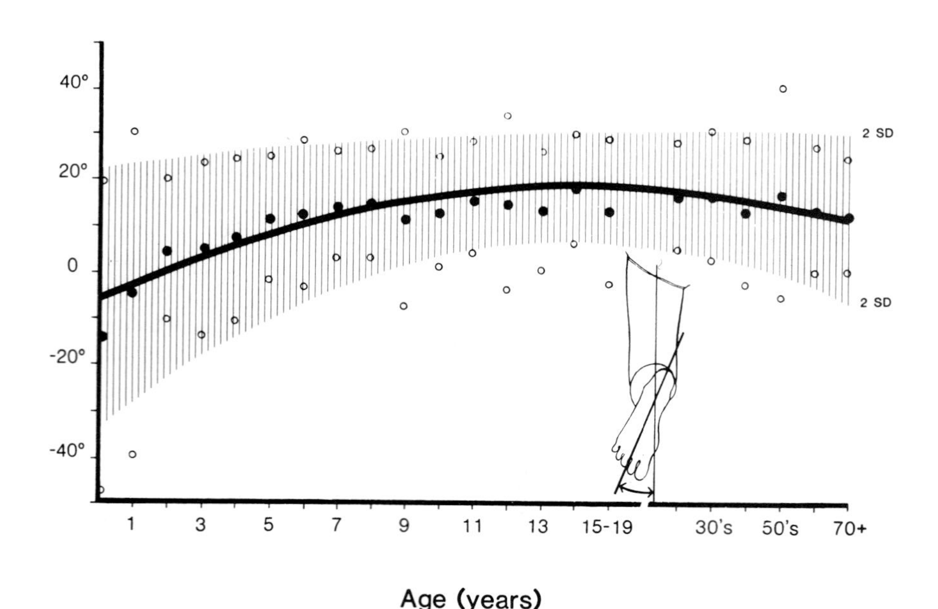

FIGURE 7–226. Thigh-foot angle.

(From Staheli, L. T., Corbett, M., Wyss, C., and King, H.: Lower extremity rotational problems in children. Normal values to guide management. J. Bone Joint Surg., 67-A:39, 1985.)

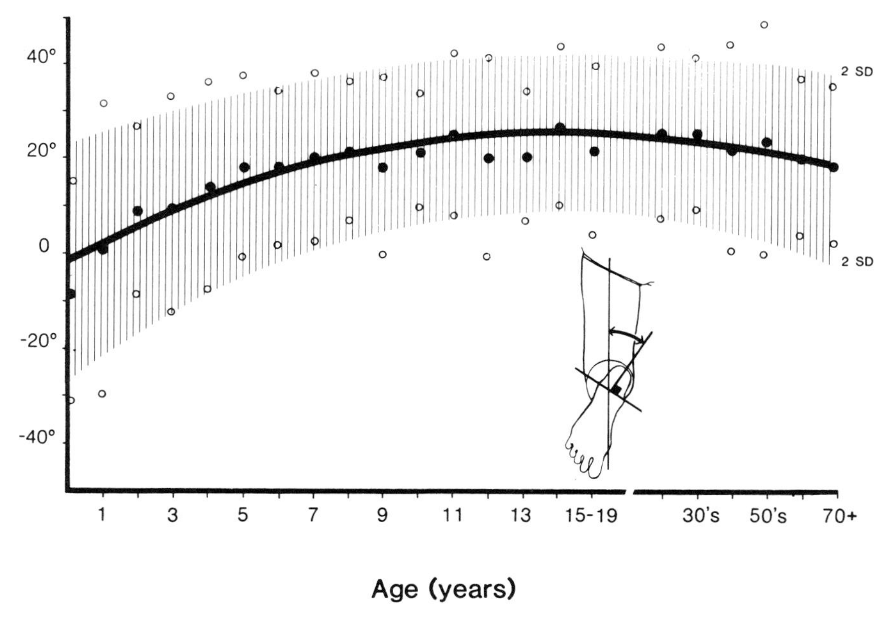

FIGURE 7–227. Angle of the transmalleolar axis.

(From Staheli, L. T., Corbett, M., Wyss, C., and King, H.: Lower extremity rotational problems in children. Normal values to guide management. J. Bone Joint Surg., *67-A*:39, 1985.)

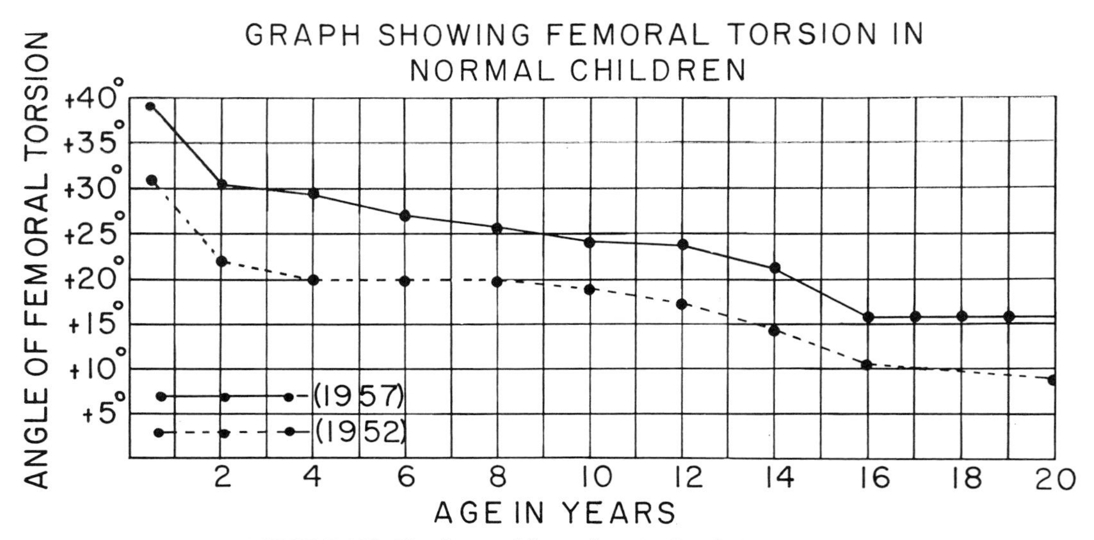

FIGURE 7–228. The degree of femoral torsion in relation to age.

The solid line on the graph (1957 study) represents the average values in 238 children with the radiograms made with the hips in 10 degrees of abduction. The broken line represents the average degree of femoral torsion determined in 215 normal children in 1952, when the radiograms were made with the hips in 35 degrees of abduction. The 1952 determinations are less accurate and their values are from 5 to 9 degrees lower than those in the 1957 study. (From Shands, A. R., Jr., and Steele, M. K.: Torsion of the femur. J. Bone Joint Surg., *40-A*:806, 1958.)

The values of the thigh-foot angle are roughly parallel to those of the angle of the transmalleolar axis; however, the values of the angle of the transmalleolar axis are greater than those of the thigh-foot angle. For practical purposes, in simple torsional problems measurement of the thigh-foot angle is adequate. For complex rotational deformities when delineation of the anatomic location of the deformity is indicated, both the thigh-foot angle and the angle of the transmalleolar axis should be measured. The angle of transmalleolar axis measures tibial torsion. The difference between the thigh-foot angle and the angle of transmalleolar axis assesses deformity of the hindfoot. The thigh-foot angle measures a combined rotation deformity of both the tibia and the hindfoot.

Foot Deformities. Angular and rotatory deformities of the foot will affect the rotational profile of the lower limb. Metatarsus varus causes in-toeing. Calcaneovalgus and flexible pes planovalgus with oblique or vertical talus cause out-toeing. The posture of the foot is inspected in stance and in prone position. Any deformity in the longitudinal or transverse axis is measured and recorded. It is important to measure passive range of motion of the ankle, as equinus deformity due to contracture of the triceps surae will cause out-toeing. In overall assessment of rotational problems of the lower limb, a manual muscle testing is performed to detect paralysis and muscle imbalance between the invertors and evertors of the foot. Invertor muscle weakness will cause out-toeing, whereas paralysis of peroneals with strong anterior and posterior tibial muscles will cause in-toeing. Ankle valgus will cause out-toeing.

Luchini and Stevens tested the validity of measurements attained in the torsional profile examination. They found significant variation in estimation of the various torsional components in each child for each examiner at different examinations. There was greater discrepancy between different examiners with the same child on the same day. They recommended that we exercise caution in interpretation of the actual numerical values obtained in assessment of torsional profile, particularly if different examiners are involved.[78] In spite of these variations this author recommends the use of the torsional profile. Table 7–16 lists the information necessary for routine assessment of ordinary rotational problems of the lower limbs. For complex problems, the degree of acetabular inclination and femoral and tibial torsion is determined by computed tomography. If instability of the hip is suspected by positive Trendelenburg test, standing anteroposterior and true lateral radiograms of both hips should be made. For complex rotational problems of the lower limb, this author recommends the recording of information given in Table 7–17.

Table 7–16. *Torsion Profile (Recommended by Staheli for Routine Use for Simple Rotational Problems of the Lower Limbs in Children)*

	R	L
FPA (Foot progression angle)		
MRH (Medial rotation of the hip)		
LRH (Lateral rotation of the hip)		
TFA (Thigh-foot angle)		
Foot deformity		

FEMORAL TORSION

Exaggerated anterior torsion of the femur is a common developmental deformity that affects rotational alignment of the lower limb and causes toeing-in. It occurs twice as frequently in girls as in boys. Increased femoral antetorsion is often familial; it is encountered in several siblings.

The Natural Course

Femoral antetorsion usually decreases with age. Shands and Steele determined the degree of femoral torsion in 238 normal children ranging in age from 3 months to 16 years.[111] The degree of femoral torsion in relation to age is shown in Figure 7–228. Between 3 and 12 months of age the average extent of normal femoral torsion is 39 degrees, and at the end of the second year, 31 degrees. From that age on, the torsion decreases 1 to 2 degrees every two years until the tenth year, when the average is 24 degrees. From the fourteenth to the sixteenth year, it decreases from 21 to 16 degrees, the latter figure corresponding to the femoral torsion of + 15.3 degrees found by Pearson and Bell in the adult English skeleton.[97] Shands and Steele consider a variation of 10 degrees above or below the average normal value to be within the limits of normal torsion.[111] The normal values of Ryder and Crane are almost identical to those of Shands and Steele (Fig. 7–229).[106]

Fabry et al. presented a 20-year follow-up study of the natural course of femoral antetorsion in 1148 hips, using the Dunlap-Shands radiographic method for determination of femoral torsion. The femoral antetorsion was about 40 degrees at birth and 32 degrees at the age of one year; then it decreased rapidly, reaching a plateau at the age of eight years. Then it decreased slowly, to an average of 16 degrees by the age of 16 years.[37]

Factors in regression of femoral antetorsion with normal growth and development are (1) weight-bearing, (2) muscular and capsular ligamentous tension, (3) gravitational forces, and (4) longitudinal growth of the femur. Galbraith et al. determined the degree of femoral antetorsion in a group of obese adolescents and in a group of adolescents of normal weight. The degree of femoral antetorsion was calculated by computed tomography or magnetic resonance imaging. The degree of femoral antetorsion was markedly less in the obese children as compared with the children of normal weight. In the obese adolescent the greater biomechanical forces exerted across the hip joint remodel the femoral neck and decrease torsion by resorption or by apposition of bone tissue on the endosteal and periosteal surfaces of the femur, and within the cortex by haversian remodeling.[42]

Table 7–17. Information Necessary for Assessment of Complex Rotational Problems of the Lower Limbs in Children

	R	L
FPA (Foot progression angle		
MRH (Medial rotation of hip)		
LRH (Lateral rotation of hip)		
Degree of femoral antetorsion as determined clinically (Ryder test)		
Degree of femoral torsion as determined by CT scan		
Instability of the hip as shown by Trendelenburg test		
Instability or subluxation of the hip as shown by standing AP radiograms of the hips		
Break in Shenton's line		
Lateral uncoverage of femoral head		
TFA (Thigh-foot angle)		
ATMA (Angle of transmalleolar axis)		
Degree of tibial torsion as determined clinically (relationship of transverse axis of knee to transmalleolar axis of ankle)		
Degree of tibial torsion as determined by CT scan		
Foot deformity		
Metatarsus varus		
Calcaneovalgus		
Flexible pes planovalgus		
Congenital convex pes valgus		
Equinus of ankle (contracture of triceps surae)		

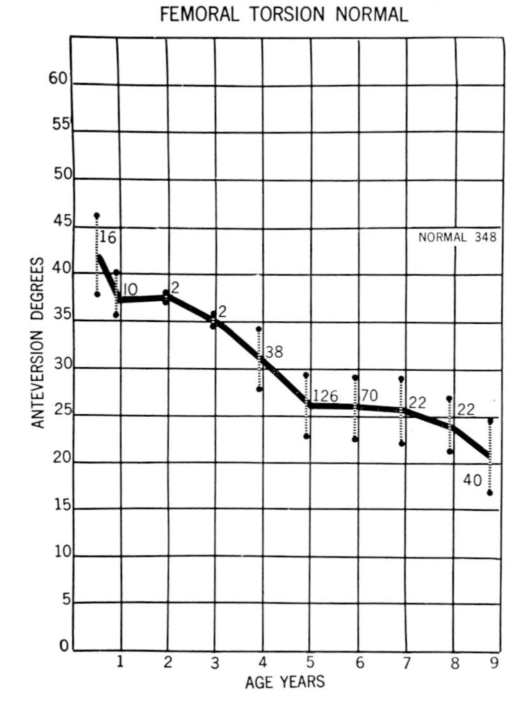

FIGURE 7–229. The degree of normal femoral torsion in relation to age.

The solid lines represent the mean; the vertical lines represent standard deviation. (From Crane, L.: Femoral torsion and its relation to toeing-in and toeing-out. J. Bone Joint Surg., *41-A*:423, 1959.)

Clinical Features

The excessive femoral antetorsion is usually present at birth; however, it is overlooked until two to three years of age, usually one or two years after the child starts to walk. The chief presenting complaint is that the child is pigeon-toed. The gait is clumsy; the thighs are rotated medially as a result, and the knees and patellae are turned inward. The appearance of the lower limbs is unsightly and disturbing, especially to a girl, while the primary concern of a boy is the loss of agility in athletic activities.

In stance also, the patellae face inward and the legs appear bowed when the feet are aligned so that they point straight forward with the knees in full extension (Fig. 7–230 A). When the thighs are rotated laterally at the hip joints so that the patellae are facing to the front, the

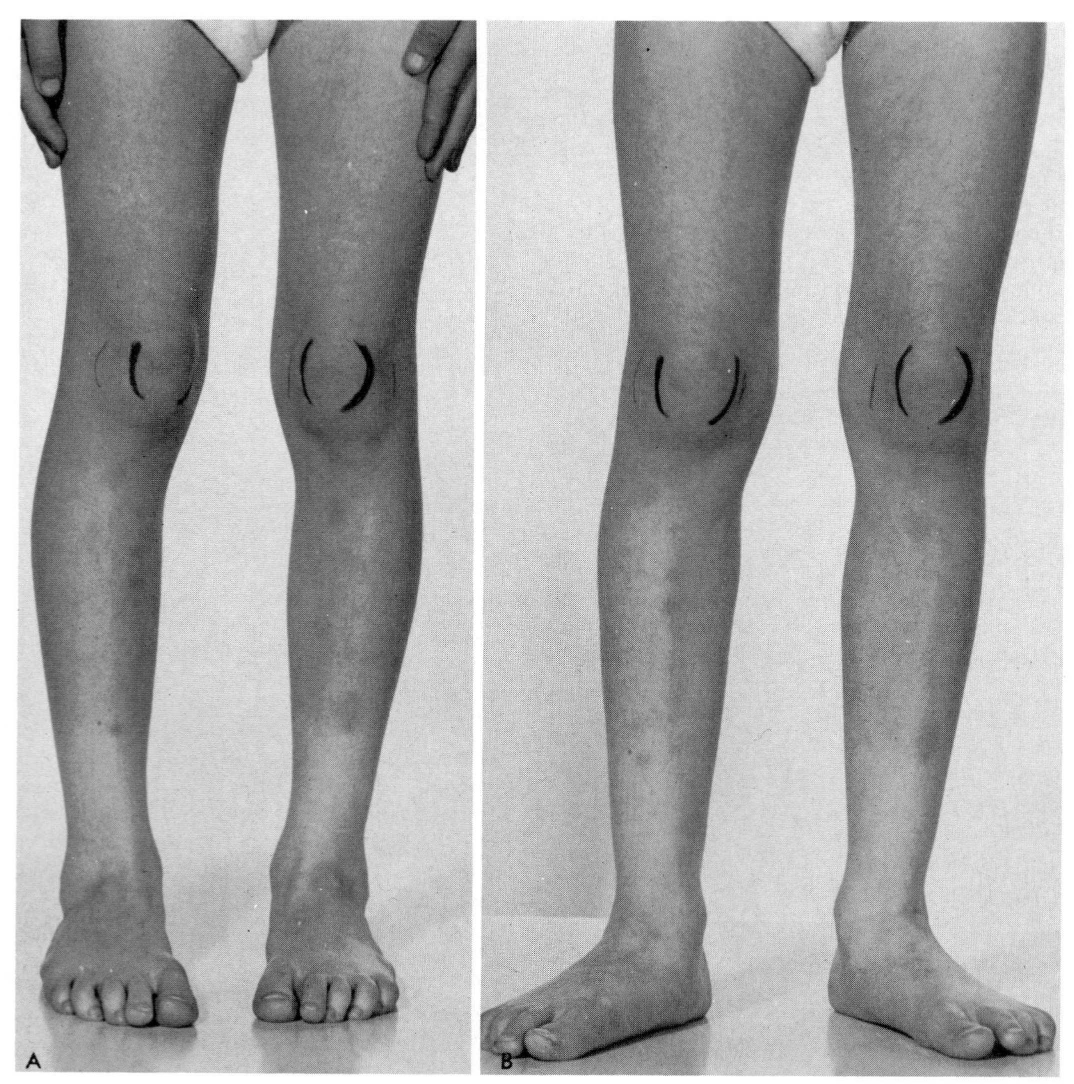

FIGURE 7–230. Clinical appearance of excessive femoral torsion in a girl.

A. With the knees in full extension and the feet aligned (pointing straight forward) the legs appear bowed and the patellae face inward. **B.** Upon lateral rotation of the hips so that the patellae are facing to the front, the feet and legs point outward and the bowleg appearance is corrected.

feet and legs point outward and the bowleg appearance is corrected (Fig. 7–230 B). A compromise between the two positions is reached by slight flexion of the knees.

Limitation of lateral rotation of the hips in extended position is the principal physical finding. Medial rotation of the hip in extension is exaggerated and may be as much as 90 degrees, whereas lateral rotation is restricted, usually to neutral position (Fig. 7–231). When the hip is in 90 degrees of flexion, lateral rotation of the hip is increased to as much as 45 degrees. This is explained by the fact that in extension of the hip, the anterior capsule and Bigelow's ligament become taut; in flexion they are relaxed, permitting lateral rotation of the hip. Thus, the importance of testing the degree of rotation of the hip in extension in femoral antetorsion cannot be overemphasized. Crane has determined the normal range of rotation of the hip in extension in various age groups (Fig. 7–232).[24]

The range of rotation of the hip in extension depends upon the inclination of the acetabulum, the angle of torsion of the proximal femur, and contracture of soft tissues—capsule, ligaments, and the muscles and fasciae about the hip, particularly the iliotibial band. It should be stressed that the degree of femoral torsion is only one factor in determining the range of medial and lateral rotation of the hip. To distinguish between soft-tissue and bony obstacles to joint motion, the hip is passively rotated laterally 10 to 20 times; by thus stretching soft-tissue contracture, the range of rotation will be increased. In childhood, medial and lateral rotation of the hips in extension ranges from about 35 to 45 degrees. In normal adults, lateral rotation of the hips exceeds medial rotation by approximately 10 degrees.

Certain adaptive changes take place in response to excessive abnormal femoral antetorsion in an attempt to compensate for the lack of lateral rotation of the hips. Soon lateral torsion of the tibia develops. The hind foot assumes a valgus posture.

As stated previously, in the fetus and newborn, the acetabulum faces in a more forward direction than in the adult. With exaggerated femoral antetorsion, this fetal direction of the acetabulum may persist and may itself be a cause of toeing-in. In the series of McSweeny, femoral torsion was found to be normal in one third of those children whose in-toeing did not correct itself, suggesting acetabular antetorsion as the cause of the toeing-in.[81]

This author has observed increased acetabular antetorsion in relation to excessive femoral antetorsion in computed tomographic studies.

The compensatory excessive lateral tibial torsion in femoral antetorsion will lead to a high quadriceps angle (Q-angle) and torsional malalignment syndrome of the patellofemoral joint and chondromalacia of the patella.[51, 52]

The stresses of marked femoral antetorsion may cause degenerative arthritic changes of the hip in adult life.

Methods of Measurement

CLINICAL METHOD

Femoral antetorsion can be assessed clinically by determining the relative positions of the midpoint of the lateral surface of the greater trochanter and the transverse axis of the femoral condyles.

The Ryder method of clinical estimation of femoral torsion is as follows: (1) The greater trochanter is palpated, (2) the lower limb is laterally rotated until the greater trochanter reaches the most lateral position, and (3) the degree of rotation of the femoral transcondylar plane from 0 degrees (neutral position) is estimated—this is the angle of femoral torsion. In antetorsion the leg is laterally rotated at the end of Step 2 and the greater trochanter lies posteriorly when the patella faces straight forward, whereas in femoral retroversion the leg is medially rotated at the end of Step 2.

IMAGING METHODS

Computed Tomography. This is the most accurate imaging method and has replaced the previous radiographic methods. The child is placed supine. In order to prevent motion the pelvis and lower limbs are secured with straps to the table top. The femoral neck and femoral condyles of both lower limbs are examined. The axial images best depicting the femoral necks and femoral condyles are selected. The degree of femoral antetorsion is calculated as follows: (1) Mark three points midway between the anterior and posterior surfaces of the femoral neck at the head, midneck, and trochanteric region. (2) Draw a line connecting these three points. (3) Determine the distal femoral transcondylar axis by the table top method. (4) The angle between the femoral neck axis and the transcondylar axis is the angle of femoral antetorsion. Intra- and interobserver variations in measurement are less than 3 degrees.[121]

Magnetic Resonance Imaging. The technique of measurement is similar to computed tomography. It is as accurate as the CT scan method.

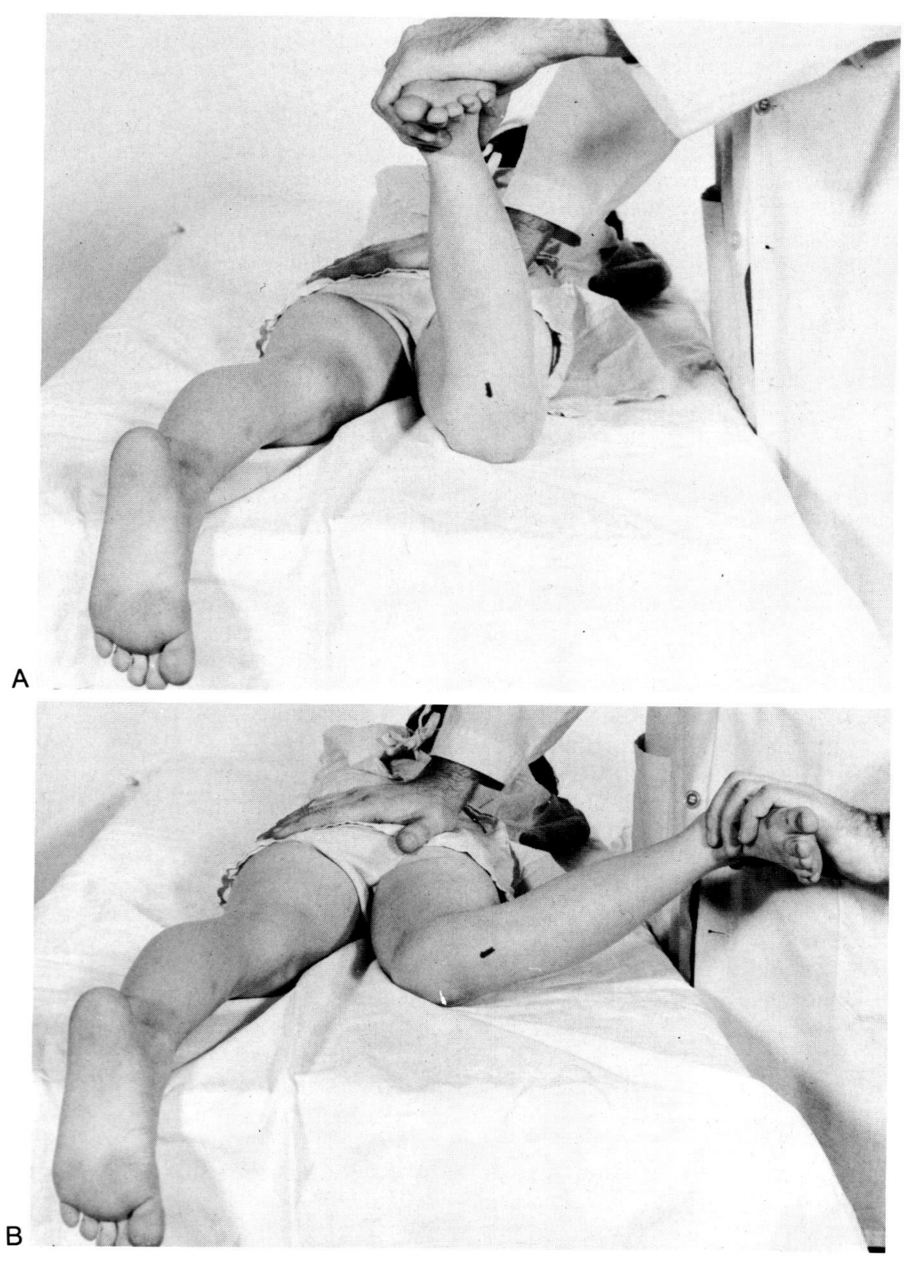

FIGURE 7–231. Range of rotation of the hip in excessive femoral antetorsion.

A. Lateral rotation of the hip in extension is exaggerated. **B.** Medial rotation of the hip in extension is limited to neutral.

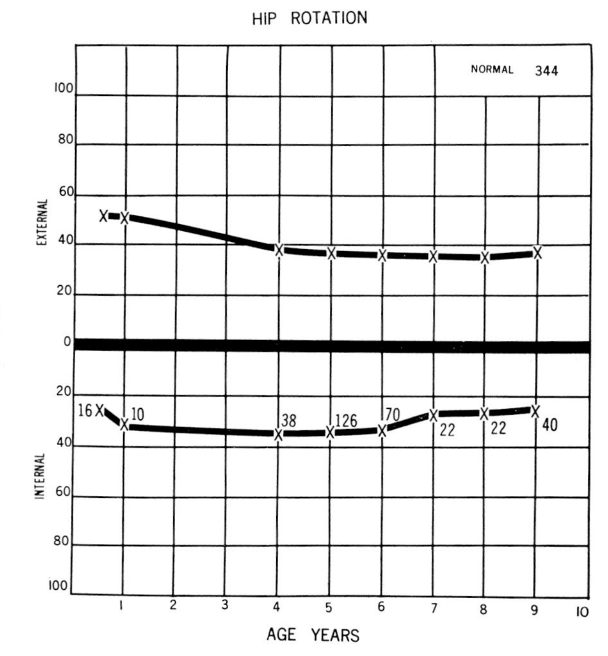

FIGURE 7–232. The range of internal and external rotation of the hips in extension in 344 normal hips.

Figures on the chart designate the number of hips examined. (From Crane, L.: Femoral torsion and its relation to toeing-in and toeing-out. J. Bone Joint Surg., *41-A*:423, 1959.)

Ultrasonography. Ultrasonography has been attempted to measure femoral antetorsion and found not to be as accurate as radiographic methods.[98]

RADIOGRAPHIC METHODS

A number of techniques are available for the measurement of upper femoral torsion. The reader is referred to the original descriptions by Dunn, by Dunlap et al., by Magilligan, and by Shands and Steele.[28, 29, 82, 111]

The essential features of radiographic technique are as follows: (1) The apparent angle of inclination or shaft-neck angle is measured in an anteroposterior or posteroanterior radiogram of the pelvis. The hips should be in full extension and neutral rotation, achieved by flexing the knees 90 degrees (over the end of the table when the patient is supine). (2) Torsion of the proximal femora is determined on a lateral radiogram of each hip. A frame is used to position the lower limbs, with the hips and knees each flexed 90 degrees and the thighs abducted 10 to 30 degrees. In the Dunlap and Shands technique, the transcondylar axis of the femur is determined by placing a radiopaque reference bar just lateral to the greater trochanter and attaching a second radiopaque bar at right angles to the first bar; the second bar represents the transcondylar axis of the femur (Fig. 7–233).[28] In the Ryder and Crane technique, the baseline of the lateral radiogram is used to represent the transcondylar plane, and a line parallel to this is drawn in the region of the femoral shaft (Fig. 7–234).[106] The apparent angle of torsion is that angle formed by the intersection of the transcondylar plane with the neck axis. (3) The true angle of torsion is then determined from the angle of measured torsion and the angle of measured inclination by using a graph prepared from special mathematical formulas (Figs. 7–235 and 7–236).

A simple method to determine the degree of anteversion of the proximal femur is to place the patient in prone position and, under image intensifier fluoroscopy, to measure the length of the femoral neck (intertrochanteric line to capital physis) with the hip in varying degrees of rotation. The hips should be in full extension. Flexion of the knees to right angles will assist in determining the degree of hip rotation. The degree of femoral antetorsion is the degree of medial rotation of the hip beyond which the relative length of the femoral neck does not increase.

Treatment

CONSERVATIVE MEASURES

This consists of reassurance of the parents and periodic observation. It is explained to the parents that excessive femoral antetorsion will most probably correct itself spontaneously by the age of seven or eight years. The child is examined at six-month intervals to assess the

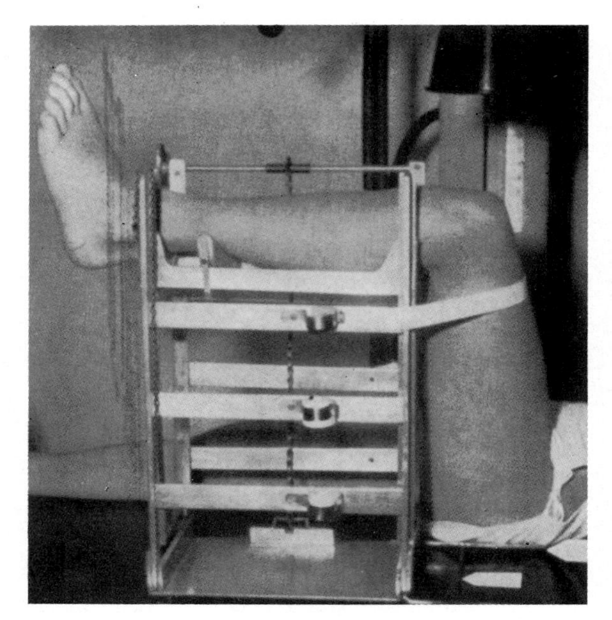
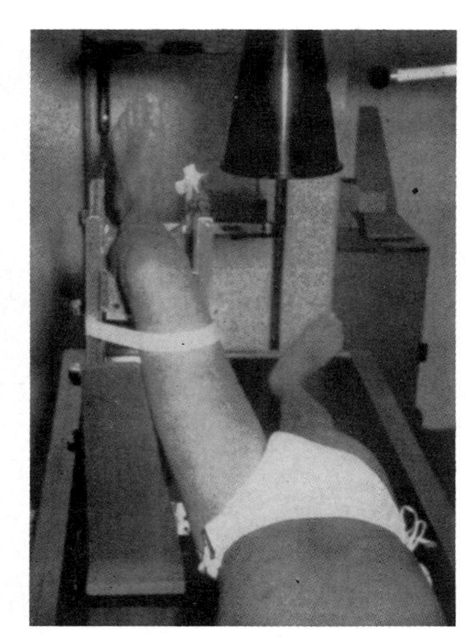

FIGURE 7–233. The apparatus used by Dunlap et al. and Shands and Steele for making lateral radiograms of each hip. (From Shands, A. R., Jr., and Steele, M. K.: Torsion of the femur. J. Bone Joint Surg., *40*-A:804, 1958.)

improvement in the range of lateral rotation of the hip in extension. It is not necessary to make radiograms of the hip or to perform antetorsion studies unless there is clinical evidence of instability of the hip as shown by positive delayed or immediate Trendelenburg test.

Nonoperative measures are ineffective in the treatment of femoral antetorsion. In the past it was customary to prescribe special orthopedic shoes with lateral sole and heel wedges. The documented study by Knittel and Staheli has conclusively demonstrated that shoe modifications have no effect on femoral torsion and intoeing gait.[69] They should not be employed.

Twister cables rotating the feet and legs laterally do not exert active corrective forces on the hips and thighs; they do not diminish femoral antetorsion. Splinting of the hips in forced lateral rotation is ineffective; this may be harmful, causing anterior uncoverage of the femoral heads and subluxation of the hips, and should not be employed.

Denis Browne splints, forcing the feet into lateral rotation, are ineffective in correcting excessive femoral antetorsion; they should not be used. They may cause secondary deformities in the segments distal to the hip joint: namely, pes valgus, lateral torsion of the tibia, and genu valgum. The deforming influence and harmful effects of the Denis Browne splint in the treatment of femoral antetorsion cannot be overemphasized.

In the study by Fabry et al., the degree of correction of femoral antetorsion obtained by Denis Browne splint and/or twister cables was not greater than that of spontaneous derotation with no treatment.[37]

It is strongly recommended by this author that children with femoral antetorsion not be subjected to ineffective and sometimes expensive methods of conservative management. Improvement of torsional deformity takes place spontaneously, consistent with the natural history of femoral antetorsion. It is not due to the "conservative" treatment prescribed by the physician.

Alteration of sitting posture is recommended by many surgeons. The child is encouraged to sit in the tailor's position and is not allowed to sit in reverse tailor's (W or TV squat) position. Posture is the effect and not the cause of femoral antetorsion. Changing of sleeping or sitting posture will not improve excessive femoral torsion. When femoral antetorsion is accompanied by excessive medial tibial torsion, it is advisable that the child sit on a chair with the knees flexed or cross-legged (Indian fashion). Sleeping prone with the legs medially rotated or sitting W fashion may prevent spontaneous derotation of the medial torsion deformity of the tibia.

OPERATIVE MEASURES

Derotation femoral osteotomy is the only effective method of correcting excessive femoral

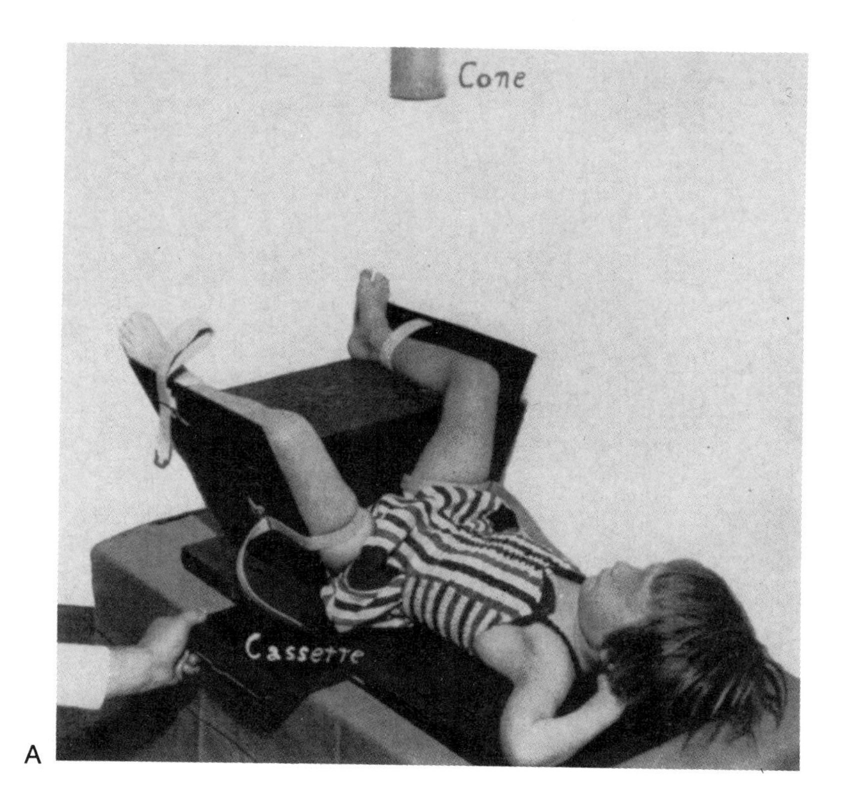

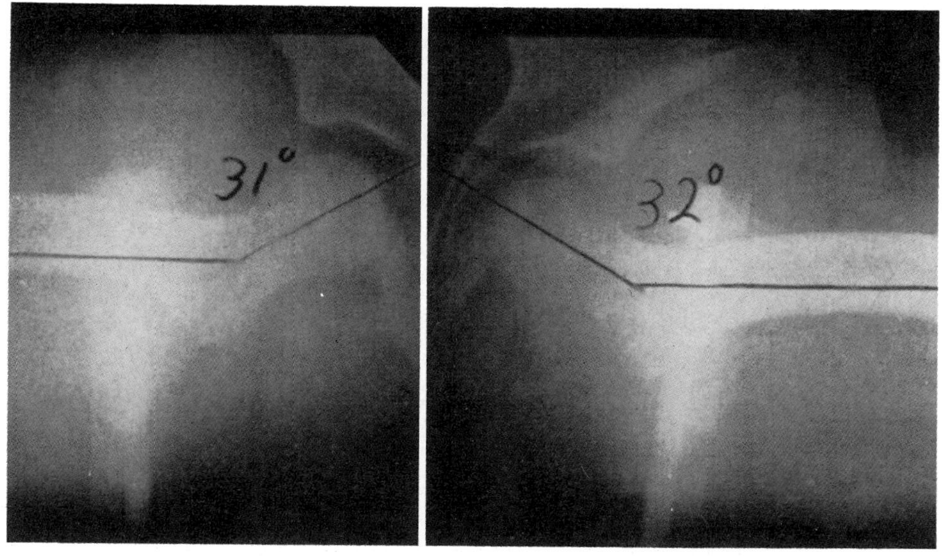

FIGURE 7–234. Ryder and Crane method of measuring femoral torsion.

A. Modified flexion-abduction frame. **B.** Radiograms of both hips made with the lower limbs positioned in the flexion-abduction frame. The baseline of the radiograms represents the transcondylar plane, and a line parallel to it is drawn in the region of the femoral shaft. The angle formed by the intersection of the neck axis and the transcondylar plane is the projected angle of anteversion. The true, or corrected, angle of torsion is determined from a special chart (see Fig. 7–236). (From Crane, L.: Femoral torsion. J. Bone Joint Surg., *41-A*:425, 1959.)

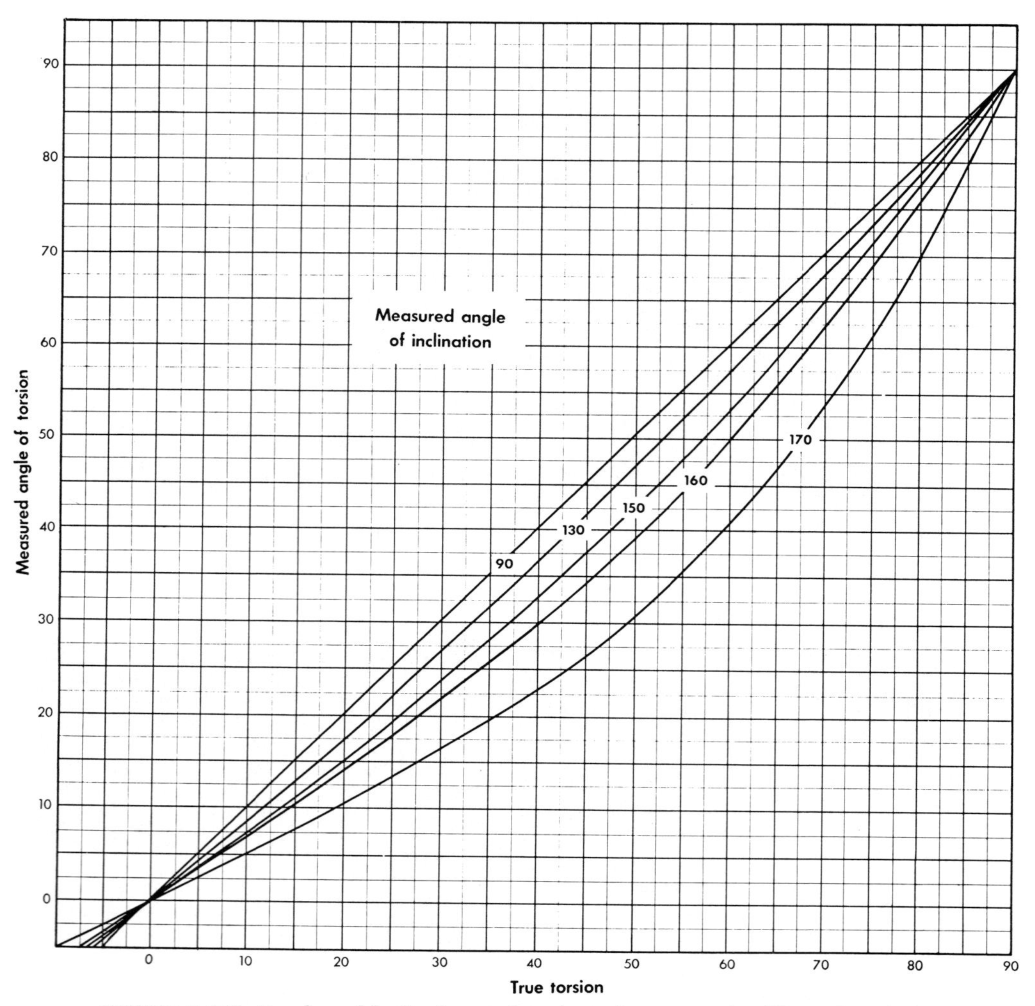

FIGURE 7–235. Graph used by Dunlap et al. to determine true angle of femoral torsion.

The measured angle of torsion and the measured angle of inclination are determined from the radiogram. The angle of hip abduction is 10 degrees. The graph is prepared from the Weber Formula No. 1. (From Dunlap, K., et al.: A new method for determination of torsion of the femur. J. Bone Joint Surg., 35-A:299, 1953.)

projected inclination \ projected anteversion	0	5	10	15	20	25	30	35	40	45	50	55	60	65	70	75	80	85	90
80	0	3	7	12	16	20	24	29	33	38	43	47	53	59	65	71	77	84	
90	0	4	9	13	17	22	27	31	36	41	46	51	56	62	67	73	79	84	
95	0	5	9	14	18	23	28	32	37	42	47	52	58	63	68	74	79	85	
100	0	5	10	14	19	24	29	34	39	44	49	54	59	64	69	74	80	85	90
105	0	5	10	15	20	25	30	35	40	45	50	55	60	65	70	75	80	85	90
110	0	5	10	16	21	26	31	36	41	46	51	56	61	66	71	76	80	85	90
115	0	5	11	16	22	27	32	38	43	48	53	57	62	67	72	76	81	85	90
120	0	6	11	17	23	28	34	39	44	49	54	59	63	68	72	77	81	86	90
125	0	6	12	18	24	30	35	41	46	51	56	60	65	69	73	78	82	86	90
130	0	6	13	19	25	31	37	42	47	52	57	62	66	70	74	78	82	86	90
135	0	7	14	20	27	33	38	44	48	54	58	63	67	71	75	79	83	86	90
140	0	7	14	21	28	34	40	46	50	56	60	64	68	72	76	80	83	87	90
145	0	8	16	23	30	36	42	48	53	58	62	66	70	74	77	80	84	87	90
150	0	9	17	25	32	39	45	50	55	60	64	68	72	75	78	81	84	87	90
155	0	10	19	27	35	42	48	54	58	63	67	70	73	77	79	82	85	87	90
160	0	11	22	31	39	46	52	58	62	65	70	73	76	78	81	83	86	88	90
165	0	13	26	36	45	52	57	62	66	70	73	76	78	80	82	84	86	88	90
170	0	18	33	45	53	60	65	69	72	75	77	79	81	83	84	86	87	89	90
175	0	29	48	59	67	71	75	77	79	81	82	84	85	86	87	88	88	89	90
180	0	90	90	90	90	90	90	90	90	90	90	90	90	90	90	90	90	90	90

ANTEVERSION

FIGURE 7–236. Chart used by Ryder and Crane to calculate the true angle of femoral torsion.

(From Ryder, C. T., and Crane, L.: Measuring femoral anteversion. J. Bone Joint Surg., 35-A:324, 1953.)

antetorsion. However, the indications for surgical correction of excessive femoral antetorsion are not clearly delineated; there is some controversy. It is difficult to lay down definite guidelines as to indications for surgery; each case should be individualized. Surgery should not be performed before the age of eight years because of the likelihood of spontaneous correction. The natural history of femoral antetorsion is such that after the age of eight years, a significant degree of spontaneous correction will not take place. Also, the surgery should *not* be postponed until late adolescence because of the possible development of increasing fixed lateral tibial torsion.

It is this author's recommendation that the eight-year-old child be observed with thorough assessment of the torsional deformity for at least one, and preferably two, years to determine whether the deformity is improving. Parents and patient should be informed of the benign natural history of the deformity and told that the surgical procedure is major and carries a significant complication rate. Asymmetrical growth stimulation and lower limb length disparity is a potential problem. The extent of the operative scars should be clearly understood. There is no definitive evidence that increased femoral antetorsion causes degenerative arthritis of the hip or knee, resulting in pain and functional disability in the adult.

The author recommends a derotation osteotomy of the femur when the child is nine years or older when (1) the degree of femoral antetorsion exceeds 45 degrees, as measured by CT scan or magnetic resonance imaging; (2) the hip cannot be rotated laterally beyond neutral position and medially rotates 90 degrees; (3) lateral tibial torsion does not exceed 35 degrees; and (4) the functional disability and unsightliness are so severe that *parents and patient demand* that something be done. Derotation osteotomy may be performed in the intertrochanteric, subtrochanteric, mid-diaphyseal, or supracondylar area. This author prefers performing the lateral derotation osteotomy at the subtrochanteric level. The technique of derotation osteotomy to correct excessive antetorsion has been described in Chapter 2. As a general rule, the distal segment of the femur should be rotated laterally to such a degree that there is equal range of medial and lateral rotation of the hip in extension to provide normal foot progression angle.

Osteotomy in the supracondylar level is technically simpler to perform than subtrochanteric osteotomy. The operative technique is as follows: Make a 2-cm. longitudinal incision over the medial aspect of the distal femur, about 1.5 cm. proximal to the superior border of the patella. The subcutaneous tissue and fascia are incised in line with the skin incision. By sharp and dull dissection in the plane between the vastus medialis and adductor longus tendon, the periosteum is exposed. Under image intensification the exact level of the osteotomy is verified. It should be 1.5 to 2.0 cm. proximal to the distal femoral physis. A 1-cm.-long incision is made in the periosteum. With an electric power drill, multiple drill holes are made in a transverse fashion through both cortices in a medial to lateral direction, under image intensifier x-ray control. The osteotomy is completed with a sharp narrow osteotome. Then the distal femoral segment is rotated laterally to the planned degree, with the hip and knee in full extension. The position of the osteotomized fragments is verified, and a double hip spica is applied with the knees and hips in full extension. Internal fixation is ordinarily not necessary in children between eight and nine years of age.[79]

Problems and complications of distal femoral osteotomy by this technique are loss of alignment due to inadequacy of fixation, errors in the degree of derotation, knee stiffness, and valgus deformity of the knee; the last-named appears to be due to medial femoral overgrowth. Fonseca and Bassett reported two cases of genu valgum deformity following derotation osteotomy to correct medial femoral torsion; both these patients required secondary surgical procedures to correct the deformity.[40] This complication has similarities to the tibia valga deformity following a fracture of the proximal tibial metaphysis. Another possible pathogenic factor is the loss of the normal mechanical restraint provided medially by the periosteum. Experimentally in rabbits, hemicircumferential division of the periosteum can produce valgus deformity.[47]

In order to prevent loss of alignment and recurrence of deformity, this author recommends the use of corticotomy and Orthofix or Ilizarov external fixator. With the use of these fixators, cast immobilization is not required. Some surgeons may prefer to use two or three threaded Steinmann pins, inserted under image intensifier radiographic control. The pins should avoid the distal femoral physis. They are inserted percutaneously and cut subcutaneously. The pins are removed when the hip spica cast is removed.

An alternative way of performing derotation osteotomy is at the midshaft level, with fixation by an intramedullary interlocking nail.[101]

Medial rotation osteotomy of the tibia may be required if there is marked secondary lateral tibial torsion. It is best to delay this for three to six months following lateral rotation osteotomy of the femur.

It has been suggested that the stresses of marked femoral antetorsion may cause degenerative arthritic changes of the hip in adult life.[45] This has not been clearly documented. In excessive medial femoral torsion with compensatory lateral tibiofibular torsion, there may be torsional malalignment of the patellofemoral joint and chondromalacia of the patella.[6, 12, 20, 38, 75, 131, 135] In patellofemoral joint instability and chondromalacia a torsional assessment should be performed; however, in children and adolescents a preventive operation to realign the knee is not indicated.

TIBIAL TORSION

The degree of tibial torsion depends upon the age of the child and is variable among individuals. The natural course of tibial torsion is to rotate laterally with increasing age. Le-Damany measured the torsion of the tibia in anatomic specimens using Broca's instrument and found that in the fetus the medial malleolus was located behind the lateral malleolus and that there was medial torsion of the tibia; at birth, the tips of the malleoli were level; and by the time walking was fully established, the medial malleolus was situated in front of the lateral malleolus and there was 20 degrees of lateral torsion of the tibia. In the normal adult tibia, tibial torsion was lateral with a mean average of 23.7 degrees.[76]

Staheli and Engel studied the degree of tibial torsion in 160 normal children and 20 adults by measuring the transmalleolar axis with the knee flexed. They found that it increased with age; during the first year of life it averaged 5 degrees of lateral rotation; during midchildhood, 10 degrees of lateral rotation; and in older children and adults, 14 degrees.[122] When transmalleolar axis is measured with the knee in full extension it measures 20 degrees of lateral rotation in the normal adult. Other studies of tibial torsion on post-mortem anatomic specimens in various age groups have given approximately the same findings.[30, 50] The torsion in the normal adult tibia was found to be 20 degrees lateral by

Dupuis, and 22.1 degrees lateral by Hutter and Scott.[30, 50] Clinical mensuration of torsion by the use of tropometer in the normal adult tibia was reported as 20 degrees lateral by Wynne-Davies and by Jaffres, and 19 degrees lateral by Smillie and Turner.[55, 113, 141]

Khermosh, Lior, and Weissman measured tibial torsion in 230 normal newborn babies and young children up to five years of age. In the early postnatal period (birth to three months), most babies had mild lateral torsion with a mean value of 2.2 degrees; only 9 per cent had no torsion (0 degrees), and 12 per cent had medial torsion (0 to 8 degrees). A gradual increase in the torsional angle with age at an average rate of 1.3 degrees per year was noted. Tibial torsion was 3.5 degrees in the 4- to 9-month age group and 4.3 degrees in the 10- to 21-month age group. The angle increased at a greater rate in the 22- to 27-month age group, in which the mean value was 6.1 degrees. There was no significant increase in the torsional angle in the 30- to 40-month age group; in the 41- to 60-month age group, it increased gradually to a mean value of 9.1 degrees. There was no statistically significant difference in the degree of torsion between the left and right tibiae in all age groups, or between the sexes.[61]

LeDamany also measured torsion of the tibiae of human specimens dating from the prehistoric age, when shoes did not exist; the average lateral tibial torsion was +25 degrees—apparently shoes played no role in the development of progressive lateral tibial torsion.[76]

The incidence of medial tibial torsion in 200 adults was determined by Hutter and Scott. They found medial tibial torsion in 5 per cent of the 100 women examined, and in 3 per cent of the men. The medial torsion was severe enough to cause difficulty in walking in 2 per cent of the female patients and in 1 per cent of the males.[50]

Measurement of Tibial Torsion

In anatomic specimens the degree of tibial torsion can be measured quite accurately by inserting a pin through the center of the condylar articulating surface of the proximal end of the tibia, and a second pin through the center of the distal end of the tibia, parallel to a line between the centers of the medial and lateral malleoli. Rotation of the tibia on its longitudinal axis is assessed by means of a tropometer. One pin inserted in the distal end of the tibia holds it upright; another pin through the upper end of the tibia is fixed to the vertical standard, and the degree of tibial torsion is measured on a protractor placed underneath the distal pin (Fig. 7–237). Inserting pins through the tibia of a living person to measure torsion is not justifiable.

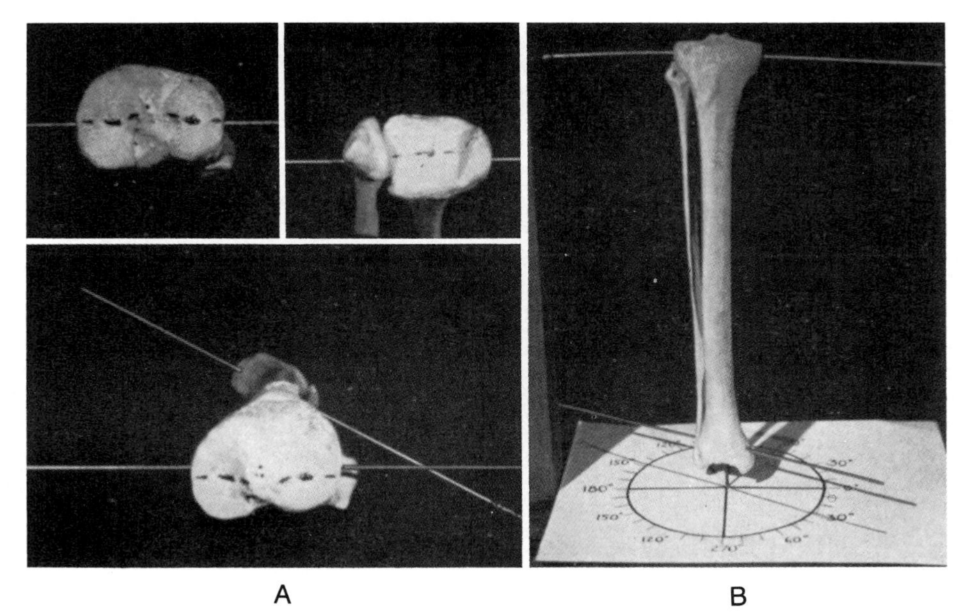

FIGURE 7–237. Method of determining the degree of tibial torsion in an anatomic specimen.

A. Pins are inserted through the articular axes of the upper and lower ends of the tibia. The angles formed by the two pins in the coronal plane is the degree of tibial torsion. **B.** A model demonstrating the method of obtaining tropometric measurements. (From Hutter, C. G., Jr., and Scott, W.: Tibial torsion. J. Bone Joint Surg., *31-A*:512, 1949.)

CLINICAL METHODS

Clinical measurement of tibial torsion by visual inspection is difficult; one can only estimate approximate values that should be measured in 5-degree increments. There is a wide range of interobserver error. *Medial* torsion is designated by minus value and *lateral* torsion by positive value; this author prefers to use the term medial or lateral instead of minus or plus.

Wynne-Davies designed an instrument for clinical measurement of tibial torsion.[140] Her apparatus was later slightly modified by Khermosh, Lior, and Weissman (Fig. 7–238).[61] The reader is referred to the original articles for description of the instruments. These clinical methods are not accurate, however, as the relative positions of the malleoli are used for measurement, not the tibia itself; thus any motion between the tibia and fibula will give a false value.

A simple clinical method employed by the author is illustrated in Figure 7–239. The child is seated on the edge of a table with his knee flexed 90 degrees, or the infant is placed in prone position and his knee is flexed to a right angle. By proper positioning of the limb, the tibial transcondylar line (axis of the knee joint) is made parallel either to the edge of the table (when sitting) or to the top of the table (when lying prone). The transmalleolar line (axis of the ankle) is determined by placing the thumb on the distal tip of the medial malleolus and the index finger on the distal tip of the fibular malleolus. The degree of tibial torsion is determined by the angle formed between the transcondylar tibial axis and the axis of the ankle joint (bimalleolar axis). It should be noted that when the bimalleolar axis is the distal line of reference, tibiofibular and not tibial torsion is measured. An alternative method of determining tibial torsion is to have the child seated with his legs hanging over the edge of the table and to determine the angle formed by the proximal tibial tuberosity and the second metatarsal ray of a normal foot supported in neutral position; if the foot is deformed into varus or valgus, the distal point of reference is the midpoint between the medial and lateral malleoli noted by observing the longitudinal axis of the tibia.

The *thigh-foot angle* is another method of determining tibial torsion. The patient is placed prone with the knees together and flexed to 90 degrees and the feet at right angles to the tibia. Tibial torsion is measured by the angle between the thigh and longitudinal axis of the foot.[118]

PLAIN RADIOGRAPHIC METHODS

For the adolescent or adult patient, several radiologic techniques are available to measure tibial torsion; radiographic methods cannot be applied to infants or young children, however, because of the lack of contrast shadows projected by their cartilaginous epiphyses. Ordinarily, radiographic measurement of tibial torsion is not indicated in children. It is of limited clinical value, and radiation exposure is not justified.

Nachlas Method. With the proximal tibial tubercle maintained in neutral position, true anteroposterior and lateral radiograms of the tibia, including the knee and ankle joints, are made. The relative positions of the medial and lateral malleoli are compared. In medial tibial torsion the medial malleolus lies posterior to the lateral malleolus, whereas in lateral tibial torsion it is located anterior to the fibular malleolus.[90] This technique provides only a rough estimate that is not inherently any more accurate than clinical methods of evaluation.

Hutter and Scott Method. The cassette is placed beneath the soles of both feet. The patient sits with his knees flexed 90 degrees and the medial borders of his feet parallel to the medial borders of his thighs. The x-ray tube is placed above the knees, and the exposure is made with the beam parallel to the longitudinal axis of the tibia. An image of the malleoli and the feet is projected on the film. Lines are drawn between the tips of the malleoli and along the medial border of the radiographic shadows of the bony structures of the foot, with the latter line approximately at a right angle to the articular axis of the knee. The intersection of these two lines forms an angle that, when subtracted from 90 degrees, will give the measurement of tibial torsion in degrees (Fig. 7–240).[50]

Rosen and Sandick Method. Two arbitrary pairs of points are marked on the leg: (1) The upper lateral point is marked at the prominent junction of the anterior and lateral aspects of the proximal end of the head of the fibula. (2) The upper medial point is marked at the most prominent medial part of the inner condyle. (3) The lower lateral point marks the prominence of the junction of the lateral and posterior margins of the fibular malleolus. (4) The lower medial point is made at the prominence of the junction of the anterior medial margins of the medial malleolus. Transverse lines are drawn between the upper two points (transcondylar

A

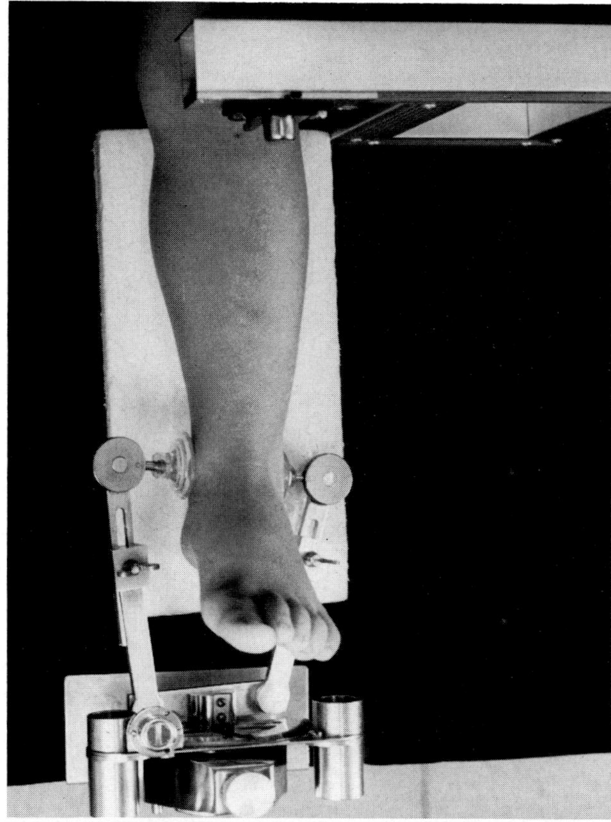

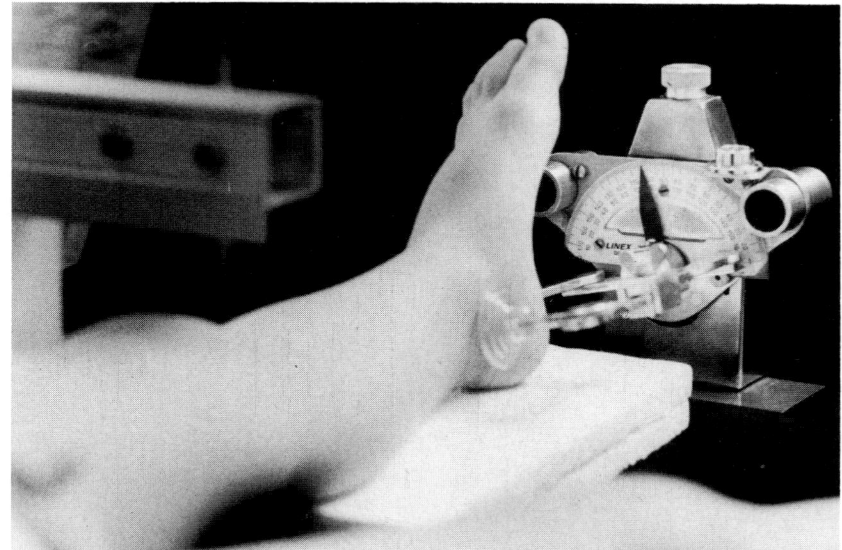

B

FIGURE 7–238. Instrument used for measuring tibial torsion (designed by Khermosh et al.).

A. The vertical pointer is directed toward the proximal tibial tubercle. The two distal discs are placed in contact with the center of the medial and lateral malleoli, while the leg is comfortably elevated and supported on a polyurethane foam plate. **B.** The pointer indicates the degree of torsion on the protractor, which is fixed at the end of the table. Medial torsion is recorded as minus (−), while lateral torsion is recorded as plus (+). (From Khermosh, O., Lior, G., and Weissman, S. L.: Tibial torsion in children. Clin. Orthop., 79:26, 1971.)

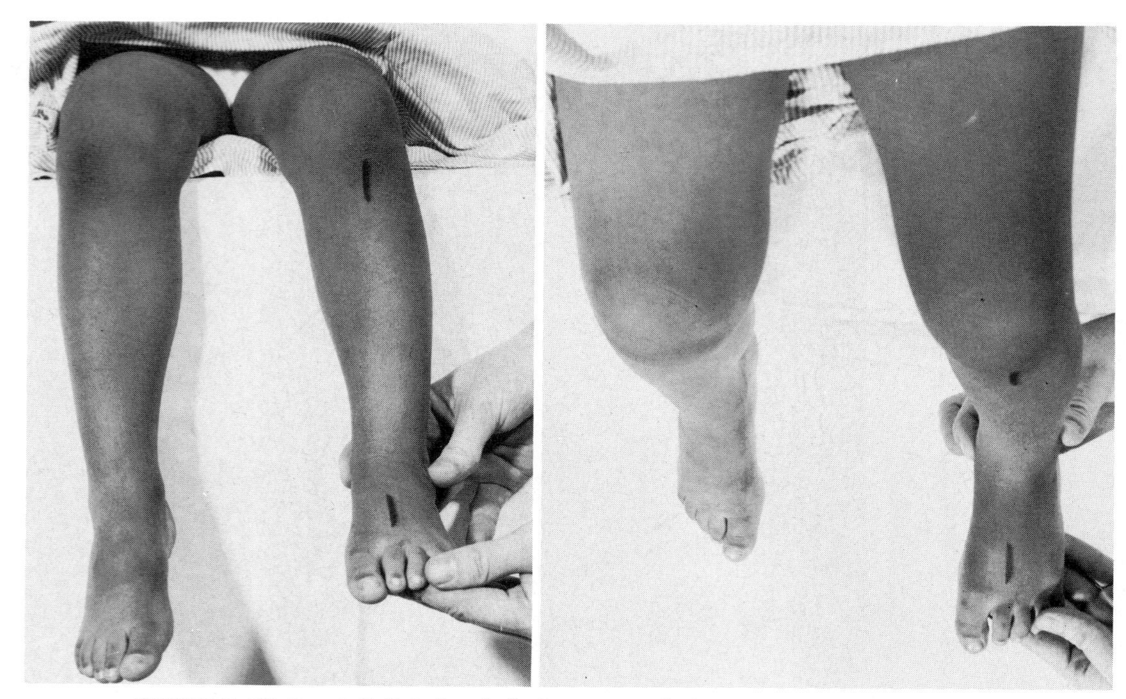

FIGURE 7–239. Practical clinical method of measuring tibial torsion (see text for explanation).

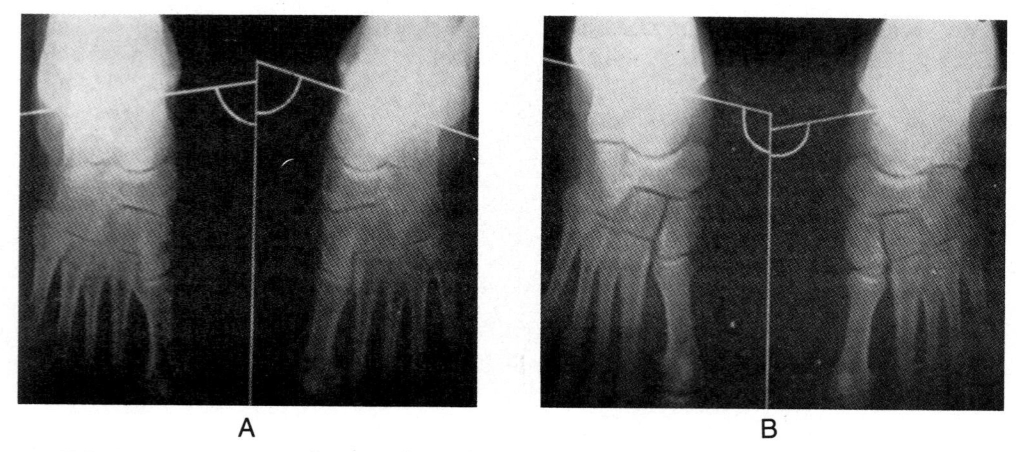

FIGURE 7–240. Hutter and Scott radiographic method of measuring the degree of tibial torsion.

Radiograms made according to the technique described in the text. **A.** Internal tibial torsion; minus 10 degrees on the right and minus 18 degrees on the left. **B.** External tibial torsion: plus 13 degrees on the right and plus 12 degrees on the left. (From Hutter, C. G., Jr., and Scott, W.: Tibial torsion. J. Bone Joint Surg., *31-A*:515, 1949.)

axis) and between the lower two points (transmalleolar axis). The angle formed by these axes represents the degree of tibiofibular torsion.[105] The Rosen and Sandick method measures tibiofibular torsion and not isolated tibial torsion.

CALCULATION OF TIBIAL TORSION BY COMPUTED TRANSVERSE TOMOGRAPHY

Transverse tomograms of the upper and lower juxta-articular areas are made with the patient supine on the sliding tables of the whole-body scanner. Motion during the procedure is avoided by strapping the lower limbs onto a Plexiglas or other support. The proximal reference line is the axis through the widest transverse condylar diameter; the distal reference line is the transverse axis through the inferior end of the tibia that bisects the anteroposterior diameter and also passes through the anterior half of the lateral malleolus. These lines are drawn on the tomographic picture. The angle formed by these two axes gives the tibiofibular torsion. The accuracy of measurement of tibial torsion by CT scanning is ±5 degrees.[56]

The mean value of tibiofibular torsion in the normal adult tibia is 30 degrees lateral. With the use of tibia and fibula together for the distal measurement, the value of tibiofibular torsion is increased.

MEASUREMENT OF TIBIAL TORSION BY ULTRASOUND[58]

In this method the posterior margins of the proximal and distal articular surfaces of the tibia are utilized as reference lines. With the patient in prone position, the posterior margin of the proximal articular surface of the tibia is identified by first locating the femoral condyles and then moving the ultrasound scanner probe distally until the first image of the tibia is obtained. By the use of longitudinal scans the distal articular surface of the tibia is identified; then a transverse scan is made. The degree of tibial torsion is measured by the angle subtended between the posterior margin of the upper and lower ends of the tibia. During the procedure it is vital that the child not move his limb. The probe should be aligned identically for both scans, and the proper bony landmarks should be scanned. Measurement of tibial torsion by ultrasound is not as accurate as by computed axial tomography. The advantage of ultrasound over CT scan is that there is no radiation. The ultrasound technique measures tibial torsion and not tibiofibular torsion. The mean value obtained by ultrasound mensuration of the degree of tibial torsion is about 40 degrees lateral—this is higher than that obtained by other methods.[58]

MEDIAL TIBIAL TORSION

In infants, abnormal medial tibial torsion is usually associated with congenital metatarsus varus or developmental genu varum. As an isolated deformity, its incidence is not common. Exaggerated medial tibial torsion may occur in combination with or independent of abnormal femoral antetorsion.

The child is usually brought to the orthopedic surgeon between the ages of 6 and 12 months with the presenting complaint that he is pigeon-toed or bowlegged. Often the condition is overlooked until the child begins to walk; then the chief complaint is that he toes-in.

On examination, both in supine position and in stance the feet point inward. In the pure form there is no varus deformity of the metatarsals. The medial malleolus is located posterior to the lateral malleolus. Involvement is usually symmetrical. In stance, because the toes are pointed inward at an angle of from 35 to 15 degrees, the center of gravity of the body falls lateral to the second metatarsal, which is the center ray of the foot. The older child will compensate for this malalignment of the body's center of gravity by everting and abducting the forefoot and/or laterally rotating the hip.

Kite distinguishes between the congenital and acquired forms of medial torsion of the legs. In his rotation test, the ankles are grasped and the limbs rotated medially and laterally at the hip joints; in the congenital form of medial torsion, the patellae can be turned medially and laterally to the same degree as in the normal child, whereas in the acquired form of medial tibial torsion, the patellae can be turned medially 90 degrees or more, but they cannot be rotated laterally past neutral position.[63–66] It should be emphasized, however, that the determination made by Kite's rotation test is the range of rotation at the hip. As stated earlier, abnormal femoral antetorsion or contracture of soft tissues in the medial and anterior aspects of the hip joint will restrict lateral rotation of the hip in extension. Kite also states that there is very little deformity of the femora in those with congenital medial torsion; also, the child with acquired medial torsion usually sits on his legs with his toes turned in; if his legs are unfolded, in a few seconds he will sit on his feet again because this is the position of comfort.[63] This author does not recommend Kite's rotation test; it is best to perform Staheli's torsion profile.

It is very important to determine whether

the older siblings and the parents have persistent abnormal medial tibial torsion, as the subdivision into hereditary and nonhereditary forms is of practical significance in the prognosis and treatment of medial tibial torsion. If the tibiae of the parents and the adolescent siblings have normal alignment, the probability of spontaneous correction by the age of seven to eight years of age is very great; however, if there is a familial incidence of persistent abnormal medial tibial torsion, the prognosis for spontaneous correction is guarded and aggressive therapeutic measures should be considered.

ABNORMAL LATERAL TIBIAL TORSION

This is usually an acquired deformity that is secondary to contracture of the iliotibial band, although it does occur occasionally as a congenital or primary developmental deformity.[3] The deformity may be unilateral or bilateral. In the congenital forms, both tibiae are usually symmetrically affected.

In stance, with the patellae facing straight forward, the feet point outward (Fig. 7–241). The center of gravity is medial to the first metatarsal. The lateral malleolus lies posterior to the medial malleolus. Any associated knock-knee deformity is noted. Ober's test should always be performed for detection of iliotibial band contracture (see Fig. 1–22, p. 30). Lateral tibial torsion may be secondary and compensatory to abnormal femoral antetorsion. The range of rotation of the hips is tested in full extended position; in abnormal femoral antetorsion, lateral rotation of the hip is restricted, whereas in iliotibial band contracture, it is the medial rotation of the hip that is limited.

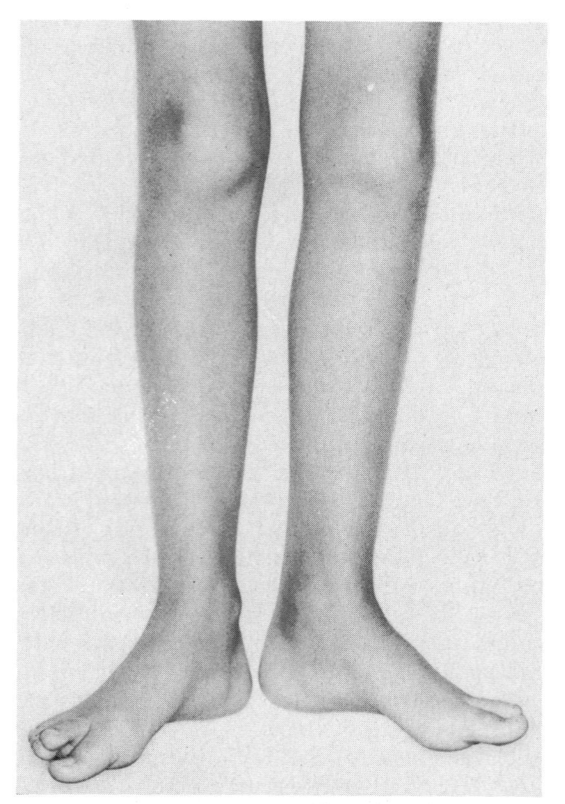

FIGURE 7–241. Exaggerated lateral tibial torsion.

In stance, with the patellae facing straight forward, the feet point outward.

In gait, the child toes out, the feet pointing in opposite directions. Triceps surae contracture, a common cause of toeing-out in children, is ruled out by testing the range of passive dorsiflexion of both ankles.

Differential Diagnosis

In-toeing may be due to a variety of abnormalities of congenital or acquired origin. It may stem from fixed bony deformity, soft-tissue contracture, muscle paralysis and imbalance, or a change in the planes of articulation. The level of pathologic involvement may be in the hip, femur, knee, leg or ankle, or foot.

In Table 7–18 the various causes of toeing-in and toeing-out are listed. In the author's experience, the most common cause of toeing-in is protective in-toeing due to pronated feet and developmental genu valgum; next, in order of decreasing frequency, are abnormal femoral antetorsion, metatarsus varus, excessive medial torsion, forward inclination of the acetabulum, and paralytic acquired causes such as spasticity of the hip adductors or of the posterior tibial muscle in cerebral palsy.

Treatment

The modality of treatment is determined according to the patient's age, the severity of the deformity, whether excessive torsional deformity is medial or lateral, and the presence or absence of familial incidence.

In infants, usually no treatment is required.

Medial Tibial Torsion. With growth, the medial tibial torsion will correct itself spontaneously. Passive stretching exercises are indicated in some cases, primarily to appease the anxious parents or grandparents. The foot is manipulated into abduction and eversion 15 to 20 times in several daily sessions. These will help to correct any associated soft-tissue contracture, such as that of the posterior tibial and/or abductor hallucis muscles. More aggressive programs of therapy are ordinarily not indicated. As stated earlier, Denis Browne splints force the feet into abduction and cause genu

Table 7–18. Etiology of Toeing-In and Toeing-Out in Children

Level of Affection	*Toe-In*	*Toe-Out*
Feet-ankles	Pronated feet (protective toeing-in) Metatarsus varus Talipes varus and equinovarus	Pes valgus due to contracture of triceps surae muscle Talipes calcaneovalgus Congenital convex pes planovalgus
Leg-knee	Tibia vara (Blount's disease) and developmental genu varum Abnormal medial tibial torsion Genu valgum—developmental (protective toeing-in to shift body center of gravity medially) Congenital or acquired hypoplasia of the tibia with relative overgrowth of the fibula	Lateral tibial torsion Congenital absence or hypoplasia of the fibula
Femur-hip	Abnormal femoral antetorsion Spasticity of medial rotators of hip (cerebral palsy)	Abnormal femoral retroversion Flaccid paralysis of medial rotators of hip
Acetabulum	Maldirected—facing anteriorly	Maldirected—facing posteriorly

valgum. Unfortunately, they are indiscriminately used for treatment of toeing-in in children, most of whom do not have actual abnormal medial tibial torsion. The use of a Denis Browne splint is recommended only in cases in which medial tibial torsion exceeds 40 degrees in a child who has a positive family history of persistent abnormal medial tibial torsion and in whom spontaneous correction is *not* taking place. Often in these children this author does not apply a Denis Browne splint until the child is 24 months of age. The length of the bar used to spread the legs should not exceed 10 cm.

Some surgeons utilize corrective casts to force the legs and feet into lateral rotation. If the primary deformity is metatarsus varus, a corrective cast is indicated to correct the foot deformity. If there is associated soft-tissue contracture, particularly of the posterior tibial, gracilis, and medial hamstring muscles, a stretching cast may again be used. However, the torsional bony deformity in the tibia itself will not be corrected by maintaining the feet in forced eversion in an above-knee or below-knee cast for a period of four to eight weeks. At least 6 to 18 months is required for such passive force to change the shape of a bone. Immobilization of the limbs of a child for such a prolonged period is not justified. The only occasional instance in which the author makes use of a corrective cast is for stretching soft-tissue contracture; later, night splints are used during sleeping hours to correct the torsional deformity with growth and development.

If abnormal medial tibial torsion persists past eight years of age, derotation osteotomy may be indicated when the deformity is severe and functionally disabling. The operative technique follows the same principles as those of correction of the tibia vara and is illustrated in Figure 7–254 and described on page 2843.

Lateral Tibial Torsion. This does not correct itself with growth. Early treatment is recommended. Soft-tissue contracture, such as taut iliotibial band or triceps surae, is stretched by passive exercises performed with the help of the parents several times a day. If the lateral tibial torsion is excessive (more than 25 degrees in the infant and the young adult) a Fillauer bar or Denis Browne foot-leg splint, holding the feet-ankles medially rotated, is worn at night during sleep.

Surgical intervention, in the form of medial rotation osteotomy of the tibia and fibula, is indicated when conservative measures fail to correct the deformity. It is best to wait and observe the child until the age of 10 to 12 years before osteotomy is performed. This author prefers proximal tibial osteotomy at the metaphyseal-diaphyseal juncture; an alternative level, preferred by some surgeons, is the supramalleolar level.

References

1. Altmann, F.: Untersuchungen uber die torsio femoris. Zeit Anat. Entwick., *75*:82, 1924.
2. Appleton, A. B.: Positional deformities and bone growth. An experimental study. Lancet, *1*:451, 1934.
3. Ardito, S., et al.: Idiopathic external torsion of the tibia. Ital. J. Orthop. Traumatol., *4*:205, 1978.
4. Arkin, A. M., and Katz, J. F.: Effects of pressure on epiphyseal growth. The mechanism of plasticity of growing bone. J. Bone Joint Surg., *38-A*:1056, 1956.
5. Bailey, W. H., and Woolley, D.: Femoral anteversion and toeing in—preliminary report. J. Bone Joint Surg., *58-B*:143, 1976.
6. Bandi, W.: Der Orthopade. Berlin, Springer-Verlag, 1974. [English translation.]
7. Banks, S. W., and Evans, E. A.: Simple transverse osteotomy and threaded pin fixation for controlled correction of torsion deformities of the tibia. J. Bone Joint Surg., *37-A*:193, 1955.
8. Bardeen, C. R., and Lewis, W. H.: Development of the limbs, body-wall and back in man. Am. J. Anat., *1*:, 1901.
9. Beals, R. K., and Skyhar, M.: Growth and development of the tibia, fibula, and ankle joint. Clin. Orthop., *182*:289, 1984.

10. Bennett, J. T., Bunnell, W. P., and MacEwen, G. D.: Rotational osteotomy of the distal tibia and fibula. J. Pediatr. Orthop., *5*:294, 1985.
11. Bernbeck, R.: Zur pathologischen Anatomie und funktionellen Pathologie der Huftuerrenkung und des Luxationsbeckens. Arch. Orthop. Unfallchir., *45*:268, 1952.
12. Blaimont, P., and Schoon, R.: A propos de 2 cas de gonarthrose associée à un vice de torsion interne du tibia. Acta Orthop. Belg., *43*:476, 1977.
13. Blount, W. P.: Bow leg. Wis. Med. J., *40*:484, 1941.
14. Blumel, J., Eggers, G. W. N., and Evans, B.: Eight cases of hereditary bilateral medial tibial torsion in four generations. J. Bone Joint Surg., *39-A*:1198, 1957.
15. Böhm, M.: Infantile deformities of the knee and hip. J. Bone Joint Surg., *15*:574, 1933.
16. Boone, D. C., and Azen, S. P.: Normal range of motion of joints in male subjects. J. Bone Joint Surg., *61-A*:756, 1979.
17. Boone, D. C., Azen, S. P., Lin, C.-M., Spence, C., Baron, C., and Lee, L.: Reliability of goniometric measurements. Phys. Ther., *58*:1355, 1978.
18. Brookes, M., and Wardle, E. N.: Muscle action and the shape of the femur. J. Bone Joint Surg., *44-B*:398, 1962.
19. Browne, D.: Congenital malformations. Practitioner, *131*:20, 1933.
20. Brunelli, G.: Trapezoidal Z osteotomy in static arthrosis of the knee. Sicot XIth Congress, October 1969, Mexico, Imprimerie des Sciences, pp. 457–462.
21. Budin, E., and Chandler, E.: Measurement of femoral neck anteversion by a direct method. Radiology, *69*:209, 1957.
22. Castle, M. E.: Tibial rotational osteotomy. Clin. Orthop., *118*:73, 1976.
23. Coon, V., Donato, G., Houser, C., and Bleck, E. E.: Normal ranges of hip motion in infants six weeks, three months and six months of age. Clin. Orthop., *110*:256, 1975.
24. Crane, L.: Femoral torsion and its relation to toeing-in and toeing-out. J. Bone Joint Surg., *41-A*:421, 1959.
25. Dega, W.: Ricerche anatomische e meccaniche sull'anca fetale rivolte a chiarire l'etiologia e la patogenesi della lussazione congenita. Chir. Organi Mov., *18*:425, 1933.
26. Delpech, J. M.: De L'Orthomorphie, Par Rapport à L'Espece Humaine. Paris, Gabon, 1829, p. 301.
27. Dorius, L. K., et al.: Dynamic stimulation of the leg in torsion. J. Biomed., *17*:1, 1984.
28. Dunlap, K., Shands, A. R., Jr., Hollister, L. C., Jr., Gaul, J. S., Jr., and Streit, H. A.: A new method for determination of torsion of the femur. J. Bone Joint Surg., *35-A*:289, 1953.
29. Dunn, D. M.: Anteversion of the neck of the femur. J. Bone Joint Surg., *340-B*:181, 1952.
30. Dupuis, P. V.: La Torsion Tibiale. Sa Mesure–Son Interet Clinique, Radiologique et Chirurgical. Paris, Masson & Cie, 1951.
31. Durham, H. A.: Anteversion of the femoral neck in the normal femur. J.A.M.A., *65*:223, 1915.
32. Dutoit, M., and Caron, J.-C.: Lamellar rotation osteotomy of the tibia in children. Int. Orthop., *8*:263, 1985.
33. Ekstrand, J., Wiktorsson, M., Obert, B., and Gillquist, J.: Lower extremity goniometric measurements. A study to determine their reliability. Arch. Phys. Med. Rehabil., *63*:171, 1982.
34. Elftman, H.: Torsion of the lower extremity. Am. J. Phys. Anthrop., *3*:255, 1945.
35. Engel, G. M., and Staheli, L. T.: The natural history of torsion and other factors influencing gait in childhood. A study of the angle of gait, tibial torsion, knee angle, hip rotation, and development of the arch in normal children. Clin. Orthop., *99*:12, 1974.
36. Fabry, G.: Torsion of the femur. Acta Orthop. Belg., *43*:454, 1977.
37. Fabry, G., MacEwen, G. D., and Shands, A. R., Jr.: Torsion of the femur. A follow-up study in normal and abnormal conditions. J. Bone Joint Surg., *55-A*:1726, 1973.
38. Ficat, R. P., and Hungerford, D. S.: Disorders of the Patello-Femoral Joint. Baltimore, Williams & Wilkins, 1977.
39. Fitzhugh, M. L.: Faulty alignment of the feet and legs in infancy and childhood. Physiother. Rev., *21*:239, 1941.
40. Fonseca, A. S., and Bassett, G. S.: Valgus deformity following derotation osteotomy to correct medial femoral torsion. J. Pediatr. Orthop., *8*:295, 1988.
41. Fukubayashi, T., Torzilli, P. A., Sherman, M. F., and Warren, R. F.: An in vitro biomechanical evaluation of anterior-posterior motion of the knee. Tibial displacement, rotation, and torque. J. Bone Joint Surg., *64-A*:258, 1982.
42. Galbraith, R. T., Gelberman, R. H., Hajek, P. C., Baker, L. A., Sartoris, D. J., Rab, G. T., Cohen, M. S., and Griffin, P. P.: Obesity and decreased femoral anteversion in adolescence. J. Orthop. Res., *5*:523, 1987.
43. Haas, S. L.: Longitudinal osteotomy. J.A.M.A., *92*:1656, 1929.
44. Haas, S. S., Epps, C. H., Jr., and Adams, J. P.: Normal ranges of hip motion in the newborn. Clin. Orthop., *91*:114, 1973.
45. Halpern, A. A., Tanner, J., and Rinsky, L.: Does persistent fetal femoral anteversion contribute to osteoarthritis? A preliminary report. Clin. Orthop., *145*:213, 1979.
46. Hernandez, R. J., Tachdjian, M. O., Poznanski, A. K., and Dias, L. S.: CT determination of femoral torsion. A.J.R., *137*:97, 1981.
47. Houghton, C. R., and Rooker, G. D.: The role of the periosteum in the growth of long bones. An experimental study in the rabbit. J. Bone Joint Surg., *61-B*:218, 1979.
48. Hueter, C.: Anatomische Studien an den Extremitatengelenken Neugelborener und Erwachsener. Virchows Arch., *25*:572, 1862.
49. Husby, O. S., Sudmann, B., Gjerdet, N. R., Hitland, S. U., and Sudmann, E.: Spontaneous correction of femoral torsion. Diaphyseal osteotomies studied in kittens. Acta Orthop. Scand., *58*:113, 1987.
50. Hutter, C. G., Jr., and Scott, W.: Tibial torsion. J. Bone Joint Surg., *31-A*:511, 1949.
51. Hvid, I., and Andersen, L. I.: The quadriceps angle and its relation to femoral torsion. Acta Orthop. Scand., *53*:577, 1982.
52. Insall, J., Falvo, K. A., and Wise, D. W.: Chondromalacia patellae. A prospective study. J. Bone Joint Surg., *58-A*:1, 1976.
53. Jacquemier, M., Chrestian, P., Ramaherison, P., Faure, F. and Bouyala, J. M.: Analysis of torsion defects in the child using tomodensitometry. Rev. Chir. Orthop., *68*:24, 1982.
54. Jackson, J. P., and Waugh, W.: The technique and complications of upper tibial osteotomy. J. Bone Joint Surg., *56*:236, 1974.
55. Jaffres, R.: La marche en rotation interne des jeunes enfants. Rev. Rhum. Mal. Osteoartic., *37*:317, 1970.
56. Jakob, R. P., Haertel, M., and Stussi, E.: Tibial torsion calculated by computerized tomography and compared to other methods of measurement. J. Bone Joint Surg., *62-B*:238, 1980.
57. Jend, H. H., Heller, M., Dallek, M., and Schoettle, H.: Measurement of tibial torsion by computer tomography. Acta Radiol. [Diagn.] (Stockh.), *22*:271, 1981.
58. Joseph, B., Carver, R. A., Bell, M. J., Sharrard, W. J. W., Levick, R. K., Aithal, V., Chacko, V., and

Murthy, S. V.: Measurement of tibial torsion by ultrasound. J. Pediatr. Orthop., *7*:317, 1987.
59. Kate, B. R., and Robert, S. L.: The angle of femoral torsion. J. Anat. Soc. India, *12*:8, 1963.
60. Katz, J. L.: The effects of remodeling on the elastic properties of bone. Calcif. Tissue Int., *36*(Suppl. 1):S31, 1984.
61. Khermosh, O., Lior, G., and Weissman, S. L.: Tibial torsion in children. Clin. Orthop., *79*:25, 1971.
62. Kingsley, P. C., and Olmsted, K. L.: A study to determine the angle of anteversion of the neck of the femur. J. Bone Joint Surg., *30-A*:745, 1948.
63. Kite, J. H.: Torsion of the lower extremities in small children. J. Bone Joint Surg., *36-A*:511, 1954.
64. Kite, J. H.: Torsion of the legs in small children. J. Med. Assoc. Ga., *43*:1035, 1954.
65. Kite, J. H.: Flat feet and lateral rotation of legs in young children. J. Int. Coll. Surg., *25*:77, 1956.
66. Kite, J. H.: Torsion of the legs in young children. Clin. Orthop., *16*:152, 1960.
67. Kling, T. F., Jr., and Hensinger, R. N.: Angular and torsional deformities of the lower limbs in children. Clin. Orthop., *176*:136, 1983.
68. Knight, R. A.: Developmental deformities of the lower extremities. J. Bone Joint Surg., *36-A*:521, 1954.
69. Knittel, G., and Staheli, L. T.: The effectiveness of shoe modifications for intoeing. Orthop. Clin. North Am., *7*:1019, 1976.
70. Kobyliansky, E., Weissman, S. L., and Nathan, H.: Femoral and tibial torsion: a correlation study in dry bones. Int. Orthop., *3*:145, 1979.
71. Kumar, S. J., and MacEwen, G. D.: Torsional abnormalities in children's lower extremities. Orthop. Clin. North Am., *13*:629, 1982.
72. Laage, H., Barnett, J. G., Brady, J. M., Dulligan, P. J., Fett, H. C., Jr., Gallagher, T. F., and Schneider, B.A.: Horizontal lateral roentgenography of the hip in children. A preliminary report. J. Bone Joint Surg., *35-A*:387, 1953.
73. Laasonen, E. M., Jokio, P., and Lindholm, T. S.: Tibial torsion measured by computed tomography. Acta Radiol. [Diagn.] (Stockh.), *25*:325, 1984.
74. Lanier, J. C.: The intoeing child. Treatment with a simple orthopedic appliance. J. Fla. Med. Assoc., *58*:19, 1971.
75. Larson, R. L., Cabaud, H. E., Slocum, D. B., James, S. L., Keenan, T., and Hutchinson, T.: The patellar compression syndrome. Clin. Orthop., *134*:158, 1978.
76. LeDamany, P.: La torsion du tibia, normal, pathologique, experimentale. J. Anat. Physiol., *45*:598, 1909.
77. Lenneis, H. R.: Orthotics measurement board for tibial torsion and toe-out. Artificial limbs. Washington, D.C., National Research Council, 11/2:42, 1967.
78. Luchini, M., and Stevens, D. B.: Validity of torsional profile examination. J. Pediatr. Orthop., *3*:41, 1983.
79. MacEwen, G. D., and Shands, A. R., Jr.: Rotational and angulation deformities of the lower extremity in childhood. Orthopedics, *2*:66, 1960.
80. McCullough, C. J., and Burge, P. D.: Rotatory instability of the load-bearing ankle. An experimental study. J. Bone Joint Surg., *62-B*:460, 1980.
81. McSweeny, A.: A study of femoral torsion in children. J. Bone Joint Surg., *53-B*:90, 1971.
82. Magilligan, D. J.: Calculation of the angle of anteversion by means of horizontal lateral roentgenography. J. Bone Joint Surg., *38-A*:1231, 1956.
83. Magnusson, R.: Rotational osteotomy. J. Bone Joint Surg., *28-A*:262, 1946.
84. Mahboubi, S., and Horstmann, H.: Femoral torsion: CT measurement. Radiology, *160*:843, 1986.
85. Malekafzali, S. S., and Wood, M. B.: Tibial torsion—a simple clinical apparatus for its measurement and its application to a normal adult population. Clin. Orthop., *145*:154, 1979.
86. Meade, J. B., et al.: Bone remodeling due to continuously applied loads. Calcif. Tissue Int., *36*(Suppl. 1):S25, 1984.
87. Micheli, A. A., et al.: Tibiotalar torsion: bioengineering paradigm. Orthop. Clin. North Am., *7*:929, 1976.
88. Moreland, M. S.: Morphological effects of torsion applied to growing bone. An in vivo study in rabbits. J. Bone Joint Surg., *62-B*:230, 1980.
89. Nachlas, I. W.: Medial torsion of the leg. Arch. Surg., *28*:909, 1934.
90. Nachlas, I. W.: Common defects of the lower extremity in infants. South. Med. J., *41*:302, 1948.
91. Netz, P.: The diaphyseal bone under torque. An experimental study on dogs. Acta Orthop. Scand. (Suppl.), *176*:1, 1979.
92. Netz, P., Eriksson, K., and Stromberg, L.: Torsional strength and geometry of diaphyseal bone. An experimental study on dogs. Acta Orthop. Scand., *49*:430, 1978.
93. Netz, P., Eriksson, K., and Stromberg, L.: Material reaction of diaphyseal bone under torsion. An experimental study on dogs. Acta Orthop. Scand., *51*:223, 1980.
94. O'Donoghue, D. H.: Controlled rotation osteotomy of the tibia. South. Med. J., *33*:1145, 1940.
95. Ogden, J. A.: Radiology of postnatal skeletal development. IX. Proximal tibia and fibula. Skeletal Radiol., *11*:169, 1984.
96. Oni, O. O., and Keswani, H.: Idiopathic or primary windswept deformity: the etiological significance of the radiological finding. J. Pediatr. Orthop., *4*:293, 1984.
97. Pearson, K., and Bell, J.: A Study of the Long Bones of the English Skeleton. Draper's Company Research Memoirs. Biometric series X and XI. Part I. London, Cambridge University Press, 1919.
98. Phillips, H. O., Greene, W. B., Guilford, W., Mittelstaedt, C. A., Gaisie, G., Vincent, L. M., and Durell, C.: Measurement of femoral torsion: comparison of standard roentgenographic techniques with ultrasound. J. Pediatr. Orthop., *5*:546, 1985.
99. Pick, J. W., Stack, J. K., and Anson, B. J.: Measurements on the human femur. I. Length, diameters, and angles. Q. Bull. Northwest. Med. Sch., *15*:281, 1941.
100. Pitkow, R. V.: External rotation contractures of the extended hip. Clin. Orthop., *110*:139, 1975.
101. Rang, M.: Personal communications, 1988.
102. Reikeras, O., Bjerkreim, I., and Kolbenstvedt, A.: Anteversion of the acetabulum and femoral neck in normals and in patients with osteoarthritis of the hip. Acta Orthop. Scand., *54*:18, 1983.
103. Ritter, M. A., DeRosa, G. P., and Babcock, J. L.: Tibial torsion? Clin. Orthop., *120*:159, 1976.
104. Rogers, S. P.: A method for determining the angles of torsion of the neck of the femur. J. Bone Joint Surg., *13*:821, 1931.
105. Rosen, H., and Sandick, H.: Measurement of tibiofibular torsion. J. Bone Joint Surg., *37-A*:847, 1955.
106. Ryder, C. T., and Crane, L.: Measuring femoral anteversion: The problem and a method. J. Bone Joint Surg., *35-A*:321, 1953.
107. Salter, R.: The present state of innominate osteotomy in congenital dislocation of the hip. J. Bone Joint Surg., *48-B*:853, 1966.
108. Schoenhaus, H. D., and Poss, K. D.: The clinical and practical aspects in treating torsional problems in children. J. Am. Podiatr. Assoc., *67*:620, 1977.
109. Schwartz, R. P., Heath, A. L., Morgan, D. W., and Towns, R. C.: A quantitative analysis of recorded variables in the walking pattern of normal adults. J. Bone Joint Surg., *46-A*:324, 1964.
110. Scrutton, D. S., and Robson, P.: The gait of 50 normal children. Physiotherapy, *54*:363, 1968.

111. Shands, A. R., Jr., and Steele, M. K.: Torsion of the femur. J. Bone Joint Surg., *40-A*:803, 1958.
112. Sikorski, J. M., Peters, J., and Watt, I.: The importance of femoral rotation in chondromalacia patellae as shown by serial radiography. J. Bone Joint Surg., *61-B*:435, 1979.
113. Smillie, I. S., and Turner, M. S.: The influence of tibial torsion on the pathology of the knee. First Congress of the International Society of The Knee, 1979.
114. Somerville, E. W.: Persistent foetal alignment. J. Bone Joint Surg., *39-B*:106, 1957.
115. Somerville, E. W.: Rotational abnormalities of the lower limbs. J. Bone Joint Surg., *45-B*:627, 1963.
116. Sorrells, R. B.: A simple means of determining lower extremity torsion. J. Arkansas Med. Soc., *74*:196, 1977.
117. Soutter, R., and Bradford, E. H.: Twists in normal and in congenital dislocated femora. N.Y. Med. J., *78*:1071, 1903.
118. Staheli, L. T.: Torsional deformities. Pediatr. Clin. North Am., *24*:799, 1977.
119. Staheli, L. T.: Medial femoral torsion. Orthop. Clin. North Am., *11*:39, 1980.
120. Staheli, L. T., Clawson, D. K., and Hubbard, D. D.: Medial femoral torsion: experience with operative treatment. Clin. Orthop., *146*:222, 1980.
121. Staheli, L. T., Corbett, M., Wyss, C., and King, H.: Lower extremity rotational problems in children. Normal values to guide management. J. Bone Joint Surg., *67-A*:39, 1985.
122. Staheli, L. T., and Engel, G. M.: Tibial torsion. A method of assessment and a survey of normal children. Clin. Orthop., *86*:183, 1972.
123. Staheli, L. T., Lippert, F., and Denotter, P.: Femoral anteversion and physical performance in adolescent and adult life. Clin. Orthop., *129*:213, 1977.
124. Stewart, S. F., and Karschner, R. G.: Congenital dislocation of the hip. A method of determining the degree of antetorsion of the femoral neck. A.J.R., *15*:258, 1926.
125. Stirling, R. I.: Derotation of the tibia. Br. Med. J., *1*:581, 1936.
126. Swanson, A. B., Greene, P. W., and Allis, H. D.: Rotational deformities of the lower extremity in children and their clinical significance. Clin. Orthop., *27*:157, 1963.
127. Syllivan, J. A., and Hitch, M.: Lower extremity torsional evaluation: examination of the child for intoe gait and commonly presenting foot abnormalities. O.N.A.J., *6*:376, 1979.
128. Terjesen, T., Benum, P., Anda, S., and Svenningsen, S.: Increased femoral anteversion and osteoarthritis of the hip joint. Acta Orthop. Scand., *53*:571, 1982.
129. Thelander, H. E., and Fitzhugh, M. L.: Posture habits in infancy affecting foot and leg alignments. J. Pediatr., *21*:306, 1942.
130. Tohno, S.: Torsion of the lower extremity. *In* Proceedings of the XIIth Congress of Societé Internationale de Chirurgie Orthopedique et de Traumatologie. Amsterdam, Excerpta Medica Foundation, International Congress Series, *291*:596, 1973.
131. Turner, M. S., and Smillie, I. S.: The effect of tibial torsion of the pathology of the knee. J. Bone Joint Surg., *63-B*:396, 1981.
132. Volkmann, R.: Chirurgische Erfahrungen uber Knochenverbiegungen und Knochenwacsthum. Arch. Pathol. Anat., *24*:512, 1862.
133. Wagner, K. S.: The effects of simulated tibial deformities on the ankle joint during the gait cycle. Foot Ankle, *5*:131, 1984.
134. Wangermez, J., and Labarbe, P.: Mesure de la torsion tibio-fibulaire sur radiolographie de profil. Relations avec la forme de la voute plantaire. Bull. Assoc. Anat. (Nancy), *59*:1013, 1975.
135. Weber, U.: Zum Torsionsproblem des distalen Femurs. Z. Orthop., *115*:707, 1977.
136. Weinmann, J. P., and Sicher, H.: Bone and Bones. Fundamentals of Bone Biology. St. Louis, C. V. Mosby, 1947.
137. Widjaja, P. M., Ermes, J. W. L. M., Sijbrandij, S., Damsma, H., and Klinkhaner, A. C.: Technique of torsion measurement of the lower extremity using computed tomography. J. Comput. Assist. Tomogr., *9*:466, 1981.
138. Wilkinson, J. A.: Femoral anteversion in rabbit. J. Bone Joint Surg., *44-B*:386, 1962.
139. Winter, W. G., Jr., and Lafferty, J. F.: The skiing sequelae of tibial torsion. Orthop. Clin. North Am., *7*:231, 1976.
140. Wynne-Davies, R.: Talipes equinovarus. A review of 84 cases after completion of treatment. J. Bone Joint Surg., 46B:464, 1969.

Angular Deformities of the Long Bones of the Lower Limbs

PHYSIOLOGIC EVOLUTION OF ALIGNMENT OF THE LOWER LIMBS

Mild to moderate medial bowing of the lower limbs, involving both the tibia and the femur, is a common and normal finding in the newborn and the young infant. It probably represents persistence of the in utero position of the lower limbs. Bowlegs are usually associated with varying degrees of medial tibial torsion.

With the development of upright stance and locomotion, the medial deviation of the legs is spontaneously corrected, provided that extraneous factors do not interfere. The "pendulum" swings toward genu valgum between two and three years of age, and finally the knock-knees are spontaneously corrected between the ages of four and ten years. Böhm, in 1933, was the first to describe this normal physiologic evolution of the shape of the lower limbs.[9] Figure 7–242 illustrates the physiologic evolution of the alignment of the lower limbs at various ages in infancy and childhood.

Vankka and Salenius defined the natural course of angular alignment of the lower limbs by studying the development of the tibiofemoral angle by clinical and radiographic mensuration in 1,480 normal children (Fig. 7–243). The findings were similar in boys and girls. In the

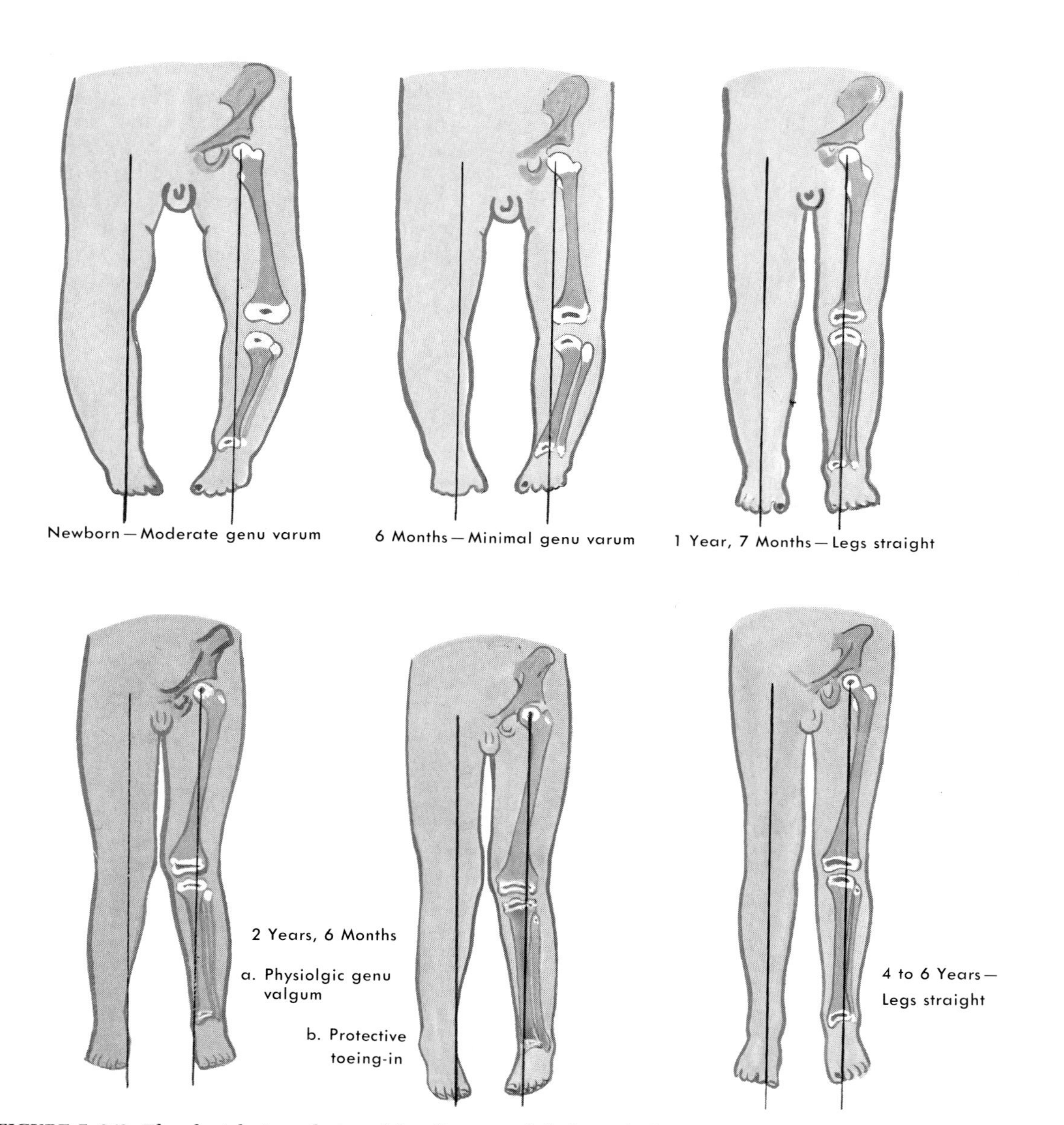

FIGURE 7–242. The physiologic evolution of the alignment of the lower limbs at various ages in infancy and childhood.

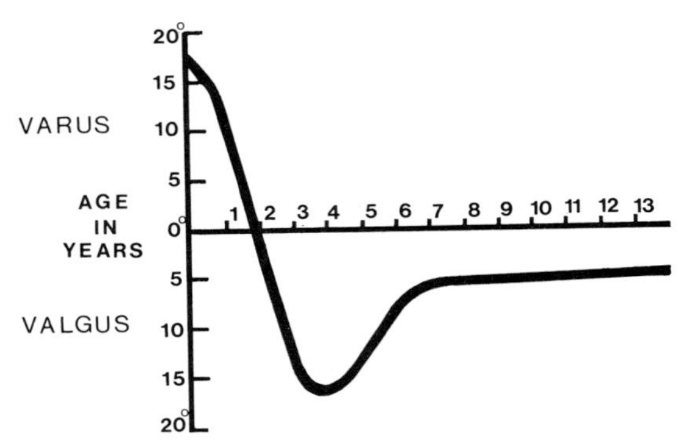

FIGURE 7–243. Development of the tibiofemoral angle during growth.

newborn and infant up to one year of age, the tibiofemoral angle was in marked varus, deviating medially 15 degrees. At about the age of one-and-one-half years the tibiofemoral angle straightened to 0 degrees. During the second and third years the tibiofemoral angle deviated laterally toward marked valgus (12 degrees). Then by age seven years, the valgus alignment gradually corrected to that of the normal adult (8 degrees in the female and 7 degrees in the male).[74]

Previously Sherman studied the natural history of bowlegs in 30 infants. The deformity corrected itself spontaneously. Only three infants had bowlegs at 16 to 18 months of age; one of these was corrected, and the other two had slight knock-knees at five years of age.[65]

Morley studied the natural history of knock-knee by performing 1,000 examinations on unselected normal children (451 children aged one to four years, 318 children aged five to eleven years). The degree of knock-knee was measured by the distance between the medial malleoli (with the patellae facing straight forward, the medial surfaces of the knees just touching, and the ankles dorsiflexed to neutral position). Four grades of knock-knees were specified: *Grade I*—intermalleolar distance of less than 2.5 cm. (1 inch); *Grade II*—2.5 cm. (1 inch) but less than 5.0 cm. (2 inches); *Grade III*—5 cm. (2 inches) but less than 7.5 cm. (3 inches); and *Grade IV*—7.5 cm. (3 inches) and over.[50]

The incidence of genu valgum was found to increase until three to three-and-one-half years of age, and then it declined. Between three and three-and-one-half years of age, only 26 per cent of children had Grade I knock-knees; 52 per cent had Grade II; and 22 per cent had Grade III or IV (2 inches or more). Only 2 per cent of children aged seven years or older had an equivalent amount of genu valgum. There was no sex difference in the incidence of knock-knees in children under five years of age. The mean weight of children with knock-knees was greater than the mean weight of comparable children without knock-knees. Morley concluded that developmental genu valgum in children under seven years of age can probably be safely ignored unless it is very severe or unless an underlying cause such as renal rickets or asymmetrical physeal damage from fracture or infection is present.[50]

The study by Morley is not longitudinal; also, the mensuration of angular alignment of the lower limbs was made by the determination of the distance between the femoral condyles for genu varum and between the medial malleoli for genu valgum. This clinical method of determination of tibiofemoral angle is not accurate and not reproducible; also it does not allow for the normal variation of the lower limb length.

PHYSIOLOGIC GENU VARUM

As already stated, a minimal or moderate degree of bowlegs is normal in infancy. Usually orthopedic attention is not sought until the child begins to stand and walk. The parents are concerned because of the appearance of the lower limbs with the wide space between the knees, the rolling gait, and the toeing-in, which is due to associated medial tibial torsion. The abnormality of gait and malalignment of the lower limbs are more noticeable when the child is tired or has walked a long distance. In taking the history the physician should enquire as to familial incidence of bowlegs and other deformities of the lower limbs (Fig. 7–244). Is there a history of trauma, milk allergy, or special dietary habits? When was the deformity first noted? What has been its progression and response to prior treatment? History of rapid progression suggests a pathologic and not a physiologic condition.

On examination, the alignment of the lower limbs is inspected in stance and gait. Medial rotation of the lower limbs exaggerates the appearance of bowlegs. It is important to align the legs so that the patellae face straight forward and to measure the degree of genu varum according to the distance between the medial femoral condyles with the medial malleoli touching. The lateral thigh-leg angle is determined. In stance, where does the center of gravity fall when projected downward from the anterior superior iliac spine? Normally it passes between the first and second metatarsals. In genu varum it passes laterally toward the third to fifth metatarsal. The feet may be normal,

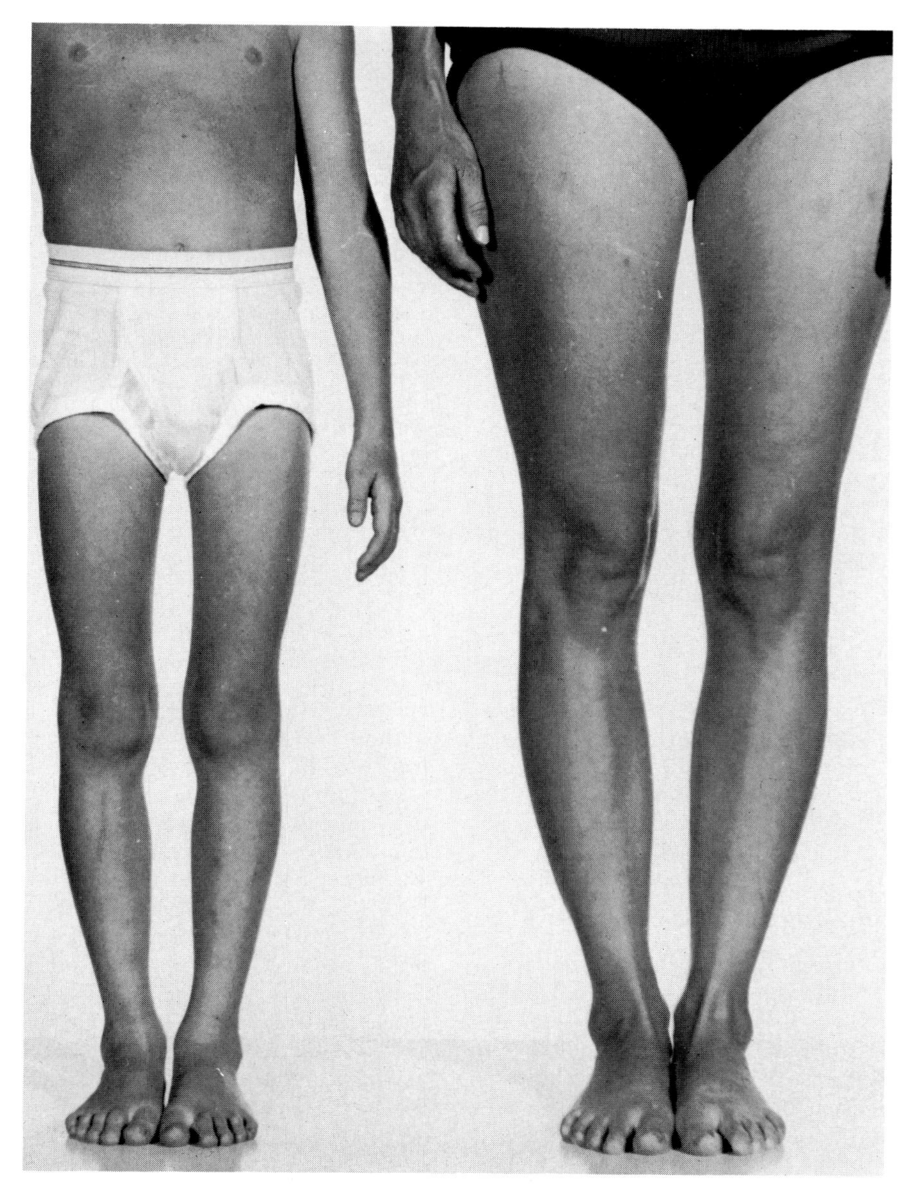

FIGURE 7–244. Bilateral genu varum in mother and son.

Note the associated medial tibial torsion. In the familial form prognosis should be guarded.

pronated, or in postural metatarsus varus. Next, the child is asked to walk and the foot progression angle is noted; it is usually medial.

In the stance phase of gait one should observe for the presence of lateral thrust. In physiologic genu varum a lateral thrust at the knee is ordinarily not present; the presence of thrust indicates incompetence of lateral ligaments of the knee and high risk of potential for progression of deformity.[39, 40] The ligamentous stability of the medial and lateral collateral and cruciate ligaments of the knee is determined.

In prone position, the range of rotation of the hips in extension, the degree of femoral antetorsion, and the thigh-foot angle are determined. The degree of tibial torsion is noted.

Radiographic Features

Ordinarily, radiograms are unnecessary. Radiologic findings, shown in Figure 7–245, are as follows: (1) The transverse planes of the knee and ankle joints are tilted medially; (2) the tibia is angulated medially at the junction of its proximal and middle thirds, and the femur at its distal third; (3) the medial cortices of tibia and femur are thickened and sclerosed; (4) the epiphysis, physis, and metaphysis have a normal appearance, and there is no evidence of intrinsic bone disease; and (5) involvement is usually symmetrical.

The metaphyseal-diaphyseal angle is determined; in physiologic genu varum it is less than 11 degrees. If the metaphyseal-diaphyseal angle is greater than 11 degrees, radiographic changes of tibia vara (Blount's disease) are likely to develop.[45]

Differential Diagnosis

In the differential diagnosis a number of pathologic conditions must be considered (Table 7–19). *Tibia vara,* Blount's disease, is the most common cause of pathologic varus deformity of the leg in children. It is characterized by steep medial angulation of the tibia in its proximal metaphyseal region. In Blount's disease the lateral cortex of the proximal tibial shaft remains nearly straight, whereas the medial cortex of the proximal tibial metaphysis angulates sharply medially. In physiologic genu varum both the medial and the lateral cortices of the tibia curve gently medially. In Blount's disease the femur is normal, except late in the course of the disease. The varus deformity is restricted to the upper tibia, whereas in physiologic genu varum the femur is often bowed medially. The proximal metaphyseal-diaphyseal angle of the tibia in physiologic genu varum is less than 11 degrees, whereas in potential Blount's disease it is greater than 11 degrees. In physiologic genu varum the proximal medial tibial metaphysis is normal, whereas in Langenskiöld Stage I Blount's disease there is fragmentation (irregular rarefaction) of the proximal medial tibial metaphysis. As Blount's disease progresses the proximal tibial epiphysis slopes medially, the medial upper tibial physeal line becomes irregular, and the lateral physeal line widens. Further changes in the course of Blount's disease are described in the section on tibia vara. Involvement in physiologic genu varum is bilateral and symmetrical, whereas in Blount's disease it may be unilateral and asymmetrical (Table 7–20).

Table 7–19. *Pathologic Conditions That Cause Genu Varum or Tibia Vara*

Metabolic Bone Disease
Vitamin D deficiency
Vitamin D–refractory rickets (hypophosphatemia)
Hypophosphatasia

Asymmetrical Growth Arrest or Retardation
Tibia vara (Blount's disease)
Trauma
Infection
Tumor

Bone Dysplasia
Metaphyseal dysplasia, camptomelic dwarfism, achondroplasia, enchondromatosis

Metal Intoxication
Specifically *fluorosis*—due to excessive fluoride intake in pregnancy

Congenital
Congenital *longitudinal deficiency of the tibia* with relative overgrowth of the fibula
Congenital *tibia vara*—angulation at middle third of the tibia, often positive family history; prognosis for spontaneous cure should be guarded

One must differentiate between physiologic genu varum and a *congenital form of tibia vara* in which moderate or marked medial angulation takes place at the junction of the middle and distal thirds; often in the latter there is a positive family history, with parents and siblings being similarly affected. In this form the prognosis for spontaneous correction should be guarded. In congenital longitudinal deficiency of the tibia with relative overgrowth of the fibula, the leg is bowed medially.

In the differential diagnosis one should also consider various types of *rickets*. The direction of axial deviation of the legs in metabolic bone disease depends upon the child's age and de-

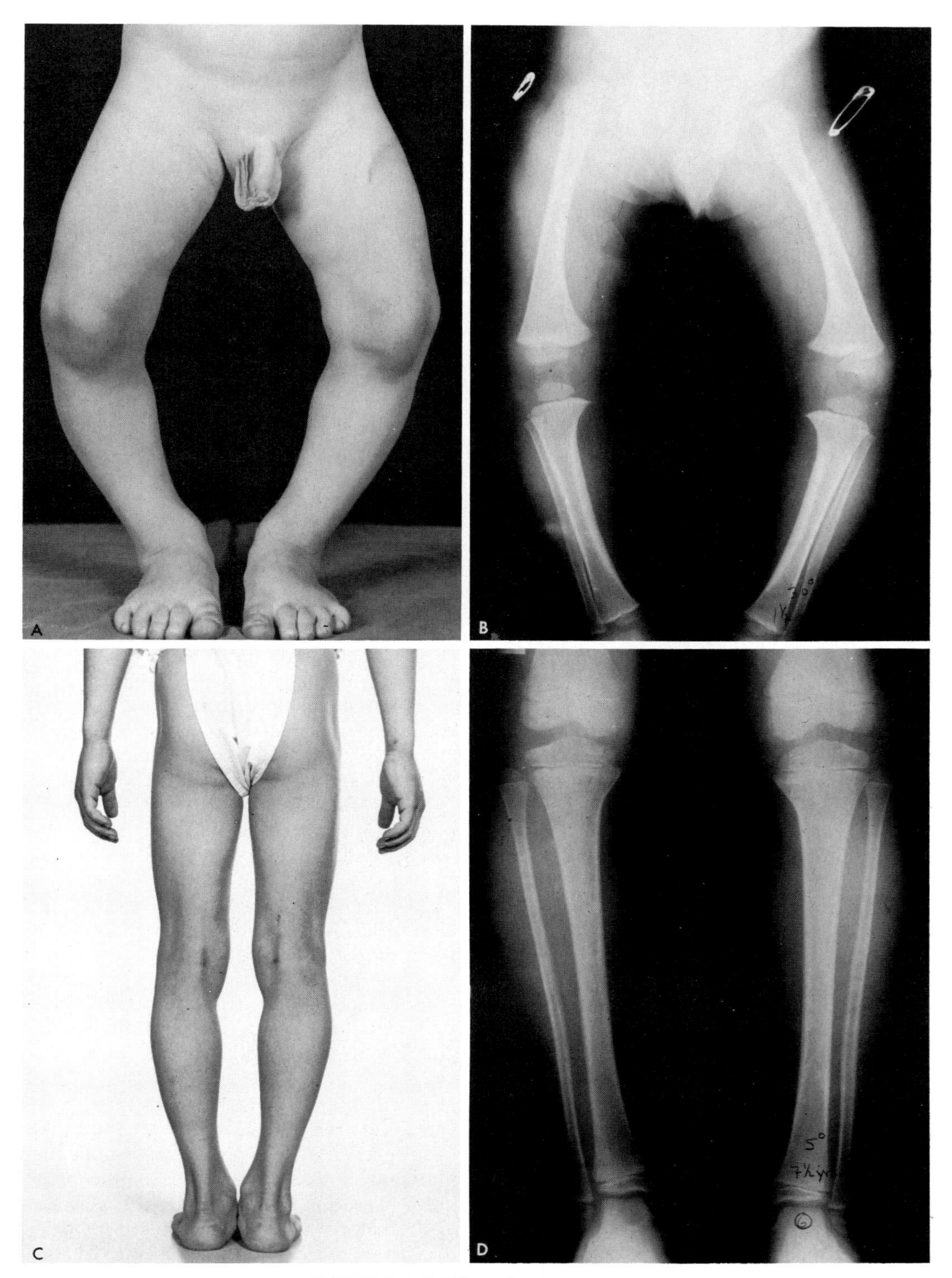

FIGURE 7–245. Bilateral genu varum.

A and **B.** At age one and one half years. **C** and **D.** At seven years, showing spontaneous correction without treatment.

Table 7–20. *Differential Diagnosis Between Tibia Vara (Blount's Disease) and Physiologic Genu Varum*

	Physiologic Genu Varum	***Tibia Vara (Blount's Disease)***
Involvement	Bilateral and usually symmetrical	Often asymmetrical; may be unilateral or bilateral
Site of medial angulation in tibia	At junction of proximal and middle thirds—gentle curve	At proximal tibial metaphysis, angulation is sharp
Femur	Bowed medially in its lower third	Normal, except late in the course of the disease
Lateral thrust—in stance phase of gait	Absent	Often present
Metaphyseal-diaphyseal angle of proximal tibia	Less than 11 degrees	Greater than 11 degrees
Medial upper tibial metaphysis	Normal	Irregular rarefaction (fragmentation)
Upper tibial epiphysis	Normal	Slopes medially
Upper tibial physis	Normal	Irregular narrowing medially and widening laterally
Lateral cortex of tibial shaft	Curves medially gently	Nearly straight
Medial cortex of tibial shaft	Curves medially gently	Sharply angulates medially

velopmental phase of angular alignment of the lower limbs. When the rickets has its onset in infancy (bowleg phase), the lower limbs will be in severe genu varum with excessive medial rotation of the tibia; this is the deformity in vitamin D deficiency/vitamin D–refractory or hyperphosphatemic rickets, and hypophosphatasia (an inborn error of metabolism manifesting in the newborn or infant). In renal osteodystrophy rickets there is a later onset in the valgus phase of the evolution of alignment of the lower limbs; therefore the pattern of limb deformity is genu valgum. In rickets the entire physis is affected and skeletal involvement is generalized. The distinguishing features of these conditions are described in Chapter 3.

Fluorosis, due to excessive fluoride intake during pregnancy, may result in severe bowlegs in infancy and can cause tibia valga in the older child.

Asymmetrical growth disturbance of medial distal femoral or medial proximal tibial physis due to trauma or infection will cause genu varum or tibia vara deformity. In these conditions, involvement is usually unilateral and radiographic features are distinctive.

Bone dysplasias, such as metaphyseal dysplasia, achondroplasia, camptomelic dwarfism, and enchondromatosis, can present with varus deformity of the leg or the knee.

Treatment

No special treatment is necessary. Parents should be assured that the bowleg appearance is normal and that it will spontaneously correct itself with weight-bearing and skeletal growth. It should also be mentioned to the parents that the child will probably, at the age of three years, temporarily develop knock-knees that will be corrected spontaneously by the age of seven years. The use of Denis Browne splints for developmental genu varum is definitely contraindicated, as it will exaggerate the physiologic knock-knees and pronation of the feet that develop normally in these children.

Some persistent parents may pressure the orthopedic surgeon to prescribe special orthopedic shoes. In a physiologic condition that resolves spontaneously, such treatment may be perceived to be "effective" by the parents or the treating physician. There is no scientific documentation that special shoes or active or passive exercises can modify the natural course of the physiologic evolution of alignment of the lower limbs in children. They should not be prescribed.

It is best to follow the natural course of physiologic genu varum. Parents are advised to bring the child back in six months for reassessment to determine whether the varus alignment of the lower limbs is improving or not. Offering the family such a return visit will allay the apprehension of nervous, demanding parents and prevent them from seeking advice from unknowledgeable health care personnel who may prescribe unnecessary treatment.

Osteotomy of the tibia or asymmetrical physeal arrest of the lateral side of the distal femoral physis or proximal tibia is not necessary in developmental genu varum.

The congenital familial severe form of tibia vara may fail to correct itself with growth. In the *adolescent,* when the malalignment is severe, surgical correction of the deformity may be indicated: It consists of osteotomy of the tibia and fibula at the apex of angulation—usually located at the junction of the middle third of the tibia. As medial tibial torsion is commonly exaggerated in this form of tibia vara, the distal fragment is derotated as well as angulated laterally. When the patient is seen at the appropriate skeletal age, asymmetrical arrest of the lateral part of the proximal tibial physis with osteotomy of the fibula will correct the deformity.

DEVELOPMENTAL GENU VALGUM

A minimal to moderate degree of knock-knees is a normal physiologic finding in children two to six years of age. When the genu valgum is *marked*, the child walks awkwardly, rubbing his knees and keeping his feet apart (Fig. 7–246). He may swing one leg around the other to avoid banging his knees. He may be easily fatigued. The feet are pronated, and the uppers of the shoes bulge and collapse medially over the medial longitudinal arch. The child will toe-in to shift the center of gravity of the body over the center of the foot, which is the second ray. If the triceps surae muscle and iliotibial band are contracted, he will toe-out. Pain in the calf and the anterior aspect of the thigh is common. In severe knock-knees, because of the malalignment of the quadriceps mechanism, the patellae may subluxate laterally. Because they are inactive, children with knock-knees are usually obese. Abnormal weight-bearing stretches the medial collateral ligaments of the knee, and in middle-aged or older adults, this excess wear and tear on the knees eventually leads to degenerative arthritis.

In the *differential diagnosis*, intrinsic bone disease and pathologic genu valgum should be ruled out if the condition is asymmetrical or unilateral; if it is excessive (the distance between the medial malleoli is greater than 9 or 10 cm.); if the child is of short stature for his age (suggesting the possibility of epiphyseal dysplasia or endocrine disease); or if there is a positive family history of marked genu valgum. Developmental tibia valga occurs in metaphyseal dysplasia.

Primary tibia valga, similar but opposite to tibia vara (Blount's disease), does occur but is uncommon. Radiograms will disclose irregular

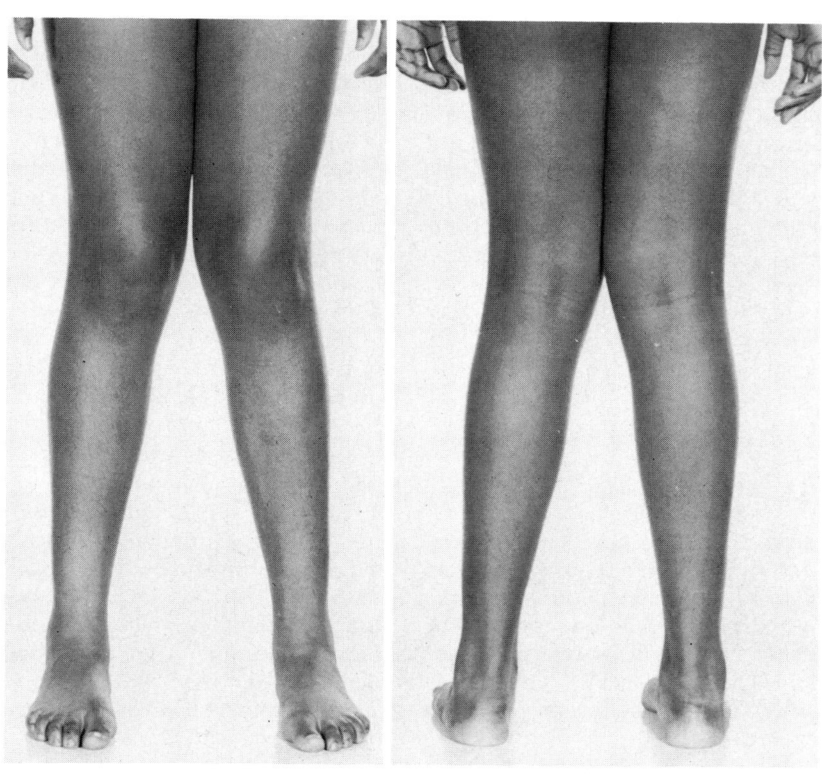

FIGURE 7–246. Bilateral genu valgum in an adolescent.

rarefaction of the lateral metaphysis and distal depression of the lateral part of the physis of the proximal tibia.

Solitary osteochondroma, multiple exostosis, multiple enchondromatosis, or subacute osteomyelitis of the distal femur or proximal tibia can cause asymmetrical growth and valgus deformity at the knee. In these conditions the radiographic changes are obvious and distinctive.

In children with renal osteodystrophy, genu valgum is a common deformity; the prognosis of the patients has markedly improved with kidney transplantation and improved medical management. The valgus deformity may be so severe as to interfere with gait. Alignment of the lower limbs in children with renal osteodystrophy should be carefully monitored during growth, as correction of deformity by asymmetrical growth arrest at the appropriate skeletal age is much simpler than varus osteotomy of the distal femur or proximal tibia.

In congenital longitudinal deficiency of the fibula, valgus deformity of the knee is common. Diagnosis is made by determination of the relative length of the fibula to the tibia in the anteroposterior and lateral radiograms of the leg, including the knee and ankle.

Trauma and premature growth arrest of the lateral part of the physis of the proximal tibia or distal femur will result in genu valgum deformity due to asymmetrical growth. Greenstick fracture of the medial part of the proximal tibial metaphysis, a "benign" injury, may cause tibia valga deformity.

Contracture of the iliotibial band, a common deformity in neuromuscular paralytic diseases such as myelomeningocele, will cause genu valgum deformity. Iliotibial band contracture may also occur in normal children owing to intrauterine malposture. In genu valgum it is important to perform the Ober test to rule out hip abduction contracture due to a taut iliotibial band.

Treatment

In the two- to six-year age group, the parents should be assured that in 95 per cent of cases the knock-knees will spontaneously correct themselves, making treatment unnecessary. This is particularly true if the child toes-in while walking. If the iliotibial band or triceps surae muscles are contracted and act as deforming forces, they should be stretched by passive manipulative exercises.

Sometimes genu valgum persists and does not resolve spontaneously, or it may develop later in the juvenile patient and gradually increase in adolescence. In these cases of excessive genu valgum and pronated feet, the center of gravity is medial to the first ray of the foot. To prevent foot strain, longitudinal arch supports and 1/8- to 3/16-inch medial heel wedges to the shoes may be prescribed. The shank of the shoes should be semiflexible. These shoe alterations will also promote toeing-in. Developmental genu valgum in children will usually resolve spontaneously, provided that the child toes-in.

In severe genu valgum, particularly in the eight-year-old and older obese child and in pathologic genu valgum, this author recommends the use of a "knock-knee" orthosis during the day. The orthosis consists of a double upright knee-ankle-foot orthosis with free ankles, drop-lock knee, and knock-knee pad with thigh and calf cuffs. The objective of the orthosis is to prevent development of ligamentous instability by protecting the knees and to unload the lateral part of the proximal tibial and distal femoral physis from abnormal stresses of weight-bearing. There is no definitive documentation in the literature that orthosis corrects genu valgum. This author uses it in the 8- to 11-year age group for developmental genu valgum and also in the younger age group for pathologic genu valgum, with explanation to the parents that it may not be effective and that surgical correction in adolescence may be required. The orthoses are used only for a period of one to two years. The psychologic drawbacks of wearing the brace in school should be carefully weighed against the probable correction that may be obtained. The use of the orthosis at night when weight-bearing is not a consideration is controversial; this author ordinarily does not use it.

In adolescence, excessive genu valgum requires more aggressive management. When significant valgus deformity at the knee persists in the immediate preadolescent years (the skeletal age of 11 years in girls and 12 years in boys), it will not correct spontaneously. In the experience of Howorth, genu valgum deformity did not correct with time when at the age of ten years the intermalleolar distance was greater than 7.5 cm. as measured with the medial femoral condyles touching each other. He recommended operative correction if the intermalleolar distance with the knees together is 7.5 to 10 cm.[34] Excessive genu valgum causes an awkward gait; the patients, especially those who are obese, walk with flat feet and laterally rotate their legs to prevent their knees from knocking together. Functionally these children are handicapped. Valgus at the knee may cause lateral compartment arthritis. The increased Q-angle of the patellar tendon may predispose to recurrent lateral subluxation of the patellofemoral joint and chondromalacia of the patella.

Several methods of surgical correction are available, including medial physeal retardation or arrest of the distal femur and/or the proximal tibia if there is sufficient growth remaining to obtain correction by asymmetrical growth. In the skeletally mature patient, varus osteotomy of the distal femur or of the proximal tibia and fibula by either modified cuneiform or close-up wedge resection is performed. Most often the valgus deformity is greater in the lower end of the femur than in the upper end of the tibia. Standing radiograms of the lower limbs with the patellae facing straight forward should be made to verify this. The tibiofemoral angles are measured between intersecting lines drawn through the axes of the femora and tibiae. The adult female has a broader pelvis than the male; therefore, a clinically straight-appearing knee has a valgus range of 5 to 9 degrees in women and 4 to 7 degrees in men (Fig. 7–247).

MEDIAL PHYSEAL RETARDATION BY STAPLING AND GROWTH ARREST BY EPIPHYSIODESIS OF THE DISTAL FEMUR AND/OR PROXIMAL TIBIA

Stapling is recommended by Howorth, Pistevos and Duckworth, and Zuege et al.[34, 56, 76] It is an effective method to correct genu valgum provided that the physes are still open and there is sufficient longitudinal growth remaining to correct the deformity. Pistevos and Duckworth recommend stapling of the medial distal femur when the intermalleolar separation is up to 12.5 cm., with an optimum age for surgery of 11½ years for boys and girls. Stapling of both

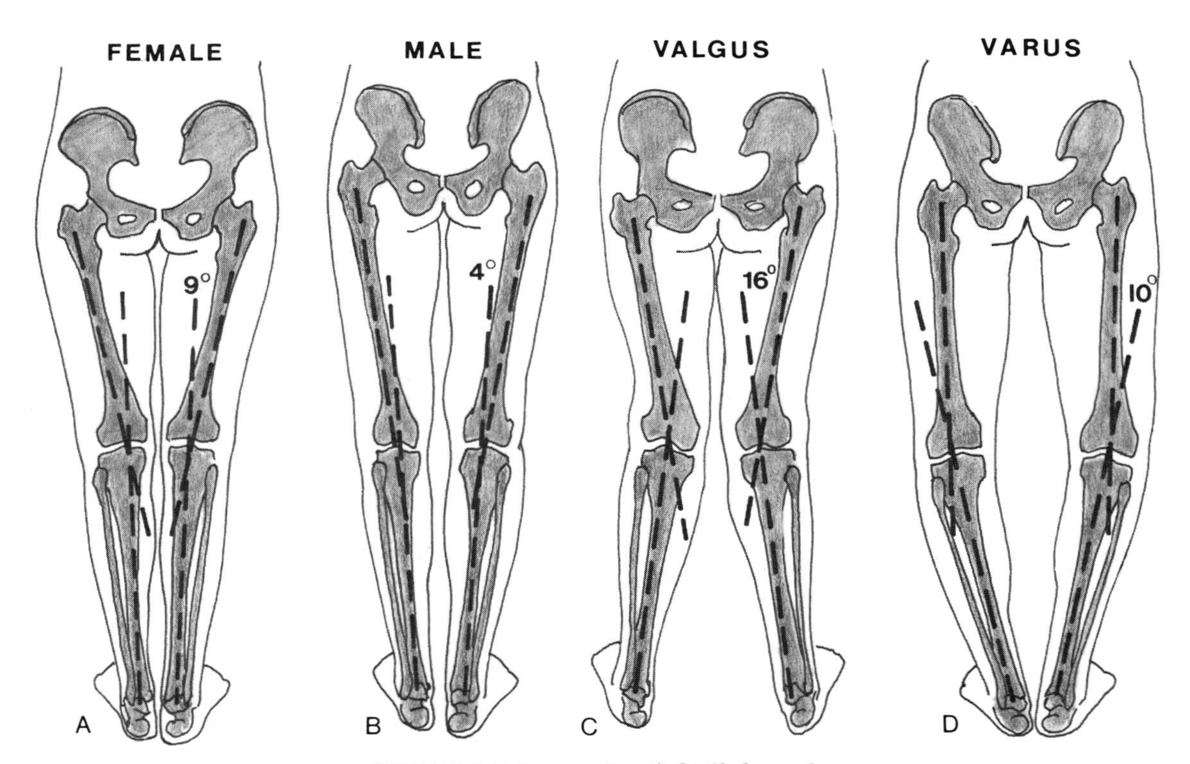

FIGURE 7–247. Mensuration of tibiofibular angle.

A. An adult woman with a broad pelvis may have straight legs with as much as 9 degrees of valgus. With 4 degrees of valgus her legs would appear slightly bowed. **B.** The legs of an adult man are slightly bowed or straight with 4 degrees of valgus. With more than 7 degrees they are knock-kneed. To look straight, standing radiograms of a man usually show a tibiofemoral angle of between 4 and 7 degrees; of a woman, 5 and 9 degrees. **C.** Valgus of 16 degrees in the radiogram of a female represents a pathologic knock-knee. The angulation is in the distal ends of the femora. Clinically the deformity would be 7 to 11 degrees. **D.** When the tibiofemoral angle reaches zero degrees, further varus is designated "minus" for purposes of tabulation. To a varus of minus 10 degrees in a male, 4 to 7 degrees must be added to explain the clinical appearance of 14 to 17 degrees of bowleg. (Redrawn after Zuege, R. C., Kempken, T. G., and Blount, W. P.: Epiphyseal stapling for angular deformity at the knee. J. Bone Joint Surg., *61-A*:320, 1979.)

distal femur and proximal tibia was performed when the valgus deformity was greater than 12.5 cm. intermalleolar separation or when the patient presented late, i.e., between 13 and 14½ years of age. In their experience with 49 patients, the results were cosmetically satisfactory in all cases. However, they noted a tendency for the surgical scars to be broad and conspicuous.[56] Zuege et al. reported the long-term results of physeal stapling in treatment of angular deformities of 82 knees in 56 patients; there were 64 cases of genu valgum and 18 of genu varum. In 12 patients with concomitant lower limb length disparity the longer lower limbs were stapled asymmetrically at a younger skeletal age than the shorter limb in order to equalize limb lengths and simultaneously correct genu valgum. The results were satisfactory or improved in 87 per cent of the deformities. When the staples were removed, a rebound-increased growth occurred in 22 patients with 35 deformities. Therefore, Zuege et al. recommended allowing for 5 degrees of rebound, of which 1 to 2 degrees will be corrected after closure of the physis. Ten revisions of staples were necessary because of extrusion or shifting. These investigators recommend that physeal stapling for correction of angular deformity not be performed before the skeletal age of 11 years in girls and 12 years in boys. Also, they advised against leaving the staples in place for longer than one year because longitudinal growth may not resume following removal of the staples.[76]

The problems of asymmetrical growth arrest by physeal stapling are (1) the unpredictability of growth after the staples have been removed; (2) the possibility of asymmetrical growth retardation in the stapled growth regions, as a result of which genu recurvatum or flexion deformity of the knee may develop; (3) widening and loosening of the tips of the staples, with eventual extrusion of the staples; and (4) irregular pattern of initial growth retardation after stapling. Growth retardation may be correlated to skeletal age—the more advanced the skeletal age at the time of stapling, the more pronounced and rapid the initial growth retardation and the lower the basal growth rate.[76] In addition, (5) a second surgical procedure may be necessary to remove the staples; and (6) the operative scars are large and unsightly.

The amount of correction can be related mathematically to the transverse width of the physis, the length of the leg distal to the growth plate to be arrested, and growth that will occur on the unarrested side of the physis based on skeletal age.

Bowen et al. developed a chart based on the Green-Anderson Growth Remaining Table that can be used to predict the degree of correction of angular malalignment that can be gained from asymmetrical growth arrest of the distal femoral or proximal tibial physis.[10]

Following medial physeal arrest, it is the continued lateral growth that will correct the valgus deformity. In calculation of the degree of angular correction, the lateral growth represents the arc of a circle with the radius equal to the transverse width of the physis. The relation between physeal length, angle of deformity, and the arc of continued growth is expressed in the formula

$$\frac{\text{arc of normal growth}}{\text{angle of deformity}} = \frac{2\pi r}{360}$$

By the use of this formula, a chart was constructed (Table 7–21) that related the amount of growth remaining (Y axis) to the angular change for varying physeal distances (X axis). Then, the angle of deformity for each physeal length was combined with the Green-Anderson Growth Remaining Chart; this allowed the angular deformity to be related to the linear growth remaining for the patient's skeletal age (Fig. 7–248). It should be stressed that this table should be used as a guideline and that after medial epiphysiodesis, if the desired correction is obtained while the lateral physis still remains open, combined epiphysiodesis should be performed to prevent overcorrection. The importance of regular and frequent follow-up cannot be overemphasized. It is crucial that these patients be seen at two-month intervals to assess the degree of correction.

The advantage of osteotomy is that the deformity is fully corrected at the time of surgery. However, peroneal nerve palsy and compartment syndrome are definite possible complications of osteotomy and occur more frequently at the proximal tibial than at the distal femoral level. The surgical procedure is of greater magnitude, and a second operation is required to remove the internal fixation device. Medial physeal arrest by epiphysiodesis or growth retardation by stapling is a simple procedure, with no potential of injury to the peroneal nerve. The valgus deformity is corrected gradually over a period of one or two years. Unfortunately, the degree of correction that will be obtained at the end of the growth period cannot be predicted with certainty; a second operation is often required to remove the staples, or when medial epiphysiodesis is performed, the lateral part of the physis should be arrested when the

*Table 7–21. Degree of Angular Change Based Upon Linear Growth Remaining**

Growth Remaining (cm)	Width of Bone at Physis (cm)							
	9.0	8.5	8.0	7.5	7.0	6.5	6.0	5.5
4.0	25.5	27.0	28.6	30.6	32.7	35.3	38.2	41.7
3.5	22.3	23.6	25.1	26.7	28.6	30.9	33.4	36.5
3.0	19.1	20.2	21.5	22.9	24.6	26.0	28.6	31.3
2.5	16.0	16.9	18.0	19.0	20.5	22.0	23.9	26.0
2.0	13.0	13.5	14.3	15.3	16.4	17.6	19.1	20.8
1.5	10.0	10.1	10.7	11.5	12.3	13.2	14.3	15.6
1.0	6.4	6.7	7.2	7.6	8.2	8.8	9.5	10.4
0.5	3.2	3.4	3.6	3.8	4.1	4.4	4.8	5.2

*From Bowen, J. R., et al.: Partial epiphysiodesis to correct angular deformity. Clin. Orthop. Rel. Res., *198*:184, 1985. Reprinted by permission.

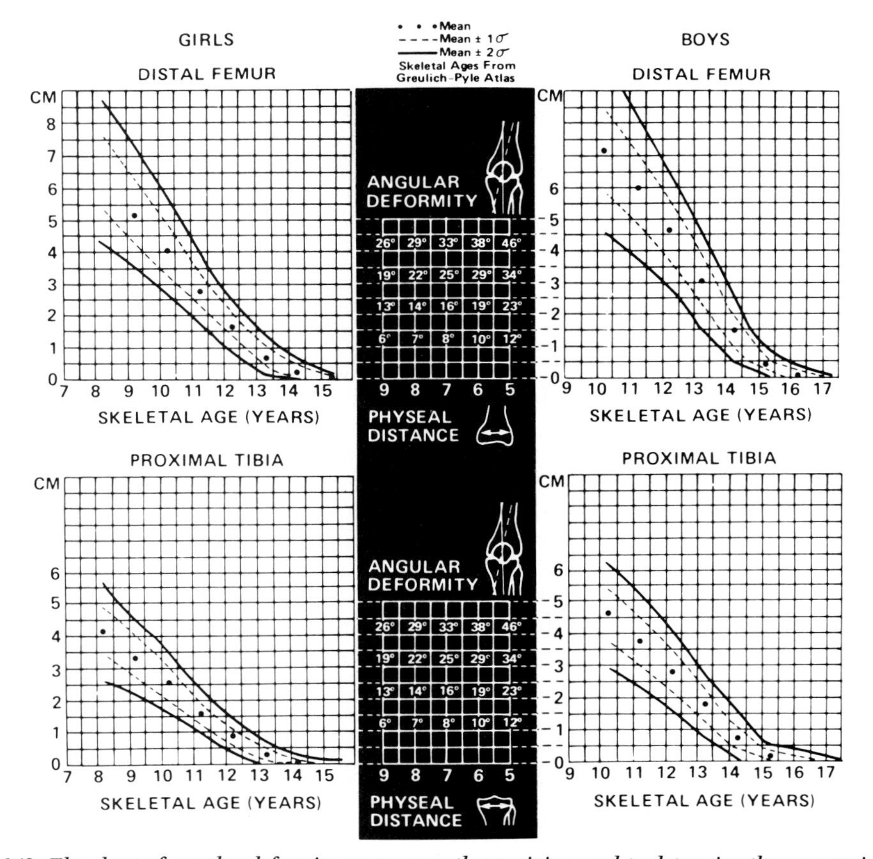

FIGURE 7–248. The chart of angular deformity* versus *growth remaining used to determine the appropriate timing for partial epiphysiodesis.

Based on the Green-Anderson growth remaining chart. (From Anderson, M., Green, W. T., and Messner, M. B.: Growth and predictions of growth in the lower extremities. J. Bone Joint Surg., *45-A*:10, 1963. From Bowen, J. R., et al.: Partial epiphysiodesis to correct angular deformity. Clin. Orthop. Rel. Res., *198*:184, 1985. Reprinted by permission.)

alignment of the lower limbs is straight. It is obvious that each case should be individually assessed. This author recommends the following plan of operative treatment: When there is sufficient growth remaining, epiphysiodesis of the medial physis of the distal femur and/or of the proximal tibia, depending upon the maximal site and degree of the valgus deformity, should be performed. This author prefers epiphysiodesis over staple growth retardation because the results are more predictable. Bowen's chart is used to determine the skeletal age at which physeal arrest should be performed. It should be clear that methods of prediction for correction of genu valgum *are not precise*. Bowen's chart is used as a general guideline. As a general rule, when the amount of knock-knee is 7.5 to 10 cm., medial growth arrest of the distal femur is performed between the skeletal ages of 10 and 11 years in girls, and 12 and 13 years in boys. It is vital to follow the patient frequently in the postoperative period (every two months the first year) to avoid overcorrection. Sometimes it is surprising how rapid the genu valgum corrects following medial epiphysiodesis.

In correction of genu valgum in multiple hereditary exostosis, the author recommends stapling. The metaphyseal-physeal area in these children is enlarged, and growth prediction is very difficult. Following removal of staples, rebound growth occurs, making timing of asymmetrical arrest difficult. When the legs straighten, the growth arrest is completed by lateral and also medial (if open) epiphysiodesis.

The operative technique of stapling of the medial side of the distal femoral condyle is as follows:

The distal femoral epiphysis is approached medially through a 5-cm. longitudinal incision between the anterior and posterior margins of the femoral condyles beginning 1 cm. superior to the knee joint line. The subcutaneous tissue is divided in line with the skin incision. The deep fascia and the patellar retinaculum are divided and each marked with 00 sutures for separate closure later. The epiphyseal plate is identified by probing with a straight Keith needle; the plate is softer than adjacent cancellous bone. With the needle inserted in the growth plate, radiograms are made in the anteroposterior and lateral planes for definite localization of the site of the physis. Vitallium staples should be used because they cause less reaction, bend minimally, and almost never break. The growth plate of the distal end of the femur is convex distally, and there is abrupt posterior tilting of the distal femoral condyle. With a staple holder, three staples are partially driven into bone, one in the center of the transverse diameter of the physis, one at the junction of the posterior one fourth and anterior three fourths, and another at the junction of the anterior one fourth and posterior three fourths.

The cross-member of the staple must be parallel to the bone surface and perpendicular to the growth plate. The legs of the staple must be equidistant from the epiphyseal plate and point to the center of the bone. Both legs of the staple must be placed in bone; a common mistake is to leave the proximal leg of the posterior staple buried in the soft tissue. Meticulous attention should be paid to avoiding technical errors. The position of the staples is verified by anteroposterior and lateral radiograms of the distal femur; once this is established as being correct, the staples are securely driven into bone. The patellar retinaculum is closed with interrupted sutures; the deep fascia is closed separately with continuous sutures. The importance of separate closure of the patellar retinaculum and deep fascia cannot be overemphasized, as they should not be caught by the staples. Otherwise, the patellar retinaculum will be bound down, with resultant restriction of knee motion, local swelling, and pain. The subcutaneous tissue and skin are closed in the usual manner, and an above-knee cylinder cast is applied. The cast is removed in two to three weeks, and the patient is allowed to ambulate freely without restriction.

When, in addition to distal femoral stapling, retardation of growth of the medial aspect of the proximal tibia is indicated (because of skeletal maturity of the patient), the author prefers epiphysiodesis to stapling.

The operative technique of epiphysiodesis of the distal femur and proximal tibia is described and illustrated in the section on limb lengthening (see Plates 113 and 114 on pp. 2878 to 2885).

In correction of genu valgum only the medial part of the physis is arrested. Be sure not to injure the growth plate beyond the midline!

OSTEOTOMY

This is performed when the patient is seen late and it is too late to obtain correction by medial epiphysiodesis (ordinarily over 14 years of age in boys and 12 years in girls). *Varus osteotomy of the proximal tibia* is indicated when the valgus deformity is in the proximal tibia below the knee joint; there should be no superolateral tilt of the knee joint line. When proximal tibial varus osteotomy is performed, peroneal nerve palsy, vascular insufficiency due to kinking of tibial vessels, and anterior compartment syndrome are potential serious complications; this should be made very clear to the parents and the adolescent patient. This author strongly recommends correction of tibia valga by metaphyseal-diaphyseal juncture corticotomy and the use of the Orthofix or Ilizarov fixator. The valgus deformity is corrected slowly by asymmetrical distraction-compression. Associated lateral torsional deformity is corrected at the same time. If the iliotibial band is taut and is a deforming force, it is released. Immobilization in a cast is not required. Neural and vascular status is closely monitored, and appropriate adjustments are made as necessary.

Hemichondrodiatasis may be performed by some surgeons; its advantage is that limb length inequality can be corrected simultaneously. The disadvantages of hemichondrodiatasis are its potential for knee stiffness and the risk of sepsis.

Osteotomy of the Distal Femur. Valgus deformity of the knee is often associated with a superolateral tilt of the knee joint line in the anteroposterior plane; in order to correct this abnormal sloping of the knee joint, the osteotomy should be performed proximal to the knee. An osteotomy of the proximal tibia does not correct this superolateral tilt of the joint, and the proximal tibia may gradually displace laterally. If the genu valgus deformity is greater than 12 to 15 degrees, and the superolateral tilt of the joint line from the horizontal is more than 10 degrees, the level of varus osteotomy should be in the distal femur and not the proximal tibia.

The operative technique is as follows: With the patient in supine position, the entire lower limb and the ipsilateral hip are prepared and draped. It is important to have the anterior superior iliac spine in the sterile field. A sterile tourniquet is used. A medial approach is used to expose the distal femur. A longitudinal medial straight incision is made along the femur, beginning from the joint line and extending proximally for 10 to 15 cm. The subcutaneous tissue and fascia are divided in line with the skin incision. The vastus medialis is dissected from the medial intermuscular septum and reflected anteriorly and laterally to expose the anterior and medial part of the distal femoral shaft, metaphysis, and epiphysis. The knee joint is opened medially for exposure, visualization, and control of guide pins.

Image intensifier radiographic control is utilized for determination of the proper level of osteotomy and placement of guide pins. First, the axis of the knee joint is determined under image intensifier x-ray control. If necessary, a guide wire is passed medial to lateral through the medial arthrotomy, transversely across the joint, and parallel to the distal articular surface of the femur. Second, a guide pin is inserted about 1 cm. proximal to the femoral articular surface under image intensifier x-ray control. It is important to ensure, by an anteroposterior radiogram, that this guide wire is parallel to the articular surface. Next, drill holes are made in the medial part of the femoral cortex 2 to 2.5 cm. proximal from the femoral articular surface along the line where the chisel will be inserted; this will prevent comminution of the medial cortex. Then, a plate holder is used to guide the chisel in order to obtain correct apposition of the plate to the long axis of the femur. The chisel is driven into the anterior one half of the medial femoral condyle and anteroposterior and lateral radiograms are made to determine the position of the chisel. It is important that the chisel not penetrate the intercondylar notch or the anterior part of the femoral articular surface.

Prior to compression of the osteotomy, two large threaded Steinmann pins are passed percutaneously from the lateral side—one in the distal fragment and one in the proximal segment. These pins will serve to ensure the correct rotational alignment of the femur after compression of the osteotomy. The femoral osteotomy is performed with the help of an oscillating saw. The lateral part of the femoral cortex is drilled and the osteotomy completed with a small osteotome. This will prevent lateral displacement of the proximal segment. Then a wedge of bone is resected medially, the width of wedge dependent upon the degree of genu valgum to be corrected.

After completion of the osteotomy and correction of the deformity, the two large threaded Steinmann pins are drilled across the osteotomy site, fixing the two bony fragments together firmly. If necessary, the proximal cortical fragment can be impacted into the cancellous bone of the distal fragment. This is easily carried out because the diameter of the femur proximal to the osteotomy is narrower than that distal to the osteotomy. This increases the angle of the osteotomy, if necessary; it also provides more stability and promotes more rapid healing.

Radiograms in the anteroposterior and lateral projections are made to determine the degree of correction, and if the correction is adequate, a 90 degree offset dynamic compression blade plate is inserted for internal fixation. An alternative method of fixation is with a Cobra plate and screws.

The wound is closed in layers, the threaded

Steinmann pins are removed, and a compression dressing is applied. On the third postoperative day, knee exercises are performed and walking with toe-touch gait is permitted. The osteotomy will usually heal in six weeks, at which time full weight-bearing is permitted.

References

1. Aldegheri, R., and Marcer, M.: Treatment of angular deformities of the leg by external distraction. Chir. Organi Mov., *66:*203, 1981.
2. Arkin, A. M., and Katz, J. F.: The effects of pressure on epiphyseal growth. J. Bone Joint Surg., *38-A:*1056, 1956.
3. Asher, C.: Knock knee (genu valgum). *In* Postural Variations in Childhood. London, Butterworths, 1975, pp. 54–72.
4. Ballerio, A.: Lassita congenita dei legamenti collaterali esterni in ginocchio valgo epifisario. Arch. Putti Chir. Organi Mov., *6:*431, 1955.
5. Balthazar, D. A., and Pappas, A. M.: Acquired valgus deformity of the tibia in children. J. Pediatr. Orthop., *4:*538, 1984.
6. Beals, R. K., and Skyhar, M.: Growth and development of the tibia, fibula and ankle joint. Clin. Orthop., *182:*289, 1984.
7. Bell, S. N., Campbell, P. E., Cole, W. G., and Menelaus, M. B.: Tibia vara caused by focal fibrocartilaginous dysplasia. Three case reports. J. Bone Joint Surg., *67-B:*780, 1985.
8. Bigongiari, L. R.: Pseudotibiotalar slant: a positioning artifact. Radiology, *122*(Suppl.):669, 1977.
9. Böhm, M.: Infantile deformities of the knee and hip. J. Bone Joint Surg., *15:*574, 1933.
10. Bowen, J. R., Leahey, J. L., Zhang, Z. H., and MacEwen, G. D.: Partial epiphysiodesis at the knee to correct angular deformity. Clin. Orthop., *198:*184, 1985.
11. Brittain, H. A.: Treatment of genu valgum. Br. Med. J., *2:*385, 1948.
12. Brueckmann, F. R., and Kettelkamp, D. B.: Proximal tibial osteotomy. Orthop. Clin. North Am., *13:*3, 1982.
13. Caldwell, G. A., Shorkey, R. L., and Duncan, T. L.: Treatment of mild knock knees and pronated feet in childhood (results in 63 cases). New Orleans Med. Surg. J., *104:*304, 1952.
14. Canale, S. T., Russell, T. A., and Holcomb, R. L.: Percutaneous epiphysiodesis: experimental study and preliminary clinical results. J. Pediatr. Orthop., *6:*150, 1986.
15. Carlson, R. L., Lohse, C. L., Eld, L. A., and Hughbanks, F. G.: Correction of angular limb deformities by physeal stapling. Mod. Vet. Pract., *53:*41, 1972.
16. Carvell, J. E.: The relationship of the periosteum to angular deformities of long bones. Experimental operations in rabbits. Clin. Orthop., *173:*262, 1983.
17. Cassarino, A., and Rappalardo, S.: High domed tibial osteotomy in the treatment of angular deviations of the knee. A new system of surgical instrumentation. Ital. J. Orthop. Traumatol., *11:*331, 1985.
18. Currarino, G., and Kirks, D. R.: Lateral widening of epiphyseal plates in knees of children with bowed legs. A.J.R., *129:*309, 1977.
19. Editorial: Genu valgum due to fluoride toxicity. Nutr. Rev., *33:*76, 1975.
20. Engel, G. M., and Lippert, F. G., III: Valgus tibial osteotomy: avoiding the pitfalls. Clin. Orthop., *160:*137, 1981.
21. Foreman, K. A., and Robertson, W. W., Jr.: Radiographic measurement of infantile tibia vara. J. Pediatr. Orthop., *5:*452, 1985.
22. Gentile, G.: Measurement of valgus and varus deformity in the lower limb. Ital. J. Orthop. Traumatol., *4:*183, 1978.
23. Geppert, T. V.: Physiological knock-knee. Am. J. Dis. Child., *83:*154, 1952.
24. Girdlestone, G. R.: Night splint for knock knees. Lancet, *1:*312, 1944.
25. Gorji, J.: Genu valgum: treatment by osteotomy (Letter). Clin. Orthop., *81:*178, 1971.
26. Griffin, P. P.: The lower limbs. *In* Lovell, W. W., and Winter, R. B. (eds.): Pediatric Orthopedics. Philadelphia, J. B. Lippincott, 1986, pp. 865–875.
27. Griffiths, H., and Wandtke, J.: Tibiotalar tilt—a new slant. Skeletal Radiol., *6:*193, 1981.
28. Hall, B. D., and Spranger, J. W.: Familial congenital bowing with short bones. Radiology, *132:*611, 1979.
29. Hansson, L. I., and Zayer, M.: Physiological genu varum. Acta Orthop. Scand., *46:*221, 1975.
30. Harper, M. C., and Canale, S. T.: Angulation osteotomy. A trigonometric analysis. Clin. Orthop., *166:*173, 1982.
31. Healy, W. L., Anglen, J. O., Wasilewski, S. A., and Krackow, K. A.: Distal femoral varus osteotomy. J. Bone Joint Surg., *70-A:*102, 1988.
32. Herring, J. A., and Kling, T. F.: Genu valgus. J. Pediatr. Orthop., *5:*236, 1985.
33. Holt, J. F., Latourette, H. B., and Watson, E. H.: Physiological bowing of the legs in young children. J.A.M.A., *154:*390, 1954.
34. Howorth, M. B.: Knock knees: with special reference to the stapling operation. Clin. Orthop., *77:*233, 1971.
35. Hueck, H.: Osteotomy for genu valgum adolescentium. Dtsch. Z. Chir., *160:*245, 1920.
36. Jackson, J. P., and Waugh, W.: The technique and complications of upper tibial osteotomy: A review of 226 operations. J. Bone Joint Surg., *56-B:*236, 1974.
37. Junghans, H.: End results of supracondylar wedge osteotomy of femur for genu valgum. Dtsch. Z. Chir., *209:*394, 1928.
38. Kellgren, H. A.: Treatment of postural abnormalities of legs in children. J. R. Inst. Public Health, *3:*97, 1940.
39. Kling, T. F., Jr.: Angular deformities of the lower limbs in children. Orthop. Clin. North Am., *18:*513, 1987.
40. Kling, T. F., Jr., and Hensinger, R. N.: Angular and torsional deformities of the lower limbs in children. Clin. Orthop., *176:*136, 1983.
41. Knight, R. A.: Developmental deformities of the lower extremities. J. Bone Joint Surg., *36-A:*521, 1954.
42. Krishnamachari, K. A. V. R., and Krishnaswamy, K.: Genu valgum and osteoporosis in an area of endemic fluorosis. Lancet, *2:*877, 1973.
43. Kummel, B.: Tibiofemoral incongruity in association with patellar instability. Clin. Orthop., *155:*97, 1981.
44. Lelièvre, J.: Genu varum. *In* Pathologie du Pied. 2nd. Ed. Paris, Masson et Cie., 1961, pp. 404–407.
45. Levine, A. M., and Drennan, J. C.: Physiologic bowing and tibia vara. The metaphyseal-diaphyseal angle in the measurement of bowleg deformities. J. Bone Joint Surg., *64-A:*1158, 1982.
46. Litt, R., and Albassir, A.: The tibial component in severe valgus. Its treatment in children. Acta Orthop. Belg., *47:*74, 1981.
47. Lloyd, E. I.: Night splint for knock knees in children. Br. Med. J., *1:*676, 1939.
48. Lloyd, E. I.: Knock knees and bowlegs. Practitioner, *150:*238, 1943.
49. McDermott, A. G. P., Kinklestein, J. A., Farine, I., Boynton, E. L., MacIntosh, D. L., and Gross, A.: Distal femoral varus osteotomy for valgus deformity of the knee. J. Bone Joint Surg., *70-A:*110, 1988.
50. Morley, A. J. M.: Knock knees in children. Br. Med. J., *2:*976, 1957.
51. Morris, H. D.: Treatment of infantile bowlegs and knock knees with special consideration for the thera-

peutic use of large doses of activated ergosterol. Analysis of 58 cases. South. Med. J., *44*:435, 1951.
52. Newell, R. L., and Durbin, F. C.: The aetiology of congenital angulation of tubular bones with constriction of the medullary canal and its relationship to congenital pseudarthrosis. J. Bone Joint Surg., *58-B*:444, 1976.
53. Pappas, A. M., Anas, P., and Toczylowski, H. M., Jr.: Asymmetrical arrest of the proximal tibial physis and genu recurvatum deformity. J. Bone Joint Surg., *66-A*:575, 1984.
54. Parker, C. A.: Treatment of bowlegs and knock knees. Surg. Clin., *4*:705, 1920.
55. Perthes, G.: Curvilinear osteotomy of tibia in genu valgum and genu varum. Zentralbl. Chir., *50*:891, 1923.
56. Pistevos, G., and Duckworth, T.: The correction of genu valgum by epiphyseal stapling. J. Bone Joint Surg., *59-B*:72, 1977.
57. Porter, R. W.: The effect of tension across a growing epiphysis. J. Bone Joint Surg., *60-B*:252, 1978.
58. Ramsey, P. L., and Hamilton, W.: Changes in tibiotalar area of contact caused by lateral talar tilt. J. Bone Joint Surg., *58-A*:356, 1976.
59. Rang, M.: The Growth Plate and Its Disorders. Baltimore, Williams & Wilkins, 1969, pp. 103–109.
60. Reichelt, A., and Imping, G.: Operative Probleme bei Achsenabweichungen der Beine. II. Mitteilung: Das Genu valgum. Z. Orthop., *3*:200, 1973.
61. Richardson, B. D., and Walker, B. F.: Radiological studies of bowing and knock knee in South African Black school children (Letter). S. Afr. Med. J., *48*:2385, 1974.
62. Robertson, W. W., Jr.: Distal tibial deformity in bowlegs. J. Pediatr. Orthop., *7*:324, 1987.
63. Ryoppy, S., and Karaharju, E. O.: Alteration of epiphyseal growth by an experimentally produced angular deformity. Acta Orthop. Scand., *45*:490, 1974.
64. Seiger, H. W.: A night splint for correction of genu valgum. J. Bone Joint Surg., *28*:178, 1946.
65. Sherman, M.: Physiologic bowing of the legs. South. Med. J., *53*:830, 1960.
66. Shopfner, C. E., and Cramer, R.: Growth remodelling of long bone. Br. J. Radiol., *46*:512, 1973.
67. Smith, D. N., and Harrison, M. H.: The correction of angular deformities of long bones by osteotomy-osteoclasis. J. Bone Joint Surg., *61-B*:410, 1979.
68. Stelling, F. H., and Meyer, L. C.: Bowlegs and knock knees in children. Pediatr. Clin. North Am., *2*:1053, 1955.
69. Takatori, Y., and Iwaya, T.: Orthotic management of severe genu varum and tibia vara. J. Pediatr. Orthop., *4*:633, 1984.
70. Tarr, R. R., Resnick, C. T., Wagner, K. S., and Sarmiento, A.: Changes in tibiotalar joint contact areas following experimentally induced angular deformities. Clin. Orthop., *199*:72, 1985.
71. Taussig, G.: Les genu valgum pathologiques de l'enfant. Rev. Chir. Orthop., *60*:247, 1974.
72. Thelander, H. E., and Fitzhugh, M. L.: Posture habits in infancy affecting foot and leg alignments. J. Pediatr., *21*:306, 1942.
73. Thompson, G. H., Carter, J. R., and Smith, C. W.: Late-onset tibia vara: a comparative analysis. J. Pediatr. Orthop., *4*:185, 1984.
74. Vankka, E., and Salenius, P.: Spontaneous correction of severe tibiofemoral deformity in growing children. Acta Orthop. Scand., *53*:567, 1982.
75. Williams, A. T.: Tibial realignment by oblique wedge osteotomy. A new method based on accurate measurement. Int. Orthop., *10*:171, 1986.
76. Zuege, R. C., Kempken, T. G., and Blount, W. P.: Epiphyseal stapling for angular deformities at the knee. J. Bone Joint Surg., *61-A*:320, 1979.

TIBIA VARA

Tibia vara (or Blount's disease) is a growth disorder of the medial part of the proximal tibial physis, epiphysis, and metaphysis. It is characterized by acute medial angulation and medial rotation of the tibia in the proximal metaphyseal region immediately below the knee.

Erlacher reported the first case of tibia vara in 1922.[28] W.P. Blount, in 1937, presented 13 new cases and reviewed the 15 cases in the literature; he delineated the similarities between infantile and adolescent tibia vara and emphasized the differences in their etiology.[12] Blount suggested the name *tibia vara,* which at present is the generally accepted term. The eponym *Blount's disease* is used quite often. The name *osteochondrosis deformans tibiae* is not accurate, as no avascular necrosis is present; it should not be used.

Langenskiöld, in 1952, classified tibia vara into six progressive radiographic stages, from mild to moderate to severe.[45] Langenskiöld and Riska, in 1964, published a large series of cases and established the guidelines for prognosis and treatment.[50]

Classification

Tibia vara is differentiated into two types: *infantile* (or *early onset*) and *late onset.* In the infantile type, deformity is noted in the first few years of life (three years and younger) and is frequently bilateral. The late-onset type is subdivided into a *juvenile form,* with onset between four and ten years of age, and a *true adolescent form,* with onset in the 11-years-and-older age group. In the past, tibia vara was classified into infantile and adolescent types; however, recently the juvenile form has been delineated.[86]

Smith classified tibia vara into the following four progressive grades, in an attempt to correlate the grade of deformity with the need for treatment; the higher the grade of deformity, the poorer the prognosis and the worse the long-term results of surgery.[79]

I. *Grade A—Potential Tibia Vara*
   This grade encompasses those children with bowlegs who demonstrate the following features:
   1. Varus angulation of not more than 15 degrees
   2. Radiographic changes as follows:
      a. Sclerosis of the medial part of the tibial diaphysis, significantly more severe than of the lateral part

b. Severe beaking of the medial part of the proximal tibial metaphysis
c. Radiolucencies in the medial part of the proximal tibial metaphysis

II. *Grade B—Mild Tibia Vara*
This grade represents all those patients in whom the diagnosis is definite but the pathologic changes are mild.
1. Any or all of the findings in Grade A
2. Femorotibial varus angulation of mild or moderate degree (15 to 30 degrees)
3. Radiographic fragmentation or stippling medially in the proximal epiphysis and/ or metaphysis

III. *Grade C—Advanced Tibia Vara*
This grade represents a more severe form of tibia vara.
1. Any or all of the findings in Grade A or B
2. The following radiographic changes:
   a. Epiphyseal fragmentation and deformity
   b. Open physis of the medial proximal part of the tibia

IV. *Grade D—Physeal Closure*
The most advanced stage of tibia vara.
1. Any or all of the findings of Grade A, B, or C
2. Closure of the medial part of the proximal tibial physis, with a bone bridge evident radiographically between the epiphysis and the metaphysis
3. Marked deficiency of the medial part of the tibial plateau and tibial epiphysis
4. Rapidly increasing varus angulation of the knee

Etiology

The pathogenesis of tibia vara seems to be repetitive trauma on the medial-posterior proximal tibial physeal-epiphyseal area from walking on a varus knee. Blount's disease is not encountered in nonambulatory children and is not initially diagnosed prior to two years of age. At least one year of walking and weight-bearing seems necessary for the deformity to develop.[21] Children with tibia vara have severe "physiologic" bowing of the legs and usually began to walk at an early age.[6]

Progressive varus deformity of the proximal tibia is produced by a combination of abnormal stress and asymmetrical growth of the upper medial and posterior parts of the tibial physis and epiphysis.[6, 35, 40] Epiphyseal compression inhibits growth, and distraction stimulates growth. When stress is removed from a growing physis, it will have a tendency to overgrowth (Delpech's law).

In their experimental work in immature rabbits, Arkin and Katz demonstrated that when a growing epiphysis is subjected to stress the rate and direction of growth are modified, yielding to the exerted stress. Increase in compression decreases growth rate, whereas increase in tension increases growth rate.[2]

Strobino et al., in their experimental work with calves, showed that abnormal pressure forces across the physes stopped growth.[83] Porter showed that tension across the physis accelerates growth.[64] Arkin and Katz believed that the effect of pressure across the physes is not an all-or-none phenomenon; there is no threshold.[2]

Tibia vara is much more common in black Jamaican than in white English children. According to Bateson, this racial preponderance seems to be due to two factors: First, Jamaican children have more severe physiologic genu varus as infants than do English children; and second, they begin walking at a much younger age, thereby exerting abnormal stress on the medial upper tibia and predisposing them to progressive tibia vara.[6, 7] Most children with the infantile type of tibia vara are obese, with a physical habitus suggestive of dystrophia adiposogenitalis.

Golding and McNeil-Smith have also called attention to the relatively high incidence and severity of this disease in the West Indies and West Africa.[35] They also noted that the black children of these two areas have excessive ligamentous laxity and begin to walk at an earlier age than do Caucasians. Both of these are factors in abnormal excessive tibiofemoral motion. The resultant effect is a change of direction of weight-bearing forces on the upper tibial epiphysis from perpendicular to oblique. The obliquity of this force tends to displace the tibial epiphysis laterally. The trabecular pattern of the metaphyseal region in tibia vara curves medially to align itself to the deviation of stress at the same time the epiphyseal line curves down so that it is at right angles to the line of stress. Thus a vicious circle is established, as longitudinal growth becomes directed not along the axis of the tibia, but at an angle, so that the medial side of the shaft becomes shorter than the lateral side. Consequently, the alteration in growth tends to increase the varus deformity.[35]

Golding further explains why the great majority of children with bowlegs do not develop tibia vara. The usual response to the increased weight borne by the inner side of the knee in a child with bowlegs is a relative increase in the rate of growth of the medial distal femoral and proximal tibial epiphyses. It is only when the loss in rate of growth due to a change in alignment is greater than the effect of stimulation that tibia vara develops. Golding concludes that tibia vara is caused by failure of growth of the posteromedial part of the upper tibial epiphysis and physis; the varus deformity results from marked alteration of the lines of forces acting on the medial portion of the upper tibial epiphysis.[33] The lateral part of the distal femoral and proximal tibial physis is widened in some cases of Blount's disease.[22] The clinical evidence is strong that abnormal pressure due to weight-bearing on the medial aspect of the proximal tibial physis, growth retardation, and asymmetrical growth are definite factors in the etiology and progression of tibia vara.

In tibia vara the fibula is overgrown in relation to the medial longitudinal half of the tibia; in addition, the upper fibula is in a more posterolateral position; according to Kessel, this is a factor in the causation of progressive varus and medial rotation deformity of the upper tibia.[40]

Cook et al. performed a biomechanical analysis of the etiology of tibia vara by investigating the stresses occurring in the physis during one-legged stance in children by finite element analysis. Forces were assigned to the medial and lateral plateaus and the lateral ligament. Increasing varus resulted in increasing compressive stress in the level of the medial tibial physis seven times normal at 30 degrees of varus. In the overweight child the changes were more severe. Their data supported the physical basis of the pathogenesis of tibia vara.[21]

The resemblance of tibia vara to infantile coxa vara because of the presence of a triangular bony fragment in the metaphyseal area has been noted by Langenskiöld.[45, 46]

Sevastikoglou and Erickson have suggested heredity as a possible etiologic factor, basing their contention on the incidence of four typical cases of tibia vara in the same family, of which two occurred in identical twins.[69] Trauma, infection, and aseptic necrosis of bone are not causative factors.

The pathogenesis of *late-onset tibia vara* (both the juvenile and the adolescent forms) is similar to that of the infantile form. The varus deformity of the upper tibia is produced by growth retardation due to asymmetrical compressive and shear forces acting across the proximal tibial physis. Suppression and deviation of normal enchondral ossification results in tibia vara.[19, 21, 92] In some cases of adolescent tibia vara there is a history of trauma; the tomographic studies of Langenskiöld have demonstrated the presence of an osseous bridge between the upper medial tibial epiphysis and metaphysis.[49] An osseous bridge is not present in all cases of adolescent tibia vara.

Pathology

A study of biopsy specimens from the medial tibial condyle in the infantile variety (nine cases by Langenskiöld and six cases by Golding and McNeil-Smith) have shown that the histologic changes are principally localized in the zone of resting cartilage in the medial part of the proximal tibial physis; they consist of (1) islands of densely packed cells that exhibit a greater degree of hypertrophy than would be expected from their topographical position, (2) islands of almost acellular fibrous cartilage, and (3) abnormal groups of capillary vessels. The presence of aseptic necrosis of bone and inflammation could not be demonstrated.[35, 47]

Langenskiöld did not take specimens from any of the adolescent type.[47] Carter et al. reported biopsy findings from the medial tibial physis from late-onset tibia vara (adolescent type); the histopathologic findings were similar to those of the infantile form.[19] The histopathologic studies of Carter et al. included the entire growth plate (medial and lateral) and adjacent structures; two of the specimens were from juvenile-onset and three from adolescent-onset disease. These authors could not find an osseous bridge across the medial portion of the physis; instead there was disorganization and misalignment of the physis and evidence of disruption of normal enchondral ossification. These histopathologic findings support the vicious circle of varus–growth suppression–further varus pathogenesis of tibia vara. The varus deformity in infantile tibia vara is more severe than in the adolescent type because the secondary ossification center in the young child is more pliable than the ossified proximal tibial epiphysis of the adolescent.

Clinical Picture

In the *infantile type*, the children are early walkers, usually at nine to ten months of age. At the onset of the disease, it is often difficult to differentiate between tibia vara and severe physiologic bowlegs. Involvement is bilateral in 50 to 75 per cent of the cases. It is predominant in the female and in the black race. The usual presenting complaint is bowing of the legs during the first year of life; however, instead of gradual spontaneous correction and progression to physiologic genu valgum, the bowing usually increases. Soon the tibia is acutely deflected inward just below the knee (Fig. 7–249). A nontender bony prominence or "beak" may be palpable over the medial aspect of the proximal tibial condyle. Pain is not a complaint. Obesity, excessive medial tibial torsion, pronated feet, and a minimal amount of shortening of the involved leg (in unilateral cases) are common associated findings.

The *juvenile type* has its onset between four and ten years of age. Involvement is often bilateral. The *adolescent type* does not develop until the age of 11 years or older; involvement is unilateral in 80 per cent of the cases, with the involved leg usually shorter than the opposite normal leg by as much as 2 to 3 cm. The

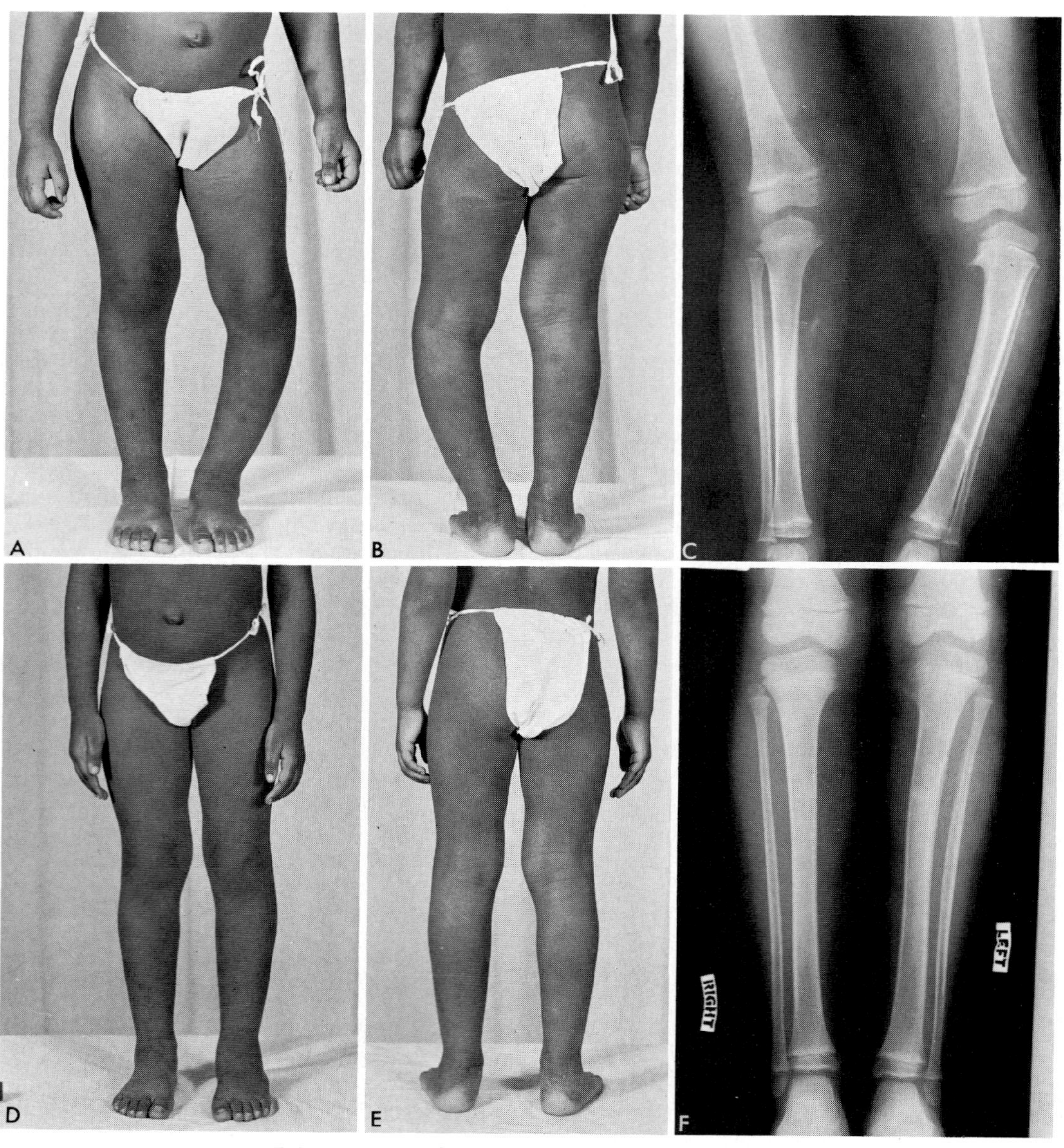

FIGURE 7–249. Blount's disease in a five-year-old girl.

A to **C.** Preoperative photographs and radiograms. Note the acute medial deflection of the tibia just below the knee. **D** to **F.** Postoperative photographs and radiograms showing correction of the deformity.

degree of varus deformity is not marked, usually not exceeding 20 degrees. The body habitus is normal. Excessive medial torsion and pes planovalgus are not accompanying features. Pain and tenderness are often present over the medial prominence of the proximal tibia.

Radiographic Features

Infantile Type. The principal finding on the radiograms is the abrupt medial angulation of the medial cortical wall of the proximal tibial metaphysis; the lateral cortical wall of the upper tibial metaphysis is nearly straight (Figs. 7–249 C and 7–250 C and D).[17]

Early differentiation between infantile tibia vara and physiologic bowlegs, prior to appearance of the typical radiographic changes of tibia vara, can be made by measurement of the metaphyseal-diaphyseal angle of the proximal tibia; this is formed by the intersection of a line through the transverse plane of the proximal tibial metaphysis with a line perpendicular to the long axis of the tibial diaphysis. Levine and Drennan found consequent development of radiographic changes of tibia vara in 29 of 30

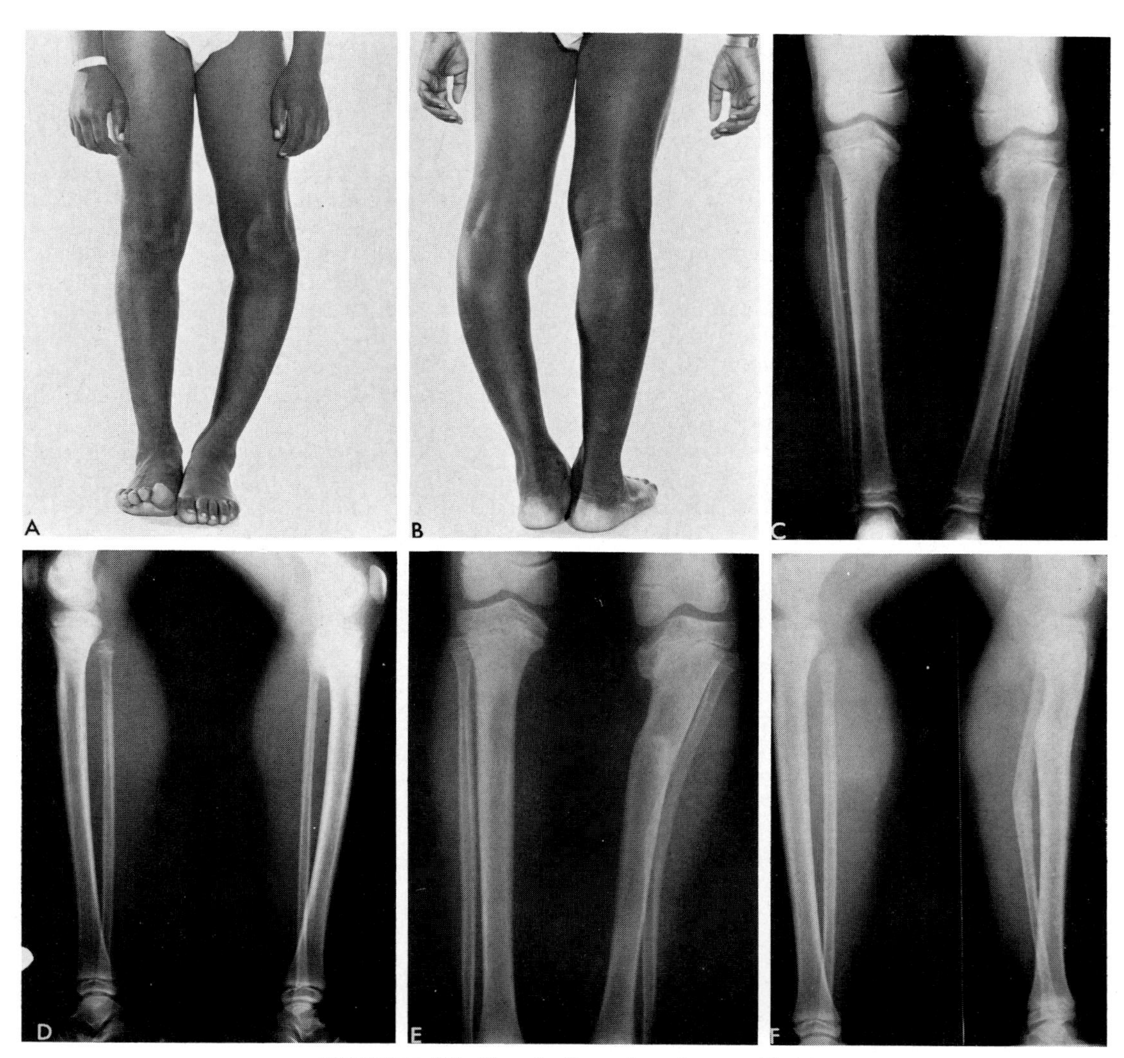

FIGURE 7–250. Blount's disease in a six-year-old girl.

A and **B.** Clinical appearance. Note the marked inward bowing of the tibia just below the knee joint. **C** and **D.** Anteroposterior and lateral radiograms of both tibiae. Note the severity of sloping of medial tibial plateau and the metaphyseal changes. An osteotomy was performed to correct the deformity. There was some instability of the knee. **E** and **F.** Postoperative radiograms. The deformity of the medial tibial plateau persists.

affected limbs with an initial metaphyseal-diaphyseal angle of more than 11.0 degrees; however, only 3 of the 58 limbs with a metaphyseal-diaphyseal angle of 11.0 degrees or less later developed radiographic changes of tibia vara.[52]

The relationship between the tibiofemoral and proximal tibial metaphyseal-diaphyseal angle determines the maximal site of varus deformity in physiologic bowlegs versus tibia vara. The tibiofemoral angle measures the deformity at the knee of the involved limb; the proximal tibial metaphyseal-diaphyseal angle shows the varus deformity within the proximal tibia. The ratio of the metaphyseal-diaphyseal angle to the tibiofemoral angle depicts the percentage of the total varus deformity contributed by the proximal part of the tibia. In their study, Levine and Drennan found that approximately 20 to 25 per cent of the varus deformity takes place in the upper tibia in physiologic bowlegs versus 60 to 65 per cent of the varus deformity in tibia vara.[52]

A number of changes are found in the proximal tibial metaphysis and epiphysis, depending upon the degree of skeletal maturation and development. The typical diagnostic radiographic features are fragmentation of the medial metaphysis of the proximal tibia and acute varus angulation of the tibia immediately below the metaphyseal beak (Fig. 7–249 C).[17] The severity and natural course of the disease vary greatly; in some patients, the radiologic changes disappear completely by the age of three to four years; spontaneous resolution of tibia vara does occur but is uncommon.[49] Often, the varus deformity of the upper tibia is progressive. Marked changes are still present by the age of 10 to 13 years. Langenskiold has subdivided the radiographic findings into six progressive stages (Fig. 7–251):[45–50]

Stage I (Two to Three Years). This stage is one of a progressive increase in the degree of varus deformity and is characterized by irregularity of the entire ossification zone of the metaphysis, with radiolucent zones separating islands of calcified tissue from the bony metaphysis. There is a delay in development of the medial portion of the epiphysis. The medial part of the metaphysis protrudes and is beaked medially and distally.

Stage II (Two and One-Half to Four Years). A marked propensity for healing is evident in this stage. A sharp lateromedial depression in the ossification line of the medial third of the metaphysis forms the characteristic "beak." The upper portion of the beak is more radiolucent than are other parts of the metaphysis. The medial part of the bony epiphysis becomes more wedge-shaped and still is less developed than its lateral part.

Stage III (Four to Six Years). Stage III is characterized by deepening of the depression filled by cartilage in the metaphyseal beak, with the radiolucent area giving the appearance of a "step" in the metaphysis. The medial part of the bony epiphysis is still wedge-shaped and is less distinct; on occasion, small areas of calcification may be present beneath the medial border.

Stage IV (Five to Ten Years). With increasing bone maturation the thickness of the epiphyseal growth plate narrows and the bony epiphysis enlarges. Consequently, the "step" in the metaphysis increases in depth, and the bony epiphysis occupies the depression in the medial part of the metaphysis. There is marked irregularity

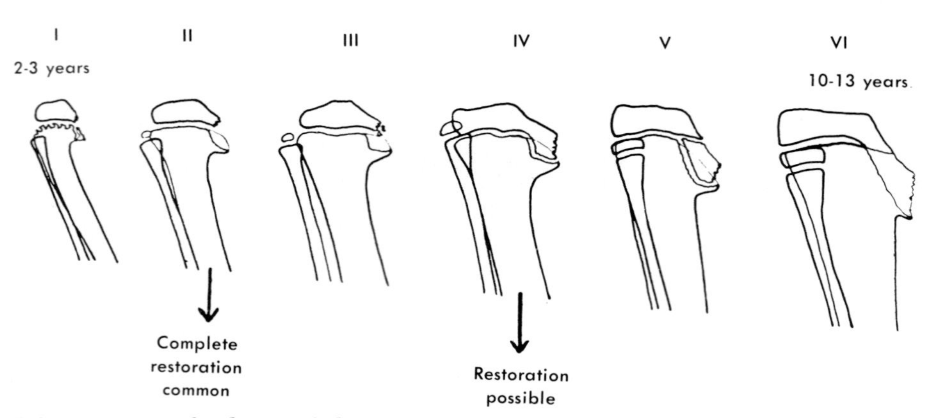

FIGURE 7–251. ***Infantile type of tibia vara—the six progressive stages develop with increasing age.***

(From Langenskiöld, A.: Tibia vara. Acta Chir., *103*:9, 1952.)

of the medial border of the bony epiphysis. A definite tendency to regression is still noted in this stage. The radiographic appearance in the partially healed Stage IV of the infantile type of tibia vara resembles that in the late stages of the adolescent type.

Stage V (9 to 11 Years). A clear band traverses medially from the lateral portion of the epiphyseal plate to the articular cartilage, separating the bony epiphysis into two portions and giving the appearance of a "partially double epiphyseal plate." There is some irregularity of the triangular area of the bony epiphysis against the joint cartilage and the cartilage covering its medial aspect. The medial articular surface of the upper end of the tibia is deformed, sloping medially and distally from the intercondylar area.

Stage VI (10 to 13 Years). The branches of the double medial part of the epiphyseal plate ossify, whereas growth continues in its normal lateral part. Stages V and VI connote irreparable structural deformity. The infantile type of tibia vara is not seen after the age of 13 years.

Adolescent Type. The radiographic findings in this type differ considerably from those in the infantile type. The middle part of the medial half of the epiphyseal plate is narrowed, with increased bone density on its other side. The bony epiphyses are normal in shape, and there is no "step" in the epiphyseal line.

Differential Diagnosis

Physiologic bowing of the tibia, if unusually marked, represents a difficult differential diagnostic problem. Both it and tibia vara may be bilateral and accompanied by excessive medial tibial torsion. The radiographic appearance in the early stages of the disease may be similar in both conditions, with medial beaking of the metaphysis and medial angulation of the tibia.

As stated earlier, in tibia vara the varus angulation is acute, taking place immediately below the medial metaphyseal beak; the metaphyseal-diaphyseal angle is greater than 11 degrees; in physiologic bowing of the tibia, however, the varus curve is much flatter and the metaphyseal-diaphyseal angle is less than 11 degrees. Langenskiöld has observed three patients in whom the development of tibia vara from a stage of physiologic bowlegs was verified radiographically.[49] Not infrequently, these patients with exaggerated physiologic genu varum have to be observed at periodic intervals for 6 to 12 months before a definitive diagnosis can be made. The diagnostic finding on the radiogram is the medial metaphyseal fragmentation. In physiologic genu varum the deformity reverses to one of physiologic genu valgum as a result of weight-bearing stresses; the legs straighten out by age six years. In tibia vara the natural course is one of steady progression (see Table 7–20).

The following conditions also must be differentiated from tibia vara. In *congenital bowing of the tibia,* angulation may take place in the middle part of the tibia. The radiographic appearance of the proximal tibia and distal femur remains normal.

Rickets in its active untreated stage is not difficult to diagnose; however, a case of mild healed rickets with residual bowing may be difficult to differentiate from Stage II of the infantile type of tibia vara. The characteristic generalized and symmetrical affection of the skeleton in rickets, as well as the absence of the clear area in the medial part of the proximal metaphyses of the tibia, will establish the diagnosis, with the appropriate laboratory studies.

Ollier's multiple enchondromatosis and a cartilaginous exostosis situated in the upper end of the tibia may clinically suggest tibia vara but is not difficult to diagnose from the radiogram.

Fractures of the proximal tibial physis may be mistaken for tibia vara, especially if the patient is first seen several weeks following injury, when callus formation is present and the medial displacement of the fracture fragment persists. On the radiograms, it will appear that there is a medially directed beak, and the distal segment will be angulated medially. On serial radiograms, however, evidence of healing of the fracture and remodeling changes will settle the diagnosis.

Osteomyelitis of the proximal tibia metaphysis may disturb growth and cause tibia vara.

Focal fibrocartilaginous dysplasia of the medial aspect of the proximal tibia may cause tibia vara. Involvement is usually unilateral. It seems that the lesion is a developmental abnormality of the mesenchymal anlage of the tibial metaphysis at the insertion of pes anserinus. Histologic findings consist of dense fibrous tissue reminiscent of tendon in its structure and arrangement, with foci in which the fibroblasts lie in lacunae, producing an appearance that resembles fibrocartilage. The histologic appearance is distinct from that of metaphyseal fibrous defect.[10]

Treatment

Treatment depends upon the degree of deformity and the age of the patient.

INFANTILE TYPE

In the *infantile type* the degree of angular deformity may vary from 10 to 60 degrees. Langenskiöld's studies of the natural history of tibia vara have shown the first four years of life to be the main period of progression, after which time the deformity either increases slowly or remains unchanged for several years. From the age of nine years until the end of the adolescent growth spurt, the usual course of the untreated disease is one of gradual increase of the deformity. In the experience of Langenskiöld, spontaneous straightening was observed in only 2 of his 61 cases of the typical infantile type. Namely, in one child, bilateral varus deformity of 20 degrees at the age of two years straightened to 0 degrees at the age of three-and-one-half years; in another patient, unilateral tibia vara of 10 degrees at the age of eight years straightened to 5 degrees at 21 years.[49, 50]

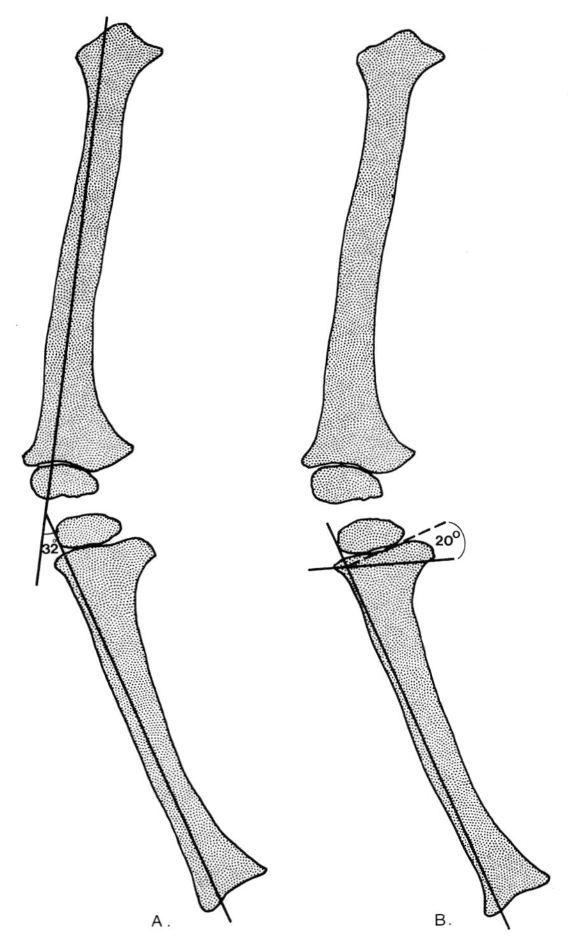

FIGURE 7–252. Radiographic measurement of angular deformity of the lower limb.

A. Tibiofemoral angle. **B.** Proximal metaphyseal-diaphyseal angle.

Nonsurgical Treatment

Observation. In the first two years of life, treatment consists of simple observation. The severity of varus deformity is graded by determination of the tibiofemoral angle as measured on standing anteroposterior radiograms that include the ankles, knees, and most of the femora (Fig. 7–250 C and D and 7–252 A); the metaphyseal-diaphyseal angle (M-D) (Fig. 7–252 B); and the epiphyseal-metaphyseal (E-P) angle (Fig. 7–253). It is imperative to supervise proper positioning of the child. Lateral radiograms of both knees are taken to demonstrate the osseous changes. Clinically the degree of deformity is determined by measuring the distance between the medial femoral condyles when the medial malleoli are gently pressed together and recording the medial thigh-leg angle by goniometer. At three- to four-month intervals the course of the deformity is observed, and radiograms are repeated at three- to six-month intervals. If the angular deformity is lessening or remains unchanged, simple observation is continued.

Orthotic Treatment. When the varus deformity is increasing or when a child in the 24- to 36-month age group presents with a metaphyseal-diaphyseal angle of greater than 11 degrees, an epiphyseal-metaphyseal angle of 25 to 30 degrees, and a tibiofemoral angle of greater than 15 degrees, treatment by an orthotic device may be tried. Radiologically the tibia vara should be Stage I or II. The effectiveness of orthotic devices is open to question. The proponents of orthotic treatment believe that excessive weight-bearing stress on physiologic bowlegs is an important factor in the pathogenesis of tibia vara, and they employ orthosis to relieve the excessive stress on the medial epiphysis and physis of the tibia to provide mediolateral stability of the knee and to correct medial rotation and angulation of the tibia. Tibia vara can resolve spontaneously—this benign course of some cases of Blount's disease makes it difficult to scientifically document the effectiveness of orthotic treatment.[79]

This author recommends the use of a knee-ankle-foot orthosis (KAFO) with free knee and ankle joints, varus correcting knee pad, and thigh-calf cuffs. The foot-ankle part of the orthosis is manufactured of plastic material and designed with a 15-degree toe-out with respect to the knee axis. The uprights of the orthosis may be single medial or double with a locking knee hinge. The brace is designed to provide

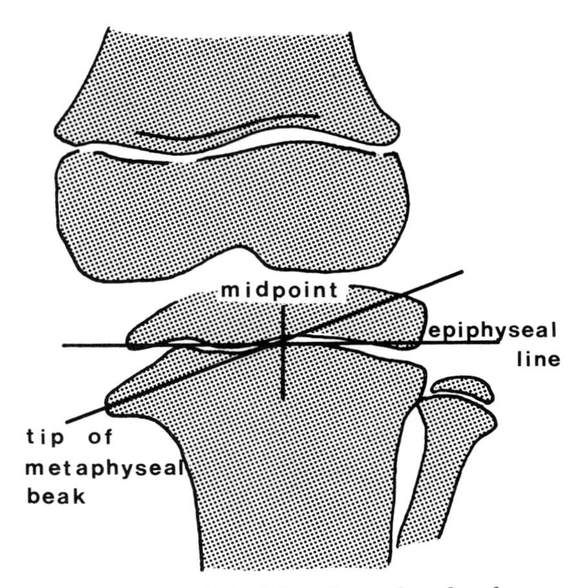

FIGURE 7–253. Epiphyseal-metaphyseal angle.

lateral rotation of the leg. The knee joint may be unlocked; however, if the lateral thrust at the knee during gait cannot be checkreined, the knee joint should be locked. In the very fat or stocky child, stability and control of the thigh may be difficult to provide with a KAFO; in such instances a hip-knee-ankle-foot orthosis (HKAFO) with a pelvic band is utilized. With such extensive bracing, however, the child has difficulty in walking; it is usually not tolerated. A HKAFO is converted to KAFO as soon as possible.

The orthosis is worn until the varus deformity is corrected, with satisfactory clinical alignment of the lower limbs and radiographic resolution of the disease.

Operative Treatment

If the deformity does not improve with orthotic treatment and radiographically the disease progresses to advanced Stage II or Stage III (Langenskiöld), surgical correction of tibia vara should be performed. The pitfall is procrastination.

Surgery is recommended primarily when a child four years or older is seen initially with advanced Stage II or Stage III deformity, with a tibiofemoral angle greater than 15 degrees, metaphyseal-diaphyseal angle of 14 degrees or greater, and epiphyseal-metaphyseal angle of 30 degrees or more. Orthotic management is unsuccessful at this stage of tibia vara deformity. Absolute definite indications for surgery are depression of the tibial plateau, impending closure of the medial physis of the upper tibia (Stage IV), and ligamentous laxity of the knee.

The critical age for a satisfactory result by surgical correction of the deformity by simple osteotomy is eight years. In patients operated after the age of eight years there is considerable recurrence of deformity and the prognosis is guarded.[45, 46, 49, 50] The importance of early surgery for prevention of arthritis due to joint incongruity and instability in adult life cannot be overemphasized. The operative technique, illustrated in Figure 7–254, is as follows: First, an oblique osteotomy of the fibula is performed through a separate 3-to 4-cm. lateral incision at the juncture of its proximal and distal thirds. Avoid injury to the peroneal nerve. Then, through an anterolateral incision, the proximal metaphysis and upper portion of the tibial diaphysis are subperiosteally exposed. It is crucial to stay in a subperiosteal plane to avoid vascular injury. The level of osteotomy is below the insertion of the patellar tendon. Do not damage the proximal tibial physis and the anterior apophyseal extension of the proximal tibial tuberosity. If in doubt, it is best to confirm the level of osteotomy by radiograms. Next, a threaded Steinmann pin of appropriate diameter is inserted through the midshaft of the tibia, parallel to the ankle joint, and another threaded Steinmann pin through the proximal tibial metaphysis parallel to the knee joint. With a "starter" and drill holes, the line of a cuneiform osteotomy is outlined; the medial limb of the buttress is in the proximal fragment to assure locking of the fragments (Fig. 7–254 B). The osteotomy is completed with sharp chisels. The distal fragment is angulated laterally and rotated outward, correcting both the varus and the medial rotation deformity. With medial sliding of the upper end of the shaft in the concave surface of the metaphyseal fragment, stable contact of the osteotomized fragments is obtained. It is important to obtain mild valgus angulation of 5 to 10 degrees. Do not place the tibia in marked valgus.[12, 13, 49] Next, the osteotomized tibial fragments are transfixed with crisscross threaded Steinmann pins (Fig. 7–254 C), and anteroposterior and lateral radiograms are made with the knee in full extension (including the knee and ankle) in order to document the degree of correction into physiologic valgus. Obtain long films to assess alignment: In unilateral tibia vara, the two limbs should be carefully compared to see that they are symmetrical. In bilateral involvement, each knee and tibia should be placed in physiologic

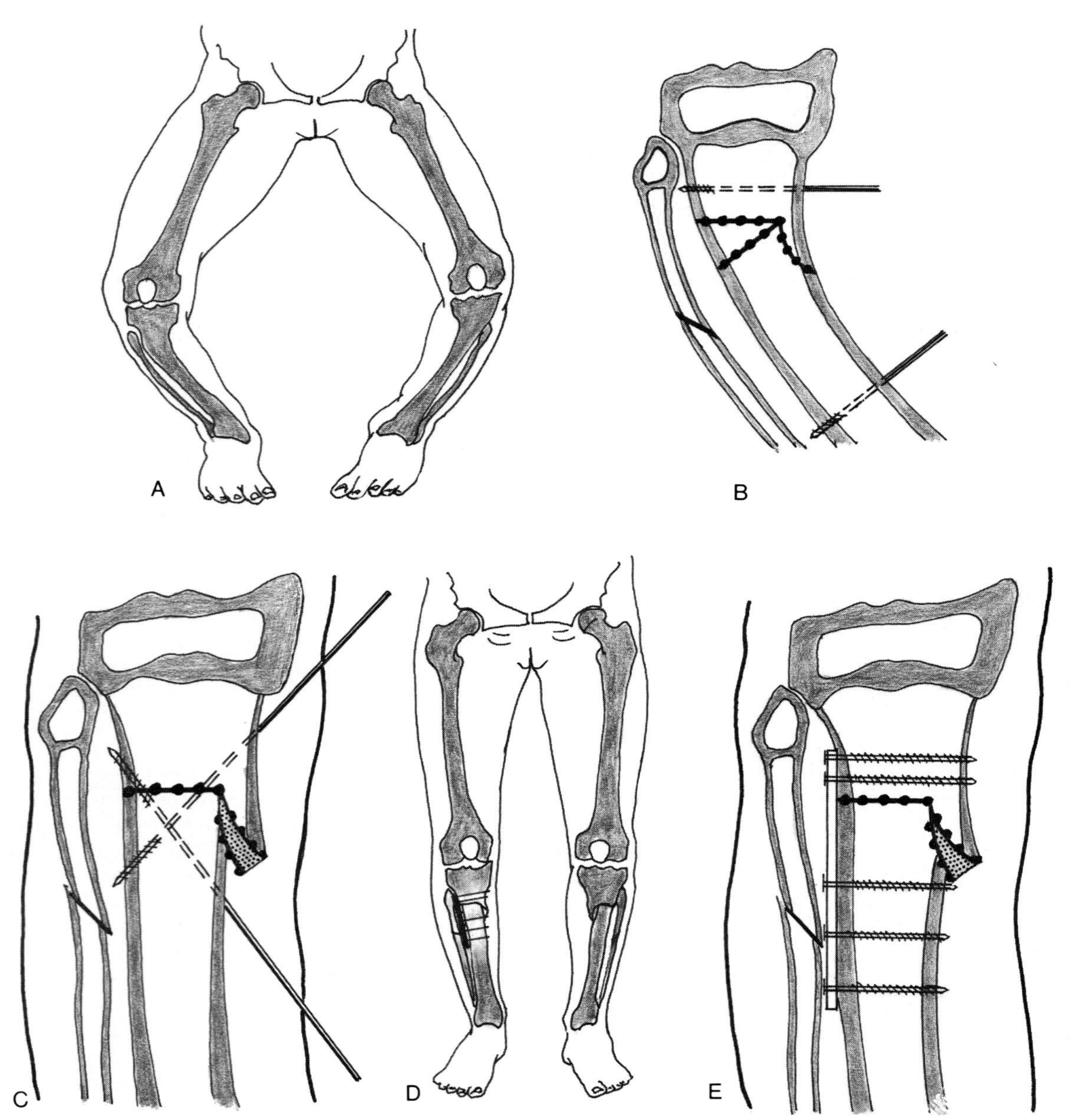

FIGURE 7–254. Operative technique of correction of bilateral tibia vara.

genu valgum. It is important to provide symmetry to the limbs.

This author recommends internal fixation with an AO five-hole compression plate that is placed laterally (Fig. 7–254 D). Some surgeons may prefer to place the plate medially because of the simplicity of its application; this author has found subcutaneous position of the plate bothersome to some patients. Prior to internal fixation the tourniquet should be released and circulatory status of the limb carefully ascertained; entrapment of the anterior tibial artery where it passes through the interosseous membrane is ruled out.[81] If there is circulatory compromise, the limb should be immediately replaced in the uncorrected position. Peroneal nerve injury is ordinarily not a problem following proximal tibial osteotomy to correct varus.

If the circulation of the limb is normal, the tibial fragments are fixed with the AO compression plate. The excised wedge is used as bone graft to fill in the defect created medially.

Next, an anterior fasciotomy is performed in order to prevent compartment syndrome. After complete hemostasis a Hemovac drain is inserted, and the wound is closed in routine manner. An above-knee cast is applied, incorporating the foot-ankle in neutral position and the knee flexed 30 to 45 degrees. The region of the fibular head-neck should be well padded to relieve pressure on the common peroneal nerve.

In the postoperative period the neurovascular status is carefully observed for compromise: This is a definite potential hazard.

Ordinarily, the osteotomy will heal in eight weeks. Five to six weeks postoperatively, if there is enough callus to prevent change or loss of position, the cast is removed and an above-knee cast is applied with the knee in full extension and the ankle-foot free, allowing partial to gradual full weight-bearing.

Some surgeons prefer internal fixation with crisscross threaded Steinmann pins. They find this method of fixation adequate; however, it is important that the knee in the cast be in full extension to immobilize the proximal fragment. The percutaneous Steinmann pins are removed four weeks after radiograms disclose enough callus to prevent change or loss of position. Another above-knee cast is applied for an additional three to four weeks, at which time usually the osteotomy will have healed.

This author uses internal fixation with AO plate and screws because it is more secure and loss of position due to inadequacy of fixation and pin breakage does not occur. The plate and screws are removed six to nine months after surgery. After plate and screw removal the limb is protected by an above-knee walking cast. These are the principal drawbacks of internal fixation with plate-screws.

In unilateral tibia vara, 1 to 2 cm. of shortening of the tibia is the usual finding. A cuneiform or dome-shaped osteotomy preserves length, whereas a closing-wedge osteotomy shortens the tibia further. When the limb shortening is significant, an open-wedge osteotomy with full-thickness iliac bone graft may be performed. This will correct the deformity and elongate the leg.[27] It is important to fix open-up osteotomies with a rigid plate until the bone graft is completely reconstituted.

An alternative method of management of unilateral tibia vara with significant limb length disparity is the use of the Orthofix (DeBastiani) or Ilizarov apparatus.[24, 71] In the DeBastiani callotasis technique, two or three screws are inserted proximally on the medial side of the proximal tibial metaphysis and upper shaft parallel to the knee joint, and two screws are placed distally in the diaphysis parallel to the ankle joint. After corticotomy the articulated Orthofix lengthener is utilized. Further details of operative technique and postoperative care of lengthening are described in the section on limb lengthening. The Ilizarov axial fixator is an alternative method of correcting axial deviation and elongating the limb. The Ilizarov fixator is technically more difficult to apply, but effectively corrects both varus and medial torsion deformity as it elongates the tibia. Lengthening of the tibia is fraught with problems and complications; the disability and rehabilitation periods are prolonged. Tibial lengthening should be considered only when shortening is 4 cm. or greater. It is simpler to arrest the growth of the contralateral tibia to equalize limb lengths.

Asymmetrical physeal distraction (hemichondrodiatasis) either by the DeBastiani or by the Ilizarov technique should not be tried in children.[24, 32] It is indicated in the adolescent with tibia vara who is near skeletal maturity.

Varus deformity can recur after valgization osteotomy. Factors in recurrence of deformity are age of the patient, stage in the course of the disease, and health of the proximal tibial physis. In general, the older the patient and the more advanced the stage of the disease, the more likely that the varus deformity will recur after corrective osteotomy. Langenskiöld states that the critical age is eight years, before which time, as a rule, a single osteotomy with complete correction of deformity prevents progression and recurrence.[49] In the retrospective study of Schoenecker et al., the critical age was five years; one osteotomy achieved complete and permanent correction of the deformity in 83 per cent of the children when it was performed before five years of age.[68] In children between five and eight years of age, the stage of the disease is important in prognosis. When the radiographic stage is II or III (Langenskiöld), one osteotomy will provide permanent correction in a high percentage of cases, although this author has seen occasional recurrence of deformity. The family should be informed of such a possibility before surgery. When the radiographic stage is IV, there is a greater chance for recurrence.

Children between five and nine years of age can present with Stage V or VI radiographic changes. In such a instance, SPEC imaging with technetium-99m and computed axial and linear tomography studies are performed to determine the status of the proximal tibial physis. If the medial physis is fused prematurely and the lateral physis is open with potential for further growth, this author recommends resection of the medial physeal bone bridge, interposition of autogenous fat as spacer to prevent bone reformation, and concomitant valgization osteotomy of the proximal tibia and fibula. The results of such a method of treatment are satisfactory.[9, 68]

When medial physeal growth does not resume after bony bridge resection, lateral epiphysiodesis of the proximal tibia and proximal fibula is performed. Lower limb length disparity is corrected by ipsilateral tibial lengthening or contralateral proximal tibial epiphysiodesis.

ADOLESCENT TYPE

Orthotic devices are ineffective in controlling the varus deformity, which progresses slowly until completion of skeletal growth. Treatment is surgical, the method depending upon the stage of the disease and the skeletal age of the patient. If there is spontaneous bridging and early closure of the medial part of the proximal tibial physis, if the lateral part of the tibial physis is open, and if the patient is near completion of skeletal growth, treatment consists of epiphysiodesis of the lateral side of the tibia and proximal fibula and valgus osteotomy of the proximal tibia and fibula. In a girl with skeletal age of 13 years, and a boy with a bone age of 14.5 years, further growth remaining from the proximal tibia is only 0.5 cm.; in such an instance, physeal bony bridge resection is meaningless. However, if the bone age in a girl is 11 to 12 years, or in a boy is 13 to 14 years, valgus osteotomy of the tibia is combined with bony bridge resection and fat interposition.

Following surgery, lower limb lengths and the status of the opposite proximal tibial-fibular physis should be assessed, because epiphysiodesis may be indicated to equalize limb lengths. When the patient is near skeletal maturity and epiphysiodesis of the longer leg will not achieve limb length equalization, an "open-up" wedge valgus osteotomy of the proximal tibia with a double cortical iliac bone graft will provide leg length. One should ensure that normal valgus alignment of 7 to 10 degrees is provided.

In the younger patient in whom the proximal tibial physis is still open, the level of osteotomy is below the insertion of the patellar tendon to prevent growth injury. In the skeletally mature patient the tibial osteotomy may be carried out through the old physeal "scar"; at the higher level one should be very cautious to avoid intra-articular fracture. Neurovascular compromise is a definite hazard.

In neglected cases, there may be marked ligamentous laxity of the knee with depression of the anterior aspect of the knee, extreme sloping and depression of the anteromedial plateau of the tibia, and hypermobility of the medial meniscus.[77] These pathologic findings are documented by arthrography of the knee.[23] This author also recommends arthroscopy of the knee for further delineation of the intra-articular pathology. In such cases one should perform transepiphyseal osteotomy and elevation of the anteromedial plateau of the medial condyle of the tibia with iliac bone grafting.[45, 49, 50, 67, 76, 82] The procedure will provide joint congruity and ligamentous stability of the knee and prevent degenerative arthritis in adult life.

The operative technique is as follows: A 6 to 7 cm. long incision is made on the anteromedial aspect of the upper tibia, beginning 1 cm. above the joint line immediately medial to the patellar tendon and extending distally and somewhat posteriorly toward the medial cortex of the tibia. Incision is carried through the subcutaneous tissues and deep fascia; avoid injury to the infrapatellar branch of the saphenous nerve. The periosteum is incised. The medial collateral ligament and pes anserinus are elevated subperiosteally and reflected posteriorly, exposing the medial condyle and metaphyseal region of the anteromedial upper tibia. Next, the capsule is incised and the joint cavity is exposed and inspected. With a straight-blade power saw the

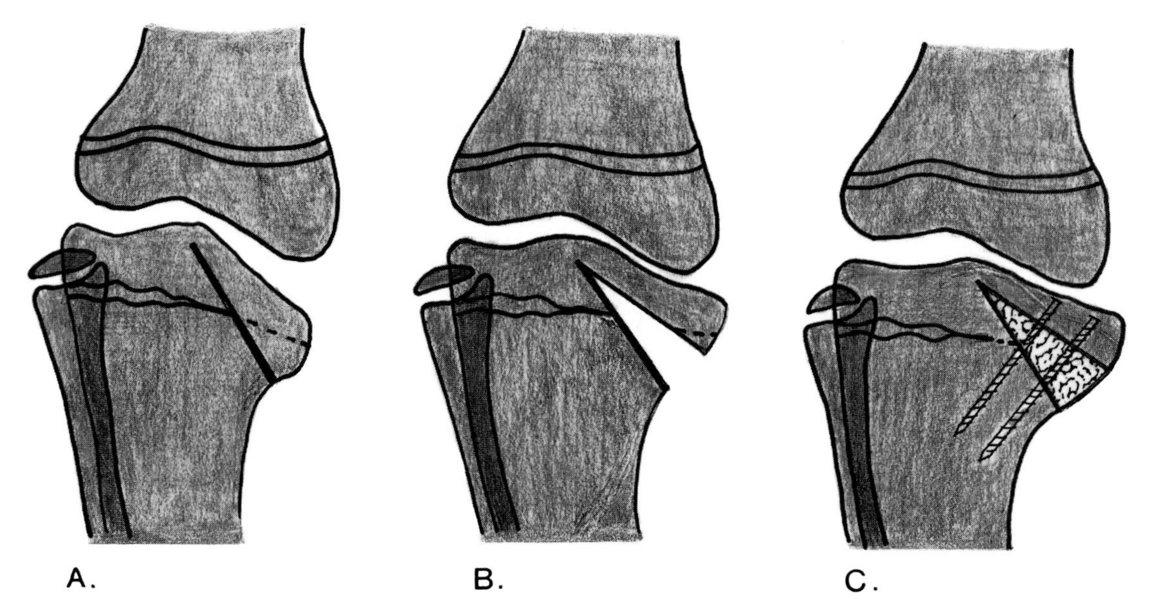

FIGURE 7–255. ***Operative technique for transphyseal osteotomy for elevation of the anteromedial upper tibial plateau.***

A. Line of osteotomy. Note it extends immediately distal to the medial beak of the metaphysis across the closed physis and stops just below the subchondral bony plate of the intercondylar area. **B.** The anteromedial tibial plateau is gently elevated. An intra-articular fracture should be avoided. **C.** Several pieces of triangular double-cortical bone grafts are inserted into the created gap.

anteromedial part of the medial condyle of the tibia is divided under direct vision; the osteotomy line extends from immediately distal to the beak of the metaphysis, across the closed tibial physis, stopping just short of the subarticular bony plate of the intercondylar area (Fig. 7–255 A). Then, with wide osteotomes and periosteal elevators the depressed anteromedial tibial plateau is gently elevated (Fig. 7–255 B). Observe the joint surface and do not cause an intra-articular fracture. Next, three or four triangular wedges of double cortical iliac bone grafts are firmly inserted into the resulting gap. The elevated medial condyle of the tibia is secured in place by internal fixation with two cancellous screws or threaded Steinmann pins (Fig. 7–255 C). Anteroposterior, oblique, and lateral radiograms of the upper tibia, including the knee joint, are made to ascertain adequacy of correction. The medial collateral ligament and pes anserinus are sutured in place; it is vital that the medial collateral ligament be reattached very tautly. If the lateral tibial physis is still open, hemiepiphysiodesis of the lateral tibial physis and epiphysiodesis of the proximal fibula are simultaneously performed. Simultaneous valgus osteotomy of the proximal tibia is not recommended by this author. It is performed before or staged after elevation of the medial tibial plateau. The periosteum and wound are closed. An above-knee cast is applied with the knee in complete extension and the foot-ankle in neutral position. Ordinarily the osteotomy heals in six weeks, at which time the cast is removed and exercises are performed to rehabilitate the knee. If threaded Steinmann pins are used for internal fixation, they are removed four weeks postoperatively, whereas if cancellous screws are used, they are not removed until three to four months postoperatively.

In adolescent tibia vara, another method of correcting varus deformity and elongating the limb simultaneously is hemichondrodiatasis (DeBastiani).[24] This is illustrated in Figure 7–256.

ADULT TIBIA VARA

Blount's disease does not have its onset in adulthood; when it is encountered in the adult it is a sequela of the infantile, juvenile, or adolescent type of tibia vara.

Zayer, in a report of 133 knees in 86 patients with Blount's disease, found that in individuals under 30 years of age there was none with degenerative joint disease, whereas in patients

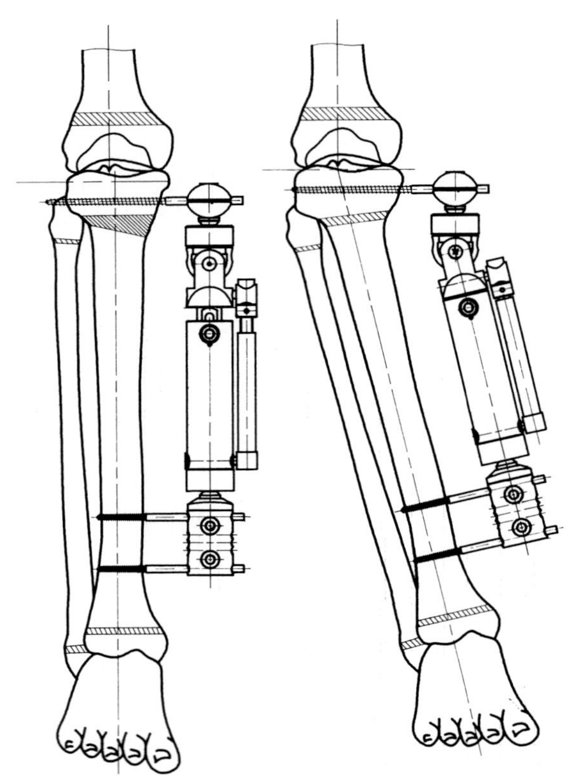

FIGURE 7–256. Hemichondrodiatasis for tibia vara.

A. Note that the epiphyseal screws are parallel to the articular plane and the diaphyseal screws are at right angles to the longitudinal axis of the tibia. The fixator body is parallel to the diaphyseal axis of the tibia. A dynamic axial fixator is fitted with an articulated body for hemichondrodiatasis.

B. Following correction of the tibia vara deformity, note that the normal anatomic axis of the tibia is restored in relation to the knee and ankle joint. (Courtesy of Professor G. DeBastiani and Dr. Franco Lavini.)

over 30 years of age, 41 per cent had radiographic evidence of degenerative changes (11 of 27 knees).[95]

Hoffmann et al. reported a 12-year follow-up of Blount's disease in 12 patients with 19 involved knees. The patients were 17 to 25 years old, the average age being 22 years. The mean follow-up was at 12 years after the initial surgery. Twelve of the 19 knees (63 per cent) were symptomatic, and eight of the symptomatic knees showed early degenerative changes by arthroscopy or arthrotomy. The poor results were due to physeal damage and subsequent joint incongruity.[37]

These long-term follow-up studies emphasize the importance of early surgical correction of tibia vara, prior to permanent damage to the proximal tibial physis and development of joint incongruity and instability.

References

1. Aberle-Horstenegg, W.: Tibia vara. Z. Orthop., *87:*414, 1956.
2. Arkin, A. M., and Katz, J. F.: The effects of pressure on epiphyseal growth. The mechanism of plasticity of growing bone. J. Bone Joint Surg., *38:*1056, 1956.
3. Barber, G. C.: Osteochondrosis deformans tibiae. Am. J. Roentgenol. Radium Ther. Nucl. Med., *42:*498, 1939.
4. Barber, G. C.: Osteochondrosis deformans tibiae. Nonrachitic bow leg in children. Am. J. Dis. Child., *64:*831, 1942.
5. Bardier, M., Senie, J. N., Fabre, J., and Gaubert, J.: Temporary epiphyseal stapling of the lower limbs in children suffering from Blount's disease. An experimental study based on a hundred and sixty cases. Ann. Chir., *36:*396, 1982.
6. Bateson, E. M.: The relationship between Blount's disease and bow legs. Br. J. Radiol., *41:*107, 1968.
7. Bateson, E. M.: Nonrachitic bow leg and knock-knee deformities in young Jamaican children. J. Radiol., *39-B:*92, 1978.
8. Bathfield, C. A., and Beighton, P. H.: Blount disease. A review of etiological factors in 110 patients. Clin. Orthop., *135:*29, 1978.
9. Beck, C. L., Burke, S. W., Roberts, J. M., and Johnston, C. E., II: Physeal bridge resection in infantile Blount's disease. J. Pediatr. Orthop., *7:*161, 1987.
10. Bell, S. N., Campbell, P. E., Cole, W. G., and Menelaus, M. B.: Tibia vara caused by focal fibrocartilaginous dysplasia. J. Bone Joint Surg., *67-B:*780, 1985.
11. Beskin, J. L., Burke, S. W., Johnston, C. E., and Roberts, J. M.: Clinical basis for a mechanical etiology in adolescent Blount's disease. Orthopedics, *9:*365, 1986.
12. Blount, W. P.: Tibia vara. Osteochondrosis deformans tibiae. J. Bone Joint Surg., *19:*1, 1937.
13. Blount, W. P.: Tibia vara, osteochondrosis deformans tibiae. Curr. Pract. Orthop. Surg., *3:*141, 1966.
14. Blount, W. P.: A mature look at epiphyseal stapling. Clin. Orthop., *77:*158, 1971.
15. Bright, R. W.: Surgical correction of partial growth plate closure—a clinical study of 24 consecutive cases. Orthop. Trans., *1:*82, 1977.
16. Butenandt, O.: Growth inhibiting therapy in osteochondrosis tiibae—Blount disease. Fortschr. Med., *99:*1490, 1981.
17. Caffey, J. P.: Pediatric X-ray Diagnosis. 7th Ed. Chicago, Year Book Medical Publishers, 1978, p. 1382.
18. Canale, S. T., Russell, T. A., and Holcomb, R. L.: Percutaneous epiphysiodesis: Experimental study and preliminary clinical results. J. Pediatr. Orthop., *6:*150, 1986.
19. Carter, J. R., Leeson, M. C., Thompson, G. H., Kalamchi, A., Kelly, C. M., and Makley, J. T.: Late-onset tibia vara: A histopathologic analysis. A comparative evaluation with infantile tibia vara and slipped capital femoral epiphysis. J. Pediatr. Orthop., *8:*187, 1988.
20. Catonne, Y., Pacault, C., Azaloux, M., Tire, J., Ridarch, A., and Blanchard, P.: Radiological appearance in Blount's disease. J. Radiol., *61:*171, 1980.
21. Cook, S. E., Lavernia, C. J., Burke, S. W., Skinner, H. B., and Haddad, R. J., Jr.: A biomechanical analysis of the etiology of tibia vara. J. Pediatr. Orthop., *3:*449, 1983.
22. Currarino, G., and Kirks, D. R.: Lateral widening of

epiphyseal plates in knees of children with bowed legs. Am. J. Roentgenol., *129:*309, 1977.
23. Dalinka, M. K., Coren, G., Hensinger, R., and Irani, R. N.: Arthrography in Blount's disease. Radiology, *113:*161, 1974.
24. DeBastiani, G., Aldegheri, R., and Renzi-Brivio, L.: The correction of axial limb deviations during growth by controlled asymmetric distraction of the growth plate (hemichondrodiatasis). Presented at the International Orthopaedic Symposium on Leg Length Inequality. Utrecht, The Netherlands, May 23–25, 1984.
25. DeMoraes, F., and Perricone, G.: Tibia vara (genu varum par osteochondrose tibiale). Acta Orthop. Belg., *25:*285, 1959.
26. Dietz, W. H., Jr., Gross, W. L., and Kirkpatrick, J. A., Jr.: Blount disease (tibia vara): Another skeletal disorder associated with childhood obesity. J. Pediatr., *101:*735, 1982.
27. Dunstan, T. S.: Open wedge osteotomy in the treatment of tibia vara. J. Bone Joint Surg., *54-A:*1332, 1972.
28. Erlacher, P.: Deformerierende Prozesse der epiphysengegend bei Kindern. Arch. Orthop. Unfallchir., *20:*81, 1922.
29. Evensen, A., and Steffensen, J.: Tibia vara (osteochondrosis deformans tibiae). Acta Orthop. Scand., *26:*200, 1957.
30. Foreman, K. A., and Robertson, W. W.: Radiographic measurement of infantile tibia vara. J. Pediatr. Orthop., *5:*452, 1985.
31. Gailey, H. A., Jr.: Osteochondrosis deformans tibiae—Blount's disease. J. Bone Joint Surg., *38-A:*1396, 1956.
32. Ganel, A., Heim, M., and Farine, I.: Asymmetrical epiphyseal distraction in treatment of Blount's disease. Orthop. Rev., *15:*237, 1986.
33. Golding, J. S. R.: Tibia vara. J. Bone Joint Surg., *44-B:*216, 1962.
34. Golding, J. S. R., Bateson, E. M., and McNeil-Smith, G. J. D.: Infantile tibia vara (Blount's disease or osteochondrosis deformans tibiae). *In* Rang, M. (ed.): The Growth Plate and Its Disorders. Edinburgh, Livingston, 1969, p. 10.
35. Golding, J. S. R., and McNeil-Smith, J. D.: Observations on the etiology of tibia vara. J. Bone Joint Surg., *45-B:*320, 1963.
36. Hansson, L. I., and Zayer, M.: Physiologic genu varum. Acta Orthop. Scand., *46:*221, 1975.
37. Hoffmann, A., Jones, R. E., and Herring, J. A.: Blount's disease after skeletal maturity. J. Bone Joint Surg., *64-A:*1004, 1982.
38. Holt, J. F., Latourette, H. B., and Watson, E. H.: Physiological bowing of the legs in young children. J.A.M.A., *154:*390, 1954.
39. Ippolito, E. G., Mickelson, M. R., and Ponseti, I. V.: A histochemical study of slipped capital femoral epiphysis. J. Bone Joint Surg., *63-A:*1109, 1981.
40. Kessel, L.: Annotations on the etiology and treatment of tibia vara. J. Bone Joint Surg., *52-B:*93, 1970.
41. Kettelkamp, D. B., and Chao, E. Y.: A method for quantitative analysis of medial and lateral compression forces on the knee during standing. Clin. Orthop., *83:*202, 1972.
42. Klasen, R. A., and Peterson, H. A.: Resection of epiphyseal bars. Orthop. Trans., *6:*134, 1982.
43. Kling, T. F., Jr.: Angular deformities of the lower limbs in children. Orthop. Clin. North Am., *18:*513, 1987.
44. Kling, T. F., and Hensinger, R. N.: Angular and torsional deformities of the lower limbs in children. Clin. Orthop., *176:*136, 1983.
45. Langenskiöld, A.: Tibia vara. Osteochondrosis deformans tibiae. A survey of 23 cases. Acta Chir. Scand., *103:*1, 1952.
46. Langenskiöld, A.: Tibia vara. Acta Chir. Scand., *103:*9, 1952.
47. Langenskiöld, A.: Aspects of the pathology of tibia vara. Ann. Chir. Gynaecol. Fenn., *44:*58, 1955.
48. Langenskiöld, A.: An operation for partial closure of an epiphyseal plate in children, and its experimental basis. J. Bone Joint Surg., *57-B:*325, 1975.
49. Langenskiöld, A.: Tibia vara: osteochondrosis deformans tibiae. Blount's disease. Clin. Orthop., *158:*77, 1981.
50. Langenskiöld, A., and Riska, E. B.: Tibia vara (osteochondrosis deformans tibiae). J. Bone Joint Surg., *46-A:*1405, 1964.
51. Leonard, D. W., and Cohen, L.: Nonrachitic bowlegs in childhood. Osteochondrosis deformans tibiae. J. Pediatr., *29:*477, 1946.
52. Levine, A. M., and Drennan, J. C.: Physiologic bowlegs and tibia vara. J. Bone Joint Surg., *64-A:*1158, 1982.
53. Lichtblau, P., and Wasman, B.: Blount's disease: Review of the literature and description of a new surgical procedure. Contemp. Orthop., *3:*524, 1981.
54. Lovejoy, J. F., Jr., and Lovell, W. W.: Adolescent tibia vara associated with slipped capital femoral epiphysis. Report of two cases. J. Bone Joint Surg., *52-A:*361, 1970.
55. Michail, J., Theodoroy, S., and Chouliaras, K.: Remarques sur l'osteochondrose deformante du tibia ou maladie d'Erlacher-Blount (tibia vara). Contribution à son étude avec 9 nouveaux cas. Acta Orthop. Belg., *25:*695, 1959.
56. Mitchell, E., Chung, S., Dao, M., and Gregg, J.: A new radiographic grading system for Blount's disease. Evaluating the epiphyseal-metaphyseal angle. Orthop. Rev., *9:*27, 1980.
57. Monticelli, G.: A new method of treating the advanced stages of tibia vara (Blount's disease). Ital. J. Orthop. Traumatol., *10:*295, 1984.
58. Mycoskie, P. J.: Complications of osteotomies about the knee in children. Orthopedics, *4:*1005, 1981.
59. O'Neill, D. A., and MacEwen, G. D.: Early roentgenographic evaluation of bowlegged children. J. Pediatr. Orthop., *2:*547, 1982.
60. Oni, O. O.: Blount's disease (Letter). Clin. Orthop., *172:*309, 1983.
61. Oyemade, G. A.: Nonrachitic deformities of the knees in Nigerian children. J. Trop. Med. Hyg., *80:*213, 1977.
62. Oyemade, G. A.: Advanced tibia vara (Blount disease) in adolescent Nigerians. J. Natl. Med. Assoc., *73:*339, 1981.
63. Pitzen, P., and Marquardt, W. O.: Beinbildung durch umschriebene epiphysenwachstumsstrotung (tibia vara bildung). Z. Orthop., *69:*174, 1939.
64. Porter, R. W.: The effect of tension across a growing epiphysis. J. Bone Joint Surg., *57-A:*259, 1975.
65. Pritchard, A. E.: Epiphyseal stapling in idiopathic knock-knee. *In* Proc. Br. Orthop. Assoc. J. Bone Joint Surg., *39-B:*581, 1957.
66. Salenius, P., and Vankka, E.: The development of the tibiofemoral angle in children. J. Bone Joint Surg., *57-A:*259, 1975.
67. Sasaki, T., Yagi, T., Monji, J., Yasuda, K., and Kanno, Y.: Transepiphyseal plate osteotomy for severe tibia vara in children: Follow-up study of four cases. J. Pediatr. Orthop., *6:*61, 1986.
68. Schoenecker, P. L., Meade, W. C., Pierron, R. L., Sheridan, J. J., and Capelli, A. M.: Blount's disease: A retrospective review and recommendations for treatment. J. Pediatr. Orthop., *5:*181, 1985.
69. Sevastikoglou, J. A., and Erickson, I.: Familial infantile osteochondrosis deformans tibiae: Idiopathic tibia vara. Acta Orthop. Scand., *38:*81, 1967.

70. Sherman, M.: Physiologic bowing of the legs. South. Med. J., *53*:830, 1960.
71. Shevtsov, V. I., and Maer, V. I.: Ambulatory treatment of children with Erlacher-Blount disease by Ilizarov's transosseous osteosynthesis method. Orthop. Travmatol. Protez., *1*:53, 1980.
72. Shopfner, C. E., and Cramer, R.: Growth remodelling of long bone. Br. J. Radiol., *46*:512, 1973.
73. Sibert, J. R., and Bray, P. T.: Probable dominant inheritance in Blount's disease. Clin. Genet., *11*:394, 1977.
74. Siegling, J. A., and Gillespie, J. B.: Adolescent tibia vara. Radiology, *32*:483, 1939.
75. Siffert, R. S.: Blount's disease—mechanism and management of intra-articular varus deformity. Orthop. Trans., *4*:58, 1980.
76. Siffert, R. S.: Intraepiphyseal osteotomy for progressive tibia vara: Case report and rationale of management. J. Pediatr. Orthop., *2*:81, 1982.
77. Siffert, R. S., and Katz, J. F.: The intra-articular deformity in osteochondrosis deformans tibiae. J. Bone Joint Surg., *52-A*:800, 1970.
78. Simon, L.: Tibia vara "epiphysarea." Paediatr. Danub., *4*:93, 1948.
79. Smith, C. F.: Tibia vara (Blount's disease). J. Bone Joint Surg., *64-A*:630, 1982.
80. Smith, D. N., and Harrison, M. H. M.: The correction of angular deformities of long bones by osteotomy-osteoclasis. J. Bone Joint Surg., *61-B*:410, 1979.
81. Steel, H. H., Sandrow, R. E., and Sullivan, P. D.: Complications of tibial osteotomy in children for genu varum and valgum: Evidence that neurologic changes are due to ischemia. J. Bone Joint Surg., *53-A*:1629, 1971.
82. Storen, H.: Operative elevation of the medial tibial joint surface in Blount's disease. One case observed for 18 years after operation. Acta Orthop. Scand., *40*:788, 1970.
83. Strobino, L. J., French, G. O., and Colonna, P. C.: The effect of increasing tensions on the growing epiphyseal bone. Surg. Gynecol. Obstet., *95*:694, 1952.
84. Takatori, Y., and Iwaya, T.: Orthotic management of severe genu varum and tibia vara. J. Pediatr. Orthop., *4*:633, 1984.
85. Tarr, R. R., Resnick, C. T., Wagner, K. S., and Sarmiento, A,: Changes in tibiotalar joint contact areas following experimentally induced angular deformities. Clin. Orthop., *199*:72, 1985.
86. Thompson, G. H., Carter, J. R., and Smith, C. W.: Late-onset tibia vara: A comparative analysis. J. Pediatr. Orthop., *4*:185, 1984.
87. Tobin, W. J.: Familial osteochondritis dissecans with associated tibia vara. J. Bone Joint Surg., *39-A*:1091, 1957.
88. Van Olm, T. M. J., and Gillespie, R.: Proximal tibial osteotomy for angular knee deformities in children. Orthop. Trans., *7*:443, 1983.
89. Vena, P., and Bisogno, L.: Blount's disease. Chir. Organi Mov., *66*:779, 1980.
90. Wah, L., and von Torklus, D.: Osteochondrosis tibiae—Blount's disease. Fortschr. Med., *99*:1484, 1981.
91. Wellens, F., Dewindt, J. S., and Carias, H. F.: Genua vara, genua valga, medial and lateral Blount's disease. A frequent orthopaedic disorder in the Netherlands Antilles. Acta Orthop. Belg., *46*:130, 1980.
92. Wenger, D. R., Mickelson, M., and Maynard, J. A.: The evolution and histopathology of adolescent tibia vara. J. Pediatr. Orthop., *4*:78, 1984.
93. Yagi, T., Kato, T., Sasaki, T., Susuda, K., and Aoki, Y.: Experience for treatment of Blount's disease. Knee, *7*:56, 1981.
94. Zayer, M.: Natural history of osteochondritis tibiae. Mb. Blount. Lund, Gleerups, 1976.
95. Zayer, M.: Osteoarthritis following Blount's disease. Int. Orthop., *4*:63, 1980.

Limb Length Discrepancy

Discrepancy in limb lengths (anisomelia) is a common orthopedic problem, arising from either shortening or overgrowth of one or more bones in the limb. It may be caused by a multitude of conditions. Any correction of limb length disparity must be performed after thorough analysis and assessment of its etiology, pathophysiology, and clinical consequences. Any change in limb length interferes with the dynamics of the locomotor system and its compensatory mechanisms.

In the past, poliomyelitis was the most common cause of limb length disparity; however, the widespread use of prophylactic vaccination has greatly reduced the incidence of poliomyelitis. In the modern world, marked limb shortening usually is caused either by congenital or developmental abnormalities or by growth arrest of the physis due to trauma or infection. Limb length discrepancy of lesser magnitude may be caused by overriding or malposition of fracture fragments of long bones. Overgrowth of a limb occurs in congenital hemihypertrophy or may be due to hyperemia in vascular malformations such as arteriovenous fistula or aneurysm in a growing child. Inflammatory processes adjacent to the physis (such as in rheumatoid arthritis of the knee or metaphyseal osteomyelitis) will increase the blood supply to the growth plate and stimulate growth. A healing fracture or osteotomy of a long bone may cause overgrowth that is due to hyperemia of the physis. The various causes of limb length disparity are summarized in Table 7–22.

Minor lower limb length inequality due to asymmetry between right and left sides is very common. The etiology of mismatching of sides is unknown. Such minor differences are of no clinical significance and are well compensated for by pelvic tilt. For example, discrepancies of a few millimeters to 2 cm. are observed in about two thirds of U.S. Army recruits.[402] Shortening of the right lower limb is more frequent than of the left.

There is no correlation between lower limb length inequality and disorders of the vertebral column except for a minimal functional scoliosis that is asymptomatic and of no consequence.

Table 7–22. *Causes of Lower Limb Length Inequality*

I. Due to shortening by growth retardation
  A. Congenital anomalies of musculoskeletal system
    1. Proximal focal femoral deficiency
    2. Congenital short femur
    3. Congenital dislocation of the hip
    4. Congenital longitudinal deficiency of the long bones in the lower limb—fibular hemimelia, tibial hemimelia
    5. Congenital hemiatrophy
    6. Other severe congenital malformations of the foot, such as talipes equinovarus
  B. Developmental and tumorous affections of the skeleton
    1. Fibrous dysplasia—Albright's syndrome
    2. Enchondromatosis—Ollier's disease
    3. Multiple hereditary exostosis
    4. Punctate epiphyseal dysplasia
    5. Dysplasia epiphysealis hemimelica (Trevor's disease)
    6. Neurofibromatosis
  C. Infections of bones and joints (produce shortening by destroying the growth plate)
    1. Osteomyelitis—femur or tibia
    2. Tuberculosis of the hip, knee, or ankle
    3. Septic arthritis
  D. Trauma
    1. Injury to physis may cause its premature fusion and shortening
    2. Overlapping and malposition of fracture fragments of the shaft of the femur or tibia will cause shortening
    3. Severe burns
  E. Neuromuscular diseases—asymmetrical paralysis causes shortening
    1. Poliomyelitis
    2. Cerebral palsy
    3. Myelomeningocele
    4. Lesions of brain and spinal cord, such as neoplasms or abscesses
    5. Peripheral nerve injuries such as sciatic, femoral, or peroneal nerve palsy
  F. Others
    1. Slipped capital femoral epiphysis
    2. Legg-Perthes disease
    3. Prolonged immobilization by weight-relieving orthoses
    4. Radiation therapy and arrest of physeal growth

II. Due to lengthening by growth stimulation
  A. Congenital anomalies of musculoskeletal system
    1. Congenital hemihypertrophy
    2. Localized gigantism with or without congenital vascular malformations
  B. Developmental and tumorous affections of skeleton and soft-tissue malformations
    1. Neurofibromatosis
    2. Hemangiomatosis of soft tissues
    3. Arteriovenous fistulae
  C. Infections and inflammatory conditions of bones and joints (by increasing blood supply to the epiphyseal and metaphyseal regions)
    1. Metaphyseal or diaphyseal osteomyelitis
    2. Rheumatoid arthritis
    3. Hemarthrosis due to hemophilia
  D. Trauma
    1. Metaphyseal or diaphyseal fractures may increase blood supply to the physis and stimulate growth
    2. Traumatic arteriovenous aneurysm or fistula
    3. Operations on the diaphysis-metaphysis of the femur or tibia (iatrogenic trauma)
      a. Stripping of the periosteum
      b. Osteosynthesis
      c. Taking of bone graft

Basic features of longitudinal growth of long bones and patterns of skeletal growth are reviewed next.

Longitudinal Growth of Long Bones

A long bone is divided into a middle portion (the shaft) and two end regions. The shaft is divided into the diaphysis and metaphysis; the end regions have an epiphysis and a physis (the cartilaginous growth plate).

Two types of epiphyses, *pressure* and *traction*, are found in the limbs. A *pressure epiphysis* is an articular epiphysis because it is located at the end of a long bone and enters into the formation of a joint. A greater portion of the longitudinal growth of a long bone takes place at the pressure epiphyses. *Traction epiphyses* are nonarticular; they serve as sites of origin or insertion for muscles, such as the lesser trochanter of the femur for the iliopsoas muscle; therefore, they are subject to traction rather than pressure, and their contribution to longitudinal growth of long bones is insignificant.

The major long bones—the femur, tibia, fibula, humerus, radius, and ulna—have an epiphysis and physis at both their proximal and their distal ends. In the short tubular bones (the phalanges, metatarsals, and metacarpals), there is only one epiphysis and one physis; these are located proximally in the phalanges, first metacarpal, and first metatarsal, whereas in the other metacarpal and metatarsal bones they are distal in location.

Long bones grow in length at the cartilaginous area of their extremities. This was shown by Stephen Hales in 1731. He marked the shafts of the limb bones of newly hatched chicks with two holes. Two months later when the chickens were sacrificed, the limb bones had increased considerably in length; however, the distance between the two "marker" holes had not increased.[216]

In 1736, Belchier discovered a new method of marking osseous tissue in pigs by feeding them madder root.[48, 49] Several years later, Duhamel, in his studies of bone growth, demonstrated that only the osseous tissue formed during the time when the animal was fed madder turned red, while that formed before and afterward was of normal color. In addition to confirming the findings of Hales that longitudinal growth of long bones takes place at the extremities, Duhamel proposed that interstitial growth also occurs to a varying extent in the diaphysis. He also demonstrated that transverse growth of the diaphysis occurs by appositional bone formation from the periosteum and not by interstitial growth in the bone tissue.[145–149] The experiments of Hales and Duhamel were repeated by John Hunter, who showed that appositional bone formation is accompanied by resorption of previously formed bony tissue.[244, 245] Flourens found that resorption of bony tissue is not confined to the endosteal aspect of the diaphysis, but also occurs in most parts of bony tissue.[165–167]

In management of lower limb length disparity it is vital to determine past growth and to predict future growth.

Patterns of Skeletal Growth

A knowledge of the fundamental principles and factors that control future bone growth is a prerequisite in the management of limb length inequality. These are reviewed briefly here; the reader is advised to study carefully the cited references, particularly the writings of Green and Anderson.[24–28, 196–201]

RATE OF GROWTH

The rate of growth varies with each age level (Fig. 7–257). Growth during infancy is very rapid, but it progressively decreases during the years of the first decade until the period of the "adolescent growth spurt," when it is again accelerated. The duration of this so-called adolescent growth spurt is one to two years, the age at its occurrence depending primarily upon the sex of the child; in girls, it takes place between 10 and 12 years; in boys, it usually occurs between the ages of 12 and 14. During this rapid growth period in adolescence, the rate of growth of the long bones often doubles;

FIGURE 7–257. Rate of growth at various ages.

A. Pattern of growth in a boy from the age of 1 to 18 years. Note, during the first decade, the decreasing rate of growth of stature and of length of femur, tibia, and trunk. In the second decade, there is a definite short period of accelerated growth—the "adolescent growth spurt." This general pattern of growth is similar in all children. (From Green, W. T., and Anderson, M.: A.A.O.S. Instructional Course Lectures, Vol. 17. St. Louis, Mosby, 1960, p. 200.)

B. Average yearly rates of growth derived from completely longitudinal series. (From Anderson, M., Green, W. T., and Messner, M. B.: Growth and prediction of growth in the lower limbs. J. Bone Joint Surg., *45-A*:5, 1963.)

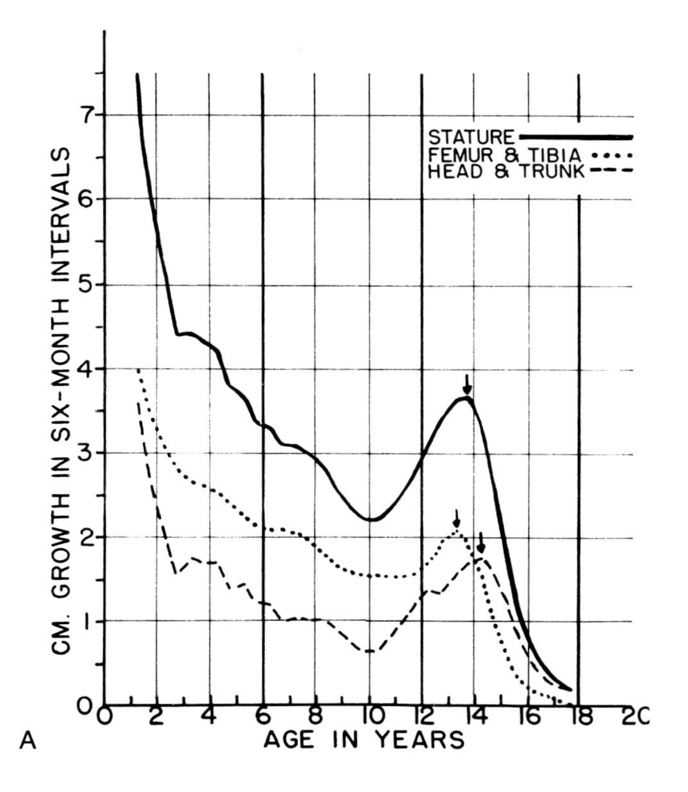

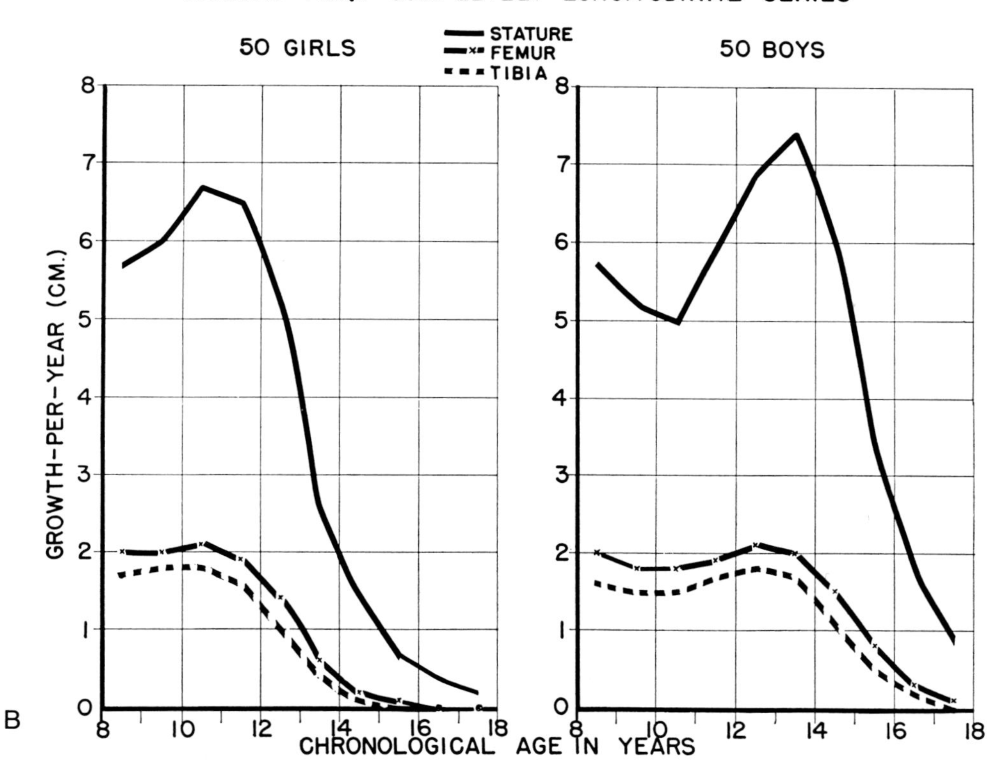

FIGURE 7–257. *See legend on opposite page*

in the ensuing four years or so, the rate of growth tapers off to zero. During all the years preceding the adolescent growth spurt, the lower limbs grow more rapidly than does the trunk, whereas following this spurt, the trunk grows more rapidly than the lower limbs. After cessation of growth in the long bones, the vertebral column continues to grow for about two years.

In the first decade of life, growth rates are similar in boys and girls, but during the adolescent growth spurt there are definite differences between the rates of growth for males and females. In general, girls are two years ahead of boys in the onset of their adolescent growth spurt and in the completion of growth. Significant growth in the lower limbs is usually terminated by the age of 14 years in girls and 16 years in boys.

In a normal lower limb, between the age of four years and maturity, the femur usually increases its total length by 2 cm. per year, while the average rate of growth of the tibia is 1.6 cm. per year.

According to Digby, 65 per cent of the growth of the entire lower limb takes place around the knee (distal femoral physis, 35 per cent; proximal tibial physis, 30 per cent), and 35 per cent of the total growth occurs in the proximal femur (15 per cent) and the distal tibia (20 per cent). These figures are only approximate, since Digby calculated the proportional growths from dry bones and did not consider sex, age, growth spurt, and relative height.[142]

Longitudinal bone growth has been studied by the temporarily arrested growth lines, which are sharply delineated transverse zones of increased radiopacity oriented parallel to the physis toward the end of the diaphysis. The mechanism of formation of growth arrest lines is as follows: In children, during periods of illness or starvation, there is a failure of cartilaginous growth and longitudinal columns of cartilage are not formed; osteoblasts, however, continue to manufacture osseous tissue and the newly formed bone accumulates, depicted as radiopaque transverse striations on the radiogram.[220, 357] Green and Anderson, using growth arrest lines as points of reference, found that between 10 and 15 years of age on the average, 71 per cent of the total femoral increment occurred at its distal epiphysis, whereas 57 per cent of the total tibial growth took place at its proximal epiphysis.[25, 200] The mean percentage of growth of each epiphysis in the lower limb is given in Table 7–23. In general, 1 cm. of growth per year takes place in the distal femur and 0.6 cm. in the proximal tibia.

Table 7–23. *Mean Average of Percentage of Growth of Epiphyses of Major Long Bones in the Lower Limbs*

	Femur		*Tibia*	
	Proximal	*Distal*	*Proximal*	*Distal*
Green-Anderson (1947, 1963)	29	71	57	43
Gill-Abbott (1942)	30	70	60	40
Wilson-Thompson (1939)	30	70	60	40
Digby (1916)	31	69	57	43

RELATIVE SIZE

The relative height and length of the femur and the tibia in relation to skeletal age are important factors in predicting future growth (Tables 7–24 to 7–26; Figs. 7–258 and 7–259). It is obvious that a child destined to be a tall adult has relatively greater yearly increments of growth; and consequently the ultimate lower limb length discrepancy will be greater in a tall child than in a short one.

The height of the parents or of the elder siblings is of some assistance in assessing the future adult size of a child, provided there is no variation in the family pattern.

RELATIVE MATURITY

This is determined by the skeletal age. Todd, and later, Greulich and Pyle have thoroughly standardized the radiographic appearance of the bones in the hands and wrists for boys and girls from birth through 18 years.[203, 441] By comparing radiograms of the wrist and hand of a given child with standard films of the same area, the skeletal age is determined. Assessment of bone age from the knee may be of some help in borderline or difficult cases.[381]

In 1976, Tanner, Waterhouse, et al. published an atlas that assesses skeletal maturity in eight stages. The assumption is made that maturation stages of each bone provide a suitable invariant sequence that is similar in all populations and is unaffected even by starvation. Three scoring systems are proposed: (1) RUS, composed of radius, ulna, and finger bones I, III, and V (13 bones); (2) carpals only (seven bones); and (3) ½ RUS and ½ carpals (20 bones, termed TW2). In skeletal maturity, girls and boys are rated separately. The Tanner-Waterhouse atlas provides the most objective criteria of progressive skeletal maturation in the growing child.[438] It is used in complex cases; ordinarily this author uses the Greulich-Pyle atlas.

Skeletal age is an excellent indicator of maturity; in predictions of future growth, it is

Text continued on page 2864

Table 7–24. *Variation in Size and Relative Maturity at Consecutive Chronological Ages**
(Values for stature, length of femur and tibia, and skeletal age derived from completely longitudinal series of fifty girls and fifty boys)

50 Girls

	***Stature** (cm.)*		***Femur** (cm.)*		***Tibia** (cm.)*		***Skeletal Age** (yr.)*	
***Age** (yr.)*	*Mean*	σ	*Mean*	σ	*Mean*	σ	*Mean*	σ
8	128.1	4.78	33.1	1.63	26.3	1.39	7.6	1.02
9	133.8	4.78	35.0	1.71	28.0	1.50	8.7	1.02
10	139.9	5.24	37.0	1.82	29.8	1.67	9.9	1.03
11	146.6	5.93	39.2	2.00	31.6	1.84	11.1	1.07
12	153.2	6.36	41.1	2.12	33.2	1.95	12.5	1.12
13	158.3	6.14	42.4	2.12	34.2	1.94	13.8	1.06
14	160.8	6.16	43.1	2.15	34.5	1.97	14.8	1.05
15	162.3	6.02	43.2	2.18	34.6	1.98	15.8	1.00
16	162.9	6.10	43.3	2.20	34.6	2.00	16.4	0.92
17	(163.8)	(6.37)	(43.3)	(2.21)	(34.7)	(2.00)	(17.1)	(0.85)
18	(164.9)	(6.10)	(43.3)	(2.21)	(34.7)	(2.00)	(17.8)	(0.46)

Figures in parentheses based on 21–42 girls only, since data were not available on all subjects at these ages.

50 Boys

	***Stature** (cm.)*		***Femur** (cm.)*		***Tibia** (cm.)*		***Skeletal Age** (yr.)*	
***Age** (yr.)*	*Mean*	σ	*Mean*	σ	*Mean*	σ	*Mean*	σ
8	127.6	5.94	(32.8)	(1.53)	(25.9)	(1.55)	(7.8)	(1.00)
9	133.3	6.15	(34.6)	(1.78)	(27.1)	(1.86)	(8.8)	(1.04)
10	138.5	6.58	36.4	1.87	28.6	1.89	9.9	0.96
11	143.5	6.94	38.2	2.07	30.1	2.07	11.0	0.88
12	149.4	7.72	40.2	2.23	31.8	2.27	12.1	0.76
13	156.3	9.13	42.3	2.52	33.6	2.49	13.1	0.80
14	163.7	9.54	44.3	2.58	35.3	2.54	14.1	0.93
15	169.8	8.68	45.8	2.38	36.4	2.34	15.1	1.14
16	173.2	7.74	46.6	2.27	36.9	2.21	16.3	1.20
17	175.0	7.41	46.9	2.30	37.1	2.21	17.3	1.10
18	175.9	7.37	47.0	2.35	37.1	2.22	(18.0)	(0.89)

Figures in parentheses based on 31–49 boys only, since data were not available on all subjects at these ages.

Bone lengths, measured from orthoroentgenograms, include both proximal and distal epiphyses. Skeletal ages read according to Greulich-Pyle Atlas (1950).

*From Anderson M., Green, W. T., and Messner, M. B.: Growth and prediction of growth in the lower extremities. J. Bone Joint Surg., *45-A*:3, 1963.

Table 7–25. *Boys: Lengths of the Long Bones Including Epiphyses:* Orthoroentgenographic Measurements from Longitudinal Series of Sixty-seven Children*

Femur

No.	Age	Mean	σ^d	σ_m	Distribution $+2\sigma_d$	$+1\sigma_d$	$-1\sigma_d$	$-2\sigma_d$
21	1	14.48	0.628	0.077	15.74	15.11	13.85	13.22
57	2	18.15	0.874	0.107	19.90	19.02	17.28	16.40
65	3	21.09	1.031	0.126	23.15	22.12	20.06	19.03
66	4	23.65	1.197	0.146	26.04	24.85	22.45	21.26
66	5	25.92	1.342	0.164	28.60	27.26	24.58	23.24
67	6	28.09	1.506	0.184	31.10	29.60	26.58	25.08
67	7	30.25	1.682	0.205	33.61	31.93	28.57	26.89
67	8	32.28	1.807	0.221	35.89	34.09	30.47	28.67
67	9	34.36	1.933	0.236	38.23	36.29	32.43	30.49
67	10	36.29	2.057	0.251	40.40	38.35	34.23	32.18
67	11	38.16	2.237	0.276	42.63	40.40	35.92	33.69
67	12	40.12	2.447	0.299	45.01	42.57	37.67	35.23
67	13	42.17	2.765	0.338	47.70	44.95	39.40	36.64
67	14	44.18	2.809	0.343	49.80	46.99	41.37	38.56
67	15	45.69	2.512	0.307	50.71	48.20	43.19	40.67
67	16	46.66	2.224	0.274	51.15	48.90	44.42	42.17
67	17	47.07	2.051	0.251	51.17	49.12	45.02	42.97
67	18	47.23	1.958	0.239	51.15	49.19	45.27	43.31

Tibia

No.	Age	Mean	σ_d	σ_m	Distribution $+2\sigma_d$	$+1\sigma_d$	$-1\sigma_d$	$-2\sigma_d$
61	1	11.60	0.620	0.074	12.84	12.22	10.98	10.36
67	2	14.54	0.809	0.099	16.16	15.35	13.73	12.92
67	3	16.79	0.935	0.114	18.66	17.72	15.86	14.92
67	4	18.67	1.091	0.133	20.85	19.76	17.58	16.49
67	5	20.46	1.247	0.152	22.95	21.71	19.21	17.97
67	6	22.12	1.418	0.173	24.96	23.54	20.87	19.46
67	7	23.76	1.632	0.199	27.02	25.39	22.13	20.50
67	8	25.38	1.778	0.217	28.94	27.16	23.60	21.82
67	9	26.99	1.961	0.240	30.91	28.95	25.02	23.06
67	10	28.53	2.113	0.258	32.76	30.64	26.42	24.30
67	11	30.10	2.301	0.281	34.70	32.40	27.80	25.50
67	12	31.75	2.536	0.310	36.82	34.29	29.21	26.68
67	13	33.49	2.833	0.346	39.16	36.32	30.66	27.82
67	14	35.18	2.865	0.350	40.91	38.04	32.32	29.45
67	15	36.38	2.616	0.320	41.61	39.00	33.76	31.15
67	16	37.04	2.412	0.295	41.86	39.45	34.63	32.22
67	17	37.22	2.316	0.283	41.85	39.54	34.90	32.59
67	18	37.29	2.254	0.275	41.80	39.54	35.04	32.78

*From Anderson, M., Messner, M. B., and Green, W. T.: Distribution of lengths of the normal femur and tibia in children from one to eighteen years of age. J. Bone Joint Surg., *46-A*:1198, 1964.

Table 7–26. *Girls: Lengths of the Long Bones Including Epiphyses:** *Orthoroentgenographic Measurements from Longitudinal Series of Sixty-seven Children*

Femur (cm.)

No.	Age (yr.)	Mean	σ_d	σ_m	Distribution $+2\sigma_d$	$+\sigma_d$	$-1\sigma_d$	$-2\sigma_d$
30	1	14.81	0.673	0.082	16.16	15.48	14.14	13.46
52	2	18.23	0.888	0.109	20.01	19.12	17.34	16.45
63	3	21.29	1.100	0.134	23.49	22.39	20.19	19.09
66	4	23.92	1.339	0.164	26.60	25.26	22.58	21.24
66	5	26.32	1.437	0.176	29.19	27.76	24.88	23.45
66	6	28.52	1.616	0.197	31.75	30.14	26.90	25.29
67	7	30.60	1.827	0.223	34.25	32.43	28.77	26.95
67	8	32.72	1.936	0.236	36.59	34.66	30.78	28.85
67	9	34.71	2.117	0.259	38.94	36.83	32.59	30.48
67	10	36.72	2.300	0.281	41.32	39.02	34.43	32.12
67	11	38.81	2.468	0.302	43.75	41.28	36.34	33.87
67	12	40.74	2.507	0.306	45.75	43.25	38.23	35.73
67	13	42.31	2.428	0.310	47.17	44.74	39.88	37.45
67	14	43.14	2.269	0.277	47.68	45.41	40.87	38.60
67	15	43.47	2.197	0.277	47.86	45.67	41.27	39.08
67	16	43.58	2.193	0.268	47.97	45.77	41.39	39.19
67	17	43.60	2.192	0.268	47.98	45.79	41.41	39.22
67	18	43.63	2.195	0.269	48.02	45.82	41.44	39.24

Tibia (cm.)

No.	Age (yr.)	Mean	σ_d	σ_m	Distribution $+2\sigma_d$	$+1\sigma_d$	$-1\sigma_d$	$-2\sigma_d$
61	1	11.57	0.646	0.082	12.86	12.22	10.92	10.28
67	2	14.51	0.739	0.090	15.99	15.25	13.77	13.03
67	3	16.81	0.893	0.109	18.60	17.70	15.92	15.02
67	4	18.86	1.144	0.140	21.15	20.00	17.72	16.57
67	5	20.77	1.300	0.159	23.37	22.07	19.47	18.17
67	6	22.53	1.458	0.178	25.45	23.90	21.07	19.61
67	7	24.22	1.640	0.200	27.50	25.86	22.58	20.94
67	8	25.89	1.786	0.218	29.46	27.68	24.10	22.32
67	9	27.56	1.993	0.243	31.55	29.55	25.57	23.57
67	10	29.28	2.193	0.259	33.67	31.47	27.09	24.89
67	11	31.00	2.384	0.291	35.77	33.38	28.62	26.23
67	12	32.61	2.424	0.296	37.46	35.03	30.19	27.76
67	13	33.83	2.374	0.290	38.58	36.20	31.46	29.08
67	14	34.43	2.228	0.272	38.89	36.66	32.20	29.97
67	15	34.59	2.173	0.265	38.94	36.76	32.42	30.24
67	16	34.63	2.151	0.263	38.93	36.78	32.48	30.33
67	17	34.65	2.158	0.264	38.97	36.81	32.49	30.33
67	18	34.65	2.161	0.264	38.97	36.81	32.49	30.33

*From Anderson, M., Messner, M. B., and Green, W. T.: Distribution of lengths of the normal femur and tibia in children from one to eighteen years of age. J. Bone Joint Surg., *46-A*:1199, 1964.

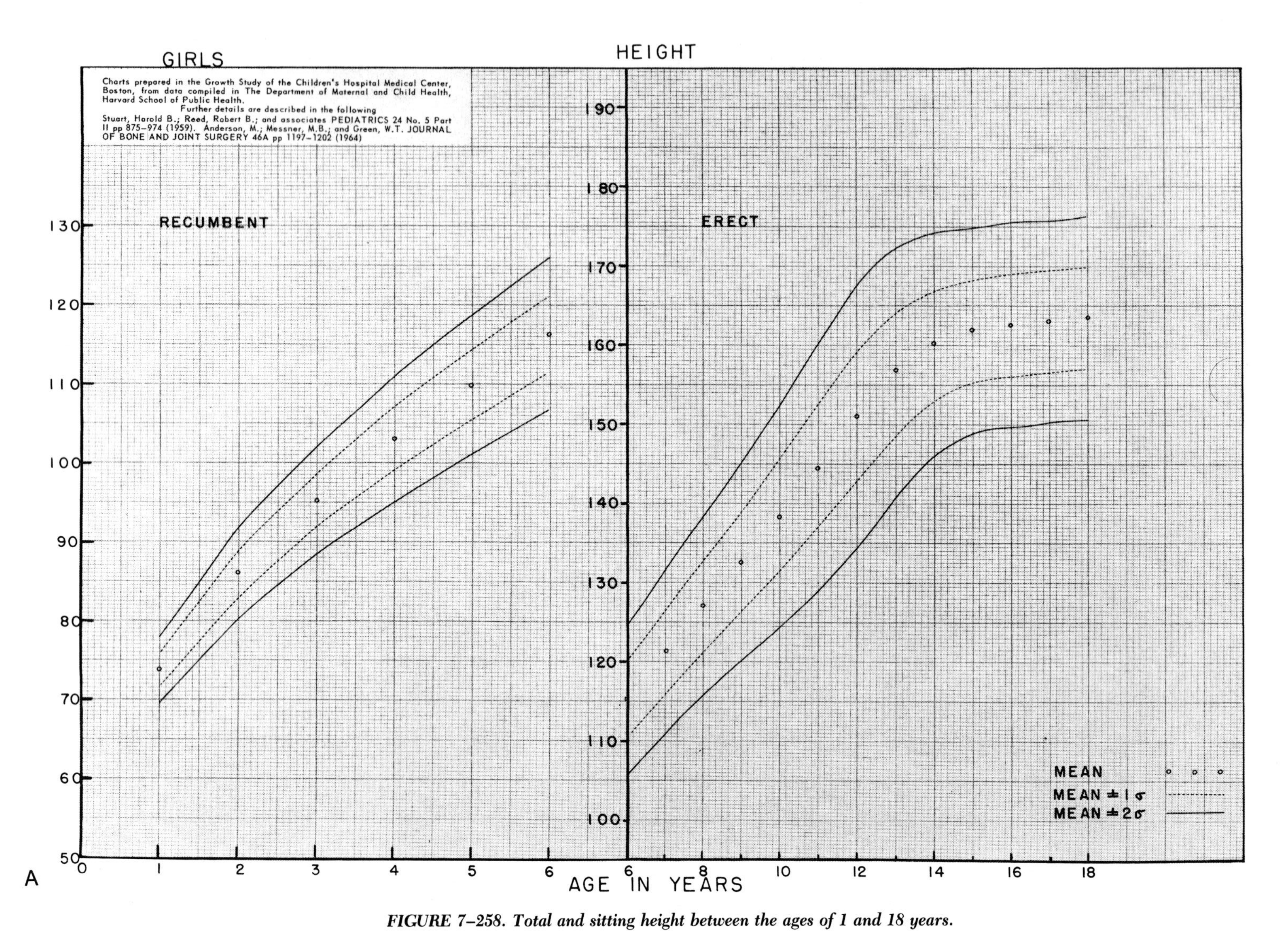

FIGURE 7–258. Total and sitting height between the ages of 1 and 18 years.

A. Total height in girls. (Chart prepared in the Growth Study of the Children's Hospital Medical Center, Boston, from data compiled in The Department of Maternal and Child Health, Harvard School of Public Health, Boston, Massachusetts. Courtesy of R. B. Reed, M. Anderson, et al.)

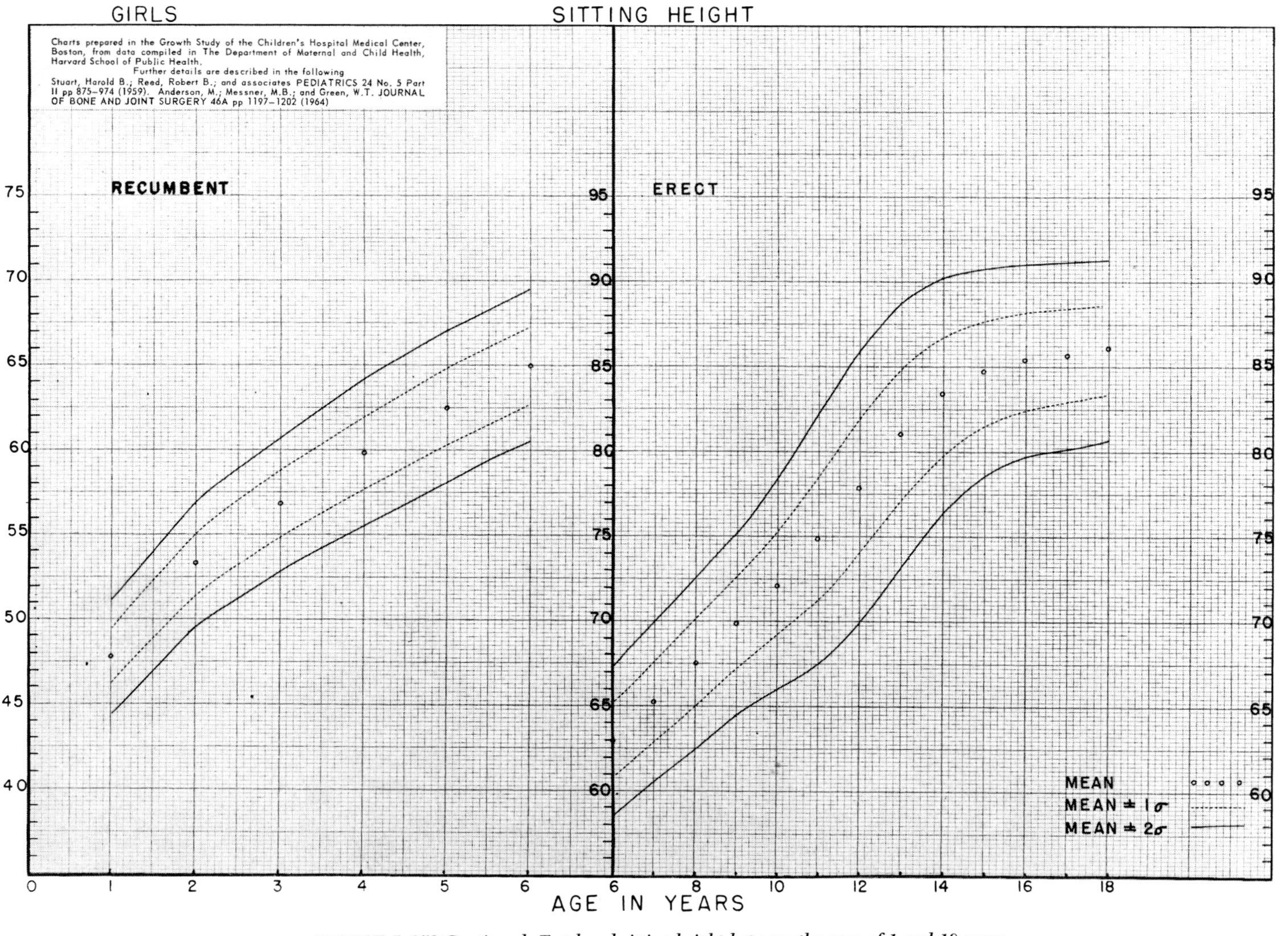

FIGURE 7–258 ***Continued. Total and sitting height between the ages of 1 and 18 years.***

B. Sitting height in girls. (Chart prepared in the Growth Study of the Children's Hospital Medical Center, Boston, from data compiled in The Department of Maternal and Child Health, Harvard School of Public Health, Boston, Massachusetts. Courtesy of R. B. Reed, M. Anderson, et al.)

Illustration continued on following page

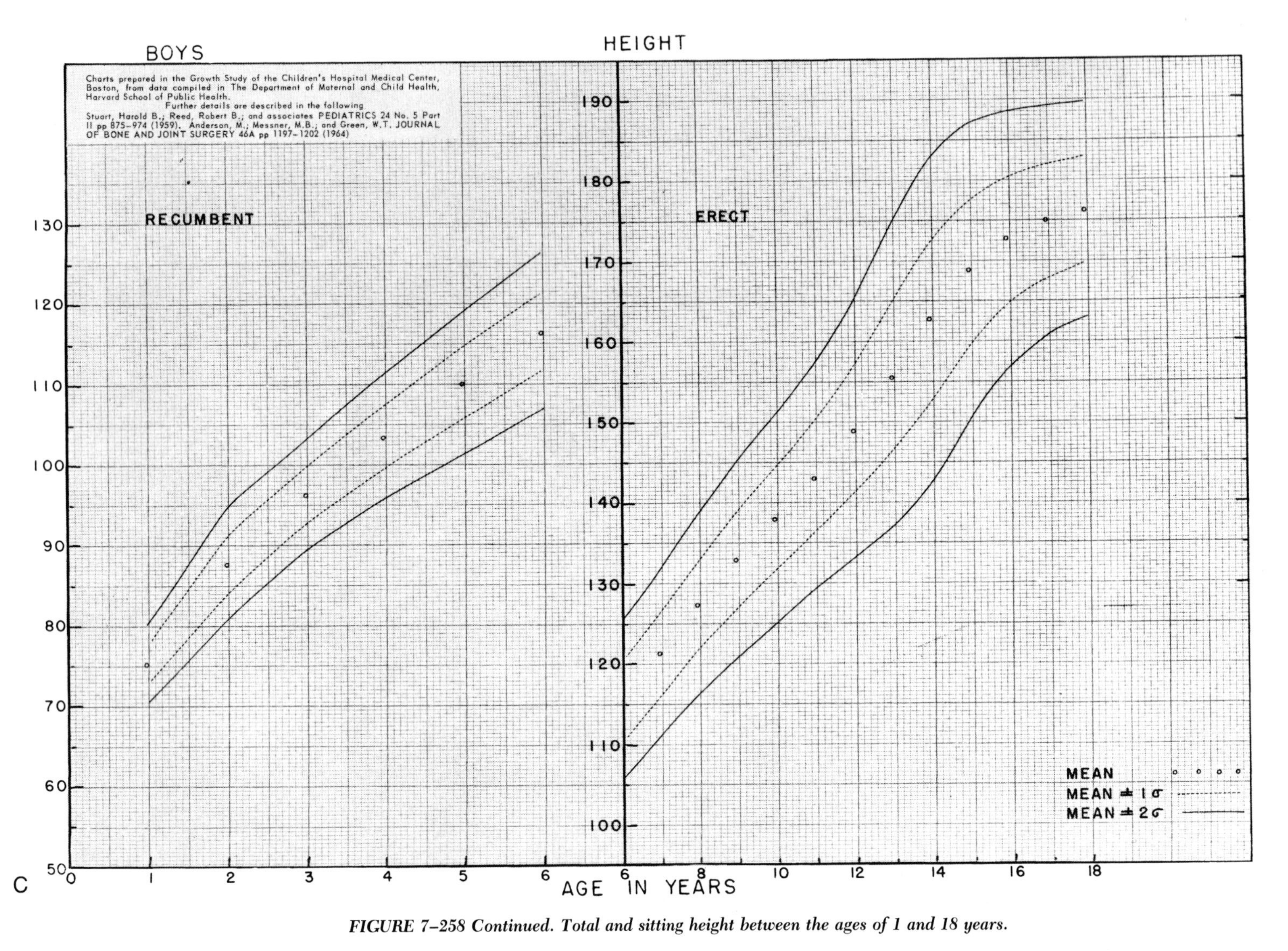

FIGURE 7–258 ***Continued. Total and sitting height between the ages of 1 and 18 years.***

C. Total height in boys. (Chart prepared in the Growth Study of the Children's Hospital Medical Center, Boston, from data compiled in The Department of Maternal and Child Health, Harvard School of Public Health, Boston, Massachusetts. Courtesy of R. B. Reed, M. Anderson, et al.)

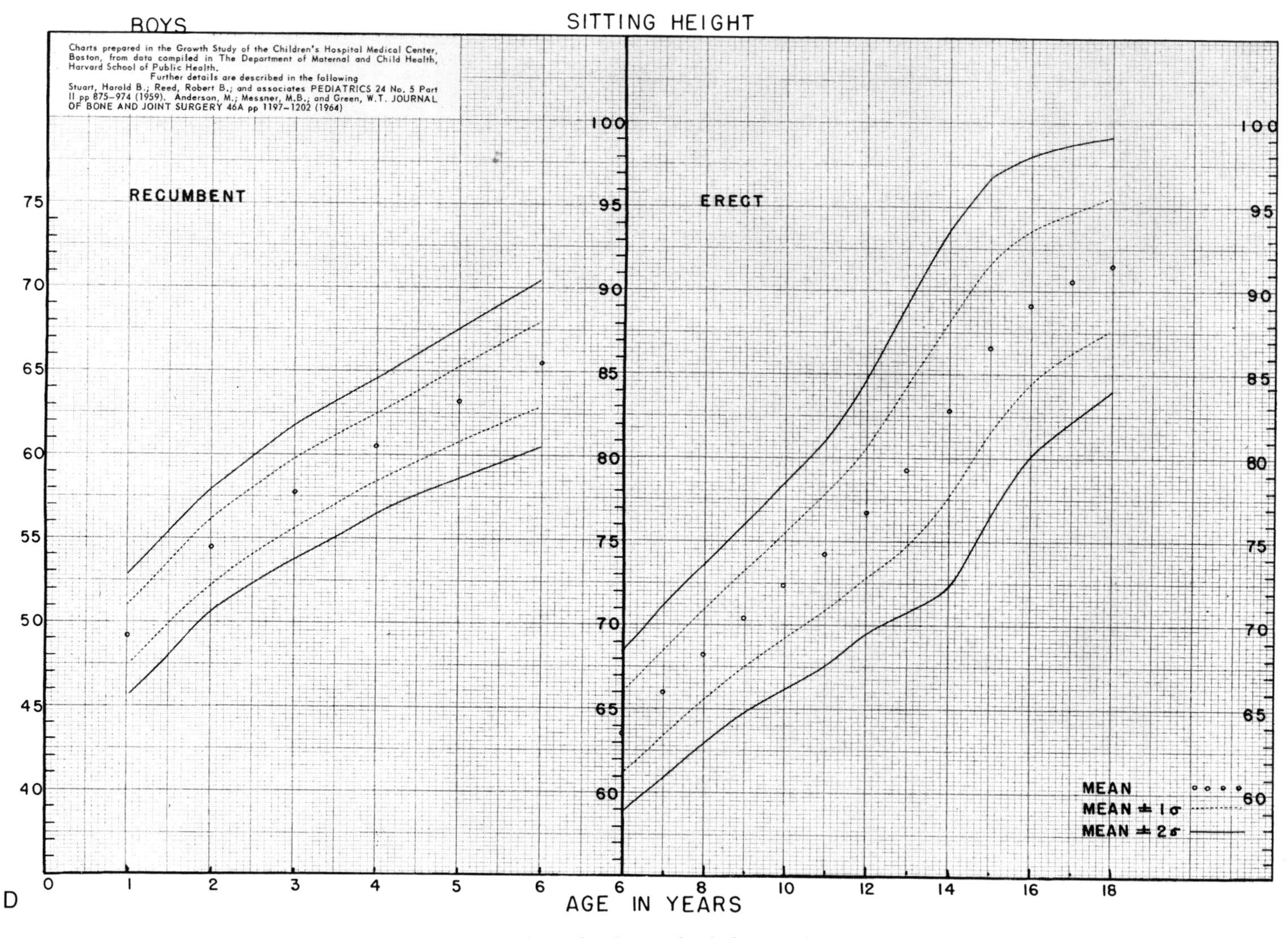

FIGURE 7–258 Continued. Total and sitting height between the ages of 1 and 18 years.

D. Sitting height in boys. (Chart prepared in the Growth Study of the Children's Hospital Medical Center, Boston, from data compiled in The Department of Maternal and Child Health, Harvard School of Public Health, Boston, Massachusetts. Courtesy of R. B. Reed, M. Anderson, et al.)

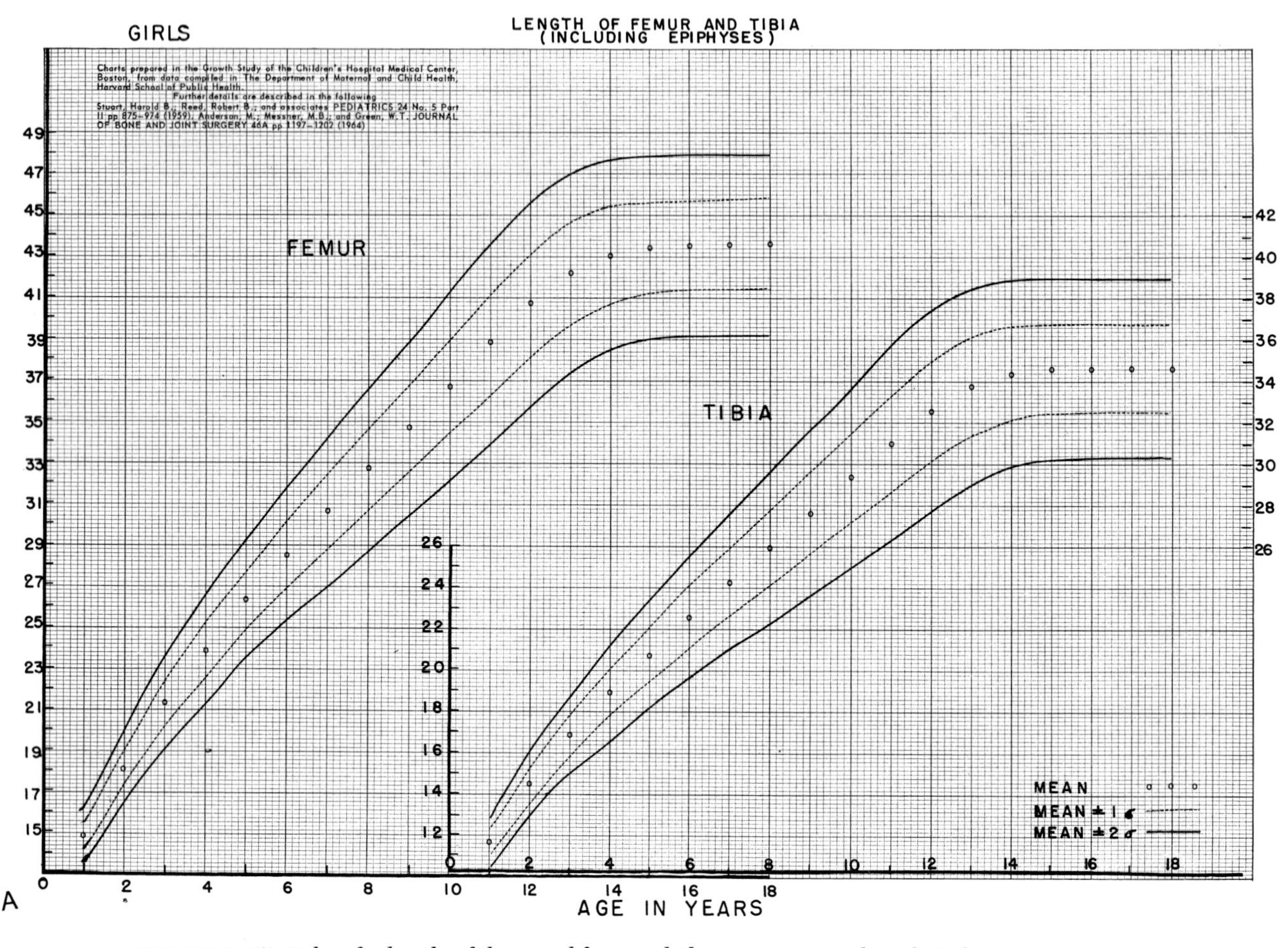

FIGURE 7–259. Values for lengths of the normal femur and tibia at consecutive chronological ages from 1 through 18 years.

A. In girls. (Courtesy of Drs. M. Anderson, M. B. Messner, and W. T. Green.)

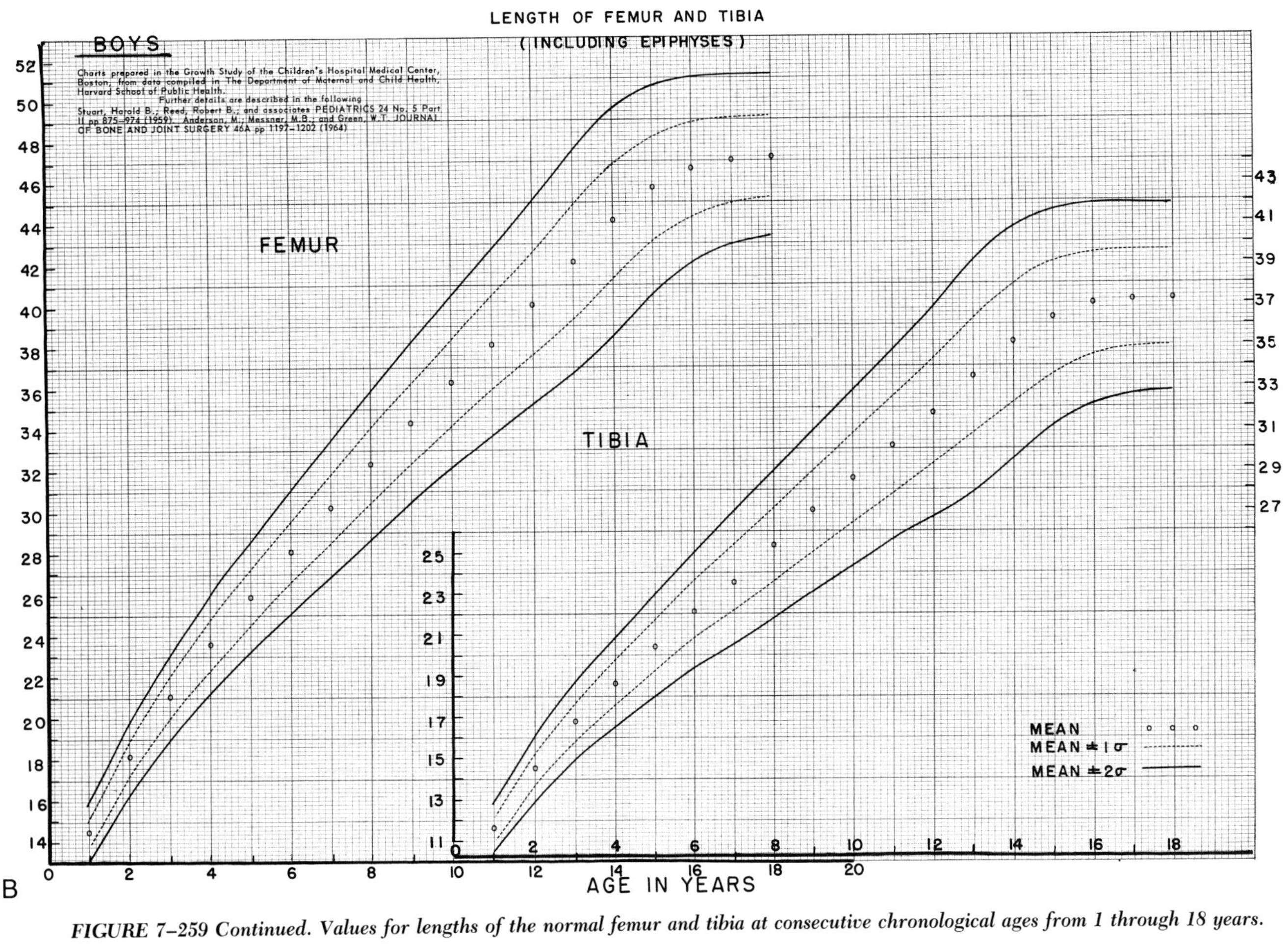

FIGURE 7–259 Continued. Values for lengths of the normal femur and tibia at consecutive chronological ages from 1 through 18 years.

B. In boys. (Courtesy of Drs. M. Anderson, M. B. Messner, and W. T. Green.)

skeletal rather than chronological age that should be considered. Another clue to skeletal maturity is the development of secondary sex characteristics, the appearance of pubic hair, voice change, breast development, and menarche. These outward physical indicators, however, do exhibit great individual variation in the order and significance of their appearance, and are only rough tools at best.

The rate of growth is another factor to consider in assessing maturation; the completion of the adolescent growth spurt indicates greater maturity.

Growth Prediction Chart

Epiphysiodesis for arrest of growth should be carried out at a very carefully selected period in the child's growth if lower limb length disparity is to be corrected with any degree of accuracy. In order to do so, the amount of growth that may occur in a normal distal femur and proximal tibia following specific skeletal ages should be known. In 1947, Green and Anderson presented such a growth prediction chart, which was revised in 1963. The revision was derived from completely "longitudinal" data on 50 boys and 50 girls, each subject being represented at every consecutive skeletal age. The 1950 edition of the Greulich-Pyle atlas was used for the assessment of the maturational levels.[25, 196]

In the new chart at each skeletal age, 8³⁄₁₂ to 15³⁄₁₂ years in girls and 10³⁄₁₂ to 17³⁄₁₂ years in boys, the mean values as well as the range of one and two standard deviations are given (Fig. 7–260). In Table 7–27 are shown the values for five percentile levels, the means, and the standard deviations. For example, the chart shows that the expected correction to be obtained from distal femoral epiphysiodesis in a boy at the skeletal age of 12 years on the mean average will amount to 5 cm. (fiftieth percentile); the broken lines on the chart indicate the range of *one standard deviation* (in 68 per cent of the boys at this age), which gives a correction between 4 and 6 cm.; the solid lines on the chart give the range of *two standard deviations*

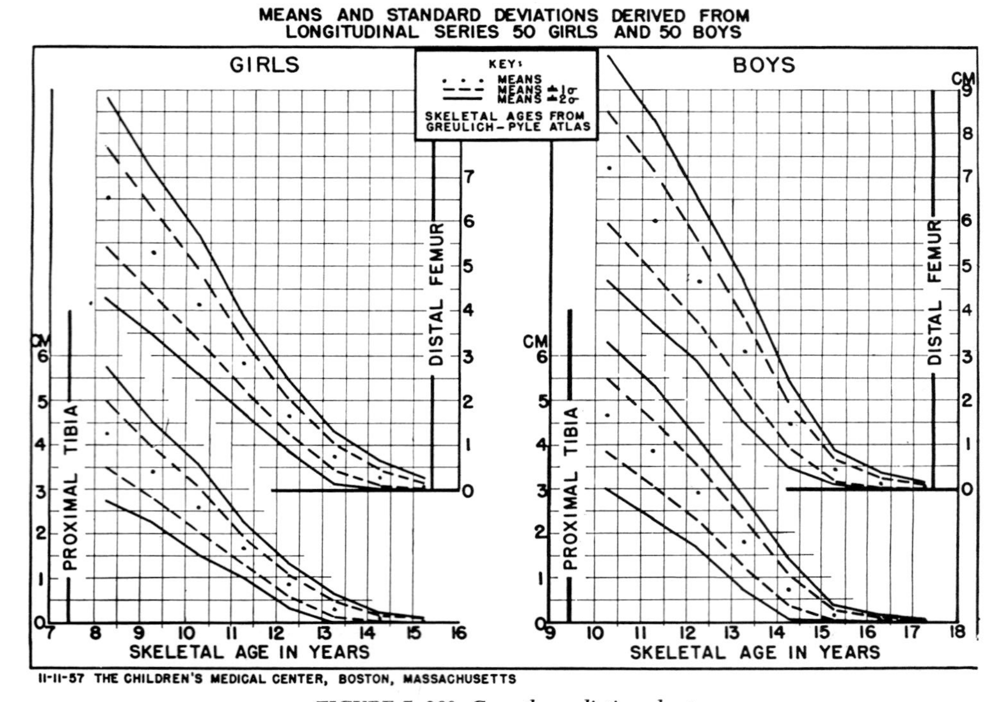

FIGURE 7–260. Growth prediction chart.

The chart is to be used as a guide in estimating the amounts of growth that may be inhibited in the distal end of the normal femur or the proximal end of the normal tibia by epiphyseal arrest at the skeletal ages indicated on the baseline. (From Anderson, M., Green, W. T., and Messner, M. B.: Growth and predictions of growth in the lower extremities. J. Bone Joint Surg., 45-A:10, 1963.)

Table 7–27. *Growth in Distal End of Normal Femur and Proximal End of Normal Tibia Observed in Longitudinal Series Following Given Skeletal Ages*†
(Growth recorded in centimeters; skeletal ages assessed from Greulich-Pyle Atlas)

	50 Girls								***50 Boys***							
	*8^3**	*9^3*	*10^3*	*11^3*	*12^3*	*13^3*	*14^3*	*15^3*	*10^3*	*11^3*	*12^3*	*13^3*	*14^3*	*15^3*	*16^3*	*17^3*
Distal End of the Femur (Total Growth Femur × 71%)																
Mean	6.54	5.30	4.15	2.82	1.66	0.75	0.27	0.05	7.21	6.01	4.65	3.09	1.48	0.45	0.15	0.04
σ	1.14	0.92	0.78	0.53	0.40	0.30	0.18	0.08	1.28	1.14	0.91	0.78	0.50	0.23	0.12	0.06
Extreme	9.8	8.6	7.2	4.7	2.8	1.5	0.7	0.4	9.7	8.4	7.2	5.7	3.0	1.0	0.6	0.2
90th	8.4	6.7	5.0	3.4	2.1	1.1	0.6	0.1	8.9	7.8	5.7	4.2	2.2	0.8	0.3	0.1
Percentiles 75th	7.2	5.8	4.6	3.2	1.9	1.0	0.4	0.1	8.3	6.7	5.2	3.5	1.8	0.6	0.2	0.1
Percentiles 50th	6.5	5.2	4.1	2.8	1.7	0.7	0.3	0.0	7.2	6.1	4.8	2.9	1.4	0.4	0.1	0.0
Percentiles 25th	5.8	4.8	3.7	2.4	1.4	0.6	0.1	0.0	6.3	5.2	4.1	2.6	1.2	0.3	0.1	0.0
Percentiles 10th	5.0	4.3	3.3	2.2	1.1	0.4	0.0	0.0	5.3	4.4	3.4	2.3	1.0	0.2	0.0	0.0
Extreme	4.1	3.1	2.2	1.6	0.7	0.1	0.0	0.0	4.8	3.8	2.8	1.6	0.4	0.1	0.0	0.0
Proximal End of the Tibia (Total Growth Tibia × 57%)																
Mean	4.25	3.39	2.58	1.65	0.86	0.32	0.09	0.02	4.65	3.83	2.92	1.80	0.74	0.16	0.04	0.01
σ	0.74	0.58	0.50	0.32	0.26	0.17	0.06	0.03	0.83	0.75	0.62	0.53	0.35	0.12	0.06	0.02
Extreme	6.0	5.1	4.3	2.8	1.5	0.8	0.3	0.1	6.7	5.6	4.7	3.4	2.2	0.7	0.3	0.1
90th	5.5	4.2	3.2	1.9	1.2	0.6	0.2	0.1	5.8	4.8	3.6	2.5	1.1	0.3	0.1	0.0
Percentiles 75th	4.6	3.7	2.7	1.8	1.0	0.4	0.1	0.1	5.3	4.3	3.3	2.0	0.8	0.2	0.0	0.0
Percentiles 50th	4.1	3.3	2.6	1.6	0.8	0.3	0.0	0.0	4.6	3.8	3.0	1.8	0.7	0.2	0.0	0.0
Percentiles 25th	3.8	3.0	2.3	1.5	0.7	0.2	0.0	0.0	4.0	3.2	2.6	1.4	0.5	0.0	0.0	0.0
Percentiles 10th	3.3	2.8	2.0	1.2	0.6	0.1	0.0	0.0	3.4	2.7	2.0	1.1	0.3	0.0	0.0	0.0
Extreme	2.5	1.9	1.1	0.9	0.3	0.0	0.0	0.0	3.0	2.3	1.6	1.0	0.1	0.0	0.0	0.0

*Figures indicate skeletal ages in years and months. Thus, 8^3 is eight years and three months.

†From Anderson, M., Green, W. T., and Messner, M. B.: Growth and prediction of growth in the lower extremities. J. Bone Joint Surg., *45-A*:3, 1963.

(in 95 per cent) and show an expected correction between 3 and 7 cm.

It should be emphasized that the growth prediction chart is to be considered as a guide rather than as an accurate prediction device.[25, 196] Various factors modify the actual correction of limb length discrepancy following epiphysiodesis. In addition to the effectiveness of the surgery itself and the sex and relative maturity of the individual, the following should be considered:

The Growth of the Long Bones of the Contralateral Short Lower Limb. Correction of limb length discrepancy is provided by the growth of the short limb; if this is not normal, certain adjustments must be made. It is obvious that if limb length inequality is caused by premature fusion of the proximal tibial physis following trauma, it will not be corrected by epiphysiodesis of the proximal tibia on the opposite normal side; all that will accomplish is to halt further shortening. The percentage of growth inhibition should be computed according to the method of Green and Anderson: The change in discrepancy in bone lengths in a given time interval is divided by the growth of the bone on the normal side during the same interval, and the resultant quotient is multiplied by 100, the formula being:

$$\text{Per cent of growth inhibition} = \frac{(\text{Growth normal}) - (\text{Growth involved})}{(\text{Growth normal})}$$

These computations should be based on a period of observation of at least three years' duration or on a measured growth of the unaffected side amounting to 5 cm. or more. The degree of inhibition is graded as follows: *mild,* 0 to 10 per cent; *moderate,* 11 to 20 per cent; *marked,* 21 to 30 per cent; and *severe,* over 31 per cent. Depending upon the rate of inhibition, individual adjustments should be made toward the lower value on the chart in the prediction of correction to be obtained from physeal arrest. For example, in a girl with a skeletal age of 11 years with moderate (11 to 20 per cent) growth inhibition, 2.5 cm. rather than 3 cm. correction is predicted; if the degree of growth inhibition is marked (21 to 30 per cent), 2 cm. correction is predicted; and if it is severe, a maximum correction of only 1.5 cm. will be achieved at skeletal maturity.

Relative Size of the Individual and the Long Bones (Femur and Tibia). This also is an important consideration. It is obvious that a tall child will grow more over a number of years than a short child. The height and the femoral and tibial lengths as related with the standards are given in Tables 7–24 and 7–25 and Figures 7–257 and 7–258. In the growth prediction chart, adjustments are made for the upper value in a tall child and for the lower value in a small child. For example, growth remaining in the distal end of the femur in a boy with a skeletal age of 14 years and 3 months varies according to the length of the femur: 10th percentile is 1.0 cm.; 50th percentile, 1.4 cm.; and 90th percentile, 2.2 cm.

Clinical Factors. Several practical variables must be considered: Foremost is balance of the head, neck, and trunk over the pelvis. Any list of the spine toward the short side and the height of the lift needed under the short limb to correct it are noted. Is there any structural scoliosis? The important consideration is the provision of a balanced trunk and compensated spine in weight-bearing. Provision of equal lower limb lengths is not desirable if it will decompensate the spine.

Is there any abnormality in gait? How disabling is the short leg limp? How coordinated is the child? Does he walk and run well without a lift?

If the patient wears an above-knee orthosis on the short limb, it is preferable that the leg with the orthosis be 1 to 1.5 cm. shorter than the opposite limb, as the patient will clear the leg with the orthosis in the swing-through phase of gait with much more ease and less strain.

Is the leg length discrepancy increasing? What is the predicted total shortening at skeletal maturity? An epiphysiodesis may be indicated to check further shortening only.

What is the predicted eventual total height of the child? This can be determined by the tables provided by Bayley and Pinneau for predicting adult height from skeletal age.[46] In a child destined to be of short stature, if the shortening of the affected limb exceeds 7.5 cm., it is undesirable to cause further reduction of limb length and height by epiphysiodesis. It is better to lengthen the short limb or to provide a prosthesis than to arrest growth on the long side. The total child should be assessed; each case is individually assessed and discussed with the patient and his parents.

The importance of following the disparity in the rates of relative growth of the two lower limbs prior to epiphysiodesis cannot be overemphasized. Any child with asymmetrical growth of lower limbs should be assessed annually in early childhood, then semiannually in the juvenile period, and every three months later when the time approaches for epiphysiodesis. The annual visits should coincide approximately with the child's birth date. An adequate record, preferably in the form of a work sheet, should be kept.

The following data are tabulated: (1) anthropometric measurements of the standing and sitting heights and lower limb lengths (both actual and apparent); (2) true lengths of the tibiae and femora as measured on the orthoroentgenograms or the CT scans; (3) the limb length disparity, total, femoral, and tibial, as measured clinically and radiographically; (4) relative maturity as shown by the skeletal age (determined by radiograms of hands and wrists); radiographic appearance and bone maturity of each ossification center in the femur and tibia; (5) appearance of secondary sex characteristics; (6) lifts needed under the short limb to level the pelvis and to balance the trunk (centering of head, neck, and shoulders over pelvis); and (7) miscellaneous information such as wearing of an above-knee orthosis, or previous and future contemplated surgery on the lower limbs and for spinal deformity. Serial standing photographs of the child (anteroposterior and posteroanterior views) with and without a lift under the short leg are desirable.

Radiographic Methods of Measuring Length of Long Bones

Clinical measurements of lower limb lengths are by nature grossly inaccurate. More thorough determinations of the length of the femora and tibiae by the use of radiographic methods are essential in the treatment of significant limb length discrepancy. Various available methods are reviewed here. Each has its advantages and disadvantages. At present, CT scan is the most accurate method of mensuration of bone length of the femora and tibiae.

Historically, Thoms, in 1929, described a method of roentgenometry of the pelvis in which a constant scale was obtained by superimposing a grid on the x-ray plate when the part is exposed to the rays.[440]

TELEOROENTGENOGRAPHY

In this technique, radiograms are made on one film with a single exposure for the entire lower limbs, or on two films with separate exposures for the femora and the tibiae (Fig. 7–261). The distance of the x-ray tube from the film is 6 feet. This method provides a fairly accurate measurement of the relative length of the two limbs at a single examination. Its disadvantages lie in the magnification produced by the divergent rays. Factors that produce distortion are changes in position of centering of the tube, the length of the bone, and the distance of the bone from the film (as the posterior body structures get thicker, this decreases). Mathematical correction of magnification by triangulation is time-consuming and inaccurate. A radiopaque ruler placed on each side parallel to the bones may improve the accuracy of measurement of teleoroentgenograms. One of its advantages is that the entire length of the femora and tibiae of both lower limbs is visualized on a single film with minimal radiation to the patient, but the technique is not satisfactory for serial mensurations and bone detail is much less than that seen on spot orthoroentgenograms or CT scan.

At present, teleoroentgenography is used only in the infant and young child; the magnification is approximately 15 per cent.

SLIT SCANOGRAPHY

This technique, developed by Millwee in 1937, reduced magnification to a minimum by rapid movement of the x-ray tube from one end of the table to the other.[322] Gill and Abbott, in 1942, described a technique in which teleoroentgenograms were made by the slit method with a tube-to-plate distance of 6 feet; the exact length of bones was determined by this technique, which also gave good bone detail.[85]

ORTHOROENTGENOGRAPHY

Green, Wyatt, and Anderson, in 1946, described the following method: On a single long film, three successive exposures are made, centered exactly over the hips, knees, and ankles. The target-to-film distance is 6 feet, each exposure including about one third of the entire lower limb (Fig. 7–261 B). They had originally used a long cassette tunnel that incorporated two sliding metal shields in order to restrict the area of film irradiated on the three successive exposures.[201] Later they reported using a rectangular beam collimator that permitted the film to be made on the table top without the use of any cassette tunnel or other special equipment (Fig. 7–262). With this latter method, measurements of bone length were strictly comparable with those made with the earlier used tunnel device; also, the patient received less radiation (total radiation, measured in air, varied from 35 mR for a young child to 84 mR for a young adult), and bone detail was greatly improved.[28]

The advantages of orthoroentgenography are

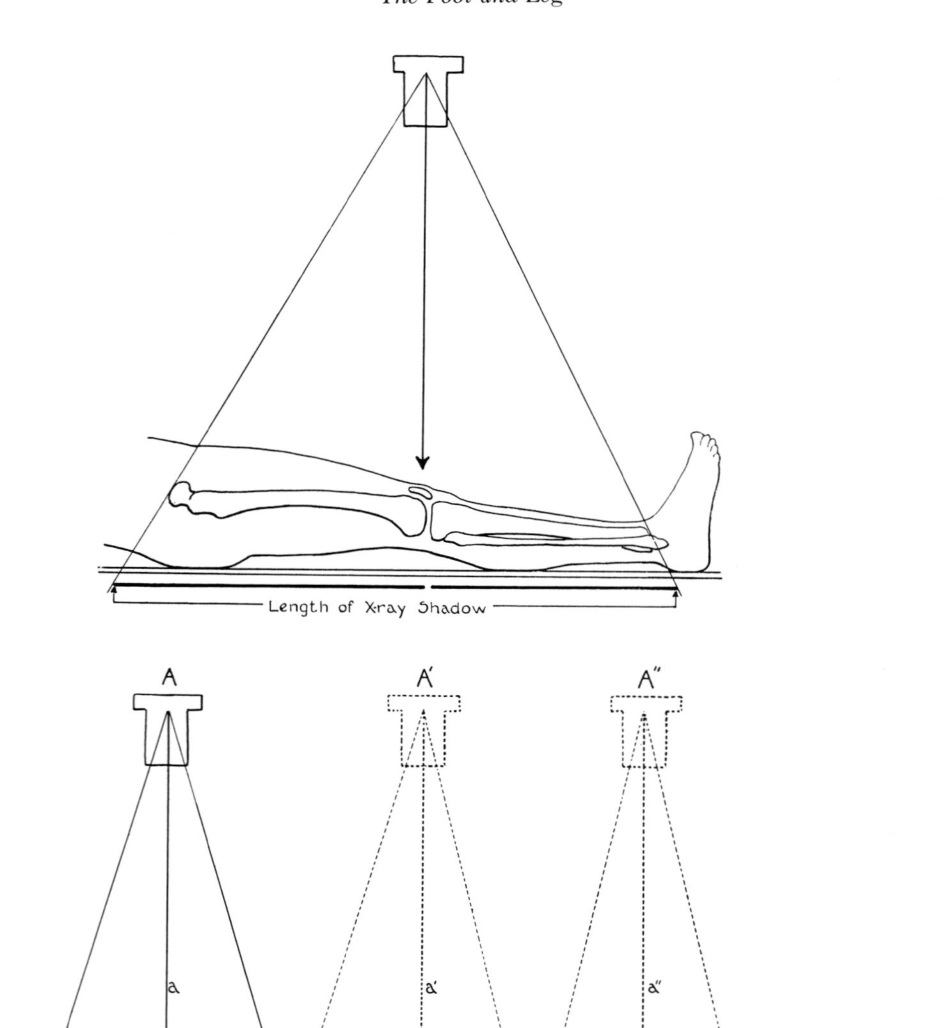

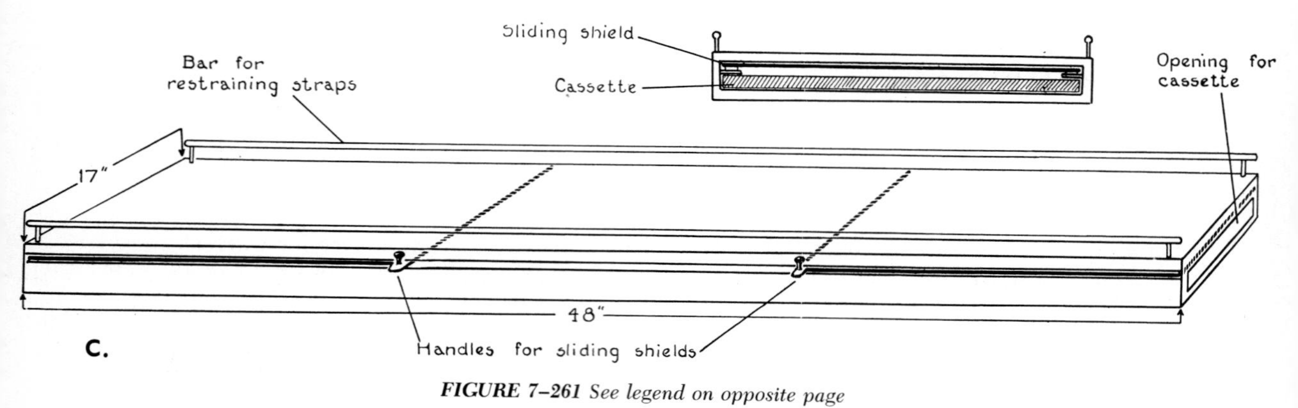

FIGURE 7–261 *See legend on opposite page*

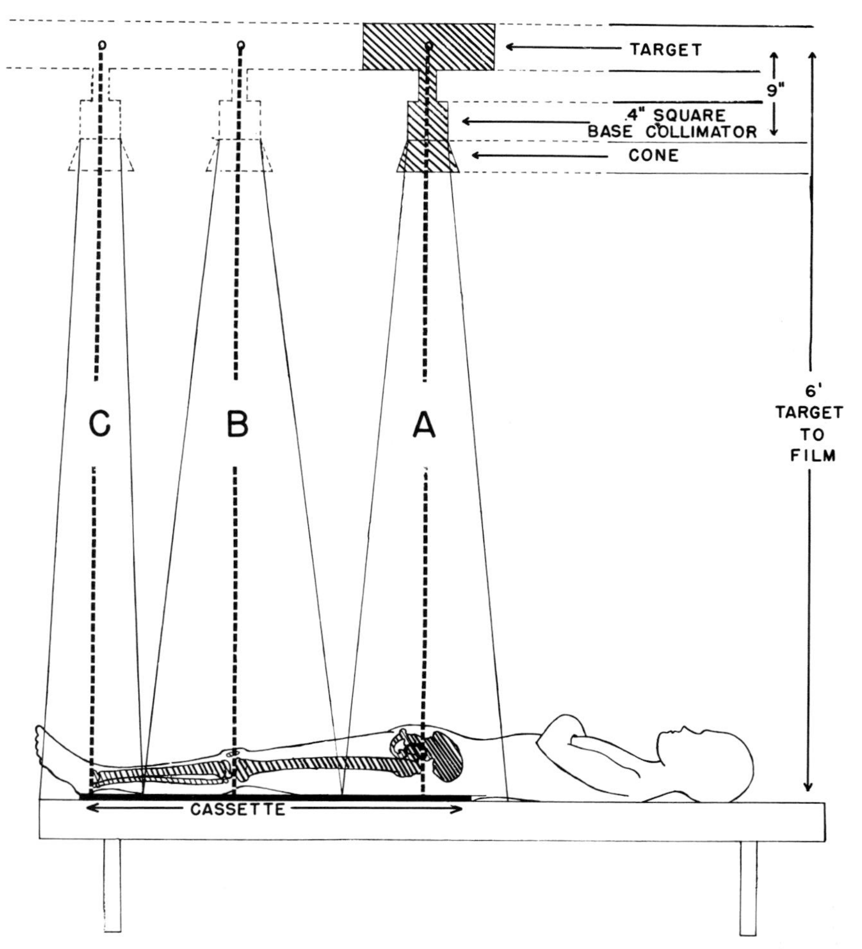

FIGURE 7–262. Diagram of the three consecutive exposures of lower limbs made on a single long film with the rectangular beam collimator.

The tube is focused precisely over the selected joint space so that the central ray passes directly through the end of the long bone. No metal is necessary to shield the parts of the film beyond the area of exposure. The size of each field can be varied according to the length of the child's limb and the desired portion of the shaft to be visualized. (From Anderson, M., Horton, B. G., and Green, W. T.: Orthoroentgenography for accurate long bone measurement. Personal communication, 1971.)

that the true length of each bone can be measured, because magnification due to divergence of rays is eliminated by directing only perpendicular rays at the ends of the long bones. Details of the osseous structure, epiphyseal plates, and contour of the bones are visualized, enabling one to evaluate the factors of the deformity. Overlapping of the shadows at the junction of the shields obscures only the region of the midshafts, where it is of little consequence.

Certain precautions should be taken to en-

FIGURE 7–261. Schematic representation of teleoroentgenogram and orthoradiogram.

A. *Teleoroentgenogram*—radiograms are made on one film with a single exposure for both entire lower limbs (or on two films with separate exposures for the femora and the tibiae). In this one-exposure technique the divergent rays produce magnification.

B. *Orthoradiogram*—on a single long film three successive exposures are made, centered exactly over the hips, knees, and ankles. Note the perpendicular rays intersect the ends of the bones, recording the true length.

C. Diagram of the cassette tunnel. The two sliding metal shields restrict the area of film irradiated on three successive exposures.

(From Green, W. T., Wyatt, G. M., and Anderson, M.: Orthoroentgenography as a method of measuring the bones of the lower extremity. J. Bone Joint Surg., *28*:61, 1946.)

sure the accuracy of orthoroentgenography: (1) The tube should be centered over the articular ends of the long bones and the exact points of focus recorded on each film with a metal marker. (2) The position of the limbs should not change between exposures. Immobilization is secured by tightening the Velcro straps, one over the midthigh and the other over the midcalf. Sandbags are placed on each side of the feet. The technician should gently explain to the patient that he should not move and should be careful that movement does not occur. (3) The knees and hips should be in full extension. If there is fixed flexion contracture of the knee or hip, lateral radiograms of the femur and tibia are made; or two posteroanterior views are made, one of the femora by focusing over the hips and then the knees, and the other of the tibia by focusing over the knees and then the ankles. In either way, accurate length of the bones can be obtained. (4) In the presence of marked leg length inequality, proper centering of the x-ray tube may be difficult, with resultant divergence of rays and distortion. In such an instance, separate x-ray exposures of each limb are made.[201]

The author recommends orthoroentgenography as the method of choice for measuring leg lengths for routine office use when CT scan mensuration is not readily available. The technique shows the entire length of both lower limbs from the iliac crests to the soles of the feet, with excellent detail of bone and soft tissue throughout; it gives an accurate measurement of true length of the bones; technically, the procedure is simple, both in making the exposure and in the measurement of the bones' shadows; radiation to the patient is minimal; and the cost is slight. Orthoroentgenography has been criticized because of the inherent difficulty of handling the long films and the matter of storage; if space is a problem, this objection can be eliminated by cutting the film into halves, taping the edges back together, and folding the films at the tape.

CT SCAN

Recently, CT scan determination of limb lengths has been developed (Fig. 7–263). This technique is simple and accurate and visualizes the entire pelvis and lower limb, and the scans are easy to store. Its drawbacks are availability and degree of radiation, which is not much more than orthoroentgenography, and its cost.[10, 186, 227]

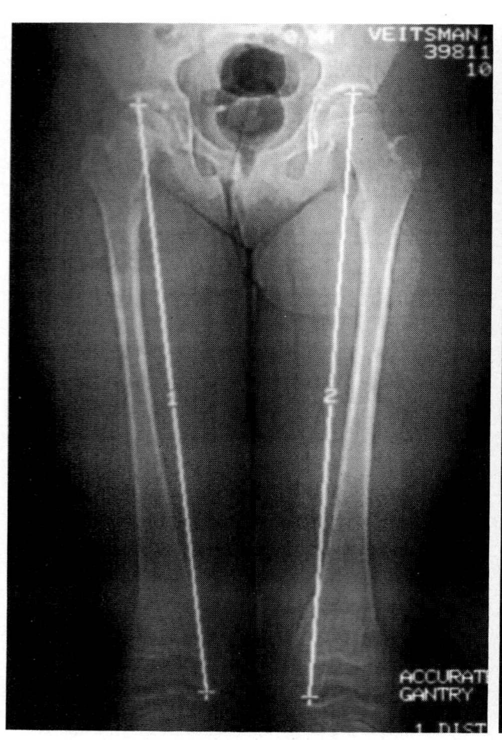

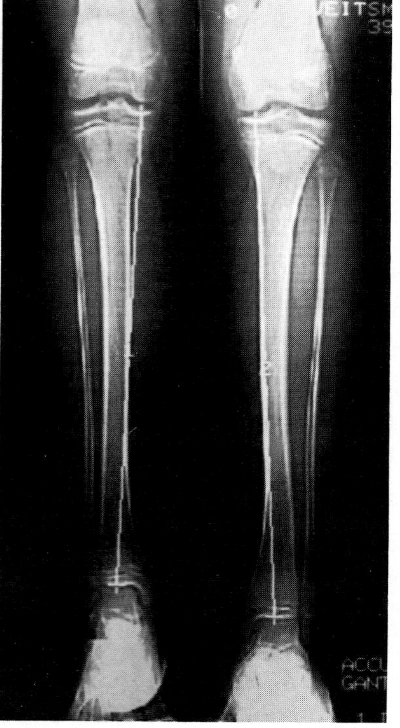

FIGURE 7–263. Radiographic mensuration of limb length discrepancy by CT scan.

Treatment

Discrepancy in length of the lower limbs can be corrected by any one of the following methods: (1) permanent arrest of growth of the longer limb—by *epiphysiodesis;* (2) retardation of growth of the longer limb—by *epiphyseal stapling;* (3) *shortening* of the longer limb; or (4) *lengthening* of the shorter limb by osteotomy and distraction or by stimulation of physeal growth.

When the lower limb length disparity is minimal and amounts to no more than 1 to 2 cm., it usually is of no clinical consequence. If there is a lateral decompensation of the spine with lowering of the pelvis on the short side or if there is a noticeable short leg limp, treatment consists of a lift to the heel of the shoe (in part or in total to make up the discrepancy). In prescribing a lift to the shoe, the objective should be balance of the trunk and not exact equalization of limb lengths. The lift should be light—part could be inside the heel and part outside. A lift in the shoe of the short limb is particularly desirable in the growing child; however, parents should be assured that a short leg will not of itself cause a structural scoliosis; such reassurance will relieve them of many years of anxiety. Adolescents and adults will usually discard the lift in the shoe because it is unsightly and a psychological handicap.

At the extreme, when the discrepancy is very severe or the leg or foot is deformed, prosthetic fitting with or without a Syme amputation may be the procedure of choice.

ARREST OR RETARDATION OF GROWTH OF THE LONGER LIMB BY EPIPHYSIODESIS

In 1933, Phemister described his method of complete arrest of longitudinal growth at the physis; premature fusion of one or more physes of the longer limb allows the short limb to grow at a relatively more rapid rate than the long limb. Limb length discrepancy is corrected by the normal growth process.[367] In the skeletally immature child, epiphysiodesis is a simple and safe method of equalizing leg lengths, provided the procedure is carefully timed and correctly executed. *Indications* for epiphysiodesis are projected lower limb disparity of 2 to 5 cm. and the desire of the patient and parents. *Prerequisites* are acceptable total height and sufficient growth remaining to give adequate correction. Limb length disparity greater than 5 cm. in a short-statured patient (less than the 25th percentile) is a *relative contraindication.* In a normal-statured patient with a lower limb length disparity of greater than 7.5 cm., this author recommends elongation of the short limb.

Methods of Calculation of the Timing for Physeal Arrest. At present there are three methods: (1) Green-Anderson growth remaining; (2) White-Menelaus "rule of thumb"; and (3) Moseley's straight-line graph. This author recommends the use of all three methods whenever possible.

Green–Anderson Growth Remaining Method.[25] The principles and steps involved in using the growth prediction chart have already been outlined. This author has utilized this method for the past 30 years and found it to be reliable and accurate. Information required is the general population data for height (see Fig. 7–258), length of femur and tibia (see Fig. 7–259), and the growth prediction chart of Green and Anderson, i.e., growth remaining in the normal distal femur and proximal tibia following consecutive skeletal age levels (see Fig. 7–260).

Data required on the individual patient are his (1) chronological age, (2) skeletal age, (3) height, (4) length of femora and tibiae of both lower limbs, (5) percent of growth inhibition, (6) growth percentage, and (7) projected limb length disparity at skeletal maturity.

Time of epiphysiodesis by the Green–Anderson growth remaining method is calculated as follows:

1. Calculate the past growth of the femur and of the tibia separately—which is equal to their present length minus first-measured length (over longest interval). Add the growths of the femur and tibia to obtain the past total growth of the lower limbs.
2. Calculate the *present disparity in length*—which is equal to the length of the long lower limb minus the length of the short lower limb.
3. Calculate *percent growth inhibition*—which is 100 times growth of the long lower limb minus the growth of the short lower limb divided by growth of the long limb. Also, calculate the growth inhibition separately for the femur and tibia. Depending upon the rate of inhibition, make appropriate adjustments toward lower values on the growth chart (see earlier).
4. Relate the length of the femur and tibia of the *long* lower limb to fit the individual patient into the Green-Anderson data. Relate the length of the femur and tibia to skeletal age for the appropriate sex (see Table 7–27). This is the growth percentage.
5. Predict the long limb length at skeletal maturity as follows:

A. Determine the mean length of the long lower limb (femur and tibia) at skeletal maturity for the population (of the appropriate sex) by reference to the Green-Anderson data.
B. Predict the length of the long limb by multiplying the mean length of population by growth percentage. A simple way is to use the graphs for the length of the femur and tibia (see Fig. 7–259).

6. Calculate future growth of the long lower limb—which is equal to the length at skeletal maturity minus present length.
7. Calculate future increase in discrepancy—which is equal to future growth of the long lower limb multiplied by growth inhibition divided by 100.
8. Calculate the predicted discrepancy at maturity—which is equal to present discrepancy plus future increase in discrepancy.
9. Predict the amount of correction by epiphysiodesis of the distal femur and proximal tibia (or both) by referring to the Green-Anderson growth remaining graph for the appropriate sex and skeletal age.

The White-Menelaus "Rule of Thumb" Method.[316, 467, 473] This is based on two assumptions: first, that the distal femoral physis provides 1 cm. (3/8 inch), and the proximal tibial physis 0.6 cm. (1/4 inch), of longitudinal growth of the lower limb each year; second, that the growth of these physes stops at the chronological age of 14 years in girls and 16 years in boys. Calculations are based on chronological rather than skeletal age and on the assumption that the relationship between rate of growth and age from onset of puberty is a straight line. These assumptions are not always true. Bone age should always be determined; whenever there is marked disparity between chronological and skeletal age, the timing of physeal arrest according to the Menelaus method is likely to be inaccurate and not reliable. Another drawback of the Menelaus method is that it does not consider the actual bone length of the femur and tibia; the amount of growth remaining varies according to the length of the long bone. It also does not consider percentage of growth inhibition. Following epiphysiodesis of the long limb, it is the growth of the short leg that will correct limb length disparity. Despite these deficiencies this author recommends the use of the Menelaus method of calculation of the timing of physeal arrest in conjunction with the Green-Anderson tables and the Moseley straight-line graph. The Menelaus method is simple, is easy to calculate, and provides a rough estimate as to the timing of epiphysiodesis. It is recommended that the growth rate, future growth, and limb length discrepancy at maturity be calculated when using the White-Menelaus rule of thumb method. The following are the steps as outlined by Moseley.[337]

1. Calculate in years the longest time interval of data.
2. Calculate in centimeters the past growth of the lower limbs by subtracting the first-measured length (over longest interval from the present length).
3. Calculate the growth rates of the lower limbs—which is growth divided by time.
4. Calculate the years of growth remaining.
5. Calculate the future growth of the lower limbs (future growth = growth rate times years remaining).
6. Predict the lower limb lengths at skeletal maturity—which is present length plus future growth.
7. Calculate the lower limb lengths at maturity—which is predicted length of the long lower limb minus predicted length of the short lower limb.
8. Predict the amount of correction by epiphysiodesis—which is equal to growth rate of the physis, or physis multiplied by years of growth remaining. (Correction by distal femoral arrest is 1.0 cm. per year, by proximal tibial arrest 0.6 cm. per year, and by combined arrest 1.6 cm. per year.)
9. Calculate the result of epiphysiodesis—which is discrepancy at maturity minus correction.

Moseley's Straight-Line Graph.[336] In this method it is assumed that the longitudinal growth line of the long and short lower limbs is straight. The limb length is related to skeletal age; thereby a correctional factor is provided for the growth percentile.

A requirement for this method is the straight-line graph (Fig. 7–264). At each office visit the following three data are obtained: (1) the skeletal age as determined by anteroposterior radiogram of the left hand and wrist; (2) the length of the long lower limb; and (3) the length of the short lower limb. The length of the lower limbs is measured on orthoroentgenograms or CT scan from the most superior point of the femoral head to the middle of the subchondral bony plate of the tibia at the ankle.

A. *Steps for Depiction of Past Growth* (Fig. 7–265 A)
   1. Plot the length of the long lower limb on the printed line for the long limb, at the appropriate length.

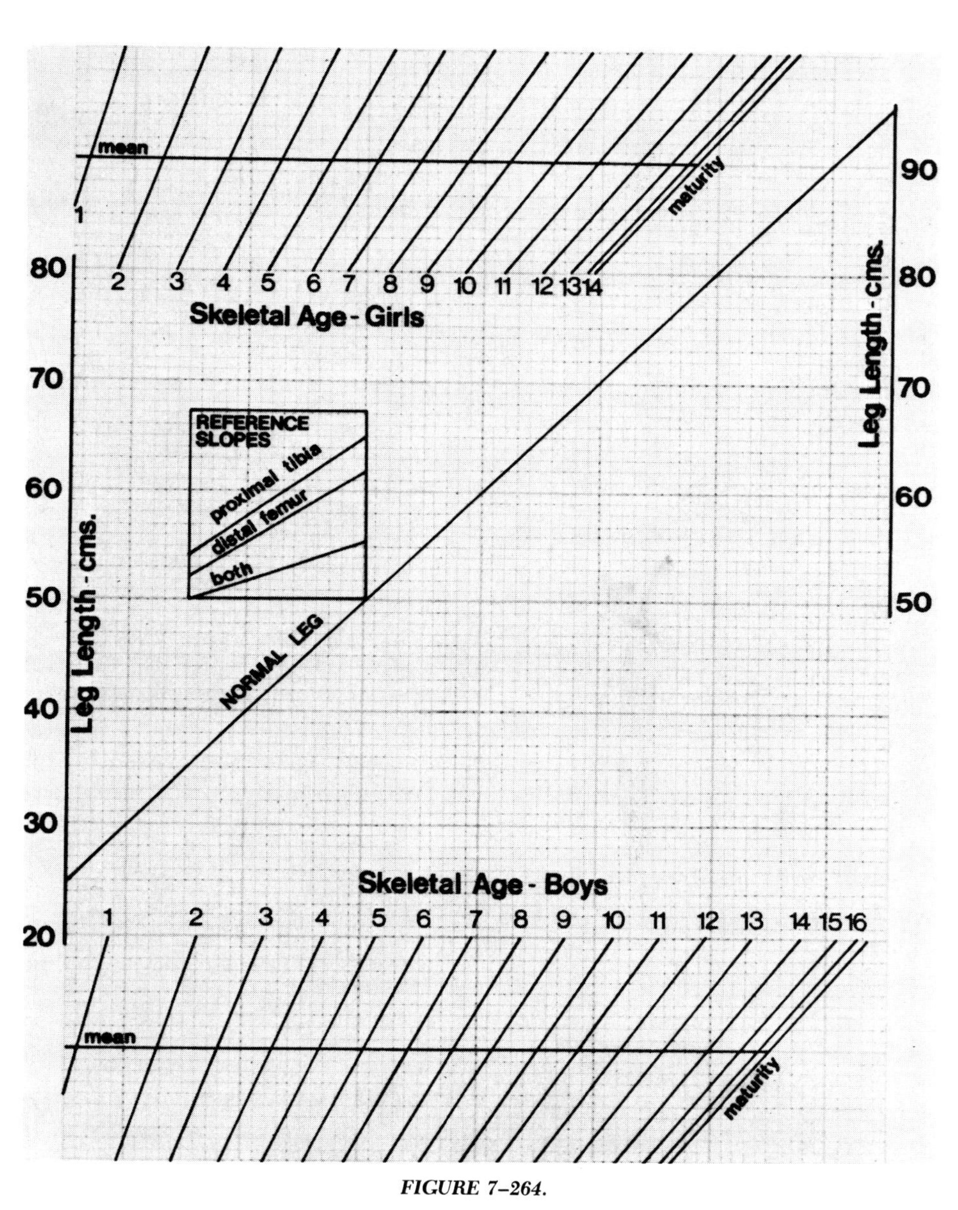

FIGURE 7–264.

(From Moseley, C. F.: A straight-line graph for leg-length discrepancy. J. Bone Joint Surg., 59-A:174, 1977.)

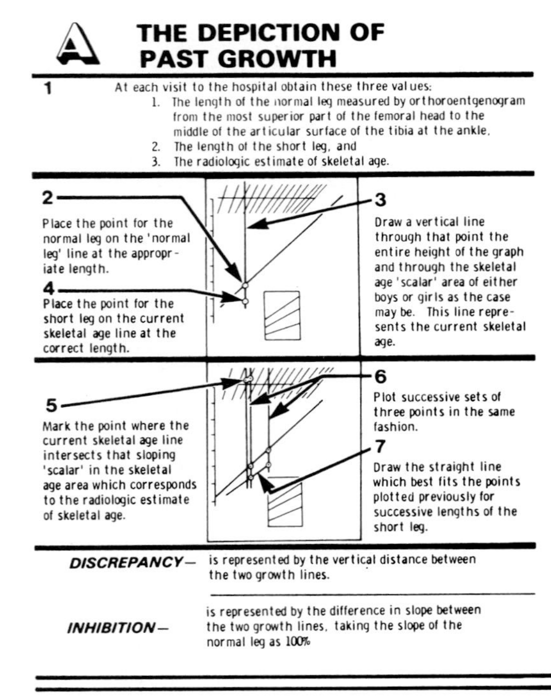

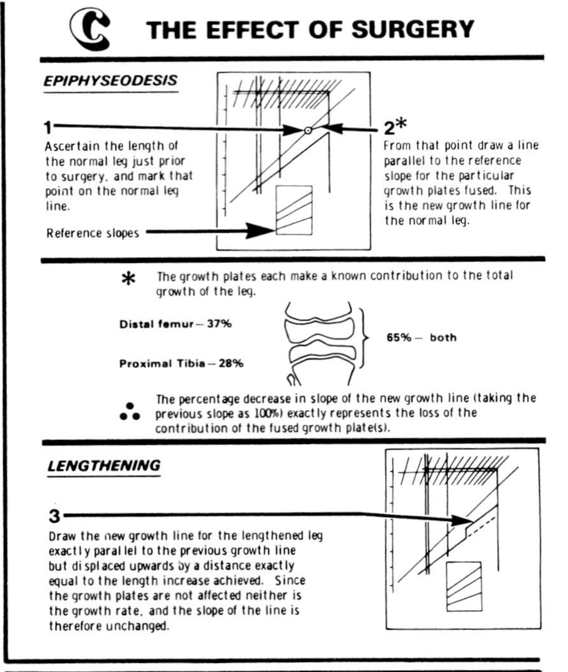

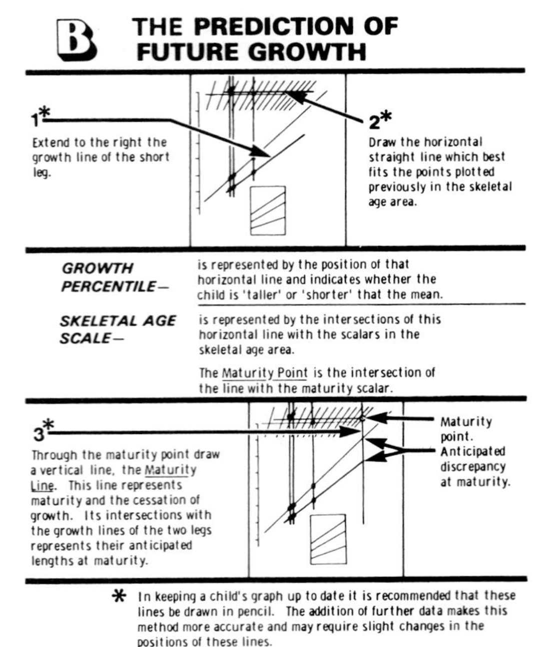

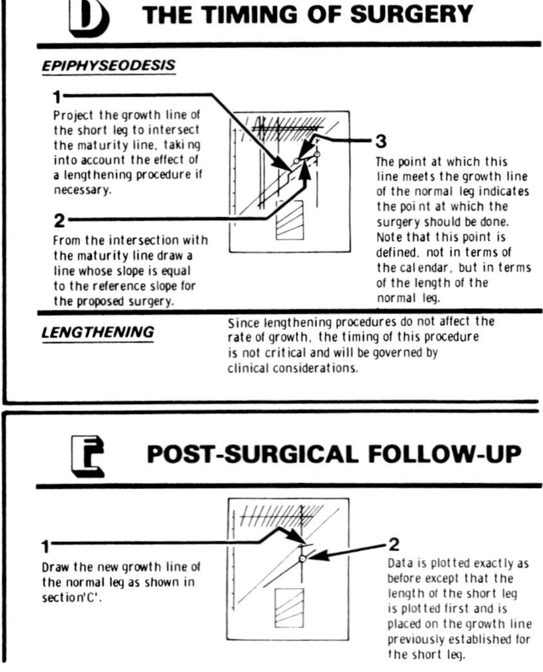

FIGURE 7–265.

(From Moseley, C. F.: A straight-line graph for leg-length discrepancy. J. Bone Joint Surg., 59-A:174, 1977.)

2. Draw a *vertical line* from the point for the long limb (which was just plotted) to and through the skeletal age area for the appropriate sex (girls upward and boys downward). All points for this visit are plotted on this vertical line, which represents the current skeletal age.
3. Plot the length of the short limb on the vertical line (current skeletal age line) just drawn, at the appropriate length.
4. Plot the point for current skeletal age, which lies on the same vertical line, placed in reference to the sloping lines for skeletal age; it may be interpolated between two of those lines if necessary.
5. Repeat these steps on each subsequent visit. On plotting the three points on the graph a series of vertical lines will be displayed, each one representing one visit.

B. *The Prediction of Future Growth* (Fig. 7–265 B)

1. Draw and extend the growth line of the short limb to the right. It should be a straight line; if the plotted points do not fit accurately, most probably there is a measurement error, either in the radiographic technique (e.g., movement during the scanogram or improper focusing) or in choosing inconsistent landmarks when measuring length on the film.

   The growth line of the short limb lies inferior to that of the long limb. The vertical distance between the two lines represents the limb length disparity. Also, the growth line of the short limb may diverge from that of the long limb; the difference in slope of the two growth lines represents the percentage of growth inhibition. The slope of the normal long limb is designated as 100 percent.
2. Draw the horizontal straight line that best fits the points previously plotted in the skeletal age area. This line may not fit these points accurately owing to error in determination of skeletal age. In such an instance, ignore the early skeletal age points and consider the recent points, which are more valid, and draw a straight line. Project this line to the right until it intersects the sloping line of mature skeletal age. The *growth percentile* is represented by the position of this horizontal line; it indicates whether the child is "taller" or "shorter" than the mean.

   The *skeletal age scale* is represented by the intersection of the horizontal straight line with the scalers in the skeletal age area. The *maturity point* is the intersection of this line with the maturity scaler.
3. Draw the *maturity line* by dropping a vertical straight line through the maturity point inferiorly to intersect the growth lines of the two lower limbs. The intersection points represent the predicted limb lengths at maturity. The distance between the two points represents the anticipated lower limb length disparity at skeletal maturity.

C. *Determination of Effect of Epiphysiodesis* (Fig. 7–265 C)

The distal femur contributes 37 percent to the total growth of the lower limb, proximal tibia 28 percent, and both 65 percent. The original slope of the growth line of the long limb is taken to be 100 percent; the percentage decrease in the slope of the new growth lines represents the loss of the contribution of the fused growth plates.

1. Determine the length of the long limb immediately prior to surgery and mark that point on the long leg growth line.
2. From that point of the long leg growth line, draw a line parallel to the reference slope for the particular growth plate proposed to be fused (the three possible epiphysiodesis sites are the distal femur, the proximal tibia, or both). This will become the new growth line for the long limb.

   A simple way to draw parallel lines to the reference slopes is as follows:
   a. Place the long edge of a rectangular transparent ruler on the chosen reference slope.
   b. Place the long edge of a second ruler against the left end of the first.
   c. Hold the second ruler steady and slide the first ruler along it; with their edges apposed, all lines drawn along the first will be parallel to the reference slope. Extend the new altered growth line of the long limb to the right until it intersects the vertical maturity line; the point of intersection represents the length of the long limb at maturity if subjected to growth arrest. When this point of intersection is the same as that of the short limb, exact limb length equalization is achieved.
3. *To predict the effect of lengthening*, draw a new growth line for the lengthened short limb as follows: First, on the ver-

tical line drawn at the last visit, elevate the point of the length of the short limb by a distance exactly equal to the length proposed; second, draw the new growth line for the lengthened short limb exactly parallel to the "old" growth line of the short limb. This assumes that the lengthening procedure does not affect the physis and that growth rate is unchanged; therefore, the slope of the growth line of the lengthened short limb remains unchanged.

If the lengthening is exactly equal to the projected disparity at maturity, the "new" growth line of the lengthened short limb will meet the maturity line at exactly the same point as the growth line of the long limb. If there is growth inhibition and the lengthening is equal to the present discrepancy, the two growth lines will not meet; therefore, it will be necessary to overlengthen the short limb.

The operative technique of distal femoral epiphysiodesis is described and illustrated in Plate 113 and that of the proximal tibia and fibula in Plate 114.

Figures 7–266 and 7–267 are two examples of adequate correction of leg length discrepancy by epiphysiodesis.

Percutaneous Epiphysiodesis. In this technique developed by Canale, through a small incision under image intensifier radiographic control and guide pin, the medial and lateral periphery of the distal femur or proximal tibia is identified.[94] A very small block of bone is removed, and with a small curet, the physis is completely destroyed using x-ray control. At the completion of the procedure, 50 percent diluted Renografin is instilled at the site of the curetted growth plate medially and laterally, and permanent radiograms are made to ensure and record that the physis is completely destroyed. Postoperative cast immobilization is not required. The knee is supported in a removable immobilizer for a period of three weeks. Rehabilitation is relatively simple as compared with the traditional Phemister-Green technique. The operative scars are small and cosmetically very acceptable. The procedure is not recommended for growth arrest of the proximal fibula because of a high rate of common peroneal nerve injury.

Some surgeons strongly believe in percutaneous epiphysiodesis, whereas others support the traditional epiphysiodesis. In the experience of this author, the growth arrest performed through this small incision by the Canale technique is not always symmetrical. This author recommends percutaneous epiphysiodesis in adolescent girls for cosmetic reasons provided they and their parents understand the higher number of failures and complications and the possibility of requiring future surgery.

Complications of Epiphysiodesis. Significant complications occur in 5 to 10 percent of epiphysiodesis procedures. They may result from miscalculation, from technical errors during surgery, or from postoperative wound infection.

Miscalculation. Undercorrection will result if epiphysiodesis is performed too late. It occurred in 3 percent (7 of 237 patients) in the series of Green and Anderson.[199] Overcorrection of discrepancy is caused either by overestimation of the growth potential of the longer limb or by underestimation of the growth potential of the shorter limb. It is imperative to follow the asymmetrical growth of the lower limbs prior to performing epiphysiodesis. In the series of Green and Anderson, overcorrection occurred in 3 percent; in five of these patients, distal femoral arrest on the originally short side was performed in order to prevent what appeared to be imminent overcorrection; in two patients of the entire group the original shorter limb became as much as ½ inch longer than its opposite member.[199]

Technical Problems During Surgery. Asymmetrical fusion between the medial and lateral parts of the growth plate will cause genu varum or valgum. It occurred in 2.6 percent (6 of 237 patients) in the series of Green and Anderson.[199] Failure of fusion of the medial or lateral side can be detected by careful follow-up during the postoperative period and corrected by repeat epiphysiodesis. If the patient is seen too late with a disturbing angular deformity, an osteotomy or asymmetrical physeal distraction is warranted for its correction.

Neurovascular dysfunction is usually a complication of epiphysiodesis of the tibia and fibula. Paralysis may result either from laceration or compression of the common peroneal nerve or from ischemia of muscles in the anterior tibial compartment. Constant vigilance by the surgeon will decrease the incidence of this serious complication, which occurred in 0.8 percent in the series of Green and Anderson.[199] It is vital to stay anterior when performing proximal fibular arrest. Do not compress the common peroneal nerve by vigorous posterior retraction! Always divide the deep fascia in order to prevent anterior compartment syndrome! Release the tourniquet and obtain complete hemostasis prior to wound closure!

A stiff knee joint may result from the patellar retinaculum being sutured to the periosteum or

Text continued on page 2887

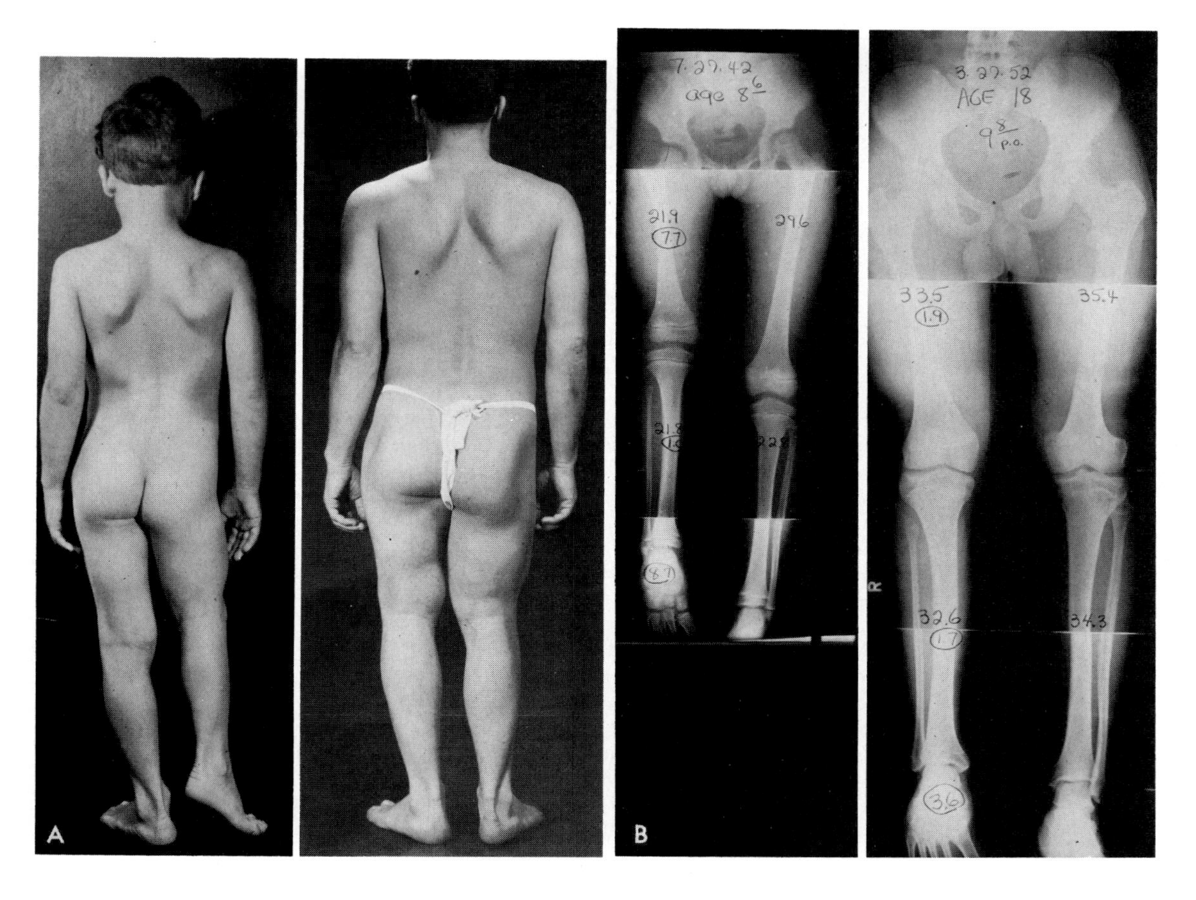

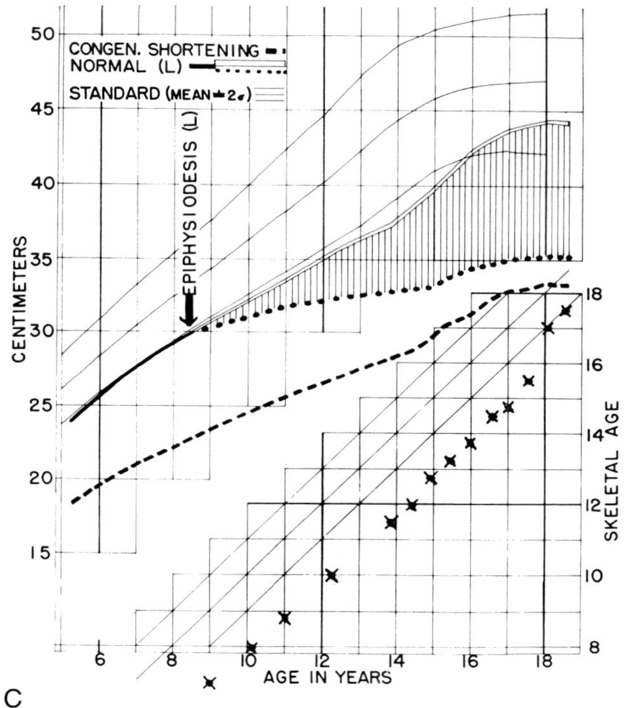

FIGURE 7–266. A boy with a congenitally short right femur.

Between the ages of five and eight years, the right femur as compared with the normal left femur had shown 26 per cent inhibition. The long bones in the normal side measured two standard deviations below average. At age eight years and five months, the total shortening of the long bones of the right limb measured 8.7 cm. (the femur 7.7 cm. short and the tibia 1 cm. short). The predicted total leg length discrepancy at skeletal maturity was 11 cm. His skeletal age was retarded two years. At age eight years and five months distal femoral epiphyseodesis of the normal left limb was performed.

A. Photographs taken at the age of eight years and at 26 years, showing the functional correction obtained. **B.** Orthoradiograms made at eight years and at skeletal maturity. **C.** Chart of progress in length of femora and skeletal age, demonstrating how distal femoral epiphyseodesis corrected the discrepancy in femoral lengths by 5.8 cm. At maturity, this boy still had 3.6 cm. shortening but he could get by with good gait without any lift in the shoe. (From Green, W. T., and Anderson, M.: Skeletal age and the control of bone growth. A.A.O.S. Instructional Course Lecture. Vol. 17. St. Louis, Mosby, 1960, p. 209.)

Epiphysiodesis of Distal Femur (Green Modification of Phemister Technique)

OPERATIVE TECHNIQUE

A. The knee is supported in 20 to 30 degrees of flexion and the joint line is identified. First, the medial aspect of the distal femur is exposed. Beginning 1 cm. superior to the joint line, a longitudinal incision about 5 to 7 cm. long is made midway between the anterior and posterior margins of the femoral condyles. The subcutaneous tissue and deep fascia are divided in line with the skin incision.

B. Following the anterior surface of the medial intermuscular septum, the vastus medialis muscle is lifted anteriorly with a blunt periosteal elevator. The suprapatellar pouch should not be entered. In the inferior margin of the wound, the capsule and reflected synovial membrane of the knee joint are gently elevated and retracted with blunt instruments distally. Caution! Do not open the joint. If the synovial membrane is inadvertently divided, which will be indicated by oozing of synovial fluid, it is closed by 00 Vicryl continuous suture. The superior medial genicular vessels traverse the wound; it is best to coagulate them to prevent troublesome bleeding later.

C. A midline longitudinal incision is made in the periosteum, starting proximally and extending throughout the extent of the wound.

D. The medial distal femoral physis is exposed by raising anterior and posterior flaps of periosteum by subperiosteal dissection; it appears as a white, glistening transverse line that is softer than adjacent cancellous bone. Some surgeons prefer to make a longitudinal I-shaped incision in the periosteum to expose the growth plate; the author, however, prefers a simple longitudinal incision, as it permits a more taut periosteal closure. The periosteum is gently retracted by 00 Tycron sutures on its borders. Rough traction and shredding of the periosteum should be avoided. If necessary, Chandler elevators are placed subperiosteally on the anterior and posterior aspects of the distal femur for adequate exposure. Dull right-angled retractors are used for proximal and distal retraction.

E and **F.** With matched pairs of osteotomes, a rectangular piece of bone 1⅛ to 1½ inches long and ½ to ⅝ inch wide is excised. The epiphyseal plate should be at the junction of the distal one third and proximal two thirds of the length of bone graft resected, at a point equidistant between the anterior and posterior surfaces of the femur. The posterior cortex of the femur should not be broken. The depth of the bone graft is ½ to ¾ inch (the blood at the tip of the osteotome will mark its depth of penetration into bone). Because of the flare of the femoral condyles, the anterior and posterior osteotomes should be tilted somewhat distally so that they are perpendicular to the medial surface of the femur. Following removal of the osteotomes, the completeness of osteotomy is checked with a thin (⅜- or ¼-inch) osteotome. Then with curved osteotomes the graft is removed. Breakage of the graft at the physis is prevented by straddling the growth plate with the osteotomes.

Plate 113. Epiphysiodesis of Distal Femur (Green Modification of Phemister Technique)

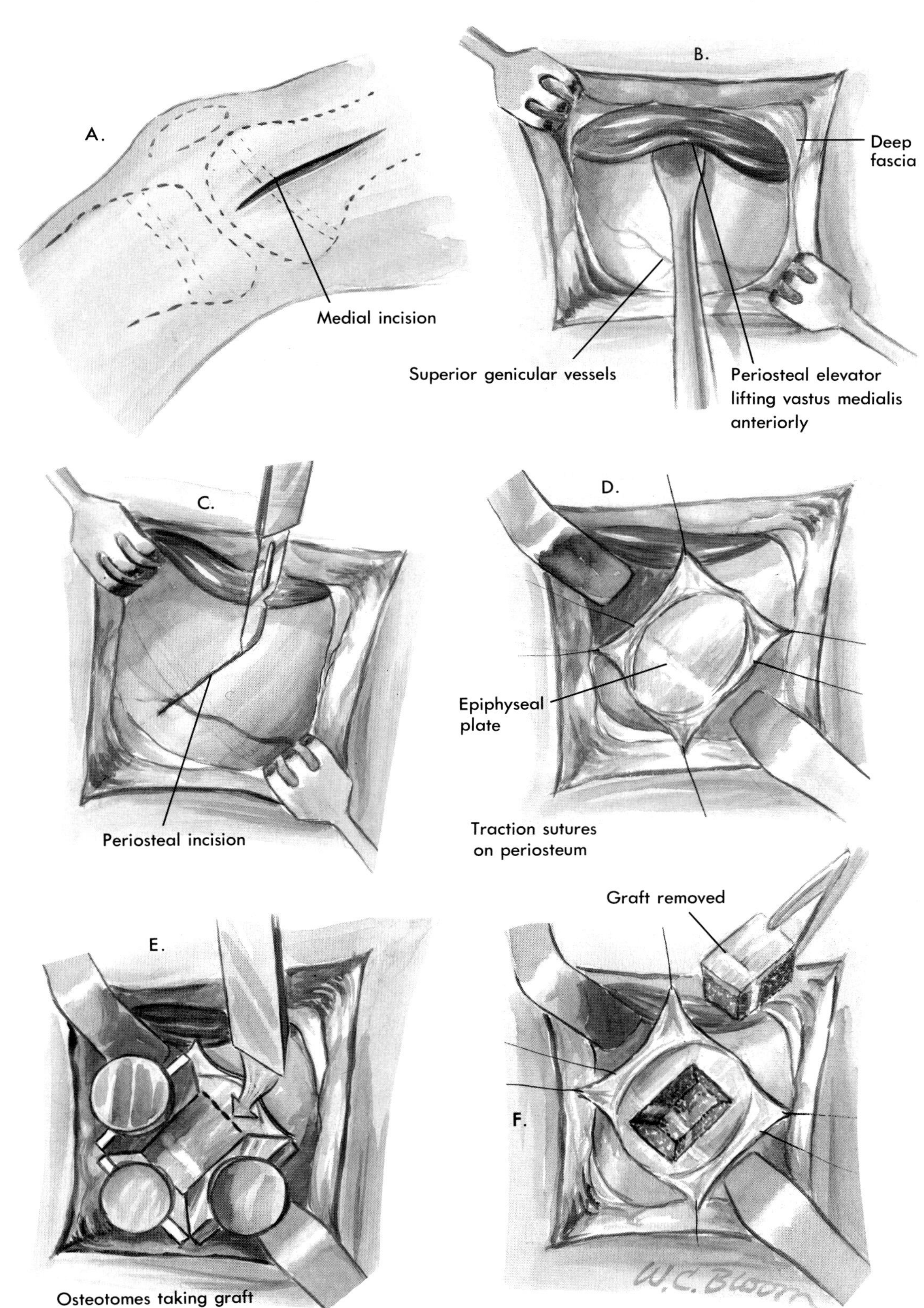

Epiphysiodesis of Distal Femur (Green Modification of Phemister Technique) (Continued)

G. The growth plate is drilled with diamond-shaped drills of increasing size in anterior, posterior, and distal directions. A hand drill provides better control and feel of depth. It should be remembered that the distal femoral physis is pointed inferiorly. The softness of the cartilaginous plate serves as a guide to its direction. Then, with a small curet, removal of the growth plate is completed, the debris of cartilage and bone being saved for later packing around the proximal end of the graft. Curettage should extend to the periphery of the growth plate, avoiding the popliteal vessels posteriorly.

H. Cancellous bone graft is taken from the proximal bed and packed into the defect created by removal of the growth plate.

I. The bone graft is then reinserted into its original bed, with its ends reversed by 180-degree rotation.

J. With an impacter and mallet, the bone graft is securely seated in the bony defect. It should be tapped in a distal direction, as the growth plate is inferior in location.

K. The periosteum is tightly closed with interrupted sutures. It is important not to include the patellar retinaculum with the periosteum, as this will bind it down, restricting knee motion. Suture the periosteum with the knee in complete extension.

L. The same procedure is repeated on the lateral side. Before closure of the wounds the position of the medial bone graft is checked to be sure it has not been dislodged by the tapping on the opposite side.

POSTOPERATIVE CARE

The limb is immobilized in an above-knee cylinder cast with the knee in neutral position or 5 degrees of flexion for a total of four weeks. The foot and ankle are left out of the cast and the patient is allowed to walk with crutches (three-point gait) as soon as he is comfortable. Because the long leg is in an extended position in the cast, appropriate lifts are placed on the shoe on the short side so that the patient can clear his leg with the cast.

Before the patient is discharged, it is best to make radiograms of the distal femur, taken through the cast, to record the integrity of bony continuity and the position of the reversed bone plugs. The cast usually becomes loose in 10 to 14 days. The cast and sutures are removed two weeks after surgery, and a new snug cast is applied. A common pitfall is the failure to extend the cast proximally enough on the thigh. Torsional stress on the distal femur should be prevented.

Following removal of the cast, the knee is mobilized by side-lying flexion-extension exercises to develop motor strength in the quadriceps femoris muscle. Crutch support is discontinued when there is 90 degrees of knee flexion and the quadriceps muscle is fair in motor power. Radiograms of the distal femur are made six weeks and three months following surgery to be sure that fusion of the growth plate has taken place. Lower limb length studies are performed at three-month intervals during the first year, and then at six-month intervals until completion of growth.

Plate 113. Epiphysiodesis of Distal Femur (Green Modification of Phemister Technique)

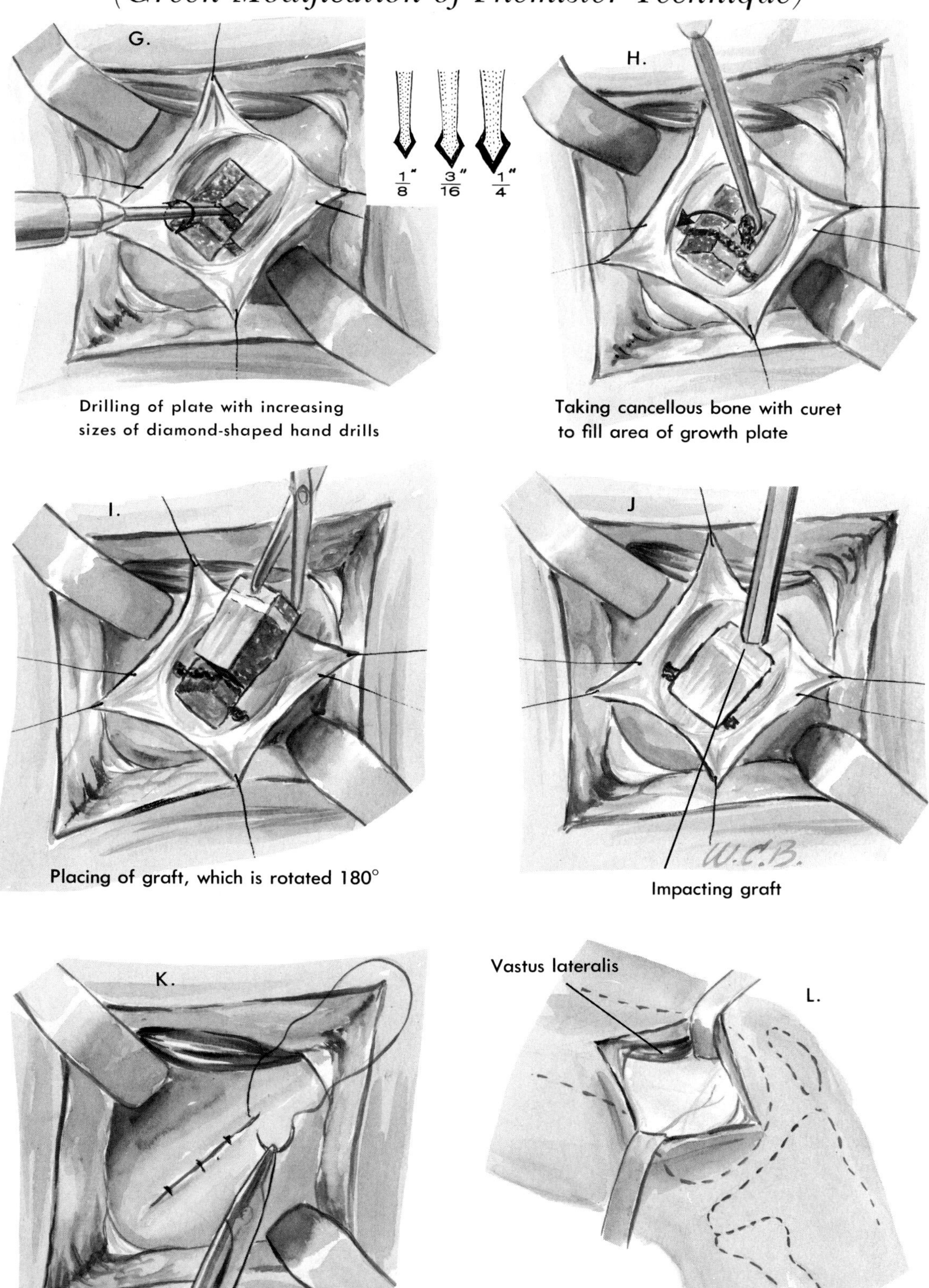

Drilling of plate with increasing sizes of diamond-shaped hand drills

Taking cancellous bone with curet to fill area of growth plate

Placing of graft, which is rotated 180°

Impacting graft

Tight closure of periosteum

Lateral exposure

Epiphysiodesis of Proximal Tibia and Fibula (Green Modification of Phemister Technique)

Growth arrest of the proximal fibula is performed first, since this provides more adequate exposure and facilitates proper identification of the common peroneal nerve. After 20 to 30 minutes of tourniquet ischemia, stimulation of the common peroneal nerve will fail to produce contraction of the innervated muscles. If the lateral side of the proximal tibial physis is arrested first, normal details of anatomy will be obscured by blood and distorted by the dissection.

OPERATIVE TECHNIQUE

A. The patient is placed in semilateral position with the lateral-side surgically prepped leg up and the knee flexed 30 degrees. A sandbag or a sterile folded sheet is placed under the knee for support. The knee joint line, the head of the fibula, and the proximal tibial tubercle are identified. A 30-degree slanted oblique incision is made midway between the proximal tibial tubercle and the fibular head; it begins proximally 1 cm. inferior to the joint line and 1 cm. anterior to the fibular head and extends distally and forward for a distance of 5 cm. The subcutaneous tissue is divided, and the wound flaps are widely undermined and retracted.

B and **C.** The head of the fibula is in line with the proximal growth plate of the tibia. (In the illustration, the head of the fibula is abnormally high.) The capsule of the knee joint, the insertion of the biceps tendon, and the fibular collateral ligament of the knee are identified.

The common peroneal nerve lies close to the medial border of the biceps femoris muscle in the popliteal fossa; then it passes distally and laterally between the lateral head of the gastrocnemius and the biceps tendon. Behind the fibular head it is subcutaneous. At the site of origin of the peroneus longus muscle at the head and neck of the fibula, the common peroneal nerve winds anteriorly around the fibular neck and then passes deep to the peroneus longus muscle and branches into the superficial and deep peroneal nerves.

D. The origins of the toe extensors, extensor hallucis longus, and anterior tibial muscles, along with a cuff of periosteal flap, are elevated from the arcuate line. With a periosteal elevator, the origin of the peroneus longus muscle is detached from the head of the fibula; keeping the dissection anterior to the fibular head will prevent injury to the nerve.

Plate 114. Epiphysiodesis of Proximal Tibia and Fibula (Green Modification of Phemister Technique)

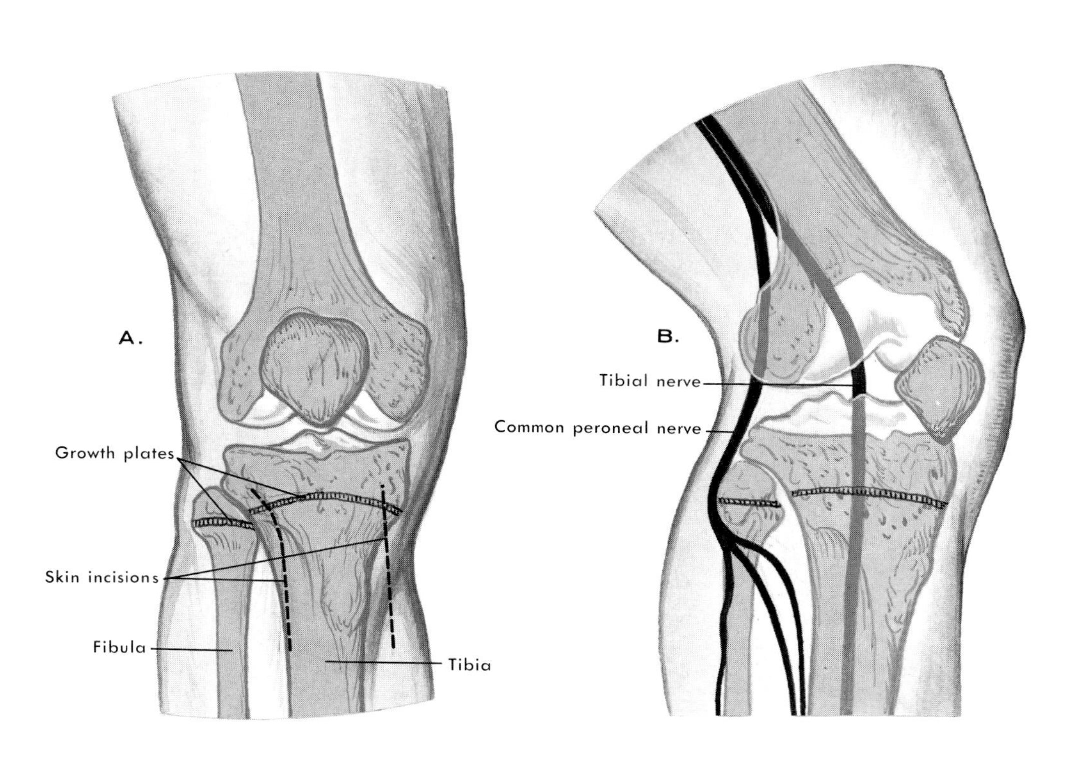

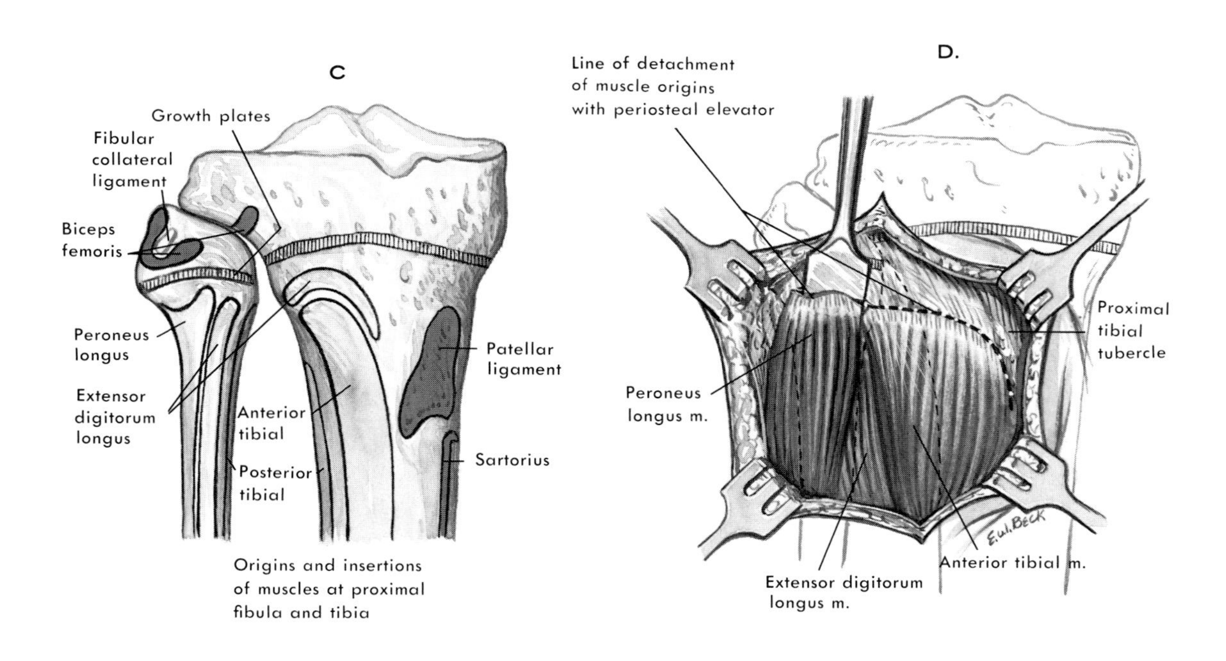

Epiphysiodesis of Proximal Tibia and Fibula (Green Modification of Phemister Technique) (Continued)

E and **F.** With a straight needle, the site of the growth plate of the proximal fibula is identified. Next, a longitudinal incision is made on the anterior aspect of the fibular head and is extended distally to include the growth plate. A rectangular piece of bone (¼" wide and ½" long) is removed from the proximal fibula, straddling the physis. Three fourths of the length of the bone graft includes the fibular head, so that only one fourth of the graft length includes the metaphysis. The growth plate is thoroughly curetted, the ends of the bone graft are reversed (180 degrees), and the piece of bone is placed securely back in the graft bed. At times, this author simply curets the growth plate but dispenses with the latter steps.

Note: A nerve stimulator should always be available in the operating room; if one has doubts about whether a strand of tissue is fibrous or neural, one should determine its nature positively by stimulation.

The lateral aspect of the proximal tibial physis is already exposed for the fibular epiphysiodesis. A longitudinal incision is made midway between the anterior and posterior borders of the lateral tibia. The periosteum is elevated, and a rectangular piece of bone is resected in a manner similar to that described for the bone graft technique with the distal femur. The growth plate is drilled with diamond-shaped drill bits of increasing size in the anterior, posterior, and *proximal* directions. A hand drill is used. The steps of the epiphysiodesis are the same as those outlined in Plate 113, *G* to *K*, for epiphysiodesis of the distal femur.

G and **H.** The medial side of the proximal tibial physis is exposed by a longitudinal incision about 5 cm. long, beginning 1 cm. distal to the joint line and continuing distally midway between the proximal tibial tubercle and the posteromedial margin of the tibia. The subcutaneous tissue and deep fascia are divided in line with the skin incision. The anterior margins of the sartorius tendon and tibial collateral ligament are partially elevated and retracted posteriorly.

The steps for growth arrest of the proximal tibial physis follow the steps described for distal femoral epiphysiodesis. The rectangular piece of bone graft removed from the tibia, usually ½" wide and ¾" long, is smaller than that removed from the femur. Prior to closure of the wound, the tourniquet is released and complete hemostasis is secured (otherwise, bleeding in the anterior tibial compartment will cause muscle ischemia and paralysis).

POSTOPERATIVE CARE

Following closure of the wound, the region of the fibular head is well padded, and the limb is immobilized in an above-knee cast that includes the foot and ankle. The knee is in 30 degrees of flexion, and the foot and ankle are in neutral position. The postoperative care is the same as that following distal femoral epiphysiodesis.

Plate 114. Epiphysiodesis of Proximal Tibia and Fibula (Green Modification of Phemister Technique)

EPIPHYSIODESIS OF PROXIMAL TIBIA AND FIBULA (continued)

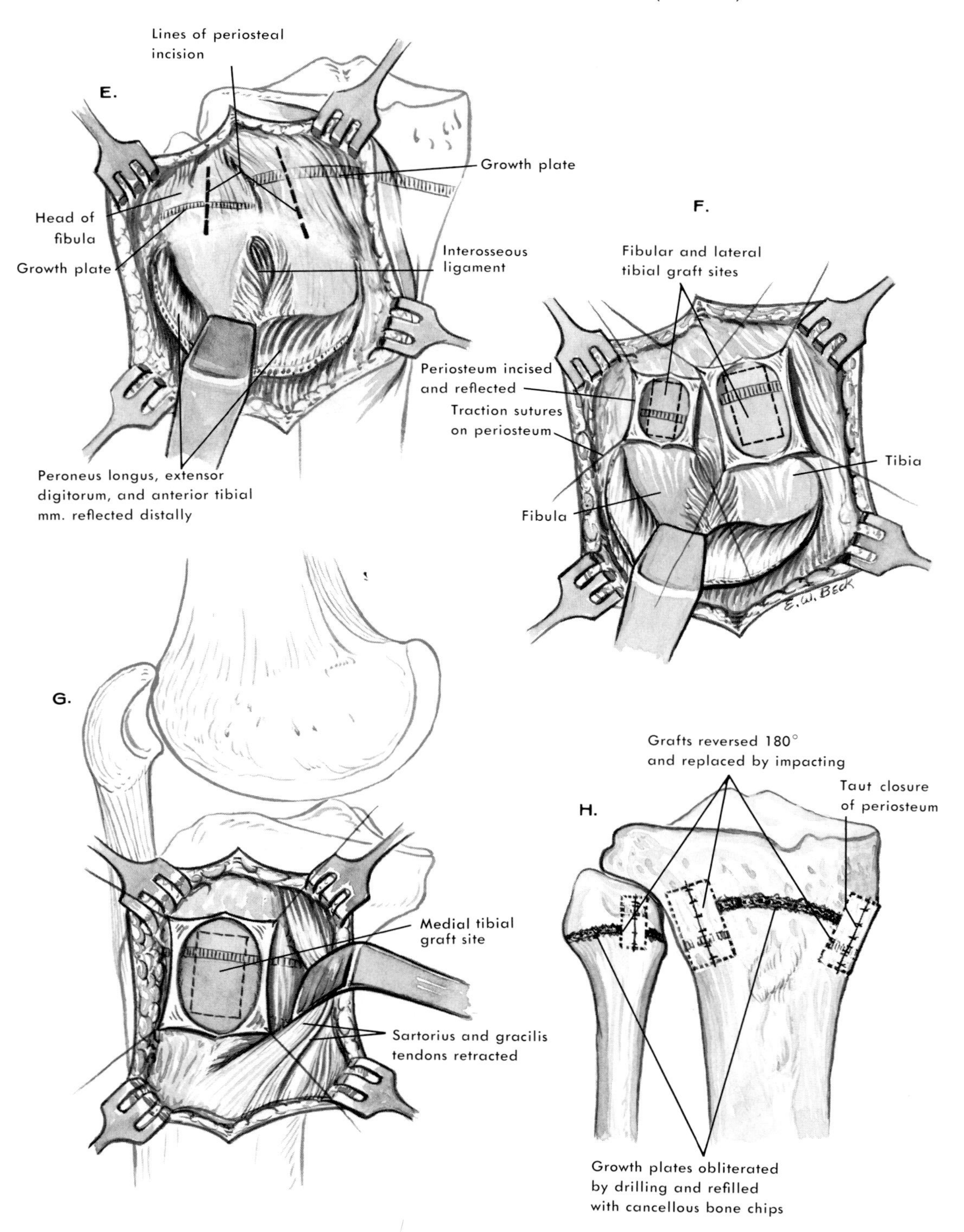

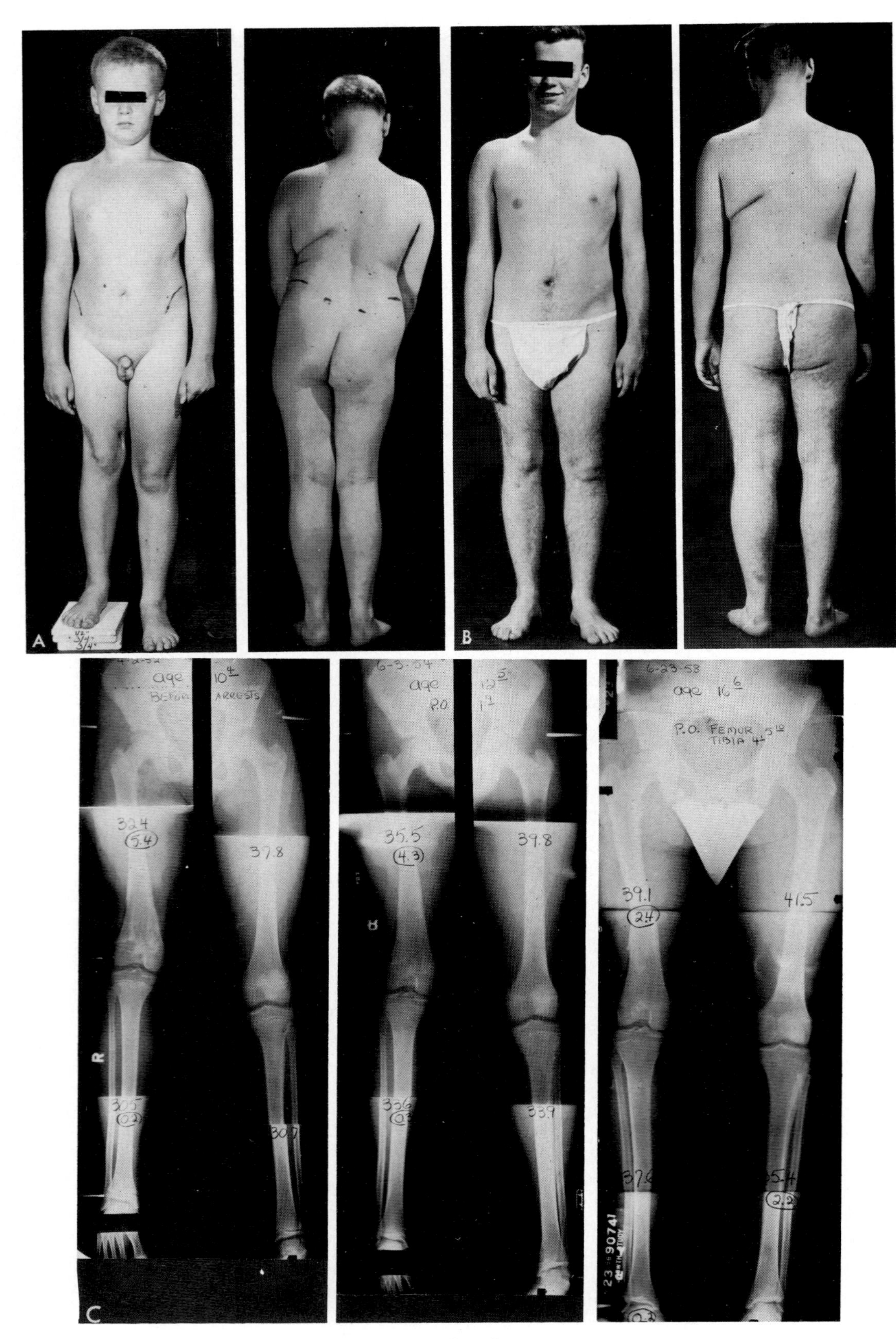

Figure 7–267 *See legend on opposite page*

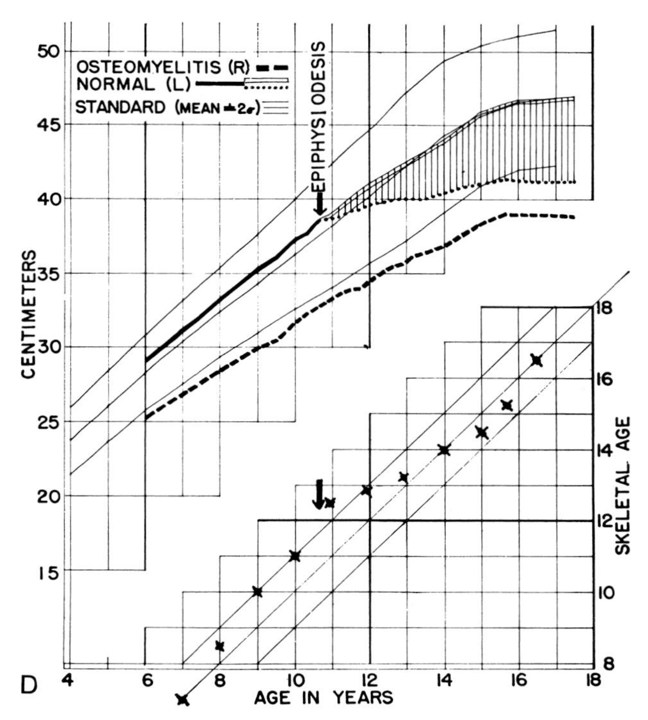

FIGURE 7–267 Continued. Short right femur due to marked growth inhibition following osteomyelitis of right lower femur in infancy.

D. The composite chart showing the progress in length of femora and in skeletal age.

from hemarthrosis. This usually takes place when epiphysiodeses of the distal femur and proximal tibia and fibula are performed simultaneously.

Partial extrusion of a loosely fitted graft may result in a bothersome bony prominence at the operative site. Exostosis may develop at the site of the transplanted physis. Always destroy the physis by curettage.

Postoperative Wound Infection and Osteomyelitis. This complication occurred in 0.8 percent of Green and Anderson's patients.[199] When infection complicates epiphysiodesis, the wound is reopened and irrigated by closed suction, and appropriate antibiotics are given.

GROWTH RETARDATION BY PHYSEAL STAPLING

Retardation of longitudinal growth of limbs by the insertion of rigid staples across the epiphyseal plate was introduced by Blount.[69] Several years earlier, Haas had interrupted the growth of an epiphysis by a wire loop, and had demonstrated that growth resumed following removal of the wire.[211] The principle of temporary arrest of linear growth theoretically was a good one, as the process was reversible; when the leg length discrepancy was corrected, the staples could be removed and growth would resume. The procedure was received with great enthusiasm. Unfortunately, many errors in surgical technique and judgment were committed. The original staples, made of 3/32-inch steel rod, were mechanically ineffective. The Vitallium staples, introduced several years later, proved to be far superior. The original technique suggested "blind" stapling, but soon it was found that radiographic control was imperative to ensure correct positioning of the staples. Experience demonstrated that the periosteum and

FIGURE 7–267. Short right femur due to marked growth inhibition following osteomyelitis of right lower femur in infancy.

At 10 and a half years of age the total shortening on the right amounted to 5.8 cm. Left distal femoral epiphyseodesis was performed at 10 years and 8 months of age, followed by arrest of left proximal tibia and fibula 20 months later. The total correction of discrepancy from the two procedures was 5.9 cm. (3.4 cm. from the femur and 2.5 cm. from the tibia). **A.** Preoperative photograph. **B.** At 18 years of age when all growth is completed. Note the improved balance. **C.** Orthoradiograms before femoral arrest, before tibial arrest, and at skeletal maturity.

Table 7–28. *Complications of Epiphyseal Stapling*

	Blount[68, 69]	***Brockway, Craig, Cockrell***[80]	***Green, Anderson***[199]	***May, Clements***[315]	***Pilcher***[369]	***Poirier***[370]
No. of stapling operations	200	62	83	76	35	33
Complications			*Number of Patients*			
Asymmetrical growth—genu valgum, varum, or recurvatum	7	13	2	11	30	15
Laxity of knee ligaments	—	?	—	—	6	20 (6 marked)
Stiff knee	—	—	—	—	—	—
Infection, metal reaction	—	—	1	3	12	—
Extrusion of staples	—	15	24	24	—	8
Buried staple	—	10	—	—	—	—
Broken staples	—	7	7	—	3	—
Failure to control growth	—	—	2	—	31	3
Slow arrest of growth	—	?	11	—	—	—
Loss of correction after removal of staples	—	?	—	4	—	—
Aneurysm	—	—	—	—	—	—
Peroneal nerve palsy	—	—	—	2	—	—

epiphyseal vessels should be left intact, if permanent interruption in growth was to be prevented. Sinking of the cross-member of the staple into the bone will cause it to be buried, making its removal very difficult. During removal of the staple, the periosteum should not be incised and the physis should not be disturbed. The incidence of complications of physeal stapling is summarized in Table 7–28.

Green and Anderson observed that stapling does not inhibit growth as immediately as does epiphysiodesis. They also noted that one cannot have absolute faith in the resumption of growth following removal of the staples; in some cases, growth may resume normally, but in others premature fusion of the physis may take place. In others after staple removal, there may be rebound longitudinal growth. For practical reasons, stapling must be considered as a method of complete arrest.[200] This author does not recommend physeal stapling for equalization of leg lengths, as epiphysiodesis is more reliable and simpler and has far fewer complications. Complications are much more frequent after stapling of the proximal tibial epiphysis than after stapling of the distal femoral epiphysis. In surgical management of lower limb length inequality, the only instance in which this author considers physeal stapling is when there is difficulty in predicting the amount of correction to be obtained by epiphysiodesis, such as in limb length inequality in multiple hereditary exostosis or other skeletal dysplasias with marked irregularity of skeletal maturation. In order to minimize complications, meticulous attention should be paid to the technical details of the procedure. During removal of the staples, the physis should not be injured by incising and elevating the periosteum.

SHORTENING OF THE LONG LIMB

Resection of a segment of the femur or of the tibia for equalization of limb lengths is performed after skeletal maturity is reached. It is not performed in a growing child, however, because epiphysiodesis at the appropriate skeletal age is a much simpler and safer method.

Tibial Shortening. Leveling of the knees is an important cosmetic consideration. When leg length discrepancy is due to a short tibia, it is logical to shorten the tibia of the longer limb. Tibial shortening, however, is not recommended by this author for the following reasons: (1) If more than 3 cm. is resected from the tibia, the muscles of the leg controlling the foot and ankle become markedly relaxed and weakened. A 5 to 7 cm. long segment of the femur can be removed without residual weakness of the thigh muscles. Because of marked loss of tension of the leg muscles and the peculiar vascular anatomy of the tibia, delayed union or nonunion is common following tibial shortening. (2) In femoral shortening, only one bone is resected, whereas in the lower leg, segments from both the tibia and the fibula must be removed. (3) Ischemic necrosis of the muscles of the anterior compartment of the leg can occur following resection of the tibia.

When tibial shortening is performed, it should not exceed 3 cm. A step-cut resection is performed in the proximal metaphyseal area through an anteromedial approach. The fibula is divided at the junction of the middle and distal thirds through a separate longitudinal incision, and its fragments are allowed to overlap. Two transfixing screws are used for internal fixation of the tibial fragments. An alternative method preferred by the author is excision of a complete segment of the tibia of the desired length and internal fixation with an AO compression plate. Risk of vascular compromise is much less when the bone segment is resected distally at the metaphyseal-diaphyseal juncture. The resected bone fragments are divided into matchstick bone grafts that will straddle the osteotomy site on the posterior and lateral surfaces of the tibia.

An above-knee plaster of Paris cast is applied with the knee in 30 degrees of flexion and the ankle in neutral position. In three weeks, the cast and sutures are removed, and an above-knee, snug, well-molded cast is applied. The knee should be in 15 to 20 degrees of flexion and the ankle slightly equinus. Gradual weight-bearing is begun with the protection of a three-point crutch gait to stimulate osteogenesis. Periodic radiograms are taken to check alignment of the fragments and healing. Union is usually firm within 10 to 12 weeks. Following removal of the cast, the motor strength of the leg muscles is evaluated; temporary support by a below-knee dynamic dorsiflexion-assist orthosis may be indicated.

Femoral Shortening. Since Rizzoli's first report of femoral shortening by overriding (cited by Goff), many techniques of reduction in the length of the femur for equalization of leg lengths have been described in the literature (Fig. 7–268).[188] The principal methods are: (1) oblique osteotomy and resection of the medial two thirds of the upper end of the distal fragment, using its lateral cortex as an intramedullary bone peg (Calvé and Galland);[89] (2) simple overriding of the osteotomized fragments and internal fixation with three or four transversely inserted screws (White);[472] (3) step-cut osteotomy and resection of bone from both fragments and internal fixation with intramedullary rod and screws (Merle D'Aubigné and Dubousset);[317] (4) simple transverse osteotomy, resection of a segment of bone and intramedullary fixation with a rod;[317] (5) V-osteotomy in which the "M" fragments are cut in half and the bone pieces are screwed to the shaft; (6) oblique, sliding osteotomy;[188] (7) shortening in the subtrochanteric region and internal fixation with a blade plate (Blount);[68] and (8) supracondylar shortening (R.D. Moore).[333]

Indications for femoral shortening are lower limb disparity (primarily in the femur) in an older adolescent near skeletal maturity or a young adult with adequate stature.

In a growing child, the surgical procedure of femoral shortening may stimulate growth, increasing length by 1 to 1.5 cm. This is not absolute, however, and because of its uncertainty, it is best to postpone shortening of long bones until completion of growth. Although a 7.5 to 10 cm. segment of the femur can be resected without significant permanent weakening of the thigh musculature, relaxation of the muscles during the period of bone healing may cause delayed union because of lack of compression of the osteotomized bone fragments. Thus, the importance of primary compression plating cannot be overemphasized. In some cases, additional support in the form of a single hip spica cast may be necessary.

This author favors midshaft femoral shortening with excision of the mid-diaphyseal segment of appropriate length and internal fixation with intramedullary rod such as Grosskemp or a similar device with screw fixation distally and proximally to control rotation. If a Küntscher or Schneider rod is used for internal fixation, it is desirable to use compression plating with a unicortical screw to control rotation and enhance healing. The procedure is technically simple and effective. Its disadvantage is that it takes a longer time for bone union.

"Closed" mid-diaphyseal femoral shortening has been advocated by Winquist et al.[479, 480] In this technique, by the use of an intramedullary circular saw, double osteotomy of the femur is performed at the midshaft, the excised fragment is displaced, and the femur is fixed with an intramedullary rod. The advantage of the closed technique is that there is no scar on the lateral midthigh, which may be cosmetically important in an adolescent girl. Its principal disadvantage is difficulty of control of rotation of fragments. Technically the procedure is difficult to perform, special instrumentation is required, and the learning curve for the surgeon is steep. "Closed" femoral shortening carries a definite risk of vascular injury. The displaced bone fragment may form an ugly mass on the lateral aspect of the thigh, which may be more objectionable than the cutaneous scar. For these reasons, this author does not recommend closed femoral shortening.

Subtrochanteric femoral shortening is indicated when there is associated coxa valga or vara that can be corrected by wedge osteotomy. The procedure is effective, and the proximal

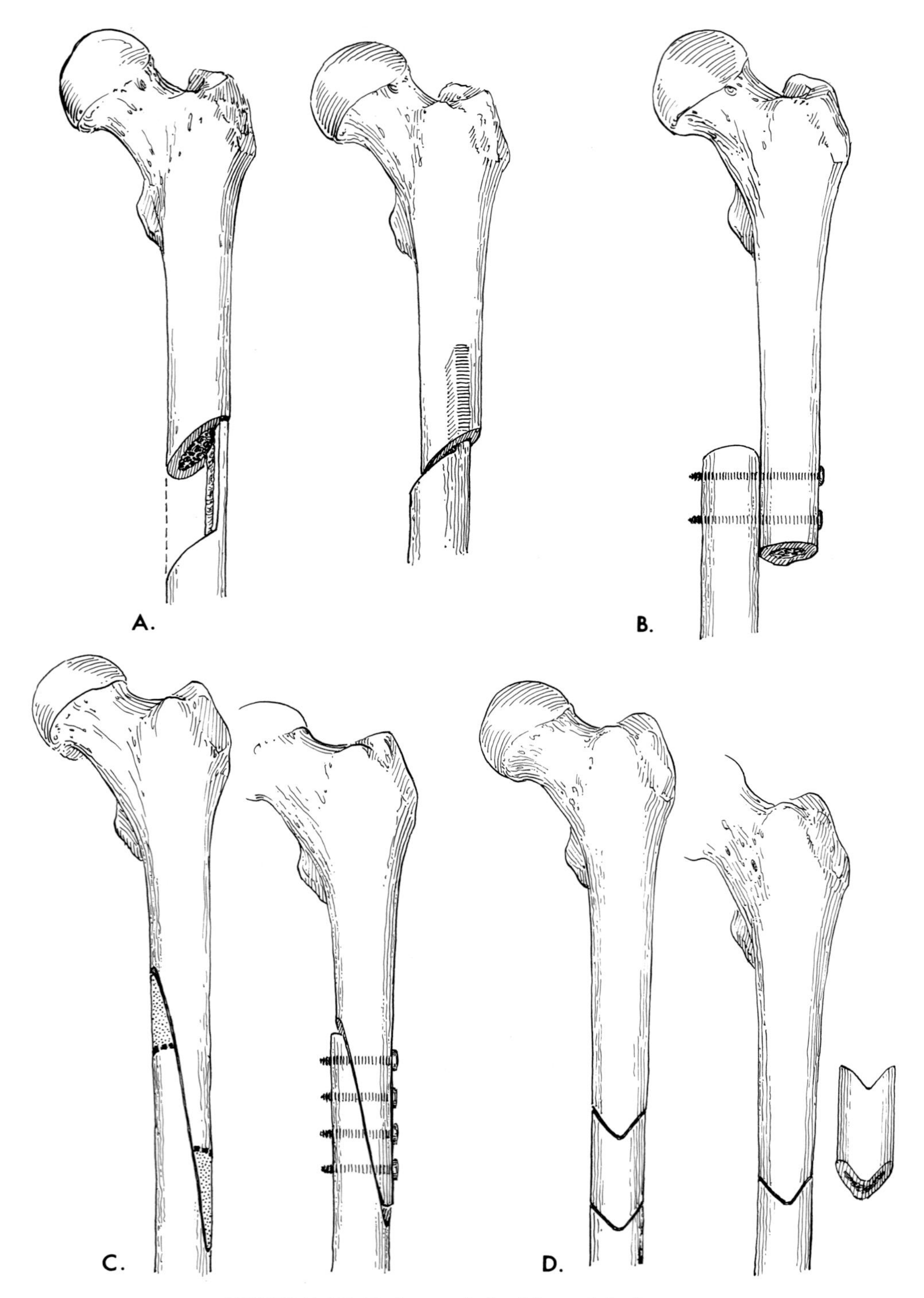

FIGURE 7–268. Various methods of femoral shortening.

A. Oblique osteotomy and resection of medial two thirds of the upper end of the distal fragment, using its lateral cortex as an intramedullary bone peg (Calvé and Galland). **B.** Simple overriding of the osteotomized fragments and internal fixation with transversely inserted screws (White). **C.** Oblique sliding osteotomy. **D.** V-osteotomy in which the "M" fragments are cut in half and the bone pieces are screwed to the shaft.

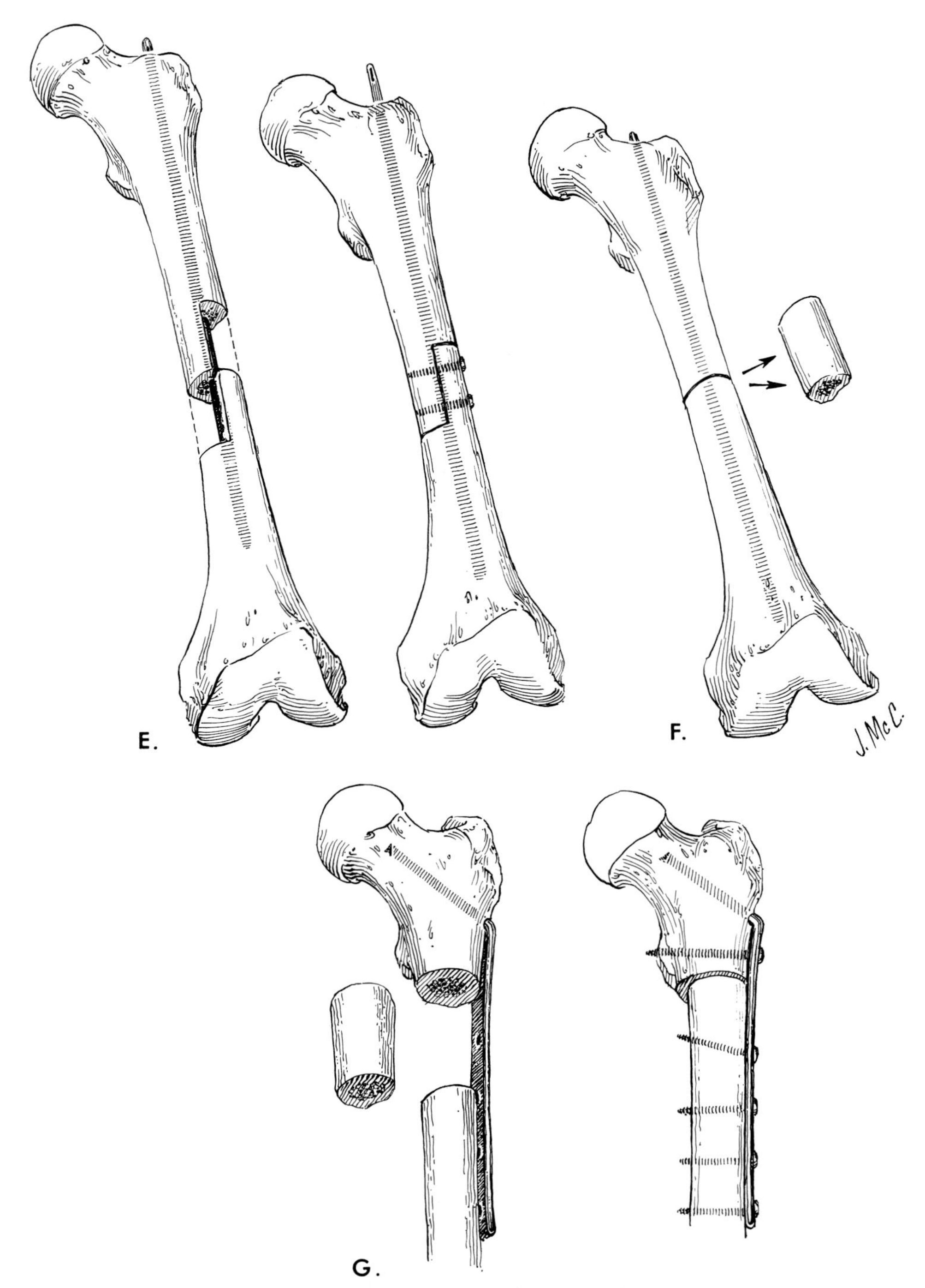

FIGURE 7–268 Continued. Various methods of femoral shortening.

E. Step-cut osteotomy with resection of bone from both fragments and internal fixation with intramedullary rod and screws (Merle D'Aubigné and Dubousset). **F.** Simple transverse osteotomy, resection of a segment of bone, and intramedullary fixation with a rod. **G.** Shortening in the subtrochanteric region and internal fixation with a blade plate (Blount).

position of the operative scar on the thigh is more pleasing cosmetically. Technically it is easy to perform, bony union takes place rapidly, and internal fixation devices are readily available. The only disadvantage is the nail or screws in the femoral head-neck, with potential for compromise of circulation and avascular necrosis. *The fixation device should not be placed in the superolateral quadrant of the femoral head.*

Supracondylar shortening of the femur is indicated when there is associated genu varum or valgus or recurvatum that requires simultaneous correction. A metaphyseal trapezoid segment of bone is resected. Bony union takes place within eight weeks. The disadvantages are technical difficulty of internal fixation and potential problems with the knee, particularly stiffness if a cast is utilized for immobilization for additional support.

Simultaneous shortening of the long femur and lengthening of the short femur is indicated when there is severe femoral shortening. Internal fixation is performed with an intramedullary rod. The healing period and convalescence are briefer than for standard femoral lengthening; however, the grafted elongated segment may take a long time to heal. Another advantage is that the reduction of the overall length of the long femur is reduced by 50 percent. Its disadvantages are difficulty of instantaneous lengthening of the short femur and the potential risk of neurovascular injury. The maximum amount that a femur can be lengthened instantaneously with a reasonable degree of safety is about 3 cm. During the lengthening procedure the hip should be extended and the knee in flexion, in order to minimize stretching of the sciatic nerve.

Complications of femoral shortening are quadriceps femoris weakness with extension lag of the knee, genu recurvatum due to hamstring muscle weakness, delayed union or nonunion, proximal migration of the intramedullary nail, and infection.

Hardware removal may pose problems. It is best to explain to the patient and family that it is desirable to remove the hardware and that although an attempt will be made to do so, it may not be feasible. Also, after hardware removal the femur should be protected for a period until there is adequate healing in order to prevent stress fracture through screw holes.

LENGTHENING OF THE SHORT LIMB

Theoretically, the ideal method of equalizing limb lengths is to lengthen the short limb.

History. In the literature, many techniques of tibial or femoral lengthening by osteotomy and mechanical distraction of the short bone have been described.

Femoral lengthening was first attempted by Codivilla in 1905. He performed an oblique osteotomy of the femoral shaft, and with the patient under anesthesia, applied skeletal traction through the calcaneus. A hip spica plaster cast was applied immediately to maintain the reduction. Codivilla reported the results in 26 cases, with a gain in length varying between 3 and 8 cm.[111] He also discussed the indications for, and contraindications to, leg lengthening.

Magnuson, in 1913, used a Hawley table to apply traction.[309] Putti, in 1921, applied traction and countertraction with one pin proximal to the site of osteotomy and one distal to it. In Putti's technique, the pin was inserted through only the lateral aspect of the thigh, but through both cortices of the femur. The two pins were connected with a telescoping tube and a spring extension mechanism.[379]

Abbott and Crego, in 1928, found control of the osteotomized fragments by Putti's technique unsatisfactory since the pins pulled out of the cortex. Better control of the fragments was secured by Abbott, who inserted four pins, two above and two below. The pins are inserted through the entire femur and thigh to prevent them from pulling out. The proximal pins are inserted in a vertical plane to avoid puncture of major vessels. Abbott also devised a single-unit extension mechanism by means of coil springs on parallel threaded bars.[2] Compere, in 1936, recommended simultaneous bone grafting to decrease the incidence of nonunion. He also discussed the indications for and against leg lengthening.[118]

McCarroll, in 1950, described a subtrochanteric Z-type of osteotomy and the use of a slotted blade plate for control of the fragments as length was increased. He also applied traction above and below the knee by means of one threaded pin through the distal femoral metaphysis and another through the upper portion of the tibia. This redistributed traction forces across the knee joint, protecting against compression of articular cartilaginous surfaces and overstretching of the capsule, and provided ligamentous support of the knee, thus decreasing the possibility of a stiff or unstable joint.[304] Bost, in 1944, advised decreasing the resistance of these soft tissues by extensive release by lengthening of the hamstrings, hip adductors, and quadriceps femoris.[74]

Bost and Larsen, in 1956, used an intramedullary rod to control the alignment of the osteotomized fragments and in addition to the conventional step-cut or oblique osteotomies, they described a transverse osteotomy. The combination of intramedullary rod fixation and transverse osteotomy made the technique of femoral lengthening easy and afforded the best means for control of the fragments.[75] Westin, in 1967, modified the Bost-Larson technique, constructing a periosteal sleeve to cover the gap in the bone.[468]

Merle d'Aubigné and Dubousset described a one-stage bilateral procedure for equalization of the femora, which they recommended as the best method to correct discrepancies of 10 cm. or more in older children and young adults with shortening primarily in the femur. The short femur is lengthened in two stages—first, an intramedullary rod is inserted in the short femur and, at a level 5 cm. distal to the lower margin of the greater trochanter, the femoral shaft is osteotomized. The fascia lata, the iliotibial band, the straight head of the rectus femoris, the intermuscular septa, and the muscles originating in the proximal segments are divided or lengthened to release the soft-tissue resistance to lengthening. Next, the osteotomized fragments are distracted with a spreader and a metal block is inserted to hold the fragments apart. The long femur is shortened over an intramedullary rod by a step-cut osteotomy and removal of two hemisegments of appropriate length; the bone fragments are impacted and transfixed with two screws, one anterior and the other posterior to the nail. Then the lengthening of the short femur is completed by spreading the osteotomized fragments farther apart and by placing the hemisegments from the long femur in the defect (one anteromedially and the other posterolaterally).[317]

Merle d'Aubigné and Dubousset reported the results of their femoral equalization procedure in 13 patients with an average preoperative leg length inequality of 14.6 cm. Of the 13 patients, 5 had corrections of 9 cm.; 1, a correction of 8 cm.; 2, correction of 6 cm.; and 1, a correction of 5 cm. They caution that if this operation is performed, the technical details must be observed strictly. Oscillometry should be used to monitor circulation in the limb, and the knee should be maintained in flexion during and after the operation to avoid tension on the sciatic nerve. They also warn that very strict aseptic technique should be maintained during surgery, as the wounds are large and the operation is lengthy.[317]

Tibial Lengthening. Abbott introduced the procedure for tibial lengthening in 1927, though various methods of femoral lengthening had been tried since the turn of the twentieth century.[1] The sound logic of lengthening the short limb rather than shortening the normal one initially stimulated great enthusiasm for the procedure. But in the ensuing two decades, the popularity of tibial lengthening waned and the operation fell into disrepute because of the numerous serious complications including shock, paralysis, sepsis, amputation, and even death. These complications were summarized by Compere in 1936.[118] Sofield, Blair, and Millar stressed another important drawback of the procedure—namely, the undesirable loss of muscle power in the lengthened limb.[426] Then, in 1952, Anderson modified Abbott's original technique. The essential features of his method are (1) fibular osteotomy; (2) distal tibiofibular synostosis to prevent valgus deformity of the ankle; (3) subcutaneous division of the tibia into proximal and distal segments by percutaneous drilling and osteoclasis to minimize trauma to soft tissues; and (4) daily distraction of the tibial segments by means of transfixing pins held in a screw distraction apparatus.[29, 30] As a result of the encouraging results of Anderson's technique, interest in tibial lengthening was restimulated.

Anderson's method does have definite advantages: (1) Soft-tissue damage is minimal; (2) periosteal stripping is avoided; (3) the periosteal tube is preserved; and (4) the hematoma remains localized.

Current Techniques of Limb Lengthening

BIOLOGIC PRINCIPLES

The experimental and clinical studies of Professor Ilizarov on controlled mechanical distraction osteogenesis have shown the following factors to be optimal for new "regenerate" bone formation[247–262]:

1. *Preservation of intramedullary circulation, bone marrow, and periosteum.* In experiments on dogs, Ilizarov compared open osteotomy of bone, periosteum, and endosteum with percutaneous corticotomy that spared the endosteum and periosteum. The consolidation rate of the regenerate bone was slower in the open osteotomy than in the closed corticotomy group, even though stable fixation with a circular fixator had been achieved in both groups. Subsequently, in experimental work in dogs, DeLafortrie showed that despite damage to the

intramedullary vessels, recanalization occurs within the first weeks following corticotomy and that subsequent regenerate bone formation is not significantly hampered if the periosteum is preserved.[137]

The following recommendations are made: Perform osteotomy by corticotomy and preserve, as much as possible, the integrity of bone marrow, intramedullary vessels, endosteum, and periosteum. Divide the bone by a sharp osteotome rather than a power saw, which will burn the cortex and traumatize soft tissues inside and outside the bone.[247] Despite meticulous attention to these technical details, damage to the endosteum and periosteum nevertheless occurs. Therefore, distraction should begin after a latency period of three to five days to allow soft-tissue healing and recanalization.

2. *Stability of external fixation.* Instability of fixation causes marked delay in consolidation time or nonunion. The Ilizarov, Orthofix, and Wagner external fixators provide stable fixation, provided they are properly applied.

3. *The rate and rhythm of distraction.* The rate is the amount of distraction and the rhythm is the frequency of distraction per day. The following rates and rhythms of distraction were employed by Ilizarov—rates of 0.5, 1, 1.5, and 2 mm. per day and rhythm of once per day, twice per day, and four times per day. The rate of osteogenesis was directly related to distraction rate and rhythm. Elongation at a daily rate of 1.5 or 2 mm. per day caused the development of local ischemia, which slowed down osteogenesis. When the rate of distraction was slower than the rate of formation, 0.5 mm. per day, premature consolidation of the regenerate bone occurred, preventing further distraction. *The optimal rate was determined to be 1 mm. per day.*

The greater the rhythm of distraction, the shorter the consolidation time—the use of a motorized autodistractor producing a quasicontinuous distraction rate (0.016 mm., 60 × per day) decreases the consolidation time markedly. Decreasing the rate while increasing the rhythm of distraction reduces the measured tension across the distraction gap.

In clinical practice the rate and rhythm of distraction depend upon the radiographic appearance of calcification of the regenerated bone in the elongated segment. Initially it is always 1 mm. per day, but four weeks postoperatively, it is increased or decreased as needed, to ensure adequate consolidation of the bone while trying to minimize the time in the fixator.

4. *The level of osteotomy.* At the metaphyseal level, bone regeneration is more rapid than at the mid-diaphysis.

INDICATIONS

A lower limb length disparity should be 5 cm. or more in a patient of normal stature; for less than this amount, this author recommends epiphysiodesis to equalize limb lengths, and in the skeletally mature patient, shortening of the long bone. Limb lengthening in a dwarf is a very controversial problem. This author strongly believes that the total patient should be considered and that the limbs of dwarfs should not be lengthened only to make them taller. There should be definite functional impairment, such as shortening of the upper limbs to such a degree that the patient is unable to attend to his toilet needs, or the presence of a deformity that needs to be corrected, at which time a simultaneous limb lengthening may be performed. It is very crucial that in dwarfs a thorough psychological assessment be performed and the strategy of limb lengthening be carefully planned.

REQUISITES

First, the joints proximal and distal to the elongated bone should be stable; when the femur is being lengthened, the hip and knee should be stable. If the acetabulum is dysplastic with subluxation, it is imperative to provide adequate coverage of the femoral head prior to lengthening. The second requisite is that neuromuscular function be normal. Third, circulation should be normal. Fourth, there should be no problems with skin or soft tissues. Fifth, the bone structure should be normal. Sixth, psychologically the patient should be stable and seventh, the patient should be at an age to be cognizant of the complications of the limb lengthening procedure and to cooperate in the postoperative program.

CONTRAINDICATIONS

Joint instability is a contraindication; for example, congenital short femur is often associated with absence of cruciate ligaments and knee joint instability. The second contraindication is paralysis. Bone lengthening makes the musculature weak. For example, a short upper limb in obstetrical brachial plexus palsy should not be lengthened because the partially paralyzed muscles will become weaker and there will be loss of function. The third contraindication is poor bone structure, such as a site of prepseudarthrosis of the tibia. The fourth is mental instability, and the fifth is lack of motivation and unfeasibility of adequate postoperative care. As a rule, this author does not recommend limb lengthening in a child under six years of age.

Professor Wagner recommends that all deformities of the limb be corrected first and that muscle function and bone structure be restored to as nearly normal as possible. For example, prior to femoral lengthening, if there is a flexion deformity of the knee due to posterior tilting of the femoral condyles, a supracondylar extension osteotomy of the distal femur should be performed first, and limb lengthening should be carried out one to two years later, when the knee has full range of motion with normal muscle function and osseous structure is restored to normal. Adduction contracture of the hip, if marked, should be corrected by an adductor myotomy; severe coxa valga and antetorsion of the proximal femur is corrected by varization derotation osteotomy of the proximal femur. If the ankle cannot be dorsiflexed to neutral position, the equinus deformity is corrected by heel cord lengthening. Violation of this basic rule, that is, correction of deformities of the limb one or two years prior to limb lengthening, will cause serious loss of function and related problems. Femoral lengthening can be performed if the hip is ankylosed.[458–460]

Professor Ilizarov, however, feels that deformities of the limbs can be simultaneously corrected during the lengthening procedure.[455] This is an individual decision of the surgeon as to whether he wants to correct the deformity first and then lengthen. This author strongly advocates Wagner's basic requisite of "correct the deformity first and then lengthen the bone; never sacrifice function for length."[458–460]

In acquired cases of limb length inequality, only the bone is significantly shortened; the soft tissues have relatively normal length. Therefore, in limb length equalization, the femur is restored to its normal length. The problem is totally different in congenital limb length inequality.

In congenital shortening, such as in congenital absence or hypoplasia of the fibula with a short tibia or a congenitally short femur, in addition to the bone, the fascia, intermuscular septa, interosseous membrane, muscles, and vessels are markedly shortened. Therefore, it is mandatory to first perform an extensive soft-tissue release and, 6 to 12 months later, to lengthen the shortened bone. This is strongly recommended by Professor Wagner and this author. Professor Ilizarov, however, believes that his technique of limb lengthening elongates soft tissues as well as bone; therefore prelengthening soft-tissue release is not indicated. A definite drawback of soft-tissue release is the size of the operative scar, which may be cosmetically objectionable.

The *technique of soft-tissue release in the congenitally short femur* is as follows: A longitudinal incision is made from the greater trochanter to the tip of the lateral epicondyle of the femur. The subcutaneous tissues are divided in line with the skin incision. Great care is exercised to protect the veins going from the deep fascia to the skin. The iliotibial tract is identified and isolated by two longitudinal incisions on its anterior and posterior borders. The deep fascia is excised in the middle two thirds of the thigh, anteriorly and posteriorly. The vastus lateralis muscle is gently elevated anteriorly and the biceps femoris muscle posteriorly. The lateral intramuscular septum is carefully dissected and excised. At the upper end of the lateral intramuscular septum is the insertion of the gluteus maximus tendon, which is very thickened and fibrotic; it is partially excised, to its normal size. If there is an associated flexion deformity of the knee, and if the hamstrings are taut, a fractional lengthening of both medial and lateral hamstrings is performed at their musculotendinous juncture. A long oblique incision is made in the iliotibial tract and is sutured in its lengthened position. The subcutaneous tissue is closed in the usual fashion with running subcuticular sutures. The patient is allowed to be up and walking within a day or two.

In *fibular hemimelia with shortening of the tibia*, the preliminary soft-tissue release should be very extensive. A midlateral, longitudinal incision is made from the head of the fibula to the ankle joint level. The subcutaneous tissue is divided. The deep fascia and the fibrous or cartilaginous anlage of the fibula are completely excised. The fibular anlage is a severe deforming force; if left intact, it will pull the distal tibial segment into valgus during limb lengthening. The anterior and posterior intramuscular septa are excised proximally. The common peroneal nerve and its branches are carefully identified, and all fascia covering the nerve is removed to prevent compression during the process of tibial lengthening. If the foot cannot be dorsiflexed to neutral position, a heel cord lengthening is performed.

Methods of Limb Lengthening

Limb lengthening may be performed through bone or by physeal distraction. This author does not recommend limb lengthening by physeal distraction because of its high rate of joint stiffness and other complications; therefore, it will not be discussed. The reader is referred to the cited references.[133, 139, 140, 153]

Limb lengthening through bone may be performed by the following techniques: (1) diaphyseal bone lengthening with bone grafting and plating of the distraction gap (Wagner technique); (2) metaphyseal limb lengthening with corticotomy and gradual lengthening without bone grafting of the distraction gap (Ilizarov technique and DeBastiani technique of callotasis); and (3) limb lengthening with cortical allografting of the distraction gap with a thin flexible unreamed intramedullary nail (Wasserstein technique).

The hardware used for external distraction is of two types: (1) large-diameter pin with cantilever system—the Wagner distraction apparatus and the DeBastiani Orthofix axial compression-distraction apparatus; and (2) small wire transfixion system with wires placed under tension and supported by external fixator rings (Ilizarov system).

The Wagner diaphyseal, DeBastiani callotasis, and Ilizarov methods of distraction-osteogenesis without bone grafting will be described.

Wagner, in 1978, developed a technique of limb lengthening that consisted of mid-diaphyseal complete osteotomy of the bone, transecting periosteum, cortex, endosteum, and contents of the medullary cavity. The fixation was by thick Schanz screws and a specially designed stable lengthening device. The screws are monolateral, acting as cantilevers. An initial acute diastasis of 0.5 to 1.0 cm. is created, and lengthening at the rate of 1.0 mm. per day is carried out beginning on the first postoperative day. When the desired amount of lengthening is achieved, the distraction gap is grafted with cancellous bone and internal fixation is provided by rigid osteosynthesis plate. When the graft is consolidated and good cortex is formed in the elongated area, the rigid plate is removed and replaced by semiflexible tubular plate. Finally, when there is normal canalization of the medullary cavity and normal cortex formation, the semitubular plate is removed. During this period, weight-bearing is partial, protecting with crutches.[458] The Wagner technique of femoral and tibial lengthening is described and illustrated in Plates 115 and 116. A case illustrating the Wagner technique of femoral lengthening is shown in Figure 7–269.

LIMB LENGTHENING BY CALLOTASIS (CALLUS DISTRACTION) (DEBASTIANI TECHNIQUE)[135]

Callotasis (or callus distraction) is a technique of limb lengthening developed by DeBastiani in which the callus formed in response to a proximal submetaphyseal corticotomy is slowly distracted by the use of a dynamic axial fixator (Orthofix). The distraction begins 10 to 14 days post corticotomy. When the required lengthening is obtained, the fixator is held rigid until radiographic evidence of good consolidation of the callus is seen. At this time the locking screw of the fixator is released, and dynamic axial loading is started and continued until corticalization is demonstrated radiographically; then the device and screws are removed.

The level of corticotomy is in the proximal area of the diaphysis—in the femur it is immediately distal to the insertion of the iliopsoas; in the tibia, distal to the insertion of the patellar tendon; and in the humerus, distal to the insertion of the deltoid. The fixator is applied on the lateral aspects of the femur and humerus and the anteromedial aspect of the tibia.

The operative technique of femoral lengthening by callotasis is shown in Plate 117 and tibial lengthening by callotasis in Plate 118. An example of lengthening by callotasis is shown in Figure 7–270.

ILIZAROV METHOD: LIMB LENGTHENING WITH DISTRACTION OSTEOGENESIS WITHOUT BONE GRAFTING

Professor Gavrill A. Ilizarov, in 1951, developed an external fixator that is often referred to as the compression-distraction apparatus. The Ilizarov fixator distracts and simultaneously compresses the divided ends of two bone segments. The operative technique is described and illustrated in Plate 119. An example of tibial lengthening with simultaneous lengthening of the foot is shown in Figure 7–271.

Wasserstein, in 1963, introduced limb lengthening with segmental cortical allografting of the distraction gap (Fig. 7–272). The technique consisted of an open subperiosteal diaphyseal osteotomy and insertion of a thin flexible unreamed intramedullary nail. Distraction with the external fixator is performed immediately after surgery at the rate of 1.0 to 2.0 mm. per day. When the desired amount of lengthening

Text continued on page 2991

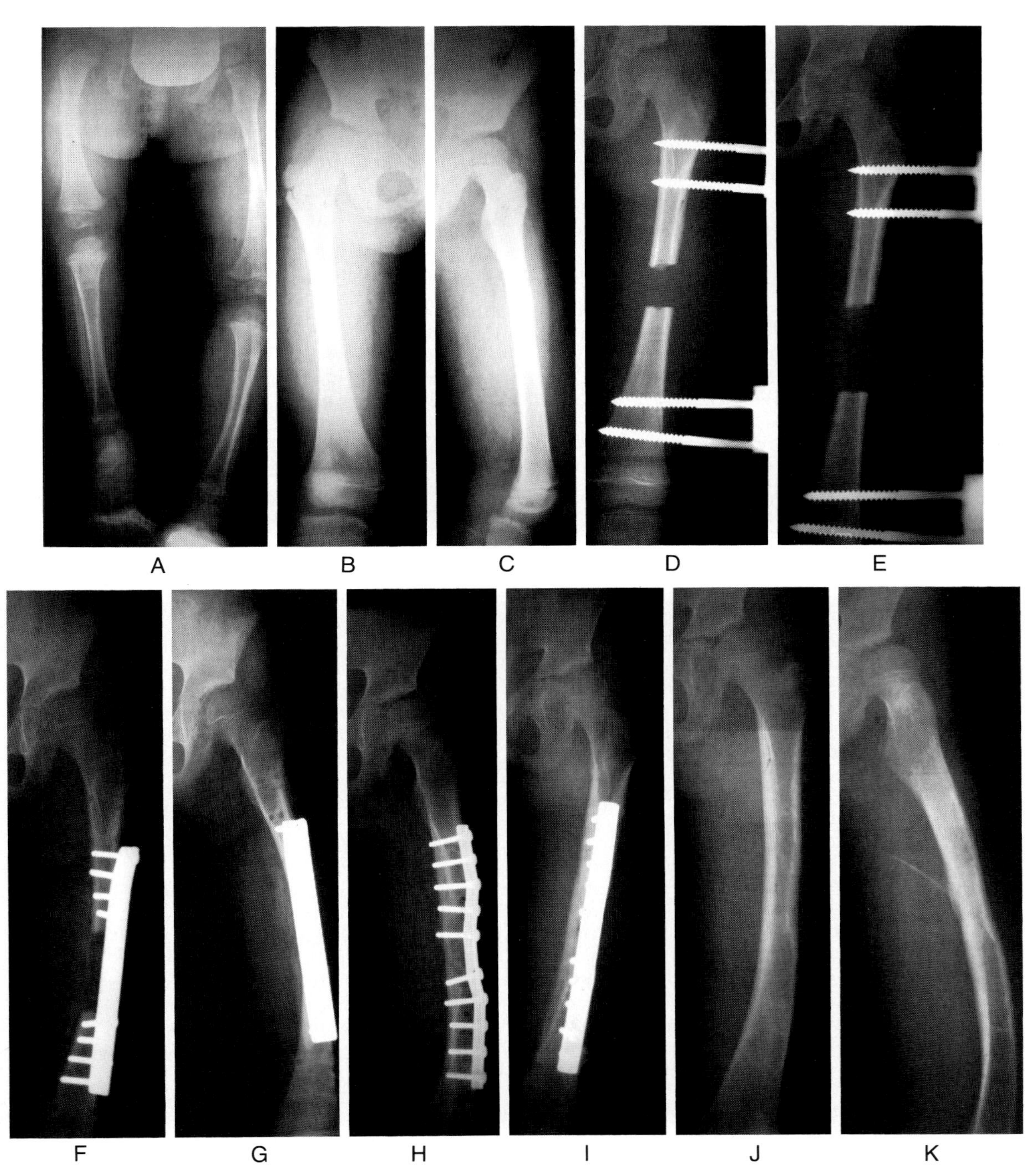

FIGURE 7–269. ***Wagner technique of diaphyseal lengthening in a congenital short femur.***

A. Anteroposterior radiogram of both lower limbs at age two years showing the congenital short left femur. **B** and **C.** Anteroposterior and lateral radiograms of the left femur at age seven years. Note that the hip is stable but that there is slight posterior subluxation of the knee joint with congenital absence of the anterior cruciate ligament. **D.** Fourteen days following femoral osteotomy and lengthening. **E.** Four weeks postoperative. Note the 6 cm. lengthening and the new bone formation in the elongated segment. **F** and **G.** Anteroposterior and lateral radiograms following plating with Wagner osteosynthesis plate and autogenous bone graft from the ilium. **H** and **I.** Seven months following surgery. Note that the Wagner osteosynthesis plate has been removed and replaced with a flexible semitubular plate. **J** and **K.** Three years postoperative anteroposterior and lateral radiograms of the left femur showing healing of the elongated segment. There is slight subluxation of the left hip, but the knee is stable.

Wagner Method of Femoral Lengthening

A and **B.** The Wagner limb-lengthening external distraction apparatus can be distracted or compressed by turning the handle at its upper end counterclockwise or clockwise. Screws inserted into the apparatus's holding pieces are anchored by bolts and washers. By tilting the holding pieces, realignment of 20 degrees in each direction is possible, for a total of 40 degrees. The screws (Schanz screws) act as a cantilever; they transmit force from the fixator body (which is not bulky) to the bone—in this specific case, the femur, osteotomized in its mid-diaphysis by open surgery. The use of unilateral pins decreases the extent of soft-tissue trapping and muscle fixation by the screws. Well-tolerated by most patients, the apparatus permits daily lengthening of the femur.

The Wagner limb-lengthening apparatus is available in two sizes. The large size is used for the femur in children and for the tibia in adults, and the small size is used for the tibia or upper limb in children.

C. After the desired length is achieved, the bone is plated with a specially designed rigid osteosynthesis plate, and the elongated segment is grafted with autogenous bone from the ilium. The external fixator is removed. When there is sufficient evidence of cortex formation on the opposite side of the plate and of medullary canalization, the rigid plate is removed and the elongated segment is internally fixed with a flexible semitubular plate. The final step of the Wagner technique is removal of the semitubular plate.

There are four phases of Wagner limb-lengthening. The first phase entails insertion of the Schanz screws; application of the distraction apparatus; mid-diaphyseal osteotomy; and lengthening. The second phase involves plating with the rigid osteosynthesis plate; grafting of autogenous iliac bone; and removal of the external distractor apparatus. The third phase consists of exchanging the rigid plate for a flexible semitubular plate. (The fourth phase, removal of the semitubular plate, is not illustrated here.)

Note: Limb-lengthening surgery should be preceded by extensive soft-tissue releases in the congenitally short limb (three to six months prior to lengthening).

In preparation for the first phase of Wagner femoral lengthening, the patient is placed in supine position, and the entire lower limb and ipsilateral pelvis are surgically prepped. The patient is so draped that the hip and knee can be freely manipulated through their full range of motion without contamination. A sterile folded sheet is placed under the knee to hold it in flexion, and to facilitate determination of the knee joint axis. Radiographic image intensification is utilized for proper orientation in placement of Schanz screw sites and level of osteotomy. The larger Wagner apparatus is used for femoral lengthening; it is placed on the lateral aspect of the thigh, where there is more space (and where the skin and soft tissues are relatively less sensitive) than on the medial side of the thigh.

The first phase of Wagner limb lengthening (D *to* W) *consists of screw insertion* (D *to* K); *apparatus application* (L); *osteotomy* (M *to* S); *and actual bone lengthening* (T *to* W).

Plate 115. Wagner Method of Femoral Lengthening

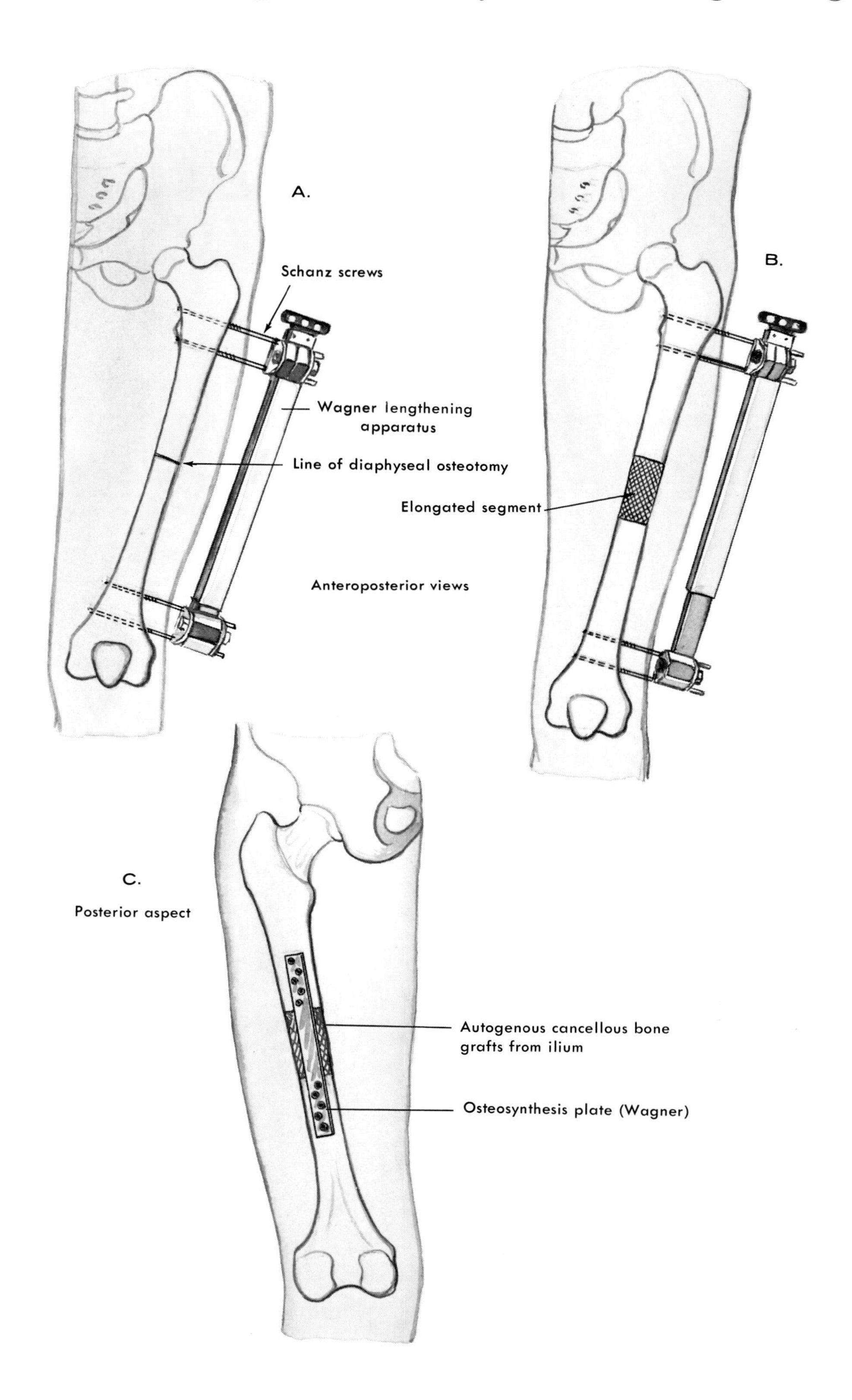

Wagner Method of Femoral Lengthening (Continued)

Percutaneous Insertion of Schanz Screws (D to K)

D. Two pairs of Schanz screws are inserted percutaneously, one pair distally at the supracondylar region of the femur, the other pair proximally at the level of the lesser trochanter. The screws should be far away from the center of the bone to allow adequate space for internal fixation later on. Caution should be exercised so as not to disturb the growth of the distal femoral physis or the greater trochanteric apophysis, if they are still open. Another factor to consider is the stability of screw anchorage on the cortex; the cortical thickness in the metaphyseal area should be at least one half of the thickness of the diaphyseal cortex. The direction of the screws is parallel to the knee joint axis. The most distal screw is inserted first. A 1- to 1½-cm.-long incision is made through the skin and subcutaneous tissues.

E. A second clean scalpel is used to divide the fascia lata longitudinally in the direction of its fibers. Upon flexion of the knee, the fascia lata moves posteriorly; therefore, a transverse incision extending anteriorly for 2 cm. is made in the fascia lata to provide adequate space for the screw, and to prevent mechanical pressure on the soft tissues. With Metzenbaum scissors or blunt scissors, the muscle fibers of the vastus lateralis are split longitudinally, deep to the bone. With a periosteal elevator, the aperture in the fascia lata and muscle fibers is enlarged, and the periosteum is split. The importance of the provision of adequate space around the screws cannot be overemphasized. Without such space, factors such as soft-tissue shift and mechanical pressure by the screw(s) will cause soft-tissue necrosis, and outside contamination of the necrotic tissue by the pin tract will lead to sepsis and drainage.

F. Now a drill sleeve is introduced through the incision. By touching the bone and identifying the anterior and posterior margins of the femoral cortex, the drill sleeve is placed exactly in the midlateral position. The posterior part of the femur should be left free for internal fixation with a plate. Because the lower Schanz screws will move distally with elongation of the limb, they are to be placed through the proximal end of the wounds. The drill sleeve should therefore be at the upper margin of the incision.

Plate 115. Wagner Method of Femoral Lengthening

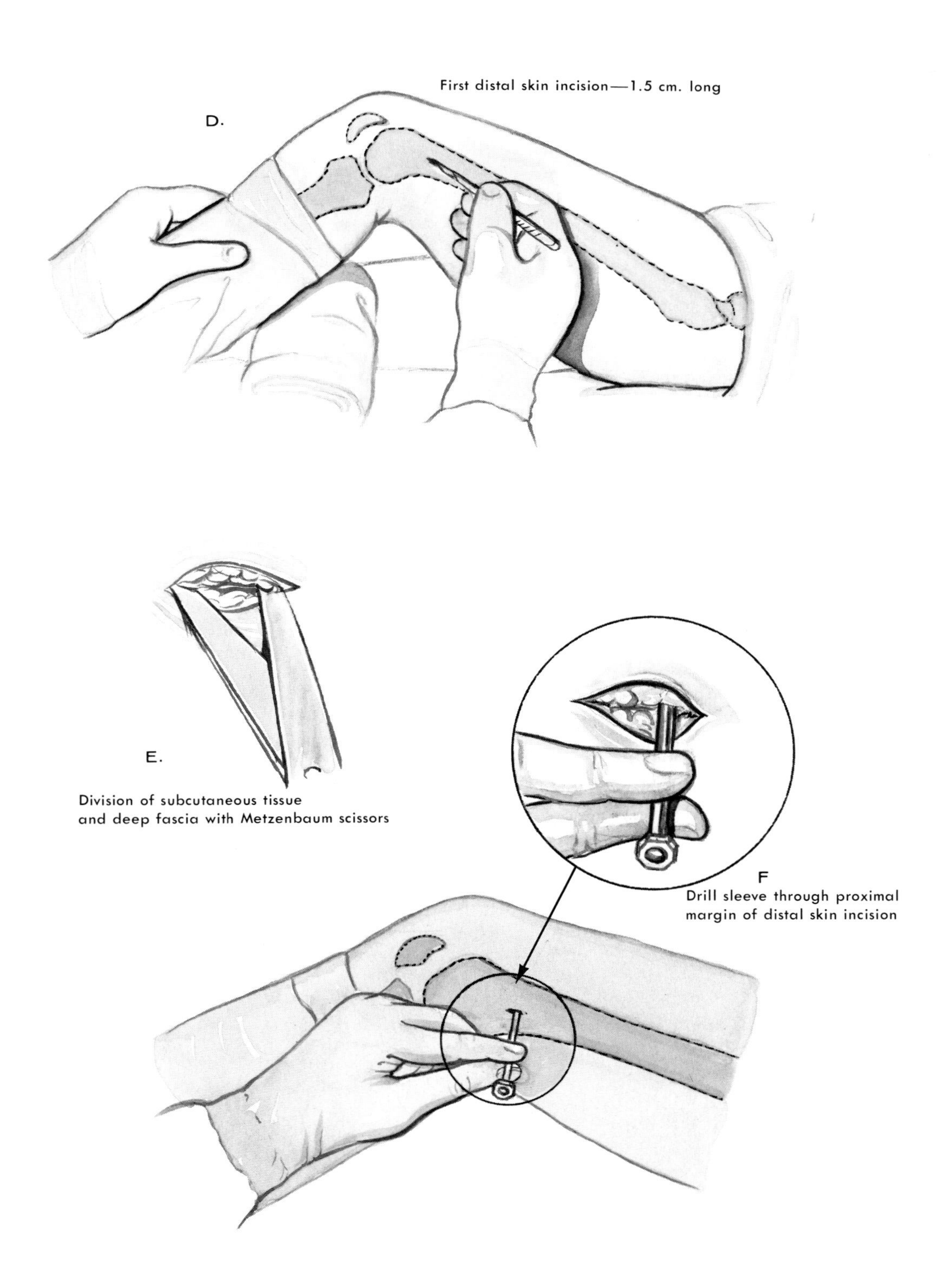

Wagner Method of Femoral Lengthening (Continued)

G. A hole for a Schanz screw is made with an electric drill through both cortices with a 3.6-mm. drill bit. The direction of the Schanz screw should be parallel to the axis of the knee joint.

H. A Schanz screw of adequate length is secured on a universal chuck. The end of this screw and of each succeeding screw should be 6 to 7 cm. away from the skin in order to allow 3 cm. of space between the skin and the holding piece of the Wagner apparatus. The ends of the screws should protrude 1 to 2 cm. from the holding piece to facilitate later removal. The Schanz screws are self-tapping. The "T" part of the handle of the universal chuck should be exactly parallel to the tip of the screw. Upon penetration of the medial cortex, the tip of the screw should be vertical (i.e., parallel to the longitudinal axis of the femur) for adequate anchorage of the threads of the screw on the medial femoral cortex in the direction of the distraction forces. Because the screw has no threads on its flat side, the screw should *not* be inserted in a horizontal position, in that the screw will have to penetrate deeper by two or three turns in order to have adequate bony purchase above and below. An additional problem is that the tip of the screw will irritate soft tissues and cause discomfort.

The drill hole is located blindly by moving the Schanz screw up and down. The Schanz screw is inserted. On penetration of the medial cortex, one can feel the tapping of the tip of the screw; as it goes through it, two additional turns are made and the chuck handle is removed.

I. With a drill guide, the correct site for placement of the second Schanz screw is determined. There are three holes in the drill guide; it is best to use the holes farthest apart for greatest stability. The holes in the drill guide are large enough to accommodate the Schanz screws. With a drill sleeve, the skin is marked for the site of insertion of the second screw. The drill guide is removed. An incision 1½ cm. long is made with the hole for the second Schanz screw in its upper end.

J. Following the details of technique described above, the second Schanz screw is inserted, parallel to the first screw, through the drill guide.

Plate 115. Wagner Method of Femoral Lengthening

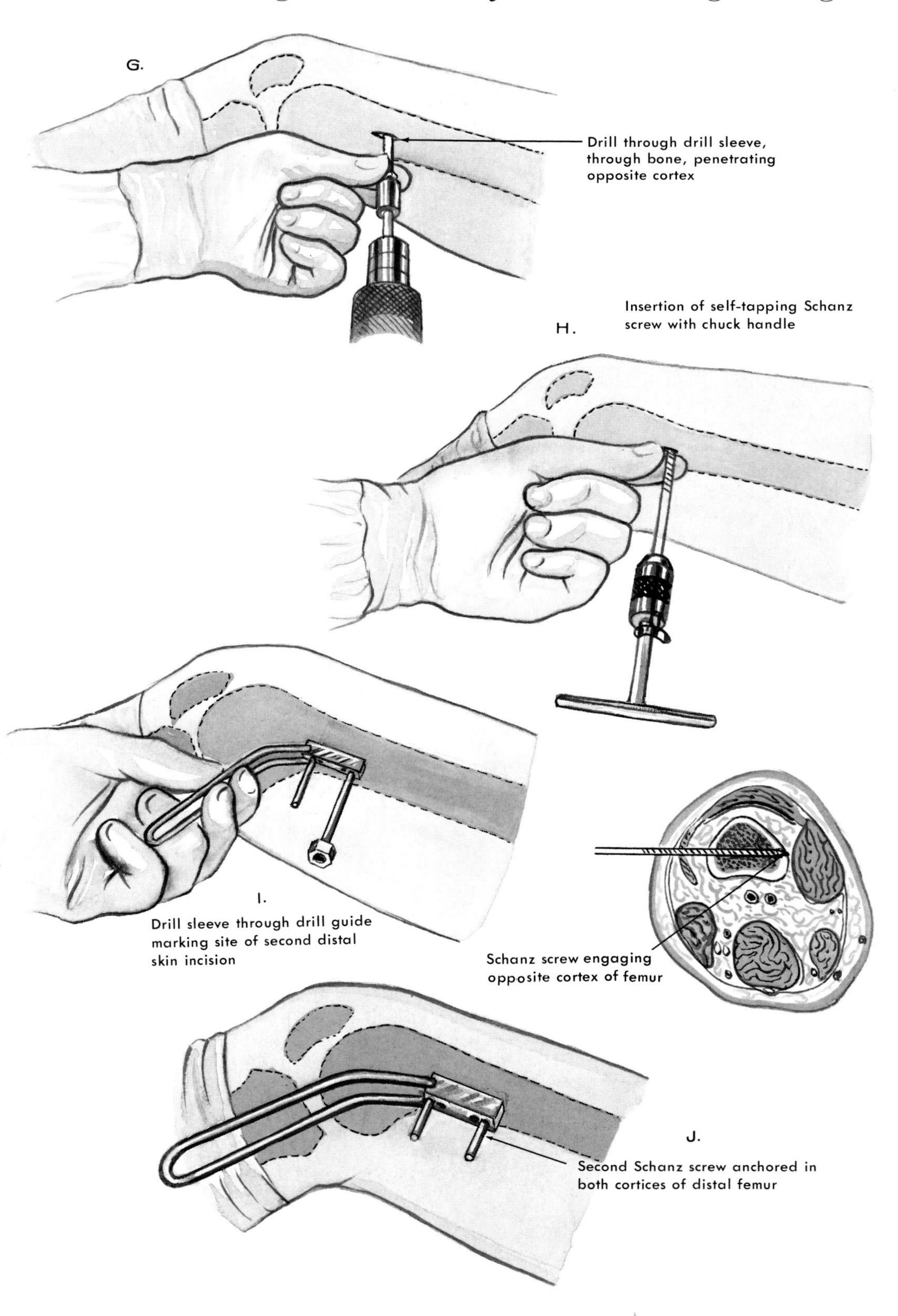

Wagner Method of Femoral Lengthening (Continued)

K. The technique covered above is utilized for the second pair of Schanz screws. The screws are anchored through the proximal femur at the level of the lesser trochanter. The uppermost screw is level with the upper half of the lesser trochanter. It should not penetrate too deeply, as it may hook the iliopsoas tendon and cause inability of the patient to sit. The position and length of the screw are double-checked by radiographic image intensification in anteroposterior and lateral projections, and adjustments are made if necessary.

The distal screws are always parallel to the axis of the knee joint, and normally, the proximal pair of screws are parallel to the distal pair. However, if rotational deformities are present, they can be corrected by changing the direction of the proximal pair of screws, keeping the distal pair always parallel to the knee joint axis. Angular deformities, valgus and varus, or anterior or posterior bowing can be corrected at the same time that the limb is lengthened, provided they are located in the center of the femoral shaft. As stated before, major deformities of valgus or varus, and those located near the hip or knee, should be realigned one or two years before limb lengthening to enable the soft tissues, muscle function, and bone structure to be restored to normal. When rotational realignment is corrected, the apparatus is applied after the osteotomy. In all other situations, the apparatus is applied *before* the osteotomy.

***Application of the Wagner Lengthening Apparatus* (L)**

L. Screws are inserted through the holes of the holding piece, preferably with the lateral tips of the screws protruding out of the lateral margin of the holding piece by 1½ to 2 cm. When fluid gets inspissated between the holding piece and the screws, it may be difficult to disconnect them unless the tips of the screws are protruding. Also, there should be enough space (2 to 3 cm.) between the skin and the apparatus to prevent skin pressure. Remember: When the patient is awake and sits down, the soft tissues become more protuberant and bulkier than when the patient is positioned for surgery and under anesthesia. One must be sure that the skin does not touch the apparatus. Proximally, the handle of the apparatus should be well clear of the greater trochanter and pelvis.

Now the lengthening apparatus is connected to the holding piece and covered with the washer, and the bolt tightened. Attention should be paid to the length of the apparatus, and to whether there is the required distance between the two holding pieces for telescoping when the limb is lengthened. For femoral lengthening, the apparatus is applied anteriorly with the holes for the screws posteriorly, giving adequate space for posterior exposure of the femur. The bolts are tightened to prevent sliding of the holding piece. The Schanz screws have a diameter of 6 mm.; if subjected to distraction forces, the screws may bend. Upon elongation, the upper screw is subjected to tension forces and the lower screw to compression forces; elongation may thus cause the screws to move or at least shift. Therefore, it is imperative to tighten the nuts firmly to increase stability and guarantee the security of the fixation of the screws to the apparatus. To achieve this, an AO screwdriver (with a 5.6-mm. diameter) or a long Schanz screw is placed into the additional free hole of the holding piece; with a wrench on the nut the two instruments are firmly closed together manually. This provides a very firm fixation of the screws to the holding piece and to the apparatus. The bolts are tightened. Sterile gauze (moistened with Betadine solution) is split and straddled around the screws. Blood should not seep into the holes of the apparatus.

To liberate entrapped tissues such as the vastus lateralis and the fascia lata from the screws, the knee is manipulated into full flexion. This is very important, because otherwise active exercise will be painful. Distraction is applied on the apparatus by turning the handle counterclockwise three to five times, and again the knee is flexed fully.

***Transverse Osteotomy of the Femoral Shaft* (M *to* S)**

M. With the knee at 45 to 90 degrees of flexion, the hip is flexed, medially rotated, and adducted for a posterolateral approach to the femoral shaft. If the hip is ankylosed, it cannot be flexed and medially rotated; in such a case, the patient is appropriately draped so that he can be turned from the supine position, which allows the Schanz screws and apparatus to be applied, to a lateral position, permitting a posterior approach to the femur. (A prone position is not recommended for the patient because the soft tissues will shift when he is turned back to the supine position, and will cause problems.) A 7- to 10-cm.-long longitudinal incision is made, centered between the upper and lower pairs of Schanz screws over the interval between the vastus lateralis and the biceps femoris, about four finger-breadths posterior to the Schanz screws. The linea aspera is almost subcutaneous in this location. The subcutaneous tissue and deep fascia are divided in line with the skin incision.

Plate 115. Wagner Method of Femoral Lengthening

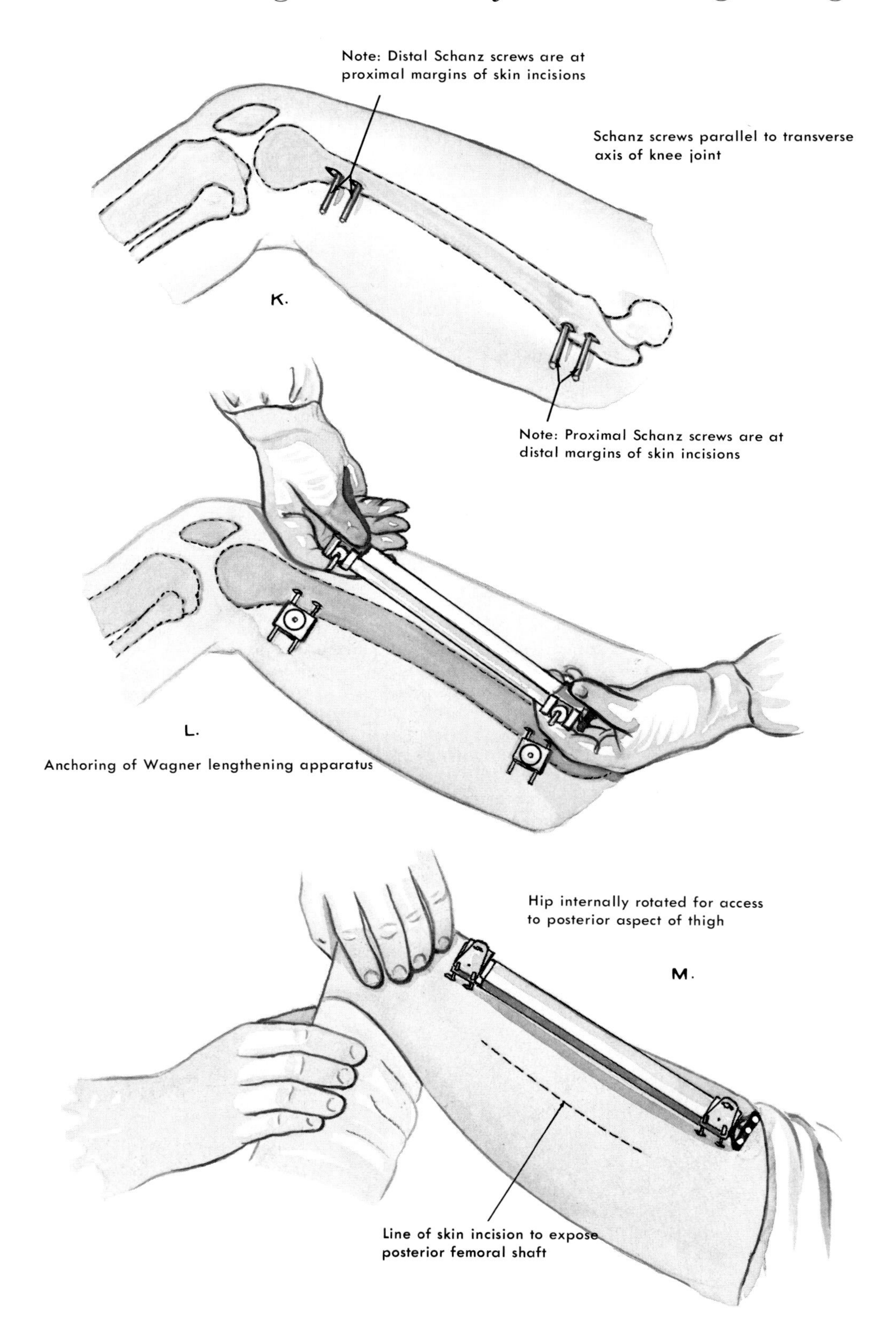

Wagner Method of Femoral Lengthening (Continued)

N. The vastus lateralis muscle is gently elevated from the lateral intermuscular septum and retracted anteriorly with two Hibbs retractors. The periosteum is longitudinally divided. With the help of a sharp periosteal elevator, two large Chandler elevators are inserted subperiosteally to expose the anterior and lateral aspects of the femoral shaft.

O. Exposure of the posterior aspect of the femur may cause troublesome hemorrhage from the perforating vessels. Bleeding can be avoided if sharp osteotomes and a mallet are used to elevate part of the cortical wall with the periosteum. Exposure of the posterior aspect of the femur by such decortication prevents injury to the vessels.

P. Two large Chandler elevators are placed posteriorly; adequate space is provided for a reciprocating saw by twisting the elevators. The level of femoral osteotomy should be midway between the two pairs of Schanz screws. This is measured with a ruler to ensure that there are equally long bone fragments for internal fixation. The periosteum is thin in the adolescent and not important in bone healing; it is sectioned transversely at the level of the osteotomy. If the periosteal tube is left intact, it will tear during distraction and may be the source of pain.

Plate 115. Wagner Method of Femoral Lengthening

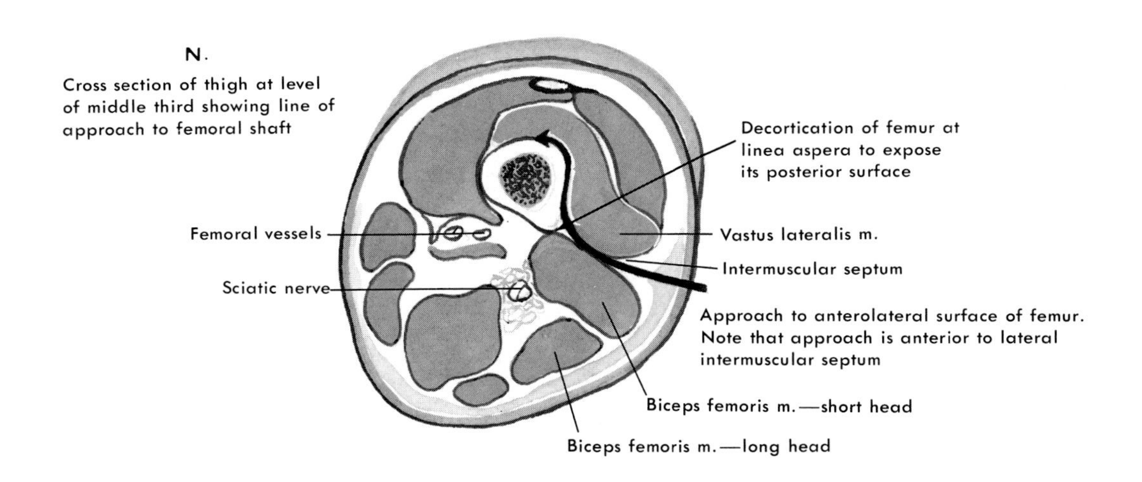

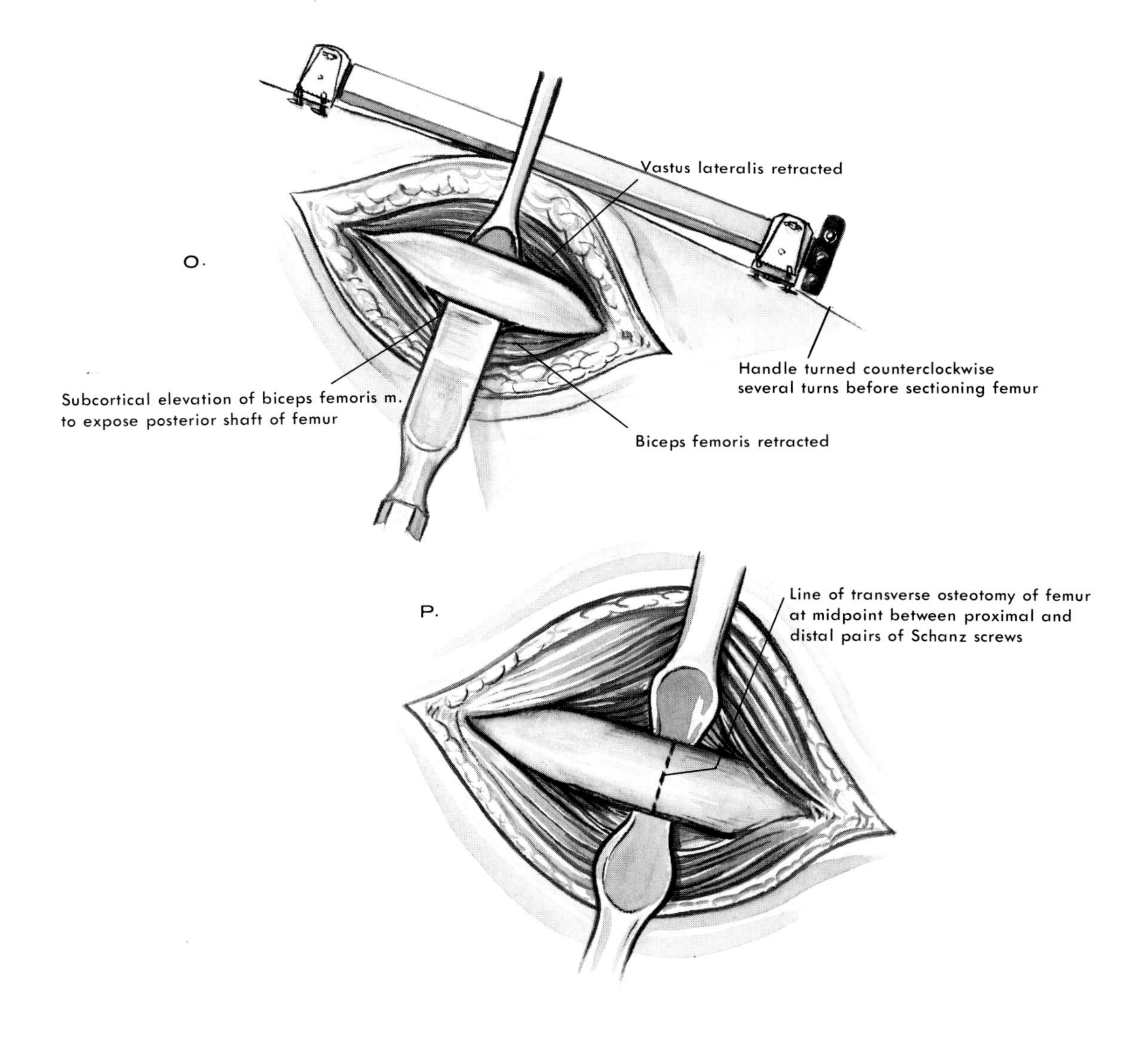

Wagner Method of Femoral Lengthening (Continued)

Q. To put the femur under further tension just before the osteotomy is performed, the handle at the upper end of the apparatus is turned counterclockwise a couple of turns. Then, with an electric reciprocating saw, a transverse osteotomy is made through the femoral shaft under normal saline irrigation. Z-pattern osteotomies or other complicated geometric configurations are not recommended. Upon completion of the osteotomy, the previously applied tension on the femur provides further stability and prevents malalignment. In the past, the handle on the limb-lengthening apparatus was turned counterclockwise several more turns, elongating the femur by 10 to 15 mm. The resulting soft-tissue tension further stabilized the osteotomized fragments and prevented painful contact between bone ends.

At present, this author recommends corticotomy as described by Ilizarov (Plate 119) and DeBastiani (Plate 117) and not osteotomy with a reciprocating saw. Do not disturb the endosteal blood supply! The lengthening of the femur is begun three to five days postoperatively.

R and **S.** The knee is flexed fully once or twice. The osteotomy site is drained by two closed-suction tubes. The fascia lata and the wound are closed in the usual fashion; the skin is closed with a subcuticular running 00 nylon suture. A fine mesh gauze is applied over the incision. The soft tissue channels around the Schanz screws are reinspected to ensure that there is no mechanical pressure. Elastic compression by Ace bandage dressing is applied. Final radiograms are made in the operating room to double-check the anatomic alignment of the femoral fragments. Any angular or axial deviation is corrected by realigning the Schanz screws and the holding piece in their anchorage to the lengthening apparatus. Fixation by the Wagner limb-lengthening apparatus is very stable, and external support by plaster of Paris cast is not necessary. The knee, ankle, and hip can be moved freely.

Plate 115. Wagner Method of Femoral Lengthening

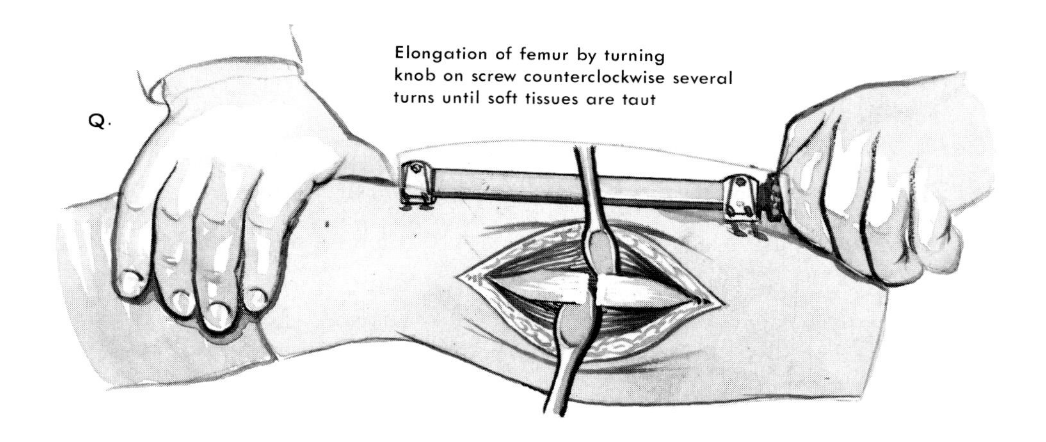

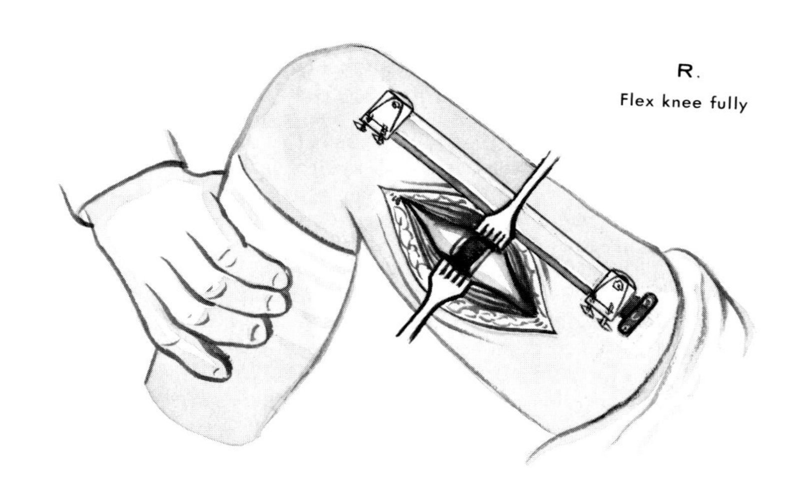

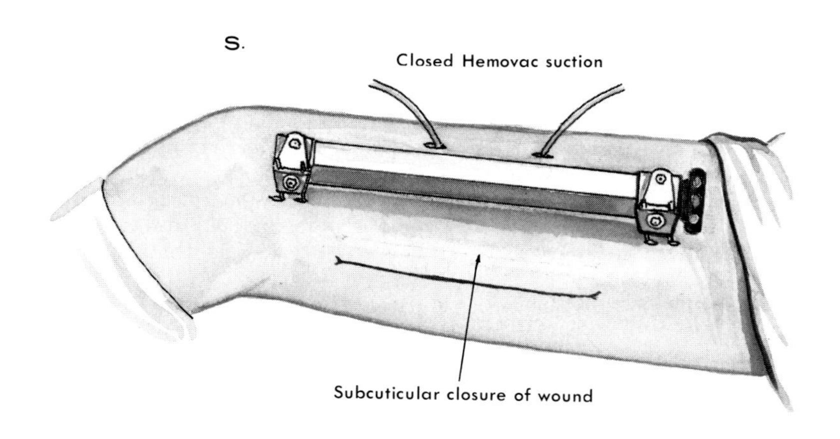

Wagner Method of Femoral Lengthening (*Continued*)

***Daily Lengthening of the Femur; Exercise Program; Wound Care* (T *to* W)**

T. Limb lengthening is carried out by the patient himself under direct supervision of the surgeon, the orthopedic nurse, or the parents. Initially it is preferable to keep the patient in the hospital for close observation. Ten to 14 days postoperatively the patient is discharged from the hospital, provided that he is reliable and can be observed closely as an outpatient. When problems and complications develop, he is readmitted to the hospital. (No special attire is required; many patients undergoing femoral lengthening can even wear blue jeans, "customized" only in that they are split on the lateral side of the femur.)

The knob is turned counterclockwise a quarter-turn at a time; six quarter-turns per day (to distract) and two quarter-turns clockwise once a day (to compress) provide a gain of 1.5 mm. of length per day, or 1.0 cm. per week. Function of the limb should be maintained during the process of limb lengthening. *Function is never sacrificed for length.*

U to **W.** The patient is instructed to walk with crutches in a three-point gait with partial weight-bearing on the lengthened limb. He is allowed to be up and around one or two days postoperatively. The amount of body weight borne should not exceed the weight of the limb distal to the site of the osteotomy. Falls should be avoided. Suction-drainage tubes are removed two days after surgery. Physical therapy is directed toward maintaining a functional range of knee motion. If the knee cannot be actively flexed more than 60 degrees, or if loss of complete knee extension is greater than 15 degrees, limb lengthening is discontinued. Exercises are kept up to increase range of knee motion; if a range of 60 degrees of knee flexion is reobtained, limb lengthening is resumed. If functional range of knee motion cannot be restored after two weeks of exercises, limb lengthening is stopped and internal fixation is carried out. (It should be explained to the patient and family that after two or three years, a limb lengthening can be repeated.) One cannot overemphasize the need for preservation of joint function. Experience has shown that, if the limits of the arc of knee motion (60 degrees of knee flexion to minus 15 degrees of knee extension) are maintained within a year, the full range of knee motion will be recovered. Individuals with ligamentous laxity do not usually present a problem. The difficulty is with those patients with congenital shortening of the femur and those with stiff joints. Should persistent flexion contracture of the knee develop, it may be corrected by fractional lengthening of the hamstrings. A hip adductor myotomy may be required in an occasional case if the hip adductors are very taut and pull the distal femoral segment into varus deformity. These soft-tissue releases are performed with the Wagner apparatus still anchored to the femur. If major soft-tissue contractures are corrected one year prior to femoral lengthening, one usually is not confronted with these problems.

Exercises are performed twice a day. The exercises are active and gravity-assisted; passive and forceful exercises are avoided, because overly aggressive exercise programs will cause irritation of the soft tissues by the Schanz screws, especially the distal ones. Manipulation of the knee with the patient under general anesthesia is fraught with danger and is not recommended except in occasional situations. Side-lying knee flexion-extension utilizes the principle of reciprocal innervation of agonist-antagonist muscles. On active flexion of the knee, the quadriceps muscle relaxes.

The most useful exercise—especially if the patient is relaxed (even listening to music or reading a book)—is sitting knee flexion, assisted by gravity forces.

The channels in the soft tissue around the Schanz screws are kept clean the first three postoperative days by application of Betadine solution three times a day. Thereafter, sponges dipped in alcohol are used for cleaning three times a day. (Professor Wagner does not apply any dressings as of two or three days postoperatively, and uses an antibiotic spray.)

There is a large amount of soft tissue coverage on the lateral aspect of the thigh, and soft tissues do shift. The distal screws in the femur can cause trouble by exerting mechanical pressure on the soft tissues. The screws migrate through the incision during the course of distraction. The lower screws migrate distally; the upper screws migrate proximally. As soon as the screws touch or press the opposite ends of the skin, the skin incision should be enlarged.

Any swelling, inflammatory reaction, or pain calls for emergency relief of mechanical pressure and tension in the soft tissues. The problem area is sterilized with a disinfectant such as Betadine solution and anesthetized. An incision then made with a scalpel will relieve pain, allow swelling to subside and prevent pin tract infection. Limb lengthening is actually not painful; whenever the patient develops pain, the screw tracts must be inspected. Schanz screws removed because of infection should be replaced with screws inserted at more distal or proximal sites. Replacement will require general anesthesia and radiographic control.

Radiograms obtained at weekly intervals may reveal bending of screws due to tension. Commonly, tension pulls the distal femoral segment into adduction, sometimes posteriorly,

Plate 115. Wagner Method of Femoral Lengthening

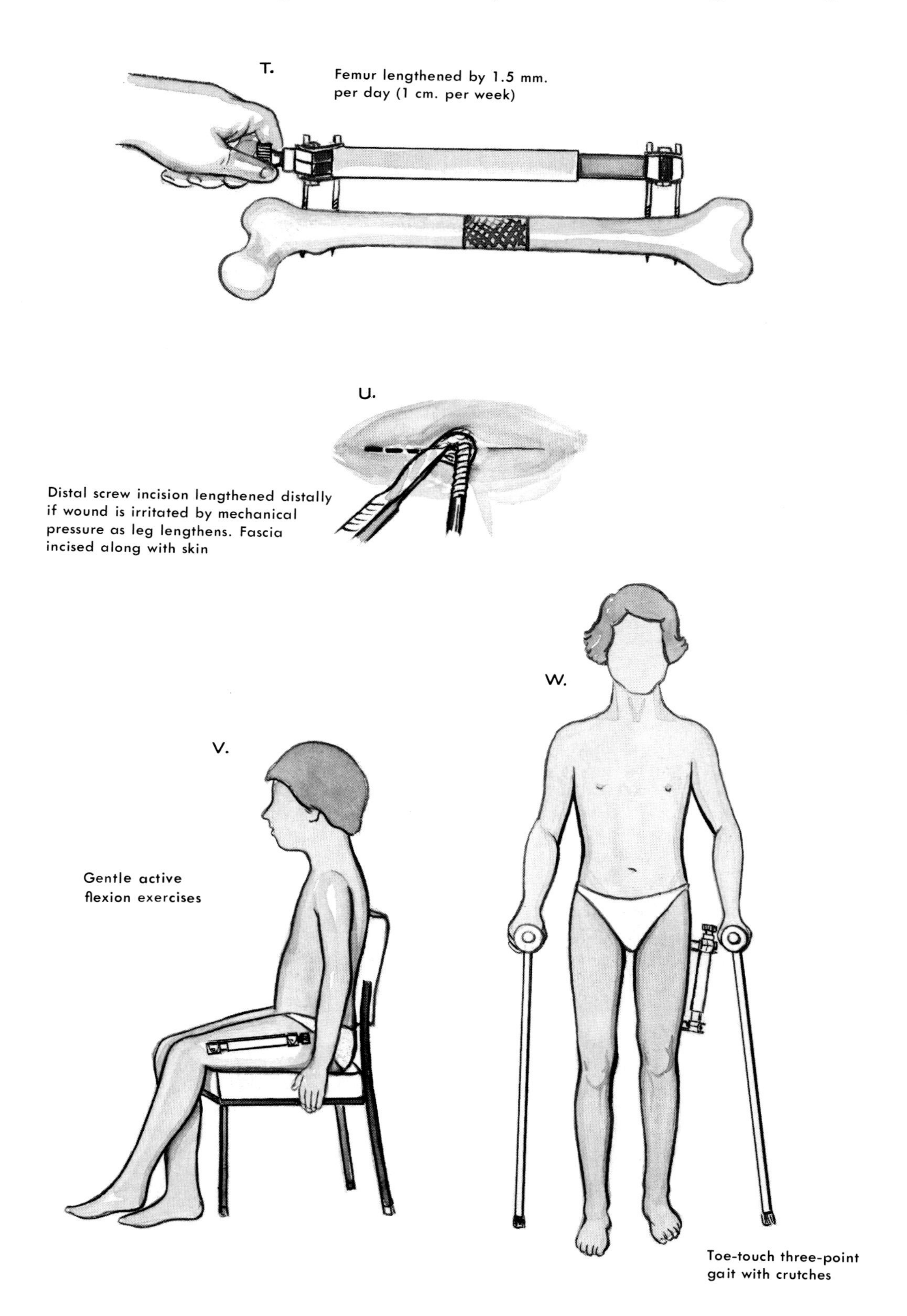

Wagner Method of Femoral Lengthening (*Continued*)

causing lateral or anterior bowing of the femur. If the angular deformity is less than 20 degrees, realignment can be performed at the time of internal fixation. However, if the varus deformity is greater than 20 degrees, the soft tissues do not elongate on the medial side, becoming instead progressively tauter and causing greater varus. In such an instance, it is best to realign during the period of distraction. In the cooperative and mature patient, general anesthesia is not required. With the patient supine and his knee in full extension, gentle traction (of about 10 to 15 lb.) is applied on the lower leg. Clockwise turns on the handle of the lengthening apparatus will decrease its distraction force to zero. The distal nuts are then opened, and the bone segments are realigned by adjusting the screws and the holding piece of the apparatus. Since straightening makes the femur longer, a further compensatory decrease in distraction force may be necessary. If medial soft tissues are taut, a slight overcorrection into some valgus may be desirable. Realignment is double-checked by radiograms. A long radiopaque pin may be used as an index to radiographic distortion, especially when image intensification is used. Tightening the nuts will once again secure stability of the fragments. If there is medial or lateral displacement of the fragments, the distal nuts are opened and the screws are shifted medially or laterally for proper realignment. When there is anterior or posterior bowing, the distal bolts are loosened and the upper end of the distal segment is tilted posteriorly or anteriorly.

After realignment, distraction is applied gradually; the original length is reobtained within 24 to 48 hours. Measurements of length made with a Bell Thompson ruler on leg-length scanograms are preferred over readings from the scale on the limb-lengthening apparatus (the latter is not reliable because of elasticity of the screws). The true length obtained may be 1 or 2 cm. shorter than the amount registered on the scale.

At the completion of the required lengthening, radiograms are carefully studied for evidence of malalignment (varus or valgus, anterior or posterior bowing) and for clues to the adequacy of the callus at the elongation site.

*The second phase of Wagner limb lengthening (*X *to* EE*) involves osteosynthesis by plating, to which bone grafting may or may not be added.*

If there is continuity of bone between the femoral fragments, there is a possibility of spontaneous consolidation. In such an instance, desired length is maintained and physical therapy is continued. The decision as to internal fixation by plating should be made at the end of distraction, and should not be delayed for two or three months, when local wound conditions and bone atrophy may make osteosynthesis by plating very difficult. There are a number of alternatives available: (1) keeping external fixation by the apparatus until spontaneous consolidation has taken place; (2) internal fixation with plating but without bone grafting; and (3) internal fixation with plating and with simultaneous bone grafting. Factors determining the option chosen are the surgeon's expertise, local wound conditions, the adequacy of consolidation and callus as seen on the radiograms, and the stability of the fragments.

If it is decided not to plate—i.e., to allow spontaneous consolidation with external fixation by the apparatus—a minimal compression force is applied by turning the handle clockwise a few quarter-turns. Pin tract care is continued. At four weeks, radiograms are again obtained. If healing and stability are adequate, compression force is applied and increasing weight-bearing permitted. Up to a 2-cm. loss in length is allowed on the scale of the limb-lengthening apparatus. A greater than 2-cm. loss in length will result in instability of fixation, collapse of the callus, and loss of alignment. When there are signs of homogeneous canalization of the medullary cavity and of normal cortication (it will take 9 to 12 months for these signs to appear), the Wagner apparatus and screws are removed. First, the Wagner apparatus is removed; the Schanz screws are left in place. Stress is applied on the screws. If stability of the elongated segment is demonstrated, the screws are removed.

Ordinarily, immediate plating upon completion of limb lengthening is recommended; it is reliable and less fraught with potential problems.

Plate 115. Wagner Method of Femoral Lengthening (Repeat of Parts T, U, V, and W)

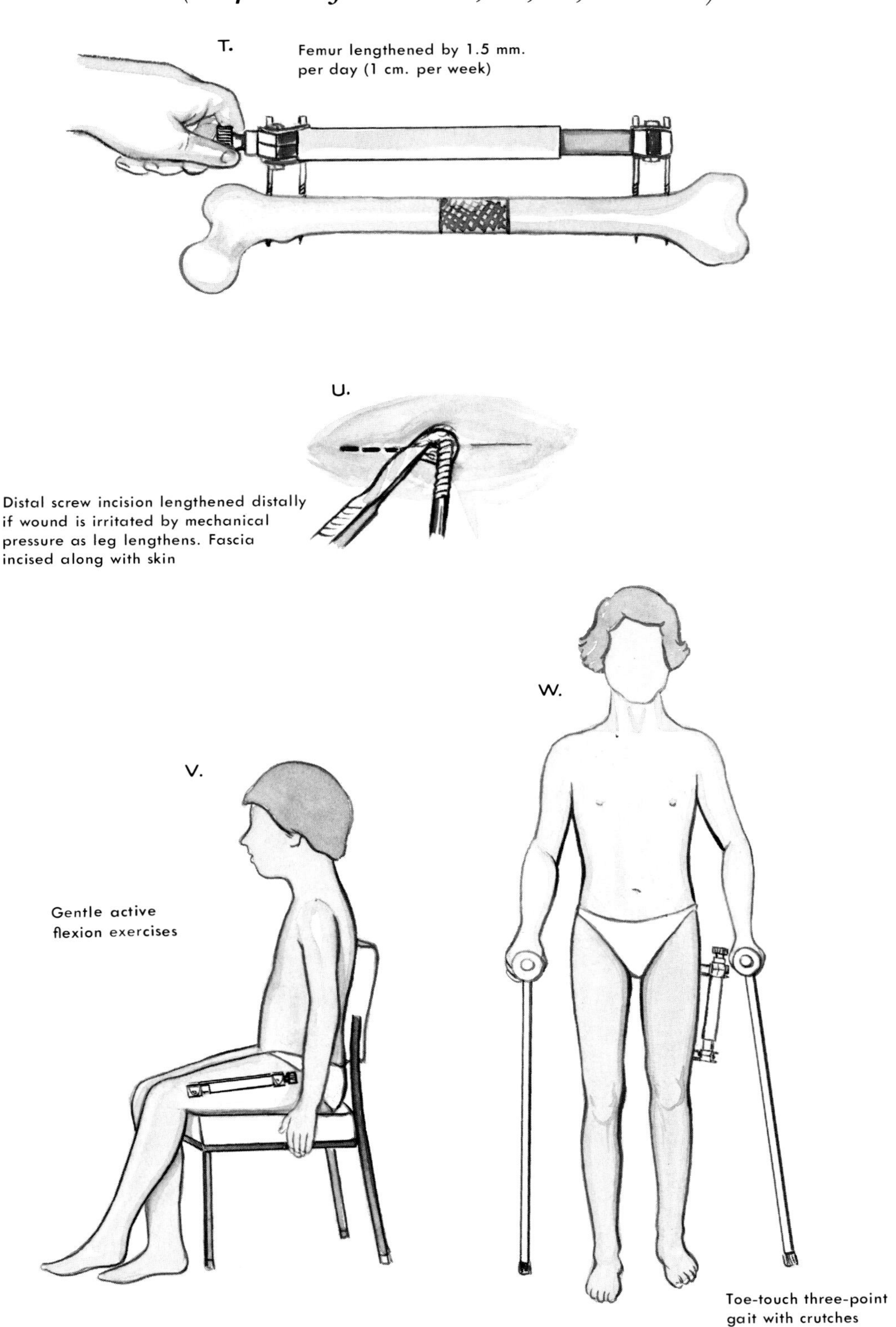

Wagner Method of Femoral Lengthening (Continued)

X. The patient is placed in a prone position under general anesthesia. The pin tracts are carefully cleansed and shielded. The entire lower limb is surgically prepared; then the Wagner apparatus is draped out with elastic Ace bandage(s) and self-adhering drape(s). For a second time, the entire lower limb and pelvis are surgically prepared; the posterior ilium, from which bone grafts are to be obtained, should be in the sterile field. It is imperative to pay utmost attention to antisepsis. The draping should be done in such a way that the surgeon can reach the handle of the lengthening apparatus and make necessary adjustments during surgery. The previous skin incision is used for exposure of the posterior aspect of the femur. The scar is excised. The subcutaneous tissue and deep fascia are divided in line with the skin incision.

Y. The lateral intermuscular septum and vastus lateralis are gently retracted anteriorly, and the biceps femoris is retracted posteriorly. In the course of the surgical approach *the screw tracts, sealed in fibrous granulation tissue, should not be opened,* as they are potentially contaminated. Excessive callus, if present on the linea aspera, is removed tangentially with an osteotome in order to provide a flat surface for attachment of the plate.

Z and **AA.** The femoral segments are connected with an osteosynthesis plate. Designed by Professor Wagner, the plate is wide, sturdy, and relatively rigid. The plate has five holes proximally and five holes distally, with an intervening solid segment that straddles the elongated femoral segment. The screw holes are close together and obliquely zig-zagged, making it possible to insert five screws instead of four. The intervening solid part comes in varying lengths, depending upon the extent of lengthening.

Plate 115. Wagner Method of Femoral Lengthening

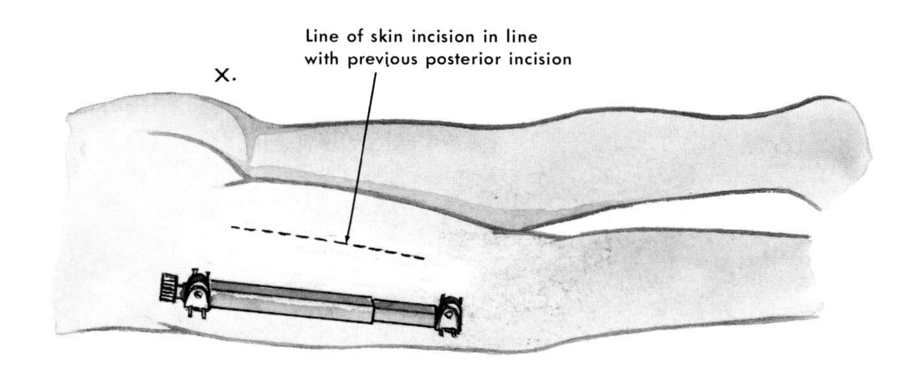

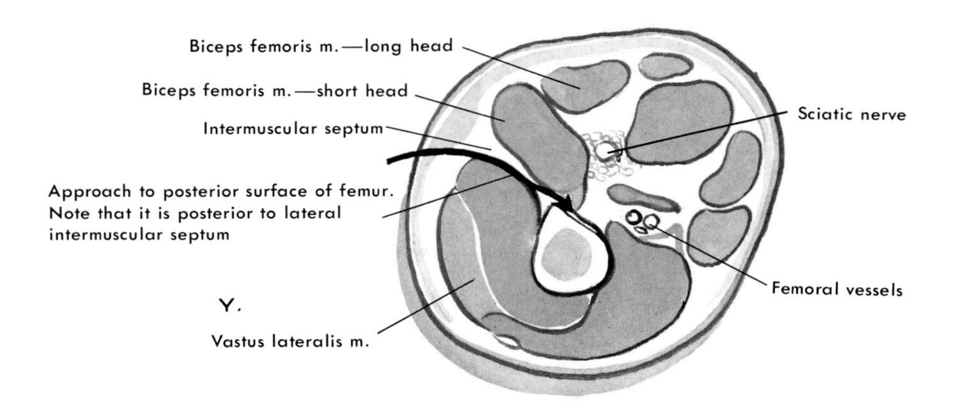

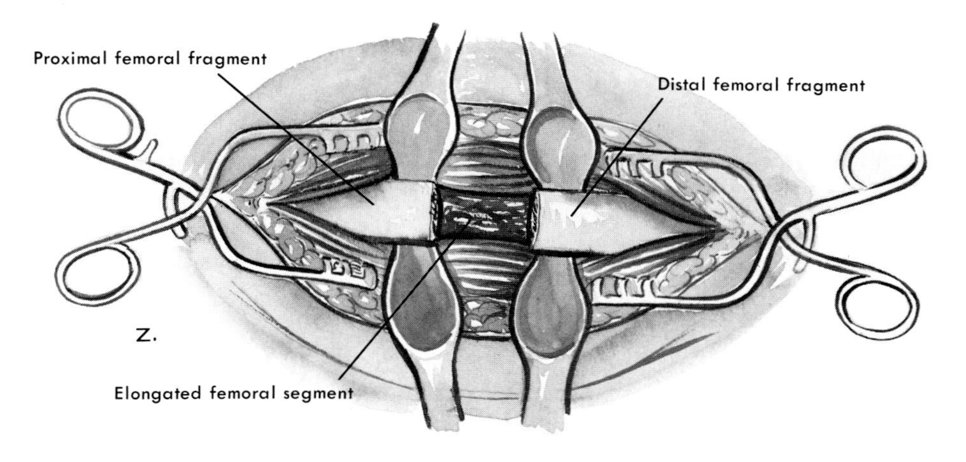

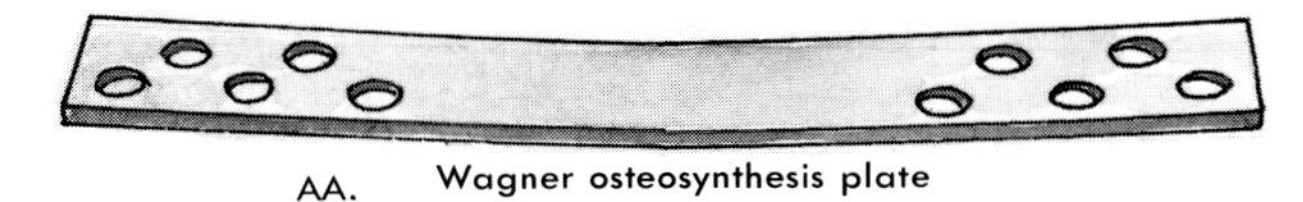

AA. Wagner osteosynthesis plate

Wagner Method of Femoral Lengthening (Continued)

BB. The plate should be applied on the *posterior* aspect of the femur; if the plate is secured on the lateral aspect of the femur, bending into varus deformity will ensue. By application of the plate on the posterior aspect of the femur, the adduction forces are on the lateral edge of the plate. It is important to bend the plate with its convexity anteriorly into antecurvatum. The muscle forces acting at the weak elongated segment of the femur tend to bend the plate posteriorly. If the plate is bent forward and placed on the posterior surface of the femur, the muscle forces will tend to straighten the plate and make it longer, but these effects are offset by the resistance of the soft tissue. The counter-tensions thus prevent untoward bending of the plate.

CC. The plate is securely fixed to the femur with screws in the usual fashion. If the distraction gap is filled with hyperemic cartilaginous tissue, bone grafting is not necessary. If the tissue in the elongated segment is fibrous and exhibits no hyperemia, it is best to bone graft. This author recommends bone grafting to expedite consolidation.

DD and **EE.** Strips of autogenous cancellous bone, harvested from the ilium, are used for onlay bone grafting. Closed-suction drainage tubes are inserted, the wound is closed in the usual fashion, and the Wagner elongation apparatus is then removed. Within 24 to 48 hours, the patient is allowed to be up and around with the help of crutches and to begin partial weight-bearing on the lengthened limb. Knee exercises are continued. Increased weight-bearing is permitted as the radiograms disclose progressive healing. Full weight-bearing is allowed when the medullary cavity shows complete homogeneous canalization and when a thick cortex is remodeled in the wall of the elongated segment opposite the plate. Then, after a month or two, the plate is removed. If after one year the cortical wall is not of solid density and the medullary canal is not homogeneously canalized, it is best to replace the rigid plate with a smaller semi-flexible AO plate to prevent a stress fracture at the distal or proximal end of the rigid plate. The rigid plate protects the elastic femur from biological forces, but excessive stress protection may cause fatigue fracture. By exchanging plates, the incidence of fatigue fracture is greatly diminished.

Plate 115. Wagner Method of Femoral Lengthening

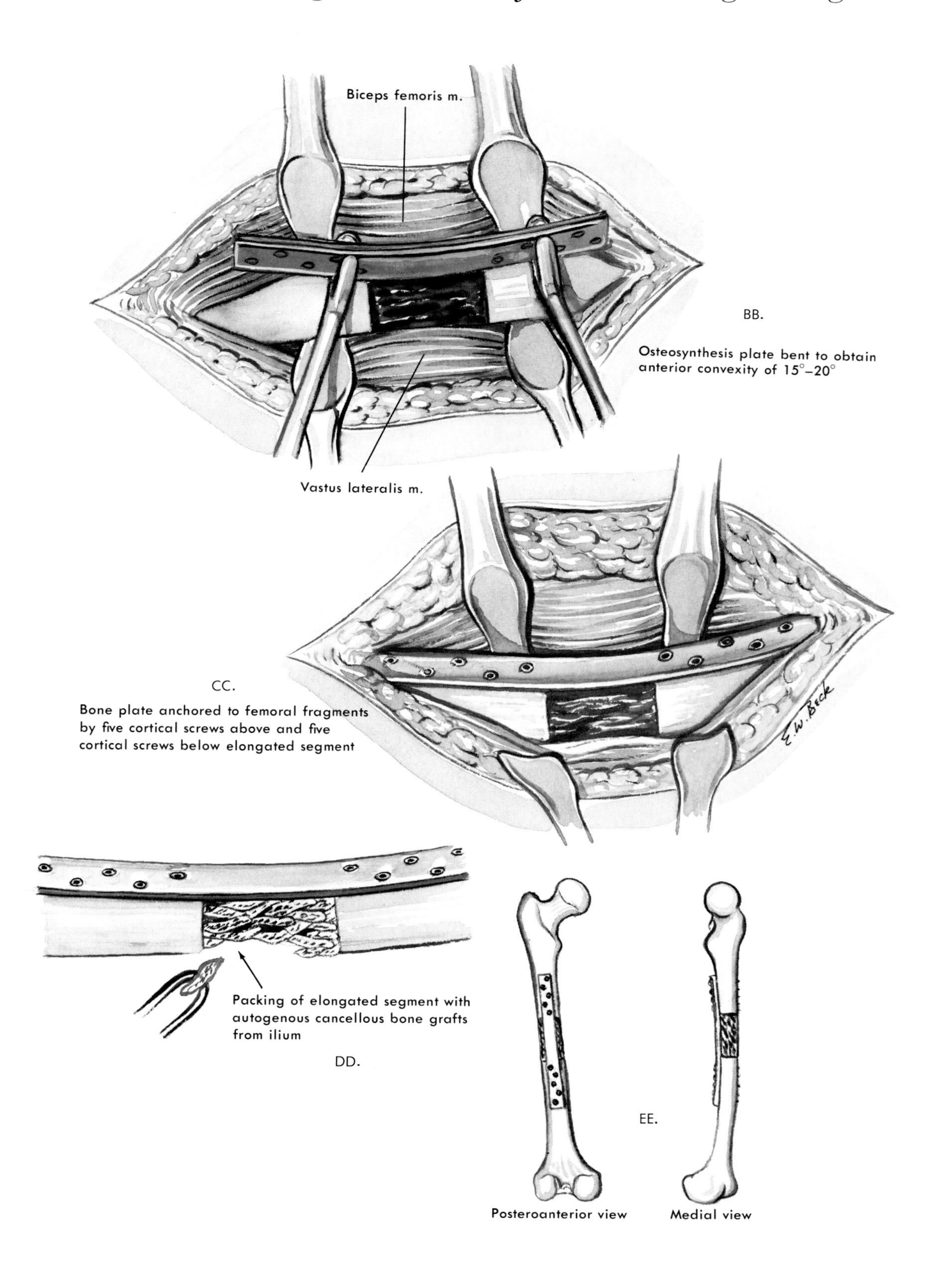

Wagner Method of Femoral Lengthening *(Continued)*

The third phase of Wagner limb lengthening entails exchanging the rigid plate for a flexible semitubular plate.

The Wagner rigid osteosynthesis plate is exchanged for a flexible semitubular plate 9 to 12 months postoperatively provided there is strong cortex formation on the opposite side of the plate and there is canalization of the medulla. It is imperative to change the plate to prevent stress fractures above and below the rigid plate. The semitubular plate is removed three to six months later.

With the patient placed in prone position, the elongated lower limb and hip are prepared and draped sterile in the usual fashion.

FF. The previous skin incision on the posterolateral aspect of the femur is used for exposure of the femur. The subcutaneous tissue and deep fascia are divided in line with the skin incision. The lateral intermuscular septum and vastus lateralis are retracted anteriorly. The biceps femoris muscle is retracted and elevated posteriorly, exposing the posterior surface of the femur and the rigid plate and screws. The screws and plate are removed. The screw holes are curetted, and with the help of sharp osteotomes and rongeurs, all the bony ridges are removed, preparing the bed for the semitubular plate.

GG. The semitubular plate is placed on the posterolateral aspect of the femur immediately next to the site of the rigid plate. First, the top screw is inserted, then the distal one.

Plate 115. Wagner Method of Femoral Lengthening

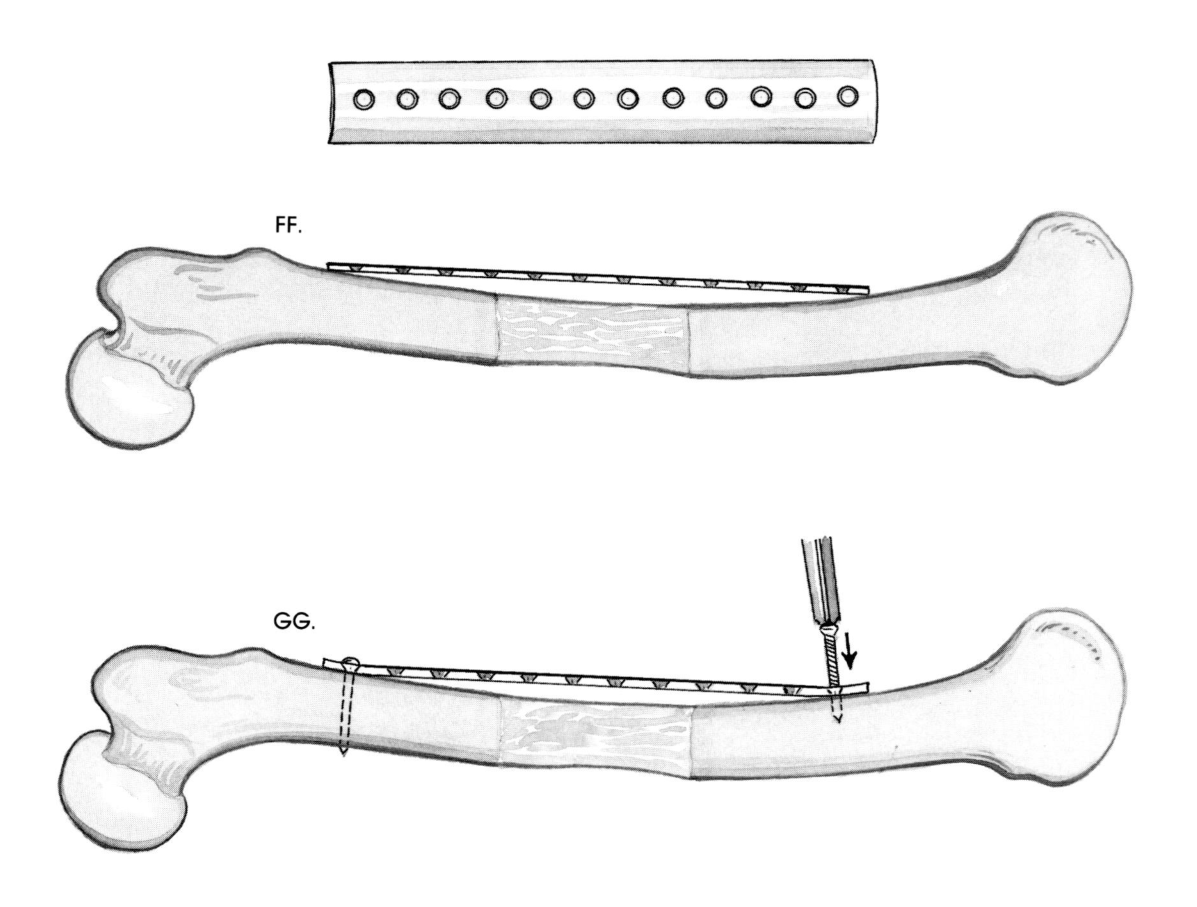

Wagner Method of Femoral Lengthening *(Continued)*

HH and **II.** Then the other screws are inserted anchoring the plate to the femur. Anteroposterior and lateral radiograms are made to check the position of the plate and screws. The wound is copiously irrigated with normal saline solution and is closed in the usual fashion. The patient is discharged to home within a few days with a three-point crutch gait protecting the elongated limb.

Plate 115. Wagner Method of Femoral Lengthening

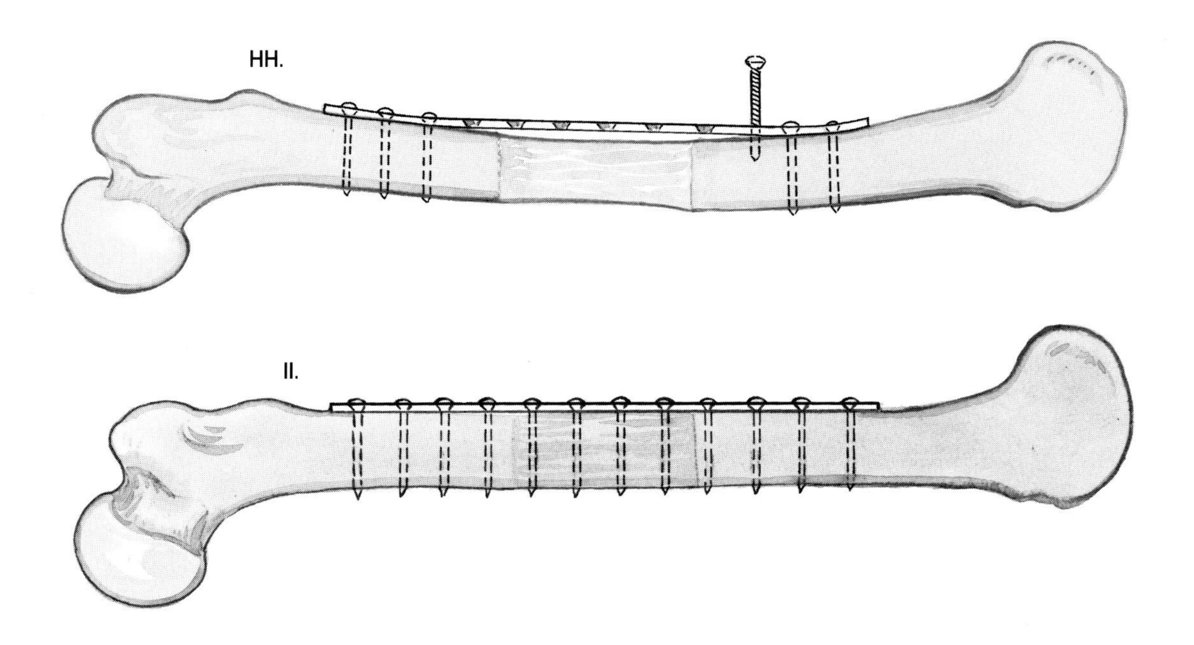

Wagner's Tibial Diaphyseal Lengthening

Tibial lengthening differs from femoral lengthening in a few respects.

OPERATIVE TECHNIQUE

A to **C.** In tibial lengthening, the apparatus is applied on the anteromedial aspect of the leg, where skin is less sensitive and the tibia is subcutaneous. Because of the thinness of the soft-tissue coverage, pin tract problems are minimized. The tibia is not, of course, the only bone affected by tibial lengthening. Since the traction forces of the bars of the apparatus pull on the soft tissues, the distal physis and proximal physis of the fibula must be protected. Bony fusion of the distal tibia and fibula is not recommended, because the resultant rigidity of the ankle mortise will cause degenerative arthritis of the ankle later in life. Therefore, the fibula is transfixed to the tibia by two cortical screws immediately above and below the osteotomy site; these are positional screws with threads penetrating all four cortices, preventing approximation of osteotomized fibular segments to the tibia. The positional screws are removed after bone healing.

The tibial lengthening apparatus is *not* put on distraction prior to division of the fibula. Rather, the fibula is first divided and then tension force is applied on the apparatus (after which the tibia is osteotomized). As the apparatus is on the medial aspect of the leg, tethering forces of the intact fibula will cause valgus deviation of the osteotomized tibial segments.

Anterior angulation and pressure on the skin are problems created by the strong pull of the triceps surae muscle; therefore, it is best to fix the tibial segments in slight posterior angulation after the initial osteotomy. It is vital to check alignment very closely; frequent adjustments may be required in order to prevent anterior bowing and valgus deformity.

Plate 116. Wagner's Tibial Diaphyseal Lengthening

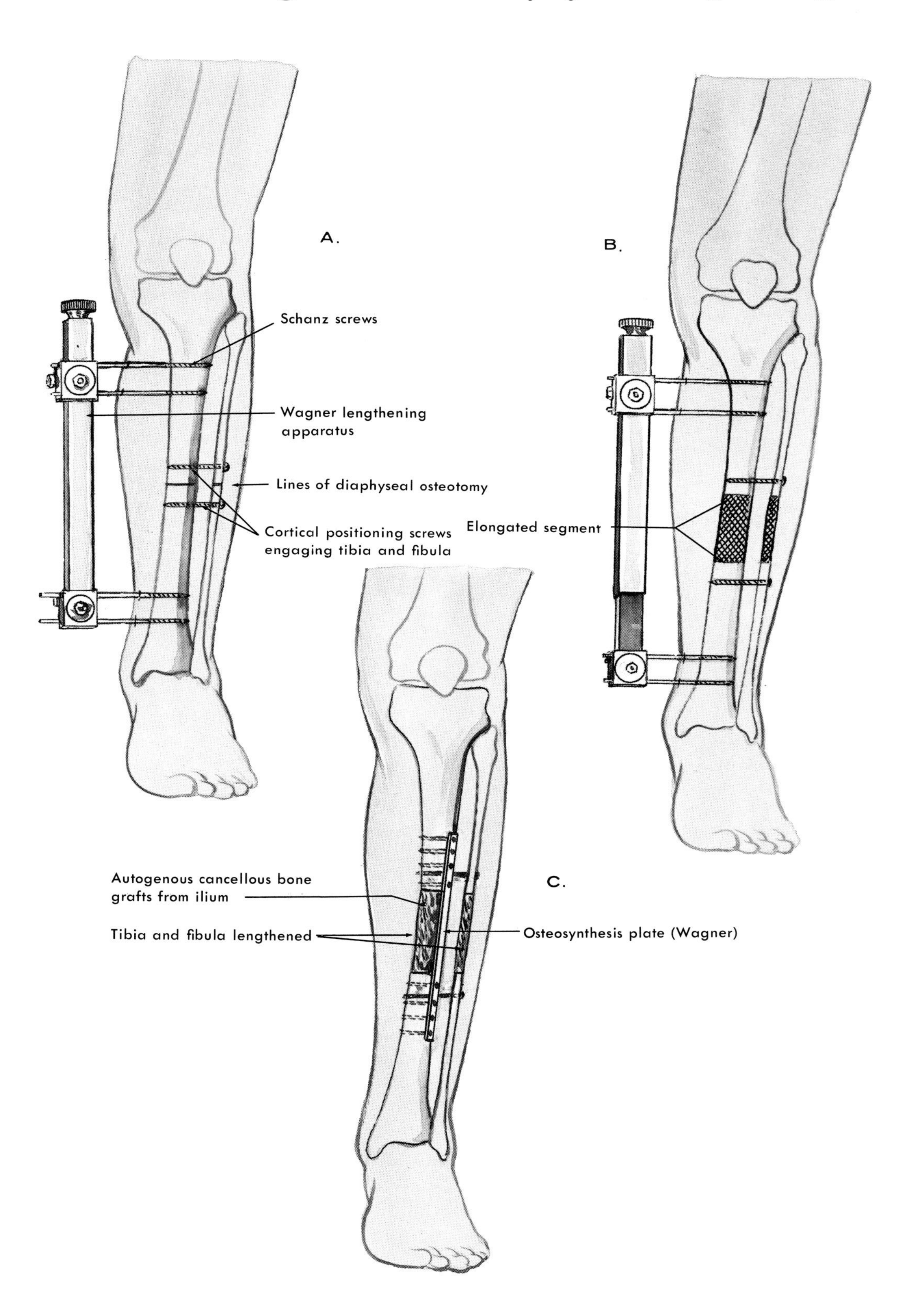

Wagner's Tibial Diaphyseal Lengthening (Continued)

The first phase of Wagner's tibial diaphyseal lengthening procedure entails insertion of Schanz screws (D *to* M); *application of the apparatus* (N *and* O); *osteotomy* (P *to* W); *and lengthening* (Z *and* AA).

D to **O.** Under image intensifier x-ray control, two pairs of Schanz screws are inserted parallel to the knee and ankle joint axes through medial incisions into the proximal and distal ends of the tibial metaphysis. The technique is similar to that described for femoral lengthening. The upper Schanz screws are distal to the proximal tibial tubercle. The proximal physis and distal physis of the tibia must not be injured. Additionally, staying a distance of 2 cm. from the growth plate will provide safety from pin tract infection. The position and depth of the screws are checked on anteroposterior and lateral radiograms. The tibial lengthening apparatus is applied posteriorly to provide space anteriorly for surgical exposure of the tibial shaft. Tension forces are not applied on the apparatus at this stage.

Plate 116. Wagner's Tibial Diaphyseal Lengthening

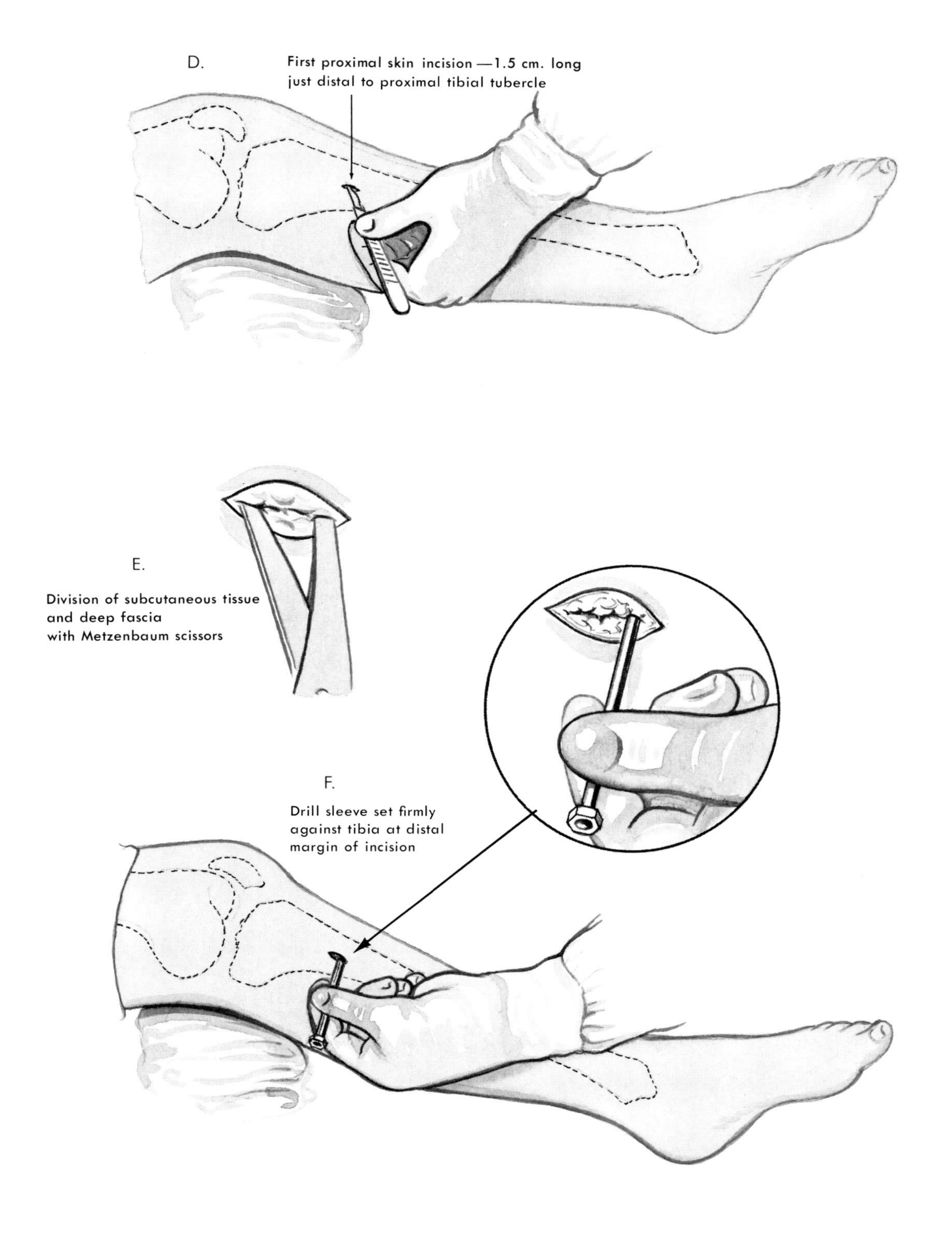

Wagner's Tibial Diaphyseal Lengthening (*Continued*)

The first phase of Wagner's tibial diaphyseal lengthening procedure entails insertion of Schanz screws (D *to* M)*; application of the apparatus* (N *and* O)*; osteotomy* (P *to* W)*; and lengthening* (Z *and* AA).

D to **O.** Under image intensifier x-ray control, two pairs of Schanz screws are inserted parallel to the knee and ankle joint axes through medial incisions into the proximal and distal ends of the tibial metaphysis. The technique is similar to that described for femoral lengthening. The upper Schanz screws are distal to the proximal tibial tubercle. The proximal physis and distal physis of the tibia must not be injured. Additionally, staying a distance of 2 cm. from the growth plate will provide safety from pin tract infection. The position and depth of the screws are checked on anteroposterior and lateral radiograms. The tibial lengthening apparatus is applied posteriorly to provide space anteriorly for surgical exposure of the tibial shaft. Tension forces are not applied on the apparatus at this stage.

Plate 116. Wagner's Tibial Diaphyseal Lengthening

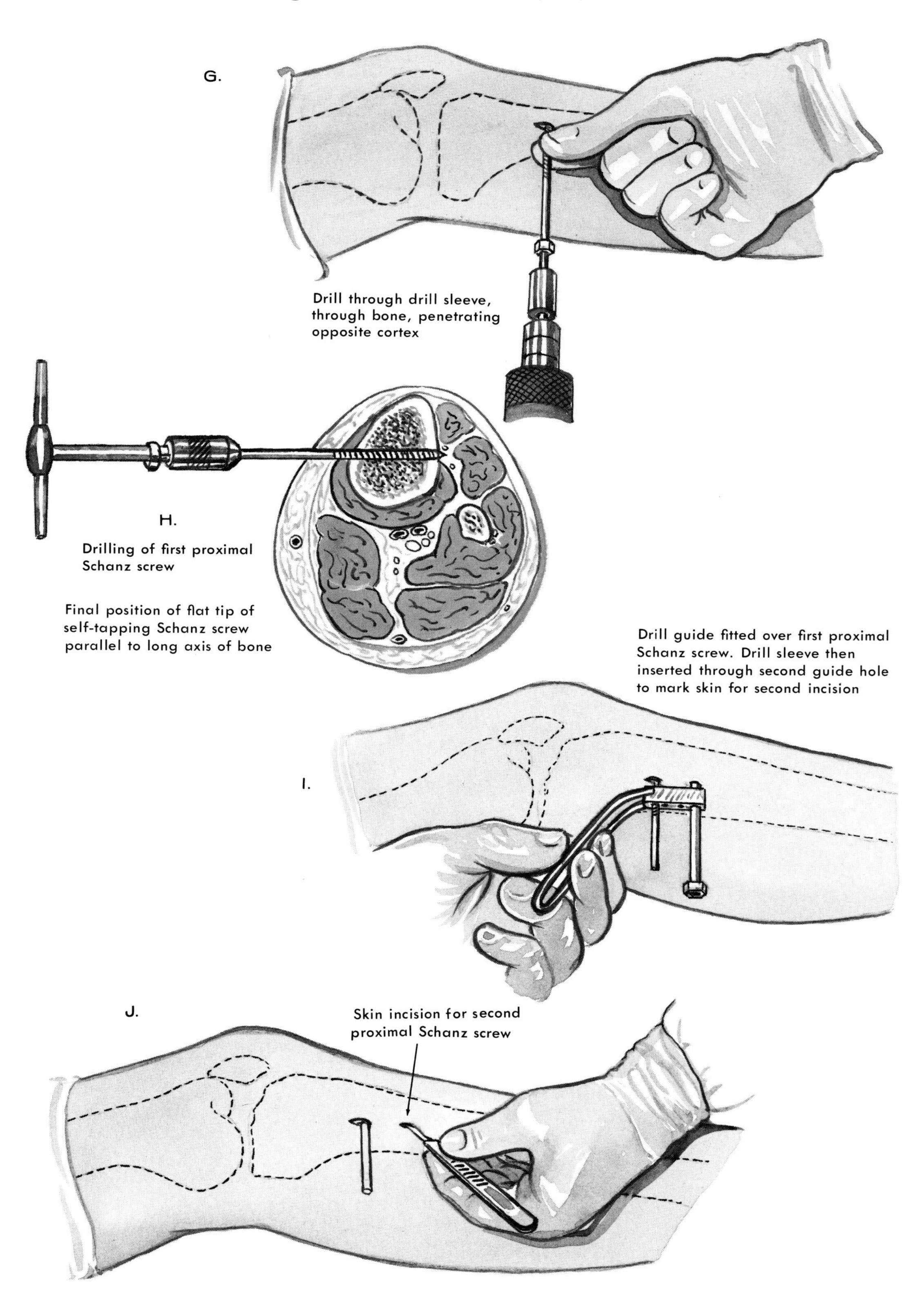

Wagner's Tibial Diaphyseal Lengthening (*Continued*)

The first phase of Wagner's tibial diaphyseal lengthening procedure entails insertion of Schanz screws (D *to* M)*; application of the apparatus* (N *and* O)*; osteotomy* (P *to* W)*; and lengthening* (Z *and* AA).

D to **O.** Under image intensifier x-ray control, two pairs of Schanz screws are inserted parallel to the knee and ankle joint axes through medial incisions into the proximal and distal ends of the tibial metaphysis. The technique is similar to that described for femoral lengthening. The upper Schanz screws are distal to the proximal tibial tubercle. The proximal physis and distal physis of the tibia must not be injured. Additionally, staying a distance of 2 cm. from the growth plate will provide safety from pin tract infection. The position and depth of the screws are checked on anteroposterior and lateral radiograms. The tibial lengthening apparatus is applied posteriorly to provide space anteriorly for surgical exposure of the tibial shaft. Tension forces are not applied on the apparatus at this stage.

Plate 116. Wagner's Tibial Diaphyseal Lengthening

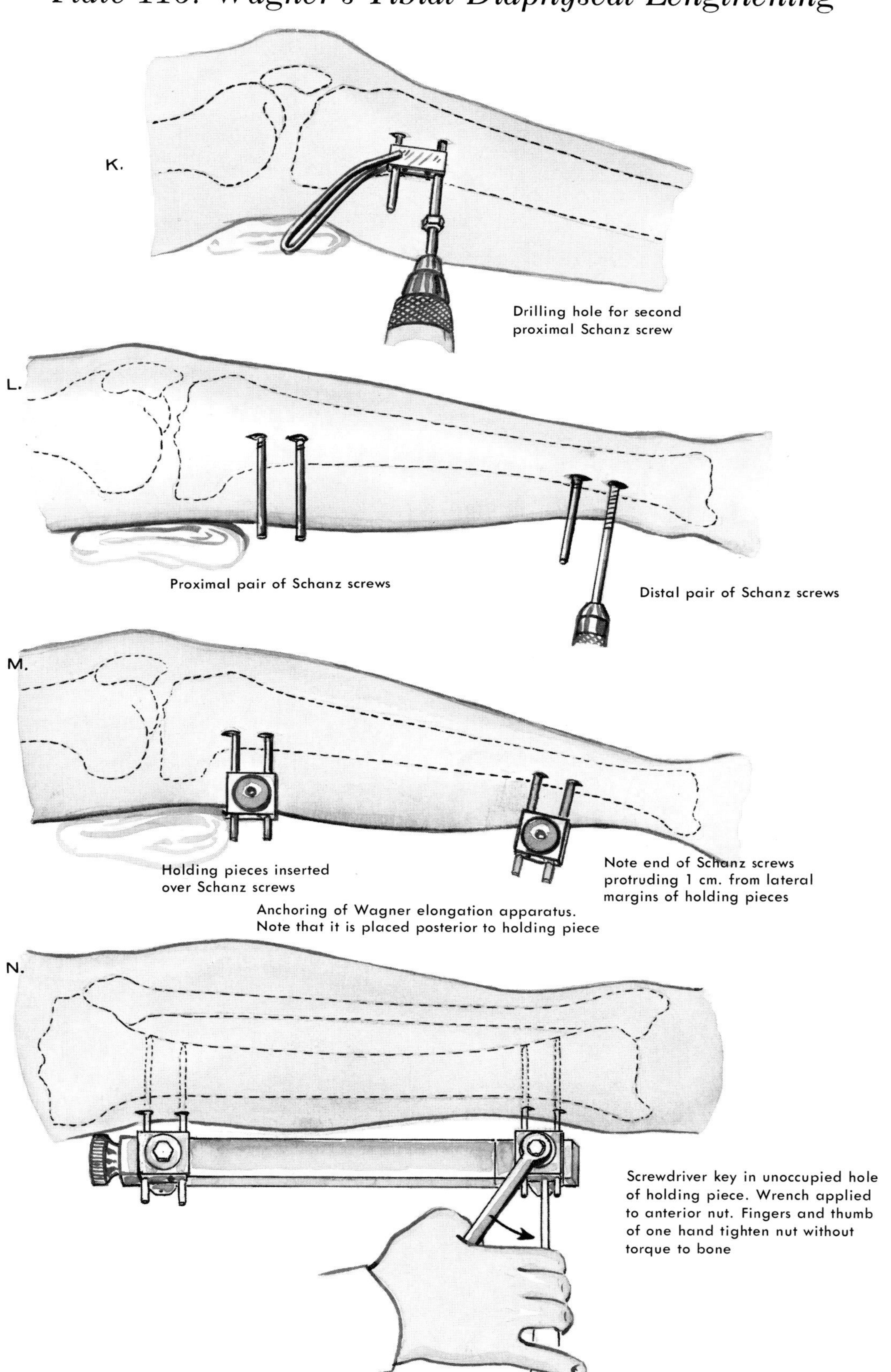

Wagner's Tibial Diaphyseal Lengthening (*Continued*)

The first phase of Wagner's tibial diaphyseal lengthening procedure entails insertion of Schanz screws (D *to* M); *application of the apparatus* (N *and* O); *osteotomy* (P *to* W); *and lengthening* (Z *and* AA).

D to **O.** Under image intensifier x-ray control, two pairs of Schanz screws are inserted parallel to the knee and ankle joint axes through medial incisions into the proximal and distal ends of the tibial metaphysis. The technique is similar to that described for femoral lengthening. The upper Schanz screws are distal to the proximal tibial tubercle. The proximal physis and distal physis of the tibia must not be injured. Additionally, staying a distance of 2 cm. from the growth plate will provide safety from pin tract infection. The position and depth of the screws are checked on anteroposterior and lateral radiograms. The tibial lengthening apparatus is applied posteriorly to provide space anteriorly for surgical exposure of the tibial shaft. Tension forces are not applied on the apparatus at this stage.

P. A 7- to 10-cm. longitudinal incision is made in the middle third of the fibula. The subcutaneous tissue and fascia are divided in line with the skin incision.

Q. The peroneal muscles are gently elevated from the posterior intermuscular septum and retracted anteriorly.

Plate 116. Wagner's Tibial Diaphyseal Lengthening

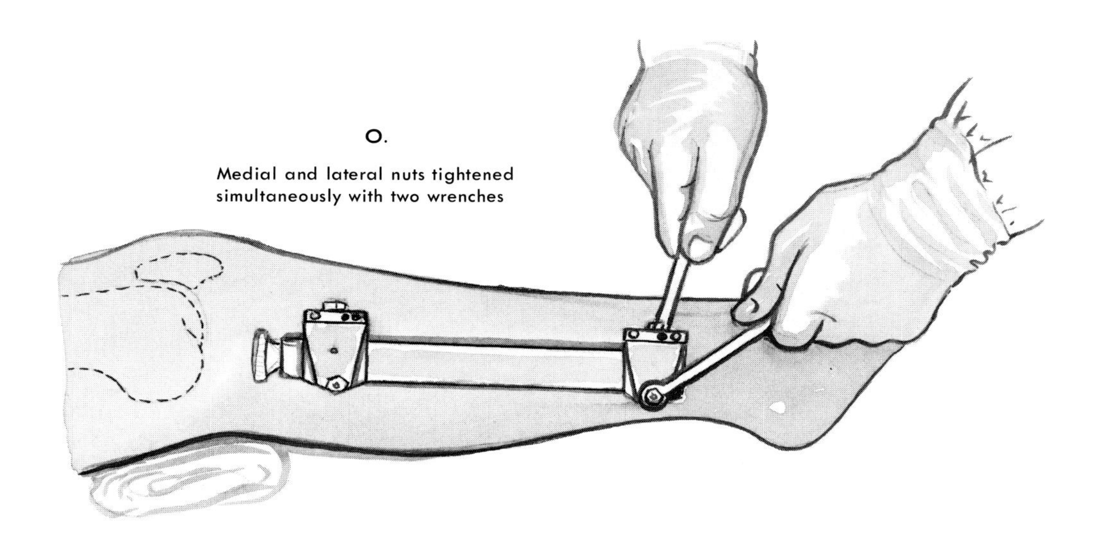

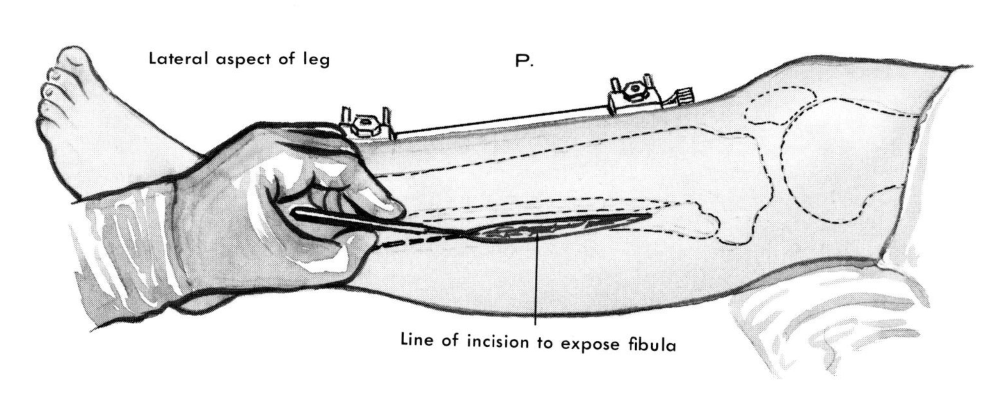

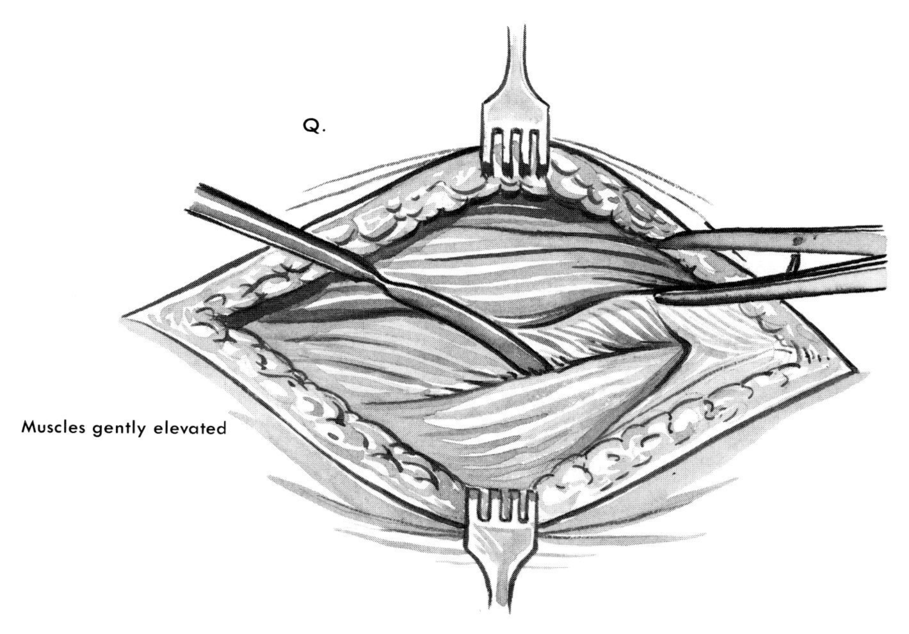

Wagner's Tibial Diaphyseal Lengthening (*Continued*)

R. The anterior intermuscular septum is sectioned and with a periosteal elevator is released from the interosseous border of the fibula.

S. The interosseous membrane is sectioned from the lateral (or interosseous) border of the tibia. Injury to the interosseous vessels and nerves should be avoided. On the posterior surface of the interosseous membrane, there are numerous vessels that may cause troublesome bleeding.

At this time the site of the osteotomy of the fibula should be determined. Measured with a ruler, the site should be exactly midway between the upper and lower pairs of the Schanz screws. A smooth Kirschner wire is inserted into the fibula to mark the site of the osteotomy. Leverage is applied to the fibula to elevate it anteriorly, and the fibula is transfixed to the tibia. Next, a flat lever retractor is introduced on the posterior surface of the fibula, the anterior surface of the interosseous membrane, and the posterior surface of the tibia. Posterior depression of the interosseous membrane will keep vessels and nerves out of harm's way and provide space for screw fixation and osteotomy.

T. The sites for the positioning screws are marked. One site should be 11 mm. to one side of the Kirschner wire; the other site should be 11 mm. to the other side of the wire. The Kirschner wire marks the site of the osteotomy of the tibia and fibula. The locations of the transfixing screws do not interfere with the screws of the Wagner osteosynthesis plate on the tibia during the second phase of the operation.

A 3.2-mm. drill is used to drill holes across both bones; the holes are tapped. To prevent splitting of the fibula, the edges of its drill holes are flattened by countersinking.

Plate 116. Wagner's Tibial Diaphyseal Lengthening

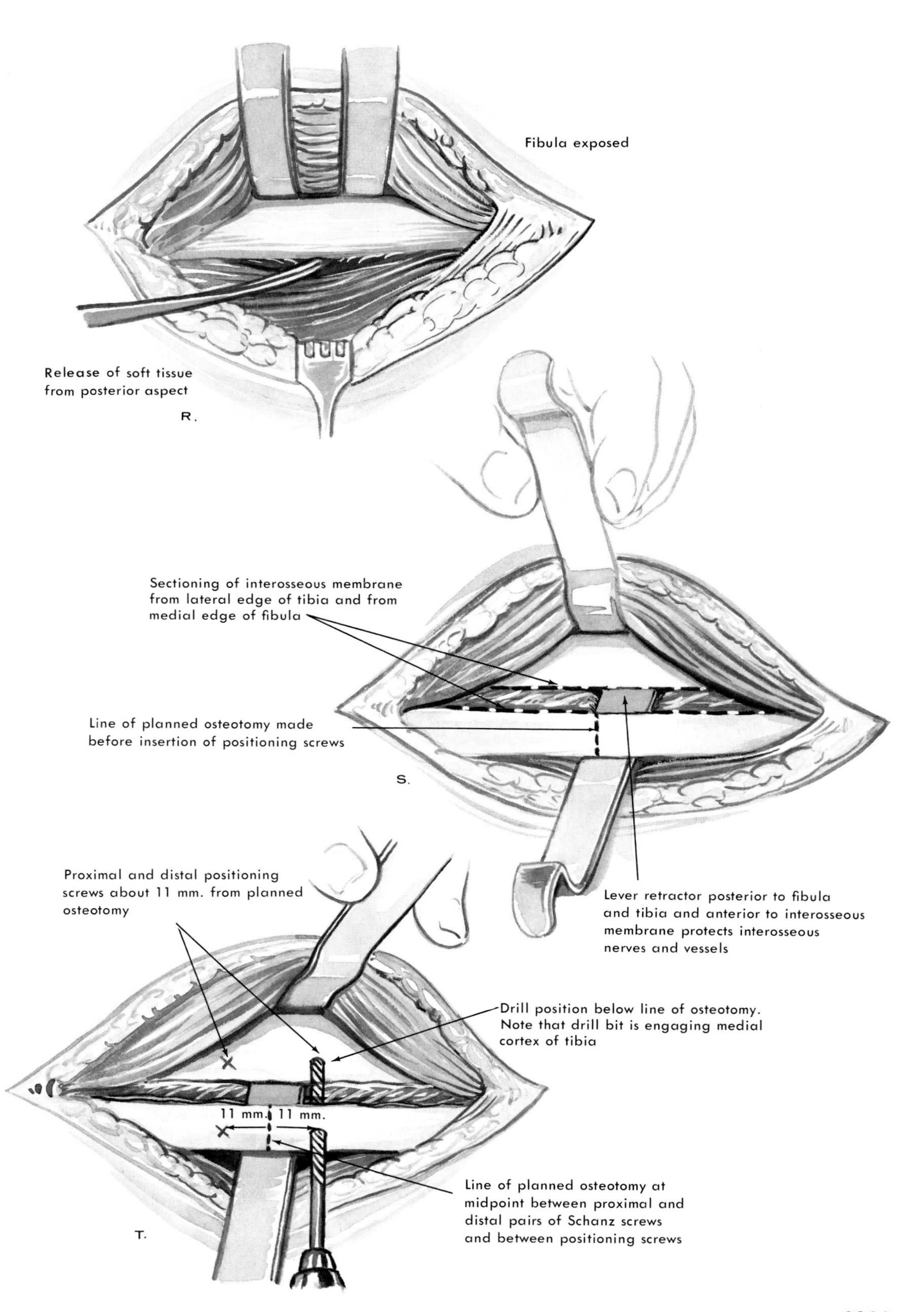

Wagner's Tibial Diaphyseal Lengthening *(Continued)*

U. The positioning screws are inserted, and their site and length are double-checked on anteroposterior and lateral radiograms.

The Kirschner wire marking the site of the osteotomy of the fibula is removed, and the fibula is divided transversely with a reciprocating saw under normal saline irrigation. Biologically it is preferable to perform corticotomy of the fibula with sharp osteotomes, thereby preserving its endosteal blood supply.

Distraction force is applied on the lengthening apparatus by turning its handle counter-clockwise three, four, or five turns.

V. An incision is made 1 cm. from the lateral edge of the anterior border on the crest of the tibia. The subcutaneous tissue and deep fascia are divided longitudinally in line with the skin incision. The antecrural muscles are elevated from the lateral surface of the tibia. The lateral surface of the tibia is exposed. A Chandler elevator is placed on the anterior aspect of the tibia.

W. Through the anterior wound, the positioning fibulotibial screws are visualized; a transverse osteotomy of the tibia is then carried out midway between the two positioning screws with a reciprocating saw under irrigation. Upon completion of the osteotomy, the gap between the two tibial segments springs open. It is this author's current preference to perform corticotomy of the tibia with sharp osteotomes and not to disturb the endosteal blood supply.

Plate 116. Wagner's Tibial Diaphyseal Lengthening

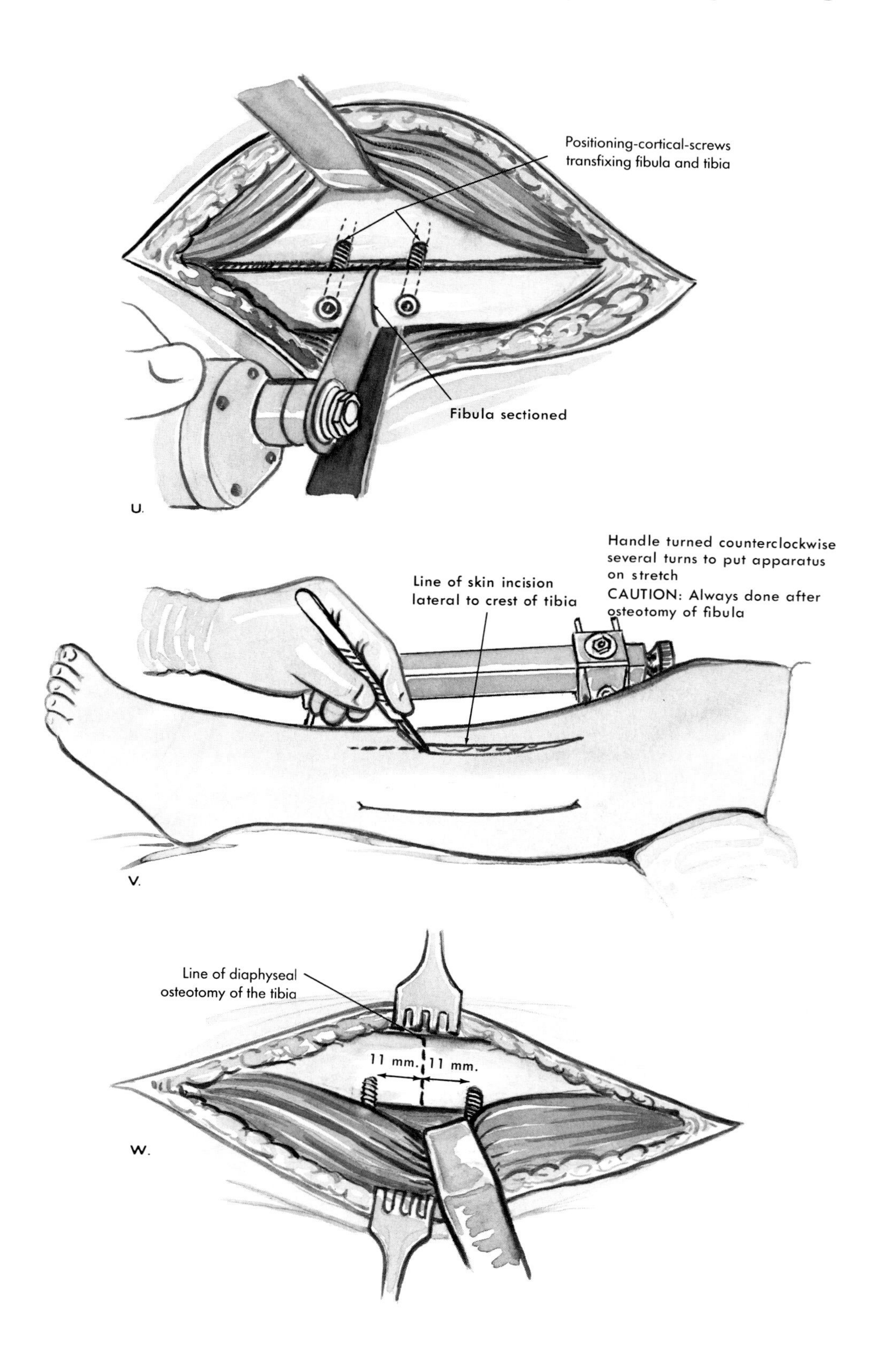

Wagner's Tibial Diaphyseal Lengthening (Continued)

X and **Y.** To avoid anterior compartment syndrome, the deep fascia is left open or elongated in alternating oblique cuts. Sometimes, if the fascia is taut, it is best to extend the skin incision proximally and excise the fascia, thereby preventing possible compression of the superficial peroneal nerve. Suction-drainage tubes are inserted. Only the subcutaneous tissues and skin are closed. Betadine-treated dressings are applied over the sites of the Schanz screws. A posterior below-knee cast and compression dressing are applied.

Lengthening of the tibia is commenced on the third to fifth day after surgery. The rate of lengthening recommended by this author is a quarter-turn eight times a day: six turns counterclockwise (distracting) and two turns clockwise (compressing). Biologically it is preferable to employ dynamized distraction and compression. That is, three successive lengthening (counterclockwise) quarter-turns are followed by a compressive (clockwise) quarter-turn and then by three successive counterclockwise turns (distraction) followed by one one-quarter turn clockwise (compression). The time schedule is set so that lengthening is performed during waking hours.

Screw tract care is similar to that required with femoral lengthening. Starting on the third day postoperatively, the screw sites are cleaned three times a day with sponges dipped in alcohol. The dressings that are applied are disinfected with alcohol (continued use of Betadine will corrode the apparatus). Tenting of the skin edges is relieved by incisions when indicated. Radiograms obtained once a week allow one to check alignment; a radiopaque Bell Thompson ruler placed next to the tibia aids in determining the amount of lengthening that has been achieved.

Z and **AA.** The patient is allowed to ambulate, and physical therapy is performed to maintain the range of motion of the knee and ankle joints. During the process of tibial lengthening, the triceps surae will shorten, and significant equinus deformity may develop. As a rule, preoperatively, if the ankle cannot be dorsiflexed to neutral position, lengthening of the heel cord is performed (usually three to six months prior to tibial lengthening). Lengthening of the Achilles tendon during the process of tibial lengthening is indicated when there is progressive equinus and restriction of ankle motion. *If the range of ankle motion is less than 20 degrees,* elongation of the heel cord should be performed immediately. Range of motion is more important than the degree of equinus. Rigidity of the ankle joint must be avoided; ankle motion and function must be preserved. If equinus develops but the range of motion of the ankle is greater than 20 degrees, lengthening of the heel cord is performed at the time of internal fixation. Professor Wagner recommends the following technique for lengthening of the heel cord.

With the apparatus in place, the patient in a prone position, and a pneumatic tourniquet on the proximal thigh, the lower limb is carefully prepared and draped. A longitudinal incision is made on the medial border of the tendo Achillis. The incision should be long, extending from the junction of the upper and middle thirds of the leg to the insertion of the Achilles tendon at the os calcis. The subcutaneous tissue and the paratenon are divided in line with the skin incision. Injury to the veins should be avoided. The Achilles tendon is divided by a very long incision in the coronal plane. It begins anteriorly in the distal part and ends posteriorly in the proximal part, so that the muscle fibers stay with the upper part. A capsulotomy of the ankle or subtalar joints is unnecessary if dorsiflexion of the ankle to neutral position was possible preoperatively.

The position for suturing of the tricep surae's split tendons is one in which the ankle is dorsiflexed 15 to 20 degrees beyond neutral. The wound is closed in the usual fashion. No cast is applied. Ambulation is allowed with partial weight-bearing of 10 to 15 pounds on the lower limb the day after surgery. There is usually no pain and no swelling.

Percutaneous lengthening of the heel cord is not recommended.

Plate 116. Wagner's Tibial Diaphyseal Lengthening

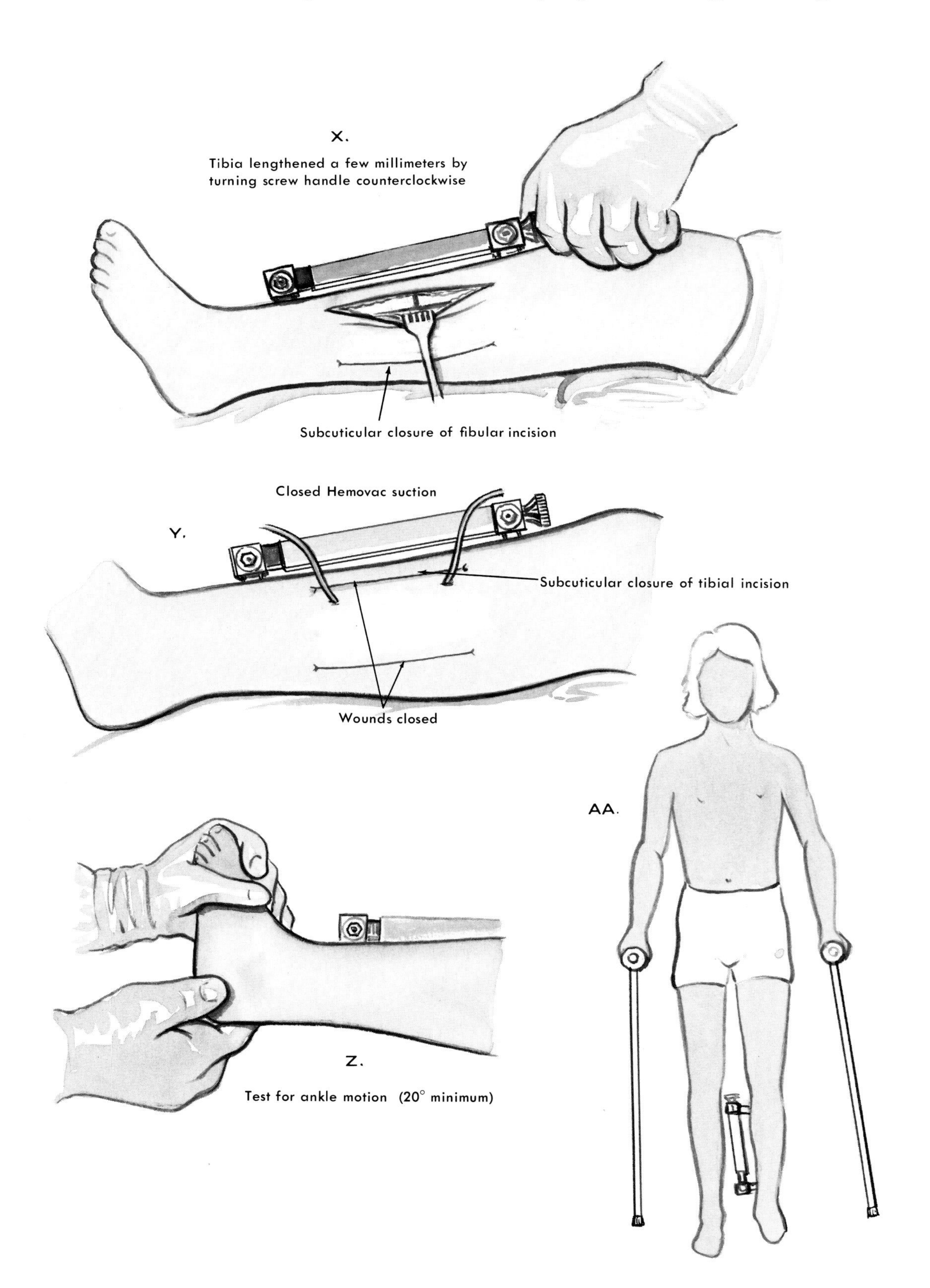

Wagner's Tibial Diaphyseal Lengthening (*Continued*)

The second phase of the Wagner procedure involves plating the elongated tibial segment with the Wagner osteosynthesis plate (BB *to* DD) *and bone grafting* (EE).

BB. The anterolateral surface of the tibia is exposed through the incision used for the tibial osteotomy.

CC. When the elongated segment is identified, two Chandler retractors are placed over the proximal tibial segment; two Chandler retractors go over the distal tibial segment as well. It is imperative not to enter the channel of the screw tracts because of possible contamination.

DD. The distracted area is plated with a four-hole Wagner osteosynthesis plate; four cortical screws are inserted above, and three or four cortical screws are inserted below. The plate is straight (not bent), and it is anchored on the lateral surface of the tibia.

Plate 116. Wagner's Tibial Diaphyseal Lengthening

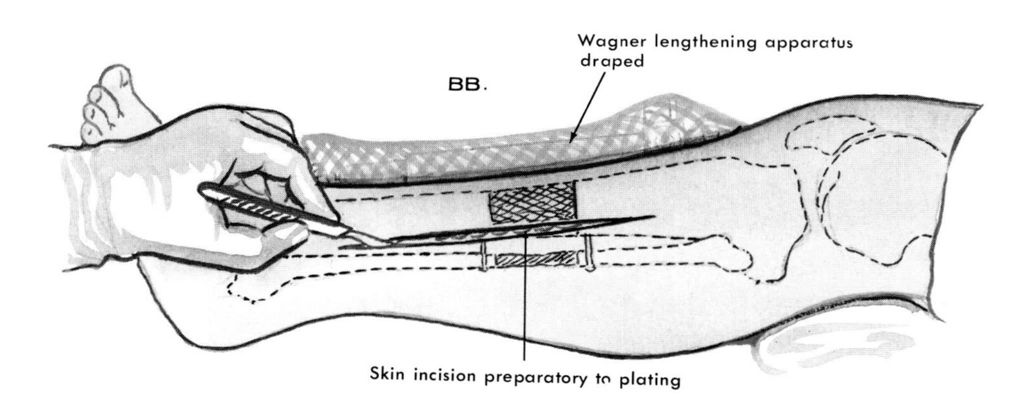

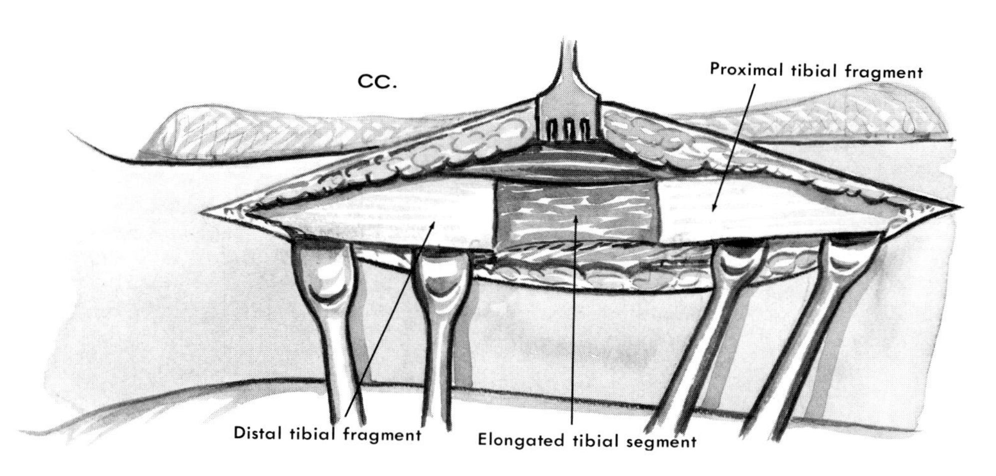

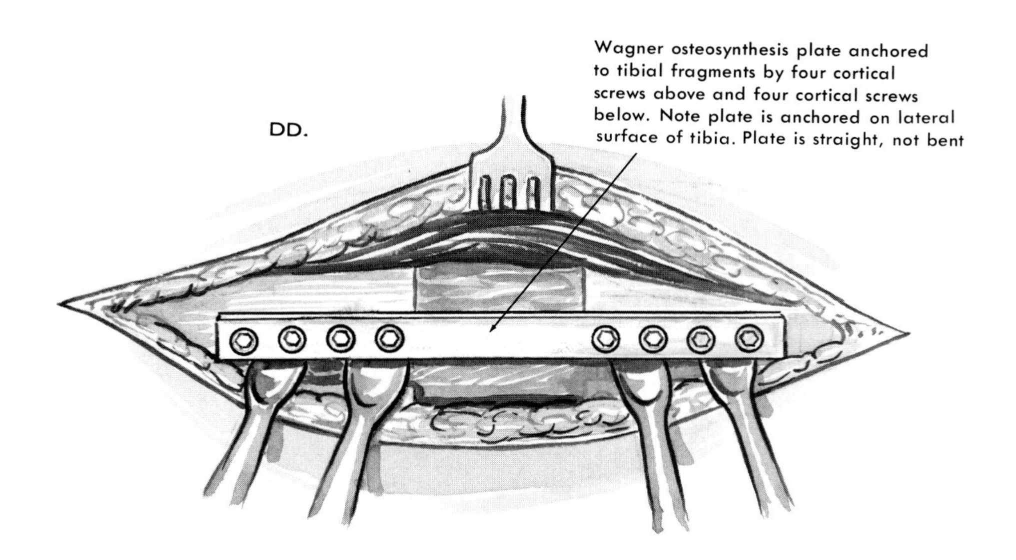

Wagner's Tibial Diaphuseal Lengthening (*Continued*)

EE. The elongated segment is packed with autogenous cancellous bone grafts harvested from the ilium. The skin and subcutaneous tissue are closed over closed-suction drains. The positional screws fixing the tibia to the fibula are not removed. If there is delayed healing of the fibula, it may be grafted at this time.

FF. The Schanz screws and the Wagner external fixation apparatus are removed. Immobilization in a cast is not required.

POSTOPERATIVE CARE

As soon as the patient is comfortable, he is permitted to be up and around—using a three-point crutch gait and toe-touch on the lengthened limb—until there is progressive consolidation.

The third phase of the Wagner tibial lengthening procedure—the exchange of the rigid plate for a flexible semitubular plate—is the same as that described for Wagner's femoral lengthening procedure (see Plate 115).

Plate 116. Wagner's Tibial Diaphyseal Lengthening

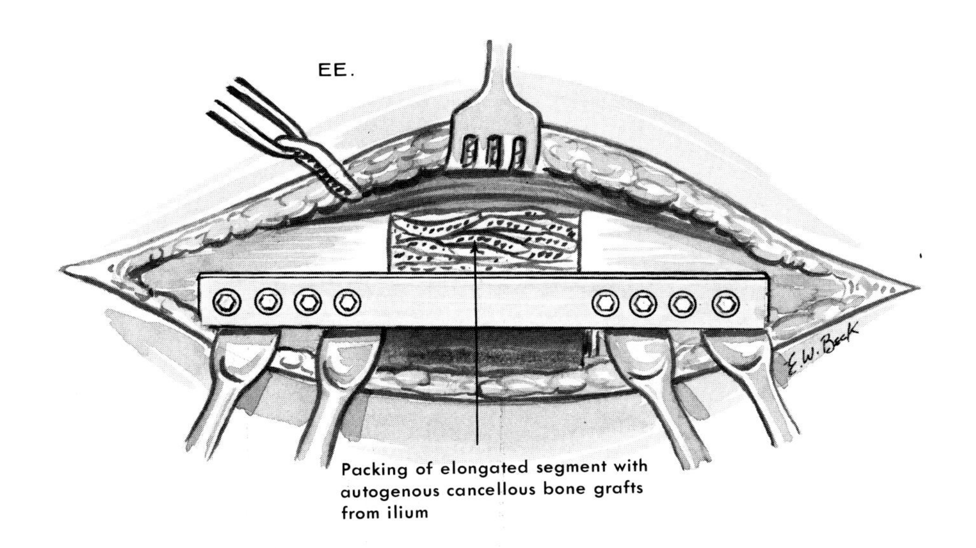

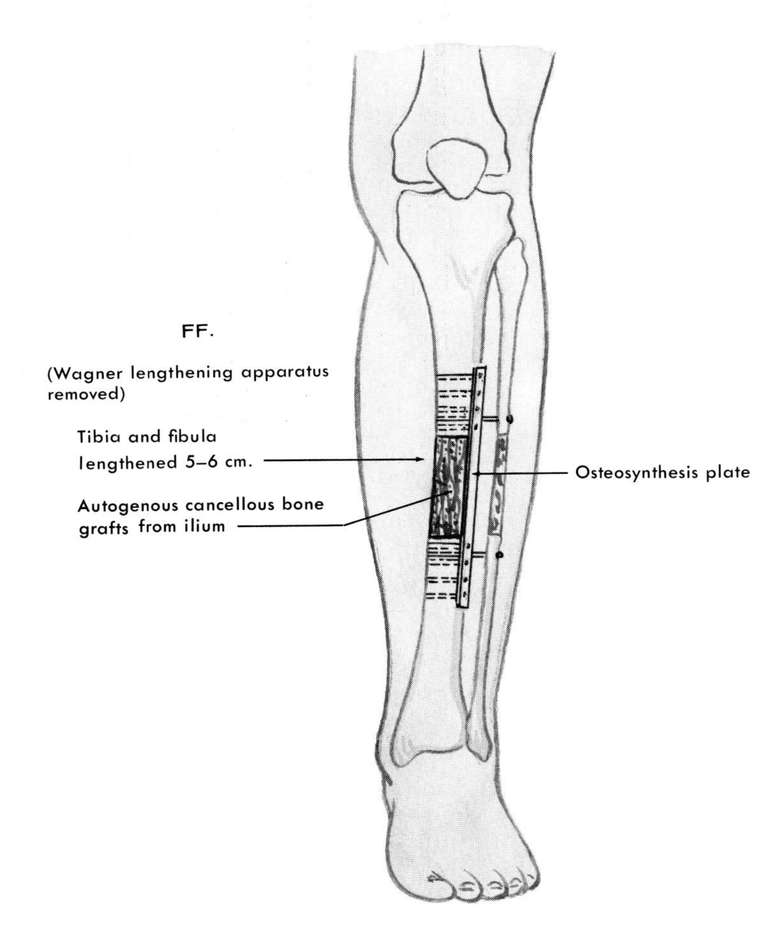

Femoral Lengthening by Callotasis (DeBastiani Technique)

In this technique, the Orthofix lengthening device is placed on the lateral aspect of the femur. Radiographic image intensification is utilized during the procedure. The first stage of the operation is insertion of screws.

OPERATIVE TECHNIQUE

A. The most proximal screw is inserted first, immediately above the lesser trochanter and perpendicular to the longitudinal axis of the femur. Under image intensifier control the proper level of the screw is determined. A longitudinal skin incision 1 cm. long is made.

B. With a pair of blunt Metzenbaum scissors the wound is spread apart.

C. The midline of the lateral cortex of the femur is determined with a trocar inserted into the correct screw guide; the screw guide should be placed on bone, perpendicular to the longitudinal axis of the femur and midline in position.

Plate 117. Femoral Lengthening by Callotasis (DeBastiani Technique)

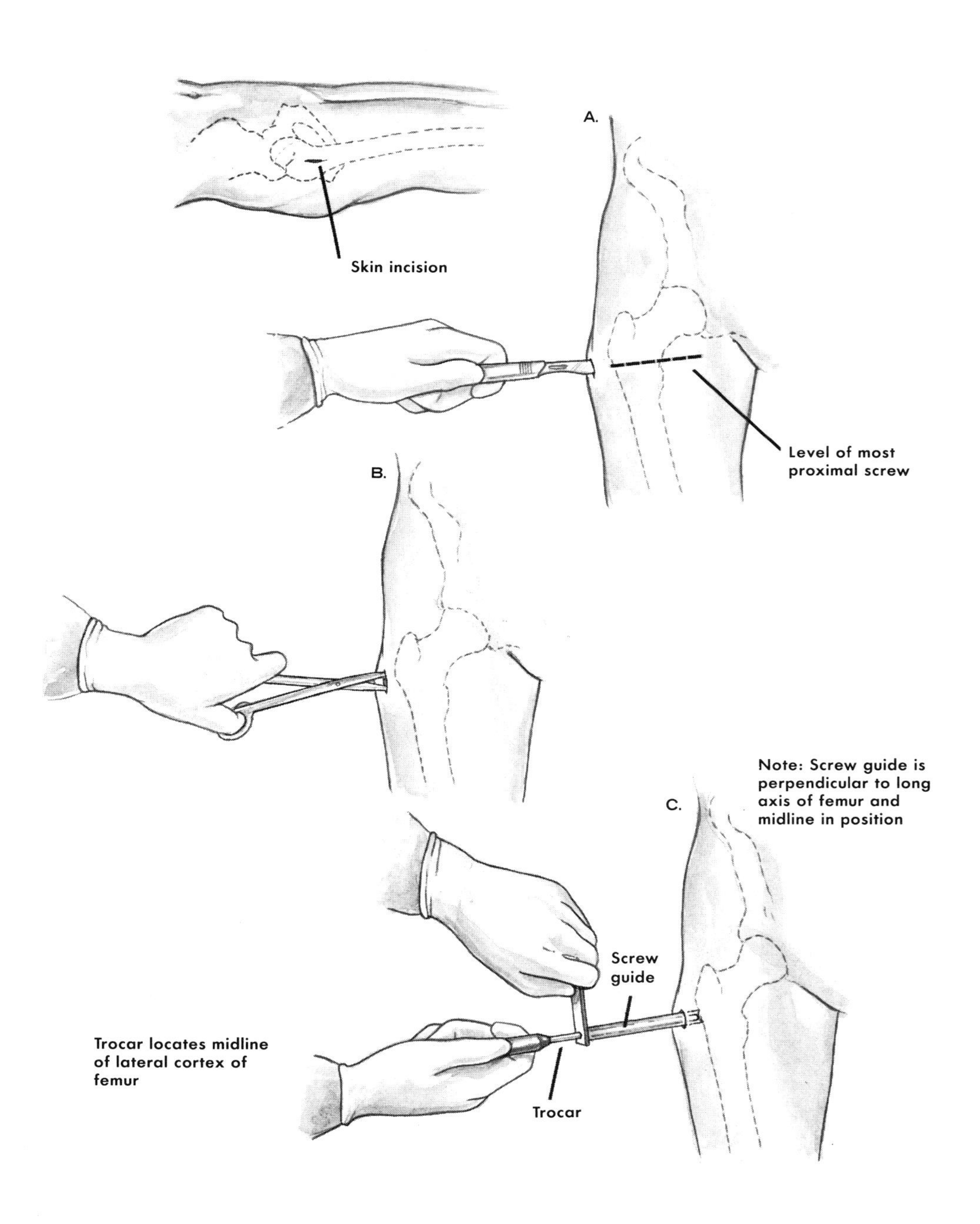

Femoral Lengthening by Callotasis (DeBastiani Technique) (Continued)

D. With the screw guide firmly pressed on bone (by pressure exerted on the handle); remove the trocar from the screw guide.

E. With a hammer, the screw guide is gently tapped to engage its teeth on the cortex.

F. A drill guide is inserted into the screw guide. Drill size should be appropriate to screw size. For cortical screws (used for femoral lengthening), a 4.8-mm. drill is used. When the diameter of the femur is 15 mm. or less, 4.5-mm. or 3.5-mm. screws are used; the correct-size drill for the smaller screws is usually 3.2 mm. For cancellous screws, a 3.2-mm. drill is used.

Plate 117. Femoral Lengthening by Callotasis (DeBastiani Technique)

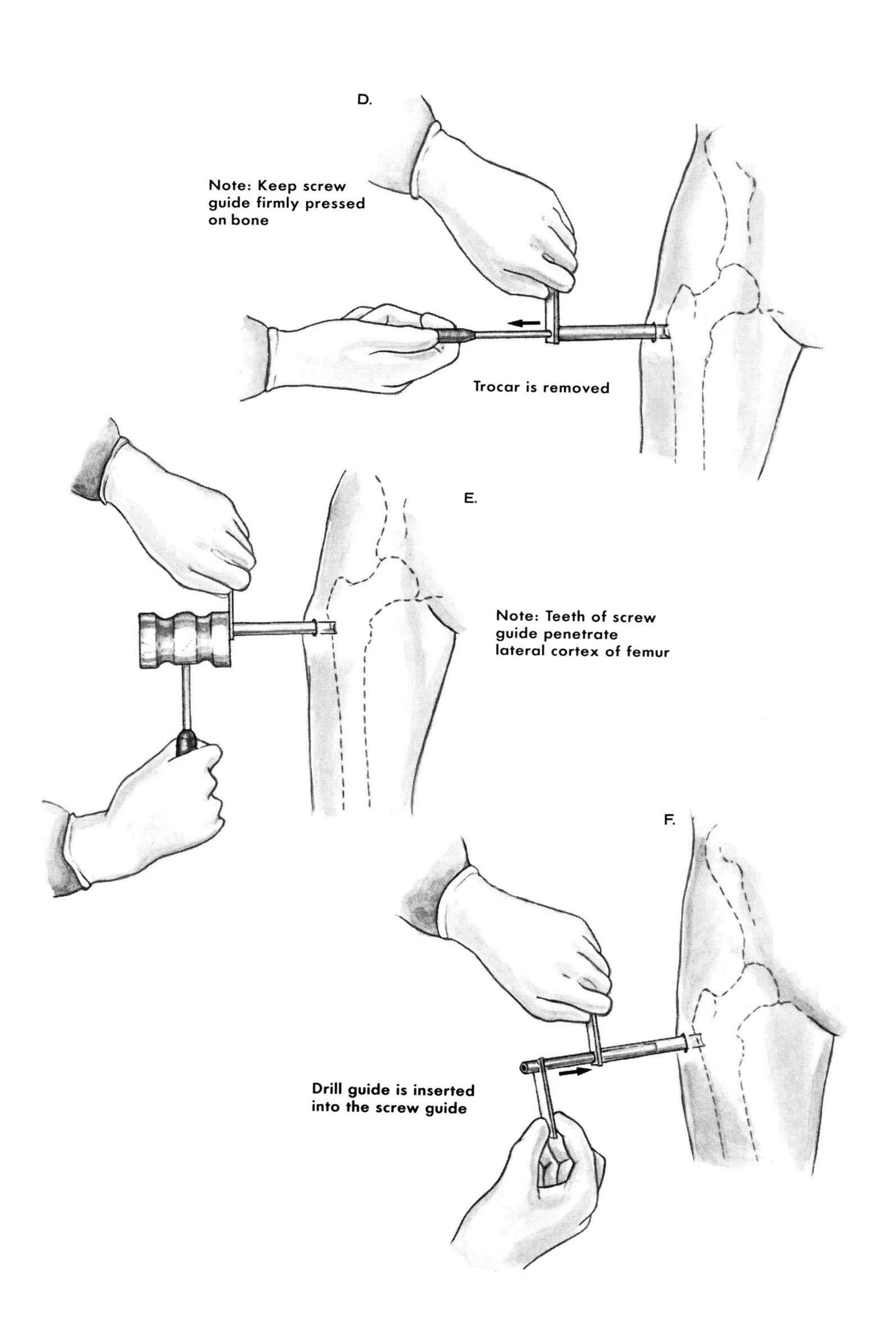

Femoral Lengthening by Callotasis (DeBastiani Technique) (Continued)

G. A drill bit of the correct size is fitted with a drill stop and inserted into the drill guide. The drill should be perpendicular to the femur.

H. With a low-speed power drill, the first cortex is drilled up to the second cortex.

I and **J.** Next, the drill stop is offset by 5 mm. for drilling through the second cortex, which should be completely penetrated by the drill. Offsetting the drill stop will prevent overpenetration of the drill and thus protect against damage to the soft tissues.

Plate 117. Femoral Lengthening by Callotasis (DeBastiani Technique)

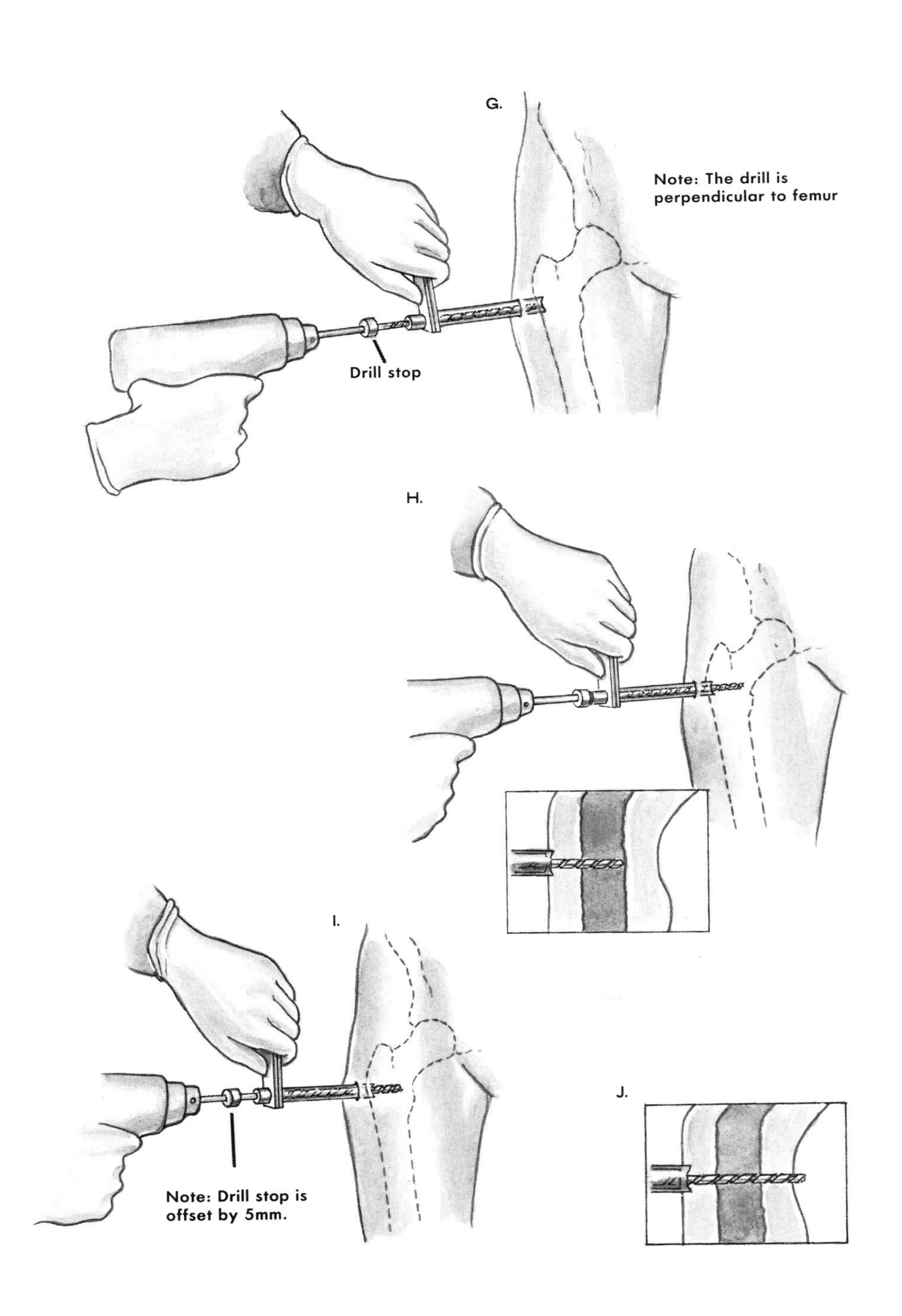

Femoral Lengthening by Callotasis (DeBastiani Technique) (Continued)

K. The drill bit and drill guide are removed. Be sure to maintain the screw guide in place by applying firm pressure on the screw guide handle.

L. A screw of appropriate size and length is selected, fitted to a "T" wrench, and inserted into the screw guide. The screw is self-tapping and requires minimum force for insertion. The screw should penetrate the first cortex, traverse the medullary canal, and penetrate the second cortex, at which point increased resistance should be felt. Screw penetration should be confirmed on radiographic image intensification.

M. The screw is turned clockwise slowly under image intensifier x-ray control. By seven or eight further half-turns—be careful not to overpenetrate!—at least two threads of the screw should protrude beyond the second cortex. Caution: The threads of the screw are tapered; turning the screw counterclockwise will loosen its purchase.

Plate 117. Femoral Lengthening by Callotasis (DeBastiani Technique)

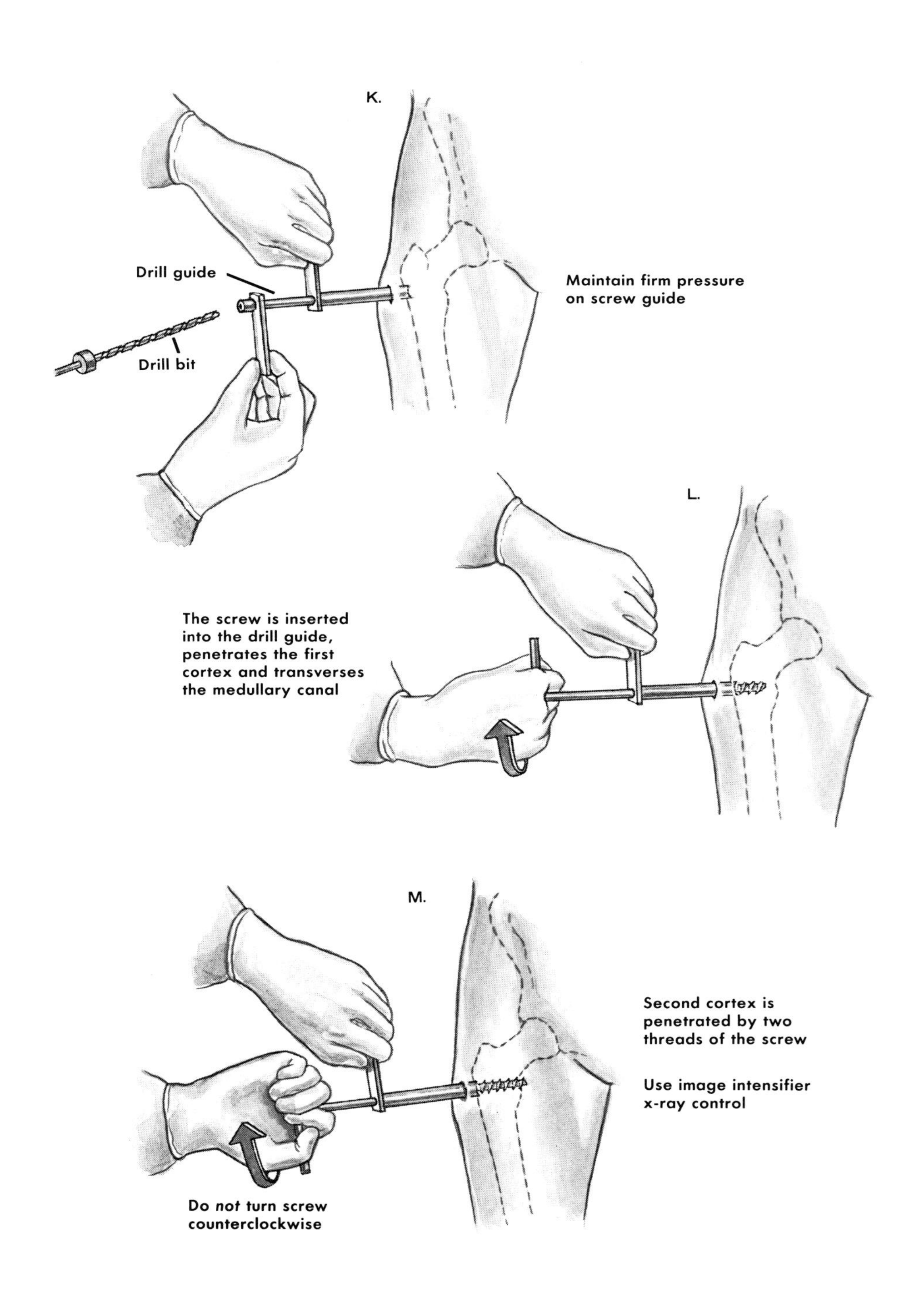

Femoral Lengthening by Callotasis (DeBastiani Technique) (Continued)

N. The lengthening device's rigid template is positioned on the lateral side of the thigh, in line with and parallel to the femoral shaft. The screw guide is left in place, and one end of the template is applied to it. The first screw should be in the most proximal hole of the template.

O. The second screw is placed in the most distal hole. The grooves on the template can be used as a guide to mark the second skin incision. The screw insertion follows the steps already spelled out (*A* to *M*).

Plate 117. Femoral Lengthening by Callotasis (DeBastiani Technique)

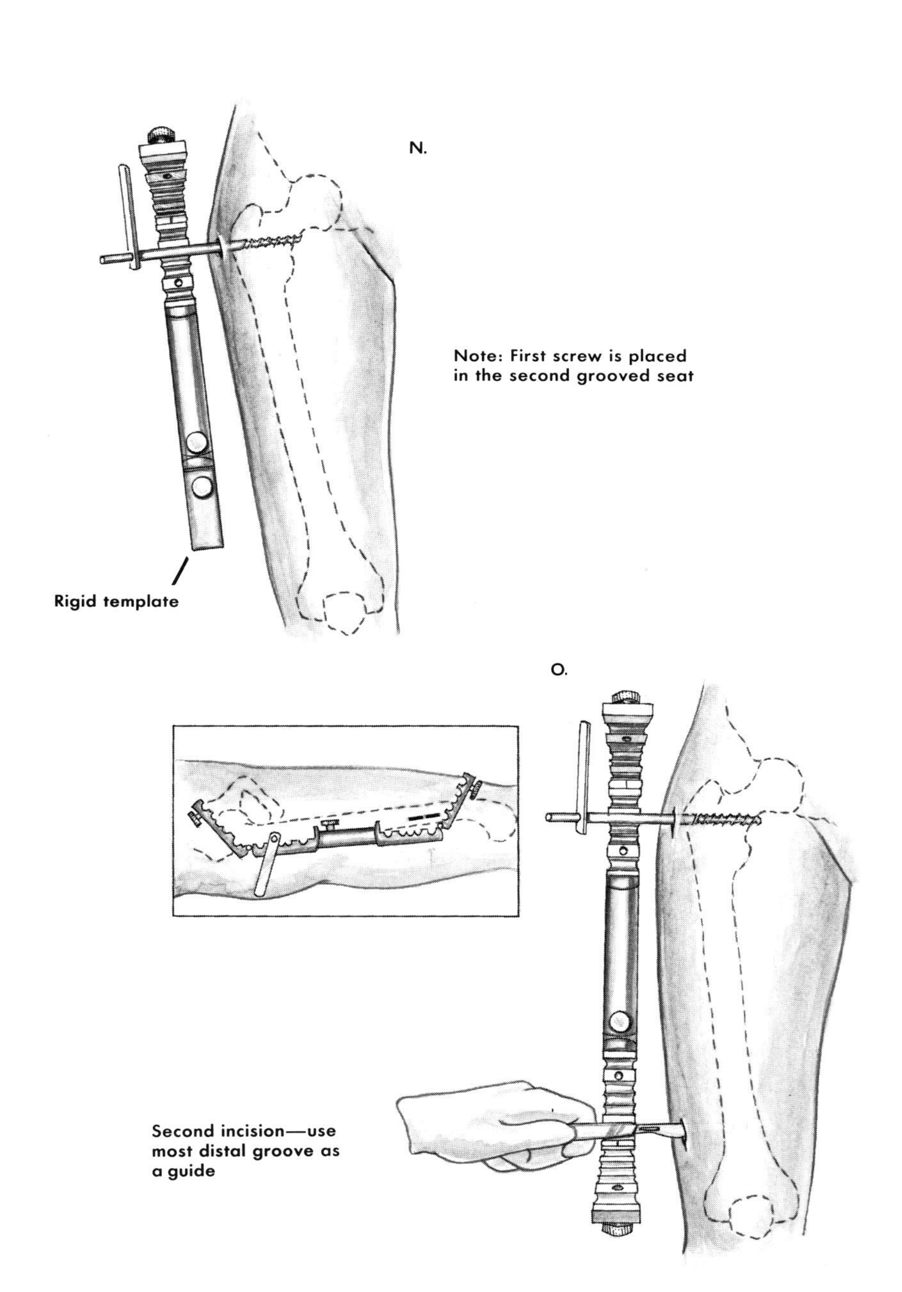

Femoral Lengthening by Callotasis (DeBastiani Technique) (Continued)

P. The third screw is placed into the fourth hole distal from the first screw.

Q. The fourth screw is placed in the hole closest to the most distal screw. Normally only two screws per clamp are required in the younger child. In the adolescent and in patients with bone of poor quality, three screws in the proximal clamp and two screws in the distal clamp are recommended.

Plate 117. Femoral Lengthening by Callotasis (DeBastiani Technique)

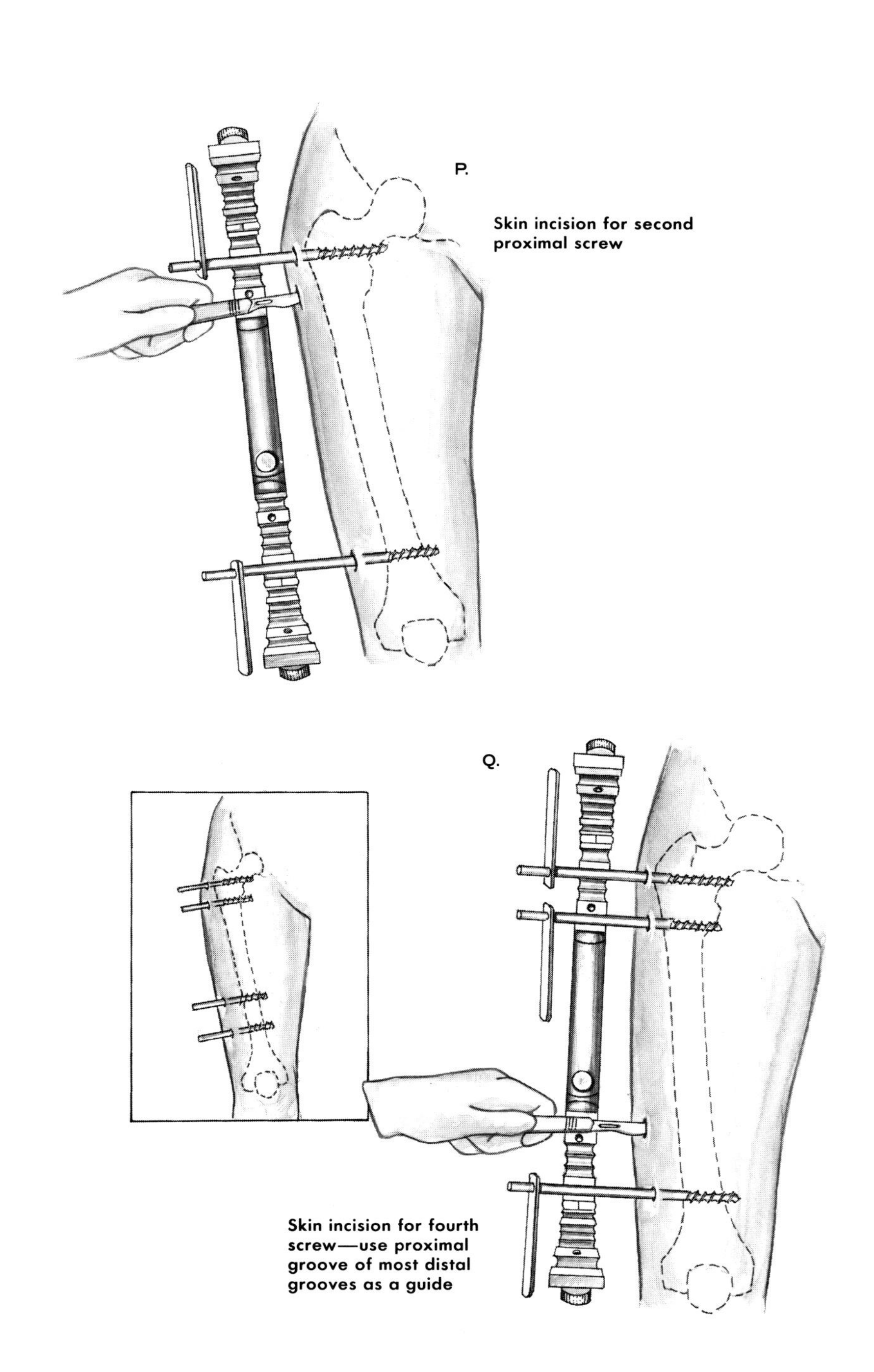

Femoral Lengthening by Callotasis (DeBastiani Technique) (Continued)

The next stage of the callotasis is corticotomy. *In the femur the level of corticotomy corresponds to the distal point of insertion of the iliopsoas muscle—usually 1 cm. inferior to the most distal of the proximal set of screws. Verify the level on x-ray image intensification.*

R and **S.** The template is removed. A 4- to 5-cm.-long longitudinal skin incision is made on the anterior aspect of the upper thigh. The subcutaneous tissue and fascia are divided in line with the skin incision. The interval between the sartorius muscle and the tensor muscle of the fascia lata is widened. The fibers of the rectus femoris muscle are separated from the vastus intermedialis muscle by gentle blunt dissection, exposing the periosteum on the anterior aspect of the femur. A longitudinal incision is made in the periosteum. Elevating the periosteum exposes the upper femoral diaphysis.

T. A 4.8-mm. drill is inserted into a short Orthofix screw guide. The drill stop is adjusted so that the tip of the drill protrudes 5 mm. beyond the end of the screw guide.

U. Holes are drilled into the medial, anterior, and lateral cortices. The drill stop will prevent the drill from penetrating the medullary cavity and damaging the marrow and intramedullary circulation.

Plate 117. Femoral Lengthening by Callotasis (DeBastiani Technique)

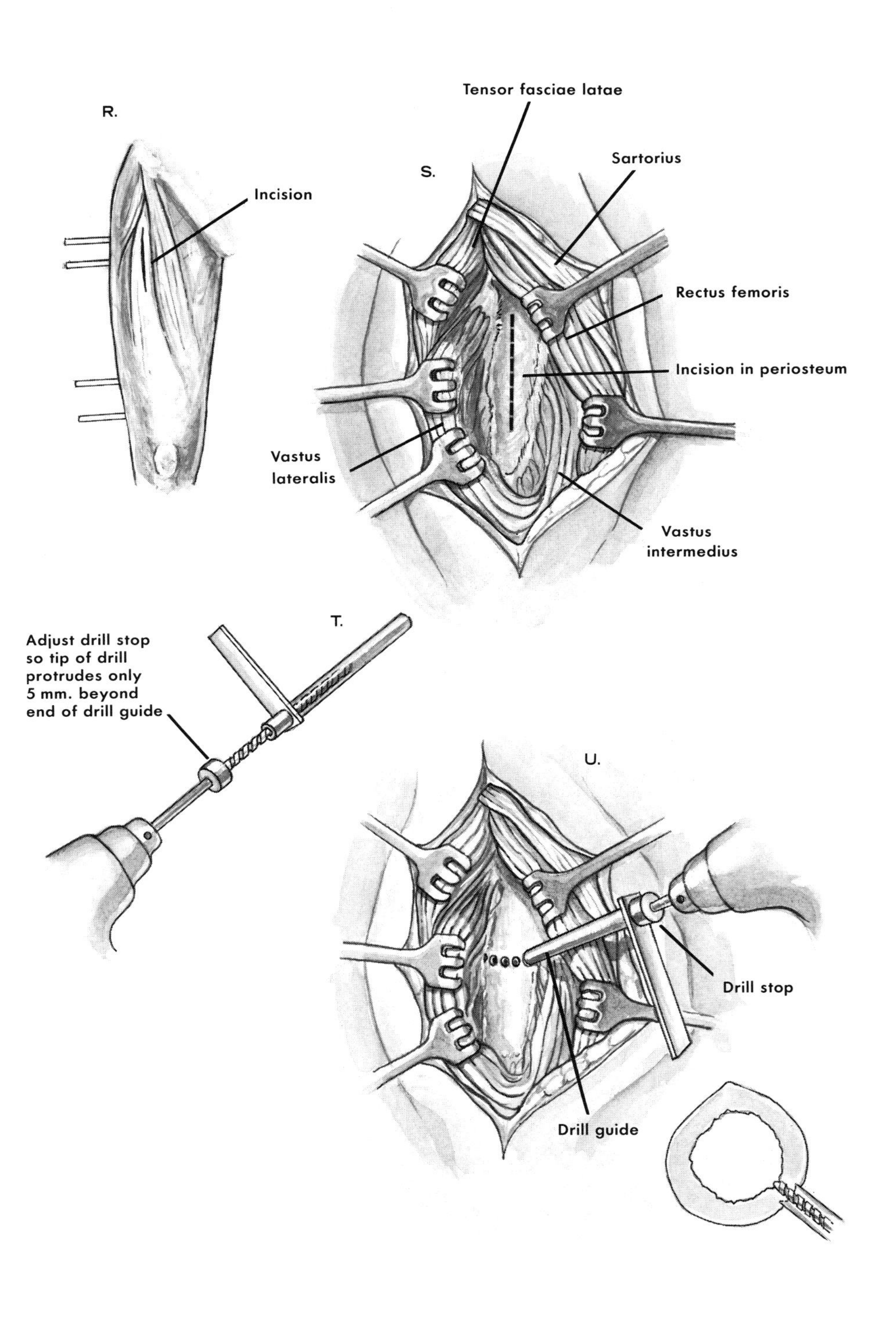

Femoral Lengthening by Callotasis (DeBastiani Technique) (Continued)

V. By the use of a small sharp-edged bone chisel, the drill holes are joined and the corticotomy completed. The medullary cavity and marrow should not be penetrated. The periosteum on the posterior aspect of the femur usually remains intact.

W. The Orthofix Dynamic Axial Fixator is anchored to the screws. The body-locking screw should be on the outside. The dot and arrow on the cam mechanism and the screws on the clamps should face upward.

The fixator should be 3 cm. away from the skin in order to allow space for postoperative swelling and cleansing of the screw sites. The body of the lengthening device should be parallel to the diaphysis of the femur. By the use of an Allen wrench the clamp screws are tightened. In order to prevent stresses when locking the clamp screws, it is wise to insert dummy screws in empty (unused) outer clamp holes.

Plate 117. Femoral Lengthening by Callotasis (DeBastiani Technique)

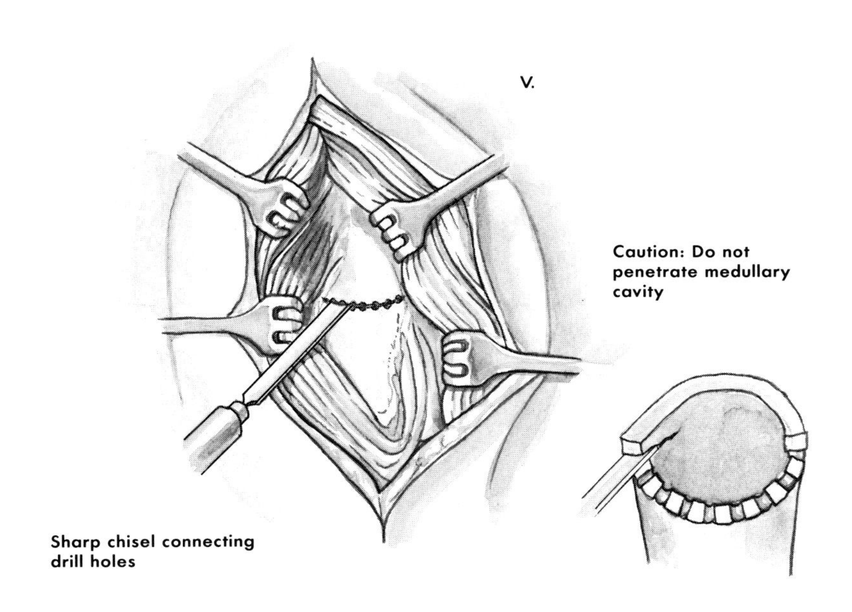

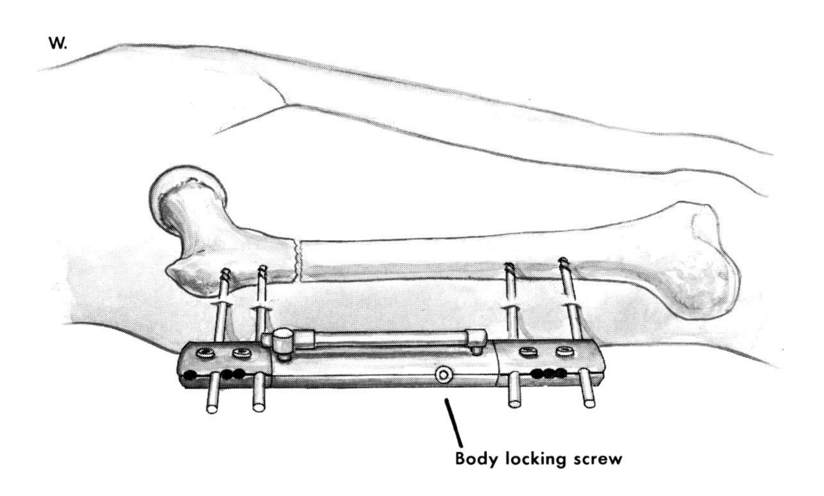

Femoral Lengthening by Callotasis (DeBastiani Technique) (Continued)

X. The cams and body-locking screw are locked by the use of a torque wrench. A click indicates the correct torque.

Y. The completeness of the corticotomy is confirmed by distracting the bony segments under image intensifier radiographic control, and the segments are then returned to their original position. The periosteum is sutured, and the wound is closed in the usual fashion. A Hemovac suction drain is left in situ for 24 to 48 hours. Any tension on the skin around the screws is relieved. The range of hip and knee motion is tested to ensure that movement is unrestricted and full.

POSTOPERATIVE CARE

Partial weight-bearing is allowed as soon as the patient is comfortable after surgery. Physical therapy is performed several times a day to maintain the range of hip and knee motion and to preserve motor strength in the muscles of the hip and knee.

Pin site care: Immediately postoperatively and several times a day thereafter, the wounds are cleaned with Betadine solution. Three days after surgery the pin sites are cleansed with alcohol twice a day. It is important to keep a crust from forming at the pin's junction with the skin. Sterile gauze, impregnated with alcohol, is used for local dressing.

Distraction commences when callus formation is seen on radiograms, about 10 to 15 days postoperatively. With the distraction attachment in place, the body-locking screw is released. Turning the screw 90 degrees (a quarter-turn) counterclockwise achieves 0.25 mm. of distraction. The sequence used to achieve a total of 1.00 mm. of distraction is incremental: three successive quarter-turns counterclockwise (distraction), followed by a single quarter-turn clockwise (compression), are spaced over the course of eight hours; three more quarter-turns counterclockwise and a final quarter-turn clockwise then follow, again carried out over eight hours. Thus, in a sixteen-hour period (the patient's waking hours), six distractive quarter-turns are "countered" by two compressive quarter-turns, yielding four advances in distraction of 0.25 mm. each—for a total gain of 1.00 mm. of distraction. The rate of distraction is reduced when it causes pain or muscle spasm. Hip and knee range of motion are checked for stiffness and to detect subluxation.

Seven days after distraction is begun, anteroposterior and lateral radiograms of the upper femur are obtained to confirm the separation of the corticotomy with callus continuity. Follow-up radiograms are obtained at three- to four-week intervals. If the callus response is poor, callus distraction is stopped for seven days and then restarted. If the distraction is excessive and a gap develops in the callus, compression is started at the same rate as that of previous distraction. (To achieve compression, the screw is turned clockwise; a 360-degree clockwise turn achieves one mm. of compression.) When callus continuity is re-established, distraction is restarted; in the beginning it is best to distract 1.50 mm. and compress 0.50 mm. With distraction-compression, osteogenesis is enhanced as, gradually, the bone is being lengthened.

When the desired length is obtained, the body-locking screw is tightened and the distraction attachment removed. Full weight-bearing is allowed. When radiograms show good consolidation of the callus, the body-locking screw is loosened; dynamic axial loading is started and continued until adequate cortex is formed all around the elongated segment. At this time the stability of the elongated segment is tested clinically with the fixator removed and the body-locking screw tightened.

If the elongated segment is stable, the screws are left in place for 4 to 6 days and then removed. Removal will require appropriate sedation or, in the case of the apprehensive child or adolescent, general anesthesia.

If the elongated segment is mechanically unstable, the fixator is reapplied and dynamic axial loading restarted.

All during this period, physical therapy is performed daily to maintain function of the elongated limb. Again, function is never sacrificed for length.

Healing index is an expression of the number of days required to achieve 1 cm. of lengthening; the figure is obtained by dividing the overall treatment time in days by the total amount of lengthening achieved in centimeters. The healing index, in the experience of Professor DeBastiani, is 36 days for the femur, 41 days for the tibia, and 24 days for the humerus.

Plate 117. Femoral Lengthening by Callotasis (DeBastiani Technique)

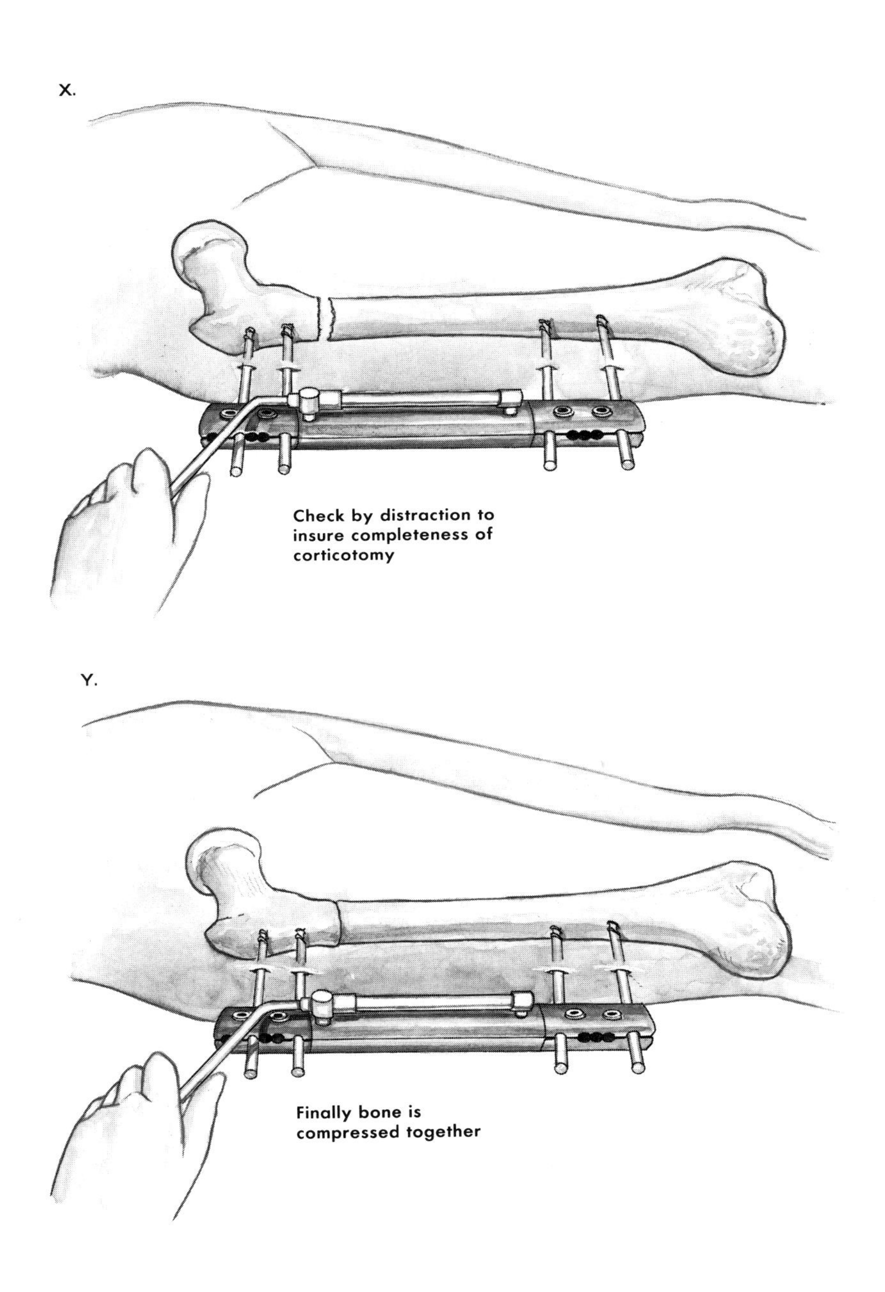

Callotasis (Callus Distraction) for Lengthening of the Tibia

The choice of Orthofix limb-lengthener for tibial elongation depends upon the length of the diaphysis and the amount of distraction planned. The 5-cm. lengthener is used when the minimum tibial length is 12 cm.; it allows maximum lengthening of 5 cm. The 5.5-cm lengthener allows maximum lengthening of 5.5 cm. and is used when the minimum tibial length is 19.5 cm. The 10-cm. leg lengthener allows 10 cm. of maximum lengthening and is used when the minimum tibial length is 24 cms. It is feasible to begin with a small device and later substitute a larger lengthener if extra distraction is necessary.

Preparatory to the steps detailed below, a 2-cm.-long segment of the diaphysis in the lower third of the fibula is excised through a separate incision in the usual fashion.

OPERATIVE TECHNIQUE

A and **B.** The screws and lengthening device are placed on the anteromedial side of the tibia. The technique for insertion of the individual screws is described in Plate 117; the only difference is that the most superior screw in the proximal tibia is cancellous. The other three screws are cortical. The cortical screws are 6 mm. in diameter; the cancellous screw is 5 mm. in diameter. When the diameter of the tibia is less than 15 mm. and the 5-cm. leg-lengthener is utilized, the cortical screws that are to be used should be 4.5 mm. in diameter; the cancellous screw should have a diameter of 3.5 mm. Screw length and thread length are estimated by assessing the radiograms and subtracting the 15 percent magnification factor in the radiograms.

The first screw (which is cancellous) is inserted perpendicular to the longitudinal axis and two cm. inferior to the tibial plateau; it should be extracapsular. In the growing skeleton the most proximal tibial screw is one cm. distal to the proximal tibial physis.

Next, the rigid template is placed in line with and parallel to the anteromedial aspect of the leg. The first screw belongs in the most proximal hole of the template, the second (a cortical screw) in the most distal hole.

Plate 118. Callotasis (Callus Distraction) for Lengthening of the Tibia

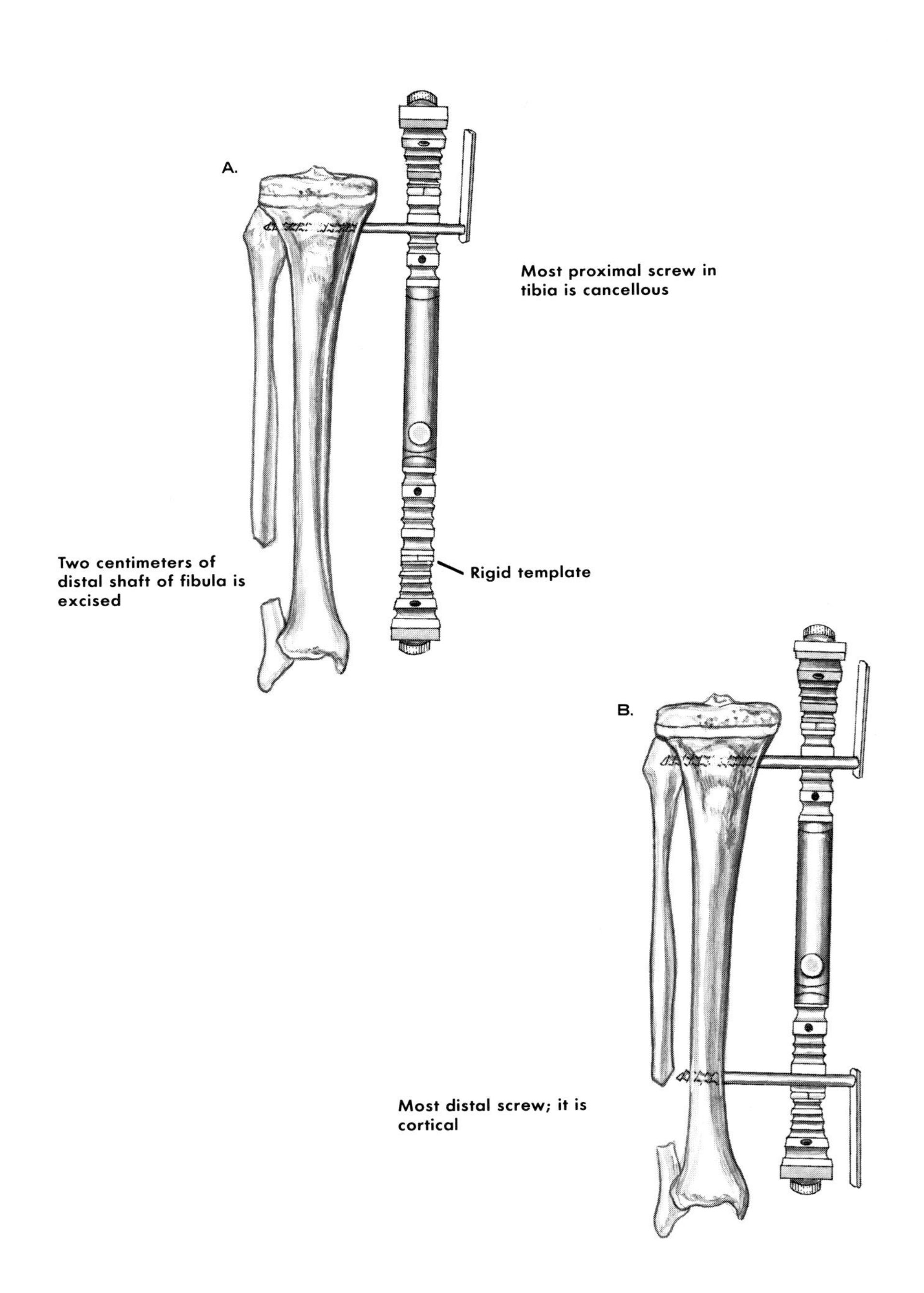

Callotasis (Callus Distraction) for Lengthening of the Tibia (Continued)

C. The third screw (also a cortical screw) is inserted into the fourth hole distal from the first screw.

D. The fourth screw (the final cortical screw) is placed in the superior hole of the distal set of the screws. If the leg is large or the tibia fairly skeletally mature, it is advisable to insert three screws in the proximal set.

Plate 118. Callotasis (Callus Distraction) for Lengthening of the Tibia

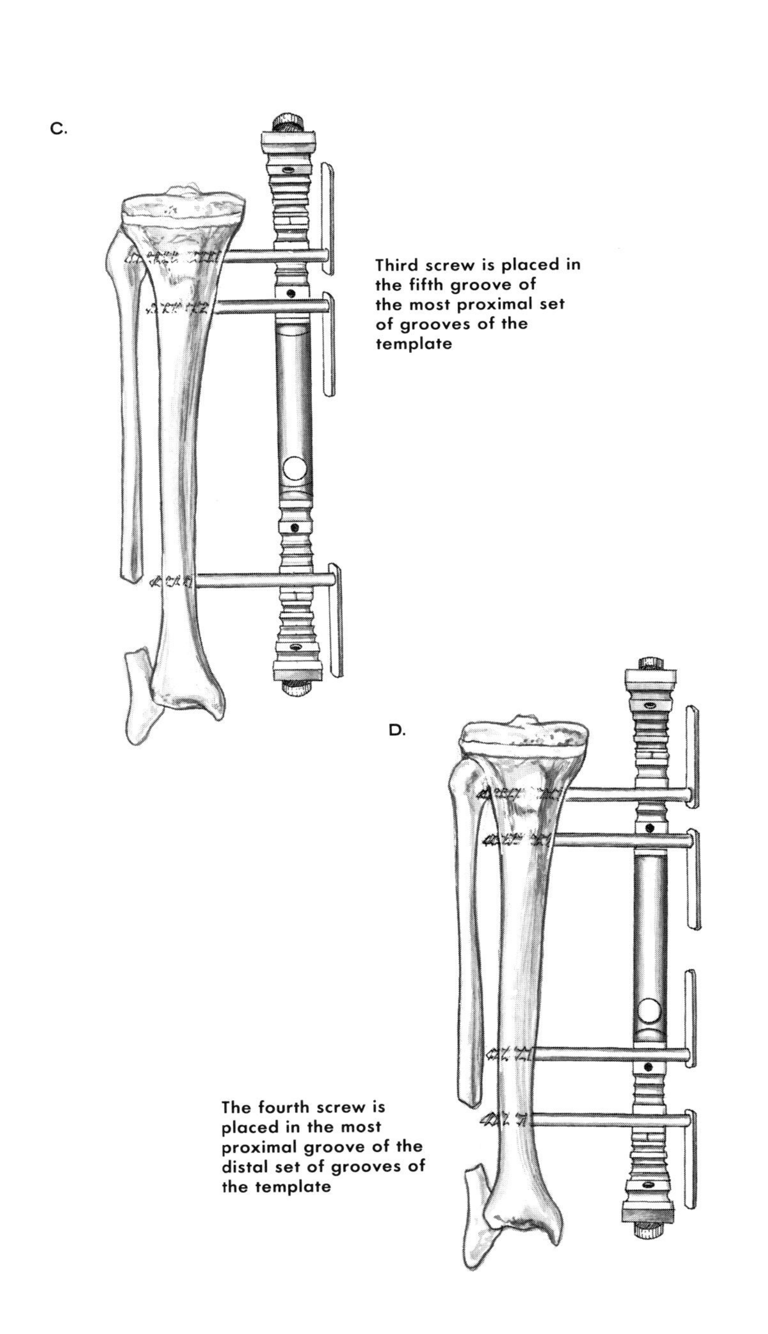

Callotasis (Callus Distraction) for Lengthening of the Tibia (Continued)

E. The rigid template is removed. An Orthofix leg-lengthener of appropriate size is then applied.

F. *Corticotomy* is performed 1 cm. inferior to the most distal of the proximal set of screws. A longitudinal incision is made on the anterolateral aspect of the leg. The periosteum is exposed, longitudinally incised, and elevated.

Plate 118. Callotasis (Callus Distraction) for Lengthening of the Tibia

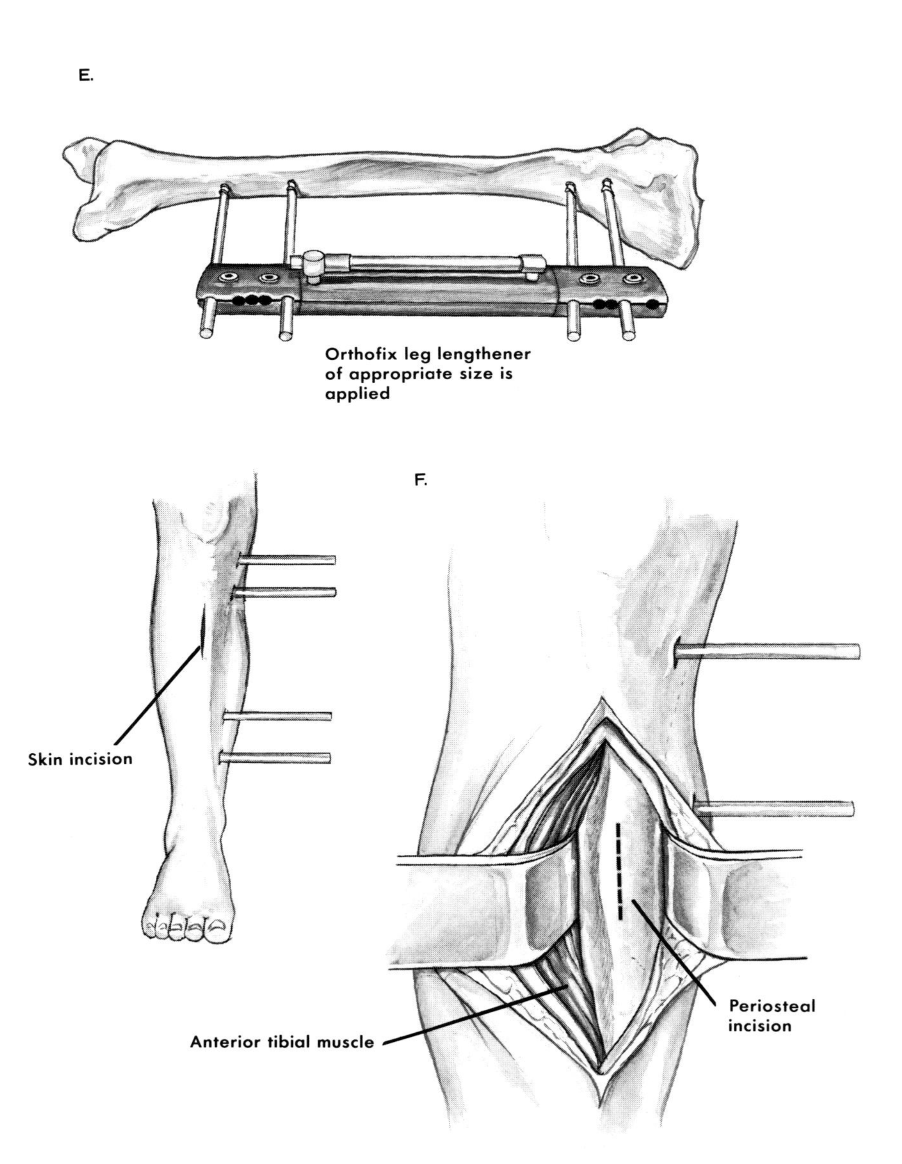

Callotasis (Callus Distraction) for Lengthening of the Tibia (Continued)

G. A 4.8-mm. drill is inserted into a short Orthofix screw guide. The drill stop is adjusted so that the tip of the drill guide protrudes 5 mm. beyond the end of the screw guide. A drill bit of the appropriate size is inserted into the drill guide.

H. Holes are drilled into the medial, lateral, and anterior cortices, with damage to the bone marrow being prevented by the drill stop. The stop is removed for drilling through the cortices medially and laterally.

I. Next, the holes are joined by chiseling the bone *without* penetrating the marrow. Be sure that the medial and lateral cortices of the tibia are completely osteotomized. The posterior cortex is broken by flexing the leg. Caution: Do not use the screws as a lever to achieve acute flexion at the corticotomy site, because loosening of the screws may occur.

Plate 118. Callotasis (Callus Distraction) for Lengthening of the Tibia

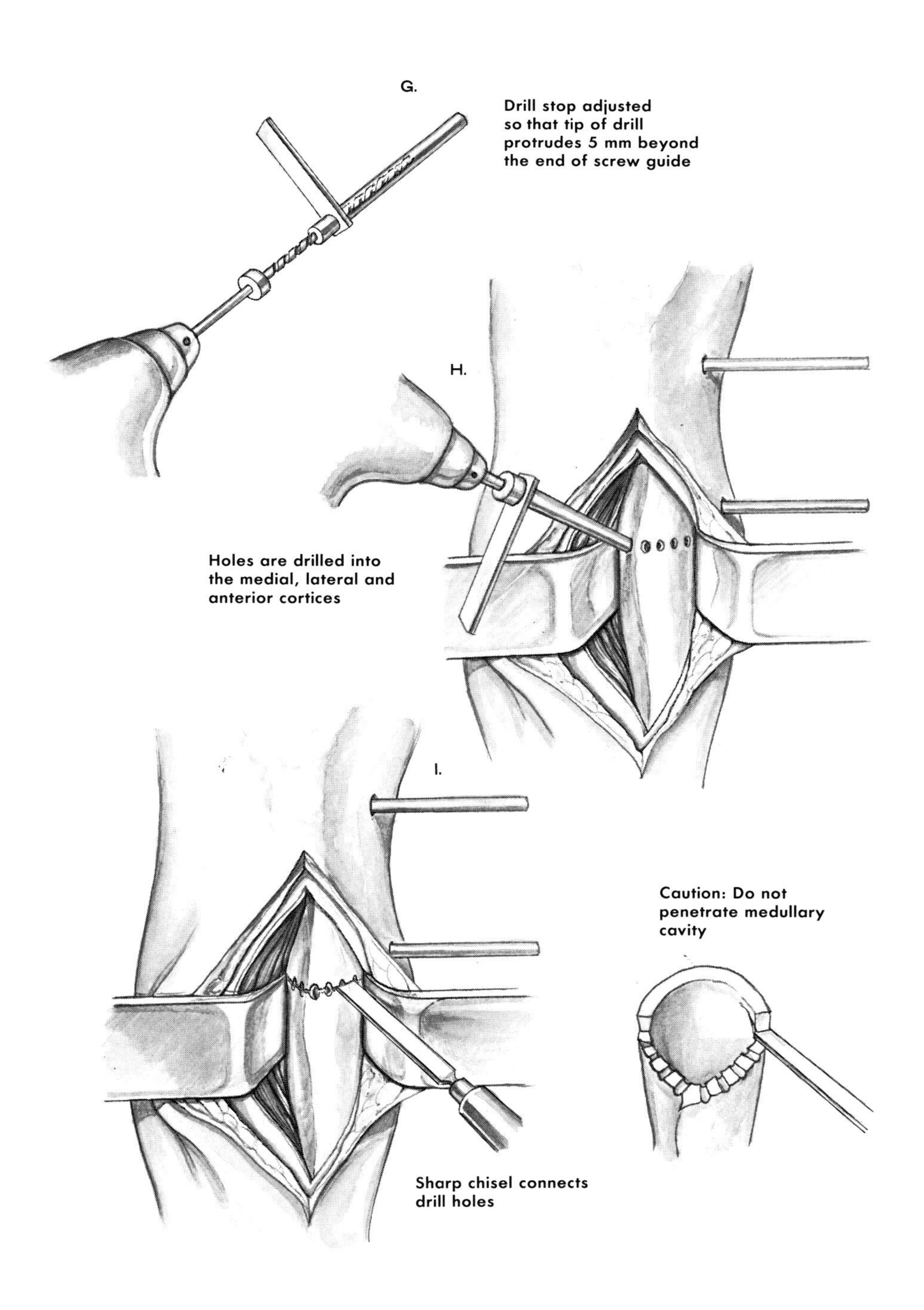

Callotasis (Callus Distraction) for Lengthening of the Tibia (Continued)

J. The periosteum is closed meticulously with interrupted sutures. **K.** The Orthofix leg-lengthener is placed on the previously inserted screws. The body of the device should be parallel with the tibial shaft.

Plate 118. Callotasis (Callus Distraction) for Lengthening of the Tibia

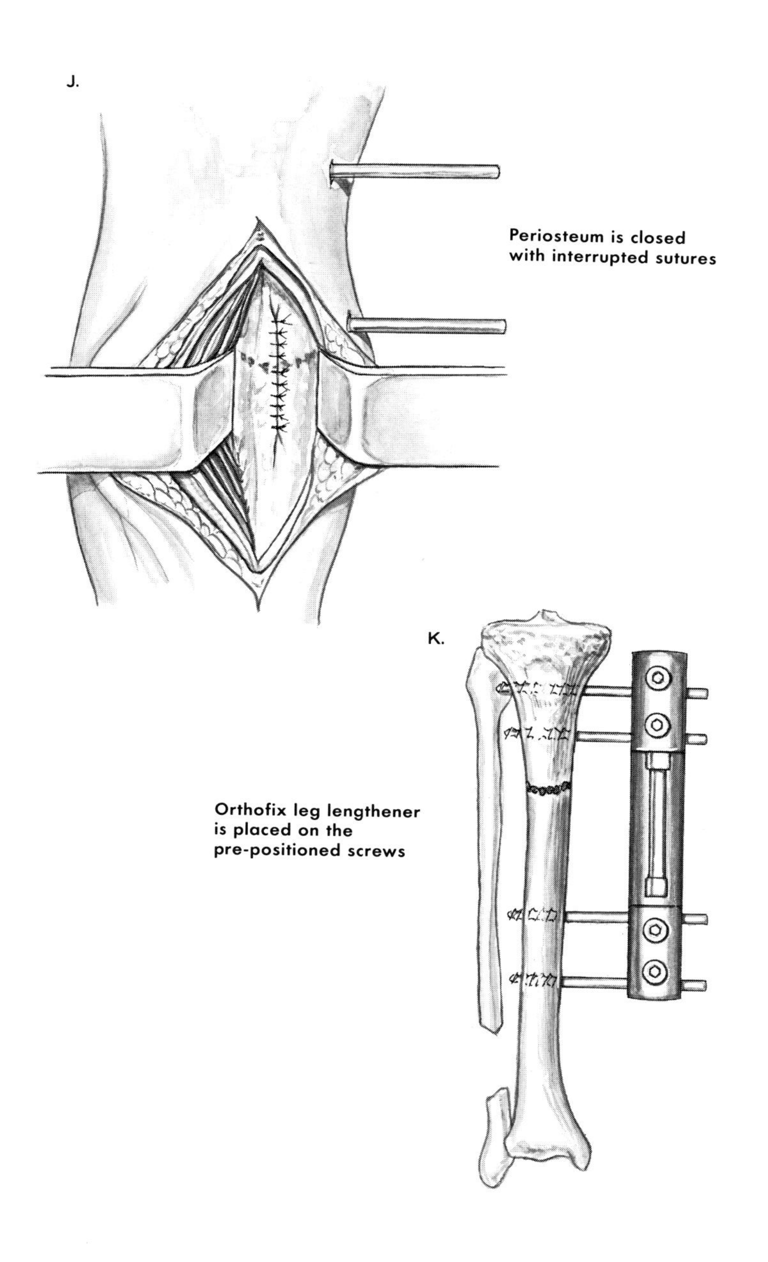

L and **M.** Any slack in the system is tightened, and the separation of the corticotomy is double-checked by distracting the bony fragments (if the corticotomy is proved complete this way, the osteotomized fragments are then returned to their original positions).

POSTOPERATIVE CARE

The wound is drained for 24 to 48 hours postoperatively, and routine screw tract care is provided as outlined in the femoral lengthening section.

Distraction is begun 10 to 14 days after the corticotomy if by this time radiograms show evidence of early callus formation. The rate of distraction is the same as that outlined for femoral lengthening. Seven days after the start of distraction, radiograms are obtained in order to confirm separation of the corticotomy with callus continuity. Radiographic follow-up is scheduled for every 14 to 21 days thereafter. If the response of the callus in the elongated segment is poor, distraction is stopped for 7 days and then recommenced. If a gap develops in the callus, compression should be applied—at the rate used for distraction—until the gap is eliminated. A wait of 7 days should precede resumption of distraction.

During the lengthening process, any axial displacement that may take place is corrected by adjusting the axial position of the lengthener.

Plate 118. Callotasis (Callus Distraction) for Lengthening of the Tibia

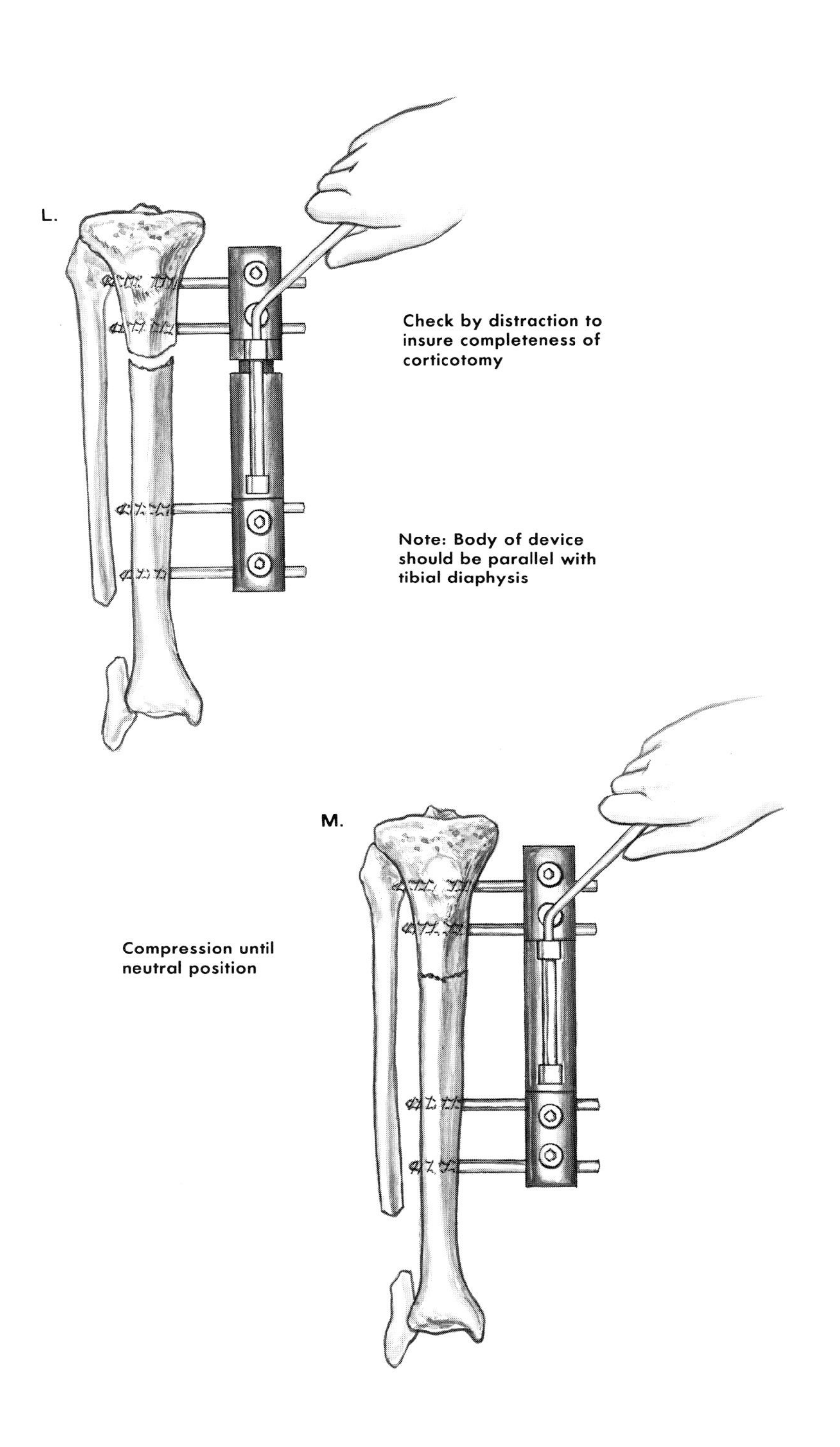

Ilizarov Leg Lengthening for Two-Level Tibial Lengthening

*OPERATIVE TECHNIQUE**

The Ilizarov apparatus is a circular external fixator utilizing smooth nonthreaded Ilizarov wires fixed to the rings under tension to stabilize the bone and limb segment. The wires are either 1.5 mm. or 1.8 mm. in diameter and are of a transfixion type crossing the ring by passing through bone and soft tissues from one side of the limb to the other. The wires are placed at multiple levels in several planes and orientations to achieve firm circumferential stability against the forces of bending, torsion, and translational displacement and shear. However, by the nature of their orientation they allow cyclic, elastic, axial micromotion of a magnitude proportional to the load applied. Cyclic axial dynamization has been proved both experimentally and clinically to stimulate bone regeneration and remodeling.

Prior to the actual application of the frame for limb lengthening, considerable preoperative evaluation and planning are required. There must be a combined clinical and radiographic assessment of the length and shape of the bone and limb. The goal of the procedure is not only to lengthen the limb but also to correct any existing angulatory, rotational, or translational deformity. Furthermore, the biomechanical axis of the limb should be restored to normal.

The following is a detailed description of the Ilizarov procedure carried out for double-level lengthening of the tibia, as modified by D. Paley.

Preassembly of the Apparatus

A to **C**. In order to save time in the operating room the frame can be assembled prior to surgery under nonsterile conditions according to measurements of the patient's leg obtained by clinical mensuration and derived from the radiographic findings.

First, the *appropriate ring diameter* for the leg is chosen. It should be just large enough to allow a clearance of two fingerbreadths from the skin at the widest part of the leg. The greatest diameter of the leg is measured directly on the patient's leg. Three rings of appropriate diameter are chosen. Each ring consists of two half-rings (of the same size) joined by two bolts and nuts.

Second, the distance between the proximal and distal ring is measured. The proximal ring should be placed just distal to the proximal tibial physis and the distal ring just proximal to the distal tibial physis. The distance between the levels of these two rings should be measured directly on the leg and confirmed radiographically (15 per cent x-ray magnification should be taken into account).

The fixator is then preassembled so that the middle ring lies about midway between the proximal and distal rings. It is important to place the proximal ring in slight varus and recurvatum in order to counter the valgus and procurvatum forces that develop during lengthening. If this measure is not taken, it will lead to deformity. Preventive measures should also be taken against the procurvatum of the distal fragment caused by the strong pull of the tendo Achillis on this short segment.

Next, put together two half-rings of the predetermined size to make a whole ring. It is important for each ring at each level to occupy a uniform plane, i.e., no half-ring should be connected upside down. Two properly connected half-rings should form a whole ring *on a single plane.* Upside-down construction will be evidenced by half-rings that each lie in a slightly different plane. Only when the half-rings are satisfactorily put together should the long bolt and nut connecting them be tightened.

Assembly of the Threaded and Telescoping Rods to the Rings

When all three rings have been constructed, the middle ring and the distal ring can be connected. A threaded rod is connected with locking nuts first to one ring (either distal or middle) at the hole adjacent to the joint between the ring's halves and then to the other ring at its corresponding hole. The distance between the rings should be half the overall distance measured from the proximal to the distal ring. A second threaded-rod-and-locking-nut connection is then made between the distal and middle rings in the manner just described, this time at the hole 180 degrees on the other side of each ring. The distance between the rings is measured to ensure that they remain parallel circumferentially.

Next, connect the distal and middle rings to the proximal ring, which should be fixed

*Written with Dror Paley, M.D., Assistant Professor of Orthopedic Surgery, University of Maryland Medical School; Attending Orthopedic Surgeon, University of Maryland Hospital, Baltimore, Maryland.

Plate 119. Ilizarov Leg Lengthening for Two-Level Tibial Lengthening

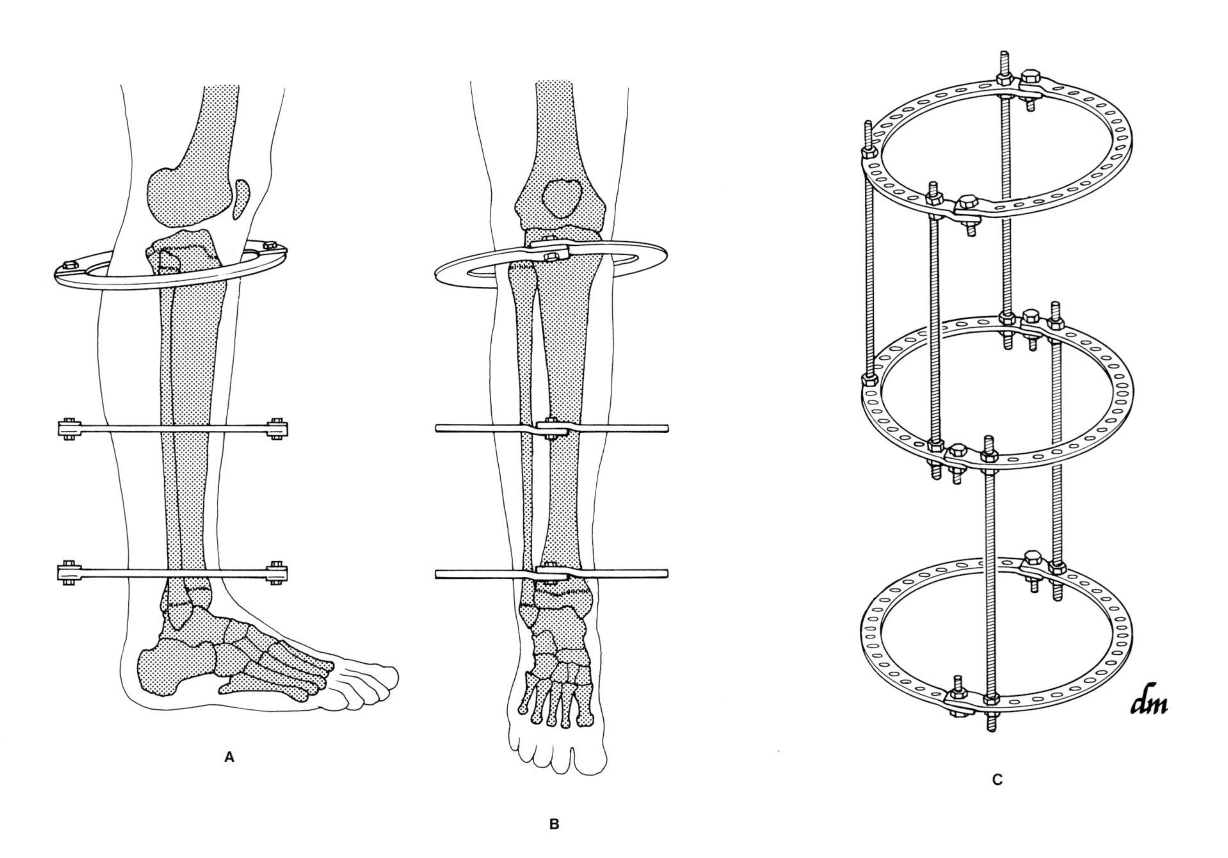

Ilizarov Leg Lengthening for Two-Level Tibial Lengthening (Continued)

in 5 degrees of varus and 5 degrees of recurvatum, to the long axis of the tibia. It may appear to be in valgus and procurvatum relative to the more distal rings, but it is the alignment relative to the tibia that counts. A simple way to achieve this is to draw two lines the diameter of the chosen rings at a 5 degree angle to each other and to directly measure the distance between the lines at one end with the other ends fixed together. When constructing the frame, connect the rings by two 180 degree counteropposed threaded rods; one anterior and the other posterior. The distance at the rod level between the rings should be different by the amount calculated to subtend an angle of 5 degrees. The anteroposterior difference places the ring in slight recurvatum. To produce the varus required, place a threaded rod laterally compressing the rings and shorten them by half the distance calculated above to produce an angle of 5 degrees. This will tilt the ring in the varus valgus plane so that the ring will tilt inferiorly on the lateral side in a degree equal to the superior tilt of the ring on the medial side (the total displacement being the amount calculated). This will cause the threaded rods to bend slightly, which is not a problem since the 0.25 mm. threaded rod is quite flexible. Assuming the distance calculated to subtend an angle of 5 degrees is 1 cm., a measurement of the spread between the rings anteriorly will be 1 cm. more than posteriorly and the spread medially will be 1 cm. more than the spread laterally. The same can be achieved using hinges in order to avoid the need for a third rod and for bending of the rod. This does, however, take more time. For distal procurvatum prophylaxis, the distal ring is fixed in a 5 degree inferior tilt anteriorly opposite the tilt of the proximal ring. Varus and valgus prophylaxis is usually not necessary in the distal ring. Distally, the tendency is frequently into varus rather than valgus. Once the frame is preassembled, it is sterilized in an autoclave and is ready for use (much the same way as the body of any external fixator).

Plate 119. Ilizarov Leg Lengthening for Two-level Tibial Lengthening (Parts A, B, and C repeated)

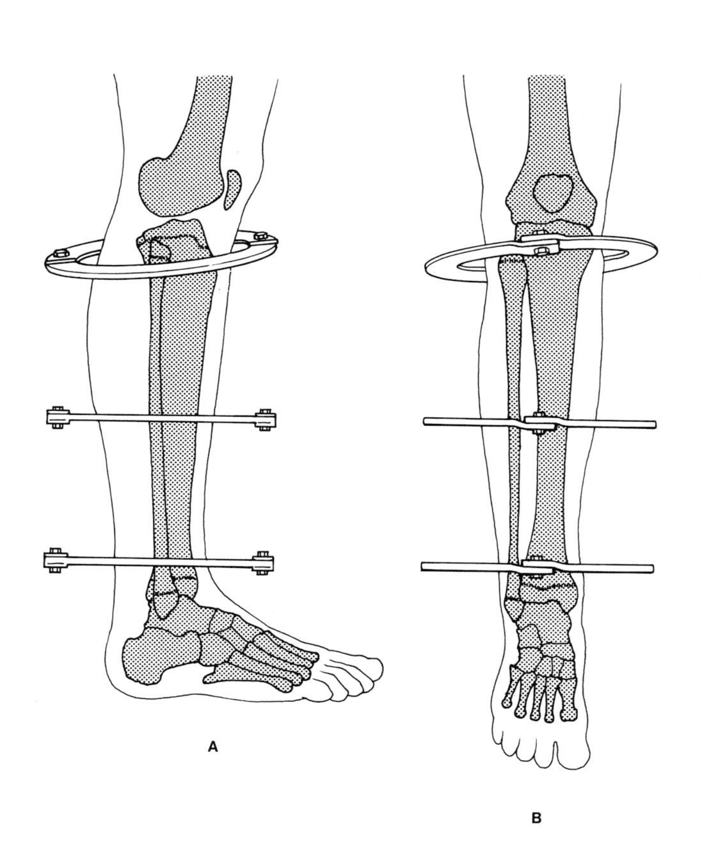

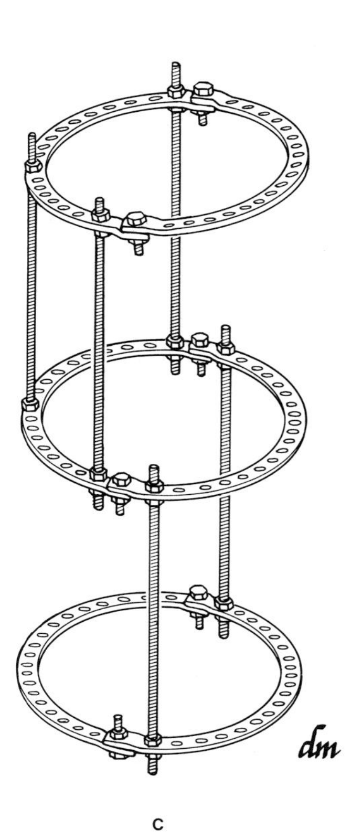

Ilizarov Leg Lengthening for Two-Level Tibial Lengthening (Continued)

Wire Insertion. **D** and **E.** The frame is then applied to the leg by first inserting the limb through it. Under image intensification with the patient on a radiolucent operating table, the length of the frame is examined relative to the tibia. The proximal ring should be immediately distal to the proximal tibial physis; the distal ring should be immediately proximal to the distal tibial physis. There should be enough space for the thickness of a wire to pass safely between the ring and the physis.

Next, a two-hole post is threaded onto the protruding end of the long bolt used to connect the two halves of the ring. The same step is repeated for the distal ring. The frame is oriented so that the posts are anterior and over the crest of the tibia. A 2-mm. nonthreaded Steinmann pin is drilled perpendicular into the crest anteroposteriorly for fixation of the Steinmann pin to the proximal post with a slotted wire fixation bolt so that the proximal and distal rings are between the two physes. Initially this pin is only fixed loosely in order to align the frame to the soft-tissue contour of the leg and bony anatomy of the tibia. The combination of the post and pin forms a very simple universal joint providing rotation in three axes. Two fingerbreadths are allowed circumferentially between the skin and the frame. The distal ring should appear on the image to be parallel to the distal physis on the anteroposterior view (as long as there is no varus valgus tilt of this ring). The middle ring is positioned perpendicular to the shaft of the tibia; and the proximal ring in 5 degrees of varus and recurvatum to the proximal tibial physis. On inspection, the anterior line of the fixator should be parallel to the anterior border of the tibia in the lateral projection. Once the position is obtained, a second 2 mm. Steinmann pin is inserted and fixed to the distal post. The 2 mm. Steinmann pins are inserted only unilaterally and are only temporary.

A stand preconstructed from parts of the Ilizarov apparatus is attached to the posterior aspect of the proximal ring, and the leg is elevated for wire insertion. If the frame has been correctly positioned on the leg, the use of image intensifier irradiation is minimized during the operative procedure.

Plate 119. Ilizarov Leg Lengthening for Two-level Tibial Lengthening

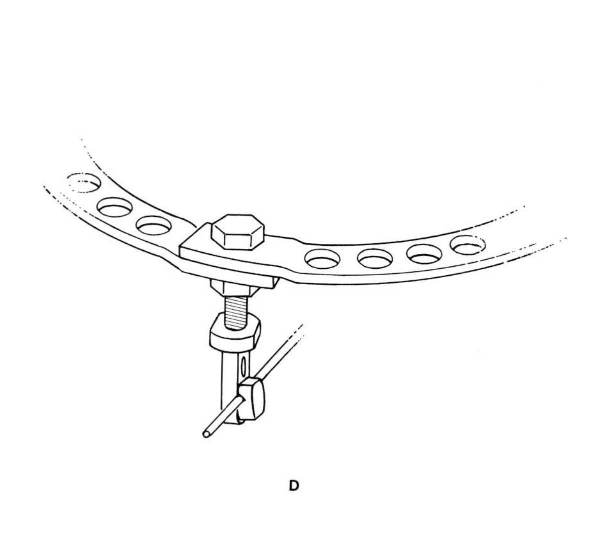

D

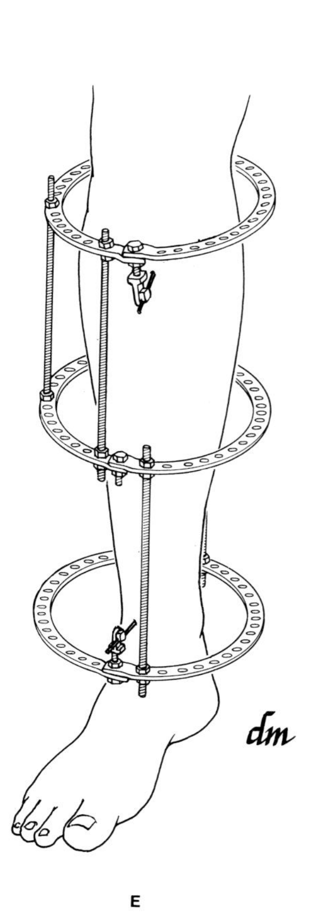

E

Ilizarov Leg Lengthening for Two-Level Tibial Lengthening (Continued)

F. The frame is used as the drill guide so that the wires that are to be inserted will lie where appropriate in relation to a particular ring.

The Ilizarov wires are of three different types. One type is bayonet point (cortical) wire, available in the following diameters and lengths: 1.5 mm. × 170 mm.; 1.5 mm. × 300 mm.; and 1.8 mm. × 370 mm. A second type, trocar point (cancellous) wire, is available in the range of sizes just cited. The third type is bayonet point wire with an attached stopper or "olive." Wire of this type, which may be referred to simply as "olive wire," comes in two sizes: 1.5 mm. × 300 mm. and 1.8 mm. × 400 mm. The "olive" wire provides interfragmentary compression and increases the stability of the assemblage. The choice of the diameter and length of any of the wires depends upon the size of the bone being operated upon and the age and weight of the patient.

Insert an olive wire horizontally along the distal surface of the proximal ring from the lateral side. A power drill is used to drill the wire through bone; first, however, the wire is poked through the skin down to bone and then drilled. No incision is made except in the case of an olive wire, where a small stab incision is made after insertion to allow the olive to pass down to bone. Initially chuck up the drill close to the skin, and gradually chuck it back during the drilling process. The image intensifier is used to determine the position of the wires. Since the wire will pass through the anterior compartment muscles, the ankle and toes are plantar flexed prior to insertion to minimize entrapment. This is particularly important in limb lengthening, since the increasing stretch on the muscles is accommodated by transfixing the muscles in their lengthened state, thus avoiding contractures of the muscles in their shortened state. As the wire exits the bone to enter into the posterior compartment, the ankle and toes are dorsiflexed and the wire advanced by tapping it in with a mallet rather than drilling across soft tissues. The latter maneuver minimizes the chance of injury to vessels and nerves, since a nonrotating wire pushes such structures out of harm's way rather than perforating them. Release pin sites if they are tenting the skin after tensioning the wire. If there are open spaces created around the incised pin sites, close the wound with 0000 Vicryl sutures.

A cube of open-cell sponge is placed on each wire where it exits the skin, followed by a rubber stopper to push down on the sponge. These are used in postoperative pin site care. The tips of the wire are wrapped in gauze or bent to prevent cutting through the surgical gloves. Throughout the operation, the surgeon and assistants should exercise great care not to puncture their skin.

G. The second wire inserted is also a horizontal olive wire with the olive lateral. This lies on the distal ring. Both these wires are fixed to the rings by means of wire fixation bolts and nuts.

Tensioning of the Wires

This is performed using a calibrated wire tensioning device. The wire is inserted into the cannulation in the tensioner, and the handle is then turned clockwise to tension the wire within the range marked 50 to 130 kg. Non-olive wires should first be fixed to the ring at one side and tensioned from the other side. The olive wires can also be tensioned this way fixing the olive end to the ring and tensioning from the other side. Use two tensioners and tension the olive wires simultaneously from both ends to ensure even forces across both sides of the olive in order to decrease the incidence of pressure necrosis of bone from the olive. The tension applied should be between 90 and 130 kg. It is safer to use only 90 kg., since the lengthening process itself generates approximately 30 to 40 kg. of stress on the wires, thereby minimizing the risk of wire breakage. After tensioning and fixing the wire, cut off only the sharp tip and leave the wire long. The protruding portion is then bent in a smooth arc around the ring to be available to retensioning if necessary. The ends of the wires with the olives are marked by bending one end in a different manner; this measure will prevent accidental pulling of the wire in the wrong direction. The wires should be fixed to the rings so that they need not be displaced in order to fix them. If a wire lies several millimeters off the ring, spacer washers on the wire fixation bolt should be used in order to fix the wire in situ. In this manner there is no prestress on the wire when it is tensioned. Any prestress can lead to either displacement of bone fragments or lysis of the bone around the pin with increased risk of pin tract infection.

Plate 119. Ilizarov Leg Lengthening for Two-level Tibial Lengthening

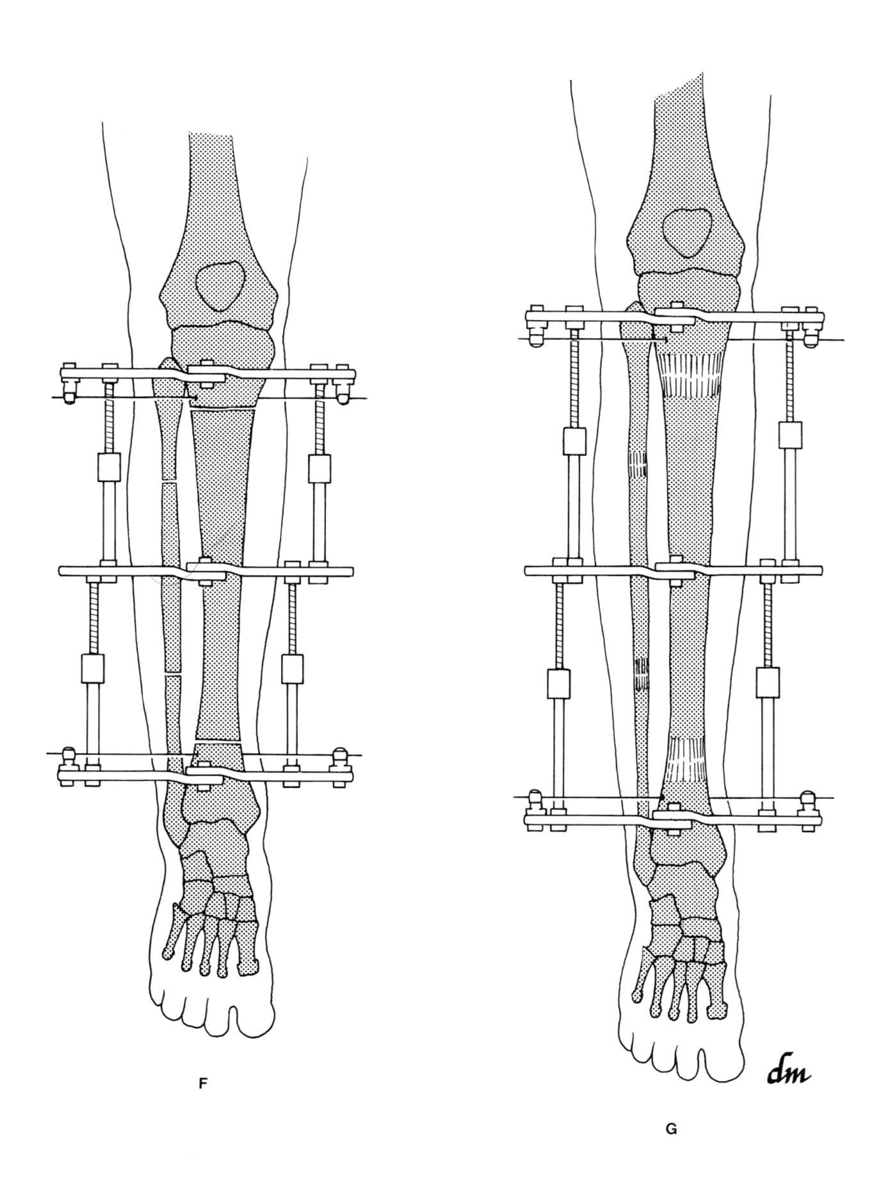

Ilizarov Leg Lengthening for Two-Level Tibial Lengthening (Continued)

H. Proximally, three more 1.50-mm. pins are added. One regular wire is passed through the head of the fibula to exit anteriorly through the anteromedial tibia. A second regular wire is passed anterolateral to the tibial crest to exit through the posteromedial corner of the tibia; in the passage of this wire, the belly of the gastrocnemius muscle is to be avoided. The third wire is of the olive type and is inserted approximately 2 cm. off the ring and supported off two posts. The olive should be medial in this case, and the wire should be virtually horizontal but for a slight slope in a posteromedial to anterolateral direction. The end result is three wires lying on the ring and one suspended below the ring. Of the three wires that are on the ring, it is preferable to have two on its superior surface and one on its inferior surface. Sponge-and-rubber-stopper placement, wire fixation, and wire tensioning are carried out as previously described.

Distal-ring wiring resembles the arrangement detailed above. One regular wire is inserted through the fibula and the tibia, and is fixed on the ring. Another regular wire is inserted immediately lateral to the tibialis anterior tendon and medial to the extensor hallucis longus and is directed from the anterolateral tibial cortex to the posteromedial tibial cortex. An olive wire is inserted off the ring with the olive on the medial aspect of the tibia.

Finally, two regular wires are inserted and fixed to the middle ring. The first wire passes through the fibula from posterior to anterior to include the tibia. The second is placed almost horizontal, going through the middle of the muscle mass of the anterior compartment.

Plate 119. Ilizarov Leg Lengthening for Two-level Tibial Lengthening

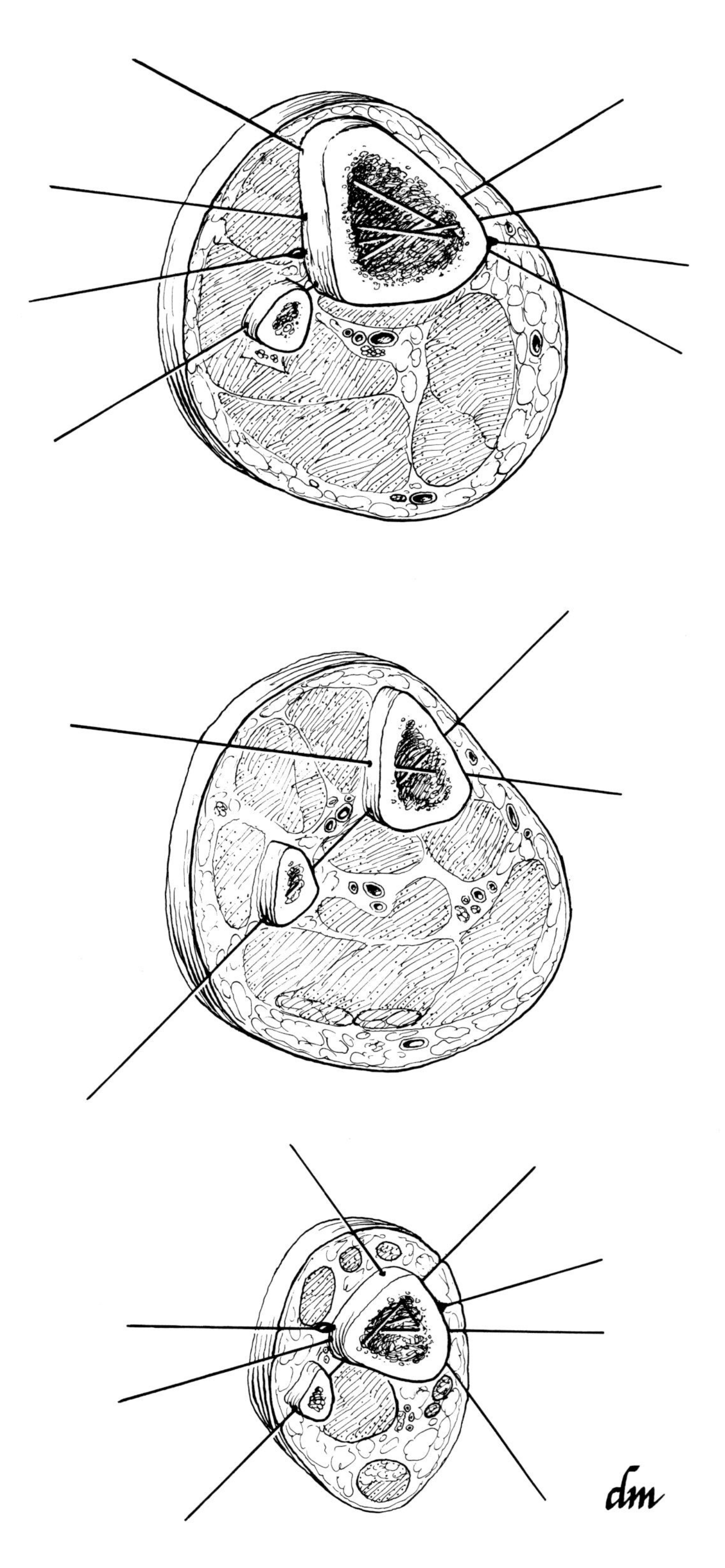

H

Ilizarov Leg Lengthening for Two-Level Tibial Lengthening (Continued)

OSTEOTOMY OF THE FIBULA AND CORTICOTOMY OF THE TIBIA

I. Once all of the wires are in place, the fibula is osteotomized at two levels—i.e., between each pair of rings. A small incision is made to expose the fibula in areas away from the peroneal nerve. A subperiosteal dissection is carried out and, under the protection of periosteal elevators or small Homan retractors, the fibula is cut with an oscillating saw. An osteotome may be used if desired, after one first carries out pre-drilling. The advantage of using the saw is that it burns the bone, thus slowing the regeneration of the fibula and lessening the risk of premature consolidation. The wounds made for osteotomy of the fibula are then closed.

The next step is the corticotomy of the tibia. The proximal and distal osteotomy levels should be as close to the metaphysis as possible. One skin incision, 1 cm. long, is made anteriorly at the level of the wire that is suspended off the proximal ring; another 1-cm.-long skin incision is made anteriorly at the level of the wire suspended off the distal ring. The corresponding osteotomes required are one immediately distal to the proximal ring's "off" wire (drop wire) and another immediately proximal to the distal ring's drop wire. (1) Through a 1-cm. longitudinal incision made just lateral to the tibial crest, cut down to and through periosteum. Insert a periosteal elevator medially and laterally to elevate the periosteum at the level of the osteotomy. A 1-cm. osteotome is inserted into the rent in the periosteum and turned 90 degrees (as shown). (2) The osteotome is used to cut into the anterior cortex of the tibia. (3) Although the osteotome should be used to create a groove, the cut should extend to but not through the medullary cavity. (4) The 1-cm. osteotome is removed, and a periosteal elevator is inserted on the lateral side. The elevator should reach around the posterolateral cortex. With the elevator lying flat against the bone, the direction of the cut can be appreciated.

A 5-mm. osteotome is inserted under the protection of the elevator and is used to cut the cortex down to and through the posterolateral corner. The osteotome should neither slide out of the cortex nor penetrate deeply into the medullary cavity. Excessive slippage of the osteotome during removal can be avoided by slightly twisting it from side to side to loosen it in the bone; broad to-and-fro maneuvers are ill-advised, as they may damage the medullary cavity. (5) The same steps are repeated on the medial side. In this case, one cuts to and through the posteromedial cortex. (6) The bone chisel, which is located in the posteromedial corner, is twisted 90 degrees to spread the osteotomized bone apart as if separated by a laminar spreader and to begin the osteoclasis of the posterior cortex. (7) The same maneuver may need to be repeated several times on the medial and lateral sides until the posterior cortex is broken. Undue movements of the osteotome are to be avoided in order to prevent disruption of medullary contents and vessels.

Plate 119. Ilizarov Leg Lengthening for Two-level Tibial Lengthening

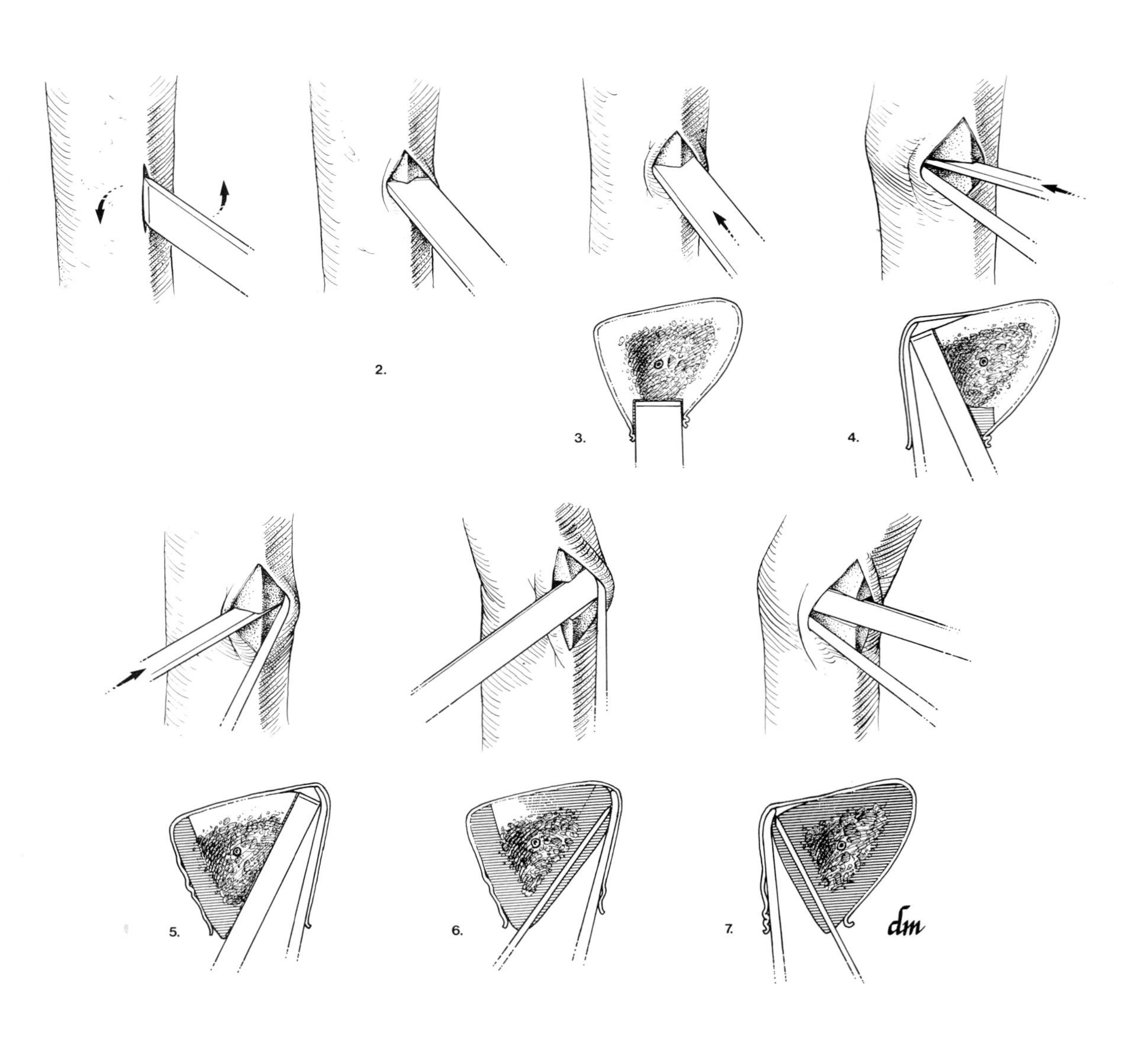

Ilizarov Leg Lengthening for Two-Level Tibial Lengthening (Continued)

J. Once the bone has cracked, one should make sure that the fracture is complete. This is done by rotating one fixator ring relative to the other. In the proximal tibia it is important not to rotate internally since this can potentially stretch the peroneal nerve. The completeness of corticotomy is also confirmed on image intensification. To ensure that the bone ends are in an undisplaced relationship after the corticotomy, it is important to reattach the connecting rods as they were before.

Plate 119. Ilizarov Leg Lengthening for Two-level Tibial Lengthening

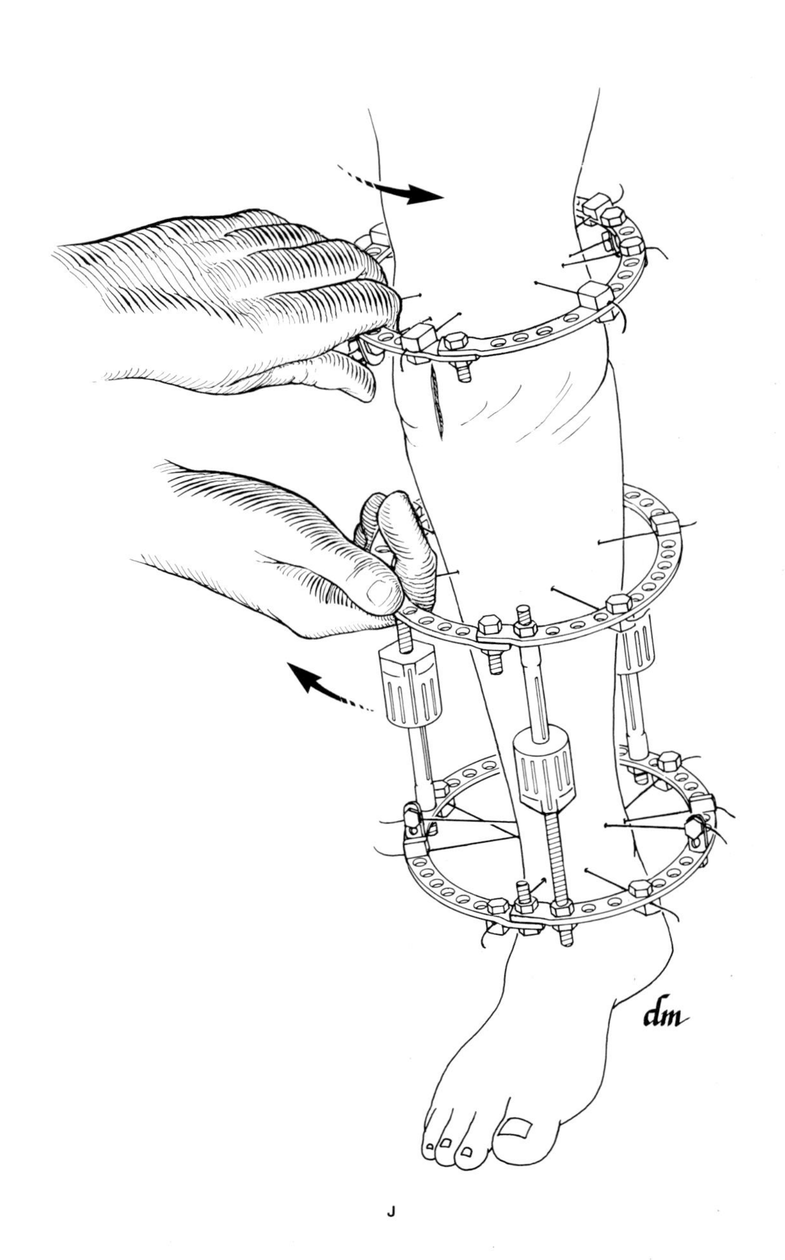

J

Ilizarov Leg Lengthening for Two-Level Tibial Lengthening (Continued)

UTILIZATION OF THE APPARATUS

K. *Final adjustments.* The last step is to pre-stress the proximal ring to effect the antivalgus-antiprocurvatum prophylaxis. This is simply done by connecting the proximal ring to the middle ring so that they are parallel to one another. This will not open up the osteotomy if the wider part of the spread between the rings is closed rather than the narrow part opened. Thereby a force is produced in the ring that will tend to spring back into varus and recurvatum, thus resisting the forces pulling the tibia into valgus and procurvatum.

Replace the connecting rods for the first corticotomy level and repeat the same steps of removing the connecting rods, tibial corticotomy, and replacement of connecting rods for the second corticotomy level. For single-level lengthenings the exact same procedure is carried out minus the middle ring but using twice the amount of proximal ring prophylaxis, i.e., 10 degrees of varus and 10 degrees of recurvatum, for the proximal ring.

The threaded rod should be inserted well into the telescoping rod (at least 35 mm.) to maintain stability—this technical detail is important in both the telescoping and graduated telescoping rods. In bilevel lengthenings two sets of telescoping rods are required.

Lengthening. Distraction begins 3 to 10 days postoperatively, depending upon the age of the patient and the extent of vascular and soft-tissue disruption at corticotomy. In children and adolescents, a 3- to 5-day wait is adequate; in the older patient, a 7- to 10-day wait is preferable. The start of distraction is delayed when there has been disruption of the medullary circulation and of the endosteal and periosteal soft tissues, as manifested by displacement of the bone ends. Distraction totaling 1.00 mm. per day is achieved in incremental gains—e.g., four advances of 0.25 mm. each daily. The lengthening can be performed with two wrenches, advancing one nut a fixed amount after the other nut is loosened. The different nuts and the direction each should be turned must be clearly marked for the patient. For a reference point, colored nail polish is used to mark the ring and the driving nut so that the amount of each turn can be measured. One full turn of the nut on the rod is equivalent to 1.00 mm. Patients perform 0.25 mm. of lengthening four times a day. (With the newer telescopic rod, advancements can be made by hand by "clicking" through 0.25 mm. of distraction at a time. The markings on the side of the rod indicate the length of the advancement. Presently available in Russia and Europe is a motorized auto-distractor that achieves a quasi-continuous distraction rate of 0.016 mm. 60 times a day.)

It may be necessary to change the rate of distraction. It is slowed to 0.75 mm. or 0.50 mm. per day when consolidation of new bone is delayed. The rate may need to be increased to 1.25 mm. or 1.50 mm. per day if consolidation takes place prematurely. With a two-level lengthening, a "standard" rate of gain of 1.00 mm. daily may not be tolerated by soft tissues. The rate of distraction is decreased to 0.75 mm. of lengthening at each level after the initial 2 cm. of lengthening.

A device that Paley has found helpful in avoiding contractures of the knee and ankle is a resting splint. Contractures result from a state of imbalance of muscles across a joint when lengthening leaves some muscles in their shortened position for too long a time, as is the case with the triceps surae. Contractures could be avoided if the ankle and knee were to be maintained in extension for some time and the muscles stimulated to grow at *that* resting length rather than solely while in their shortened length in equinus and knee flexion. The resting splints, used only at night and during those parts of the day when the patient is relatively inactive and sitting, thus have their rationale.

If a contracture does develop, a very useful maneuver, reported by Paley, is to overlengthen the limb by 1.00 cm. and then shorten the limb by 1.50 cm. The overlengthening leads to further lengthening of the already contracted muscles, which upon shortening are left loose, eliminating the contracture. In addition, reversing the tension of "distraction osteogenesis" causes the bone that has been newly formed in response to such tension to consolidate very rapidly, decreasing (favorably) the healing index.

Pin site care, according to Paley, consists of the application of a solution of chlorhexidene and isopropyl alcohol once a day to the sponges, which are changed once a week. Polysporin ointment is applied to any pin site that is red or inflamed; this is done on a daily basis until the inflammation resolves. If inflammation or infection persists, the skin around the pin site is injected radially and down the tract with a solution of 100 mg./cc. of cephalosporin. The tension of the wire is also checked; if loosened, the wire is re-tensioned as necessary. According to Paley, this routine has been consistently successful in care of the pin tract.

Plate 119. Ilizarov Leg Lengthening for Two-level Tibial Lengthening

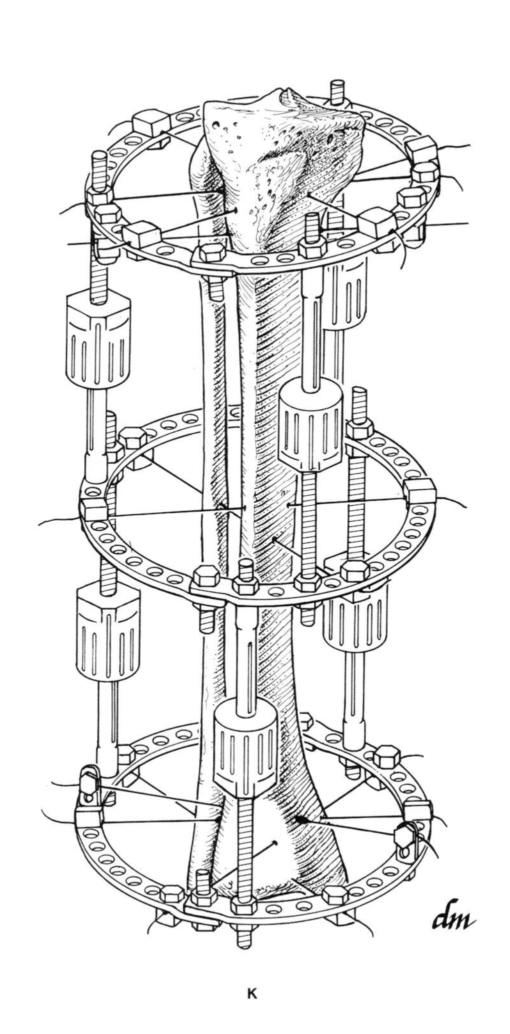

K

Ilizarov Leg Lengthening for Two-Level Tibial Lengthening (Continued)

This author's preference is to use Betadine-soaked sponges (2″ by 2″) over the pin sites and to change the sponges three times a day. Two to three days later, the pin sites should be healed; they can then be cleansed with isopropyl alcohol three times a day.

Physical therapy is performed several times a day to maintain and increase adjacent joint range and to increase muscle strength. When complications develop during elongation they are managed as outlined below. Radiograms obtained once or twice a month are checked for signs of translational and rotational malalignments; hinges are used to correct such problems if necessary. The distraction is stopped when the desired length is achieved. Early weight-bearing, as tolerated, is essential for stimulation of new bone formation. Fixation by the Ilizarov method is very stable.

Removal of the apparatus proceeds when three standards are met. (1) *Radiographically*, the regenerated bone should be normotrophic, exhibiting normal cortex formation and medullary cavitation along the elongated segment. (2) With the connecting rods of the apparatus removed, the regenerated bone should be stable when tested *clinically*. (3) With the connecting rods removed, the patient should *subjectively* feel that the limb is firm under the stress of loading; there should be no pain on weight-bearing or walking.

After removal of the fixator there is a definite risk of stress fracture of the newly generated bone, even after minor trauma. This author recommends protecting the limb in a plastic knee-ankle-foot orthosis (KAFO) with an anterior plastic shell. (The KAFO is appropriate after tibial lengthening, but a hip-knee-ankle-foot orthosis [HKAFO] is called for after femoral lengthening. The hip and knee joints are freed with a droplock, allowing motion, and the ankle joint is also allowed motion.)

The patient is weaned from the orthosis gradually. If the regenerate bone fractures, the limb should be immobilized in a cast. The fracture will heal rapidly, and the new bone stimulated by the fracture is better than the previous regenerate bone.

Plate 119. Ilizarov Leg Lengthening for Two-level Tibial Lengthening (Part K repeated)

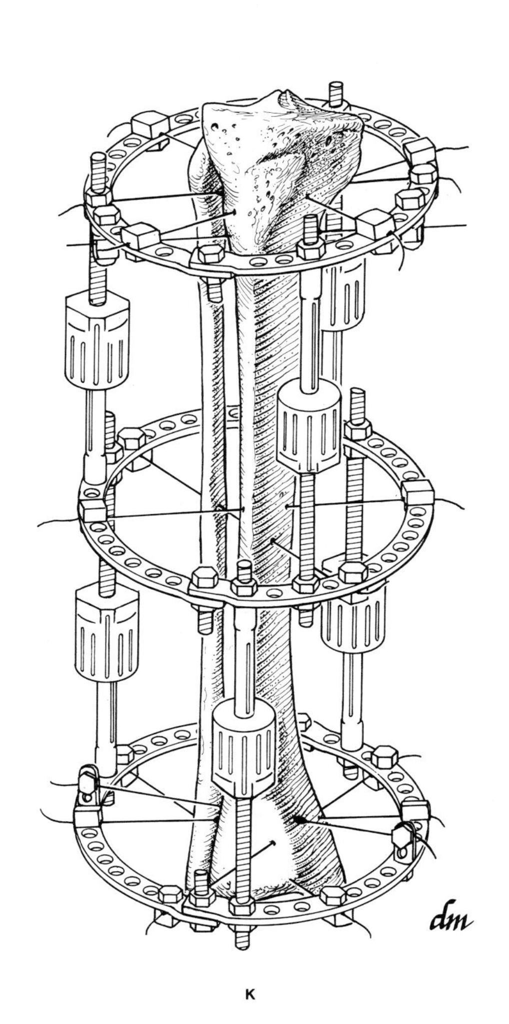

K

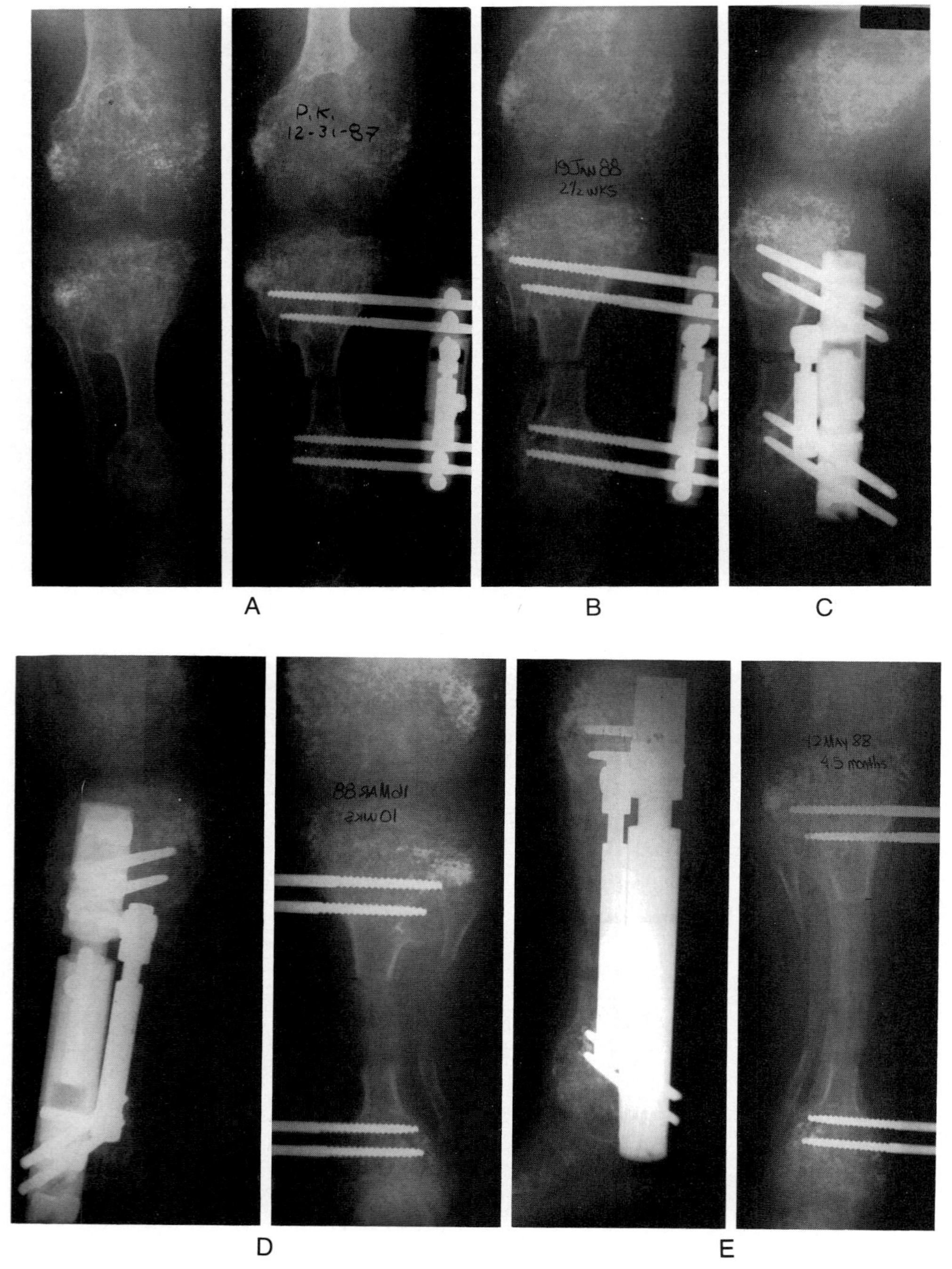

FIGURE 7–270. Callotasis technique of tibial lengthening with the Orthofix apparatus in a ten-year-old boy with severe achondroplasia.

A. Preoperative anteroposterior radiogram of the right lower limb. **B.** Immediate postoperative anteroposterior radiogram of the right tibia. Note the corticotomy of the tibia and osteotomy of the fibula. **C.** Anteroposterior and lateral radiograms of the right tibia and fibula two and one-half weeks postoperatively. Note the early callus formation at the corticotomy site. At this time the lengthening was commenced. **D.** Anteroposterior and lateral radiograms of the right tibia and fibula ten weeks after surgery. Five cm. of lengthening was achieved. Note the "fluffy" new bone formation at the distraction site. At this time a percutaneous Achilles tenotomy was performed to correct severe equinus deformity of the ankle. **E.** Lateral and anteroposterior radiograms of the tibia and fibula showing early trabecular formation at the distraction site; 10.6 cm. of lengthening was achieved. Note the neutral position of the ankle.

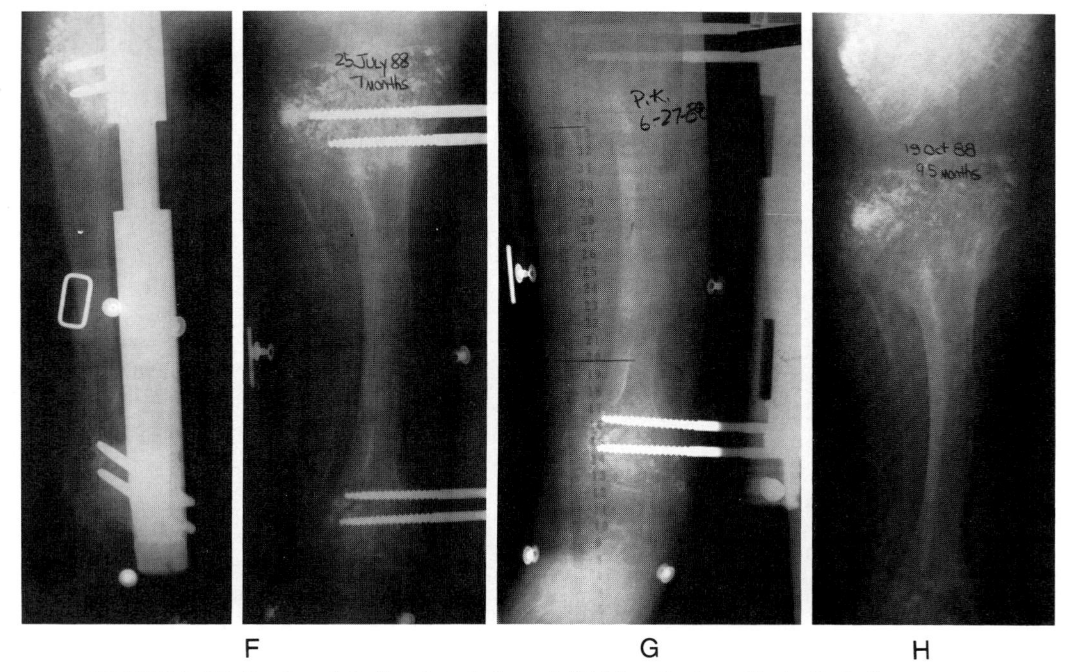

FIGURE 7–270 Continued. Callotasis technique of tibial lengthening with the Orthofix apparatus in a ten-year-old boy with severe achondroplasia.

F. Six months postoperative anteroposterior radiogram of the right tibia-fibula showing 13.6 cm. lengthening. Note the new osteogenic bone. At this time the fixator was locked for one month. **G.** Seven months postoperative anteroposterior and lateral radiograms of the leg. Note the strong cortex formation and significant remodeling of the elongated segment. The fixator was retained for an additional month. At that time the fixator was dynamized for two months; then the fixator was removed, but the pins were kept in place for one week and the child was allowed to walk on the leg. The pins were removed on an outpatient basis. **H.** Nine and one-half months postoperative radiogram of the tibia showing that the elongated tibia is fully healed by distraction osteogenesis using the DeBastiani technique. (Courtesy of Dr. Alvin Crawford.)

is obtained, the periosteal tube of the distraction gap is incised; a previously fashioned correct length of diaphyseal cortical allograft is fitted in the elongated segment, which fits over the intramedullary nail. By use of external fixation the segmental allograft is compressed between the two bone ends of the distraction gap. Union of the allograft is rapid, as it is placed in a vascular, highly osteogenic bed. Union usually takes place within two months, at which time the external fixator is removed.[462]

Problems and Complications

A distinction is made between problems and complications. *Problems* are difficulties that develop during lengthening; they are expected and often cannot be avoided. Problems do not interfere with the overall result, and they are managed by making appropriate alterations in management. For example, migration of screws or pins and mechanical pressure on skin and soft tissues is foreseen; it is a problem and is treated by extending the incision to relieve pressure. *Complications* are not expected. Preventive measures should be taken to avoid them; however, they cannot always be prevented. A wound infection, for example, is a complication and not a problem.

A complication is *minor* when it does not interfere with the treatment course or in achieving treatment objectives, whereas a *major* complication leaves permanent residua and interferes with obtaining the original treatment goals. Delayed union is a relatively minor complication in the child, whereas in the adolescent or adult it is a problem that is anticipated, discussed with the patient ahead of time, and treated by bone grafting. A nonunion is a complication.

Problems and complications are very common in limb lengthening (Table 7–29). This high rate of complications should be discussed with the parents and patient preoperatively. The etiology, prevention, and management of these complications will be presented sequen-

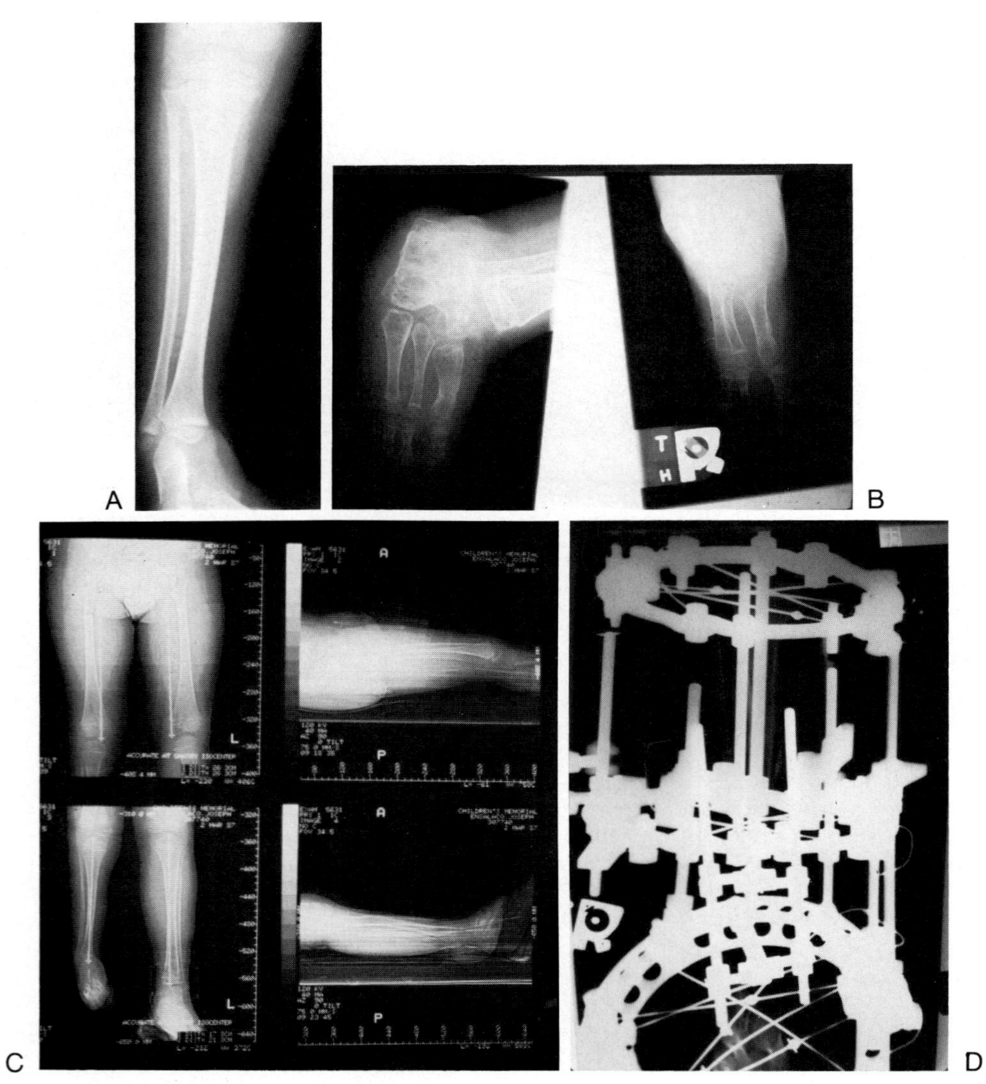

FIGURE 7–271. Ilizarov lengthening of the hypoplastic tibia and fibula with equinovarus deformity of the hypoplastic foot with congenital absence of the central ray in a seven-year-old boy.

A and **B.** Preoperative anteroposterior radiograms of the left tibia and foot showing the deformity. **C.** Preoperative CT scanogram of the lower limbs. The left tibia is 4.6 cm. short and the left femur is 1.2 cm short. **D.** Postoperative radiograms of the leg following Ilizarov apparatus application. Note the one level tibial lengthening with simultaneous correction of equinovarus deformity of the foot.

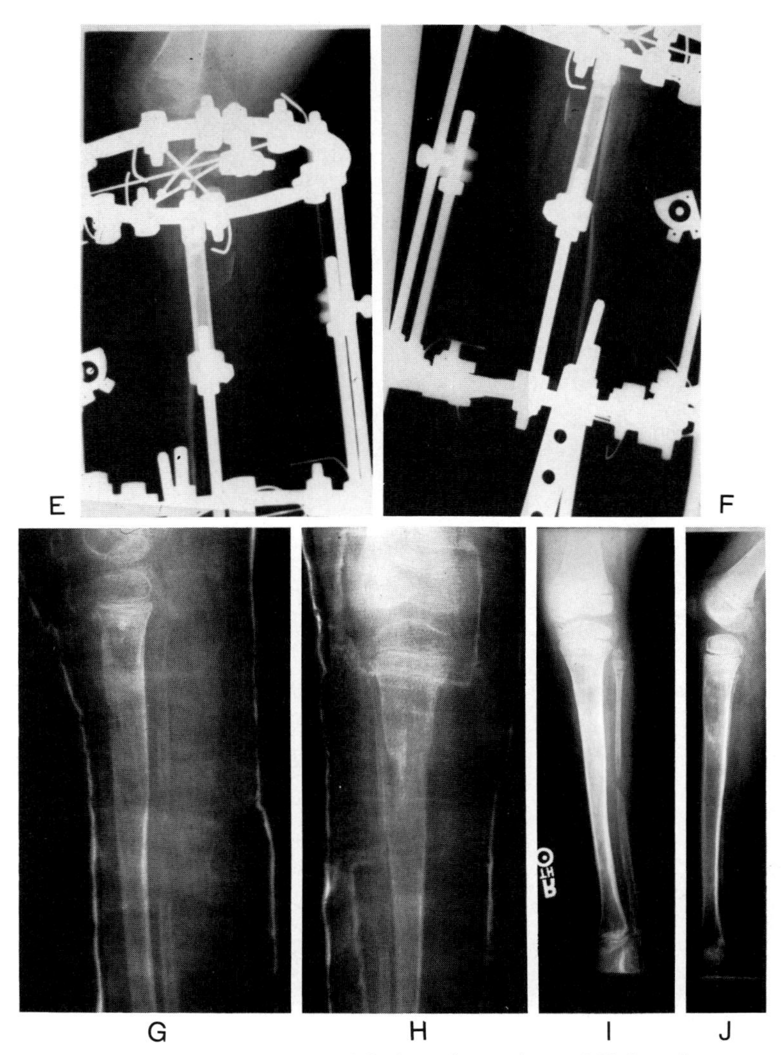

FIGURE 7–271 Continued. Ilizarov lengthening of the hypoplastic tibia and fibula with equinovarus deformity of the hypoplastic foot with congenital absence of the central ray in a seven-year-old boy.

E and **F.** Anteroposterior and lateral radiograms four months post surgery. Note the distraction osteogenesis. **G** and **H.** Anteroposterior and lateral radiograms six months postoperatively. The Ilizarov apparatus was removed and the tibia was supported in an above-knee walking cast. **I** and **J.** Anteroposterior and lateral radiograms one year postoperatively showing complete healing of the elongated segment. The patient is walking without any limp.

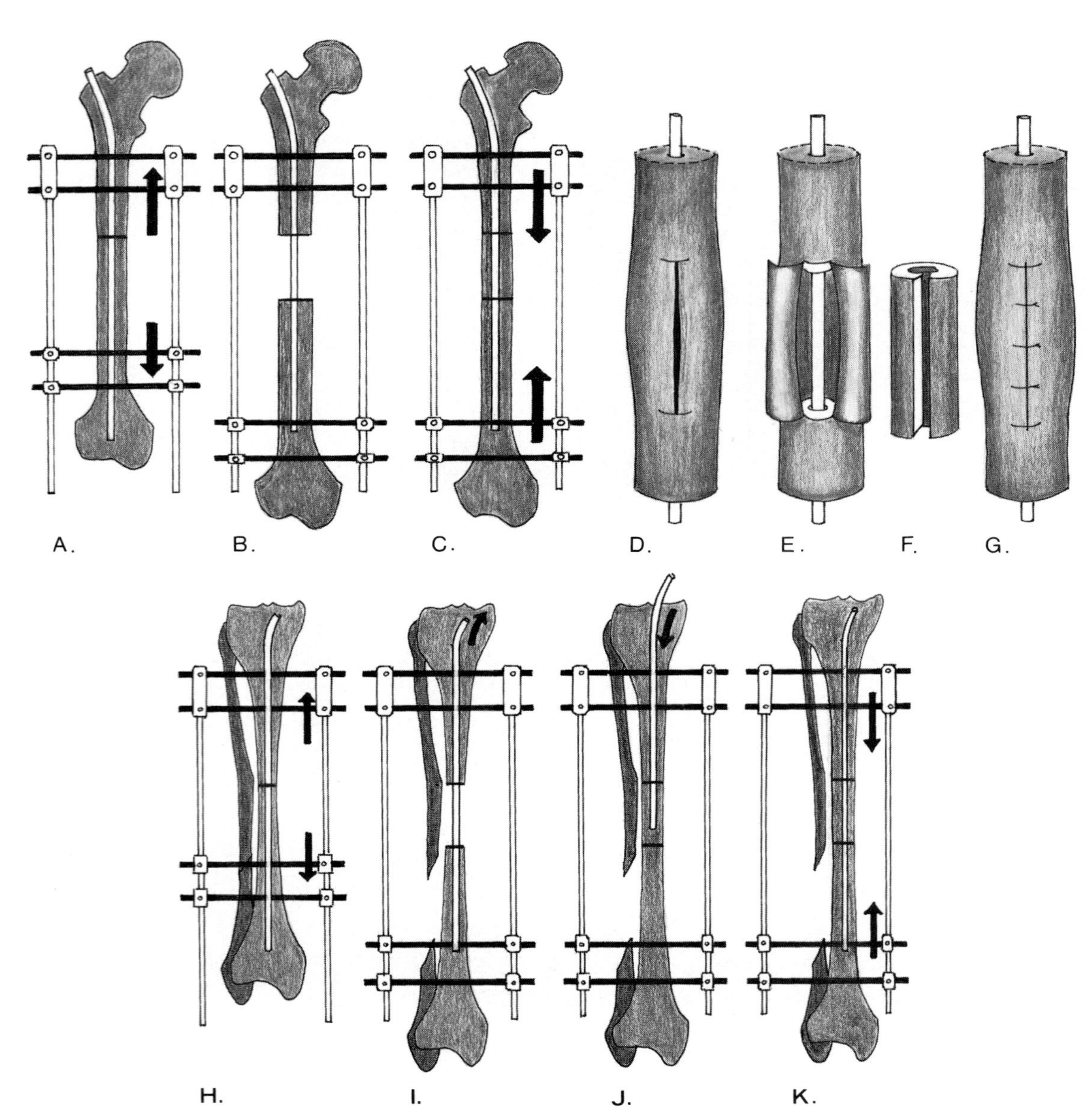

FIGURE 7–272. Wasserstein technique of lengthening of the femur and tibia.

Note that a circular external fixator is used for distraction; an unreamed, thin, intramedullary nail is inserted for alignment; and cortical segmental allografting is placed to fill the distraction gap. **A** to **G.** Lengthening of the femur. **H** to **K.** Lengthening of the tibia. (Redrawn after Professor I. Wasserstein, Eberbach, Federal Republic of Germany.)

Table 7–29. Problems and Complications of Limb Lengthening

I. *Intraoperative*
   A. *Pin insertion*—Injury to nerves and vessels by penetration of the pins or screws
   B. *Corticotomy*
      1. Disturbance of endosteal and medullary blood supply
      2. Oblique or comminuted fracture at site of osteotomy
      3. Stretching and paresis of common peroneal nerve
II. *Immediate Postoperative Period*
   A. Compartment syndrome
   B. Skin necrosis and slough
   C. Wound infection
III. *During Distraction Period*
   A. *Screw or pin tract problems*
      1. Soft-tissue necrosis
      2. Soft-tissue infection
      3. Osteomyelitis
   B. *Contracture of muscles*
   C. *Muscle weakness*
   D. *Neurologic compromise*
      1. Common peroneal nerve—due to compression by taut fascial band
      2. Lateral popliteal nerve—due to physeal separation of proximal fibular epiphysis
      3. Femoral or sciatic nerve—extremely rare, usually not encountered when distraction is gradual—less than 2 mm./day
   E. *Vascular problems*
      1. Hypertension
      2. Late erosion of the vessels by the pins
      3. Deep vein thrombosis
      4. Sudeck's atrophy
      5. Edema and hypertrophic swelling of the soft tissues of the limb
   F. *Joint subluxation-dislocation*
   G. *Joint stiffness*
   H. *Axial deviations*
      1. Tibia
         a. Valgus and anterior angulation (procurvatum) when elongated segment is proximal metaphysis or midshaft
         b. Varus and procurvatum—when elongated segment is proximal metaphysis and midshaft
      2. Femur
         a. Varus or procurvatum—when elongated segment is proximal metaphysis and midshaft
         b. Valgus and procurvatum when elongated segment is distal metaphysis
      3. Humerus
         a. Varus and flexion—when elongated segment is proximal metaphysis
         b. Flexion—when elongated segment is midshaft or distal metaphysis
      4. Forearm—flexion in both radius and ulna
IV. *Delayed Consolidation*
V. *Stress Fracture and Plastic Bowing of the Elongated Segment*
VI. *Mental Disturbance—Psychosis*

tially as they develop during surgery and during the various stages of limb lengthening.

INTRAOPERATIVE

During predrilling or insertion of screws or pins, it is possible to penetrate vessels or nerves. This is particularly true in the leg and forearm. The surgeon should be knowledgeable about the cross-sectional anatomy.

In the Ilizarov technique it is best to press the wire down to bone; after drilling through the bone, the end of the wire is gently hammered through the soft tissues on the other side of the limb. Despite these preventive measures, percutaneous transfixation or perforation of vessels or nerves may occur. During surgery, while the patient is still anesthetized, the tourniquet should be released and circulation assessed. In suspected cases the wake-up test and determination of nerve function are appropriate. Nerve function may be monitored intraoperatively by somatosensory evoked potentials. When there is suspicion of neurovascular penetration, the pins or screws should be removed and replaced at another site.

Problems During Corticotomy. *First,* endosteal and medullary circulation should be disturbed as minimally as possible. Only the cortex should be penetrated by the drill or osteotome. The *second* problem while performing corticotomy is the creation of an oblique or comminuted fracture. It is crucial to weaken the bone prior to performing closed osteoclasis. This author prefers multiple controlled drilling of the cortex prior to osteotomy (DeBastiani technique). The *third* problem during corticotomy is stretching of the common peroneal nerve. In the Ilizarov technique, when completing the fracture of the posterior cortex of the tibia, the two assembled rings are rotated in opposite directions; in order to avoid damage to the peroneal nerve, rotate the ring on the distal segment of the tibia laterally and not medially.

IMMEDIATE POSTOPERATIVE PERIOD

Compartment syndrome is a serious complication that can result from corticotomy or damage to vessels during screw or pin insertion. There should be complete hemostasis prior to wound closure. If necessary, extend the incision and coagulate or ligate bleeding vessels. Fasciotomy should be performed after all tibial lengthening; this is difficult in the Ilizarov technique, in which corticotomy is performed through a 1 cm. long small incision. Always drain the wound with medium-sized tubes and closed Hemovac suction. In the immediate postoperative period, neurovascular function should be closely monitored. If symptoms and signs of compartment syndrome develop, compartment pressure studies and appropriate treatment should be carried out.

Skin necrosis and slough is a possible complication in tibial and ulnar lengthening because the corticotomy site is subcutaneous.

Wound infection may develop. The operative field should be sterile. Because corticotomy is performed through a small incision and pins or screws are inserted percutaneously, nonchalant performance should not be tolerated.

DURING DISTRACTION PERIOD

Screw or Pin Tract Problems. These result from soft-tissue necrosis by the mechanical pressure of the migrating screws or pins. The necrotic soft tissue may be secondarily infected, and infection, if untreated, may eventually spread to bone, causing osteomyelitis. In limb lengthening, serous discharge around the screw or pin tracts is almost universal. The rate of pin or screw tract problems increases with greater depth of soft tissue between skin and bone, increase in diameter of pin or screw, instability of pin fixation, and motion between skin-pin interspace. The screw or pin sites should be carefully chosen at surgery; this is particularly important in femoral lengthening. When the patient is upright, sitting, or in supine or prone position, the screws or pins should not exert undue pressure on soft tissues. In femoral lengthening when inserting the distal screws or pins, the fascia lata should be divided horizontally and vertically, permitting full flexion of the knee. The proximal screws are placed in the lower part of the skin incision, whereas the distal screws are placed in the upper part of the incision; this allows some degree of migration of screws during lengthening. Daily care of the pin sites as outlined in the operative technique is important.

When mechanical pressure on skin develops, the skin incision is enlarged to relieve it; this can be performed under local anesthesia. The inflamed screw sites are dressed with Betadine solution. When soft tissues are infected, cultures are taken and appropriate antibiotics are administered orally. The screw or pin site may require debridement; in such an instance it is best to radially inject an antibiotic solution, such as cephalosporin around the pin site. Most screw inflammations and infections respond to these measures. If pin tract infection does not resolve and persists, it is best to remove the screw or pin and reinsert a new pin at a more proximal or distal site; this is best performed under general anesthesia under strict aseptic conditions.

Chronic osteomyelitis due to pin or screw tract infection is extremely rare; if it develops, it is treated by open curettage and debridement of the infected bone and soft tissues. In the Wagner technique of diaphyseal lengthening, persisting soft-tissue and bone infections may contraindicate internal fixation and bone grafting of the elongated segment.

Contracture of Muscles. During limb lengthening, disparity of relative length of bone and muscle develops—bone length becomes greater than muscle length and the muscles gradually develop contracture. The tendency toward contractural deformity is more common in two-joint muscles and in agonist muscles, which are stronger than their antagonist muscle groups. In tibial lengthening, equinus of the ankle and flexion deformity of the knee develop as a result of contracture of the triceps surae, which is a biarticular muscle and much stronger than its antagonist ankle dorsiflexors. During femoral lengthening the hip adductor and quadriceps femoris muscles develop contractural deformity, causing anterolateral angulation of the femur and limitation of knee flexion.

In the Ilizarov method of limb lengthening, other factors in the etiology of muscle contracture are pin placement and transfixation of muscles and possible differential rate of histogenesis of muscle versus osseous tissue.

Prevention. In congenital short limbs (such as congenital short femur or congenital short tibia with longitudinal deficiency of the fibula), in addition to the bone, the fascia, intermuscular septa, interosseous membrane, muscles, nerves, and vessels are also markedly shortened. Therefore, this author recommends routine extensive soft-tissue release and excision of fascia three to six months prior to bone lengthening. Ilizarov states that this preliminary soft-tissue resection-release is not necessary with his technique because soft tissues elongates as well as bone.

During limb elongation, *physical therapy* is vital. Several times during the day passive stretching exercises are performed, lengthening the muscles that have a tendency toward contracture. For example, in tibial lengthening, ankle dorsiflexion and knee extension exercises are performed simultaneously, stretching the triceps surae both proximally and distally. In femoral lengthening, hip abduction and knee flexion exercises are carried out in order to stretch the hip adductors and quadriceps femoris. An additional way to stretch the quadriceps muscle is to sit in a high chair with weights on the ankle for one or two hours of the day—gravity and ankle weights will stretch the quadriceps. Also, this author, in femoral lengthening, employs unilateral split Russell's traction on the leg that is being lengthened. Unilateral traction will tilt the ipsilateral pelvis inferiorly, and traction on the leg will stretch the hip adductors. This type of traction will also prevent hip and knee subluxation. The vertical force of the split Russell's traction is placed underneath the proximal tibia, thereby preventing posterior subluxation of the knee.

Ankle dorsiflexion and knee extension orthoses can be used to prevent development of muscle contracture. Ordinarily the patient uses the splint only at night, while sleeping. If necessary, the orthosis can also be used several hours of the day. These orthotic devices keep the muscles in elongated position.

In Ilizarov limb lengthening a pin may be inserted in the calcaneus and connected to the most distal ring of the Ilizarov fixator (Fig. 7–273); this measure will keep the ankle out of equinus; however, stiffness of the ankle is a potential problem with this technique.

Treatment. When fixed contracture of muscles is established and becomes a deforming force, musculotendinous lengthening by open surgery is indicated. Tendon lengthening causes motor weakness of the muscle. Do not perform heel cord lengthening indiscriminately, as overlengthening may result in triceps surae muscle weakness, calcaneus deformity, and greater functional disability. Fascial release allows the muscle to stretch out more readily, and it does

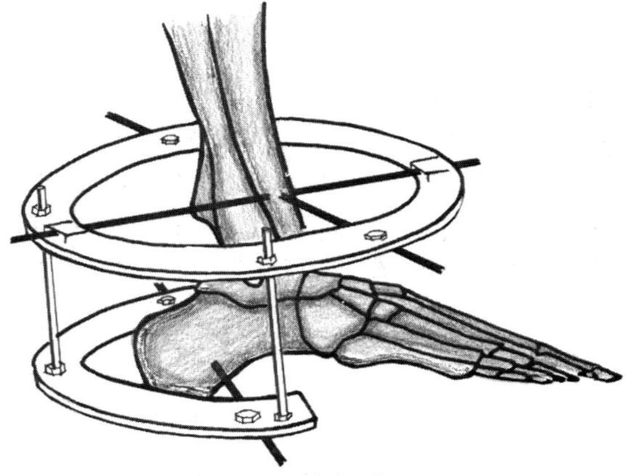

FIGURE 7–273. Extension of the Ilizarov device to the os calcis to control lateral subluxation and equinus of the ankle in tibial lengthening.

not weaken the muscle as much as muscle-tendon lengthening.

Prior to surgical fascial release and open musculotendinous lengthening, overlengthening and shortening may be attempted, as recommended by Paley.[349] Overlengthening the bone causes the soft tissues to lengthen; on shortening the bone the lengthened soft tissues will maintain some of their overelongated length. This distraction-compression process also stimulates consolidation of the regenerate bone.

Muscle Weakness. An overlengthened muscle due to bone lengthening may become weak in motor function, following the rules of the Blix curve. In femoral lengthening the possibility of quadriceps muscle weakness and knee extension lag is always a potential problem.

Neurologic Compromise. As stated above, neurologic compromise may occur during pin insertion. The neurovascular structures may be perforated or skewered by the pin, or the nerves may be eroded by the pin later, during distraction. The patient will complain of acute persisting pain and paresthesia in the distribution of the nerve. Tapping the pin will precipitate or aggravate the symptoms.

Nerve damage may also occur during corticotomy and/or when compartment syndrome develops.

During distraction the common peroneal nerve is most often affected. This is usually due to compression by the taut fascial band, which becomes tauter as the limb is being lengthened. Distraction should stop immediately when signs of impending nerve damage develop. The bone is shortened and nerve function reassessed. If neuropathy persists, the nerve is decompressed by release of the taut fascia by open surgery. In congenital short limbs this author recommends open surgical fascial release prior to limb lengthening.

Physeal separation of the upper fibula may cause lateral popliteal nerve palsy. Femoral or sciatic nerve paresis is ordinarily not caused by gradual distraction of less than 2 mm. per day. Instantaneous limb lengthening or distraction at a very rapid rate may stretch the nerve and cause paresis.

In the upper limb, radial nerve palsy may develop during lengthening of the humerus; in the forearm, ulnar and median nerve neuropathy can occur.

Vascular Problems. *Hypertension* can develop as a result of stretching the sympathetic nerve fibers. The blood pressure of the patient should be monitored once a day. If hypertension develops, distraction should stop for a few days. Ordinarily the blood pressure will return to normal; then the distraction is resumed at a slower rate and increased rhythm.

During distraction, particularly in the Ilizarov technique, there may be *late erosion of the vessels by the pin.* If the problem is pin related, the pin should be removed. Vascular consultation is obtained, as it may be necessary to perform angiography and vascular anastomosis or bypass.

Other vascular problems during distraction are deep vein thrombosis and Sudeck's atrophy with a cold cyanotic limb. These are very rare—but can occur. They are appropriately managed by the vascular surgeon.

Edema and excessive hypertrophy of the soft tissues of the limb may develop. This is quite common in the Ilizarov technique and may persist in 20 per cent of the cases.

Joint Subluxation and Dislocation

Etiology. Preoperative joint instability: The stability of the joints proximal and distal to the bone to be lengthened should be thoroughly assessed prior to lengthening. An unstable dysplastic hip should be stabilized by appropriate pelvic and/or femoral osteotomy. In congenital short femur, knee joint instability is commonly present owing to absence of the cruciates. During lengthening of the femur, posterior subluxation or dislocation of the knee is a definite problem, which is addressed during lengthening by split Russell's traction with the vertical traction force on the proximal tibia and exercises to increase motor strength of the quadriceps femoris muscle.

Marked knee joint instability is a relative contraindication to femoral lengthening. Preoperatively the parents and patient should be informed of the great risk of such a problem and the possibility of extension of the apparatus across the knee joint with a desubluxating hinge, which will permit knee motion while preventing posterior translation of the upper tibia in relation to the femoral condyles. In congenital short tibia with longitudinal deficiency of the fibula, posterolateral subluxation and dislocation of the ankle commonly occur during tibial lengthening. This is an anticipated problem; prior to lengthening the tibia a posterolateral release with excision of the fibular anlage should be performed. During lengthening an ankle-foot orthosis is worn at night to prevent posterolateral displacement of the talus under the tibia. In spite of these preventive measures, posterolateral subluxation of the ankle frequently develops because of the tensile mechanical forces of lengthening. It is vital to detect the problem early and extend the limb lengthening device across to the hindfoot. When the Ilizarov apparatus is being used, wires are inserted in the calcaneus with the "olive" laterally. Preoperatively, this author explains to the patient and parents the high frequency of ankle subluxation when congenital short tibia with longitudinal deficiency of the fibula exists. They should understand that the ankle joint will be stiff and subluxated and will require reconstruction and arthrodesis. Ankle joint stabilization is anticipated as a phase in the course of tibial lengthening in most of these cases.

Lengthening of the short fibula with an unstable and valgus ankle may be considered in some cases. Lowering the fibular malleolus to normal position will prevent lateral subluxation of the ankle. This author finds lengthening of the fibula difficult; distal tibiofibular synostosis is much simpler and more effective in preventing ankle valgus.

Dynamic imbalance and contracture of muscles across the joint may cause joint subluxation. A dysplastic but stable hip may become unstable when hip adductor contracture develops during femoral lengthening. Ipsilateral traction on the lower limb will tilt the pelvis inferiorly and stretch out the contracted hip adductors. Adductor myotomy of the hip is performed if the contractural deformity is not corrected by traction. In tibial lengthening when a progressive equinus deformity of the ankle develops, heel cord lengthening should be performed. Hamstrings should be lengthened if their contractural pull is causing posterior subluxation of the knee.

Treatment. Subluxation should be detected before dislocation develops. The importance of close clinical and radiographic observation of the joints proximal and distal to the elongated bone cannot be overemphasized. Mild subluxation can be reduced by stopping the lengthening, shortening the limb, and traction. Lengthening of contracted fascia and muscles may be indicated. Ordinarily these measures, with aggressive physical therapy, are successful in correcting minimal subluxations.

When there is moderate to marked subluxation the lengthening apparatus should be extended across the joint. Reduce the joint by the use of appropriate hinges and traction. A dislocated joint such as the hip will require open reduction. When marked subluxation or dislocation occurs limb lengthening should be discontinued. Never sacrifice function for length!

Joint Stiffness. This is almost a universal problem. It is caused by muscle contracture and increased pressure across the joints. Scarring of muscles transfixed by the Ilizarov wires causes permanent shortening of the muscles. Physical therapy in the form of active and passive exercises is performed one to two hours a day to maintain and increase range of joint motion. According to Wagner, the minimal range of motion in the knee is 45 degrees and the ankle 15 degrees.[458, 460] With less than this amount of range of motion, limb lengthening should stop and active and passive exercises be performed. When range of motion does not improve, the limb may be shortened to decompress the joint and a continuous passive motion machine (knee or ankle) may be applied. Passive manipulation of the stiff joint under general anesthesia may be attempted; however, this is fraught with risk of fracture-separation of the physis. Occasionally the joint stiffness persists; in such cases, hinged extensions are added to the lengthening apparatus, bridging the joint; the bones are distracted and the joint moved by a passive motion machine.

In the experience of this author, when knee motion is 60 degrees or greater and ankle motion 30 degrees or greater, full range of joint motion will return in three to six months. When the arc of motion is between 45 and 60 degrees at the knee and at 15 to 30 degrees at the ankle, there will be some permanent loss of range of motion, varying between 10 and 20 degrees at the ankle and 20 and 30 degrees at the knee. Extensor lag of the knee is a problem that may require treatment by patellar retinacular release and distal advancement or shortening of the patellar tendon.

Axial Deviations. These occur because of the imbalance of the muscular and fascial tensile forces across the elongated segment. The bone tends to deviate toward the side of greater tensile strength. In the *tibia* the greater muscle mass is posterior and lateral; therefore, when the elongated segment is in the proximal metaphysis and midshaft of the tibia, the deviation is toward valgus and procurvatum (anterior angulation); when it is in the distal tibia, the deviation is toward varus and procurvatum. In the femur, when the elongated segment is in the proximal metaphysis or midshaft, the axial deviation during elongation is toward varus and procurvatum. When it is in the distal femoral metaphysis, the deviation is toward procurvatum and valgus (the latter is caused by the pull of the fascia lata). In humeral lengthenings when the elongated segment is proximal, the axial deviation is toward varus and flexion; in midshaft and distal metaphyseal elongations of the humerus, the axial deviation is toward flexion alone. In forearm lengthenings, in both the ulna and the radius, the tendency of axial deviation is toward flexion.

Instability and rigidity of the biomechanical forces exerted by the hardware is another etiologic factor. In general, axial deviations are more frequent and more difficult to control with the monolateral thick-pin, cantilever-system fixators (Wagner or DeBastiani Orthofix) than with the circular thin-pin transfixation systems (Ilizarov). The monolateral thick-pin cantilever systems are strongest in the plane of the pins and weakest in the plane at a right angle to the pins. Therefore, the angle of insertion of the pins is an important consideration. When the Orthofix or Wagner system is used to elongate the tibia, it is best to place the pins and fixator anteriorly to prevent anterior angulation; however, anterior position of the pins-fixator does not prevent valgus deviation, as the plane of deformity is perpendicular to the plane of the pins, which is the weakest plane for the fixator. Therefore, the recommendation for prevention of anterolateral axial deviation in lengthening of the tibia using the Orthofix system is to place the pins and the fixator anterolaterally.

When using the Ilizarov technique, the circular thin-pin fixators are placed at angles to prevent anterolateral angulation when the site of corticotomy is the proximal tibia. The ring proximal to corticotomy is in varus and recurvatum, whereas the ring distal to the corticotomy is perpendicular to the tibia. When the two rings are aligned after corticotomy, a force against anterolateral angulation (i.e., valgus and procurvatum) is provided. When the site of the corticotomy is in the distal tibia, the ring distal to the level of corticotomy is placed in valgus and recurvatum and the ring proximal to the corticotomy is perpendicular to the tibia; thereby, upon aligning the ring after corticotomy, force against varus and procurvatum is provided. An additional measure can be employed in distal tibial corticotomies; i.e., place a ring on the hind foot with a pin in the calcaneus and the stopper (olive) on the medial side. Thereby equinus and varus deformity of the ankle is checkreined. In lengthening the femur by the Ilizarov technique when the level of corticotomy is proximal, the metaphyseal-diaphyseal region anterolateral angulation (i.e., varus and procurvatum axial deviation) is prevented by placing the ring proximal to the corticotomy into valgus and recurvatum; the distal ring is placed parallel to the knee in single-level corticotomy. When the two rings are aligned parallel following corticotomy, forces are provided to prevent varus and procurvatum deviation of the elongated segment.

In femoral lengthening with the monolateral thick-pin fixator, it is difficult to control varus and procurvatum deviation of the elongated segment. When these deformities develop, the patient is taken to the operating room and under appropriate sedation (or general anesthesia in the apprehensive patient) the deformity is corrected by closed manipulation and the fixator readjusted.

With the Ilizarov circular fixator, correction of axial deviation is much simpler. Modularity of the system makes it very versatile, enabling correction of any deformity at any time during treatment. By asymmetrical distraction—more on the concave and less on the convex side—a varus or valgus angulation is easily straightened. If the angular deformity is moderate, it is best to place hinges over the apex of the deformity, which is ordinarily at the level of corticotomy and distract on the concave side, thereby correcting the deformity. When an axial deformation is associated with translation, olive wires may be inserted for pulling on the deformity and reducing it. Olive wires also may be utilized as fulcrums for hinge correction.

It is vital to recognize and correct axial deviations during distraction. At the end of lengthening the anatomic alignment of the limb should be normal; for example, in the lower limb the biomechanical axis should be such that the centers of the hip, knee, and ankle are in line with each other. In the upper limb the carrying angle of the elbow should be restored to normal.

Premature Consolidation. This occurs more commonly in children than in adolescents or adults. It may be caused by an unduly prolonged latency period or incomplete corticotomy, or in the tibia, the fibula may heal prematurely.

It is important to section the fibula with a saw, instead of performing corticotomy, and transfix it proximally and distally to the tibia with screws as described in the Wagner technique. In the DeBastiani Orthofix technique a segment of the distal fibular shaft is excised. It is vital to ensure and document by radiography that a complete corticotomy is performed at the time of surgery.

Initial *treatment* of premature consolidation is to continue distraction at an increased rate until a "pop," due to sudden fracture of the consolidated osseous tissue in the elongated segment, is heard or felt by the patient, who is warned that the pop may be painful. Following the closed osteoclasis, the bone is reshortened by the amount of excessive lengthening and gradual elongation is resumed. Because of the potential problems that can be caused by excessive lengthening it is best to readmit the patient to the hospital for close observation.

If the foregoing simple method fails, closed osteoclasis may be performed under general anesthesia. In the Ilizarov method, the distraction rods are removed, and the circular rings with the fixator pins proximal and below the elongation site are rotated relative to each other. Caution! In the tibia rotate the distal ring laterally and not medially in order to prevent stretching and paresis of the common peroneal nerve. With the monolateral thick-pin cantilever system the fixator is removed, the elongated segment is broken by closed manipulation, and then the fixator is reapplied. Following closed osteoclasis the distraction rate is increased to 1.5 mm. per day for seven to ten days to prevent recurrence of premature consolidation.

Open osteotomy of the consolidated elongated segment is rarely required.

DELAYED CONSOLIDATION AND NONUNION

This is more common in the adolescent and adult patient than in children; also, it is more frequent in congenitally short limbs than in limbs with acquired shortening. The bone that is to be lengthened should have normal healing potential; for example, in congenital pseudarthrosis of the tibia with short leg, the lengthening should be performed at the proximal metaphyseal level, not at the old pseudarthrosis site, which is now healed. Nutrition of the patient should be normal.

Etiologies of delayed consolidation during lengthening are disturbance of endosteum and medullary circulation during corticotomy, initial diastasis and interruption of medullary blood vessels, too rapid distraction, instability of the fixation-lengthening device, and infection. Most of these causes can be prevented.

It is important to detect early problems of delayed consolidation. Within three weeks of lengthening, calcification in the distraction gap should take place. This is best visualized by ultrasonography, which shows calcification of the new bone from either side and the presence of cystic areas in the interzone.

Treatment. When delayed consolidation occurs, distraction should stop and the distraction gap compressed to stimulate osteogenesis. If a cystic area has developed, the elongated segment is compressed until the cyst is eliminated; then distraction is commenced at an increased rhythm. The technique recommended is distraction-compression (back and forth) eight to ten times a day.

In the Wagner method, the elongated segment is primarily grafted with autogenous bone and plated for internal fixation. With the DeBastiani callostasis and Ilizarov techniques, bone grafting is employed only when frank nonunion develops. In the latter, the technique of Wasserstein is recommended; this provides immediate stability and fixation and allows earlier removal of the fixator.

STRESS FRACTURE AND PLASTIC BOWING OF THE ELONGATED BONE

Stress fracture is quite common. In the Wagner diaphyseal lengthening method, it may occur at the ends of the plate; the osteosynthesis plate may fracture, or fracture may occur following removal of the plate. In the Ilizarov and DeBastiani methods, fracture occurs less frequently than in the Wagner method. Following removal of the external fixator it is the author's recommendation to protect the limb with a plastic orthosis and partial weight-bearing with crutches. Following these precautionary measures, the incidence of fracture has markedly decreased. Plastic bowing of the elongated bone may develop after removal of the fixator.

MENTAL DISTURBANCE

The patient may become depressed, irritable, hyperkinetic, and uncooperative during or following lengthening. Acute psychosis has developed. It is mandatory that a preoperative psychological assessment be carried out in a potential patient considered for limb lengthening. Parents should be involved in this evaluation. The expectations of the patient and parents are often very high for this type of surgery. In most congenitally short limbs and in dwarfs, limb length inequality is only a part of the disability. The body image of the patient is important. Parents and patients should fully understand the details of surgery, magnitude of operative scars, potential problems and complications, the prolonged postoperative course, and the great possibility of numerous other operative procedures that may be required. During the course of limb lengthening the psychologist or psychotherapist is called in for help as necessary.

In spite of all these problems and complications, the end result of limb lengthening is satisfactory.

References

1. Abbott, L. C.: The operative lengthening of the tibia and fibula. J. Bone Joint Surg., *9*:128, 1927.
2. Abbott, L. C., and Crego, C. H.: Operative lengthening of the femur. South. Med. J., *21*:823, 1928.
3. Abbott, L. C., and Gill, G. G.: Surgical approaches to the epiphyseal cartilages of the knee and ankle joint. Arch. Surg., *46*:591, 1943.
4. Abbott, L. C., and Saunders, J. B.: The operative lengthening of the tibia and fibula. Preliminary report on further development of principles and technic. Ann. Surg., *110*:961, 1939.
5. Accinno, M. A., and Parker, M. V.: Leg length inequality treated by epiphyseal arrest and stimulation. A preliminary report. J. Med. Assoc. Alabama, *24*:38, 1954.
6. Acheson, R. M.: The Oxford method of assessing skeletal maturity. Clin. Orthop., *10*:19, 1957.
7. Acheson, R. M.: The environment and the growth of children. Ir. J. Med. Sci., *6*:397, 1959.
8. Agerholm, J.: The zig-zag osteotomy. Acta Orthop. Scand., *29*:63, 1959.
9. Ahmadi, B., et al.: Experience with 141 tibial lengthenings in poliomyelitis and comparison of 3 different methods. Clin. Orthop., *145*:150, 1979.
10. Aitken, A. G., et al.: Leg length determination by CT digital radiography. A.J.R., *144*:613, 1985.
11. Aitken, A. P.: Overgrowth of the femoral shaft following fracture. Am. J. Surg., *49*:147, 1940.
12. Aldegheri, R., DeBastiani, G., and Renzi-Brivio, L.: Allungamento diafisario dell'arto inferiore (Studio di 78 casi). Chir. Organi Mov., *70*:111, 1985.
13. Aldegheri, R., and Pizzoli, A.: External fixation devices in children. Chir. Organi Mov., *64*:301, 1978.
14. Aldegheri, R., Renzi-Brivio, L., and Agostini, S.: The callotasis method of limb lengthening. Clin. Orthop., *241*:137, 1989.
15. Aldegheri, R., Trivella, G., and Lavini, F.: Epiphyseal distraction. (Chondrodiatasis-hemichondrodiatasis.) In press.

15a. Aldegheri, R., Trivella, G., and Lavini, F.: Epiphyseal distraction. Chondrodiatasis. Clin. Orthop., *241*: 117, 1989.

16. Alho, A., Berg, G., Karaharju, E., and Armond, I.: Filling of a bone defect during experimental osteotaxis distraction. Acta Orthop. Scand., *53*:29, 1982.
17. Allan, P. G.: Bone lengthening. J. Bone Joint Surg., *30-B*:490, 1948.
18. Allan, P. G.: Simultaneous femoral and tibial lengthening. J. Bone Joint Surg., *45-B*:206, 1963.
19. Allioux, J. J., Rigault, P., Padovani, J. P., Finidori, G., Touzet, Ph., and Mallet, J. F.: Allongement extemporané du femur chez l'enfant et l'adolescent. Etude de 25 cas. Rev. Chir. Orthop., *74*:252, 1988.
20. Amako, T., and Honda, K.: An experimental study of the epiphyseal stapling. Kyushu J. Med. Sci., *8*:131, 1957.
21. Amstutz, H. C.: One-stage femoral lengthening. J. Hosp. Spec. Surg., *1*:57, 1975.
22. Amstutz, H. C., and Sakai, D. N.: Equalization of leg length (Editorial). Clin. Orthop., *136*:2, 1978.
23. Anderson, L., Westin, G. W., and Oppenheim, W. L.: Syme amputation in children: indications, results and long-term follow-up. J. Pediatr. Orthop., *4*:550, 1984.
24. Anderson, M., and Green, W. T.: Length of femur and tibia: Norms derived from orthoroentgenogram of children from 5 years of age until epiphyseal closure. Am. J. Dis. Child., *75*:279, 1948.
25. Anderson, M., Green, W. T., and Messner, M. B.: Growth and prediction of growth in the lower extremities. J. Bone Joint Surg., *45-A*:1, 1963.
26. Anderson, M., Messner, M. B., and Green, W. T.: Distribution of lengths of the normal femur and tibia in children from one to eighteen years of age. J. Bone Joint Surg., *46-A*:1197, 1964.
27. Anderson, M., Green, W. T., and Messner, M. B.: The classic. Growth and prediction of growth in the lower extremities by Margaret Anderson, M. S., William T. Green, M. D., and Marie Blail Messner, A. B., from the Journal of Bone and Joint Surgery, *45-A*:1, 1963. Clin. Orthop., *136*:7, 1978.
28. Anderson, M., Horton, B. G., and Green, W. T.: Orthoroentgentography for accurate long bone measurement. Modification of technique possible with use of rectangular bone collimator. Personal communication, 1960.
29. Anderson, W. V.: Leg lengthening. J. Bone Joint Surg., *34-B*:150, 1952.
30. Anderson, W. V.: Lengthening of the lower limb: Its place in the problems of limb length discrepancy. *In* Graham, W. D. (ed.): Modern Trends in Orthopedics, Vol. V. London, Butterworth & Co., 1967.
31. Armour, P. C., et al: Equalisation of leg length. J. Bone Joint Surg., *63-B*:587, 1981.
32. Armstrong, W. D.: Bone growth in paralyzed limbs. Proc. Soc. Exp. Biol. Med., *61*:358, 1946.
33. d'Aubigne, R. M., and Dubousset, J.: Surgical correction of large discrepancies in the lower extremities of children and adults: an analysis of twenty consecutive cases. J. Bone Joint Surg., *53-A*:411, 1971.
34. Bagnoli, G., Penna, G., Landini, A., Confalonieri, N., Torri, G., and Pietrogrande, V.: Experimental study on bone formation under straining forces: clinical and radiologic features. Il Policlinico (Italian), *91*:908, 1984.
35. Baldwin, B. T.: The physical growth of children from birth to maturity. Ames, University of Iowa Publication, *1*:1921.
36. Ball, R. M.: Equalization of leg length (Letter). Clin. Orthop., *146*:308, 1980.
37. Barford, B., and Christensen, J.: Fractures of the femoral shaft in children with special reference to subsequent overgrowth. Acta Chir. Scand., *116*:235, 1958.
38. Barr, J. S., Lingley, J. R., and Gall, E. A.: The effects of roentgen irradiation on epiphyseal growth: Experimental studies upon the albino rat. A.J.R., *49*:104, 1943.
39. Barr, J. S., and Ober, F. R.: Leg lengthening in adults. J. Bone Joint Surg., *15*:674, 1933.
40. Barr, J. S., Stindfield, A. J., and Reidy, J. A.: Sympathetic ganglionectomy and limb length in poliomyelitis. J. Bone Joint Surg., *32-A*:793, 1950.
41. Baumann, F., and Harms, J.: The extension nail. A new method for lengthening of the femur and tibia. Arch. Orthop. Unfallchir., *90*:139, 1977.
42. Bayer, L. M., and Bayley, N.: Growth Diagnosis. Chicago, University of Chicago Press, 1959.
43. Bayley, N.: Table for predicting adult height and skeletal age and present height. J. Pediatr., *28*:49, 1946.
44. Bayley, N.: Growth curves of height and weight by age for boys and girls. Scaled according to physical maturity. J. Pediatr., *48*:187, 1956.
45. Bayley, N.: Individual patterns of development. Child Dev., *27*:45, 1956.
46. Bayley, N., and Pinneau, S. R.: Tables for predicting adult height from skeletal age: Revised for use with the Greulich-Pyle Hand Standards. J. Pediatr., *40*:423, 1952.
47. Beals, R. K.: Hemihypertrophy and hemihypotrophy. Clin. Orthop., *166*:199, 1982.
48. Belchier, J.: An account of the bones of animals being changed to a red color by aliment only. Phil. Trans. R. Soc., *39*:287, 1735–1736.
49. Belchier, J.: A further account of the bones of animals being made red by aliment only. Phil. Trans. R. Soc., *39*:299, 1735–1736.

50. Bell, J. S., and Thompson, W. A.: Modified spot scanography. A.J.R., *63*:915, 1950.
51. Bender, T. J., Jr.: A method of femoral shortening for leg length discrepancy. Clin. Orthop., *123*:108, 1977.
52. Bensahel, H., Huguenin, P., and Briard, J. L.: Transepiphyseal lengthening of the tibia. A propos of a case. Rev. Chir. Orthop., *69*:245, 1983.
53. Berchiche, R., and Wittek, F.: Lengthening of the leg skeleton using distraction epiphysiolysis. Treatment of lower limb inequality. Acta Orthop. Belg., *49*:321, 1983.
54. Bertrand, P.: Technique d'allongenement du femur dans les grands raccourcissements. Rev. Chir. Orthop., *37*:530, 1951.
55. Bertrand, P., and Trillat, A.: Le traitement des inegalités de longueur des membres inferieurs pendant la croissance. Rev. Orthop., *34*:264, 1948.
56. Bianco, A. J., Jr.: Femoral shortening. Clin. Orthop., *136*:49, 1978.
57. Bier, A.: Hyperemia as a Therapeutic Agent. Authorized translation. Glech, G. M. (ed.). Chicago, A. Robertson & Co., 1905.
58. Birnstingl, M.: Congenital arteriovenous fistula with increased limb growth. Proc. R. Soc. Med., *55*:797, 1962.
59. Bisgard, J. D.: Effects of sympathetic ganglionectomy upon bone growth. Proc. R. Exp. Biol., *29*:229, 1931.
60. Bisgard, J. D.: Longitudinal bone growth, the influence of sympathetic deinnervation. Ann. Surg., *97*:374, 1933.
61. Bisgard, J. D.: Longitudinal overgrowth of long bones with special reference to fractures. Surg. Gynecol. Obstet., *62*:823, 1936.
62. Bisgard, J. D., and Bisgard, M. E.: Longitudinal growth of long bones. Arch. Surg., *31*:568, 1935.
63. Blachier, D., Trevoux, L., and Carlioz, H.: Allongements progressifs du femur selon la technique de Wagner. Rev. Chir. Orthop., *72*:495, 1986.
64. Blair, V. P., III, Walker, S. J., Sheridan, J. J., and Schoenecker, P. L.: Epiphysiodesis: a problem of timing. J. Pediatr. Orthop., *2*:281, 1982.
65. Bliskunov, A.: Intramedullary limb lengthening. Presented at Sixteenth Pediatric Orthopedic International Seminar, San Francisco, May 23–24, 1988.
66. Blomqvist, E., and Rudstrom, P.: Uber Femurfrakturen bei Kindern unter besonder Berucksichtigung des gesteigerten Langenwachstums. Acta Chir. Scand., *88*:267, 1943.
67. Blount, W. P.: Unequal leg length in children. Surg. Clin. North Am., *38*:1107, 1958.
68. Blount, W. P.: Unequal leg length. A.A.O.S. Instructional Course Lectures, Vol. 17. St. Louis, C.V. Mosby, 1960.
69. Blount, W. P., and Clark, G. R.: Control of bone growth by epiphyseal stapling. Preliminary report. J. Bone Joint Surg., *31-A*:464, 1949.
70. Blount, W. P., and Zeier, E.: Control of bone length. J.A.M.A., *148*:451, 1952.
71. Bohlman, H. R.: Experimental with foreign materials in the region of the epiphyseal cartilage plate of growing bones to increase their longitudinal growth. J. Bone Joint Surg., *11*:365, 1929.
72. Bonini, C. A., Terzi, A., and Deimichel, R.: Personal strategies in the technic of leg lengthening. Minerva Chir., *37*:1489, 1982.
73. Bos, C. F., et al.: Treatment of failed open reduction for congenital dislocation of the hip. A 10-year follow-up of 14 patients. Acta Orthop. Scand., *55*:531, 1984.
74. Bost, F. C.: Operative lengthening of the bones of the lower extremity. A.A.O.S. Instructional Course Lectures, Vol. 1. Ann Arbor, J.W. Edwards, 1944, p. 50.
75. Bost, F. C., and Larsen, L. J.: Experiences with lengthening of the femur over an intramedullary rod. J. Bone Joint Surg., *38-A*:567, 1956.
76. Bosworth, D. M.: Skeletal distraction of the tibia. Surg. Gynecol. Obstet., *66*:912, 1938.
77. Bright, R. W.: Applications and limitations of the Orthofix hardware. Presented at the Sixteenth Pediatric Orthopedic International Seminar, San Francisco, May 23–24, 1988.
78. Brockway, A.: Clinical resume of 46 leg-lengthening operations. J. Bone Joint Surg., *17*:969, 1935.
79. Brockway, A., and Fowler, S. B.: Experience with 105 leg lengthening operations. Surg. Gynecol. Obstet., *75*:252, 1942.
80. Brockway, A., Craig, W. A., and Cockrell, B. R., Jr.: End result study of sixty-two stapling operations. J. Bone Joint Surg., *36-A*:1063, 1954.
81. Brodin, H.: Longitudinal bone growth. The nutrition of the epiphyseal cartilages and the local blood supply. Acta Orthop. Scand., Suppl. 20, 1955.
82. Broman, B., Dahlberg, G., and Lichtenstein, A.: Height and weight during growth. Acta Pediat., *30*:1, 1942.
83. Brooke, R.: Bone shortening for inequality of length in the lower limbs. Proc. R. Soc. Med., *30*:441, 1937.
84. Brooks, M.: Femoral growth after occlusion of the principal nutrient canal in day-old rabbits. J. Bone Joint Surg., *39-B*:563, 1957.
85. van Bruggen, J. P.: Surgical leg lengthening: a preliminary report. Ned. Tijdschr. Geneeskd., *125*:1958, 1981.
86. Burdick, C. G., and Siris, L. E.: Fractures of the femur in children. Ann. Surg., *77*:736, 1923.
87. Burwell, R. G.: Studies in the transplantation of bone VII: The fresh composite homograft-allograft of cancellous bone. An analysis of factors leading to osteogenesis in marrow transplants and in marrow containing bone grafts. J. Bone Joint Surg., *46-B*:110, 1964.
88. Bylander, B., Selvik, G., Hansson, L. I., and Aronson, S.: A roentgen stereophotogrammetric analysis of growth arrest by stapling. J. Pediatr. Orthop., *1*:81, 1981.
89. Calvé, J., and Galland, M.: A new procedure for compensatory shortening of the unaffected femur in case of considerable asymmetry of the lower limbs, fractures of the femur, coxalgia. Am. J. Orthop. Surg., *16*:211, 1918.
90. Cambras, R. A., Puente, J. J., Perez, H. B., Angulo, M. A., and Concepcion, T. P.: Limb lengthening in children. Orthopedics, *7*:468, 1984.
91. Cameron, B. M.: A technique for femoral-shaft shortening. A preliminary report. J. Bone Joint Surg., *39-A*:1309, 1957.
92. Cameron, N., Tanner, J. M., and Whitehouse, R. H.: A longitudinal analysis of the growth of limb segments in adolescence. Ann. Hum. Biol., *9*:211, 1982.
93. Canadell, J., and dePablos, J.: Breaking bony bridges by physeal distraction. A new approach. Int. Orthop., *9*:223, 1985.
94. Canale, S. T., Russell, T. A., and Holcomb, R. L.: Percutaneous pinning: Experimental study and clinical results. J. Pediatr. Orthop., *6*:150, 1986.
95. Carlioz, H., and Filipe, G.: Allongements progressifs du femur selon la technique de Wagner et étude critique des 30 premiers cas. Rev. Chir. Orthop., *66*:473, 1980.
96. Carlson, W. O., and Wenger, D. R.: A mapping method to prepare for surgical excision of a partial physeal arrest. J. Pediatr. Orthop., *4*:232, 1984.
97. Carpenter, E. B., and Dalton, J. B., Jr.: A critical evaluation of epiphyseal stimulation. J. Bone Joint Surg., *38-A*:1089, 1956.
98. Carroll, N. C.: Experimental observations on the effects of leg lengthening by the Wagner method. Clin. Orthop., *160*:250, 1981.
99. Cartwright, L. J.: Orthoroentgenography as applied to the lower extremities of children. Radiography, *15*:234, 1949.

100. Catagni, M., Paley, D., Cattaneo, R., and Villa, A.: Lengthening of the congenitally short tibia by the Ilizarov technique. Personal communication, 1987.
101. Caton, J., Dumont, P., Bernard, J., and Michel, C. R.: Etude des resultats moyen terme d'une serie de 33 allongements des membres inferieurs selon la technique de Wagner. Rev. Chir. Orthop., *71*(Suppl. 11):48, 1980.
102. Cattaneo, R.: The experience of the hospital of Lecco in extensive limb lengthening with Ilizarov's method. First International Conference on Human Achondroplasia, Rome, November 19–21, 1986.
103. Cattaneo, R., Paley, D., Catagni, M., and Villa, A.: Forearm lengthening by the Ilizarov technique. Personal communication, 1987.
104. Cattaneo, R., Villa, A., Catagni, M., and Tentori, L.: Limb lengthening in achondroplasia by Ilizarov's method. Int. Orthop. *12*:173, 1988.
105. Cattaneo, A., Villa, A., Catagni, M., and Tentori, L.: Traitement des inegalites du femur par la methode d'Ilizarov. Rev. Chir. Orthop., *71*:405, 1985.
106. Cattaneo, R., Villa, A., Catagni, M., Tentori, L., and Cassi, M.: Application de la methode d'Ilizarov dans l'allongement de l'humerus. Rev. Chir. Orthop., *72*:303, 1986.
107. Cauchoix, J., et al.: One stage femoral lengthening. Clin. Orthop., *136*:66, 1978.
108. Chache, P. B., and Chong, K. C.: Experience with tibial lengthening in Singapore. Clin. Orthop., *125*:100, 1977.
109. Chapchal, G., and Zeldenrust, J.: Experimental research for promoting longitudinal growth of lower extremities by irritation of growth region of femur and tibia. Acta Orthop. Scand., *17*:371, 1948.
110. Chirkova, A. M., and Dyachkova, G. V.: Dynamics of the morphologic changes in fascio-muscular apparatus of the leg lengthened by the method of Ilizarov. *In* Questions on Transosseous Osteosynthesis by Ilizarov Method. Booklet 7. Kurgan, 1981, pp. 100–105.
111. Codivilla, A.: On the means of lengthening in the lower limbs, the muscles and the tissues which are shortened through deformity. Am. J. Orthop. Surg., *2*:353, 1905.
112. Cole, W. M.: Leg lengthening for shortening due to infantile paralysis. Minn. Med., *13*:904, 1930.
113. Coleman, S. S.: Lower limb length discrepancy. *In* Lovell, W. W., and Winter, R. B. (eds.): Pediatric Orthopaedics. Philadelphia, J. B. Lippincott, 1986, p. 781.
114. Coleman, S. S.: Simultaneous femoral and tibial lengthening for limb length discrepancies. Arch. Orthop. Trauma. Surg., *103*:359, 1985.
115. Coleman, S. S., and Noonan, T. D.: Anderson's method of tibial lengthening by percutaneous osteotomy and gradual distraction. Experiences with thirty-one cases. J. Bone Joint Surg., *49-A*:263, 1967.
116. Coleman, S. S., and Stevens, P. M.: Tibial lengthening. Clin. Orthop., *136*:92, 1978.
117. Colville, J., and MacAuley, P.: Leg lengthening: a clinical review of 45 cases. Ir. Med. J., *71*:42, 1978.
118. Compere, E. L.: Indications for and against the leg lengthening operations. J. Bone Joint Surg., *18*:692, 1936.
119. Compere, E. L., and Adams, C. O.: Studies of longitudinal growth of long bones: the influence of trauma to the diaphysis. J. Bone Joint Surg., *19*:922, 1937.
120. Connolly, J. F., Huurman, W. W., Lipiello, L., and Pankaj, R.: Epiphyseal traction to correct acquired growth deformities. Clin. Orthop., *202*:258, 1986.
121. Coursley, G., Ivins, J. C., and Barker, N. W.: Congenital arteriovenous fistula in the extremities. An analysis of 69 cases. Angiology, *7*:201, 1956.
122. Cuny, C., Lepelley, M., Jolly, A., Guillaumot, M., Legras, B., Prevot, J., and Beau, A.: 148 epiphysiodesis in the management of leg length inequality. Chir. Pediatr., *21*:245, 1980.
123. Dal Monte, A., and Donzelli, O.: Tibial lengthening according to Ilizarov in congenital hypoplasia of the leg. J. Pediatr. Orthop., *7*:135, 1987.
124. Dal Monte, A., Valdiserri, L., and Donzelli, O.: Lengthening of the femur in children (considerations on 34 operated cases). Chir. Organi Mov., *66*:439, 1980.
125. Dal Monte, A., Valdiserri, L., and Donzelli, O.: Lengthening of the tibia in children (considerations on 24 operated cases). Chir. Organi Mov., *66*:451, 1980.
126. Dalton, J. B., Jr., and Carpenter, E. B.: Clinical experience with epiphyseal stapling. South. Med. J., *47*:544, 1954.
127. D'Aubigne, R. M., and Dubousset, J.: Surgical correction of large length discrepancies in the lower extremities of children and adults. J. Bone Joint Surg., *53-A*:411, 1971.
128. David, V. C.: Shortening and compensatory overgrowth following fractures of the femur in children. Arch. Surg., *9*:438, 1924.
129. DeBastiani, G.: Lengthening of the lower limbs in achondroplasts. First International Conference on Human Achondroplasia, Rome, November 19–21, 1986.
130. DeBastiani, G., Aldegheri, R., and Renzi-Brivio, L.: Indicazioni particolari dei fisatori esterni. G. Ital. Fissatore Esterno, *504*:31, 1979.
131. DeBastiani, G., Aldegheri, R., and Renzi-Brivio, L.: Fissatore esterno assiale. Chir. Organi Mov., *65*:287, 1979.
132. DeBastiani, G., Aldegheri, R., and Renzi-Brivio, L.: The treatment of fractures with a dynamic axial fixator. J. Bone Joint Surg., *66-B*:538, 1984.
133. DeBastiani, G., Aldegheri, R., Renzi-Brivio, L., and Trivella, G.: Limb lengthening by distraction of the epiphyseal plate. A comparison of two techniques in the rabbit. J. Bone Joint Surg., *68-B*:545, 1986.
134. DeBastiani, G., Aldegheri, R., Renzi-Brivio, L., and Trivella, G.: Chondrodiatasis-controlled symmetrical distraction of the epiphyseal plate. Limb lengthening in children. J. Bone Joint Surg., *68-B*:550, 1986.
135. DeBastiani, G., Aldegheri, R., Renzi-Brivio, L., and Trivella, G.: Limb lengthening by callus distraction (callotasis). J. Pediatr. Orthop., *7*:129, 1987.
136. DeBastiani, G., and Trivella, G.: Limb lengthening by chondrodiatasis. The Behaviour of the Growth Plate Conference, Ottawa, May 13–15, 1987.
137. dePablos, J.: Histology of physeal distraction and the effect of the rate of distraction on physeal preservation. Presented at the Sixteenth Pediatric Orthopedic International Seminar, San Francisco, May 23–24, 1988.
138. dePablos, J., and Canadell, J.: Elongacion de miembros inferiores. Experiencia en la clinica Universitaria de Navarra. Rev. Med. Univ. Navarra, *31*:43, 1987.
139. dePablos, J., and Canadell, J.: Bone lengthening by physeal distraction: an experimental study. Orthop. Trans., *10*:370, 1986.
140. dePablos, J., Villas, C., and Canadell, J.: Bone lengthening by physial distraction. Int. Orthop., *10*:163, 1986.
141. Dickerson, R. C., and Duthie, R. B.: The diversion of arterial blood flow to bone. A preliminary report. J. Bone Joint Surg., *45-A*:356, 1963.
142. Digby, K. H.: The measurement of diaphyseal growth in proximal and distal direction. J. Anat. Physiol., *50*:187, 1915–1916.
143. DiLeo, P., et al.: Growth disturbances following fractures of the femur and tibia in children. Ital. J. Orthop. Traumatol., *11*:127, 1985.

144. Downie, G. R.: Limb deficiencies and prosthetic devices. Orthop. Clin. North Am., *7*:465, 1976.
145. Duhamel, H. L.: Sur une racine qui a la faculté de teindre en ronge les os des animaux vivants. Mem. Acad. R. Sci., 1–13, 1739.
146. Duhamel, H. L.: Sur le developpement et la crue des os des animaux. Mem. Acad. R. Sci., 354–370, 1742.
147. Duhamel, H. L.: Quatrième memoire sur les os. Mem. Acad. R. Sci., 87–111, 1743.
148. Duhamel, H. L.: Cinquième memoire sur les os. Mem. Acad. R. Sci., 111–146, 1743.
149. Duhamel, H. L.: Sixième memoire sur les os. Mem. Acad. R. Sci., 288–317, 1743.
150. Dyachkova, G. V., Ilizarov, G. A., Zuzmanovich, F. N., and Marchashov, A. M.: Radiologic studies of muscles. Methodologic Recommendations (Russian). Kurgan, 1983.
151. Dyachkova, G. V., and Utenkin, A. A.: Extensibility of superficial fascia in elongation of the leg in experiment. Ortop. Travmatol. Protez., *41*:44, 1980.
152. Elo, J. O.: The effect of subperiosteally implanted autogenous whole-thickness skin grafts on growing bone. An experimental study. Acta Orthop. Scand., Suppl. 45, 1960.
153. Eydelshtein, B. M., Udalova, N. I., and Bochkarev, G. F.: Dynamics of reparative regeneration after lengthening by the method of distraction epiphysiolysis. Acta Chir. Plast., *15*:194, 1973.
154. Eyre-Brook, A. L.: Bone shortening for inequality of leg lengths. Br. Med. J., *1*:222, 1951.
155. Eyring, E. J.: Staged femoral lengthening. Clin. Orthop., *136*:83, 1978.
156. Fahey, J. J.: The effects of lumbar sympathetic ganglionectomy on longitudinal bone growth as determined by the teleroentgenographic method. J. Bone Joint Surg., *18*:1042, 1936.
157. Fassett, F. J.: On inquiry as to the practicability of equalizing unequal legs by operation. Am. J. Orthop. Surg., *16*:277, 1918.
158. Fedotova, R. G.: Long-term results of operative elongation of the shortened lower extremity in children and adolescents. Ortop. Travamatol. Protez., *33*:8, 1972.
159. Fedotova, R. G.: Growth of the crural and hip bones after elongation for congenital shortening of the lower limb in children and adolescents. Ortop. Travmatol. Protez., *10*:55, 1974.
160. Ferguson, A. B.: Surgical stimulation of bone growth by a new procedure. J.A.M.A., *100*:26, 1933.
161. Filipe, G., Bercovy, M., and Carlioz, H.: Epiphysiodesis in the treatment of discrepancies in length of the lower extremity (author's transl.). Chir. Pediatr., *19*:227, 1978.
162. Fischenko, P. J., Karimova, L. F., and Pilipenko, N. P.: Roentgenographic imaging of the regenerate formation in distraction epiphysiolysis. Ortop. Traumatol. Protez., *37*:29, 1976.
163. Fishbane, B. M., and Riley, L. H.: Continuous transphyseal traction. A simple method of bone lengthening. Johns Hopkins Med. J., *138*:79, 1976.
164. Fishbane, B. M., and Riley, L. H.: Continuous transphyseal traction: experimental observations. Clin. Orthop., *136*:120, 1978.
165. Flourens, P.: Recherches sur le developpement des os et des dents. Arch. Museum d'Histoire Naturelle, *2*:315, 1841.
166. Flourens, P.: Recherches sur le developpement des os. Coll. R. Acad. Sci. Paris, *15*:875, 1842.
167. Flourens, P.: Theorie experimentale de la formation des os. Paris, Ballière, 1847.
168. Flourens, P.: Note sur le developpement des os en longueur. Coll. R. Acad. Sci. Paris, *52*:186, 1861.
169. Forgon, M.: Bone growth accelerated by stimulation of the epiphyseal plate with electric current. Arch. Orthop. Trauma. Surg., *104*:121, 1985.
170. Franke, J.: Moglichkeiten und Probleme der Beinverlangerung mittels Distraktionsepiphysiolysen. Illisarow. Beitr. Orthop. Traumatol., *24*:638, 1977.
171. Freiberg, A. H.: Codibilla's method of lengthening of the lower extremity. Surg. Gynecol. Obstet., *14*:614, 1912.
172. Frejka, B., and Fait, M.: Clinical evaluation of linear growth stimulation. *In* Septième Congres International de Chirurgie Orthopedique. Barcelona, September 16–21, 1957. Bruxelles, Imprimerie des Sciences, 1958, pp. 644–661.
173. Fries, J. B.: Growth following epiphyseal arrest. A simple method of calculation. Clin. Orthop., *114*:316, 1976.
174. Gage, J. R., and Cary, J. M.: The effects of trochanteric epiphyseodesis on growth of the proximal end of the femur following necrosis of the capital femoral epiphysis. J. Bone Joint Surg., *62-A*:785, 1980.
175. Ganel, A., Horoszowski, H., Kamhin, M., and Farine, I.: Leg lengthening in achondroplastic children. Clin. Orthop., *144*:194, 1979.
176. Garbarino, J. L., Clancy, M., Harcke, H. T., Steel, H. H., and Cowell, H. R.: Congenital diastasis of the inferior tibiofibular joint: A review of the literature and report of two cases. J. Pediatr. Orthop., *5*:225, 1985.
177. Gay, W. I.: A method for surgical lengthening of the femur of the dog. Milit. Med., *123*:283, 1958.
178. Gekeler, J., Dietz, J., and Schuler, T. M.: Prognosis of leg length differences in congenital fibula defect. Z. Orthop., *120*:729, 1982.
179. Gelbke, H.: Influence of pressure and tension on growing bone in experiments with animals. J. Bone Joint Surg., *33-A*:947, 1951.
180. Giles, L. G.: Lumbosacral facetal "joint angles" associated with leg length inequality. Rheumatol. Rehabil., *20*:233, 1981.
181. Giles, L. G.: Low-back pain associated with leg length inequality. Spine, *6*:510, 1981.
182. Giles, L. G.: Lumbar spine structural changes associated with leg length inequality. Spine, *7*:159, 1982.
183. Gill, G. G.: Cause of discrepancy in length of the limbs following tuberculosis of the hip in children: arrest of growth from premature central closure of the epiphyseal cartilage about the knee. J. Bone Joint Surg., *26*:272, 1944.
184. Gill, G. G.: A simple roentgenographic method for the measurement of bone length: a modification of Millwee's method of slit scanography. J. Bone Joint Surg., *26*:767, 1944.
185. Gill, G. G., and Abbott, L. C.: Practical method of predicting growth of the femur and tibia in the child. Arch. Surg., *45*:286, 1942.
186. Glass, R. B., et al.: Leg length determination with biplanar CT scanograms. Radiology, *156*:833, 1985.
187. Goff, C. W.: Growth determination. A.A.O.S. Instr. Course Lect., *7*:160, 1951.
188. Goff, C. W.: Surgical Treatment of Unequal Extremities. Springfield, Ill., Charles C Thomas, 1960.
189. Goldstein, L. A., and Dreisinger, F.: Spot roentgenography—a method for measuring the length of the bones of the lower extremities. J. Bone Joint Surg., *32-A*:449, 1950.
190. Goldstrohm, G. L.: The results of 39 fractures complicated by major segmental bone loss and/or leg length discrepancy. J. Trauma, *24*:50, 1984.
191. Goodship, A., and Kenright, J.: The influence of induced micromotion upon the healing of experimental tibial fractures. J. Bone Joint Surg., *67-B*:650, 1985.
192. Gotz, J., and Schellmann, W. D.: Continuous lengthening of the femur with intramedullary stabilization. Arch. Orthop. Unfallchir., *82*:305, 1975.
193. Gracheva, V. I.: Leg lengthening by distraction epi-

physeolysis. *In* Methodologic Recommendations (Russian). Kurgan, 1976, p. 24.
194. Graf, R., and Millner, M.: Experiences with lengthening the lower leg in dysplasia using the Wagner apparatus. Z. Orthop., *121*:183, 1983.
195. Granieri, P.: Results with epiphysiodesis in the treatment of leg length discrepancy. Bull. Hosp. Spec. Surg., *1*:33, 1958.
196. Green, W. T., and Anderson, M.: Experiences with epiphyseal arrest in correcting discrepancies in length of the lower extremities in infantile paralysis. J. Bone Joint Surg., *29*:659, 1947.
197. Green, W. T., and Anderson, M.: Discrepancy in length of the lower extremities. A.A.O.S. Instr. Course Lect., *8*:294, 1951.
198. Green, W. T., and Anderson, M.: The problem of unequal leg lengths. Pediatr. Clin. North Am., *2*:1137, 1955.
199. Green, W. T., and Anderson, M.: Epiphyseal arrest for the correction of discrepancies in length of the lower extremities. J. Bone Joint Surg., *39-A*:353, 1957.
200. Green, W. T., and Anderson, M.: Skeletal age and the control of bone growth. A.A.O.S. Instr. Course Lect., *17*:199, 1960.
201. Green, W. T., Wyatt, G. M., and Anderson, M.: Orthoroentgenography as a method of measuring the bones of the lower extremity. J. Bone Joint Surg., *28*:60, 1946.
202. Greiff, J., et al: Growth disturbance following fracture of the tibia in children. Acta Orthop. Scand., *51*:315, 1980.
203. Greulich, W. W., and Pyle, S. I.: Radiographic Atlas of Skeletal Development of the Hand and Wrist. 2nd Ed. Stanford, Stanford University Press, 1959.
204. Grill, F.: Distraction of the epiphyseal cartilage as a method of limb lengthening. J. Pediatr. Orthop., *4*:105, 1984.
205. Gross, R. H.: An evaluation of tibial lengthening procedures. J. Bone Joint Surg., *53-A*:693, 1971.
206. Gualtieri, I., et al: Lengthening of the femur with an external fixer. (Personal technique with results.) Ital. J. Orthop. Traumatol., *8*:283, 1982.
207. Gullickson, G., Jr., Olson, M., and Kottke, F. J.: Effect of paralysis of one lower extremity in bone growth: preliminary report. Arch. Phys. Med., *13*:392, 1950.
208. Haas, S. L.: The relation of the blood supply to the longitudinal growth of bone. Am. J. Orthop. Surg., *15*:157, 305, 1917.
209. Haas, S. L.: The localization of the growing point in the epiphyseal cartilage plate of bones. Am. J. Orthop. Surg., *15*:563, 1917.
210. Haas, S. L.: Interstitial growth in growing long bones. Arch. Surg., *12*:887, 1926.
211. Haas, S. L.: Retardation of bone growth by a wire loop. J. Bone Joint Surg., *27*:25, 1945.
212. Haas, S. L.: Mechanical retardation of bone growth. J. Bone Joint Surg., *30-A*:506, 1948.
213. Haas, S. L.: Restriction of bone growth by pins through the epiphyseal cartilaginous plate. J. Bone Joint Surg., *32-A*:338, 1950.
214. Haas, S. L.: Stimulation of bone growth. Am. J. Surg., *95*:125, 1958.
215. Hahnet, H.: Die Distraktionsepiphysiolyse-erste Erfahrungen bei der operativen Beinverlangerung nach Illisarow. Beitr. Orthop. Traumatol., *24*:594, 1977.
216. Hales, S.: Statistical essays: Containing vegetable staticks: or, an account of some statistical experiments on the sap in vegetables. Vol. 1., 2nd Ed. London, Innys, Woodward and Peele, 1731.
217. Hansson, L. I.: Daily growth in length of diaphysis measured by oxytetracycline in rabbit normally and after medullary plugging. Acta Orthop. Scand., Suppl. 101, 1967.
218. Hardy, A. E.: Shortening and angulation of femoral shaft fractures treated by cast brace application and early ambulation. Clin. Orthop., *168*:139, 1982.
219. Harmon, P. H., and Krigsten, W. M.: The surgical treatment of unequal leg length. Surg. Gynecol. Obstet., *71*:482, 1940.
220. Harris, H. A.: Bone Growth in Health and Disease: The Biological Principles Underlying the Clinical, Radiological and Histological Diagnosis of Perversion of Growth and Disease in the Skeleton. London, Oxford University Press, 1933.
221. Harris, R. I., and McDonald, J. L.: The effect of lumbar sympathectomy upon the growth of legs paralyzed by anterior poliomyelitis. J. Bone Joint Surg., *18*:35, 1936.
223. Harsha, W. N.: Distracting effects placed across the epiphysis of long bones. J.A.M.A., *179*:776, 1962.
224. Hart, G. H.: Femoral shortening for equalization of leg lengths. Lancet, *78*:1, 1958.
225. Hatcher, C. M.: Growth increment curve for the femur and tibia. *In* Campbell, W. C.: Operative Orthopaedics. St. Louis, C. V. Mosby, 1939, p. 954.
226. Hechard, P., and Carlioz, H.: Practical method of prediction of leg length inequality. Rev. Chir. Orthop., *64*:81, 1978.
227. Hellstadius, A.: Investigation by experiments on animals of the role played by epiphyseal cartilage in longitudinal growth. Acta Chir. Scand., *95*:156, 1947.
228. Hellstadius, A.: On the importance of epiphyseal cartilage to growth in length. Acta Orthop. Scand., *20*:84, 1950.
229. Hellstadius, A.: A reply in consideration of Walter Duben and Heinz Gelbke's article: animal experiments concerning the problem of epiphyseal or interstitial osseous growth in length, conclusion on the articles of A. Hellstadius and P. Macroix. Acta Orthop. Scand., *25*:26, 1955.
230. Helms, C. A., et al.: CT scanograms for measuring leg length discrepancy. Radiology, *151*:802, 1984.
231. Hendryson, I. E.: An evaluation of the estimated percentage of growth from the distal epiphyseal line. J. Bone Joint Surg., *27*:208, 1945.
232. Herndon, C. H., and Spencer, G. E.: An experimental attempt to stimulate linear growth of long bones in rabbits. J. Bone Joint Surg., *35-A*:758, 1953.
233. Herron, L. D., Amstutz, H. C., and Pakai, D. N.: One stage femoral lengthening in the adult. Clin. Orthop., *136*:74, 1978.
234. Hewitt, D.: Some familial correlations in height, weight and skeletal maturity. Ann. Hum. Genet., *22*:26, 1957.
235. Hickey, P. M.: Teleoroentgenography as an aid in orthopedic measurements. A.J.R., *11*:232, 1924.
236. Hiertonn, T.: Arteriovenous anastomoses and acceleration of bone growth. Acta Orthop. Scand., *26*:322, 1957.
237. Hodgen, J. T., and Franz, C. H.: Arrest of growth of epiphyses. Arch. Surg., *53*:664, 1946.
238. Hofman, A., and Wenger, D. R.: Posteromedial bowing of the tibia. Progression of discrepancy in leg lengths. J. Bone Joint Surg., *63-A*:384, 1981.
239. Hood, R. W., and Riseborough, E. J.: Lengthening of the lower extremity by the Wagner method: a review of the Boston Children's Hospital experience. J. Bone Joint Surg., *63-A*:1122, 1981.
240. Hootnick, D., Boyd, N. A., Fixsen, J. A., and Lloyd Roberts, G. C.: The natural history and management of congenital short tibia with dysplasia or absence of the fibula. J. Bone Joint Surg., *59-B*:267, 1977.
241. Houghton, G. R., and Duriez, J.: Allongement tibial par elongation du cartilage de croissance tibial superieur. Etude experimentale chez le lapin. Rev. Chir. Orthop., *136*:120, 1978.
242. Howard, R. C.: A case of congenital arteriovenous

aneurysm involving the femur. J. Bone Joint Surg., *41-B*:358, 1959.
243. Howorth, M. B.: Leg-shortening operation for equalizing leg length. Arch. Surg., *44*:543, 1942.
244. Hunter, J.: Experiments and observations on the growth of bones from the papers of the late Mr. Hunter. By Everard Home, Read October 4, 1798. Transactions of the Society for Improvement of Medical and Chirurgical Knowledge, *2*:277, 1800.
245. Hunter, J.: Experiments and observations on the growth of bones, from papers of the late Mr. Hunter. *In* Palmer, J. F. (ed.): The Works of John Hunter with Notes, Vol. IV. London, Longman, Rees, Orme, Brown, Green and Longman, 1835, pp. 315–318.
246. Hunter, L. Y., and Hensinger, R. N.: Premature monomelic growth arrest following fracture of the femoral shaft. A case report. J. Bone Joint Surg., *60-A*:850, 1978.
247. Ilizarov, G. A.: Basic principles of transosseous compression and distraction osteosynthesis. Orthop. Travmatol. Protez., *32*:7, 1971.
248. Ilizarov, G. A.: *In* Bianchi-Maiocchi, A. (ed.): L'osteosintesi Transossea Secundo GA Ilizarov (Italian). Milan, Medi Surgical Video, June 1985.
249. Ilizarov, G. A.: Experimental, theoretical and clinical aspects of transosseous osteosynthesis developed in KNIIEKOT Institute (Russian). 1986, pp. 18–20.
250. Ilizarov, G. A.: L'osteosintesi transossea nelle fratture e pseudoartrosi dell'avambraccio. Milan, Medi Surgical Video, 1986.
251. Ilizarov, G. A.: Some theoretical and clinical aspects of transosseous osteosynthesis. *In* Abstracts of Second International Symposium on Experimental, Theoretical and Clinical Aspects of Transosseous Osteosynthesis Method Developed in KNIIEKOT (Russian). Kurgan, September 3–5, 1986.
252. Ilizarov, G. A.: Correction of hyperlordosis in achondroplasia through hip extension osteotomy. First International Conference on Human Achondroplasia, Rome, November 19–21, 1986.
253. Ilizarov, G. A., and Berko, V. G.: Roentgenographic dynamics of the bone regenerate development in limb elongation: an experimental and clinical study. Ortop. Travmatol. Protez., *32*:25, 1976.
254. Ilizarov, G. A., and Berko, V. G.: Morphologic characteristic of the regenerate formed in elongation of the hip in experiment. Ortop. Travmatol. Protez., *41*:54, 1980.
255. Ilizarov, G. A., and Deviatov, A. A.: Operative elongation of the leg with simultaneous correction of the deformities. Ortop. Travmatol, Protez., *30*:32, 1969.
256. Ilizarov, G. A., and Deviatov, A. A.: Operative elongation of the leg. Ortop. Travmatol. Protez., *32*:20, 1971.
257. Ilizarov, G. A., Kuznetsova, A. B., Peschansky, V. S., Shchudlo, M. M., Khanes, G. S., and Migalkins, N. S.: Blood vessels under various regimens of the extremity distraction. Anat. Histol. Embryol., *86*:49, 1984.
258. Ilizarov, G. A., Palienko, L. A., Schreiner, A. A., and Bogomjagkov, V. S.: Dynamics of the number of colony forming cells for fibroblasts in the bone marrow and its relationship with the activity of osteogenesis upon reparative regeneration under the conditions of crus elongation in dogs. Ontogenez, *15*:146, 1984.
259. Ilizarov, G. A., Schreinen, A. A., Imerlishvili, I. A., Bakhlykov, Y. N., Onirkova, A. M., and Marterl, I. I.: On the problem of improving osteogenesis conditions in limb lengthening. *In* Abstracts of First International Symposium on Experimental and Clinical Aspects of Transosseous Osteosynthesis in the Method Developed in KNIIEKOT (Russian). Kurgan, September 20–22, 1983, pp. 4–5.
260. Ilizarov, G. A., and Soybelman, L. M.: Some clinical and experimental data on the bloodless lengthening of lower limbs. Exp. Khir. Anes., *4*:27, 1969.
261. Ilizarov, G. A., Soybelman, L. M., and Chirkova, A. M.: Some roentgenographic and morphologic data on bone tissue regeneration in distraction epiphyseolysis in experiment. Ortop. Travmatol. Protez., *31*:26, 1970.
262. Ilizarov, G. A., and Trohova, V. G.: Operative elongation of the femur. Ortop. Travmatol. Protez., *34*:51, 1973.
263. Ingalls, M. W.: Bone growth and pathology as seen in the femur (and tibia): studies on the femur. Arch. Surg., *26*:787, 1933.
264. Irani, R. N., Nicholson, J. T., and Chung, S. M. K.: Long-term results in the treatment of femoral shaft fractures in young children by immediate spica immobilization. J. Bone Joint Surg., *58-A*:945, 1976.
265. Ireland, J., et al.: Hip adduction/abduction deformity and apparent leg length inequality. Clin. Orthop., *153*:156, 1980.
266. Janes, J. M., and Jennings, W. K.: Effect of induced arteriovenous fistula on leg length. 10 year observations. Proc. Mayo Clin., *36*:1, 1961.
267. Janes, J. M., and Musgrove, J. E.: Effect of arteriovenous fistula on growth of bone. Preliminary report. Proc. Mayo Clin., *24*:405, 1949.
268. Janes, J. M., and Musgrove, J. E.: Effects of arteriovenous fistula on growth of bone. Surg. Clin. North Am., *30*:1191, 1950.
269. Jani, L.: Die Distraktionsepiphysiolyse. Z. Orthop., *113*:189, 1975.
270. Jani, L.: Tierexperimentelle Studie uber Tibiaverlangerung durch Distraktions epiphysiolyse. Z. Orthop., *111*:627, 1973.
271. Janovac, M., and Fait, M.: Elongation of the leg by distraction of the proximal growth cartilage (author's transl.). Acta Chir. Orthop. Traumatol. Cech., *48*:150, 1981.
272. Johansson, J. E., and Barrington, T. W.: Femoral shortening by step-cut osteotomy for leg length discrepancy in adults. Clin. Orthop., *181*:132, 1981.
273. Jones, D. C., and Moseley, C. F.: Subluxation of the knee as a complication of femoral lengthening by the Wagner technique. J. Bone Joint Surg., *67-B*:33, 1985.
274. Judet, J., Judet, R., Rigault, P., and Plumerault, J.: Les allongements du membre inferieur chez l'enfant. Mem. Acad. Chir., *95*:532, 1969.
275. Judet, J., Judet, R., Lord, G., and Rigault, P.: Greffes osteoperiostées pediculées (decortication osteo-musculaire) dans l'allongement des os de membres. Mem. Acad. Chir., *92*:428, 1966.
276. Kalamchi, A., Cowell, H. R., and Kim, K. I.: Congenital deficiency of the femur. J. Pediatr. Orthop., *5*:129, 1985.
277. Kawamura, B.: Limb lengthening. Orthop. Clin. North Am., *9*:155, 1978.
278. Kawamura, B., Mosono, S., and Takahashi, T.: The principles and technique of limb lengthening. Int. Orthop., *5*:69, 1981.
279. Kawamura, B., Mosono, S., Takahashi, T., Yano, T., Kobayashi, Y., Shibata, N., and Shinoda, Y.: Limb lengthening by means of subcutaneous osteotomy: Experimental and clinical studies. J. Bone Joint Surg., *50-A*:851, 1986.
280. Keck, S. W., and Kelly, P. J.: The effect of venous stasis on intraosseous pressure and longitudinal bone growth in the dog. J. Bone Surg., *47-A*:539, 1965.
281. Kelly, P. J., Janes, J. M., and Peterson, L. P. A.: The effect of arteriovenous fistulae on the vascular pattern of the femora of immature dogs: microradiographic study. J. Bone Joint Surg., *41-A*:1101, 1959.
282. Kempf, I., Grosse, A., and Beck, G.: Closed locked

intramedullary nailing. Its application to comminuted fractures of the femur. J. Bone Joint Surg., *67-A*:709, 1985.
283. Kenwright, J.: Complications of diaphyseal limb lengthening in prevention and escape from disasters. Presented at the Sixteenth Pediatric Orthopedic International Seminar, San Francisco, May 23–24, 1988.
284. Key, J. A.: Survival and growth of an epiphysis after removal and replacement. J. Bone Joint Surg., *31-A*:150, 1949.
285. Khoury, S. C., Silberman, F. S., and Cabrini, R. L.: Stimulation of the longitudinal growth of long bones by periosteal stripping. J. Bone Joint Surg., *45-A*:1679, 1963.
286. Klenerman, L.: Unequal legs (Editorial). Br. Med. J. (Clin. Res.), *286*:1302, 1983.
287. Kunkle, H. M., and Carpenter, E. B.: A simple technique for x-ray measurement of limb-length discrepancies. J. Bone Joint Surg., *36-A*:152, 1954.
288. LaCroix, P.: Remarques sur le mechanisme de l'allongement des os. Arch. Biol., *56*:185, 1945.
289. LaCroix, P.: Excitation de la croissance in longueur du tibia pas decollement de son perioste diaphysaire. Rev. Orthop., *33*:3, 1947.
290. LaCroix, P.: The Organization of Bones. London, Churchill, 1951.
291. Laing, P. G.: The blood supply of the femoral shaft. An anatomical study. J. Bone Joint Surg., *35-B*:462, 1953.
292. von Llangenbeck, B.: Oeber Krankhaftes langenwachsthum der Rohrenknochen und seine Verwerthung fur die chirurgie. Praxis Berlin Klin. Wochenschr., *6*:265, 1869.
293. Langenskiöld, A.: Growth and disturbances appearing 10 years after roentgen ray injury. Acta Chir. Scand., *105*:350, 1953.
294. Langenskiöld, A.: Inhibition and stimulation of growth. Acta Orthop. Scand., *26*:308, 1957.
295. Langenskiöld, A., and Edgren, W.: The growth mechanism of the epiphyseal cartilage in the light of experimental observation. Acta Orthop. Scand., *19*:19, 1949.
296. LeCoeur, P.: Egalisation des members inferieurs par allongement avec fixation immediate. Rev. Chir. Orthop., *49*:217, 1963.
297. Lefort, J.: Utilization of a coefficient of residual growth in prediction of lower limb discrepancies (author's transl.). Rev. Chir. Orthop., *67*:753, 1981.
298. Leong, J. C., Ma, R. Y., Clark, J. A., Cornish, L. S., and Yau, A. C.: Viscoelastic behavior of tissue in leg lengthening by distraction. Clin. Orthop., *139*:102, 1979.
299. Letts, R. M., and Meadows, L.: Epiphysiolysis as a method of limb lengthening. Clin. Orthop., *133*:230, 1978.
300. Lewis, D. de W.: Congenital arteriovenous fistulae. Lancet, *2*:621, 1930.
301. Lewis, O. J.: The blood supply of developing long bones with special reference to the metaphyses. J. Bone Joint Surg., *38-B*:928, 1956.
302. Liedberg, E., and Persson, B. M.: Technical aspects of midshaft femoral shortening with Kuntscher nailing. Clin. Orthop., *136*:62, 1978.
303. Lorenzi, G. L., et al.: Growth disturbances following fractures of the femur and tibia in children. Ital. J. Orthop. Traumatol., *11*:133, 1985.
304. McCarroll, H. R.: Trials and tribulations in attempted femoral lengthening. J. Bone Joint Surg., *32-A*:132, 1950.
305. McGibbon, K. C., Deacon, A. E., and Raisbeck, C. G.: Experiences in growth retardation with heavy Vitallium staples. J. Bone Joint Surg., *44-B*:86, 1962.
306. Macewen, W.: The Growth of Bone. Observations on Osteogenesis. An Experimental Inquiry into the Development and Reproduction of Diaphyseal Bone. Glasgow, Maclehose, 1912.
307. Macnicol, M. F., and Catto, A. M.: Twenty-year review of tibial lengthening for poliomyelitis. J. Bone Joint Surg., *64-B*:607, 1982.
308. Magnuson, P. B.: Lengthening shortened bones of the leg by operation. Ivory screws with removable heads as a means of holding the two bone fragments. Univ. Pa. Med. Bull., *21*:103, 1908–1909.
309. Magnuson, P. B.: Lengthening of shortened bones of the leg by operation. Surg. Gynecol. Obstet., *17*:63, 1913.
310. Malan, E., and Puglionisi, A.: Congenital angiodysplasias of extremities. J. Cardiovasc. Surg., *5*:87, 1964.
311. Manning, C.: Leg lengthening. Clin. Orthop., *136*:105, 1978.
312. Maresh, M. M.: Growth of the major long bones in healthy children: a preliminary report on successive roentgenograms of the extremities from early infancy to 12 years of age. Am. J. Dis. Child., *66*:227, 1943.
313. Marin, G. A.: A case of congenital arteriovenous aneurysm involving the femur. Guys Hosp. Rep., *109*:169, 1960.
314. Marsh, H. O., Adas, E., and Laboia, K.: Experimental attempt to stimulate growth by a distracting force across the lower femoral epiphysis. Am. Surg., *27*:615, 1961.
315. May, V. R., Jr., and Clemens, E. L.: Epiphyseal stapling: With special reference to complications. South. Med. J., *58*:1203, 1965.
316. Menelaus, M. B.: Correction of leg length discrepancy by epiphyseal arrest. J. Bone Joint Surg., *48-B*:336, 1966.
317. Merle D'Aubigné, R., and Dubousset, J.: Surgical correction of large length discrepancies in the lower extremities of children and adults. J. Bone Joint Surg., *53-A*:411, 1971.
318. Merrill, O. E.: A method for the roentgen measurement of the long bones. A.J.R., *48*:405, 1942.
319. Mezhenina, E. P., Roulla, E. A., Pechersky, A. G., Babich, V. D., Shadrina, E. L., and Mizhevich, T. V.: Methods of limb elongation with congenital inequality in children. J. Pediatr. Orthop., *4*:201, 1984.
320. Miller, A., and Rosman, M. A.: Hypertensive encephalopathy as a complication of femoral lengthening. Can. Med. Assoc. J., *124*:296, 1981.
321. Millins, M. B., and Hall, J. E.: Transiliac lengthening of the lower extremity. A modified innominate osteotomy for the treatment of postural imbalance. J. Bone Joint Surg., *61-A*:1182, 1979.
322. Millwee, R. H.: Slit scanography. Radiology, *28*:483, 1937.
323. Mirovsky, Y., Axer, A., and Hendel, D.: Residual shortening after osteotomy for Perthes disease. A comparative study. J. Bone Joint Surg., *66-B*:184, 1984.
324. Mitchell, G. P.: L'elongation du tibia. Rev. Chir. Orthop., *49*:205, 1963.
325. Montgomery, W. S., and Ingram, A. J.: Experimental studies and clinical evaluation of linear growth stimulation. South. Med. J., *49*:793, 1956.
326. Monticelli, G., and Spinelli, R.: Distraction epiphysiolysis as a method of limb lengthening. I. Experimental study. Clin. Orthop., *154*:254, 1981.
327. Monticelli, G., and Spinelli, R.: Limb lengthening by epiphyseal distraction. Int. Orthop., *5*:85, 1981.
328. Monticelli, G., and Spinelli, R.: Allungamento di arti mediante corticotomia a cielo chiuso. Ital. J. Orthop. Traumatol., *9*:139, 1983.
329. Monticelli, G., Spinelli, R., and Bonucci, E.: Distraction epiphysiolysis as a method of limb lengthening. II. Morphologic investigations. Clin. Orthop., *154*:262, 1981.

330. Moore, B. H.: A bone lengthening apparatus. J. Bone Joint Surg., *13:*170, 1931.
331. Moore, B. H.: A critical appraisal of the leg lengthening operation. Am. J. Surg., *52:*415, 1941.
332. Moore, J. R.: Tibial lengthening and femoral shortening. Pa. Med. J., *36:*751, 1933.
333. Moore, R. D.: Supracondylar shortening of the femur for leg length inequality. Surg. Gynecol. Obstet., *84:*1087, 1947.
334. Morel, G., Servant, J., Valle, A., Jegou, D., and Teillet, J.: Extemporaneous femoral lengthening by the Cauchoix technic in children and adolescents. Rev. Chir. Orthop., *69:*195, 1983.
335. Mosca, V., and Moseley, C. F.: Complications of Wagner leg lengthening and their avoidance. Orthop. Trans., *10:*462, 1986.
336. Moseley, C. F.: A straight-line graph for leg-length discrepancies. J. Bone Joint Surg., *59-A:*174, 1977.
337. Moseley, C. F.: A straight-line graph for leg-length discrepancies. Paper presented at the Sixteenth Pediatric Orthopedic International Seminar, San Francisco, 1988.
338. Mueller, W. K., and Higgason, J. M.: Spot scanography: Method of determining bone measurements. A.J.R., *61:*402, 1949.
339. Murphy, J. P.: "Short leg" and sciatica (Letter). J.A.M.A., *242:*1257, 1979.
340. Nahoda, J.: Comments on the stimulation of growth in the long bones. Acta Chir. Orthop. Traumatol. Cech., *50:*241, 1983.
341. Nettleblad, H., Randolph, M. A., and Weiland, A. J.: Free microvascular epiphyseal-plate transplantation. An experimental study in dogs. J. Bone Joint Surg., *66-A:*1421, 1984.
342. Newton, S.: Leg lengthening in children. O.N.A.J., *5:*113, 1978.
343. Nisbet, N. W.: Congenital arteriovenous fistula in the extremities. Br. J. Surg., *41:*658, 1954.
344. Noble, J., Diamond, R., Stirrat, C. R., and Sledge, C. B.: Breaking force of the rabbit growth plate and its application to epiphyseal distraction. Acta Orthop. Scand., *53:*13, 1982.
345. Noble, J., Sledge, C. B., Walker, P. S., Diamond, R., Stirratt, C. R., and Sosman, J. L.: Limb lengthening by epiphysial distraction. J. Bone Joint Surg., *60-B:*139, 1978.
346. Ollier, L.: Traite experimental et clinique de la regeneration des os et de la production artificielle du tissu osseux. Paris, V. Masson et Fils, 1867.
347. Ombredanne: Allongement d'un femur sur un membre trop court. Bull. Mem. Soc. Chir., *39:*1177, 1913.
348. Paley, D.: Hinges: Theoretical Aspects. Abstracts from the International Conference on the Ilizarov Techniques for Management of Difficult Skeletal Problems. New York, Hospital for Joint Disease, No. 1–3, 1987.
349. Paley, D.: Current techniques of limb lengthening. J. Pediatr. Orthop., *8:*73, 1988.
350. Paley, D.: The biomechanical principles and considerations of the Ilizarov external fixation. *In* The Ilizarov External Fixator. In press.
351. Paley, D., Fleming, B., Pope, M., and Kristiansen, T.: A comparative study of fracture gap motion and shear in external fixation. *In* Advances in External Fixation Abstracts. Riva del Garda, September 28–30, 1986, p. 54.
352. Paley, D., Young, M. C., Wiley, A. M., Fornasier, V. L., and Jackson, R. W.: Percutaneous bone marrow grafting of fractures and bony defects. An experimental study. Clin. Orthop., *208:*300, 1986.
353. Papaioannou, T., et al.: Scoliosis associated with limb-length inequality. J. Bone Joint Surg., *64-A:*59, 1982.
354. Pappas, A. M.: Congenital abnormalities of the femur and related lower extremity malformations: Classification and treatment. J. Pediatr. Orthop., *3:*45, 1983.
355. Pappas, A. M., et al: Leg length discrepancy associated with hypertrophy. Clin. Orthop., *144:*198, 1979.
356. Park, E. A.: Bone growth in health and disease. Arch. Dis. Child., *29:*269, 1954.
357. Park, E. A., and Richter, C. P.: Transverse lines in bone; mechanism of their development. Bull. Johns Hopkins Hosp., *93:*234, 1953.
358. Parker, S. G.: Regulation of longitudinal bone growth. Arch. Surg., *59:*1100, 1949.
359. Parrini, L., et al.: Growth disturbances following fractures of the femur and tibia in children. Ital. J. Orthop. Traumatol., *11:*139, 1985.
360. Pavlov, H., et al: Infantile coxa vara. Radiology, *135:*631, 1980.
361. Pearse, H. E., Jr., and Morton, J. J.: The stimulation of bone growth by venous stasis. J. Bone Joint Surg., *12:*97, 1930.
362. Pease, C. N.: Local stimulation of growth of long bones, a preliminary report. J. Bone Joint Surg., *34-A:*1, 1952.
363. Peck, M. E.: Obstructive anomalies of the iliac vein associated with growth shortening in the ipsilateral extremity. Ann. Surg., *146:*619, 1957.
364. Peixinko, M., et al.: Correction of leg inequality in Klippel-Trenaunay-Weber syndrome. Int. Orthop., *6:*45, 1982.
365. Peterson, H. A.: Operative correction of post-fracture arrest of the epiphyseal plate. Case report with ten-year follow-up. J. Bone Joint Surg., *62-A:*1018, 1980.
366. Phalen, G. S., and Chatterton, C. C.: Equalizing lower extremities: a clinical consideration of leg lengthening versus leg shortening. Surgery, *12:*678, 1942.
367. Phemister, D. B.: Operative arrestment of longitudinal growth of bones in the treatment of deformities. J. Bone Joint Surg., *15:*1, 1933.
368. Phemister, D. B.: Bone growth and repair. Ann. Surg., *102:*261, 1935.
369. Pilcher, M. F.: Epiphyseal stapling: 35 cases followed to maturity. J. Bone Joint Surg., *44-B:*82, 1962.
370. Poirier, H.: Epiphysial stapling and leg equalization. J. Bone Joint Surg., *50-B:*61, 1968.
371. Pouliquen, J. C., Beneux, J., Judet, R., and Cogan, D.: Tibia lengthening in children. Results and complications. Rev. Chir. Orthop., *62*(Suppl. 2):125, 1978.
372. Pouliquen, J. C., and Etienne, W.: Segmentary growth of the lower limb after surgical lengthening in the child (author's transl.). Chir. Pediatr., *19:*179, 1978.
373. Pouliquen, J. C., Gorodischer, S., Verneret, C., and Richard, L.: Allongement du femur chez l'enfant et l'adolescent. Etude comparative d'une serie de 82 cas. Rev. Chir. Orthop. In press.
374. Pous, J. G.: Wagner's method of equalization surgery in congenital malformations. Chir. Pediatr., *19:*359, 1978.
375. Prett, C.: An advance in the treatment of leg inequality. Nurs. Times, *75:*26, 1979.
376. Price, C.: Early experience with lengthening in achondroplasia. Presented at Sixteenth Pediatric Orthopedic International Seminar, May 23–24, 1988.
377. Pugh, D. G., and Winkler, N. T.: Scanography for leg length measurements: an easy satisfactory method. Radiology, *87:*130, 1966.
378. Pujadas, G. M.: A method of measuring the length of the bones. J. Int. Coll. Surg., *22:*308, 1954.
379. Putti, V.: The operative lengthening of the femur. J.A.M.A., *77:*934, 1921.
380. Putti, V.: Operative lengthening of the femur. Surg. Gynecol. Obstet., *58:*318, 1934.
381. Pyle, S. L., and Hoerr, N. L.: Radiographic Atlas of

Skeletal Development of the Knee. Springfield, Ill., Charles C Thomas, 1955.
382. Pyle, S. L., Reed, R. B., and Stuart, H. C.: Patterns of skeletal development in the hand. Pediatrics, *24*(Suppl.):886, 1959.
383. Ratcliff, A. H. C.: The short leg in poliomyelitis. J. Bone Joint Surg., *41-B:*56, 1959.
384. Regan, J. M., and Chatterton, C. C.: Deformities following surgical epiphyseal arrest. J. Bone Joint Surg., *28:*265, 1946.
385. Reid, M. R.: Studies on abnormal arteriovenous communications, acquired and congenital. I. Report of a series of cases. Arch. Surg., *10:*601, 1925.
386. Reidy, J. A., Lingley, J. R., Gall, E. A., and Barr, J. S.: The effect of roentgen irradiation on epiphyseal growth. II. Experimental studies upon the dog. J. Bone Joint Surg., *29:*853; discussion, 873, 1947.
387. Rezaian, S. M.: Tibial lengthening using a new extension device. Report of thirty-two cases. J. Bone Joint Surg., *58-A:*239, 1976.
388. Ricciardi, L.: Monocompartmental epiphyseal distract. Ital. J. Orthop. Traumatol., *10:*57, 1984.
389. Richard, L.: Les allongements des membres par corticotomie et fixateur externe chez l'enfant et l'adolescent (These). Paris, Fac. Med. Xavier Bichat, 1988.
390. Rigault, P., and Bouyala, J. M.: Les grandes hypoplasies et aplasies squelettiques congenitales des membres inferieurs chez l'enfant. Chir. Pediatr., *19:*291, 1978.
391. Rigault, P., Boucquay, P., Padovani, J. P., Raux, P., and Findori, G.: Progressive femoral lengthening in children. A propos of 36 cases. Rev. Chir. Orthop., *66:*13, 1980.
392. Rigault, P., Dolz, G., Padovani, J. P., Touzet, P., Mallet, J. F., Finidori, G., and Raux, P.: Progressive tibial lengthening in children (author's transl.). Rev. Chir. Orthop., *67:*461, 1981.
393. Ring, P. A.: Shortening and paralysis in poliomyelitis. Lancet, *2:*980, 1957.
394. Ring, P. A.: Experimental bone lengthening by epiphysial distraction. Br. J. Surg., *46:*169, 1958.
395. Ring, P. A.: Prognosis of limb inequality following paralytic poliomyelitis. Lancet, *2:*1306, 1958.
396. Ring, P. A.: Congenital short femur. J. Bone Joint Surg., *41-B:*73, 1959.
397. Ring, P. A., and Ward, B. C. H.: Paralytic bone lengthening following poliomyelitis. Lancet, *2:*551, 1958.
398. Robinow, M., et al.: Standards for limb bone length ratios in children. Radiology, *143:*433, 1982.
399. Rook, F. W.: Modified osteotomy of the tibia. Surg. Gynecol. Obstet., *109:*771, 1959.
400. Royle, N. D.: The treatment of inequality of length in the lower limbs. Med. J. Aust., *1:*716, 1923.
401. Rubin, P.: Dynamic Classification of Bone Dysplasias. Chicago, Year Book Medical Publishers, 1964.
402. Rush, W. A., and Steiner, H. A.: A study of lower extremity length inequality. A.J.R., *56:*616, 1946.
403. Sadofeva, V. I., Karimova, L. F., Koniukhov, M. P., Ovsiankin, N. A., and Sosnenko, E. G.: State of the growth zone after distraction epiphysiolysis. Vestn. Khir., *124:*93, 1980.
404. Sadovnik, A. P.: Determination of the degree of severity and of the evolution of shortening of the extremities in children. Ortop. Travmatol. Protez., *9:*28, 1981.
405. Salai, M., Chechick, A., Ganel, A., Blankstein, A., and Horoszowski, H.: Subluxation of the hip joint during femoral lengthening. J. Pediatr. Orthop., *5:*642, 1985.
406. Sandaa, K.: Orthoroentgenographic measurements of long bones. Acta Orthop. Scand., *22:*76, 1952.
407. Selye, H.: On the mechanism controlling the growth in length of the long bones. J. Anat., *68:*289, 1934.
408. Sevastikoglou, J.: A simple application of orthoroentgenography. Acta Orthop. Scand., *22:*80, 1952.
409. Shanda, A.: Shortening of the long leg. Int. J. Surg., *30:*273, 1917.
410. Shapiro, F.: Ollier's disease: An assessment of angular deformity, shortening and pathologic fracture in twenty-one patients. J. Bone Joint Surg., *64-A:*95, 1982.
411. Shapiro, F.: Developmental patterns in lower-extremity length discrepancies. J. Bone Joint Surg., *64-A:*639, 1982.
412. Shapiro, F.: Legg-Calvé-Perthes' disease: a study of lower extremity length discrepancies and skeletal maturation. Acta Orthop. Scand., *53:*437, 1982.
413. Shapiro, F.: Longitudinal growth of the femur and tibia after diaphyseal lengthening. J. Bone Joint Surg., *69-A:*684, 1987.
414. Shchurov, V. A., Gracheva, V. I., Maltsev, V. D., and Bogomiagkov, V. S.: Dynamics of the functional indices of the lengthened leg using Ilizarov's mono- and bilocal distraction osteosynthesis. Ortop. Travmatol. Protez., *4:*15, 1983.
415. Shchurov, V. A., Kudrin, B. I., and Shein, A. P.: Correlation of the biomechanical and functional characteristics of soft tissue after crural bone lengthening by the Ilizarov method. Ortop. Travmatol. Protez., *10:*30, 1981.
416. Shtin, V. P., and Nikitenko, E. T.: Basing the term of beginning of distraction in operation lengthening of the leg in experiment. Ortop. Travmatol. Protez., *35:*48, 1974.
417. Shtin, V. P., and Nikitenko, E. T.: The rate of the distraction in elongation of the long tubular bones. Ortop. Travmatol. Protez., *36:*10, 1975.
418. Shurov, V. A., Gracheva, V. V., Maltzev, V. D., and Bogomyagkov, V. S.: Dynamics of some functional indices of elongated leg in use of mono and bifocal distraction osteosynthesis after Iliazarov. Ortop. Travmatol. Protez., *44:*15, 1983.
419. Sollogoub, I.: La methode d'Ilizarov appliquée aux allongements des membres inferieurs chez l'enfant. Thèse Médecine, Fac. Med. Tours, 1986.
420. Siffert, R. S.: Roentgenographic evidence of growth plate closure. Clin. Orthop., *155:*302, 1981.
421. Sijbrandij, S.: Leg length inequality. Ned. Tijdschr. Geneeskd., *125:*1971, 1981.
422. Simon, S., Whiffen, J., and Shapiro, F.: Leg-length discrepancies in monoarticular and pauciarticular juvenile rheumatoid arthritis. J. Bone Joint Surg., *63-A:*209, 1981.
423. Sledge, C. B., and Noble, J.: Experimental epiphyseal distraction. Clin. Orthop., *136:*111, 1978.
424. Smirnova, L. A., Belenko, L. I., Mazhara, N. N., and Yakovlev, V. M.: Morphologic changes of large nerve trunks and neuromuscular apparatus of the leg during its closed elongation. Ortop. Travmatol. Protez., *43:*37, 1972.
425. Sofield, H. A.: Leg lengthening. Surg. Clin. North Am., *19:*69, 1939.
426. Sofield, H. A., Blair, S. J., and Millar, E. A.: Leg lengthening. A personal follow-up of 40 patients some years after the operation. J. Bone Joint Surg., *40-A:*311, 1958.
427. Speed, K.: Longitudinal overgrowth of long bones. Surg. Gynecol. Obstet., *36:*787, 1923.
428. Spriggins, T., Kenright, J., and Whittle, M.: Distraction epiphyseolysis in an experimental model. Annual Report of the Oxford Orthopedic Engineering Centre, *12:*52, 1985.
429. Stamp, W. G., and Lansche, W. E.: Treatment of discrepancy in leg length. South. Med. J., *53:*764, 1960.
430. Startzeva, I. A., and Gorkunova, Z. I.: Effect of the distraction epiphyseolysis on the growth of the elon-

gated bone (experimental study). Ortop. Travmatol. Protez., *43*:36, 1982.
431. Stein, A. H., Morgan, H. C., and Porras, R.: The effect of an arteriovenous fistula on intramedullary bone pressure. Surg. Gynecol. Obstet., *109*:287, 1959.
432. Stephens, D. C.: Femoral and tibial lengthening. J. Pediatr. Orthop., *3*:424, 1983.
433. Stephens, D. C., Herrick, W., and MacEwen, G. D.: Epiphysiodesis for limb length inequality: results and indications. Clin. Orthop., *136*:41, 1978.
434. Stinchfield, A. J., Reidy, J. A., and Barr, J. S.: Prediction of unequal growth of the lower extremities in anterior poliomyelitis. J. Bone Joint Surg., *31-A*:478, 1949.
435. Stout, J. A., and Gibbs, K. R.: The child undergoing a leg-lengthening procedure. Am. J. Nurs., *81*:1152, 1981.
436. Straub, L. R., Thompson, T. C., and Wilson, P. D.: The results of epiphysiodesis and femoral shortening in relation to equalization of leg length. J. Bone Joint Surg., *27*:254, 1945.
437. Sveshnikov, A. A., Smotrova, L. A., and Grigench, I. S.: The use of 99m Tc colloid to study the lymph flow in a leg stretch after GA Ilizarov technique. Ortop. Travmatol. Protez., *42*:21, 1981.
438. Tanner, J. M., Whitehouse, R. H., Marshall, W. A., Healy, N. J. R., and Goldstein, H.: Assessment of Skeletal Maturity and Prediction of Adult Height (TW2 Method). London, Academic Press, 1975.
439. Thompson, T. C., Straub, L. R., and Campbell, R. D.: An evaluation of femoral shortening with intramedullary nailing. J. Bone Joint Surg., *36-A*:43, 1954.
440. Thoms, H.: A new method for roentgen pelvimetry. J.A.M.A., *92*:1515, 1929.
441. Todd, T. W.: Atlas of Skeletal Maturation. St. Louis, C. V. Mosby, 1937.
442. Torode, I. P., and Gillespie, R.: Anteroposterior instability of the knee: a sign of congenital limb deficiency. J. Pediatr. Orthop., *3*:467, 1983.
443. Torri, G., Bagoli, G. F., Penna, G. F., Pietrogrande, L., Landini, A., Confalarieri, N., and Pietrogrande, V.: Experimental study on bone formation under straining forces. Histologic findings. Il Policlinico, *91*:925, 1984.
444. Troupp, H.: Nervous and vascular influence on longitudinal growth of bone. An experimental study of rabbits. Acta Orthop. Scand., Suppl. 51, 1961.
445. Truesdell, E. D.: Inequality of the lower extremities following fractures of the shaft of the femur in children. Ann. Surg., *74*:498, 1921.
446. Trueta, J.: The influence of the blood supply in controlling bone growth. Bull. Hosp. Joint Dis., *14*:147, 1953.
447. Trueta, J.: Trauma and bone growth. Septième Congres International de Chirurgie Orthopedique. Barcelona, 1957. Bruxelles, Imprimerie de Sciences, 1958, pp. 329–353.
448. Trueta, J., and Amato, V. P.: The vascular contribution to osteogenesis. III. Changes in the growth cartilage caused by experimentally induced ischaemia. J. Bone Joint Surg., *42-B*:571, 1960.
449. Tupman, G. S.: Treatment of inequality of the lower limbs. The results of operation for stimulation of growth. J. Bone Joint Surg., *42-B*:489, 1960.
450. Tupman, G. S.: A study of bone growth in normal children and its relationship to skeletal maturation. J. Bone Joint Surg., *44-B*:42, 1962.
451. Vanderhoeft, P. J., Kelly, P. J., Janes, J. M., and Peterson, L. F. A.: Growth and structure of bone distal to an arteriovenous fistula. Quantitative analysis of tetracycline-induced transverse growth patterns. J. Bone Joint Surg., *45-B*:582, 1963.
452. Vesely, D. G., and Mears, T. M.: Surgically induced arteriovenous fistula. Its effect upon inequality of leg lengths. South. Med. J., *57*:129, 1964.
453. Villarubias, J.: Techniques and complications in extensive limb lengthening. First International Conference on Human Achondroplasia, Rome, November 19–21, 1986.
454. Villarubias, J., Ginebeda, J., and Cavaliere, P.: Hyperlordosis and hip flexion during growth: Prevention and reduction technique. First International Conference on Human Achondroplasia, Rome, November 19–21, 1986.
455. Vizkelety, T.: Elongation of the leg with the Kawamura-method (author's transl.). Magy Traumatol. Orthop. Helyreallito Sebesz., *23*(4):309, 1980.
456. Vorobev, V. N.: Distraction epiphysiolysis for lengthening of the extremities in children with the hip and knee tuberculosis. Vestn. Khir., *120*:79, 1978.
457. Waddell, G.: Femoral shortening with intramedullary fixation. Coll. Surg. Edinb., *22*:367, 1977.
458. Wagner, H.: Operative lengthening of the femur. Clin. Orthop., *136*:125, 1978.
459. Wagner, H.: Surgical lengthening of the femur. Report of fifty-eight cases (author's transl.). Ann. Chir., *43*:263, 1980.
460. Wagner, H.: Personal communication, 1988.
461. Walker, G.: Congenital arteriovenous fistula within the tibia. J. Bone Joint Surg., *53-B*:108, 1971.
462. Wasserstein, I.: Distraktions-Kompressions Methode zur verlangerung von verkurtzen extremitaten unter verwendung von zylindrisheen homologen knochentransplantaten. Verhand lungsband der 1 traumatologich-orthopadishen. Konferenz der Estlandishchen SSR Kochtia-Jawe, 1963.
463. Wasserstein, I.: Distraction compression method of elongation of the lower extremity with use of bone tubular homograft. Ortop. Travmatol. Protez., *29*:44, 1968.
464. Wasserstein, I.: Segmental cortical allografting. Presented at the Sixteenth Pediatric Orthopedic International Seminar, San Francisco, May 23–24, 1988.
465. Wasserstein, I., and Correll, J.: The distraction compression method for elongation of shortened extremities with homologous cylindric bone grafts. Orthopadie, *8*:425, 1984.
466. Weinmann, D. T., Kelly, P. J., and Owen, C. A., Jr.: Blood flow in bone distal to a femoral arteriovenous fistula in dogs. J. Bone Joint Surg., *46-A*:1676, 1964.
467. Westh, R. N., and Menelaus, M. B.: A simple calculation for the timing of epiphysial arrest: a further report. J. Bone Joint Surg., *63-B*:117, 1981.
468. Westin, G. W.: Femoral lengthening using a periosteal sleeve. Report of 26 cases. J. Bone Joint Surg., *49-A*:83, 1967.
469. Wevdenskogo, S. P.: Distraction epiphysiolysis of crural bones. Ortop. Traumatol. Protez., *10*:53, 1974.
470. White, A., Punjabi, M., and Southwick, W.: The four biomechanical stages of fracture repair. J. Bone Joint Surg., *59-A*:188, 1977.
471. White, J. W.: A simplified method for tibial lengthening. J. Bone Joint Surg., *12*:90, 1930.
472. White, J. W.: Femoral shortening for equalization of leg length. J. Bone Joint Surg., *17*:597, 1935.
473. White, J. W.: A practical graphic method of recording leg length discrepancies. South. Med. J., *33*:946, 1940.
474. White, J. W.: Overlapping procedure for shortening bone defects. A.A.O.S., Instructional Course Lectures, Vol. 2. Ann Arbor, J. W. Edwards, 1944, p. 48.
475. White, J. W.: Leg length discrepancies. A.A.O.S. Instructional Course Lectures. Ann Arbor, J. W. Edwards, 1949, p. 201.
476. Whitehill, R., and Hakala, M. W.: Arterial hypertension induced by femoral lengthening. A canine model. J. Bone Joint Surg., *60-A*:815, 1978.
477. Wilk, L. H., and Badgley, C. E.: Hypertension,

another complication of leg lengthening procedure. Report of a case. J. Bone Joint Surg., *45-A*:1263, 1963.

478. Wilson, P. D., and Thompson, T. C.: A clinical consideration of the method of equalizing leg length. Ann. Surg., *110*:992, 1939.
479. Winquist, R. A.: Closed intramedullary osteotomies of the femur. Clin. Orthop., *212*:155, 1986.
480. Winquist, R. A., Hansen, S. T., Jr., and Pearson, R. E.: Closed intramedullary shortening of the femur. Clin. Orthop., *136*:54, 1978.
481. Witt, A. N., Jager, M., and Hilderbrandt, J. J.: Results of animal experiments with an implantable femur distractor for operative leg lengthening. Arch. Orthop. Unfallchir., *88*:273, 1977.
482. Wolf, J., White, A., Punjabi, M., and Southwick, W.: Comparison of cyclic loading versus constant compression in the treatment of long-bone fractures in rabbits. J. Bone Joint Surg., *63-A*:805, 1981.
483. Wray, J., and Goodman, H. O.: Postfracture vascular phenomenon and long-bone overgrowth in the immature skeleton of the rat. J. Bone Joint Surg., *43-A*:1047, 1961.
484. Wu, Y. K., and Miltner, L. J.: A procedure for stimulation of longitudinal growth of bone. An experimental study. J. Bone Joint Surg., *19*:909, 1937.
485. Yabsley, R. H., and Harris, W. R.: The effect of shaft fractures and periosteal stripping on the vascular supply to epiphyseal plates. J. Bone Joint Surg., *47-A*:551, 1965.
486. Yaroshevskaya, E. N., and Dzakhov, S. D.: Morphological characteristic of muscles of the elongated lower extremity. Ortop. Travmatol. Protez., *30*:63, 1969.
487. Yosipovitch, Z. H., and Palti, Y.: Alterations in blood pressure during leg-lengthening. A clinical and experimental investigation. J. Bone Joint Surg., *49-A*:1352, 1967.
488. Zanasi, R.: Surgical equalisation of leg length: shortening of the long femur and lengthening of the short in one operation. Ital. J. Orthop. Traumatol., *8*:265, 1982.
489. Zavijalov, P. V., and Plaskin, J. T.: Elongation of crural bones in children using a method of distraction epiphysiolysis. Vest. Khir. Grekova, *103*:67, 1967.
490. Zavijalov, P. V., and Plaskin, J. T.: Distraction epiphyseolysis in lengthening of the lower extremity in children. Khirurgija (Moskva) (Russian), *44*:121, 1968.
491. Ziv, I., et al.: Femoral intramedullary nailing in the growing child. J. Trauma, *24*:432, 1984.

8. Fractures and Dislocations

Fractures in children differ from those in adults in several ways: (1) *Growth disturbance:* Injuries may involve the physis and *disturb growth,* producing progressive shortening and angular deformity. (2) *Bone remodeling:* The normal process of *bone remodeling* in the growing child will realign the malunited fragments and make accurate anatomic reduction of somewhat less importance than in the adult. Bone remodels in response to the stresses of body weight and the pull of muscles. Asymmetrical growth of the physis corrects the deformity resulting from malunion. Angular deformity is realigned (straightened out) by asymmetrical growth of the physis.[78] Periosteal resorption corrects the bump of a fracture. On the concave (compression) side, negative potential developed by the loaded bone stimulates periosteal new bone formation, which fills the concavity; on the convex side, the bone resorbs in accordance to Wolff's law.[136, 151] In general, the younger the child and the closer the fracture site to the physis, the greater is the potential for spontaneous correction. Fractures in the middle of the shaft of a long bone will remodel little, if any. Angular deformities in the plane of motion of an adjacent hinge joint, such as the knee, ankle, or elbow, are corrected readily, whereas spontaneous correction of angular deformities in other directions, such as cubitus varus following supracondylar fracture of the humerus, is minimal if it takes place at all. Rotational deformities do not correct themselves spontaneously. Displaced intra-articular fractures and displaced fractures traversing the physis at right angles do not remodel. (3) *Bone overgrowth:* Fractures through the diaphyseal metaphysis of a long bone stimulate longitudinal growth by increasing the blood supply to the physis and epiphysis; thus, some degree of overriding with bayonet or side-to-side apposition is desirable in certain age groups, particularly in the long bones of the lower limb. (4) *Rate of healing:* Bone healing is rapid in childhood because of the thickened periosteum and abundant blood supply. The younger the child, the more rapid is the union; for example, in the neonatal period, a fracture of the femoral shaft heals in two to three weeks; during early childhood, in four weeks; in the period from seven to ten years, in six weeks; whereas, in adolescence, in eight to ten weeks. In the young child reduction should be achieved early. There is no time for deliberation. (5) *Nonunion:* This usually does not occur because of the tremendous osteogenic activity of the thick periosteum of children. Displaced intra-articular fractures may not heal; also, union may be delayed or fail to occur when soft tissues (such as muscle tendons or periosteum) are interposed between fracture fragments. With few exceptions, open surgical reduction of fractures is not indicated in children; such intervention merely delays normal healing and predisposes to nonunion.

ANATOMIC AND BIOMECHANICAL DIFFERENCES

The fractures may involve the physis, epiphysis, metaphysis, or diaphysis of a long bone. Diaphyseal (or shaft) fractures may be complete, greenstick, torus (or buckle), and bowed by plastic deformation. In complete fracture, the direction of the fracture is determined by the direction of the breaking force. In *transverse* fractures, produced by angulation, the fracture is perpendicular to the longitudinal axis and the bone fragments tear the periosteum on one side. Transverse fractures usually occur in infants and young children. A common example is physeal-epiphyseal separation. *Oblique* fracture results from axial overload; the shear force produces a fracture line angled 30 to 45 degrees in relation to the longitudinal axis of the long bone. This is frequently seen in the tibia, femur, or both bones of the forearm. The oblique fractures are usually unstable because of the extensive tear of the periosteum. In *spiral* fractures, produced by twisting forces, the oblique fracture line partially encircles the diameter of the shaft. An intact periosteal hinge renders these fractures stable after clockwise or counterclockwise rotation provided they are immobilized in a cast that controls rotation. They usually occur in the older child; the femoral and humeral shafts are common sites. A *butterfly* fracture is comminuted, with the fracture line traversing in various directions as a result of axial overload and angulation. The periosteum is completely torn on the side opposite the butterfly fragments; this type of fracture is very unstable.

Greenstick fracture is an incomplete fracture in which the bone is completely broken on the tension side but the cortex and periosteum remain intact on the compression side. Angular deformity commonly occurs due to plastic deformation of the intact cortical bone. In treatment it is vital to convert the fracture from incomplete to complete. Greenstick fractures are common in children.

Torus (or buckle) fracture is produced by an impaction compression force. It occurs frequently in the metaphyseal region of long bones in children, an anatomic site where the porosity of the bone is marked due to relative abundance of laminar bone in proportion to rigid lamellar bone. It is also commonly seen in the osteoporotic bones of paralytic limbs of the adolescent.

In traumatic bowing of long bones, plastic deformation of bone results from microfractures due to shear forces on the concave side of a long bone. The ulna and fibula are common sites. Injury to the physis warrants special detailed discussion since it presents unique problems in the diagnosis and management of fractures in children.

The Normal Physis and Its Response to Trauma

The physis (also referred to in the literature as the epiphyseal plate, epiphyseal cartilage, and epiphyseal growth plate) is separated from the epiphysis by the *bone plate,* which is a rudimentary cortex formed by a variable number of lamellae, usually six to eight, its thickness being about one fifth that of the physis (Fig. 8–1A). The bone plate has openings through which vessels penetrate. It remains visible in the radiogram until late in life after epiphyseal closure.

The physis proper consists of four zones. The first, a zone of *undifferentiated* or *resting cartilage cells,* is located immediately adjacent to the bone plate. The chondrocytes are arranged in irregular clusters separated from one another by abundant cartilage matrix (Fig. 8–1B). This is the germinal layer that supplies the developing cartilage cells. The source of its cells, in turn, is from the perichondral ring at its periphery, which grows by apposition. Injury to this zone of resting cells will result in cessation of growth.

The second, the *zone of proliferating cartilage,* is the site where length is provided to the tubular bone by active growth of cartilage cells (Fig. 8–1 C). The former concept of these cartilage cells being lined up in linear columns parallel to the long axis of the shaft is incorrect; they are best visualized as a stack of coins, i.e., flattened and largest at their transverse diameter. Each row of cartilage cells is separated from its neighboring abundant cartilage matrix containing bundles of collagen fibrils. The number of cells in the zone of proliferation reflects the activity of the growth plate; the greater their number, the greater is the productivity of the plate. The zone of resting cells and the zone of proliferation together constitute approximately half the physis.

The third, the *zone of vacuolization,* or *hypertrophic cell zone,* is the layer in which the

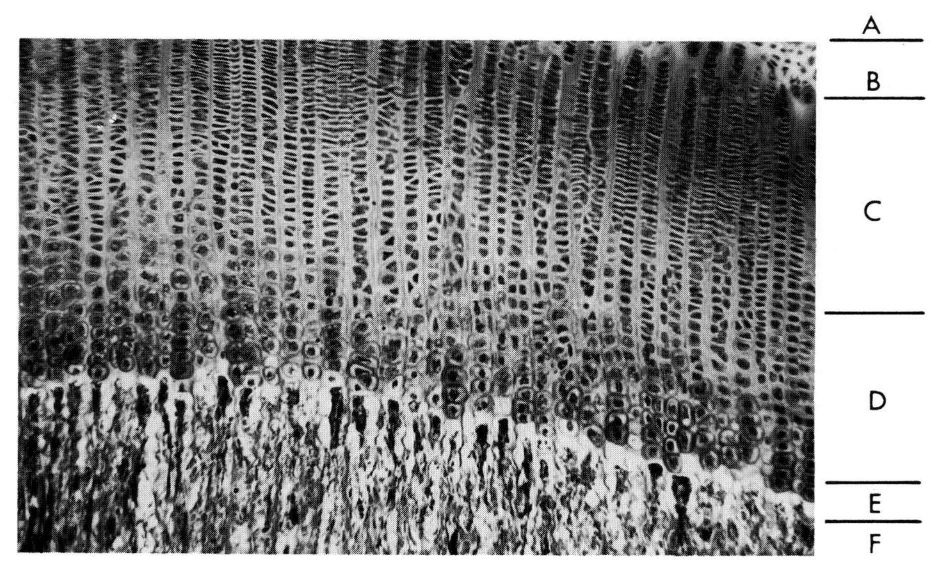

FIGURE 8–1. The growth plate from the upper epiphyseal cartilage of a rabbit's tibia.

A. Bone plate. **B.** Zone of resting cartilage cells. **C.** Zone of proliferation. **D.** Zone of hypertrophic or giant cells. **E.** Zone of cell degeneration or provisional calcification. **F.** The layer of bone formation. (× 40) (Courtesy of J. Trueta.)

chondrocytes become swollen and vacuolated in the process of maturation leading to cell death (Fig. 8–1D). There is no active growth in this zone; length is added to the bone passively by hypertrophy of the cells. As the chondrocytes swell, the intercellular cartilage matrix diminishes.

The fourth, the *zone of provisional calcification*, or *cell degeneration*, is the area where, with the death of chondrocytes and the production of alkaline phosphatase, the longitudinal bars of cartilage matrix become calcified. Dead cells are soon absorbed by invasion of vascular mesenchyme.

Injury to the germinal cells of the physis by direct trauma, circulatory loss, or compression will arrest longitudinal bone growth.

Direct Trauma

Experimental investigations on the effects of injury to the physis are numerous: Ollier, in 1867, performed experiments in immature rabbits and cats by making linear incisions across the physis. Superficial cuts did not affect growth, whereas deep cuts arrested growth. He also found that growth was not disturbed as a result of multiple needle punctures of the plate.[102] Vogt was unable to produce any disturbance of growth by separating the epiphysis through the natural line of cleavage in the epiphyseal plates of goats and sheep.[143] The strength of the physis is provided by the intercellular cartilage matrix. In the first two zones of the physis, there is abundant cartilage matrix and the growth plate is strong; whereas, in the third zone (hypertrophic cell zone), the chondrocytes enlarge to the detriment of their extracellular support, making this zone the weakest portion of the physis. This weakness is to shearing, bending, and tension stresses, not to compression. The fourth zone is reinforced by the addition of calcification. The region of trabecular formation in the metaphysis also contributes to the strength of the physis. The bone matrix laid about the spurs of calcified intercellular substance firmly unites the diaphyseal side of the fourth zone with the metaphysis (Fig. 8–1F).

The weakest part of the physis is the third layer (or the zone of cartilage cells). This was first demonstrated by Haas, who found that when the periosteum about the periphery of a physis was incised, the epiphysis could be easily detached from the metaphysis by gentle pressure. The plane of cleavage was constant, passing through the layer of hypertrophic cartilage cells.[57] Harris designed an apparatus to determine the shearing strength of the upper tibial epiphysis in the rat, and confirmed the finding of Haas that, when the epiphysis separates from the diaphysis, the plane of cleavage consistently passes through the third layer of the physis.[64] The clinical significance of these findings is that the growing cartilage cells in the physis remain adherent to the epiphysis.

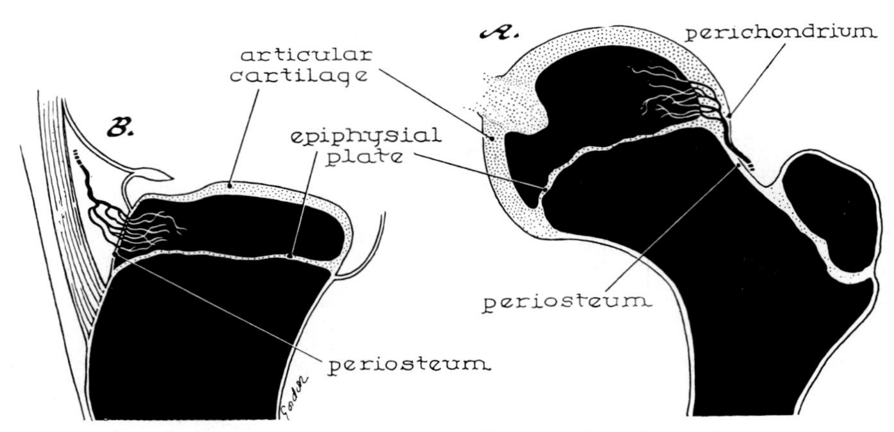

FIGURE 8–2. Two basic patterns of blood supply to the epiphysis.

A. *Epiphysis is entirely covered by articular cartilage* (the upper femoral epiphysis). The blood vessels enter the epiphysis by traversing the perichondrium at the periphery of the epiphyseal plate. During epiphyseal displacement these vessels are vulnerable to rupture. **B.** *Epiphysis is partly covered by articular cartilage.* The vessels enter bone by penetrating the cortex at the side of the epiphysis (proximal tibial epiphysis). In this type epiphyseal separation could occur without serious damage to vessels. (From Dale, G. G., and Harris, W. R.: Prognosis in epiphyseal separations. J. Bone Joint Surg., *40-B*:117, 1958.)

From the circulatory point of view, epiphyses can be subdivided into two types: those that are entirely covered by articular cartilage, and those that are only partially covered. In the former (Type A), the artery enters the epiphysis by traversing the perichondrium at the periphery of the physis. Examples of this type are the proximal radial and upper femoral epiphyses. In the second type (Type B), those that are only partially covered, the nutrient vessels enter the bone by penetrating the cortex at the side of the epiphysis, like the blood supply of the diaphysis of a long bone. Frequently, more than one vessel enters the epiphysis or a single vessel may branch into many tributaries. The majority of the epiphyses in the body are classified as Type B (Fig. 8–2).[43]

Harris and Hobson studied the histologic changes in experimentally displaced upper femoral epiphyses in rabbits. As previously stated, this epiphysis is intra-articular and is entirely covered by articular cartilage; its nutrient vessels must enter it by being closely applied to the periphery of the epiphyseal plate. Their being so situated makes them vulnerable to injury and they inevitably become damaged in epiphyseal separation. In the study of Harris and Hobson, complete displacement of the upper femoral epiphysis resulted in aseptic necrosis, which was slowly repaired by growth of callus and blood vessels from the stump of the femoral neck. As the bulk of the physis remains attached to the epiphysis, it acted as a barrier to successful revascularization. Deliberate removal of the physis permitted earlier revascularization.[66]

Dale and Harris demonstrated that when a Type B epiphysis (such as the proximal tibial epiphysis) is separated from the metaphysis, the nutrient vessels are not damaged and its capacity for growth is not disturbed. Enchondral ossification is temporarily interfered with, as evidenced by the increased thickness of the physis; however, healing takes place rapidly within three weeks and avascular necrosis does not occur. Thus, the prognosis of an epiphyseal separation is dependent upon the degree of damage to its blood supply rather than the mechanical disturbance of the physis.[43]

Brashear produced fractures through the distal femoral epiphysis of rats by applying a varus angulation force. This resulted in distraction on the lateral side of the physis. On the distraction side, the cleavage plane passed through the zone of hypertrophic cartilage cells; whereas on the compression side, the fracture line passed through the metaphyseal trabeculae. A combination of shearing and compression stresses crushed the metaphyseal bone into the physis, damaging all layers of cells.[23]

Depending upon the level of fracture within the physis, three types of healing are observed: (1) If the fracture is proximal in the hypertrophic zone, healing takes place by resorption of the proximal cartilage and fracture debris, a process that temporarily delays enchondral bone formation and causes moderate widening of the physis. After resorption of the proximal cartilage

Table 8–1. *Operations on Immature Dogs**

Group	*Operation*	*Line Drawing of Operation*	*No. of Operations*	*General Effect on Growth*
1	Resection of the margin of the epiphyseal plate, epiphysis, and adjoining metaphysis	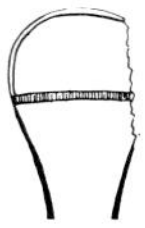	6	Minimum angulation
2	Longitudinal osteotomy through the distal radial and femoral epiphysis crossing the plate in a plane perpendicular to it	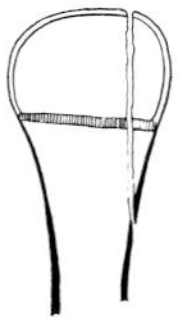		
	a. No internal fixation		5	Minimum retardation
	b. Internal fixation—one screw transversely across the metaphysis		15	Minimum retardation
	c. Detachment of all soft tissues from fragment, with replacement and fixation		5	Maximum retardation
	d. Detachment of soft tissues, insertion in 90 per cent alcohol for ten minutes, replacement, and fixation		3	Maximum retardation
3	Longitudinal osteotomy in the metaphysis of the radius extending distally to the epiphyseal plate with separation across the plate in the line of cleavage	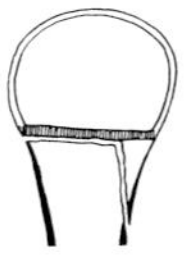	15	Variable retardation (none to moderate)
4	Drilling of holes longitudinally across the distal epiphyseal plate of the radius and femur	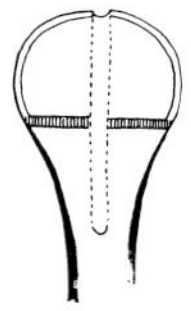		
	a. One hole, 1/4 inch in diameter		2	Maximum retardation
	b. One hole, 5/32 inch in diameter		13	Minimum retardation
	c. One hole, 5/32 inch in diameter, with the insertion of beeswax		5	Minimum retardation
	d. Eight to ten holes, 0.45 mm. in diameter		5	No retardation
5	Longitudinal insertion of cortical-bone graft (homogenous), 5/32 inch in thickness, through a drill hole across the distal epiphyeal plate of the femur	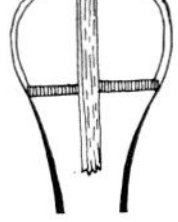	8	Arrest
6	Longitudinal insertion of smooth metallic pins extending from the articular surface of the epiphysis into the metaphysis of the distal part of the femur and radius	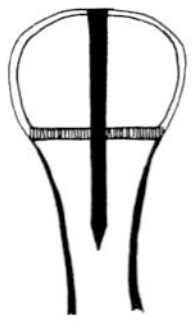		
	a. Steinmann pin, 5/32 inch		14	Minimum retardation
	b. Five Kirschner pins, 0.045 cm.		4	Variable retardation (none to minimum)
7	Longitudinal insertion of threaded metallic pins (1/4 inch and 5/32 inch) from the articular surface of the epiphysis into the metaphysis of the distal part of the femur	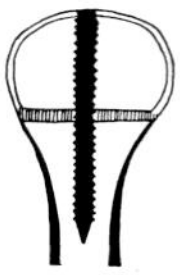	17	Arrest

*From Campbell, C. J., Grisolia, A., and Zanconato, G.: The effects produced in the cartilaginous epiphyseal plate of immature dogs by experimental surgical traumata. J. Bone Joint Surg., *41-A*:1221, 1959. Reprinted with permission.

and debris, normal enchondral ossification is resumed. This healing process is usually completed by the end of the third week. (2) If the fracture is more distal or deeper in the hypertrophic zone, there is considerable delay in resorption of the proximal cartilage, with marked widening of the physis distal to the fracture. The cells in the middle of this wide plate mature and are invaded by avascular tissue. This results in a split epiphyseal line—a second healing process, which may not be completed until after the fifth week. (3) If the injury involves the entire depth of the growth plate, the healing process will be incomplete. It occurs either by hyperplasia of the few scattered remaining cartilage cells of the resting zone or by narrowing of the defect by encroachment of the normal epiphyseal cartilage on all sides. If the defect is very large, healing cannot take place and growth in that segment of the epiphysis ceases.[23]

Campbell, Grisolia, and Zanconato studied the histologic effects and growth disturbances caused by surgical trauma to the physis of immature dogs (Table 8–1). Their conclusions are as follows:

1. After epiphyseal injury in an immature animal of specified age and growth potential, the amount of retardation of growth is roughly proportional to the amount of destruction of the region or zone of the epiphyseal plate which is responsible for replenishing the cells of the cartilage columns.
2. A defect in the cartilaginous epiphyseal plate caused by trauma which extends from the epiphysis to the metaphysis is not repaired by cartilage with the structural pattern of the normal epiphyseal plate. If there is nothing to obstruct the ingrowth of tissue, the defect is filled at first by an undifferentiated mesenchymal tissue which later forms a cancellous-bone bridge.
3. A bone may continue to grow in length normally if a relatively small cancellous-bone bridge connects the epiphysis to the metaphysis. When retardation occurs, the amount of retardation is usually proportional to the size and stability of the bone bridge. A cortical-bone graft, when placed across an epiphyseal plate, causes growth arrest if it unites to the bone of the epiphysis and metaphysis and does not break or is not absorbed.
4. Smooth metallic pins or nails of small gauge inserted from the epiphysis into the metaphysis at an angle perpendicular to the epiphyseal plate may cause less growth retardation than a cancellous-bone bridge of equal size. With growth, the epiphysis may glide over the pin if there is sufficient growth potential left in the epiphyseal plate.
5. Threaded pins or screws placed across the epiphyseal plate cause growth arrest if the threads are of sufficient gauge so that the epiphysis is me-

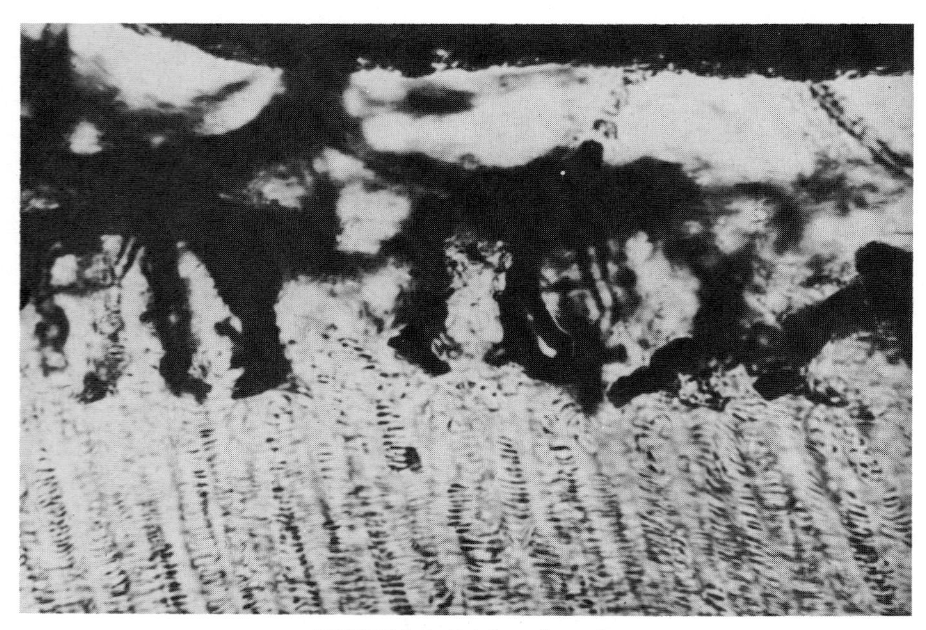

FIGURE 8–3. Epiphyseal vessels.

After progressive branching and anastomosis, the epiphyseal arteries reach the bone plate, cross it, and expand into terminal loops or tufts underneath the bone plate, giving the appearance of a rake. These vessels supply the germinal layer or the zone of resting cells. The bone plate is seen as being white in this illustration and the injected vessels as black (× 35). (From Trueta, J., and Morgan, J. D.: The vascular contribution to osteogenesis. J. Bone Joint Surg., *42-B*:103, 1960.)

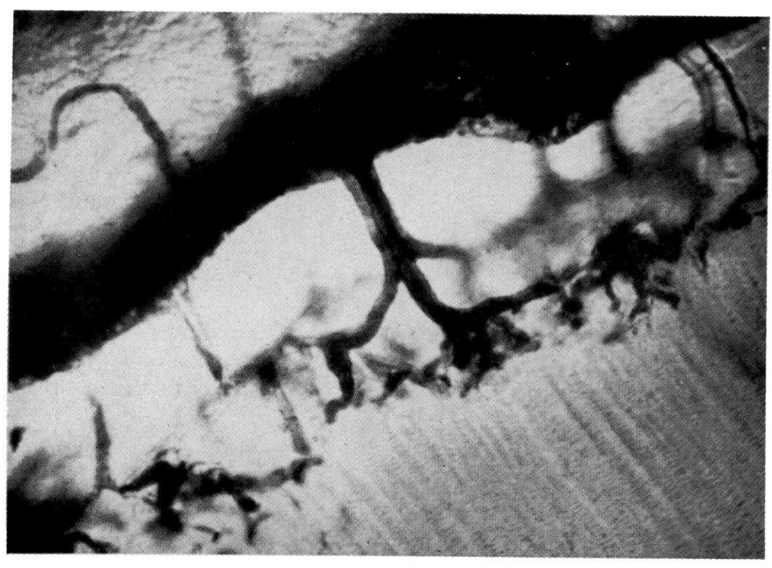

FIGURE 8–4. The epiphyseal vessels traverse the bone plate through canals toward the zone of "resting" cartilage cells (× 40).

(From Trueta, J., and Morgan, J. D.: The vascular contribution to osteogenesis. J. Bone Joint Surg., *42-B*:102, 1960.)

chanically fixed to the metaphysis until the epiphyseal plate is closed.*

Loss of Circulation

The normal vascular supply of the physis has been described by Trueta and Morgan.[140] There are two separate systems of circulation to the growth plate, one that supplies its epiphyseal surface (or E side), and the other, its metaphyseal surface (or M side).

Vascular Supply to the Epiphyseal Side of the Physis. Numerous branches of the epiphyseal artery reach to the bone plate, traverse it through canals, expand into terminal loops and tufts underneath the bone plate, and return to the epiphysis as large veins, not always through the same canal.

A former erroneous belief was that a rich blood supply existed *only* on the metaphyseal side of the growth plate. On the contrary, circulation underneath the bone plate is very rich, the vascular expansions forming a "ceiling" of blood with their endothelium in close contact with the "resting" chondrocytes, thus serving as an abundant vascular supply to the reproductive side of the growth plate (Figs. 8–3 to 8–5).

Vascular Supply to the Metaphyseal Side of the Physis. The terminal ramifications of the nutrient artery constitute about four fifths of the vessels that reach the growth plate from the metaphyseal side; their branches are evenly distributed over the central three fourths or more of the growth plate. The periphery of the growth plate on its metaphyseal side is supplied from a system of large periosteal vessels known as the perforating vessels of the metaphysis (Fig. 8–6).

Effect of Ischemia on the Physis. This has been studied by Trueta and Amato on the tibiae of rabbits. Through a small drill hole (made with a fine dental drill on the medial side of the proximal epiphysis of the right tibia and thus avoiding any direct injury to the physis), a flat spatula was introduced to the center of the epiphysis. A cavity was made parallel to the plane of the physis, and a strip of polyethylene film was placed in the cavity to prevent revascularization near the growth plate. The lateral side of the epiphysis was left intact to serve as a control. In the left tibia, using a similar technique, the polyethylene film was placed on the metaphyseal side of the physis and at a sufficient distance to prevent any direct damage. Groups of rabbits were sacrificed at varying intervals after operation to study the changes in the growth plate produced by ischemia. In

*From Campbell, C. J., Grisolia, A., and Zanconato, G.: The effects produced in the cartilaginous epiphyseal plate of immature dogs by experimental surgical traumata. J. Bone Joint Surg., *41-A*:1221, 1959. Reprinted with permission.

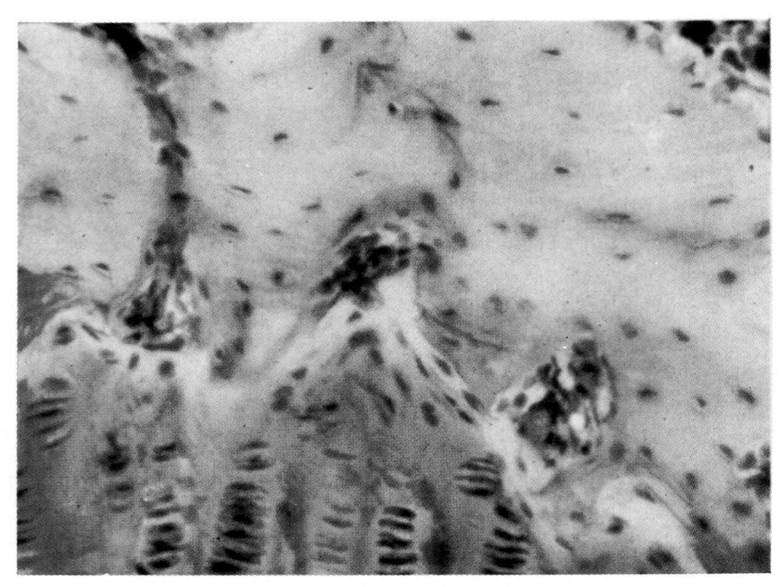

FIGURE 8–5. Epiphyseal vascular ends under the bone plate.

Each terminal bulging of a vessel covers the space corresponding to form four to ten cell columns. Note the close contact of the vascular endothelium to the "resting" cartilage cells (× 240). (From Trueta, J., and Morgan, J. D.: The vascular contribution to osteogenesis. J. Bone Joint Surg., *42-B*:102, 1960.)

other groups of rabbits, the polyethylene film was removed at varying intervals after the first operation, and then the rabbits were killed at 2 to 24 days after the second operation to study the revascularization that had occurred. The results of this investigation showed that the epiphyseal vessels are responsible for the nourishing blood supply of the reproductive cells of the physis; any extensive interruption of the epiphyseal vessels will result in irreparable damage to the growth plate. The principal role of the metaphyseal vessels—carrying calcium and vitamin D in the serum and phosphates in the erythrocytes—is calcification of the matrix, the removal of degenerate cells, and the deposition of lamellar bone along the inner side of the empty tubes. Thus, the metaphyseal vessels are of no nutritional importance to the prolif-

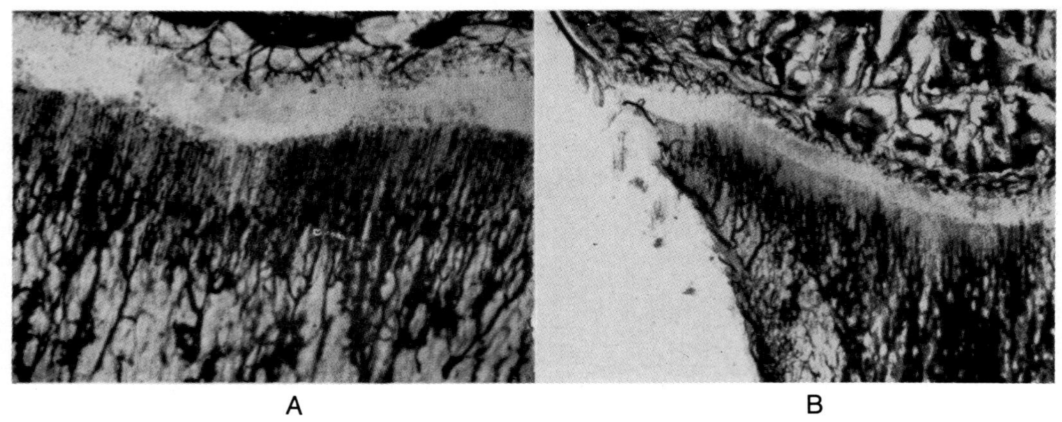

FIGURE 8–6. Metaphyseal vessels.

The nutrient artery supplies about four fifths of the vessels reaching the growth plate from its metaphyseal side, and the loops of its branches cover the central three fourths or more of the physis (**A** × 8 and **B** × 15). (From Trueta, J., and Morgan, J. D.: The vascular contribution to osteogenesis. J. Bone Joint Surg., *42-B*:104, 1960.)

erative chondrocytes of the physis. The absence of calcification will keep the cartilage cells alive.[139]

Compression

Trueta and Trias, in their studies of the effect of pressure on the epiphyseal cartilage of the rabbit, came to the following conclusions: (1) Persistent compression affects the growth plate by interference with the blood flow on one or both sides of the physis. (2) Despite exertion of the same pressure upon both sides of the growth plate, only the metaphyseal side is readily affected in the early stages: as long as no damage is caused to the epiphyseal side of the growth plate, the lesions are fully reversible. (3) Interference with growth is directly proportionate to the damage caused by compression to the epiphyseal side of the growth plate, and, in general, to the duration of compression. (4) Severe continuous compression of the epiphyseal plate will affect its growth by interrupting its blood supply.[141] Trueta and Trias summarized their findings, designating the following four stages of compression injury:

Stage one: up to seven days of compression there is an inhibition of degeneration of the hypertrophic cells at the end of the growth columns. This allows the cells to survive for an, as yet, indefinite number of days: in some of our experiments, up to more than twelve days. During all this time cells from the proliferative section of the columns continue to develop into hypertrophic cells while the rate of cell division at the proliferative level of the columns remains apparently normal. In these circumstances the growth cartilage at the area of greatest pressure may develop to about four times its normal height.

Stage two: at approximately eight to ten days after the initiation of compression, the continuous accumulation of the new cartilage cells and their lack of subsequent removal at the metaphyseal end of the epiphyseal cartilage causes the compression to increase. This occurs despite the increase in the distance between the pins, because of compression of the springs of the clamp. In about ten days changes appear in the epiphyseal end of the growth cartilage. From then on, the suffering cartilage cells and their organization become progressively greater until the next phase is reached.

Stage three: at about 14 days or more the disorganization is, in general, severe and mostly reversible. The bone plate covering the epiphyseal side of the cartilage has dead cells and appears broken into fragments. The new addition of cells by division of the proliferative section is interrupted and shortly after this, irregular vascular invasion occurs from both ends, despite the continuation of compression.

Stage four consists of fusion of the growth cartilage by bone formation following the vascular invasion of the previous phase, beginning by establishing a narrow bone bridge across the growth plate.*

Noteworthy, in the initial period, is the protection of the hypertrophic cells and the lack of action on the proliferative segment of the physis.

Classification

Fractures involving the physis have been classified by several authors:

Foucher divided them into three classes: (1) pure separations of the epiphysis from the diaphysis (divulsion épiphysaire) without any osseous tissue adhering to it; (2) separation of the epiphysis with a thin, finely granular layer of osseous material attached to it (fracture épiphysaire); and (3) solution of continuity of the diaphysis in the midst of the osseous spongy tissue near the epiphysis (fracture pre-épiphysaire).[52]

Poland subdivided fractures involving the physis into the following types: *Type A*, pure and complete separation; *Type B*, partial separation with fracture of the diaphysis; *Type C*, partial separation with fracture of the epiphysis; and *Type D*, complete separation with fracture of the epiphysis (Fig. 8–7).[106]

Aitken designated the three types of fractures involving the epiphyseal cartilage plate as: *Type I*, an avulsion type of fracture due to shearing or twisting force in which the fracture line passes through the zone of degenerating cartilage cells and emerges through a portion of the metaphyseal bone. Displacement in this type of fracture may be marked, but ultimate deformity due to displacement or growth disturbance is rare.

Type II, a compression type of fracture caused by a combination of crushing or shearing force, commonly involves the distal tibial epiphysis, but rarely the distal femoral epiphysis. The line of fracture originates in the joint and may emerge between the bony epiphysis and the zone of the degenerative cartilage cells of the physis; or the fracture line may cross the physis and emerge between it and the diaphysis. In the former, growth disturbance will not occur; whereas in the latter, premature arrest of growth and deformity will follow.

Type III is a compression type of injury in which the physis has been crushed between the bony epiphysis and the diaphysis. In this type,

*From Trueta, J., and Trias, A.: The vascular contribution to osteogenesis. J. Bone Joint Surg., *43-B*:800, 1961. Reprinted with permission.

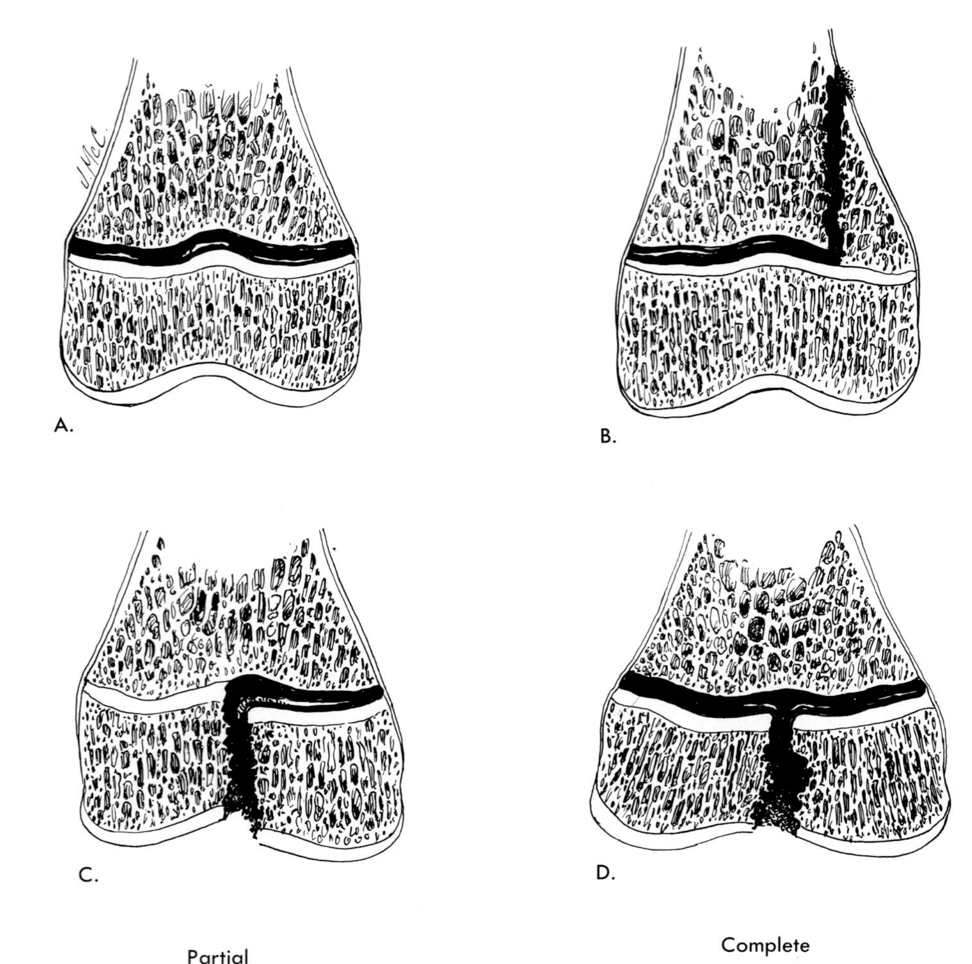

FIGURE 8–7. Poland's classification of epiphyseal separation.

A. Pure and complete separation. **B.** Partial separation with fracture of the diaphysis. **C.** Partial separation with fracture of the epiphysis. **D.** Complete separation with fracture of the epiphysis. (Redrawn after Poland, J.: Traumatic separation of the epiphysis. London, Smith, Elder & Co., 1898, p. 80.)

the fracture line may be so small as to be overlooked or may be considered of no clinical importance.[2–5]

Salter and Harris presented the following thorough and practical classification of physeal injuries based on the mechanism of injury, the relationship of the fracture line to the germinal layer of the physis, and the prognosis concerning disturbance of growth.

Type I. This is produced by a shearing or avulsion force and is commonly encountered in infants whose physes are relatively thick. It may also occur in pathologic fractures such as those seen in rickets, scurvy, or osteomyelitis. The epiphysis separates from the metaphysis without any bony fragment, and the plane of cleavage is through the zone of the hypertrophying cells, with the germinal cells of the physis remaining with the epiphysis (Fig. 8–8 A). Displacement of fragments is checked by the intact thick periosteal attachments. Reduction is usually unnecessary. Growth is not disturbed, unless there is associated aseptic necrosis and premature closure of the physis due to interruption of its blood supply; for example, in acute traumatic separation of the capital femoral epiphysis.

Type II. A shearing or avulsion force causes this fracture, which is the most common type of physeal injury. It frequently occurs in children over ten years of age. The line of separation extends along the hypertrophic zone of the physis to a variable distance and then out through a portion of the metaphyseal bone (Fig. 8–8 B). In the radiogram, a triangular metaphyseal fragment is readily visible, which is re-

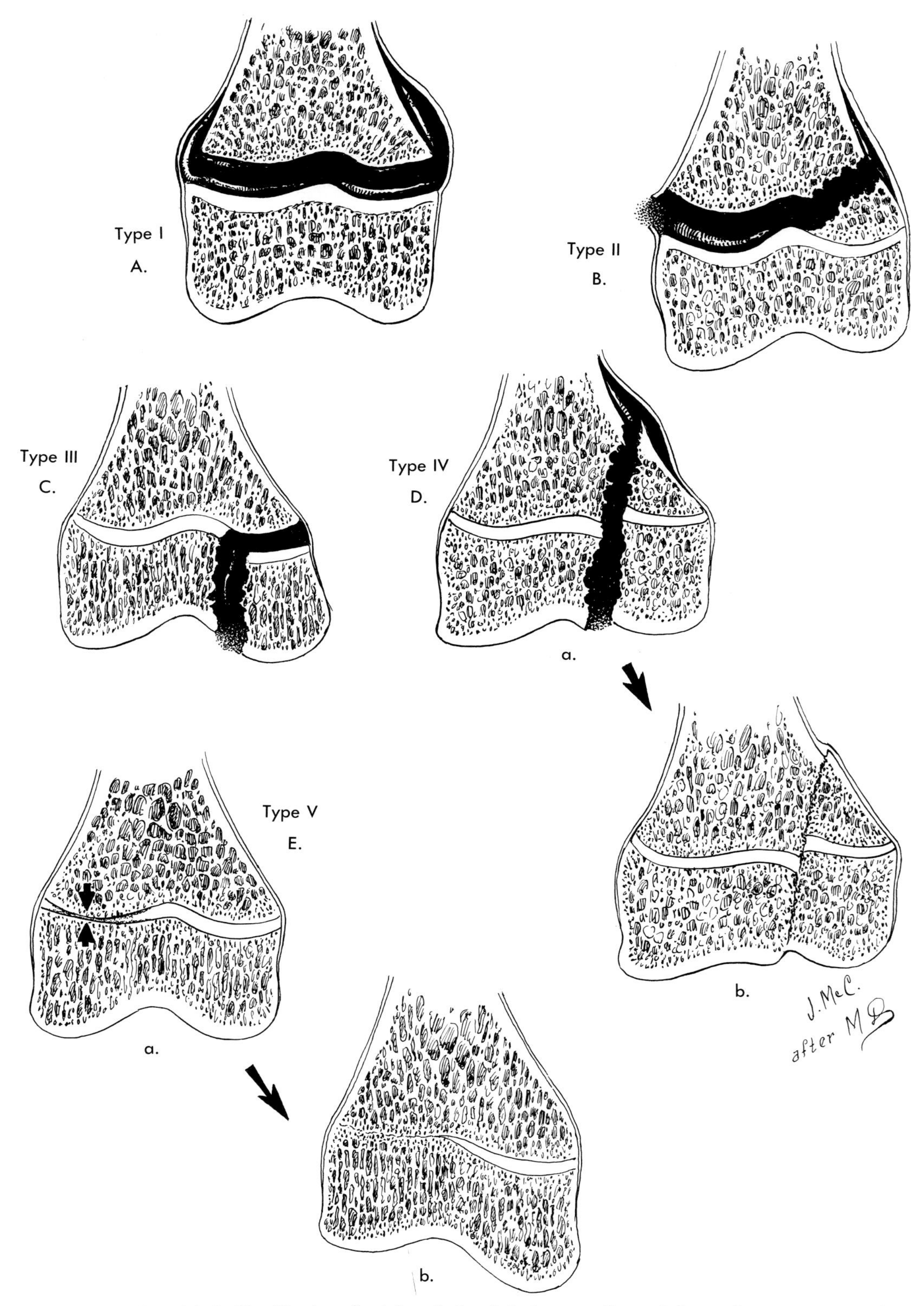

FIGURE 8–8. Classification of epiphyseal plate injuries according to Salter and Harris.

(Redrawn after Salter, R. B., and Harris, W. R.: Injuries involving the epiphyseal plate. J. Bone Joint Surg., *45-A*:587, 1963.)

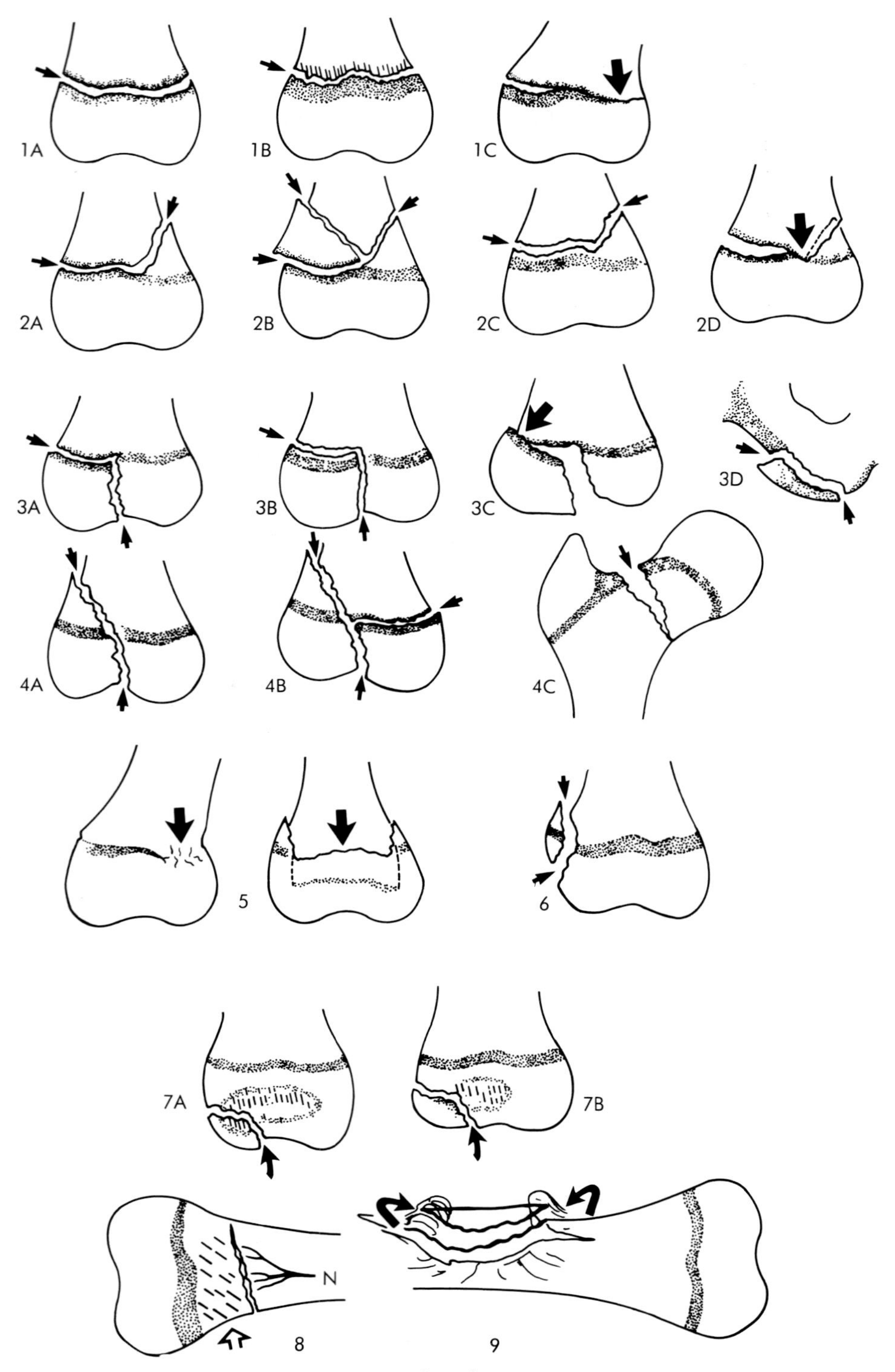

FIGURE 8–9 *See legend on opposite page*

ferred to as "Thurston Holland's sign." The periosteum is intact on the concave side of the angulation (i.e., the side with the metaphyseal fragment), whereas on the convex side the periosteum is stripped and torn from the diaphysis, but still remains attached to the epiphysis. This is accounted for not only by the thickness, the great vascularity, and the loose connection of the periosteum with the diaphysis, but also by the intimate connection of the periosteum with the perichondrium of the epiphysis. In Type II physeal injury, reduction is ordinarily achieved and maintained with relative ease. The intact periosteal hinge on the concave side and the metaphyseal bone fragment prevent over-reduction. Growth is not disturbed, as the germinal layer of chondrocytes remains attached to the epiphysis and circulation to the epiphysis is not interrupted.

Type III. This rare injury is caused by an intra-articular shearing force, which usually occurs in the proximal or distal tibial epiphysis. There is an intra-articular fracture of the epiphysis, with the plane of cleavage extending from the joint surface to the weak zone of hypertrophic cells of the physis and then extending parallel with the growth plate to its periphery (Fig. 8–8 C). Restoration of the congruous articular surface is essential in its treatment; in markedly displaced fractures, open surgery is often necessary to obtain accurate anatomic reduction. Prognosis for future growth is good, provided there is no impairment of circulation to the separated fragment of the epiphysis.

Type IV. This injury is most commonly seen at the lower end of the humerus in fractures of the lateral condyle. The fracture line begins at the articular surface and extends through the epiphysis, across the full thickness of the physis, and then through a segment of the metaphysis. There is a complete vertical split that involves the important germinal layer of the physis (Fig. 8–8 D). The fracture fragments may be undisplaced or separated to a varying extent. It is imperative to achieve perfect anatomic reduction in order to restore a smooth articular surface and also to prevent osseous bridging across the physis with consequent local premature growth arrest. Only fine smooth Kirschner wires should be used for internal fixation; they should traverse the plate perpendicularly and be removed after four to six weeks.

Type V. This rare injury usually occurs in the knee or ankle—articulations that normally move only in one plane into flexion and extension. On the application of marked abduction or adduction strain, a severe compression force is transmitted through the epiphysis to a segment of the physis, crushing the germinal layer of the chondrocytes (Fig. 8–8 E). Displacement of the epiphysis is minimal in this type of physeal injury. Often the seriousness of the condition is not suspected and the injury is misdiagnosed as a simple sprain. In treatment, the part is supported in a cast, and weight-bearing is avoided for at least three weeks. The prognosis in Type V physeal injury is poor, since premature arrest of growth almost always occurs.[121]

The Salter-Harris classification is simple and easy to use in daily clinical practice. However, it does not include injuries to the zone of Ranvier or to epiphyseal hyaline cartilage, or complex combined injuries. Ogden has devised a more comprehensive classification of injuries to the growth mechanism, which is given in Figure 8–9.[96, 97]

Injuries to the Perichondral Ring (Type 6 of Ogden's classification of injury to the growth mechanism). The perichondral ring is a circumferential fibrous band of collagen fibers that encircle the physis. At the metaphyseal junction the perichondral ring attaches to the perios-

FIGURE 8–9. Ogden's classification of injuries to the growth mechanism.

1A. Propagation across the physeal cartilage. **1B.** Propagation across the diseased primary spongiosa (e.g., leukemia, thalassemia), with the physeal interface variably involved. **1C.** Disruption of a localized segment of the physis. **2A.** Partial propagation across both the physis and the metaphysis. **2B.** Free and attached metaphyseal fragments. **2C.** Propagation across both the primary spongiosa and the metaphysis. **2D.** Localized disruption of the physis at the point of propagation into metaphysis. **3A.** Epiphyseal fragment with propagation through the physis. **3B.** Epiphyseal fragment with propagation through the primary spongiosa. **3C.** Crushing injury to peripheral physis. **3D.** Nonarticular cartilage avulsion (e.g., ischial tuberosity). **4A.** Combined epiphyseal-physeal-metaphyseal fragments. **4B.** Epiphyseal-physeal-metaphyseal fragment combined with Type 3A or 3B lesion. **4C.** Propagation through a nonarticular epiphyseal region (e.g., intraepiphyseal cartilage of the developing femoral neck). **5.** Longitudinal growth retardation of a major physeal segment. **6.** Avulsion or crushing of the peripheral physis (zone of Ranvier). **7A.** Osteochondral fragment involving the physis of the secondary ossification center. **7B.** Chondral fragment involving hypertrophic cells of the physis of the secondary ossification center. **8.** A metaphyseal fracture temporarily cuts off the nutrient artery (N), causing transient ischemia to the metaphyseal segment between the fracture and the physis. **9.** Damage to periosteum, with or without discrete osseous injury, disrupts normal membranous ossification.

teum, whereas at the epiphyseal side it is connected to the zone of Ranvier—a wedge-shaped group of cells contiguous with the germinal cartilage cells of the physis. The cells at the zone of Ranvier supply cells to the external surface of the germinal layers of the growth plate and increase the latitudinal dimension of the physis by appositional growth.

Injuries to the perichondral ring are rare; they are produced by localized contusions or avulsions of overlying skin and soft tissues, such as may occur from lawn mower injuries or severe burns. Rupture of the perichondral ring often results in osseous bridging between the epiphysis and metaphysis, leading to progressive angular deformity.[111] Displacement of the perichondral ring causes a traumatic exostosis.[110]

Injuries to the Cartilaginous Growth Plate of the Epiphysis (Type 7 of Ogden's classification of injury to the growth mechanism). This injury is not uncommon. The fracture is totally intraepiphyseal and does not involve the physis. The fracture line extends from the articular surface through the epiphyseal cartilage into the secondary ossification center of the epiphysis, which may be cartilaginous or ossified, depending upon the skeletal maturation of the child. Ogden subclassified Type 7 injury to the growth mechanism into two subtypes: in *Type 7A*, the fracture line propagates through the epiphyseal and articular cartilage into the bone of the secondary ossification center; in *Type 7B*, the fracture line is through the epiphyseal and articular cartilage but does not involve the ossified secondary center of ossification of the epiphysis—the lesion is entirely cartilaginous and difficult to diagnose. An example of Type 7A injury is an osteochondral fracture such as that of the femoral condyle or the dome of the talus. Type 7B injury takes place in the distal tibia and in nonarticular areas such as the proximal tibial tuberosity (Osgood-Schlatter disease), the greater trochanter, or the base of the fifth metatarsal.

Ogden classifies injuries to the metaphyseal growth and remodeling mechanism as Type 8, and that to the diaphyseal growth mechanism as Type 9.[97, 98]

Incidence

Approximately 15 per cent of all fractures in children involve the physis.[121] The relative incidence of physeal fractures is given in Table 8–2. The distal radius, humerus, tibia, and fibula are the common sites.

Principles of Management of Fractures Involving the Physis

These are well outlined by Salter and Harris.[121]

All reductions, whether closed or open, should be performed with the utmost gentleness in order to prevent damage to the delicate cartilage of the physis. Forceful manipulations are condemned. During open reduction, direct pressure on the physis by blunt instruments should be avoided.

Epiphyseal separations should be *reduced immediately*, as each day of delay will make reduction progressively more difficult. In fact, after ten days, Types I and II physeal injuries cannot be reduced without exerting undue force and damaging the cartilaginous growth plate.

Table 8–2. *Incidence of Epiphyseal Fractures*

Site	*Per Cent**	*Per Cent†*	*Per Cent‡*
Distal radius	46	30	26
Distal humerus	14	6	13
Distal fibula	13	6	3
Distal tibia	11	18	14
Distal ulna	5	4	2
Proximal radius	5	0.2	1
Proximal humerus	3	5	6
Distal femur	1	5	0.2
Proximal ulna	1	–	0.6
Proximal tibia	0.8	2	2
Proximal fibula	0.2	–	0.4

*From Neer, C. S., II, and Horwitz, B. S.: Fractures of the epiphyseal plate. Clin. Orthop., *41*:24, 1965. Reprinted with permission.

†From Peterson, C. A., and Peterson, H. A.: Analysis of the incidence of injuries to the epiphyseal growth plate. J. Trauma, *12*:275, 1972. Reprinted with permission.

‡From Ogden, J. A.: Injury to the growth mechanism of the immature skeleton. Skeletal Radiol., *6*:237, 1981. Reprinted with permission.

When a Type I or Type II fracture is seen late (i.e., after seven to ten days), it is better to accept malunion than to cause growth arrest by forceful manipulation or open surgery. In Type III or IV physeal injuries, congruity of articular surfaces is essential; in such cases, delayed reduction is performed, if indicated.

As stated, reduction of Type I and Type II fractures involving the physis can be readily obtained and maintained. In Type III physeal injuries, open reduction may be indicated to restore a congruous articular surface, particularly in weight-bearing joints. Open reduction is required in almost all cases of Type IV fractures of the physis. Caution must be exercised in order to prevent injury to the circulation of the epiphysis. Only smooth Kirschner wires must be used for internal fixation, and under no circumstances should screws or threaded wires be inserted across the physis. The internal fixation device is removed when the fracture has healed.

Type III and Type IV physeal injuries require accurate anatomic reduction. In Type I and Type II fractures of the physis, perfect reduction is desirable, but not mandatory. Bone remodeling will correct moderate residual deformities. In general, one can accept a greater degree of deformity in multiplane joints (such as the shoulder) than in single plane joints (such as the knee and ankle).

Types I, II, and III injuries consolidate very rapidly, usually in about half the time required for a fracture through the metaphysis of the same bone. Type IV injuries require the same period for union as metaphyseal fractures.

Fractures involving the physis should be closely followed for possible development of growth disturbance. Parents should be warned of potential complications, but without causing much anxiety. As already indicated, the factors that determine the prognosis are: the type of physeal injury, the age of the child at the time of fracture, the integrity of the blood supply to the epiphysis, the method of reduction, and whether the fracture is open or closed.

References

1. Ahstrom, J. P., Jr.: Epiphyseal injuries of the lower extremity. Surg. Clin. North Am., *1*:119, 1965.
2. Aitken, A. P.: The end results of the fractured distal radial epiphysis. J. Bone Joint Surg., *17*:302, 1935.
3. Aitken, A. P.: The end results of the fractured distal tibial epiphysis. J. Bone Joint Surg., *18*:685, 1936.
4. Aitken, A. P.: End results of fractures of the proximal humeral epiphysis. J. Bone Joint Surg., *18*:1036, 1936.
5. Aitken, A. P.: Fractures of the epiphysis. Clin. Orthop., *41*:19, 1965.
6. Aitken, A. P., and Magill, H. K.: Fractures involving the distal femoral epiphyseal cartilage. J. Bone Joint Surg., *34-A*:96, 1952.
7. Arguelles, F., Gomar, F., Garcia, A., and Esquerdo, J.: Irradiation lesions of the growth plate in rabbits. J. Bone Joint Surg., *59-B*:85, 1977.
8. Arkin, A. M., and Katz, J. F.: The effects of pressure on epiphyseal growth. J. Bone Joint Surg., *38-A*:1056, 1956.
9. Banks, S. W., and Compere, E. L.: Regeneration of epiphyseal cartilage. An experimental study. Ann. Surg., *114*:1076, 1941.
10. Barnhard, H. J., and Geyer, R. W.: Effects of x-radiation on growing bone. Radiology, *78*:207, 1962.
11. Barr, J. S., Lingley, J. R., and Gall, E. A.: The effects of roentgen irradiation on epiphyseal growth. I. Experimental studies upon the albino rat. A.J.R., *49*:104, 1943.
12. Bennett, R. B., and Blount, W. P.: Destruction of epiphyses by freezing. J.A.M.A., *105*:661, 1935.
13. Benum, P.: Autogenous transplantation of apophyses. Acta Orthop. Scand., Suppl. 156, 1974.
14. Bisgard, J. D., and Bisgard, M. E.: Longitudinal growth of long bones. Arch. Surg., *31*:508, 1935.
15. Bisgard, J. D., and Hunt, H. B.: Influence of roentgen rays and radium on epiphyseal growth of long bones. Radiology, *26*:56, 1936.
16. Blount, W. P.: Fractures in Children. Baltimore, Williams & Wilkins, 1955.
17. Bohler, L.: The Treatment of Fractures. 5th English Ed. (Translated from German 13th Ed. by Hans Tretter et al.) New York, Grune & Stratton, 1956–1958.
18. Bonnin, J. G.: A Complete Outline of Fractures. 2nd Ed. London, William Heinemann, 1946.
19. Bouyala, J. M., and Rigault, P.: Les traumatismes du cartilage de conjugalson. Rev. Chir. Orthop., *65*:259, 1979.
20. Bowen, D. R.: Epiphyseal separation-fracture. Interstate Med. J., *17*:607, 1915.
21. Brashear, H. R., Jr.: Epiphyseal fractures of the lower extremities. South. Med. J., *51*:845, 1958.
22. Brashear, H. R., Jr.: Epiphyseal fractures. A microscopic study of the healing process in rats. J. Bone Joint Surg., *41-A*:1055, 1959.
23. Brashear, H. R., Jr.: Epiphyseal avascular necrosis and its relation to longitudinal bone growth. J. Bone Joint Surg., *45-A*:1423, 1963.
24. Bright, R. W.: Surgical correction of partial epiphyseal plate closure in dogs by bone bridge resection and use of silicone rubber implants. J. Bone Joint Surg., *54-A*:1133, 1972.
25. Bright, R. W.: Operative correction of partial epiphyseal plate closure by osseous-bridge resection and silicone-rubber implant. J. Bone Joint Surg., *56-A*:655, 1974.
26. Bright, R. W., and Elmore, S. M.: Some effects of immunosuppressive drugs on the epiphyseal plates of rats. Surg. Forum, *18*:485, 1967.
27. Bright, R. W., and Elmore, S. M.: Physical properties of epiphyseal plate changes. Surg. Forum, *19*:463, 1968.
28. Bright, R. W., Burstein, H., and Elmore, M.: Epiphyseal-plate cartilage. A biomechanical and histological analysis of failure modes. J. Bone Joint Surg., *56-A*:688, 1974.
29. Brinn, L. B., and Moseley, J. E.: Bone changes following electrical injury. A.J.R., *97*:682, 1966.
30. Brodin, H.: Longitudinal bone growth. The nutrition of the epiphyseal cartilages and the local blood supply. Acta Orthop. Scand., Suppl. 20, 1955.
31. Brooks, B., and Hillstrom, H. T.: Effect of roentgen rays on bone growth and bone regeneration. Am. J. Surg., *20*:599, 1933.

32. Campbell, C. J.: The healing of cartilage defects. Clin. Orthop., *64*:45, 1969.
33. Campbell, C. J., Grisolia, A., and Zanconato, G.: The effects produced in the cartilaginous epiphyseal plate of immature dogs by experimental surgical traumata. J. Bone Joint Surg., *41-A*:1221, 1959.
34. Cassidy, R. H.: Epiphyseal injuries of the lower extremities. Surg. Clin. North Am., *38*:1125, 1958.
35. Cave, E. F. (ed.): Fractures and Other Injuries. Chicago, Year Book, 1958.
36. Charnley, J.: The Closed Treatment of Common Fractures. Edinburgh, E. S. Livingstone, 1950.
37. Compere, E. L.: Growth arrest in long bones as a result of fractures that include the epiphysis. J.A.M.A., *105*:2140, 1935.
38. Compere, E. L., Banks, S. W., and Compere, C. L.: Pictorial Handbook of Fracture Treatment. 5th Ed. Chicago, Year Book, 1963.
39. Conwell, H. E., and Reynolds, F. C.: Key and Conwell's Management of Fractures, Dislocations and Sprains. 7th Ed. St. Louis, Mosby, 1961.
40. Cooper, A.: A Treatise on Dislocations and on Fractures of Joints. 2nd Ed. London, the author, 1823; Boston: T. R. Marvin, 1844.
41. Cotton, F. J.: Dislocations and Joint Fractures. Philadelphia, Saunders, 1924.
42. Dahl, B.: Effects des rayons-x sur les os longs in developement. J. Radiol. Electr., *18*:131, 1934.
43. Dale, G. G., and Harris, W. R.: Prognosis of epiphyseal separation. J. Bone Joint Surg., *40-B*:116, 1958.
44. Delpech, J. M.: De l'orthomorphie par rapport a l'espice humaine. Paris, Gabon, 1829.
45. DePalma, A. F.: The Management of Fractures and Dislocations. An Atlas. 2nd. Ed. Philadelphia, Saunders, 1970.
46. Desjardins, A. U.: Osteogenic tumor: Growth injury of bone and muscular atrophy following therapeutic irradiation. Radiology, *14*:296, 1930.
47. Dreyfuss, J. R., and Glimcher, M. J.: Epiphyseal injury following frostbite. N. Engl. J. Med., *253*:1065, 1955.
48. Eliason, E. L., and Ferguson, L. K.: Epiphyseal separation of the long bones. Surg. Gynecol. Obstet., *58*:85, 1934.
49. Ford, L. T., and Canales, G. M.: A study of experimental trauma and attempts to stimulate growth by the lower femoral epiphysis in rabbits. Ill. J. Bone Joint Surg., *42-A*:439, 1960.
50. Ford, L. T., and Key, J. A.: A study of experimental trauma to the distal femoral epiphysis in rabbits. J. Bone Joint Surg., *38-A*:84, 1956.
51. Foucher, M.: De la divulsion des epiphyses. Cong. Med. France, Paris, *1*:63, 1863.
52. Foucher, M.: Annales du Congrés Medical de Rouen, 1863. Quoted in Poland, J.: Traumatic Separation of the Epiphyses. London, Smith, Elder, & Co., 1898, p. 72.
53. Friedenberg, Z. B.: Reaction of the epiphysis to partial surgical resection. J. Bone Joint Surg., *39-A*:332, 1957.
54. Furlong, R. (ed.): Fractures and Dislocations. Washington, D.C., Butterworth, 1966.
55. Groves, E. W. H.: On Modern Methods of Treating Fractures. Bristol, England, John Wright & Sons, 1916.
56. Haas, S. L.: Transplantation of the articular end of bone, including the epiphyseal cartilage line. Surg. Gynecol. Obstet., *23*:301, 1916.
57. Haas, S. L.: The localization of the growing point in the epiphyseal cartilage plate of bones. Am. J. Orthop. Surg., *15*:563, 1917.
58. Haas, S. L.: The relation of the blood supply to the longitudinal growth of bone. Am. J. Orthop. Surg., *15*:157, 305, 1917.
59. Haas, S. L.: The changes produced in growing bones after injury to the epiphyseal cartilage. J. Orthop. Surg., *1*:67, 166:226, 1919.
60. Haas, S. L.: Further observations on the transplantation of the epiphyseal cartilage plate. Surg. Gynecol. Obstet., *52*:958, 1931.
61. Haas, S. L.: Restriction of bone growth by pins through the epiphyseal cartilage plate. J. Bone Joint Surg., *32-A*:338, 1950.
62. Hall-Craggs, E.: Influence of epiphyses on the regulation of bone growth. Nature, *221*:1245, 1969.
63. Hamilton, F. H.: A Practical Treatise on Fractures and Dislocations. 5th Ed. Philadelphia, Henry C. Lea, 1875.
64. Harris, W. R.: The endocrine basis for slipping of the upper femoral epiphysis. J. Bone Joint Surg., *32-B*:5, 1950.
65. Harris, W. R.: Epiphyseal injuries. A.A.O.S. Instr. Course Lect., *15*:206, 1958.
66. Harris, W. R., and Hobson, K. W.: Histological changes in experimentally displaced upper femoral epiphysis in rabbits. J. Bone Joint Surg., *38-B*:914, 1956.
67. Harris, W. R., Martin, R., and Tile, M.: Transplantation of epiphyseal plates. An experimental study. J. Bone Joint Surg., *47-A*:897, 1965.
68. Harsha, W. N.: Effects of trauma upon epiphyses. Clin. Orthop., *10*:140, 1957.
69. Hellstadius, A.: An investigation by experiments in animals of the role played by the epiphyseal cartilage in longitudinal growth. Acta Chir. Scand., *95*:156, 1947.
70. Heuter, C.: Anatomische Studien an der Extremitatengelenken Neugeborner und Erwachsener. Virchows Arch., *25*:572, 1862.
71. Hirsch, C., and Evans, F. G.: Studies on some physical properties of infant compact bone. Acta. Orthop. Scand., *35*:300, 1965.
72. Holden, C. E. A.: The role of blood supply to soft tissue in the healing of diaphyseal fractures. An experimental study. J. Bone Joint Surg., *54-A*:993, 1972.
73. Holland, C. T.: Radiographical note on injuries to the distal epiphyses of radius and ulna. Proc. R. Soc. Med., *22*:695, 1929.
74. Huller, T., and Nathan, H.: Does the periosteum contribute to bone strength? Isr. J. Med. Sci., *6*:630, 1970.
75. Hutchinson, J.: Lectures on injuries to the epiphysis and their results. Br. Med. J., *69*:669, 1894.
76. Imbert, R.: Pathologie experimentale de l'appareil de croissance des os longs. Marseille Chir., *3*:581, 1951.
77. Judet, R., Judet, J., and LaGrange, J.: Les Fractures des Membres chez l'Enfant. Paris, Librairie Maloine, 1958.
78. Karaharju, E. O., Ryoppy, S. A., and Makinen, R. J.: Remodelling by asymmetrical epiphyseal growth. J. Bone Joint Surg., *58-B*:122, 1976.
79. Key, J. A.: Survival and growth of an epiphysis after removal and replacement. J. Bone Joint Surg., *31-A*:150, 1949.
80. Key, J. A., and Ford, L. T.: Study of experimental trauma to the distal femoral epiphysis in rabbits. II. J. Bone Joint Surg., *40-A*:887, 1958.
81. Landells, J. W.: The reaction of injured human articular cartilage. J. Bone Joint Surg., *39-B*:548, 1957.
82. Langenskiold, A., and Edgren, W.: The growth mechanism of the epiphyseal cartilage in the light of experimental observations. Acta Orthop. Scand., *19*:19, 1950.
83. McLaughlin, H. L.: Trauma. Philadelphia, Saunders, 1960.
84. Malgaigne, J. F.: Traite des Fractures et des Luxations. Paris, Bailliere, 1847.
85. Morgan, J. D.: Blood supply of growing rabbits' tibia. J. Bone Joint Surg., *41-B*:185, 1959.

86. Morscher, E.: Posttraumatische Zapfenepiphyse. Arch. Orthop. Unfallchir., *61*:128, 1967.
87. Morscher, E.: Strength and morphology of growth cartilage under hormonal influence of puberty. Animal experiments and clinical study on the etiology of local growth disorders during puberty. Reconstr. Surg. Traumatol., *10*:3, 1968.
88. Morscher, E., Desaulles, P. A., and Schenk, R.: Experimental studies on tensile strength and morphology of the epiphyseal cartilage at puberty. Ann. Paediatr., *205*:112, 1965.
89. Neer, C. S., II, and Horwitz, B. S.: Fractures of the epiphyseal plate. Clin. Orthop., *41*:24, 1965.
90. Nordentoft, E. L.: Experimental epiphyseal injuries. Acta Orthop. Scand., *40*:176, 1969.
91. O'Brien, T. R., Morgan, J. P., and Suter, P. F.: Epiphyseal plate injury in the dog: A radiographic study of growth disturbance in the forelimb. J. Small Anim. Pract., *12*:19, 1971.
92. O'Donoghue, D. H.: Treatment of Injuries to Athletes. 2nd Ed. Philadelphia, Saunders, 1970.
93. Ogden, J. A.: Injury to the immature skeleton. *In* Touloukian, R. (ed.): Pediatric Trauma. New York, John Wiley & Sons, 1978.
94. Ogden, J. A.: The development and growth of the musculoskeletal system. *In* Albright, J. A., and Brand, R. A. (eds.): The Scientific Basis of Orthopaedics. New York, Appleton-Century-Crofts, 1979.
95. Ogden, J. A.: Chondro-osseous development and growth. *In* Urist, M. R. (ed.): Fundamental and Clinical Bone Physiology. Philadelphia, Lippincott, 1981.
96. Ogden, J. A.: Injury to the growth mechanism of the immature skeleton. Skeletal Radiol., *6*:237, 1981.
97. Ogden, J. A.: Skeletal Injury in the Child. Philadelphia, Lea & Febiger, 1981.
98. Ogden, J. A.: Skeletal growth mechanism injury patterns. J. Pediatr. Orthop., *2*:371, 1982.
99. Ogden, J. A..: Pocket Guide to Pediatric Fractures. Baltimore, Williams & Wilkins, 1987.
100. Ogden, J. A., and Southwick, W. O.: Electrical injury involving the immature skeleton. Skeletal Radiol., *6*:187, 1981.
101. Ohyoshi, K., and Miura, T.: Five cases of the epiphyseal detachment of long bone. Hokkaido Igaku Zasshi, *5*:37, 1959.
102. Ollier, L.: Traite Experimental et Clinique de la Regeneration des Os et de la Production Artificielle du Tissue Osseux. Paris, Masson et Fils, 1867, Vol. I, pp. 236, 386.
103. Pauwels, F.: Grundniss einer Biomechanik der Frakturheilung Verhandlungen. Dtsch. Orthop. Gesellschaft, *34*:62, 1940.
104. Pauwels, F.: Über die mechanische Bedeutung der groberan Kortikalisstruktur beim normal und pathologisch verbogenen Rohrenknochen. Anat. Nachr., *1*:53, 1950.
105. Peterson, C. A., and Peterson, H. A.: Analysis of the incidence of injuries to the epiphyseal growth plate. J. Trauma, *12*:275, 1972.
106. Poland, J.: Traumatic Separation of the Epiphyses. London, Smith, Elder, & Co., 1898.
107. Poland, J.: Traumatic separation of the epiphyses in general. Historical. Clin. Orthop., *41*:7, 1965 (reprinted from Pediatrics, *4*:49, 1897).
108. Pollen, A. G.: Fractures and Dislocations in Children. Edinburgh, Churchill-Livingstone, 1973.
109. Porter, R. W.: The effect of tension across a growing epiphysis. J. Bone Joint Surg., *60-B*:252, 1978.
110. Rang, M.: The Growth Plate and Its Disorders. Baltimore, Williams & Wilkins, 1969.
111. Rang, M.: Children's Fractures. Philadelphia, Lippincott, 1974.
112. Ray, S. K., Connolly, J. F., and Huurman, W. W., Jr.: Distraction treatment of deformities due to physeal fractures. Surg. Forum, *29*:543, 1978.
113. Redell, G.: Retardation of growth after traumatic epiphyseal separation. Acta Orthop. Scand., *25*:97, 1955.
114. Reed, H.: Fractures and dislocations of the extremities in children. J. Trauma, *17*:351, 1977.
115. Ring, P. A.: The effects of partial or complete excision of the epiphyseal cartilage of the rabbit. J. Anat., *89*:79, 1955.
116. Ring, P. A.: Excision and reimplantation of the epiphyseal cartilage of the rabbit. J. Anat., *89*:231, 1955.
117. Ring, P. A.: Transplantation of epiphyseal cartilage. J. Bone Joint Surg., *37-B*:642, 1955.
118. Rockwood, C. A., Wilkins, K. E., and King, R. E. (eds.): Fractures in Children. Philadelphia, Lippincott, 1984.
119. Ryoppy, S., and Karaharju, E. O.: Alteration of epiphyseal growth by an experimentally produced angular deformity. Acta Orthop. Scand., *45*:490, 1974.
120. Salter, R. B.: Textbook of Disorders and Injuries of the Musculoskeletal System. Baltimore, Williams & Wilkins, 1970.
121. Salter, R. B., and Harris, W. R.: Injuries involving the epiphyseal plate. J. Bone Joint Surg., *45-A*:587, 1963.
122. Scudder, C. L.: The Treatment of Fractures. 7th Ed. Philadelphia, Saunders, 1938.
123. Serafin, J.: Effect of longitudinal transection of the epiphysis and metaphysis on cartilaginous growth. Am. Dig. Orthop. Lit., *1*:17, 1970.
124. Sharrard, W. J. W.: Paediatric Orthopaedics and Fractures. Oxford, Blackwell, 1979.
125. Siegling, J. A.: Growth of the epiphysis. J. Bone Joint Surg., *23*:39, 1941.
126. Siffert, R. S.: The effect of staples and longitudinal wires on epiphyseal growth. J. Bone Joint Surg., *38-A*:1077, 1956.
127. Siffert, R. S., and Barash, E. S.: The potential for growth of experimentally produced hemi-epiphyses. J. Bone Joint Surg., *48-A*:1548, 1966.
128. Siffert, R. S., and Katz, J. F.: Experimental intra-epiphyseal osteotomy. Clin. Orthop., *82*:234, 1972.
129. Smith, M. K.: The prognosis in epiphyseal line fractures. Ann. Surg., *79*:273, 1924.
130. Snyder, C. H.: Deformities resulting from unilateral surgical trauma to the epiphyses. Ann. Surg., *100*:335, 1934.
131. Solomon, L.: Diametric growth of the epiphyseal plate. J. Bone Joint Surg., *48-B*:170, 1966.
132. Speed, K.: A Textbook of Fractures and Dislocations. Covering Their Pathology, Diagnosis and Treatment. Philadelphia, Lea & Febiger, 1942.
133. Spira, E., and Farin, I.: The vascular supply to the epiphyseal plate under normal and pathologic conditions. Acta Orthop. Scand., *38*:1, 1967.
134. Steinert, V.: Epiphysenlosung und Epiphysenfrakturen. Arch. Orthop. Unfallchir., *58*:200, 1965.
135. Stimpson, L. A.: Fractures and Dislocations. Philadelphia, Lea & Febiger, 1910.
136. Stimpson, L. A.: A Manual of Fractures and Dislocations. 2nd Ed. Philadelphia, Lea & Febiger, 1947.
137. Treharne, R. W.: Review of Wolff's law and its proposed means of operation. Orthop. Review, *10*:35, 1981.
138. Trueta, J.: Studies of the Development and Decay of the Human Frame. Philadelphia, Saunders, 1968.
139. Trueta, J., and Amato, V. P.: The vascular contribution of osteogenesis. III. Changes in the growth of cartilage caused by experimentally induced ischaemia. J. Bone Joint Surg., *42-B*:571, 1960.
140. Trueta, J., and Morgan, J. O.: The vascular contribution to osteogenesis. I. Studies by the injection method. J. Bone Joint Surg., *42-B*:97, 1960.

141. Trueta, J., and Trias, A.: The vascular contribution to osteogenesis. IV. The effect of pressure upon the epiphyseal cartilage of the rabbit. J. Bone Joint Surg., *43-B*:800, 1961.
142. Tschantz, P., and Ruttishauser, E.: La surcharge mecanique de l'os vivant. Ann. Anat. Pathol., *12*:223, 1967.
143. Vogt, P.: Die traumatische Epiphysenntreimung und deren Einfluss auf des Langenwachsthum der Rohrenknochen. Arch. Klin. Chir., *22*:343, 1978.
144. Volkmann, R.: Chirurgische Erfahrungen über Knochenverbiegungen und Knochenwachstum. Arch. Pathol. Anat., *24*:512, 1862.
145. Watson-Jones, R., Sr.: Fractures and Joint Injuries. 4th Ed. Baltimore, Williams & Wilkins, 1962.
146. Weber, B. G.: Epiphysenfugen-Verletzungen. Helv. Chir. Acta, *31*:103, 1964.
147. Weber, B. G.: Operative Treatment of Fractures in Children. New York, Springer Verlag, 1979.
148. White, A. A., Punjabi, M. M., and Southwick, W. O.: The four biomechanical stages of fracture repair. J. Bone Joint Surg., *59-A*:188, 1977.
149. Whitesides, E. S.: Normal growth in a transplanted epiphysis. J. Bone Joint Surg., *59*:A:546, 1977.
150. Wiles, P.: Fractures, Dislocations and Sprains. 2nd. Ed. Baltimore, Williams & Wilkins, 1969.
151. Wilson, C., and Percy, E. C.: Experimental studies on epiphyseal stimulation. J. Bone Joint Surg., *38-A*:1096, 1956.
152. Wolff, J.: Das Gesetz der Transformation der Knochen. Berlin, Hirschwald, 1892.
153. Yabsley, R. H., and Harris, W. R.: The effect of shaft fractures and periosteal stripping on the vascular supply to epiphyseal plates. J. Bone Joint Surg., *47-A*:551, 1965.
154. Yoshida, H.: Experimental studies on the repair of injured epiphyseal cartilage plate. J. Jpn. Orthop. Assoc., *33*:993, 1959.

The Upper Limb

Injuries to the Region of the Shoulder

FRACTURES OF THE CLAVICLE

The term *clavicle* is derived from the Latin word "clavis" (key); the clavicle is also referred to as the *collar bone.* Extending from the acromion process of the scapula to the upper border of the manubrium sterni, it serves as the only connection between the arm and trunk, and is consequently subjected to all medially directed forces exerted upon the upper limb. The clavicle is the most frequently broken bone in children.

In the superior view, this long bone has a double curve in the horizontal plane, being convex forward in its medial two thirds and concave forward in its lateral third. Biomechanically the point of juncture of the two curves is the weakest point. The shape of the clavicle is prismatic in its medial two thirds with anterior, posterior, and inferior surfaces; in its lateral third, it is flattened with superior and inferior surfaces. The lateral third of the clavicle provides attachment to the trapezius muscle posterosuperiorly and the deltoid muscle anteriorly. In its medial two thirds, the clavicular portion of the sternocleidomastoid muscle is inserted above and the pectoralis major muscle is attached in front and below. The superior surface of the clavicle is subcutaneous throughout its whole length. On its inferior surface, the costal tuberosity provides attachment for the strong costoclavicular ligaments medially; the conoid and trapezoid ligaments are inserted laterally, and the subclavius muscle originates in a groove in its middle two thirds. The subclavian vessels and branches of the brachial plexus traverse beneath the clavicle. Directly underneath the midclavicle are the medial and lateral cords of the brachial plexus; the thin subclavius muscle and clavipectoral fascia are the only structures interposed between the clavicle and nerves. Fortunately, fractures of the clavicle occur at the distal part of the insertion of the subclavius; when they occur at the middle third of the clavicle the brachial plexus and subclavian vessels are protected by the subclavius muscle.

The clavicle is the first bone in the body to ossify, doing so in membrane without going through a prior enchondral stage; cartilaginous growth areas develop later at both its ends; however, in late adolescence, usually at about the age of 16 to 18 years, a single ossification center develops at the medial end of the clavicle, fusing with the shaft by 25 years of age.[55] Occasionally an ossification center may develop at the acromion process, in which case it unites with the shaft immediately.[20] These ossification centers should not be mistaken for fractures. In some radiographic views the double curve of the clavicle may mimic a fracture.

Mechanism of Injury

In the newborn, the breaking force may arise from compression of the shoulders during a difficult delivery at birth. The usual cause in a child is a fall, either from a high chair or out of bed onto the outstretched hand, elbow, or side of the shoulder. The fracture may occasionally

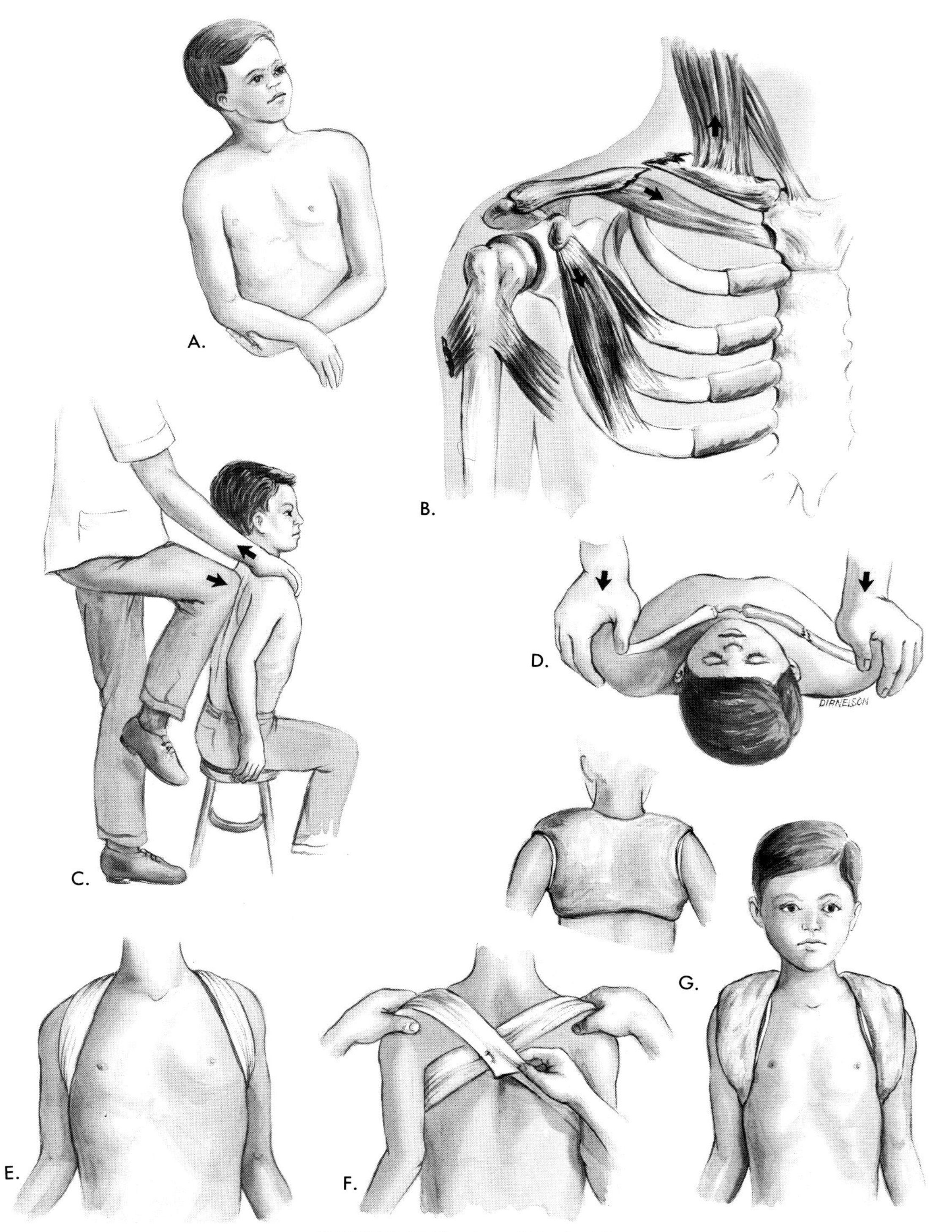

FIGURE 8–10. Fracture of the clavicle.

A and **B.** Deformity of fractured clavicle at the junction of its middle and outer thirds. Note the downward, forward, and inward drop of the affected shoulder because of the weight of the limb and the pull of the pectoral muscles. The medial fragment is pulled upward and backward by the pull of the sternocleidomastoid muscle. **C** and **D.** Method of reduction (see text for explanation). **E** and **F.** Figure-of-eight bandage used for immobilization. It is made of stockinette and orthopedic white felt. **G.** Figure-of-eight bandage made of plaster of Paris cast is used in children over six years of age.

be produced by direct violence applied from in front and above, the clavicle being forced against the upper ribs. An open fracture may occur following a direct blow, but this is extremely rare because of the mobility of the overlying skin and also because the fracture commonly results from indirect force.

Pathologic Anatomy

The most frequent site of the fracture is the junction of the middle and lateral thirds of the bone. In the infant or young child, the break is often incomplete, being of the greenstick type. In older children and in adolescents, the fracture is frequently complete; the fragments may be undisplaced, but are bowed anteriorly, shortening the bone and increasing its normal anterior convexity. When there is overriding of the fragments, the affected shoulder drops downward and inward, taking along the lateral fragment. This displacement is caused partially by the weight of the limb and partially by the pull of the pectoralis and trapezius muscles. The medial end of the lateral fragment is tilted posteriorly. The medial fragment is pulled upward and backward by the sternocleidomastoid muscle with the costoclavicular ligaments serving as a checkrein on the displacement (Fig. 8–10 A and B). The skin is then stretched over the lateral end of the medial fragment by the lowered shoulder.

If the breaking force is great, and particularly if it is direct, the fracture is comminuted. Occasionally, small, sharp fragments of bone may penetrate the skin or lacerate the subclavian vessels.

Fractures of the lateral third of the clavicle are infrequent and usually result from direct violence. The fracture is commonly transverse and may be comminuted. If the coracoclavicular ligaments are intact, displacement is minimal or negligible, the outer fragment being fixed to the acromion by the acromioclavicular ligaments and the inner fragment being bound to the coracoid process by the conoid and trapezoid ligaments. If the coracoclavicular ligaments are torn, the small lateral fragment is displaced with the acromion and the fracture acts like an acromioclavicular dislocation. The distal fragment, acromion, and shoulder are displaced downward and inward.

The medial third of the clavicle fractures very rarely and then as a result of direct violence. The fragments are usually held together by the intact costoclavicular ligaments.

Diagnostic Features

*BIRTH FRACTURES**

The clinical diagnosis of fractured clavicle in the newborn is made very occasionally, since the majority of these fractures are asymptomatic. Farkas and Levine reported a radiographic survey of 300 consecutive living newborns; five were delivered with fractured clavicles (1.7 per cent). In none of the cases had the fracture been suspected following the routine pediatric examination in the delivery room and the nursery. On re-examination, however, Farkas and Levine were able to demonstrate crepitations at the fracture site. The break is usually complete, with overriding of the fragments. Involvement is usually unilateral, with no report of bilateral fractures. The injury occurs during delivery of the shoulders, with fracture of the anteriorly positioned clavicle predominating over that of the posterior clavicle.[19] Occasionally, fracture of the clavicle in the newborn may be misdiagnosed as congenital muscular torticollis.[34]

In clinically symptomatic cases, attention is drawn to the injury by the "pseudoparalysis"—i.e., lack of spontaneous movement of the upper limb ôn the affected side. This should be distinguished from obstetrical brachial plexus paralysis and from acute osteomyelitis of the humerus. Brachial plexus paralysis and fractured clavicle may coexist. On careful inspection and palpation, crepitation, local swelling, and tenderness will be found, suggesting the presence of a fractured clavicle. The diagnosis is confirmed by radiograms.

INFANCY AND CHILDHOOD

In infants and young children, a fractured clavicle of the greenstick type may escape notice until the appearance of the developing callus (Fig. 8–11). In such an instance, the condition should not be mistaken for congenital pseudarthrosis of the clavicle, which, likewise, is painless. The radiographic findings of congenital pseudarthrosis of the clavicle are characteristic: There is a definite wide zone of radiolucency with smooth margins at the site of the defect and no evidence of callus formation across the fracture site. When the fracture is complete, with displacement, the clinical appearance is typical (see Fig. 8–10 A). The shoulder on the affected side is lower than the opposite normal

---

*See references 5, 9, 11, 14, 15, 19, 27, 37, 42, 48, 64, 66, 71, 73, 80, and 84.

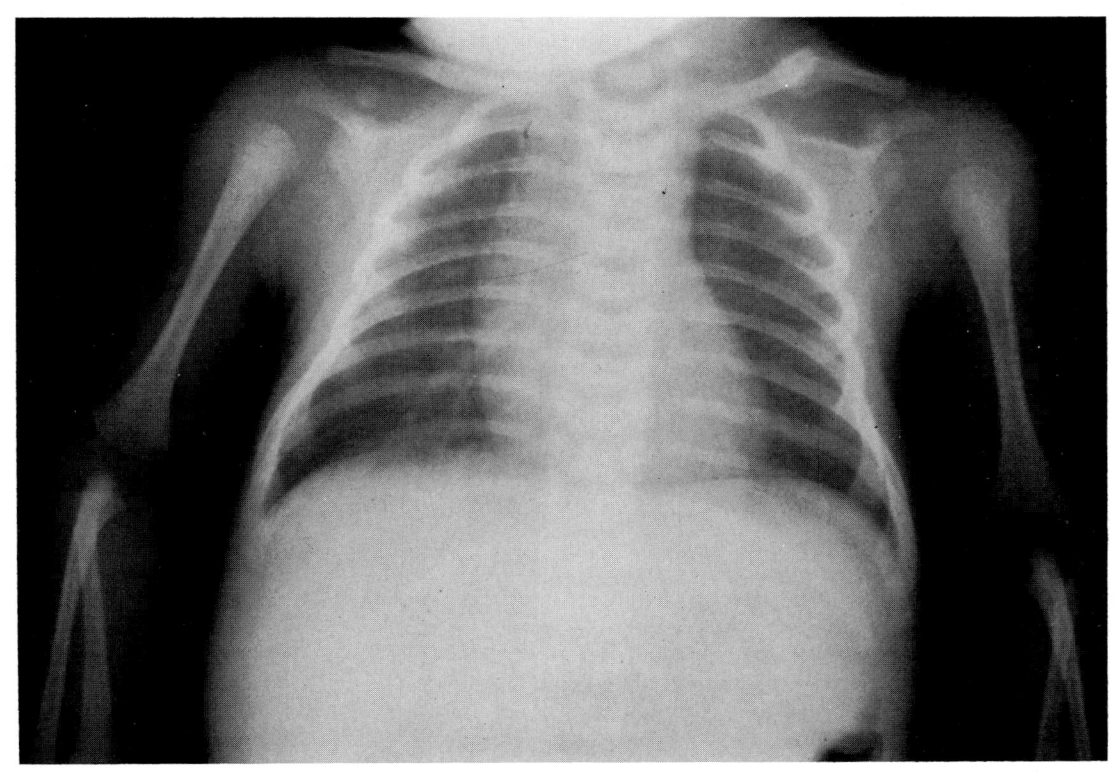

FIGURE 8–11. Fracture of left clavicle in a newborn.

This injury usually escapes notice until the development of callus.

one, and it is drooped forward and inward. The patient rests the involved arm against his body and supports it at the elbow with the opposite hand. The tension on the sternocleidomastoid muscle tilts the head toward the affected side and rotates the chin toward the opposite side. Any change in position of the upper limb or of the cervical spine is painful. On palpation, there is local swelling, tenderness, and crepitation over the fracture site.

Fractures in the middle third of the clavicle will be clearly depicted in the anteroposterior radiogram (Fig. 8–12). To demonstrate fractures of the medial and lateral end of the clavicle, however, special oblique, lateral, or lordotic (40-degree cephalic tilt) views may be required.

Treatment

BIRTH FRACTURES

An asymptomatic fracture in the neonate or young infant may be ignored. It will unite without external immobilization and any malalignment will correct itself with growth. The nurses and parents are instructed to handle the infant gently, avoiding direct pressure over the broken clavicle. While the patient sleeps in prone position, soft padding may be placed under the affected shoulder to prevent it from drooping too far forward (this is done only when the fracture is grossly unstable and only for a few days).

When the fracture is painful and accompanied by "pseudoparalysis," it is best to protect it by splinting the arm for two weeks. A soft cotton pad is placed in the axilla, and with the elbow in acute flexion, the upper limb is loosely anchored across the front of the chest with two or three turns of elastic bandage. It is not necessary to encircle the elbow and clavicle with the bandage; and it is not advisable to apply a sling to hang from the opposite shoulder. The parents are instructed to reapply the bandage after each bath and skin care. Within 10 to 14 days, the pain will completely subside, the fracture will be united clinically, and the splint is removed.

Muscle function in the upper limb is assessed by the reflex stimulation method to rule out associated obstetrical brachial plexus paralysis. Occasionally a birth fracture of the clavicle is accompanied by fracture of the upper humeral epiphysis involving the physis. In the initial

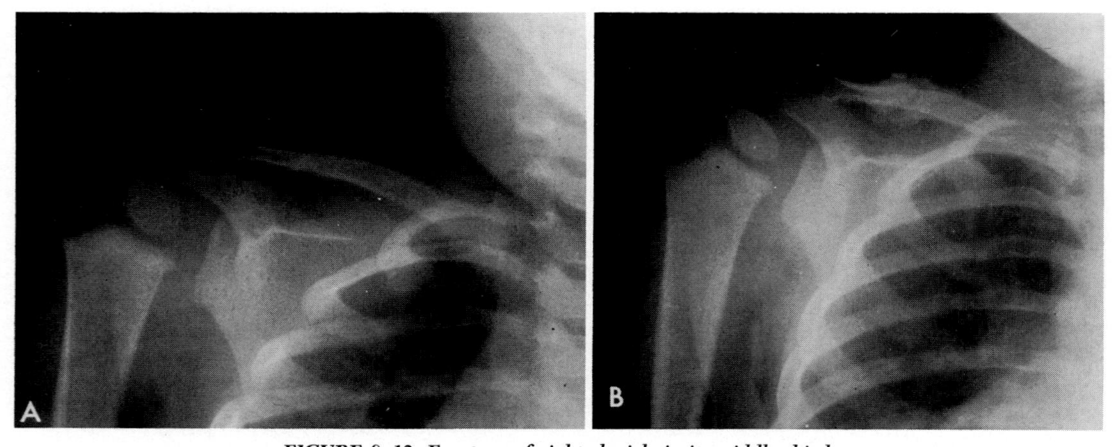

FIGURE 8–12. Fracture of right clavicle in its middle third.

A. Initial radiogram. **B.** Two weeks later, showing massive callus.

radiograms, often this is not diagnosed; however, in the follow-up films, massive subperiosteal new bone formation will be seen and the condition may be mistaken for osteomyelitis. In the newborn with acute infection, there may be no systemic reaction. Osteomyelitis should be suspected if there is an area of rarefaction (bone destruction) in the metaphysis, if the pain is persistent, or if the swelling of the arm is marked and diffuse.

YOUNG CHILDREN

In children under six years of age, displaced fractures of the clavicle do not require reduction. Gross malalignment and the "bump" of the massive callus will remodel and disappear within six to nine months. The child is made comfortable by applying a figure-of-eight bandage (see Fig. 8–10 E and F). A 2- or 3-inch-wide stockinette is stuffed with orthopedic white felt. The patient is seated on a stool with the surgeon standing behind him; an assistant holds the upper limbs in the position of surrender. The bandage is applied in the following manner: Beginning posteriorly, the stockinette is passed in front of the normal clavicle, through the axilla, across the back, over the top of the fractured clavicle, through the axilla, and across the back, and then is anchored by two or three large safety pins to the other end of the stockinette. Tension is applied on the stockinette as it passes through the axilla of the involved side with the shoulder held upward and backward. It is imperative not to embarrass circulation. A circle of adhesive strapping on the back of the figure-of-eight bandage will maintain its tightness. Large pads of soft cotton may be placed over the superior and anterior aspects of the clavicle, reaching into the axilla; these are particularly indicated if the fracture fragments are overriding and unstable; the length and alignment of the clavicle are maintained by the weight of the arm over the axillary pads, which serve as fulcrums. Soft, well-padded, pre-made, figure-of-eight clavicular supports are available commercially. The clavicular splints do not immobilize the fracture; their purpose is to provide comfort to the patient by holding the shoulders backward. If there is associated torticollis, the affected limb is supported with a sling suspended from the opposite shoulder.

The fracture is immobilized for three to four weeks. During this period tautness of the figure-of-eight bandage should be maintained. The parents are shown how to tighten the bandage by applying tension on the stockinette over the broken clavicle and securing it with an additional safety pin. They should be cautioned against excessive pressure on the axillary vessels and consequent circulatory embarrassment; they should also check the skin for irritation and pressure sores. The surgeon should examine the patient seven to ten days following injury, assess neurovascular function, and if necessary, make radiographs of the clavicle. Efficacy of reapplication of the figure-of-eight bandage by the parents is double-checked. Exuberant callus forms within two to three weeks.

OLDER CHILDREN AND ADOLESCENTS

In children over six years of age and in adolescents, angulated greenstick fractures seldom, if ever, warrant reduction (Figs. 8–13 and

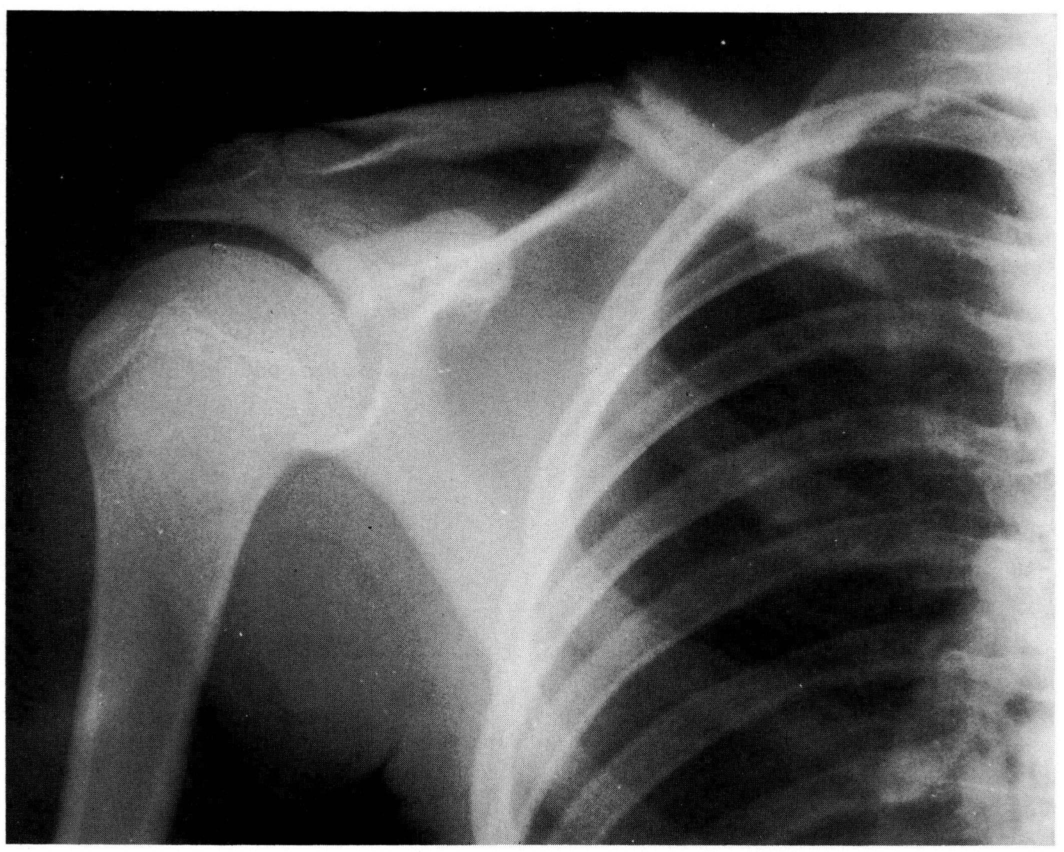

FIGURE 8–13. Angulated greenstick fracture of right clavicle.

8–14). If the fracture is complete and markedly displaced with overriding or angulation, closed reduction may be required. Local anesthesia is utilized in the cooperative patient; under strict aseptic precautions, several milliliters of 1 per cent procaine is injected into the hematoma. General anesthesia usually is not required. Reduction is performed with the patient sitting on a stool. The operator places his knee between the scapulae and pulls the shoulders backward and upward. If the child is apprehensive, the fracture might be more comfortably reduced in the supine, recumbent position. The child's lower limbs and pelvis are anchored on the table with sheets; a padded sandbag is placed posteriorly between the shoulders, and the affected arm is allowed to hang in extended position at the side of the table. The weight of the arm alone will reduce the fracture, and this is less painful for the patient. If necessary, the operator can gently but firmly push the shoulders back to restore length and alignment to the fractured fragments. Radiograms are made to check reduction.

For the older child, immobilization is best provided by application of one of the commercially available, well-padded, figure-of-eight harnesses. This type of harness does not stretch as the stockinette does; therefore, frequent tautening of the harness is not required.

Occasionally in the uncooperative child or unreducible situation, one may have to immobilize the fracture by applying a plaster of Paris cast in a manner similar to the figure-of-eight bandage just described. With the child sitting on the table, felt padding and sheath wadding are applied in figure-of-eight fashion. Both the felt and sheath wadding should extend beyond the margins of the plaster cast. Then while an assistant pushes the shoulders upward and backward by pressure on the flexed elbows and the surgeon applies posterior counterpressure with his knee on the upper dorsal spine, a 4-inch-wide plaster of Paris cast is applied. As soon as the plaster turns are completed, the patient is replaced in supine position, and using the sandbag as counterpressure, the operator pushes the shoulders posteriorly with the palms of his hands (see Fig. 8–10 G).

If the arm becomes swollen because of pres-

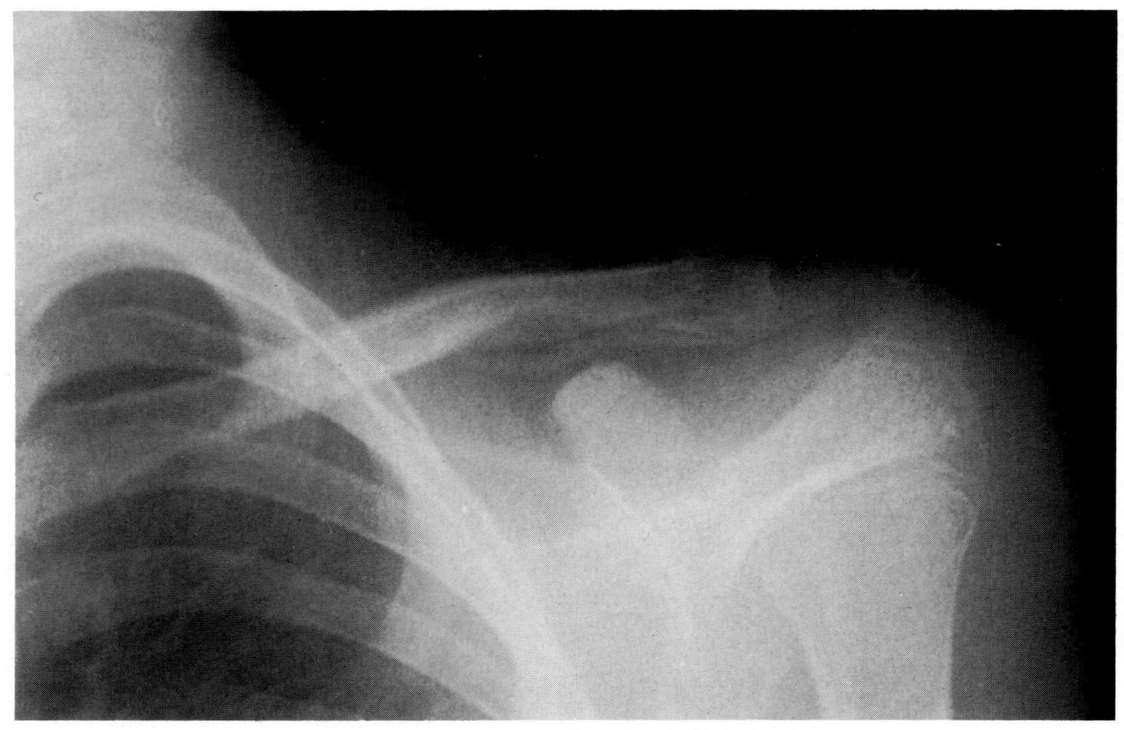

FIGURE 8–14. Fracture of lateral end of left clavicle.

sure of a tight splint against the axillary vessels, the cast is trimmed to relieve pressure from the cast. Four to six weeks of immobilization in the cast are required in the adolescent for osseous union to take place.

RECUMBENT TREATMENT

Fractures of the clavicle in the child with multiple injuries who is forced to rest in bed because of other major trauma (such as fractured femur, ruptured spleen, or subdural hematoma) are best managed by maintaining recumbent supine posture on a firm mattress. A small but firm pillow is placed between the scapulae, and the weight of the upper limb will gradually reduce the fracture. For comfort, a stockinette and felt figure-of-eight bandage can be applied if necessary. In an adolescent girl, the cosmetic end-result of a displaced and overriding fracture may be improved by lateral arm skin traction, similar to modified Dunlop, with the shoulder in 90 degrees of abduction and 90 degrees of lateral rotation. Care is taken not to stretch the brachial plexus in a semicomatose or agitated patient. Bony union ordinarily occurs within three to four weeks.

Open reduction of a fractured clavicle is rarely, if ever, indicated in children. In the adolescent, accept angulation and deformity of malunion. Do not perform open reduction. The operative scar is often more displeasing than the bony prominence of the malunited fracture. The only justification for open surgery is the repair of subclavian vessels that have been lacerated by the sharp bone fragments of a comminuted fracture. Open reduction of a fractured clavicle may result in nonunion.

Complications

Neurovascular complications are extremely rare; they are usually the result of direct force and comminuted fracture. Laceration of a subclavian artery or vein can occur; the thick periosteum of a child protects the vessels from the sharp bone fragments.[31, 58] The presence of subclavian vessel laceration is suggested by the development of a large, rapidly increasing hematoma. Surgical intervention for repair of the torn vessel should be immediate, as the patient may die of extravasation or shock.[17, 76]

Subclavian vein compression following greenstick fracture of the clavicle with inferior bowing has been reported in a child.[43] Venous congestion and swelling of the involved arm suggest the possibility of such a complication.

Nonunion of fracture of the clavicle is extremely rare; it usually results from surgical intervention.[24, 49, 53, 61, 74, 78, 81] Open reduction and internal fixation of clavicle fracture should be performed only when there are associated neurovascular complications.

References

1. Ali Kahn, M. A., and Lucas, H. K.: Plating of fractures of the middle third of the clavicle. Injury, 9:263, 1978.
2. Alkalaj, I.: Internal fixation of a severe clavicular fracture in a child. Isr. J. Med. Sci., 9:306, 1960.
3. Bagnoli, F., Bruchi, S., Sardelli, S., Vispi, L., Buonocore, G., Franchi, F., and Bracci, R.: Calcitonin and parathyroid hormone in newborn infants with fracture of the clavicle. Calcif. Tissue Int., *36*:357, 1984.
4. Bearn, J. G.: Direct observation of the function of the capsule of the sternoclavicular joint in clavicular support. J. Anat., *101*:159, 1967.
5. Bianchi, G., and Bertoni, G. P.: Bilateral fracture of the clavicle in the newborn. Minerva Pediatr., *19*:2226, 1967.
6. Billington, R. W.: A new plaster yoke for fracture of the clavicle. South. Med. J., *24*:667, 1931.
7. Bonnet, J.: Fracture of the clavicle. Arch. Chir. Neerlandicum, *27*:143, 1975.
8. Brooks, A., and Henning, G.: Injury to the proximal clavicular epiphysis. J. Bone Joint Surg., *54-A*:1347, 1972.
9. Calandi, C., and Bartolozzi, G.: On 110 cases of fracture of the clavicle in the newborn. Riv. Clin. Pediatr., *64*:541, 1959.
10. Cappelo, N., and Longhi, G.: Fractures of the clavicle in children and adults. Minerva Med., *54*:408, 1963.
11. Cohen, A. W., and Otto, S. R.: Obstetric clavicular fractures. J. Reprod. Med., *25*:119, 1980.
12. Conwell, H. E.: Fractures of the clavicle. Simple fixation dressing with summary of the treatment and results attained in 92 cases. J.A.M.A., *90*:838, 1928.
13. Cooper, S. B.: Fractures of the clavicle in infants and young children. Orth. Nurses Assoc. J., *4*:187, 1977.
14. Curiel, P., and Serra, E.: Obstetrical clavicular fractures. Riv. Obstet. Ginecol., *22*:181, 1967.
15. DeBlasio, A., and Iafusco, F.: Fracture of the clavicle in newborn infants. Pediatria (Napoli), *68*:815, 1960.
16. D'Eramo, B.: Open therapy of fractures of the clavicle. Acta Chir. Ital., *24*:489, 1968.
17. Dickson, J. W.: Death following fractured clavicle. Lancet, *2*:666, 1952.
18. Eliason, E. L.: Fractures of the clavicle. J.A.M.A., *91*:1974, 1928.
19. Farkas, R., and Levine, S.: X-ray incidence of fractured clavicle in vertex presentation. Am. J. Obstet. Gynecol., *59*:204, 1950.
20. Fawcett, J.: The development and ossification in the human clavicle. J. Anat. Physiol., *47*:225, 1913.
21. Fedotov, V. K.: Comparative characteristics of some methods of conservative therapy in clavicular fractures in children. Vestn. Khir., *107*:109, 1972.
22. Fedotov, V. K.: Method of closed juxtaposition of fragments of the clavicle in children. Orthop. Travmatol. Protez., *35*:68, 1974.
23. Fitisenko, I.: On the treatment of clavicular fracture in children. Khirurgiia (Mosk.), *39*:36, 1963.
24. Ghormley, R. K., Black, J. R., and Cherry, J. H.: Ununited fractures of the clavicle. Am. J. Surg., *51*:343, 1941.
25. Gibbon, J. H.: Lucas-Championniere and mobilization in the treatment of fractures. Surg. Gynecol. Obstet., *43*:271, 1926.
26. Gilchrist, D. A.: A stockinette-Velpeau for immobilization of the shoulder girdle. J. Bone Joint Surg., *45-A*:1382, 1963.
27. Golfieri, C., Babini, L., and Petocchi, T.: Intranatal fracture of the clavicle. Clin. Pediatr. (Bologna), *48*:335, 1966.
28. Greenwood, H. H.: Treatment of fractures of the clavicle. Br. Med. J., *1*:1021, 1928.
29. Heppenstall, R. B.: Fractures and dislocations of the distal clavicle. Orthop. Clin. North Am., *6*:477, 1975.
30. Houston, H. E.: An unusual complication of clavicular fracture. J. Ky. Med. Assoc., *75*:170, 1977.
31. Howard, F., and Shafer, S.: Injuries to the clavicle with arteriovenous complications. J. Bone Joint Surg., *47-A*:1335, 1965.
32. Jablon, M., Sutker, A., and Post, M.: Irreducible fracture of the middle third of the clavicle. Report of a case. J. Bone Joint Surg., *61-A*:296, 1979.
33. Jit, I., and Kulkarni, M.: Times of appearance and fusion of epiphysis at the medial end of the clavicle. Indian J. Med. Res., *64*:773, 1976.
34. Kato, T., Kanbara, H., Sato, S., and Tanaka, I.: Five cases of clavicular fracture misdiagnosed as congenital muscular torticollis. Orthop. Surg. (Tokyo), *19*:729, 1968.
35. Key, J. A., and Conwell, H. E.: Fractures of the clavicle. *In* Key, J. A., and Conwell, H. E. (eds.): The Management of Fractures, Dislocations and Sprains. St. Louis, C. V. Mosby, 1946, pp. 495–512.
36. Konovalov, A. M., and Fedotov, V. K.: Plastic splint in the treatment of clavicle fractures in children. Vestn. Khir., *103*:129, 1969.
37. Lehmacher, K., and Lehmann, C.: Clavicular fracture in newborn infants after spontaneous delivery in the occipital position. Z. Geburtschilfe Gynaek., *158*:134, 1962.
38. Lemire, L., and Rosman, M.: Sternoclavicular epiphyseal separation with adjacent clavicular fracture. J. Pediatr. Orthop.,. *4*:118, 1984.
39. Lester, C. W.: Treatment of fractures of the clavicle. Ann. Surg., *89*:600, 1929.
40. McCally, W. C., and Kelly, D. A.: Treatment of fractures of the clavicle, ribs, and scapulae. Am. J. Surg., *50*:558, 1940.
41. Manske, D. J., and Szabo, R. M.: The operative treatment of mid-shaft clavicular non-unions. J. Bone Joint Surg., *67-A*:1367, 1985.
42. Marinoni, R., and Blini, V.: Contribution to the knowledge and treatment of fractures of the clavicle in the newborn. Osped. Maggiore, *49*:506, 1961.
43. Mital, M., and Aufrane, O.: Venous occlusion following greenstick fracture of the clavicle. J.A.M.A., *206*:1301, 1968.
44. Molski, K., and Wasilewski, Z.: Komza's plaster cast in treatment of mid-clavicle fractures in children. Chir. Narzadow Ruchu Ortop. Pol., *37*:651, 1972.
45. Montgomery, S. P., and Lloyd, R. D.: Avulsion fracture of the coracoid epiphysis with acromioclavicular separation. J. Bone Joint Surg., *59-A*:963, 1977.
46. Mosely, H. F.: The clavicle: Its anatomy and function. Clin. Orthop., *58*:17, 1968.
47. Mourigan, H.: Fractures de la clavicula en el recien nacido. Arch. Pediatr. Uruguay, *25*:539, 1954.
48. Nasso, S., and Verga, A.: La frattura della clavicola nel neonato. Minerva Pediatr., *6*:593, 1954.
49. Neer, C. S., II: Nonunion of the clavicle. J.A.M.A., *172*:1006, 1960.
50. Neer, C. S., II: Fractures of the distal third of the clavicle. Clin. Orthop., *58*:43, 1968.
51. Neviaser, J.: Injuries of the clavicle and its articulations. Orthop. Clin. North Am., *11*:233, 1980.
52. Neviaser, R. J., Neviaser, J. S., and Neviaser, T. J. S.: A simple technique for internal fixation of the clavicle. A long term evaluation. Clin. Orthop., *109*:103, 1975.
53. Nogi, J., Heckman, J. D., Hakala, M., and Sweet, D. E.: Non-union of the clavicle in a child. Clin. Orthop., *110*:19, 1975.

54. Ogden, J. A.: Distal clavicular physeal injury. Clin. Orthop., *188*:68, 1984.
55. Ogden, J. A., Conlogue, G. J., and Bronson, M. L.: Radiology of postnatal skeletal development. III. The clavicle. Skeletal Radiol., *4*:196, 1979.
56. Paffen, P. J., and Jansen, E. W. L.: Surgical treatment of clavicular fracture with Kirschner wires: A comparative study. Arch. Chir. Neerlandicum, *30*:43, 1978.
57. Parkes, J. C., and Deland, J. T.: A three-part distal clavicle fracture. J. Trauma, *23*:437, 1983.
58. Penn, I.: The vascular complication of fractures of the clavicle. J. Trauma, *4*:819, 1964.
59. Phillips, S. B., and Ogden, J. A.: Radiology of postnatal skeletal development. VII. The scapula. Skeletal Radiol., *9*:157, 1983.
60. Picchio, A. A.: Fractures of the clavicle in infants. Minerva Ortop., *3*:124, 1952.
61. Pyper, J. B.: Non-union of fractures of the clavicle. Injury, *9*:268, 1978.
62. Rang, M.: Clavicle. *In* Rang, M.: Children's Fractures. 2nd. Ed. Philadelphia, Lippincott, 1983.
63. Rockwood, C. A.: Fractures of the outer clavicle in children and adults. J. Bone Joint Surg., *64-B*:642, 1982.
64. Rolandi, L.: Fractures of the clavicle in the newborn. Osped. Maggiore, *48*:651, 1960.
65. Rowe, C. R.: An atlas of anatomy and treatment of mid-clavicular fractures. Clin. Orthop., *58*:29, 1968.
66. Sanford, H. N.: The Moro reflex as a diagnostic aid in fracture of the clavicle in the newborn infant. J. Dis. Child., *41*:1304, 1931.
67. Sayre, L.: A simple dressing for fracture of the clavicle. Am. Pract., *4*:1, 1871.
68. Simurda, M. A.: Retrosternal dislocation of the clavicle: A report of 4 cases and a method of repair. Can. J. Surg., *11*:487, 1968.
69. Snyder, L. A.: Loss of the accompanying soft tissue shadow of the clavicle with occult fracture (letter). South. Med. J., *72*:243, 1979.
70. Sorrells, R. B.: Fractures of the clavicle. J. Arkansas Med. Soc., *71*:253, 1975.
71. Spina, G. M.: Clinical aspects and therapy of obstetric fractures of the clavicle. Minerva Ortop., *12*:160, 1961.
72. Stubbins, S. G., and McGaw, W. H.: Suspension case for acromioclavicular separation and clavicular fractures. J.A.M.A., *169*:672, 1959.
73. Swolinzky, K., and Borell, H.: Clavicular fracture in newborn infants. Geburtshilfe Frauenheilkd., *21*:749, 1961.
74. Taylor, A. R.: Non-union of fractures of the clavicle. A review of thirty-one cases. *In* Proceedings of the British Orthopaedic Association. J. Bone Joint Surg., *51-B*:568, 1969.
75. Tessore, A., and Ussi, G.: Rare traumatic findings: Fracture of the inner third of the clavicle in a child. Beitr. Orthop. Traumatol., *17*:172, 1970.
76. The Death of Sir Robert Peal. Lancet, 2:19, 1850.
77. Todd, T. W., and DiErrico, J., Jr.: The clavicular epiphyses. Am. J. Anat., *41*:25, 1928.
78. Tregonning, G., and MacNab, I.: Post-traumatic pseudarthrosis of the clavicle. *In* Proceedings of the New Zealand Orthopaedic Association. J. Bone Joint Surg., *58-B*:264, 1976.
79. Trinchi, E., Vangelista, D., and Campacci, R.: On fractures of the clavicle. Fracastoro, *61*:149, 1968.
80. Wechselberg, K.: Studies on diagnosis and prognosis of clavicle fractures at birth. Med. Monatsschr., *26*:498, 1972.
81. Wilkens, R. M., and Johnston, R. M.: Un-united fractures of the clavicle. J. Bone Joint Surg., *65-A*:773, 1983.
82. Wong, P. C.: Fractures of the clavicle in children of Singapore. J. Singapore Paediatr. Soc., *8*:55, 1966.
83. Yates, D. W.: Complications of fractures of the clavicle. Injury, 7:189, 1976.
84. Zardini, V.: On the semeiology of clavicle fracture in the newborn. Minerva Ortop., *13*:491, 1962.
85. Zenni, E. J., Kreig, J. K., and Rosen, M. J.: Open reduction and internal fixation of clavicular fractures. J. Bone Joint Surg., *63-A*:147, 1981.

PHYSEAL SEPARATION OF THE MEDIAL (STERNAL) END OF THE CLAVICLE

The epiphysis at the medial end of the clavicle does not begin to ossify until the eighteenth year; it fuses with the shaft between the twenty-second and twenty-fifth years. The acromial end of the clavicle has no epiphysis.

Traumatic separation of the physis of the sternal end of the clavicle is a rare injury; Poland could collect only six cases; three of them were separations of an ossified epiphysis (ages 20, 18, and 17 years) and three were separations of cartilaginous epiphysis (ages 14, 11, and 3 years).[29] Karlen, in 1943, reported a case in a boy 12 years of age; Denham and Dingley reported four patients, all under 18 years of age (three 14 and one 16 years old).[9, 18] Wheeler and associates reported traumatic fracture separation of the medial physis of the clavicle in an infant; the displacement was anterosuperior.[35]

If the injury occurs before ossification has taken place in the medial epiphysis, the condition is often mistaken for dislocation of the sternoclavicular joint. Physeal separation of the medial end of the clavicle mimics sternoclavicular dislocation.[1–36] Injury after the age of 25 years causes dislocation, whereas prior to the age of 20 years trauma to the sternoclavicular joint results in physeal separation; the mean age of the patient at injury is 18.6 years.[6]

The medial end of the clavicle is attached to the sternum and first rib by a heavy sheath of fibrous tissue. The injury is commonly caused by indirect violence, such as a fall or blow upon the anterolateral aspect of the shoulder causing the clavicle to be driven medially and posteriorly. The displacement is anterior and superior where the indirect force is exerted on the posterolateral aspect of the shoulder. It may occasionally be produced by direct mechanism in which a direct anteroposterior force is applied on the anteromedial end of the clavicle; this describes the second case of Denham and Dingley, in which a wagon loaded with wood ran over the patient's chest. The physeal cartilage remains attached to the intact intra-articular disc and sternoclavicular ligaments. The costoclavicular ligaments are partially torn. It is the metaphysis of the clavicle that displaces. In complete displacement the clavicular metaphysis may pull out of its periosteal tube, which is left in place with its attaching sternoclavicular and costoclavicular ligaments—this makes reduction unstable.

On clinical examination, in anterior displacement prominence of the sternal end of the clavicle may be sharp and palpable immediately beneath the skin. The clavicular part of the sternocleidomastoid muscle is pulled anteriorly with the bone and is in spasm, causing the patient's head to tilt toward the affected side.

In posteromedial displacement there is local swelling, tenderness, and depression at the medial end of the clavicle; in severe displacements compression of the trachea may cause dyspnea and hoarseness; pressure on the brachial plexus and subclavian vessels will lead to vascular insufficiency with diminution or absence of radial pulse as well as paresthesia and paresis.[6, 14]

Imaging Findings. A routine anteroposterior radiogram of the clavicle will appear normal. It is important to make Rockwood's 45 degree superiorly projected lordotic view and compare the position of the medial end of the injured and uninjured clavicles. The displacement of the bony metaphysis of the sternal end of the clavicle may be anterosuperior or posteromedial. Remember that the epiphysis of the medial end of the clavicle begins to ossify at 18 years of age; the unossified epiphysis of the child will not be depicted in the radiogram.

This author recommends computed tomography of the sternoclavicular articulation; it will clearly visualize this physeal fracture separation (Fig. 8–15).[10, 16]

Treatment. Anterior displacements are treated by immobilization in a sling for three weeks. Ordinarily, closed reduction is not necessary. The local bony prominence will disappear in three to six months by remodeling from the periosteal tube and medial epiphysis of the clavicle. Results are excellent, with no residual deformity or disability.

Posterior displacements are also treated conservatively. An attempt at closed reduction is made when displacement is moderate or severe, preferably with the patient appropriately sedated or under general anesthesia. *Medial displacement must be reduced before the posterior displacement can be reduced.* When there is

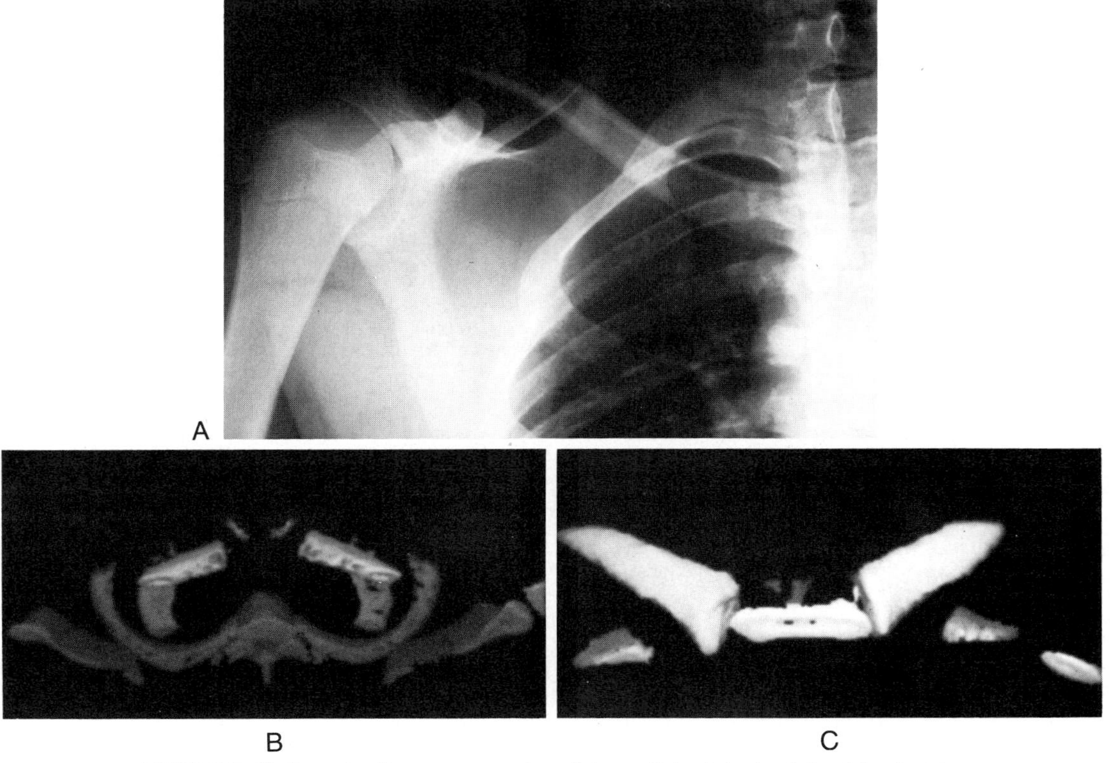

FIGURE 8–15. Posterior fracture separation of the medial epiphysis of the right clavicle.

A. Anteroposterior radiogram. **B.** CAT scan showing posterior displacement. **C.** Three-dimensional reconstruction showing that the fracture is reduced.

evidence of compression of the trachea and neurovascular structures, reduction should be performed immediately as an emergency procedure. The technique of manipulative reduction is as follows: *First,* with the patient in supine position, place a thick bolster (5 to 7 cm. thick) between the shoulder (raising the shoulders from the bed enables full retraction of the shoulders); *second,* push the clavicle laterally by applying direct pressure on the anterior aspect of the shoulder and forcing it into complete retraction. During this maneuver the arm should be adducted to the side of the trunk. The axis of motion of the clavicle is at its sternal end. When the patient is supine with his arm at the side of his chest, the clavicle is elevated 20 degrees from the horizontal. Abducting the arm at right angles elevates the axis of the clavicle 50 degrees above the horizontal. Therefore, when traction is applied with the shoulder in 90 degrees of abduction, the lateral pull exerted on the clavicle is an oblique angle and relatively inefficient. Also, the pectoralis major is stretched when the arm is in abduction, which tends to draw the clavicle medially. When the arm is adducted to the side of the trunk, the clavicle is at an angle of about 20 degrees to the horizontal and the pectoralis major is relaxed; therefore, a more effective lateral pull is exerted on the clavicle by retraction of the shoulder. *Third,* grasp the clavicle percutaneously and elevate it anteriorly into position. In an occasional instance in which the medial end of the clavicle is inferior, the clavicle is elevated superiorly and anteriorly.[6] Following reduction, the shoulder is immobilized in a figure-of-eight clavicular splint for four to six weeks. Lordotic radiograms and computed axial tomographic studies are made to determine the reduction.

Open reduction is rarely indicated. It is performed when there is compression of the trachea or neurovascular structures and closed manipulative reduction under general anesthesia fails to reduce the medial end of the clavicle. In such an instance, open reduction is performed through a skin incision 1 cm. above the clavicle; when the skin incision is placed on the clavicle, the scar is ugly. Following anatomic reduction, the medial part of the shaft of the clavicle is sutured through a hole in the metaphysis to its epiphysis with 0 Tycron suture. The torn periosteum is repaired. It is best to drill a Kirschner wire obliquely through the anterior cortex of the clavicle, across the growth plate, and into the epiphysis to stabilize the fragments. The lateral end of the wire is bent bent to prevent its migration. A Velpeau dressing is applied. The wire is removed in six weeks.

References

1. Asher, M. A.: Dislocations of the upper extremity in children. Orthop. Clin. North Am., *7*:583, 1976.
2. Barth, E., and Hagen, R.: Surgical treatment of dislocations of the sternoclavicular joint. Acta Orthop. Scand., *54*:746, 1983.
3. Beckman, T.: A case of simultaneous luxation of both ends of the clavicle. Acta Chir. Scand., *56*:156, 1923.
4. Borowieck, B., Charow, A., Cook, W., Rozychi, D., and Thaler, S.: An unusual football injury. Arch. Otolaryngol., *95*:185, 1972.
5. Brooks, A. L., and Henning, G. D.: Injury to the proximal clavicular epiphysis. J. Bone Joint Surg., *54-A*:1347, 1972.
6. Buckerfield, C. T., and Castle, M. E.: Acute traumatic retrosternal dislocation of the clavicle. J. Bone Joint Surg., *66-A*:379, 1984.
7. Clark, R. L., Milgram, J. W., and Yawn, D. H.: Fatal aortic perforation and cardiac tamponade due to a Kirschner wire migrating from the right sternoclavicular joint. South Med. J., *67*:316, 1974.
8. Collins, J. J.: Retrosternal dislocation of the clavicle. J. Bone Joint Surg., *54-A*:203, 1972.
9. Denham, R. H., Jr., and Dingley, A. F., Jr.: Epiphyseal separation of the medial end of the clavicle. J. Bone Joint Surg., *49-A*:1179, 1967.
10. Deutsch, A. L., Resnick, D., and Mink, J. H.: Computed tomography of the glenohumeral and sternoclavicular joints. Orthop. Clin. North Am., *16*:497, 1985.
11. Elting, J. J.: Retrosternal dislocation of the clavicle. Arch. Surg., *104*:35, 1972.
12. Fawcett, J.: The development and ossification in the human clavicle. J. Anat. Physiol., *47*:225, 1913.
13. Ferry, A. M., Rook, F. W., and Masterson, J. H.: Retrosternal dislocation of the clavicle. J. Bone Joint Surg., *39-A*:905, 1957.
14. Gangahar, D. M., and Flogaite, T.: Retrosternal dislocation of the clavicle producing thoracic outlet syndrome. J. Trauma, *18*:369, 1978.
15. Greenlee, D. P.: Posterior dislocation of the sternal end of the clavicle. J.A.M.A., *125*:426, 1944.
16. Hatfield, M. K., Gross, B. H., Glazer, G. M., and Martel, W.: Computed tomography of the sternum and its articulations. Skeletal Radiol., *11*:197, 1984.
17. Howard, F. M., and Shafer, S. J.: Injuries to the clavicle with neurovascular complications. J. Bone Joint Surg., *47-A*:1335, 1965.
18. Karlen, M. A.: Traitamiento quirurgivo de la epifiseolosis clavicular. Bol. Soc. Cir. Uruguay, *14*:94, 1943.
19. Kennedy, J. L.: Retrosternal dislocation of the clavicle. J. Bone Joint Surg., *31-B*:74, 1949.
20. Lee, F. A., and Gwinn, J. L.: Retrosternal dislocation of the clavicle. Radiology, *110*:631, 1974.
21. Lemire, L., and Rosman, M.: Sternoclavicular epiphyseal separation with adjacent clavicular fracture. J. Pediatr. Orthop., *4*:118, 1984.
22. Leonard, J. W., and Gifford, R. W.: Migration of a Kirschner wire from the clavicle into the pulmonary artery. Am. J. Cardiol., *16*:598, 1965.

22a. Levinsohn, E. M., Bunnell, W. P., and Yuan, H. A.: Computed tomography in the diagnosis of dislocations of the sternoclavicular joint. Clin. Orthop., *140*:12, 1979.

23. Louri, J. A.: Tomography in the diagnosis of posterior dislocation of the sternoclavicular joint. Acta Orthop. Scand., *51*:579, 1980.
24. Lucas, G. L.: Retrosternal dislocation of the clavicle. J.A.M.A., *193*:850, 1965.

25. Nettles, J. S., and Linscheid, R. L.: Sternoclavicular dislocations. J. Trauma, *8*:158, 1968.
26. Neviaser, J.: Injuries of the clavicle and its articulations. Orthop. Clin. North Am., *11*:233, 1980.
27. Paterson, D. C.: Retrosternal dislocation of the clavicle. J. Bone Joint Surg., *43-B*:90, 1961.
27a. Peacock, H. K., Brandon, J. R., and Jones, O. L., Jr.: Retrosternal dislocation of the clavicle. South. Med. J., *63*:1324, 1970.
28. Ogden, J. A., and Phillips, S. B.: Radiology of postnatal skeletal development. VII. The scapula. Skeletal Radiol., *9*:157, 1983.
29. Poland, J.: Traumatic Separation of the Epiphyses. London, Smith, Elder, & Co., 1898.
29a. Rockwood, C. A., Jr.: Fractures and dislocations of the shoulder. *In* Rockwood, C. A., Jr., and Green, D. P. (eds.): Fractures. Philadelphia, J. B. Lippincott, 1975.
30. Rodrigue, M. H.: Case of dislocation inwards of the internal extremity of the clavicle. Lancet, *1*:309, 1843.
30a. Savastano, A. A., and Stutz, S. J.: Traumatic sternoclavicular dislocation. Int. Surg., *63*:10, 1978.
31. Selesnick, H., Jablon, M., Frank, C., and Post, M.: Retrosternal dislocation of the clavicle. Report of four cases. J. Bone Joint Surg., *66-A*:287, 1984.
32. Simurda, M. A.: Retrosternal dislocation of the clavicle: A report of 4 cases and a method of repair. Can. J. Surg., *11*:487, 1968.
32a. Stankler, L.: Posterior dislocation of the clavicle. A report of 2 cases. Br. J. Surg., *50*:164, 1962.
32b. Stein, A. H., Jr.: Retrosternal dislocation of the clavicle. J. Bone Joint Surg., *39-A*:656, 1957.
33. Tyer, H., Sturrock, W., and Callow, F.: Retrosternal dislocation of the clavicle. J. Bone Joint Surg., *45-B*:132, 1963.
34. Weber, B. G.: Epiphyseal injuries: Internal fixation of fractures of Aitken type 2 and 3. Proceedings of the Twelfth Congress of Fractures of the International Society of Orthopaedic Surgery and Traumatology, Tel Aviv, October 9–12, 1972.
35. Wheeler, M. E., Llaaveg, S. J., and Sprague, B. L.: S-C joint disruption in an infant. Clin. Orthop., *139*:68, 1979.
36. Worman, L. W., and Leagus, C.: Intrathoracic injury following retrosternal dislocation of the clavicle. J. Trauma, *7*:416, 1967.

ACROMIOCLAVICULAR DISLOCATION

Injury to the acromioclavicular joint is very rare in children because the force of direct violence or a direct blow will instead fracture the clavicle. In adolescents, however, dislocation of the acromioclavicular joint is a quite common occurrence in sports. Three grades of injury are recognized: sprain of the acromioclavicular ligament; rupture of the acromioclavicular ligament; and rupture of the acromioclavicular, conoid, and trapezoid ligaments.

Clinical findings depend on the severity of the lesion. Immediately following injury, the patient will complain of pain on all motions of the shoulder, particularly forward rotation. There is definite local tenderness over the acromioclavicular joint. When the joint is dislocated, the upriding prominent lateral end of the clavicle can be palpated. Radiograms should be made with the patient standing and holding weight in each hand and the central beam passing anteroposteriorly through the joint. In subluxation the acromion process is depressed in relation to the lateral end of the clavicle, whereas in dislocation there will be complete discontinuity of the articular ends. An associated fracture of the lateral end of the clavicle should be ruled out.

Treatment depends upon the degree of injury to the joint. In a sprain of the acromioclavicular ligament, simple strapping and a sling are all that is necessary. In subluxation, strapping and a plaster jacket are applied—the clavicle is depressed by a padded strap across the clavicle and the acromion is elevated by pushing the humerus upward with strapping. The acromioclavicular joint is immobilized for three weeks. Dislocations of the acromioclavicular joint require open reduction, capsular repair, and internal fixation with a threaded wire. For details of operative technique and other methods of treatment, the reader is referred to the cited literature.[1–50]

References

1. Allmann, F. L.: Fractures and ligamentous injuries of the clavicle and its articulation. J. Bone Joint Surg., *49-A*:774, 1967.
2. Asher, M. A.: Dislocation of the upper extremity in children. Orthop. Clin. North Am., *7*:583, 1976.
3. Beckman, T.: A case of simultaneous luxation of both ends of the clavicle. Acta Chir. Scand., *56*:156, 1923.
4. Bednarek, J., Kaczan, Z., and Krochmalski, M.: Results of treatment of dislocations of the acromioclavicular joint. Chir. Narzadow Ruchu Ortop. Pol., *46*:13, 1981.
5. Bernard, T. N., Jr., Brunet, M. E., and Haddad, R. J., Jr.: Fractured coracoid process in acromioclavicular dislocations. Report of four cases and review of the literature. Clin. Orthop., *175*:227, 1983.
6. Berson, B. L., Gilbert, M. S., and Green, S.: Acromioclavicular dislocations: Treatment by transfer of the conjoined tendon and distal end of the coracoid process to the clavicle. Clin. Orthop., *135*:157, 1978.
7. Bjerneld, H., Hovelius, L., and Thorling, J.: Acromioclavicular separations treated conservatively. A 5-year follow-up study. Acta Orthop. Scand., *54*:743, 1983.
8. Eidman, D. K., Siff, S. J., and Tullos, H. S.: Acromioclavicular lesions in children. Am. J. Sports Med., *9*:150, 1981.
9. Ejeskar, A.: Coracoclavicular wiring for acromioclavicular joint dislocation. A ten year follow-up study. Acta Orthop. Scand., *45*:652, 1974.
10. Falstie-Jensen, S., and Mikkelsen, P.: Pseudodislocation of the acromioclavicular joint. J. Bone Joint Surg., *64-B*:368, 1982.
11. Fleming, R. E., Tornberg, D. N., and Kiernan, H.: An operative repair of acromioclavicular separation. J. Trauma, *18*:709, 1978.
12. Fritschy, D.: Results of various treatment methods in acromio-clavicular luxations. Z. Unfallmed. Berufskr., *69*:37, 1976.
13. Fukuda, K., Craig, E. V., An, K. N., Cofield, R. H.,

and Chao, E. Y. S.: Biomechanical study of the ligamentous system of the acromioclavicular joint. J. Bone Joint Surg., *68-A*:434, 1986.
14. Gardner, E., and Gray, D. J.: Prenatal development of the human shoulder and acromioclavicular joints. Am. J. Anat., *92*:219, 1953.
15. Gerli, A., Odella, F., and Percudani, W.: Surgical treatment of acromioclavicular dislocation. Chir. Ital., *31*:113, 1979.
16. Hastings, D. E., and Horne, J. G.: Anterior dislocation of the acromioclavicular joint. Injury, *10*:285, 1979.
17. Heitemeyer, U., Hierholzer, G., Schneppendahl, G., and Haines, J.: The operative treatment of fresh ruptures of the acromioclavicular joint. (Tossy III). Arch. Orthop. Trauma. Surg., *104*:371, 1986.
18. Hohlbach, G., Vatankhan, M., and Naser, M.: Surgical treatment of fresh acromioclavicular luxation with the Bosworth screw. Unfallchirurgie, *9*:6, 1983.
19. Holz, U., and Weller, S.: Luxation of the acromioclavicular joint. Hefte Unfallheilkd., *160*:222, 1982.
20. Horn, J. S.: The traumatic anatomy and treatment of acute acromioclavicular dislocations. J. Bone Joint Surg., *36-B*:194, 1954.
21. Imatani, J., Hanlon, J., and Cady, W.: Acute, complete acromioclavicular separation. J. Bone Joint Surg., *57-A*:328, 1975.
22. Jacobs, B., and Wade, P. A.: Acromio-clavicular joint injury. An end-result study. J. Bone Joint Surg., *48-A*:475, 1966.
23. Kawabe, N., Watanabe, R., and Sato, M.: Treatment of complete acromioclavicular separation by coracoacromial ligament transfer. Clin. Orthop., *185*:222, 1984.
24. Kennedy, J. G., and Cameron, H.: Complete dislocation of the acromioclavicular joint. J. Bone Joint Surg., *36-B*:202, 1954.
25. Larsen, E., Bjerg-Nielsen, A., and Christensen, P.: Conservative or surgical treatment of acromioclavicular dislocation. A prospective, controlled, randomized study. J. Bone Joint Surg., *68-A*:552, 1986.
26. Leithe, J., Starke, W., Amon, K., and Schilling, H.: Dynamic stabilization of acromioclavicular joint dislocation. Chirurg., *53*:48, 1982.
27. Lichtblau, P. D.: Shoulder dislocation in the infant. Case report and discussion. J. Fla. Med. Assoc., *64*:313, 1977.
28. Lindsey, R. W., and Gutowski, W. T.: The migration of a broken pin following fixation of the acromioclavicular joint. A case report and review of the literature. Orthopedics, *9*:413, 1986.
29. Meixner, J.: Diagnosis and treatment of dislocations with para-articular fractures of the acromioclavicular joint in childhood. Zentralbl. Chir., *108*:793, 1983.
30. Montgomery, S. P., and Lloyd, R. D.: Avulsion fracture of the coracoid epiphysis with acromioclavicular separation. Report of two cases in adolescents and review of the literature. J. Bone Joint Surg., *59-A*:963, 1977.
31. Neu, K., and Kramer, H.: The pseudoluxation of the acromio-clavicular joint—a special type of epiphyseolysis (author's transl.). Z. Kinderchir., *34*:80, 1981.
32. Neviaser, J. S.: Acromioclavicular dislocation treated by transference of the coraco-acromial ligament. A long-term follow-up in a series of 112 cases. Clin. Orthop., *58*:57, 1968.
33. Petersson, C. J.: Resection of the lateral end of the clavicle. A 3- to 30-year follow-up. Acta Orthop. Scand., *54*:904, 1983.
34. Petersson, C. J., and Redlund-Johnell, I.: Radiographic joint space in normal acromioclavicular joints. Acta Orthop. Scand., *54*:431, 1983.
35. Powers, J. A., and Bach, P. J.: Acromioclavicular separations. Closed or open treatment? Clin. Orthop., *104*:312, 1974.
36. Richards, R. R., Herzenberg, J. E., and Goldner, J. L.: Bilateral nontraumatic anterior acromioclavicular joint dislocation. A case report. Clin. Orthop., *209*:255, 1986.
37. Rosenorn, M., and Pedersen, E. B.: The significance of the coracoclavicular ligament in experimental dislocation of the acromioclavicular joint. Acta Orthop. Scand., *45*:346, 1974.
38. Saga, J.: Recurrent inferior dislocation of the clavicle at the acromioclavicular joint. A case report. Am. J. Sports Med., *10*:145, 1982.
39. Shoji, H., Roth, C., and Chuinard, R.: Bone block transfer of coracoacromial ligament in acromioclavicular injury. Clin. Orthop., *208*:272, 1986.
40. Siegling, C. W., and Jahn, K.: Therapy of acromioclavicular luxation. Zentralbl. Chir., *107*:858, 1982.
41. Simmons, E. H., and Martin, R. F.: Acute dislocation of the acromioclavicular joint. Can. J. Surg., *11*:473, 1968.
42. Sondergard-Petersen, P., and Mikkelsen, P.: Posterior acromioclavicular dislocation. J. Bone Joint Surg., *64-B*:52, 1982.
43. Thelen, E., and Rehn, J.: Acromioclavicular divulsions—results of operative and conservative treatment in 162 cases. Unfallheilkunde, *79*:417, 1976.
44. Tossy, J. D., Mead, N. C., and Sigmond, H. M.: Acromioclavicular separations: Useful and practical classification for treatment. Clin. Orthop., *28*:111, 1963.
45. Urist, M. R.: Complete dislocation of the acromioclavicular joint. J. Bone Joint Surg., *28*:813, 1946.
46. Urist, M. R.: Follow-up notes to articles previously published in The Journal. Complete dislocation of the acromioclavicular joint. J. Bone Joint Surg., *45-A*:1750, 1963.
47. Vainionpaa, S., Kirves, P., and Laike, E.: Acromioclavicular joint dislocation—surgical results in 36 patients. Ann. Chir. Gynaecol., *70*:120, 1981.
48. Vartanian, S. G.: Apparatus for treating dislocation of the acromial end of the clavicle. Ortop. Travmatol. Protez., *5*:48, 1981.
49. Waldrop, J. I., Norwood, L. A., and Alvarez, R. G.: Lateral roentgenographic projections of the acromioclavicular joint. Am. J. Sports Med., *9*:337, 1981.
50. Weaver, J. K., and Dunn, H. K.: Treatment of acromioclavicular injuries, especially complete acromioclavicular separation. J. Bone Joint Surg., *54-A*:1187, 1972.

*FRACTURES OF THE SCAPULA**

The scapula is a flat triangular bone located between pads of muscles in the posterior upper thorax. Its borders are thickened and it is freely mobile on the chest wall. These anatomic features make injuries to the scapula very rare. Almost any part of the bone may be broken.

The scapula is ossified from seven or more centers: one for the body, two for the acromion, two for the coracoid process, one for the vertebral border, and one for the inferior angle.

At birth, the scapula is composed of a large osseous plate (consisting of its body and spine) and a cartilaginous mass comprising the coracoid process, the acromion, the glenoid, and the edge of the scapular spine. Between 15 and

*See references 1 to 70.

18 months of age, the ossification center for the *middle of the coracoid process* appears. The base of the coracoid process that rests on the glenoid fossa begins to ossify between the seventh and tenth years; it is sometimes called the subcoracoid bone. When fully ossified, it is pyramidal in shape. Shortly following its appearance, the subcoracoid bone first joins posteriorly with the body of the scapula, and later (between the fourteenth and sixteenth years) with the middle of the ossified portion of the coracoid process. Frequently, a scalelike ossification nucleus appears on the tip of the coracoid process at about the fourteenth year, and joins on at the eighteenth year. Occasionally, an additional point of ossification in the form of a cap appears at the seventeenth year, joining the body of the process between the twentieth and twenty-fifth years. This cap-shaped-apophysis does not unite with the scalelike-apophysis.

Ossification of the acromion process originates from two centers, one being at its base and the other at its apex. These begin to ossify between the fourteenth and sixteenth years, and coalesce to form one apophysis at about the nineteenth year, connecting with the scapular spine from the twenty-second to the twenty-fifth years. Sometimes bony union may fail to take place between the acromion and the spine of the scapula, the junction created consisting only of fibrous tissue. Such tardy union or failure of osseous union should not be mistaken for fracture.

The glenoid fossa is composed of four segments: the subcoracoid bone on its upper third; a portion of the coracoid process internally; a part from the body of the scapula; and a cartilaginous plate in the lower part of the glenoid, which joins the body of the scapula between the twentieth and the twenty-fifth years. In its early stages of development, the glenoid fossa is convex, but later becomes flat and then concave.

The ossification center for the inferior angle of the scapula appears at the fifteenth year and fuses by the twentieth year; and that of the vertebral border of the scapula appears by the seventeenth year, fusing by the twenty-fifth year.

Fractures of the Body of the Scapula

These are the result of direct violence such as a crushing injury in an automobile accident or a fall from a height. The blade of the scapula is often comminuted, the fracture lines running in various directions, but at times, the bone may split throughout its length in a transverse or oblique line. The spine of the scapula may be fractured with the body of the scapula. The intraspinous portion is more frequently fractured than the supraspinous one. Usually there is little if any displacement of the fractured fragments, as they are held together by the surrounding muscles. The fracture is rarely open, but the direct trauma may cause severe damage to the overlying soft parts. Frequently there are extensive crushing injuries of the thorax with multiple fractures of the ribs or the vertebral column, pneumothorax, and subcutaneous emphysema. Because of the gravity of the accompanying conditions, the scapular fracture is often missed. In order to demonstrate the fracture, it is necessary to obtain oblique tangential views in addition to the routine anteroposterior radiograms. Computed axial tomography will clearly depict the fracture.

The primary objective of treatment is to make the patient comfortable. It is not necessary to reduce the fracture or to immobilize the entire arm and shoulder. If the soft-tissue condition permits, the scapula is fixed against the chest wall by criss-cross moleskin adhesive strapping across the shoulder and down over the patient's back to the level of his waist. If the patient is ambulatory, he can be made more comfortable by suspending his arm in a sling. The fracture will heal within four weeks and any resultant irregularity of bony contour will be remodeled and will disappear with growth. Shoulder stiffness is not a problem in children.

Fractures of the Scapular Neck

These are usually caused by a direct blow to the front or back of the shoulder. The fracture line usually begins in the suprascapular notch and runs downward and laterally to the axillary border of the scapular neck inferior to the glenoid. The capsular attachments of the glenohumeral joint and the articular surface of the glenoid remain intact. Depending upon the force of inury, the fracture may be undisplaced, minimally displaced, markedly displaced, or comminuted. If the coracoclavicular and acromioclavicular ligaments are intact, there is little, if any, displacement of the articular fragment; however, if these ligaments are torn, or if the fracture line is lateral to the coracoid process, the articular fragment is displaced downward and inward by the weight of the limb and the muscle pull. In severe crushing injuries, the fracture line may include the acromion, scapular spine, and glenoid.

Treatment. It consists of support of the shoulder and arm in a triangular sling for a period of three to four weeks. Circumduction and pendulum exercises for the shoulder can be performed 14 days after injury when the patient is more comfortable.

Markedly displaced fractures of the scapular neck are treated by skeletal traction with a pin through the base of the olecranon; the shoulder is abducted to 90 degrees and the forearm is flexed to right angles. Gradually the glenoid fragment will be repositioned in normal anatomic alignment. After two to three weeks the traction is removed and circumduction shoulder exercises are performed to maintain range of motion of the shoulder. Open reduction of markedly displaced fracture of the scapular neck is occasionally indicated.

Fractures of the Glenoid Cavity of the Scapula

These are produced either by direct or indirect force. Direct violence, such as a fall on the lateral side of the shoulder, will usually produce a stellate fracture, which may be minimally displaced or comminuted with separation of the fragments. In indirect injuries, such as a fall on the flexed elbow, the breaking force is transmitted up the shaft of the humerus, shearing off a fragment of the glenoid. When the shoulder is in extended and abducted position during the fall, the anterior part of the glenoid is fractured; whereas when the shoulder is in flexion and abduction, a fragment from the posterior part of the glenoid is detached. The humeral head may subluxate if the fracture fragment is large and markedly displaced. Avulsed fracture of the glenoid bone may result from acute traumatic dislocation of the shoulder. Sudden severe contraction of the long head of the triceps may cause avulsion fracture of the inferior brim of the glenoid cavity.

Fractures of the glenoid should be managed conservatively. The shoulder joint is immobilized in a triangular sling and swathe. After two to three weeks, pendulum and circumduction exercises are performed within tolerance of pain. Immobilization is discontinued after four weeks. Stellate fractures with marked displacement are treated with lateral arm skeletal traction with a Kirschner wire through the base of the olecranon. After two weeks, traction is removed and a triangular sling is applied for an additional two weeks. Open reduction of a fracture of the glenoid cavity is difficult and its results disappointing. Functional results of conservative treatment are good, despite gross irregularity of the joint. If avulsed fragments become symptomatic, they are excised at a later date.

When a large fragment of the anterior or posterior portion of the glenoid fossa is fractured and widely separated and causes the humeral head to subluxate, open reduction and internal fixation with a screw are indicated. Any tears of the capsule are repaired to stabilize the joint.

Fractures of the Acromion

The acromion process breaks occasionally from direct violence or from indirect force transmitted vertically by the humeral head. The line of fracture is usually lateral to the acromioclavicular joint, though occasionally it occurs at its base adjacent to the spine of the scapula. The shoulder is flattened, and there is localized pain, swelling, and tenderness. Abduction of the shoulder is very painful and restricted. Treatment consists of immobilization in a circular strapping (pushing the flexed elbow upward and the lateral part of the clavicle downward) and a sling for a period of three to four weeks. If, later, abduction of the shoulder is limited by a downward projecting malunited acromion, partial acromionectomy is performed to improve range of shoulder motion.

Fracture of the Coracoid Process

This isolated injury is a rare lesion. It may be caused by sudden muscular action of the short head of the biceps and the coracobrachialis muscles or by direct violence. Treatment consists of immobilization for a period of three weeks. Results are excellent, even in the presence of nonunion of the coracoid process.

Fracture-Separation of Epiphyses of Acromion and Coracoid Process

These occasionally occur in adolescents and young adults. Their treatment is the same as that of a fracture of a bone. Traumatic dislocation of the scapulocostal joint is a very rare injury.

References

1. Armstrong, C. P., and Van der Spuy, J.: The fractured scapula: Importance and management based on a series of 62 patients. Injury, *15*:324, 1984.

2. Aulicino, P. L., Reinert, C., Kornberg, M., and Williamson, S.: Displaced intra-articular glenoid fractures treated by open reduction and internal fixation. J. Trauma, *26*:1137, 1986.
3. Benchetrit, E., and Friedman, B.: Fracture of the coracoid process associated with subglenoid dislocation of the shoulder. A case report. J. Bone Joint Surg., *61-A*:295, 1979.
4. Benton, J., and Nelson, C.: Avulsion of the coracoid process in an athlete: Report of a case. J. Bone Joint Surg., *53-A*:356, 1971.
5. Bernard, T. N., Jr., Brunet, M. E., and Haddad, R. J., Jr.: Fractured coracoid process in acromioclavicular dislocations. Report of four cases and review of the literature. Clin. Orthop., *175*:227, 1983.
6. Boyer, D. W., Jr.: Trapshooter's shoulder: Stress fracture of the coracoid process: Case report. J. Bone Joint Surg., *57-A*:862, 1975.
7. Brower, A. C., Neff, J. R., and Tillema, D. A.: An unusual scapular stress fracture. A.J.R., *129*:519, 1977.
8. Crenshaw, A. H.: Approaches to the shoulder joint. *In* Edmonson, A. S., and Crenshaw, A. H. (eds.): Campbell's Operative Orthopaedics. St. Louis, Mosby, 1980, pp. 81–90.
9. DePalma, A. F.: Fractures and dislocations of the scapula. *In* Surgery of the Shoulder. 3rd Ed. Philadelphia, Lippincott, 1983, pp. 362–371.
10. DeRosa, G. P., and Kettelkamp, D. B.: Fracture of the coracoid process of the scapula: A case report. J. Bone Joint Surg., *59-A*:696, 1977.
11. Fery, A., and Sommelet, J.: Fractures de l'apophyse coracoide: A propos de 10 observations (English abstract). Rev. Chir. Orthop., *65*:403, 1979.
12. Froimson, A. I.: Fracture of the coracoid process of the scapula. J. Bone Joint Surg., *60-A*:710, 1978.
13. Gambrioli, P. L., Maggi, F., and Randelli, M.: Computerized tomography in the investigation of scapulohumeral instability. Ital. J. Orthop. Traumatol., *11*:223, 1985.
14. Ganz, R., and Noesberger, B.: Die Behandlung der Scapula-Frakturen. Hefte Unfallheilkd., *126*:59, 1975.
15. Garcia-Elias, M., and Salo, J. M.: Non-union of a fractured coracoid process after dislocation of the shoulder. A case report. J. Bone Joint Surg., *67-B*:722, 1985.
16. Germain, M., and Poilleux, F.: Fracture de l'apophyse coracoide. Rev. Chir. Orthop., *57*:555, 1971.
17. Goldberg, R. P., and Vicks, B.: Oblique angled view for coracoid fractures. Skeletal Radiol., *9*:195, 1983.
18. Hall, R. H., Issac, F., and Booth, C. R.: Dislocation of the shoulder with special reference to accompanying small fractures. J. Bone Joint Surg., *41-A*:489, 1959.
19. Hardegger, F. H., Simpson, L. A., and Weber, B. G.: The operative treatment of scapular fractures. J. Bone Joint Surg., *66-B*:725, 1984.
20. Heyse-Moore, G. H., and Stoker, D. J.: Avulsion fractures of the scapula. Skeletal Radiol., *9*:27, 1982.
21. Hollinshead, R., and James, K. W.: Scapulothoracic dislocation (locked shoulder). J. Bone Joint Surg., *61-A*:1102, 1979.
22. Houghton, G. R.: Avulsion of the cranial margin of the scapula: A report of two cases. Injury, *11*:45, 1979.
23. Imatani, R. J.: Fractures of the scapula: A review of 53 fractures. J. Trauma, *15*:473, 1975.
24. Ishizuki, M., Yamaura, I., Isobe, Y., Furuya, K., Tanabe, K., and Nagatsuka, Y.: Avulsion fracture of the superior border of the scapula. Report of five cases. J. Bone Joint Surg., *63-A*:820, 1981.
25. Judet, R.: Traitement chirurgicales fractures de l'omoplate. Acta Orthop. Belg., *30*:673, 1964.
26. Kelbel, J. M., Jardon, O. M., and Huurman, W. W.: Scapulothoracic dissociation. A case report. Clin. Orthop., *209*:210, 1986.
27. Lasada, N. A., and Murray, D. G.: Fracture separation of the coracoid process associated with acromioclavicular dislocation conservative treatment—a case report and review of the literature. Clin. Orthop., *134*:222, 1978.
28. Liberson, R.: Os acromiale: A contested anomaly. J. Bone Joint Surg., *19*:683, 1937.
29. McClure, J. G., and Raney, B.: Anomalies of the scapula and related research. Clin. Orthop., *110*:22, 1975.
30. McGahan, J. P., and Rab, G. T.: Fracture of the acromion associated with an axillary nerve deficit: A case report and review of the literature. Clin. Orthop., *147*:216, 1980.
31. McGahan, J. P., Rab, G. T., and Dublin, A.: Fractures of the scapula. J. Trauma, *20*:880, 1980.
32. McLennan, J. G., and Ungersma, J.: Pneumothorax complicating fracture of the scapula. J. Bone Joint Surg., *64-A*:598, 1982.
33. Magerl, F.: Osteosynthesen in Bereich der Schulter: Pertuberkulare Humerusfrakturen, Scapulahalsfrakturen. Helv. Chir. Acta, *41*:225, 1974.
34. Mathews, R. E., Cocke, T. B., and D'Ambrosia, R. D.: Scapular fractures secondary to seizures in patients with osteodystrophy. Report of two cases and review of the literature. J. Bone Joint Surg., *65-A*:850, 1983.
35. Mick, C. A., and Weiland, A. J.: Pseudarthrosis of a fracture of the acromion. J. Trauma, *23*:248, 1983.
36. Moneim, M. S., and Balduini, F. C.: Coracoid fracture as a complication of surgical treatment by coracoclavicular tape fixation. A case report. Clin. Orthop., *168*:133, 1982.
37. Montgomery, S. P., and Loyd, R. D.: Avulsion fracture of the coracoid epiphysis with acromioclavicular separation. Report of two cases in adolescents and review of the literature. J. Bone Joint Surg., *59-A*:963, 1977.
38. de Mourgues, G., Machenaud, A., Fischer, L., Schnepp, J., Contet, J. J., and Vidalain, J. P.: Fractures de l'omoplate: A propos d'une serie de 130 cas traites orthopediquement. Lyon Chir., *69*:47, 1973.
39. Muller-Farber, J.: Die Skapulafrakturen konservative oder operative Behandlung. Unfallheilkunde, *79*:293, 1976.
40. Neer, C. S., II: Fractures about the shoulder. *In* Rockwood, C. A., and Green, D. P. (eds.): Fractures. Philadelphia, Lippincott, 1975, pp. 585–623.
41. Nettrour, L. F., Krufky, E. L., Mueller, R. E., and Raycroft, J. F.: Locked scapula: Intrathoracic dislocation of the inferior angle. J. Bone Joint Surg., *54-A*:413, 1972.
42. Oppenheim, W. L., Dawson, E. G., Quinlan, C., and Graham, S. A.: The cephaloscapular projection. A special diagnostic aid. Clin. Orthop., *195*:191, 1985.
43. Oreck, S. L., Burgess, A., and Levine, A. M.: Traumatic lateral displacement of the scapula: A radiographic sign of neurovascular disruption. J. Bone Joint Surg., *66-A*:758, 1984.
44. Ovesen, J., and Nielsen, S.: Experimental distal subluxation in the glenohumeral joint. Arch. Orthop. Trauma. Surg., *104*:78, 1985.
45. Pate, D., Kursunoglu, S., Resnick, D., and Resnick, C. S.: Scapular foramina. Skeletal Radiol., *14*:270, 1985.
46. Peraino, R. A., Weinman, E. J., and Schloeder, F. X.: Fractures during convulsions in two patients with renal osteodystrophy. South. Med. J., *70*:595, 1977.
47. Pettersson, H.: Bilateral dysplasia of the neck of the scapula and associated anomalies. Acta Radiol. [Diagn.], *22*:81, 1981.
48. Piulachs, P., Nogue-Tutor, R., and Piulachs, J.: Fractura de la apofisis coracoides. Cir. Esp., *29*:485, 1975.
49. Protass, J. J., Stampfli, F. W., and Osmer, J. C.: Coracoid process fracture diagnosis in acromioclavicular separation. Radiology, *116*:61, 1975.
50. Randelli, M., and Gambrioli, P. L.: Glenohumeral osteometry by computed tomography in normal and unstable shoulders. Clin. Orthop., *208*:151, 1986.
51. Randelli, M., Odella, F., and Gambrioli, P. L.: Clinical

experience with double contrast medium computerized tomography (arthro-CT) in instability of the shoulder. Ital. J. Orthop. Traumatol., *12*:151, 1986.
52. Rask, M. R., and Steinberg, L. H.: Fracture of the acromion caused by muscle forces. A case report. J. Bone Joint Surg., *60-A*:1146, 1978.
53. Rounds, R. C.: Isolated fracture of the coracoid process. J. Bone Joint Surg., *31-A*:662, 1949.
54. Rowe, C. R.: Fractures of the scapula. Surg. Clin. North Am., *43*:1565, 1963.
55. Rubenstein, J. D., Ebraheim, N. A., and Kellam, J. F.: Traumatic scapulothoracic dissociation. Radiology, *157*:297, 1985.
56. Sandrock, A. R.: Another sports fatigue fracture: Stress fracture of the coracoid process of the scapula. Radiology, *117*:274, 1975.
57. Smith, D. M.: Coracoid fracture associated with acromioclavicular dislocation: A case report. Clin. Orthop., *108*:165, 1975.
58. Solheim, L. F., and Roaas, A.: Compression of the suprascapular nerve after fracture of the scapular notch. Acta Orthop. Scand., *49*:338, 1978.
59. Sutro, C. J.: Dentated articular surface of the glenoid: An anomaly. Bull. Hosp. Joint Dis., *28*:104, 1967.
60. Taga, I., Yoneda, M., and Ono, K.: Epiphyseal separation of the coracoid process associated with acromioclavicular sprain. A case report and review of the literature. Clin. Orthop., *207*:138, 1986.
61. Tarquinio, T., Weinstein, M. E., and Virgilio, R. W.: Bilateral scapular fractures from accidental electric shock. J. Trauma, *19*:132, 1979.
62. Thompson, D. A., Flynn, T. C., Miller, P. W., and Fischer, R. P.: The significance of scapular fractures. J. Trauma, *25*:974, 1985.
63. Varriale, P. L., and Adler, M. L.: Occult fracture of the glenoid without dislocation. A case report. J. Bone Joint Surg., *65-A*:688, 1983.
64. Weber, B. G., Brunner, C. H., and Freuler, F.: Treatment of Fractures in Children and Adolescents. Berlin, Springer-Verlag, 1980, pp. 94–95.
65. Wilber, M. C., and Evans, E. B.: Fractures of the scapula. An analysis of forty cases and a review of the literature. J. Bone Joint Surg., *59-A*:358, 1977.
66. Wolf, A. W., Shoji, H., and Chuinard, R. G.: Unusual fracture of the coracoid process. A case report and review of the literature. J. Bone Joint Surg., *58-A*:423, 1976.
67. Wong-Pack, W., Bobechko, P. E., and Becker, E. J.: Fractured coracoid with anterior shoulder dislocation. J. Can. Assoc. Radiol., *31*:278, 1980.
68. Zaricznyj, B.: Reconstruction for chronic scapuloclavicular instability. Am. J. Sports Med., *11*:17, 1983.
69. Zettas, J. P., and Muchnic, P. D.: Fractures of the coracoid process based in acute acromioclavicular separation. Orthop. Rev., *5*:77, 1976.
70. Zilberman, Z., and Rejovitzky, R.: Fracture of the coracoid process of the scapula. Injury, *13*:203, 1981.

FRACTURES INVOLVING THE PROXIMAL HUMERAL PHYSIS

(Fracture-Separation of Upper Epiphysis of Humerus)

The proximal epiphysis of the humerus develops from three centers of ossification: one major central one for the head, which usually appears between the ages of four and six months (sometimes before birth); one for the greater tuberosity, which ossifies by three years; and one for the lesser tuberosity, which is visible on the radiograph by the age of five years. These ossification nuclei coalesce into a single center by the age of seven years. The physis is concave inferiorly; in its medial half, it follows the line of the anatomic neck and then passes laterally and downward to the distal border of the greater tuberosity. Fusion of the upper humeral epiphysis with the shaft takes place between 20 and 22 years of age. About 80 per cent of the longitudinal growth of the humerus is contributed by its proximal physis.

The supraspinatus, infraspinatus, and teres minor muscles are inserted on three flat impressions on the greater tuberosity, whereas the subscapularis muscle is inserted on an impression on the lesser tuberosity. In the metaphyseal and proximal diaphyseal regions, the pectoralis major tendon inserts to the crest of the greater tuberosity; the teres major is attached to the crest of the lesser tubercle of the humerus; and the floor of the intertubercular groove gives insertion to the latissimus dorsi muscle.

Fracture-separations of the upper humeral epiphysis may take place at any age while the physis is open, the period of greatest frequency being between the ages of 11 and 15 years. It can occur at birth, and the oldest patient reported in the literature is a 23-year-old man with pituitary gigantism, in whom epiphyseal closure was delayed secondarily to the endocrine lesion. It is three times more frequent in boys than in girls in the series of Smith, of Neer and Horwitz, and of Dameron and Reibel.[19, 47, 67] Bourdillon reports preponderance in the male with a male to female ratio of 4:1.[11]

Mechanism of Injury

Fractures that involve the proximal humeral physis usually result from indirect violence, the force being exerted up through the humeral shaft with the arm in an adducted, extended, and laterally rotated position. A common accident is a fall backward in which the person extends his elbow in an attempt to break the fall with his hand and gets the hand caught under his buttock. A direct blow or a fall on the lateral aspect of the shoulder may also cause a fracture. Neer and Horwitz reported a direct blow to the shoulder as the etiologic agent in 59 of their 89 cases; they believed the fracture is characteristically produced by a posterolateral shearing force that adducts the humeral shaft and displaces it forward.[47]

Pathologic Anatomy

Dameron and Reibel performed experimental studies on 12 anatomic specimens of the proximal ends of the humeri from stillborn infants. They could not fracture the humerus through the physis without displacing the metaphysis posteriorly or laterally; the fracture fragments were maintained in position by the thick periosteal envelope. By forceful manipulation it was extremely difficult to displace the metaphysis posteriorly at the physis; however, when the arm was extended and adducted, the metaphysis could be displaced anteriorly with relative ease. The upper end of the metaphysis ruptured the periosteum immediately lateral to the tendon of the long head of the biceps. (The anterior rather than the posterior displacement of the metaphysis is partly due to asymmetrical configuration of the dome of the metaphysis, with its apex posterior and medial to its center, and partly due to firmer attachment of the periosteum along the posterior surface of the periphery of the epiphysis.) Once the periosteum was torn and began to strip distally, the fracture became progressively less stable. In all stillborn specimens, the fracture occurred at the physis without any metaphyseal bone fragment.[19]

This Salter-Harris Type I physeal injury is typical of that encountered in infants and young children. In older children and adolescents, a fragment of metaphysis usually remains attached to the posterior medial epiphysis (Type II physeal injury). Thus, the cartilage cells contributing to the longitudinal growth of the humerus are spared. Types III, IV, and V physeal injuries are not encountered in the upper end of the humerus; this is accounted for by the fact that the glenohumeral joint is the most mobile and multiplane joint in the body, and for mechanical reasons, crushing or splitting injuries of its physis are very unlikely.

The degree of displacement depends upon the force causing the injury and upon the direction of muscle pull. There may be simple loosening of the epiphysis with practically no displacement, or the displacement may be partial or complete. Neer and Horwitz have graded the degree of displacement as: *Grade I*, less than 5 mm.; *Grade II*, to one third of the shaft; *Grade III*, to two thirds of the shaft; and *Grade IV*, greater than two thirds of the shaft, including total displacement.[47]

In grades III and IV displacement there is always a varying degree of angulation. Partial displacement occurs more frequently than complete displacement. The epiphysis remains in the glenoid fossa, but is rotated into abduction and lateral rotation by the pull of attached muscles, so that its articular surface is tilted inferiorly. The upper end of the humeral shaft is drawn upward, forward, and inward by the combined action of the pectoralis major, latissimus dorsi, and teres major muscles. The arm is abducted to a varying degree by the pull of the deltoid muscle. The periosteum is stripped off the lateral aspect of the humeral diaphysis to a varying extent. The intact portion of the periosteum on the posteromedial aspect holds the fragments together, making closed reduction difficult; it also forms a mold for the callus and later for the new bone produced by the physis. Occasionally the fracture is impacted with the upper end of the metaphysis driven into the epiphysis.

Diagnosis

This should be the first lesion to be considered in injuries to the shoulder region in children between ages 9 and 15 years. Disability is great, with marked swelling and local tenderness.

With complete displacement of the fracture fragments, the presenting deformity is characteristic. The arm is shortened and is held in a varying degree of abduction and extension. There is a prominence in the front of the axilla near the coracoid process caused by the upper end of the distal fragment, which can be palpated and even seen. The anterior axillary fold is distorted, with a characteristic puckering of the skin caused by the lower fragment hooking into it. The humeral head is palpable in its normal position. On grasping the head of the humerus between the fingers and thumb of one hand while holding the flexed elbow with the other hand, the surgeon may be able to demonstrate motion and crepitus between the fracture fragments. When the displacement is slight, most of these physical findings will be absent, the diagnosis being confirmed by radiograms in both the anteroposterior and lateral views (Fig. 8–16).

Treatment

In infants and young children (up to five years of age), the usual epiphyseal injury is Type I (Salter and Harris). It is difficult to delineate the position of the upper humeral epiphysis since it is mostly cartilaginous. If the arm is shortened and abducted, an attempt is made to restore length and alignment by apply-

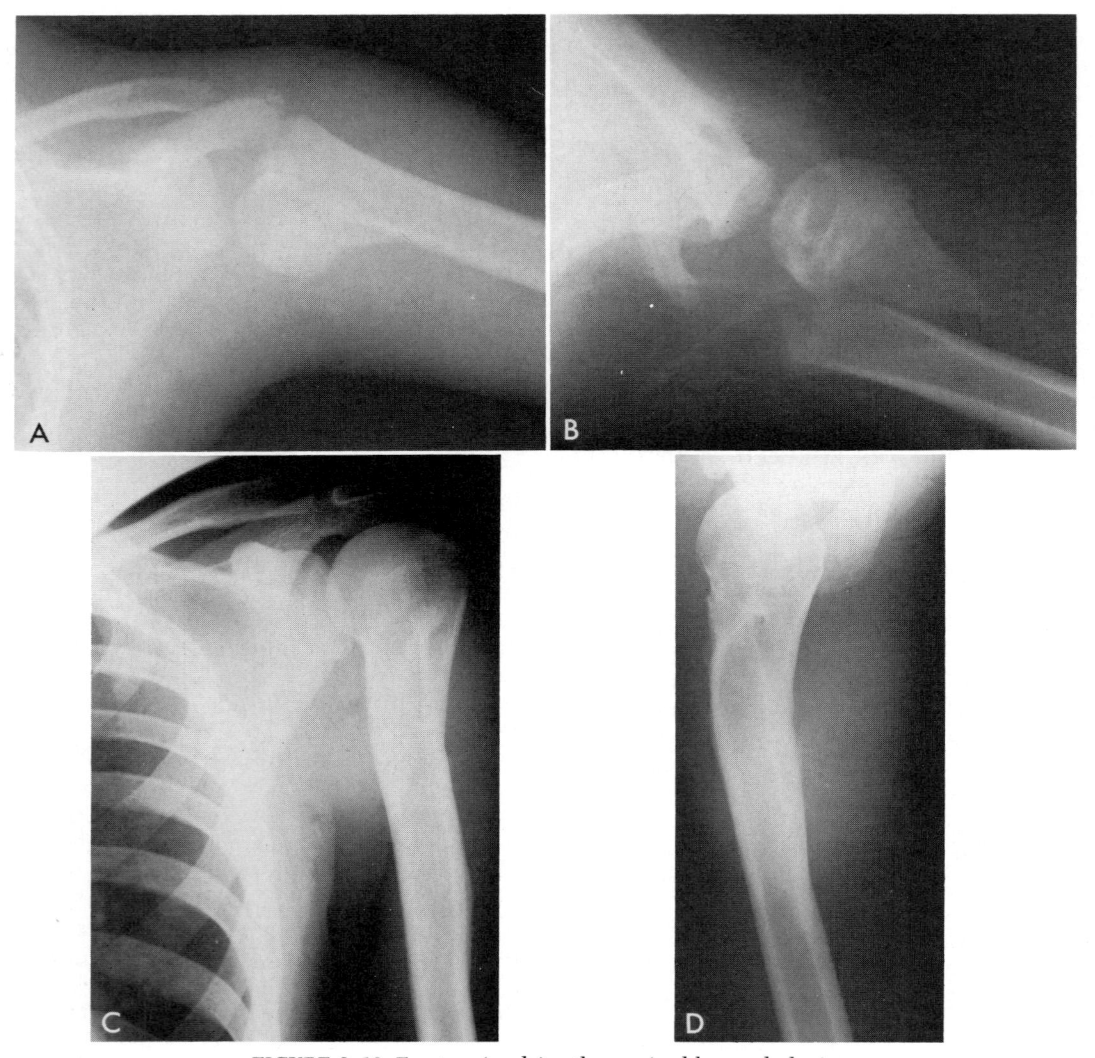

FIGURE 8–16. Fracture involving the proximal humeral physis.

A and **B**. Initial radiograms. **C** and **D**. Radiograms taken six years later, showing remodeling of malunion. (Courtesy of Dr. John J. Fahey.)

ing longitudinal traction with the arm in 90 degrees of abduction, 90 degrees of flexion, and 15 to 25 degrees of lateral rotation. Exact apposition of the fragments is not necessary and administration of a general anesthetic is not justified. The shoulder and upper limb are immobilized in a modified Velpeau bandage. Within three to four weeks, solid union will take place. Any malalignment and angular deformity will correct itself with growth and remodeling.

In children over six years of age and in adolescents the usual fracture is a Salter-Harris Type II epiphyseal injury. When there is no displacement, a modified Velpeau bandage is applied for four weeks, by which time the fracture will be firmly consolidated.

When there is minimal displacement with the degree of angulation less than 20 degrees, a gentle closed reduction is attempted without general anesthesia. Again, it is not necessary to reduce the fracture into normal anatomic alignment. Remodeling will correct any deformity and will have excellent functional and cosmetic results.

When the fracture is moderately angulated (more than 20 degrees) or completely displaced, it should be manipulated into an acceptable position. This is best carried out under general anesthesia. In a cooperative patient, local anesthesia with supplemental analgesia may be adequate, however. The longer its duration following injury, the more difficult this fracture is to reduce. The time for easiest manipulative reduction is during the first few hours after trauma. The prime difficulty of reduction is the position assumed by the upper humeral epiphysis, which is small, mobile, and difficult to grasp and stabilize during manipulation. The proximal fragment is abducted and laterally rotated; to permit reduction it is essential to place the distal fragment in line with the proximal fragment. Thus, traction is exerted with the arm in 90 degrees of abduction, 90 degrees of flexion, and slight lateral rotation. During the maneuver, an assistant grasps and stabilizes the humeral head between his thumb and fingers. The metaphysis is forced back through the defect in the anterior periosteum and impacted into the epiphysis. Radiograms are made in anteroposterior and lateral views to check anatomic alignment. If reduction is stable, a modified Velpeau bandage is applied; if unstable, a shoulder spica cast is applied with the arm in 90 degrees of abduction, 60 degrees of forward flexion, and neutral rotation.

Closed reduction may be difficult or, at times, impossible. If the preceding manipulation fails, a heavy smooth Kirschner wire is inserted (under strict aseptic operating room conditions and radiographic control) in a superoinferior direction from the acromion into the upper humeral epiphysis, transfixing the two. The pin should not engage the metaphysis, however; this is documented by taking multiple views under image intensifier radiographic control. The shoulder is positioned in abduction and flexion prior to fixing the humeral head to the acromion. The manipulative reduction is repeated. If it is successful and the fracture is stable, a modified Velpeau bandage is again applied; if it is successful but unstable, a shoulder spica cast is applied in the degree of abduction and flexion that affords the greatest stability. Osseous union will occur in four to six weeks. Alignment of fracture fragments is checked by periodic radiograms since it may be lost, even in a shoulder spica cast. A hanging cast, so commonly used in adults, is not effective in children, as the fragments become displaced when the arm is adducted to the sides of the trunk.

Perfect anatomic reduction is not essential since gross malalignment is compatible with excellent functional result. This is because the shoulder is the most mobile articulation in the human skeleton and is not a weight-bearing joint. The greater the growth potential of the proximal humerus, the more acceptable the malalignment. In general, in boys under 15 years of age and in girls under 13 years of age, 50 per cent bayonet apposition of the fragments will be corrected with growth and remodeling; however, one should be cautious in accepting angulation of more than 20 degrees (Fig. 8–17).

Only very occasionally is open reduction indicated in an older adolescent in whom conservative measures have failed to achieve adequate reduction. The tendon of the long head of the biceps may be caught between the fragments, or more frequently, a patient is seen several days after injury and the fragments are bound firmly together by the thickened reactive periosteum. Before embarking on open surgery, the consequences of the blemish of an unsightly scar should be weighed. In the author's experience, angulation can ordinarily be corrected if it is less than 20 degrees, and the marked overriding and shortening are acceptable. The protruding bony prominence of the upper end of the humeral shaft may restrict medial rotation and adduction to a varying degree; however, over a period of several years, the bony block will be absorbed by remodeling with excellent functional range of shoulder motion.

Side arm or overhead arm traction with a pin in the olecranon may be attempted, but usually fails. Instead of disengaging the fragments, it stretches the capsule and subluxates the humeral head.

Nilsson and Svartholm reported excellent results in 43 of 44 cases of fractures of the upper end of the humerus. They found considerable displacement does not in itself necessarily lead to any significant disability and advised open reduction only in those cases of serious displacement that cannot be treated with closed methods; i.e., dislocation of the upper humeral epiphysis or serious rotational displacement.[49] Dameron and Reibel, in an end-result study of 69 patients (46 of whom returned for end-result evaluation) with an average follow-up of seven years, concluded that more than the usual displacement and angulation can be accepted in the treatment of this physeal injury, and believed open reduction is not indicated.[19] Neer and Horwitz, in a study of 89 fractures of the proximal humeral physis presented the end-results in 62 patients with a minimum follow-up of 4.8 years. Shortening of the humerus of from 1 to 3 cm. occurred in 9 per cent of the patients with fractures of Grade I and Grade II displacement and in 33 per cent of those with Grade IV displacement. In children under 11 years of age, permanent shortening was not

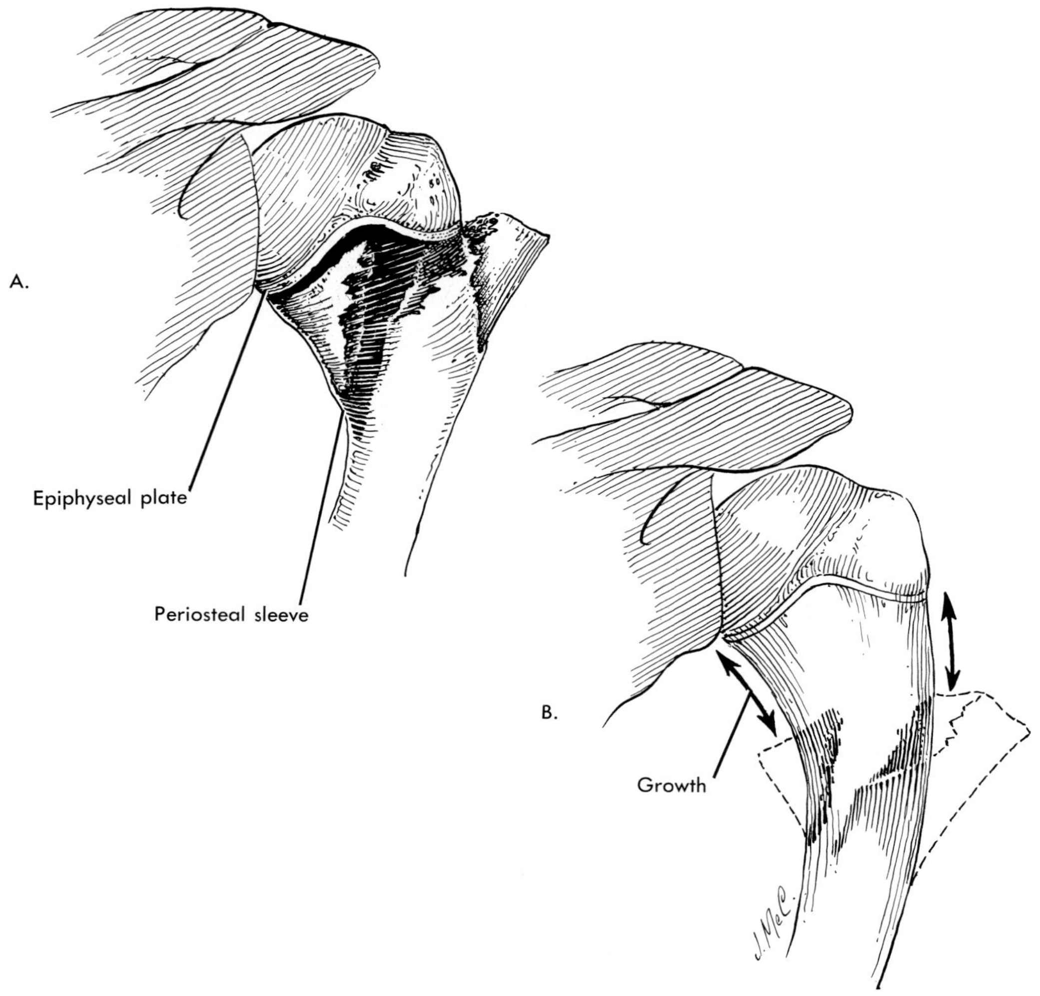

FIGURE 8–17. Diagram showing remodeling process of a malunited fracture involving the proximal humeral physis.

noted. In children 11 years of age and older, length and axis deformities of moderate degree were not infrequent; however, the functional results in all these cases were very satisfactory because of the compensation provided by the great mobility of the glenohumeral joint and because discrepancies in length are clinically less significant in the upper limb than in the lower limb. They concluded that the remodeling powers of the epiphysis of the proximal humerus are so great that the hazards of operative reduction are rarely, if ever, justified. It is advisable, however, to warn the parents of children over 11 years of age that growth and remodeling may not fully correct the inequality, and some permanent shortening and angulation may occur. This is especially true in cases with marked displacement.[47]

References

1. Aitken, A. P.: End results of fractures of the proximal humeral epiphysis. J. Bone Joint Surg., *18*:1036, 1936.
2. Aitken, A. P.: Fractures of the proximal humeral epiphysis. Surg. Clin. North Am., *43*:1573, 1963.
3. Arzinger-Jonasch, H.: Proximal humerus injuries in childhood and adolescence. Hefte Unfallheilkd., *160*:195, 1982.
4. Astedt, B.: A method for treatment of humerus fractures in the newborn using the S. Von Rosen splint. Acta Orthop. Scand., *40*:234, 1969.
5. Aufranc, O. E., Jones, W. N., and Bierbaum, B. E.: Epiphyseal fracture of the proximal humerus. J.A.M.A., *207*:727, 1969.
6. Aufranc, O. E., Jones, W. N., and Butler, J. E.: Epiphyseal fracture of the proximal humerus. J.A.M.A., *213*:1476, 1970.
7. Austin, L. J.: Fractures of the morphological neck of the humerus in children. Can. Med. Assoc. J., *40*:546, 1939.
8. Baxter, M. P., and Wiley, J. J.: Fractures of the

proximal humeral epiphysis. Their influence on humeral growth. J. Bone Joint Surg., *68-B*:570, 1986.
9. Blount, W.: Fractures in Children. Baltimore, Williams & Wilkins, 1955.
10. Bonelli, A., and Schiavetti, E.: Considerazioni su alcuni aspetti delle frature di gomito nel bambino. Chir. Organi Mov., *52*:286, 1963.
11. Bourdillon, J. F.: Fracture separation of the proximal epiphysis of the humerus. J. Bone Joint Surg., *32-B*:35, 1950.
12. Bovill, E. G., Jr., Schneider, F. R., and Day, L.: Fracture of the proximal humerus with displacement in a child. J.A.M.A., *216*:1188, 1971.
13. Butterworth, R. D., and Carpenter, E. B.: Bilateral slipping of the proximal epiphysis of the humerus. J. Bone Joint Surg., *30-A*:1003, 1948.
14. Callahan, D. J.: Anatomic considerations: Closed reduction of proximal humeral fractures. Orthop. Rev., *13*:79, 1984.
15. Campbell, J., and Almond, G. A.: Fracture-separation of the proximal humeral epiphysis. J. Bone Joint Surg., *59-A*:262, 1977.
16. Charry, V.: Un cas de fracture irreductible du col chirurgical de l'humerus chez un adolescent. Rev. Chir. Orthop., *24*:244, 1937.
17. Ciaramella, G., and Rulfoni, R.: Le complicazioni neurologiche nelle fratture dell'artro superiore. Chir. Ital., *14*:569, 1962.
18. Conwell, H. E.: Fractures of the surgical neck and epiphyseal separations of the upper end of the humerus. J. Bone Joint Surg., *8*:508, 1926.
19. Dameron, T. B., Jr., and Reibel, D. B.: Fractures involving the proximal humeral epiphyseal plate. J. Bone Joint Surg., *51-A*:289, 1969.
20. Divis, G.: Epiphyseolysis humeri unter beträchtlicher Dislokation des Gelenkskopfes: Unblütige Reposition. Arch. Orthop. Unfallchir., *25*:342, 1927.
21. Fischer, L., Noirclerc, J. A., Neidhardt, J. H., Spay, G., and Comtet, J. J.: Anatomo-radiographic study of the importance of different ligaments in the vertical retention of the head of the humerus. (Origin of Ch. Clavel Gleno-humeral dislocation). Lyon Med., *223*:629, 1970.
22. Fraser, R. L., Haliburton, R. A., and Barber, J. R.: Displaced epiphyseal fractures of the proximal humerus. Can. J. Surg., *10*:427, 1967.
23. Friedlander, H. L.: Separation of the proximal humeral epiphysis: A case report. Clin. Orthop., *35*:163, 1964.
24. Gassan, I. U. P., Zhukov, M. D., Golovin, V. T., Avessolomov, A. M., and Bondarenko, T. F.: Treatment of fractures of the eminentia capitata of the humerus in children. Ortop. Travmatol. Protez., *7*:75, 1977.
25. Gerard, Y., and Segal, P.: Traitement chirurgical des decollements epiphysaires de l'extremite superieure de l'humerus chez l'adolescent. Rev. Chir. Orthop., *59*:205, 1973.
26. Giebel, G., and Suren, E. G.: Injuries of the proximal humeral epiphysis. Indications for surgical therapy and results. Chirurg. *54*:406, 1983.
27. Gilchrist, D.: A stockinette-Velpeau for immobilization of the shoulder girdle. J. Bone Joint Surg., *45-A*:1382, 1963.
28. Guibert, L., Allouis, M., Bourdelat, D., Catier, P., Bracq, H., and Babut, J. M.: Fractures and slipped epiphyses of the proximal humerus in children. Place and methods of surgical treatment. Chir. Pediatr., *24*:197, 1983.
29. Hawkins, R. J., Bell, R. H., and Gurr, K.: Fractures of the proximal part of the humerus. The three-part operative treatment. J. Bone Joint Surg., *68-A*:1410, 1986.
30. Hohl, J. C.: Fractures of the humerus in children. Orthop. Clin. North Am., *7*:557, 1976.
31. Jaschke, W., Hopf, G., Gerstner, C., and Hiemer, W.: Proximal humerus fracture with dislocation in childhood. Transacromial percutaneous osteosynthesis using Kirschner wires. Zentralbl. Chir., *106*:618, 1981.
32. Jeffery, C. C.: Fracture separation of the upper humeral epiphysis. Surg. Gynecol. Obstet., *96*:205, 1953.
33. Judet, J., and Judet, R.: Fractures du col chirurgical l'humerus. Acta Orthop. Belg., *30*:243, 1964.
34. Kohler, R., and Trillaud, J. M.: Fracture and fracture separation of the proximal humerus in children. Report of 136 cases. J. Pediatr. Orthop.. *3*:326, 1983.
35. Kristiansen, B., and Christensen, S. W.: Plate fixation of proximal humeral fractures. Acta Orthop. Scand., *57*:320, 1986.
36. Langenskiold, A.: Adolescent humerus varus. Acta Chir. Scand., *105*:353, 1953.
37. Lee, H. G.: Operative reduction of an unusual fracture of the upper epiphyseal plate of the humerus. J. Bone Joint Surg., *26*:401, 1944.
38. Lemberg, R., and Liliequist, B.: Dislocation of the proximal epiphysis of the humerus in newborns. Acta Paediatr. Scand., *59*:377, 1970.
39. Levin, G. D.: A valgus angulation fracture of the proximal humeral epiphysis. Clin. Orthop., *116*:155, 1976.
40. Lorenzo, F. T.: Osteosynthesis with Blount's staples in fractures of the proximal end of the humerus. A preliminary report. J. Bone Joint Surg., *37-A*:45, 1955.
41. Lucas, L., and Gill, J. H.: Humerus varus following birth injury to the proximal humerus. J. Bone Joint Surg., *29*:367, 1947.
42. McBride, E. D., and Sisler, J.: Fractures of the proximal humeral epiphysis and the juxta-epiphyseal humeral shaft. Clin. Orthop., *38*:143, 1965.
43. McKibbon, B., and Holdsworth, F.: The dual nature of epiphyseal cartilage. J. Bone Joint Surg., *49-B*:351, 1967.
44. Michel, L.: Le decollement obstetrical de l'epiphyse superieure l'humerus. Rev. Orthop., *24*:201, 1937.
45. de Mourgues, G., and Fischer, L. P.: Resultats lointains des decollements, epiphysaires de l'extremite superieure de l'humerus chez l'adolescent. Rev. Chir. Orthop., *53*:241, 1971.
46. Neer, C. S., II: Displaced proximal humeral fractures. I. Classification and evaluation. J. Bone Joint Surg., *52-A*:1077, 1970.
47. Neer, C. S., II, and Horwitz, B. S.: Fractures of the proximal humeral epiphyseal plate. Clin. Orthop., *41*:24, 1965.
48. Neer, C. S., II, and Rockwood, C. A., Jr.: Fractures of the proximal humerus. *In* Rockwood, C. A., Jr., and Green, D. P. (eds.): Fractures. Philadelphia, Lippincott, 1975, pp. 585–610.
49. Nilsson, S., and Svartholm, F.: Fracture of the upper end of the humerus in children. Acta Chir. Scand., *130*:433, 1965.
50. Olszewski, W., and Skolowski, J.: Anatomical obstacles in reduction of fractures of the humeral head in children. Chir. Narzadow Ruchu Ortop. Pol., *38*:127, 1973.
51. Olszewski, W., Sokolowski, J., and Swiecki, M.: Fractures and epiphyseolysis of the proximal end of the humerus in children. Chir. Narzadow Ruchu Ortop. Pol., *39*:569, 1974.
52. Paavolainen, P., Bjorkenheim, J. M., Slatis, P., and Paukku, C. P.: Operative treatment of severe proximal humeral fractures. Acta Orthop. Scand., *54*:374, 1983.
53. Plaske, I. I.: Comparative evaluation of the methods for treating fractures of the capitilum humeri in children. Vestn. Khir., *111*:84, 1973.
54. Poland, J.: Traumatic Separation of the Epiphyses. London, Smith, Elder, & Co., 1898.
55. Rang, M.: Children's Fractures. Philadelphia, Lippincott, 1974.
56. Reddy, K. R., Lotke, P. A., Ecker, M. L., and Rufferi,

S.: Simple method for treatment of epiphyseal fractures of the proximal humerus, 1–8. Presented at A.A.O.S. Meeting, Las Vegas, 1981.
57. Reisig, J., Grobler, V., and Grobler, B.: Differential treatment of proximal humerus fractures in childhood. Zentralbl. Chir., *105*:25, 1980.
58. Rettig, H.: Frakturen im Kindesalter. Munich, Verlag-Bergmann, 1957.
59. Rigault, P., Padovani, J. P., and Chapuis, B.: Fractures et decollements epiphysaires de l'extremite superieure de l'humerus chez l'enfant. Forum Chir. (78e Congres Francais de Chirurgie), *7*:27, 1977.
60. Robin, G. C., and Kedar, S. S.: Separation of the upper humeral epiphysis in pituitary gigantism. J. Bone Joint Surg., *44-A*:189, 1962.
61. Roche, A. E.: The ultimate results of a case of separated upper epiphysis of the humerus. Clinical Journal, *55*:478, 1926.
62. Rotham, R. H., Marvel, J. P., Jr., and Heppenstall, R. B.: Anatomical considerations in the glenohumeral joint. Orthop. Clin. North Am., *6*:341, 1975.
63. Sabate, A. F., Rubio, I., and Olivares, M.: Desprendemientos epifisarios graves del cuello humeral. Barcelona Quirurgica, *18*:329, 1974.
64. Salter, R. B., and Harris, W. R.: Injuries involving the epiphyseal plate. J. Bone Joint Surg., *45-A*:587, 1975.
65. Scaglietti, O.: The obstetrical shoulder trauma. Gynecol. Obstet., *66*:868, 1938.
66. Sherk, H., and Probst, C. E.: Fractures of the proximal humeral epiphysis. Orthop. Clin. North Am., *6*:401, 1975.
67. Smith, F.: Fracture separation of the proximal humeral epiphysis. Am. J. Surg., *91*:627, 1956.
68. Stewart, M. J., and Hundley, J. M.: Fractures of the humerus: A comparative study in methods of treatment. J. Bone Joint Surg., *37-A*:681, 1955.
69. Sysa, N. F.: On methods of treatment of fractures of the proximal end of the humerus in children. Ortop. Travmatol. Protez., *26*:22, 1965.
70. Tondeur, G.: Les fractures recentes de l'epaule. Acta Orthop. Belg., *30*:5, 1964.
71. Truesdale, E. D.: Birth Fractures and Epiphyseal Dislocations. New York, Paul B. Hoeber, 1917.
72. Visser, J. D., and Rietberg, M.: Interposition of the tendon of the long head of biceps in fracture separation of the proximal humeral epiphysis. Neth. J. Surg., *32*:12, 1980.
73. Vivian, D. N., and Janes, J. M.: Fractures involving the proximal humeral epiphysis. Am. J. Surg., *87*:211, 1954.
74. Wahl, D.: Fractures of the proximal end of the humerus in children. Beitr. Orthop. Traumatol., *29*:379, 1982.
75. Whitman, R.: A treatment of epiphyseal displacements and fractures of the upper extremity of the humerus designed to assure definite adjustment and fixation of the fragments. Ann. Surg., *47*:706, 1908.
76. Williams, D. J.: The mechanisms producing fracture-separation of the proximal humeral epiphysis. J. Bone Joint Surg., *63-B*:102, 1981.
77. Wilson, J. N.: *In* Watson-Jones, R. (ed.): Fractures and Joint Injuries. 5th Ed. New York, Churchill-Livingstone, 1976, p. 548.
78. Zancolli, R.: Fratture dell'epifisi superiore dell'omero. Chir. Organi Mov., *12*:445, 1928.

Injuries to the Arm

*FRACTURES OF THE SHAFT OF THE HUMERUS**

Fractures of the humeral shaft in children are uncommon in comparison to the frequency with which they occur in the adult. The shaft of the humerus is roughly cylindrical in its upper half, becoming gradually broadened and flattened below. Surgically, it may be considered as extending from the upper border of the insertion of the pectoralis major muscle proximally to the supracondylar ridges distally.

Its numerous muscle attachments must be considered in the analysis of humeral shaft fractures. The deltoid, biceps brachii, and brachialis anticus muscles cover it anteriorly. The coracobrachialis muscle inserts beneath the upper half of the biceps brachii muscle. The pectoralis major inserts into the lateral lip of the bicipital groove of the humerus. The posterior surface is covered by the deltoid and triceps brachii muscles. On the lateral and medial aspects of the humerus, intermuscular septa dip down between the muscles to be attached to the bone, dividing the arm into anterior and posterior compartments. The neurovascular bundle courses along the medial aspect of the humerus in the anterior compartment, consisting of the brachial vessels and the median, musculocutaneous, and ulnar nerves. The radial nerve lies in the posterior compartment in a shallow groove in the posterior and lateral surfaces of the middle and upper thirds of the shaft of the humerus between the origins of the medial and lateral heads of the triceps brachii muscle. The radial nerve traverses obliquely downward and laterally as it passes from the axilla to the anterolateral epicondylar region.

Mechanism of Injury

The majority of the fractures of the shaft of the humerus are caused by direct violence, such as falls on the side of the arm; these tend to be transverse or comminuted and not infrequently are open. The more severe the injury, the greater is the possibility of comminution or of open fracture (Fig. 8–18). Segmental fractures occasionally occur.

Indirect violence, such as a fall on the hand or elbow, will produce an oblique spiral fracture. A forceful muscular action, such as throw-

*See references 1 to 46.

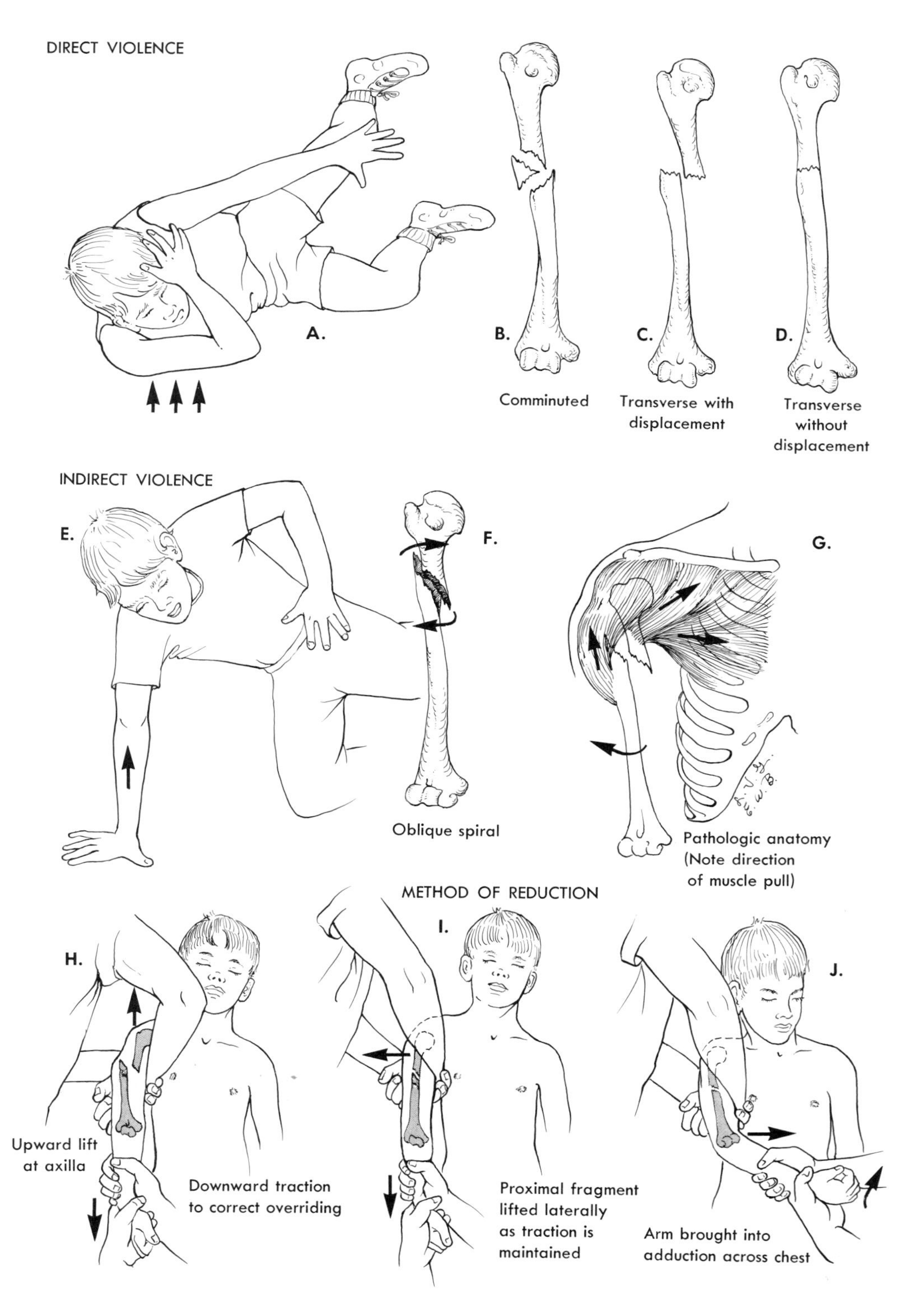

FIGURE 8–18. Fractures of the humeral shaft above insertion of deltoid and distal to attachment of pectoralis major muscles.

A to **F**. *Mechanism of injury.* Direct violence, such as falls on the side of the arm, will cause comminuted or transverse fractures (**A** to **D**). Indirect violence, such as falls on the hand, will cause oblique spiral fractures (**E** and **F**).

G. *Pathologic anatomy* when fracture site is at junction of upper and middle thirds. Note the pull of the deltoid muscle tends to displace the distal fragment laterally and upward, while the pectoralis major, latissimus dorsi, and teres major muscles will adduct and internally rotate the proximal fragment.

I and **J**. *Method of reduction* when the level of fracture is between the insertions of the pectoralis major and deltoid muscles.

ing a baseball, may also result in an oblique or spiral fracture; however, when a minor injury causes the humeral shaft to fracture, the possibility of a pathologic fracture, such as through a unicameral bone cyst, fibrous dysplasia, or metastatic lesion, should be ruled out.

Pathologic Anatomy

The direction of displacement of the fracture fragments depends on whether the level of fracture is proximal or distal to the insertion of the deltoid muscle. When the fracture occurs in the lower third or at a level of the lower and middle thirds of the humerus below the deltoid insertion, the action of the supraspinatus, deltoid, and coracobrachialis muscles will tend to pull the proximal fragment laterally and anteriorly, whereas the distal fragment is drawn upward by contraction of the biceps and brachialis muscles (Fig. 8–19 A).

If the fracture occurs in the upper and middle thirds of the humeral shaft, i.e., above the insertion of the deltoid but distal to that of the pectoralis major, the pull of the deltoid muscle will tend to displace the distal fragment laterally and upward, while the pectoralis major, latissimus dorsi, and teres major muscles will adduct and medially rotate the proximal fragment (Fig. 8–18 G).

The displacement of the fracture fragments is also influenced by gravity, the position in which the upper limb is held, and the forces causing the fracture. The distal fragment is usually internally rotated, as the arm is held across the chest while the proximal fragment remains in mid-position.

Diagnosis

The deformity, local swelling, and pain caused by humeral shaft fractures make the clinical diagnosis very obvious and simple; however, the pitfall is failure to detect associated neurovascular injury. The intimate relation of the radial nerve to the humerus in the musculospiral groove makes it especially vulnerable. Injury to nerves may result secondarily by their being stretched over the displaced fragments or primarily at the time of initial trauma by being torn or crushed between the fragments. With radial nerve paralysis, there is anesthesia over the dorsum of the hand between the first and second metacarpals and loss of motor strength of extensors of the wrist, fingers and thumb, and supinators of the forearm. The median and ulnar nerves are rarely injured. Vascular injury to brachial vessels is extremely rare.

Treatment

The preferred treatment of humeral shaft fractures in adults is a hanging cast. In children, this method of treatment is not effective, as it requires the cooperation of the patient in sleeping and staying in a semirecumbent or sitting posture without support beneath the elbow and also in the added responsibility for performing the proper exercises. A hanging cast is also not practical for the irrational or unconscious patient or for the patient who must remain recumbent in bed because of associated injuries.

Wherever there is marked displacement of the fragments, the initial step is to reduce the fracture. When the level of the fracture is between the sites of insertion of the pectoralis major and deltoid muscles with adduction and medial rotation of the proximal fragment, reduction is carried out by first applying downward traction to correct overriding and to disengage the fracture fragments, and then, while maintaining distal traction and with the surgeon's forearm in the patient's axilla, lifting the proximal fragment laterally in abduction. The reduction is completed by bringing the distal fragment into adduction and medial rotation by adducting the upper limb across the patient's chest (Fig. 8–18 H to J and Fig. 8–20).

When the level of the fracture is distal to the deltoid insertion with abduction and lateral rotation of the upper fragment, again downward traction is initially applied with the arm in abduction and lateral rotation to correct overriding of fracture fragments; then, while the assistant maintains distal traction, the surgeon lifts the upper end of the lower fragment into abduction with one hand and with his other, pushes the proximal fragment into adduction, reducing the fracture (Fig. 8–19 B and C).

Radiograms of the humerus, in both anteroposterior and lateral views, are taken to confirm the reduction, and its stability is checked clinically. It is not essential in children to obtain end-to-end anatomic alignment. Overriding of 1 to 1.5 cm. can be easily accepted, as overgrowth is common in a displaced shaft fracture of the humerus; however, angulation of more than 15 to 20 degrees is not desirable, and one should pay attention to rotational alignment.

In infants and young children, the fracture is immobilized for a period of four to six weeks by bandaging the arm to the side of the thorax in a modified Velpeau bandage or a sling and swathe (Fig. 8–19 E). In the cooperative older child and adolescent a modified stockinette Velpeau may be applied. Adequate fixation can also be provided by sugar-tong or U-slab plaster of

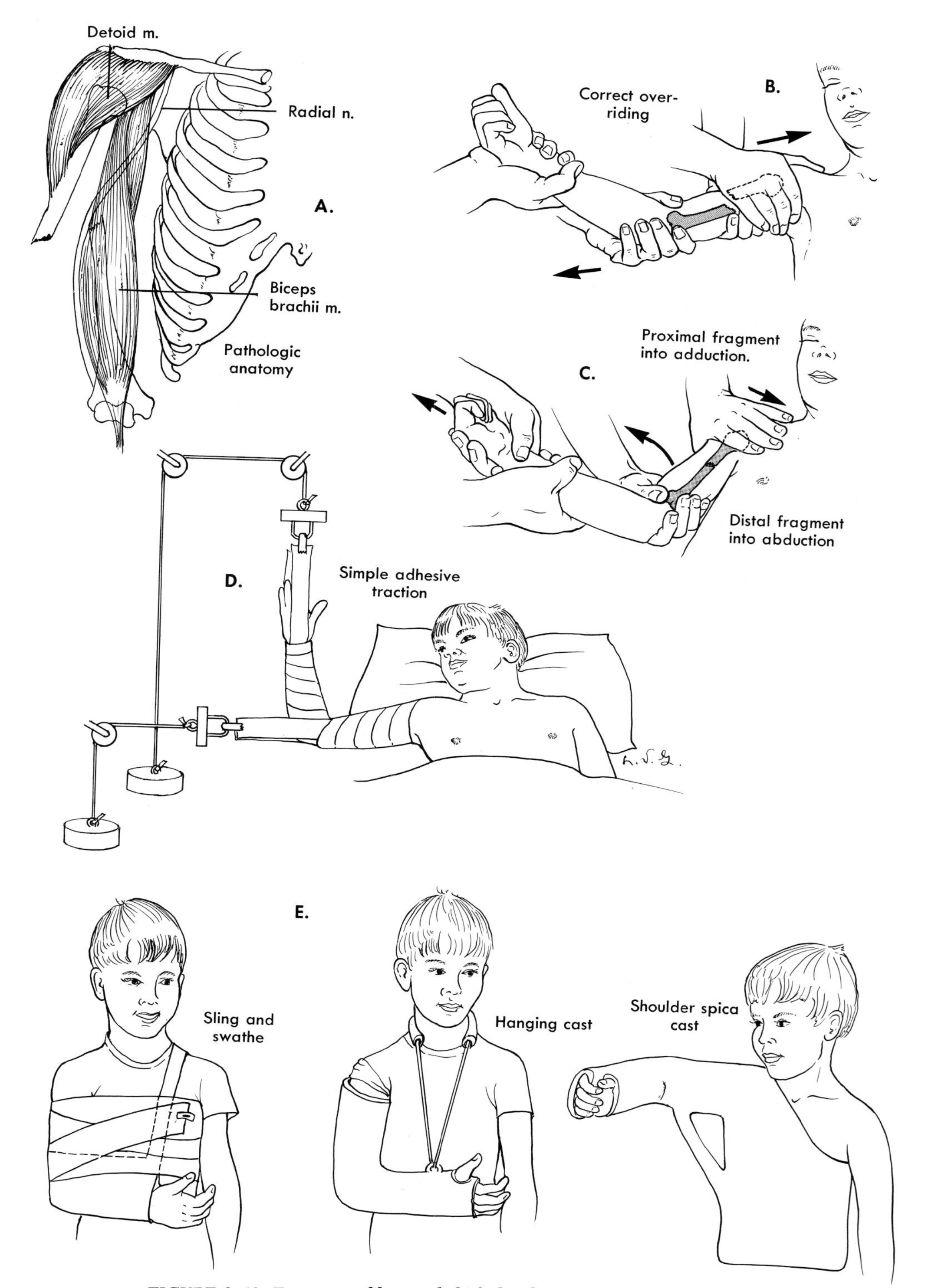

FIGURE 8–19. Fractures of humeral shaft distal to insertion of deltoid muscle.

A. *Pathologic anatomy* when site of fracture is at junction of the lower and middle thirds. Note the proximal fragment is displaced laterally by the pull of the deltoid muscle and anteriorly by the coracobrachialis muscle. The distal fragment is pulled upward by the action of the biceps and brachialis muscles.

B and **C.** *Method of reduction.* With the arm in abduction and external rotation, distal traction is applied to correct overriding; then, while an assistant maintains traction, the distal fragment is pulled into abduction with one hand and the proximal fragment is pushed into abduction with the other.

D. Traction when fracture is unstable or oblique with much overriding.

E. Methods of immobilization after reduction.

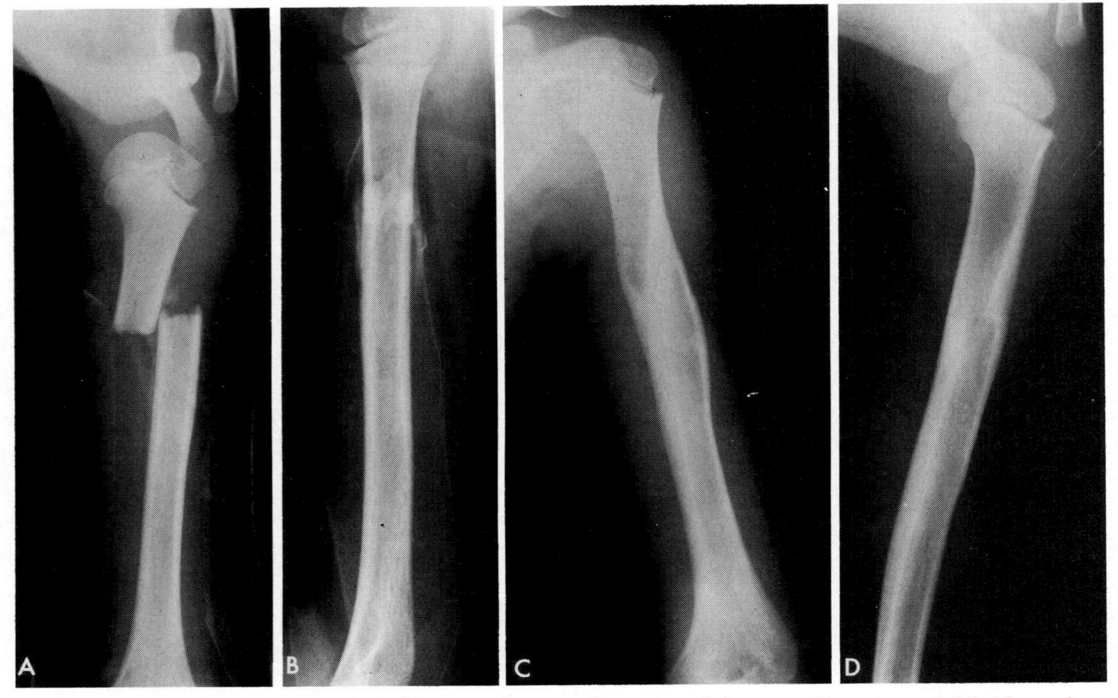

FIGURE 8–20. Fracture of humeral shaft between the sites of insertion of the pectoralis major and deltoid muscles.

Note the overriding and adduction of proximal fragment. Treated by closed reduction and plaster of Paris reinforced modified Velpeau bandage. **A** and **B.** Initial radiograms. **C** and **D.** Four months later, showing healing.

Paris cast. If the fracture is unstable or oblique, with marked overriding of the fragments, and acceptable reduction cannot be maintained, lateral adhesive skin traction is applied to maintain acceptable position of the fracture fragments for a period of two to three weeks until callus is demonstrable in the radiograms, and then it is immobilized as just described until healing is completed (Fig. 8–19 D).

In the older child or adolescent with an unstable fracture, following reduction, a shoulder spica cast is used for immobilization. This should extend distally to include the pelvis and should be well molded above the iliac crests (Fig. 8–19 E).

Skeletal traction with a Kirschner wire through the olecranon and suspension of the forearm and hand are indicated either when the local skin and soft-tissue conditions do not permit adhesive skin traction, when the fracture is open, or when there is marked comminution and displacement of the fracture fragments in a patient who must remain in bed because of associated trauma, such as head injury.

In the older adolescent who is cooperative, the hanging cast is the best method of treatment, as it permits him to be ambulatory and active. An above-elbow cast is applied from the metacarpal heads to the axilla with the elbow in 90 degrees of flexion and the forearm in neutral rotation. In fractures in the distal third of the humeral shaft, the forearm is placed in full pronation, however. Supinating force of the biceps brachii muscle is lost by a break in continuity of the humerus at this level, and the elbow joint rotated into pronation by the unopposed action of the pronators. Since the joint is fixed in pronation, attempts to place the forearm in supination will result in varus deformity at the fracture site. A collar and cuff are attached to a plaster loop at the wrist and passed around the patient's neck. The weight of the cast should be slight; if it is excessive, the bone fragments will be distracted.

Improper length of the collar and cuff is a common error. If it is too long and the wrist drops below the horizontal plane, the distal fragment of the humerus will tilt posteriorly and anterior angulation of the fracture will result. Conversely, a short collar and cuff will cause posterior bowing. A pad of rolled sponge is attached to the medial aspect of the cast to serve as a fulcrum for the arm as it presses against the chest wall.

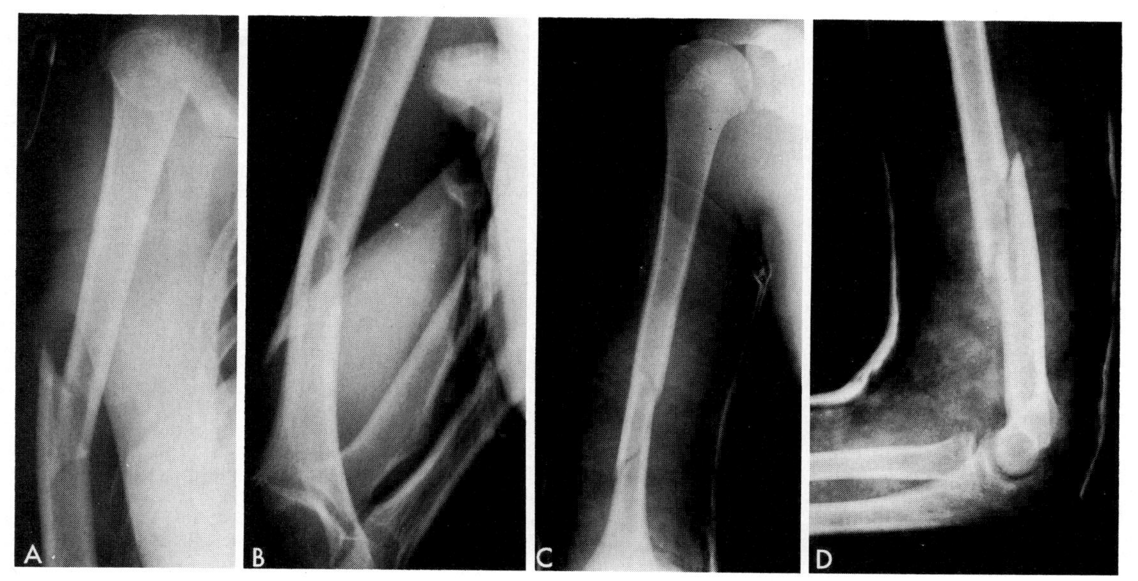

FIGURE 8–21. ***Long spiral fracture of lower third of right humerus.***

Hanging cast is best method of treatment in the cooperative adolescent patient. **A** and **B.** Initial radiograms. **C** and **D.** Radiograms in cast, showing the satisfactory anatomic alignment.

The patient sleeps in semirecumbent position. Erect position is maintained during the day as much as possible. There should be no support under the elbow. Pressure from clothing, as from a buttoned coat over the cast, or anything that might compress the arm against the body must be avoided, as it interferes with traction.

Circumduction and pendulum exercises for the shoulder are demonstrated and begun early. The patient assumes a forward and laterally inclined position; he is then asked to swing the arm in increasingly larger circles through all motions of the shoulder to the limit of tolerance. The arm with the cast should hang free vertically, the wrist still supported by the collar and cuff.

The hanging cast method of treatment is ideal, particularly for long spiral oblique fractures and in comminuted fractures of the lower two thirds of the humeral shaft (Fig. 8–21).

Radial nerve paralysis, which is not uncommon in adults, is rare in children. Complete severance of the nerve in closed fractures is very unlikely, and nerve function almost always recovers if the fracture is managed by conservative methods. Primary open reduction of a closed fracture of the humeral shaft is not indicated. The wrist and hand are splinted in functional position, and passive exercises are performed to maintain full range of motion of the joint. Electromyographic studies are helpful in following the return of nerve function. If, after three to four months, there is no evidence of nerve regeneration, the nerve is explored.

References

1. Astedt, B.: A method for the treatment of humerus fractures in the newborn using the S. von Rosen splint. Acta Orthop. Scand., *40*:234, 1969.
2. Avellan, W. H.: Über Frakturen des unteren Humerusendes bei Kindern. Acta Chir. Scand. (Suppl.), 27, 1933.
3. Bell, M. J., Beauchamp, C. G., Kellam, J. K., and McMurtry, R. Y.: The results of plating humeral shaft fractures in patients with multiple injuries. The Sunnybrook experience. J. Bone Joint Surg., *67-B*:293, 1985.
4. Bohler, L.: Conservative treatment of fresh closed fractures of the shaft of the humerus. J. Trauma, 5:464, 1965.
5. Bonelli, A., and Schiavetti, E.: Considerazioni su alcuni aspetti delle fratture di gomita nel bambino. Chir. Organi Mov., *52*:286, 1963.
6. Bostman, O., Bakalim, G., Vainionpaa, S., Wilppula, E., Patiala, H., and Rokkanen, P.: Immediate radial nerve palsy complicating fracture of the shaft of the humerus: When is early exploration justified? Injury, *16*:499, 1985.
7. Bostman, O., Bakalim, G., Vainionpaa, S., Wilppula, E., Patiala, H., and Rokkanen, P.: Radial palsy in shaft fracture of the humerus. Acta Orthop. Scand., *57*:316, 1986.
8. Brumback, R. J., Bosse, M. J., Poka, A., and Burgess, A. R.: Intramedullary stabilization of humeral shaft fractures in patients with multiple trauma. J. Bone Joint Surg., *68-A*:960, 1986.
9. Cartner, M. J.: Immobilization of fractures of the shaft of the humerus. Injury, 5:175, 1973.
10. Casiano, E.: Reduction and fixation by pinning "ban-

derillero" style fractures of the humerus in children. Milit. Med., *125*:363, 1960.
11. Chapman, M. W.: The role of intramedullary fixation in open fractures. Clin. Orthop., *212*:26, 1986.
12. Comfort, T. H.: The Surgartong splint in humeral shaft fractures. Minn. Med., *56*:363, 1973.
13. Derian, P. S.: Extremity fractures in children. II. Upper extremity. Postgrad. Med., *48*:132, 1970.
14. Flemming, J. E., and Beals, R. K.: Pathologic fracture of the humerus. Clin. Orthop., *203*:258, 1986.
15. Gainer, B. J., and Metzler, M.: Humeral shaft fracture with brachial artery injury. Clin. Orthop., *204*:154, 1986.
16. Gilchrist, D. K.: A stockinette-Velpeau for immobilization of the shoulder girdle. J. Bone Joint Surg., *49-A*:750, 1967.
17. Griswold, R. A., Goldberg, H., and Robertson, J.: Fractures of the humerus. Am. J. Surg., *43*:31, 1939.
18. Hall, R. F., Jr., and Pankovich, A. M.: Technique and results of closed intramedullary rodding of diaphyseal fractures of the humerus. Orthop. Trans., *6*:359, 1982.
19. Harper, M. C.: Localized acquired hypertrichosis associated with fractures of the arm in young females. A report of two cases. Orthopedics, *9*:73, 1986.
20. Hedstrom, O.: Growth stimulation of long bones after fracture or simple trauma: A clinical and experimental study. Acta Orthop. Scand. (Suppl.), *122*:7–41, 55–62, 102–105, 1969.
21. Holm, C. L.: Management of humeral shaft fractures. Fundamental nonoperative techniques. Clin. Orthop., *71*:132, 1970.
22. Holstein, A., and Lewis, G. B.: Fractures of the humerus with radial-nerve paralysis. J. Bone Joint Surg., *45-A*:1382, 1963.
23. Hosner, W.: Fractures of the shaft of the humerus. Reconstr. Surg. Traumatol., *14*:38, 1974.
24. Hunter, S. G.: The closed treatment of fractures of the humeral shaft. Clin. Orthop., *164*:192, 1982.
25. Kamhin, M., Michaelson, M., and Waisbrod, H.: The use of external skeletal fixation in the treatment of fractures of the humeral shaft. Injury, *9*:245, 1978.
26. Klenerman, L.: Fractures of the shaft of the humerus. J. Bone Joint Surg., *48-B*:105, 1966.
27. Korzh, A. A., Bondarenko, N. S., and Vasilevski, N. N.: Basic principles of treatment of fractures of bones of the upper extremity in children. Ortop. Travmatol. Protez., *30*:9, 1969.
28. Lange, R. H., and Foster, B. J.: Skeletal management of humeral shaft fractures associated with forearm fractures. Clin. Orthop., *195*:173, 1985.
29. Macnichol, M. F.: Roentgenographic evidence of median-nerve entrapment in a greenstick humeral fracture. J. Bone Joint Surg., *60-A*:998, 1978.
30. Magilligan, D. J.: Unusual regeneration of bone in a child. J. Bone Joint Surg., *28*:873, 1946.
31. Nagy, A.: Treatment of childhood humeral fractures by wire fixation. Magy. Traumatol. Orthop., *20*:182, 1977.
32. Ormandy, L.: Olecranon screw for skeletal traction of the humerus. Am. J. Surg., *127*:615, 1974.
33. Packer, W., Foster, R., Garcia, A., and Grantham, S.: The humeral fracture with radial nerve palsy: Is exploration warranted? Clin. Orthop., *88*:34, 1972.
34. Pollen, A. G.: Fractures and Dislocations in Children. Edinburgh, Churchill-Livingstone, 1973.
35. Pollock, F. H., Drake, D., Bovill, E. G., Day, L., and Trafton, P.: Treatment of radial neuropathy associated with fractures of the humerus. J. Bone Joint Surg., *63-A*:239, 1981.
36. Ricciardi-Pollini, P. T., and Falez, F.: The treatment of diaphyseal fracture by functional bracing. Results in 36 cases. Ital. J. Orthop. Traumatol., *11*:199, 1985.
37. Rogers, J. F., Bennett, J. B., and Tullos, H. S.: Management of concomitant ipsilateral fractures of the humerus and forearm. J. Bone Joint Surg., *66-A*:552, 1984.
38. Rush, L. V., and Rush, H. L.: Intramedullary fixation of fractures of the humerus by longitudinal pin. Surgery, *27*:268, 1950.
39. Sakvarelidze, M. V.: Indications for and methods of surgical treatment of inveterate and complicated fractures of the humerus and the forearm bone in children. Ortop. Travmatol. Protez., *3*:42, 1978.
40. Sarmiento, A., Kinman, P. B., Galvin, E. G., Schmitt, R. H., and Phillips, J. G.: Functional bracing of fractures of the shaft of the humerus. J. Bone Joint Surg., *59-A*:596, 1977.
41. Schneider, P.: Humeral fractures and their treatment in children. Ther. Umsch., *26*:136, 1969.
42. Shah, J. J., and Bhatti, N. A.: Radial nerve paralysis associated with fracture of the humerus. A review of 62 cases. Clin. Orthop., *172*:171, 1983.
43. Trotter, D. H., and Dobozi, W.: Nonunion of the humerus: Rigid fixation, bone grafting and adjunctive bone cement. Clin. Orthop., *204*:162, 1986.
44. VanderGriend, R., Tomasin, J., and Ward, E. F.: Open reduction and internal fixation of humeral shaft fractures. Results using AO plating techniques. J. Bone Joint Surg., *68-A*:430, 1986.
45. Wessely, J.: Basic indications for osteosynthesis in juvenile shaft fractures. Hefte Unfallheilkd., *129*:383, 1977.
46. Wolfe, J. S., and Eyring, E. J.: Median-nerve entrapment within a greenstick fracture. J. Bone Joint Surg., *56-A*:1270, 1974.

SUPRACONDYLAR FRACTURE OF THE HUMERUS

A supracondylar fracture of the humerus lies within the metaphysis of the distal humerus and proximal to the transverse physeal line. It is the most common type of elbow fracture in children and adolescents. According to most series, it accounts for between 50 and 60 per cent of elbow fractures and is seen most frequently in children between the ages of three and ten years. The peak incidence is between five and eight years; the incidence in males is twice as frequent as in females, and the left arm is involved more commonly than the right arm.[115]

The high incidence of deformities in the elbow and the potential neurovascular complications that result from supracondylar fractures make it a serious injury.

Mechanism of Injury and Classification

Two types of supracondylar fracture are designated, according to the position of the forearm in relation to the arm at the time of injury, and the displacement of the distal fragment.

The more common *extension type* accounts for approximately 95 per cent of cases. It is caused by a fall on the outstretched hand with hyperextension of the elbow. The distal fragment may be tilted posteriorly with the anterior cortex fractured but the posterior cortex intact (incomplete or greenstick fracture); or the fracture may be complete with the distal fragment displaced posterior to the proximal fragment (Fig. 8–22). In the totally displaced fractures the distal fragment lies medial or lateral to the lower end of the proximal fragment. Medial displacement is much more common than lateral displacement; this is due to the pull of triceps brachii and biceps brachii muscles, which originate and lie more medially on the

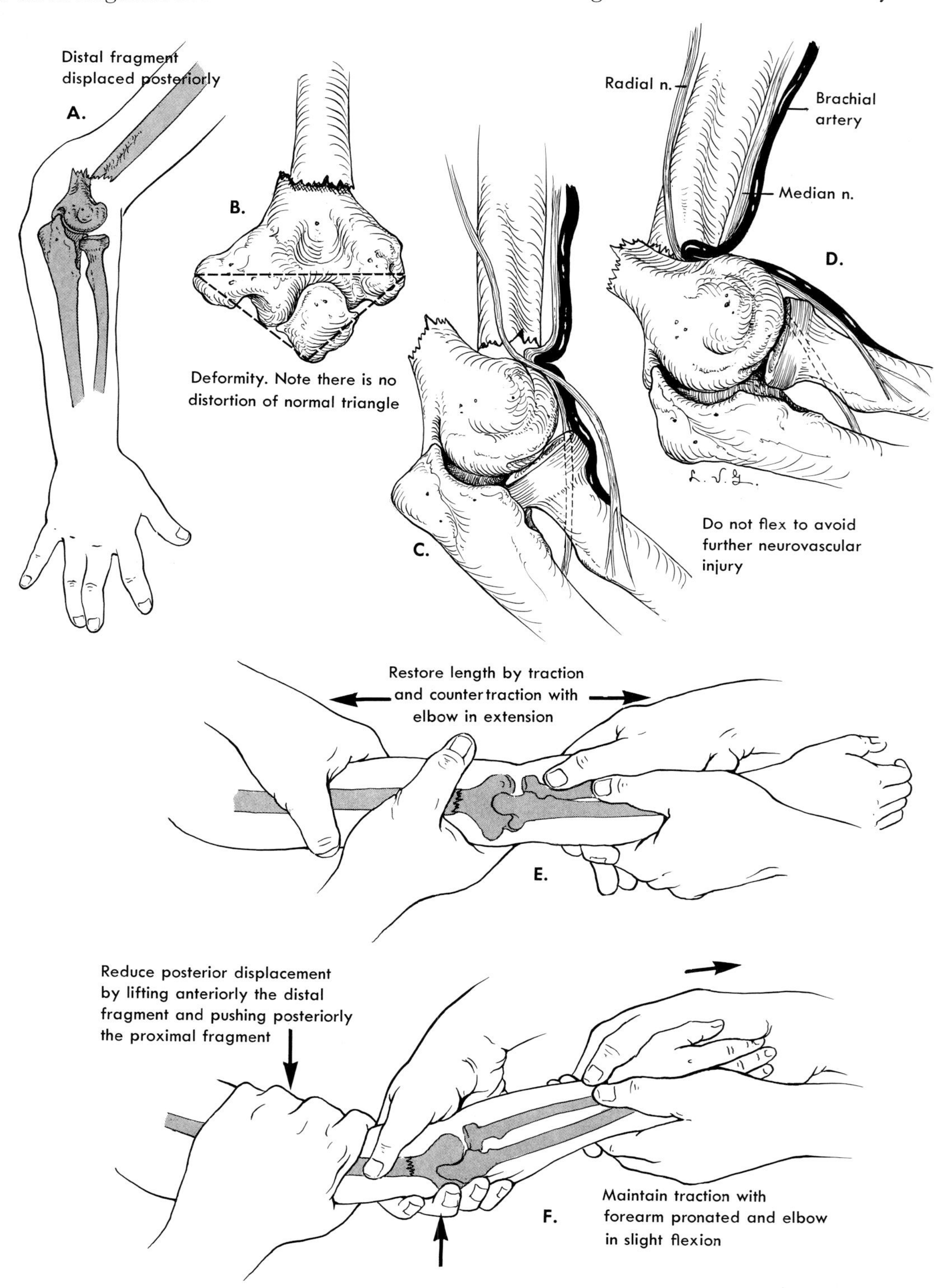

FIGURE 8–22. Supracondylar fracture of the humerus—extension type (see text for explanation).

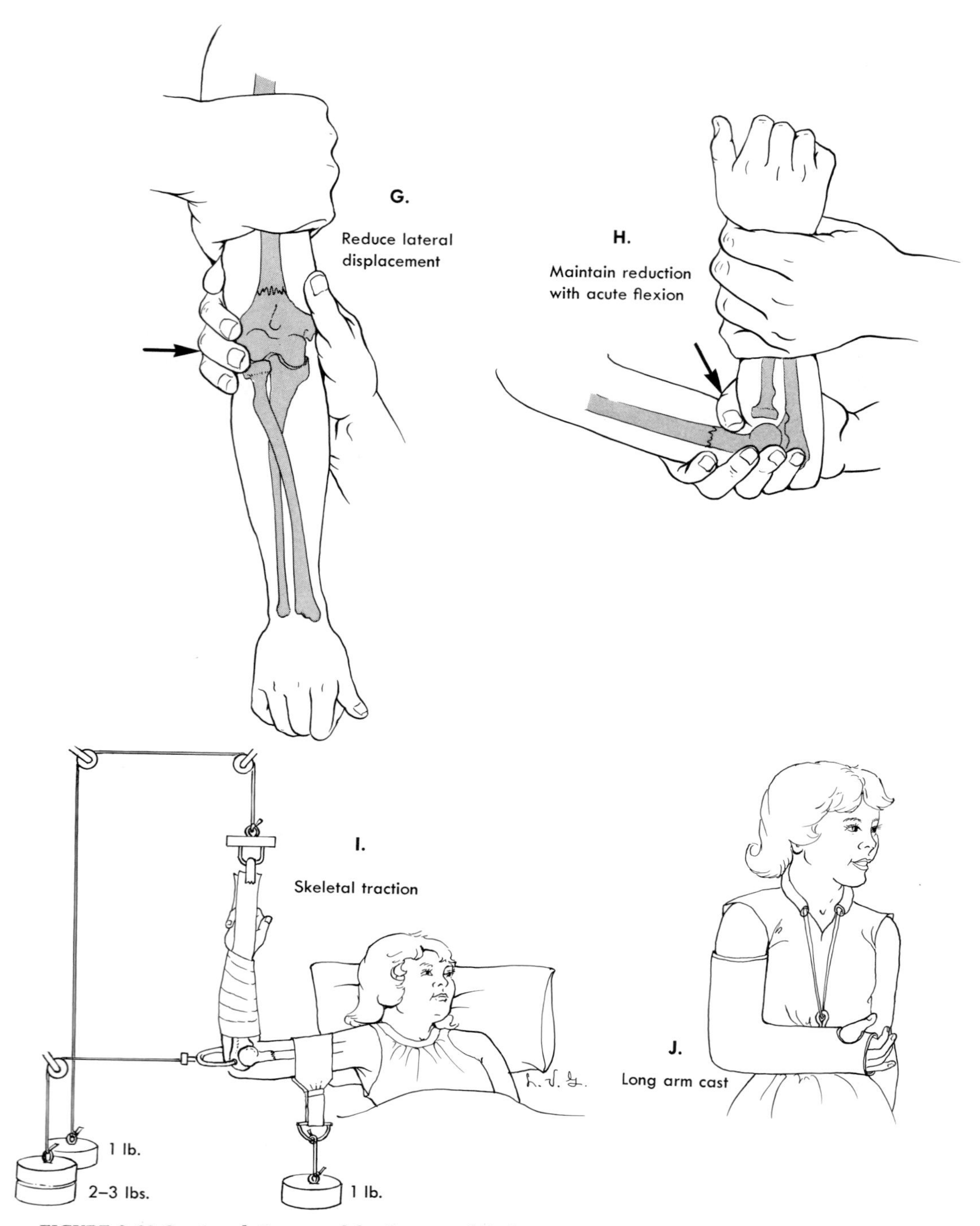

FIGURE 8–22 Continued. Supracondylar fracture of the humerus—extension type (see text for explanation).

shaft of the humerus.[125] Another factor to consider is the direction of the fracturing force, which is more adduction than abduction.[102, 103]

The *flexion type* is rare, occurring in about 5 per cent of cases. It usually is caused by a fall in which a direct blow on the posterior aspect of the flexed elbow is sustained. The result is anterior angulation or displacement of the distal fragment (Fig. 8–23). Again, the fracture may be incomplete (greenstick) with the anterior cortex intact or complete.

According to the degree of displacement of the fragments, three grades of supracondylar fractures of the humerus are recognized: (1)

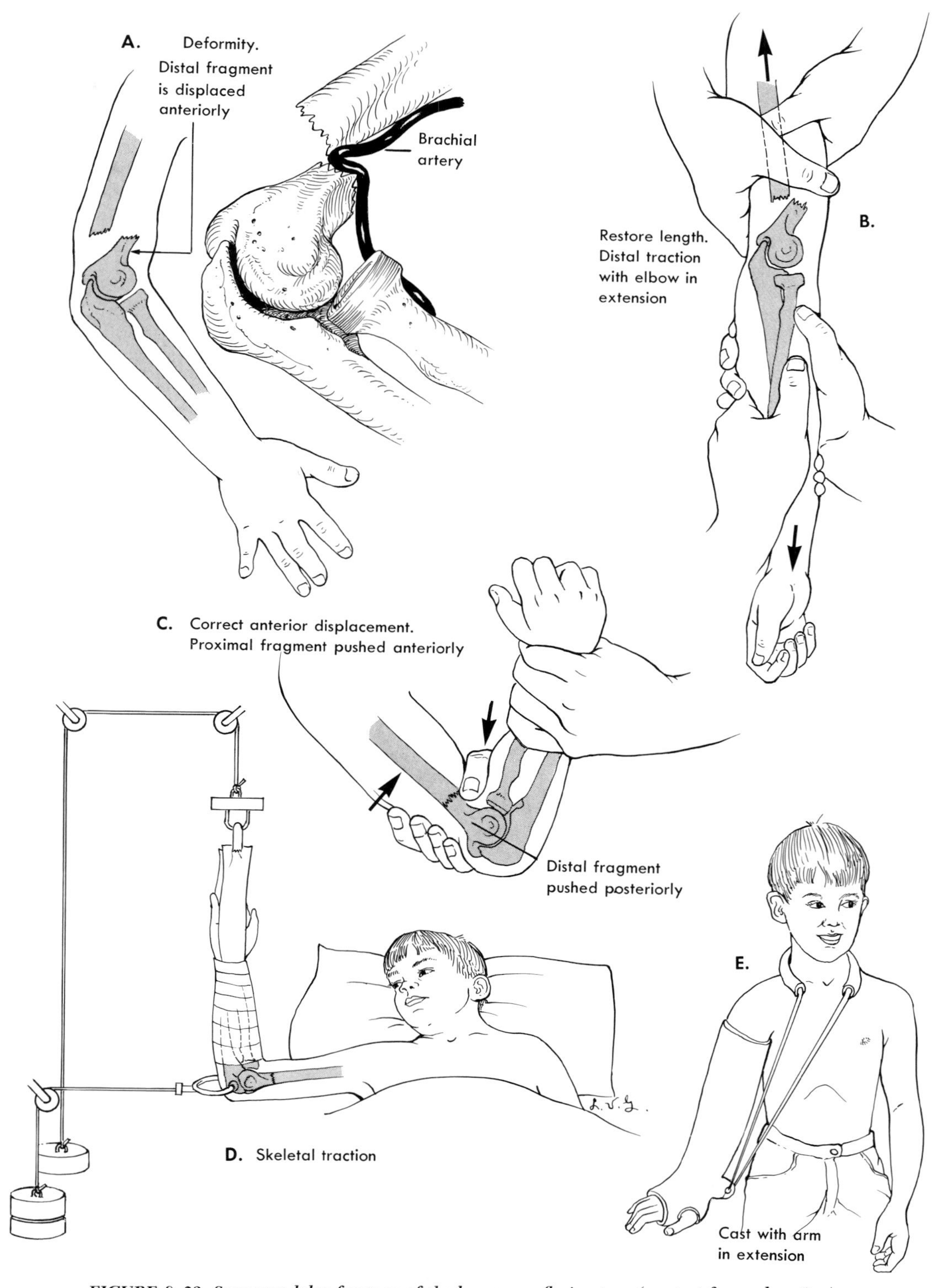

FIGURE 8–23. Supracondylar fracture of the humerus—flexion type (see text for explanation).

fracture with no displacement; (a) without comminution of medial or lateral cortex; (b) with comminution of medial or lateral cortex; (2) fracture with angulation of the distal fragment; the posterior cortex is intact in the extension type and the anterior cortex is intact in the flexion type; and (3) fracture with moderate or severe displacement in which there is no contact between the cortices of the two fragments. In the extension type the displacement may be posteromedial or posterolateral.

It is important that in supracondylar fractures the exact type and the degree and direction of the displacement be delineated, since the method of treatment varies accordingly.

Pathologic Anatomy

EXTENSION TYPE

The fracture line extends immediately proximal to the epicondyles and distal to the termination of the distal diaphysis. In the sagittal plane, it traverses obliquely upward and backward, and in the frontal plane, it is frequently transverse (Fig. 8–22 A and B). The older the patient, the more oblique the fracture line tends to be in the frontal plane. As a rule, transverse fractures are more stable than oblique ones. When the fracture line is transverse, simple rotation does not angulate the distal fragment, whereas if the fracture line is oblique, rotation will angulate the distal fragment.

Posteromedially displaced fractures tend to angulate into varus; posterolaterally displaced fractures angulate into valgus.[13] A medially displaced distal fragment tends to rotate posteromedially. In the posterolateral displacement the distal fragment is rotated laterally. The fracture is often complete, and sometimes greenstick, with the posterior cortex intact.

The distal fragment is displaced proximally and posteriorly by the fracturing force transmitted upward through the bones of the forearm and because of the pull of the triceps muscle. It is often tilted laterally or medially and rotated medially.

The lower end of the proximal fragment projects anteriorly and stretches or pierces the periosteum, forcing its way into the brachialis anticus and biceps brachii. The periosteum is stripped from both the anterior surface of the distal fragment and the posterior surface of the proximal fragment. The degree of displacement of the fracture fragments is limited by the extent of periosteal stripping.

In the experimental production of hyperextension supracondylar fractures in monkeys, Abraham and associates found three progressive stages of periosteal changes: *Stage I*—The periosteum is stretched but still intact and not torn. This takes place in minimally displaced fractures. *Stage II*—With progressive displacement of the fracture the periosteum stretches farther and becomes partially torn by the sharp anterior edge of the proximal fragment. *Stage III*—The periosteum is completely torn anteriorly and stripped posteriorly from the proximal fragment for a variable distance. A variable portion of the periosteum remains attached to the distal fragment, which may become interposed between the fracture fragments.[1]

There is a considerable amount of local bleeding and swelling. The hematoma that infiltrates the antecubital fossa may compress neurovascular structures. The brachialis muscle shields the anterior neurovascular structures from injury. In severely displaced fractures the sharp spikes of the bone ends perforate the brachialis muscle and contuse, occlude, or lacerate vessels and nerves (Fig. 8–22 C and D). Medially the brachial vessels and median nerve are at high risk. In medially displaced fractures the supratrochlear artery will bind the brachial vessels, which will tether across the spike and become completely occluded.[249] The median nerve may become compressed or lacerated by the sharp edge of the anteromedial bony spike of the proximal fragment. The brachial vessels and median nerve can occasionally become trapped and compressed between the fracture fragments.[281] Laterally the radial nerve may be injured by the anterolateral spike.

In severe displacements the skin may be penetrated by the sharp bony spike and the fracture may be open.

FLEXION TYPE

In the sagittal plane, the fracture line courses from below upward and forward. The proximal fragment is displaced posteriorly, whereas the distal fragment is displaced anteriorly and upward (Fig. 8–23 A). There may be a varying degree of medial or lateral tilting and rotation. The periosteum is stripped from the posterior surface of the distal fragment and from the anterior surface of the proximal fragment. Soft-tissue swelling and damage are usually much less than in the extension type. The problem occurs when the fracture fragments are displaced—the ulnar nerve is at high risk; it tents over the posterior margin of the proximal fragment. The brachial vessels may be kinked between the fracture fragments.

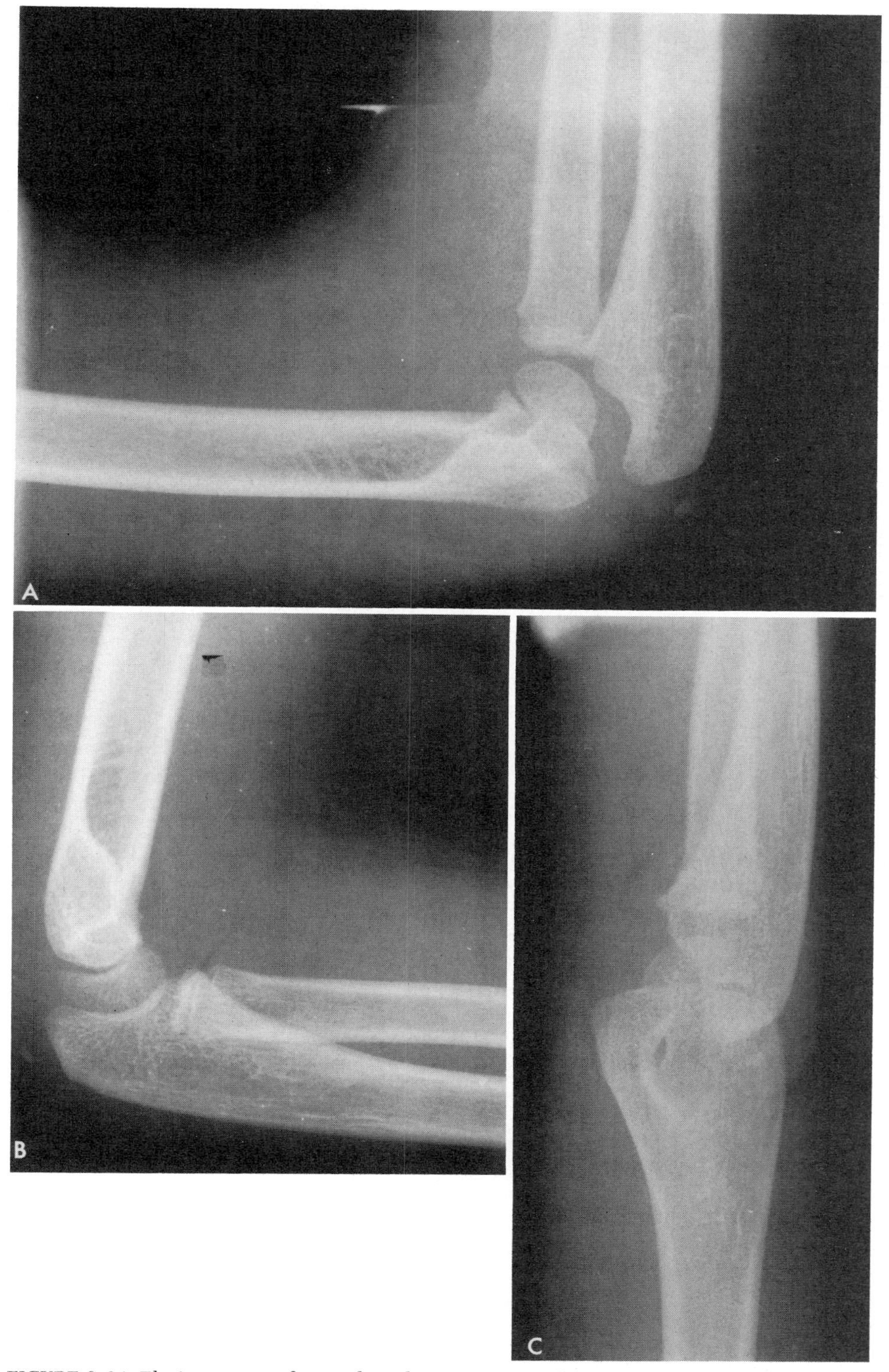

FIGURE 8–24. The importance of a true lateral view in suspected supracondylar fracture of humerus.

A. An oblique view of distal humerus suggesting supracondylar fracture and anterior tilting of distal fragment. **B** and **C.** A true lateral radiogram of the distal humerus and a semioblique view show that there is no fracture. These radiograms emphasize the importance of a true lateral view of the distal humerus; when in doubt, one should make comparative views of the opposite uninjured elbow.

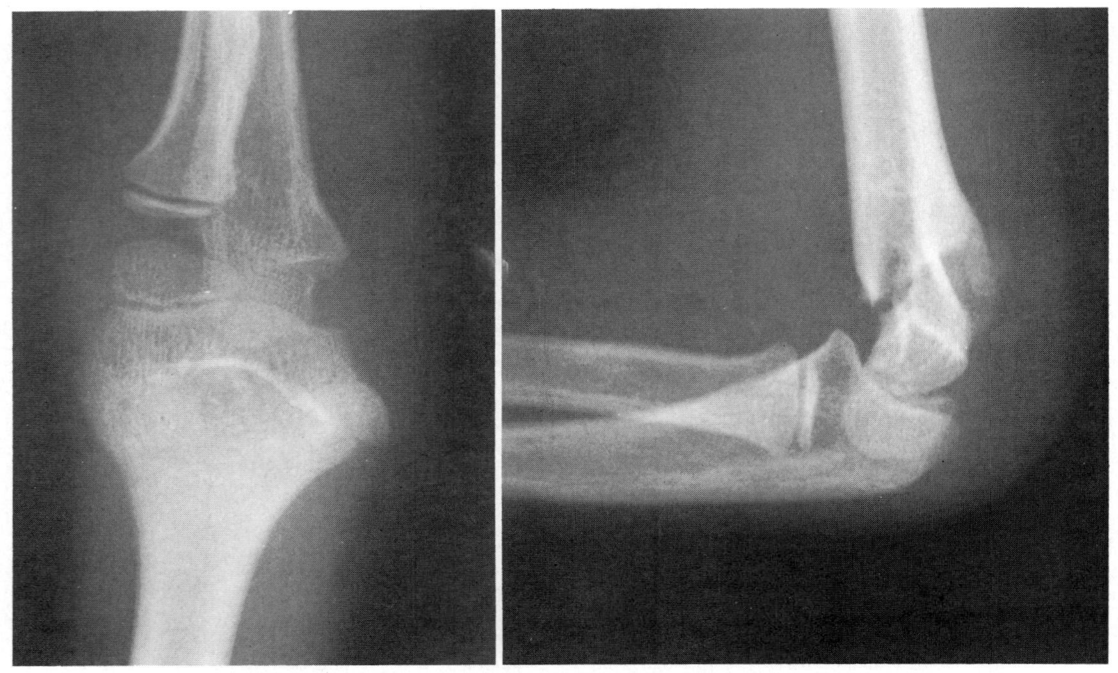

FIGURE 8–25. Radiograms showing undisplaced supracondylar fracture of the humerus.

Diagnosis

Supracondylar fracture of the humerus is diagnosed by the history, by clinical findings, and by radiographic studies. In the simple undisplaced supracondylar fracture seen soon following injury, swelling may be minimal, and the most characteristic finding will be tenderness over the supracondylar region of the humerus. In supracondylar fracture of the humerus the local tenderness and swelling are both medial and lateral over the supracondylar ridges, whereas in lateral condylar fractures they are lateral, and in medial epicondylar fractures, medial. In radial neck fracture the tenderness is over the radial neck posterolaterally.

In the presence of more violent injury with displacement of the fragments, swelling and deformity of the elbow become more characteristic. In general, the amount of swelling depends on the severity of the fracture and the time that has elapsed between the occurrence of the injury and the examination of the patient; in a patient seen several hours following trauma, tension develops in the antecubital area owing to the extravasation of blood, and skin changes in the form of blebs may occur. There is usually severe pain, and examination of the posterior aspect of the lower humerus will reveal a discontinuity of the bone. In the *extension type* the anteriorly displaced proximal fragment is often palpable beneath the skin. In the presence of overriding, there will be shortening of the involved arm and an S-shaped configuration of the upper limb in the region of the elbow joint. In the rare *flexion type* the elbow is held in flexion; posteriorly the prominence of the olecranon is less than normal because of anterior angulation or displacement of the distal fragment.

In hyperextension injuries the distal fragment is usually displaced posteromedially and rotated medially. The forearm follows the distal fragment of the humerus; therefore, the elbow and forearm are rotated medially and tilted into varus. In the more rare posterolateral displacement of the distal fragment, the elbow and forearm are rotated laterally and tilted into valgus.

Clinically, supracondylar fractures of the humerus may be mistaken for acute dislocation of the elbow—in the latter the tip of the olecranon is far posterior to the epicondyles of the humerus, and the bony prominence on the anterior aspect of the elbow joint is smooth (because it is produced by humeral condyles) and more distal than in supracondylar fractures.

Most important in the physical examination is the careful assessment of the vascular and neural function in the injured limb. Any neu-

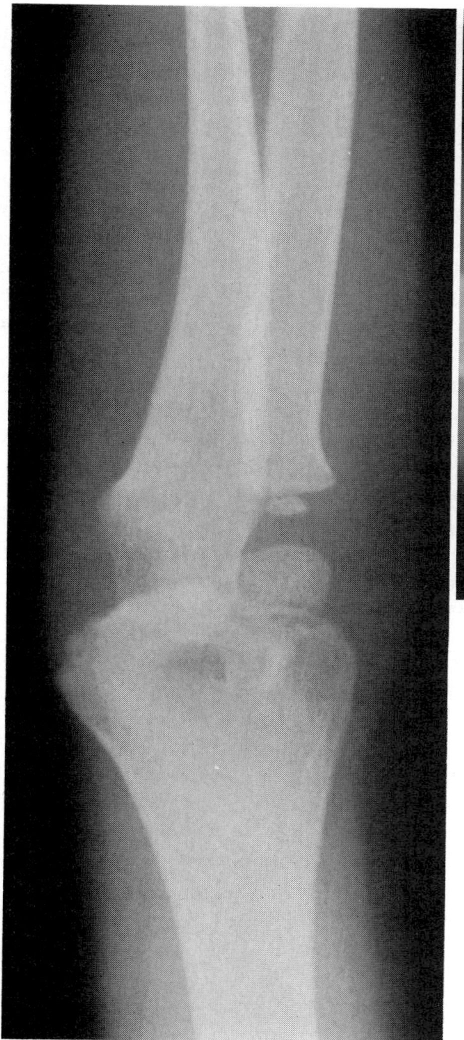

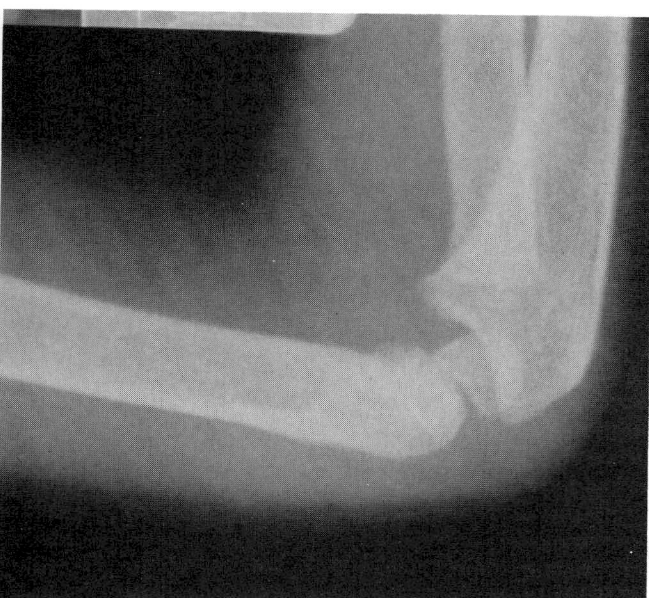

FIGURE 8–26. Supracondylar fracture—extension type.

The fracture is minimally displaced and is treated by simple immobilization in a posterior plaster of Paris mold.

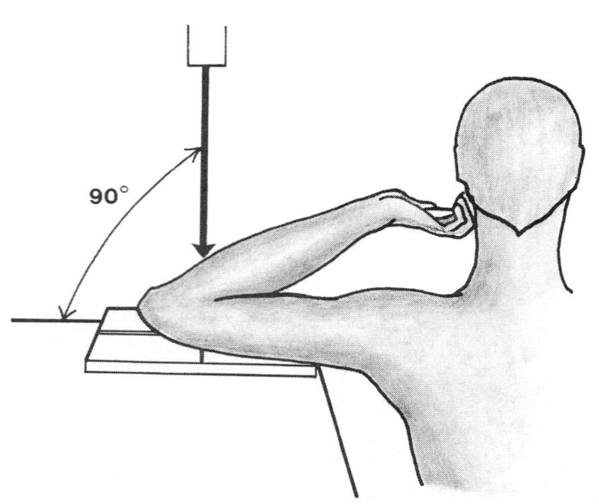

FIGURE 8–27. Jones axial radiographic view of the elbow.

(Redrawn after Rockwood, C. A., Wilkins, K. E., and King, R. E. (eds.): Fractures in Children. Philadelphia, J. B. Lippincott, 1984, p. 373.)

rovascular deficit should be recorded. Failure to detect vascular injuries will be disastrous, resulting in permanent deformity and disability.

The treating physician should be constantly alert for any signs of pain, pallor, cyanosis, absence of pulse, coldness, or paralysis, any of which may indicate the possibility of impending Volksmann's ischemia.

Radiographic Findings. The diagnosis is confirmed by radiographic examination (Figs. 8–24 to 8–26). The injured elbow is painful and difficult to straighten into full extension; therefore, the Jones axial view is made for the anteroposterior view of the distal humerus (Fig. 8–27). It is vital that the x-ray tube be directed perpendicular to the film in the cassette and not tilted cephalad. The superimposed upper radius and ulna may make visualization of the distal humerus difficult; in such an instance medial and lateral oblique views are made.

A true lateral view of the distal humerus is made, preferably with the elbow in 90 degrees of flexion. It is a mistake to rotate the upper limb medially or laterally to take a true lateral projection. Place the arm at the side of the chest with the elbow flexed to right angles, and insert the cassette with the film between the chest and elbow. When a nondisplaced or minimally displaced supracondylar fracture of the humerus is suspected, the importance of obtaining an exact lateral projection cannot be overemphasized. When a supracondylar fracture is suspected, a true lateral projection of the distal humerus should be obtained; often a false diagnosis of fracture is made by the finding on an oblique view of anterior tilting of the distal humeral epiphysis. When in doubt, one should make radiograms of both elbows for comparison. In an oblique view the distal humeral epiphysis may appear tilted anteriorly, and often a false diagnosis of supracondylar fracture is made (see Fig. 8–24).

In the anteroposterior projection the angle between the physeal line of the lateral condyle of the humerus and a line perpendicular to the long axis of the humeral shaft is determined. This is referred to as Baumann's angle, which is a reliable method of assessing angular deformity of the distal humerus (Fig. 8–28). However, if the x-ray tube is angulated in the cephalocaudal direction greater than 20 degrees, Baumann's angle may change and become inaccurate. Another method of determining the alignment of the distal humerus is measurement of the angle between the distal humeral articular surface (a line drawn parallel to the ossification margin of the distal humerus) and the longitudinal axis of the humeral shaft.

In the lateral projection one should carefully scrutinize the "fat pad sign."[215] The *anterior "fat pad"* is a triangular radiolucency ventral to the distal humerus; it is clearly visualized, and in the presence of effusion into the elbow joint it is displaced anteriorly. The *posterior "fat pad"* is not visible when the elbow is flexed at right angles; however, if there is effusion into the joint by intra-articular fracture or a dislocation that is spontaneously reduced, it is visualized. Distal humeral fractures will cause subperiosteal bleeding and elevate the posterior fat pad.

In the true lateral radiogram of the elbow the configuration and alignment of the distal hu-

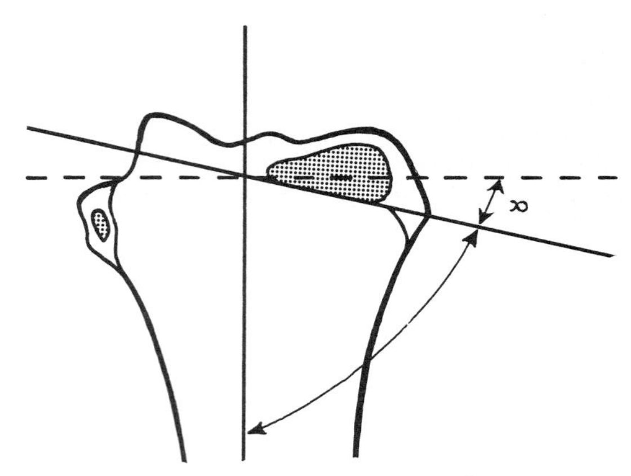

FIGURE 8–28. Baumann's angle.

(Redrawn after Rockwood, C. A., Wilkins, K. E., and King, R. E. (eds.): Fractures in Children. Philadelphia, J. B. Lippincott, 1984, p. 373.)

merus should be carefully assessed: (1) In the normal elbow the distal humerus will project as a "teardrop"; the lower part of the teardrop is formed by the ossific center of the capitellum (Fig. 8–29 A); (2) the angle formed by the long axis of the humerus and the long axis of the lateral condyle is about 40 degrees (Fig. 8–29 B). In supracondylar fractures with posterior tilting of the distal fragment the humerolateral condylar lateral angle will diminish, whereas with anterior tilting of the distal fragment it will increase; (3) the anterior humeral line, i.e., the line drawn through the anterior cortex of the distal humerus, will pass through the middle third of the ossific nucleus of the capitellum (Fig. 8–29 C). In supracondylar fractures the anterior humeral line will be abnormal.[246] (4) The coronoid line—a line drawn projected superiorly along the anterior border of the coronoid process—will just touch the anterior border of the lateral condyle of the humerus (Fig. 8–29 D). In supracondylar fractures in which the distal fragment is tilted posteriorly the coronoid line passes anterior to the anterior border of the lateral condyle.

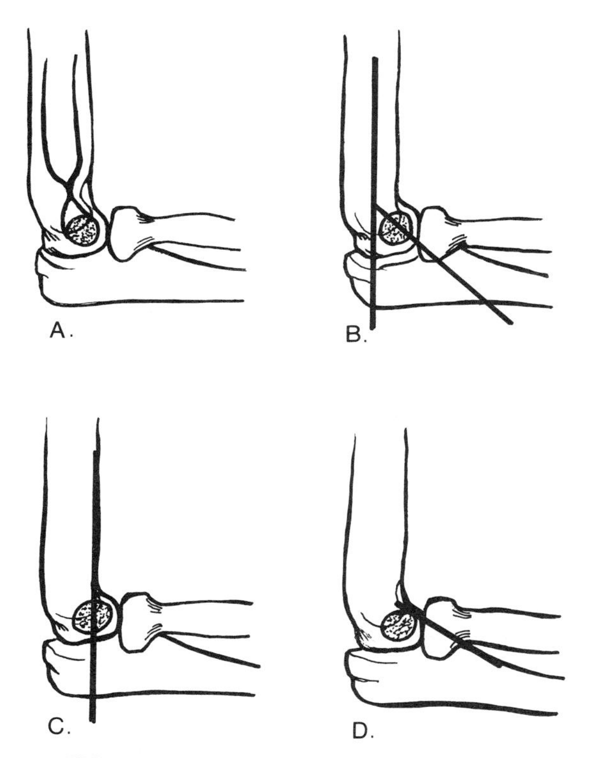

FIGURE 8–29. Drawings of the lateral x-ray of the normal distal humerus showing the lateral radiographic lines.

A. The "teardrop" of the normal distal humerus in lateral radiogram of the elbow; its distal part is formed by the ossific center of the capitellum. **B.** The angle formed by the long axis of the humerus and the long axis of the lateral condyle. In the normal elbow it is about 40 degrees. **C.** The "anterior-humeral line," i.e., the line drawn through the anterior cortex of the distal humerus. In the normal elbow it should pass through the middle third of the ossific nucleus of the capitellum. When the distal humerus is angulated posteriorly, the anterior humeral line passes in the anterior third or anterior to the ossific center of the capitellum. **D.** The "coronoid line" is the line drawn along the anterior border of the coronoid process. In the normal elbow it will just touch the anterior border of the lateral condyle. (Redrawn after Rockwood, C. A., Wilkins, K. E., and King, R. E. (eds.): Fractures in Children. Philadelphia, J. B. Lippincott, 1984.)

Instructions on the x-ray requisition should specify that anteroposterior and true lateral projections of the distal humerus, including the elbow joint, be made. An anteroposterior view of the elbow will reveal whether the fracture line is transverse or oblique, and whether the distal fragment is medially or laterally angulated. Look for comminution and compression of the medial or lateral cortices of the distal humerus. A lateral view of the elbow will show whether the distal fragment is displaced posteriorly or anteriorly. If a nondisplaced or minimally displaced fracture is clinically suspected and anteroposterior and lateral radiograms do not demonstrate the fracture, make oblique views and comparative views of the opposite elbow.

The anatomic level of the fracture line should be carefully studied. A common mistake is to include fractures through the distal diaphysis of the humerus as supracondylar fracture. A fracture to be classified as supracondylar should be a metaphyseal fracture. Distal diaphyseal fractures of the humerus are unstable, and reduction is difficult to maintain. Another error is to miss involvement of the distal humeral physis. Transcondylar and T-fractures of the distal humerus are very rare in children.

When a child is anesthetized for closed reduction, it is advisable to repeat the radiograms if necessary to delineate the exact level of the fracture and to ascertain whether the physis is involved. Occasionally after reduction and immobilization in cast, one may have to make computerized axial tomographic studies for accurate delineation of the pathology.

Treatment

EMERGENCY SPLINTING

Proper splinting of the limb before sending the patient to the radiography department and while awaiting definitive treatment is very important. In extension type fractures, flexion of the elbow should be avoided, as it may cause further damage to neurovascular structures (see Fig. 8–22 D). The limb is immobilized in a simple splint (aluminum or padded board with loosely applied bandage) in the deformed position that it lies in, preferably with the elbow in extension and the forearm in pronation. Circulation should always be checked prior to and following application of the splint. The radial pulse should be assessed to determine whether it is normal and whether capillary return is good. Sensation and motor function are also carefully checked and recorded.

The method of treatment is dependent upon the degree of displacement of the fracture fragments and the amount of soft-tissue swelling, and whether there is any disturbance of neurovascular function.

Supracondylar fractures in children should be managed as acute emergencies. The most effective method of preventing local swelling (or decreasing it if the elbow is already swollen) is to achieve immediate reduction and restore normal alignment.

UNDISPLACED OR MINIMALLY DISPLACED FRACTURES

Treatment of undisplaced or minimally displaced hyperextension type supracondylar fractures of the humerus consists of application of a posterior plaster splint with the elbow flexed at 90 degrees and the forearm in pronation (Figs. 8–25 and 8–26). The plaster splint is kept on for four weeks. Follow-up radiograms are taken after a week and again at the time the posterior splint is removed. It is important that the status of circulation be assessed in the first 24 to 48 hours and the family of the patient be educated to recognize the signs and symptoms of circulatory embarrassment. In a mildly displaced fracture with moderate swelling, it is advised that the child be admitted to the hospital for a period of one or two days for observation.

The average time required for bony union to take place is three weeks; full range of movement in the elbow usually returns in about eight weeks.

Cubitus varus can occur owing to collapse of the medial cortex of the distal humerus following minimally displaced fractures treated by simple plaster immobilization. Two such cases were reported by Fahey, who cautioned that one must be on the alert for the possibility of such an unfavorable outcome, even when the displacement does not appear to be of such magnitude that reduction is required.[79] If there is compression on the medial side, the fracture should be manipulated and medial tilting and rotation of the distal fragment corrected first, followed by flexion of the elbow to correct posterior tilting of the distal fragment. Clinically the carrying angle of the elbow, and radiographically Baumann's angle, should always be matched with the contralateral normal side.

MODERATELY DISPLACED FRACTURES WITH INTACT POSTERIOR CORTEX

When local swelling is minimal and neurovascular function normal, the moderately displaced extension type supracondylar fracture with intact posterior cortex is treated by closed reduction performed under general anesthesia. The technique is as follows: (1) Length should first be restored by traction and countertraction with the elbow in extension but *not hyperextension* to prevent pulling and injury of the brachial vessels (see Fig. 8–22 E). (2) Next, while maintaining traction (with the forearm pronated and the elbow in slight flexion), reduce posterior displacement of the distal fragment by lifting it anteriorly and by pushing the proximal fragment posteriorly (see Fig. 8–22 F). (3) Then reduce lateral displacement by pushing the distal fragment medially; any rotational deformity is also corrected at this time (see Fig. 8–22 G). (4) The elbow is hyperflexed to 90 degrees to tighten the posterior hinge of the periosteum and to maintain the reduction.

In supracondylar fractures, the biceps brachii muscle loses its supinating action because of the break in continuity of the humerus. The unopposed action of the strong pronator teres muscle swings the proximal radioulnar joint into pronation. Since the joint is fixed by the pronators, varus deformity at the fracture site will result. The direction of original displacement of the distal fragment is another consideration in deciding the position of the forearm when it is immobilized in the cast; if it was *displaced medially*, the forearm is *pronated* in order to tighten the medial hinge and to close the fracture line on the lateral side, thus preventing any cubitus varus deformity; but if the distal fragment was *displaced laterally*, *supination* of the forearm will tighten the lateral periosteal hinge and close the fracture line on the medial side, thus preventing cubitus valgus.

Next, radiograms are made in the anteroposterior and lateral projections to determine the adequacy of reduction (Figs. 8–30 and 8–31). *Any medial or lateral tilting of the distal fragment must be completely corrected;* if not corrected, it will result in cubitus varus or valgus

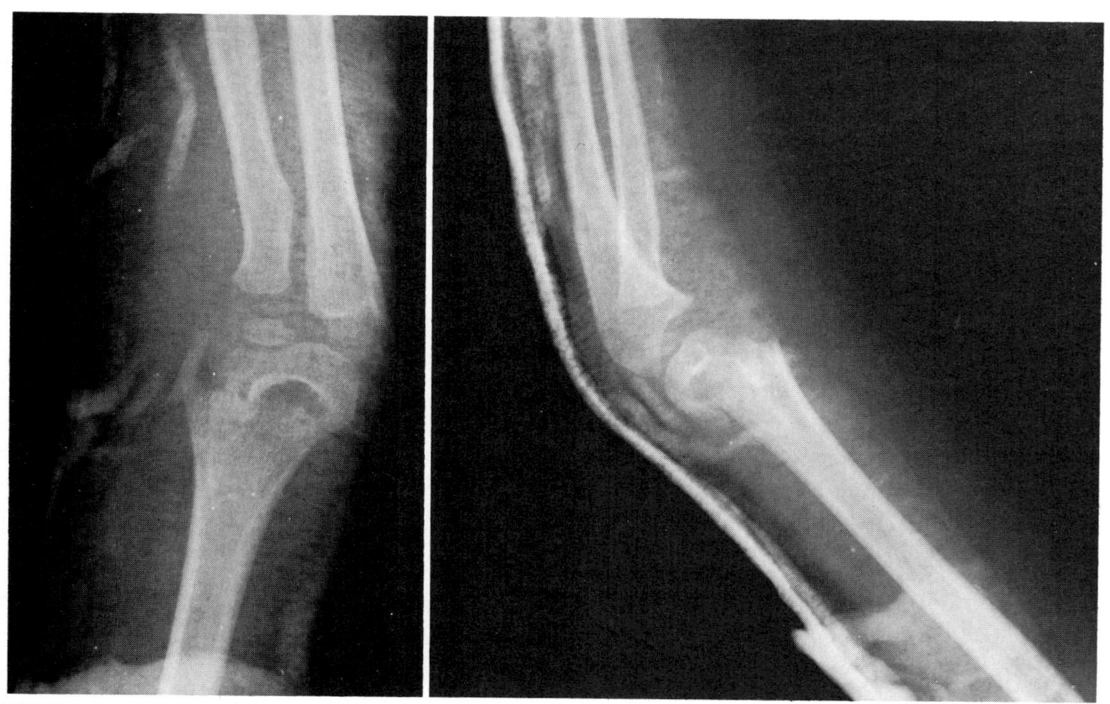

FIGURE 8–30. Moderately displaced extension type of supracondylar fracture of the humerus with some bony contact.

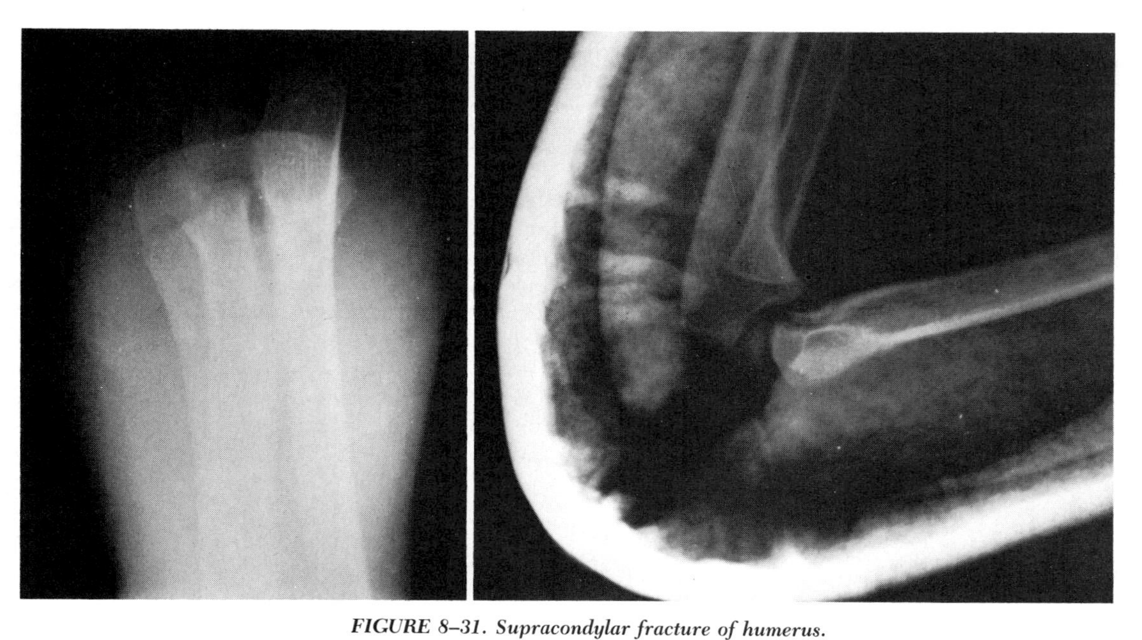

FIGURE 8–31. Supracondylar fracture of humerus.

Radiographic views immediately following reduction show accurate anatomic alignment.

deformity. Appositional malalignments are inconsequential, as they will correct themselves spontaneously by extensive remodeling and have no effect on the carrying angle or final range of motion of the elbow. Rotation of the distal fragment is not corrected by remodeling and may look bizarre in the radiogram, but it will be compensated clinically by rotation at the shoulder. Posterior angulation of the distal fragment will result in hyperextension at the elbow and anterior angulation in flexion deformity; however, these deformities are in the plane of motion of the elbow and spontaneously correct themselves.[14, 268]

Vigorous manipulations and remanipulations should be avoided, as they may cause further damage to vessels, nerves, and soft tissues.

Following satisfactory reduction, peripheral circulation is again assessed. If it is normal, an above-elbow cast is applied for immobilization. The cast should not constrict the soft tissues in the antecubital area. A window is cut out in the region of the radial artery at the wrist to check circulation.

Following manipulative reduction the intact posterior cortex may break, making the fracture unstable. In such an instance, percutaneous pinning may be advisable.

In the presence of marked swelling and skin blistering, closed reduction is carried out as just outlined, but instead of immobilization in the cast, Dunlop skin traction is applied to the injured limb for several days until the swelling subsides. Peripheral circulation is also closely observed. It is not necessary to apply skeletal traction when the original fracture was only moderately displaced with intact posterior cortex and when anatomic stable reduction has been achieved. After the swelling subsides, the elbow is immobilized in an above-elbow cast, as previously described. Some surgeons prefer to elevate the injured arm in traction prior to attempting closed reduction, but as already stated, early reduction of the fracture will promote decrease of the swelling.

Radiograms are made periodically (at four and ten days) following injury to check maintenance of reduction, and then again at three weeks. The total period of immobilization is about four to six weeks.

The *flexion type of supracondylar fracture of the humerus* (the reverse type with the distal fragment displaced forward) is a simpler injury to treat when the fracture is greenstick with anterior cortex intact or when minimally displaced (see Fig. 8–23). Closed reduction is carried out by longitudinal traction with the elbow in extension; the distal fragment is displaced posteriorly followed by correction of lateral tilting and displacement by manual pressure. The elbow is immobilized in extension. Occasionally the fragments are severely displaced, and the fracture may require treatment by percutaneous pinning or skeletal traction as described next. Ulnar nerve injury may necessitate open reduction and internal fixation.

SEVERELY DISPLACED FRACTURES

A completely displaced supracondylar fracture of the humerus is best treated by *closed manipulative reduction* followed by maintenance of reduction, preferably by *closed percutaneous pinning.*

When the elbow is very swollen, skeletal traction is applied for an initial period of 10 to 14 days to maintain the reduction, followed by immobilization in a cast (Figs. 8–32 and 8–33). When satisfactory reduction cannot be achieved by closed manipulation, two options are available—primary open reduction and internal fixation, or an attempt at closed reduction by skeletal traction followed by retention in cast.

Closed Manipulative Reduction. This should be performed under general anesthesia with the child completely relaxed. Axillary or regional block anesthesia or local hematoma infiltration with lidocaine is not adequate; either will aggravate the apprehension of the child who is in acute pain. In addition, the anesthesiologist may be blamed for any neurovascular compromise when such residual loss complicates the picture.

Image intensifier radiographic control is essential. Take further radiograms if the preoperative radiograms were not adequate to delineate the degree and direction of fracture and to determine whether the physis is involved. Initially attempt reduction by manipulation as described on page 3068. When adequate reduction cannot be obtained, this author recommends manipulation with skeletal traction with a threaded pin through the olecranon. The same pin may be used for skeletal traction, if necessary.

The technique of pin insertion through the olecranon is as follows: The child's arm is suspended by an assistant while the surgeon inserts a threaded Kirschner wire (3/32 inch in diameter) through the crest of the ulna about 2.5 to 3 cm. distal to the tip of the olecranon process and 1 to 1.5 cm. anterior to its posterior border. The level of the pin in the olecranon should be immediately proximal to the coronoid process; if it is distal to it, the traction force tends to

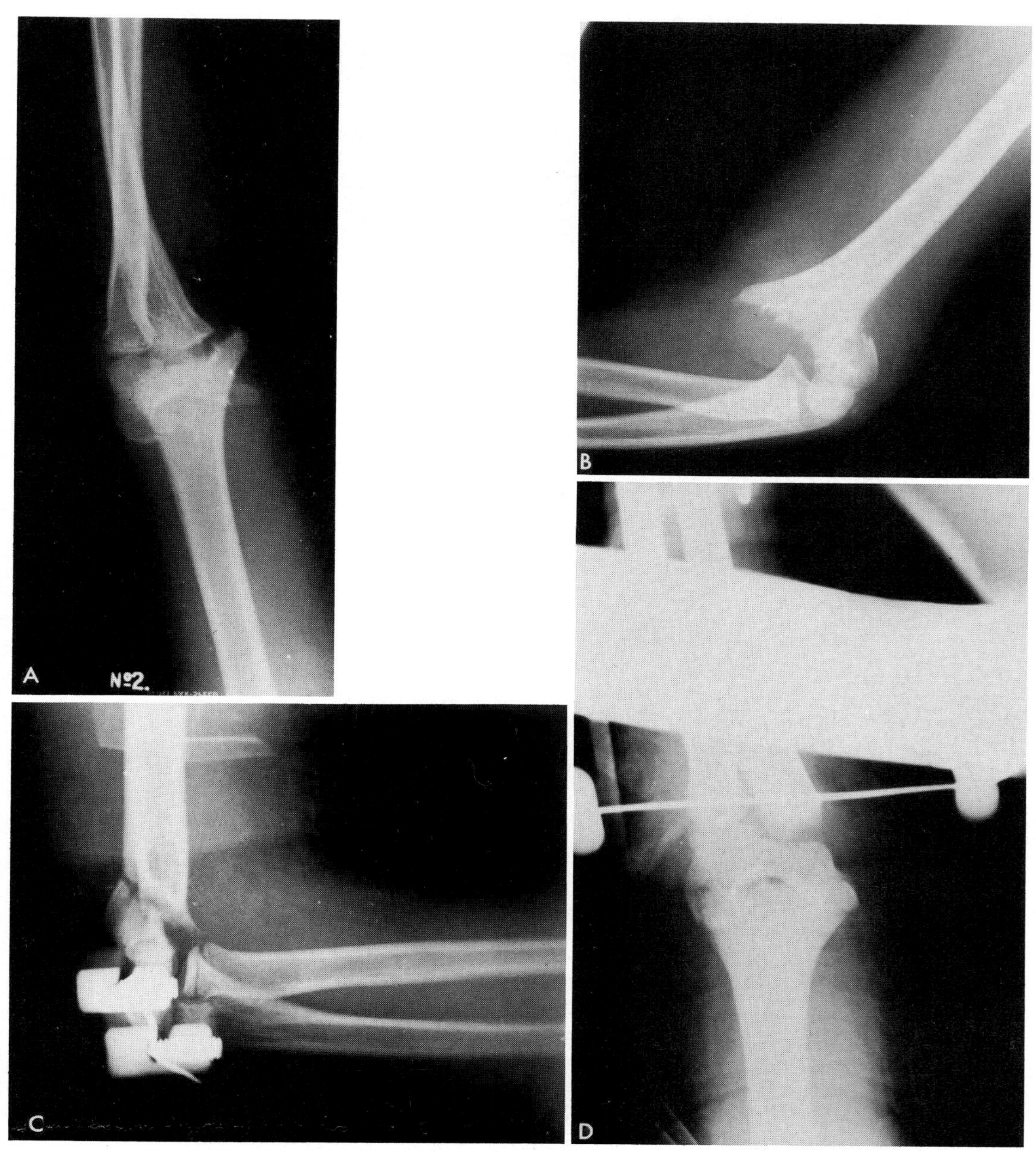

FIGURE 8–32. Supracondylar fracture of the humerus—markedly displaced.

The fracture was treated by insertion of threaded Kirschner wire through olecranon, closed manipulative reduction, and skeletal traction for 18 days followed by immobilization in plaster of Paris cast for two more weeks. **A** and **B.** Initial radiograms. **C** and **D.** Radiograms while in traction, showing satisfactory alignment.

Illustration continued on following page

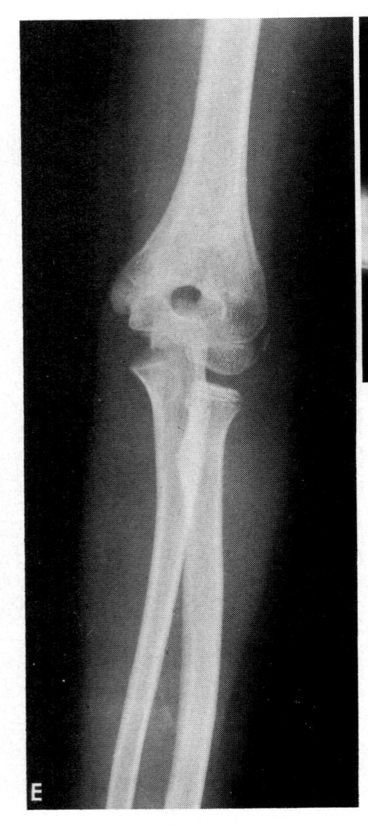

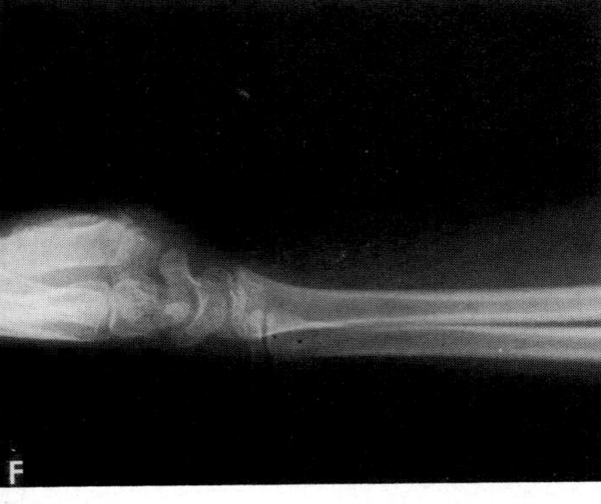

FIGURE 8–32 Continued. Supracondylar fracture of the humerus—markedly displaced.

E and **F.** Radiograms three months later, showing healing in good position.

extend rather than flex the elbow.[104] Bony landmarks about the elbow are carefully identified, and the wire is drilled from the medial to the lateral side so as to avoid injury to the ulnar nerve. The assistant should not acutely flex the elbow in an attempt to increase the prominence of the olecranon. A threaded Kirschner wire is used to prevent it from becoming loose and causing pin tract infection. A traction bow is fastened to the wire, and the fracture is manipulated as previously described. The relationship of the bony prominence on the posterior aspect of the elbow is determined. As stated, any lateral or medial tilting of the distal fragment is unacceptable. The result is good if the reduction of the fracture is good. Do not accept borderline reduction! Radiograms are made to determine the accuracy of reduction. The circulation is checked. The fracture is internally fixed by percutaneous pinning by two crisscrossed smooth pins, one inserted through the medial epicondyle and the other through the lateral epicondyle. Smooth pins do not disturb growth; however, they must engage the opposite cortex of the proximal fragment of the distal humerus. Crisscross pins provide secure fixation. It is best to pin with the patient in prone position. The use of image intensifier radiographic control and a power drill driver has made percutaneous pinning relatively simple.

When there is marked swelling of the elbow, two pins are inserted parallel to the lateral condyle, avoiding injury to the ulnar nerve by the medial pin (Fig. 8–34). After pinning, the elbow is extended fully with the forearm in full supination, and alignment of the distal arm and elbow is determined—the carrying angle of the elbow should match the contralateral side. Radiograms are made. When reduction and internal fixation are satisfactory, the tips of the pins are bent and cut subcutaneously, thereby minimizing the risk of pin tract infections. Some surgeons may prefer to leave the tips of the pins protruding to facilitate later removal. As a rule, this author prefers to cut pins subcutaneously when they cross the physis. An above-elbow cast is applied with the elbow in 45 to 60 degrees of flexion and the forearm in 45 degrees of pronation. Extreme position of the forearm and elbow is not required because of stability of fixation by the pins. The pins are removed three to four weeks postoperatively.

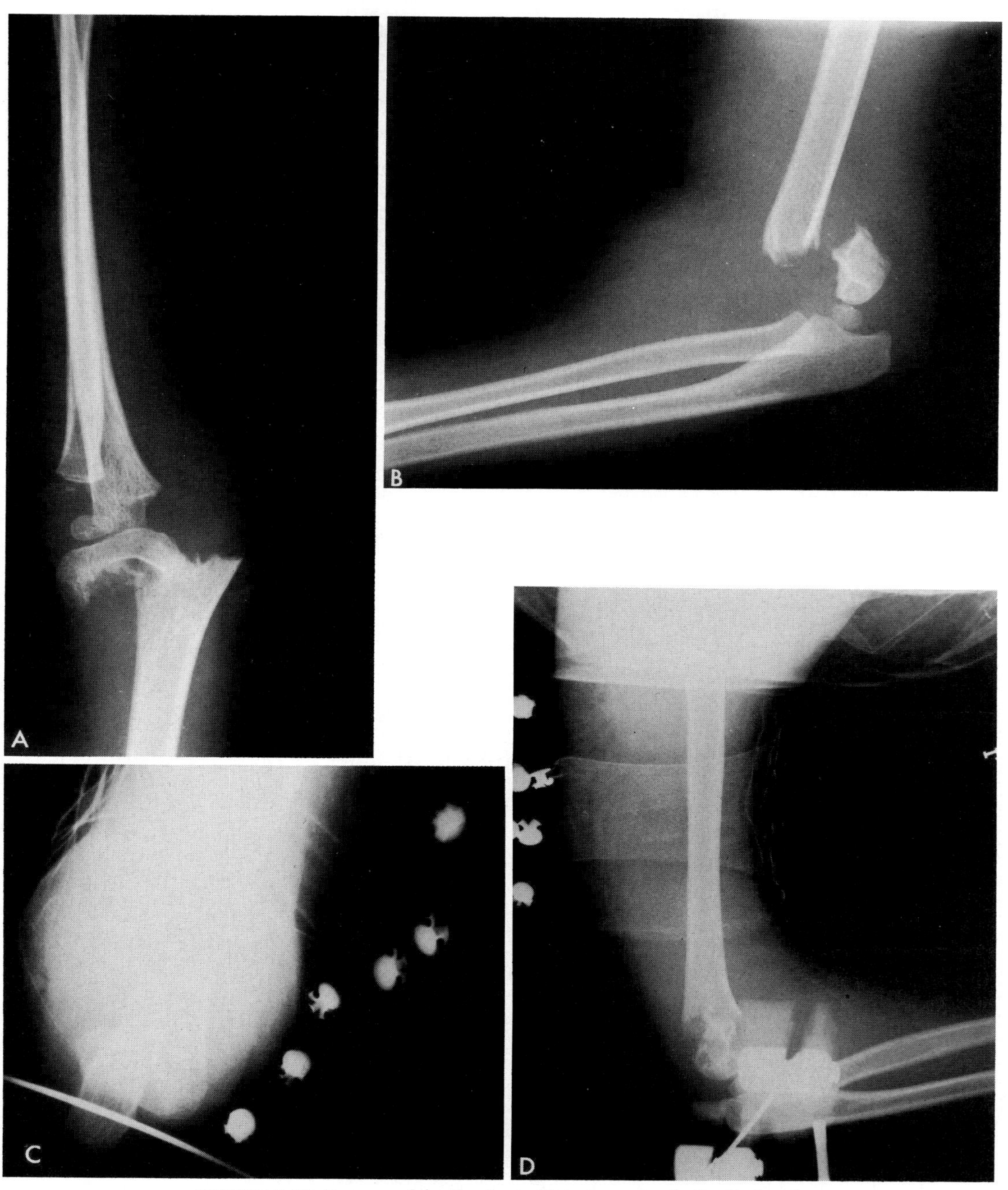

FIGURE 8–33. Supracondylar fracture of humerus—markedly displaced.

Note the anterior displacement of lower end of the proximal fragment. This patient had impending Volkmann's contracture with absence of radial pulse, pain on extension of the digits, and pallor of fingertips. Immediate reduction was carried out. Ten minutes later, the radial pulse returned. **A** and **B.** Initial radiograms. **C** and **D.** Radiograms in traction, showing satisfactory alignment.

Illustration continued on following page

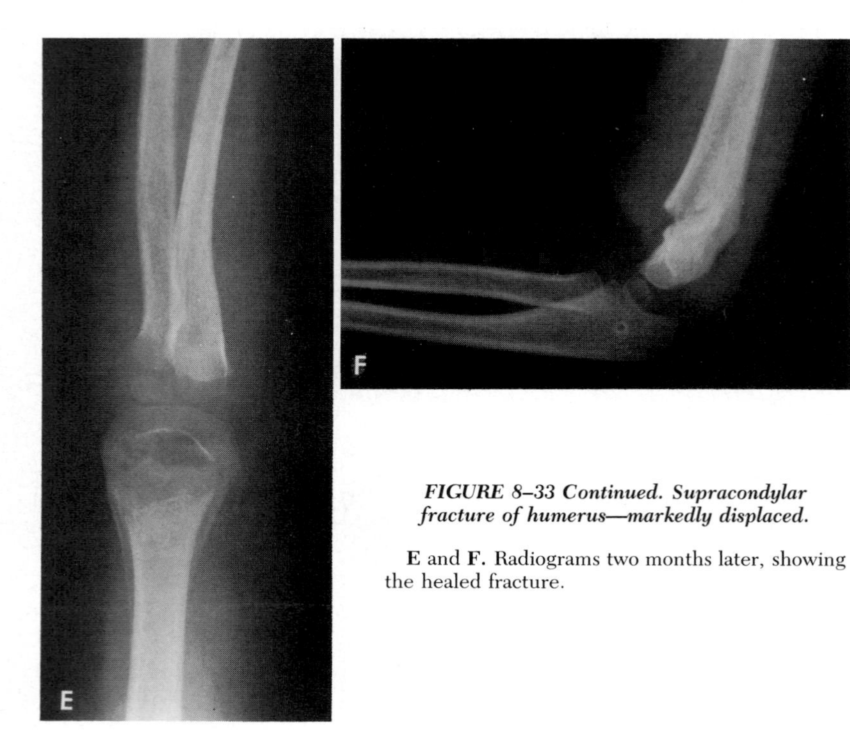

FIGURE 8–33 Continued. Supracondylar fracture of humerus—markedly displaced.

E and **F**. Radiograms two months later, showing the healed fracture.

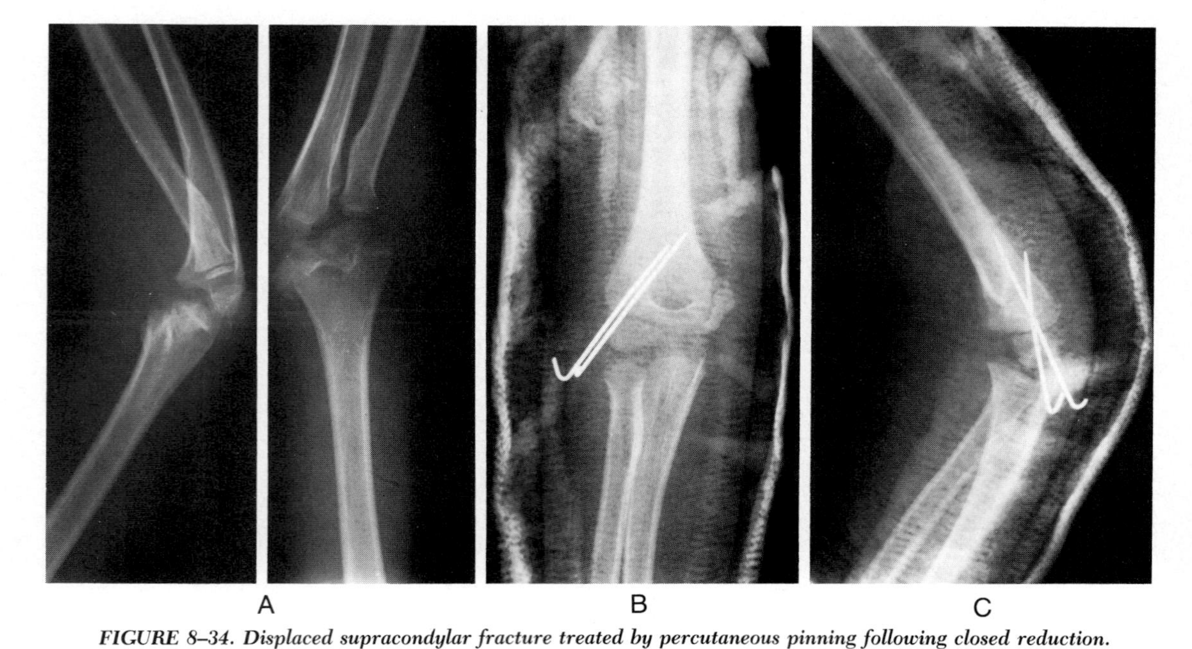

FIGURE 8–34. Displaced supracondylar fracture treated by percutaneous pinning following closed reduction.

A and **B**. Preoperative radiograms showing the displaced fracture. **C**. Following reduction and percutaneous pinning.

Another cast is applied for an additional two to three weeks, depending upon the radiographic state of healing.

Results of percutaneous pin fixation following reduction of displaced supracondylar fractures are good; it is the preferred, the generally accepted, and the popular method of maintaining reduction.[52, 84, 85, 109, 139, 195, 220] It provides secure fixation; the cost effectiveness due to the short period of hospitalization is very appealing to the third-party payer. The apprehensive child is much more comfortable following percutaneous pinning than in skeletal traction. Loss of alignment is less likely after pinning than in skeletal traction. Also, because acute flexion of the elbow is not required for maintenance of reduction the chance of circulatory embarrassment is minimized. Despite these advantages, percutaneous pinning has its problems and complications. There is definite risk of ulnar nerve injury from the medial pin. Pin tract infection may develop, with the possibility of physeal involvement and growth disturbance. The pin may slip or migrate, and alignment may be lost. In the literature cited above the incidence of cubitus varus was 5 per cent, in spite of initial adequate reduction.

MAINTENANCE OF REDUCTION BY LATERAL SKELETAL TRACTION

Lateral skeletal traction is indicated when the elbow is very swollen, obscuring bony landmarks, and the skin is blistered from the tense subcutaneous hematoma. This author has had extensive experience with the skeletal traction method of maintenance of reduction. The results are equally good as those of percutaneous pinning. Its drawbacks are the prolonged stay in the hospital and the initial period of relative discomfort to the child.

Lateral skeletal traction is applied with the shoulder abducted 60 degrees and the arm elevated 20 degrees above the horizontal (see Fig. 8–22 I). This position provides maximum venous drainage of the upper limb. Also, it curtails the patient's movements in bed, thus obviating the possibility of vascular damage by inadvertent increase in the degree of elbow flexion. A hyperactive child is placed on a Bradford frame. The posterior aspect of the elbow is not obscured; all the surgeon has to do is to kneel down to inspect the bony prominences; this author finds that with lateral traction it is very simple to use the visual method of treatment, as advocated by Lyman Smith (Fig. 8–35). In the *overhead skeletal traction method*, advocated by Smith, the humerus is suspended vertically with distal traction applied using a pin through the olecranon. Skin traction is applied on the forearm, which is suspended across the chest with weights hanging on the contralateral side of the bed. A sling is applied on the anterior aspect of the lower arm, exerting a posteriorly directed force on the posteriorly displaced proximal fragment of the fracture. Overhead traction is employed by many surgeons.* The disadvantage of overhead traction is that it does not provide adequate control over the proximal fragment if the patient moves about in bed; thus, it is possible for him to force the elbow into acute flexion and cause circulatory embarrassment. Such an instance was reported by Staples.[279]

Fahey prefers the use of a screw through both cortices of the ulna for skeletal traction because of difficulties encountered in introducing a Kirschner wire in the presence of a swollen elbow and the possibility of damaging the ulnar nerve.[79] This has not been a problem in the experience of this author.

In lateral skeletal traction a 3 to 5 lb. weight is applied on the lateral traction bow, and the forearm is suspended by adhesive strapping traction with 1 or 2 lb. of weight. In the extension type supracondylar fracture, in which the proximal fragment is anteriorly displaced, a sling with a 1 or 2 lb. weight is applied on the upper arm, pulling it posteriorly. Circulation and neural function are closely checked and recorded. The maintenance of reduction is determined by periodic radiograms. In two or three weeks, the fracture is stable enough to remove the Kirschner wire and continue immobilization in an above-elbow cast for an additional two to three weeks. Then the cast is removed, and active exercises are instituted to restore range of motion of the elbow joint (Fig. 8–36). Passive stretching exercises are never performed, and weights should not be used to stretch the elbow into full extension.

OPEN REDUCTION

Indications. *Absolute* indications for primary open reduction are the following: (1) *acute vascular injury*—entrapment, laceration, or compression. In such an instance, when the brachial vessels are explored, the fracture is reduced and fixed internally with crisscross pins. (2) *Irreducible fracture* with marked separation of the fracture fragments, buttonholing of the brachialis muscle by anterior spike of the lower end of the proximal fragment, and puncturing of the overlying skin. Often these se-

*See References 22, 35, 36, 60, 70, 104, 114, 163, 267, 269, 270, 279, and 280.

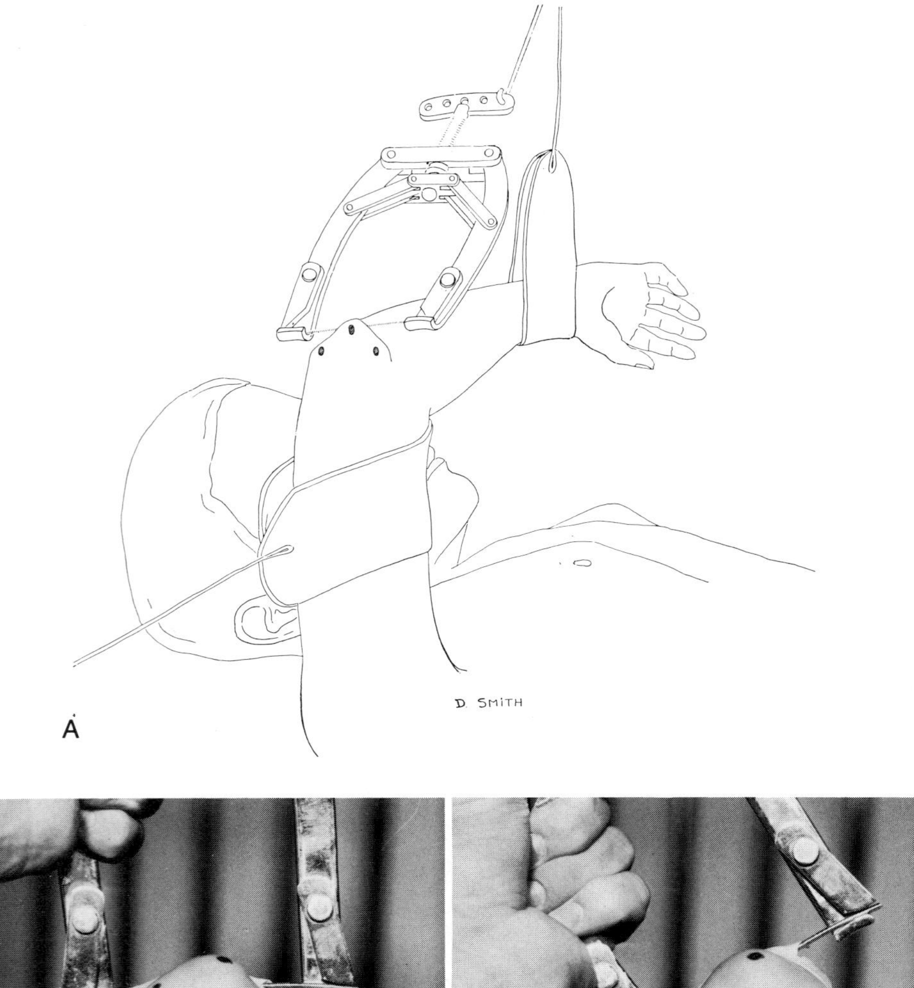

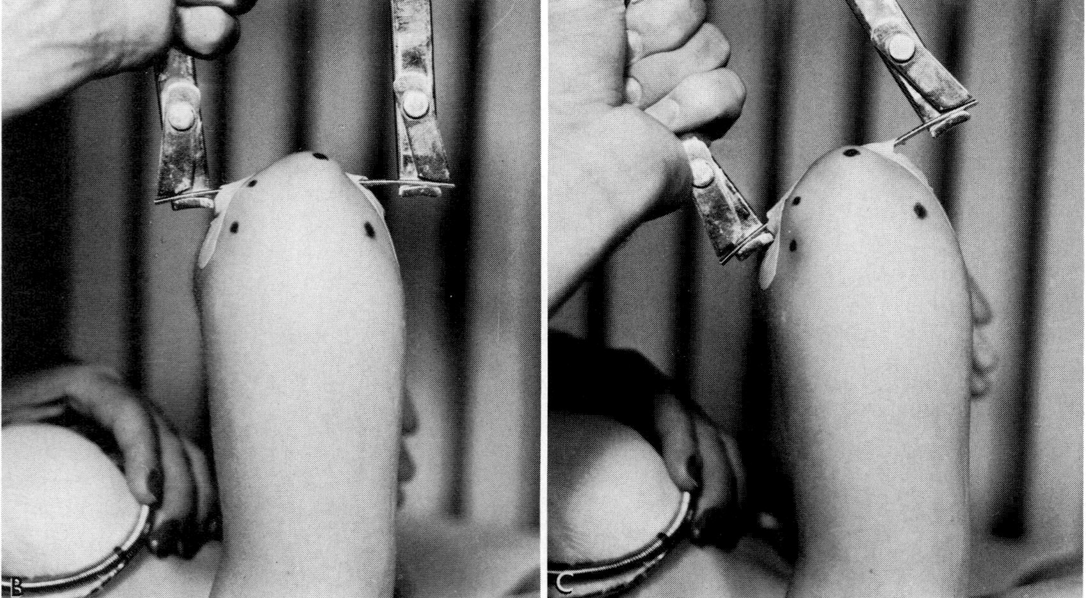

FIGURE 8–35. Overhead skeletal traction through a pin in the olecranon for treatment of markedly displaced supracondylar fractures of the humerus.

A. Traction arrangement. **B.** Bony prominences are aligned like those of the contralateral normal elbow. **C.** The distal fragment has, for demonstration purposes, been tilted into valgus deformity. (From Smith, L.: Deformity following supracondylar fractures of the humerus. J. Bone Joint Surg., *42-A*:244 and 246, 1960.)

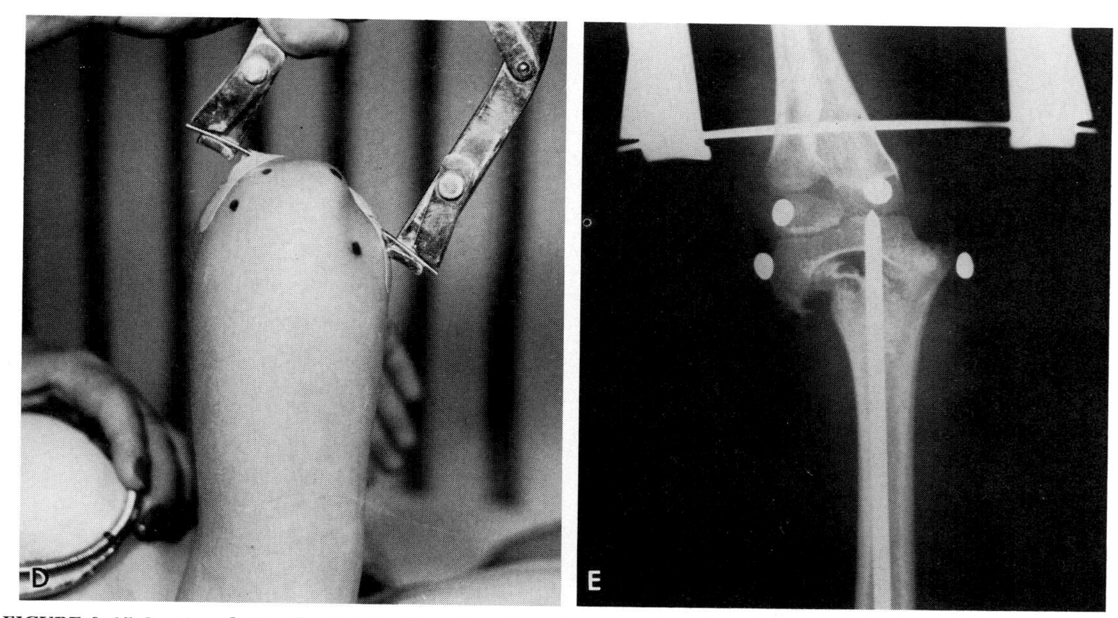

FIGURE 8–35 Continued. Overhead skeletal traction through a pin in the olecranon for treatment of markedly displaced supracondylar fractures of the humerus.

D. The distal fragment has been tilted into varus position. **E.** Radiographic appearance of the elbow as it is in **B.** Lead dots are placed on the ink markings and a wire taped along the long axis of the humerus. The lateral displacement of the distal fragment will have no effect on the carrying angle or function. (From Smith, L.: Deformity following supracondylar fractures of the humerus. J. Bone Joint Surg., *42-A*:244 and 246, 1960.)

verely displaced fractures are accompanied by a weak radial pulse that disappears on an attempt at closed reduction. Do not repeatedly manipulate these fractures, as you will cause more soft-tissue injury. (3) *Open fractures.* These result from severe injuries. When the wound is debrided, the fracture is openly reduced and fixed internally. With meticulous surgical technique and antibiotic coverage, the postoperative infection rate has become very low.

Relative indication is failure to achieve satisfactory reduction by closed methods. In the past this author has recommended the use of skeletal traction for gradual reduction of the difficult fractures and nonoperative management because the results of such closed nonoperative management have been functionally and cosmetically good. At present, this author favors primary open reduction, after a thorough discussion with the family and patient concerning the advantages and disadvantages of the open versus closed method of treatment. *Advantages* of primary open reduction are (1) greater likelihood of obtaining excellent anatomic reduction as opposed to the closed skeletal traction method. The latter often requires repeated adjustments and radiograms, and there is still the possibility that a satisfactory reduction cannot be achieved and that a secondary corrective angular rotation osteotomy of the distal humerus may be required. (2) At surgery any soft-tissue obstacles to reduction are easily removed, entrapped neurovascular structures liberated, and the large hematoma evacuated. The marked swelling of the elbow will subside rapidly, and the patient will be comfortable soon after surgery. (3) The hospital stay will be only a few days—besides its financial benefits, the psychological stress to the child and family will be less. Open reduction, however, has definite drawbacks, *problems, and complications,* including (1) loss of range of elbow motion. This develops almost universally following open reduction.[56, 125, 303] Range of flexion is more restricted than extension. When a posterior surgical approach is used, the degree of joint stiffness is greater than with anteromedial or anterolateral approaches.[49, 105] (2) *Cubitus varus* of varying degrees is reported in about one third of the cases treated by open reduction.[60, 305] This is due to inadequacy of reduction and insecure internal fixation at the time of open reduction; it can be avoided. (3) Postoperative *infection* is a calculated risk of surgery. In the literature the overall incidence

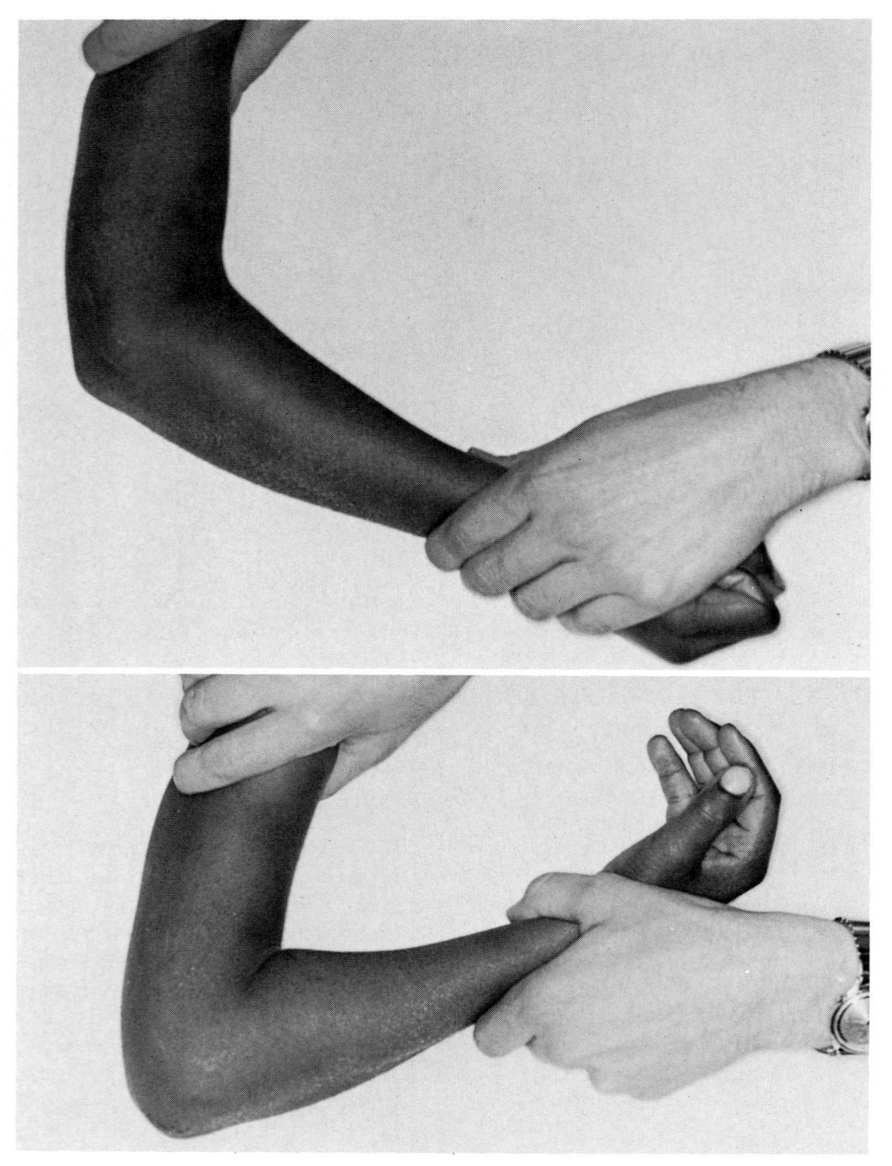

FIGURE 8–36. Active exercises to develop range of motion of elbow joint.

The left hand of the therapist is used to guide the forearm into extension and flexion; motion is performed actively by the patient. Passive stretching exercises and lifting of weights should not be performed.

of infection following open reduction is approximately 2 per cent.[49, 105, 240, 264, 305] With appropriate antibiotic treatment, infection will clear. (4) Growth disturbance due to physeal injury is more probable with open methods. (5) *Myositis ossificans* develops more often when open reduction versus closed reduction is carried out. (6) *Nerve and vessel injury* may occur inadvertently at the time of open reduction.

Open reduction should be performed soon after failure of attempt at closed reduction. Delay of surgery will cause greater joint stiffness. Ordinarily the anterolateral surgical approach is relatively easy, and the anterior soft-tissue pathology and radial nerves are well visualized; however, if there is evidence of ulnar or median nerve or brachial vessel injury, the anteromedial approach is used. *The posterior approach should not be employed.* Internal fixation is with crisscross smooth pins. An above-elbow cast is applied with the elbow in 45 degrees of flexion. The cast and pins are removed three to four weeks postoperatively. The fracture is metaphyseal; it will heal rapidly. Nonunion or delayed union is ordinarily not a problem unless complicated by a low-grade indolent infection. A posterior removable above-elbow splint is applied for an additional two weeks. The splint is removed several times a day, and active assisted gentle range of motion exercises are performed. Forceful manipulations are avoided. After removal of the splint the elbow is protected in a sling during outdoor activities for an additional one or two weeks.

Preoperatively it is explained to the parents that joint stiffness is a problem—not a complication of the treatment—and that it will take 6 to 12 months to regain joint motion. The possible use of a continuous passive elbow machine is mentioned to the parents.

Complications

MALUNION AND CHANGES IN CARRYING ANGLE

The carrying angle is the lateral angle that the longitudinal axis of the *fully supinated* forearm makes with the longitudinal axis of the upper arm when the elbow is *completely extended.* The carrying angle tends to disappear with pronation of the forearm and with flexion of the elbow. With progressive flexion of the elbow from complete extension, the carrying angle becomes less and less evident until complete flexion is reached, at which time the arm is covered by the forearm and there is no apparent angular deviation at the elbow. Changes in the carrying angle cannot be detected when one examines the flexed elbow from the front. However, if the flexed elbow is examined posteriorly and compared with the opposite normal elbow, changes in the carrying angle will become quite apparent. The bony relations of the medial and lateral epicondyles and the olecranon process are palpated. The examiner grasps the child's left elbow with his left hand and places his right thumb on the tip of the lateral condyle, the long finger on the tip of the medial epicondyle, and the index finger on the olecranon process. When examining the right elbow, the surgeon reverses his hand positions for convenience.

With the elbow flexed to a right angle, the three points make a fairly symmetrical equilateral triangle and tend to lie in a plane parallel with the plane of the posterior surface of the upper arm. In some children, the capitellum becomes quite prominent in 90 degrees of flexion and disturbs the symmetry of the lateral segment of the triangle. When the elbow is in complete extension, three bony points are almost in a straight line.

It is important to remember that the carrying angle is subject to considerable normal individual variation. Lyman Smith studied the carrying angle of 150 normal children, 80 girls and 70 boys, aged 3 to 11 years (the age when supracondylar fracture is most common). He found the average carrying angle to be 6.1 degrees cubitus valgus in the girls, with a range of 0 to 12 degrees, and 5.4 degrees in boys, with a range of 0 to 11 degrees. Some of the children (9 per cent) had no carrying angle or cubitus rectus, and 48 per cent had a carrying angle of 55 degrees or less.[268]

In measurements of the carrying angle of 100 subjects, Aebi found the average value for men to be 6.5 degrees, with a range of 0 to 14 degrees; in women, the averge was 13 degrees, with a range of 4 to 20 degrees.[2]

The effect on the carrying angle caused by various types of displacement of the distal fragment in supracondylar fractures was experimentally studied by Smith. He simulated a transverse supracondylar fracture in an articulated upper limb by an osteotomy through the supracondylar region, the fragments being held together by spring wiring. Medial and lateral displacement of the distal fragment did not change the carrying angle (Fig. 8–37 B and C). Medial rotation of the distal fragment also had no effect on the degree of the carrying angle (Fig. 8–37 D). Only medial or lateral tilt of the distal fragment changed the carrying angle (Fig. 8–37 E and F). Clinically the direction, obliquity, and course of the fracture line are factors in angulation. When the fracture line is transverse, the fracture does not angulate by pure rotation of the distal fragment, whereas when the fracture line is oblique, rotation causes angulation. Posteromedially displaced fractures develop varus angulation, whereas posterolaterally displaced fractures deviate into valgus.

The compressional forces of normal muscle tone, particularly biceps and triceps brachii, and of the elasticity of soft tissues surrounding the fracture fragments will angulate the distal fragment when there is medial and lateral displacement and instability of the fracture. Again, posteromedially displaced fractures tend to develop varus angulation and posterolaterally displaced fractures valgus deviation. This can best be prevented by traction on the distal fragment in the direction of the longitudinal axis of the distal part of the humerus.

Cubitus varus or valgus deformity results from malunion; it is not caused by physeal growth disturbance (Figs. 8–38 and 8–39). Oc-

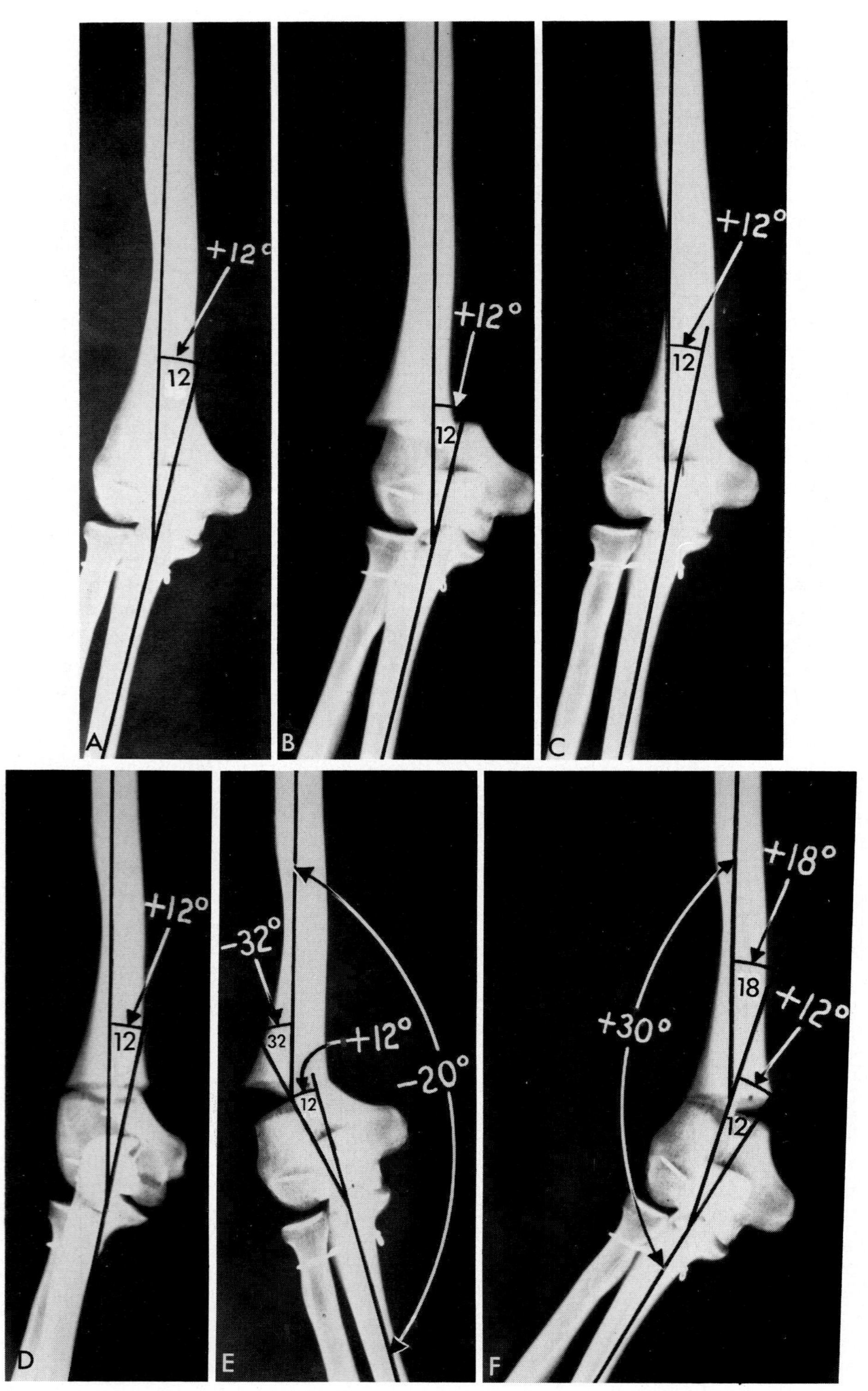

FIGURE 8–37. The effect on the carrying angle of various types of displacement of the distal fragment in supracondylar fractures of the humerus.

A. The carrying angle of the elbow—12 degrees. **B.** Following medial displacement of the distal fragment, the carrying angle did not change from its 12 degrees. **C.** Upon lateral displacement, the carrying angle again did not change. **D.** Fifteen-degree medial rotation of distal fragment did not change the carrying angle. **E.** Upon 32-degree medial tilting of the distal fragment, the carrying angle changed to 20 degrees varus. **F.** The distal fragment was tilted laterally 18 degrees, and the carrying angle increased to 30 degrees valgus. (From Smith, L.: Deformity following supracondylar fractures of the humerus. J. Bone Joint Surg., *42-A*:238, 239, 1960.)

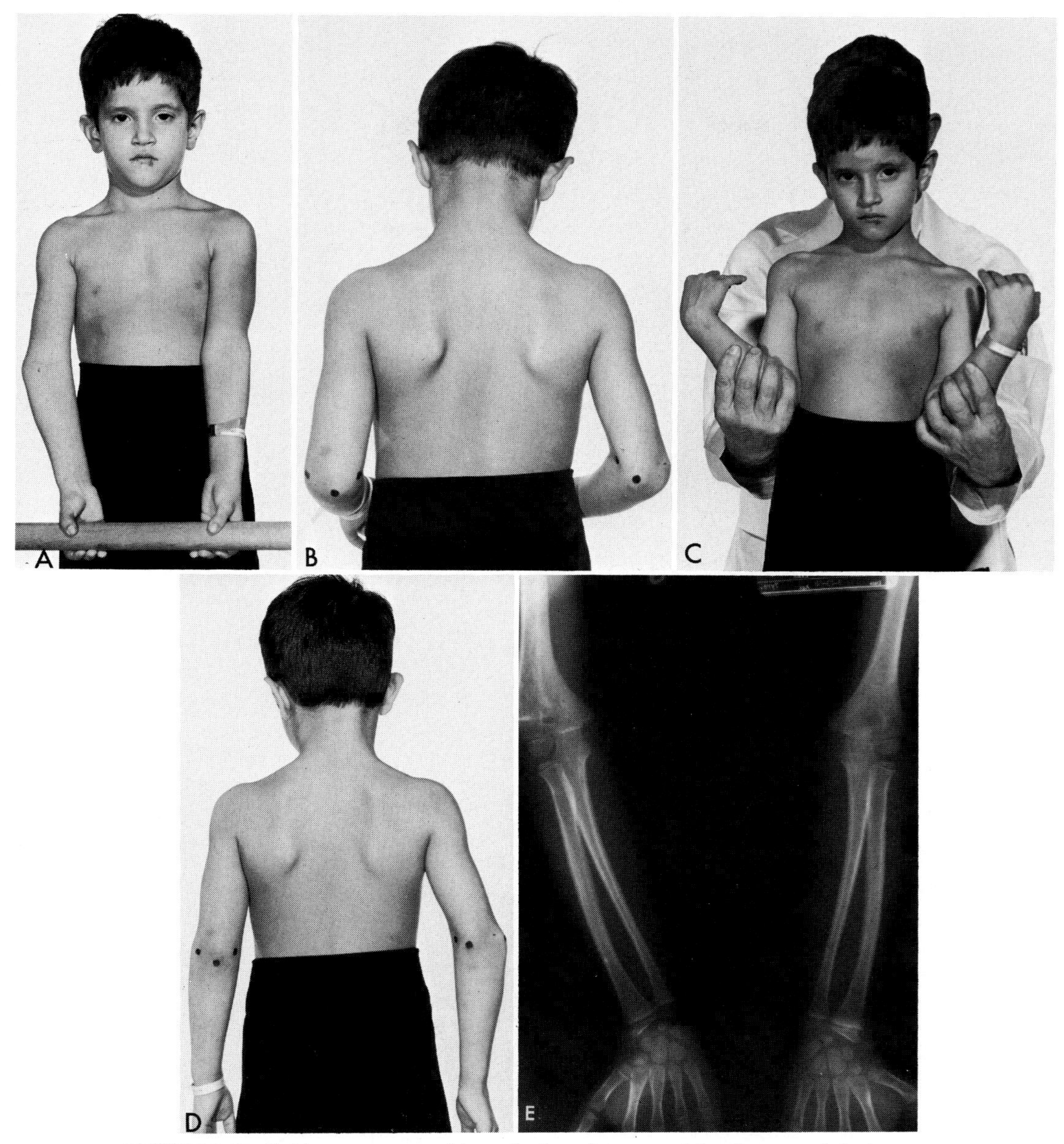

FIGURE 8–38. Cubitus varus caused by malunion of supracondylar fracture of the humerus.

Deformity on the right is due to medial tilting of the distal fragment. **A** to **D.** Clinical appearance. **E.** Anteroposterior radiogram with the elbows in extension.

casionally a transcondylar T-fracture is mistaken for supracondylar fracture; in such an instance the fracture may involve the physis and asymmetrical growth will cause cubitus valgus or varus. Cubitus varus deformity is much more common than cubitus valgus. If the varus or valgus deformity of the elbow is severe and causes cosmetic and functional problems, it is corrected by supracondylar osteotomy of the humerus. Ordinarily, cubitus valgus is cosmetically acceptable but can cause tardy ulnar nerve palsy. The operative technique of osteotomy of the distal humeral shaft to correct cubitus varus is described in Plate 120 and Figure 8–40.

NEURAL COMPLICATIONS

The radial, ulnar, and median nerves may be injured at the time of fracture, during attempts at reduction, or by compression during Volkmann's ischemia. Ordinarily, radial nerve injury occurs when the distal fragment is displaced posteromedially and median nerve paralysis de-

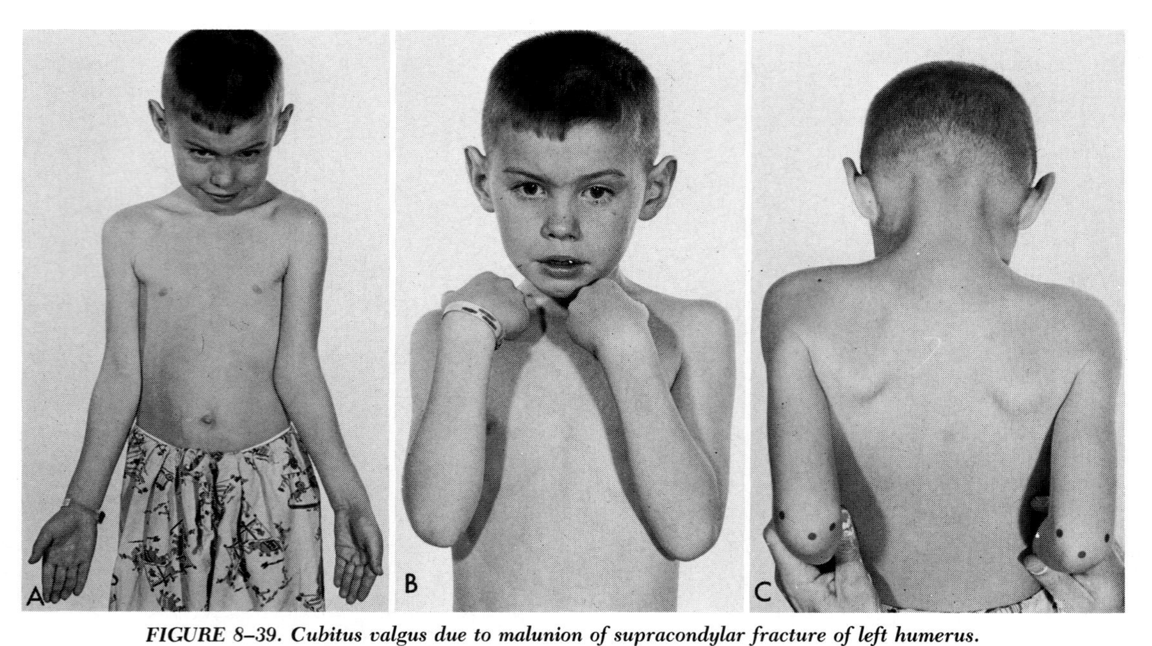

FIGURE 8–39. Cubitus valgus due to malunion of supracondylar fracture of left humerus.

Deformity on the left is caused by lateral tilting of the distal fragment. **A** to **C.** Clinical appearance.

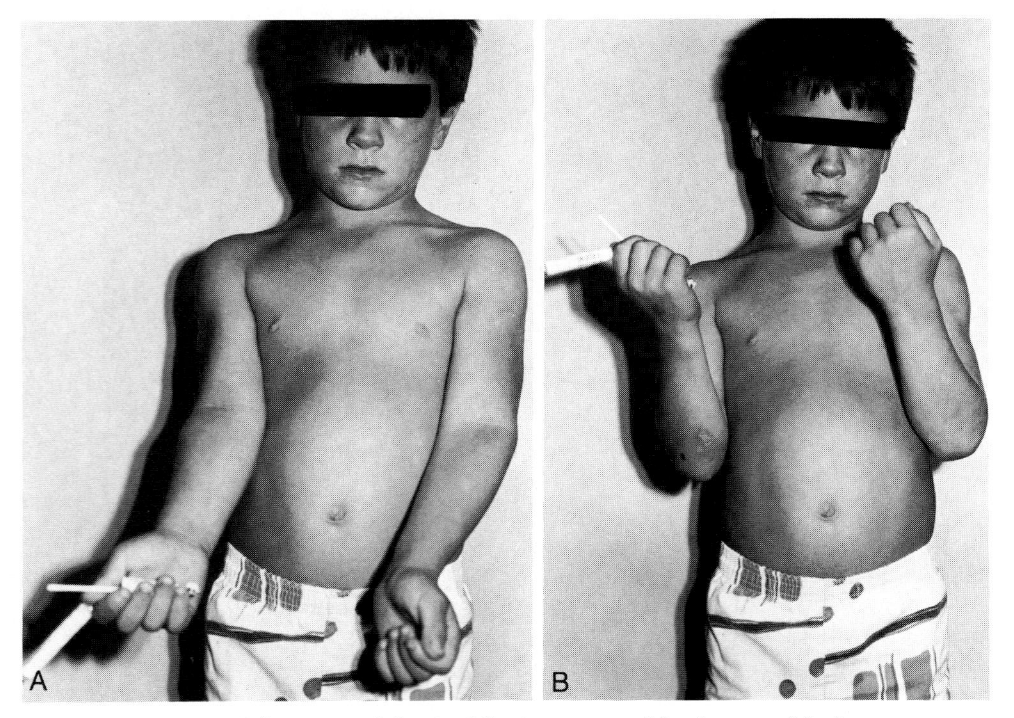

FIGURE 8–40. Cubitus varus deformity following supracondylar fracture of the humerus.

A. Preoperative photograph. **B.** Postoperative photograph following valgus angulation osteotomy and internal fixation with crisscross pins.

velops with posterolateral displacement of the distal fragment.[126] Siris, in 1939, reported a series of 330 supracondylar fractures of the humerus, with 11 cases of nerve paralysis (seven of the radial nerve and four of the ulnar nerve).[266] Sorrel and Sorrel-Dejerine found an incidence of 7 per cent (16 of 207 supracondylar fractures)—seven ulnar, four radial, four median, and one combined median and ulnar nerve paralysis.[273] Both Siris and Sorrel recommended exploration when there are no signs of improvement in 15 days.[266, 273]

Bailey reviewed 71 cases of supracondylar fractures of the humerus in children and found six cases of nerve injury (8 per cent); four had radial nerve involvement only, one had involvement of the median nerve alone, and one had involvement of all three nerves—the radial, median, and ulnar. In two of the cases, paralysis was present prior to attempts at reduction; in the remaining four cases, the nerves were injured during attempted reduction of the fracture. In all six cases the nerves were compressed or contused, and partial return of function in the paralyzed muscle took place before the end of two months and complete recovery before the end of 14 weeks.[16]

Lipscomb and Burleson reported a 16 per cent incidence of nerve injury in supracondylar fractures (in 17 of 108 patients).[181] Trauma to the radial nerve was most common. Five of the 17 patients were treated expectantly; partial return or full return of function occurred in two to three weeks. In four patients, the nerve injury accompanied trauma to the brachial artery, and surgical exploration was performed because of the vascular lesion. In one patient with radial nerve palsy, open reduction of the fracture was performed early, and tension on the nerve was released. Four patients with nerve palsy were observed for a period of three to four weeks. Because there was no recovery of nerve function, exploration was performed. In no patient was a nerve found to be divided, but the nerves were compressed by old hemorrhage, bound down by fibrous tissue, or stretched over a bone fragment. Complete recovery was obtained by neurolysis. In one patient with palsy of all three nerves, partial return of function was obtained by neurolysis. Lipscomb and Burleson advised observation of nerve palsies for a few weeks after adequate reduction of the fracture. If no improvement occurred after this period, they advised surgical exploration.[181]

Spinner and Schreiber reported six cases of anterior interosseous nerve paralysis as a complication of supracondylar fractures of the humerus in children.[276] They proposed traction as the mechanism of the paralysis, the distracting elements being the proximal fragment of the humerus and a tethering structure in the forearm. They believed that the paralysis is caused by contusion of the nerve by the anteriorly displaced proximal fragment of the humerus at the level of the fracture. The characteristic physical finding of anterior interosseous nerve paralysis is loss of flexion power of the distal phalanx of the thumb and the index finger, with all other median nerve functions intact. In all six of their patients, spontaneous recovery occurred in six to eight weeks. They recommended exploration of the median nerve from the distal part of the humerus through the pronator teres, should clinical or electromyographic recovery not take place in six to eight weeks following surgery.[276]

A complete evaluation of radial, ulnar, and median nerve function should be performed before and after reduction of supracondylar fracture of the humerus. As stated, manipulation should be gentle to avoid injury to the nerves. If there is paralysis, passive exercises are performed to maintain range of motion of the digits, and the hand is splinted in functional position. Nerve function is periodically determined. If, within six to eight weeks, function has not returned, nerve conduction and electromyographic studies are performed, the nerves are explored, and neurolysis is performed. It is best to transpose the ulnar nerve anteriorly. If the nerve palsy is associated with Volkmann's ischemia, neurolysis is performed along with fasciotomy and epimysiotomy.

VASCULAR INJURY

Circulatory compromise occurs in about 5 per cent of supracondylar fractures of the humerus.[218] The vascular injury may be induced directly by the fracture or indirectly in the forearm by compression in a taut compartment. *Direct injury* by the fracture fragments may be complete transection of the brachial artery, intimal tear, false aneurysm, or spasm due to compression. The brachial vessels may be entrapped in the fracture fragments. In the severely displaced fracture the anteroinferior sharp edge of the proximal fragment may transect and rupture the brachial artery. This is more common in open fractures.[85, 181, 218, 219, 275] When the level of transection is proximal to the inferior ulnar collateral artery, rich collateral circulation will provide adequate blood supply to the forearm and hand; however, increasing

Text continued on page 3092

Osteotomy of the Distal Humerus for Correction of Cubitus Varus

OPERATIVE TECHNIQUE

A. A longitudinal incision is made over the anterolateral aspect of the distal third of the arm, with the anterior margin of the brachioradialis muscle serving as an anatomic landmark. The incision begins 1 cm. proximal and anterior to the lateral epicondyle of the humerus and extends proximally for a distance of approximately 7 cm.

B. The subcutaneous tissue and fascia are divided in line with the skin incision. The skin flaps are mobilized and retracted. The anterior margin of the brachioradialis muscle laterally and the lateral margin of the biceps muscle medially are identified, and by blunt dissection in the loose areolar tissue between these two muscles, the radial nerve is located. A moist hernia tape is passed around the radial nerve for gentle handling and traction.

The biceps muscle is retracted medially, exposing the lateral half of the brachialis muscle beneath it. By blunt dissection with a periosteal elevator, the lateral one third to one half of the muscle fibers of the brachialis are raised, exposing the periosteum on the front of the lower end of the humerus. The periosteum is incised longitudinally, as shown in the illustration, its distal end stopping 1 cm. proximal to the capsule of the elbow joint.

C. The periosteum is reflected with a periosteal elevator, and the lower end of the shaft of the humerus is exposed. It is essential not to disturb the growth of the distal humeral physis and to keep out of the elbow joint.

Plate 120. Osteotomy of the Distal Humerus for Correction of Cubitus Varus

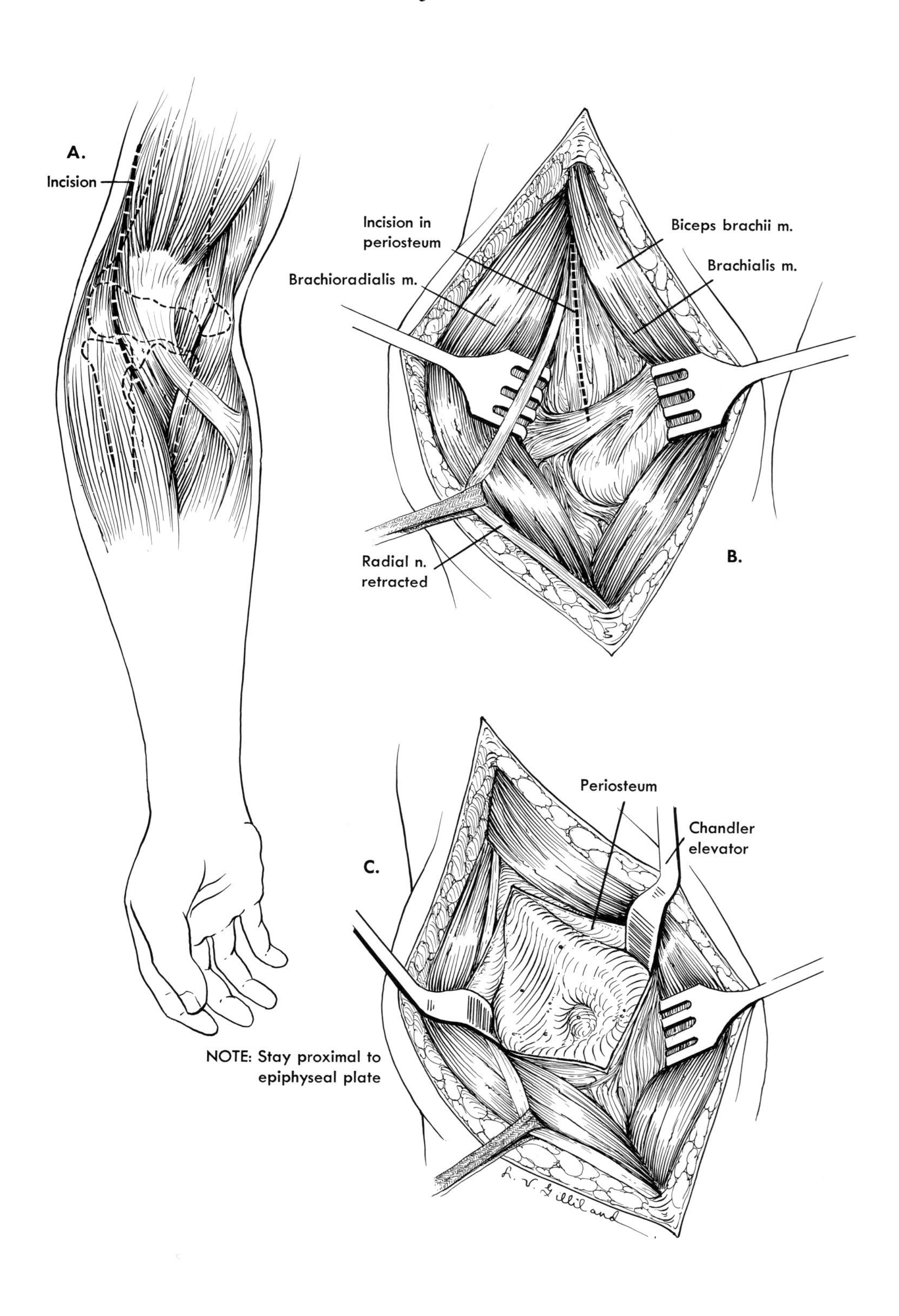

Osteotomy of the Distal Humerus for Correction of Cubitus Varus (Continued)

D. With a starter and drill, the line of a dome-shaped osteotomy is outlined with drill holes through both anterior and posterior cortices. The medial arch of the dome should be deeper and 1 to 1.5 cm. longer than the lateral arch, which is almost transverse. With sharp, thin osteotomes and/or oscillating electric saw, the osteotomy is completed, great care being taken not to split the medial cortex of the dome of the proximal fragment.

E. The bone fragments are manipulated, and angular and rotational deformities are corrected. If necessary, a wedge of bone may be removed from the lateral side of the distal fragment with a rongeur. The osteotomy fragments are fixed with crisscross Steinmann pins inserted through stab wound separate from the skin incision. The periosteum and the wound are closed in the usual manner.

F. The upper limb is immobilized in an above elbow cast, with the elbow in 90 degrees of flexion and the forearm in 45 degrees of pronation.

Plate 120. Osteotomy of the Distal Humerus for Correction of Cubitus Varus

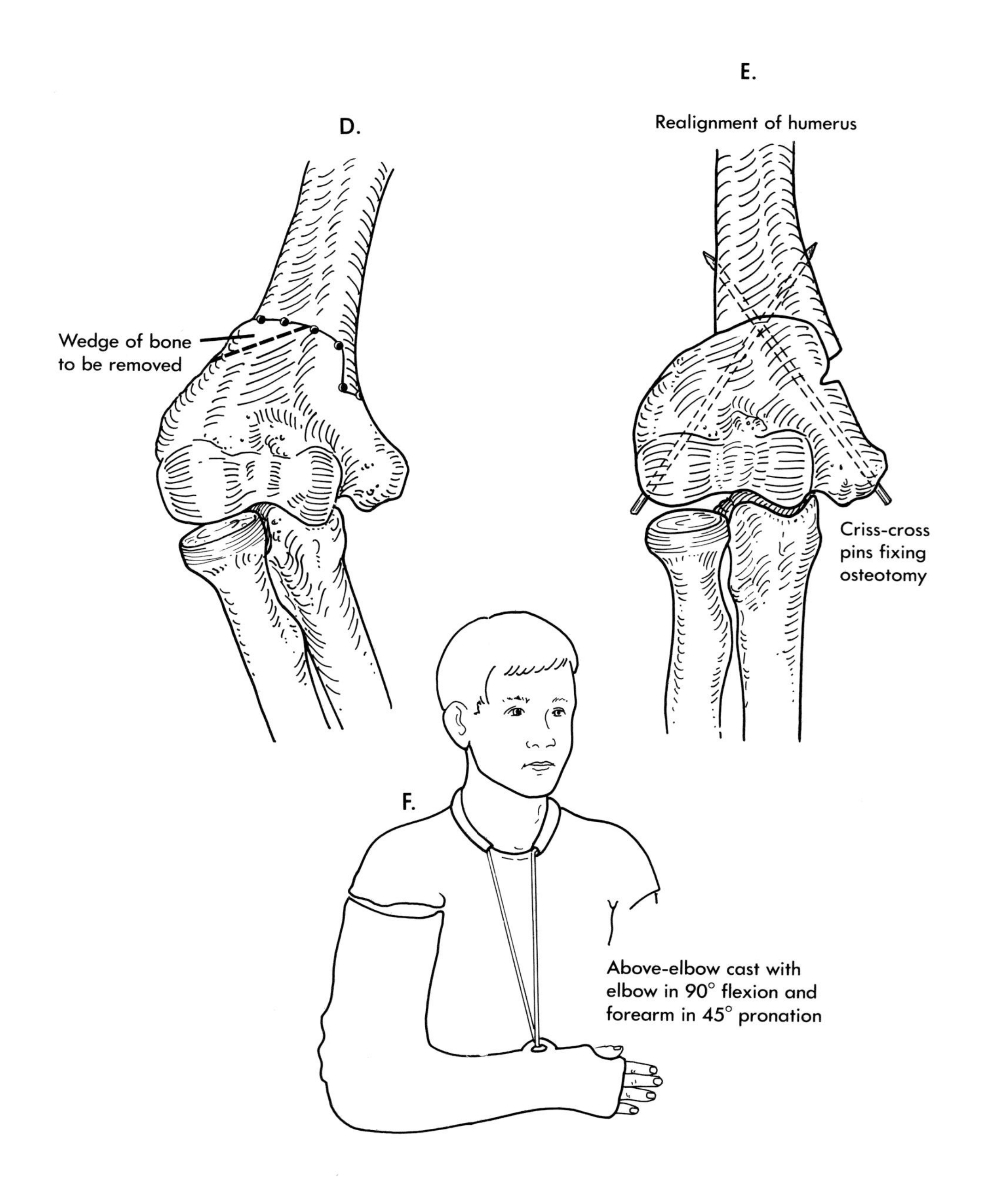

Osteotomy of the Distal Humerus for Correction of Cubitus Varus (Continued)

An alternative method is to perform a closing wedge osteotomy through the posterior approach.

G. The patient is placed in prone position, and the skin incision begins immediately above the tip of the olecranon and extends proximally for a distance of 7 to 10 cm. The subcutaneous tissue and fascia are opened in line with the skin incision.

H. The wound flaps are mobilized and retracted, exposing the lower one third of the tendon of triceps muscle.

I. The ulnar nerve is identified directly above the ulnar groove, dissected proximally, and retracted with silicone (Silastic) tubing posteriorly and inferiorly to protect it from injury. The triceps tendon is split longitudinally and each half is retracted, thus exposing the posterior surface of the humerus.

It is not necessary to expose the radial nerve as long as dissection does not extend more proximally than does the junction of the middle and distal thirds of the humerus.

Plate 120. Osteotomy of the Distal Humerus for Correction of Cubitus Varus

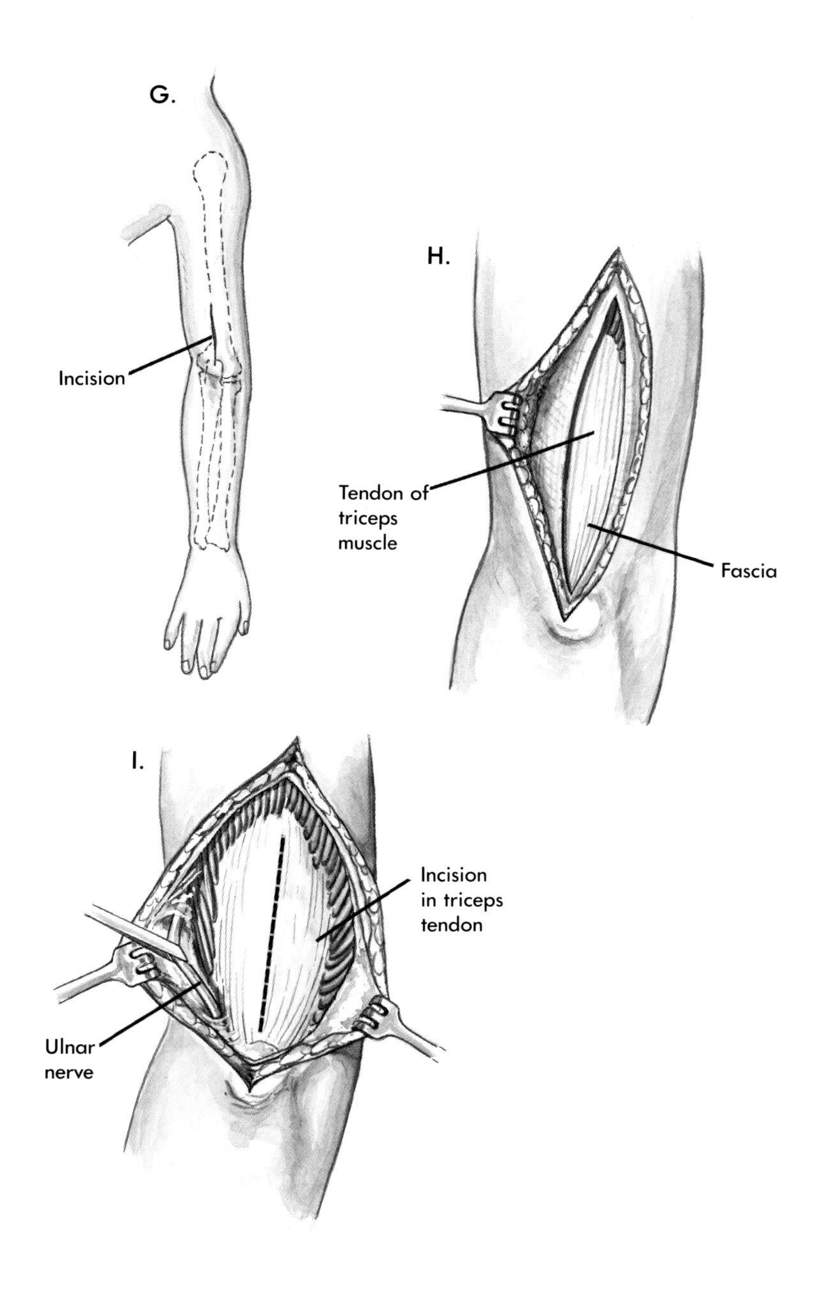

Osteotomy of the Distal Humerus for Correction of Cubitus Varus (Continued)

J and **K.** The periosteum on the posterior surface of the humerus is divided by a T-incision. Stay proximal to the olecranon fossa and distal humeral physis. A wedge osteotomy from the distal humeral methaphysis based laterally is resected. The osteotomized fragments are approximated and fixed internally with two or three criss-cross pins inserted through the stab wound separate from the skin incision.

The wound is closed in the usual fashion and an above-elbow cast is applied, with the elbow in 90 degrees of flexion and the forearm in 45 degrees of pronation.

POSTOPERATIVE CARE

Radiograms are made after five days and again at two weeks to check maintenance of anatomic alignment of the fracture fragments. The osteotomy usually heals in six weeks. The cast and pins are removed, and *active* exercises are begun to restore range of motion of the elbow. Passive exercises are *not* performed. Weights should not be lifted for two months.

Plate 120. Osteotomy of the Distal Humerus for Correction of Cubitus Varus

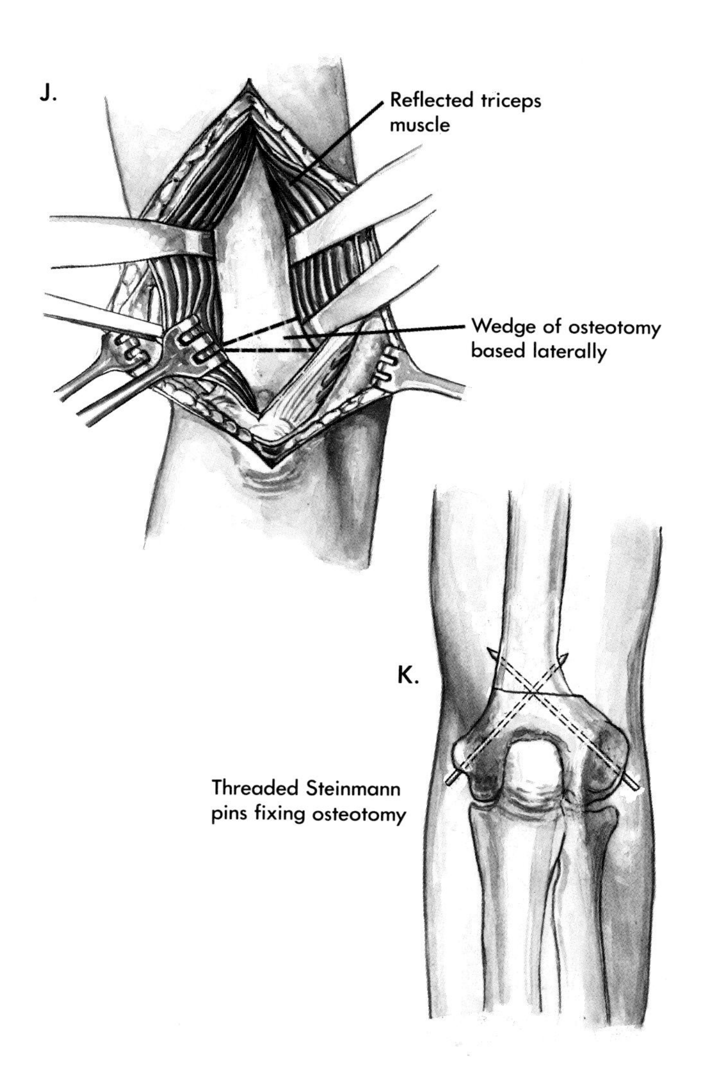

compartment pressure may compromise this collateral circulation. The possibility of *brachial artery laceration* is suspected by the rapidly enlarging hematoma at the puncture site and lack of circulation in the forearm and hand. Treatment is by repair or vessel graft, performed by a peripheral vascular surgeon. The *entrapment of brachial vessels* requires open reduction and liberation of the vessels. The extent of vascular injury is assessed and appropriately treated by the vascular surgeon. *Spasm* of the brachial artery and *intimal lesions* require arteriography for delineation of pathology. Arterial spasm may be relieved by stellate ganglion block and/or local application of papaverine. Resection of the spasmodic segment and vessel graft may be required. All these procedures are performed by the vascular surgeon.

The brachial vessels may be compressed by the hematoma when the swollen elbow is acutely flexed; in such an instance, extension of the elbow will decompress the vessels. The displaced fracture fragments may compress the brachial vessels; reduction of the fracture will liberate the vessels. Prolonged compression and occlusion may result in thrombosis. Partial tear of the brachial artery may cause aneurysm—this will manifest as a painful, red, warm swelling over the fracture site. A bruit will suggest aneurysm. Arteriography will confirm the diagnosis. Treatment consists of resection of the aneurysm and vessel graft or primary repair performed by a vascular surgeon.

Volkmann's Ischemia. This develops in about 1 per cent of the cases. Its pathogenesis and treatment are described separately on page 3099.

Joint Stiffness. Loss of motion almost always occurs in supracondylar fractures; however, it usually does not exceed 5 to 10 degrees.[57, 118] Occasionally, when posterior angulation is not corrected, there may be significant (20 to 30 degrees) hyperextension deformity of the elbow. Loss of elbow flexion due to anterior impingement gradually corrects with remodeling.[105, 169]

Myositis Ossificans. This is a rare complication that may follow closed or open reduction.[3, 60] It should be suspected when marked progressive stiffness of the elbow develops following cast removal. Bone scan with ^{99m}technetium will show increased uptake prior to radiographic changes. Within three to four weeks ossification and calcification in the brachialis muscle become visible in the radiogram. Treatment consists of rest and gentle motion. Forceful passive exercises should not be performed. Nonsteroidal anti-inflammatory drugs (such as Naprosyn or Tolectin) can be given during the acute inflammatory painful phase. Prognosis is good—within two years the joint stiffness and calcification will probably disappear. This author has not excised a mature myositis ossificans. Radiation is not recommended.

References

1. Abraham, E., Powers, T., and Wilt, P.: Experimental hyperextension supracondylar fractures in monkeys. Clin. Orthop., *171*:309, 1982.
2. Aebi, H.: Der Ellbogenwinkel, seine Beziehungen zu Geschlect, Korperbay und Huftbreite. Acta Anat., *3*:228, 1947.
3. Aitken, A. P., Smith, L., and Blackett, C. W.: Supracondylar fractures in children. Am. J. Surg., *59*:161, 1943.
4. Alcott, W. H., Bowden, B. W., and Miller, P. R.: Displaced supracondylar fractures of the humerus in children: Long-term follow-up of 69 patients. J.A.M.A., *76*:910, 1977.
5. Ali, E.: Supracondylar fracture of the humerus in children in Guyana. West Indian Med. J., *30*:34, 1981.
6. Allen, P. D., and Gramse, A. E.: Transcondylar fractures of the humerus treated by Dunlop traction. Am. J. Surg., *67*:217, 1945.
7. Alonso-Llames, M.: Bilaterotricipital approach to the elbow. Its application in the osteosynthesis of supracondylar fractures of the humerus in children. Acta Orthop. Scand., *43*:479, 1972.
8. Andersen, J. C., and Berge, T.: Dislocated supracondylar humeral fractures in children treated by reduction and fixation with Steinman pins. Tidsskr. Nor. Laegeforen., *100*:1785, 1980.
9. Arino, V. L., Lluch, E. E., Ramirez, A. M., Ferrer, J., Rodriquez, L., and Baixault, F.: Percutaneous fixation of supracondylar fractures of the humerus in children. J. Bone Joint Surg., *59-A*:914, 1977.
10. Arnold, J. A., Nasca, R. J., and Nelson, C. L.: Supracondylar fractures of the humerus: The role of dynamic factors in prevention of deformity. J. Bone Joint Surg., *59-A*:589, 1977.
11. Arnold, K., Schumacher, D., and Reinbacher, L.: Supracondylar humeral fracture in childhood. Z. Arztl. Fortbild. (Jena), *66*:659, 1972.
12. Aronson, D. D., and Prager, B. I.: Supracondylar fractures of the humerus in children. A modified technique for closed pinning. Clin. Orthop., *219*:174, 1987.
13. Ashhurst, A. P. C.: An Anatomical and Surgical Study of Fractures of the Lower End of the Humerus. Philadelphia, Lea & Febiger, 1910.
14. Attenborough, C. G.: Remodelling of the humerus of the supracondylar fractures in childhood. J. Bone Joint Surg., *35-B*:386, 1953.
15. Aufranc, D. E., Jones, W. N., and Bierbaum, B. E.: Open supracondylar fracture of the humerus. J.A.M.A., *208*:682, 1969.
16. Bailey, G. G., Jr.: Nerve injuries in supracondylar fractures of the humerus in children. N. Engl. J. Med., *221*:260, 1939.
17. Bakalim, G., and Wilppuia, E.: Supracondylar humeral fractures in children. Causes of changes in the carrying angle of the elbow. Acta Orthop. Scand., *43*:366, 1972.
18. Balenty, P. V., Iliescu, G., Brazda, A., Semenescu,

V., and Iancu, N.: On the migration of the Kirschner wires following osteosynthesis of a supracondylar fracture. Beitr. Orthop. Traumatol., *14*:8, 1967.
19. Basom, W. C.: Supracondylar and transcondylar fractures in children. Clin. Orthop., *1*:43, 1953.
20. Bates, E. H., and Taylor, T. K.: Supracondylar fractures of the humerus in children. Minn. Med., *54*:445, 1971.
21. Baumann, E.: Über Regenerationserscheinungen am verletzten Ellbogen. Schweiz. Med. Wochenschr., *54*:1057, 1924.
22. Baumann, E.: Beitrage zur Kenntnis der Frakturen am Ellbogengelenk. Unter besonderer Berucksichtigung der Spatfolgen. Allgeneines und Fractura und supra condylica. Beitr. Klin. Chir., *146*:1, 1929.
23. Baumann, E.: Zur Behandlung der Knochenbruche am Ellbogengelenk. Langenbecks Arch. Chir., *295*:300, 1960.
24. Baumgartner, R., Herzog, B., and Jani, L.: Covered drill tread osteosynthesis, a simple method for treatment of dislocated supracondylar humerus fractures among children. Helv. Chir. Acta, *42*:15, 1975.
25. Beck, A.: Therapy of supracondylar fracture in children. Zentralbl. Chir., *60*:2242, 1933.
26. Bellemore, M. C., Barrett, I. R., Middleton, R. W., Scougall, J. S., and Whiteway, D. W.: Supracondylar osteotomy of the humerus for correction of cubitus varus. J. Bone Joint Surg., *66-A*:566, 1984.
27. Bender, J.: Cubitus varus after supracondylar fracture of the humerus in children: Can this deformity be prevented? Reconstr. Surg. Traumatol., *17*:100, 1979.
28. Bender, J., and Busch, C. A.: Results of treatment of supracondylar fractures of the humerus in children with special reference to the cause and prevention of cubitus varus. Arch. Chir. Neerl., *30*:29, 1978.
29. Bertola, L.: On supracondylar fractures of the humerus in childhood. Minerva Ortop., *10*:543, 1959.
30. Bezes, H., Massart, P., and Darmon, C.: Supracondylar fractures of the elbow in children and osteosynthesis by "open sky" double wiring using J. Seror's method. Apropos of 100 cases. J. Chir. (Paris), *120*:521, 1983.
31. Bhuller, G. S., and Connolly, J. F.: Ipsilateral supracondylar fractured humerus and fractured radius. Nebr. Med., J., *67*:85, 1982.
32. Bialik, B., Weiner, A., and Fishman, J.: Scoring system for assessing the treatment of supracondylar fractures of the humerus. Isr. J. Med. Sci., *19*:173, 1983.
33. Blount, W. P.: Fractures in Children. Baltimore, Williams & Wilkins, 1955, p. 26.
34. Boettcher, I., Sailer, R., and Kovacicek, S.: Treatment of supracondylar humeral fractures in children. Chirurg, *40*:28, 1969.
35. Bohler, L.: The Treatment of Fractures. 5th Ed. New York, Grune & Stratton, 1956–58. (Translation of *Technik der Knochenbruchbehandlung im Frienden und im Kriege*, 1885.)
36. Bohler, L.: Behandlung der supracondylaren Oberarmbruche bei Kindern und Jugenlichen. Monatschr. Unfallheilkd., *64*:1, 1961.
37. Bondarenko, N. S.: Transcondylar and supracondylar fractures of the humerus in children. Ortop. Travmatol. Protez., *10*:77, 1975.
38. Bondarenko, N. S., Dovgan, B. L., and Kazitski, V. M.: Determination and elimination of rotational displacement in transcondylar and supracondylar humeral fractures in children. Ortop. Travmatol. Protez., *8*:40, 1979.
39. Bongers, K. J., and Ponsen, R. J.: Use of Kirschner wires for percutaneous stabilization of supracondylar fractures of the humerus in children. Arch. Chir. Neerl., *31*:203, 1979.
40. Bradic, I., Vracun, D., and Pasini, M.: Percutaneous medial transcondylar osteosynthesis in supracondylar fractures of the humerus. Acta Chir. Iugosl., *26*:49, 1979.
41. Brandberg, R.: Treatment of supracondylar fractures by reduction followed by fixation in plaster splint. Acta Chir. Scand., *82*:400, 1939.
42. Brewster, A. H., and Karp, M.: Fractures in the region of the elbow in children. Surg. Gynecol. Obstet., *71*:643, 1940.
43. Brezina, L., and Prasil, J.: Contribution to the treatment of supracondylar fractures of the humerus in children (author's transl.). Acta Chir. Orthop. Traumatol. Cech., *43*:528, 1976.
44. Broudy, A. S., Jupiter, J., and May, J. W., Jr.: Management of supracondylar fracture with brachial artery thrombosis in a child: Case report and literature review. J. Trauma, *19*:540, 1979.
45. Brown, A.: Supracondylar fractures of the humerus. Nurs. Times, *71*:2016, 1975.
46. Buhl, O., and Hellberg, S.: Displaced supracondylar fractures of the humerus in children. Acta Orthop. Scand., *53*:67, 1982.
47. Bulle, G.: Treatment of supracondylar humeral fracture in children. Bruns. Beitr. Klin. Chir., *218*:646, 1971.
48. Cameron, S. M.: The aetiology and prevention of cubitus varus from supracondylar fractures in children. *In* Proceedings. J. Bone Joint Surg., *57-B*:255, 1975.
49. Carcassonne, M., Bergoin, M., and Hornung, H.: Results of operative treatment of severe supracondylar fractures of the elbow in children. J. Pediatr. Surg., *7*:676, 1972.
50. Carli, C.: Wire traction for supracondylar fracture of the elbow in children. Chir. Organi Mov., *18*:311, 1933.
51. Celoria, F.: Rupture of humeral artery in supracondylar fracture of the elbow. Rev. Soc. Pediatr. Litoral., *11*:133, 1946.
52. Childress, H. M.: Transarticular pin fixation in supracondylar fractures at the elbow in children. A case report. J. Bone Joint Surg., *54-A*:1548, 1972.
53. Christensen, L. O.: Method for bandaging of supracondylar extension fracture in children. Ugeskr. Laeger, *97*:1216, 1935.
54. Cooper, A., Sr.: A Treatise on Dislocations and Fractures of Joints. Philadelphia, Carey & Lea, 1825.
55. Corkery, P. H.: The management of supracondylar fractures of the humerus in children. Br. J. Clin. Pract., *18*:583, 1964.
56. Coventry, M. B., and Henderson, C. C.: Supracondylar fractures of the humerus—49 cases in children. Rocky Mt. Med. J., *53*:458, 1956.
57. Crawford, A. H., and Oestreich, A. E.: Danger of loss of reduction of supracondylar elbow fracture during radiography. J. Pediatr. Orthop., *3*:523, 1983.
58. Crawley, D. B., and Reckling, F. W.: Supracondylar fracture of the humerus in children. Am. Fam. Physician, *5*:113, 1972.
59. Cregan, J. C. F.: Prolonged traumatic arterial spasm after supracondylar fracture of the humerus. J. Bone Joint Surg., *33-B*:363, 1951.
60. D'Ambrosia, R. D.: Supracondylar fractures of humerus—prevention of cubitus varus. J. Bone Joint Surg., *54-A*:60, 1972.
61. Danielsson, L., and Pettersson, H.: Open reduction and pin fixation of severely displaced supracondylar fractures of the humerus in children. Acta Orthop. Scand., *51*:249, 1980.
62. Denis, R., and Guilleret, F.: Supracondyloid fractures of the elbow irreducible by external maneuvers. Lyon Chir., *36*:620, 1940.
63. Deutschlander, K.: Zur Behandlung der suprakondylaren Überstreckungsbruchen des Oberarmes. Chirurg, *6*:733, 1934.

64. Djorcevic, L. J., Dimisrijevic, A., Popovic, M., and Vasiljevic, M.: Current status and experience with treatment of supracondylar fractures in children. Srp. Arh. Celok. Lek., *93*:711, 1965.
65. Doder, A., and Andelic, M.: Surgical treatment of comminuted supracondylar and transcondylar fractures of the humerus. Med. Arh., *22*:23, 1968.
66. Dodge, H. S.: Displaced supracondylar fractures of the humerus in children—treatment by Dunlop's traction. J. Bone Joint Surg., *54-A*:1408, 1972.
67. Donchess, J. C.: Treatment of supracondylar fracture of the humerus. J. Indiana Med. Assoc., *42*:717, 1949.
68. Dowd, G. S., and Hopcroft, P. W.: Varus deformity in supracondylar fractures of the humerus in children. Injury, *10*:297, 1979.
69. Dunlop, J.: Transcondylar fractures of the humerus in childhood. J. Bone Joint Surg., *21*:59, 1939.
70. Edman, P., and Lohr, G.: Supracondylar fractures of the humerus treated with olecranon traction. Acta Chir. Scand., *126*:505, 1963.
71. Eid, A. M.: Reduction of displaced supracondylar fracture of the humerus in children by manipulation in flexion. Acta Orthop. Scand., *49*:39, 1978.
72. Eilenberger, S., and Betzler, H. J.: Experiences with percutaneous Bohr-wire fixation in supracondylar fractures of the humerus in childhood. Med. Welt, *25*:992, 1974.
73. Ekesparre, W. V.: Die Behandlung der suprakondylaren Humerusfraktur im Kindesalter. Dtsch. Med. J., *9*:168, 1958.
74. Ekesparre, W. V.: Treatment of supracondylar fractures of the humerus in children. Ann. Chir. Infant, *11*:213, 1970.
75. El-Ahwany, M. D.: Supracondylar fractures of the humerus in children with a note on the surgical correction of late cubitus varus. Injury, *6*:45, 1974.
76. El-Sharkawi, A. H., and Fattah, H. A.: Treatment of displaced supracondylar fractures of the humerus in children in full extension and supination. J. Bone Joint Surg., *47-B*:273, 1965.
77. Eliason, E. L.: Dressing for supracondylar fractures of the humerus. J.A.M.A., *82*:1934, 1924.
78. Elstrom, J. A., Pankovich, A. M., and Kassab, M. T.: Irreducible supracondylar fracture of the humerus in children. A report of two cases. J. Bone Joint Surg., *57-A*:680, 1975.
79. Fahey, J. J.: Fractures of the elbow in children. A.A.O.S. Instr. Course Lect., *17*:13, 1960.
80. Felsenreich, F.: Kindliche suprakondylare Frakturen und posttraumatische Deformitaten des Ellenbogengelenkes. Arch. Orthop. Unfallchir., *29*:555, 1931.
81. Ferro, R., Perquis, P., Bergeron, J., Reymondon, L., and Honorat, M.: Results of treatment of a series of 150 cases of supracondylar fractures in children at the Hospital Principal of Dakar. Bull. Soc. Med. Afr. Noire Llang. Fr., *17*:19, 1972.
82. Finochietto, R., and Ferre, R. L.: Fractures del codo. Cubito varo posttraumatico. Prensa Med. Argent., *12*:598, 1937.
83. Finochietto, R., and Liambias, A.: Supracondylar fractures of elbow in children. Semana Med., *2*:1837, 1933.
84. Flynn, J. C., Matthews, J. G., and Benoit, R. L.: Blind pinning of displaced supracondylar fractures of the humerus in children. Sixteen years' experience with long-term follow-up. J. Bone Joint Surg., *56-A*:263, 1974.
85. Fowles, J. V., and Kassab, M. T.: Displaced supracondylar fractures of the elbow in children. A report on the fixation of extension and flexion fractures by two lateral percutaneous pins. J. Bone Joint Surg., *56-B*:490, 1974.
86. French, P. R.: Varus deformity of the elbow following supracondylar fractures of the humerus in children. Lancet, 1:439, 1959.
87. Ganul, V. P.: Certain characteristics of the method and technique of permanent traction in the treatment of extension supra and transcondylar fractures of the humerus in children. Ortop. Travmatol. Protez., *35*:20, 1974.
88. Ganul, V. P.: Break plane and its influence on the treatment procedure using a skeletal traction method for trans- and supracondylar humeral fractures in children. Ortop. Travmatol. Protez., *2*:47, 1978.
89. Garneir, C.: Surgical reduction of supracondylar fractures in children. Sem. Hop. Paris, *23*:455, 1947.
90. Gartland, J. J.: Management of supracondylar fractures of the humerus in children. Surg. Gynecol. Obstet., *109*:145, 1959.
91. Ger, E.: Supracondylar fractures of the humerus in children. Reasons for unsatisfactory results. S. Afr. Med. J., *48*:1709, 1974.
92. Gerner, T., Benum, P., and Schistad, G.: Supracondylar fractures of the humerus in children treated with traction. Tidsskr. Nor. Laegforen., *95*:1587, 1975.
93. Gerstner, C., Hartmann, C., Jaschke, W., Hopf, G., and Hiemer, W.: Percutaneous osteosynthesis of supracondylar humerus fractures with Kirschner wires in childhood (author's transl.). Zentralbl. Chir., *106*:603, 1981.
94. Giannestras, N. J.: Displaced supracondylar fractures in children. Am. J. Orthop., *7*:92, 1963.
95. Giannini, S., Maffel, G., Girolami, M., and Ceccarelli, F.: The treatment of supracondylar fractures of the humerus in children by closed reduction and fixation with percutaneous Kirschner wires. Ital. J. Orthop. Traumatol., 9:181, 1983.
96. Gignal, R., and Bragoszewski, T.: Evaluation of the results of conservative treatment of supracondylar fractures in children. Chir. Narzadow Ruchu Ortop. Pol., *45*:127, 1980.
97. Gille, P., Sava, P., Guyot, J., and Mourot, M.: Anterior interosseous nerve syndrome following supracondylar fractures in children (author's transl.). Rev. Chir. Orthop., *64*:131, 1978.
98. Gjerloff, C., and Sojbjerg, J. O.: Percutaneous pinning of supracondylar fractures of the humerus. Acta Orthop. Scand., *49*:597, 1978.
99. Gottschalk, E., and Ackermann, A.: Collar and cuff in childhood supracondylar humeral fractures. Beitr. Orthop. Traumatol., *24*:206, 1977.
100. Goudarzi, Y. M.: Treatment of supracondylar fractures of the humerus in children and adolescents (author's transl.). Aktuel. Traumatol., *10*:153, 1980.
101. Gradinger, R., and Biehl, T.: Elbow joint-near fractures in the child. I. Classification, supracondylar humeral fracture, epicondylar rupture fracture. Fortschr. Med., *101*:165, 1983.
102. Graham, H. A.: Supracondylar fractures of the elbow in children. Part I. Clin. Orthop., *54*:85, 1967.
103. Graham, H. A.: Supracondylar fractures of the elbow in children. Part II. Clin. Orthop., *54*:93, 1967.
104. Griffin, P. P.: Supracondylar fractures of the humerus. Treatment and complications. Pediatr. Clin. North Am., *22*:477, 1975.
105. Gruber, M. A., and Hudson, O. C.: Supracondylar fracture of the humerus in childhood. End result study of open reduction. J. Bone Joint Surg., *46-A*:1245, 1964.
106. Gruss, J. D., Daum, R., and Gruss, B.: Treatment of supracondylar fractures of the humerus in children. Presse Med., *78*:1845, 1970.
107. Gruss, J. D., Daum, R., and Suy, R.: Supracondylar fracture in children. Acta Orthop. Belg., *38*:335, 1972.
108. Guther, R.: Innervation disorders following supracon-

dylar fractures in children (author's transl.). Zentralbl. Chir., *104*:1410, 1979.
109. Haddad, R. J., Jr., Saer, J. K., and Riordan, D. C.: Percutaneous pinning of displaced supracondylar fractures of the elbow in children. Clin. Orthop., *71*:112, 1970.
110. Hagen, R.: Skin-traction-treatment of supracondylar fractures of the humerus in children. Acta Orthop. Scand., *35*:138, 1964.
111. Hagen, R.: On the treatment of supracondylar humeral fractures in children. Chirurg, *39*:414, 1968.
112. Hamilton, D. R.: The treatment of supracondylar fracture of the humerus: With special reference to the advantages of skin traction. Papua New Guinea Med. J., *24*:198, 1981.
113. Hammond, G.: The management of supracondylar fractures of the humerus in children. Surg. Clin. North Am., *32*:747, 1952.
114. Hamsa, R. W., Sr.: A method for aligning supracondylar fractures of the humerus. Clin. Orthop., *123*:104, 1977.
115. Hanlon, C. R., and Estes, W. L.: Fractures in children. A statistical anlaysis. Am. J. Surg., *87*:312, 1954.
116. Hart, G. M., Wilson, D. W., and Arden, G. P.: The operative management of the difficult supracondylar fracture of the humerus in the child. Injury, *9*:30, 1977.
117. Hart, V. L.: Reduction of supracondylar fracture in children. Surgery, *11*:33, 1942.
118. Henrikson, B.: Supracondylar fracture of the humerus in children. A late review of end-results with special reference to the cause of deformity, disability and complications. Acta Chir. Scand. Suppl., 369, 1966.
119. Hesoun, P.: Die suprakondylare Oberarmfraktur im Kindesalter. Auswertung von 99 suprakondylaren Oberarmfrakturen aus den Jahren 1965 bis 1975. Unfallheilkunde, *79*:213, 1976.
120. Hey-Groves, E. W.: Direct skeletal traction in the treatment of fractures. Br. J. Surg., *16*:149, 1928.
121. Hierholzer, G., Horster, G., and Hax, P. M.: Supracondylar corrective osteotomies of the humerus in childhood. Aktuel. Probl. Chir. Orthop., *20*:101, 1981.
122. Hirt, H. J., Vogel, W., and Reichmann, W.: Die suprakondylare Humerusfraktur im Kindesalter. M.M.W., *118*:705, 1976.
123. Hofmann, V.: Behandlung der suprakondylaren Humerusfraktur im Kindesalter. Zentralbl. Chir., *93*:1678, 1968.
124. Hofmann, V.: Causes of functional disorders following supracondylar fractures in childhood. Beitr. Orthop. Traumatol., *15*:25, 1968.
125. Holmberg, I.: Fractures of the distal end of the humerus in children. Acta Chir. Scand. (Suppl.), 103, 1945.
126. Hordegen, K. M.: Neurologische Komplikationen bei kindlichen suprakondylaren Humerusfrakturen. Arch. Orthop. Unfallchir., *68*:294, 1970.
127. Hoyer, A.: Treatment of supracondylar fracture of the humerus by skeletal traction in an abduction splint. J. Bone Joint Surg., *34-A*:623, 1952.
128. Huegel, A., and Bijan, A.: Zur dringlichen primaroperativen Versorgung kindlicher suprakondylarer Oberarmfrakturen. Klin. Chir., *221*:633, 1974.
129. Ippolito, E., Caterini, R., and Scola, E.: Supracondylar fractures of the humerus in children. Analysis at maturity of fifty-three patients treated conservatively. J. Bone Joint Surg., *68-A*:333, 1986.
130. Izadpanah, M.: Die modifizierte blountsche Methode bei suprakondylaren Humerusfrakturen im Kindesalter. Arch. Orthop. Unfallchir., *77*:348, 1973.
131. Jachimowicz, B., and Groyecki, A.: Supracondylar fractures of the humerus in children. Chir. Narzadow Ruchu Ortop. Pol., *45*:207, 1980.
132. Jarvis, J. G., and D'Astous, J. L.: The pediatric T-supracondylar fracture. J. Pediatr. Orthop., *4*:697, 1984.
133. Jaschke, W., and Stojanovic, R.: Adequate treatment of supracondylar fracture of the humerus with associated brachial artery and nerve injury in childhood (author's transl.). Z. Kinderchir., *32*:353, 1981.
134. Jefferiss, C. D.: "Straight lateral traction" in selected supracondylar fractures of the humerus in children. Injury, 8:213, 1977.
135. Jewett, E. L.: New closed method of treating supracondylar fractures. Am. J. Surg., *44*:572, 1939.
136. Jonasch, E.: V-Osteotomie bei cubitus varus nach suprakondylaren Oberarmbruchen bei Kindren. Arch. Orthop. Unfallchir., 48:659, 1957.
137. Jones, D.: Transcondylar fractures of the humerus in children: Definition of an acceptable reduction. Proc. R. Soc. Med., *70*:624, 1977.
138. Jones, E. T., and Louis, D. S.: Median nerve injuries associated with supracondylar fractures of the humerus in children. Clin. Orthop., *150*:181, 1980.
139. Jones, K. G.: Percutaneous pin fixation of fractures of the lower end of the humerus. Clin. Orthop., *50*:53, 1967.
140. Judet, H.: Exact immediate nonsurgical reduction of transverse supracondylar fracture in children. Bull. Soc. Chir. Paris, *28*:542, 1936.
141. Judet, J.: Traitment des fractures sus-condyliennes transversales de l'humerus chez l'enfant. Rev. Chir. Orthop., *39*:199, 1953.
142. Kagan, N., and Herold, H. Z.: Correction of axial deviations after supracondylar fractures of the humerus in children. Int. Surg., *58*:735, 1973.
143. Kamal, A. S., and Austin, R. T.: Dislocation of the median nerve and brachial artery in supracondylar fractures of the humerus. Injury, *12*:161, 1980.
144. Karlsson, J., Thorsteinsson, T., Thorleifsson, R., and Arnason, H.: Entrapment of the median nerve and brachial artery after supracondylar fractures of the humerus in children. Arch. Orthop. Trauma. Surg., *104*:389, 1986.
145. Katzman, H.: Zur Behandlung suprakondylarer Oberarmfrakturen bei Kindern. Zentralbl. Chir., *90*:2089, 1965.
146. Kawada, T.: Treatment of supracondylar fracture of the humerus. Orthop. Surg. (Tokyo), *20*:491, 1969.
147. Kazmin, A. I., Ter-Egiazarov, G. M., and Mogian, G. H. H.: Varus deformities of the elbow joint in children after trans- and supracondylar fractures of the humerus and their treatment. Ortop. Travmatol. Protez., *35*:1, 1974.
148. Kekomaki, M., Luoma, R., Rikalainen, M., and Vilkki, P.: Operative treatment of supracondylar fracture of the humerus in childhood. Duodecim, 99:598, 1983.
149. Kekomaki, M., Luoma, R., Rikalainen, H., and Vilkki, P.: Operative reduction and fixation of a difficult supracondylar extension fracture of the humerus. J. Pediatr. Orthop., *4*:13, 1984.
150. Keller, E.: Supracondylar fractures in children and their treatment with special consideration of muscular mechanism. Arch. Klin. Chir., *192*:702, 1938.
151. King, D., and Secor, C.: Bow elbow (cubitus varus). J. Bone Joint Surg., *33-A*:572, 1951.
152. Klages, F.: Supracondyloid fractures in child. Dtsch. Med. Wochenschr., *58*:810, 1932.
153. Klinefelter, E. W.: Influence of position on measurement of projected bone angle. A.J.R., *55*:722, 1946.
154. Kocher, T.: Beitrage zur Kenntnis einiger praktisch wichtiger Fracturformen. Basel und Leipzig, Carl Sallmann, 1896.
155. Kolesnikov, I. O. P.: Results of the conservative treatment of transcondylar fractures of the humerus in children. Khirurgiia (Mosk.), *43*:109, 1967.

156. Konradt, J., Braunsdorf, M., and Waldschmidt, J.: Concomitant injuries and complications of supracondylar humerus fracture in childhood. Med. Welt, *27*:978, 1976.
157. Kopecky, J., Simecek, O., and Richter, V.: Percutaneous fixation of adverse dislocated supracondylar fractures of the humerus in children. Rozhl. Chir., *57*:303, 1978.
158. Koszla, M. M., and Czarnecka-Kupis, I.: Treatment of humeral supracondylar fractures in children. Chir. Narzadow Ruchu Ortop. Pol., *34*:757, 1969.
159. Kramhoft, M., Keller, I. L., and Solgaard, S.: Displaced supracondylar fractures of the humerus in children. Clin. Orthop., *221*:215, 1987.
160. Krasznai, I., Ficzere, O., and Kovalkovits, I.: Emergency care of supracondylar humeral fractures in childhood. Orv. Hetil., *117*:1452, 1976.
161. Krebs, B.: Surgical treatment of supracondylar humeral fractures in children. Ugeskr. Laeger, *142*:871, 1980.
162. Krezel, T., and Zelaznowski, W.: Spontaneous growth correction in supracondylar fractures of the humerus in children. Chir. Narzadow Ruchu Ortop. Pol., *32*:531, 1967.
163. Kristensen, J.L., and Vibild, O.: Supracondylar fractures of the humerus in children. Acta Orthop. Scand., *47*:375, 1976.
164. Kroener, D.: The care of childhood supracondylar humerus fractures with crossed drill wires. Chirurg, *41*:188, 1970.
165. Labelle, H., Bunnell, W. P., Duhaime, M., and Poitras, B.: Cubitus varus deformity following supracondylar fractures of the humerus in children. J. Pediatr. Orthop., *2*:539, 1982.
166. Laburthe-Tolra, Y.: Epiphyseal atrophy following supracondylian fractures of the humerus in children. Ann. Chir., *27*:1211, 1973.
167. von Laer, L.: The supracondylar fracture of the humerus in children (author's transl.). Arch. Orthop. Trauma. Surg., *95*:123, 1979.
168. LaGrange, J., and Rigault, P.: Fractures supracondyliennes. Rev. Chir. Orthop., *48*:337, 1962.
169. LaGrange, J., and Rigault, P.: Treatment of supracondylar fractures of the humerus in children. Presse Med., *78*:2382, 1970.
170. Langenskiold, A.: Adolescent humerus varus. Acta Chir. Scand., *105*:353, 1953.
171. Langenskiold, A., and Kivilaakso, R.: Varus and valgus deformity of the elbow following supracondylar fracture of the humerus. Acta Orthop. Scand., *38*:313, 1967.
172. Lanz, T. V., and Wachsmuth, W.: Praktische Anatomie, 2. Aufl., Bd. I/III. Berlin, Springer, 1959.
173. Lavik, K.: Supracondylar fracture of the humerus in children treated with traction using Semb's abduction splint. Nord. Med., *63*:422, 1960.
174. Lawrence, W.: Supracondylar fractures of the humerus in children. Br. J. Surg., *44*:143, 1956.
175. Lefort, J.: Supracondylar fractures in children: Treatment techniques and indications. Ann. Chir., *36*:293, 1982.
176. Levai, J. P., Tanguy, A., Collin, J. P., and Teinturier, P.: Recurrent posterior dislocation of the elbow following malunion of supracondylar fracture of the humerus. Report of a case (author's transl.). Rev. Chir. Orthop., *65*:457, 1979.
177. Leveuf, J.: Treatment of supracondylar fractures in children. Rev. Orthop., *32*:263, 1946.
178. Leveuf, J., and Godard, H.: Open reduction of supracondyloid fractures in children. Fixation by transplanted bone. J. Chir., *45*:358, 1935.
179. Liebling, G.: Treatment of supracondylar humeral fractures in children with special reference to Blount's collar and cuff technic. Z. Arztl. Fortbild. (Jena), *77*:639, 1983.
180. Lim Khai Liang: A review of recent supracondylar fractures of the humerus in children. Singapore Med. J., *11*:264, 1970.
181. Lipscomb, P. R., and Burleson, R. J.: Vascular and neural complications in supracondylar fractures of the humerus in children. J. Bone Joint Surg., *37-A*:487, 1955.
182. Lobova, M. A.: The ossificates in supracondylar fractures of the humerus and their outcomes in children. Ortop. Travmatol. Protez., *27*:48, 1966.
183. Lonnroth, H.: Measurement of rotational displacement in supracondylar fractures of the humerus. Acta Radiol. (Stochkh.), *57*:65, 1962.
184. Loup, J.: Surgical treatment of 13 cases of supracondylar fracture of the humerus in children. Ann. Chir., *30*:391, 1976.
185. Lubinus: Ueber den Entstehungsmechanismus und die Therapie der suprakondylaren Humerusfrakturen. Dtsch. Z. Chir., *186*:289, 1924.
186. Lund-Kristensen, J., and Vibild, O.: Supracondylar fractures of the humerus in children. A follow-up with particular reference to late results after severely displaced fractures. Acta Orthop. Scand., *47*:375, 1976.
187. Lusk, W. C.: Reduction of supracondylar fractures of the humerus. Ann. Surg., *37*:433, 1908.
188. Macaffe, A. L.: Infantile supracondylar fractures. J. Bone Joint Surg., *49-B*:768, 1967.
189. McGraw, J. J., Akbarnia, B. A., Hanel, D. P., Keppler, L., and Burdge, R. E.: Neurological complications resulting from supracondylar fractures of the humerus in children. J. Pediatr. Orthop., *6*:647, 1986.
190. Madsen, E.: Supracondylar fractures of the humerus in children. J. Bone Joint Surg., *37-B*:241, 1955.
191. Magerl, F.: Ellenbogenfraktur beim Erwachsenen—ein dorsaler kombinierter Zugang zum Humerus. Z. Unfallmed. Berufskr., *2*:59, 1973.
192. Magerl, F.: Suprakondylare Korrekturosteotomien am Humerus bei Erwachsenen. Z. Unfallmed. Berufskr., *2*:87, 1973.
193. Malgaigne, J. F.: Treatise on Fractures. Philadelphia, Lippincott, 1859.
194. Mann, T. S.: Prognosis in supracondylar fractures. J. Bone Joint Surg., *45-B*:516, 1963.
195. Marsh, H. O., and Navarro, L.: The fractured elbow. Supracondylar fractures of the humerus in children. J. Kans. Med. Soc., 67:351, 1966.
196. Matsuno, S., and Kondo, Y.: Treatment of supracondylar fracture of the humerus. Orthop. Surg. (Tokyo), *20*:482, 1969.
197. Matzen, P. F., and Hein, W.: Treatment of supracondylar overstretching fractures of the humerus in childhood. Beitr. Orthop. Traumatol., *24*:200, 1977.
198. Maylahn, D. J., and Fahey, J. J.: Fractures of the elbow in children. J.A.M.A., *166*:220, 1958.
199. Micheli, L. J., Skolnick, M. D., and Hall, J. E.: Supracondylar fractures of the humerus in children. Am. Fam. Physician, *19*:100, 1979.
200. Miller, E. M., Fell, E. H., Brock, C., Todd, M. C., and Requarth, W. H.: Progress in the management of severe supracondylar fractures of the elbow. Ann. Surg., *113*:1098, 1941.
201. Minne, J.: Late results of orthopaedic and surgical therapy of transverse supracondylar fractures in children. Echo Med. Nord., *1*:129, 1936.
202. Mitchell, W. J., and Adams, J. P.: Supracondylar fractures of the humerus in children. A 10-year review. J.A.M.A., *175*:573, 1961.
203. Mitchell, W. J., and Adams, J. P.: Effective management for supracondylar fractures of the humerus in children. Clin. Orthop., *23*:197, 1962.
204. Moehring, H. D.: Irreducible supracondylar fracture of the humerus complicated by anterior interosseous nerve palsy. Clin. Orthop., 206:228, 1986.
205. Morier-Genoud, J., and Lavanchy, P.: Treatment of

a supracondylar fracture of the humerus in a child. Rev. Med. Suisse Romande, *99*:371, 1979.
206. Morkos, N.: Conservative treatment of supracondylar humeral fractures in children using Blount's bandage. Zentralbl. Chir., *94*:565, 1969.
207. Moroz, P. F.: Reconstructive surgery in incorrectly united supra- and transcondylar fractures of the humerus in children. Ortop. Travmatol. Protez., *35*:63, 1974.
208. Morris, P. K.: Supracondylar fracture of the humerus involving the elbow joint. Proc. Mine. Med. Off. Assoc., *50*:33, 1970.
209. Morwood, J. B.: Supracondylar fracture with absent radial pulse: Report of 2 cases. Br. Med. J., *1*:163, 1939.
210. Muller, M. E., Allgower, M., Schneider, R., and Willenegger, H.: Manual of Internal Fixation. 2nd. Ed. New York, Springer, 1979.
211. Nacht, J. L., Ecker, M. L., Chung, S. M., Lotke, P. A., and Das, M.: Supracondylar fractures of the humerus in children treated by closed reduction and percutaneous pinning. Clin. Orthop., *177*:203, 1983.
212. Nand, S.: Management of supracondylar fracture of the humerus in children. Int. Surg., *57*:893, 1972.
213. Nasser, A., and Chater, E.: Open reduction and Kirschner wire fixation for supracondylar fracture of the humerus. J. Bone Joint Surg., *58-B*:135, 1976.
214. Nielsen, C. M., Rasmussen, P. C., and Stecher, J. E.: Supracondylar fracture of the humerus in children. Ugeskr. Laeger, *143*:203, 1981.
215. Norell, H. G.: Roentgenographic visualization of extracapsular fat: its importance in the diagnosis of traumatic injuries to the elbow. Acta Radiol., *42*:205, 1954.
216. Norman, O.: Roentgenological studies on dislocation in supracondylar fractures of the humerus. Ann. Radiol. (Paris), *18*:395, 1975.
217. Olszewski, W., and Kijas, Z.: Results of conservative treatment of supracondylar fractures of the humerus in children. Chir. Narzadow Ruchu Ortop. Pol., *46*:541, 1981.
218. Ottolenghi, C. E.: Acute ischemic syndrome: Its treatment. Prophylaxis of Volkmann's syndrome. Am. J. Orthop., *2*:312, 1960.
219. Ottolenghi, C. E.: Prophylaxic du syndrome de Volkmann dans des fractures supracondyliennes du condo chez l'enfant. Rev. Chir. Orthop., *57*:517, 1971.
220. Palmer, E. E., Niemann, K. M., Vesely, D., and Armstrong, J. H.: Supracondylar fracture of the humerus in children. J. Bone Joint Surg., *60-A*:653, 1978.
221. Papavasiliou, V. A., and Beslikas, T. A.: T-condylar fractures of the distal humeral condyles during childhood: An analysis of six cases. J. Pediatr. Orthop., *6*:302, 1986.
222. Papp, G.: Conservative treatment of supracondylar humerus fractures in children with Blount's method (author's transl.). Magy. Traumatol. Orthop., *22*:81, 1979.
223. Parmeggiani, G., and Lommi, G.: Supracondyloid fractures of the humerus in childhood. Minerva Ortop., *16*:490, 1965.
224. Pesula, E., and Wondrak, E.: Late sequelae of dislocated supracondylar fractures of the humerus in children. Rozhl. Chir., *61*:607, 1982.
225. Petrov, N., Gucev, S., Kirkov, L. J., Dajljevik, S., and Ruso, B.: Supracondylar fractures in children. Acta Chir. Iugosl., *29*:229, 1982.
226. Piggot, J.: Supracondylar fractures of the humerus in children. Analysis at maturity of fifty-three patients treated conservatively (letter). J. Bone Joint Surg., *68-A*:1304, 1986.
227. Piggot, J., Graham, H. K., and McCoy, G. F.: Supracondylar fractures of the humerus in children. Treatment by straight lateral traction. J. Bone Joint Surg., *68-B*:577, 1986.
228. Pirone, A. M., Graham, H. K., and Krajbuch, J. I.: Management of displaced extension-type supracondylar fractures of the humerus in children. J. Bone Joint Surg., *70-A*:641, 1988.
229. Piroth, P., Gharib, M., and Langer, I.: Supracondylar humeral fractures in infants and small children. Z. Kinderchir., *32*:347, 1981.
230. Plemencic, M., Romcevic, B., Kolombo, E., and Ranic, V.: Supracondylar fractures in children and their treatment. Acta Chir. Iugosl., *24*:Suppl. 2:153, 1977.
231. Podrazhanski, V. A.: Surgical treatment of supra- and transcondylar fractures of the humerus in children. Ortop. Travmatol. Protez., *35*:62, 1974.
232. Poigenfurst, J.: Consequences of delayed surgery in juvenile upper arm condyle fractures. Arch. Orthop. Unfallchir., *60*:364, 1966.
233. Poitras, B., Labelle, H., Tchelebi, H., Duhaime, M., Rivard, C. H., Labelle, P., Simoneau, R., Morin, B., and Fassier, F.: Supracondylar fractures of the humerus in children. Review of 217 cases. Union Med. Can., *112*:325, 1983.
234. Pompner, K.: Severe open supracondylar humeral fracture in childhood. Zentralbl. Chir., *98*:1622, 1973.
235. Post, M., and Haskell, S. S.: Reconstruction of the median nerve following entrapment in supracondylar fracture of the humerus. J. Trauma, *14*:252, 1974.
236. Pouliquen, J. C.: Supra-condylar fractures in the child. J. Chir. (Paris), *112*:165, 1976.
237. Prietto, C. A.: Supracondylar fractures of the humerus. A comparative study of Dunlop's traction versus percutaneous pinning. J. Bone Joint Surg., *61-A*:425, 1979.
238. Prins, J. G., and Vermaak, J. C.: Extension therapy with Von Ekesparre darts of supracondylar fractures of the humerus in children. Arch. Chir. Neerl., *26*:140, 1974.
239. Raganowicz, M., and Slaskie, P.: The treatment of supracondylar fracture of humerus in children (author's transl.). Przegl. Lek., *36*:355, 1979.
240. Ramsey, R. H., and Griz, J.: Immediate open reduction and internal fixation of severely displaced supracondylar fractures of the humerus in children. Clin. Orthop., *90*:130, 1973.
241. Reinaerts, H. H., and Cheriex, E. C.: Assessment of dislocation in the supracondylar fracture of the humerus treated by overhanging traction. Reconstr. Surg. Traumatol., *17*:92, 1979.
242. Revenko, T. A., and Tsaimidanova, N. B.: Abduction splint for treatment of transcondylar fractures of the humerus in children. Ortop. Travmatol. Protez., *33*:68, 1972.
243. Richkin, J.: Treatment of supracondylar fractures. South Afr. Med. J., *12*:742, 1938.
244. Ritter, G., and Sarvestani, M.: Problems and therapy of the supracondylar upper-arm fracture in childhood. Fortschr. Med., *91*:671, 1973.
245. Rocher, H. L.: Surgical reduction of supracondylar transverse fracture of elbow in children. Bordeaux Chir., *3*:431, 1932.
246. Rogers, L. F., Malave, S., Jr., White, H., and Tachdjian, M. O.: Plastic bowing, torus and greenstick supracondylar fractures of the humerus: Radiographic clues to obscure fractures of the elbow in children. Radiology, *128*:145, 1978.
247. Rosman, M.: A fracture board to facilitate the management of supracondylar humeral fractures in children. J. Trauma, *15*:153, 1975.
248. Rouffet, F., Pourcher, J., Fingerhut, A., Nataf, G., Elberg, J. F., and Huguet, J. C.: Treatment of supracondylar fractures in children. Apropos of 30 cases. Acta Orthop. Belg., *43*:110, 1977.

249. Rowell, P. J.: Arterial occlusion in juvenile humeral supracondylar fracture. Injury, *6*:254, 1975.
250. Ruster, D., and Wolf, W.: Errors before and during percutaneous wire fixation of juvenile supracondylar upper arm fractures. Beitr. Orthop. Traumatol., *23*:111, 1976.
251. Salter, R. B.: Supracondylar fractures in childhood. J. Bone Joint Surg., *41-B*:881, 1959.
252. Samimi, P., and Abel, R.: Results of conservative treatment of supracondylar humeral fractures in childhood. Monatsschr. Unfallheilkd., *69*:313, 1966.
253. Sandegard, E.: Fractures of the lower end of the humerus in children. Treatment and end results. Acta Chir. Scand., *89*:1, 1943.
254. Satter, P., Schulte, H. D., and Door, B.: The results of treatment of supracondylar humeral fractures in children with special consideration to Blount's method. Zentralbl. Chir., *96*:125, 1971.
255. Schickendanz, H., Maag, G., and Schurer, E.: Supracondylar humerus fractures in children. Beitr. Orthop. Traumatol., *29*:12, 1981.
256. Schink, W.: Die Fractura supracondylica humeri und die ischanische Kontraktur im Kindesalter. Chirurg, *39*:417, 1968.
257. Schmeider, H., and Hofmann, S.: Supracondylar upper arm and forearm fractures as combination injuries in the child. Monatsschr. Unfallheilkd., *72*:299, 1969.
258. Schwencke, K.: Our experiences in 71 supracondylar humeral fractures treated with crossed drill wires. Monatsschr. Unfallheilkd., *71*:221, 1968.
259. Sebestik, V., and Neubauer, M.: Supracondylar fractures of the humerus in children. Rozhl. Chir., *55*:781, 1976.
260. Seewald, H.: Rush pinning of children's supracondylar humeral fractures. Zentralbl. Chir., *96*:468, 1971.
261. Seghini, G.: Outcome of therapy of supracondylar fractures. Arch. Chir. Ortop., *20*:33, 1955.
262. Sgrosso, J. A.: Skeletal traction in therapy of supracondylar fractures in childhood. Rev. Ortop. Traumatol., *5*:381, 1936.
263. Shevtson, V. I., and Znamenskii, G. B.: Treatment of trans- and supracondylar fractures of the humerus in children (review of the literature). Ortop. Travmatol. Protez., *11*:68, 1982.
264. Shifrin, P. G., Gehring, H. W., and Iglesias, L. J.: Open reduction and internal fixation of displaced supracondylar fractures of the humerus in children. Acta Orthop. Belg., *38*:157, 1972.
265. Shifrin, P. G., Gehring, H. W., and Iglesias, L. J.: Open reduction and internal fixation of displaced supracondylar fractures of the humerus in children. Orthop. Clin. North Am., *7*:573, 1976.
266. Siris, I. E.: Supracondylar fracture of the humerus. An analysis of 330 cases. Surg. Gynecol. Obstet., *68*:201, 1939.
267. Smith, F. M.: Kirschner wire traction in elbow and upper arm injuries. Am. J. Surg., *74*:770, 1947.
268. Smith, L.: Deformity following supracondylar fractures of the humerus. J. Bone Joint Surg., *42-A*:235, 1960.
269. Smith, L.: Deformity following supracondylar fractures of the humerus. J. Bone Joint Surg., *47-A*:1668, 1965.
270. Smith, L.: Supracondylar fractures of the humerus treated by direct observation. Clin. Orthop., *50*:37, 1967.
271. Smyth, E. H. J.: Primary rupture of brachial artery and median nerve in supracondylar fracture of the humerus. J. Bone Joint Surg., *38-B*:736, 1956.
272. Sojbjerg, J. O., and Blom, L.: Percutaneous fixation of supracondylar fractures of the humerus in children. Ugeskr. Laeger, *145*:1775, 1983.
273. Sorrel, E.: A propos des fractures supracondyliennes de l'humerus chez l'enfant. Rev. Orthop., *32*:383, 1946.
274. Sorrel, E., and Longuet, Y.: La voie trans-brachial anterieure dans la chirurgie des fractures supra-condyliennes de l'humerus chez l'enfant (indication et technique). Rev. Chir. Orthop., *32*:3, 1946.
275. Spear, H. C., and Janes, J. M.: Rupture of the brachial artery accompanying dislocation of the elbow or supracondylar fracture. J. Bone Joint Surg., *33-A*:889, 1951.
276. Spinner, M., and Schreiber, S.: Anterior interosseous nerve paralysis—a complication of supracondylar fractures of the humerus in children. J. Bone Joint Surg., *51-A*:1584, 1969.
277. Spissak, L., Kirnak, J., and Majesky, I.: Use of extension in the treatment of supracondylar humeral fractures in children. Indications and results. Acta Chir. Orthop. Traumatol. Cech., *36*:172, 1969.
278. Spitzer, A. G., and Paterson, D. C.: Acute nerve involvement in supracondylar fractures of the humerus in children. J. Bone Joint Surg., *55-B*:227, 1973.
279. Staples, O. S.: Supracondylar fractures of the humerus in children. Complications and problems associated with traction. J.A.M.A., *168*:730, 1958.
280. Staples, O. S.: Complications of traction treatment of supracondylar fracture of the humerus in children. J. Bone Joint Surg., *41-A*:369, 1959.
281. Staples, O. S.: Dislocation of the brachial artery. A complication of supracondylar fracture of the humerus in childhood. J. Bone Joint Surg., *47-A*:1525, 1965.
282. Stare, J.: Surgical results in severe supracondylar fractures of the forearm in childhood. Acta Chir. Iugosl., *24*:139, 1977.
283. Suire, P., Hakim, H., and Desrouffet, J.: Treatment of supracondylar humeral fractures with extensive displacement in the child. Ann. Chir., *23*:619, 1969.
284. Suzuki, K., Takahashi, S., Takimune, A., and Ono, S.: Management of supracondylar fracture of the humerus. Orthop. Surg. (Tokyo), 20:486, 1969.
285. Swenson, A. L.: Treatment of supracondylar fractures of humerus by Kirschner wire transfixation. J. Bone Joint Surg., *30-A*:993, 1948.
286. Symeonides, P. P., Paschaloglou, C., and Pagalides, T.: Radial nerve enclosed in the callus of a supracondylar fracture. J. Bone Joint Surg., *57-B*:523, 1975.
287. Ter-Egiazarov, G. M., Pavlova, G. A., Travkin, A. A., and Markulov, V. N.: Neurological complications of the supra- and transcondylar fractures of the humerus in children. Ortop. Travmatol. Protez., *11*:37, 1982.
288. Teutsch, W., and Schmidt, H.: Results of follow-up examination following conservatively treated supracondylar humeral fractures in children. Zentralbl. Chir., *92*:2874, 1967.
289. Thompson, V. P.: Supracondylar fractures of the humerus in children. J.A.M.A., *146*:609, 1951.
290. Thorgersen, E.: Supracondylar fractures treated by Bohler method in children. Norsk. Mag. Laegevidensk., *96*:121, 1935.
291. Turra, S., Pavaninio, G., and Pasquon, P. G.: Complications of supracondylar fractures of the humerus in children. Clin. Orthop., *25*:222, 1974.
292. Twedt, B.: Skeletal traction for supracondylar fractures of humerus. O.N.A.J., *4*:9, 1977.
293. Ulrikh, E. V.: Modification of fixation of fragments in open reposition of transcondylar fractures of the humerus in children. Ortop. Travmatol. Protez., *35*:59, 1974.
294. Urmonas, V. K.: A splinting device for the treatment of transcondylar fractures of the humerus in children. Ortop. Travmatol. Protez., *27*:66, 1966.
295. Vahvanen, V., and Aalto, K.: Supracondylar fracture of the humerus in children. Acta Orthop. Scand., *49*:225, 1978.
296. Van der Hoff, H. L. M.: One hundred uncomplicated supracondylar fractures in children. Acta Chir. Scand., *88*:99, 1943.

297. Van Gorder, G. W.: Surgical approach in supracondylar "T" fractures requiring open reduction. J. Bone Joint Surg., *22*:278, 1940.
298. Verde, D.: Osteosynthesis in supracondylar fractures in child. Arch. Putti, *1*:22, 1951.
299. Virenque, J., and LaFage, J.: Les fractures supracondyliennes du coude chez l'enfant. Resultats compares des traitments orthopedique et chirurgical, a propos de 163 observations. Ann. Chir., *21*:544, 1967.
300. Wade, F. V., and Batdorf, J.: Supracondylar fractures of the humerus. A 12 year review with follow-up. J. Bone Trauma, *1*:269, 1961.
301. Wahl, D., Lent, G., and Kurth, C.: Supracondylar fractures of the humerus in children: Classification (author's transl.). Zentralbl. Chir., *104*:1393, 1979.
302. Walloe, A., Egund, N., and Eikelund, L.: Supracondylar fracture of the humerus in children: Review of closed and open reduction leading to a proposal for treatment. Injury, *16*:296, 1985.
303. Watson-Jones, R.: Fractures and Joint Injuries. 4th Ed, Vol. 2. Edinburgh, E. & S. Livingstone, 1955, p. 501.
304. Weiland, A. J., Meyer, S., Tolo, V. T., Berg, H. L., and Mueller, J.: Surgical treatment of displaced supracondylar fractures of the humerus in children. Analysis of fifty-two cases followed for five to fifteen years. Clin. Orthop., *25*:222, 1974.
305. Weiland, A. J., Meyer, S., Tolo, V. T., Berg, H. L., and Mueller, J.: Surgical treatment of displaced supracondylar fractures of the humerus in children. Analysis of fifty-two cases followed for five to fifteen years. J. Bone Joint Surg., *60-A*:657, 1978.
306. Weller, S.: Konservatierte oder operative Behandlung von suprakondylaren Oberarmfrakturen. Aktuel. Traumatol., *2*:79, 1974.
307. Wessely, J., and Decker, S.: The treatment of supracondylar fractures of the humerus in children (author's transl.). Unfallheilkunde, *81*:618, 1978.
308. Wilkins, K. E.: Supracondylar fractures of the humerus: *In* Rockwood, C. H., Wilkins, K. E., and King, R. E. (eds.): Fractures in Children. Philadelphia, J. B. Lippincott, 1984, p. 376.
309. Wilppula, E., and Bakalim, G.: Late results in supracondylar humeral fractures in children. Arch. Orthop. Trauma Surg., *104*:23, 1985.
310. Wilson, J. C., and McDonnell, D. P.: Fractures of the lower end of the humerus in children. J. Bone Joint Surg., *30-A*:347, 1948.
311. Winfeld, P., and Pilgaard, S.: Osteosyntese af suprakondylare humerus frakturer hos born. Nord. Med., *66*:1266, 1961.
312. Winkler, E.: Supracondylar humeral fracture—Fixation by percutaneous double wires. Hefte Unfallheilkd., *102*:154, 1970.
313. Witt, A. N.: Zur operativen Behandlung der supracondylaren Humerusfrakturen im Kindesalter. Chirurg, *26*:488, 1955.
314. Wojcik, T.: Reconstruction of the humerus after supracondylar fractures in children. Chir. Narzadow Ruchu Ortop. Pol., *35*:295, 1970.
315. Worlock, P.: Supracondylar fractures of the humerus. Assessment of cubitus varus by the Baumann angle. J. Bone Joint Surg., *68-B*:755, 1986.
316. Worlock, P. H., and Colton, C. L.: Displaced supracondylar fractures of the humerus in children treated by overhead olecranon traction. Injury, *15*:316, 1984.
317. Wray, J.: Management of supracondylar fracture with vascular insufficiency. Arch. Surg., *90*:279, 1965.
318. Yamamoto, I., Ishii, S., Usui, M., Ogino, T., and Kaneda, K.: Cubitus varus deformity following supracondylar fracture of the humerus. A method for measuring rotational deformity. Clin. Orthop., *201*:179, 1985.
319. Zhu, S. X.: Analysis of therapeutic effects in cases of supracondylar fracture of the humerus in children (author's transl.). Chung Hua I Hsueh Tsa Chih, *62*:170, 1982.
320. Zimmermann, H. G.: Percutaneous larding-wire osteosynthesis of supracondylar humeral fracture in childhood. Method and follow-up examination results. Chirurg, *49*:248, 1978.

VOLKMANN'S ISCHEMIC CONTRACTURE (Compartment Syndrome)

In 1881, Richard von Volkmann described an ischemic paralysis and contracture of the muscles of the forearm and hand, and less frequently of the leg, which followed the application of taut bandages in the treatment of injuries in the region of the elbow and knee. He suggested that the pathologic changes primarily resulted from obstruction of arterial blood flow, which, if unrelieved, after six hours, would result in death of the muscles.[114]

Initially supracondylar fractures of the humerus were the most common cause of Volkmann's ischemia. With improved management of the elbow fractures in children, the incidence and type of predisposing injury are changing. For example, at the Mayo Clinic, Meyerding reported the incidence of Volkmann's ischemic contracture as 0.18 per thousand new registrants prior to 1935.[74] The incidence decreased to 0.03 per thousand new registrants at the Mayo Clinic between 1955 and 1965. Eichler and Lipscomb found 35 per cent of the cases of Volkman's ischemia were caused by supracondylar and elbow fractures, 20 per cent by fractures of both bones of the forearm, and 20 per cent by soft-tissue or crush injuries without associated fractures. Other new causes noted by them were perfusion of the upper limb for treatment of malignant neoplasms, massive blood transfusion under pressure during cardiac surgery, and excision of congenital radioulnar synostosis in which compartment syndrome occurred as a complication. In the series of Eichler and Lipscomb, 70 per cent of these patients were males.[28]

In the past, there were two contending theories about the mechanism of Volkmann's ischemic contracture: one, that it resulted from arterial insufficiency, and the other, that it developed secondarily to venous occlusion and stasis. In 1940, Griffiths firmly established that the process is caused by arterial occlusion.[36]

Pathophysiology. The pathophysiology of Volkmann's ischemia as outlined by Eaton and Green is as follows:[25]

Ischemia produces anoxia in muscles, which in turn causes formation of histamine-like substances; consequently capillary permeability increases and conspicuous intramuscular edema develops. This increasing intramuscular edema causes progressive increase in the intrinsic tissue pressure of the muscles. Circular unyielding dressings on the limb and limited expansion in a taut fascial envelope increase the venous compression, which causes further increase in intrinsic tissue pressure. Pressor receptors within the compartment and within the muscle itself stimulate a reflex vasospasm affecting all vessels in this general area. This vasospasm aggravates and perpetuates the initial vascular compromise, and a destructive ischemia-edema cycle develops. Eaton and associates were able, experimentally, to produce transient yet complete spasmodic shutdown of the brachial artery by injecting a small bolus of autogenous blood beneath the volar carpal ligaments of rabbits.

The pathologic process is one of necrosis of muscle with secondary fibrosis that may develop calcification in its terminal phase. The infarct has an ellipsoid shape with its axis along the anterior interosseous artery and its central point slightly above the middle of the forearm. The flexor digitorum profundus, the flexor pollicis longus, and the median nerve are the most commonly and severely affected. During the acute stage, when the volar compartment of the forearm is surgically exposed, the deep fascia will be very taut and will spread widely when split. The muscles, which are either pale or blue-black from extravasation, will protrude through the wound. The veins are always engorged.

Circulatory embarrassment in supracondylar fractures of the humerus may result from the brachial artery being caught and kinked at the fracture site, from contusion and spasm of the artery at the moment of fracture, from compression of the brachial vessels by a tight encircling cast, or from rapidly progressive swelling in a taut fascial compartment.

Distal to the lacertus fibrosus the brachial artery branches into the radial and ulnar arteries. The radial artery is superficially located, whereas the ulnar artery is deeply situated, traversing deep to the pronator teres muscles. The ulnar artery gives origin to the common interosseous artery, which divides immediately into anterior and posterior interosseous branches. The flexor digitorum profundus and flexor pollicis longus muscles receive their blood supply through the anterior interosseous artery. The median nerve is particularly vulnerable to damage because of its course deep to the lacertus fibrosus and through the substance of the pronator teres muscle.

Diagnosis. The warning signs of Volkmann's ischemia are pain, pallor (or cyanosis), pulselessness, paresthesia, and paralysis. Of these five p's, the most important hallmark is *pain*. The possibility of Volkmann's ischemia should always be ruled out when increasing pain develops in the forearm following injury in the region of the elbow or forearm. A characteristic physical finding is exaggeration of the pain upon passive extension of the fingers. Within 6 to 12 hours, progressive swelling and firmness develop in the volar compartment of the forearm. The *radial pulse* may be present or absent. The presence of a normal radial pulse does not rule out Volkmann's ischemia, since the radial artery may not be compressed because of its superficial location and its pulsation may not disappear until the entire vascular system is in spasm. *Paleness* or cyanosis is best detected in the nailbed with delay of vascular return following compression. There is always a varying degree of *sensory loss*—the median nerve is paralyzed in most cases. When the possibility of Volkmann's ischemia is suspected, compartmental pressure studies should be performed.[78–82]

This author recommends Mubarak's wick catheter method; it is very satisfactory and simple.[78–82] Insertion of the intracath and wick into the muscle is painful. Use a local anesthetic. Caution! Do not inject the anesthetic into the fascia and muscle. Whenever possible, measure the pressure when the child is under anesthesia for reduction of the fracture. It is important to familiarize oneself with the technique. First, insert the intracath with the needle into the muscle; second, remove the needle and insert the wick catheter through the plastic sleeve; and third, tape the wick catheter to the skin and pull the plastic sleeve back. Fill the system with heparinized normal saline and measure the compartment pressure with the transducer recorder. Double-check the patency of the wick catheter by hand pressure on the muscle. Remove all external pressure on the tested muscle and measure the compartment pressure again. If the pressure exceeds 30 torr, fasciotomy is indicated.

In the Whitesides technique of tissue pressure measurement, special equipment is not required.[118] All you need is a 20 cc. syringe, a three-way tap, intravenous connecting tube, sterile normal saline, and blood pressure mercury manometer—these are readily available in any emergency room or hospital. First, assemble the syringe with the plunger at the 15 cc. mark and draw up saline to fill half the tube. Close the three-way tap to retain the normal saline in the tube. Second, anesthetize the skin with local anesthetic, but do not infiltrate the muscle. Introduce the 18-gauge needle into the muscle to be tested; connect the tubing to the mercury manometer and open the three-way tap. Third, push in the plunger and slowly increase the pressure. Read the mercury manometer. When compartment pressure is high, the mercury pressure will rise. Avoid the following pitfalls: (1) *Inject slowly*, as rapid injection will push fluid into the muscle and give a false high value; and (2) avoid drawing back on the plunger, because it will suck muscle fibers into the needle and give a false high value!

Should one measure compartment pressure routinely when clinically symptoms and signs suggest Volkmann's ischemia? Yes! It will prompt the surgeon to be decisive and to act quickly. If compartment pressures are equivocal or normal, double-check equipment and repeat pressure determination. When in doubt, depend upon your clinical judgment.

Keep accurate records. In doubtful cases ask for consultation with a colleague. These cases have potential medicolegal implications.

The destructive process of Volkmann's ischemia is progressive. The interval between injury and repair should not exceed eight hours. Within 12 to 24 hours, it becomes fully developed.

Within five to ten days, the swelling and sensitivity gradually subside and the muscles of the flexor compartment become hard and inelastic. Gradually fibrosis of the involved muscles produces fixed contractural deformity—the elbow is flexed, the forearm pronated, the wrist flexed, the metacarpophalangeal joints hyperextended, and the interphalangeal joints flexed (Fig. 8–41).

Treatment. In the acute ischemic stage, treatment should be immediate. If signs of impending Volkmann's ischemia cannot be relieved within 6 to 12 hours by extension of the elbow, removal of all tight encircling bandages, and reduction of the fracture, arteriography is performed. If a vascular surgeon is available, he should be called in consultation. If the brachial artery is in spasm only, a stellate ganglion block is performed. If, within 30 minutes, circulation does not improve, fasciotomy and epimysiotomy of the forearm and exploration of the brachial artery are indicated. The technique of epimysiotomy and fasciotomy is described by Eaton and Green as follows:[25]

A longitudinal incision is made at the flexor crease of the elbow medial to the biceps tendon and is extended along the middle of the volar surface of the forearm to the flexor crease of the wrist. Proximally the incision may be extended to expose the brachial artery without

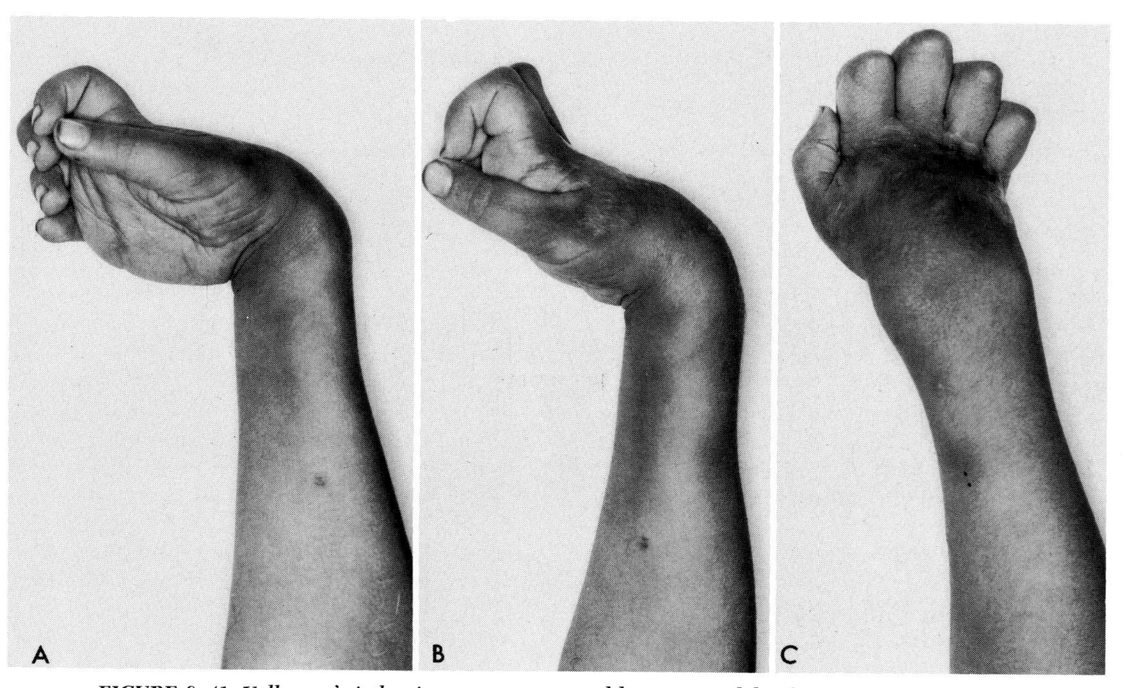

FIGURE 8–41. Volkmann's ischemic contracture caused by supracondylar fracture of the humerus.

A to **C**. Clinical appearance.

Illustration continued on following page

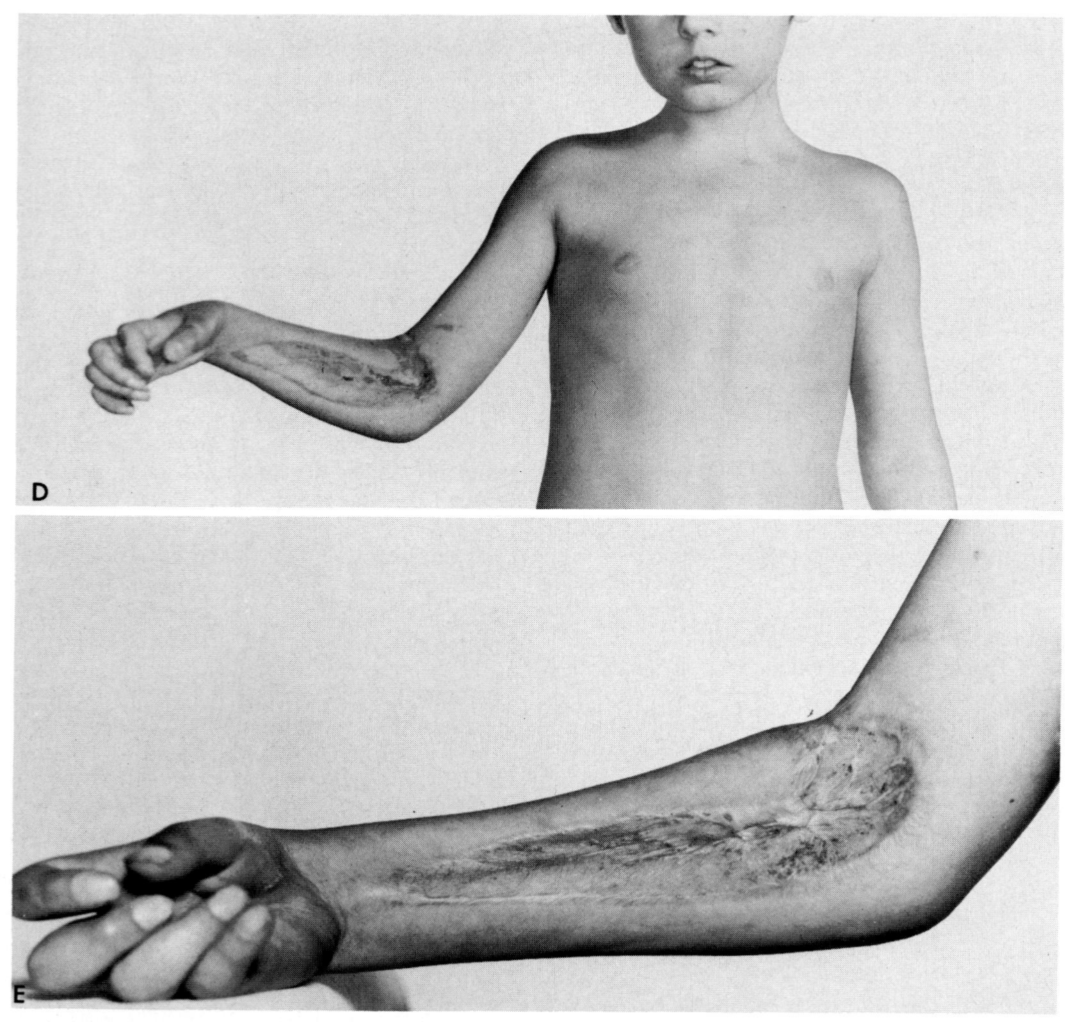

FIGURE 8–41 Continued. Volkmann's ischemic contracture caused by supracondylar fracture of the humerus.

D and **E.** This patient had decompression by fasciotomy.

crossing the flexor crease. The subcutaneous tissue is divided and the antebrachial fascia is sectioned longitudinally throughout its entire length. The fascial sheath of each muscle (the epimysium or perimysium) is carefully divided from its lower to upper margin. Muscle fibers should not be sectioned and meticulous attention should be paid to avoiding inadvertent injury to any nerve branches that penetrate the epimysium.

Following decompression by fasciotomy and epimysiotomy there will be a dramatic return of circulation unless the muscles have become grossly gangrenous. If indicated, the brachial artery is explored. The major nerves are decompressed; particularly important is decompression of the median nerve as it passes beneath the humeral and ulnar heads of the flexor carpi ulnaris muscle.

The fascia is not closed. Often muscle edema prevents approximation of the skin edges. In such an instance, the wound is left open and covered with nonadherent dressing. Skeletal traction is applied with a pin through the olecranon. A delayed closure is performed in two to three days when the edema has subsided. Relaxing incisions and skin grafts may be utilized to cover the bulging muscle bellies.

In the postoperative period, proper splinting and active and passive exercises are essential to obtain good function.

Treatment of *established* Volkmann's ischemic contracture depends upon the severity of the deformity and the period following injury.

Eaton and Green recommend that fasciotomy and epimysiotomy be performed weeks or even months following onset, as long as induration of the volar compartment is present. Two to three months postinjury, the author fractionally lengthens the contracted flexor muscles of the forearm at their muscle junction. This is combined with neurolysis of the median and ulnar nerves.

In severe late cases, both bones of the forearm may be shortened to gain relative length of the contracted muscles.

References

1. Ahstrom, J. P., Jr.: Treatment of established Volkmann's ischemic contracture of the forearm and hand. Curr. Pract. Orthop. Surg., *6*:213, 1975.
2. Allen, M. J., Steingold, R. F., Kotecha, M., and Barnes, M.: The importance of the deep volar compartment in crush injuries of the forearm. Injury, *16*:273, 1985.
3. Allen, M. J., Stirling, A. J., Crawshaw, C. V., and Barnes, M. R.: Intracompartmental pressure monitoring of leg injuries. An aid to management. J. Bone Joint Surg., *67-B*:53, 1985.
4. Arciero, R. A., Shishido, N. S., and Pau, T. J.: Acute anterolateral compartment syndrome secondary to rupture of the peroneus longus muscle. Am. J. Sports Med., *12*:366, 1984.
5. Ashton, H.: The effect of increased tissue pressure on blood flow. Clin. Orthop., *113*:15, 1975.
6. Bass, R. R., Allison, E. J., Jr., Reines, H. D., Yeager, J. C., and Pryor, W. H., Jr.: Thigh compartment syndrome without lower extremity trauma following application of pneumatic antishock trousers. Ann. Emerg. Med., *12*:382, 1983.
7. Bell, S.: Repeat compartment decompression with partial fasciectomy. J. Bone Joint Surg., *68-B*:815, 1986.
8. Blount, W. P.: Volkmann's ischemic contracture. Surg. Gynecol. Obstet., *90*:244, 1950.
9. Bonutti, P. M., and Bell, G. R.: Compartment syndrome of the foot. A case report. J. Bone Joint Surg., *68-A*:1449, 1986.
10. Bradley, E. L., III: The anterior tibial compartment syndrome. Surg. Gynecol. Obstet., *136*:289, 1973.
11. Bristow, W. R.: Myositis ossificans and Volkmann's paralysis. Notes on two cases illustrating the rare complications of supracondylar fracture of the humerus. Br. J. Surg., *10*:475, 1923.
12. Brooks, B.: Pathologic changes in muscle as a result of disturbance of circulation. Arch. Surg., 5:188, 1922.
13. Brower, T. D.: Volkmann's ischemic paralysis. Surg. Clin. North Am., *40*:491, 1960.
14. Bruce, J.: Localized Volkmann's contracture. J. Bone Joint Surg., *22*:738, 1940.
15. Bunnell, S.: Ischemic contracture, local, in the hand. J. Bone Joint Surg., *35-A*:101, 1953.
16. Bunnell, S., Coherty, E. W., and Curtis, R. M.: Ischemic contracture, local in the hand. Plast. Reconstr. Surg., *3*:424, 1948.
17. Christenson, J. T., and Wulff, K.: Compartment pressure following leg injury: The effects of diuretic treatment. Injury, *16*:591, 1985.
18. Clancey, G. J.: Acute posterior compartment syndrome in the thigh. A case report. J. Bone Joint Surg., *67-A*:1278, 1985.
19. Cohen, H. H.: Adjustable volar flexion splint for Volkmann's contracture. J. Bone Joint Surg., *24*:189, 1942.
20. Cohn, B. T., Shall, J., and Berkowitz, M.: Forearm fasciotomy for acute compartment syndrome: A new technique for delayed primary closure. Orthopedics, *9*:1243, 1986.
21. Davey, J. R., Rorabeck, C. H., and Fowler, P. J.: The tibialis posterior muscle compartment. An unrecognized cause of exertional compartment syndrome. Am. J. Sports Med., *12*:391, 1984.
22. DeBat, H.: Volkmann's syndrome. Infirm. Fr., *148*:5, 1973.
23. Decoulx, P., Razemon, J. P., and Vandevelde, D.: Treatment of the sequelae of Volkmann's syndrome. Rev. Chir. Orthop., *2*:111, 1972.
24. DeLee, J. C., and Stiehl, J. B.: Open tibial fracture with compartment syndrome. Clin. Orthop., *160*:175, 1981.
25. Eaton, R. G., and Green, W. T.: Epimysiotomy and fasciotomy in the treatment of Volkmann's ischemic contracture. Orthop. Clin. North Am., *3*:175, 1972.
26. Eaton, R. G., and Green, W. T.: Volkmann's ischaemia. A volar compartment syndrome of the forearm. Clin. Orthop., *113*:58, 1975.
27. Eaton, R. G., Green, W. T., and Stark, H. A.: Volkmann's ischemic contracture. J. Bone Joint Surg., *47-A*:1289, 1965.
28. Eichler, G. R., and Lipscomb, P. R.: The changing treatment of Volkmann's ischemic contracture from 1955 to 1965 at the Mayo Clinic. Clin. Orthop., *50*:215, 1967.
29. Fevre, M., and Judet, J.: Traitment de sequelles de la maladie de Volkmann. Rev. Chir. Orthop., *43*:437, 1957.
30. Flemming, C. W.: A case of improving Volkmann's ischaemic contracture treated by incision of the deep fascia. Lancet, *2*:293, 1931.
31. Foisie, P. S.: Volkmann's ischemic contracture. N. Engl. J. Med., *226*:671, 1942.
32. Garber, J. N.: Volkmann's contracture as a complication of fractures of the forearm and elbow. J. Bone Joint Surg., *21*:154, 1939.
33. Geary, N.: Late surgical decompression for compartment syndrome of the forearm. J. Bone Joint Surg., *66-B*:745, 1984.
34. Gibson, M. J., Barnes, M. R., Allen, M. J., and Chan, R. N.: Weakness of foot dorsiflexion and changes in compartment pressures after tibial osteotomy. J. Bone Joint Surg., *68-B*:471, 1986.
35. Graham, B., and Loomer, R. L.: Anterior compartment syndrome in a patient with fracture of the tibial plateau treated by continuous passive motion and anticoagulants. Report of a case. Clin. Orthop., *195*:197, 1985.
36. Griffiths, D. L.: Volkmann's ischaemic contracture. Br. J. Surg., *28*:239, 1940.
37. Griffiths, D. L.: Volkmann's ischaemic contracture. J. Bone Joint Surg., *33-B*:299, 1951.
38. Grosz, C. R., Shaftan, G. W., Kottmeier, P. K., and Herbsman, H.: Volkmann's contracture and femoral shaft fractures. J. Trauma, *13*:129, 1973.
39. Harmon, J. W.: The significance of local vascular phenomena in the production of ischemic necrosis in skeletal muscles. Am. J. Pathol., *24*:625, 1948.
40. Heppenstall, R. B., Scott, R. J., Shenton, D. W., and Chance, B.: Compartment syndrome. The critical role of blood pressure in the establishment of muscle ischaemia and the increased susceptibility of the traumatized compartment. Orthop. Trans., *9*:374, 1985.
41. Heppenstall, R. B., Scott, R., Sapega, A., Park, Y. S., and Chance, B.: A comparative study of the tolerance of skeletal muscle to ischemia. Tourniquet application compared with acute compartment syndrome. J. Bone Joint Surg., *68-A*:820, 1986.
42. Hernandez, J., Jr., and Peterson, H. A.: Fracture of

the distal radial physis complicated by compartment syndrome and premature physeal closure. A case report. J. Pediatr. Orthop., *6*:627, 1986.
43. Hill, R. L.: Volkmann's ischemic contracture in hemophilia. Trans. Hawaii Territor. Med. Assoc., 26, 1929.
44. Hill, R. L., and Brooks, B.: Volkmann's ischemic contracture in hemophilia. Ann. Surg., *103*:44, 1936.
45. Hodgson, N.: Volkmann's ischaemic contracture treated by transplantation of internal epicondyle. Br. J. Surg., *17*:317, 1929.
46. Holden, C. E. A.: Compartmental syndromes following trauma. Clin. Orthop., *113*:95, 1975.
47. Holden, C. E. A.: The pathology and prevention of Volkmann's ischaemic contracture. J. Bone Joint Surg., *61-B*:296, 1979.
48. Holmes, W., Highet, W. B., and Seddon, H. J.: Ischaemic nerve lesions occurring in Volkmann's contracture. Br. J. Surg., *32*:259, 1944.
49. Horwitz, T.: Significance of venous circulation about the elbow in pathomechanics of Volkmann's contracture. Surg. Gynecol. Obstet., *74*:871, 1942.
50. Imbriglia, J. E., and Boland, D. M.: An exercise-induced compartment syndrome of the dorsal forearm—a case report. J. Hand Surg., *9-A*:142, 1984.
51. Jacobsson, S., and Kjellmer, I.: Accumulation of fluid in exercising skeletal muscle. Acta Physiol. Scand., *60*:286, 1984.
52. Jepson, P. N.: Ischaemic contracture: Experimental study. Ann. Surg., *84*:785, 1926.
53. Jones, D. A.: Volkmann's ischemia. Surg. Clin. North Am., *50*:329, 1970.
54. Jones, E. B.: Volkmann's ischaemia: Observations at open operation. Br. Med. J., *1*:1053, 1940.
55. Jones, S.: Volkmann's contracture. J. Bone Joint Surg., *17*:669, 1935.
56. Kinmonth, J. B.: The physiology and relief of traumatic arterial spasm. Br. Med. J., *1*:59, 1952.
57. Kulowski, J.: Tendon lengthening for Volkmann's ischemic clawhand. South. Med. J., *53*:1241, 1960.
58. Laigle, L.: Evolution of ideas concerning Volkmann's syndrome. Medicine, *19*:893, 1938.
59. Lee, B. Y., Brancato, R. F., Park, I. H., and Shaw, W. W.: Management of compartmental syndrome. Diagnostic and surgical considerations. Am. J. Surg., *12*:383, 1984.
60. Leriche, R.: A propos du mecanisme et de la therapeutique de la maladie de Volkmann. J. Int. Chir., *3*:81, 1938.
61. Lipscomb, P. R.: The etiology and prevention of Volkmann's ischaemic contracture. Surg. Gynecol. Obstet., *103*:353, 1956.
62. Lipscomb, P. R., and Burleson, R. J.: Vascular and neural complications in supracondylar fractures of the humerus in children. J. Bone Joint Surg., *37-A*:487, 1955.
63. Lueck, R. A., and Ray, R. D.: Volkmann's ischemia of the lower extremity. Surg. Clin. North Am., *52*:145, 1972.
64. Malan, E., and Tattoni, G.: Physio-anatomo-pathology of acute ischemia of the extremities. J. Cardiovasc. Surg., *4*:212, 1963.
65. Massart, R.: La maladie de Volkmann. Rev. Orthop., *22*:385, 1935.
66. Matsen, F. A., III: Compartment syndrome. A unified concept. Clin. Orthop., *113*:8, 1975.
67. Matsen, F. A., III, and Clawson, D. K.: The deep posterior compartmental syndrome of the leg. J. Bone Joint Surg., *57-A*:34, 1975.
68. Matsen, F. A., III, Mubarak, S. J., and Rorabeck, C. H.: A practical approach to compartmental syndromes. A.A.O.S. Instr. Course Lect., *32*:88, 1983.
69. Matsen, F. A., III, Winquist, R. A., and Krugmire, R. B., Jr.: Diagnosis and management of compartmental syndromes. J. Bone Joint Surg., *62-A*:286, 1980.
70. Matsen, F. A., III, Mayo, K. A., Krugmire, R. B., Jr., Sheridan, G. W., and Kraft, G. H.: A model compartment syndrome in man with particular reference to quantification of nerve function. J. Bone Joint Surg., *59-A*:648, 1977.
71. Maurer, P.: Vascular and nervous complications of fractures of the two bones of the forearm. Volkmann's syndrome. Rev. Prat., *22*:170, 1972.
72. Meyerding, H. W.: Volkmann's ischemic contracture. J.A.M.A., *94*:394, 1930.
73. Meyerding, H. W.: Volkmann's ischemic contracture. Surg. Clin. North Am., *10*:49, 1930.
74. Meyerding, H. W.: Volkmann's ischemic contracture associated with supracondylar fractures of the humerus. J.A.M.A., *106*:1139, 1936.
75. Meyerding, H. W., and Krusen, F. H.: Treatment of Volkmann's ischemic contracture. Ann. Surg., *100*:417, 1939.
76. Middleton, D. S.: Discussion of Volkmann's ischemic contracture. Lancet, *2*:299, 1928.
77. Midgley, R. D.: Volkmann's ischemic contracture of the forearm. Orthop. Clin. North Am., *4*:983, 1973.
78. Mubarak, S. J., and Carroll, N. C.: Volkmann's contracture in children: Aetiology and prevention. J. Bone Joint Surg., *61-B*:285, 1979.
79. Mubarak, S. J., and Hargens, A. R.: Compartment Syndromes and Volkmann's Contracture. Philadelphia, Saunders, 1981.
80. Mubarak, S. J., and Hargens, A. R.: Acute compartment syndromes. Surg. Clin. North Am., *63*:539, 1983.
81. Mubarak, S. J., and Owen, C. A.: Double incision fasciotomy of the leg for decompression in compartment syndromes. J. Bone Joint Surg., *59-A*:184, 1977.
82. Mubarak, S. J., Owen, C. A., Hargens, A. R., Garetto, L. P., and Akeson, W. H.: Acute compartment syndromes. Diagnosis and treatment with the aid of the wick catheter. J. Bone Joint Surg., *60-A*:1091, 1978.
83. Nario, C. V.: La enfermedad se Volkmann experimantal. J. Int. Chir., *3*:87, 1938.
84. Nisbet, N. W.: Volkmann's ischaemic contracture benefited by muscle slide operation. J. Bone Joint Surg., *34-B*:245, 1952.
85. Osborne, A. H., Dorey, L. R., and Harvey, J. P., Jr.: Volkmann's contracture associated with prolonged external pressure on the forearm. Arch. Surg., *104*:794, 1972.
86. Ottolenghi, C. E.: Prophylaxie du syndrome de Volkmann dans des fractures supracondyliennes du coude chez l'enfant. Rev. Chir. Orthop., *57*:517, 1971.
87. Page, C. M.: Operation for relief of flexion contracture in forearm. J. Bone Joint Surg., *5*:233, 1923.
88. Parkes, W.: The treatment of established Volkmann's contracture by tendon transplantation. J. Bone Joint Surg., *33-B*:359, 1951.
89. Pavanini, G., and Volpe, A.: Diaphysary resection using Colzi's method in the treatment of Volkmann's contracture. Clin. Orthop., *26*:287, 1975.
90. Plewes, L. W.: Occlusion of brachial artery and Volkmann's ischemic contracture. Br. Med. J., *1*:1054, 1945.
91. Pollock, G. A.: Early operation for Volkmann's ischaemic contracture. Br. Med. J., *1*:783, 1944.
92. Reigstad, A., and Hellum, C.: Volkmann's ischaemic contracture of the forearm. Injury, *12*:148, 1980.
93. Rorabeck, C. H.: The treatment of compartment syndromes of the leg. J. Bone Joint Surg., *66-B*:93, 1984.
94. Rorabeck, C. H., and Clarke, K. M.: The pathophysiology of the anterior tibial compartment syndrome.

An experimental investigation. J. Trauma, *18*:299, 1978.
95. Rorabeck, C. H., and Macnab, I.: Anterior tibial-compartment syndrome complicating fractures of the shaft of the tibia. J. Bone Joint Surg., *59-A*:549, 1976.
96. Russell, W. L., Apyan, P. M., and Burns, R. P.: An electronic technique for compartment pressure measurement using the wick catheter. Surg. Gynecol. Obstet., *160*:173, 1985.
97. Russell, W. L., Apyan, P. M., and Burns, R. P.: Utilization and wide clinical implementation using the wick catheter for compartment pressure measurements. Surg. Gynecol. Obstet., *160*:207, 1985.
98. Sarokhan, A. J., and Eaton, R. G.: Volkmann's ischemia. J. Hand Surg., *8*(5 Pt. 2):806, 1983.
99. Schink, W.: Die Fractura supracondylica humeri und die ischamische Kontrakturin im Kindersalter. Chirurg, *39*:417, 1968.
100. Seddon, H. J.: Volkmann's contracture. Treatment by excision of the infarct. J. Bone Joint Surg., *38-B*:152, 1956.
101. Seddon, H. J.: L'ischemie de Volkmann. Rev. Chir. Orthop., *46*:149, 1960.
102. Seddon, H. J.: Volkmann's ischaemia. Br. Med. J., *1*:1587, 1964.
103. Shall, J., Cohn, B. T., and Froimson, A. I.: Acute compartment syndrome of the forearm in association with fracture of the distal end of the radius. Report of two cases. J. Bone Joint Surg., *68-A*:1451, 1986.
104. Sheridan, G. W., and Matsen, F. A., III: Fasciotomy in the treatment of acute compartment syndrome. J. Bone Joint Surg., *58-A*:112, 1976.
105. Sheridan, G. W., Matsen, F. A., III, and Krugmire, R. B., Jr.: Further investigations on the pathophysiology of the compartmental syndrome. Clin. Orthop., *123*:266, 1977.
106. Stanford, S.: Traumatic ischaemia in forearm and leg. Lancet, *1*:462, 1944.
107. Staples, O. C.: Dislocation of the brachial artery—a complication of supracondylar fracture of the humerus in childhood. J. Bone Joint Surg., *47-A*:1525, 1965.
108. Steindler, A.: Ischemic contracture. Surg. Gynecol. Obstet., *62*:358, 1936.
109. Strauss, M. B., Hargens, A. R., Gershuni, D. H., Greenberg, D. A., Crenshaw, A. G., Hart, G. B., and Akeson, W. H.: Reduction in skeletal muscle necrosis using intermittent hyperbaric oxygen in a model compartment syndrome. J. Bone Joint Surg., *65-A*:656, 1983.
110. Styf, J. R., and Korner, L. M.: Chronic anterior compartment syndrome of the leg. Results of treatment by fasciotomy. J. Bone Joint Surg., *68-A*:1338, 1986.
111. Sundararaj, G. D., and Mani, K.: Pattern of contracture and recovery following ischaemia of the upper limb. J. Hand Surg., *10-B*:155, 1985.
112. Sundararaj, G. D., and Mani, K.: Management of Volkmann's ischaemic contracture of the upper limb. J. Hand Surg., *10-B*:401, 1985.
113. Tarlow, S. D., Achterman, C. A., Hayhurst, H., and Ovadia, D. N.: Acute compartment syndrome in the thigh complicating fracture of the femur. A report of three cases. J. Bone Joint Surg., *68-A*:1439, 1986.
114. Volkmann, R.: Die ischaemischen Mustellahmungen und Kontrakturer. Zentralbl. Chir., *8*:801, 1881.
115. Wallenstein, R.: Results of fasciotomy in patients with medial tibial syndrome or chronic anterior-compartment syndrome. J. Bone Joint Surg., *65-A*:1252, 1983.
116. Werbel, G. B., and Shybut, G. T.: Acute compartment syndrome caused by a malfunctioning pneumatic compression boot. A case report. J. Bone Joint Surg., *68-A*:1445, 1986.
117. White, J. W., and Stubbins, S. G.: Carpectomy for intractable flexion deformities of the wrist. J. Bone Joint Surg., *26*:131, 1966.
118. Whitesides, T. E., Jr., Haney, T. C., Morimoto, K., and Harada, H.: Tissue pressure measurements as a determinant for the need of fasciotomy. Clin. Orthop., *113*:43, 1975.
119. Willhoite, D. R., and Moll, J. H.: Early recognition and treatment of impending Volkmann's ischemia in the lower extremity. Arch. Surg., *100*:11, 1970.
120. Wray, J.: Management of supracondylar fracture with vascular insufficiency. Arch. Surg., *90*:279, 1965.
121. Zancolli, E.: Tendon transfers after ischaemic contracture of the forearm. Am. J. Surg., *109*:356, 1965.

FRACTURE-SEPARATION OF THE ENTIRE DISTAL HUMERAL PHYSIS

This injury, originally thought to be extremely rare, at present is considered not so uncommon. In the past the problem was misdiagnosis due to difficulty in interpreting the radiogram, because the cartilaginous distal epiphysis of the humerus is not visible on the plain radiograms. Therefore, fracture separations of the entire distal epiphysis of the distal humerus were often mistaken for infantile supracondylar fractures or lateral condylar fractures.

Historically, Garlt in 1818 is credited by Stimson to be first to describe fracture separation of the distal humeral epiphysis.[33] One of the earliest case reports of a 12-year-old child was given by R. W. Smith, who emphasized the importance of the differential diagnosis between supracondylar fractures, dislocation, and epiphyseal separations of the elbow.[32] A critical review of six previously published cases in the literature was given by Poland, in 1898.[27] Ashhurst reported seven cases in his monograph.[2] Marmor and Bechtol described a Type I physeal injury (Salter-Harris) in a two-year-old child; Kaplan and Reckling reported a Type II physeal injury with medial displacement of the lower humeral epiphysis in an eight-year-old boy.[12, 16]

Mechanism of Injury. This depends upon the age of the patient. In the newborn and young infant, rotary shear force appears to be the causative agent. Birth trauma associated with difficult delivery and child abuse are commonly present in this type of injury. Flexion contracture of the elbow, which is normal in the newborn, prevents hyperextension forces in the distal humerus. In the five- to seven-year age group the fracture force is often indirect (a fall on the outstretched hand), and violent hyperextension of the elbow is the cause of the fracture. Occasionally the fracture force is direct (a fall on the olecranon), in which hyperflexion type of injury occurs.

Classification. The age incidence of this fracture is newborn to seven years, with most of the cases occurring under 2.5 years of age. Based upon the radiographic appearance of the distal fragment and the degree of ossification of the epiphysis of the lateral condyle, DeLee and associates classified this injury into three groups. *Group A* occurs in the newborn and young infant (less than nine months old); the secondary ossification center of the lateral condylar epiphysis has not appeared. The fracture is a Salter-Harris Type I injury. There is no metaphyseal fragment (Thurston-Holland sign). In *Group B* the ossification center of the epiphysis of the lateral condyle has appeared. It occurs in the seven-month to three-year age group. Most of the cases are Salter-Harris Type I physeal injury; some cases are Salter-Harris Type II with a small flake of metaphyseal bone. *Group C* is characterized by a large metaphyseal fragment and a well-developed ossification center of the lateral condylar epiphysis; it occurs in the three- to seven-year age group. The metaphyseal fragment is often lateral and occasionally posterior or medial.

The majority of these fractures are of the extension type, with the distal humeral epiphysis displaced posteriorly and medially; occasionally the injury is of the flexion type, with the distal humeral epiphysis displaced anteriorly and medially.

Physical Findings. The elbow is swollen with local tenderness over the distal humerus. The clinical appearance is very similar to that of elbow dislocation; however, on careful palpation the anatomic relationship of the medial and lateral condyles of the humerus and olecranon is normal. When the elbow is markedly swollen, these anatomic landmarks will be obscured and difficult to palpate.

In the newborn and young infant the local swelling may be minimal. On gentle passive manipulation one may be able to elicit abnormal motion at the fracture site and a "muffled crepitus," which Poland considers to be a sign of physeal separation. The "muffled crepitus" is produced by motion between the fracture fragments covered by soft cartilage; this is in contrast to the fracture crepitus, in which motion occurs between the osseous ends at the fracture site.[27]

Ordinarily the longitudinal alignment of the upper limb is within normal limits with little or no angular deformity; this is due to the large wide fracture surfaces that minimize the tendency for tilting and rotation. Neurovascular injury does not occur because of the minimal displacement of the fracture fragments.

Radiographic Findings. In the newborn and young infant, in whom there is no ossification center of the distal epiphysis of the humerus, the radiologic diagnosis is difficult. The location of the distal epiphysis of the humerus can be determined from the position of the ossified portions of the upper ends of the radius and ulna. Radiograms of both elbows are made in the anteroposterior, lateral, and oblique projections. In fracture separation of the cartilaginous distal humeral epiphysis, the anatomic relationship of the proximal radius and ulna with each other is normal but displaced in relation to the humerus. The displacement is almost always posteromedial; it is very rare that the displacement is anterior.[9, 36, 37]

In Group B and C fractures, the lateral condylar epiphysis is ossified and radiographic diagnosis is relatively easy (Fig. 8–42).

When radiograms are repeated one to two weeks after injury, they will show periosteal new bone formation around the distal humeral metaphysis and extending beyond the physis around the epiphysis as a result of the extensive periosteal stripping.

Differential Diagnosis. The condition is easily confused with dislocation of the elbow. The salient distinguishing feature of fracture-separation of the lower humeral epiphysis is the

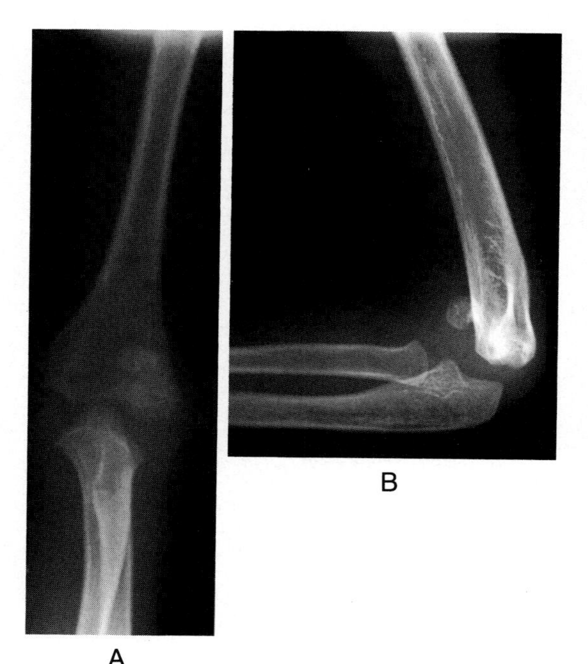

FIGURE 8–42. Fracture separation of the entire distal humeral epiphysis.

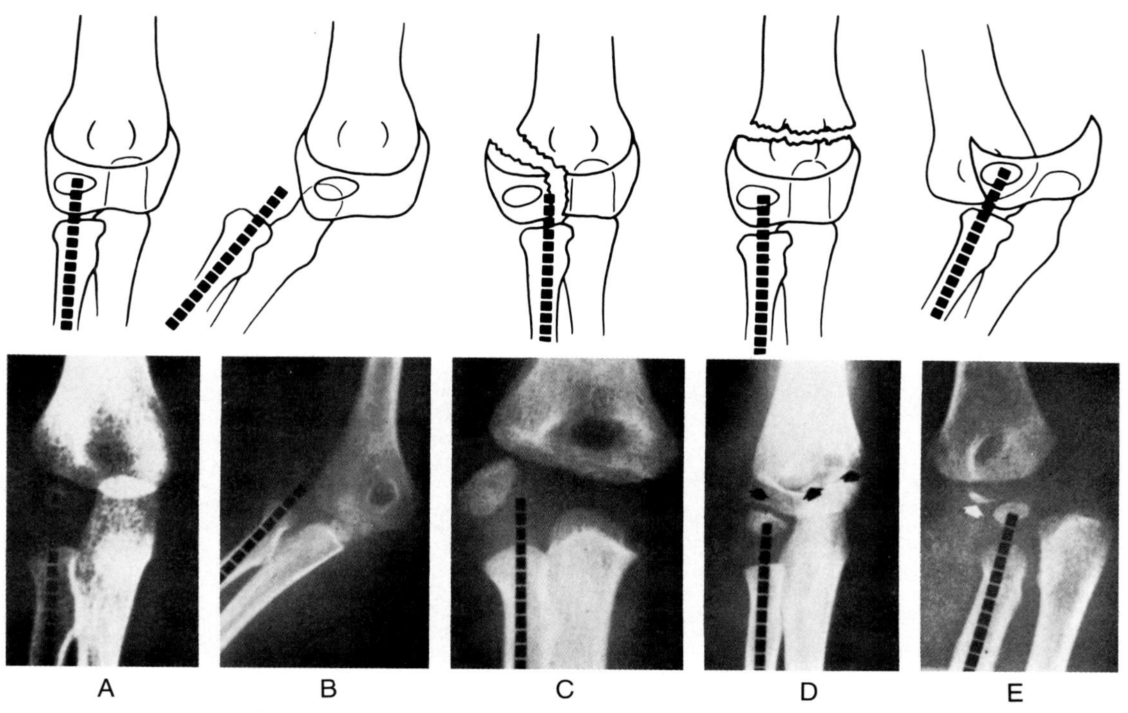

FIGURE 8–43. Radiographic differential diagnosis of the fracture separation of the entire distal humeral physis.

A. Normal elbow. Longitudinal line drawn up the radial diaphysis passes through the capitellum. **B.** Dislocation of the elbow. Note the line drawn—long axis of the radius does not pass through the capitellum. **C.** Salter-Harris Type IV physeal injury of the lateral condyle. **D.** Supracondylar fracture. Note that the fracture line is supracondylar above the distal humeral physis. **E.** Fracture separation of the distal humeral physis with a Thurston-Holland sign *(arrow)*. (From DeLee, J. C., Wilkins, K. E., Rogers, L. F., and Rockwood, C. A.: J. Bone Joint Surg., 62A:48, 1980. Reproduced by permission.)

normal relationship of the ossification center of the capitellum with the radius. A longitudinal line drawn up the shaft of the radius normally passes through the capitellum; in dislocation, however, it does not, indicating a disruption of the joint (Fig. 8–43 A and B). A Type II physeal injury (Salter-Harris) should be differentiated from a fracture of the lateral condyle of the humerus; the latter is a Type IV physeal injury, in which the fracture fragment is often displaced by the pull of the common extensor muscles of the forearm with subsequent loss of its normal relationship to the radial head.[12] Arthrography of the elbow will clearly show the cartilaginous lower end of the humerus and differentiate displaced Salter-Harris Type I fracture from elbow dislocation and Salter-Harris Type II fracture from Type IV physeal injuries.

Treatment. It consists of gentle closed reduction by traction on the forearm and repositioning of the posteromedially displaced distal fragment. The elbow is flexed to 90 degrees and the forearm pronated, and an above-elbow cast is applied for a period of three weeks. If there is marked swelling about the elbow after closed reduction, the upper limb is placed in Dunlop traction to reduce the swelling and then immobilized in an above-elbow cast.

When the patient is seen late and callus is already present, an attempt at closed reduction should not be made. Open reduction should not be performed. Residual cubitus varus and disability are usually minimal. In an occasional case in which resulting cubitus varus deformity is significant, it is best to treat it later by supracondylar humeral osteotomy—it is safer, with less risk of growth plate injury.

Postoperative Care. Malunion is rare but can occur.[11, 16] It is usually less than 10 to 15 degrees and clinically is insignificant. There is one case report in the literature of nonunion.[18] Avascular necrosis of the trochlea occurs when displacement is marked. The blood supply to the trochlea is by one or two small vessels that come from the periphery; these vessels are end-arteries isolated from the metaphyseal circulation.[20]

References

1. Akbarnia, B. A., Silberstein, M. J., Rende, R. J., Graviss, E. R., and Luisiri, A.: Arthrography in the diagnosis of fractures of the distal end of the humerus in infants. J. Bone Joint Surg., *68-A*:599, 1986.
2. Ashhurst, A. P. C.: Fractures of the Elbow. An Anatomical and Surgical Study of Fractures of the Lower End of the Humerus. Philadelphia, Lea & Febiger, 1910.
3. Barrett, W. P., Almquist, E. A., and Staheli, L. T.: Fracture separation of the distal humeral physis in the newborn. J. Pediatr. Orthop., *4*:617, 1984.
4. Beals, R. K.: The normal carrying angle of the elbow. A radiographic study of 422 patients. Clin. Orthop., *119*:194, 1976.
5. Bore Ichuk, N. V., and Baturina, V. V.: Delayed results of the treatment of fractures of the distal epimetaphysis of the humerus in children. Ortop. Travmatol. Protez., *32*:68, 1971.
6. Chand, K.: Epiphyseal separation of the distal humerus epiphysis in an infant. A case report and review of the literature. J. Trauma, *14*:521, 1974.
7. Cothay, D. M.: Injury to the lower medial epiphysis of the humerus before development of the ossific center. J. Bone Joint Surg., *49-B*:766, 1967.
8. Crabbe, W.: The treatment of fracture-separation of the capitular epiphysis. J. Bone Joint Surg., *45-B*:722, 1963.
9. DeLee, J. C., Wilkins, K. E., Rogers, L. F., and Rockwood, C. A.: Fracture-separation of the distal humeral epiphysis. J. Bone Joint Surg., *62-A*:46, 1980.
10. Freyschmidt, J., Saure, D., Suren, G., and Fritsch, R.: Radiologic diagnosis of injuries of the epiphyses in childhood. Roentgenblatter, *30*:309, 1977.
11. Holda, M. E., Manoli, A., and LaMont, R. L.: Epiphyseal separation of the distal end of the humerus with medial displacement. J. Bone Joint Surg., *62-A*:52, 1980.
12. Kaplan, S. S., and Reckling, F. W.: Fracture separation of the lower humeral epiphysis with medial displacement. Review of the literature and report of a case. J. Bone Joint Surg., *53-A*:1105, 1971.
13. Katthagen, B. D., Mittelmeier, H., and Schmitt, E.: Corrective osteotomies of the distal humerus following childhood elbow injuries. Unfallheilkunde, *86*:349, 1983.
14. McCarthy, S. M., and Ogden, J. A.: Radiology of postnatal skeletal development. VIII. The scapula. Skeletal Radiol., *10*:209, 1983.
15. McIntyre, W. M., Wiley, J. J., and Charette, R. J.: Fracture-separation of the distal humeral epiphysis. Clin. Orthop., *188*:98, 1984.
16. Marmor, L., and Bechtol, C. O.: Fracture separation of the lower humeral epiphysis: Report of a case. J. Bone Joint Surg., *42-A*:333, 1960.
17. Mauer, I., Kolovos, D., and Loscos, R.: Epiphyseolysis of the distal humerus in a newborn. Bull. Hosp. Joint Dis., *28*:109, 1967.
18. Mizuno, K., Hirohata, K., and Kashiwagi, D.: Fracture-separation of the distal humerus in young children. J. Bone Joint Surg., *61-A*:570, 1979.
19. Moroz, P. F.: Treatment of fractures of the distal epiphysis of the humerus in children. Ortop. Travmatol. Protez., *4*:70, 1976.
20. Morrissy, R. T., and Wilkins, K. E.: Deformity following distal humeral fracture in childhood. J. Bone Joint Surg., *66-A*:557, 1984.
21. Olerud, S., and Reuterski, O. G.: Interesting epiphyseal fractures. Lakartidningen, *68*:3143, 1971.
22. Omer, G. E., Jr., and Simmons, J. W.: Fracture of the distal humeral metaphyseal growth plate. South. Med. J., *61*:651, 1968.
23. Orniak, G. A.: Late results of the treatment of fractures of the humeral distal epiphysis in children. Pol. Przegl. Chir., *38*:286, 1966.
24. Paige, M. L., and Port, R. B.: Separation of the distal humeral epiphysis in the neonate. A combined clinical and roentgenographic diagnosis. Am. J. Dis. Child., *139*:1203, 1985.
25. Peiro, A., Mut, T., Aracil, J., and Martos, F.: Fracture-separation of the lower humeral epiphysis in young children. Acta Orthop. Scand., *52*:295, 1981.
26. Peterson, H. A.: Triplane fracture of the distal humeral epiphysis. J. Pediatr. Orthop., *3*:81, 1983.
27. Poland, J.: Traumatic Separation of the Epiphyses. London, Smith, Elder & Co., 1898.
28. Rogers, L. F.: The radiography of epiphyseal injuries. Radiology, *96*:289, 1970.
29. Rogers, L. F., and Rockwood, C. A., Jr.: Separation of the entire distal humeral epiphysis. Radiology, *106*:393, 1973.
30. Sakakida, K.: Clinical observations on the epiphysial separation of long bones. Clin. Orthop., *34*:119, 1964.
31. Siffert, R. S.: Displacement of the distal humeral epiphysis in the newborn infant. J. Bone Joint Surg., *45-A*:165, 1963.
32. Smith, R. W.: Observations on dysfunction of the lower epiphysis of the humerus. Dublin Quart. J. Med. Sci., *9*:63, 1850.
33. Stimson, L. A.: A Treatise on Fractures. Philadelphia, Lea & Febiger, 1883.
34. Sutherland, D. H., and Wrobel, L.: Displacement of the entire distal humeral epiphysis. *In* Proceedings of the Western Orthopaedic Association. J. Bone Joint Surg., *56-A*:206, 1974.
35. Wilkins, K. E.: Physeal fractures of the distal humerus: Avoiding the pitfalls. A.A.O.S. Instr. Course Lect., *35*:83, 1986.
36. Wilkins, K. E.: Fractures involving the entire distal humeral epiphysis. *In* Rockwood, C. A., Wilkins, K. E., and King, R. E. (eds.): Fractures in Children. Philadelphia, J. B. Lippincott, 1984, p. 465.

FRACTURES OF THE LATERAL CONDYLE OF THE HUMERUS

The ossification center of the lateral condyle appears between 18 months and two years of age. It extends medially to form the principal part of the lower articular end of the humerus. The ossific center for the medial part of the trochlea appears at 12 years of age. The lateral epicondyle ossifies at the age of 13 years and fuses with the capitellum at 16 or 17 years. The radial collateral ligament, the tendon of the supinator longus, and the common tendon of the extensor muscles of the forearm are attached to the lateral epicondyle.

Fractures of the lateral condyle of the humerus are rather common, constituting 13 to 18 per cent of all fractures in the region of the elbow in children.

The injury is a Type IV physeal injury (Salter-Harris), i.e., it is an intra-articular transepiphyseal fracture. It is mostly encountered in children between the ages of 3 and 14 years, the peak incidence being from 6 to 10 years of age. It is three to four times more common in boys than in girls.

Mechanism of Injury and Pathology

Fracture of the lateral condyle of the humerus usually results from indirect violence in a fall on the outstretched hand with the forearm in abduction and the elbow in extension. The force is transmitted up the radius; the fracture may also be produced by a traction force that thrusts the elbow into varus position. Jacob et al. applied varus strain on the extended elbow in cadaveric specimens. The pull of the lateral ligament avulsed the lateral condyle with the ulnar trochlear ridge as the fulcrum. The lateral cortex yielded to the varus strain and the bone fractured. When the intra-articular cartilage remained intact, it acted as a hinge. Upon release of the varus strain the fracture reduced. When, on increasing the varus angulation, the articular cartilage tore, the fracture displaced through 90 degrees in two planes. Upon releasing the varus pull, the lateral condyle remained displaced and did not reduce.[29]

The fracture line begins at the lateral side of the distal metaphysis of the humerus and extends obliquely downward and medially, traverses the physis, and enters the joint in the lateral portion of the trochlea. Thus, the distal fragment contains the epiphysis of the capitellum, a part of the trochlea, the lateral epicondyle, and a part of the metaphysis with the radial collateral ligament and the common tendon of the extensor muscles of the forearm attached to it.

The anatomic location of the fracture line may be one of two types, according to Milch (Fig. 8–44): in *Type A* the fracture line traverses lateral to the trochlea through the capitulotrochlear groove. The fracture will angulate but not translocate. This is a Salter-Harris Type IV fracture. In *Type B* the fracture line courses and exits through the apex of the trochlea; the fracture is unstable. It will angulate, and in addition, the proximal radius and ulna will translocate laterally.[48] These two separate courses of the fracture line were previously described by Stimson.[72]

The degree of displacement of the posterior fragment may be of three grades: *first degree*—it is undisplaced or minimally displaced with intact hyaline cartilage at the joint; the fracture is stable (Figs. 8–45A and 8–46); *second degree*—the fracture is moderately displaced; the

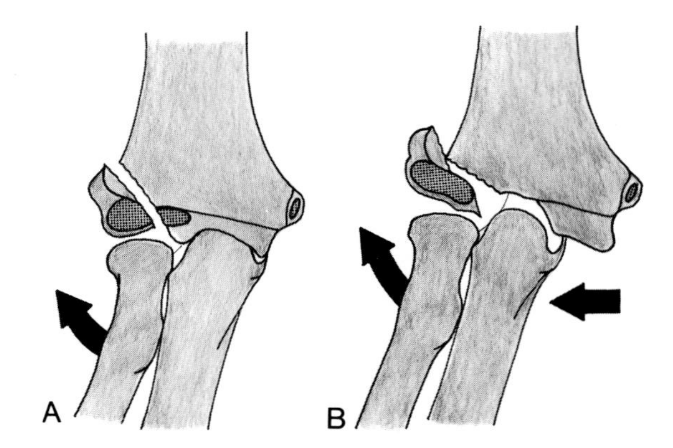

FIGURE 8–44. Anatomic location of the fracture line in lateral condylar fractures described by Milch.

A. Type A—The fracture line traverses lateral to the trochlea through the capitulotrochlear groove. The fracture fragment angulates, and the elbow joint is stable; the radial head and olecranon do not translocate laterally. **B.** Type B—The fracture line courses and exits into the elbow joint at the apex of the trochlea. In this type the elbow joint is unstable. The fracture fragment angulates, and the radial head and olecranon translocate laterally. (Redrawn after Milch, H. E.: Fractures and fracture-dislocations of the humeral condyles. J. Trauma, *4*:592, 1964.)

fracture line traverses completely through the articular cartilage surface and the fracture is unstable. Lateral translocation of the radial head and olecranon may occur (Fig. 8–45 B). The *third degree* is severe displacement of the fracture. The lateral condylar fragment is displaced laterally and proximally and rotated to a varying degree. When it is 90 degrees, the articular surface faces inward and the fractured surface, laterally; in its extreme form of 180 degree rotation around both the horizontal and the vertical axes, the distal articular surface faces cephalad toward the fracture site, the inner trochlear surface faces outward, and the lateral surface faces inward. The radial head and olecranon are translocated laterally, i.e., the elbow joint is subluxated or dislocated laterally (Fig. 8–45 C).

Diagnosis

Following injury, these patients complain of severe pain. There is marked swelling, ecchymosis, and local tenderness over the lateral aspect of the elbow. In the absence of soft-tissue swelling, one may be able to palpate the detached fragment. Ordinarily rotation of the forearm is not restricted.

The diagnosis is made by the radiographic findings. Anteroposterior, lateral, and oblique projections are obtained. Sometimes only the

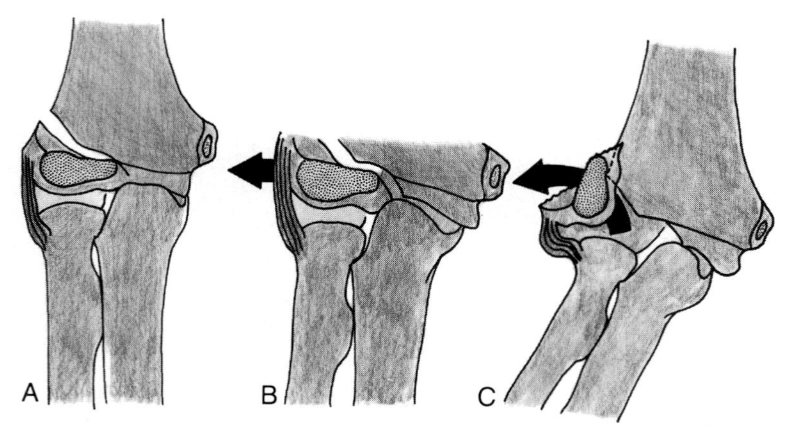

FIGURE 8–45. Degrees of displacement in lateral condylar fractures of the humerus.

A. Drawing illustrating undisplaced lateral condylar fracture—note the intact hyaline cartilage at the joint. This is first degree. **B.** Drawing illustrating moderately displaced lateral condylar fracture. The fracture line traverses completely through the articular cartilage surface. The fracture fragment is unstable. Lateral displacement of the radial head and olecranon may occur. This is second degree. **C.** Drawing illustrating severely displaced lateral condylar fracture. Note that the fragment is displaced laterally and proximally and is rotated. The radial head and olecranon are translocated laterally. (Redrawn after Jakob, R., Fowles, J. V., Rang, M., and Kassab, M. T.: Observations concerning fractures of the lateral humeral condyle in children. J. Bone Joint Surg., *57B*:430, 1975.)

oblique view will disclose displacement. Undisplaced fractures may not be diagnosed unless comparative radiograms of the opposite elbow are obtained.

In the young child it is easy to miss this fracture, because the ossific center of the lateral condyle is small. When there is clinical suggestion of lateral condylar fracture, perform arthrography of the elbow with varus stress in multiple projections. In obscure cases, computerized axial tomography is indicated. This author has no personal experience in the diagnostic use of nuclear magnetic resonance imaging in occult injuries of the elbow; it may be the way of the future.

Treatment

Fractures of the lateral condyle of the humerus are unstable; they tend to become displaced even when immobilized because of the pull of the common extensors. As the fracture line crosses the physis, accurate anatomic repositioning is imperative to decrease the likelihood of growth damage. Congruity of the joint must be restored. This fracture is intra-articular and synovial fluid bathes the fracture line, predisposing to delayed union and nonunion.

The Undisplaced Fracture. In the radiogram the fracture line traverses a more or less horizontal course. The articular cartilage is intact and acts as a hinge and provides some stability to the fracture. Treatment is simple immobilization in an above-elbow cast for a period of four weeks; the position of the elbow is 90 degrees of flexion with the forearm in full supination to minimize the pull of the extensor muscles. Do not hyperflex the elbow beyond 90 degrees, as it will tend to displace the lateral condylar fragment. Even undisplaced fractures of the lateral condyle may be unstable and may become displaced while immobilized in the cast. Repeated radiograms are made every three to four days during the first 14 days to detect further displacement. With the slightest evidence of further displacement, this author recommends immediate percutaneous pinning in situ, using image intensifier x-ray control, with the patient under general anesthesia in the operating room.

Minimally Displaced Fracture. This is the troublemaker. In the literature some authors recommend conservative closed treatment of minimally displaced fractures of the lateral condylar epiphysis. The author recommends that such fractures be internally fixed with two smooth Kirschner wires (this is easily done percutaneously under image intensifier radiographic control). Nonunion and growth arrest occur more commonly in minimally displaced fractures than in the displaced rotated fractures because the latter are treated more adequately.[17]

In the *displaced fracture*, primary open reduction and internal fixation constitute the treatment of choice. The operative technique is described and illustrated in Plate 121.

Delayed Case. A minimally displaced fracture

treated by immobilization in cast may become significantly displaced in several weeks, or occasionally a lateral condylar fracture is missed and the child presents late. Should one perform delayed open reduction or accept the deformity? In the literature the consensus is a "hands-off" policy for a fracture three weeks old or more.[22, 29, 47, 58, 71] The results of late surgery are poor because early callus and proliferative fibrous tissue formation require extensive soft-tissue dissection to obtain satisfactory reduction. The complication rate of joint stiffness, avascular necrosis, premature physeal closure, and cubitus valgus is very high.

When the fracture is left alone, nonunion and malunion will result in cubitus valgus deformity and tardy ulnar nerve palsy; however, avascular necrosis and joint stiffness do not develop. Jakob and Fowles, in their thorough study of the results of delayed surgery in lateral condylar fractures, recommended that a displaced fracture more than three weeks old should be left alone and the ulnar nerve transposed anteriorly to prevent tardy ulnar nerve palsy.[29] Rang concurs with Jakob and Fowles.[58]

This author has performed delayed open reduction in 6- to 18-month-old fractures with good results. First, circumvent extensive soft-tissue dissection exposing the distal humeral diaphysis and metaphysis through a posterior approach; following the recommendation of Böhler, perform an osteotomy of the olecranon and approach the fragment transarticularly.[7] Second, under image intensifier radiographic

Text continued on page 3116

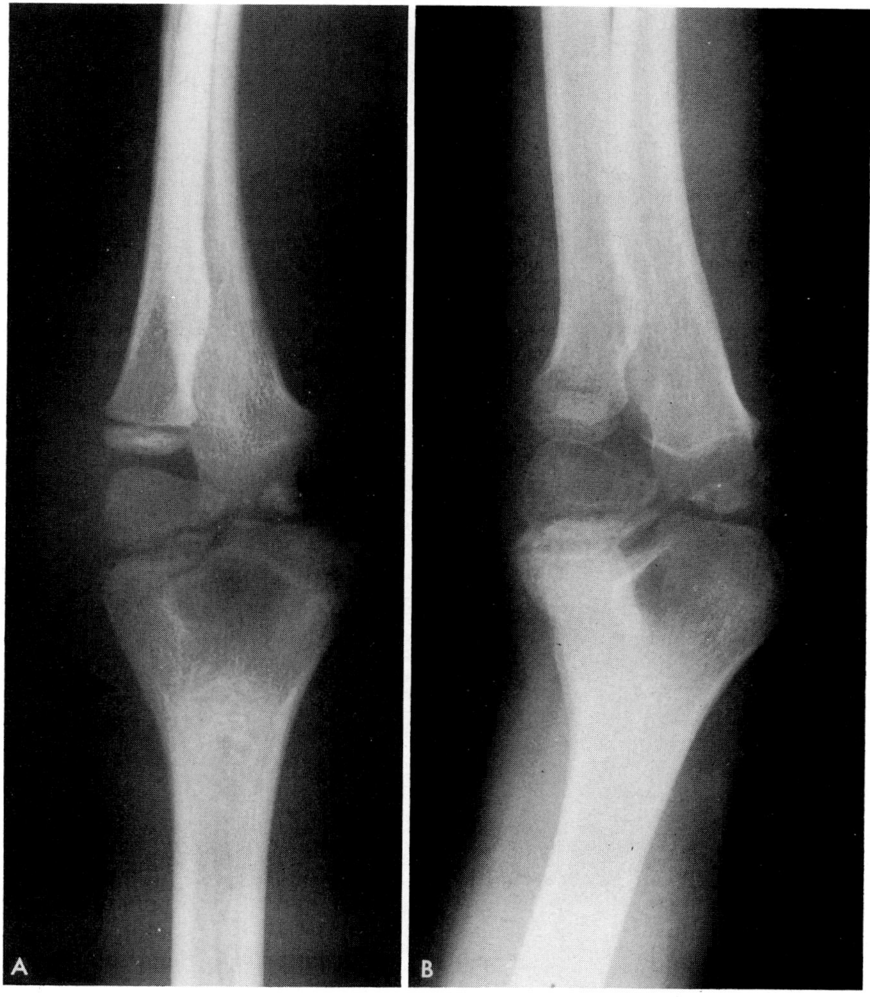

FIGURE 8–46. Undisplaced fracture of lateral condyle of humerus.

Fracture was treated by simple immobilization in long arm cast. **A.** Initial radiogram. **B.** Radiogram taken after two months, showing healing.

Open Reduction and Internal Fixation of Fracture of the Lateral Condyle

OPERATIVE TECHNIQUE

A. The incision begins 5 to 7 cm. proximal to the lateral epicondyle of the humerus and extends distally over the epicondylar ridge of the lateral epicondyle and then continues distally and posteriorly over the interval between the anconeus and the extensor carpi ulnaris muscles for a distance of 2.5 cm.

B. The deep fascia is opened in line with the skin incision. Working distally to proximally, the plane between the triceps muscle posteriorly and the brachioradialis muscle anteriorly is developed. Frequently, there is a tear in the aponeurosis of the brachioradialis muscle, which leads directly to the fracture site. One should avoid the radial nerve in the proximal end of the wound where it enters in the interval between the brachialis and brachioradialis muscles. The dissection is carried distally between the anconeus and the extensor carpi ulnaris muscles, exposing the joint capsule.

C. The periosteum is incised along the lateral epicondylar ridge and adjacent humerus, and the joint capsule is opened.

D. On exposure of the fracture site, the blood from the hematoma will flow out; the wound is irrigated with normal saline to remove small pieces of loose bone and to obtain clear visualization. Caution! Do not dissect the fracture fragment, particularly its posterior aspect, where the only blood vessels supplying the lateral condylar apophysis enter; it will increase the risk of avascular necrosis. It is vital to have a clear view of the fracture bed and the joint surface anteriorly and inferiorly. Insert a right-angled long retractor (in pediatric surgery it is called an infantile rectal retractor) or a Homan retractor into the anterior aspect of the elbow, and visualize the radial head. In order to expose the joint surface, it may be necessary to incise a small amount of the capsule and synovium. With a Freer elevator, elevate the periosteum on the humeral shaft for a distance of 0.5 to 1.0 cm.; this measure will provide a better definition of the fracture bed.

Plate 121. Open Reduction and Internal Fixation of Fracture of the Lateral Condyle

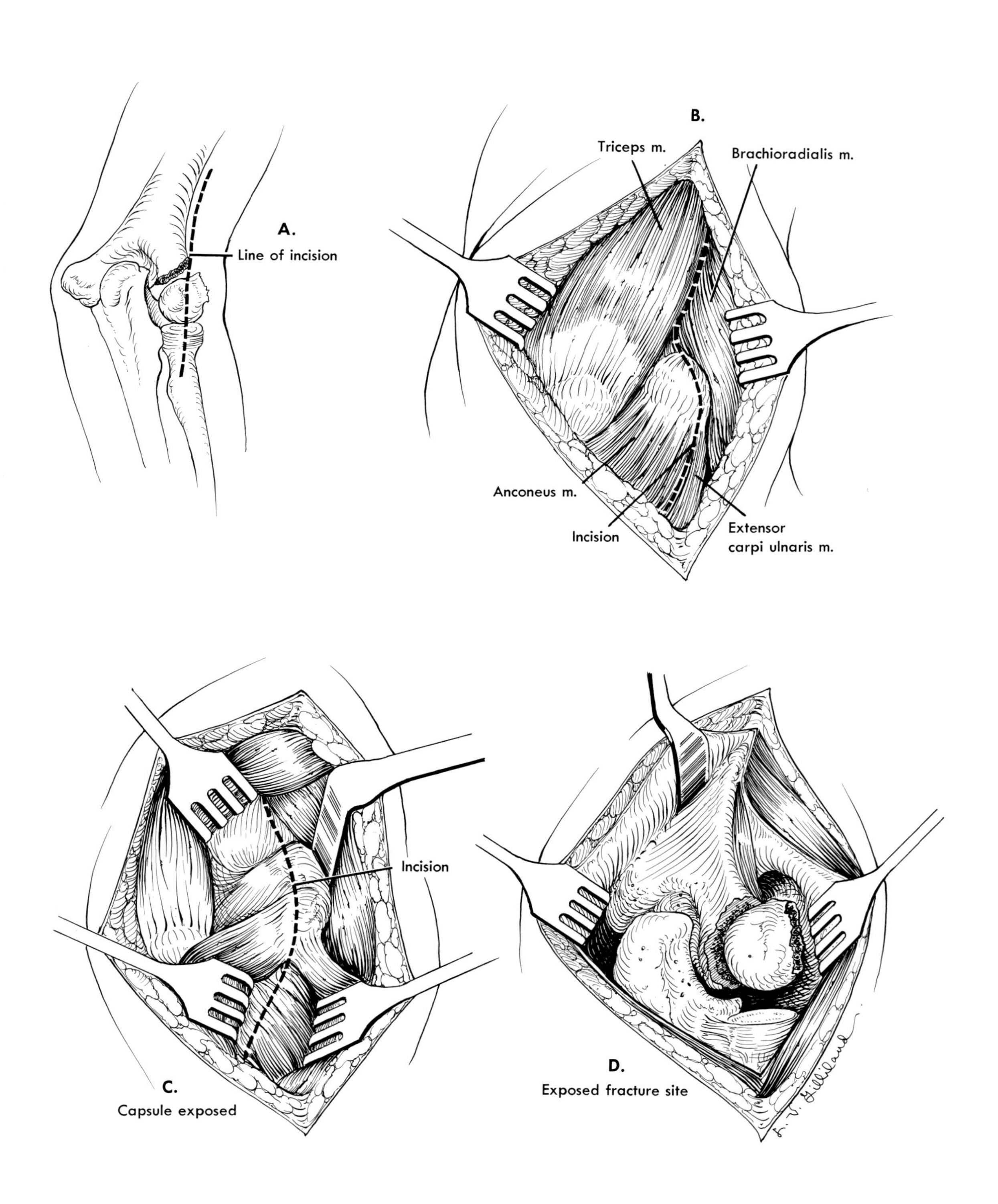

Open Reduction and Internal Fixation of Fracture of the Lateral Condyle (Continued)

E. As the lateral condyle fracture fragment is held with a bone tenaculum or a towel clip, the fracture is reduced anatomically. The articular cartilage surface should be perfectly aligned; if it is not, delayed union and joint stiffness may develop. Inspect the lateral cortex of the humerus; apposition of the fracture fragments should be anatomic. Strive for perfection! Ordinarily, it is not necessary to detach the soft tissues from the lateral epicondyle. Two smooth Kirschner wires are drilled across the fracture site through stab wounds separate from the skin incision. The wires should engage the medial cortex of the humerus. The reduction and position of the wires are checked by radiograms. The distal ends of the wires are cut off but are left protruding slightly from the skin, and their ends are bent to prevent migration.

F, G. The periosteum and the capsule of the joint are closed by interrupted sutures. The wound is closed, and the upper limb is immobilized in an above-elbow cast, with the elbow in 90 degrees of flexion and the forearm in neutral position.

POSTOPERATIVE CARE

In about three to four weeks, the pins are removed and another above-elbow cast is applied for an additional two to three weeks. Gentle, active exercises are performed to restore range of motion of the elbow joint. It is imperative to follow the patient for possible premature closure of the lateral portion of the distal humeral physis, cubitus valgus, and tardy ulnar nerve palsy.

Plate 121. Open Reduction and Internal Fixation of Fracture of the Lateral Condyle

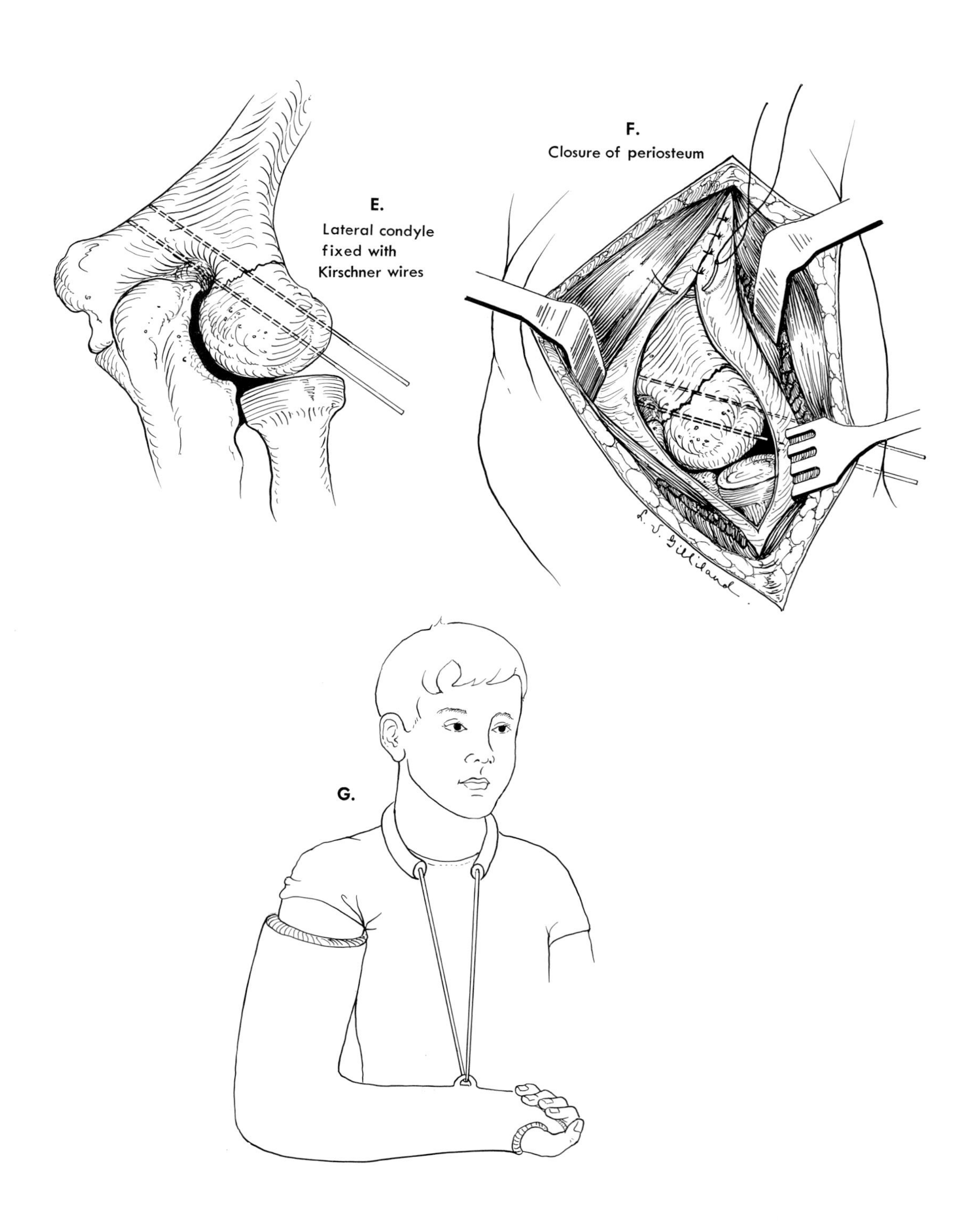

control the physis of the lateral condyle and distal humerus are located by the use of Keith needles. All fibrous and osseous bridges are meticulously excised, and the fracture fragment is reduced and internally fixed with pins (two or three). The articular cartilage surface and the physis should be anatomically aligned—do not accept "step-off." Third, with a dental burr and pituitary forceps, remove bony and soft-tissue remnants between the repositioned lateral condylar and distal humeral physes and place autogenous fat as a spacer (following Langenskiöld technique) to prevent new osseous bridge formation and closure of the physis. Fourth, three to four weeks postoperatively the cast is removed but the pins are left in place, and elbow motion and active assisted and gentle passive exercises are performed. The pins are removed six to eight weeks postoperatively. Then continuous passive motion machine is employed several hours of the day.

This author recommends the skilled, experienced pediatric orthopedic surgeon to consider delayed open reduction, provided that the foregoing technical details are executed and meticulous postoperative care is provided. A continuous passive motion machine is employed until functional range of elbow motion is restored.

Excision of the lateral condylar fragment should not be performed in children.

Problems and Complications

These include delayed union, nonunion, malunion, premature physeal arrest, cubitus valgus or varus, radial nerve paralysis sustained at injury or during open reduction, avascular necrosis, and myositis ossificans.

Delayed Union. The *causative factors* are (1) distraction-tension forces exerted by the extensor muscles of the forearm originating from the lateral epicondyle of the humerus; (2) the fracture is intra-articular, and therefore fibrin and subsequent callus formation is inhibited by the synovial fluid; (3) circulatory compromise and avascular necrosis of the lateral condyle; and (4) insecure internal fixation at open reduction; pins back out and alignment of the fracture is lost.

Treatment. If the fracture is *nondisplaced and stable*, the only finding is persistence of the radiolucent fracture line. Treatment consists of simple observation; ultimately the fracture will unite and the radiolucent line will disappear. If the fracture is *minimally displaced* and the position of the lateral condylar fragment is acceptable, long-term immobilization in an above-elbow cast and/or maintenance of the internal fixation by pins is recommended. In about two thirds of these cases the fracture will heal in three months; the remainder will fail to heal and may become further displaced—these are classified as nonunion.[16, 17]

Nonunion. When there is failure of healing three to four months postinjury, the fracture should be classified as a nonunion. In the minimally displaced nonunions this author agrees with Flynn and Jeffrey and recommends compression screw fixation across the metaphyseal fragments with autogenous bone grafting.[16, 17, 30] In the literature, however, Hardacre et al. question the value of bone grafting of these minimally displaced nonunited lateral condylar fractures; in the experience of these authors the results of two bone grafted cases were not better than those that were simply observed. This author disagrees with Hardacre, because in his experience the minimally displaced ununited fractures have become significantly displaced several years later.[22]

Nonunion occurs in displaced fractures because of initial failure to diagnose and treat or inadequate treatment of a minimally displaced fracture that becomes displaced because of inadequate treatment. Union will not take place when hyaline articular cartilage opposes the osseous bed of the fractured fragment of the distal humeral metaphysis.

Nonunion of the lateral condyle fracture results in progressive cubitus valgus and tardy ulnar nerve palsy. The lateral condylar fragment becomes progressively displaced proximally and laterally. The range of the elbow joint may be restricted, especially in full extension. Otherwise, functionally these patients perform satisfactorily. Management of nonunion is discussed under delayed open reduction.

Premature Physeal Fusion. Retardation or arrest of growth of the lateral condyle and continued normal growth of the medial condyle will result in progressive cubitus valgus. The ulnar nerve is repeatedly stretched by flexion-extension motion of the elbow over the apex of the deformity, and may become inflamed in its course behind the medial epicondyle; tardy ulnar nerve palsy will develop.

Wadsworth studied 28 children with fracture of the capitellum (8 undisplaced and 20 displaced), and found six cases of premature physeal fusion. He distinguished two types of premature fusion; in the first, the capitular epiphysis fused to the metaphysis, and in the second, the capitular and trochlear epiphyses fused together and then to the metaphysis. Both

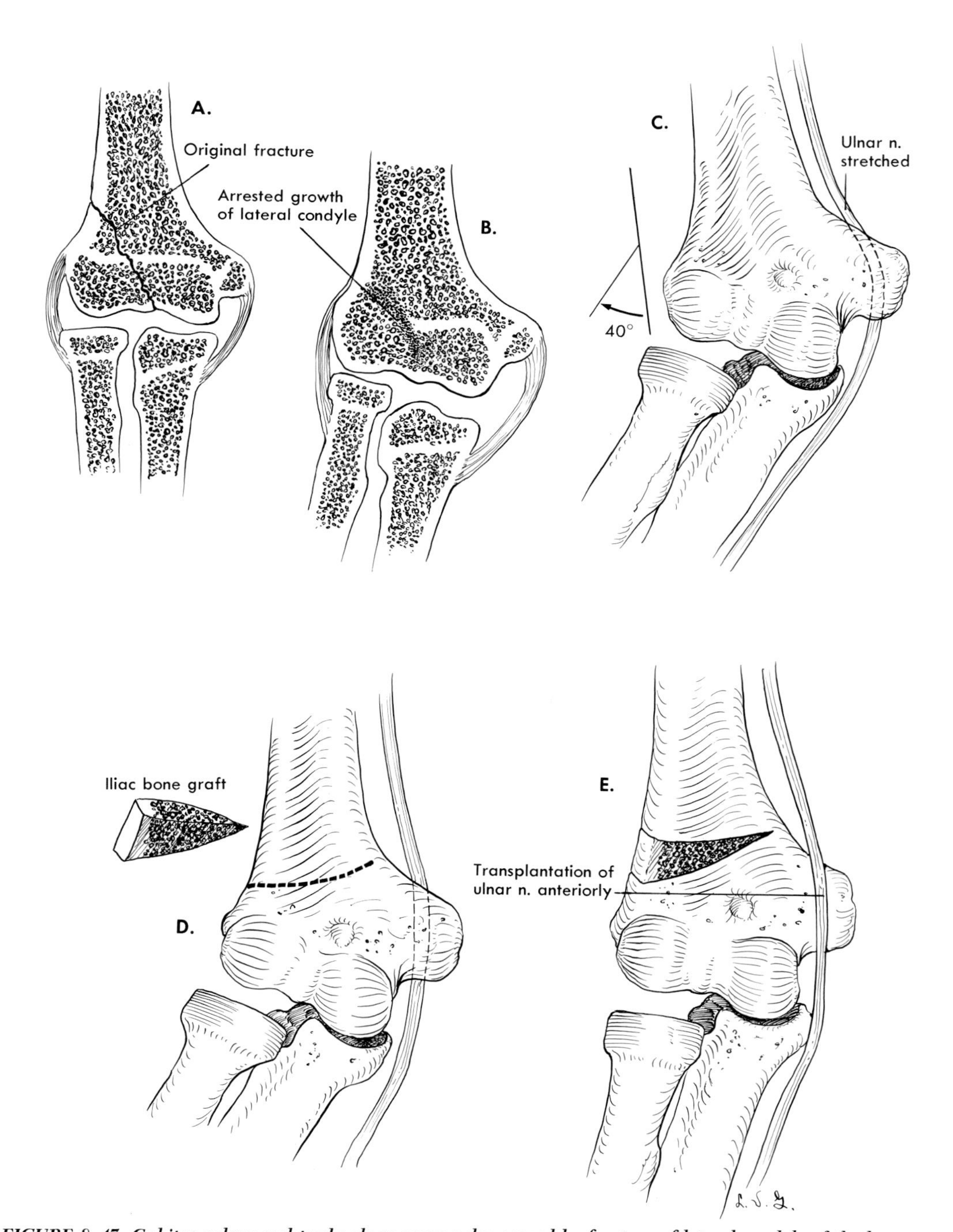

FIGURE 8–47. Cubitus valgus and tardy ulnar nerve palsy caused by fracture of lateral condyle of the humerus.

A. Original fracture is Type IV epiphyseal plate injury. **B.** Premature closure of the physis of distal humerus on the lateral side. **C.** Progressive increasing cubitus valgus deformity will stretch the ulnar nerve and cause paresis. **D** and **E.** Correction of cubitus varus deformity by open-up osteotomy with bone graft wedge. The ulnar nerve is transposed anteriorly.

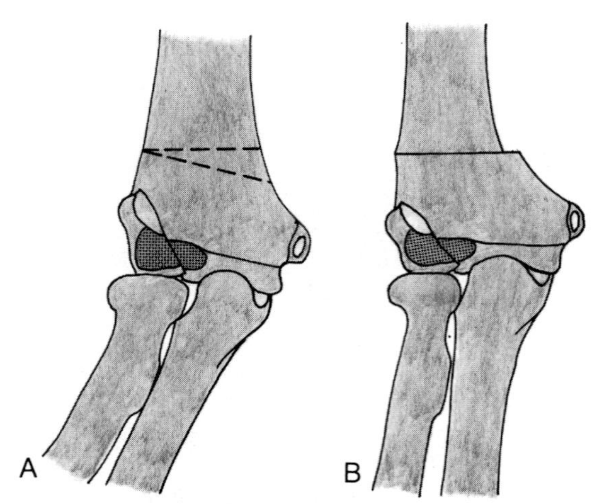

FIGURE 8–48. Closing wedge osteotomy to correct cubitus valgus when the deformity is only angular (Milch's Type A fracture pattern).

A. Preoperative drawing showing lines of osteotomy. **B.** Postoperative drawing showing correction of valgus deformity. Internal fixation is with crisscross pins. (Redrawn after Milch, H. E.: Fractures and fracture-dislocations of the humeral condyles. J. Trauma, *4*:592, 1964.)

types of premature fusion resulted in valgus deformity.[76]

Cubitus Valgus. This angular deformity of the elbow is a common complication of lateral condylar fractures of the humerus. It may be caused by malunion, nonunion, or premature physeal arrest of the lateral condyle. The problem is stretching of the ulnar nerve and tardy ulnar nerve palsy.

When there is no lateral translocation of the radial head and olecranon (i.e., Milch type A fracture pattern), the deformity of the elbow is only angular. It is corrected by open-up osteotomy of the distal humerus with a graft wedge, and the ulnar nerve is transposed anteriorly (Fig. 8–47). An alternative method is closing wedge osteotomy (Fig. 8–48).

When cubitus valgus is associated with lateral translocation of the radial head and olecranon (Milch Type B fracture pattern), correction of the deformity by opening wedge osteotomy of the distal humerus will result in an ugly medial prominence at the elbow. This is unacceptable cosmetically. The osteotomy should correct both lateral angulation and translocation. Therefore, a combined varus angulation–lateral translocation osteotomy is performed—aligning the longitudinal axes of the humerus and forearm (Fig. 8–49). Internal fixation of this type of osteotomy is difficult—often the author uses plate-screws and crisscross threaded Steinmann pins.

When cubitus valgus is due to nonunion of the lateral condyle fracture, both conditions require treatment. A posterior approach is used to expose the distal diaphysis and metaphysis of the humerus. An osteotomy of the olecranon is performed to expose the articular surface of the distal humerus and the nonunion site. The radial nerve is exposed distally, gently dissected, and retracted out of harm's way. Do not disturb circulation of the lateral condyle—avoid soft-tissue dissection, particularly on the pos-

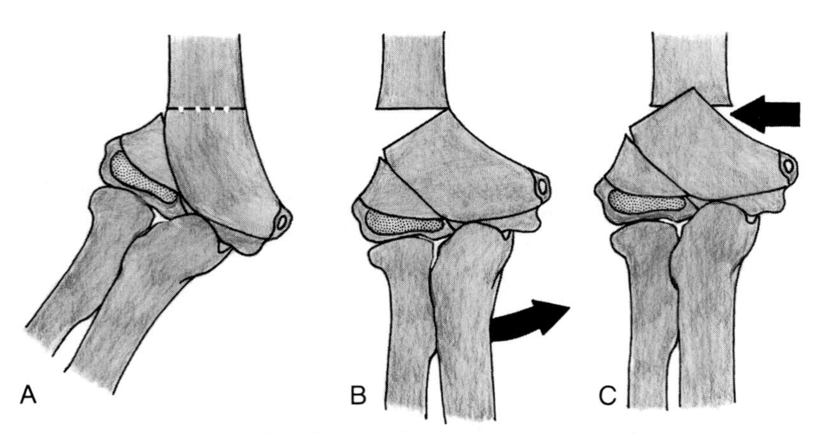

FIGURE 8–49. Combined varus angulation–lateral displacement osteotomy of the distal humerus to correct cubitus valgus and lateral translocation of the proximal radius and ulna (Type B Milch fracture pattern). The longitudinal axis of the humerus and forearm are aligned.

A. Cubitus valgus combined with lateral translocation (Milch Type II fracture pattern of Salter-Harris Type IV physeal injury of the lateral condyle of the humerus). **B.** In Milch Type B fracture pattern in which an opening wedge osteotomy of the distal humerus is performed, an ugly prominence of the medial elbow is created that is not cosmetically acceptable. **C.** When varus angulation osteotomy is combined with lateral displacement, the longitudinal axis is realigned with that of the forearm. (Redrawn after Milch, H. E.: Fractures and fracture-dislocations of the humeral condyles. J. Trauma, *4*:592, 1964.)

terior aspect of the lateral condyle. The lateral condylar fragment is fixed to the distal humeral metaphysis by a compression cancellous screw; then the cubitus valgus is corrected by a varus angulation–lateral displacement osteotomy of the distal humerus at the level of the diaphyseal-metaphyseal junction.

Cubitus Varus. Prolonged hyperemia due to delayed union may stimulate overgrowth of the lateral condyle of the humerus and result in cubitus varus. Ordinarily, this deformity is minimal and of no clinical significance. Treatment is not required.

Tardy Ulnar Nerve Palsy.[8, 21, 49] This develops from progressive cubitus valgus due to nonunion or malunion. Symptoms and signs develop gradually, with motor deficit manifesting first, followed somewhat later by sensory loss. At the earliest signs of neuritis, the ulnar nerve is transferred anteriorly to the medial epicondyle in order to prevent permanent neural deficit.

Radial Nerve Paralysis. This is very rare; it may occur owing to stretching from the displaced lateral condyle, or it may be injured by the surgeon at the time of open reduction.[42, 68]

Avascular Necrosis of the Lateral Condyle. Blood supply to the lateral condyle of the humerus may be interrupted during open reduction when extreme dissection is required to reposition the fracture fragment into its bed.[22, 29, 42, 71] In nonoperated cases, avascular necrosis of the lateral condyle is very rare; in the literature there is only one such case, which was partial and not complete avascular necrosis.[79]

References

1. Agins, H. J., and Marcus, N. W.: Articular cartilage sleeve fracture of the lateral humeral condyle capitellum: A previously undescribed entity. J. Pediatr. Orthop., *4*:620, 1984.
2. Akbarnia, B. A., Silberstein, M. J., Rende, R. J., Graviss, E. R., and Luisiri, A.: Arthrography in the diagnosis of fractures of the distal end of the humerus in infants. J. Bone Joint Surg., *68-A*:599, 1986.
3. Badger, F. G.: Fractures of the lateral condyle of the humerus. J. Bone Joint Surg., *36-B*:147, 1954.
4. Blount, W. P.: Fractures of the lateral condyle of the humerus. *In* Fractures in Children. Baltimore, Williams & Wilkins, 1954, pp. 43–45.
5. Blount, W. P.: The treatment of elbow injuries in children. Wiederherstell. Traum., 7:1, 1963.
6. Bocchi, L., Orso, C. A., and Lacovara, V.: Surgical trends in treatment of fractures of the external humeral condyle in children. Chir. Organi Mov., *64*:605, 1978.
7. Bohler, L.: Fractures of the lateral condyle of the humerus in children. *In* The Treatment of Fractures, Supplementary Volume to the 5th English edition, pp. 2490–2493. By L. and J. Bohler. Translated from the 1st German Edition by Alfred Wallner. New York and London, Grune & Stratton, 1966.
8. Brenken, M., and Kuttner, H.: Die Ulnarisspatlahmung in folge Frakhn des Condyles lateralis Humeri. Arch. Orthop. Unfallchir., *28*:182, 1930.
9. Broca, A.: Decollements epiphysaires et fractures de la region condylienne externe. J. Practiciens, *97*:117, 1914.
10. Canale, G., Beccario, L., and Orestano, U.: Detachment of the external condyle of the humerus in children. Minerva Ortop., *19*:480, 1968.
11. Conner, A. N., and Smith, M. G. H.: Displaced fractures of the lateral humeral condyle in children. J. Bone Joint Surg., *52-B*:460, 1970.
12. Crabbe, W. A.: The treatment of fracture-separation of the capitular epiphysis. J. Bone Joint Surg., *45-B*:733, 1963.
13. Editorial: Fractures of the lateral condyle of the humerus in children. Injury, *16*:363, 1985.
14. Fabian, E.: Zur Behandlung der Fractura Condyli externi Humeri mitteb. Exstirpation des freien Fragmente. Dsch. Z. Chir., 128:409, 1914.
15. Fahey, J. J.: Fractures of the elbow in children. A.A.O.S. Instr. Course Lect., *17*:13, 1960.
16. Flynn, J. C., and Richards, J. F.: Non-union of minimally displaced fractures of the lateral condyle of the humerus in children. J. Bone Joint Surg., *53-A*:1096, 1971.
17. Flynn, J. C., Richards, J. F., Jr., and Saltzman, R. I.: Prevention and treatment of non-union of slightly displaced fractures of the lateral humeral condyle in children. An end-result study. J. Bone Joint Surg., *57-A*:1087, 1975.
18. Fontanetta, P., MacKenzie, D. A., and Rosman, M.: Missed, maluniting, and malunited fractures of the lateral humeral condyle in children. J. Trauma, *18*:329, 1978.
19. Foster, D. E., Sullivan, J. A., and Gross, R. H.: Lateral humeral condylar fractures in children. J. Pediatr. Orthop., *5*:16, 1985.
20. Freeman, R. H.: Fractures of the lateral humeral condyle. J. Bone Joint Surg., *41-B*:631, 1959.
21. Gay, J. R., and Love, J. G.: Diagnosis and treatment of tardy paralysis of the ulnar nerve. J. Bone Joint Surg., *29*:1087, 1947.
22. Hardacre, J. A., Nahigian, S. H., Froimson, I., and Brown, J. E.: Fractures of the lateral condyle of the humerus in children. J. Bone Joint Surg., *53-A*:1083, 1971.
23. Hefti, F., Jakob, R. P., and von Laer, L.: Fractures of the lateral humeral condyle in children and adolescents (author's transl.). Orthopade, *10*:274, 1981.
24. Herring, J. A.: Lateral condylar fracture of the elbow. J. Pediatr. Orthop., *6*:724, 1986.
25. Heyle, J. H.: Fractures of external condyle of humerus in children. Ann. Surg., *51*:1069, 1935.
26. Holst-Nielsen, F., and Ottsen, P.: Fractures of the lateral condyle of the humerus in children. Acta Orthop. Scand., *45*:518, 1974.
27. Huurman, W. W.: Lateral humeral condylar fracture. Nebr. Med. J., *68*:300, 1983.
28. Ingersoll, R.: Fractures of the humeral condyles in children. Clin. Orthop., *41*:32, 1965.
29. Jakob, R., Fowles, J. V., Rang, M., and Kassab, M. T.: Observations concerning fractures of the lateral humeral condyle in children. J. Bone Joint Surg., *57-B*:430, 1975.
30. Jeffrey, C. C.: Non-union of the epiphysis of the lateral condyle of the humerus. J. Bone Joint Surg., *40-B*:396, 1958.
31. Johanson, J., and Rosman, M.: Fracture of the capitellum humeri in children. A rare injury often misdiagnosed. Clin. Orthop., *146*:157, 1980.
32. Jones, K. G.: Percutaneous pin fixation of fractures of the lower end of the humerus. Clin. Orthop., *50*:53, 1967.

33. Judet, H.: Fracture du Condyle Externe des L'humerus. *In* Traite des Fractures des Membres. 2nd Ed., Chap. 12. Paris, L'Expansion Scientifique Francais, 1922, pp. 139–146.
34. Kalenak, A.: Ununited fractures of the lateral condyle of the humerus. A fifty year follow-up. Clin. Orthop., *124*:181, 1977.
35. Keon-Cohen, B. T.: Fractures of the elbow. J. Bone Joint Surg., *48-A*:162, 1966.
36. Kini, M. G.: Fractures of the lateral condyle of the lower end of the humerus with complications. A simple technique for closed reduction of the capitellar fracture. J. Bone Joint Surg., *24*:270, 1942.
37. Kitlinski, H.: Fracture of lateral condyle and rupture of medial epicondyle of humerus in children. Chir. Narzadow Ruchu Orthop. Pol., *31*:143, 1966.
38. Koudela, K., and Kavan, Z.: Fracture of lateral epicondyle of humerus with elbow dislocation inward and detachment of medial epicondyle (author's transl.). Acta Chir. Orthop. Traumatol. Cech., *44*:553, 1977.
39. LaGrange, J., and Rigault, P.: Fractures du condyle externe. Rev. Chir. Orthop., *48*:415, 1962.
40. Learmonth, J. R.: A technic for transplanting the ulnar nerve. Surg. Gynecol. Obstet., *75*:792, 1942.
41. Lloyd, R. D., and Miller, W.: Fractures of the lateral humeral condyle in children, review of the literature and late results of internal fixation (resident paper). Oklahoma City, University of Oklahoma, 1973.
42. McDonnell, D. P., and Wilson, J. C.: Fractures of the lower end of the humerus in children. J. Bone Joint Surg., *30-A*:347, 1948.
43. McGowan, A. J.: The results of transposition of the ulnar nerve for traumatic ulnar neuritis. J. Bone Joint Surg., *32-B*:293, 1950.
44. McLearie, M., and Merson, R. D.: Injuries to the lateral condyle epiphysis of the humerus in children. J. Bone Joint Surg., *36-B*:84, 1954.
45. Malgaigne, J. F.: A treatise on fractures. Translated by John H. Packard. Philadelphia, Lippincott, 1859, pp. 448–451.
46. Massart, C.: Les fractures du condyle externe chez l'enfant-etude clinique et radiographique de ces fractures et de leurs resultats eloignes. Rev. Orthop., *15*:475, 1928.
47. Maylahn, D. J., and Fahey, J. J.: Fractures of the elbow in children. Review of 300 consecutive cases. J.A.M.A., *166*:220, 1958.
48. Milch, H.: Fractures of the external humeral condyle. J.A.M.A., *160*:641, 1956.
49. Miller, E. M.: Late ulnar nerve paralysis. Surg. Gynecol. Obstet., *38*:37, 1924.
50. Moorhead, E. L.: Old untreated fracture of the external condyle of humerus-factors in influencing choice of treatment. Surg. Clin., *3*:987, 1919.
51. Morrissy, R. T., and Wilkins, K. E.: Deformity following distal humeral fracture in childhood. J. Bone Joint Surg., *66-A*:557, 1984.
52. Mouchet, A.: Paralysies tardiness du nerf cubital a la suite des fractures du condyle externe de l'humerus. J. Chir. (Paris), *12*:437, 1914.
53. Murphy, J. B.: Cicatricial fixation of ulnar nerve from ancient cubitus valgus—release and transference to a new site. The Clinics of John B. Murphy, *5*:661, 1916.
54. Ogino, T., Minami, A., and Fukuda, K.: Tardy ulnar nerve palsy caused by cubitus varus deformity. J. Hand Surg., *11-B*:352, 1986.
55. Papavasiliou, V. A., and Beslikas, T. A.: Fractures of the lateral humeral condyle in children—an analysis of 39 cases. Injury, *16*:364, 1985.
56. Papavasiliou, V. A., and Beslikas, T. A.: T-condylar fractures of the distal humeral condyles during childhood: An analysis of six cases. J. Pediatr. Orthop., *6*:302, 1986.
57. Patania, S., and Letizia, G.: Contribution to the study of fractures of the external condyle of the humerus in children. Minerva Orthop., *16*:418, 1965.
58. Rang, M.: Fractures in Children. Philadelphia, J. B. Lippincott, 1983, pp. 152–196.
59. Reinders, J. F., and Lens, J.: A missed opportunity: Two fractures of the lateral humeral condyle in a girl aged 5 years. Neth. J. Surg., *35*:78, 1983.
60. Riess, J.: Fractures of the lateral humeral condyle in children. Z. Orthop., *80*:427, 1951.
61. Rocher, H. L., and Guerin, R.: Luxation ouverte du coude avec fracture du condyle externe. Arch. Franco-Belg. Chir., *32*:627, 1930.
62. Rohl, L.: On fractures through the radial condyle of the humerus in children. Acta Chir. Scand., *104*:74, 1953.
63. Rutherford, A.: Fractures of the lateral humeral condyle in children. J. Bone Joint Surg., *67-A*:851, 1985.
64. Sharp, I. K.: Fractures of the lateral humeral condyle in children. Acta Orthop. Belg., *31*:811, 1965.
65. Sherren, J.: Remarks on chronic neuritis of the ulnar nerve due to deformity in the region of the elbow-joint. Edinburgh Med. J., *23*:500, 1908.
66. Smith, F. M.: Children's elbow injuries: Fractures and dislocations. Clin. Orthop., *50*:7, 1967.
67. Smith, F. M.: An eighty-four year follow-up on a patient with ununited fracture of the lateral condyle of the humerus. A case report. J. Bone Joint Surg., *55-A*:378, 1973.
68. Smith, F. M., and Joyce, J. J.: Fractures of the lateral condyle of the humerus in children. Am. J. Surg., *87*:324, 1954.
69. Smith, M. K.: Fractures of the external condyle of the humerus with rotation. Ann. Surg., *86*:304, 1927.
70. So, Y. C., Fang, D., Leong, J. C. Y., and Bong, S. C.: Varus deformity following lateral humeral condylar fractures in children. J. Pediatr. Orthop., *5*:569, 1985.
71. Speed, J. S., and Macey, H. B.: Fractures of the humeral condyles in children. J. Bone Joint Surg., *15*:903, 1933.
72. Stimson, L. A.: A Practical Treatise on Fractures and Dislocations. 5th Ed. New York, Lea Bros. & Co., 1907, pp. 253–256.
73. Stone, J. S.: Fractures of the external condyle of the humerus in childhood with rotation of the condylar fragment. Boston Med. Surg. J., *176*:151, 1917.
74. von Laer, L., Pagels, P., and Schroeder, L.: The treatment of fracture of the radial condyle of the humerus. Unfallheilkunde, *86*:503, 1983.
75. Voshell, A. F., and Taylor, K. P. A.: Regeneration of the lateral condyle of the humerus after excision. J. Bone Joint Surg., *21*:421, 1939.
76. Wadsworth, T. G.: Premature epiphyseal fusion after injury to the capitulum. J. Bone Joint Surg., *46-B*:46, 1964.
77. Wadsworth, T. G.: Injuries of the capitular (lateral humeral condylar) epiphyses. Clin. Orthop., *85*:127, 1972.
78. Watson-Jones, R.: Displacement of the epiphysis of the lateral condyle. *In* Fractures and Joint Injuries. 4th Ed., Vol. II. Edinburgh, E. & S. Livingstone, 1955, pp. 539–542.
79. Wilson, J. N.: Fractures of the external condyle of the humerus in children. Br. J. Surg., *43*:88, 1955.
80. Wilson, P. D.: Fractures and dislocations in the region of the elbow. Surg. Gynecol. Obstet., *56*:335, 1933.
81. Wilson, P. D.: Fracture of the lateral condyle of the humerus in childhood. J. Bone Joint Surg., *18*:301, 1936.
82. Zeier, F. G.: Lateral condylar fracture and its many complications. Orthop. Rev., *10*:49, 1981.

*FRACTURES OF THE MEDIAL EPICONDYLE OF THE HUMERUS**

The ossification center of the medial epicondyle of the humerus appears at about five years of age and unites with the humeral diaphysis between 18 and 20 years of age. The common tendon of the flexor muscles of the forearm (flexor carpi radialis, flexor carpi ulnaris, flexor digitorum sublimis, palmaris longus, and part of the pronator teres) takes its origin from the anterior aspect of the medial epicondyle, which also gives attachment to the ulnar collateral ligament of the elbow joint. The ulnar nerve runs in a groove in the posterior aspect of this epicondyle—an anatomic relation responsible for the frequent occurrence of the ulnar nerve injury in this fracture. The medial epicondyle is an apophysis and does not contribute to longitudinal growth of the humerus.

Fractures of the epicondyle usually occur between 7 and 15 years of age. They constitute about 10 per cent of all fractures in the region of the elbow joint in children.

The mechanism of injury is a valgus strain of the joint, producing traction on the medial epicondyle through the flexor muscles. The epicondyle may be minimally displaced, moderately displaced to the level of the joint, markedly displaced and incarcerated into the elbow joint, or severely displaced in association with posterolateral dislocation of the elbow (Fig. 8–50). About half of the cases of fractures of the medial epicondyle are associated with dislocation of the elbow (see Fig. 8–48 C).

Incarceration of the fragment into the joint usually occurs at the time of reduction of the dislocation; or it may be pulled into the joint by the abduction force when the elbow is temporarily opened on its medial side, or while the joint is momentarily dislocated.

Diagnosis

Physical findings depend upon the degree of displacement of the medial epicondyle. The elbow is held in partial flexion and any motion is painful. There is local tenderness over the medial aspect of the joint. The pain is aggravated when valgus strain is exerted at the elbow joint.

Radiographs will disclose the absence of the medial epicondyle from its normal position. The displaced fragment may be seen in the lateral, anteroposterior, or oblique projections of the elbow. If the diagnosis is in doubt, radiograms of the opposite elbow are made for comparison. When the medial epicondyle is incarcerated into the joint, the articular cartilage space is widened on its medial aspect and the bony fragment is best visualized in the lateral views. When the elbow is dislocated posterolaterally, the medial epicondyle is usually located posterior to the trochlea. Ulnar nerve paresis is a common complication of this injury.

Treatment

If the medial epicondyle is *minimally displaced*, the joint is immobilized in an above-elbow cast with the elbow in moderate flexion and the forearm in pronation for three weeks.

If the epicondyle is moderately displaced but the elbow is stable on valgus strain, treatment again consists of simple immobilization in an above-elbow cast for three weeks. The functional result will be excellent despite the fact that healing is by fibrous union. Occasionally the fragment may fail to heal and produces symptoms due to irritation by local pressure, such as rubbing on a table while writing; in such an instance, complete relief of symptoms is obtained by excision of the loose fragment.

If the medial epicondyle is *markedly displaced* and the elbow joint is *unstable* on application of valgus strain, open reduction and internal fixation are indicated. The patient is placed in prone position with his upper limb adducted behind his back with a pneumatic tourniquet in place.

The medial longitudinal skin incision starts at the fractured medial epicondyle and extends proximally for a distance of 5 to 7 cm. parallel with the epicondylar ridge of the humerus. The subcutaneous tissue and deep fascia are divided in line with the skin incision. The ulnar nerve is identified, dissected free, and retracted posteriorly with a moist hernia tape. The fractured medial epicondyle is identified, and it is anatomically repositioned with a sharp towel clip on the common tendon of the flexor muscles.

Next, through two small stab wounds in the skin, separate from the incision, two smooth medium-sized Kirschner wires are drilled across the fracture site in a proximal and lateral direction. The pins should engage the lateral cortex. The position of the wires and the accuracy of reduction are verified by making radiograms of the elbow in the anteroposterior and lateral projections. The distal parts of the wire are bent

*See references 1 to 73.

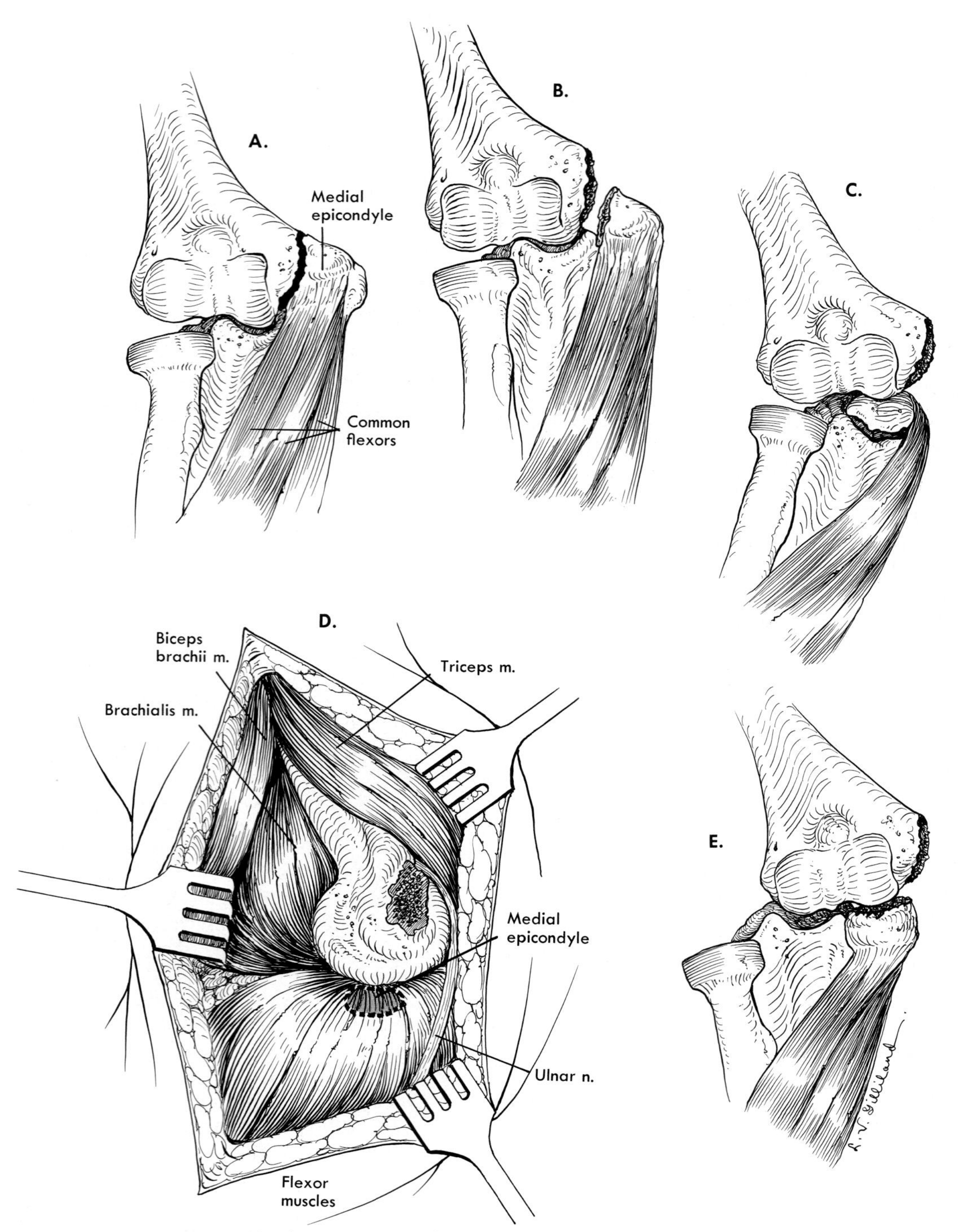

FIGURE 8–50. Fracture and displacement of medial epicondyle of the humerus.

A. Minimal displacement. **B.** Moderate displacement. **C** and **D.** Marked displacement and incarceration into the elbow joint. **E.** Fracture and displacement associated with posterolateral dislocation of the elbow joint.

to prevent migration and then are cut off with a wire cutter, leaving the ends protruding slightly through the skin. The perisoteum and capsule are repaired with interrupted sutures, giving further stability to the reduction of the fracture fragments. After closure of the wound, an above-elbow cast is applied, immobilizing the elbow in 90 degrees of flexion and the forearm in full pronation.

In about four weeks, the cast and pins are removed and active exercises are instituted to restore range of motion of the elbow.

The author does not recommend closed reduction of markedly displaced medial epicondyle fractures. Immobilization in an above-elbow cast with the elbow in acute flexion and the forearm in full pronation for six weeks (in order to maintain reduction by relieving the pull of the flexor muscle) will result in fixed flexion deformity of the elbow.

When the epicondyle is incarcerated in the joint, manipulation to dislodge the fragment should not be performed, because frequently this method is unsuccessful, and there is a definite danger of injury to the ulnar nerve, which is often incarcerated with the fragment. It is best to dislodge the trapped epicondyle by open surgery. Whether the epicondyle should be reattached or not depends upon the age of the patient and the extent of damage to the epicondyle. In children under ten years of age, the epicondyle, if normal and not crushed, is reattached to its bed of origin to avoid any underdevelopment of the medial aspect of the elbow. In the older child or in a case in which the bone fragment is damaged, it is excised. Ordinarily if the fracture is associated with dislocation, rehabilitation is prolonged, and often some fixed flexion deformity remains.

References

1. Aitken, A. P., and Childress, H. M.: Intraarticular displacement of internal epicondyle following dislocation. J. Bone Joint Surg., *20*:161, 1938.
2. Ashurst, A. P. C.: An Anatomical and Surgical Study of Fractures of the Lower End of the Humerus. Philadelphia, Lea & Febiger, 1910.
3. Bairov, G. A., and Gorely, I. V. V.: Transcutaneous temporary osteosynthesis of fractures of the inner supracondyle of the humerus in children. Ortop. Travmatol. Protez., *10*:70, 1975.
4. Bede, W. B., Lefebvre, A. R., and Rosman, M. A.: Fractures of the medial humeral epicondyle in children. Can. J. Surg., *18*:137, 1975.
5. Bensahel, H., Csukonyi, Z., Badelon, O., and Badaoui, S.: Fractures of the medial condyle of the humerus in children. J. Pediatr. Orthop., *6*:430, 1986.
6. Bernstein, S. M., King, J. D., and Sanderson, R. A.: Fractures of the medial epicondyle of the humerus. Contemp. Orthop., *6*:37, 1981.
7. Blount, W. P.: Unusual fractures in children. A.A.O.S. Instr. Course Lect., *7*:57, 1954.
8. Blount, W. P.: Fractures in Children. Baltimore, Williams & Wilkins, 1955.
9. Boyd, H. B., and Altenberg, A. R.: Fractures about the elbow in children. Arch. Surg., *49*:213, 1944.
10. Brewster, A. H., and Karp, M.: Fractures in the region of the elbow in children. An end-result study. Surg. Gynecol. Obstet., *71*:643, 1940.
11. Brodeur, A. E., Silberstein, M. J., and Graviss, E. R.: Radiology of the Pediatric Elbow. Boston, G. K. Hall, 1981.
12. Capla, D., and Kundrat, J.: Fracture of medial epicondyle of humerus (author's transl.). Acta Chir. Orthop. Traumatol. Cech., *46*:147, 1979.
13. Cataliotti, F., Giglio, A. L., and Salomone, G.: Percutaneous osteosynthesis in fracture-dislocations of the epitrochlea and of condylo-epicondyloid block in childhood. Minerva Med., *63*:4256, 1972.
14. Chacha, P. B.: Fracture of the medial condyle of the humerus with rotational displacement. J. Bone Joint Surg., *52-A*:1453, 1970.
15. Chessare, J. W., Rogers, L. F., White, H., and Tachdjian, M. O.: Injuries of the medial epicondyle ossification center of the humerus. A.J.R., *129*:49, 1977.
16. Collins, R., and Lavine, S. A.: Fracture of the medial epicondyle. Clin. Proc. Child. Hosp. D. C., *20*:274, 1964.
17. Conn, J. J., and Wade, P. A.: Injuries of the elbow: A 10 year follow-up. J. Trauma, *1*:248, 1961.
18. Cothay, D. M.: Injury to the lower medial epiphysis of the humerus before development of ossific centre. Report of a case. J. Bone Joint Surg., 49-B:766, 1967.
19. Cotton, F. J.: Elbow fractures in children. Ann. Surg., *35*:75, 242, 365, 1902.
20. Cotton, F. J.: Dislocations and Joint Fractures. 2nd ed. Philadelphia, Saunders, 1924.
21. Dahl-Iverson, E.: Fracture condylienne humerale interne. Reduction simple, sanglante. Lyon Chir., *33*:234, 1936.
22. Dunlop, J.: Traumatic separation of medial epicondyle of humerus in adolescence. J. Bone Joint Surg., *17*:577, 1935.
23. Eid, A. M.: Displacement of the medial epicondyle into the elbow joint. Egypt. Orthop. J., *10*:160, 1975.
24. El Ghawabi, M. H.: Fracture of the medial condyle of the humerus. J. Bone Joint Surg., *57-A*:677, 1975.
25. Fahey, J. J.: Fractures of the elbow in children. A.A.O.S. Instr. Course Lect., *17*:13, 1960.
26. Fahey, J. J., and O'Brien, E. T.: Fracture-separation of the medial humeral condyle in a child confused with fracture of the medial epicondyle. J. Bone Joint Surg., *53-A*:1102, 1971.
27. Fairbanks, H. A. T., and Buxton, St. J. D.: Displacement of the internal epicondyle into the elbow joint. Lancet, *2*:218, 1934.
28. Faysse, R., and Marion, J.: Fractures du condyle interne de l'humerus. Rev. Chir. Orthop., *48*:337, 1962.
29. Fevre, M., and Roudaitis, J.: La reduction non sanglante des fractures de l'epitrochlee avec interposition de ce fragment dans l'interligne articulone du coude. Rev. Chir. Orthop., *20*:300, 1933.
30. Fowles, J. V., and Kassab, M. T.: A fracture of the internal condyle of the humerus in a child. Diagnosis and treatment. Apropos of one case. Tunis. Med., *50*:189, 1972.
31. Fowles, J. V., and Kassab, M. T.: Displaced fractures of the medial humeral condyle in children. J. Bone Joint Surg., *62-A*:1159, 1980.
32. Fowles, J. V., Kassab, M. T., and Moula, T.: Untreated intra-articular entrapment of the medial humeral epicondyle. J. Bone Joint Surg., *66-B*:562, 1984.

33. Ghaweabi, M.: Fracture of the medial condyle of the humerus. J. Bone Joint Surg., *57-A*:677, 1975.
34. Granger, B.: On a particular fracture of the inner condyle of the humerus. Edinburgh Med. Surg. J., *14*:196, 1818.
35. Haraldsson S.: Vascularization of the distal end of humerus. Acta Orthop. Scand. (Suppl.), *38*:1, 1959.
36. Harrison, R. B., Keats, T. E., Frankel, C. J., Anderson, R. L., and Youngblood, P.: Radiographic clues to fractures of the unossified medial humeral condyle in young children. Skeletal Radiol., *11*:209, 1984.
37. Hasner, E., and Husby, J.: Fracture of epicondyle and condyle of humerus. Acta Chir. Scand., *101*:195, 1951.
38. Higgs, S.: Fractures of the internal epicondyle of the humerus. Br. Med. J., *1*:666, 1936.
39. Ingersoll, R. E.: Fractures of the humeral condyles in children. Clin. Orthop., *41*:32, 1965.
40. Kilfoyle, R. M.: Fractures of the medial condyle and epicondyle of the elbow in children. Clin. Orthop., *41*:43, 1965.
41. Kiss, A., and Vincze, J.: Fractures of the medial humeral epicondyle in children (author's transl.). Magy. Traumatol. Orthop. Helyreallito Sebesz., *24*:1, 1981.
42. Kolonta, I., Iuiu, G., and Sergach, V.: Surgical treatment of fractures of the humeral epicondyles. Orthop. Travmatol. Protez., *11*:77, 1978.
43. LaGrange, J., and Rigault, P.: Les fractures de l'extremite inferieure de l'humerus chez l'enfant. Rev. Chir. Orthop., *48*:4, 1962.
44. Lane, L. C.: Fractures of the bones which form the elbow joint and their treatment. Trans. Am. Surg. Assoc., *9*:431, 1891.
45. Masse, P.: Technique de reduction des luxations du coude avec fracture ou interposition de l'epitrochlee. Rev. Prat., *5*:1038, 1955.
46. Maylahn, D. J., and Fahey, J. J.: Fractures of the elbow in children. Review of three hundred consecutive cases. J.A.M.A., *18*:228, 1958.
47. Milch, H.: Isolated fractures and fracture-dislocations of the humeral condyles. *In* Societe Internationale de Chirurgie Orthopedique et de Traumatologie. Neuvieme Congres, Vienne, 1964, pp. 645—652.
48. Mitchell, W. J., and Adams, J. P.: Fracture and dislocation of the elbow in children. Curr. Pract. Orthop. Surg., *2*:102, 1964.
49. Papavasiliou, V. A.: Fracture-separation of the medial epicondylar epiphysis of the elbow joint. Clin. Orthop., *171*:172, 1982.
50. Patrick, J.: Fracture of medial epicondyle with displacement into elbow joint. J. Bone Joint Surg., *28*:143, 1946.
51. Pollosson, E., and Arnulf, G.: Fracture du condyle interne-reposition sanglante. Lyon Chir., *34*:337, 1937.
52. Potter, C. M. C.: Fracture-dislocation of the trochlea. J. Bone Joint Surg., *36-B*:250, 1954.
53. Rai, P. K., and Sharma, R. N.: Bilateral fracture of medial condyle of humerus in child. J. Indian Med. Assoc., *76*:138, 1981.
54. Roberts, N. W.: Displacement of the internal epicondyle into the elbow joint. Four cases successfully treated by manipulation. Lancet, *2*:78, 1934.
55. Rosendahl, B.: Displacement of the medial epicondyle into the elbow joint: The final result in a case where the fragment has not been removed. Acta Orthop. Scand., *28*:212, 1959.
56. Salter, R. B., and Harris, W. R.: Injuries involving the epiphyseal plate. J. Bone Joint Surg., *45-A*:587, 1963.
57. Sandegard, E.: Fracture of the lower end of the humerus in children—treatment and end results. Acta Chir. Scand., *89*:1, 1943.
58. Schmier, A. A.: Internal epicondylar epiphysis and elbow injuries. Surg. Gynecol. Obstet., *80*:416, 1945.
59. Silberstein, J. J., Brodeur, A. E., Graviss, E. R., and Atchawee, L.: Some vagaries of the medial epicondyle. J. Bone Joint Surg., *63-A*:524, 1981.
60. Smith, F. M.: Displacement of the medial epicondyle of the humerus into the elbow joint. Ann. Surg., *124*:425, 1946.
61. Smith, F. M.: Medial epicondyle injuries. J.A.M.A., *142*:396, 1950.
62. Smith, F. M.: Surgery of the Elbow. 2nd Ed. Philadelphia, Saunders, 1972.
63. Speed, J. S., and Macey, H. B.: Fractures of the humeral condyles in children. J. Bone Joint Surg., *15*:903, 1933.
64. Spi, S. S. A. L., Geryk, B., and Macek, M.: Morphological and functional results of children's fractures of humerus epicondyles (author's transl.). Acta Chir. Orthop. Traumatol. Cech., *40*:362, 1973.
65. Taverner, M.: Discussion of Dahl Iverson, M. E.: Fracture condylienne humerale interne. Reduction simple, sanglante. Lyon Chir., *33*:234, 1936.
66. Tayob, A. A., and Shively, R. A.: Bilateral elbow dislocations with intra-articular displacement of medial epicondyles. J. Trauma, *20*:332, 1980.
67. Varma, B. P., and Srivastava, T. P.: Fracture of the medial condyle of the humerus in children: A report of 4 cases including the late sequelae. Injury, *4*:171, 1972.
68. Walker, H. B.: A case of dislocation of the elbow with separation of the internal epicondyle and displacement of the latter into the elbow joint. Br. J. Surg., *15*:677, 1928.
69. Watson-Jones, R.: Displacement of the epiphysis of the medial epicondyle. *In* Fractures and Joint Injuries. Vol. 2. Edinburgh, Livingstone, 1955, p 543.
70. Wilson, J. N.: The treatment of fractures of the medial epicondyle of the humerus. J. Bone Joint Surg., *42-B*:778, 1960.
71. Wilson, J. N.: Fractures of the external condyle of the humerus in children. Br. J. Surg., *43*:88, 1955.
72. Woods, G. M., and Tullos, H. G.: Elbow instability and medial epicondyle fracture. Am. J. Sports Med., *5*:23, 1977.
73. Yelton, C. L.: Injuries about the elbow. J. Bone Joint Surg., *37*:650, 1955.

DISLOCATION OF THE ELBOW

Dislocation of the elbow is a relatively uncommon injury in children, usually occurring between 11 and 15 years of age, when the physes about the elbow begin to close. It is more frequently encountered in boys, with the left elbow being more often affected than the right.

The direction of displacement varies according to the direction of the force. The most common type of dislocation is, by far, posterior, usually accompanied by some lateral displacement. In posterior dislocations the proximal radioulnar joint is not disturbed. Rotatory luxation with total displacement of one bone and part of the other bone may occur in the posterior type when only one collateral ligament is torn. Isolated dislocations of the proximal ulna may occur. Other rare forms are anterior, lateral, and medial dislocations. Divergent dislocation of the radius and ulna is extremely rare

Table 8–3. Classification of Elbow Dislocation

I. Displacement of the radioulnar unit with its articulation intact in the distal humerus
  A. Posterior
    1. Posteromedial
    2. Posterolateral
  B. Anterior
  C. Medial
  D. Lateral
II. Divergent with disruption of radioulnar articulations
  A. Anteroposterior—with radius displaced anterior and ulna posterior
  B. Transverse—with ulna displaced medial and radius lateral

(Table 8–3).[3, 23, 36, 48, 77, 104] Dislocation of the elbow in children and adolescents is often associated with fractures; bones involved, in order of frequency, are the medial epicondyle, proximal radius, coronoid process, and olecranon. Involvement of the trochlea and lateral condylar physis is extremley rare.

Mechanism of Injury and Pathologic Anatomy

Posterior dislocation usually results from a fall on the outstretched hand with the forearm supinated and the elbow extended or partially flexed (Fig. 8–51). The coronoid process, which normally resists posterior displacement of the ulna, is relatively small in children. The anterior capsule of the elbow joint is torn by the force of the impact transmitted upward through the ulna and radius; and the momentum of the body applied to the lower end of the humerus tears the joint capsule anteriorly. The collateral ligaments are stretched or ruptured. The radius and ulna, being firmly bound by the annular ligament and the interosseous membrane, are displaced upward and posteriorly together; the coronoid process of the ulna becomes locked in the olecranon fossa of the humerus by the contraction of the biceps and triceps. In posterolateral dislocations, the biceps tendon serves as a fulcrum for rotation and valgus hinging of the forearm. The normal cubitus valgus of the elbow promotes lateral displacement. The periosteum is stripped from the posterior surface of the humerus, and the brachialis muscle becomes stretched.

As already stated, with posterior luxations, there is often a varying degree of lateral displacement of the forearm bones (Fig. 8–52). With the ulnar collateral ligament, a portion of the medial epicondyle may be avulsed and displaced posteriorly (Fig. 8–53). On reduction, the medial epicondyle may be incarcerated in the joint. With posteromedial dislocation, fracture of the lateral condyle of the humerus may occur (Fig. 8–54). Fracture-separation of the upper epiphysis of the radius is another complication. Injury to the brachial vessels or ulnar and median nerves may occur. The median nerve may become entrapped.

Anterior dislocation is a rare injury caused by a direct blow or fall on the olecranon process; the latter, with the proximal end of the radius, is displaced anteriorly to the lower end of the humerus.[10, 56, 108, 109, 124] Medial or lateral luxations usually result from direct trauma, violent twisting of the forearm, or falls upon the hand.

Diagnosis

Immediately following the injury, the patient presents with a painful and swollen elbow, which is held in partial flexion and supported at the forearm by the opposite hand. Any attempted motion of the elbow is very painful and restricted, with marked muscle spasm. When a normal elbow is extended, the olecranon process and the medial and lateral epicondyles form three points on a straight line; and when the normal elbow is flexed to 90 degrees in the lateral view, the olecranon is aligned vertically with the epicondyles; the tip of the olecranon is, however, definitely posterior to the plane of the epicondyles (Fig. 8–46 B). In posterior dislocation, the olecranon process is displaced backward from its normal position in relation to the humerus, and one can palpate the concavity of the semilunar notch (Fig. 8–46 C and D); increasing the degree of elbow flexion exaggerates the prominence of the olecranon process. The radial head can usually be palpated behind the lateral condyle of the humerus and lateral to the olecranon. In the antecubital fossa, there is definite fullness due to prominence of the humerus. From the anterior view, the forearm appears to be shortened, whereas from the posterior view, the upper arm appears to be decreased in length. The foregoing physical findings, however, are soon obscured by the development of marked soft tissue swelling in the region of the elbow.

It is imperative to assess and record neuromuscular function of the upper limb, particularly of the ulnar and median nerves. The brachial artery may be torn.

Radiographs should always be made prior to treatment; they should be meticulously scrutinized to rule out the presence of associated fractures of the medial epicondyle, coronoid process, proximal radius, or lateral condyle.

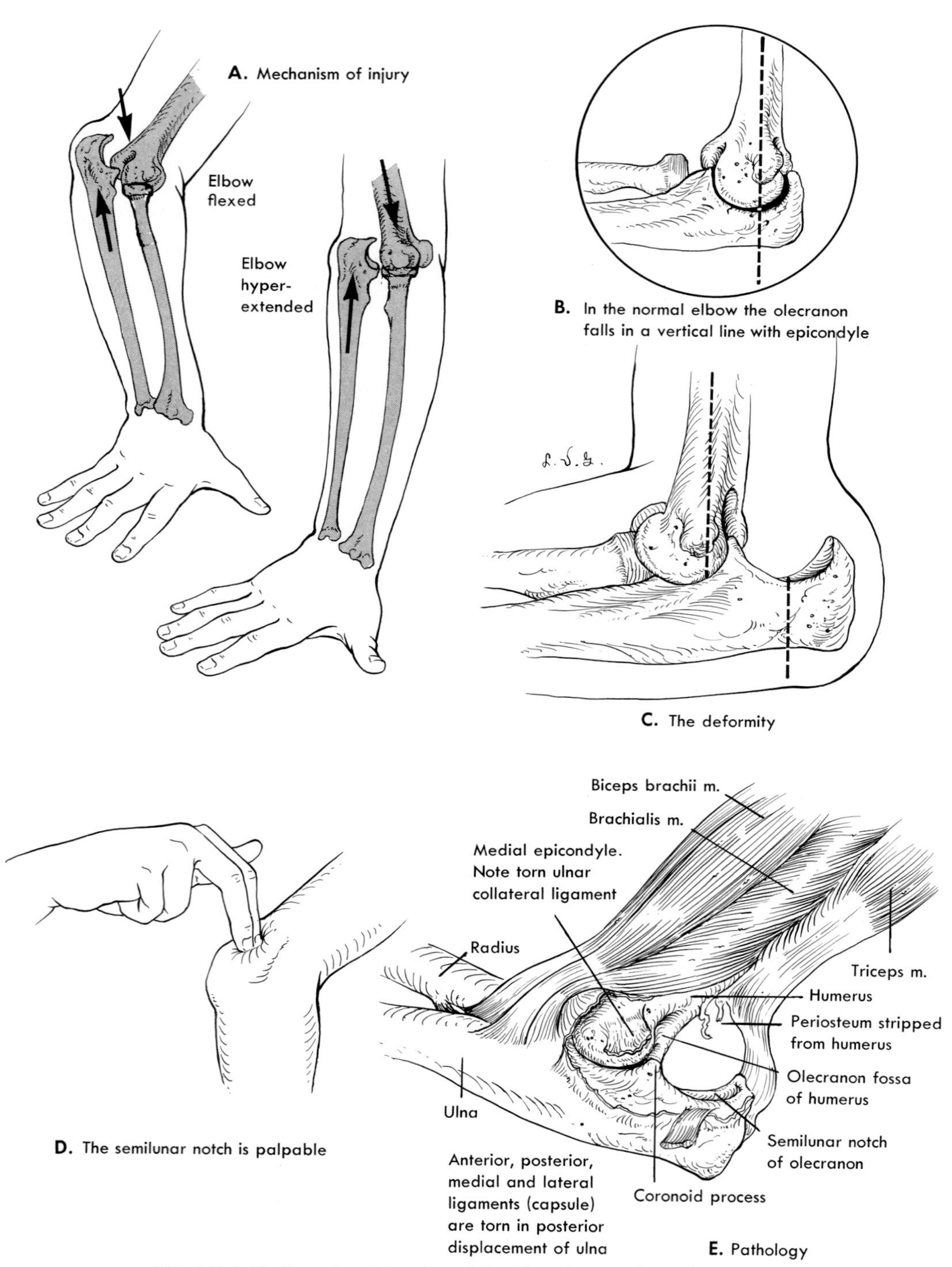

FIGURE 8–51. Posterior dislocation of the elbow (see text for explanation).

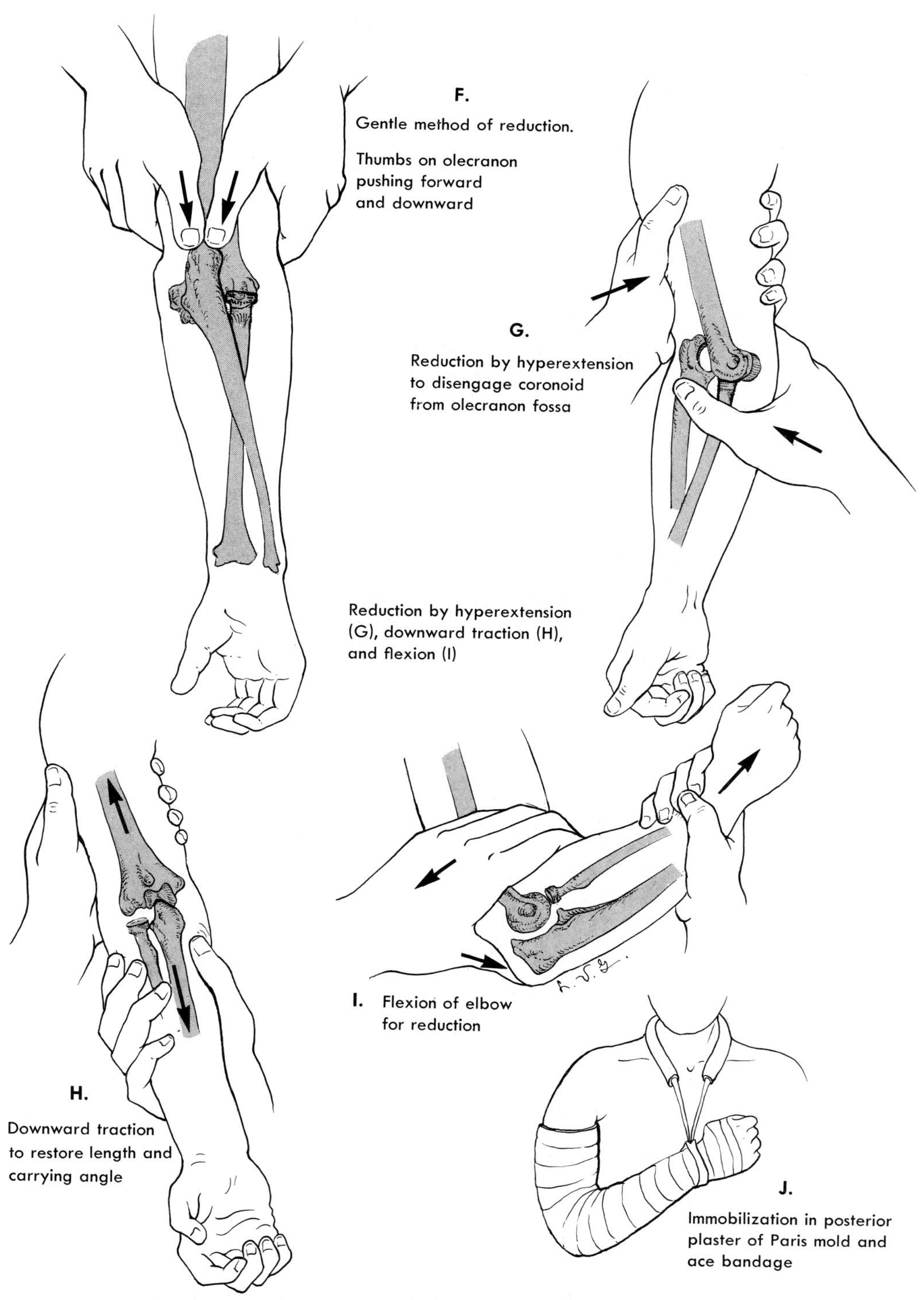

FIGURE 8–51 Continued. Posterior dislocation of the elbow (see text for explanation).

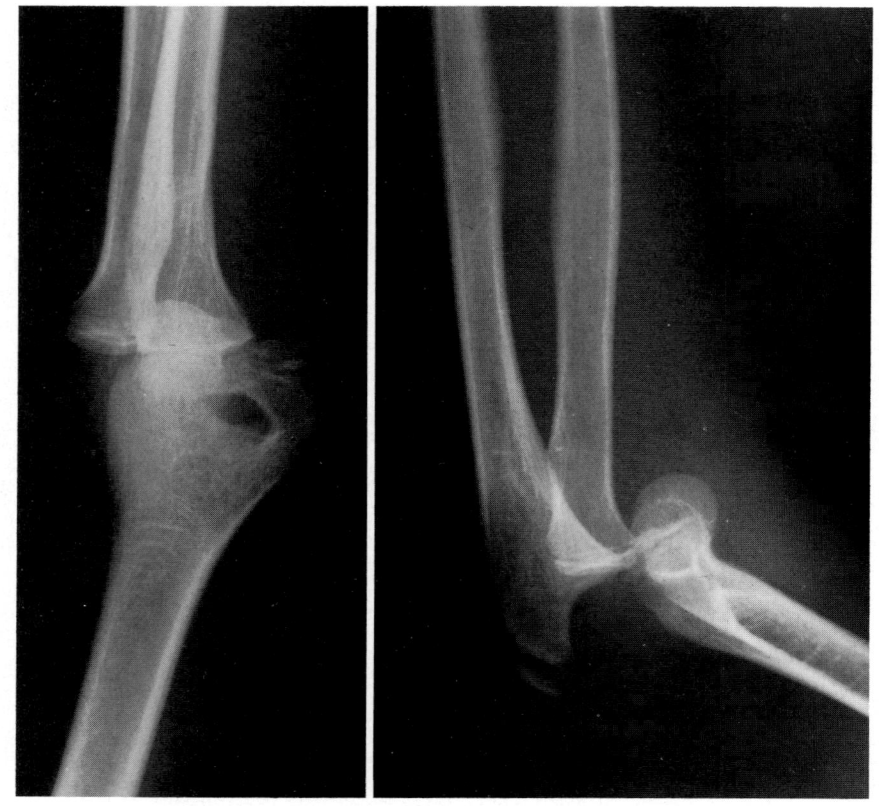

FIGURE 8–52. Radiograms of posterolateral dislocation of elbow.

Treatment

Reduction of recent *posterior dislocation* is easily accomplished. General anesthesia is usually not necessary. There are several methods available.[19, 111]

In children, a gentle and effective method is as follows: Place the patient in prone position with the injured limb hanging over the edge of the table. The weight of the arm provides distal traction in the long axis of the humerus, elongating the triceps posteriorly and the biceps and brachialis anteriorly. Sometimes it is necessary for an assistant to apply manual traction on the forearm. The surgeon encircles the patient's arm with his fingers (to give countertraction), and, with his thumbs, pushes the olecranon downward and forward (Fig. 8–51 F). Following reduction, the elbow is acutely flexed as much as swelling will permit and without causing circulatory embarrassment.

An alternate method of reduction is by hyperextension, downward traction, and flexion: (1) Hold the upper arm with one hand to apply steady countertraction (an assistant, if available, can do it). With the other hand, grasp the forearm and, with the elbow in some hyperextension, exert moderate traction to disengage the tip of the coronoid process from the olecranon fossa (Fig. 8–51 G). Marked hyperextension of the elbow should be avoided in order to avoid unnecessary strain on the already torn capsule and other soft tissues on the anterior aspect of the joint. (2) Then apply downward traction with the elbow in neutral extension to restore length. While traction is maintained, any lateral displacement and increase in the carrying angle are corrected. (3) Next, the elbow is gently flexed. Often, as the olecranon engages the articular surface of the humerus, a "click" can be palpated and heard. Postreduction radiograms are obtained to check the anatomic accuracy of reduction and, most important, to rule out the presence of associated fractures. The elbow is flexed to the degree that swelling will permit without interfering with circulation and immobilized in a posterior plaster of Paris splint and Ace bandage.

Three weeks after closed reduction, the plaster splint is removed and active exercises are instituted to restore normal range of motion of the elbow. A triangular sling may be worn for

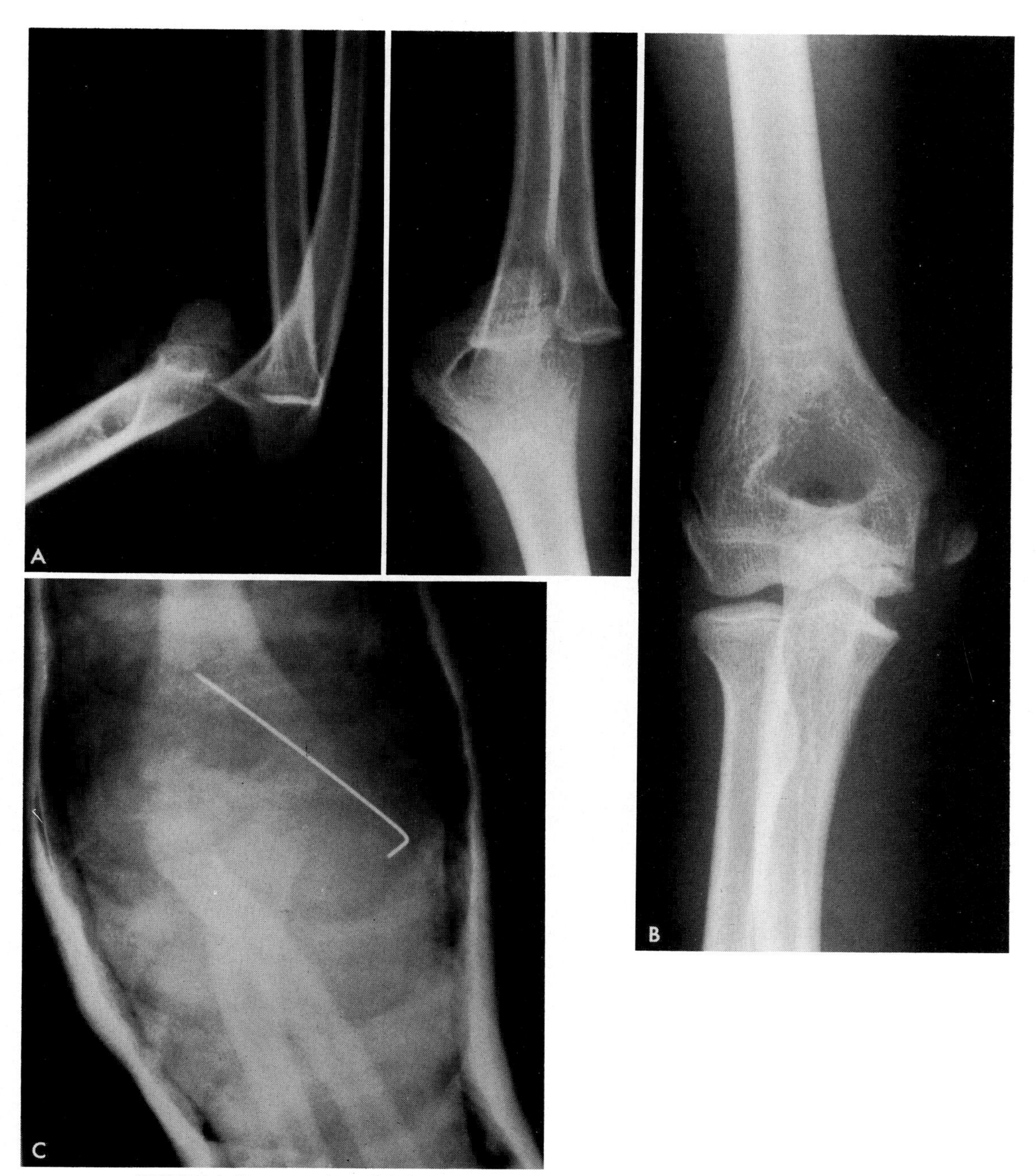

FIGURE 8–53. Posterolateral dislocation of the elbow with fracture of the medial epicondyle.

A. Initial radiograms. **B.** Immediate postreduction radiogram showing the displaced fracture of the medial epicondyle. This patient had persistent ulnar nerve paralysis. The bony fragment was excised and the ulnar nerve transposed anteriorly. **C.** An alternate method is pinning of the medial epicondyle with a Kirschner wire, as shown in this radiogram of another patient.

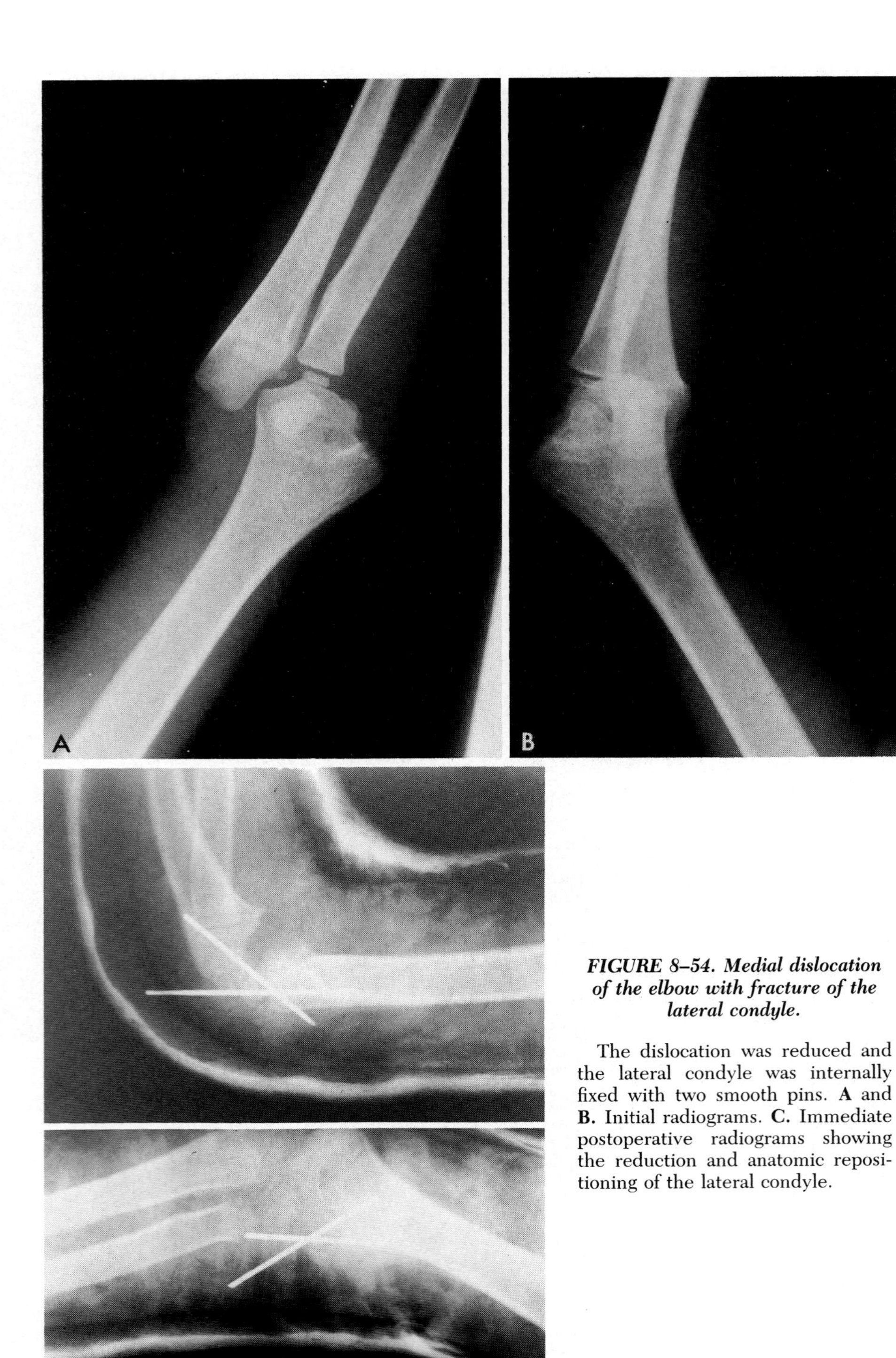

FIGURE 8–54. Medial dislocation of the elbow with fracture of the lateral condyle.

The dislocation was reduced and the lateral condyle was internally fixed with two smooth pins. **A** and **B.** Initial radiograms. **C.** Immediate postoperative radiograms showing the reduction and anatomic repositioning of the lateral condyle.

seven days for comfort. Passive exercises should *not* be performed, as they promote the development of myositis ossificans. Any lifting strain or forced hyperextension should be avoided for two months following the injury.

Anterior dislocation is a very rare injury.[10, 16, 56, 108, 109, 124] Cohn, in a review of the early literature, found only 23 cases.[16] Linscheid and Wheeler reported two cases of anterior dislocation out of 110 elbow dislocations and stated that there are fewer than 50 reported cases in the literature.[73] In anterior dislocation of the elbow, there is extensive soft-tissue damage, and often associated fractures of the olecranon or of the proximal shaft of the ulna. Reduction is accomplished as follows: (1) Apply longitudinal traction with the elbow in flexion to distract the articular surfaces; (2) then, while maintaining traction, exert firm steady pressure distally and posteriorly on the upper part of the forearm as the elbow is gradually extended. A click will indicate the achievement of reduction.

Reduction of the extremely rare medial or lateral dislocations of the elbow follows the principles outlined for treatment of posterior dislocation, i.e., first, traction in the line of deformity to disengage the articular ends of both bones of the forearm; then, while traction is maintained, correction of any lateral or medial displacement; next, as reduction is achieved, flexion of the elbow. The divergent dislocation is reduced by longitudinal traction with the elbow in semiflexion, and the proximal radius and ulna are squeezed together. There is only one case reported in a child, by DeLee.[23] The other cases described in the literature are in adults.[3, 36, 48, 77, 104, 112]

When a dislocated elbow is associated with fracture, first reduce the dislocation. In the immediate postreduction radiograms, assess the fracture and treat it as if the dislocation had not occurred.

Old dislocations of the elbow usually require open reduction.[2, 31, 70, 99, 100, 106]

Complications

VASCULAR INJURIES

These are associated with more violent injuries, and in general, are more common in cases of open dislocation than in closed dislocations. The severity of trauma to the brachial artery varies from simple contusion to laceration or rupture.[5, 27, 29, 42, 52–54, 56, 64, 75, 105, 116]

In a review of the literature up to 1937, Eliason and Brown found 20 cases in addition to their own.[29] Linscheid and Wheeler reported vascular complications in 8 of the 110 elbow dislocations seen during a 15-year period at the Mayo Clinic. In two of these patients, circulatory embarrassment consisted of loss of radial pulse until reduction was accomplished. In the remaining six patients, injury to the brachial artery was more serious. Three patients sustained lacerations of the brachial artery; ligations were performed in two, and arterial repair was attempted in one. The latter patient developed a hematoma during anticoagulant therapy, and redislocation occurred with failure of the anastomosis. Three of the six patients sustained stretching injuries of the brachial artery. In one patient this was associated with severe skin abrasions and contusions; the second patient, despite rather prompt reduction, had thrombosis of the radial artery; the third had sensory loss, and the radial pulse was absent when the cast was removed after five weeks.[73]

The author has encountered two children with Volkmann's ischemic contracture of the forearm following posterior dislocation of the elbow. Both were treated by reduction in the emergency room and were sent home after application of a solid cast. One cannot overemphasize the importance of assessing the status of circulation in the limb prior to reduction of dislocation. Following reduction, adequacy of circulation is again determined. *It is best to admit these children to the hospital for close supervision of circulation*, particularly if there is marked swelling of the elbow. If the child is sent home from the emergency room, the parents should be instructed how to check the circulation in the hand, and the physician himself should examine the child at close intervals. One should realize that Volkmann's ischemic contracture occurs as frequently with elbow dislocation as with supracondylar fractures of the humerus.

In cases with laceration of the brachial artery, immediate exploration of the antecubital area is indicated for anastomosis or reconstruction of the artery. Ligation of the artery is not recommended because of the consistent compromise of the collateral circulation.[75] In stretching vascular injuries, the stretching force should be relieved.

NEURAL INJURIES

Injury to the nerves occurs more frequently than injury to the vessels.

Ulnar Nerve Involvement. The ulnar nerve is rather firmly anchored down in the groove behind the medial epicondyle, and may be easily damaged in dislocations, particularly if there is an associated avulsion of the medial epicondyle, which, when trapped in the joint, compresses the ulnar nerve by holding taut the band of fibrous tissue that crosses the nerve.

In the report of Cotton, in 1929, the incidence of ulnar nerve injury in elbow dislocations was very high.[19] Watson-Jones described 13 ulnar nerve lesions in 97 elbow dislocations.[120] With early detection of entrapment of the medial epicondyle in elbow dislocations, and with appropriate treatment, seriousness and severity of ulnar nerve lesions have been minimized. In 1979 Galbraith and McCullough found only nine ulnar nerve lesions in their study of elbow dislocations—almost all of these were transient with complete spontaneous recovery.[32]

Linscheid and Wheeler reported neural complications in 24 of 110 elbow dislocations. The ulnar nerve only was involved in 16 patients; the involvement consisted of transient paresthesia and anesthesia in 11 of these patients (in seven, it disappeared in less than one day, and the others had full return of ulnar sensation within two months of reduction). Of the remaining five patients, only one had a persistent ulnar nerve palsy but received no further treatment. The other four patients had anterior translocation of the ulnar nerve from three weeks to two years after dislocation, with fair to good return of function in all. The dislocation was associated with avulsion of the medial epicondyle in three patients. Three patients had median nerve hypesthesia only, and four patients had both ulnar and median nerve involvement. The remaining patient with neural damage sustained a brachial plexus stretch injury.[73]

Treatment of neural complications should be conservative in the beginning, as most cases will recover spontaneously. If ulnar nerve paralysis persists, the nerve probably is entangled in dense scar tissue in the region of the medial epicondyle. Two months after reduction of the joint, it is advisable to free the nerve and transpose it anteriorly into a normal tissue bed free of scar. If ulnar nerve palsy is associated with displaced fracture of the medial epicondyle, it is best to translocate the nerve anteriorly when excising the detached medial epicondyle.

Median Nerve Injury. Entrapment of the median nerve may occur in three ways. *First*, it may be *simply kinked* in the anterior part of the elbow joint between the distal humerus and olecranon (Fig. 8–55 A). The median nerve slips posteriorly along the medial condylar ridge when the elbow is in hyperextension and the upper radius and ulna are displaced posteromedially.[88] *Second*, the median nerve may be entrapped between the fractured surface of the medial epicondyle and humerus (Fig. 8–55 B). With healing of the fracture the median nerve is encased in bone.[94, 11] *Third*, the median nerve is displaced posteriorly when the elbow joint dislocates and gets caught between the trochlea and olecranon during the process of reduction (Fig. 8—55 C).[110] During manipulative reduction, when the elbow is hyperextended with the forearm pronated, the median nerve is forced backward, making it vulnerable to entrapment.[45] Also, rupture of the ulnar collateral ligament or fracture-avulsion of the medial epicondyle enhances entrapment of the median nerve.[22, 30, 43, 78, 80, 87, 88, 90, 111]

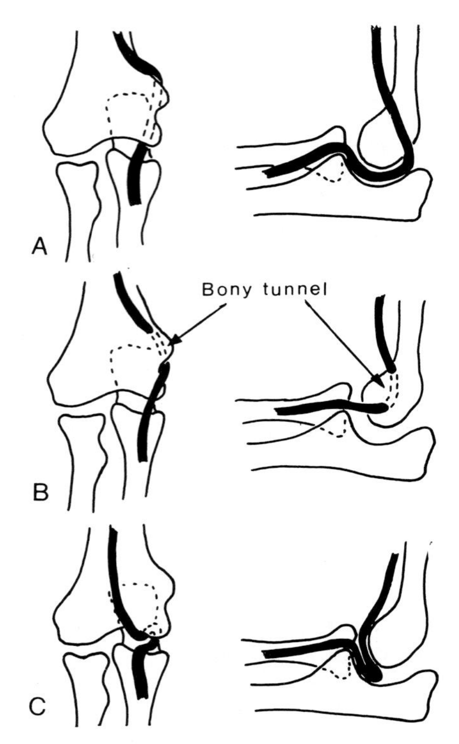

FIGURE 8–55. Types of median nerve entrapment.

A. The nerve is caught within the elbow joint traversing posterior to the distal humerus. **B.** The median nerve is entrapped between the fracture surfaces of the medial epicondylar apophysis and the medial condyle. **C.** The nerve is kinked in the anterior portion of the elbow joint. (Redrawn after Hallett, J.: Entrapment of the median nerve after dislocation of the elbow. J. Bone Joint Surg., *63-B*:408, 1981.)

Diagnosis of median nerve entrapment is difficult because the nerve lesion is not painful and motor sensory changes are subtle initially and slow in their development. When confronted with persistent median nerve palsy, one should rule out the possible presence of Volkmann's ischemic contracture. In time, persistent impingement of the median nerve over the posterior surface of the medial epicondyle will produce a depression with sclerotic margins—this is referred to as Matev's sign.[80]

Treatment of median nerve entrapment is difficult because often the incarcerated nerve is so badly damaged that it is necessary to resect the injured segment and reanastomose the nerve. This requires expert microneurosurgical technique. The results are not good, with only partial recovery of function.

HETEROTOPIC BONE FORMATION AND MYOSITIS OSSIFICANS

This disabling complication may restrict elbow motion permanently. Linscheid and Wheeler reported heterotopic bone formation in 32 of 110 elbow dislocations. The heterotopic bone is most commonly located below the medial or lateral epicondyle along the course of the collateral ligaments. In these areas, it is usually of small size, extending only a short distance. In five of their patients, the heterotopic bone developed in the region of the anterior capsule; in four of these patients, the large deposits of heterotopic bone interfered significantly with the degree of functional return. In two cases, they believed the heterotopic bone was partially caused by excessive passive manipulation and the use of heavy weights in an attempt to straighten the elbow. One patient was treated with capsulotomy and partial excision of the heterotopic mass seven months after dislocation, with improvement in extension amounting to 40 degrees.[73]

Myositis ossificans occurs within the muscle, usually the brachialis.[95] Pathogenic factors are trauma and hemorrhage within the brachialis during manipulative reduction by hyperextension of the elbow. Delay of initial reduction and vigorous passive stretching exercises following cast removal are other causes of myositis ossificans.[75] It is vital to carry out *immediate gentle reduction*, if necessary under general anesthesia, and to perform gentle active assisted exercises in the post-cast rehabilitation period. If necessary use a passive continuous motion machine, but no force and no rough passive stretching exercises!

The possible complication of heterotopic new bone formation and myositis ossificans should be suspected if, following removal of the cast, the elbow joint is unusually tender and remains so for a long time, and if the elbow joint is stiff with very slow restoration of motion. The diagnostic features and treatment of heterotopic new bone formation and myositis ossificans conscripta are discussed on page 3092.

In brief, bone scan with technetium-99m will show increased local uptake prior to plain radiograms. Computed tomography scan will delineate the location of the heterotopic new bone, whether it is within the muscle, ligament, or capsule. Partial rest and gentle active exercises to develop motion, and anti-inflammatory medications such as Naprosyn are the tools of treatment during the active phase of myositis ossificans. When the heterotopic bone is mature, use a continuous passive motion machine prior to excising the heterotopic bone. Rarely excision of mature heterotopic bone is performed in which case continuous passive motion is used to maintain and increase the range of elbow motion.

RECURRENT DISLOCATION OF THE ELBOW

This is a rare but disabling complication. The first case was reported by Albert in 1881.[1] It usually occurs in boys who first sustained dislocation when younger than 15 years of age (about 80 per cent of cases). Osborne and Cotterill discovered 18 cases in a three-year period and found reports of 30 other cases.[85] Except for two patients, all recurrent dislocations have been posterior or posterolateral.* Three cases of recurrent bilateral dislocation of the elbow have been described in the literature.[60, 82, 91]

Osborne and Cotterill proposed that the basic pathologic defect causing recurrent dislocation of the elbow is laxity of the posterolateral ligamentous and capsular structures due to failure of reattachment following a tear at the time of simple traumatic dislocation. A pocket of capsule is formed into which the radial head becomes displaced as it slides off its articulation with the capitellum.[85] An osteochondral fracture may take place with the detached bone fragment lying in the posterolateral capsule. A permanent defect or crater develops in the posterolateral margin of the capitellum, and the radial head also becomes damaged, sometimes with a crater or a "shovel-like" defect. Radiograms will often demonstrate the abnormal shape of the capitellum and of the radial head, but the radiographic changes will not be detected unless the lesions are confined to the cartilaginous surfaces.

---

*See references 15, 28, 33, 37, 49, 57, 60, 65, 67, 72, 76, 79, 82, 85, 91, 97, 107, 113, 117, 119 and 128.

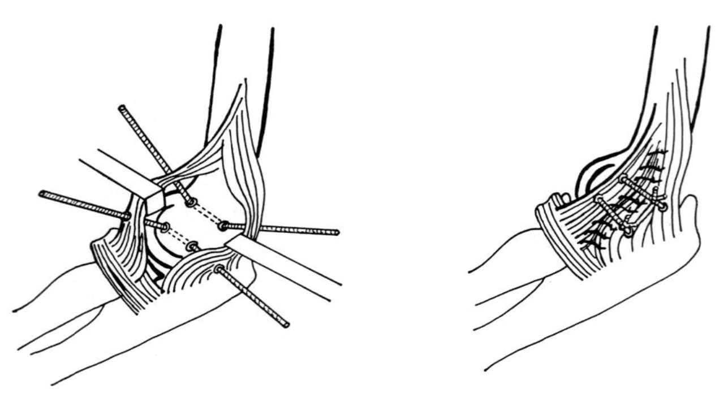

FIGURE 8–56. Osborne and Cotterill operation for repair of the lateral capsular damage in recurrent dislocation of the elbow.

(From Osborne, G., and Cotterill, P.: Recurrent dislocation of the elbow. J. Bone Joint Surg., *48-B*:344, 1966.)

A defect in the trochlea, possibly due to osteochondritis dissecans, has been described by Reichenheim and by King.[65, 92] Spring has reported loose bodies in the joint.[107]

Treatment. In childhood, if recurrence of dislocation is infrequent, one should refrain from operative treatment, since the normal process of growth may cause tightening of the capsule and ligaments, with consequent decrease of frequency and eventual cessation of dislocations. Also, occasional dislocations at intervals of once a year or so are not an indication for surgery.

Operative treatment is indicated if dislocations occur following minimal injury in the older adolescent. Several methods of surgical correction have been described in the literature, namely:

1. Transfer of the biceps tendon to the coronoid process of the ulna, reinforcing the joint anteriorly by an active tenodesis.[65, 91]

2. Increase in the depth of the coronoid process by an intra-articular bone graft.[82, 119]

3. Repair or reinforcement of soft tissues about the elbow joint, using either fascial strips or tendinous straps to reinforce the collateral ligament.[67, 107] Kapel constructed an intra-articular ligament by using portions of the biceps and triceps tendons passed through a hole in the distal humerus between the olecranon and coronoid fossa.[60] Osborne and Cotterill repaired the capsular and ligamentous laxity.[85]

The soft tissue repair described by Osborne and Cotterill is recommended by the author, as it is simple and effective. They reported successful results with no recurrence in eight patients. The author's experience is limited to only two cases, in both of which there was no recurrence and the range of motion was normal.

The operative technique of Osborne and Cotterill is as follows (Fig. 8–56):

Technique. An incision is made on the lateral side of the elbow from the lateral epicondylar ridge to the annular ligament. The elbow is opened behind the lateral ligament and any fragments of bone are removed from the postero-lateral part of the capsule. The bone of the lateral epicondyle and of the lateral side of the capitellum is cleared of soft tissue and scarified. . . . One or two transverse holes are drilled with an awl, and catgut is passed through the bone and through the postero-lateral capsule in order to tie the capsule down tightly so that it will adhere to the bone of the lower end of the humerus as close to the articular margin as possible. A similar repair of the medial ligament is done if it is necessary. A plaster cylinder is applied with the elbow at about 40 degrees for four weeks, after which the patient is allowed to recover movements gradually.*

References

1. Albert, E.: Lehrbuch der Chirurgie und Operationslehre. Vol II. Zweite Auflage. Wien, Urban & Schwarzenberg, 1881.
2. Allende, G., and Freytes, M.: Old dislocation of the elbow. J. Bone Joint Surg., *26*:691, 1944.
3. Andersen, K., Mortensen, A. C., and Gron, P.: Transverse divergent dislocation of the elbow. A report of two cases. Acta Orthop. Scand., *56*:442, 1985.
4. Arnold, K., and Lindenau, K. F.: Elbow luxation in children. Zentralbl. Chir., *95*:873, 1970.
5. Aufranc, O. E., Jones, W. N., and Turner, R. H.: Dislocation of the elbow with brachial artery injury. J.A.M.A., *197*:719, 1966.
6. Aufranc, O. E., Jones, W. N., and Turner, R. H.: Elbow dislocation with radial head fracture. J.A.M.A., *197*:1092, 1966.
7. Barquet, A.: Posterior dislocation of the ulna at the elbow with associated fracture of the radial shaft. Injury, 15:390, 1984.

*From Osborne, G., and Cotterill, P.: Recurrent dislocation of the elbow. J. Bone Joint Surg., *48-B*:340, 1966.

8. Beach, P. M., Jr., and Hewson, J. S.: Elbow dislocation with comminuted fracture of the proximal radial shaft—thoughts on the mechanism. Am. J. Surg., *112*:941, 1966.
9. Beverly, M. C., and Fearn, C. B.: Anterior interosseous nerve palsy and dislocation of the elbow. Injury, *16*:126, 1984.
10. Blatz, D. J.: Anterior dislocation of the elbow. Orthop. Rev., *10*:129, 1981.
11. Bondarenko, N. S., and Beda, I. U. F.: Multiple fractures and multiple fracture-dislocations of the elbow joint in children. Ortop. Travmatol. Protez., *4*:18, 1976.
12. Bondarenko, N. S., and Dovgan, B. L.: Fracture-dislocations in the elbow joint in children. Ortop. Travmatol. Protez., *31*:48, 1970.
13. Carey, R. P. L.: Simultaneous dislocation of the elbow and the proximal radio-ulnar joint. J. Bone Joint Surg., *66-B*:254, 1984.
14. Carlioz, H., and Abols, Y.: Posterior dislocation of the elbow in children. J. Pediatr. Orthop., *4*:8, 1984.
15. Ciaudo, O., Huguenin, P., and Bensahel, H.: Recurrent dislocation of the elbow (author's transl.). Rev. Chir. Orthop., *68*:207, 1982.
16. Cohn, I.: Forward dislocation of both bones of the forearm at the elbow. Surg. Gynecol. Obstet., *35*:776, 1922.
17. Cooper, A. P., Sr.: A Treatise on Dislocations and Fractures of the Joints. Boston, Lilly, Wait, Carter & Hendee, 1832.
18. Cotton, F. J.: Dislocations and Joint Fractures. Philadelphia, Saunders, 1924.
19. Cotton, F. J.: Elbow dislocation and ulnar nerve injury. J. Bone Joint Surg., *11*:348, 1929.
20. Cromack, P. I.: The mechanism and nature of the injury in dislocations of the elbow and a method of treatment. Aust. N.Z. J. Surg., *30*:212, 1960.
21. Crosby, E. H.: Elbow dislocations reduced by traction in four different directions. J. Bone Joint Surg., *18*:1077, 1936.
22. Danielsson, L. G.: Median nerve entrapment in elbow dislocation. A case report. Acta Orthop. Scand., *57*:450, 1986.
23. DeLee, J. C.: Transverse divergent dislocation of the elbow in a child. Case report. J. Bone Joint Surg., *63-A*:322, 1981.
24. Dimiccoli, N., and Rinaldi, E.: Free luxation of the elbow in childhood. Arch. Putti Chir. Organi Mov., *24*:253, 1969.
25. Dougherty, W.: Elbow injuries in children. J. Iowa Med. Soc., *56*:1125, 1966.
26. Durig, M., Gauer, E. F., and Muller, W.: Die operative Behandlung der residivierenden und traumatischen Luxation des Ellenbogengelenkes nach Osborne und Cotterill. Arch. Orthop. Trauma. Surg., *86*:141, 1976.
27. Ebong, W. W.: Gangrene complicating closed posterior dislocation of the elbow. Int. Surg., *63*:44, 1978.
28. Ejsted, R., Christensen, F. A., and Nielsen, W. B.: Habitual dislocation of the elbow. Arch. Orthop. Trauma. Surg., *105*:187, 1986.
29. Eliason, E. L., and Brown, R. B.: Posterior dislocation at the elbow with rupture of the radial and ulnar arteries. Ann. Surg., *106*:1111, 1937.
30. Fourrier, P., Levai, J. P., and Collin, J. P.: Incarceration du nerf median au cours d'une luxation du coude. Rev. Chir. Orthop., *63*:13, 1977.
31. Fowles, J. V., Kassab, M. T., and Douik, M.: Untreated posterior dislocation of the elbow in children. J. Bone Joint Surg., *66-A*:921, 1984.
32. Galbraith, K. A., and McCullough, C. J.: Acute nerve injury as a complication of closed fractures or dislocations of the elbow. Injury, 11:164, 1979.
33. Gayton, W.: Recurrent dislocation of the elbow. J. Bone Joint Surg., *42-B*:406, 1960.
34. Gilsson, D. J.: After-treatment of dislocation of the elbow with a note on the treatment of stiff elbows. Aust. N.Z. J. Surg., *5*:134, 1935.
35. Ginzburg, S. O.: Fracture-dislocation of the antibrachium in the elbow joint in a child. Vestn. Khir., *103*:79, 1969.
36. Ginzburg, S. O., and Bukhny, A. F.: Divergent dislocations and fracture-dislocations of the forearm and elbow joint in children. Ortop. Travmatol. Protez., *28*:33, 1967.
37. Gossman, J. A.: Recurrent dislocation of the ulna at the elbow. J. Bone Joint Surg., *25*:448, 1943.
38. Gradinger, R., and Biehl, T.: Elbow joint dislocations in the child. Fortschr. Med., *101*:221, 1983.
39. Grant, I. R., and Miller, J. H.: Osteochondral fracture of the trochlea associated with fracture dislocation of the elbow. Injury, *6*:257, 1975.
40. Green, N. E.: Entrapment of the median nerve following elbow dislocation. J. Pediatr. Orthop., *3*:384, 1983.
41. Greenspan, A., Norma, A., and Rosen, H.: Radial head-capitellum view in elbow trauma: Clinical application with radiographic-anatomic correlation. A.J.R., *143*:355, 1984.
42. Grimer, R. J., and Brooks, S.: Brachial artery damage accompanying closed posterior dislocation of the elbow. J. Bone Joint Surg., *67-B*:378, 1985.
43. Gurdjian, E. S., and Smathers, H. M.: Peripheral nerve injury in fractures and dislocations of long bones. J. Neurosurg., *2*:202, 1945.
44. Haliburton, R. A., Barber, J. R., and Fraser, R. L.: Pseudodislocation: An unusual birth injury. Can. J. Surg., *10*:455, 1967.
45. Hallett, J.: Entrapment of the median nerve after dislocation of the elbow. J. Bone Joint Surg., *63-B*:408, 1981.
46. Hankin, F. M.: Posterior dislocation of the elbow. A simplified method of closed reduction. Clin. Orthop., *190*:254, 1984.
47. Harvey, S., and Tchelebi, H.: Crossed dislocation of the elbow in children. Unusual complications. Union Med. Can., *105*:910, 1976.
48. Harvey, S., and Tchelebi, H.: Proximal radio-ulnar translocation. J. Bone Joint Surg., *61-B*:447, 1979.
49. Hassman, G. C., and Neer, C. S.: Recurrent dislocation of the elbow. J. Bone Joint Surg., *57-A*:1080, 1975.
50. Head, R. W.: Radial head-capitellum view in elbow trauma (letter). A.J.R., *140*:1273, 1983.
51. Hendel, D., Aghasi, M., and Halperin, N.: Unusual fracture dislocation of the elbow joint. Arch. Orthop. Trauma Surg., *104*:187, 1985.
52. Henderson, R. S., and Robertson, I. M.: Open dislocation of the elbow with rupture of the brachial artery. J. Bone Joint Surg., *34-B*:636, 1952.
53. Hennig, K., and Franke, D.: Posterior displacement of brachial artery following closed elbow dislocation. J. Trauma, *20*:96, 1980.
54. Hofmann, K. E., III, Moneim, M. S., and Omer, G. E.: Brachial artery disruption following closed posterior elbow dislocation in a child—assessment with intravenous digital angiography. Clin. Orthop., *184*:145, 1984.
55. Hogan, K. M., and Sawyer, J. R.: Fracture dislocation of the elbow. Am. J. Nurs., *76*:1266, 1976.
56. Jackson, J. A.: Simple anterior dislocation of the elbow joint with rupture of the brachial artery. Am. J. Surg., *47*:479–486, 1940.
57. Jacobs, R. L.: Recurrent dislocation of the elbow joint. Clin. Orthop., *74*:151, 1971.
58. Jensen, U. H., and Rud, B.: Bilateral dislocation of the elbows. Ugeskr. Laeger, *145*:1784, 1983.

59. Josefsson, P. O., Johnell, O., and Gentz, C. F.: Long-term sequelae of simple dislocation of the elbow. J. Bone Joint Surg., *66-A*:927, 1984.
60. Kapel, O.: Operation for habitual dislocation of the elbow. J. Bone Joint Surg., *33-A*:707, 1951.
61. Keyl, W.: Fractures and dislocations of the elbow joint in childhood. Fortschr. Med., *91*:136, 1973.
62. Keyl, W.: Fractures and dislocations of the elbow joint in childhood. II. Dislocations. Fortschr. Med., *91*:190, 1973.
63. Keyl, W.: Fractures and dislocations of the elbow joint in childhood—sequelae. Fortschr. Med., *91*:265, 1973.
64. Kilburn, P., Sweeney, J. G., and Silk, F. F.: Three cases of compound posterior dislocation of the elbow with rupture of the brachial artery. J. Bone Joint Surg., *44-B*:119, 1962.
65. King, T.: Recurrent dislocation of the elbow. J. Bone Joint Surg., *35-B*:50, 1953.
66. Kini, M. G.: Dislocation of the elbow and its complications. J. Bone Joint Surg., *22*:107, 1940.
67. Knoflach, J. G.: Zur Operation der habituellen Ellbogenluxation. Zentralbl. Chir., *62*:2897, 1935.
68. Koszla, M. M., and Oklot, K.: Elbow luxation in children. Wiad. Lek., *27*:2025, 1974.
69. Krishnamoorthy, S., Bose, K., and Wong, K. P.: Treatment of old unreduced dislocation of the elbow. Injury, *8*:39, 1976.
70. Lansinger, O., Karlsson, J., Korner, L., and Mare, K.: Dislocation of the elbow joint. Arch. Orthop. Trauma. Surg., *102*:183, 1984.
71. Lavine, L. S.: A simple method of reducing dislocations of the elbow joint. J. Bone Joint Surg., *35-A*:785, 1953.
72. Levai, J. P., Tanguy, A., Collin, J. P., and Teinturier, P.: Recurrent posterior dislocation of the elbow following malunion of supracondylar fracture of the humerus. Report of a case (author's transl.). Rev. Chir. Orthop., *65*:457, 1979.
73. Linscheid, R. L., and Wheeler, D. K.: Elbow dislocations. J.A.M.A., *194*:113, 1965.
74. Loomis, L. K.: Reduction and after treatment of posterior dislocation of the elbow. Am. J. Surg., *63*:56, 1944.
75. Louis, D. S., Ricciardi, J. E., and Spengler, D. M.: Arterial injury: A complication of posterior elbow dislocation. J. Bone Joint Surg., *56*:1631, 1974.
76. McKellar Hall, R.: Recurrent posterior dislocation of the elbow joint in a boy. J. Bone Joint Surg., *35-B*:56, 1953.
77. MacSween, W. A.: Transposition of radius and ulna associated with dislocation of the elbow in a child. Injury, *10*:314, 1978.
78. Mannerfelt, L.: Median nerve entrapment after dislocation of the elbow. J. Bone Joint Surg., *50-B*:152, 1968.
79. Mantle, J. A.: Recurrent posterior dislocation of the elbow. J. Bone Joint Surg., *48-B*:590, 1966.
80. Matev, I.: A radiological sign of entrapment of the median nerve in the elbow joint after posterior dislocation. A report of two cases. J. Bone Joint Surg., *58-B*:353, 1976.
81. Meyn, M. A., and Quigley, T. B.: Reduction of posterior dislocation of the elbow by traction on the dangling arm. Clin. Orthop., *103*:106, 1974.
82. Milch, H.: Bilateral recurrent dislocation of the ulna at the elbow. J. Bone Joint Surg., *18*:777, 1936.
83. Motta, A., Callea, C., and Poli, G.: Radial nerve paralysis caused by articular interposition in dislocation of the elbow. Chir. Organi Mov., *64*:113, 1978.
84. Neviaser, J. S., and Wickstrom, J. K.: Dislocation of the elbow: A retrospective study of 115 patients. South. Med. J., *70*:172, 1977.
85. Osborne, G., and Cotterill, P.: Recurrent dislocation of the elbow. J. Bone Joint Surg., *48-B*:340, 1966.
86. Prior: Severe compound dislocation of the elbow joint successfully treated. Lancet, *2*:366, 1844.
87. Pritchard, D. J., Linscheid, R. L., and Svien, H. J.: Intra-articular median nerve entrapment with dislocation of the elbow. Clin. Orthop., *90*:100, 1973.
88. Pritchett, J. W.: Entrapment of the median nerve after dislocation of the elbow. J. Pediatr. Orthop., *4*:752, 1984.
89. Quan, L., and Marcuse, E. K.: The epidemiology and treatment of radial head subluxation. Am. J. Dis. Child., *139*:1194, 1985.
90. Rana, N. A., Kenwright, J., Taylor, R. G., and Rushworth, G.: Complete lesion of the median nerve associated with dislocation of the elbow joint. Acta Orthop. Scand., *45*:365, 1974.
91. Rang, M.: Children's Fractures. Philadelphia, Lippincott, 1974, p. 190.
92. Reichenheim, P. P.: Transplantation of the biceps tendon as a treatment for recurrent dislocation of the elbow. Br. J. Surg., *35*:201, 1947.
93. Richet G: Observation de luxation en avant de l'extremite superieure des os de l'avant bras, complique de fracture du cubitus suivie de reflexions sur ces luxations. Arch. Gen., *6*:472, 1839.
94. Roaf, R.: Foramen in the humerus caused by the median nerve. J. Bone Joint Surg., *39-B*:748, 1957.
95. Roberts, P. H.: Dislocation of the elbow. Br. J. Surg., *56*:806, 1969.
96. Rubens, M. K., and Aulicino, P. L.: Open elbow dislocation with brachial artery disruption: Case report and review of the literature. Orthopedics, 9:539, 1986.
97. Schwab, G. H., Bennett, J. B., Woods, G. W., and Tullos, H. S.: Biomechanics of elbow instability: The role of the medial collateral ligament. Clin. Orthop., *146*:42, 1980.
98. Scullion, J. E.: Fracture of the neck of the radius with spontaneously reduced dislocation of the elbow. J. R. Coll. Surg. Edinb., *27*:246, 1982.
99. Silva, J. F.: Old dislocation of the elbow. Ann. R. Coll. Surg., *22*:363, 1958.
100. Silva, J. F.: The problems relating to old dislocation and the restriction of the elbow movement. Acta Orthop. Belg., *41*:399, 1975.
101. Siris, P. E.: Elbow fractures and dislocations. Surg. Gynecol. Obstet., *40*:665, 1925.
102. Smith, F. M.: Surgery of the Elbow. Philadelphia, Saunders, 1972.
103. Sorrel, E.: Luxation recidivante du coude. Bull. Mem. Soc. Nat. Chir., *61*:790, 1935.
104. Sovio, O. M., and Tredwell, S. J.: Divergent dislocation of the elbow in a child. A case report. J. Pediatr. Orthop., *6*:96, 1986.
105. Spear, H. C., and Janes, J. M.: Rupture of the brachial artery accompanying dislocation of the elbow or supracondylar fracture. J. Bone Joint Surg., *33-A*:889, 1951.
106. Speed, J. S.: An operation for unreduced posterior dislocation of the elbow. South. Med. J., *18*:193, 1925.
107. Spring, W. E.: Report of a case of recurrent dislocation of the elbow. J. Bone Joint Surg., *35-B*:55, 1953.
108. Srivastava, K. K., and Kochlar, V. L.: Forward dislocation of the elbow joint without fracture of the olecranon. Aust. N.Z. J. Surg., *44*:71, 1974.
109. Staunton, F. W.: Dislocation forward of the forearm without fracture of the olecranon. Br. Med. J., *2*:1570, 1905.
110. St. Clair Strange, F. G.: Entrapment of the median nerve after dislocation of the elbow. J. Bone Joint Surg., *64-B*:224, 1982.
111. Steiger, R. N., Larrick, R. B., and Meyer, T. L.: Median-nerve entrapment following elbow dislocation in children. J. Bone Joint Surg., *51-A*:381, 1969.
112. Stimson, L. A.: A Practical Treatise on Fractures and Dislocations. Philadelphia, Lea Brothers & Co., 1900.
113. Symeonides, P. P., Paschaloglou, C., Stavrou, Z.,

and Pangalides, T.: Recurrent dislocation of the elbow. J. Bone Joint Surg., *57-A*:1084, 1975.
114. Tayob, A. A., and Shively, R. A.: Bilateral elbow dislocation with intra-articular displacement of the medial epicondyles. J. Trauma, *20*:332, 1980.
115. Thompson, H. C., and Garcia, A.: Myositis ossificans: Aftermath of elbow injuries. Clin. Orthop., *50*:129, 1967.
116. Tomchin, I.: Two cases of open dislocation of the elbow joint with rupture of the brachial artery in children. Khirurgiia (Mosk.), *43*:130, 1967.
117. Trias, A., and Comeau, Y.: Recurrent dislocation of the elbow in children. Clin. Orthop., *100*:74, 1974.
118. Wadstrom, J., Kinast, C., and Pfeiffer, K.: Anatomical variations of the semilunar notch in elbow dislocations. Arch. Orthop. Trauma Surg., *105*:313, 1986.
119. Wainwright, D.: Recurrent dislocation of the elbow joint. Proc. R. Soc. Med., *40*:885, 1947.
120. Watson-Jones, R.: Primary nerve lesions in injuries of the elbow and wrist. J. Bone Joint Surg., *12*:121, 1930.
121. Wheeler, D. K., and Linscheid, R. L.: Fracture dislocations of the elbow. Clin. Orthop., *50*:95, 1967.
122. Wilson, P. D.: Fractures and dislocations in the region of the elbow. Surg. Gynecol. Obstet., *56*:335, 1933.
123. Winroth, G., Hedstrom, S. A., and Lidgren, L.: Posttraumatic bacterial arthritis with luxation of the elbow. A case report. Arch. Orthop. Trauma. Surg., *103*:227, 1984.
124. Winslow, R.: A case of complete anterior dislocation of both bones of the forearm at the elbow. Surg. Gynecol. Obstet., *16*:570, 1913.
125. Witvoet, J., and Tayon, B.: La luxation recidivante du coude. Rev. Chir. Orthop., *60*:485, 1974.
126. Woods, G. M., and Tullos, H. G.: Elbow instability and medial epicondyle fracture. Am. J. Sports Med., *5*:23, 1977.
127. Woods, R. S.: Backward dislocation of the elbow. Br. Med. J., *1*:15, 1935.
128. Zeier, F. G.: Recurrent traumatic elbow dislocation. Clin. Orthop., *169*:211, 1982.

FRACTURES INVOLVING THE PROXIMAL RADIAL PHYSIS AND RADIAL NECK

The disc-shaped head of the radius is of greater diameter than its neck. The shallow, cuplike, and slightly concave upper surface of the radial head that articulates with the capitellum of the humerus is covered by hyaline cartilage. The smooth radial head rotates within the annular ligament and articulates medially with the radial notch of the ulna. On the posterior aspect of the radial neck, there is a small ridge for insertion of a part of the upper fibers of the supinator muscle. The radial tuberosity for the insertion of the biceps brachii muscle is immediately distal to the neck. A great portion of the radial neck is intracapsular; therefore intra-articular effusion does not develop when fracture involves only the metaphysis.

The shape of the radial head in the child at four years of age is identical to that in the adult, with the same eccentric concavity and sharp anterolateral rim; however, they differ in size and in the amount of cartilage. Normally the radial head is tilted in relation to the radial shaft with an angle of 12.5 degrees in the anteroposterior projection and 3.5 degrees in the lateral view.

The ossification center of the upper epiphysis of the upper radius appears at the fifth year as a small sphere. Occasionally the ossification centers can be bipartite, which should not be misdiagnosed as a fracture. Another possible source of misinterpretation is the distal slope of the lateral border of the metaphysis of the radial neck prior to ossification of the radial head; this apparent tilting of the radial neck should not be mistaken for a fracture. The ossification center of the radial head fuses with the body between the ages of 16 and 18 years.

Incidence

Injuries involving the proximal radial epiphyseal plate constitute 5 per cent of all physeal injuries, and account for 4.5 to 10 per cent of fractures about the elbow in children under 16 years of age. It occurs on the average at the age of 10 years, with the upper age limit being 13 years and the lower, 5 years (i.e., after the appearance of the ossification center of the proximal radial epiphysis). Approximately three fourths of cases occur in children aged nine years or older. There is no sex predilection.[24]

Mechanism of Injury

The fracture is caused by a fall on the outstretched hand with the elbow in extension and the forearm usually supinated. The force is transmitted through the shaft of the radius, and the momentum of the body drives the capitellum against the lateral half of the radial head, tilting and displacing it laterally (Fig. 8–57). At the moment of impact, there is a valgus strain on the medial aspect of the elbow; the distraction force may rupture the medial collateral ligament, avulse the medial epicondyle, or cause fracture of the olecranon or upper shaft of the ulna. The compression force may also fracture the lateral epicondyle or condyle of the humerus. The displacement of the fragments in those associated with fracture is usually minimal. In Reidy and Van Gorder's series of 30 cases there were 11 associated injuries in 9 of the patients.[49]

The direction of tilting of the displaced head relative to the shaft of the radius depends on the rotational attitude of the radius at the time

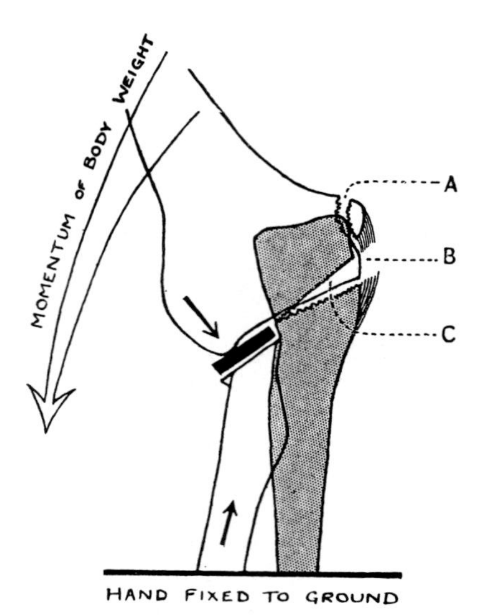

FIGURE 8–57. ***Diagram to illustrate the mechanism of fractures involving the proximal radial physis.***

The compression force on the radial side as the capitellum of the humerus is driven against the outer side of the radial head as indicated. The distraction force in the ulnar side of the joint may produce the following lesions. A, Avulsion of the medial epicondylar apophysis; B, rupture of the medial collateral ligament; C, fracture of the olecranon or upper ulna of abduction type. (From Jeffery, C. C.: Fractures of the head of the radius in children. J. Bone Joint Surg., *32-B*:314, 1950.)

of injury; if the forearm is fully supinated, the displacement is lateral; if the forearm is in neutral mid-position, it is posterior.[22]

Another mechanism of injury according to Jeffrey is as follows: The patient first falls on the hand and sustains a temporary posterior dislocation or subluxation of the elbow joint. The resultant upward force on the flexed elbow displaces the radial head posteriorly almost 90 degrees by the impact against the inferior aspect of the capitellum. Spontaneous reduction of elbow dislocation leaves the separated radial head beneath the capitellum (Fig. 8–58). This second form of injury is rare. Jeffrey reported 2 such cases in his series of 24; Reidy and Van Gorder, 1 of 30 cases; and Wood, 2 similar cases from the Royal Hospital for Sick Children, Glasgow, Scotland.[22, 49, 65]

O'Brien found two cases of posterior displacement of the proximal radial epiphysis (Fig. 8–59). He proposed a double mechanism of injury in its causation. First, a fall on the outstretched hand produces a posterior dislocation with displacement of the proximal end of the radius beneath the capitellum; second, a further blow on the forearm or the elbow spontaneously reduces the posterior dislocation, but displaces the radial epiphysis posteriorly.[42] Both mechanisms are likely to occur in different cases; i.e., the radial epiphysis may fracture and become displaced either at the time of posterior dislocation or at the time of spontaneous reduction.

Another mechanism is described by Newman: the fracture of the radial neck occurs during the process of dislocation by the capitellum pressing against the proximal tip of the radial head. In this type the radial head is displaced into the anterior part of the elbow joint; the elbow may remain dislocated or it may be located.[40] Vahvanen and Grippenberg confirmed this mechanism of injury in a report of a case in which the radial head was found free in the anterior portion of the elbow joint.[60]

In children, the proximal radial epiphysis is cartilaginous and resilient; thus, a fracture through the articular surface of the radial head is extremely rare. The site of fracture in childhood is either through the physis with a metaphyseal fragment (Type II physeal injury or Type I physeal injury in the young child according to the classification of Salter and Harris), or through the neck proper (3 to 4 mm. distal to the physis). Occasionally the valgus injury causes Salter-Harris Type IV physeal fracture with the fracture line coursing vertically through the metaphysis, physis, or epiphysis into the elbow joint. In the report of 34 cases by Jones and Esah, 50 per cent were

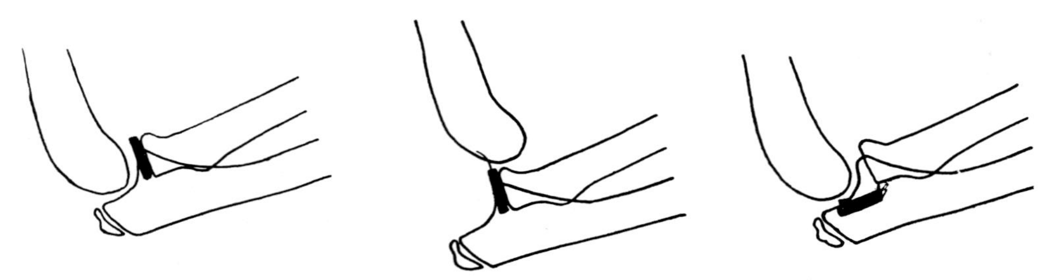

FIGURE 8–58. ***Diagrams to show the mechanism of 90-degree posterior displacement of the radial head.***

(From Jeffery, C. C.: Injuries of the head of the radius in children. J. Bone Joint Surg., *32-B*:3, 1950.)

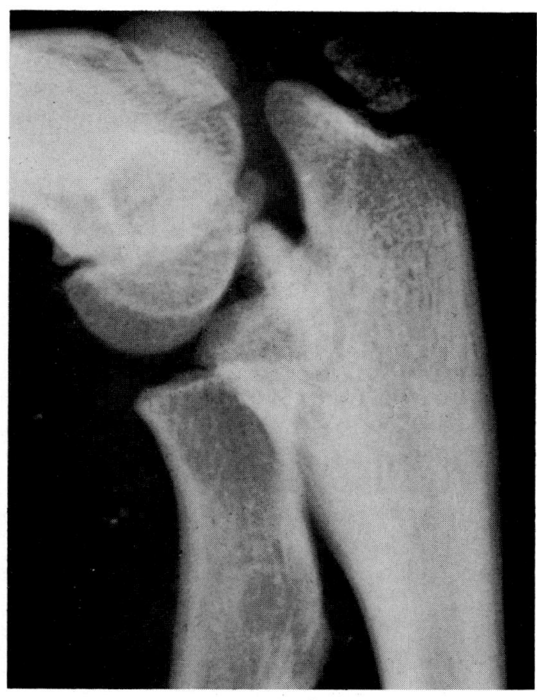

FIGURE 8–59. Posterior displacement of proximal radial epiphysis in a 12-year-old girl.

(From O'Brien, P. I.: Injuries involving the proximal radial epiphysis. Clin. Orthop., *41*:57, 1965.)

through the radial neck proper and 50 per cent were Type II fractures involving the proximal radial physis.[24]

Direct crushing of the radial head by the convex lateral condyle of the humerus will cause an intra-articular fracture of the proximal radial epiphysis (Fig. 8–60). This is extremely rare.

Classification

Fracture of the radial neck and proximal physis, according to Wilkins, can be classified based on the mechanism of injury and location of the fracture line. *The first category is valgus injury.* This can be subdivided into *Type A*, Salter-Harris Type II or I physeal injury; *Type B*, Salter-Harris Type IV injury; and *Type C*, pure fracture of the radial neck without physeal involvement.[64] Valgus injury may be simple without associated fractures or complex with associated injuries, namely (1) avulsion fracture of the medial epicondyle, (2) rupture of the medial collateral ligament, and (3) fracture of the olecranon or upper ulna of abduction type. *The second category* of fracture of the radial neck or proximal physis is caused by dislocation of the elbow. This is subdivided into *reduction injuries* (Type D), in which the upper radius is fractured during the process of spontaneous reduction with the radial head displaced and located proximal in the posterior part of the elbow joint; and, *dislocation injuries* (Type E), in which the upper radius is fractured during the process of dislocation by the compression-impact of the capitellum on the radius; in this case the radial head lies distal in the anterior part of the elbow joint. This nomenclature and anatomic description of fractures of the radial neck and proximal physis are summarized in Table 8–4.

Displacement of the radial head according to O'Brien may be subdivided into three categories based on the degree of angulation as shown in Figure 8–61: *minimal*—when the degree of downward tilting of the superior surface of the head from the horizontal is from 0 to 30 degrees (Fig. 8–62); *moderate*—when it is from 31 to 60 degrees; or *marked*—61 to 90 degrees. This gradation serves as a guide in both treatment and prognosis.[42, 49]

Diagnosis

The affected elbow is held in moderate flexion, with the opposite hand supporting the forearm, which is held in neutral rotation. There will be local swelling and ecchymosis over the lateral aspect of the elbow. When pressure is applied with the tip of the index finger, the radial head and neck are exquisitely

Table 8–4. *Mechanistic Classification of Fractures of the Radial Neck and Proximal Physis**

I. *Valgus injuries†*
- *Type A:* Salter-Harris Type II and I fracture of the proximal radial physis
- *Type B:* Salter-Harris Type IV fracture of the proximal radial physis
- *Type C:* Fracture of the radial neck without involvement of the physis

II. *Fractures caused by dislocation of the elbow*
- *Type D:* Occurring during the process of reduction (the radial head lies proximal and posterior on the elbow joint)
- *Type E:* Occurring during dislocation by the compression impact of the capitellum on the radial head (the radial head lies distal in the anterior part of the elbow joint)

*Modified from Wilkins, K.: Fractures of the neck and head of the radius. *In* Fractures in Children. Philadelphia, J. B. Lippincott, 1984, p. 502.

†Valgus injuries may be simple or complex, associated with avulsion fracture of the medial epicondyle of the humerus, rupture of the medial collateral ligament, or abduction type fracture of the olecranon or upper ulna.

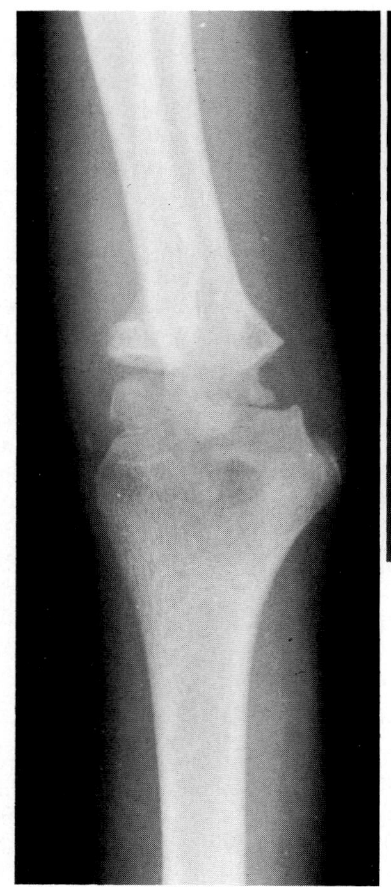

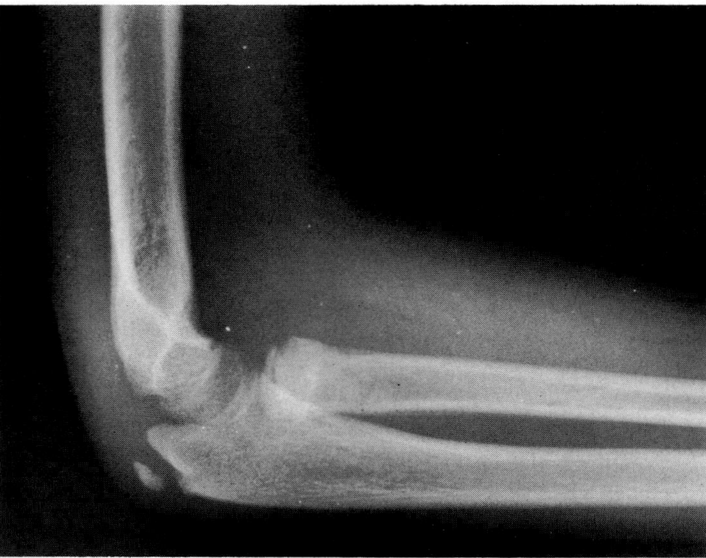

FIGURE 8–60. Intra-articular fracture of the proximal radial epiphysis caused by a direct crushing injury by the lateral condyle of the humerus.

tender; the pain may be referred to the radial side of the wrist.[50]

Gentle passive flexion and extension of the elbow are restricted in range, but are relatively less painful than pronation and supination of the forearm, which are accompanied by severe pain. Radial deviation of the forearm at the

< 30°   30°–60°   > 60°

45°

I   II   III

FIGURE 8–61. Degrees of displacement of proximal radial epiphyses.

I. Minimal displacement. II. Moderate displacement. III. Marked displacement. (From O'Brien, P. I.: Injuries involving the proximal radial epiphysis. Clin. Orthop., *41*:52, 1965.)

elbow is also very painful. Ordinarily, crepitation is absent.

Radiograms should be made of the *proximal end of the radius* in the anteroposterior and lateromedial views. When the clinical findings are suggestive but the x-rays are inconclusive, it is best to make radiographs of the normal proximal forearm held in the same degree of flexion and supination as the affected side. Caution: Do not misdiagnose a bipartite ossification center of the radial head or the minimal tilting of the radial neck as a fracture.[8]

It is also advisable to take several views with the proximal radius in various degrees of rotation. The degree of the tilting of the radial head is measured in the films that most clearly depict the profile of the radius at the fracture site. The surgeon should always look for associated fractures, particularly of the medial epicondyle and olecranon or proximal ulna.

Treatment

Factors determining modality of treatment depend upon the degree of angulation, amount

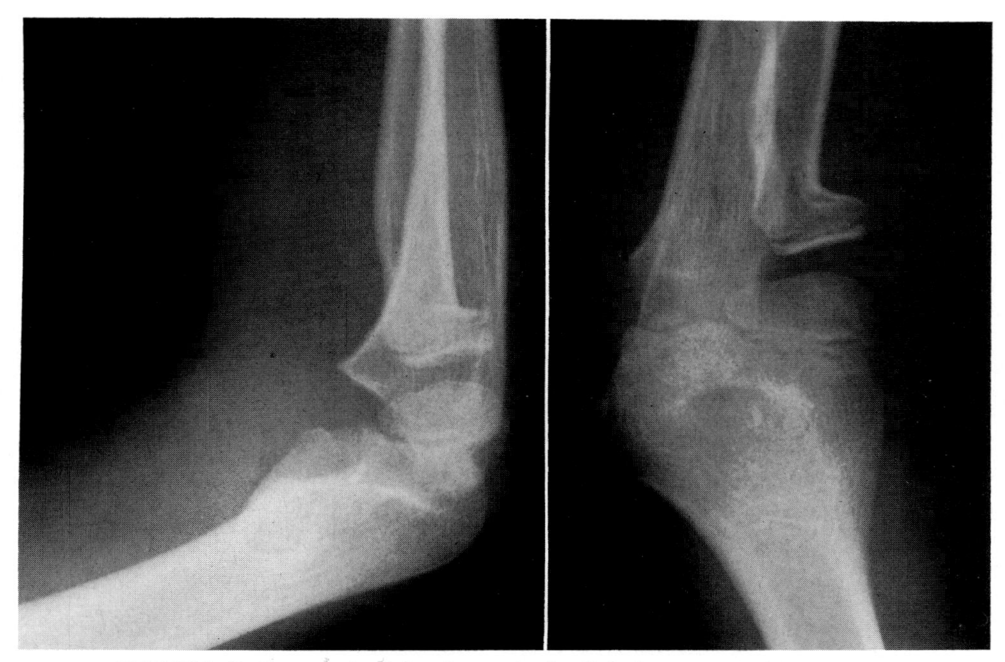

FIGURE 8–62. Fracture involving the proximal radial physis—minimal displacement.

of translocation, presence or absence of associated injuries, age of the patient and potential of remodeling of malunion with growth, and the duration of injury—whether fresh or several days old.

In *undisplaced or minimally displaced* fractures, treatment consists of simple immobilization of the elbow (in 90 degrees of flexion and neutral rotation of the forearm) in a posterior plaster splint or an above-elbow cast for two weeks. Then the elbow and forearm are gradually mobilized and partially supported in a sling. With such early use of the limb, an excellent result can be obtained. When a child is over ten years of age, it is preferable to correct the tilting of the radial head to less than 15 degrees by closed reduction. When the child is younger than ten years of age, lateral tilting of up to 30 degrees can be accepted, as it will be spontaneously corrected with remodeling.

In *moderately displaced* fractures (31 to 60 degrees of lateral tilting of the radial head), a closed reduction under general anesthesia should be attempted. The technique is as follows:

First, the elbow is completely *extended* to provide some fixation of the ulna in relation to the humerus. The forearm is then fully supinated to bring the most prominent part of the displaced radial head into a superficial location in the lateral aspect of the elbow between the common extensor muscle mass and the anconeus muscle. As emphasized by Jeffrey, it is important to determine the direction of displacement of the radial head by studying anteroposterior radiograms centered upon the head of the radius and taken in various recorded positions of rotation.[22] The manipulative reduction is then carried out with the forearm in the degree of rotation that brings the most prominent part of the displaced head farthest laterally. Distal traction is applied and the supinated forearm is forcibly deviated ulnarward to widen the lateral aspect of the radiohumeral articulation; this maneuver provides space into which the tilted radial head can be moved. Firm digital pressure is applied in an upward and inward direction upon the displaced radial head to complete the reduction.

Radiograms are made to check restoration of normal anatomic relationship of the fracture fragments. If satisfactory reduction is achieved, i.e., the degree of tilting of the radial head is corrected to less than 30 degrees, an above-elbow cast is applied with the elbow joint held in right-angle flexion and neutral mid-rotation. Angulation up to 45 to 60 degrees can be accepted if there is functionally adequate passive range of pronation-supination of the forearm (60 degrees in each direction). Translocation should be 3 mm. or less; if it is greater than 4 mm. the result may be poor with risk of proximal radioulnar synostosis.[40] In three to four weeks, bony union is usually adequate for the cast to be removed and gradual active mobilization of the elbow begun. Repeated radiograms are taken to ensure maintenance of reduction. Certain of these fractures are unstable, and the initial satisfactory reduction may be lost while in the cast; this occurred in 2 of the 7 cases of Dougall and in 3 of the 34 cases of Jones and Esah.[9, 24] If the position is lost while in the cast, closed reduction is repeated; often the second time, it can be maintained with a snug cast; however, if it is lost again, internal fixation with a Kirschner wire is required with oblique pins directed proximally from the radial neck to the head. When closed manipulative reduction is not adequate, while the patient is under general anesthesia percutaneous manipulative reduction may be attempted with a double-pronged instrument under strict aseptic conditions with image-intensifier radiographic control.[2]

Markedly displaced fractures (60 to 90 degrees of angulation and translocation greater than 4 mm.) often require open reduction. A very gentle closed manipulative reduction is attempted under general anesthesia; if unsuccessful, open reduction is immediately performed. O'Brien warns that a closed manipulation of a head tilted more than 60 degrees can cause further damage to the cartilaginous epiphysis and recommends early gentle open reduction, as it will minimize such damage and achieve stable repositioning of the radial head on the neck.[42] Complete displaced fracture with the radial head lying loose anteriorly or posteriorly should have primary open reduction.

A posterolateral approach is used for surgical exposure. The capsule is divided and the elbow joint is entered. Care is taken that the posterior interosseous nerve is not damaged. Jones and Esah recommend that the posterior interosseous nerve be exposed by separating the fibers of the supinator muscle with a blunt dissector; they also recommend retracting the soft tissues away from the nerve rather than pulling on both the tissues and the nerve. This wide exposure prevents neuropraxia of the posterior interosseous nerve and facilitates repositioning of the radial head on its neck.[24] Injury to the posterior interosseous nerve can also be avoided by staying posterior and posturing the forearm in full pronation. Sectioning of the orbicularis ligament is not performed unless it is necessary to achieve reduction. The forearm is fully pronated and supinated to test the stability of reduction. The author recommends internal fixation with one smooth Kirschner wire (of adequate diameter), which is inserted obliquely from distal to proximal from the radial neck into the head, facilitating pin removal in three to four weeks postoperatively. It is best to leave the pins protruding distally through the skin with the tips bent. One may prefer to leave the bent tips immediately under the skin in order to prevent pin tract infection.

There is variance of opinion in the literature concerning the necessity of internal fixation following open reduction. Key placed one or two sutures of fine catgut in the periosteum of the neck and then sutured the annular ligament about it. He suggested that the elbow and forearm be manipulated and placed in a position in which the radial head is fairly stable before any sutures are placed.[27] Reidy and Van Gorder do not use internal fixation except for an occasional suture.[49] O'Brien occasionally finds that he has to use a Kirschner wire to hold the radial head in place.[42] Jones and Esah recommend internal fixation particularly if the radial head is found to be detached and unstable following reduction. They introduce two Kirschner wires behind and lateral to the lateral condyle of the humerus, crossing the radial head obliquely from the margin of its articular surface into the radial shaft. The wires are removed between three and eight weeks later. They used Kirschner wires in six elbows, with functional results rated good in four and satisfactory in two.[24] Osteotomy of the upper ulna in order to visualize the articular surface is not recommended by the author.

The consensus of opinion is to avoid pins across the elbow joint inserted through the capitellum of the humerus into the center of the radial head and along half the length of the radial shaft. The complication rate of transarticular pins is high. Motion at the elbow joint and pin fatigue will result in breakage, making it very difficult, if not impossible, to retrieve the broken pin in the radius.[40, 63]

The only occasion to utilize capitellum-radial head transarticular pins is when the radial head is completely detached, lying free in the posterior or anterior part of the elbow joint. In such a situation insert a smooth Steinmann pin of adequate diameter from the capitellum into the elbow joint. As the pin transverses the radiohumeral joint, the elbow is flexed to 90 degrees and the forearm is placed in midrotation prior to transfixion of the joint. The proximal end of the wire is bent and cut but allowed to extend percutaneously in order to prevent migration and permit later removal. Immobilize the elbow in an above-elbow cast, high on the arm, and immobilize the shoulder in a Velpeau cast. In this way elbow motion is checkreined and pin breakage prevented. The pin is removed in three weeks and a new snug cast is applied for an additional one or two weeks.

In children, unlike in adults, the radial head should not be excised because of consequent growth disturbance and deformity of the wrist and elbow. When the fracture is diagnosed late, the deformity of radial head tilting can be corrected by open-up wedge osteotomy with a bone graft.

Complications

Loss of joint motion is caused by joint incongruity, enlargement of the radial head, fibrous adhesions, or proximal radioulnar synostosis. Rotation of the forearm is primarily affected—loss of pronation is greater than supination.

Malunion results from failure either to achieve adequate reduction or to maintain reduction.

Premature fusion of the upper radial physis occurs quite often in moderately and markedly displaced fractures. This will cause shortening of the radius and increased cubitus valgus, depending upon the age of the child at the time of injury and the severity of the cartilaginous damage. This occurred in about one third of the cases of O'Brien, but in none was the cubitus valgus severe enough to require osteotomy.[42] Premature fusion occurred in 11 of 30 cases reported by Reidy and Van Gorder.[49] Shortening of the radius is usually less than 0.5 cm.[40]

Avascular necrosis of the radial head occurred in about 10 per cent of the 34 cases of Jones and Esah; they were unable to relate it to the degree of initial displacement or to the age at the time of injury. The results were poor in all three cases.[24] Newman reported avascular necrosis in 9 of his 48 cases; all of them were in severely displaced fractures that required open reduction. The end results were poor.[40]

Overgrowth of the radial head due to hypervascularity and stimulation of epiphyseal growth occurs in some cases, restricting elbow motion. Vahvanen and Gripenberg reported this in 40 per cent of their cases, but functional result was good with no disability.[60]

A notch on the radial neck was found in 6 of 125 cases of O'Brien, who believed it to be caused by a taut, scarred orbicular ligament.[42]

Synostosis between the proximal radius and ulna has been reported by Fielding, Dougall, and O'Brien.[9, 13, 42] Fibrous adhesions between the radius and ulna were noted in one case by Jones and Esah.[24] These will block rotation of the forearm. Myositis ossificans may develop, particularly in the supinator muscle.[60]

Factors that have a definite influence on the prognosis are: (1) the degree of angulation, displacement, and translocation of the upper radial epiphysis (the more severe it is, the worse the prognosis); (2) association with injuries such as elbow dislocation, avulsion of the medial epicondyle, rupture of the medial collateral ligament, and fracture of the olecranon; (3) adequacy of reduction; (4) the patient's age at the time of injury; and (5) delay in effective treatment. After open operation, children under ten years of age have a higher percentage of good and excellent results than do those in the older age group. Reidy and Van Gorder correlated the results in 24 patients with maximum displacement (60 degrees or more) with age and type of treatment. Twenty had open reduction and four had closed reduction. Of the 20 with open reduction, 8 were 6 to 9 years of age and 12 were 10 to 13 years of age. Of the 8 younger patients 7 had good or excellent results and 1, a poor result. Only 4 of the 12 older patients had excellent or good results, however, and 8, a fair or poor result.[49]

In other series the overall incidence varies 15 to 23 per cent.[21, 24] It is wise to forewarn the parents of the possibility of the above complications and poor results, particularly loss of forearm rotation.

References

1. Anderson, T. E., and Breed, A. L.: A proximal radial metaphyseal fracture presenting as wrist pain. Orthopedics, 5:425, 1982.
2. Angelov, A.: A new method for treatment of the dislocated radial neck fracture in children. *In* Chapchal, G. (ed.): Fractures in Children. New York, George Thieme Verlag, 1981, pp. 192–194.
3. Aufranc, O. E., Jones, W. N., Turner, R. H., and Thomas, W. H.: Radial neck fracture in a child. J.A.M.A., *2202*:1140, 1967.
4. Bado, J. L.: The Monteggia lesion. Clin. Orthop., *50*:71, 1967.
5. Baehr, F. H.: Removal of the separated upper epiphysis of the radius. N. Engl. J. Med., *24*:1263, 1932.
6. Blount, W. P.: Fractures in Children. Baltimore, Williams & Wilkins, 1955.
7. Bohrer, J. V.: Fracture of the head and neck of the radius. Ann. Surg., 97:204, 1933.
8. Brodeur, A. E., Silberstein, M. J., and Graviss, E. R.: Radiology of the Pediatric Elbow. Boston, G. K. Hall, 1981.
9. Dougall, A. J.: Severe fractures of the neck of the radius in children. J. R. Coll. Surg. Edinb., *14*:220, 1969.
10. Dunlop, J.: Separation of medial epicondyle of humerus. Case with displaced upper radial epiphysis. J. Bone Joint Surg., *17*:584, 1935.
11. Fasol, P., and Schedl, R.: Percutaneous reduction of

fractures of the neck of the radius in children by means of a Steinmann nail. Wien. Klin. Wochenschr., *88*:135, 1976.
12. Feray, C.: Methode originale de reduction "peu sanglante" des fractures graves de la tete radiale chez l'enfant. Presse Med., *7*:2155, 1969.
13. Fielding, J. W.: Radio-ulnar crossed union following displacement of the proximal radial epiphysis. J. Bone Joint Surg., *46-A*:1277, 1964.
14. Fischer, M., and Maroske, D.: The broken Kirschner wire as a complication of transarticular fixation of the neck of the radius. Unfallheilkunde, *79*:277, 1976.
15. Fogarty, E. E., Blake, N. S., and Regan, B. F.: Fracture of the radial neck with medial displacement of the shaft of the radius. Br. J. Radiol., *56*:486, 1983.
16. Fowles, J. V., and Kassab, M. T.: Observations concerning radial neck fractures in children. J. Pediatr. Orthop., *6*:51, 1986.
17. Gasperini, E., and Parmeggiani, G.: Separation-fractures of the proximal extremity of the radius in children. Reduction with a percutaneous method. Arch. Orthop., *79*:77, 1966.
18. Gaston, S. R., Smith, F. M., and Boab, O. D.: Epiphyseal injuries of the radial head and neck. Am. J. Surg., *85*:266, 1953.
19. Gille, P., Mourot, M., Aubert, D., Lecuyer, F., and Djebar, A.: Fracture of the neck of the radius. Rev. Chir. Orthop., *64*:247, 1978.
20. Goldenberg, R. R.: Closed manipulation for the resolution of fracture of the neck of the radius in children. J. Bone Joint Surg., *27*:267, 1945.
21. Henrikson, B.: Isolated fractures of the proximal end of the radius in children. Acta Orthop. Scand., *40*:246, 1969.
22. Jeffrey, C. C.: Fractures of the head of the radius in children. J. Bone Joint Surg., *32-B*:314, 1950.
23. Jeffrey, C. C.: Fractures of the neck of the radius in children. Mechanism of causation. J. Bone Joint Surg., *54-B*:717, 1972.
24. Jones, E., and Esah, M.: Displaced fractures of the neck of the radius in children. J. Bone Joint Surg., *53-B*:429, 1971.
25. Judet, J., Judet, R., and Lefranc, J.: Fracture du col radial chez l'enfant. Ann. Chir., *16*:1377, 1962.
26. Kaplan, E. B.: Surgical approach to the proximal end of the radius and its use in fractures of the head and neck of the radius. J. Bone Joint Surg., *23*:86, 1941.
27. Key, J. A.: Treatment of fractures of the head and neck of the radius. J.A.M.A., *96*:101, 1939.
28. Key, J. A.: Survival of the head of the radius in a child after removal and replacement. J. Bone Joint Surg., *28*:148, 1946.
29. Lewis, R. W., and Thibodeau, A. A.: Deformity of the wrist following resection of the radial head. Surg. Gynecol. Obstet., *64*:1079, 1937.
30. Lindham, S., and Hugosson, C.: The significance of associated lesions including dislocation in fractures of the neck of the radius in children. Acta Orthop. Scand., *50*:79, 1979.
31. McBride, E. D., and Monnet, J. C.: Epiphyseal fractures of the head of the radius in children. Clin. Orthop., *16*:264, 1960.
32. Manoli, A.: Medial displacement of the shaft of the radius with a fracture of the radial neck. J. Bone Joint Surg., *61-A*:788, 1979.
33. Metaizeau, J. P., Prevot, J., and Schmitt, M.: Reduction et fixation des fractures et decollements epiphysaires de la tete radiale par broche centro-medullaire. Rev. Chir. Orthop., *66*:47, 1980.
34. Mommsen, U., Sauer, H. D., Bethke, K., and Schontag, H.: Fractures of the head of the radius in childhood. Langenbecks Arch. Chir., *351*:111, 1980.
35. Montgomery, A. H.: Separation of the upper epiphysis of the radius. Arch. Surg., *10*:961, 1925.
36. Mouchet, A.: Les fractures du col du radius. Rev. Chir., *21*:596, 1900.
37. Murawski, E., and Stach, O. W.: Conservative reduction of radial bone neck fractures in children. Pol. Przegl. Chir., *49*:117, 1977.
38. Murawski, E., Stachow, J., Gajewski, P., and Gawrych, E.: Treatment of radial neck fractures in children. Padiatr. Grenzgeb., *21*:463, 1982.
39. Murray, R. C.: Fractures of the head and neck of the radius. Br. J. Surg., *28*:109, 1940.
40. Newman, J. H.: Displaced radial neck fractures in children. Injury, *9*:114, 1977.
41. Nussbaum, A. J.: The off-profile proximal radial epiphysis: Another potential pitfall in the x-ray diagnosis of elbow trauma. J. Trauma, *23*:40, 1983.
42. O'Brien, P. I.: Injuries involving the proximal radial epiphysis. Clin. Orthop., *41*:51, 1965.
43. Ozga, A., and Borkowski, Z.: Results of treatment of fractures of the neck of the radius and of epiphysiolysis at the proximal end of the radius in children. Chir. Narzadow Ruchu Ortop. Pol., *35*:283, 1970.
44. Patterson, R. F.: Treatment of displaced fracture of the neck of the radius in children. J. Bone Joint Surg., *16*:695, 1934.
45. Pesudo, J. V., Aracil, J., and Barcelo, M.: Leverage method in displaced fractures of the radial neck in children. Clin. Orthop., *169*:215, 1982.
46. Poland, J.: A Practical Treatise on Traumatic Separation of the Epiphyses. London, Smith, Elder & Co., 1898.
47. Pollen, A. G.: Fractures and Dislocations in Children. Baltimore, Williams & Wilkins, 1973.
48. Poulsen, O., and Tophoj, K.: Fracture of the head and neck of the radius. Follow-up on 61 patients. Acta Orthop. Scand., *45*:66, 1974.
49. Reidy, J. A., and Van Gorder, G. W.: Treatment of displacement of the proximal radial epiphysis. J. Bone Joint Surg., *45-A*:1355, 1963.
50. Schwartz, R. P., and Young, F.: Treatment of fractures of the head and neck of the radius and slipped radial epiphysis in children. Surg. Gynecol. Obstet., *57*:528, 1933.
51. Scullion, J. E., and Miller, J. H.: Fracture of the neck of the radius in children: Prognostic factors and recommendations for management. J. Bone Joint Surg., *67-B*:491, 1985.
52. Speed, K.: Fractures of the head of the radius. Am. J. Surg., *38*:157, 1924.
53. Speed, K.: Traumatic lesion of the head of the radius. Surg. Clin. North Am., *4*:651, 1924.
54. Stankovic, P., Emmerman, H., Burkhardt, K., and Kurtsch, U.: Die Frakturen des proximalen Radius im Kindesalter. Z. Kinderchir. Suppl., *16*:77, 1975.
55. Strachan, J. C. H., and Ellis, B. V.: Vulnerability of the posterior interosseous nerve during radial head resection. J. Bone Joint Surg., *53-B*:320, 1971.
56. Svinukhov, N. P.: The outcomes of operative treatment of fractures of the neck of the radius in children. Ortop. Travmatol. Protez., *26*:13, 1965.
57. Svinukhov, N. P.: On the mechanism of injury and the method of closed repositioning of intra-articulare fractures of the neck of the radius in children. Vestn. Khir., *96*:129, 1966.
58. Svinukhov, N. P.: Degenerative-dystrophic changes in fractures of the proximal end of the radial bone in children. Ortop. Travmatol. Protez. *31*:20, 1970.
59. Tibone, J. E., and Stoltz, M.: Fractures of the radial head and neck in children. J. Bone Joint Surg., *63-A*:100, 1981.
60. Vahvanen, V., and Gripenberg, L.: Fracture of the radial neck in children. A long term follow-up study of 43 cases. Acta Orthop. Scand., *49*:32, 1978.
61. von Laer, L.: The fracture of the proximal end of the radius in adolescence. Arch. Orthop. Trauma. Surg., *99*:167, 1982.

62. Vostal, O.: Fractures of the neck of the radius in children. Acta Chir. Orthop. Traumatol. Cech., *37*:294, 1970.
63. Wedge, J. H., and Robertson, D. E.: Displaced fractures of the neck of the radius. J. Bone Joint Surg., *64-B*:256, 1982.
64. Wilkins, K.: Fractures of the neck and head of the radius. *In* Fractures in Children. Philadelphia, Lippincott, 1984, p. 502.
65. Wood, S. K.: Reversal of the radial head during reduction of fracture of the neck of the radius in children. J. Bone Joint Surg., *51-B*:707, 1969.
66. Wright, P. R.: Greenstick fracture of the upper end of the ulna with dislocation of the radio-humeral joint or displacement of the superior radial epiphysis. J. Bone Joint Surg., *45-B*:727, 1963.

FRACTURES OF THE OLECRANON

These result either from direct violence (such as a fall on the point of the elbow) or from indirect violence (as when the elbow is suddenly flexed against the opposing triceps muscle). Fractures of the olecranon also occur in association with various injuries about the elbow produced by an abduction force—such as fractures of the capitellum, radial neck, or medial epicondyle. Secondary centers of ossification of the olecranon (bipartite olecranon or patella cubiti) should not be misdiagnosed as fractures.

If the fracture is undisplaced or minimally displaced, treatment consists of simple immobilization of the elbow in a long arm cast for three or four weeks (Figs. 8–63 and 8–64). Moderately displaced fractures are immobilized with the elbow in extension. Flexion of the elbow is rapidly restored in children following removal of the cast, and extension contracture is not a problem. Markedly displaced fractures require open reduction, soft-tissue repair, and internal fixation with a wire (Fig. 8–65).

References

1. Bassett, L. W., Mirra, J. M., Forrester, D. M., Gold, R. H., Bernstein, M. L., and Rollins, J. S.: Post-traumatic osteochondral "loose body" of the olecranon fossa. An entity which can be mistaken for a normal anatomical variant or osteoid osteoma. Radiology, *141*:635, 1981.
2. Beddow, F. H., and Corkery, P. H.: Lateral dislocation of the radio-humeral joint with greenstick fracture of the upper end of the ulna. J. Bone Joint Surg., *42-B*:782, 1960.
3. Blount, W. P.: Fractures in Children. Baltimore, Williams & Wilkins, 1955.
4. Boobyer, G. N.: A new method of internal fixation of olecranon fractures. Injury, *12*:101, 1980.
5. Brodeur, A. E., Silberstein, M. J., and Graviss, E. R.: Radiology of the Pediatric Elbow. Boston, G. K. Hall, 1981.
6. Burghele, N., and Serban, N.: Fractures of the olecranon: Treatment by external fixation. Ital. J. Orthop. Traumatol., *8*:159, 1982.
7. Cotton, F. J.: Separation of the epiphysis of the olecranon. Boston Med. Surg. J., 692–994, 1900.
8. Coughlin, M. J., Slabaugh, P. B., and Smith, T. K.: Experience with the McAtee olecranon device in olecranon fractures. J. Bone Joint Surg., *61-A*:385, 1979.
9. Daland, E. M.: Fractures of the olecranon. J. Bone Joint Surg., *15*:601, 1933.
10. Fahey, J. J.: Fractures of the elbow in children. A.A.O.S. Instr. Course Lect., *17*:13, 1960.
11. Fyfe, I. S., Mossad, M. M., and Holdsworth, B. J.: Methods of fixation of olecranon fractures. An experimental mechanical study. J. Bone Joint Surg., *67-B*:367, 1985.
12. Gartsman, G. M., Sculco, T. P., and Otis, J. C.: Operative treatment of olecranon fractures. Excision or open reduction with internal fixation. J. Bone Joint Surg., *63-A*:718, 1981.
13. Grantham, S. A., and Kiernan, H. A.: Displaced olecranon fractures in children. J. Trauma, *15*:197, 1975.
14. Guerra, A., and Innao, V.: Transolecranal dislocations. Ital. J. Orthop. Traumatol., *8*:175, 1982.
15. Holdsworth, B. J., and Mossad, M. M.: Elbow function following tension band fixation of displaced fractures of the olecranon. Injury, *16*:182, 1984.
16. Horne, J. G., and Tanzer, T. L.: Olecranon fractures: A review of 100 cases. J. Trauma, *21*:469, 1981.
17. Hume, A. C.: Anterior dislocation of the head of the radius associated with undisplaced fracture of the olecranon in children. J. Bone Joint Surg., *39-B*:508, 1957.
18. Jensen, C. M., and Olsen, B. B.: Drawbacks of traction-absorbing wiring (TAW) in displaced fractures of the olecranon. Injury, *17*:174, 1986.
19. Johnson, R. P., Roether, A., and Schwab, J. P.: Olecranon fractures treated with AO screw and tension bands. Orthopedics, *9*:66, 1986.
20. Kiviluoto, O., and Santavirta, S.: Fractures of the olecranon. Analysis of 37 consecutive cases. Acta Orthop. Scand., *49*:28, 1978.
21. Macko, D., and Szabo, R. M.: Complications of tension-band wiring of olecranon fractures. J. Bone Joint Surg., *67-A*:1396, 1985.
22. Matthews, J. G.: Fractures of the olecranon in children. Injury, *12*:207, 1980.
23. Maylahn, D. J., and Fahey, J. J.: Fractures of the elbow in children. J.A.M.A., *166*:220, 1958.
24. Newell, R. L. M.: Olecranon fractures in children. Injury, *7*:33, 1975.
25. O'Donoghue, D. H., and Stanley, L.: The persistent olecranon epiphysis in the adult. J. Bone Joint Surg., *24*:677, 1942.
26. Pavlov, H., Torg, J. S., Jacobs, B., and Vigorita, V.: Nonunion of olecranon epiphysis: Two cases in adolescent baseball pitchers. A.J.R., *136*:819, 1981.
27. Porteous, C. J.: The olecranon epiphyses. Proc. J. Anat., *94*:286, 1960.
28. Rettig, A. C., Waugh, T. R., and Evanski, P. M.: Fracture of the olecranon: A problem of management. J. Trauma, *19*:23, 1979.
29. Selesnick, F. H., Dolitsky, B., and Haskell, S. S.: Fracture of the coronoid process requiring open reduction with internal fixation. A case report. J. Bone Joint Surg., *66-A*:1304, 1984.
30. Silberstein, M. J., Brodeur, A. E., Graviss, E. R., and Luisiri, A.: Some vagaries of the olecranon. J. Bone Joint Surg., *63-A*:722, 1981.
31. Smith, F. M.: Surgery of the Elbow. 2nd Ed. Philadelphia, Saunders, 1972.
32. Taylor, T. K. F., and Scham, S. M.: A posteromedial approach to the proximal end of the ulna for the internal fixation of olecranon fractures. J. Trauma, *9*:594, 1969.
33. Torg, J. S., and Moyer, R. A.: Non-union of a stress fracture through the olecranon epiphyseal plate observed in an adolescent baseball pitcher. A case report. J. Bone Joint Surg., *59-A*:264, 1977.

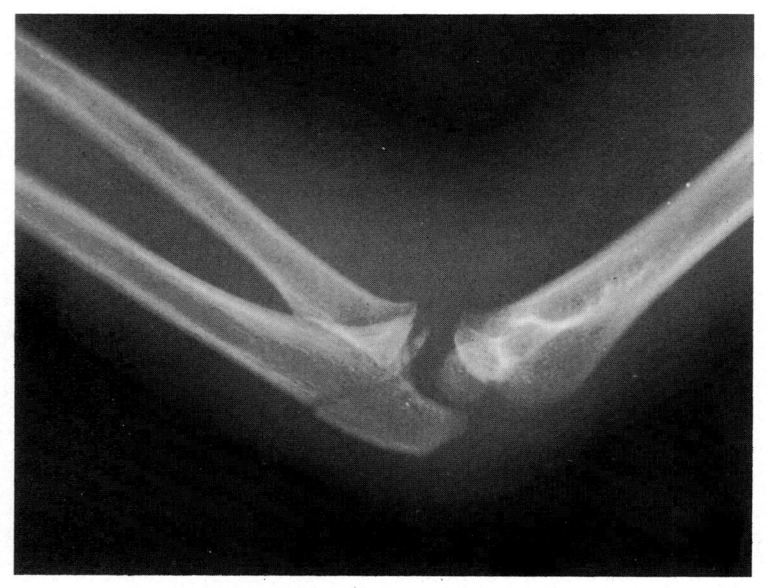

FIGURE 8–63. Undisplaced fracture of olecranon.

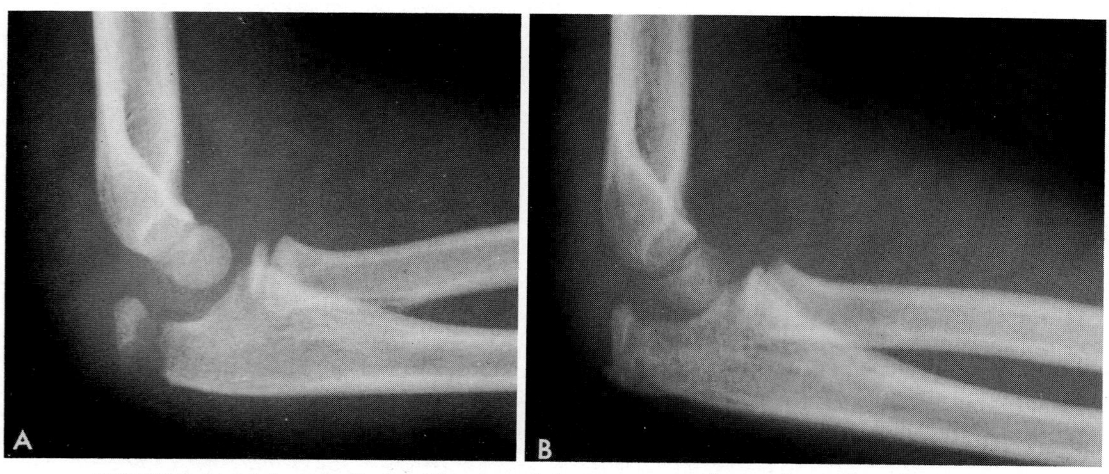

FIGURE 8–64. Moderately displaced fracture of olecranon treated by an above-elbow cast with the elbow in extended position.

A. Initial radiogram. **B.** Radiogram taken after five weeks, showing healing.

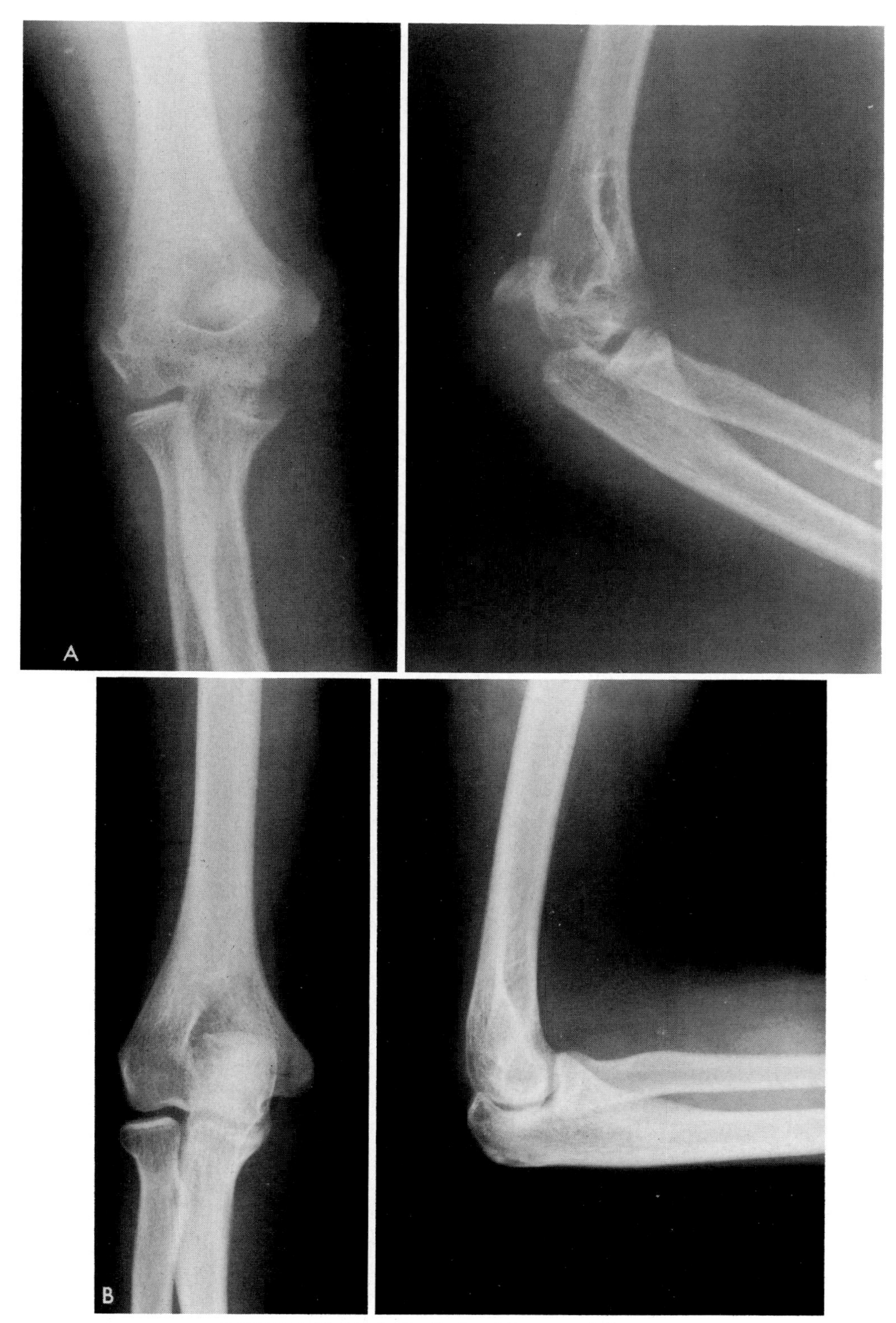

FIGURE 8–65. Markedly displaced fracture of olecranon.

Fracture was treated by open reduction, soft-tissue repair, and internal fixation with wire. **A.** Initial radiograms. **B.** Three years later, radiograms show healing and remodeling.

34. Wadsworth, T. G.: Screw fixation of the olecranon after fracture or osteotomy. Clin. Orthop., *119*:197, 1976.
35. Wainwright, D.: Fractures of the olecranon process. Br. J. Surg., *29*:403, 1942.
36. Weseley, M. S., Barenfeld, P. A., and Einstein, A. L.: The use of the Zuelzer hook plate in fixation of olecranon fractures. J. Bone Joint Surg., *58-A*:859, 1976.
37. Yates, C., and Sullivan, J. A.: Arthrographic diagnosis of elbow joint injuries in children. J. Pediatr. Orthop., *7*:54, 1987.
38. Zeitlin, A.: Traumatic origin of accessory bones at the elbow. J. Bone Joint Surg., *17*:933, 1935.
39. Zimmerman, H.: Fractures of the elbow. *In* Weber, B. G., Brunner, C., and Frueler, F. (eds.): Treatment of Fractures in Children and Adolescents. New York, Springer-Verlag, 1980.

PULLED ELBOW (SUBLUXATION OF THE RADIAL HEAD)

The term *pulled elbow* is used to denote a clinical entity in young children in whom traumatic subluxation of the radial head is produced by sudden traction on the hand with the elbow extended and the forearm pronated. This common injury was known in historic times; Van Arsdale states that Hippocrates was the first to recognize the condition, though Fournier is usually given credit for first accurately describing the injury in 1671.[15, 49]

Various eponyms and synonyms have been used to denote this traumatic lesion, some of which are subluxation of the head of the radius, subluxation of the radius by elongation, subluxation of the annular ligament at the proximal radioulnar joint, "nursemaid's elbow," "temper tantrum elbow," and Malgaigne's injury or luxation.[1–51]

Pulled elbow is one of the most common musculoskeletal injuries in children under four years of age, and is rarely, if ever, found in children over five years. The peak incidence is between the ages of one and three years. It is more frequent in boys than in girls, and the left side is more commonly subluxated than the right. In the emergency department of the Hospital for Sick Children, Toronto, 112 children with pulled elbow were seen in a period of one year, according to Salter and Zaltz.[38] This average incidence of two per week is also reported by Griffin and Snellman.[21, 42]

Mechanism of Injury and Pathologic Anatomy

The lesion is caused by sudden longitudinal traction on the wrist of a young child whose elbow is extended and forearm is pronated. Common circumstances that precipitate this injury are pulling a child as he stumbles in an attempt to keep him from falling, lifting him by the hand up a curb, pulling the child's hand through the sleeve of a dress or sweater, swinging the child around while holding him by the hand, or forcefully pulling a child away from something by his hand. Occasionally, the injury may be sustained in a fall.

In the literature, there has been much speculation about the exact etiology. One of the theories offered has been that in young children the head of the radius is not fully developed and that the perimeter of the cartilaginous head is smaller than the neck; hence, it is not firmly held in place by the annular ligament.[31] This is an error probably based on a misinterpretation of a statement by Pierseol.[38]

Ryan examined the upper end of the radius in 15 fetal specimens and found that the radial head is definitely larger than the radial neck, and that the ratio of the two does not differ greatly from that of the adult, the average of the fetal radii being 1.53, and that of the adult radii, 1.50. The smallest ratio among the fetal radii was 1.10; the smallest ratio in the adult radii was 1.25. The largest ratio in fetal radii was 1.79; the largest in the adult, 1.80.[37] This investigation was supported by Salter and Zaltz, who examined the proximal end of the radius in 12 child cadavers ranging in age from two days to nine years; in each and every specimen they found the diameter of the radial head to be larger than that of the neck by 30 to 60 per cent, the ratio varying from 1.3:1 to 1.6:1.[38] Thus, the former concept that the radial head is easily pulled through the annular ligament because it is smaller than the radial neck is erroneous and should be discarded.

Stone studied the mechanism of injury in 12 anatomic specimens, and was able to produce the lesion in six of the elbows, oberving that the annular ligament slipped over the radial head only when the forearm was pronated. He also noted that the radial head is oval in outline rather than circular, and that when the forearm is supinated, the anterior aspect of the radial head is elevated sharply from the neck; when traction was applied with the forearm in supination, the annular ligament was pulled against this sharp bony elevation. Laterally and posteriorly, the radial head rises rather gradually, so that when traction is applied with the forearm in pronation, the annular ligament lies over this part and becomes stretched until it slips over the head.[45]

In their investigations of the elbows of 25 stillborn infants, McRae and Freeman con-

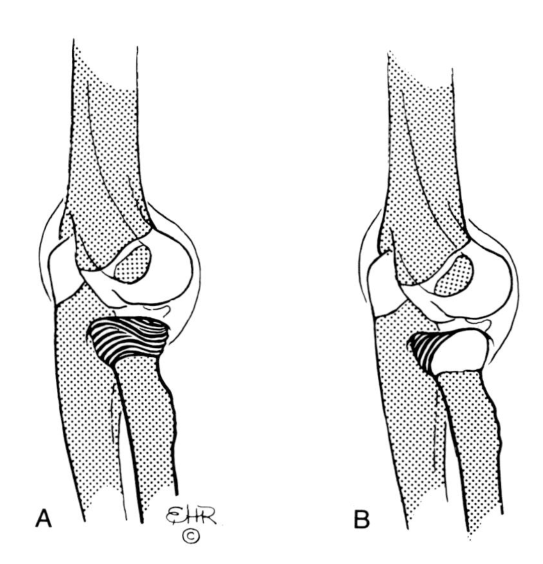

FIGURE 8–66. Diagram illustrating pathologic anatomy of pulled elbow in a young child.

A. Normal arrangement of the annular ligament, as seen from the lateral view. **B.** Lateral view of the pulled elbow. Note the tear in the distal attachment of the annular ligament through which the radial head has protruded slightly; the detached portion of the annular ligament has slipped into the radiohumeral joint where it has become trapped when traction was discontinued. (From Salter, R. B.: Disorders and Injuries of the Musculoskeletal System. Baltimore, Williams & Wilkins, 1970, p. 430.)

cluded that pulled elbow is caused by the annular ligament slipping over the radial head.[29]

Salter and Zaltz also observed that the superior surface of the radial head (viewed axially from above) is slightly oval rather than circular, and that with the forearm supinated, the sagittal diameter of the radial head is consistently greater (less than 1 mm.) than the coronal diameter. These findings were similar to the measurements of Stone.[38, 45]

Salter and Zaltz studied the pathologic anatomy in the 12 aforementioned anatomic specimens. The proximal radiohumeral and radioulnar joints were exposed, leaving the joint capsule and annular ligament intact. Sudden firm and steady traction was exerted on the extended elbow by pulling on the hand, first with the forearm in supination, and then in pronation. They could not subluxate the radial head in any of the 12 specimens when traction was applied to the extended elbow with the forearm in *supination*; but in the child cadavers under five years of age, when traction was applied on the extended elbow with the forearm in *pronation*, a transverse tear could be produced in the thin distal attachment of the annular ligament to the periosteum of the radial neck. When the forearm is pronated, the narrowest diameter of the radial head is in the anteroposterior plane. Once a transverse tear in the orbicularis ligament has occurred, the anterior portion of the radial head escapes from under the anterior part of the annular ligament, which, in turn, becomes interposed and is caught between the articular surfaces of the radial head and the capitellum when traction is discontinued (Fig. 8–66). When the interposed part of the annular ligament extended beyond the equator of the radial head, its reduction could not be achieved by passive supination of the forearm (Fig. 8–67 A); but when the proximal edge of the annular ligament did not extend beyond the equator of the radial head, the interposed annular ligament could be repositioned in its normal site by simple supination of the forearm with the elbow in slight flexion (Fig. 8–67 B).

In the anatomic specimens of children five years of age or older, a tear in the annular ligament could not be produced by firm traction with the elbow in extension and the forearm in pronation. This is because of the thicker and stronger distal attachment of the annular ligament to the periosteum of the radial neck in the older child; with continued traction, the entire elbow was dislocated.

The foregoing anatomic findings of Salter and Zaltz correlate well with the many characteristic clinical features of pulled elbow in living children.

Diagnosis

The clinical picture is characteristic. Immediately following the injury, the child cries with pain and refuses to use the affected limb. A "click" may have been heard or felt in the child's elbow by the person who pulled it.

The child will hold the injured elbow by his side, supporting the forearm with his opposite hand. The forearm is *always pronated* and the elbow partially flexed. On gentle palpation, one

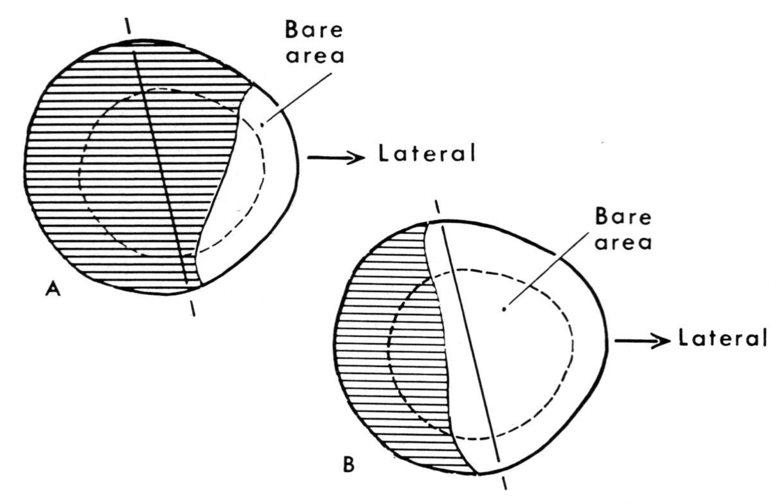

FIGURE 8–67. Diagram showing pathologic anatomy of two degrees of pulled elbow (superior axial view of radial heads).

A. The detached margin of the annular ligament has slid beyond the equator or widest part of the head. This severe degree results when the tear in the attachment of the annular ligament extends over more than half of its length. It occurs very rarely, and reduction cannot be achieved by closed manipulation. **B.** The detached margin of the annular ligament has not slid beyond the equator of the radial head. This is the common form of pulled elbow. The interposed annular ligament is readily freed from the radiohumeral joint by simply supinating the forearm with the elbow in slight flexion. (From Salter, R. B., and Zalta, C.: Anatomic investigations of the mechanism of injury and pathologic anatomy of "pulled elbow" in young children. Clin. Orthop., 77:141, 1971.)

can elicit local tenderness over the anterolateral aspect of the radial head. There is no restriction to flexion and extension of the elbow, but supination of the forearm is markedly limited and voluntarily resisted.

Radiograms of the elbow are normal. There is no distal displacement of the proximal radius from the capitellum; it is the relationship of the radius and ulna that indicates the pronated posture of the forearm. The diagnosis of subluxation of the radial head is made by the typical clinical findings.

Treatment

Often reduction of the pulled elbow is unknowingly carried out by the x-ray technician, who passively forces the forearm into full supination in an attempt to obtain a true anteroposterior projection of the elbow. If the child escapes such "treatment," the pediatrician or orthopedic surgeon performs the reduction of radial head subluxation as follows: The elbow is gently flexed to 90 degrees by holding the child's forearm above the wrist with one hand while, with the other hand, the lower end of the humerus and elbow are firmly held to prevent rotation at the shoulder; the thumb is placed in the region of the radial head for palpation and the exertion of mild pressure if necessary. Then the child's forearm is rapidly and firmly rotated into full supination. As reduction is achieved, a palpable and sometimes audible click can be felt in the region of the radial head. Another signal of reduction is the spectacular and instantaneous relief of pain. The child stops crying and begins to use the arm in a normal manner almost immediately. Should treatment have been delayed and subluxation persist following reduction, the child will still be in some discomfort and will not be anxious to use the limb for several hours or days.

Immobilization is not necessary if it is the first time that subluxation has occurred. A simple sling may be used for a week to keep the elbow out of harm's way. It is important to educate the parents to the potential danger of pulling the child by his hands.

If treatment of subluxation is delayed for more than 12 hours following reduction, the upper limb is immobilized for 10 days in a long arm posterior splint with the elbow in 90 degrees of flexion and the forearm in full supination.

Recurrence of subluxation as a result of a subsequent pull on the hand occurs in about 5 per cent of cases. Following manipulative reduction of a recurrent case, it is best to immobilize the upper limb in an above-elbow cast for at least two to three weeks.

In a very few children over four years of age, the subluxated radial head may be irreducible by closed manipulation, particularly if it is recurrent, necessitating open operation. In one such case, Salter and Zaltz had to divide the annular ligament, withdraw its ends from the radiohumeral joint, and repair it.[38]

References

1. Anderson, S. A.: Subluxation of the head of the radius, a pediatric condition. South. Med. J., *35*:286, 1942.
2. Beegel, P. M.: "Slipped elbow" in children. J. Maine Med. Assoc., *45*:293, 1954.
3. Bourquet: Mémoire sur les luxations dites incomplètes de l'extrémité. Rev. Med. Chir., *15*:287, 1854.
4. Boyette, B. P., Ahoskie, N. C., and London, A. H., Jr.: Subluxation of the head of the radius, "nursemaid's elbow." J. Pediatr., *32*:278, 1948.
5. Broadhurst, R. W., and Buhr, A. J.: The pulled elbow. Br. Med. J., *1*:1018, 1959.
6. Caldwell, C. E.: Subluxation of the radial head by elongation. Cincinnati Lancet Clinic, *66*:496, 1891.
7. Chaissaignac: Paralysie douloureuse des jeunes enfants. Arch. Gen. Med., *1*:653, 1856.
8. Corrigan, A. B.: The pulled elbow. Med. J. Aust., *2*:187, 1965.
9. Costigan, P. G.: Subluxation of the annular ligament at the proximal radioulnar joint. Alberta Med. Bull., *17*:7, 1952.
10. Cushing, H. W.: Subluxation of the radial head in children. Boston Med. Surg. J., *114*:77, 1886.
11. Davis, J. H.: Subluxation of the radial head in children (nursemaid's elbow). Med. Times, *13*:1379, 1965.
12. Dimon, J. H., III: Pulled elbow or babysitter's elbow. O.N.A.J., *6*:72, 1979.
13. Douglas, G. J.: Injuries to the elbow in children. Med. J. Aust., *2*:353, 1961.
14. Duverney, J. G.: Traité des Maladies des Os. Paris, De Bure l'aine, 1751.
15. Fournier, D.: L'Oeconomic Chirurgical, 250. Paris, Francoise Clouzier & Cie, 1671.
16. Frumkin, K.: Nursemaid's elbow: A radiographic demonstration. Ann. Emerg. Med., *14*:690, 1985.
17. Gardner, J.: On an undescribed displacement of the bones of the forearm in children. London Med. Gaz., *20*:878, 1837.
18. Gatrell, C. B.: Radiologic findings in radial head subluxation. Am. J. Dis. Child., *140*:856, 1986.
19. Gattey, P. H., and Wedge, J. H.: Unilateral posterior dislocation of the radial head in identical twins. J. Pediatr. Orthop., *6*:220, 1986.
20. Green, J. T., and Gay, F. H.: Traumatic subluxation of the radial head in young children. J. Bone Joint Surg., *36-A*:655, 1954.
21. Griffin, M. E.: Subluxation of the head of the radius in young children. Pediatrics, *15*:103, 1955.
22. Hardy, R. H.: Pulled elbow. J. R. Coll. Gen. Pract., *28*:224, 1978.
23. Hart, G. M.: Subluxation of the head of the radius in young children. J.A.M.A., *169*:1734, 1959.
24. Hudson, D. A., and DeBeer, J. D.: Isolated traumatic dislocation of the radial head in children. J. Bone Joint Surg., *68-B*:378, 1986.
25. Hutchinson, J., Jr.: On certain obscure sprains of the elbow occurring in young children. Ann. Surg., 2:91, 1885.
26. Kanter, A. J., and Bruton, O. C.: Subluxation of the head of the radius. Am. Practitioner, *31*:39, 1952.
27. Letter: Radial head subluxation. Am. J. Dis. Child., *140*:505, 1986.
28. Lindeman, S. H.: Partial dislocation of the radial head peculiar to children. Br. Med. J., *2*:1058, 1885.
29. McRae, R., and Freeman, P.: The lesion in pulled elbow. J. Bone Joint Surg., *47-B*:808, 1965.
30. McVeagh, T. C.: The slipped elbow in young children. Calif. Med., *74*:260, 1951.
31. Magill, H. K., and Aitken, A. P.: Pulled elbow. Surg. Gynecol. Obstet., *98*:753, 1954.
32. Metcalf, N. F., and Metcalf, W. K.: Letter: Pulled elbow, evidence for a genetic factor. Br. Med. J., *3*:544, 1975.
33. Moore, E. M.: Subluxation of the radius from extension in young children. Trans. N.Y. Med. Assoc., *3*:18, 1886.
34. Oberlander, J.: The so-called pseudopareses of the arm in small children (subluxation radii periannularis, Chassaignac's arm paralysis). Llandarzt., *43*:1684, 1967.
35. Poinsot, G.: Dislocations of the head of the radius downward (by elongation). N.Y. Med. J., *41*:8, 1885.
36. Quan, L., and Marcuse, E. K.: The epidemiology and treatment of radial head subluxation. Am. J. Dis. Child., *139*:1194, 1985.
37. Ryan, J. R.: The relationship of the radial head to the radial neck diameters in fetuses and adults with reference to radial head subluxation in children. J. Bone Joint Surg., *51-A*:781, 1969.
38. Salter, R. B., and Zaltz, C.: Anatomic investigation of the mechanism of injury and pathologic anatomy of "pulled elbow" in children. Clin. Orthop., *77*:134, 1971.
39. Silquini, P. L.: La pronazione dolorosa. Min. Ortop., *14*:481, 1963.
40. Silver, C. M., and Simon, S. D.: Subluxation of head of the radius in children. R.I. Med. J., *43*:722, 1960.
41. Smith, E. E.: Subluxation of the head of the radius in children. Ohio Med. J., *45*:1080, 1949.
42. Snellman, O.: Subluxation of the radial head in children. Acta Orthop. Scand., *28*:311, 1959.
43. Sorrells, R. B.: Pulled elbow. J. Arkansas Med. Soc., *72*:209, 1975.
44. Stanley, D.: Isolated traumatic anterior dislocation of the radial head—a mechanism of injury in children. Injury, *17*:182, 1986.
45. Stone, C. A.: Subluxation of the head of the radius—report of a case and anatomical experiments. J.A.M.A., *1*:28, 1916.
46. Storen, G.: Traumatic dislocation of the radial head as an isolated lesion in children. Acta Chir. Scand., *116*:144, 1959.
47. Sweetman, R.: Pulled elbow. Practitioner, *182*:487, 1959.
48. Tucker, K.: Some aspects of post-traumatic elbow stiffness. Injury, *9*:216, 1978.
49. Van Arsdale, W. H.: On subluxation of the head of the radius in children with a resume of one hundred consecutive cases. Ann. Surg., *9*:401, 1889.
50. Van Santvoordt, R.: Dislocation of the radial head downward. N.Y. Med. J., *45*:63, 1887.
51. Veseley, D. G.: Isolated traumatic dislocations of the radial head in children. Clin. Orthop., *50*:31, 1967.

MONTEGGIA FRACTURE-DISLOCATION

In 1814, Giovanni Monteggia first described two cases of fracture of the proximal third of the ulna in association with anterior dislocation of the radial head.[66]

Cooper, in 1844, described anterior, poste-

Text continued on page 3158

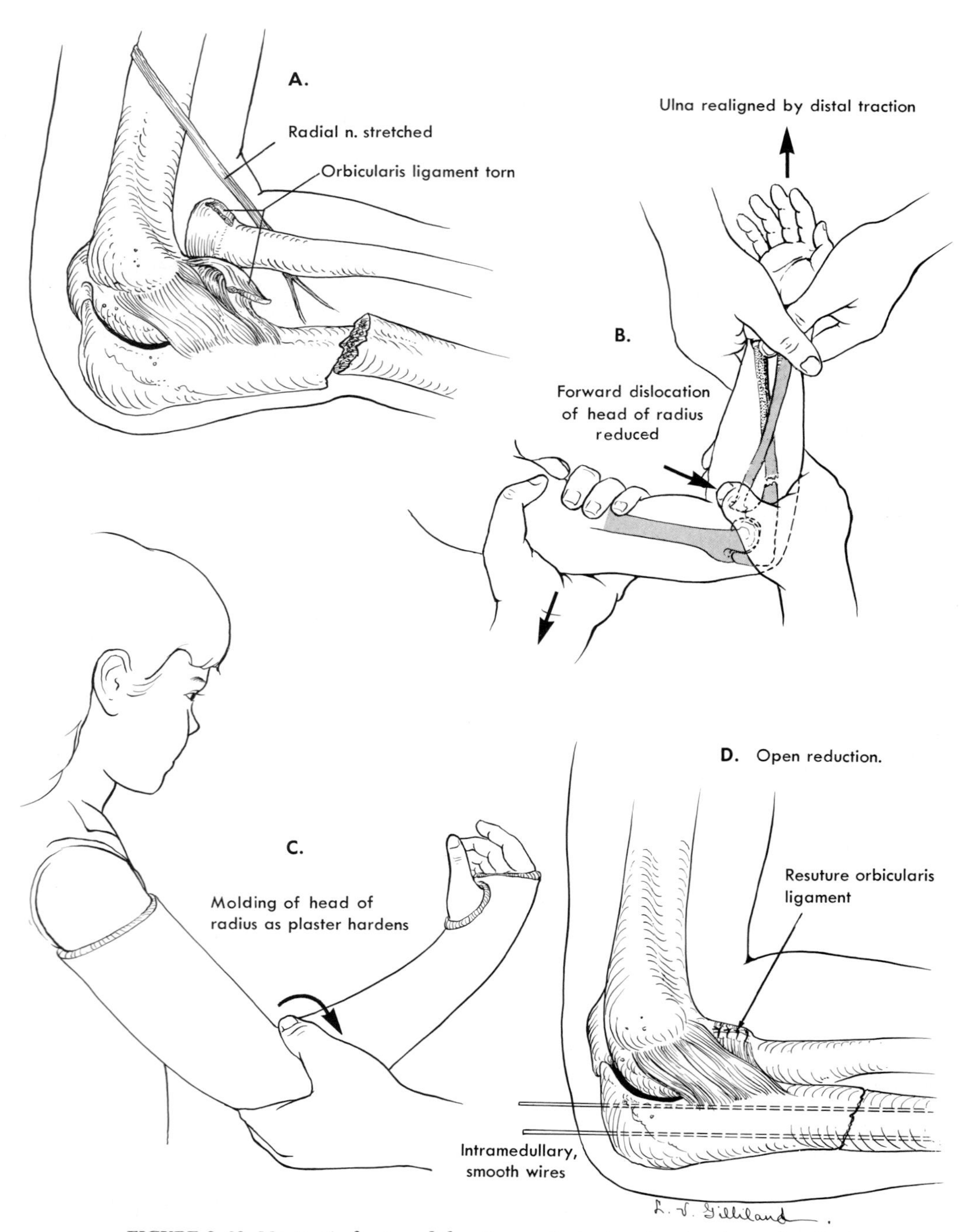

FIGURE 8–68. ***Monteggia fracture-dislocation—anterior type (see text for explanation).***

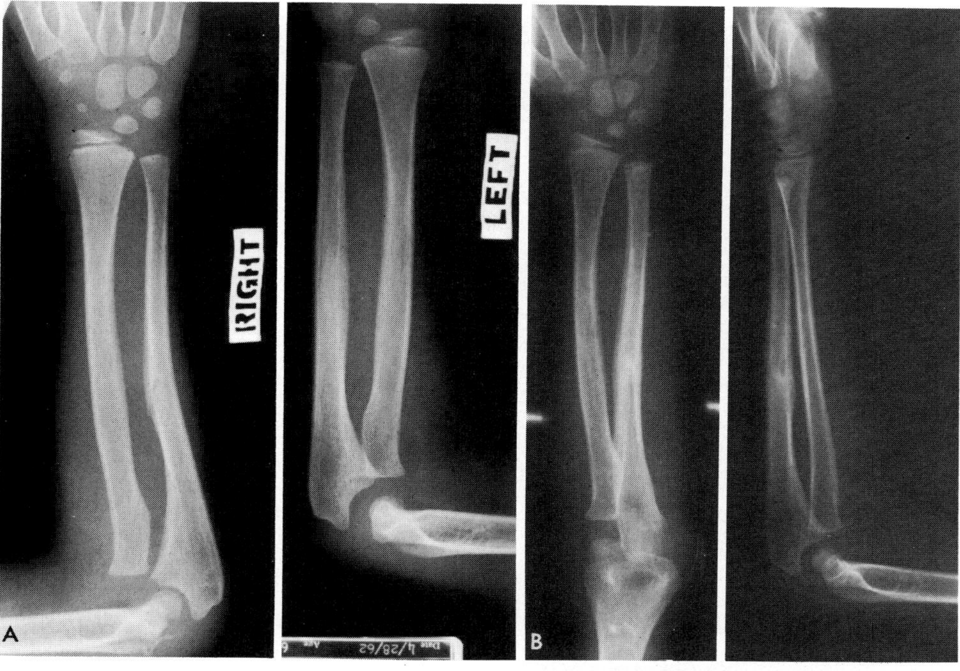

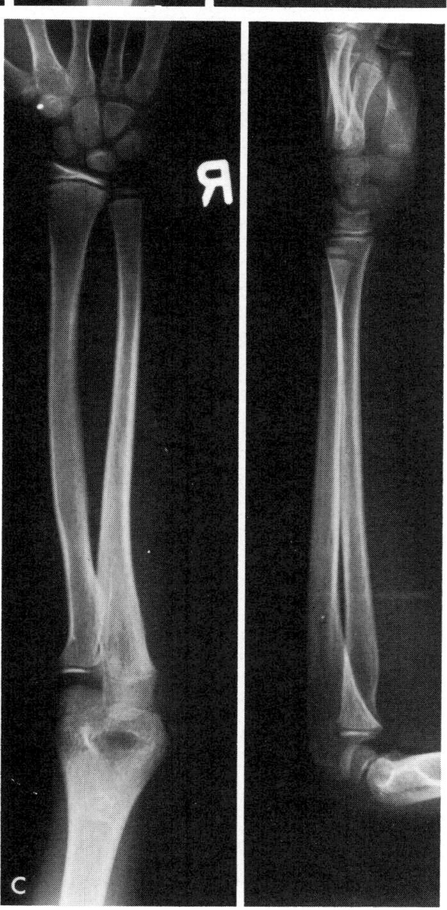

FIGURE 8–69. Monteggia fracture-dislocation—anterior type on the right.

A. Initial radiogram of both forearms including wrists and elbows (the normal left one is for comparison). Note the anterior dislocation of the radial head and anterior angulation of the greenstick fracture of the ulna in its middle third. **B.** Radiograms of right forearm three months following closed reduction. The fracture has healed and the reduction of the radial head has been maintained. **C.** Two years later, radiograms show remodeling and complete healing.

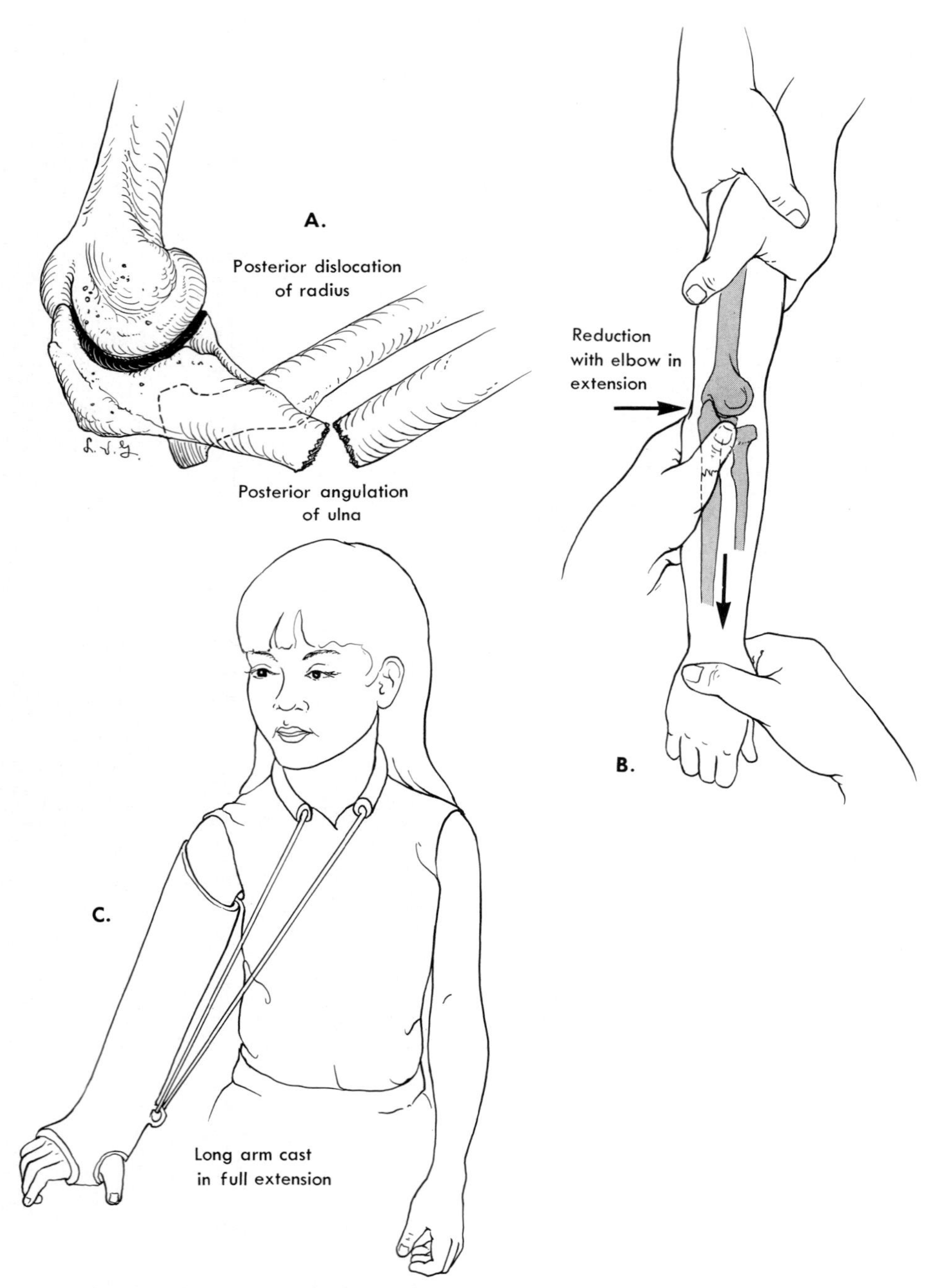

FIGURE 8–70. Monteggia fracture-dislocation—posterior type (see text for explanation).

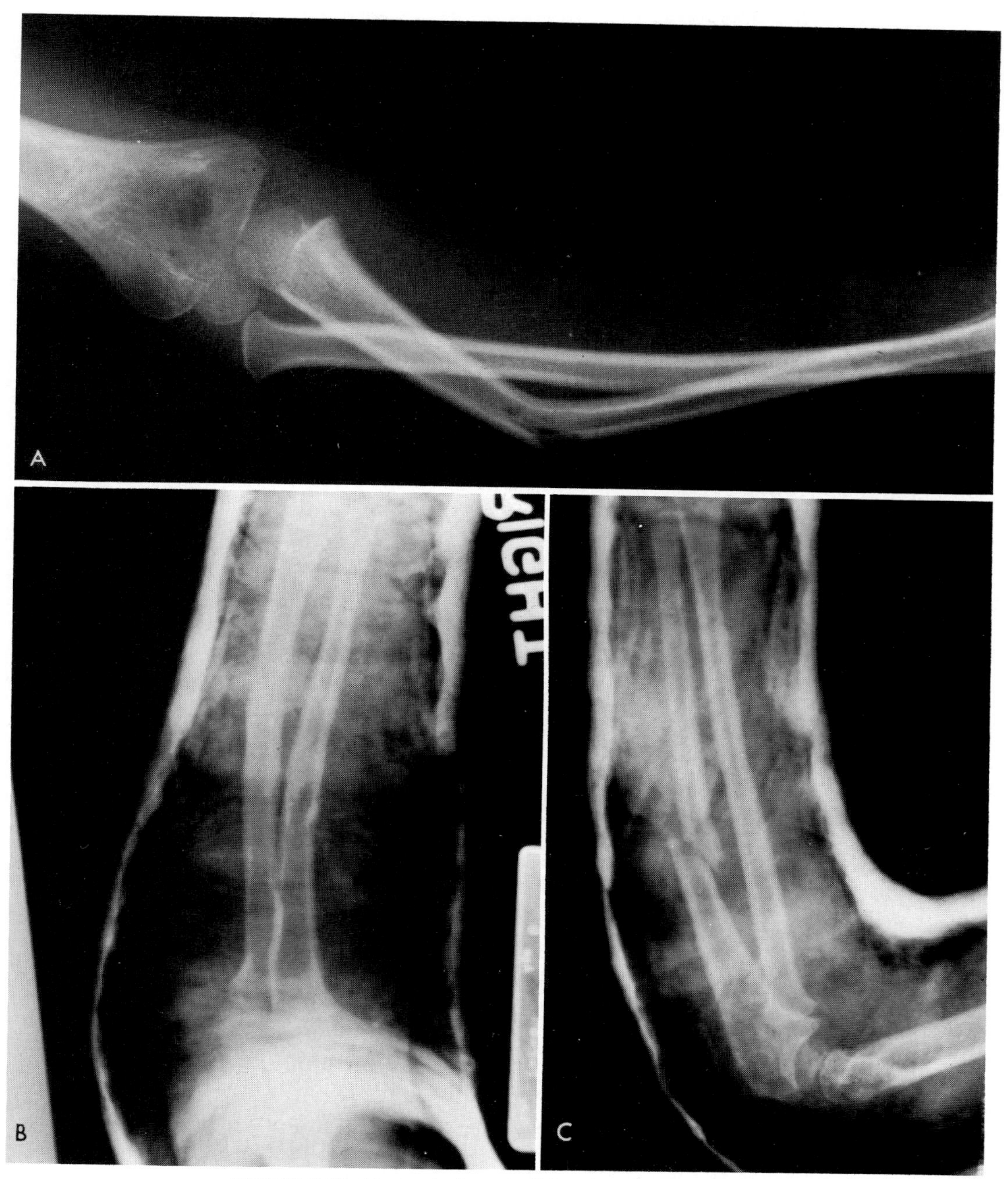

FIGURE 8–71. Monteggia fracture-dislocation—posterior type.

A. Initial radiogram. Note the posterior dislocation of the radial head and fracture of the ulna in its middle third. **B** and **C**. Postreduction views.

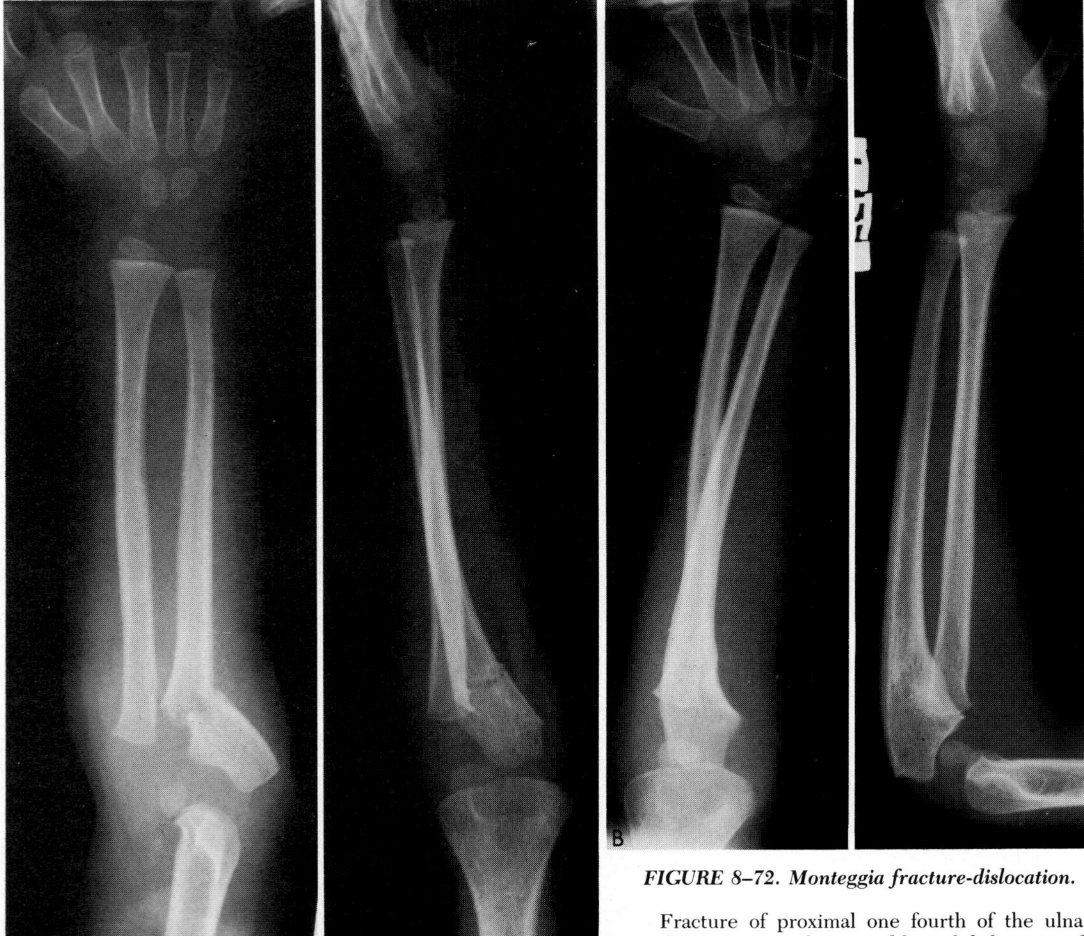

FIGURE 8–72. Monteggia fracture-dislocation.

Fracture of proximal one fourth of the ulna with anterior angulation and lateral dislocation of the radial head was treated by closed reduction. **A.** Initial radiograms. **B.** Radiograms six months later, showing healing and remodeling.

FIGURE 8–73. The role of individual structures in provision of stability to the upper end of the radius.

A. When the annular ligament is intact and all other stabilizing structures are sectioned, the radial head still maintains a normal snug relationship to the ulna in all positions of the forearm—pronation, neutral, and supination.

B. The interosseous membrane, the supinator muscle with its oblique cord, and the lateral ligament of the elbow are removed. The annular ligament is sectioned completely laterally so that the only stabilizing structure intact is the quadrate ligament. In neutral position of the forearm, the radial head fits only loosely in the radial notch. Supination provides a stable relationship as the anterior fibers of the quadrate ligament tauten. In pronation, the posterior fibers of the quadrate ligament are taut and the radial head is held firmly in the radial notch. When limits of rotation are exceeded, disruption takes place.

C and **D.** All structures are removed except the interosseous membrane and the annular ligament. In supination, the interosseous membrane is taut and the radial head is firmly maintained in the radial notch (**C**); in pronation the interosseous membrane is very lax with close approximation of the radius and ulna. The radial head still is maintained in the radial notch.

E. When all structures, except the interosseous membrane, are divided, and the forearm is supinated, the radial head still articulates with the capitellum as shown.

F. When the forearm is pronated, the interosseous membrane is lax and the radial head dislocates laterally.

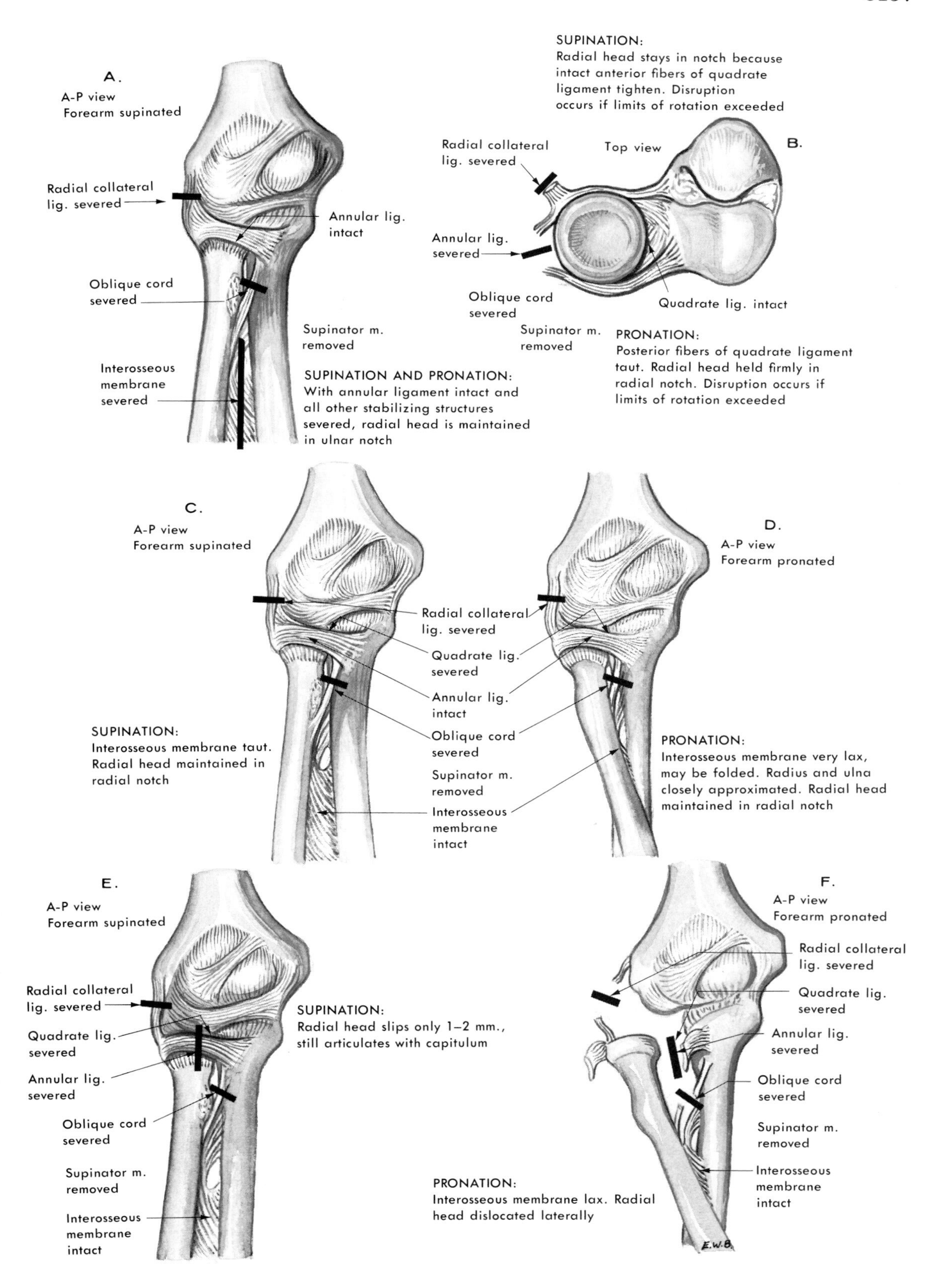
A.
A-P view
Forearm supinated
Radial collateral
lig. severed
Annular lig.
intact
Oblique cord
severed
Supinator m.
removed
Interosseous
membrane
severed
SUPINATION AND PRONATION:
With annular ligament intact and
all other stabilizing structures
severed, radial head is maintained
in ulnar notch
SUPINATION:
Radial head stays in notch because
intact anterior fibers of quadrate
ligament tighten. Disruption
occurs if limits of rotation exceeded
Radial collateral
lig. severed
Top view
B.
Annular lig.
severed
Oblique cord
severed
Quadrate lig. intact
Supinator m.
removed
PRONATION:
Posterior fibers of quadrate ligament
taut. Radial head held firmly in
radial notch. Disruption occurs if
limits of rotation exceeded
C.
A-P view
Forearm supinated
D.
A-P view
Forearm pronated
Radial collateral
lig. severed
Quadrate lig.
severed
Annular lig.
intact
Oblique cord
severed
Supinator m.
removed
Interosseous
membrane
intact
SUPINATION:
Interosseous membrane taut.
Radial head maintained in
radial notch
PRONATION:
Interosseous membrane very lax,
may be folded. Radius and ulna
closely approximated. Radial head
maintained in radial notch
E.
A-P view
Forearm supinated
Radial collateral
lig. severed
Quadrate lig.
severed
Annular lig.
severed
Oblique cord
severed
Supinator m.
removed
Interosseous
membrane
intact
SUPINATION:
Radial head slips only 1–2 mm.,
still articulates with capitulum
F.
A-P view
Forearm pronated
Radial collateral
lig. severed
Quadrate lig.
severed
Annular lig.
severed
Oblique cord
severed
Supinator m.
removed
Interosseous
membrane
intact
PRONATION:
Interosseous membrane lax. Radial
head dislocated laterally
E.W.B.

rior, and lateral dislocation of the radial head with fracture of the shaft of the ulna.[21] In 1909, Perrin suggested that the condition be called *Monteggia fracture*.[75] The eponym *Monteggia lesion* was used by Bado as a more general term to designate various types of dislocation of the radial head in association with fracture of the ulnar shaft.[3, 4] The term *Monteggia equivalent* has been used when the proximal radial epihysis is fracture-separated or the radial neck is fractured instead of the radial head being dislocated.[76] Mechanical considerations have led other authors to include, in Monteggia equivalent, fractures of the ulnar shaft associated with separation of the distal radial physis and lateral condylar fracture with ipsilateral ulnar shaft fracture.[80]

The Monteggia fracture is a rare injury, constituting about 2 per cent of fractures involving the elbow in children. Despite its rarity, this lesion has been the subject of great interest because of its inherent serious complications as a result of having been inadequately treated or having gone unrecognized.

The usual *age incidence* is between seven and ten years; however, it does occur in infants and adolescents.

Classification

There are three basic types of Monteggia fracture: *Type I*, or *extension type*, in which the head of the radius is dislocated anteriorly with volar angulation of the fractured shaft of the ulna (Figs. 8–68 and 8–69); *Type II*, or *flexion type*, in which the radial head is dislocated posteriorly, with dorsal angulation of the fractured shaft of the ulna (Figs. 8–70 and 8–71); and *Type III*, in which the radial head is dislocated laterally with fracture of the shaft of the ulna (Fig. 8–72). Type I is the most common form, accounting for about 85 per cent of cases. Type II accounts for approximately 10 per cent of cases, and Type III for 5 per cent.[24, 88]

Fracture of both bones of the forearm at the same level with anterior dislocation of the radial head is sometimes referred to as Type IV Monteggia fracture. Basically it is a Type I lesion; the radial head dislocates initially and then the radial shaft fractures under the stress of continued hyperextension force.[5]

The level of the fracture varies. In approximately two thirds of the cases, it is located at the junction of the proximal and middle thirds of the shaft; in one sixth of the cases, it is located in the middle third of the shaft; and in the remainder, it is equally distributed between the distal third of the ulnar shaft and the olecranon process.

Mechanism of Injury

The radius and ulna are firmly bound to each other at their upper and lower ends by strong ligaments and throughout their extent by a strong interosseous membrane. The radial head is maintained within the radial notch of the ulna by the strong annular ligament, which is attached to the anterior and posterior margins of the ulnar notch. The quadrate ligament, the radial collateral ligament of the elbow, and the capsule of the elbow joint are the other supporting structures. Of these ligaments the annular ligament is the most important; if all the ligaments except the annular ligament were divided, still the radial head would not dislocate. The quadrate ligament tears with excessive rotation of the forearm. The interosseous ligament is taut in supination and lax in pronation. Hyperpronation of the forearm and excessive laxity of the interosseous ligament will allow the radial head to slip off the annular ligament (Fig. 8–73).[103]

Three theories have been proposed to explain the pathogenesis of the anterior or extension type of Monteggia fracture. The *direct blow* was proposed as the cause by Speed and Boyd and subsequently by Smith.[14, 15, 84, 88]

As the ulna fractures and shortens, it puts stress on the radial head, which becomes dislocated following rupture of the annular ligament. The torn ligament may be loose or may fold in behind the radial head. In certain instances, the radial head may be pulled out from beneath the annular ligament, coming to lie anterior to an intact ligament.

The *hyperpronation theory* was proposed by Evans, who noted that in extension type Monteggia fractures, the skin over the subcutaneous border of the ulna was always intact. He believed Type I Monteggia fracture resulted from hyperpronation during a fall on the outstretched hand, with the body rotating around the fixed and pronated forearm (Fig. 8–74). In a series of experiments on cadavers, he was able to produce fracture of the middle third of the ulna with anterior dislocation of the radial head by subjecting the specimens to hyperpronation. However, Evans stripped the forearm and arm of all soft tissues, save for the capsule and ligaments of the elbow and the interosseous membrane.[28] Bado, in his monograph, supported the theory that Type I Monteggia fracture is a hyperpronation injury.[4]

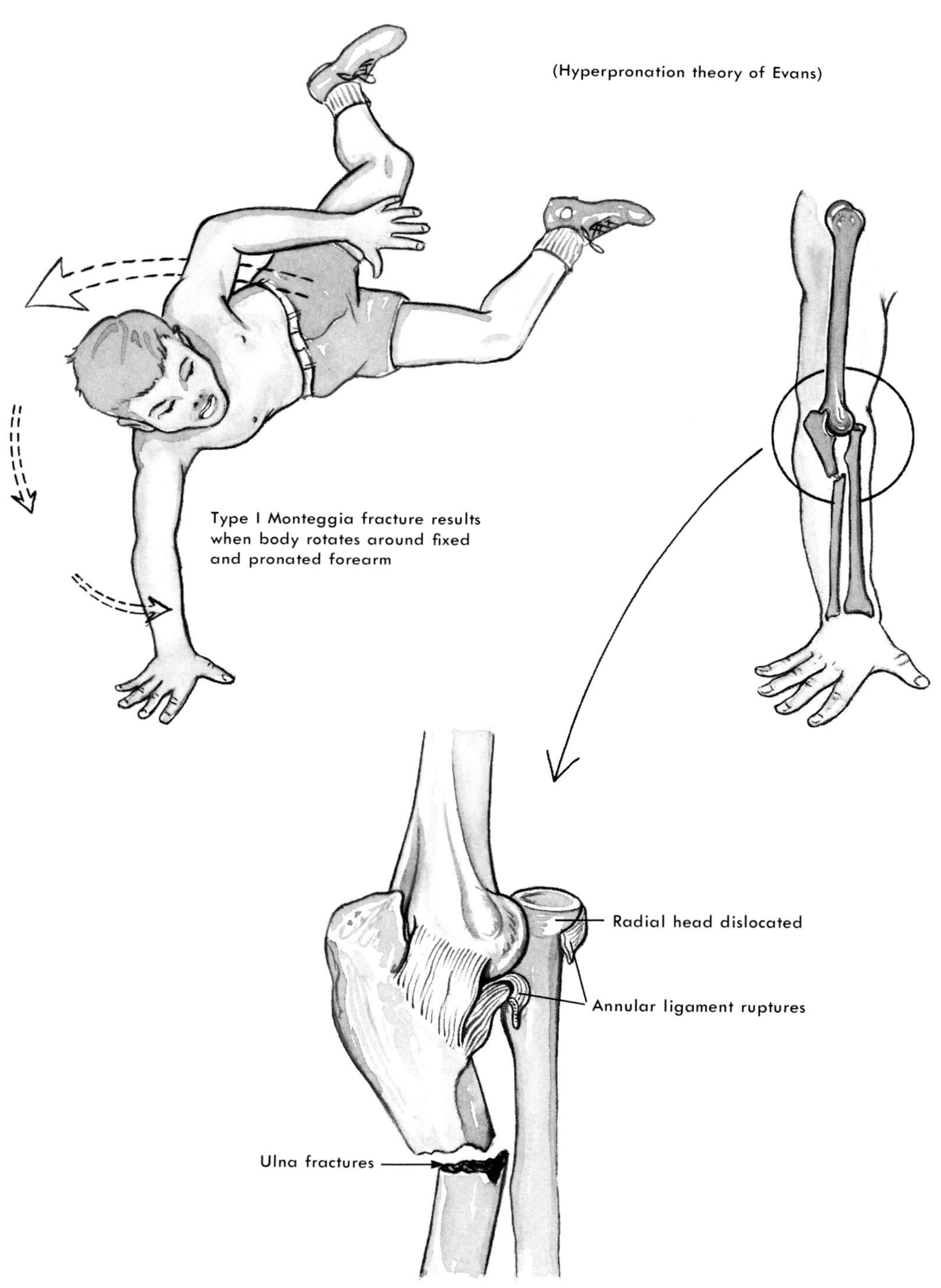

FIGURE 8–74. Mechanism of Type I extension type of Monteggia fracture dislocation.

Hyperpronation theory of Evans. (See text for explanation.)

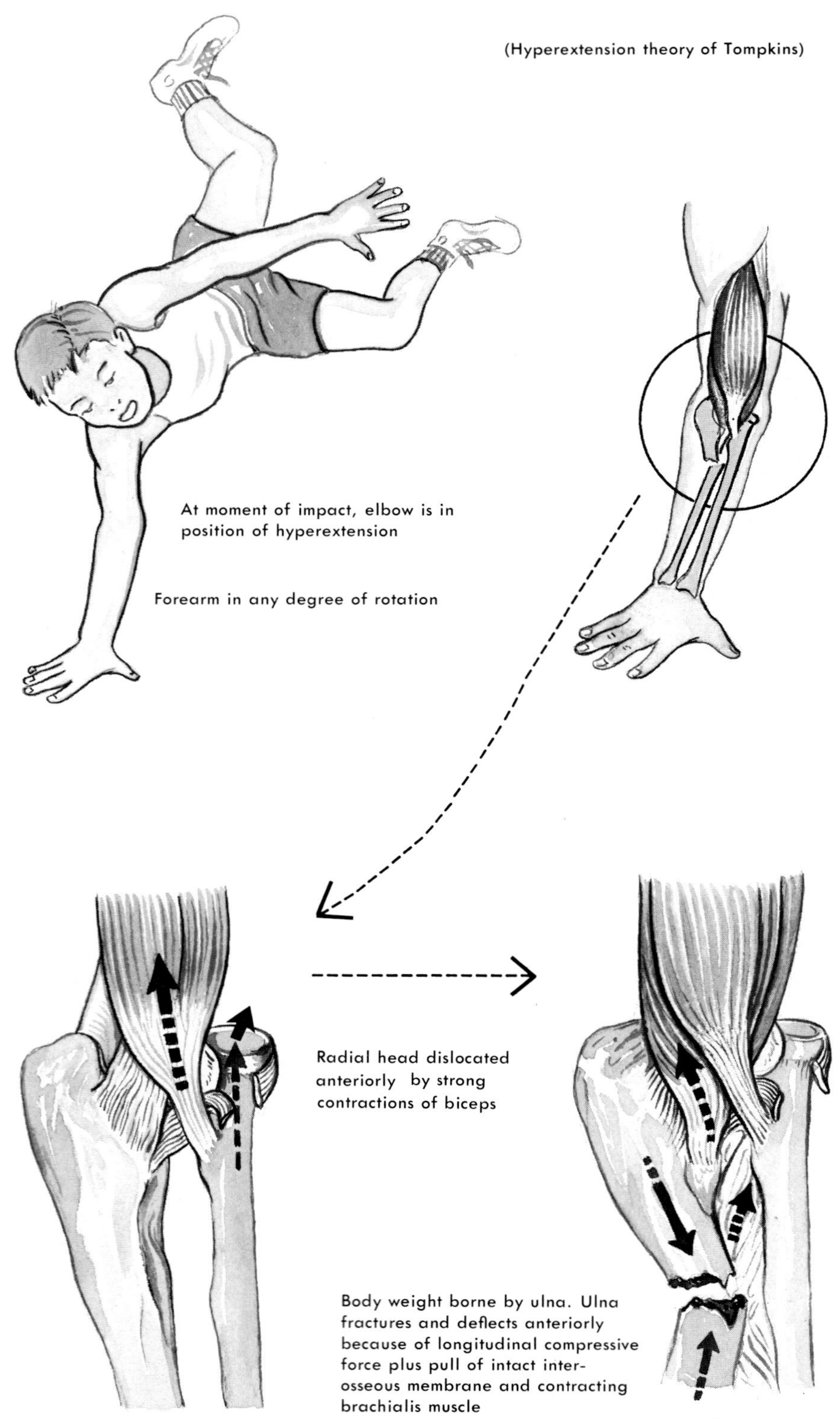

FIGURE 8–75. Hyperextension theory of Tomkins to explain pathogenesis of Type I—extension type—Monteggia fracture dislocation.

(See text for explanation.)

Tompkins objected to both the direct blow and hyperpronation theories, proposing that this fracture is a *hyperextension injury* sustained when the child falls on his outstretched hand with his forearm in any degree of rotation (Fig. 8–75). At the moment of impact, the elbow is in the position of hyperextension. The radial head is dislocated anteriorly by strong contraction of the biceps muscle. When this occurs, all the body weight is borne by the ulna, which fractures and is deflected anteriorly as the result of longitudinal compressive force coupled with the pull of the intact interosseous membrane and the simultaneous contracting brachialis muscle.[97]

The direction of the dislocation of the radial head depends upon the direction of the angulation of the ulna, i.e., with anterior angulation of the fracture of the ulna the radial head displaces anteriorly; on posterior angulation of the fractured ulna the radial head dislocates posteriorly; and on lateral angulation the radial head displaces laterally.

Type II (flexion) Monteggia fracture-dislocation occurs with the elbow in flexion; the forearm may be in pronation, neutral, or in supination.

The pathomechanics of Type III (adduction) Monteggia injury is not clear; there is controversy among authors.[8, 68, 94, 95] The deforming force is proposed to be forced supination by Bado, excessive pronation by Penrose, and forced supination in hyperextension by Wright.[3, 4, 73, 107]

Diagnosis

The patient with a Monteggia fracture usually holds his elbow partially flexed and his forearm in pronation. Any rotation of the forearm or flexion-extension of the elbow is painful and restricted. The elbow is swollen, ecchymotic, and tender. Depending upon the type of Monteggia fracture, the radial head is palpable anterior, posterior, or lateral to its normal location. Palpation of the ulnar diaphysis will reveal the deformity of the angulated fracture with local tenderness. A careful neurologic examination should be performed to rule out injury to the posterior interosseous nerve.

In order to recognize this injury, it is imperative to obtain radiograms of the forearm that include both the elbow and wrist.[16, 36] Whenever forearm radiograms show isolated greenstick or complete fracture of the ulna or when there is plastic bowing of the ulna, make separate anteroposterior and lateral radiograms centered on the elbow. Pay particular attention to detect subluxation or dislocation of the radial head! Normally a line drawn through the longitudinal axis of the radius should pass through the center of the ossification center of the capitellum of the humerus. This occurs regardless of the degree of flexion or extension of the elbow (Fig. 8–76); if it does not, then the radial

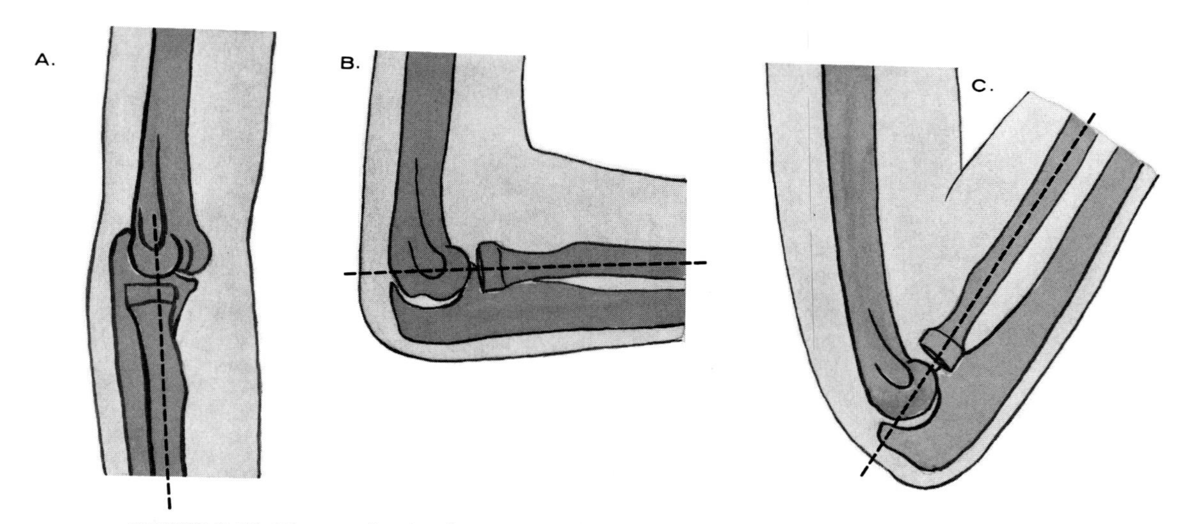

FIGURE 8–76. Diagram showing the anatomic relationship of the radial head to the capitellum of the humerus in the normal elbow.

A to **C.** A line drawn through the longitudinal axis of the radius passes through the center of the ossification center of the humerus.

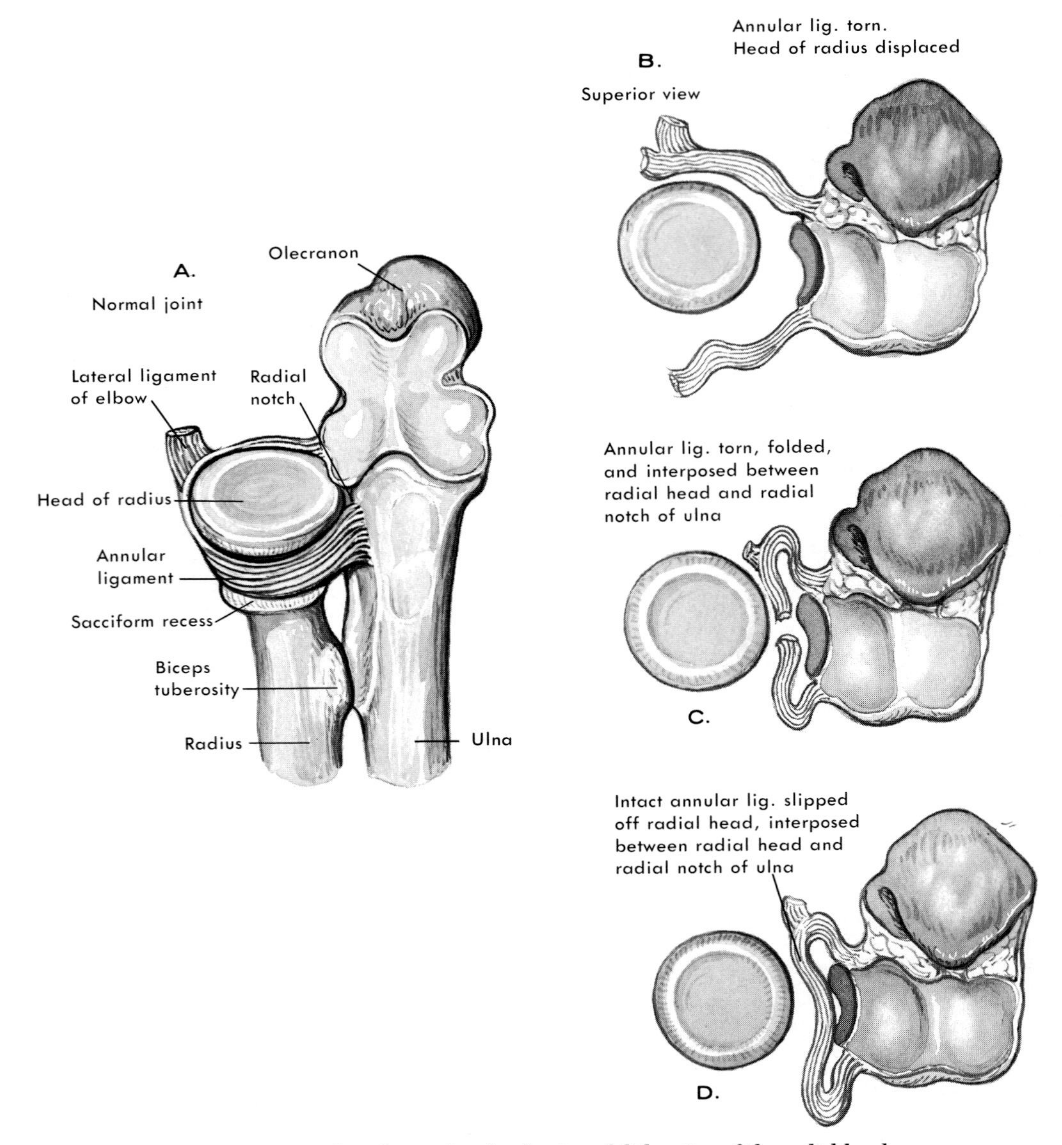

FIGURE 8–77. Obstacles to closed reduction of dislocation of the radial head.

A. Normal proximal radioulnar articulation.
B. The annular ligament is torn but is not interposed between the radial head and the radial notch of the ulna.
C. The annular ligament is torn, folded, and interposed between the radial head and the radial notch of the ulna.
D. The annular ligament is intact, but has slipped off of the radial head and is interposed between the radial head and the radial notch of the ulna.

head is dislocated. Possible associated fractures of the wrist and elbow should always be ruled out.

A diagnostic problem is the possibility of congenital dislocation of the radial head when the injury is old and missed. Congenital dislocations of the radial head are usually bilateral and frequently posterior; in the radiogram the radial head is big, elliptical, or slightly irregular. The radius is too long and the capitellum of the humerus is flattened.[19] Lloyd-Roberts and Bucknill proposed that all unilateral dislocations (particularly anterior) are acquired—post-traumatic and not congenital.[59]

Treatment

Early closed reduction is usually successful in children. This is most possibly due to the pathologic anatomy. In children it appears that either the tear of the annular ligament is transverse and not longitudinal (which occurs in the adult) and the orbicularis ligament is avulsed from the ulna rather than torn. Ordinarily reduction of Monteggia fracture-dislocation is performed under general anesthesia.

The *anterior Monteggia fracture* (Type I) is reduced as follows: With the forearm in full supination, longitudinal traction is applied first; then the elbow is gently flexed to beyond 90 degrees to relax the biceps muscle. The radial head is gently repositioned by direct manual pressure anteriorly on the bone (see Fig. 8–68 B). The angulated ulnar shaft is reduced by firm manual pressure; this is rarely difficult once the radial head has been repositioned. Following reduction, the radial head will be quite stable as long as the elbow is kept in acute flexion.

Tompkins has pointed out that, subsequent to reduction during immobilization, the ulnar fracture has a tendency to develop an increasing radial bow; this is caused by the normal slight bowing of the ulna, by the contraction of the flexor muscles in the forearm, and perhaps by the anconeus muscle. Tompkins recommends immobilization of the forearm in neutral rotation in only slight supination, with the cast carefully molded over the lateral side of the ulna at the level of the fracture (see Fig. 8–68 C). As long as the elbow is in acute flexion (110 degrees) and the biceps is relaxed, it will not be necessary to keep the forearm in full supination to maintain the reduction.[97]

Posterior (Type II) Monteggia fracture is reduced by applying traction to the forearm with the elbow in full extension. The radial head is reduced manually (see Fig. 8–70 B). The posterior angulated ulnar fracture is anatomically aligned, and an above-elbow cast is applied with the elbow in full extension and the forearm in neutral rotation (see Fig. 8–70 C).

Lateral (Type III) Monteggia fracture-dislocation is reduced with the elbow in extension. Apply direct pressure over the radial head and radial border of the ulna. Reduction is achieved by exerting longitudinal traction on the distal forearm. A well-molded above-elbow cast is applied with the elbow in 90 degrees of flexion and the forearm in supination.

Type IV Monteggia fracture is extremely rare in children. Reduction of Type IV fracture is similar to that for Type I.

Immobilization is maintained until there is union of the ulna; this ordinarily requires five to seven weeks, depending upon the age of the patient.

OPERATIVE TREATMENT

Occasionally open reduction is indicated when one is unable to achieve or maintain anatomic reduction by closed methods. The obstacles to closed reduction are (1) interposition of torn portions of the ruptured orbicularis ligament; (2) the intact annular ligament slipped off the radial head and interposed between the radial head and the radial notch of the ulna (Fig. 8–77); and (3) interposition of a cartilaginous or osteochondral fragment in the radial notch of the ulna.

In order to detect redislocation or subluxation it is important to repeat radiograms in three to four days postreduction and then again in seven to ten days postreduction. Loose casts should be changed and a snug cast should be reapplied. It is crucial to maintain anatomic reduction of the radial head. Minor angular deformities (5 to 10 degrees) of the ulna can be accepted as they will correct with remodeling.

Open reduction of the radial head is carried out through the Boyd surgical approach, and the annular ligament is repaired as shown in Plate 122. The angulated fracture of the ulna is reduced and fixed internally with one or two smooth Steinmann pins or a four-hole plate. When marked swelling of the elbow does not allow elbow flexion to 90 degrees or more, it is best to fix the radiohumeral joint by a Steinmann pin inserted percutaneously through the capitellum into the radial head. The Steinmann pin should be of adequate diameter in order to prevent breakage of the pin; also, it is safer to apply an above-elbow cast and immobilize the shoulder with a sling and Ace bandage around the

Text continued on page 3168

Surgical Exposure of the Proximal Radioulnar Joint and Repair of Avulsed Annular Ligament

OPERATIVE TECHNIQUE

A. The incision begins over the lateral epicondyle of the humerus and extends distally and posteriorly along the interval between the anconeus and the extensor carpi ulnaris muscles and ends medially at the subcutaneous margin of the upper one fourth of the ulna. The subcutaneous tissue and fascia are divided in line with the skin incision. The wound flaps are mobilized and retracted.

B. The interval between the anconeus and extensor carpi ulnaris muscles is developed, and dissection is extended down to the capsule of the elbow joint.

C. The anconeus muscle is detached partially to permit mobilization and facilitate further exposure of the joint. A longitudinal incision is made in the capsule.

D. The elbow joint is exposed, and the pathology is assessed. Note that in this drawing the annular ligament is avulsed and interposed between the radial head and the radial notch of the ulna.

Plate 122. Surgical Exposure of the Proximal Radioulnar Joint and Repair of Avulsed Annular Ligament

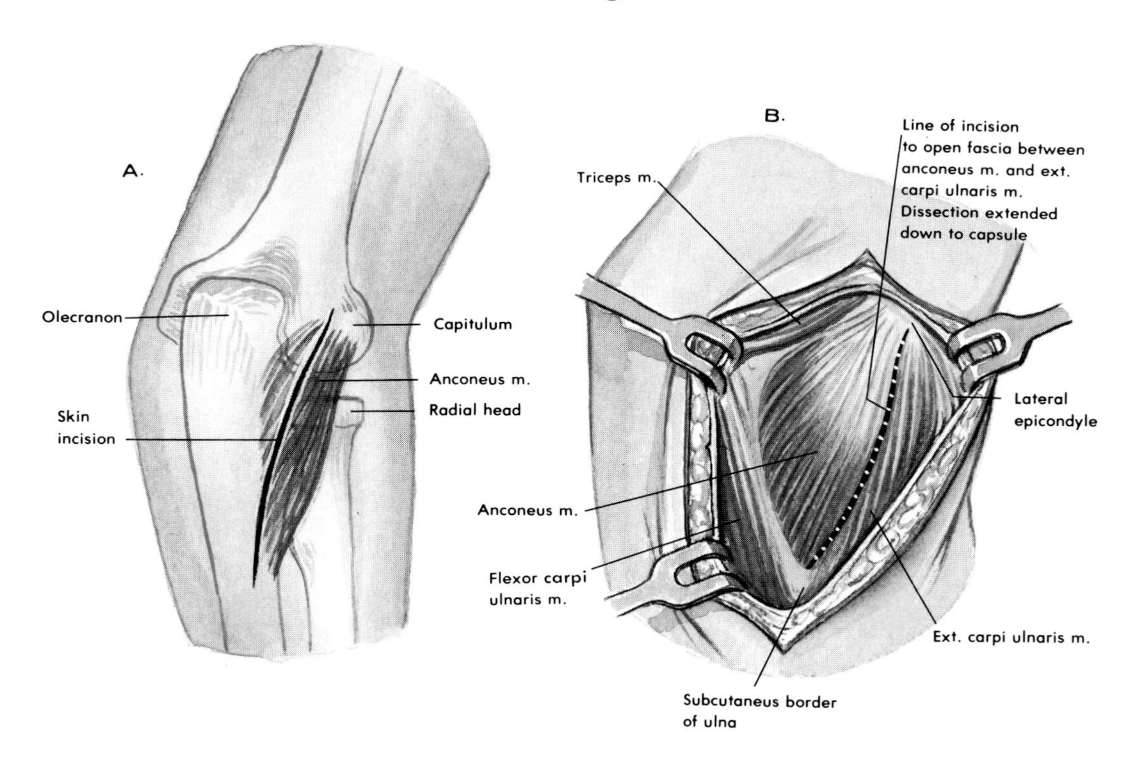

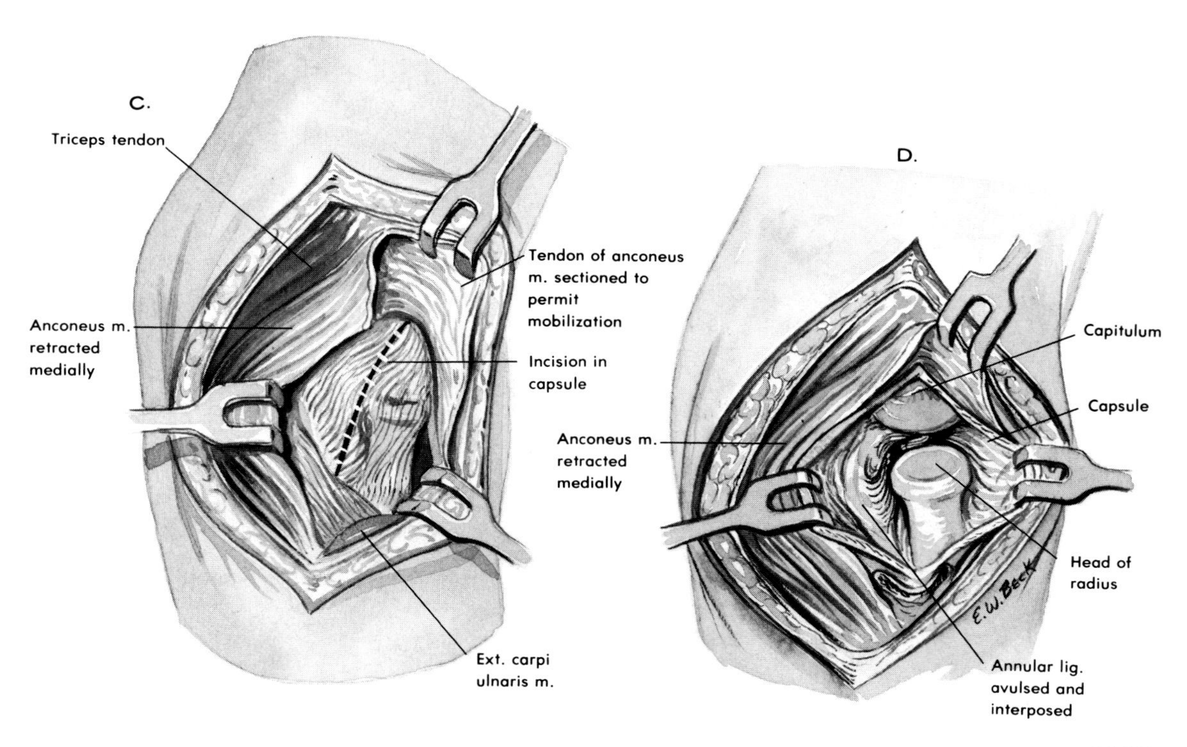

Surgical Exposure of the Proximal Radioulnar Joint and Repair of Avulsed Annular Ligament *(Continued)*

E. If the annular ligament is torn, interposed segments are freed with tissue forceps. The ends of the annular ligament are brought around the head of the radius and secured with interrupted sutures.

F. If the annular ligament is intact and interposed between the head of the radius and the radial notch of the ulna, use a Freer elevator to restore its position around the radial head.

G. If the annular ligament is intact but cannot be freed, make a vertical incision, bring the ends around the radial head, and join them with interrupted sutures.

The wound is closed in the usual fashion and an above-elbow cast is applied, with the elbow in 90 degrees of flexion and the forearm in full supination.

POSTOPERATIVE CARE

The cast is removed in four to six weeks, and gently, active-assisted exercises are performed to restore normal range of elbow motion.

Plate 122. Surgical Exposure of the Proximal Radioulnar Joint and Repair of Avulsed Annular Ligament

E.

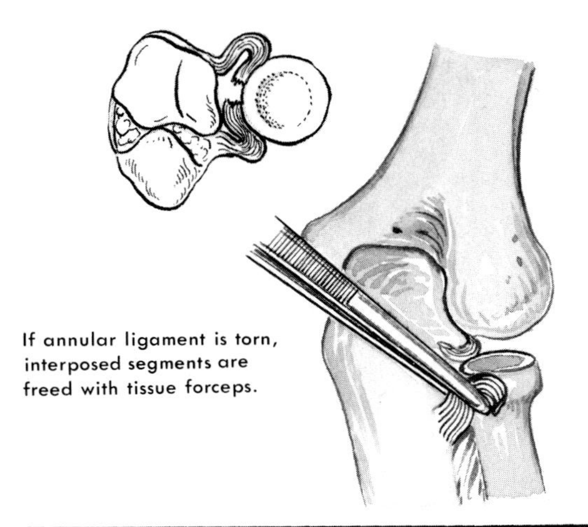

If annular ligament is torn, interposed segments are freed with tissue forceps.

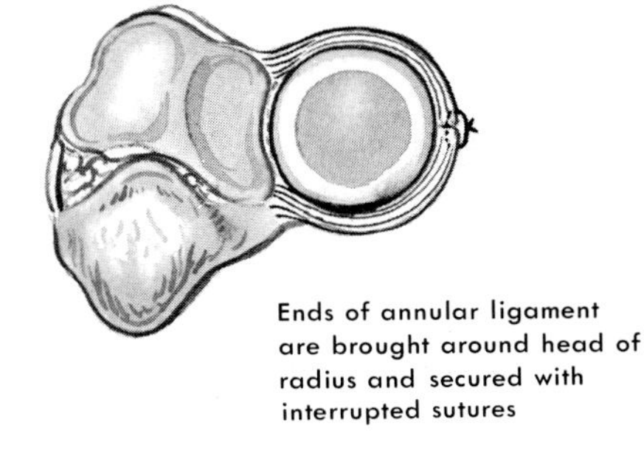

Ends of annular ligament are brought around head of radius and secured with interrupted sutures

F.

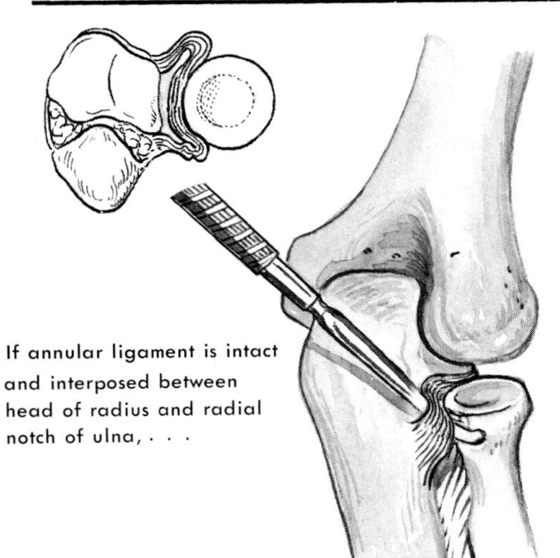

If annular ligament is intact and interposed between head of radius and radial notch of ulna, . . .

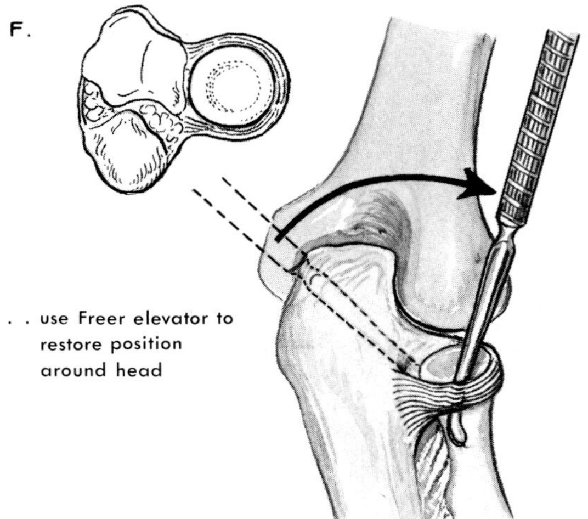

. . . use Freer elevator to restore position around head

G.

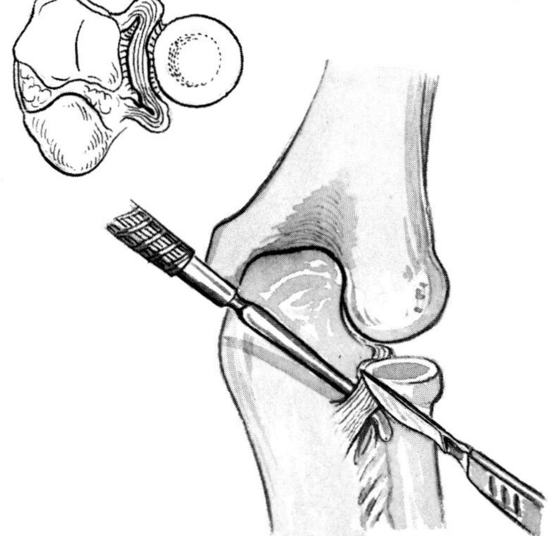

If annular ligament is intact but cannot be freed intact from interposed position, make vertical incision, bring ends around head of radius, and join ends with interrupted sutures

chest or a Velpeau cast. The Steinmann pins are removed in three weeks; a second above-elbow cast is applied with the elbow in 90 to 100 degrees of flexion for an additional two weeks. Then the cast is removed and active-assisted range of motion exercises are performed. Open reduction of the radial head and repair of the annular ligament always carry the risk of traumatic ossification.

In instances when the diagnosis of Monteggia fracture is delayed, open surgery is required to reduce the radial head. Closed reduction should not be attempted when two weeks have lapsed since the injury. Avoid the temptation of multiple attempts of closed reduction as they are harmful, resulting in traumatic myositis ossificans and ankylosis of the elbow or proximal radioulnar joint. Open surgery is gentler and safer.

In the event that more than two to three weeks have elapsed from the time of injury, adequate repair of the annular ligament is not feasible because of scar tissue formation. This author recommends a strip of the triceps fascia to repair the annular ligament, as advocated by Bell Tawse and Lloyd-Roberts.[9, 59] A central strip of the triceps tendon is utilized by Bell Tawse and a lateral strip of the triceps is recommended by Lloyd-Roberts. The operative technique is described and illustrated in Plate 123.

When the diagnosis is made late, this author recommends open reduction of the dislocated radial head with radial shortening and osteotomy of the ulna to correct its angular deformity. The annular ligament is reconstructed with a strip of triceps tendon. The operative technique is described and illustrated in Plate 124.

Another method of spontaneous closed reduction of the dislocated radius is by elongation of the ulna by the Ilizarov technique.[60, 83] This author has no personal experience in this method of treatment of Monteggia fracture-dislocation.

This author will consider reduction of Monteggia fracture-dislocation even several years following injury. Leaving the radial head dislocated anteriorly will result in progressive cubitus valgus deformity, radial collateral elbow ligament instability, limitation of flexion of the elbow, and tardy ulnar nerve palsy (Fig. 8–78).

Excision of the radial head will improve elbow flexion; however, this should not be performed in a child as it will cause cubitus valgus, prominence of the distal end of the ulna, and radial deviation of the wrist. Removal of the radial head should be deferred until completion of skeletal growth. Long-term results of radial head excision are secondary subluxation and mechanical derangement of the distal radioulnar joint.

Complications

These include (1) posterior interosseous radial nerve palsy from anterior or lateral displacement of the radial head; (2) malunion of fracture of the ulnar shaft; (3) radiohumeral fibrous ankylosis; (4) radioulnar synostosis; (5) recurrence of radial head dislocation; (6) myositis ossificans; and (7) Volkmann's ischemic contracture.

NERVE PALSY

The posterior interosseous nerve passes beneath the fibrous arch of the supinator muscle (arcade of Frohser). This is the most superior part of the superficial head of the supinator muscle, extending between the tip and medial portion of the lateral epicondyle. The sensory branch of the posterior interosseous nerve separates before the nerve courses beneath the arcade of Frohser but its motor branch is tethered under the arcade. Therefore, a pure motor deficit with intact sensation is produced by a compressive lesion, and a combined motor and sensory deficit is caused by stretching lesions.[91] Transitory posterior interosseous nerve palsy occurs in about 20 per cent of anterior or lateral Monteggia fracture-dislocations. Almost all of the nerve lesions are neurapraxia or axonotmesis and not neurotmesis. Nerve function usually returns in two to three months following injury. Therefore, surgical exploration of the nerves is not indicated; treatment should be conservative expectant observation.[1, 27, 39, 43, 58, 87, 90, 91]

In the literature there is a case report of irreducible Monteggia lesion with radial nerve entrapment.[67] When serial electromyography studies in six and ten weeks show no return of function, magnetic resonance imaging of both elbows is performed to delineate the pathology. Neurosurgical evaluation is carried out; if the nerve is compressed under the arcade of Frohser, the fibrous arch of the supinator muscle is sectioned. In the experience of this author all posterior interosseous nerve palsies secondary to Monteggia fracture-dislocations have fully recovered.

RECURRENCE OF RADIAL HEAD DISLOCATION

When this complication develops, an attempt of closed reduction may be made; if unsuccess-

Text continued on page 3178

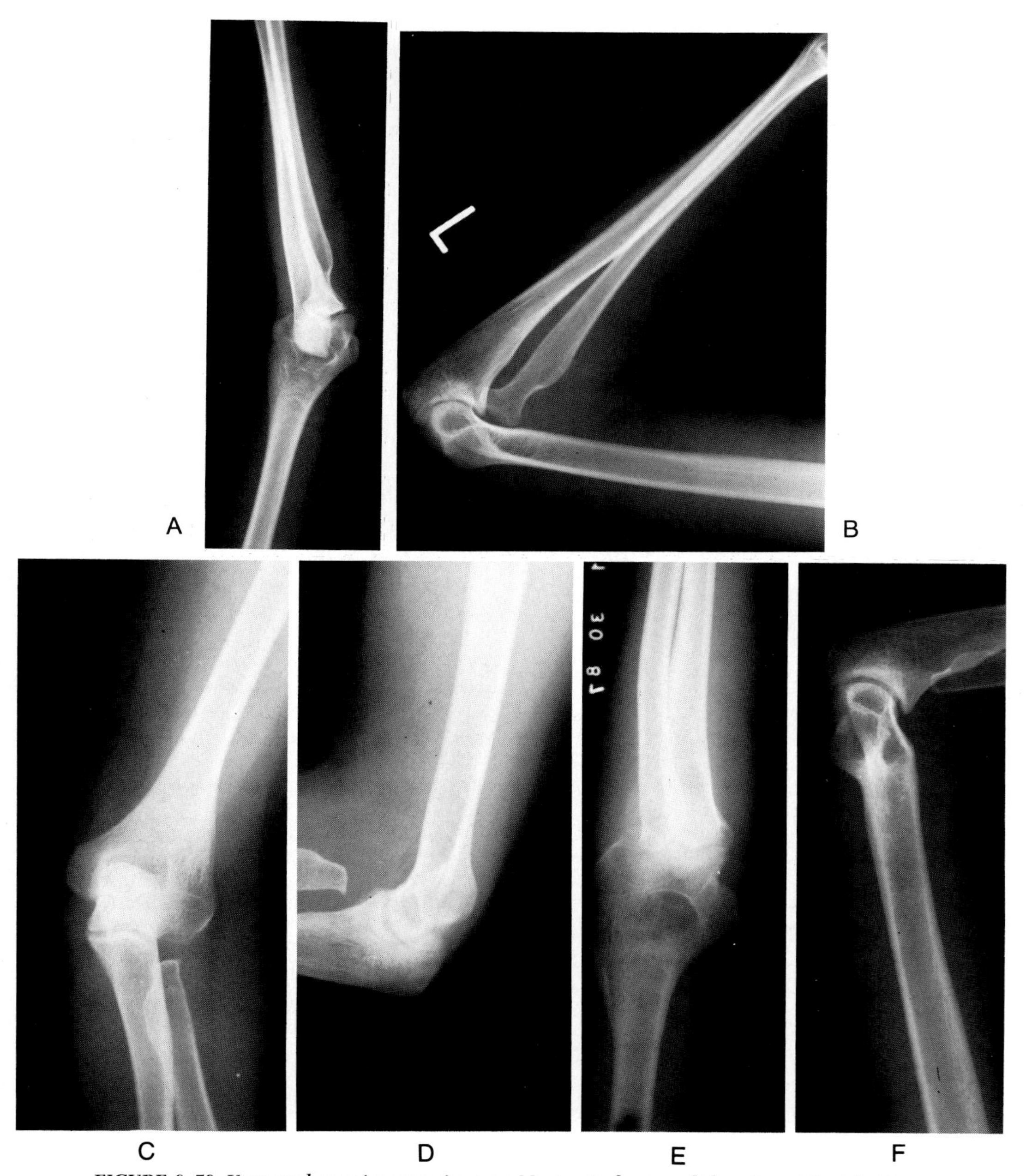

FIGURE 8–78. Untreated anterior extension type Monteggia fracture dislocation of the left elbow.

A and **B.** Anteroposterior and lateral radiograms of the left elbow. Patient had severe cubitus valgus with tardy ulnar nerve palsy.

C and **D.** Radial head was excised and ulnar nerve transposed anteriorly. Six months later a varus osteotomy of the distal humerus was performed to correct the cubitus valgus deformity.

E and **F.** Anteroposterior and lateral radiograms of the left elbow showing normal alignment. The patient is symptom free.

Open Reduction of Dislocation of the Radial Head in Monteggia Fracture-Dislocation and Reconstruction of the Annular Ligament with a Strip of Triceps Fascia

OPERATIVE TECHNIQUE

A. The incision begins 5 to 7 cm. proximal to the tip of the olecranon, curving slightly laterally at the elbow joint toward the radial neck for a distance of 5 cm. The subcutaneous tissue and fascia are divided in line with the skin incision. The wound flaps are retracted, exposing the triceps tendon, flexor carpi ulnaris, anconeus, and extensor carpi ulnaris muscles.

B. The fascia between the anconeus and extensor carpi ulnaris muscles is divided, and an incision made over the insertion of the anconeus muscle.

C. The anconeus muscle is freed from its lateral and medial attachments and elevated proximally. *Caution!* Preserve its nerve and blood supply. The extensor carpi ulnaris muscle is retracted laterally and the flexor carpi ulnaris muscle is retracted medially so that the capsule of the elbow joint is exposed. A longitudinal incision is made in the capsule.

D. The capsule is opened, and the dislocated radial head with the torn annular ligament is exposed.

Plate 123. Open Reduction of Dislocation of the Radial Head in Monteggia Fracture-Dislocation and Reconstruction of the Annular Ligament with a Strip of Triceps Fascia

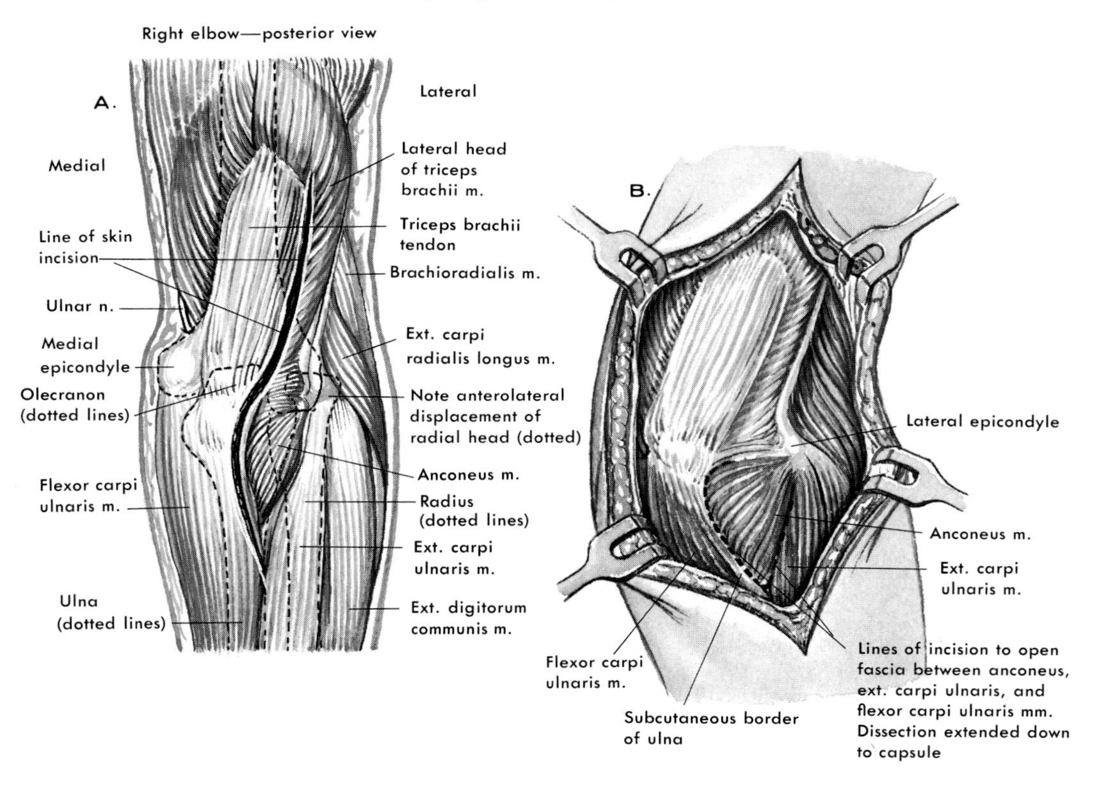

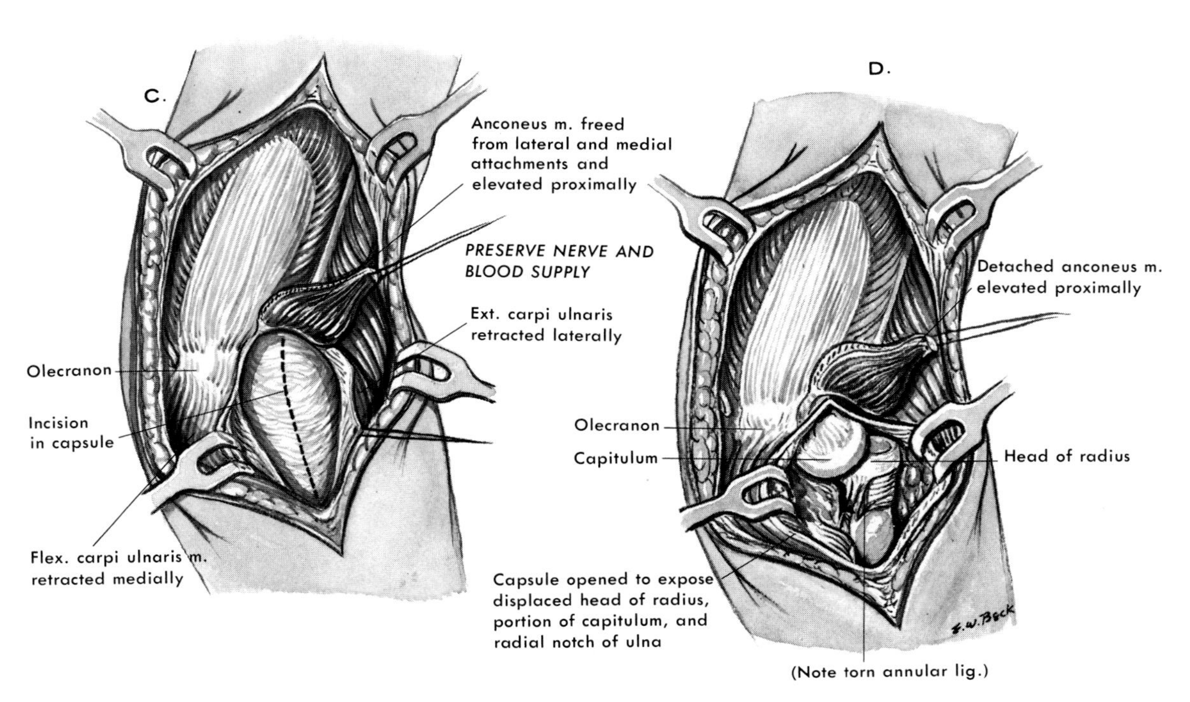

Open Reduction of Dislocation of the Radial Head in Monteggia Fracture-Dislocation and Reconstruction of the Annular Ligament with a Strip of Triceps Fascia (*Continued*)

E. The radial head is reduced, and the torn, irreparable remains of the annular ligament are excised. Next, the triceps tendon is cleared of surrounding connective tissue, and a strip, 1 cm. × 6 cm., from the lateral side of the triceps tendon is detached. Leave its distal attachments intact. The strip of triceps tendon should include the periosteum of the ulna, and the hinge should be at the level of the reduced radial neck.

F. A drill hole is made in the proximal ulna at a level with the neck of the radius.

G. The triceps tendon strip is passed around the neck of the radius through the drill hole in the ulna and sutured to the periosteum of the ulna and to itself; thereby, a new annular ligament is reconstructed.

H. The capsule is closed with interrupted sutures.

I. A stout, smooth Kirschner wire is drilled into the capitulum of the humerus into the center of the radial head and the proximal half of the radial shaft. The anconeus muscle is resutured to the periosteum of the ulna and fascia of the extensor carpi ulnaris.

The wound is closed, the tip of the Kirschner wire is bent to prevent migration, and an above-the-elbow cast is applied holding the elbow in 90 degrees of flexion.

POSTOPERATIVE CARE

The cast is removed four weeks after surgery, and the Kirschner wire is taken out. Radiograms are made to assess concentricity of reduction of the radial head in the radial notch of the ulna, and another above-the-elbow cast is applied for an additional two weeks. The cast is then removed, and active-assisted exercises are performed to restore range of motion of the elbow joint.

Plate 123. Open Reduction of Dislocation of the Radial Head in Monteggia Fracture-Dislocation and Reconstruction of the Annular Ligament with a Strip of Triceps Fascia

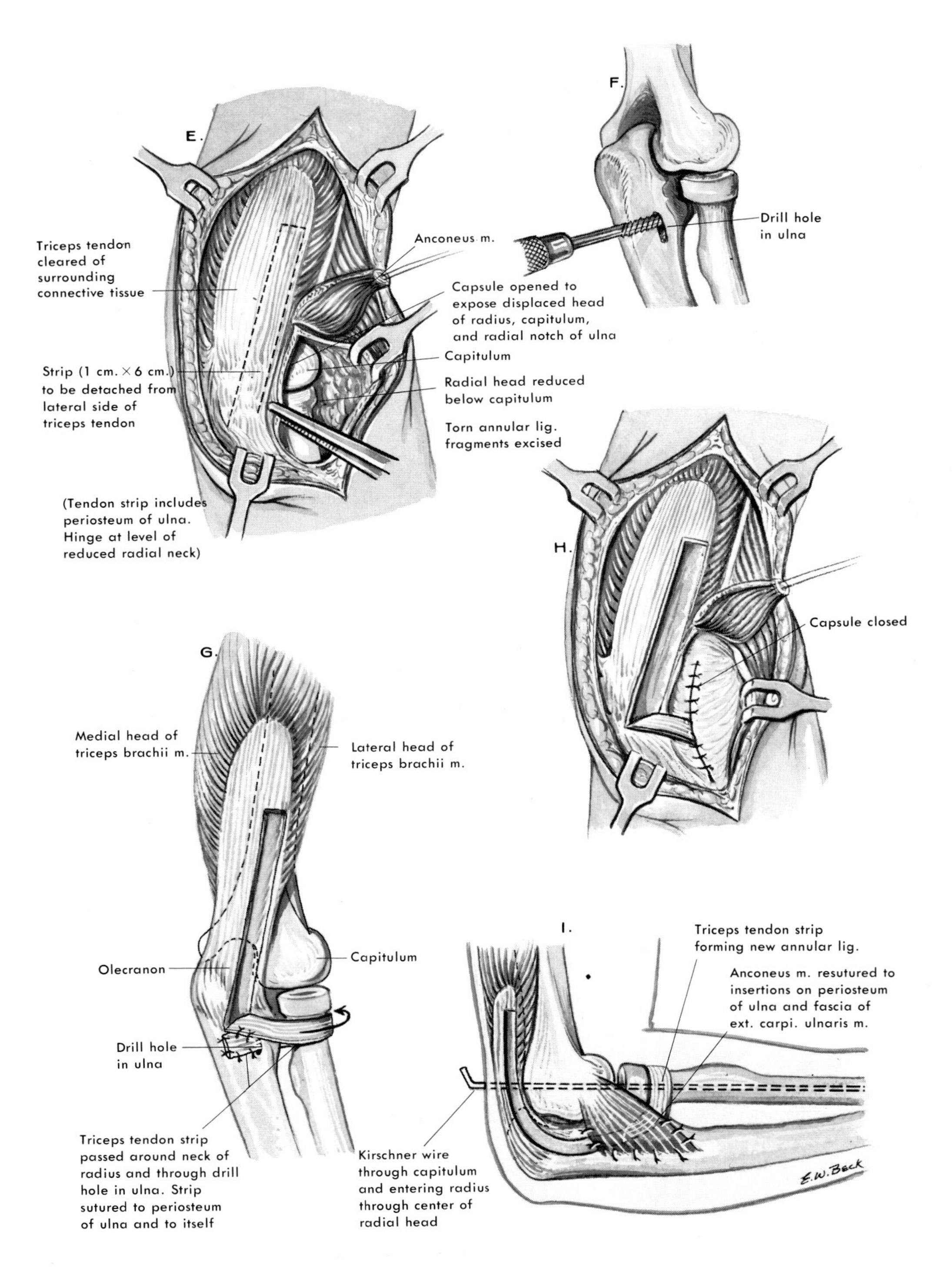

Open Reduction of Dislocated Radial Head in Monteggia Fracture-Dislocation with Reconstruction of the Annular Ligament with a Strip of Triceps Tendon and Shortening of the Radius and Osteotomy of the Ulna to Correct Angular Deformity

OPERATIVE TECHNIQUE

A. The incision is made 7 cm. above the lateral epicondyle of the humerus and extended distally to the lateral epicondyle, where it is curved posteriorly and medially toward the ulna and terminates at the middle of the ulnar shaft. The subcutaneous tissue and fascia are divided in line with the skin incision. The wound flaps are retracted.

B. The triceps tendon, anconeus, flexor carpi ulnaris, and extensor carpi ulnaris muscles are exposed. Incisions are made between the fascia of anconeus and extensor carpi ulnaris and between the anconeus and flexor carpi ulnaris muscles. Dissection is extended to the capsule of the elbow joint.

C. The anconeus muscle is detached from its lateral and medial insertions and is retracted proximally. The supinator muscle is divided from its insertion to the ulna and radius. Caution! Preserve the nerve supply to the aconeus muscle, and do not injure the posterior interosseous nerve.

D. The pathology of the proximal radioulnar joint is assessed. Often the orbicularis ligament is shredded to pieces and the interosseous ligament is torn and scarred.

Plate 124. Open Reduction of Dislocated Radial Head in Monteggia Fracture-Dislocation with Reconstruction of the Annular Ligament with a Strip of Triceps Tendon and Shortening of the Radius and Osteotomy of the Ulna to Correct Angular Deformity

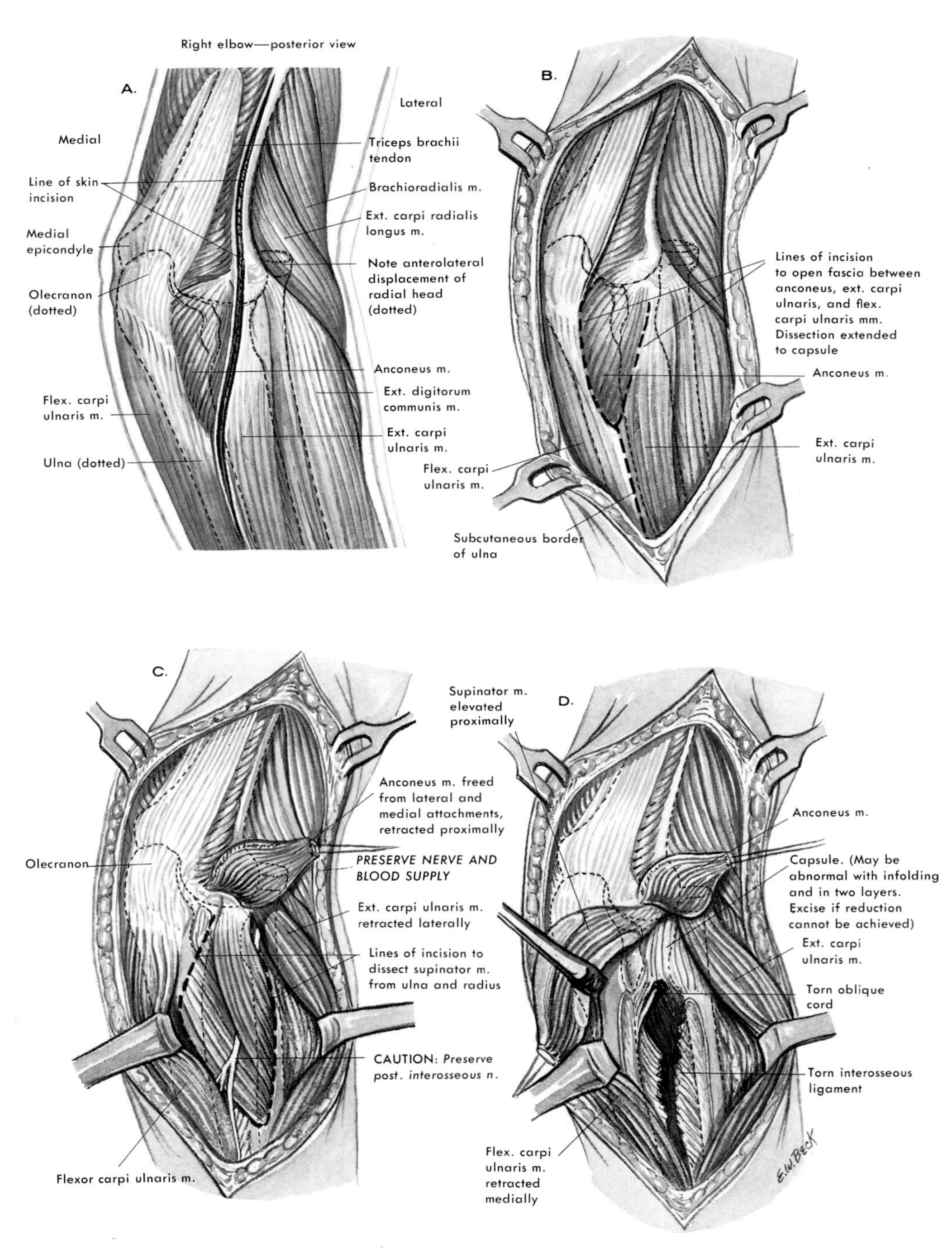

Open Reduction of Dislocated Radial Head in Monteggia Fracture-Dislocation with Reconstruction of the Annular Ligament with a Strip of Triceps Tendon and Shortening of the Radius and Osteotomy of the Ulna to Correct Angular Deformity (Continued)

E. Prior to reconstructing an annular ligament, inspect and assess the deformation of the ulna and radius. The angular deformity of the malunited ulna should be corrected first by osteotomy and internal fixation with a four-hole plate or an intramedullary Steinmann pin. If the radius is relatively long in relation to the ulna, one has two options: (1) instantaneous elongation of the ulna with simultaneous correction of the angular deformity, or (2) shortening of the radius. This author recommends shortening of the radius at its mid-diaphysis through a separate incision; internal fixation is with a four- or six-hole AO plate.

F. In this illustration, the shortening of the radius is at its proximal third and through the same incision. After the radius is shortened, the radial head is easily reduced in its anatomic position. Reconstruction of the annular ligament is similar to that described in Plate 123. Fixation is accomplished with a Kirschner wire, which is introduced retrograde through the osteotomy site of the midshaft of the radius and inserted up the radial head to its articular surface.

G. At this stage, loop the strip of triceps tendon around the radial neck, from medial to lateral; pass through a drill hole in the ulna; and suture to itself.

H, I. After the anatomic reduction of the radial head is checked, the pin is drilled through the capitellum of the humerus out through the skin. The shortened segment of the radius in its mid-diaphysis is then aligned, and the Kirschner wire is drilled into the distal segment of the radial shaft. Sometimes, in the adolescent, this author has found it simpler to fix the shortened radius at its midshaft with a four-hole plate and to fix the radius to the capitellum separately by a percutaneous pin. In the experience of this author, shortening of the radius has increased the range of pronation and supination of the forearm. The wound is closed in the usual fashion and an above-the-elbow cast is applied, with the elbow in 90 degrees of flexion and the forearm in full supination.

POSTOPERATIVE CARE

The capitellum-radius transfixation pin is removed in three to four weeks postoperatively, and the elbow is immobilized for an additional two weeks. Then active exercises are performed to restore range of motion of the elbow and forearm.

Plate 124. Open Reduction of Dislocated Radial Head in Monteggia Fracture-Dislocation with Reconstruction of the Annular Ligament with a Strip of Triceps Tendon and Shortening of the Radius and Osteotomy of the Ulna to Correct Angular Deformity

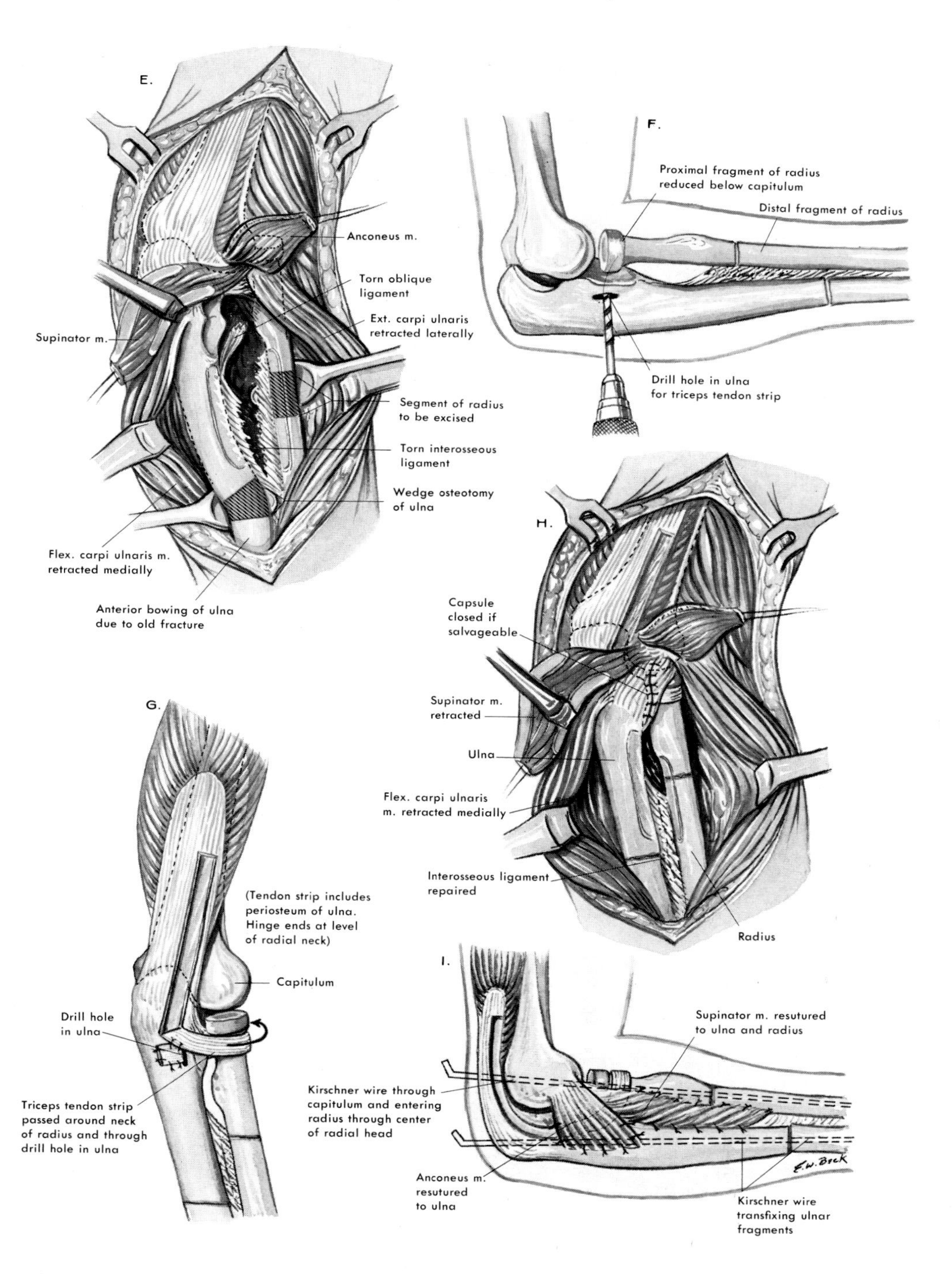

ful, one should immediately proceed to open reduction, internal fixation, and possibly a Bell Tawse procedure if necessary.

MALUNION OF THE FRACTURE OF THE ULNAR SHAFT

Anterior or posterior angulation of 10 to 15 degrees does not cause any functional impairment. Radial deviation and encroachment of the interosseous space, however, can restrict pronation-supination of the forearm. The ulna is abducted during pronation and adducted during supination.[81] Initially Bado believed that the contraction and pull of the anconeus is a deforming force in producing abduction of the ulna; however, electromyography studies by Basmajian showed only moderate periodicity of the anconeus and did not support this theory.[4, 6, 81] When there is marked radial deviation and restriction of rotation of the forearm, corrective osteotomy is indicated.

RADIOULNAR SYNOSTOSIS

This may be fibrous or bony between the proximal ulna and radius.[17] After appropriate computed tomography studies, one may attempt resection of the synostosis and fat interposition as a spacer; however, in the experience of this author the results have not been satisfactory. There has been no improvement in the range of pronation-supination of the forearm. It is best in these cases to leave the forearm in neutral rotation and allow shoulder motions to compensate for the loss of forearm rotation.

RADIOHUMERAL FIBROUS ANKYLOSIS

This occurs when repeated attempts of closed reduction are made, especially in the later diagnosed cases. Treatment consists of continuous passive motion of the elbow.

PARA-ARTICULAR ECTOPIC OSSIFICATION

This is best left alone and not resected.

VOLKMANN'S ISCHEMIC CONTRACTURE

It is the policy of this author to admit all patients with Monteggia fracture-dislocations to the hospital after reduction and observe circulatory status very closely, because Volkmann's ischemic contracture may occur.[7] At particular risk are patients treated by acute flexion of the swollen elbow after closed reduction of Type I (extension) Monteggia fracture.

PROBLEMS AND COMPLICATIONS OF TREATMENT

The transcapitellar-radial pin across the elbow joint can break or migrate (if smooth). In some cases there is no alternative approach for security of maintaining reduction; it is a calculated risk one must take. However, steps can be taken to prevent these problems: (1) use a Steinmann pin of adequate diameter, and not a Kirschner wire; (2) provide secure immobilization in a cast—the cast should extend high on the arm, and in the restless child utilize an additional soft Velpeau bandage, a sling, or an Ace bandage around the chest; (3) bend the tip of the Steinmann pin to prevent migration.

The posterior interosseous nerve can easily be divided during operation; stay posterior and pronate the forearm.

Monteggia Equivalent Lesions of the Forearm

These are variants of Type I (flexion) injury and include the following:

1. *Anterior dislocation of the radial head.* The mechanism of injury is hyperpronation. Rule out plastic bowing of the ulna by making true lateral radiograms of both forearms. Treatment consists of closed reduction under general anesthesia with the forearm in full supination and direct thumb pressure on the radial head. Immobilization is in an above-elbow cast with the elbow flexed 100 to 110 degrees. Occasionally open reduction is required.

2. *Anterior dislocation of the radial head with anterior plastic bowing of the ulna.* Treatment is the same as described for anterior dislocation. If the radial head is unstable and redislocates because of marked anterior bending of the ulna, one may have to correct the ulnar deformity by osteotomy through a percutaneous corticotomy.

3. *Anterior dislocation of the radial neck with fracture of the olecranon.* Treatment follows the same principles as outlined for Type I injury. A displaced olecranon fracture may require open reduction and intramedullary fixation.

4. *Fracture of the ulna with fracture-separation of the proximal radial epiphysis.* Instead of the radial head being dislocated, the proximal radial epiphysis is separated. Most of these radial physeal injuries are Salter-Harris Type II. In the adolescent the radial neck may fracture. Treat this as a Type I injury. Open reduction of the radial neck fracture may be required if the angulation is greater than 45 degrees.

5. *Anterior dislocation of the radial head associated with fracture of the ulna and fracture separation of the distal radial epiphysis.*[54, 95] It is vital to examine thoroughly and make radiograms of the wrist to rule out associated injuries of the distal radius (or ulna) in Monteggia fractures.

References

1. Austin, R.: Tardy palsy of the radial nerve from a Monteggia fracture. Injury, *7*:262, 1976.
2. Bachiocco, R., Sgarbi, G., DeSessa, L., and Costa, C.: Monteggia's lesions in the child. Chir. Organi Mov., *63*:31, 1976.
3. Bado, J. L.: The Monteggia Lesion. Springfield, Ill., Charles C Thomas, 1962.
4. Bado, J. L.: The Monteggia lesion. Clin. Orthop., *50*:71, 1967.
5. Barquet, A., and Caresani, J.: Fracture of the shaft of the ulna and radius with associated dislocation of the radial head. Injury, *12*:471, 1980.
6. Basmajian, J. V., and Griffin, W. R., Jr.: Function of anconeus muscle. J. Bone Joint Surg., *54-A*:1712, 1972.
7. Baumann, E.: Mutilation of hand and arm with Volkmann's ischemic contracture following a compound Monteggia fracture treated by circular plaster cast (author's transl.). Ther. Umsch., *30*:877, 1973.
8. Beddow, F. H., and Corkery, P. H.: Lateral dislocation of the radio-humeral joint with greenstick fracture of the upper end of the ulna. J. Bone Joint Surg., *42-B*:782, 1960.
9. Bell Tawse, A. J. S.: The treatment of malunited anterior Monteggia fractures in children. J. Bone Joint Surg., *47-B*:718, 1965.
10. Blount, W. P.: Fractures in Children. Baltimore, Williams & Wilkins, 1955.
11. Bondarenko, N. S.: Characteristics of Monteggia injuries in children. Vestn. Khir., *120*:112, 1978.
12. Bouyala, J. M., Christian, P., and Ramaherison, P.: Osteotomie haute du cubitus dans le traitement de la luxation anterieure residuelle apres fracture de Monteggia. Chir. Pediatr., *19*:201, 1978.
13. Boyd, H. B.: Surgical exposure of the ulna and proximal third of the radius through one incision. Surg. Gynecol. Obstet., *71*:86, 1940.
14. Boyd, H. B.: Treatment of fractures of the ulna with dislocation of the radius. J.A.M.A., *115*:1699, 1940.
15. Boyd, H. B., and Boals, J. C.: The Monteggia lesion. A review of 159 cases. Clin. Orthop., *66*:94, 1969.
16. Brodueur, A. E., Silberstein, M. J., and Graviss, E. R.: Radiology of the Pediatric Elbow. Boston, G. K. Hall, 1981.
17. Bruce, H. E., Harvey, J. P., Jr., and Wilson, J. C., Jr.: Monteggia fractures. J. Bone Joint Surg., *56-A*:1563, 1974.
18. Bryan, R. S.: Monteggia fractures of the forearm. J. Trauma, *11*:992, 1971.
19. Bucknill, T. M.: Anterior dislocation of the radial head in children. Proc. R. Soc. Med., *70*:620, 1977.
20. Coch, R.: Monteggia's fracture. Rozhl. Chir., *49*:401, 1970.
21. Cooper, A.: Dislocations and Fractures of the Joints. Boston, T. R. Marvin, 1844, pp. 391–400.
22. Creer, W. S.: Some points about the Monteggia fracture. Proc. R. Soc. Med., *40*:241, 1947.
23. Cunningham, S. R.: Fracture of the ulna with dislocation of the head of the radius. J. Bone Joint Surg., *16*:351, 1934.
24. Curry, G. J.: Monteggia fracture. Am. J. Surg., *73*:613, 1947.
25. Eady, J. L.: Acute Monteggia lesions in children. J. S.C. Med. Assoc., *71*:107, 1975.
26. Eady, J. L.: Acute Monteggia lesions in children. Orthop. Dig., *4*:15, 1976.
27. Engber, W. D., and Keene, J. S.: Anterior interosseous nerve palsy associated with a Monteggia fracture. A case report. Clin. Orthop., *174*:133, 1983.
28. Evans, E. M.: Pronation injuries of the forearm with special reference to the anterior Monteggia fracture. J. Bone Joint Surg., *31-B*:578, 1949.
29. Fahey, J. J.: Fractures of the elbow in children. A.A.O.S. Instr. Course Lect., *17*:13, 1960.
30. Fahmy, N. R. M.: Unusual Monteggia lesions in children. Injury, *12*:399, 1981.
31. Fontanesi, G., and Pelliccioni, S.: Boyd's approach in the surgical treatment of Monteggia's fracture. Chir. Organi Mov., *55*:340, 1966.
32. Fowles, J. V., Sliman, N., and Kassab, M. T.: The Monteggia lesion in children. Fracture of the ulna and dislocation of the radial head. J. Bone Joint Surg., *65-A*:1276, 1983.
33. Ginzbury, S. O.: Transarticular fixation of the head of the radius in the treatment of long-term Monteggia injuries in children. Vestn. Khir., *102*:131, 1969.
34. Gordon, M. L.: Monteggia fractures. A combined surgical approach employing a single lateral incision. Clin. Orthop., *50*:87, 1967.
35. Gottschalk, E.: Osteosynthesis of forearm in children involving the radius head, olecranon and Monteggia injury. Beitr. Orthop. Traumatol., *27*:78, 1980.
36. Guistra, P., Killoran, P., Furman, R., *et al.*: The missed Monteggia fracture. Radiology, *110*:45, 1974.
37. Hamilton, W., and Parkes, J. C., II.: Isolated dislocation of the radial head without fracture of the ulna. Clin. Orthop., *97*:94, 1973.
38. Hollwarth, M., and Hausbrandt, D.: Monteggia fractures in infants (author's transl.). Unfallheilkunde, *81*:77, 1978.
39. Holst-Nielsen, F., and Jensen, V.: Tardy posterior interosseous nerve palsy as a result of an unreduced radial head dislocation in Monteggia fractures: A report of two cases. J. Hand Surg., *9-A*:572, 1984.
40. Hume, A. C.: Anterior dislocation of the head of the radius associated with undisplaced fracture of the olecranon in children. J. Bone Joint Surg., *39-B*:508, 1957.
41. Hunt, G. H.: Fracture of the shaft of the ulna with dislocation of the head of the radius. J.A.M.A., *112*:1241, 1939.
42. Hurst, L. C., and Dubrow, E. N.: Surgical treatment of symptomatic chronic radial head dislocation: A neglected Monteggia fracture. J. Pediatr. Orthop., *3*:227, 1983.
43. Jessing, P.: Monteggia lesions and their complicating nerve damage. Acta Orthop. Scand., *46*:601, 1975.
44. Kalamchi, A.: Monteggia fracture-dislocation in children. Late treatment in two cases. J. Bone Joint Surg., *68-A*:615, 1986.
45. Kamali, M. D.: Monteggia fracture. J. Bone Joint Surg., *56-A*:841, 1974.
46. Kaplan, E. B.: The quadrate ligament of the radio-ulnar joint of the elbow. Bull. Hosp. J. Dis., *25*:126, 1964.
47. King, R. E.: The Monteggia lesion. *In* Rockwood, C. A. Jr., Wilkins, K. E., and King, R. E. (eds.): Fractures in Children. Philadelphia, Lippincott, 1984.
48. Kini, M. G.: Dislocation of the head of the radius associated with fracture of the upper third of the ulna. Antiseptic, *37*:1059, 1940.
49. Kirschner, R.: Proceedings: Fractures of the upper third of the elbow and Monteggia's fractures. Hefte Unfallheilkd., *114*:119, 1973.

50. Kirschner, R.: Osteosynthesis of the fracture of the two upper thirds of the forearm and of the Monteggia fractures (author's transl.). Acta Chir. Orthop. Traumatol. Cech., *42*:256, 1975.
51. Kolomyttsev, V. D.: Treatment of Monteggia and Galeazzi fracture dislocation of the forearm. Ortop. Travmatol. Protez., *4*:27, 1976.
52. Kovalkovits, I., Molnar, I., and Krasznai, I.: Postoperative treatment of the Galeazzi and Monteggia syndrome. Chirurg, *42*:88, 1971.
53. Kovanda, M.: Surgical therapy of Monteggia fractures (author's transl.). Acta Chir. Orthop. Traumatol. Cech., *41*:255, 1974.
54. Kristiansen, B., and Eriksen, A. F.: Simultaneous type II Monteggia lesion and fracture-separation of the lower radial epiphysis. Injury, *17*:51, 1986.
55. Letts, M., Weins, J., and Locht, R.: Monteggia fracture-dislocation in children. J. Bone Joint Surg., *67-B*:724, 1984.
56. Liang, C. R., Segura, M., and Strickland, K. P.: Monteggia fractures in children. Can. J. Biochem., *48*:580, 1970.
57. Lichtenberg, R. P.: A study of 2,532 fractures in children. Am. J. Surg., *87*:330, 1954.
58. Lichter, R. L., and Jackson, T.: Tardy palsy of posterior interosseous nerve with a Monteggia fracture. J. Bone Joint Surg., *57-A*:124, 1975.
59. Lloyd-Roberts, G. C., and Bucknill, T. M.: Anterior dislocation of the radial head in children. J. Bone Joint Surg., *59-B*:402, 1977.
60. Lyba, R. M., and Skorik, N. M.: Treatment of inveterate Monteggia's fracture-dislocations by the compression-distraction method. Ortop. Travmatol. Protez., *3*:69, 1978.
61. McGuire, T. P., and Myers, P.: Ulnar osteotomy for missed Monteggia fracture. Proceedings. J. Bone Joint Surg., *68-B*:336, 1986.
62. MacLennan, A.: Common fractures about the elbow joint in children. Surg. Gynecol. Obstet., *64*:447, 1937.
63. Mandaba, J. L., Desgrippes, Y., and Bensahel, H.: Reflections on thirty eight cases of Monteggia fracture of children (author's transl.). J. Chir. (Paris), *116*:573, 1979.
64. May, V., and Mauck, W.: Dislocation of the radial head with associated fracture of the ulna. South. Med. J., *54*:1255, 1961.
65. Maylahn, D. J., and Fahey, J. J.: Fractures of the elbow in children. J.A.M.A., *166*:220, 1958.
66. Monteggia, G. B.: Instituzione Chirurgiche, 5:130, 1814. (Translated by Helen Rang). Milan, Maspero, 1813–1815.
67. Morris, A. H.: Irreducible Monteggia lesion with radial nerve entrapment. J. Bone Joint Surg., *56-A*:1744, 1974.
68. Mullick, S.: The lateral Monteggia fracture. J. Bone Joint Surg., *59-A*:543, 1977.
69. Napieralski, K.: Accompanying injuries in Monteggia fracture. Beitr. Orthop. Traumatol., *16*:507, 1969.
70. Naylor, A.: Monteggia fractures. Br. J. Surg., *29*:323, 1942.
71. Pansecchi, V.: Considerations on a case of the anterior type of Monteggia fracture-dislocation. Minerva Ortop., *18*:670, 1967.
72. Peiro, A., Andres, F., and Fernandez-Esteve, F.: Acute Monteggia lesions in children. J. Bone Joint Surg., *59-A*:92, 1977.
73. Penrose, J. F.: The Monteggia fracture with posterior dislocation of the radial head. J. Bone Joint Surg., *33-B*:65, 1951.
74. Perfilova, N. G., and Vladikin, S. E.: Monteggia's fracture-dislocation in children. Ortop. Travmatol. Protez., *33*:61, 1972.
75. Perrin, J.: Les fractures du cubitus accompagnées de luxation de l'extremité superieur du radius. Paris, Thése de Paris, G. Steinheil, 1909.
76. Pizio, Z.: Fracture of the ulna and of the neck of the radius in a child as a specific form of Monteggia's fracture. Chir. Narzadow Ruchu Ortop. Pol., *35*:585, 1970.
77. Poinsot, G.: Dislocations of the head of the radius downward (by elongation). N.Y. State J. Med., *41*:8, 1885.
78. Poland, J.: A Practical Treatise on Traumatic Separation of the Epiphyses. London, Smith, Elder & Co., 1898.
79. Ramsey, R., and Pederson, H. E.: The Monteggia fracture-dislocation in children. J.A.M.A., *182*:115, 1962.
80. Ravessoud, F. A.: Lateral condylar fracture and ipsilateral ulnar shaft fracture: Monteggia equivalent lesions? J. Pediatr. Orthop., *5*:364, 1985.
81. Ray, R. D., Johnson, R. J., and Jameson, R. M.: Rotation of the forearm. J. Bone Joint Surg., *33-A*:993, 1951.
82. Reckling, F. W., and Cordell, L. D.: Unstable fracture-dislocation of the forearm. The Monteggia and Galleazzi lesions. Arch. Surg., *96*:999, 1968.
83. Samoilovich, E. F., and Kiselev, V. P.: Bloodless reduction of inveterate and improperly united Monteggia-type fracture-dislocations in children. Khirurgiia (Mosk.), *6*:99, 1981.
84. Smith, F. M.: Monteggia fractures: Analysis of 25 consecutive fresh injuries. Surg. Gynecol. Obstet., *85*:630, 1947.
85. Smith, F. M.: Surgery of the Elbow. 2nd. Ed. Philadelphia, Saunders, 1972.
86. Solcard, R.: Fracture de Monteggia vicieusement consolidée avec synostose radiocubitale. Rev. Orthop. Chir., *19*:36, 1932.
87. Spar, I.: A neurologic complication following Monteggia fracture. Clin. Orthop., *122*:207, 1977.
88. Speed, J. S., and Boyd, H. B.: Treatment of fractures of the ulna with dislocations of the radius. J.A.M.A., *115*:1699, 1940.
89. Spinner, M., and Kaplan, E. B.: The quadrate ligament of the elbow—its relationship to the stability of the proximal radio-ulnar joint. Acta Orthop. Scand., *41*:632, 1970.
90. Spinner, M., Freundlich, B. D., and Teicher, J.: Posterior interosseous nerve palsy as a complication of Monteggia fractures in children. Clin. Orthop., *58*:141, 1968.
91. Stein, F., Grabias, S. L., and Deffer, P. A.: Nerve injuries complicating Monteggia lesions. J. Bone Joint Surg., *53-A*:1432, 1971.
92. Stelling, F. H., and Cote, R. H.: Traumatic dislocation of the head of the radius in children. J.A.M.A., *160*:732, 1956.
93. Strube, H. D., Thummler, P., and Schweikert, C. H.: Monteggia's injury, treatment and late results. Hefte Unfallheilkd., *132*:444, 1978.
94. Thakore, H. K.: Lateral Monteggia fracture in children: Case report. Ital. J. Orthop. Traumatol., *9*:55, 1983.
95. Theodorou, S. D.: Dislocation of the head of the radius associated with fracture of the upper end of the ulna in children. J. Bone Joint Surg., *51-B*:700, 1969.
96. Thompson, H. A., and Hamilton, A. T.: Monteggia fracture: Internal fixation of fractured ulna with intramedullary pin. Am. J. Surg., *79*:579, 1950.
97. Tompkins, J. G.: The anterior Monteggia fracture. J. Bone Joint Surg., *53-A*:109, 1971.
98. Trillat, A., Marsan, C., and Llapeyre, B.: Classification and treatment of Monteggia fractures. A propos of 36 cases. Rev. Chir. Orthop., *55*:639, 1969.

99. Van Santvoordt, R.: Dislocation of the radial head downward. N.Y. State J. Med., *45*:63, 1887.
100. Vukovic, M.: Luxation of the head of the radius following treatment for Monteggia injury. Med. Arch., *32*:237, 1978.
101. Wieser, R., Scheier, H. J., Grammont, P., Chestian, P., Ramaherison, P., Bouyala, J. M., and Jani, L.: Persistent luxation of the radial head in children after Monteggia fractures (author's transl.). Orthopade, *10*:307, 1981.
102. Wiley, J. J., and Galey, J. P.: Monteggia injuries in children. J. Bone Joint Surg., *67-B*:728, 1985.
103. Wiley, J. J., Pegington, J., and Horwich, J. P.: Traumatic dislocation of the radius at the elbow. J. Bone Joint Surg., *56-B*:501, 1974.
104. Williams, E. A.: Internal stabilisation of the radial head in anterior Monteggia fracture. J. R. Coll. Surg. Edinb., *25*:17, 1980.
105. Wise, R. A.: Lateral dislocation of the head of the radius with fracture of the ulna. J. Bone Joint Surg., *23*:379, 1941.
106. Wojakowski, I., and Karkoszka, J.: Forearm tractures of the Monteggia type, complicated by fractures of the medial epicondyle of the humerus and the distal end of the radius. Chir. Narzadow Ruchu Ortop. Pol., *31*:561, 1966.
107. Wright, P. R.: Greenstick fracture of the upper end of the ulna with dislocation of the radio-humeral joint or displacement of the superior radial epiphysis. J. Bone Joint Surg., *45-B*:727, 1963.
108. Zatonski, E.: Surgical procedure and evaluation of results of treatment of inveterate isolated dislocations of the radial head and accompanying fractures of the forearm of the Monteggia type in children and adolescents. Chir. Narzadow Ruchu Ortop. Pol., *40*:15, 1975.
109. Zeitlin, A.: The traumatic origin of accessory bones at the elbow. J. Bone Joint Surg., *17*:933, 1935.
110. Zimmerman, H.: Fractures of the elbow. *In* Weber, B. G., Brunner, C., and Freuler, F. (eds.): Treatment of Fractures in Children and Adolescents. New York, Springer-Verlag, 1980.

Injuries to the Forearm and Hand

FRACTURES OF THE SHAFT OF THE RADIUS AND ULNA

The upper end of the ulna articulates with the trochlea of the humerus and provides flexion-extension of the elbow; in its lower portion the ulna splints the radius and provides stability to the forearm. The radius articulates with the carpus and through its rotatory motions of pronation and supination it provides dexterity to the hand.

In the forearm the radius and ulna are firmly bound together by the interosseous membrane, which provides a hinge mechanism for rotatory movements. The annular ligament holds together the proximal radioulnar joint; the distal radioulnar and radiocarpal joints are firmly connected by the dorsal and volar radiocarpal ligaments, and the medial ulnocarpal and lateral radiocarpal ligaments.

Fractures of the shaft of the radius and ulna may occur in their distal third, middle third, or upper third. One or both bones may be broken. The fracture may be of the greenstick type or complete; the latter may be undisplaced, minimally displaced, or markedly displaced with overriding. The fracture may be greenstick or complete in both radius and ulna, or it may be complete in one bone and greenstick in the other. Angulation may be volar, dorsal, or toward or away from the interosseous space. Traumatic bowing of one or both bones of the forearm may occur in children. When only one bone of the forearm is broken, the integrity of the proximal and distal radioulnar joints should always be determined by obtaining radiograms that include the elbow and wrist joints with the entire forearm. *Monteggia fracture*—dislocation of the radial head with fracture of the ulna—has been discussed. *Galeazzi fracture* is dislocation of the inferior radioulnar joint with a fracture of the lower third of the radius.

According to Blount, 75 per cent of the fractures of the shaft of the radius and ulna are in the distal third, 18 per cent in the middle third, and 7 per cent in the proximal third.[8–10, 12]

Mechanism of Injury and Pathologic Anatomy

In children, the common injury is by indirect violence sustained in a fall on the outstretched hand. The breaking force is transmitted to the radius. With the hand fixed on the ground, the momentum of the body rotates the humerus and ulna laterally and a fracture of the ulna results. Direct violence occasionally is the cause of "both-bone" fracture in children; often these are associated with severe soft-tissue trauma and the fracture may be open.

Once the bones break, the direction and extent of displacement of the fractured fragments depend upon the level of the fracture, muscle action, and the direction of the breaking force. In the reduction and immobilization of these fractures, the origin, insertion, and action of the forearm muscle must be considered. The biceps brachii and supinator brevis muscles insert into the proximal third of the radius; these muscles are the powerful supinators of the forearm. The pronator teres, originating above the elbow medially, inserts into the middle third of the radius. The pronator quadratus, located on the anterior aspect of the lower forearm, inserts into the distal third of the radius. The brachioradialis muscle originates from the lower end of the lateral aspect of the humerus and inserts into the lateral surface of the distal radius, immediately above the styloid process; the brachioradialis muscle assists in elbow flexion and is also a semipronator and semisupinator of the forearm, bringing it from supine or prone position to neutral rotation. The extensors of the wrist and digits have no deforming influence on the fracture fragments, but act as a dynamic posterior splint when under tension, as when the elbow is flexed. The extensors and abductors of the thumb act with the brachioradialis muscle in fractures of the distal third of the radius and pull the distal fragment of the radius proximally. The powerful flexor muscles of the forearm tend to pull the distal fragments anteriorly and produce dorsal bowing of the radius and ulna during healing.

In fractures of the *upper third* of the forearm and above the insertion of the pronator teres muscle, the *proximal fragment* of the radius is supinated and flexed because of the unopposed action of the biceps brachii and supinator brevis muscles, and the distal fragment is pronated by the action of the pronator teres and pronator quadratus muscles. Therefore, to obtain alignment of the fracture, the distal fragment should be supinated.

In fractures of the *middle third* of the forearm (below the insertion of the pronator teres), the *proximal fragment* of the radius is held in neutral rotation, as the action of the supinator muscles is counteracted by the pronator teres. The proximal fragment is drawn into flexion by the action of the biceps muscle. The *distal fragment* is pronated and drawn toward the ulna by the pronator quadratus muscle. To achieve anatomic reduction, the distal fragment is brought into neutral rotation—midway between full supination and full pronation.

In fractures of the *lower third* of the forearm, the distal fragment of the pulled radius is pronated and pulled inward by the pronator quadratus muscle. Overriding and shortening are caused by the obliquity of the fracture and the pull of the muscles.

The preservation and restoration of the interosseous space are important factors to consider in forearm fractures. Any deviation of the radius and ulna toward each other will encroach on the interosseous membrane; the result is narrowing or obliteration of the interosseous space and marked restriction or loss of rotation of the forearm. Functional handicap will be great, as the dexterity of the hand is contingent on the range and power of supination and pronation of the forearm.

Diagnosis

The history of injury, the clinical signs of local swelling and tenderness, angular deformity, pain on motion of the forearm, and the radiographic findings make the diagnosis obvious.

Treatment

Fractures of both bones of the forearm are difficult to treat, and often they are mismanaged. There are certain pitfalls that should be avoided.

The Loose Cast. In order to maintain reduction, fixation should be secure. As the swelling about a fracture site subsides and muscle atrophies, the cast becomes loose and the fracture fragments are displaced. This loss of position can occur as late as the third week following reduction. A loose cast can be detected in the radiogram. The author prefers a circular solid cast; at seven to ten days after reduction, the cast is removed if it is loose, the alignment of the fracture fragments is determined, and a new snug cast is applied. Others may prefer bandaged sugar-tong plaster splints for immobilization because they are easily adjusted and tightened as the swelling subsides. One cannot overemphasize the importance of a *snug cast* in preventing loss of alignment.

Inadequate Fixation. Displaced fractures of the radius and ulna should always be immobilized in a sturdy above-elbow cast, extending from the axilla to the metacarpal heads, with the elbow in 90 degrees of flexion. In children, stiffness of joints from prolonged immobilization is not a problem. In unstable fractures of the distal third of the radius, the plaster cast should include the proximal phalanges to immobilize the metacarpophalangeal joints; secure fixation of the proximal phalanx of the thumb is particularly important. Blount recommends the use of finger traction on a banjo splint; the author does not believe it is effective in preventing or correcting loss of position of fragments.[9, 10]

Failure to Detect and Correct Loss of Position. In unstable fractures of both bones of the forearm, the position of the fragments should be determined by radiograms at three days, seven days, and then at weekly intervals for four weeks. If satisfactory position is lost, the fracture should be remanipulated promptly. Between 10 and 14 days postfracture, the repeated reduction is apt to be more stable because of the "stickiness" of the fragments consequent to the healing process. A common error is to accept inadequate radiograms. The radiographic projection should be "true" anteroposterior and "true" lateral. Oblique views are misleading. If necessary, the surgeon himself should assist the x-ray technician in proper positioning of the forearm.

Failure of Adequate Initial Reduction. The more accurate the fracture reduction, the less is the potential for loss of alignment. Reduction of displaced overriding fractures of the distal forearm is difficult in the presence of marked local swelling. There is no emergency in the treatment of these fractures. Often such a child has a full stomach at the time of injury, obviating treatment under general anesthesia. Compression with a plaster splint is applied, and the child is admitted to the hospital and put to bed with the limb elevated. Within a day or two, the swelling will have receded and, under general anesthesia, the fracture can be manipulated under optimal conditions.

Failure to Immobilize Forearm in Position of Stability. The degree of rotation of the forearm in which fractures of the radius and ulna should be immobilized has been the subject of some controversy. The *forearm is immobilized in the position of rotation in which reduction is most stable.* The standard routine has been full supination in fractures of the upper third, neutral rotation in those of the middle third, and full pronation in the lower-third fractures. Once stable and adequate reduction is achieved, the preservation and restoration of the interosseous space is the important consideration. If reduction is stable, the author recommends the position of full supination in all fractures. As stated before, in full supination of the forearm, the radius and ulna are parallel to each other; and if a snug cast is maintained during the healing period, the pull of the muscles will not cause malalignment of a satisfactorily reduced stable fracture. However, if fractures of the middle third of the radius and ulna are stable in neutral rotation, the position of the forearm in the cast should be neutral rotation. Stability of reduction is determined clinically and by radiographic examinations.

Failure to Break the Cortex Completely. This is another common pitfall in angulated greenstick fractures. The strong advice of Blount should be followed.[9, 10] Merely to straighten the bone is not adequate; the intact cortex must be broken through as described in the following section.

Failure to Detect and Correct Rotational Deformity. Rotational deformity of the forearm can be recognized by clinical inspection and the radiographic findings. Observe the resting posture of the forearm. Are the bones properly aligned? If the proximal segment is supinated and the distal segment pronated, the latter should be supinated to reduce the fracture. In the radiogram the following observations should be made. *First,* the *position of the bicipital tuberosity* should be noted (as advocated by Evans).[38] In the normal forearm the bicipital tuberosity is located medially when the forearm is in full supination, posteriorly when in neutral (mid-position), and laterally when in full pronation (Fig. 8–79). In between, relative positions can be determined to 30 degrees. When performing closed reduction, align the distal fragment to the same degree of rotation of the proximal fragment as determined by the position of the bicipital tuberosity. It should be kept in mind that the degree of clinical loss of rotation of the forearm is directly proportional to the degree of malrotation of the fracture; i.e., 15 degrees of malrotation restricts clinical rotation of the forearm by 15 degrees. The *second* radiographic sign is *angulation* at the fracture site. Note the direction and degree of angulation. Volar bowing indicates supination deformity, whereas dorsal bowing indicates pronation deformity. Angular deformity restricts the range of widening and narrowing of the interosseous membrane, thereby limiting rotation. In general, 15 degrees of angulation limits rotation by 30 degrees. The *third* radiographic finding indicating malrotation is change in diameter or width of the cortex and smooth curve of the radius.

Circulatory Embarrassment and Volkmann's Ischemia. These can be caused by fracture of both bones of the forearm. When the forearm is swollen or when a displaced fracture is reduced by manipulation, it is wise to admit the child to the hospital, elevate the limb, and closely observe the circulation for one to three days.

Open Reduction. Rarely, if ever, should this be performed in fractures of both bones of the forearm in a child because of the definite risk of delayed union and nonunion. Radioulnar synostosis and infection are other serious complications.

Keeping the foregoing principles in mind, one treats "both-bone" fractures of the forearm as follows:

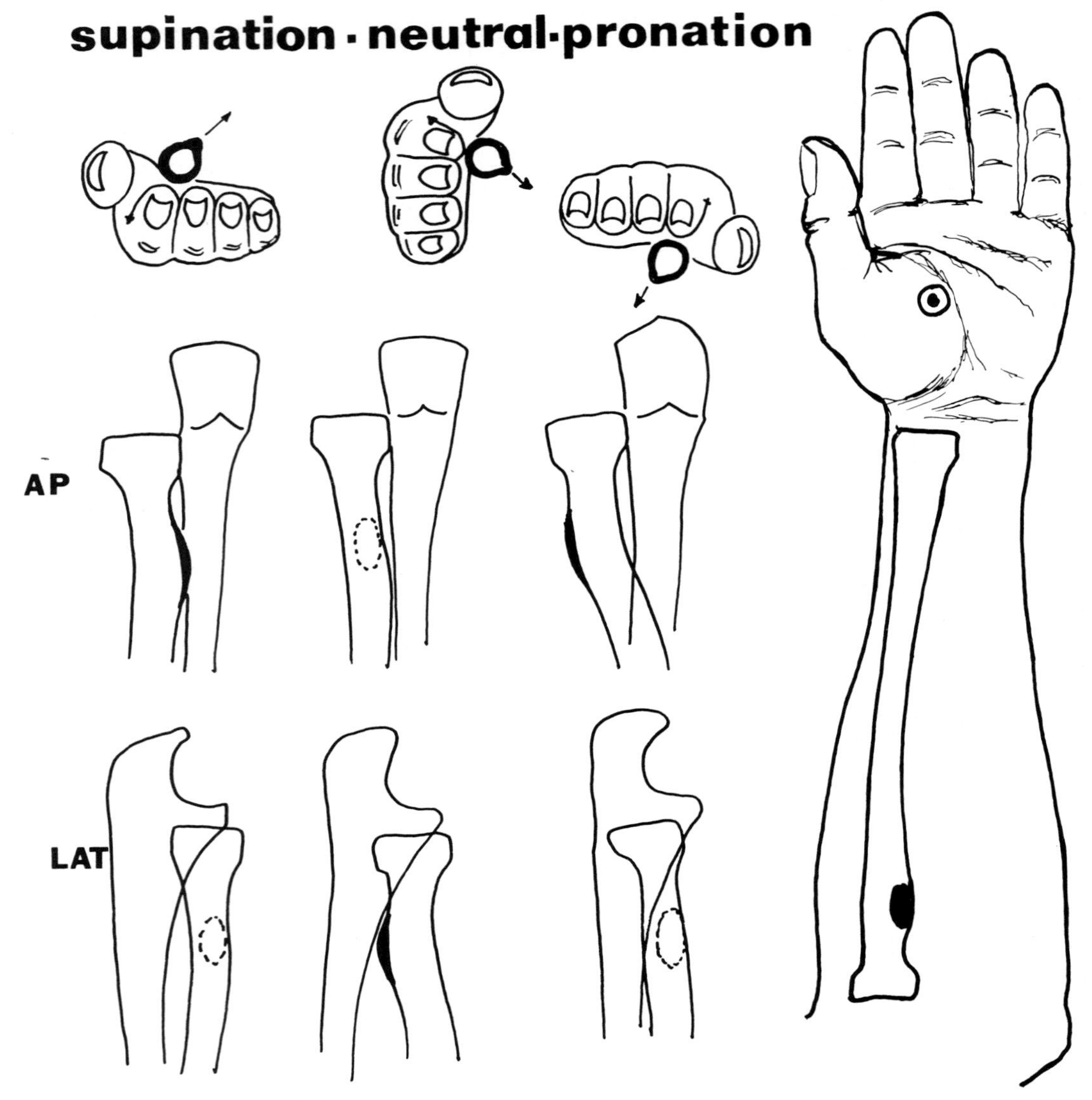

***FIGURE 8–79.** Determination of the rotation of the proximal radius in fractures of both bones of the forearm by use of the bicipital tuberosity as a guide.*

(Redrawn after Evans, E. M.: J. Bone Joint Surg., 27:373, 1945.)

GREENSTICK FRACTURES OF MIDDLE THIRD OF RADIUS AND ULNA

The usual deformity is dorsal angulation of the distal fragment with the apex of the fracture toward the volar aspect. Simple straightening of the bones and immobilization in the cast are not adequate, as the deformity will recur. The intact cortex should be completely broken through. Overcorrect slightly in order to prevent recurrence of the deformity from plastic deformation while in the cast. Ordinarily in a recent fracture, general anesthesia is not required. The technique of manipulative reduction is as follows: (1) Grasp the forearm with one hand above and one hand below the fracture site. (2) Pronate supination injuries. (3) Place the volar aspect of the apex of the forearm deformity over your knee; then suddenly reverse it and break the intact cortex on the dorsal aspect. It will be accompanied by an audible crack. This will correct the angular deformity. The periosteal tube remains intact and holds the fragments together in normal alignment. Study the position of the bicipital

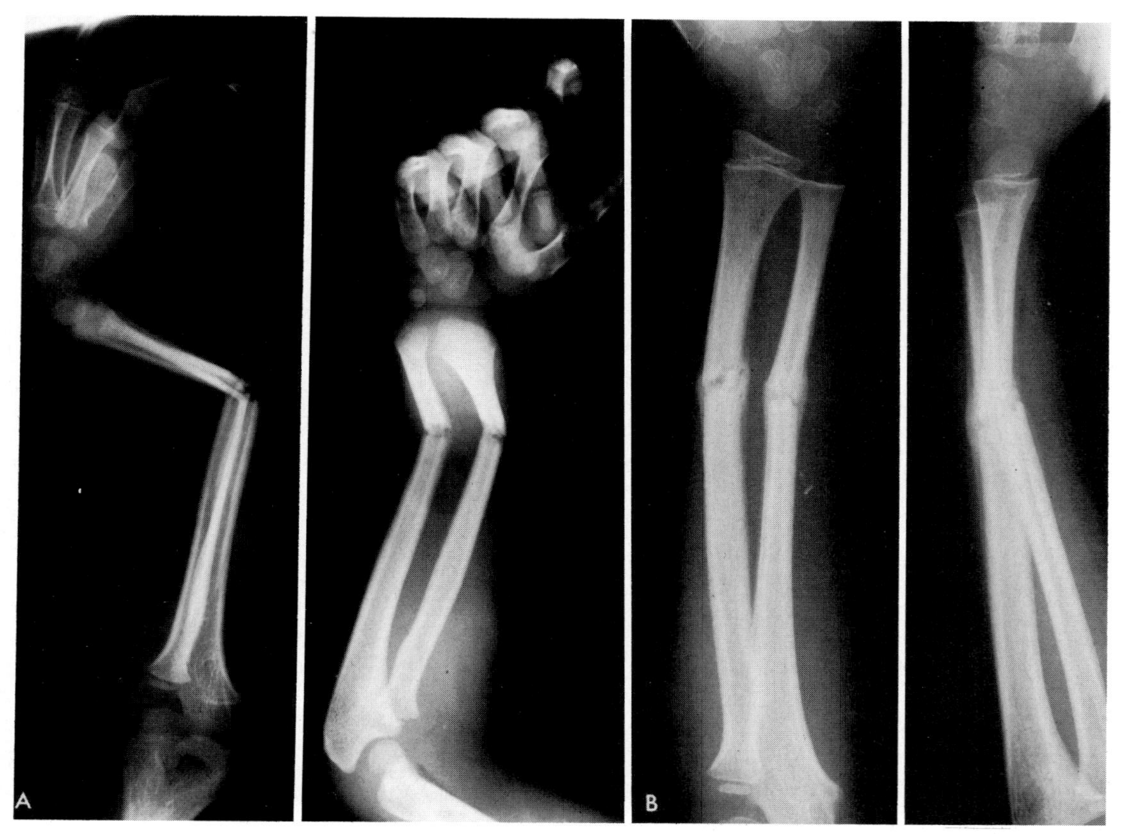

FIGURE 8–80. Fracture of both bones of forearm with marked dorsal angulation of distal fragments.

A. Initial radiogram. **B.** Four weeks after closed reduction.

tuberosity in the anteroposterior radiogram to align the distal fragment to the proximal fragment. An above-elbow cast is applied with the elbow in 90 degrees of flexion and the forearm in full supination or midway between pronation and supination. The cast should be well molded, utilizing three-point fixation. The swelling will subside and the cast will become loose. Change the cast in seven to ten days. Make serial radiograms to detect loss of alignment. The fracture will consolidate in four to six weeks; immobilize in the cast for an additional one to two weeks in order to prevent plastic deformation resulting from premature cast removal (Figs. 8–80 and 8–81).

DISPLACED FRACTURES OF MIDDLE THIRD OF BOTH BONES OF FOREARM

These require correction of angular and rotational deformities. If normal alignment is not restored, there will be restriction of pronation and supination of the forearm. Bayonet (side-to-side) cortex apposition with some overriding is acceptable, provided rotation is reduced anatomically and there is no angular deviation of the radius and ulna toward each other and no encroachment on the interosseous space. In the determination of the degree of angulation and rotation, the injured and normal forearm should be compared, both clinically by inspection and by radiograms made in symmetrical positions and several projections.

The technique of manipulative reduction is as follows: (1) With the patient supine, the elbow is flexed to right angles and the forearm is supinated. One assistant applies longitudinal traction by grasping the distal ends of the radius and ulna at the wrist, while another assistant applies countertraction at the elbow. (2) Traction forces initially are applied to increase the deformity. (3) Once the overlapping bones are hitched together, the surgeon repositions the fragments into anatomic alignment with his thumbs. The width of the interosseous space is restored by digital pressure on the soft tissues

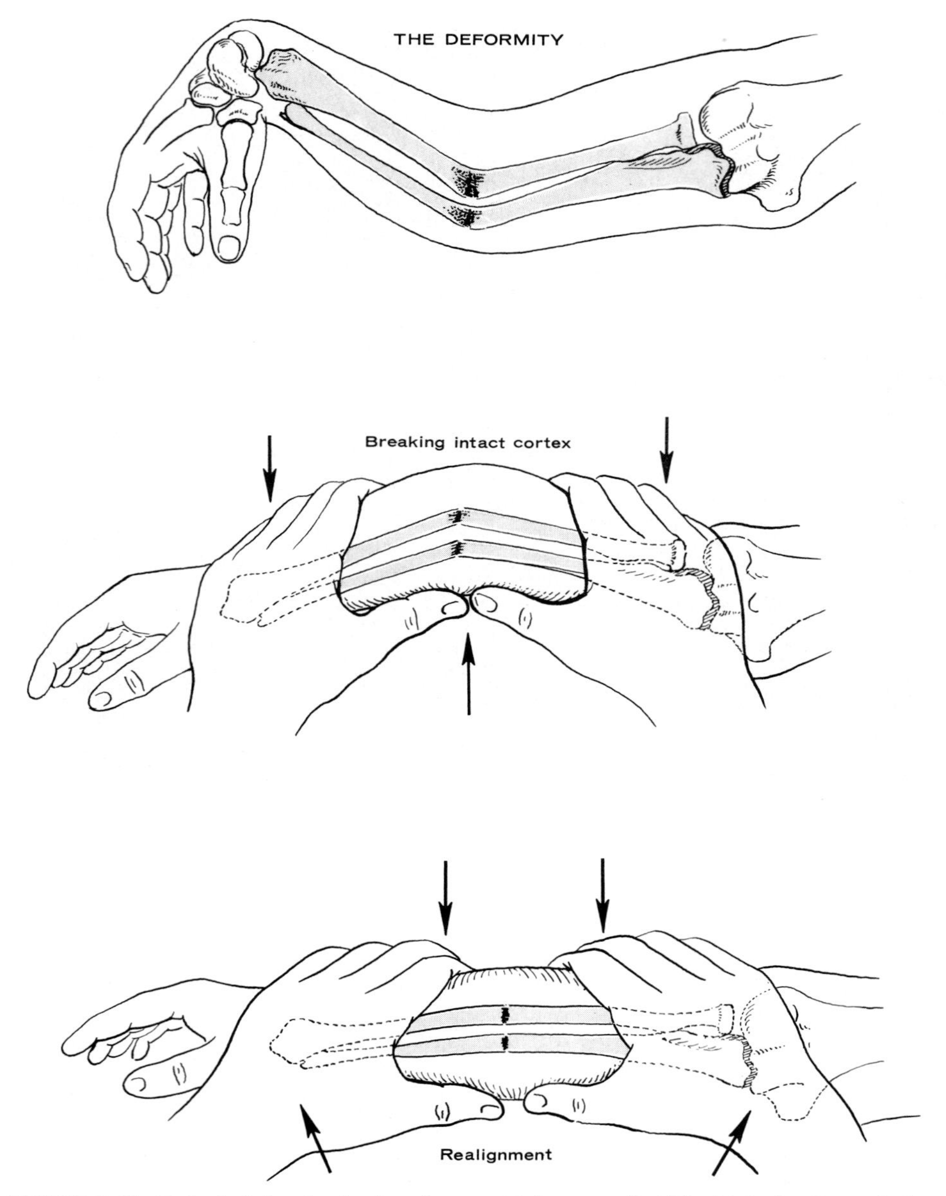

FIGURE 8–81. Method of closed reduction of greenstick fracture of middle third of radius and ulna.

between the bones. (4) While traction is maintained, a long arm cast is applied with the elbow in 90 degrees of flexion and the forearm fully supinated. The cast should be well molded over the volar aspect of the radius and also just above the elbow to prevent slipping of the cast up and down. Explain to the parents that loss of alignment may occur in the cast because of longitudinal instability, and that remanipulation and even external or internal fixation may be required. It is best to warn them.

Displaced fractures in the middle third of the radius and ulna require about six weeks to heal. Postreduction care follows the principles outlined previously—namely, a snug cast, frequent x-rays to detect loss of position, and prompt remanipulation if such loss occurs. Improvement of fracture alignment can be achieved up to three weeks following injury.

If initial closed manipulation fails to correct angular deformity, open surgical reduction should not be performed. A well-padded cast is applied for immobilization; it will also serve as a compression dressing to reduce the local swelling. After five days, the fracture is remanipulated. Often this second attempt will be

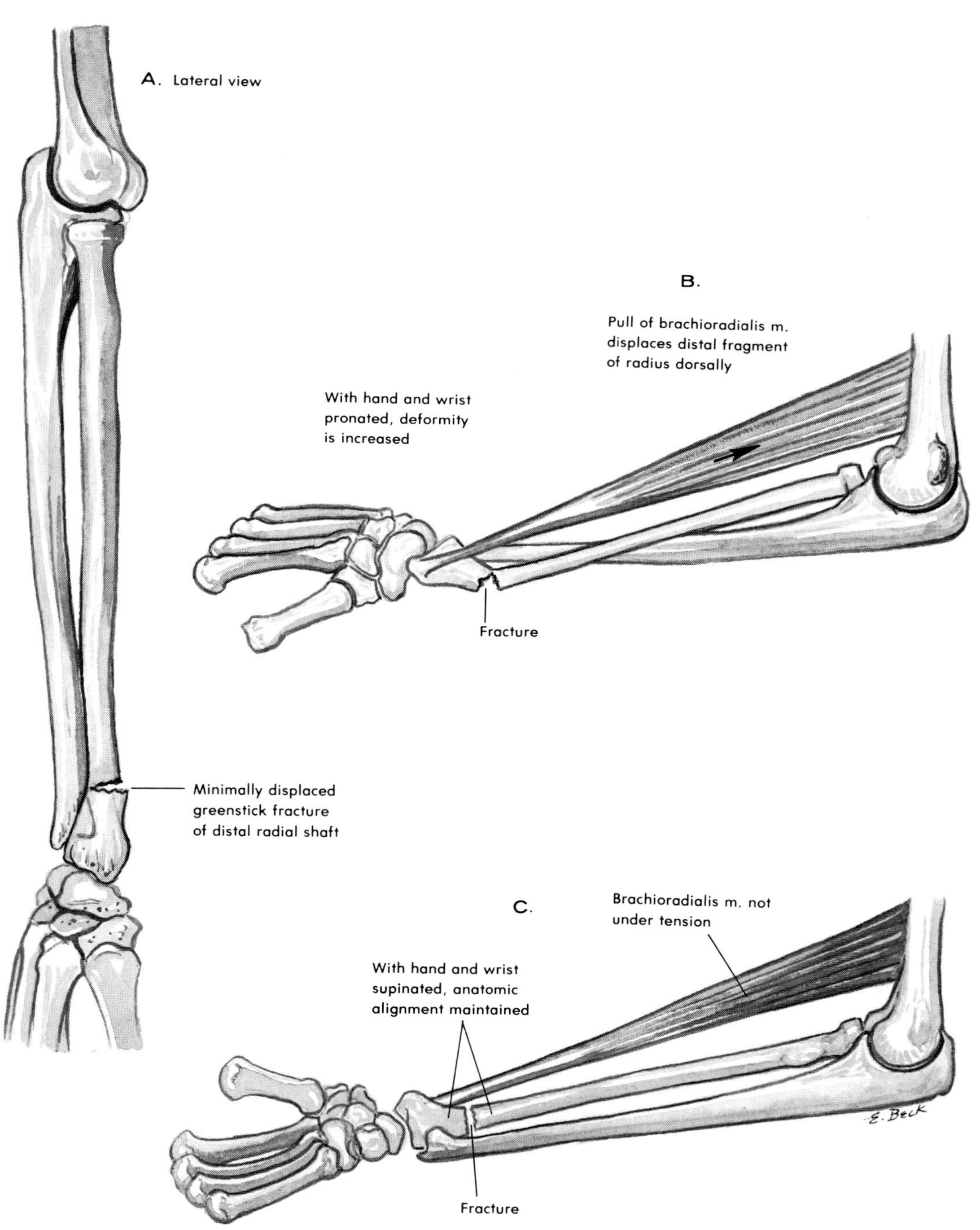

FIGURE 8–82. Minimally displaced greenstick fracture of the distal radial shaft. The tensioning effect of the pull of brachioradialis when the hand and wrist are pronated.

A. Lateral view showing the minimally displaced greenstick fracture.
B. When the hand and wrist are pronated, the brachioradialis muscle displaces the distal fragment of the radius dorsally.
C. When the hand and wrist are supinated, the brachioradialis muscle is not under tension and anatomic alignment is maintained.

successful in obtaining anatomic alignment. If unsuccessful, perform open reduction. In the past, the dictum was no open surgery. However, with modern technology of internal fixation, surgical skills, and anesthesia, the results of open reduction of both-bone fractures in children are excellent. The ulna is fixed by intramedullary fixation with the rod inserted through the olecranon. The radius is plated. Do not accept malrotation and angulation because the result is permanent loss of motion!

FRACTURES OF THE DISTAL THIRD OF THE RADIUS AND ULNA

"Torus" or Buckle Fracture of the Distal Metaphysis of the Radius and Ulna. This is the most common fracture in the lower forearm in young children. (The word *torus* is derived from the Latin *tori,* meaning a "swelling or protuberance.") The impact of the indirect violence of a fall on the outstretched hand crumples the dorsal cortex but the volar cortex remains intact. The distal fragment is angulated dorsally. Treatment consists of a below-elbow cast or volar splint for a period of three weeks.

Greenstick Fracture of the Distal Radius at the Junction of the Metaphysis and Diaphysis With Intact Ulna. This fracture is a "wolf in a lamb's clothing." It appears to be simple to treat; however, in the cast a minimally displaced fracture may become moderately angulated with an unacceptable deformity. Be cautious! The mechanism of injury is indirect violence sustained by a fall on the outstretched hand with rotation. The distal fragment of the radius is tilted dorsally and supinated with volar angulation deformity. Scrutinize the radiograms carefully. Be sure there is no associated fracture of the ulnar styloid.

Treatment. Reduction is achieved by pronation rotational force on the pronated hand-wrist, distal traction, and volar tilting of the distal fragment with thumb pressure. In the past it was customary to immobilize the fracture in an above-elbow cast with the forearm in full pronation. With this fully pronated posture of the forearm it was hoped that the intact periosteum dorsally would lock the fracture in place and also checkrein supination deformity from developing. However, often dorsal angulation and supination deformity recurred while in the cast. Pollen pointed out that the brachioradialis is the deforming force; in full pronation the pull of the brachioradialis (the long supinator) supinates and displaces the distal fracture fragment dorsally, whereas in supination the brachioradialis maintains the reduction (Fig. 8–82).[96] Therefore, it is recommended that after anatomic reduction the troublesome fracture be immobilized in an above-elbow cast with the forearm in 45 to 60 degrees of supination. Make radiograms in five and ten days! Change the loose cast in ten days. Any loss of alignment and recurrence of deformity should be corrected. Make radiograms in three weeks. The total period of immobilization is six weeks.

Greenstick Fracture of the Distal Radius and Ulna. These do not require reduction if the dorsal angulation is insignificant; however, if it exceeds 30 degrees in infants and 15 degrees in children, closed reduction is required. During manipulation the deformity is reversed; i.e., longitudinal traction is applied and the distal fragment is angulated toward the volar aspect until the intact dorsal cortex is broken through completely. Then the fracture is reduced in anatomic alignment and an above-elbow cast is applied for a period of four to six weeks. In greenstick fractures, if the intact cortex is not completely broken through, the deformity will recur.

Complete Fractures of the Distal Third of the Radius and Ulna. The distal fragments are displaced dorsally and radially with varying degrees of overriding (Fig. 8–83). The fracture of the radius may be complete and that of the ulna, greenstick. They should be reduced, preferably under general anesthesia or 1 per cent lidocaine local anesthesia. The technique of reduction is as follows. (1) With the patient supine, an assistant grasps the fingers in one hand and the thumb in the other hand, and applies strong longitudinal traction *in the line of deformity*; another assistant applies countertraction at the elbow. (2) The surgeon pushes the fragments into normal position with his thumb and fingers. The soft tissues between the distal radius and ulna are pressed to restore the width of the interosseous space. It is desirable to achieve perfect anatomic alignment; however, side-to-side bayonet apposition in good alignment is acceptable. Encroachment on the interosseous space by the fragments should be corrected, as it will restrict rotation of the forearm (Figs. 8–84 to 8–86). Minimal overriding will be remodeled. Marked overriding may occasionally require skeletal traction through the metacarpals for correction.

An above-elbow cast is applied for immobilization, which is maintained for six weeks. When both bones are fractured, neutral rotation of the forearm may provide more stability, whereas if only the radius is broken, the reduction may be more stable in pronation.

Text continued on page 3194

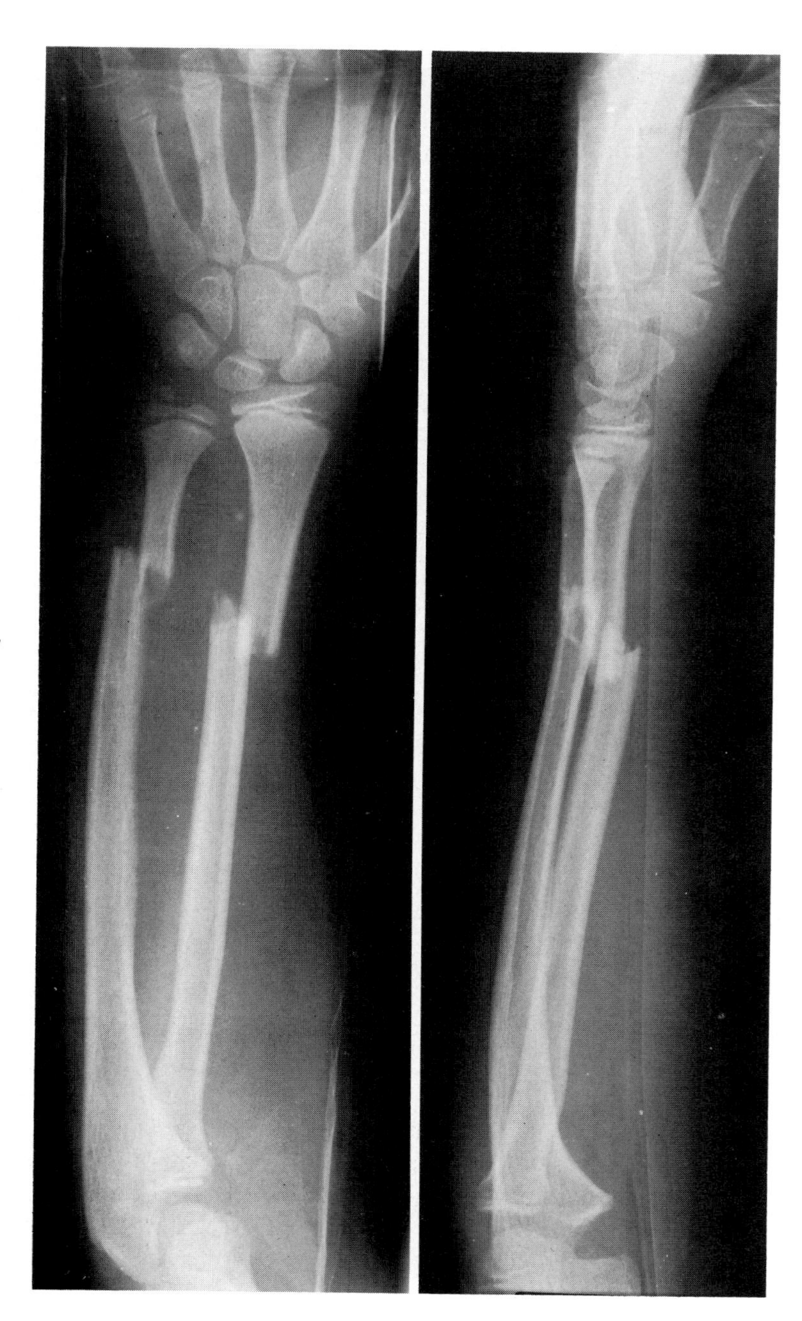

FIGURE 8–83. Fracture of radius and ulna in its distal fourth.

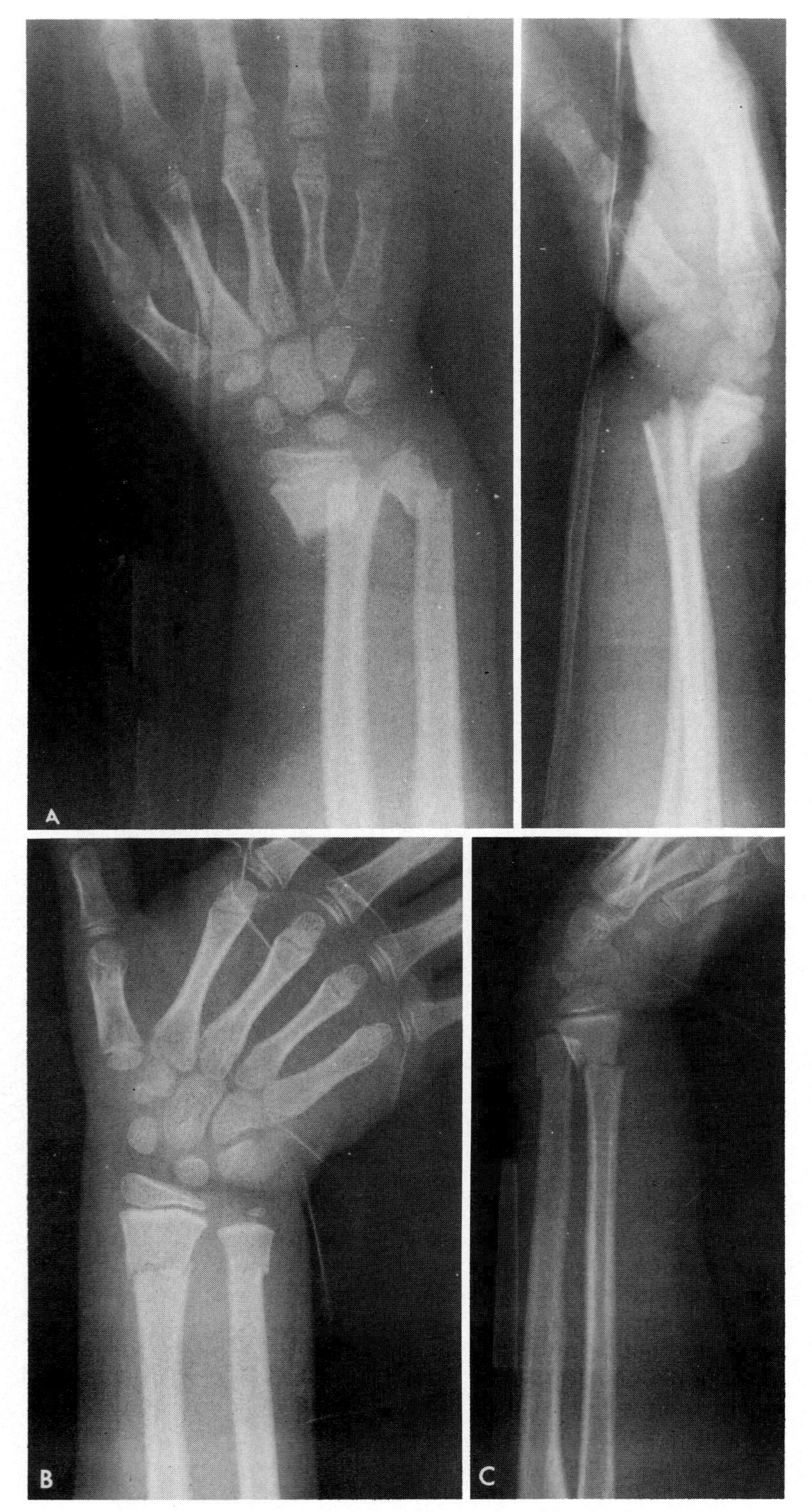

FIGURE 8–84. Fracture of the right radius and ulna at the junction of the distal metaphysis with the diaphysis.

A. Initial radiogram. **B** and **C.** Following closed reduction.

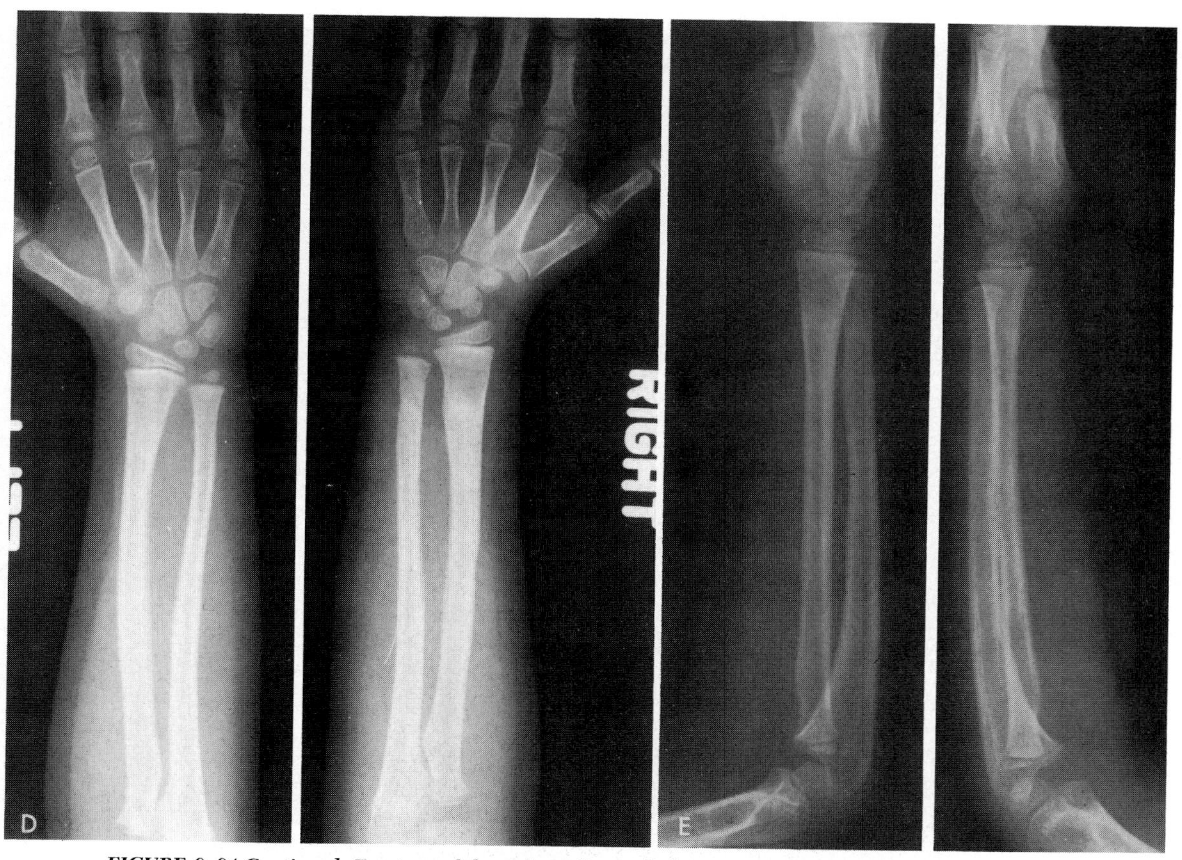

FIGURE 8–84 Continued. Fracture of the right radius and ulna at the junction of the distal metaphysis with the diaphysis.

D and **E**. Anteroposterior and lateral radiograms made eight months later, showing healing and remodeling.

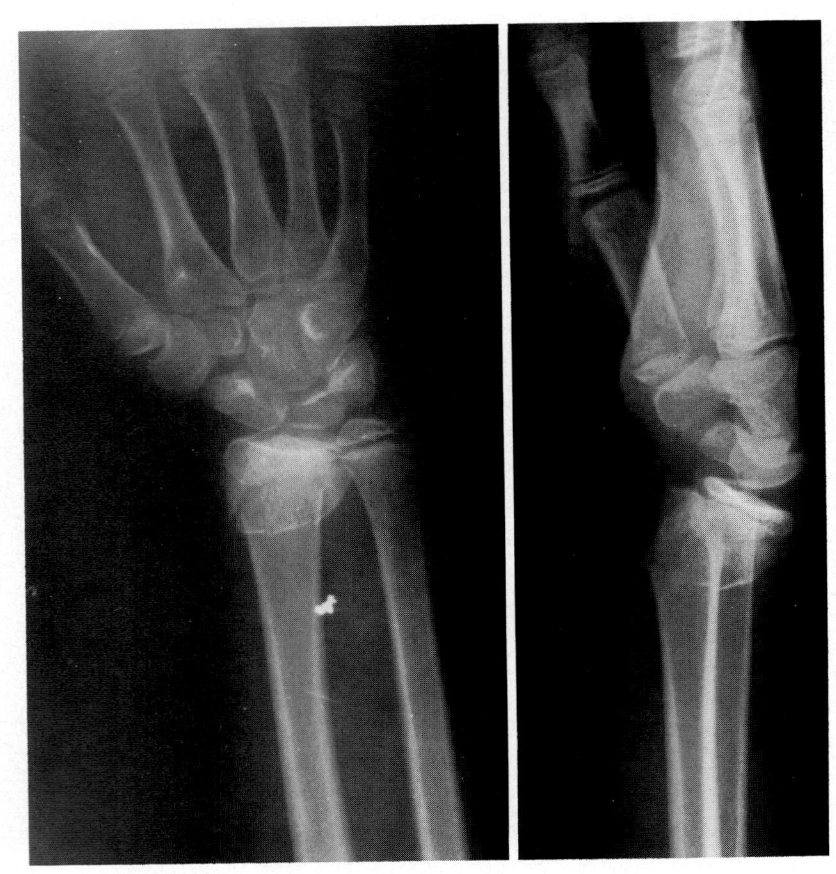

FIGURE 8–85. Fracture of lower end of diaphysis of radius.

Note marked dorsal angulation and displacement.

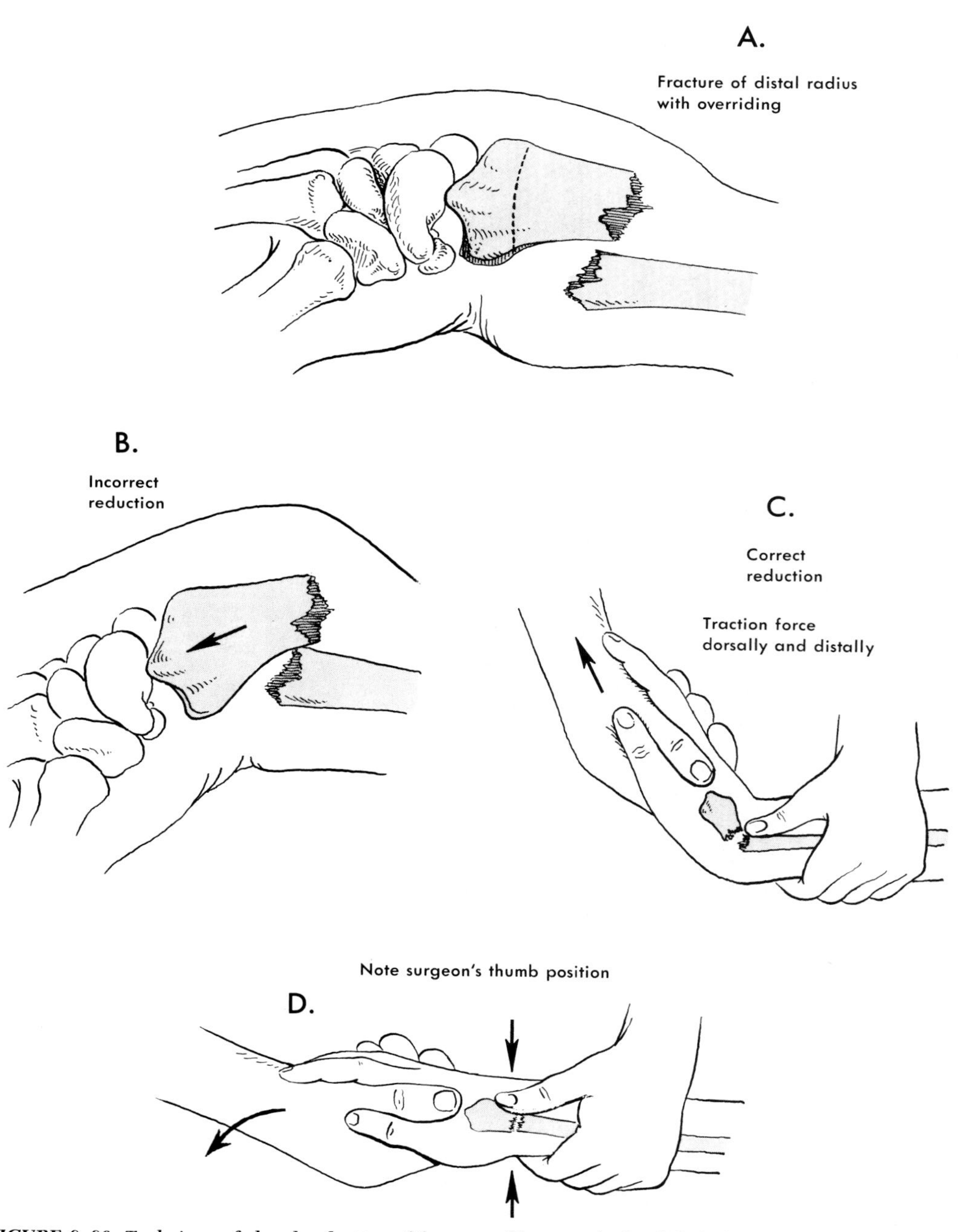

FIGURE 8–86. Technique of closed reduction of fracture of lower end of radial shaft (see text for explanation).

FRACTURES OF THE PROXIMAL THIRD OF THE SHAFT OF THE RADIUS AND ULNA

These relatively rare injuries are often caused by direct trauma. Frequently one bone is fractured. As in all fractures of the forearm, the elbow and wrist should be included in the radiogram to rule out dislocation of the radial head or of the inferior radioulnar joint (Fig. 8–87).

Isolated fracture of the proximal third of the radial shaft is reduced and immobilized with the forearm in full supination and the elbow in extension. In order to prevent the cast from slipping, apply tincture of benzoin on the skin and mold the cast well above the condyles. A cast with the elbow in flexion does not provide adequate control of the proximal segment.

PLASTIC DEFORMATION (OR TRAUMATIC BOWING) OF BOTH BONES OF THE FOREARM

Plastic deformation of the long bones occurs in children because the skeletally immature bones are porous due to the greater number and size of canals of the open osteon (haversian) systems. The modules of elasticity in tension and in bending are related to the vascular pattern in bone. When a bending force is applied to a long bone of an infant or a child, the long bone will bend to a certain degree. Tensile stress is exerted on the convex side and compression stress is produced on the concave side. Initially the deformation is *elastic*—i.e., the long bone will return gradually to its original contour when the bending forces are relieved. This stage of bone failure is called *elastic defor-*

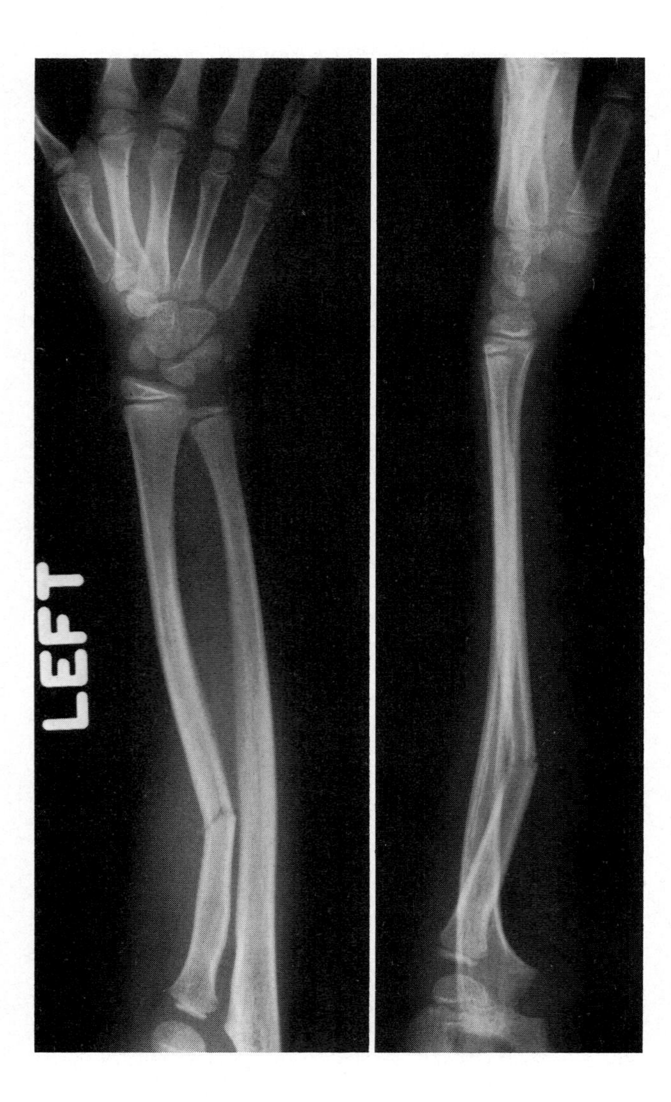

FIGURE 8–87. Greenstick fracture of the shaft of the radius at the junction of its proximal and middle thirds.

The ulna is not fractured, but the inferior radioulnar joint was subluxated. Radiograms of the entire forearm, including the elbow and wrist joints, should always be made.

mation. On continued exertion of greater longitudinal compression forces, the elastic limit is exceeded and the bending of the long bone becomes fixed. There is discontinuity of the collagen bundles of the osseous tissue and microfractures on the concave side; however, there is no gross fracture. This fixed bowing of the long bone is called *plastic deformation.*[14, 21]

Plastic deformation of the bones of the forearm was described by Borden in 1974; since then numerous reports have been published in the literature.[14, 15, 27, 32, 108, 127, 131]

Site of Involvement. One or both bones of the forearm may be involved. The ulna is the most common site followed by the radius. One bone may be traumatically bowed and the other fractured. When both bones are bowed, plastic deformation in one bone may be greater than in the other.

Clinical Picture. In the acute stage the child complains of pain and the involved bone will be locally tender on palpation. The bowing of the forearm is evident on comparison with the opposite normal forearm. Later, with healing of the bone, pain and tenderness subside but the deformity and limitation of pronation-supination of the forearm will persist.

Radiographic Findings. The bowing deformity of the ulna or radius is evident; it is best seen in the true lateral projection and when compared with that of the opposite normal forearm. It is vital to include the elbow and wrist in the radiogram in order not to miss an associated Monteggia lesion with dislocation of the radial head or Galeazzi lesion with dislocation of the distal radioulnar joint. With healing, periosteal new bone does not form. There may be cortical thickening on the concave side of the long bone.

In the acute stage of plastic deformation bone scan with technetium-99m will show increased local uptake.

Treatment. Correction of bowing of the ulna or radius, or both, is indicated if the deformity is significant and restricting normal range of pronation-supination of the forearm. Some degree of remodeling and spontaneous correction of bowing may take place in the young child (under four years of age) but it is minimal or none in the juvenile and adolescent patient.[32, 106]

Correction may be achieved by closed or open methods; either way it is performed under general anesthesia. Forewarn the parents that osteoclasis is often necessary for anatomic reduction and maintenance of reduction. First, attempt to correct by bending the bowed bone in the opposite direction with the apex of the curvature fixed against a padded firm support. Great force is necessary. Provide firm support to the wrist, elbow, and distal and proximal physes to prevent dislocation or physeal fracture-separation. Sustain the pressure for several minutes. If the bowing will straighten, it will do so gradually. In order to maintain the reduction, the deformity should be overcorrected. If one bone is fractured and the other is bowed, correct the bowed bone first. Also, if both bones are bowed, correct the bone with the greater deformity first.

In the experience of this author it is simpler and safer to perform percutaneous corticotomy at the apex of the deformed bone through a 1-cm. incision; fracture the bone and achieve anatomic reduction. At the completion of reduction there should be full range of passive pronation and supination. This author has seen a number of unhappy parents because their child was subjected to general anesthesia and, after straightening, the plastic deformation recurred in the cast.

Immobilization is in an above-elbow cast with the forearm in full supination for a period of six weeks.

REMODELING OF MALUNION OF FRACTURES OF BOTH BONES OF THE FOREARM

The degree of spontaneous correction of residual deformities by remodeling depends upon the age of the child, the distance of the fracture site from the physis, the amount of deformity, and the direction of angulation. To reiterate, narrowing of the interosseous space by angulation of the radius and ulna toward each other is not acceptable because invariably it will result in some degree of restriction of pronation-supination of the forearm. Dorsal angulation of the distal fragment (apex volar) will be remodeled rapidly. Figures 8–88 to 8–90 illustrate spontaneous correction of malunion of fractures of both bones of the forearm.

References

1. Akhundov, A. A.: Surgical treatment of antibrachial bone fractures in children. Vestn. Khir., *106*:85, 1971.
2. Alpar, E. K., Thompson, K., Owen, R., and Taylor, J.: Midshaft fractures of forearm bones in children. Injury, *13*:153, 1981.
3. Arunachalam, V. S., and Griffiths, J. C.: Fracture recurrence in children. Injury, 7:37, 1975.
4. Aufranc, O., Jones, W. N., and Stewart, W. G., Jr.: Reduced fracture of the forearm in a child. J.A.M.A., *194*:1004, 1965.
5. Bagley, C. H.: Fractures of both bones of the forearm. Surg. Gynecol. Obstet., *42*:95, 1926.

Text continued on page 3200

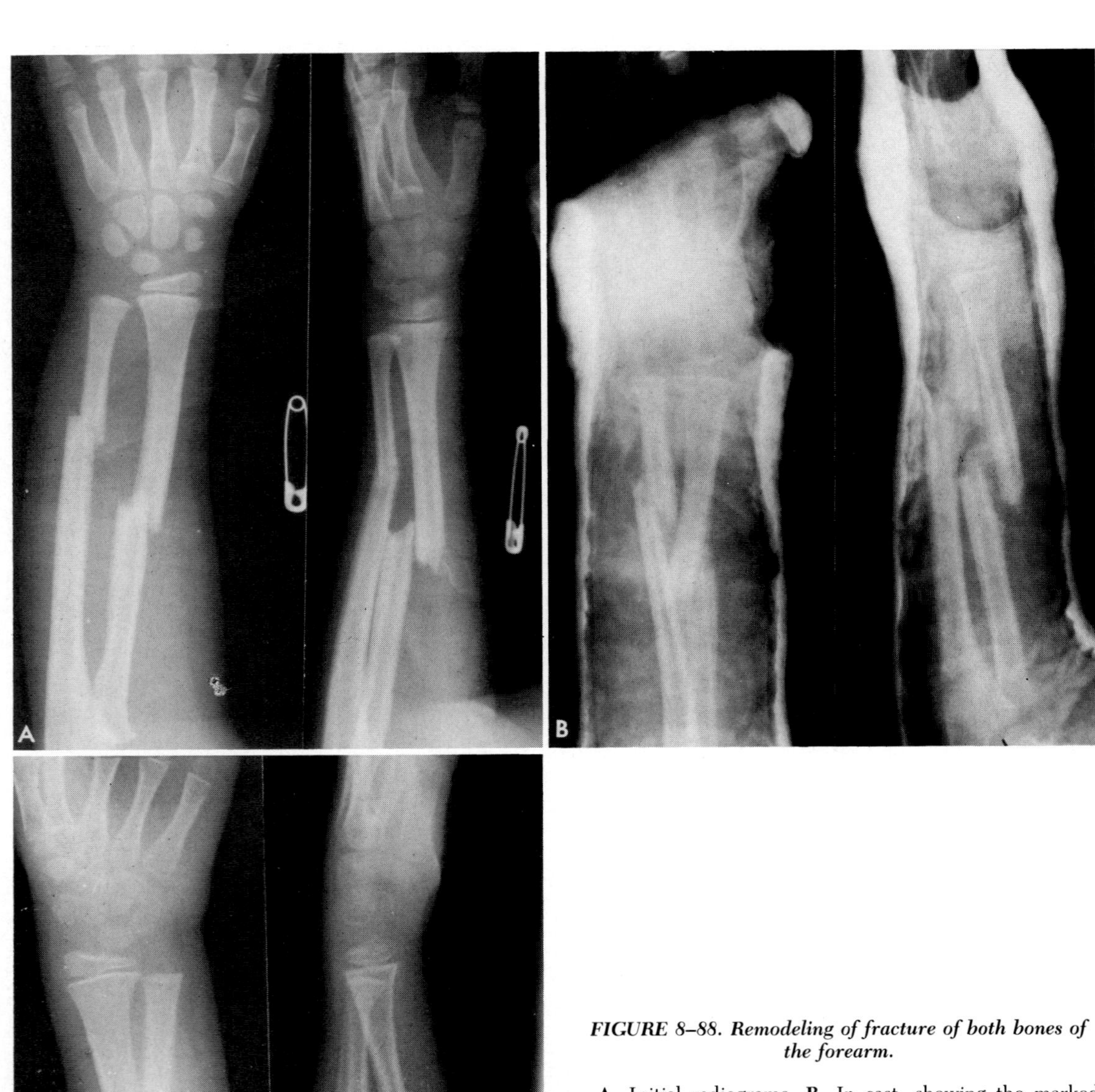

FIGURE 8–88. Remodeling of fracture of both bones of the forearm.

A. Initial radiograms. **B.** In cast, showing the marked displacement of the fragments. **C.** Four weeks later, showing the malunion.

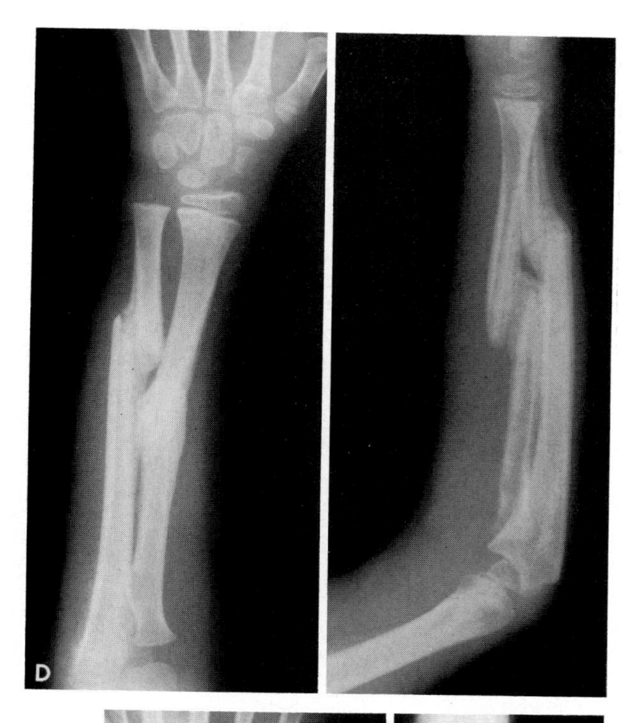

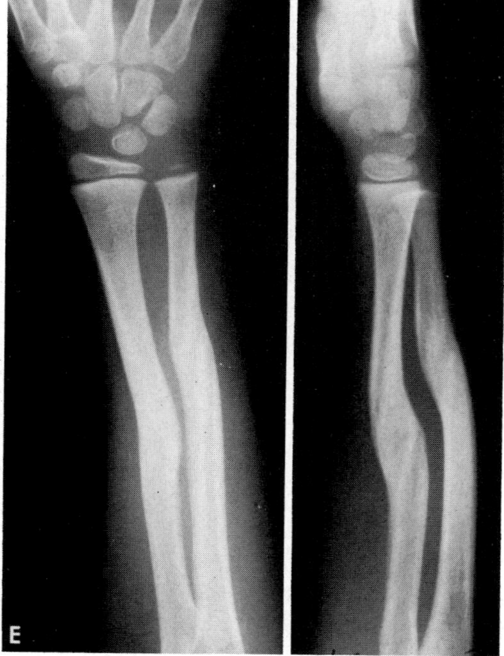

FIGURE 8–88 Continued. Remodeling of fracture of both bones of the forearm.

D. After one month there is solid bony union. Parents were unhappy and desired surgery to correct the deformity. They were assured it would be spontaneously corrected by remodeling. **E.** Six months later, alignment was good, child had normal looking arm with excellent function.

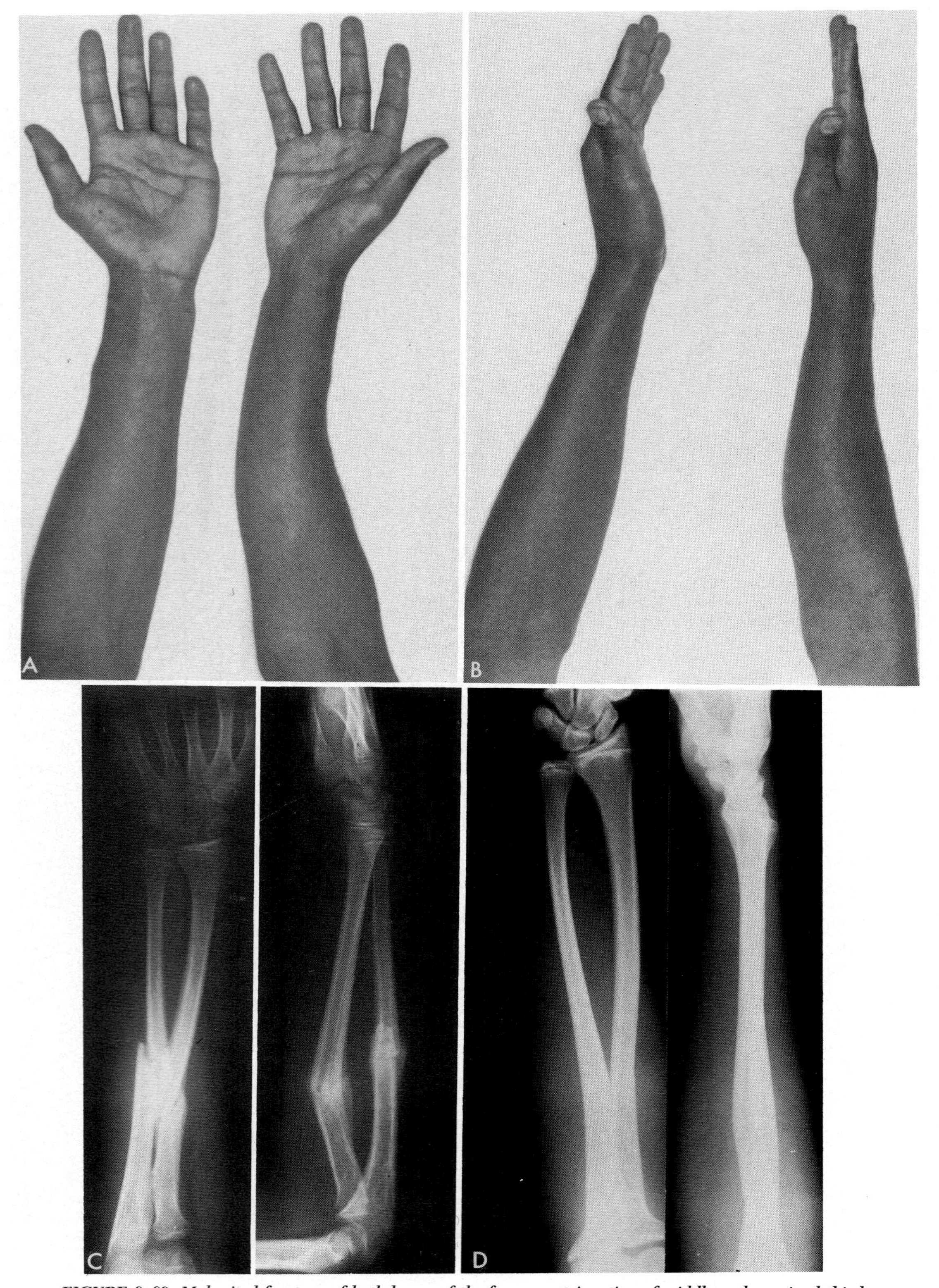

FIGURE 8–89. Malunited fracture of both bones of the forearm at junction of middle and proximal thirds.

A and **B.** Clinical appearance of the deformity. The distal fragment is angulated dorsally and radially. **C.** Radiograms showing the malalignment. **D.** Four years later. Note the spontaneous correction by remodeling.

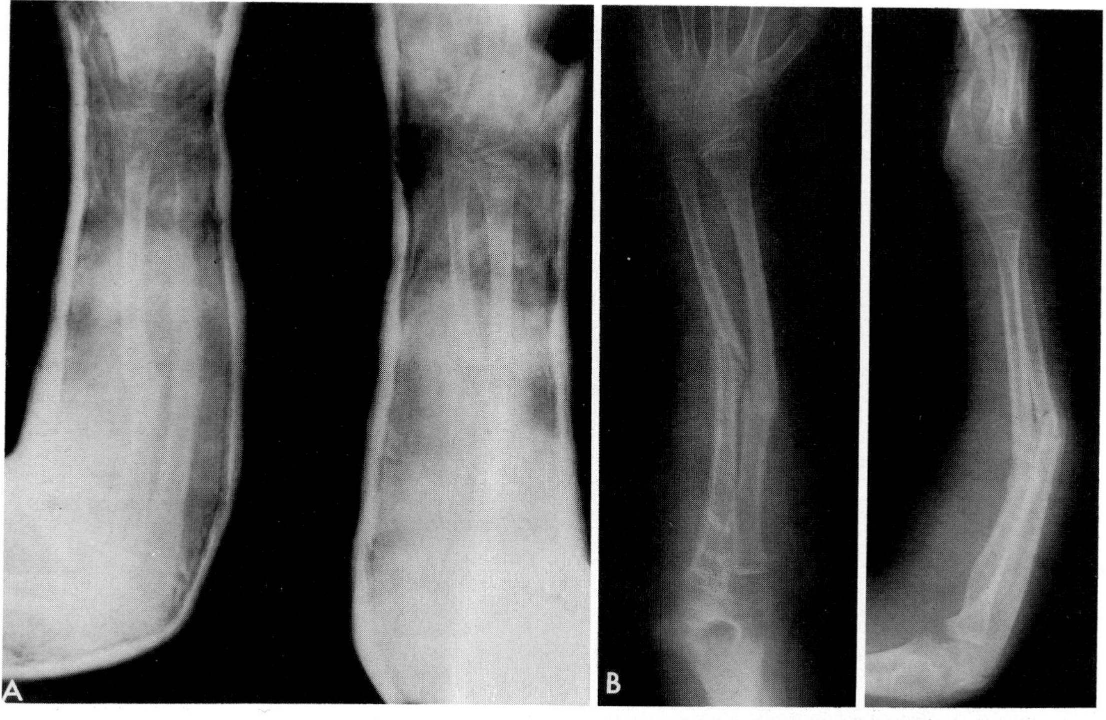

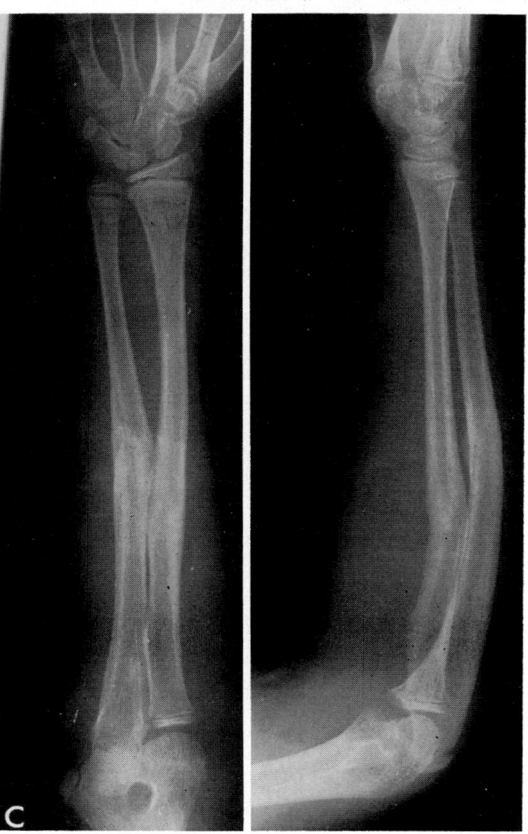

FIGURE 8–90. "Both-bone" fractures of forearm.

These views illustrate the importance of changing the cast when it becomes loose and obtaining a true lateral view. **A.** Radiograms following reduction. Alignment was interpreted to be satisfactory. Note this is an oblique and not a true lateral view. The patient was told to return in a month. **B.** On removal of the cast, the dorsal angulation of fracture fragments was noted. **C.** Six months later, remodeling has taken place.

6. Barquet, A.: Posterior dislocation of the ulna with associated fracture of the radial shaft. Injury, *15*:390, 1984.
7. Bengner, U., and Johnell, O.: Increasing incidence of forearm fractures. A comparison of epidemiologic patterns 25 years apart. Acta Orthop. Scand., *56*:158, 1985.
8. Blount, W. P.: Fractures of the forearm in children. Pediatr. Clin. North Am., *2*:1097, 1955.
9. Blount, W. P.: Fractures of the forearm in children. Indust. Med. Surg., *32*:9, 1963.
10. Blount, W. P.: Forearm fractures in children. Clin. Orthop., *51*:93, 1967.
11. Blount, W. P.: Fractures in Children. Reprinted. Huntington, N.Y., R. E. Kreiger, 1977.
12. Blount, W. P., Shaefer, A. A., and Johnson, J. H.: Fractures of the forearm in children. J.A.M.A., *120*:111, 1942.
13. Bonnemann, D., and Weigert, M.: Fractures of the forearm in children; operative treatment. Zentralbl. Chir., *104*:224, 1979.
14. Borden, S.: Traumatic bowing of the forearm in children. J. Bone Joint Surg., *56-A*:611, 1974.
15. Borden, S.: Roentgen recognition of acute plastic bowing of the forearm in children. A.J.R., *125*:524, 1975.
16. Bosworth, B. M.: Fractures of both bones of the forearm in children. Surg. Gynecol. Obstet., *72*:667, 1941.
17. Burman, M.: Primary torsional fracture of the radius or ulna. J. Bone Joint Surg., *35-A*:665, 1953.
18. Callender, G. W.: Fractures injuring joints; fractures interfering with the movement of the wrist and with those of pronation and supination. St. Bartholomew's Hosp. Rep., *1*:281, 1865.
19. Carr, C. R., and Tracy, H. W.: Management of fractures of the distal forearm in children. South. Med. J., *57*:540, 1964.
20. Catterall, A.: Fractures in children. *In* Wilson, J. N. (ed.): Watson-Jones Fractures and Joint Injuries. 5th Ed. Edinburgh, Churchill-Livingstone, 1976, p. 487.
21. Chamay, A.: Mechanical and morphological aspects of experimental overload fatigue on bone. J. Biomech., *3*:263, 1970.
22. Chapman, K. W., and Frankel, V. H.: Rotational deformity of both bones following forearm fractures. J. Bone Joint Surg., *55-B*:66, 1973.
23. Chigot, P., and Esteve, P.: Treatment of diaphyseal fractures of the forearm in children. Rev. Prat., *22*:1615, 1972.
24. Christensen, J. B., Cho, K. O., and Adams, J. P.: A study of the interosseous distance between the radius and ulna during rotation of the forearm. J. Bone Joint Surg., *45-B*:778, 1965.
25. Compere, C. L.: *In* discussion of Carr, C. R., and Tracy, H. W.: Management of fractures of the distal forearm in children. South. Med. J., *57*:540, 1964.
26. Cooper, R. R.: Management of common forearm fractures in children. J. Iowa Med. Soc., *54*:689, 1964.
27. Crowe, J. E., and Swischuk, L. E.: Acute bowing fractures of the forearm in children: A frequently missed injury. A.J.R., *128*:981, 1977.
28. Cruess, R. L.: The management of forearm injuries. Orthop. Clin. North Am., *4*:969, 1973.
29. Currey, J. D., and Butler, G.: The mechanical properties of bone tissue in children. J. Bone Joint Surg., *57-A*:810, 1975.
30. Daruwalla, J. S.: A study of radio-ulnar movements following fractures of the forearm in children. Clin. Orthop., *139*:114, 1979.
31. Davis, D. R., and Green, D. P.: Forearm fractures in children. Pitfalls and complications. Clin. Orthop., *120*:172, 1976.
32. Demos, T.: Radiologic case study. Orthopedics, *3*:108, 1980.
33. Destot, E.: De la perte des mouvements de pronation et de supination dans les fractures de l'avant bras. Lyon Med., *112*:61, 1909.
34. Destot, E.: Pronation and supination of the forearm in traumatic lesions. Presse Med., *21*:41, 1913.
35. Dodge, H. S., and Cady, G. W.: Treatment of fractures of the radius and ulna with compression plates. J. Bone Joint Surg., *54-A*:1167, 1972.
36. Dohler, R., Al-Arfaj, A. L., and Loffler, W.: Complete forearm fractures in children—possibilities and limitations of conservative therapy. An analysis of 195 cases. Unfallheilkunde, *86*:22, 1983.
37. Eliason, E. L.: Fractures of the Humerus, Radius and Ulna. New York, Appleton, 1925.
38. Evans, E. M.: Rotational deformity in the treatment of fractures of both bones of the forearm. J. Bone Joint Surg., *27*:373, 1945.
39. Evans, E. M.: Fractures of the radius and ulna. J. Bone Joint Surg., *33-B*:548, 1951.
40. Fatti, J. F., and Mosher, J. F.: An unusual complication of fracture of both bones of the forearm. J. Bone Joint Surg., *68-A*:451, 1986.
41. Fee, N. F., Dobranski, A., and Bisla, R. S.: Gas gangrene complicating open forearm fractures. Report of five cases. J. Bone Joint Surg., *59-A*:135, 1977.
42. Feldkamp, G., and Daum, R.: Long term results of forearm shaft fractures in children. Hefte Unfallheilkd., *132*:389, 1978.
43. Feoktistov, G. F.: A method of fracture fixation during open reduction in the ulnar joint region of children. Ortop. Travmatol. Protez., *32*:70, 1971.
44. Fernandez, D. L.: Conservative treatment of forearm fractures in children. *In* Chapchal, G. (ed.): Fractures in Children. New York, Thieme-Stratton, 1981.
45. Filipe, G., Dupont, J. Y., and Carlioz, H.: Recurrent fractures of both bones of the forearm in children. Chir. Pediatr., *20*:421, 1979.
46. Fink, D.: Forearm fractures in adolescents. Unfallheilkunde, *80*:479, 1977.
47. Fleischer, H.: Marrow wiring in lower-arm fractures of children. Dtsch. Med. Wochenschr., *100*:1278, 1975.
48. Friberg, K. S. I.: Remodelling after distal forearm fractures: Part 1. Acta Orthop. Scand., *50*:537, 1979.
49. Friberg, K. S. I.: Remodelling after distal forearm fractures: Part 2. Acta Orthop. Scand., *50*:731, 1979.
50. Friberg, K. S. I.: Remodelling after distal forearm fractures. Part 3. Acta Orthop. Scand., *50*:741, 1979.
51. Fuller, D. J., and McCullough, C. J.: Malunited fractures of the forearm in children. J. Bone Joint Surg., *64-B*:364, 1982.
52. Gainor, J. W., and Hardy, J. H., III: Forearm fractures treated in extension. Immobilization of fractures of the proximal bones of the forearm in children. J. Trauma, 9:167, 1969.
53. Gandhi, R. K., Wilson, P., Brown, J. J. M., and Macleod, W.: Spontaneous correction of deformity following fractures of the forearm in children. Br. J. Surg., *50*:5, 1962.
54. Giberson, R. G., and Ivins, J. C.: Fractures of the distal part of the forearm in children. Minn. Med., *35*:744, 1952.
55. Glatzer, R. L., Perlman, R. D., Michaels, G., and Matles, A.: Fractures of both bones of the distal forearm in children. Bull. Hosp. J. Dis., *28*:14, 1967.
56. Griffin, P. P.: Forearm fractures in children. Clin. Orthop., *129*:320, 1977.
57. Gruber, R., and von Laer, L. R.: The etiology of the refracture of the forearm in childhood. Aktuel. Traumatol., *9*:251, 1979.
58. Gumbs, V. L., Segal, D., Halligan, J. B., and Lower,

G.: Bilateral distal radius and ulnar fractures in adolescent weight lifters. Am. J. Sports Med., *10*:375, 1982.

59. Hanlon, C. R., and Estes, W. L.: Fractures in childhood—a statistical analysis. Am. J. Surg., *87*:312, 1954.
60. Harbison, J. S., Stevenson, T. M., and Lipert, J. R.: Forearm fractures in children. Aust. N.Z. J. Surg., *48*:84, 1978.
61. Helferich, H.: Fractures and Dislocations. Philadelphia, W. B. Saunders, 1902, p. 211.
62. Herrick, R. T.: Bilateral distal radius and ulnar shafts in adolescent weight lifters. Am. J. Sports Med., *11*:369, 1983.
63. Hey Groves, E. W.: On Modern Methods of Treating Fractures. Bristol, John Wright & Sons, 1916, p. 227.
64. Hoffer, M. M., and Schobert, W.: The failure of casual treatment for nondisplaced ulnar shaft fractures. J. Trauma, *24*:771, 1984.
65. Hogstrom, H., Nilsson, B. E., and Willner, S.: Correction with growth following diaphyseal forearm fracture. Acta Orthop. Scand., *47*:299, 1976.
66. Hohmann, D., Luther, R., and Weseloh, G.: Therapy of forearm fractures close to the elbow joint. Dtsch. Med. Wochenschr., *23*:533, 1972.
67. Holdsworth, B. J., and Sloan, J. P.: Proximal forearm fractures in children: Residual disability. Injury, *14*:174, 1982.
68. Hughston, J. C.: Fractures of the forearm in children. J. Bone Joint Surg., *44-A*:1678, 1962.
69. Ihasz, M., Salamon, A., and Korcsmar, J.: Experience with the surgical management of childhood forearm fractures. Magy. Traumatol. Orthop. Helyreallito Sebez., *27*:56, 1984.
70. Jacoby, A. W.: Note on the interosseous membrane of the forearm: The discussion of its fibers in surgical anatomy. Bull. Hosp. J. Dis., *32*:105, 1971.
71. Judet, J., Rigault, P., and Plumerault, J.: Diaphyseal fractures of the two bones of the forearm in children. Technique and results of treatment with the R. and J. Judet external fixation. Presse Med., *74*:2583, 1966.
72. Jupiter, J. B.: The management of multiple fractures in one upper extremity: A case report. J. Hand Surg., *11-A*:279, 1986.
73. Kay, S., Smith, C., and Oppenheim, W. L.: Both-bone midshaft forearm fractures in children. J. Pediatr. Orthop., *6*:306, 1986.
74. King, R. E.: Fractures of the shafts of the radius and ulna. *In* Rockwood, C. A., Wilkins, K. E., and King, R. E. (eds.): Fractures in Children. Philadelphia, Lippincott, 1984, pp. 301–362.
75. Kurz, W., Vinz, H., and Wahl, D.: Late results of osteosynthesis in forearm fractures in childhood. Zentralbl. Chir., *107*:149, 1982.
76. Kurz-Lange: Operative Behandlung von Vorarmschaftbruchen bei Kindern. Padiatr. Praxis, *10*:47, 1971.
77. Kuzmin, B. P.: Repeated fractures of both bones of the forearm in children. Ortop. Travmatol. Protez., *28*:70, 1967.
78. Lange, R. H., and Foster, R. J.: Skeletal management of humeral shaft fractures associated with forearm fractures. Clin. Orthop., *195*:173, 1985.
79. Levinthal, D. H.: Fractures of the lower one third of both bones of the forearm in children. Surg. Gynecol. Obstet., *57*:790, 1933.
80. Lanzi, F.: Evolution of fractures of the forearm in children and adolescents. Arch. Ortop., *78*:327, 1965.
81. Lindholm, R., Puronvarsi, U., Lindholm, S., and Leiviska, T.: Vorderarmschaft-bruche bei Kindern und Erwachsenen. Beitr. Orthop. Traumatol., *7*:369, 1972.
82. London, P. S.: A Practical Guide to the Care of the Injured. Edinburgh, E. & S. Livingstone, 1967.
83. London, P. S.: Observations on the treatment of some fractures of the forearm by splintage that does not include the elbow. Injury, *2*:252, 1971.
84. Lorthior, J.: Traitment des fractures chez l'enfant. Acta Orthop. Belg., *31*:611, 1965.
85. Manoli, A., II: Medial displacement of the shaft of the radius with a fracture of the radial neck. Report of a case. J. Bone Joint Surg., *61-A*:788, 1979.
86. Matthews, L., Kaufer, H., Garver, D., and Sonstegard, D.: The effect on supination-pronation of angular malalignment of fractures of both bones of the forearm. J. Bone Joint Surg., *64-A*:14, 1982.
87. Milch, H.: Roentgenographic differentiation between torsion and rotation in fractures of the forearm. Bull. Hosp. J. Dis., *10*:216, 1949.
88. Miller, J. H., and Osterkamp, J. A.: Scintigraphy in acute plastic bowing of the forearm. Radiology, *142*:742, 1982.
89. Moesner, J., and Ostergaard, A. H.: Diaphysefrakturer newborn. Nord. Med., *75*:355, 1966.
90. Morger, R., and Brunner, C.: Fractures of the forearm. Ther. Umsch., *40*:951, 1983.
91. Nilsson, B. E., and Obrant, K.: The range of motion following fracture of the shaft of the forearm in children. Acta Orthop. Scand., *48*:600, 1977.
92. Nunley, J. A., and Urbaniak, J. R.: Partial bony entrapment of the median nerve in a greenstick fracture of the ulna. J. Hand Surg., *5*:557, 1980.
93. Ogden, J. A., Conlogue, G. J., Light, T. R., and Sloan, T. R.: Fractures of the radius and ulna in a skeletally immature fin whale. J. Wildl. Dis., *17*:111, 1981.
94. Onne, L., and Sandblom, P.: Late results in fractures of the forearm in children. Acta Chir. Scand., *98*:549, 1949.
95. Patrick, J.: A study of supination and pronation with special reference to the treatment of forearm fractures. J. Bone Joint Surg., *28*:737, 1946.
96. Pollen, A. G.: Fractures and Dislocations in Children. Baltimore, Williams & Wilkins, 1973.
97. Rang, M.: Children's Fractures. Philadelphia, Lippincott, 1974.
98. Ravessoud, F. A.: Lateral condylar fracture and ipsilateral ulnar shaft fracture: Monteggia equivalent lesions? J. Pediatr. Orthop., *5*:364, 1985.
99. Ray, R. D., Johnson, R. J., and Jameson, R. M.: Rotation of the forearm. An experimental study of pronation and supination. J. Bone Joint Surg., *33-A*:993, 1951.
100. Reed, F. E., Jr., and Apple, D. F., Jr.: Ipsilateral fractures of the elbow and forearm. South. Med. J., *69*:149, 1976.
101. Rettig, A. C.: Stress fracture of the ulna in an adolescent tournament tennis player. Am. J. Sports Med., *11*:103, 1983.
102. Rigault, P.: Forearm fractures in children. Ann. Chir., *34*:810, 1980.
103. Rogers, J. F., Bennett, J. B., and Tullos, H. S.: Management of concomitant ipsilateral fractures of the humerus and forearm. J. Bone Joint Surg., *66*:552, 1984.
104. Rosenholz, U.: Treatment of biosseous fractures of the third distal segment of the forearm in children. Friuli Med. (Suppl.), *6*:1221, 1968.
105. Ryan, P., and Hayes, G.: Personal communication, 1979.
106. Rydholm, U., and Nilsson, J. E.: Traumatic bowing of the forearm. Clin. Orthop., *139*:121, 1979.
107. Salter, N., and Dareus, H. D.: The amplitude of forearm and of humeral rotation. J. Anat., *87*:407, 1953.

108. Sanders, W. E., and Heckman, J. D.: Traumatic plastic deformation of the radius and ulna. A closed method of correction of deformity. Clin. Orthop., *188*:58, 1984.
109. Sarmiento, A., Cooper, J., and Sinclair, W. F.: Forearm fractures—early functional bracing, a preliminary report. J. Bone Joint Surg., *57-A*:297, 1975.
110. Sarmiento, A., Kinman, P. B., Murphy, B., and Phillips, J. G.: Treatment of ulnar fractures by functional bracing. J. Bone Joint Surg., *58-A*:1104, 1976.
111. Schweiberer, L., and Altherr, W. F.: Forearm shaft fractures in childhood. Hefte Unfallheilkd., *132*:381, 1978.
112. Scudder, C. L.: Treatment of Fractures. 3rd Ed. Philadelphia, Saunders, 1902, p. 201.
113. Seyfarth, G.: The management of strongly displaced forearm fractures in children and juveniles. Contribution to the problem of surgical justification. Arch. Orthop. Unfallchir., *64*:64, 1968.
114. Simon, L., and Heydenreich, W.: Markdrahtungsosteosynthese bei kindlichen Unterarmschaftfrakturen. Aktuel. Traumatol., *2*:191, 1975.
115. Skillern, P. G., Jr.: Complete fracture of the lower third of the radius in childhood with greenstick fracture of the ulna. Ann. Surg., *61*:209, 1915.
116. Spissak, L., Geryk, B., and Stolcova, E.: Anatomical and functional results of conservative therapy of diaphyseal forearm fractures in children. Acta Chir. Orthop. Traumatol. Cech., *43*:441, 1976.
117. Stanitski, C. L., and Micheli, L. J.: Simultaneous ipsilateral fractures of the arm and forearm in children. Clin. Orthop., *153*:218, 1980.
118. Steinert, V.: Unterarm-frakturen im Kindesalter. Beitr. Klin. Chir., *212*:170, 1966.
119. Stern, P. J., and Drury, W. J.: Complications of plate fixation of forearm fractures. Clin. Orthop., *175*:25, 1983.
120. Stucke, K., and Schilling, H.: Infantile radius fractures. Monatsschr. Unfallheilkd., *68*:478, 1965.
121. Stuhmer, K. G.: Fractures of the distal forearm. *In* Weber, B. G., Bruner, C., and Freuler, F. (eds.): Treatment of Fractures in Children and Adolescents. New York, Springer-Verlag, 1980.
122. Tarr, R. R., Garfinkel, A., and Sarmiento, A.: The effects of angular and rotation deformities of both bones of the forearm. An in vitro study. J. Bone Joint Surg., *66-A*:65, 1984.
123. Tato, F. B., Specchiulli, F., and Tiritiello, F.: A rare injury of the forearm in childhood. Chir. Organi Mov., *67*:471, 1981.
124. Teutsch, W., and Puschert, H.: Results of follow-up studies of conservatively treated forearm fractures in children. Zentralbl. Chir., *93*:1237, 1968.
125. Thelen, E.: Analysis of treatment methods in forearm fractures. Hefte Unfallheilkd., *129*:107, 1977.
126. Thomas, E. M., Tuson, K. W. R., and Browne, P. S. H.: Fractures of the radius and ulna in children. Injury, *7*:120, 1975.
127. Thomsen, J. L.: Acute plastic bowing of bone. J. Bone Joint Surg., *64-B*:123, 1982.
128. Tischer, W.: Forearm fractures in childhood. Zentralbl. Chir., *107*:138, 1982.
129. Trukhachev, M. I.: Peculiarities of fractures of the lower third of the forearm in children and their treatment. Klin. Khir., *6*:47, 1966.
130. Undeland, K.: Rotational movements and bony union in shaft fractures of the forearm. J. Bone Joint Surg., *44-B*:340, 1962.
131. Voumard, C., Lopez, J., Queloz, J., and Landry, M.: Plastic fractures of the forearm in the child. Ann. Radiol. (Paris), *21*:551, 1978.
132. Warren, J. D.: Anterior interosseous nerve palsy as a complication of forearm fractures. J. Bone Joint Surg., *45-B*:511, 1963.
133. Watson, F. M., Jr., and Eaton, R. G.: Post-traumatic radio-ulnar synostosis. J. Trauma, *18*:467, 1978.
134. Watson-Jones, R.: Fractures and Joint Injuries. Baltimore, Williams & Wilkins, 1946, p. 516.
135. Weigert, M., and Bonnemann, D.: Surgical indications in forearm shaft fractures in children. Hefte Unfallheilkd., *132*:386, 1978.
136. Wessely, J., and Heydenreich, K.: Indications for surgery of forearm shaft fractures in children. Hefte Unfallheilkd., *132*:392, 1978.
137. Whipple, A. O., and St. John, F. B.: Study of 100 consecutive fractures of the shafts of both bones of the forearm. Surg. Gynecol. Obstet., *25*:77, 1917.
138. Wilde, C. D., Weiss, H., and Wissing, H. J.: Results of conservatively treated forearm shaft fractures in children: Complications and indications for osteosynthesis. Hefte Unfallheilkd., *132*:396, 1978.
139. Wilson, J.: Fractures of the forearm. Pediatr. Clin. North Am., *14*:664, 1967.
140. Wilson, J. C., Jr., and Krueger, J. C.: Fractures of the proximal and middle thirds of the radius and ulna in children. Study of end results with analysis of treatment and complications. Am. J. Surg., *112*:326, 1966.
141. Young, T. B.: Irreducible displacement of the distal radial epiphysis complicating a fracture of the lower radius and ulna. Injury, *16*:166, 1984.

FRACTURE-SEPARATION OF THE DISTAL RADIAL PHYSIS

Salter-Harris Type I Injuries

This injury to the distal radial physis occurs in the infant or young child. The mechanism of injury is a fall on the outstretched hand. The young child does not use the involved limb and cries in pain when the parents touch the wrist. There is local swelling and tenderness at the distal radial physis.

In the infant plain radiograms usually appear to be normal; the fat pad sign may be positive in the lateral projection—the subperiosteal hemorrhage elevates the pronator quadratus and overlying fat pad.

The ossification center of the distal radial physis usually appears at one year of age, with a range between 8 and 18 months.

In the child two years of age and older, comparison radiograms of the opposite normal wrist should be made to detect minimal displacement of the ossific nucleus of the distal radius. Occasionally the radial styloid process may have a separate ossification center—do not mistake this for a fracture!

Treatment consists of a below-elbow volar splint or cast for a period of three weeks.

Salter-Harris Type II Injuries

This fracture is the most common physeal injury, constituting about 50 per cent of the total. It usually occurs in children between the

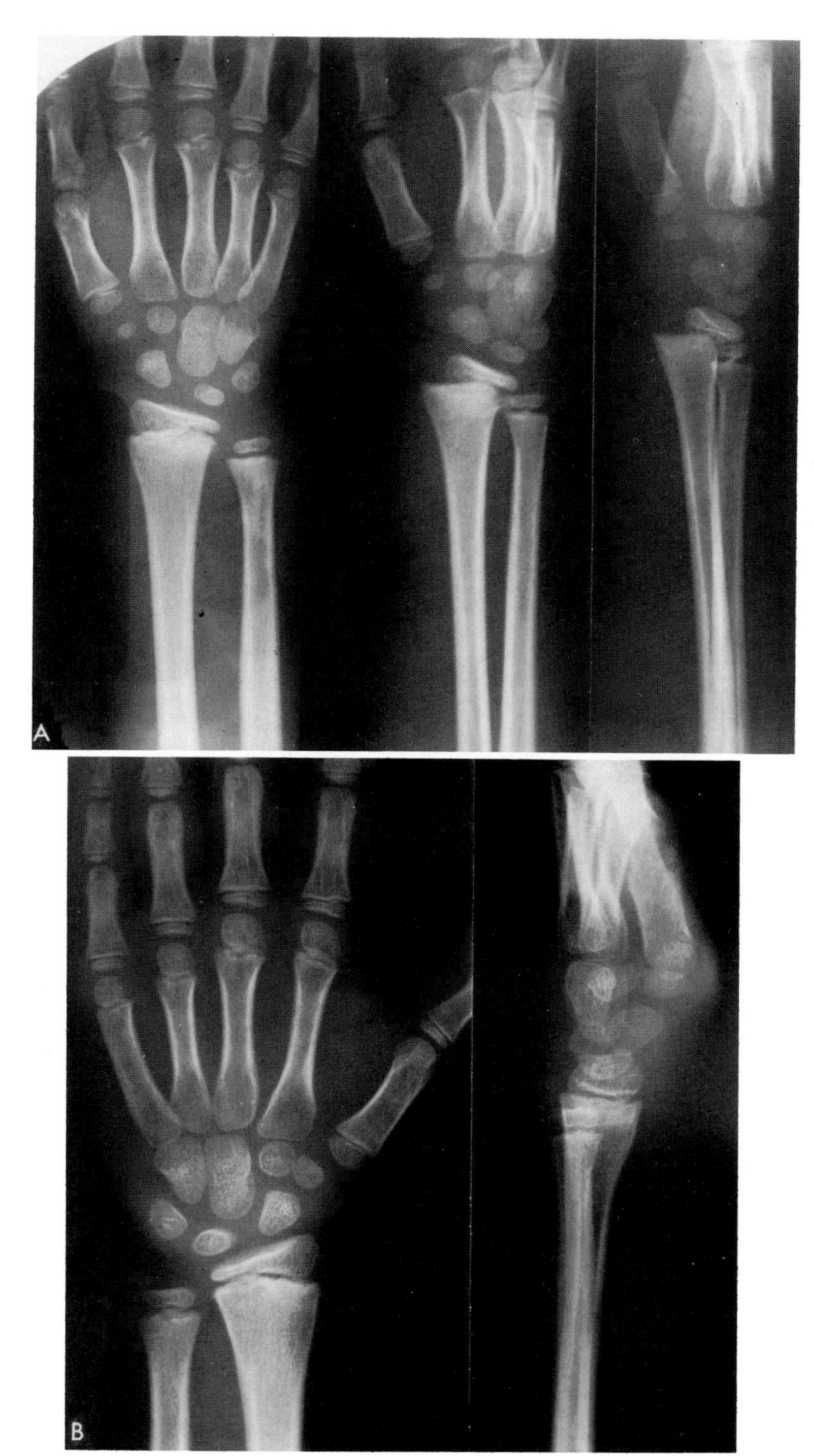

FIGURE 8–91. Fracture involving the distal radial physis.

A. Initial radiogram showing dorsal displacement of distal radial epiphysis. It was treated by closed reduction.
B. Radiogram of same wrist a year later; note the completely healed fracture with no growth disturbance.

ages of six and ten years who sustain injury by falling on an outstretched hand. The shearing forces of hyperextension and supination displace the radial epiphysis dorsally, with a small metaphyseal bone fragment attached to the dorsal or dorsoradial aspect of the epiphysis. The distal radial epiphysis may be displaced alone, or it may be associated with a greenstick fracture of the metaphysis of the ulna, separation of the distal ulnar epiphysis, or fracture of the tip of the ulnar styloid process.

Clinically, there is local pain, swelling, and "silver fork" deformity. Radiograms will establish the diagnosis by revealing posterior displacement of the epiphysis, which is best visualized in the lateral projection (Fig. 8–91). The dorsal metaphyseal bone fragment is usually small, requiring close scrutiny for detection.

Treatment consists of closed reduction and immobilization in an above-elbow cast for a period of three to four weeks. Repeated forceful manipulations should be avoided, as they cause damage to the physis. That malunion does not persist has been well demonstrated by Aitken.[3, 4] Within a maximum period of two to three years (usually five to eight months), the distal radial epiphysis will assume its normal relation to the radial metaphysis. Remodeling takes place by new bone formation on the dorsum of the distal radius so that the diaphysis is elevated to the epiphysis. The volar portion of the radius is gradually absorbed. If one or two attempts at gentle closed reduction fail, it is wise to leave the epiphysis displaced; open reduction of the markedly displaced epiphysis should not be performed.

The prognosis for a Type II physeal injury is good. Occasionally, the longitudinal forces of the impact may crush the germinal cells of the physis, producing a Type V physeal injury. This crushing of the physis cannot be detected in the early radiograms; however, within 6 to 12 months, the follow-up radiograms will disclose growth arrest by the gradual narrowing and obliteration of the radiolucent line of the physis and overgrowth of the ulna in relation to the radius.

References

1. Abbott, L. E., and Saunders, J. B.: Injuries of median nerve in fractures of the lower end of the radius. Surg. Gynecol. Obstet., *57*:507, 1933.
2. Abram, L. J., and Thompson, G. H.: Deformity after premature closure of the distal radial physis following a torus fracture with a physeal compression injury. Report of a case. J. Bone Joint Surg., *69-A*:1450, 1987.
3. Aitken, A. P.: The end results of the fractured distal radial epiphysis. J. Bone Joint Surg., *17*:302, 1935.
4. Aitken, A. P.: Further observations on fractured distal radial epiphysis. J. Bone Joint Surg., *17*:922, 1935.
5. Altissimi, M., Antenucci, R., Fiacca, C., and Mancini, G. B.: Long-term results of conservative treatment of fractures of the distal radius. Clin. Orthop., *206*:202, 1986.
6. Blount, W. P.: Fractures in Children. Baltimore, Williams & Wilkins, 1955.
7. Bragdon, R. A.: Fractures of the distal radial epiphysis. Clin. Orthop., *41*:59, 1965.
8. Eisenberg, D., Kirchner, S. G., and Green, N. E.: Stress fracture of the distal radius caused by "wheelies." South. Med. J., *79*:918, 1986.
9. Elsasser, U., Ruegsegger, P., Anliker, M., Exner, G. U., and Prader, A.: Loss and recovery of trabecular bone in the distal radius following fracture—immobilization of the upper limb in children. Klin. Wochenschr., *57*:763, 1979.
10. Friberg, K. S.: Remodelling after distal forearm fractures in children. I. The effect of residual angulation on the spatial orientation of the epiphyseal plates. Acta Orthop. Scand., *50*:537, 1979.
11. Friberg, K. S.: Remodelling after distal forearm fractures in children. II. The final orientation of the distal and proximal epiphyseal plates of the radius. Acta Orthop. Scand., *50*:731, 1979.
12. Friberg, K. S.: Remodelling after distal forearm fractures in children. III. Correction of residual angulation in fractures of the radius. Acta Orthop. Scand., *50*:741, 1979.
13. Friberg, S., and Lundstrom, B.: Radiographic measurements on the radio-carpal joint in distal radial fractures. Acta Radiol. [Diagn.] (Stockh.), *17*:869, 1976.
14. Grimault, L., and Leonhart, E.: De collement epiphyssaire de l'extremitiés inferieure du radius. Rev. Chir. Orthop., *12*:261, 1925.
15. Hanlon, C. R., and Estes, W. L.: Fractures in childhood—a statistical analysis. Am. J. Surg., *87*:312, 1954.
16. Hernandez, J., Jr., and Peterson, H. A.: Fracture of the distal radial physis complicated by compartment syndrome and premature physeal closure. J. Pediatr. Orthop., *6*:627, 1986.
17. Holland, C. T.: A radiographical note on injuries to the distal epiphyses of the radius and ulna. Proc. R. Soc. Med., *22*:695, 1929.
18. Kristiansen, B., and Eriksen, A. F.: Simultaneous type II Monteggia lesion and fracture-separation of the lower radial epiphysis. Injury, *17*:51, 1986.
19. Lee, B. S., Esterhai, J. L., Jr., and Das, M.: Fracture of the distal radial epiphysis. Characteristics and surgical treatment of premature, post-traumatic epiphyseal closure. Clin. Orthop., *185*:90, 1984.
20. Lesko, P. D., Georgis, T., and Slabaugh, P.: Irreducible Salter-Harris Type II fracture of the distal radial epiphysis. J. Pediatr. Orthop., *7*:719, 1987.
21. McLaughlin, H. L.: Trauma. Philadelphia, Saunders, 1959.
22. Manoli, A., II: Irreducible fracture-separation of the distal radial epiphysis. Report of a case. J. Bone Joint Surg., *64-A*:1095, 1982.
23. Meadoff, N.: Median nerve injuries in fractures in the region of the wrist. Calif. Med., *70*:252, 1949.
24. Mischkowsky, I., Daum, R., and Reif, W.: Injuries of the distal radial epiphysis. Arch. Orthop. Trauma. Surg., *96*:15, 1965.
25. Muller, J., Roth, B., and Willenegger, H.: Long-term results of epiphyseal fractures to the distal radius treated by percutaneous wire fixation. *In* Chapchal, G. (ed.): Fractures in Children. New York, Thieme-Stratton, 1981.
26. Peterson, C. A., and Peterson, H. A.: Analysis of the incidence of injuries to the epiphyseal growth plate. J. Trauma, *12*:275, 1972.
27. Peterson, H. A.: Partial growth plate arrest and its treatment. J. Pediatr. Orthop., *4*:246, 1984.

28. Pollen, A. G.: Fractures and Dislocations in Children. Edinburgh, Churchill-Livingstone, 1973.
29. Reichmann, W.: Distal radial fracture in childhood. Handchirurgie, *10*:179, 1978.
30. Roy, S., Caine, D., and Singer, K.: Stress changes of the distal radial epiphysis in young gymnasts. A report of 21 cases and a review of the literature. Am. J. Sports Med., *13*:301, 1985.
31. Rutt, J., Kusswetter, W., and Beck, E.: Results of treatment in epiphysiolysis of the distal forearm. Unfallheilkunde, *86*:492, 1983.
32. Salter, R. B., and Harris, W. R.: Injuries involving the epiphyseal plate. J. Bone Joint Surg., *45-A*:587, 1963.
33. Shall, J., Cohn, B. T., and Froimson, A. I.: Acute compartment syndrome of the forearm in association with fracture of the distal end of the radius. Report of two cases. J. Bone Joint Surg., *68-A*:1451, 1986.
34. Solgaard, S.: Early displacement of distal radius fracture. Acta Orthop. Scand., *57*:229, 1986.
35. Sterling, A. P., and Habermann, E. T.: Acute posttraumatic median nerve compression associated with a Salter II fracture dislocation of the wrist. Bull. Hosp. J. Dis., *34*:167, 1963.
36. Stuhmer, K. G.: Fractures of the distal forearm. *In* Weber, B. G., Bruner, C., and Freuler, F. (eds.): Treatment of Fractures in Children and Adolescents. New York, Springer-Verlag, 1980.
37. Sumner, J. M., and Khuri, S. M.: Entrapment of the median nerve and flexor pollicis longus tendon in an epiphyseal fracture-dislocation of the distal radioulnar joint: A case report. J. Hand Surg., *9*:711, 1984.
38. Sussenbach, F., and Weber, B. G.: Epiphysenfugenverletzungen am distalen Unterschenkel. Bern, Wien, Humber, 1970.
39. Teisinger, P., Vyhnanek, L., Eckert, V., and Druga, R.: Changes in the soft parts due to injuries of peripheral epiphysis of the radius. Cesk. Radiol., *24*:136, 1970.
40. Vidal, J., Buscayret, C., Fischbach, C., Brahin, B., Paran, M., and Escare, P.: Une methode originale dans le traitement des fractures comminutives de l'extremitié inferieure du radius: "le taxis ligamentaire." Acta Orthop. Belg., *43*:781, 1977.
41. Wagner, H.: Korrektureingriffe nach Verletzungen des distalen Radiusendes. Langenbecks Arch. Chir., *334*:211, 1973.
42. Watson-Jones, R.: Fractures and Joint Injuries. Edinburgh, Churchill-Livingstone, 1940.
43. Young, T. B.: Irreducible displacement of the distal radial epiphysis complicating a fracture of the lower radius and ulna. Injury, *16*:166, 1984.

FRACTURES OF THE PHALANGES AND METACARPALS IN THE HAND

Fractures of the bones in the hand are rare injuries in children, but if encountered, they are treated as in the adult.

Comminuted fracture of the distal phalanx caused by direct crushing force is frequently seen in children.[19, 50, 54, 58] The nail is trephined to release the hematoma and to relieve the intense pain due to the distended pulp. Traumatic avulsion of the fingernail may cause injury to the physis of the distal phalanx.[23] If the nailbed is injured it should be repaired in order to prevent a deformed fingernail.[5] Repositioning and fixation of the fingernail will serve as an external splint.[9, 61] When the nailbed is avulsed and irreparable, split-thickness nailbed graft may be performed.[65] A padded aluminum finger splint is applied to protect the fingertip.

When the level of fracture is proximal to the insertion of the flexor digitorum sublimis, the angulation is dorsal (Fig. 8–92 C and D). It is reduced and immobilized with the interphalangeal joints in extension. A displaced T-fracture of the distal end of the proximal phalanx requires open reduction and internal fixation with a Kirschner wire.

Fractures of the *middle phalanx* may be undisplaced or angulated. If the site of the fracture is distal to the insertion of the flexor digitorum sublimis tendon, the proximal fragment is angulated toward the palm; this is treated by manual traction and flexion of the distal fragment. It is immobilized in a below-elbow plaster cast with a volar padded aluminum splint. The interphalangeal joints are completely flexed; the metacarpophalangeal joint is partially flexed, whereas the wrist is in neutral position (Fig. 8–92 E and F).

In fractures of the midshaft of the proximal phalanx, the apex of the angulation is volar owing to the action of the intrinsic muscles (Fig. 8–92 A and B). The fracture line may be transverse or oblique. Reduction is achieved and maintained in flexion; it should never be immobilized in extension. Those fingers adjacent to the injured ones are splinted as well. Unstable fractures may require skeletal traction with a pin through the distal phalanx. Attention should be given to maintaining correct rotational alignment. Fractures involving the physis of the phalanges require accurate reduction.[14, 48] Occasionally the fracture may be irreducible by closed methods and require open reduction.[37] Asymmetrical physeal arrest will cause angular deformity. If bone bridging across the growth plate is less than 50 per cent, the bony bridge is resected and fat interposed (Langenskiold procedure). This is feasible with magnifying loops or microsurgery (Fig. 8–93). Open-up or closing wedge osteotomy may be needed to correct angular deformity.

Rotational malalignment of fracture of the proximal phalanx will cause overlapping of the fingers.[20] This may be simple to correct by metacarpal rotational osteotomy.[15]

Metacarpal fractures usually occur in adolescents who get into fist fights. The dorsally angulated fracture of the shaft of the metacarpal is easily reduced by elevation of the distal fragment (Fig. 8–94). The displaced fracture of

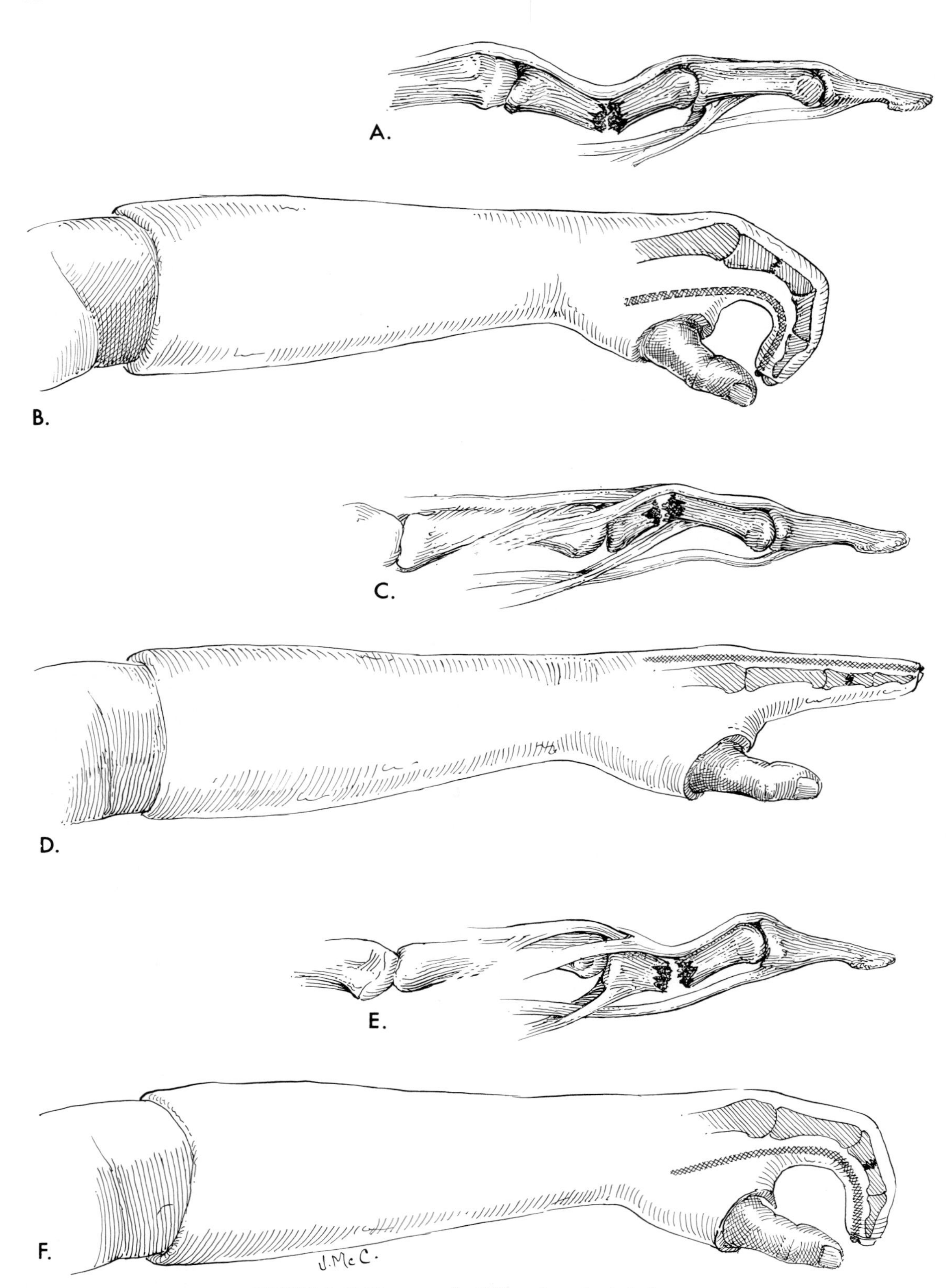

FIGURE 8–92. Fracture of middle and proximal phalanges.

A and **B.** Fracture of proximal phalanx. **C** and **D.** Fracture of middle phalanx proximal to insertion of flexor digitorum sublimis tendon. **E** and **F.** Fracture of middle phalanx distal to insertion of flexor digitorum sublimis tendon.

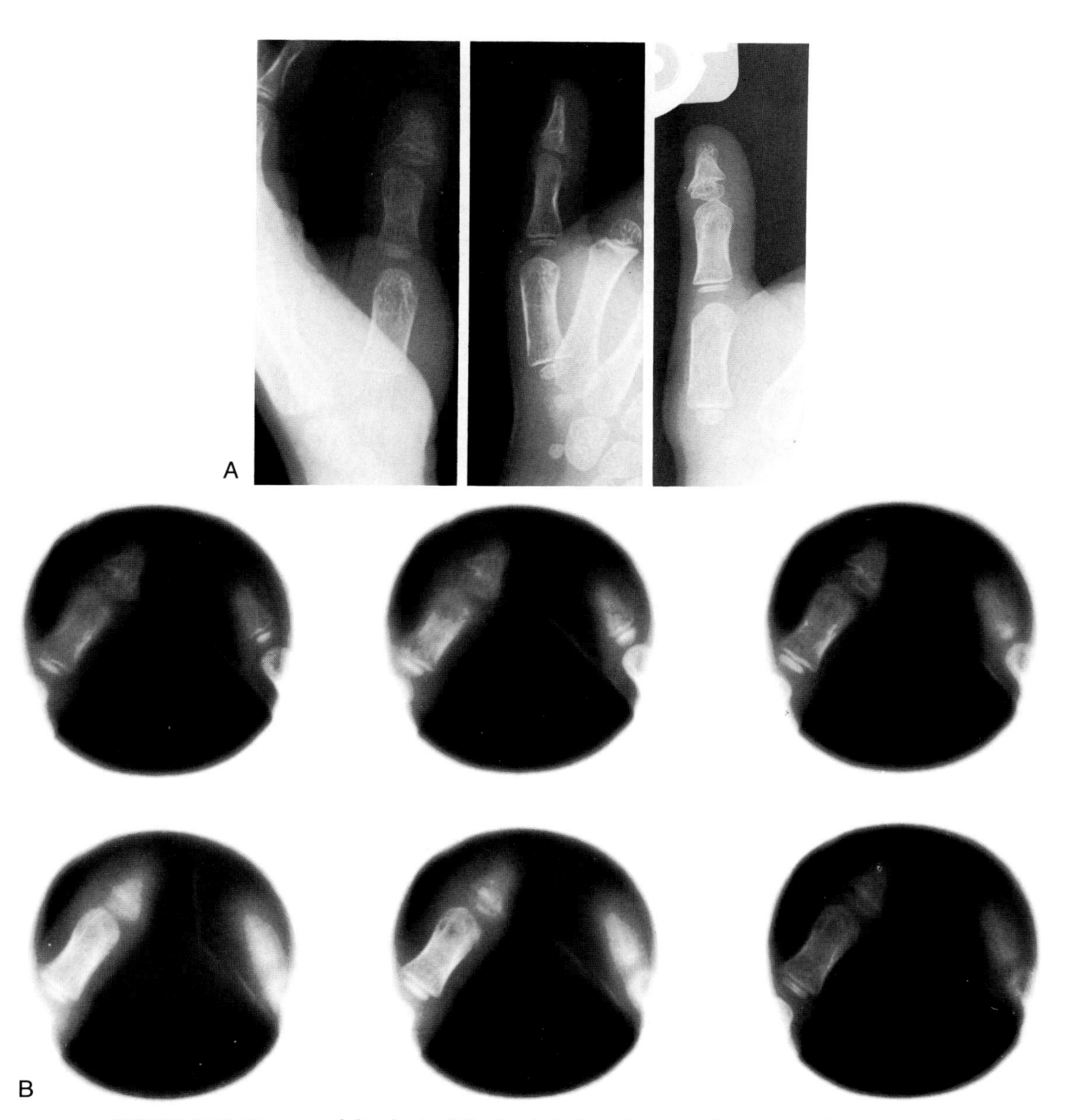

FIGURE 8–93. Fracture of the physis of the distal phalanx of the thumb with partial growth arrest and lateral angulation.

A. Preoperative radiograms. Anteroposterior, lateral, and oblique views showing the bony bridge on the radial aspect of the physis of the distal phalanx.

B. Linear tomograms showing the bony bridge extending across 65 per cent of the growth plate.

Illustration continued on following page

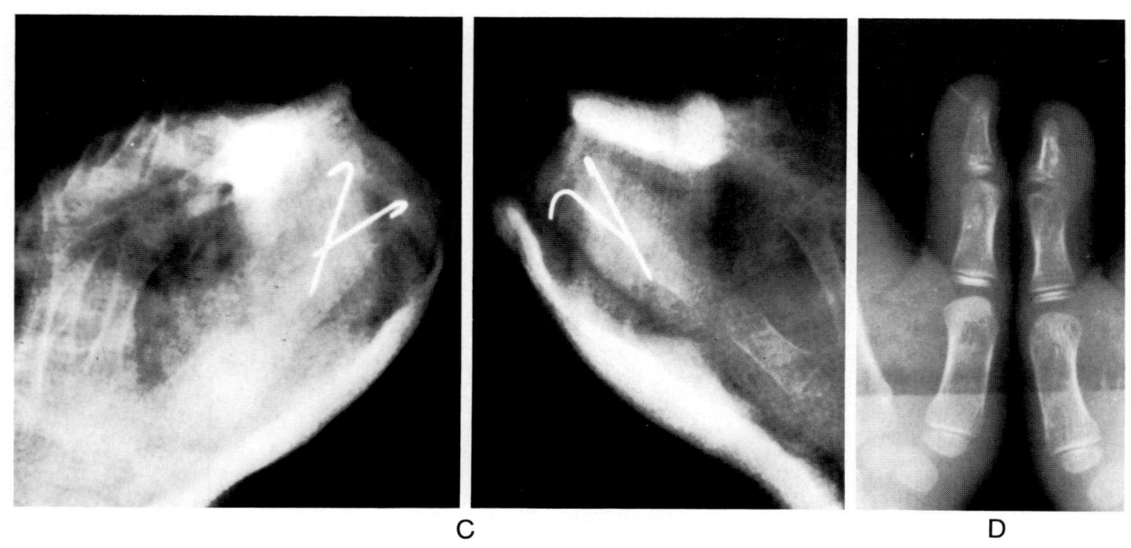

FIGURE 8–93 Continued. Fracture of the physis of the distal phalanx of the thumb with partial growth arrest and lateral angulation.

C. Immediate postoperative radiogram following resection of the bridge, open-up osteotomy, and internal fixation with two smooth pins.

D. Two years later, showing correction of deformity and open physis with normal growth of the distal phalanx.

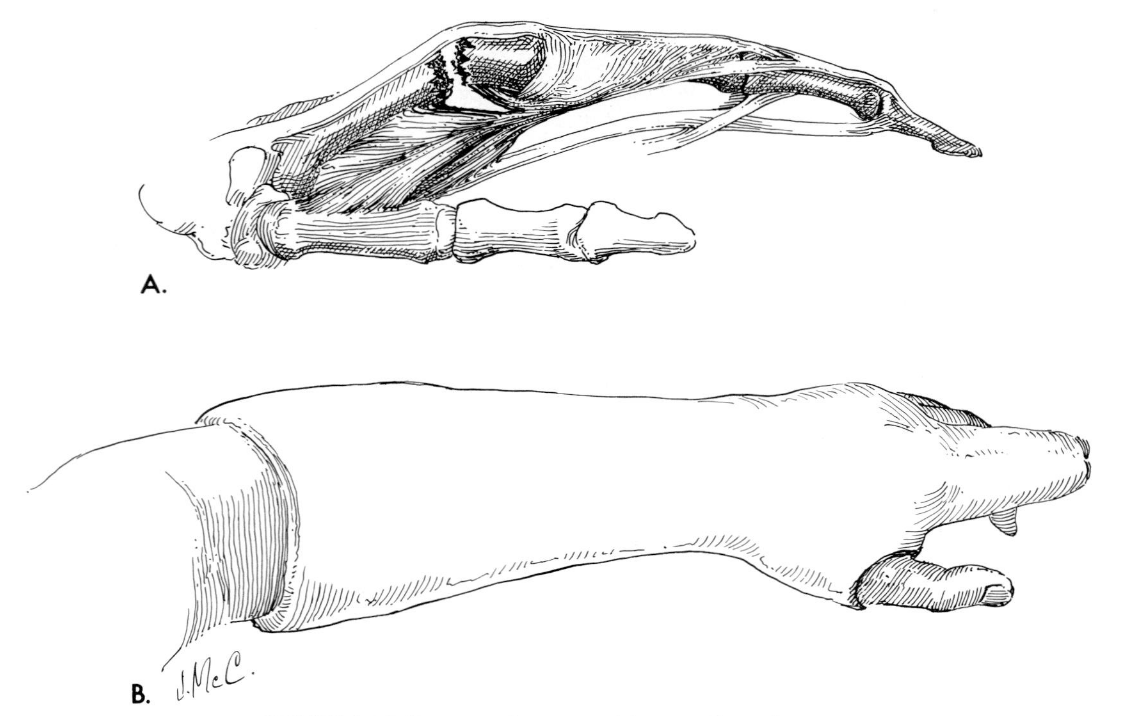

FIGURE 8–94. Fracture of metacarpal (see text for explanation).

the metacarpal neck is reduced by acute flexion of the metacarpophalangeal joint and by pushing the distal fragment dorsally along the longitudinal axis of the proximal phalanx. These fractures are immobilized in a below-elbow cast for four weeks with the finger of the affected metacarpal in moderate flexion. Occasionally they may require internal fixation with an intramedullary pin. Spiral fracture of the metacarpal shaft is rare; it is treated simply by cast immobilization.[17]

Bennett's fracture may require open reduction and internal fixation with smooth Kirschner wire.[28, 59] Metacarpophalangeal dislocation of the thumb usually results from a hyperextension force; the metacarpal head may be trapped through a buttonhole in the capsule and require open reduction.[33–36]

The carpal scaphoid may fracture in a child. Treatment is conservative by immobilization in a below-elbow cast including the thumb.[12, 18, 29, 39, 51, 67] Occasionally unstable displaced fracture of the carpal navicular may require open reduction and internal fixation with a Herbert screw.[31] Delayed union or nonunion may occur in carpal navicular fracture, requiring screw fixation and bone grafting.[47, 49, 66, 75]

References

1. Abdon, P.: Subcapital fractures of the fifth metacarpal bone. Arch. Orthop. Trauma. Surg., *103*:231, 1984.
2. Al-Aralie, K. M.: Severe mincer injuries of the hand in children in Saudi Arabia. J. Hand Surg., *9-B*:249, 1984.
3. Allieu, Y.: Treatment of fractures of the base of the first metacarpal. Acta Orthop. Belg., *39*:1063, 1973.
4. Alnot, J. Y.: Fractures of the metacarpal neck. Acta Orthop. Belg., *39*:1100, 1973.
5. Ashbell, T. S., Kleinert, H. E., and Putcha, S. M.: The deformed fingernail: A frequent result of failure to repair nailbed injuries. J. Trauma, *7*:177, 1967.
6. Aufaure, P., Benjeddou, M., and Gilbert, A.: Fractures of the wrist and hand in children. Ann. Chir., *36*:499, 1982.
7. Barton, N. J.: Fractures of the hand. J. Bone Joint Surg., *66-B*:159, 1984.
8. Becton, J. L., Christian, J. D., and Jackson, J. G., III: A simple technique for treating the complex dislocation of the index metacarpophalangeal joint. J. Bone Joint Surg., *57-A*:698, 1975.
9. Belpomme, C.: External osteosynthesis of distal fractures of the phalanges by reposition-fixation of the fingernail. Int. Surg., *60*:219, 1975.
10. Belsky, M. R.: Closed reduction and internal fixation of proximal phalangeal fractures. J. Hand Surg., *9-A*:725, 1984.
11. Black, D.: Comparison of internal fixation techniques in metacarpal fractures. J. Hand Surg., *10-A*:466, 1985.
12. Bloem, J. J.: Fracture of the carpal scaphoid in a child aged 4. Arch. Chir. Neerl., *23*:91, 1971.
13. Bogdanov, E. A., and Langovaia, V. I.: Fractures of the metacarpals and finger phalanges in children. Ortop. Travmatol. Protez., *32*:19, 1971.
14. Bora, F. W., Jr., Nissenbau, M., and Ignatius, P.: The treatment of epiphyseal fractures of the hand. Orthop. Dig., *5*:11, 1976.
15. Botelheiro, J. C.: Overlapping of fingers due to malunion of a phalanx corrected by a metacarpal rotational osteotomy—report of two cases. J. Hand Surg., *10-B*:389, 1985.
16. Burkhalter, W. E.: Closed treatment of fractures of the hand. Bull. Hosp. J. Dis. Orthop. Inst., *44*:145, 1984.
17. Capron, J. C.: Spiral fracture of the metacarpals. Acta Orthop. Belg., *39*:1045, 1973.
18. Christodoulou, A. G., and Colton, C. L.: Scaphoid fractures in children. J. Pediatr. Orthop., *6*:37, 1986.
19. Coyle, M. P., Jr., and Leddy, J. P.: Injuries of the distal finger. Primary Care, *7*:245, 1980.
20. Dixon, G. L., Jr., and Moon, N. F.: Rotational supracondylar fractures of the proximal phalanx in children. Clin. Orthop., *83*:151, 1972.
21. Duthie, G.: Meshed adhesive tape for the treatment of crushed fingers in children. J. Hand Surg., *9-B*:41, 1984.
22. Eaton, R. G.: Joint Injuries of the Hand. Springfield, Ill., Charles C Thomas, 1971.
23. Enger, W. D., and Glancy, W. G.: Traumatic avulsion of the fingernail associated with injury to the phalangeal epiphyseal plate. J. Bone Joint Surg., *60-A*:713, 1978.
24. Evrard, H., and Nokerman, B.: Centromedullary nailing in metacarpal fractures. Acta Orthop. Belg., *39*:1035, 1973.
25. Flatt, A. E.: The Care of Minor Hand Injuries. 3rd. Ed. St. Louis, Mosby, 1972.
26. Gerard, F. M.: Post-traumatic carpal instability in a young child. J. Bone Joint Surg., *62-A*:131, 1980.
27. Green, D. P.: Hand injuries in children. Pediatr. Clin. North Am., *24*:903, 1977.
28. Griffiths, J. C.: Bennett's fracture in childhood. Br. J. Clin. Pract., *20*:582, 1966.
29. Grundy, M.: Fractures of the carpal scaphoid in children. Br. J. Surg., *56*:523, 1969.
30. Hastings, H., III: Hand fractures in children. A statistical analysis. Clin. Orthop., *188*:120, 1984.
31. Herbert, T. J.: Management of the fractured scaphoid using a new bone screw. J. Bone Joint Surg., *66-B*:114, 1984.
32. Ireland, M. L., and Taleisnik, J.: Nonunion of metacarpal extraarticular fractures in children: Report of two cases and review of the literature. J. Pediatr. Orthop., *6*:352, 1986.
33. Jonasch, E.: Thumb dislocation at the metacarpophalangeal joint in children and adolescents. Monatsschr. Unfallheilkd., *77*:280, 1974.
34. Jonasch, E.: Fracture and dislocations of the fingers in children—conservative therapy and its results. Hefte Unfallheilkd., *141*:43, 1980.
35. Jones, N. F.: Irreducible palmar dislocation of the proximal interphalangeal joints associated with an epiphyseal fracture of the middle phalanx. J. Hand Surg., *10-A*:261, 1985.
36. Kaplan, E. B.: Dorsal dislocation of the metacarpophalangeal joint of the index finger. J. Bone Joint Surg., *47-A*:522, 1957.
37. Keene, J. S.: An irreducible phalangeal epiphyseal fracture-dislocation. A case report. Clin. Orthop., *186*:212, 1984.
38. Khalkhodzhaev, M., Turgunov, S. B., Tursunov, B. S., and Dzhalilov, P. S.: Open fractures of the fingers in children. Vestn. Khir., *130*:113, 1983.
39. Kristensen, O.: Fractures of the scaphoid in children. Ugeskr. Laeger, *136*:146, 1974.
40. Kucynski, K.: The proximal interphalangeal joint: Anatomy and causes of stiffness in the fingers. J. Bone Joint Surg., *50-B*:656, 1968.
41. von Laer, L., Herzog, B., and Gruber, R.: Conservative treatment of finger fractures during growth period (author's transl.). Z. Kinderchir. Grenzgeb., *30*:Suppl.:110, 1980.

42. Leonard, M. H.: Open reduction of fractures of the neck of the proximal phalanx in children. Clin. Orthop., *116*:176, 1976.
43. Leonard, M. H., and Dubravcik, P.: Management of fractured fingers in the child. Clin. Orthop., *73*:160, 1970.
44. Letter: Frisbee finger. N. Engl. J. Med., *293*:725, 1975.
45. Lewis, R. C., and Hartman, J. T.: Controlled osteotomy for correction of rotation in proximal phalanx fractures. Orthop. Rev., *2*:11, 1973.
46. Leyshon, A.: The treatment of delayed union and non-union of the carpal scaphoid by screw fixation. J. Bone Joint Surg., *66-B*:124, 1984.
47. Lindsay, W. K.: Hand injuries in children. Clin. Plast. Surg., *3*:65, 1976.
48. Mansoor, I. A.: Fractures of the proximal phalanx of the fingers. J. Bone Joint Surg., *51-A*:196, 1969.
49. Maudsley, R. H., and Chen, S. C.: Screw fixation in the management of the fractured carpal scaphoid. J. Bone Joint Surg., *54-B*:432, 1972.
50. Metcalf, W., and Whalen, W. P.: Salvage of the injured distal phalanx. Clin. Orthop., *13*:114, 1959.
51. Mussbichler, H.: Injuries of the carpal scaphoid in children. Acta Radiol. [Diagn.] (Stockh.), *56*:361, 1961.
52. Pagliughi, G., and Vespasiani, A.: Fracture-detachment of the base of the 1st metacarpus in children. Chir. Ital., *32*:162, 1980.
53. Patella, V.: The use of Hoffmann-Vidal type mini-fixateurs. Ital. J. Orthop. Traumatol., *9*:297, 1983.
54. Pfeiffer, K. M.: Advances in osteosynthesis of hand fractures. Handchirurgie, *8*:17, 1976.
55. Pritsch, M., Engel, J., and Farin, I.: Manipulation and external fixation of metacarpal fractures. J. Bone Joint Surg., *63-A*:1289, 1981.
56. von Raffler, W.: Irreducible juxta-epiphyseal fracture of a finger. J. Bone Joint Surg., *46-B*:229, 1964.
57. Recht, P.: Injuries of the terminal phalanx and nail. Handchirurgie, *8*:153, 1976.
58. Rosenthal, E. A.: Treatment of fingertip and nailbed injuries. Orthop. Clin. North Am., *14*:675, 1983.
59. Ryba, W.: Die Bennettfraktur bei Jugendlichen. Z. Kinderchir., *3*:Suppl.:394, 1967.
60. Saito, H.: Free nailbed graft for treatment of nailbed injuries of the hand. J. Hand Surg., *8*:171, 1983.
61. Sandzen, S. C.: Management of the acute fingertip injury in the child. Hand, *6*:190, 1974.
62. Segmuller, G.: Diaphyseal and articular fractures of the growing skeleton of the hand. Handchirurgie, *10*:167, 1978.
63. Seymour, N.: Juxta-epiphyseal fracture of the terminal phalanx of the finger. J. Bone Joint Surg., *48-B*:347, 1966.
64. Sharma, L. K., and O'Riain, S.: Hand injuries in childhood—a survey of fifty patients. J. Ir. Med. Assoc., *66*:598, 1973.
65. Shepard, G. H.: Treatment of nail bed avulsion with split-thickness nail bed grafts. J. Hand Surg., *8*:49, 1983.
66. Southcott, R., and Rosman, M. A.: Non-union of carpal scaphoid fractures in children. J. Bone Joint Surg., *59-B*:20, 1977.
67. Spissak, L., and Geryk, B.: Childhood fractures of the scaphoid bone. Acta Chir. Orthop. Traumatol. Cech., *38*:91, 1971.
68. Stein, F.: Skeletal injuries of the hand in children. Clin. Plast. Surg., *8*:65, 1981.
69. Steinert, V., and Knorr, P.: Metacarpal and finger fractures in childhood. Zentralbl. Chir., *96*:113, 1971.
70. Stelling, F. H., III: Surgery of the hand in the child. J. Bone Joint Surg., *45-A*:623, 1963.
71. Strickland, J. W.: Bone, nerve and tendon injuries of the hand in children. Pediatr. Clin. North Am., *22*:451, 1975.
72. Stripling, W. D.: Displaced intra-articular osteochondral fracture—cause for irreducible dislocation of the distal interphalangeal joint. J. Hand Surg., *7*:77, 1982.
73. Swanson, A. B.: Fractures involving the digits of the hand. Orthop. Clin. North Am., *1*:261, 1970.
74. Swischuk, L. E.: Significance of intraarticular fluid without visible fracture in children. A.J.R., *142*:1261, 1984.
75. Verdan, C., and Narakas, A.: Fractures and pseudarthrosis of the scaphoid. Surg. Clin. North Am., *48*:1083, 1968.
76. Wakefield, A. R.: Hand injuries in children. J. Bone Joint Surg., *46-A*:1226, 1964.
77. Wehbe, M. A.: Mallet fractures. J. Bone Joint Surg., *66-A*:658, 1984.
78. Weston, W. J.: Joint space widening with intra-capsular fractures in joints of the fingers and toes of children. Australas. Radiol., *15*:367, 1971.
79. Williams, G. S.: Hand injuries in children: Late problems and primary. Clin. Plast. Surg., *4*:503, 1977.
80. Wood, V. E.: Fractures of the hand in children. Orthop. Clin. North Am., *7*:527, 1976.
81. Wray, R. C.: Proximal interphalangeal joint sprains. Plast. Reconstr. Surg., *74*:101, 1984.

*WRINGER INJURY TO THE UPPER LIMB**

Wringer injuries of the upper limb are sustained by a child whose hand is drawn into the power-driven rollers of a washing machine. If the elbow is flexed as the forearm is drawn into the roller, the maximum damage to the soft tissues is sustained in the antecubital fossa; whereas if the elbow is extended, the maximum trauma is to the axilla. The extent of injury is increased by applying countertraction to the limb or by reversing the direction of the rollers, thus subjecting it to a second crushing. Other factors determining the severity of the damage are the length of time during which the limb was caught between the rollers, the size of the limb, the tension of the rollers, and the rapidity of their revolution.

The crushing injury is primarily to the soft tissues, i.e., the skin, subcutaneous tissue, muscles, tendons, and nerves. The bones are rarely fractured, but it is important to take radiograms to detect any possible damage.

Clinically, the limb may be found diffusely swollen and ecchymotic in some areas, especially in the antecubital fossa and in the axilla. Minor abrasions are common. Occasionally there is avulsion of the skin.

Nerve and muscle function in the crushed limb is determined. There may be disruption of nerves and tearing of tendons or muscles without a break in the skin. In the beginning, it is difficult to assess the extent of the injury, and it is wise to make a guarded prognosis. Within a day or two, what appears to be a minor

*See references 1 to 37.

injury may progress to sloughing of the regional skin and devitalization of the muscles.

Treatment

Regardless how benign the appearance of the injury, it is best to hospitalize the patient for at least two or three days to observe the progression of the damage. After proper sedation, the limb is washed with a mild antiseptic soap, a sterile compression bandage is applied, and the limb is elevated to minimize edema and further swelling.

Once a day, under aseptic precautions, the sterile compression bandage is changed and the limb is inspected for progression of injury. If there are subcutaneous collections of transudate or blood, they should be decompressed by aspiration to allow the skin to fall back into a nutritive bed. If there is sloughing of skin, the area is allowed to granulate for seven to ten days, and is then covered with a split-thickness graft. A pedicle type of graft is indicated where tendons, nerves, and bone are exposed. The joints are splinted in functional position.

References

1. Adams, J. P., and Fowler, F. D.: Wringer injuries of the upper extremity. South. Med. J., *52*:798, 1959.
2. Akbarnia, B. A., Campbell, C. J., and Bowen, J. R.: Management of massive defects in radius and ulna following wringer injury. A case study. Clin. Orthop., *116*:167, 1976.
3. Allen, H. S.: Wringer injuries of the upper extremity. Ann. Surg., *113*:1101, 1941.
4. Allen, J. E., Beck, A. R., and Jewett, T. C., Jr.: Wringer injuries in children. Arch. Surg., *97*:194, 1968.
5. Archer, R. R., and Sawyer, J. L.: Surgical management of wringer arm injuries. South. Med. J., *61*:975, 1968.
6. Beck, A. R., Jewett, T. C., Jr., and Allen, J. E.: Emergency room treatment of wringer injuries in children. Hosp. Top., *45*:6, 1967.
7. Bell, J. L., Mason, M. L., and Allen, H. S.: Management of acute crushing injuries of the hand and forearm over a five year period. Am. J. Surg., *87*:370, 1954.
8. Chamberlain, J. W., and Soltes, M.: Wringer injuries. Pediatrics, *28*:96, 1961.
9. Davis, M. W.: Wringer injuries. Minn. Med., *50*:1217, 1967.
10. Duncan, R. E., and Moseley, T.: Wringer injuries in children. An analysis of 300 cases. J. Fla. Med. Assoc., *56*:106, 1969.
11. Edgerton, M. T., and Golden, G. T.: Wringer (crush) injuries of the upper extremity. *In* Littler, J. W., Cramer, L. M., and Smith, J. W. (eds.): Symposium on Reconstructive Hand Surgery. Educational Foundation of the American Society of Plastic and Reconstructive Surgeons. St. Louis, Mosby, 1974, p. 178.
12. Entin, M. A.: Roller and wringer injuries: Clinical and experimental studies. Plast. Reconstr. Surg., *15*:290, 1955.
13. Franz, J. L., and Root, H. D.: Upper extremity wringer injury. Vasc. Surg., *9*:302, 1975.
14. Fraser, M.: The wringer injury. Am. J. Surg., *100*:646, 1960.
15. Garrick, J. A.: Wringer injuries. Minn. Med., *50*:195, 1967.
16. Golden, G. T., Fisher, J. C., and Edgerton, M. T.: Wringer arm reevaluated: A survey of current surgical management of upper extremity compression injuries. Ann. Surg., *177*:362, 1973.
17. Graham, W. P., Miller, S. H., Davis, T. S., and Schantz, J. C.: Treating wringer injuries. Pa. Med., *78*:67, 1975.
18. Groher, W., and Heidensohn, P.: Ruckenschmerzen und roentgenologische Veranderungen bei Wasserspringer. Z. Orthop., *108*:51, 1970.
19. Hardin, C. A., and Robinson, D. W.: Coverage problems in the treatment of wringer injuries. J. Bone Joint Surg., *36-A*:292, 1954.
20. Harris, N., and Wood, E.: Roller injuries of the upper extremity. J. Trauma, *18*:605, 1978.
21. Hausmann, P. F., and Everett, H. H.: Wringer injury. Surgery, *28*:71, 1950.
22. Iritani, R. I., and Siler, V. E.: Wringer injuries of the upper extremity. Surg. Gynecol. Obstet., *113*:67, 1961.
23. Luck, J. V., and Maddux, R.: Washing machine wringer injuries in children. G.P., *12*:87, 1955.
24. Lynn, R. B., and Reed, R. C.: Wringer injuries. J.A.M.A., *174*:500, 1960.
25. MacCollum, D. W.: Wringer arm. N. Engl. J. Med., *218*:549, 1938.
26. MacCollum, D. W., Bernhard, W. F., and Banner, R. L.: The treatment of wringer arm injuries. N. Engl. J. Med., *247*:750, 1952.
27. McCulloch, H., Boswick, A., Jr., and Jonas, R.: Household wringer injuries: A three year review. J. Trauma, *13*:1, 1973.
28. McGee, G. E., and Groff, D. B.: Wringer injuries of the extremities. South. Med. J., *76*:304, 1983.
29. Matev, I.: Wringer injuries of the hand. J. Bone Joint Surg., *49-B*:722, 1967.
30. Moseley, T., and Hardman, W. W., Jr.: Treatment of wringer injuries in children. South. Med. J., *58*:1372, 1965.
31. Neff, R. S., and Cohen, P. Z.: Wringer arm injuries in children. Rev. Surg., *27*:217, 1970.
32. Perry, A. W., Reeves, C., and Woolley, M.: Wringer arm injuries. Am. Surg., *35*:53, 1969.
33. Posch, J. L., and Weller, C. N.: Mangle and severe wringer injuries of the hand in children. J. Bone Joint Surg., *36-A*:57, 1954.
34. Poulos, E.: The open treatment of wringer injuries in children. Am. Surg., *24*:458, 1958.
35. Schulz, I.: Wringer injury. Surgery, *20*:301, 1946.
36. Stone, H. H., Cantwell, D. V., and Fulenwider, J. T.: Wringer arm injuries. J. Pediatr. Surg., *11*:375, 1976.
37. Trimble, C., and Delauro, J.: Treatment of wringer injury. J. Trauma, *9*:175, 1969.

The Lower Limb

TRAUMATIC DISLOCATION OF THE HIP

Seldom does a child sustain traumatic dislocation of the hip. Maffei, in a review of 1,842 cases at the Rizzoli Institute of Bologna, could find only three in children.[114] Choyce, in 1924, collected from the literature 58 cases of children with traumatic dislocation of the hip and added 6 cases of his own.[31] Mason covered the period between 1922 and 1954, studying 88 reported cases.[118] Fineschi, in 1956, presented a careful study of 150 reported cases in the world literature.[52] In 1968, the Scientific Research Committee of the Pennsylvania Orthopedic Society gave a final report based on 51 cases collected from the membership of the Society between 1959 and 1966. Earlier, they had presented the initial findings in 32 children.[137, 138] Recent literature contains many case reports with comprehensive review of the literature of traumatic hip dislocation in children, as well as general studies of traumatic dislocation of the hip in which cases in children are included.[1–189]

Types

Traumatic dislocation of the hip is classified according to the position of the displaced femoral head in relation to the acetabulum (Fig. 8–95).

Posterior
Iliac—femoral head lies posteriorly and superiorly along the lateral aspect of the ilium (Fig. 8–96 A).
Ischial—femoral head is displaced posteroinferiorly and lies adjacent to the greater sciatic notch (Fig. 8–96 B).
Anterior
Obturator—femoral head lies in the region of the obturator membrane (Fig. 8–96 D). Perineal type is the extremely inferiorly displaced form of anterior dislocation.

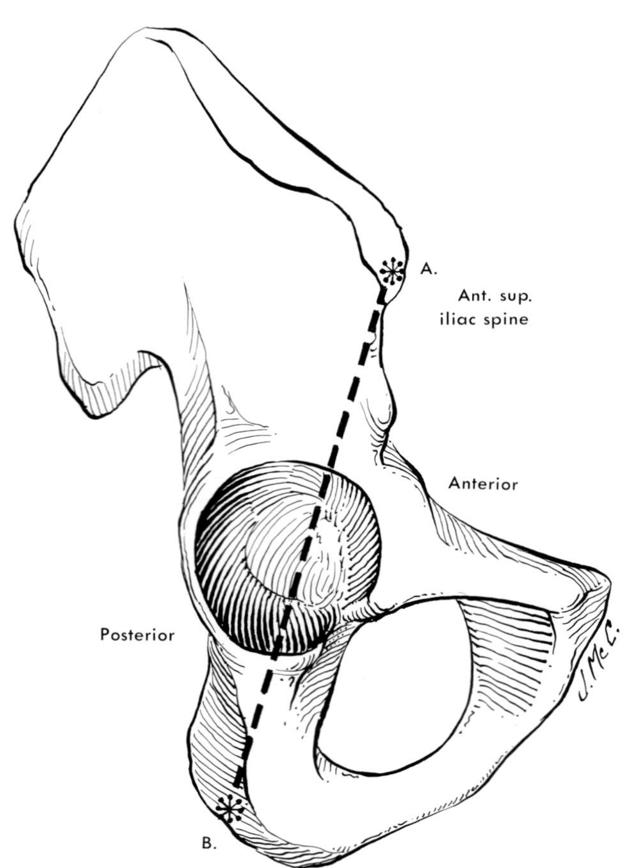

FIGURE 8–95. A line drawn from the anterior-superior iliac spine to the ischial tuberosity bisects the acetabulum, dividing anterior from posterior luxation. When the femoral head is displaced anterior to this line, the dislocation is called anterior and vice versa.

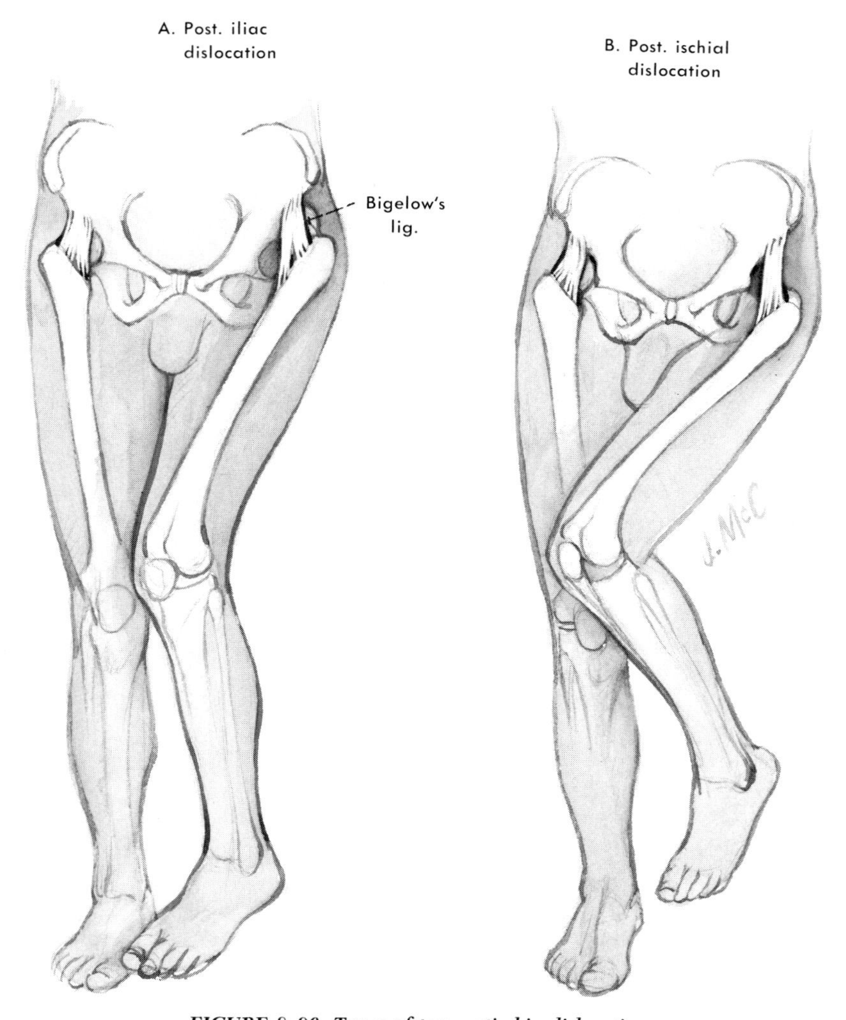

FIGURE 8–96. Types of traumatic hip dislocation.

Illustration continued on following page

Pubic—femoral head is displaced anterosuperiorly along the superior ramus of the pubic bone. Suprapubic type is the extremely superiorly displaced form of pubic dislocation (Fig. 8–96 C).

Central. There is a comminuted fracture of the central portion of the acetabulum with displacement of the femoral head and acetabular fragments into the pelvis. Central dislocations of the hip are actually fractures of the pelvis; however, as the associated hip-joint injury presents the greater disability, they are discussed with hip dislocation.

Inferior. Pure inferior dislocation is very rare.[147, 160]

Stewart and Milford have further subdivided fracture-dislocations of the hip according to the severity of the associated fracture of the acetabulum or the femoral head:

Grade I: simple dislocation without fracture or with a chip from the acetabulum so small as to be of no consequence

Grade II: dislocation with one or more large rim fragments, but with sufficient socket remaining to ensure stability after reduction

Grade III: explosive or blast fracture with disintegration of the rim of the acetabulum that produces gross instability

Grade IV: dislocation with a fracture of the head or neck of the femur

Dislocation of the hip with fracture of the femoral shaft presents a unique problem of management, and for this reason, the author recommends it be added, as a fifth grade, to the four just given.[171]

Central dislocations of the hip were classified as follows by Stewart and Milford:

Grade I Central: linear or stellate fracture through the floor of the acetabulum but without appreciable dislocation

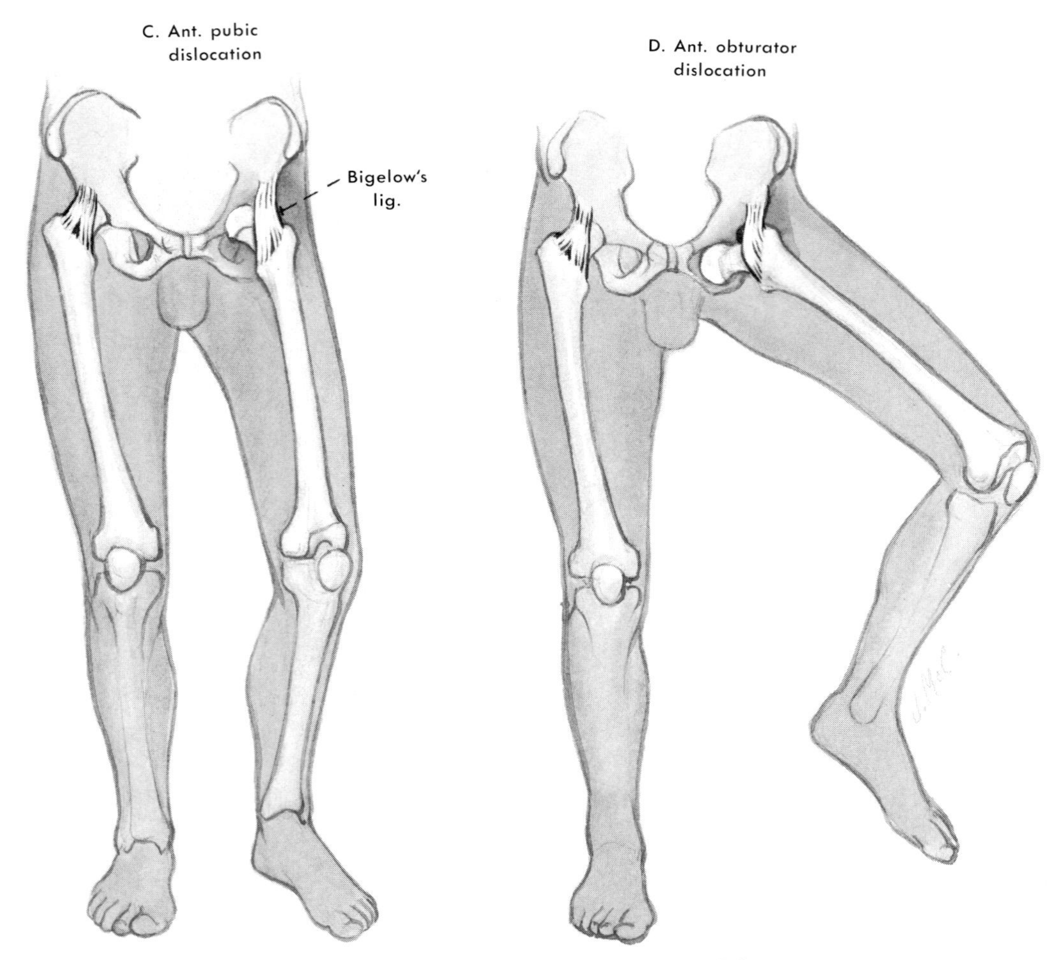

FIGURE 8–96 Continued. Types of traumatic hip dislocation.

Grade II Central: comminuted fracture with mild to moderate central displacement of the femoral head and acetabular fragments

Grade III Central: marked displacement of the fragments and protrusion of the head of the femur into the pelvis, with or without comminution of the superior portion of the acetabulum

Grade IV Central: dislocation with an associated fracture of the head or neck of the femur.[171]

In children, the majority of traumatic dislocations of the hip are of the posterior type. In the 1968 study of 51 patients by the Pennsylvania Orthopedic Society, 80 per cent of the dislocations were of the posterior type, 16 per cent anterior, and 4 per cent central.[138]

There is a definite predilection for males, the injury being four times more common in boys than in girls. It may occur in any age group, but there are two peak periods of incidence—between 4 and 7 years, and between 11 and 15 years. The right and left hips are involved equally. Very rarely are both hips dislocated.[14, 54, 169]

Mechanism of Injury

Because the femoral head may become displaced out of the acetabular socket only as a result of very extreme force, hip dislocation is found in persons who have been subjected to severe trauma, as in a serious automobile collision. *Posterior dislocation* is produced when the flexed knee strikes against the dashboard with the hip flexed and adducted. The driver of the car is more likely to sustain an associated fracture of the posterior wall of the acetabulum, because on applying the brakes, his hip is in semiflexed position and the femoral head is displaced posterosuperiorly by the impact (Fig. 8–97 A); whereas the passenger's hip is more often in hyperflexion at the moment of the impact and the femoral head is driven downward and backward, with the acetabulum sus-

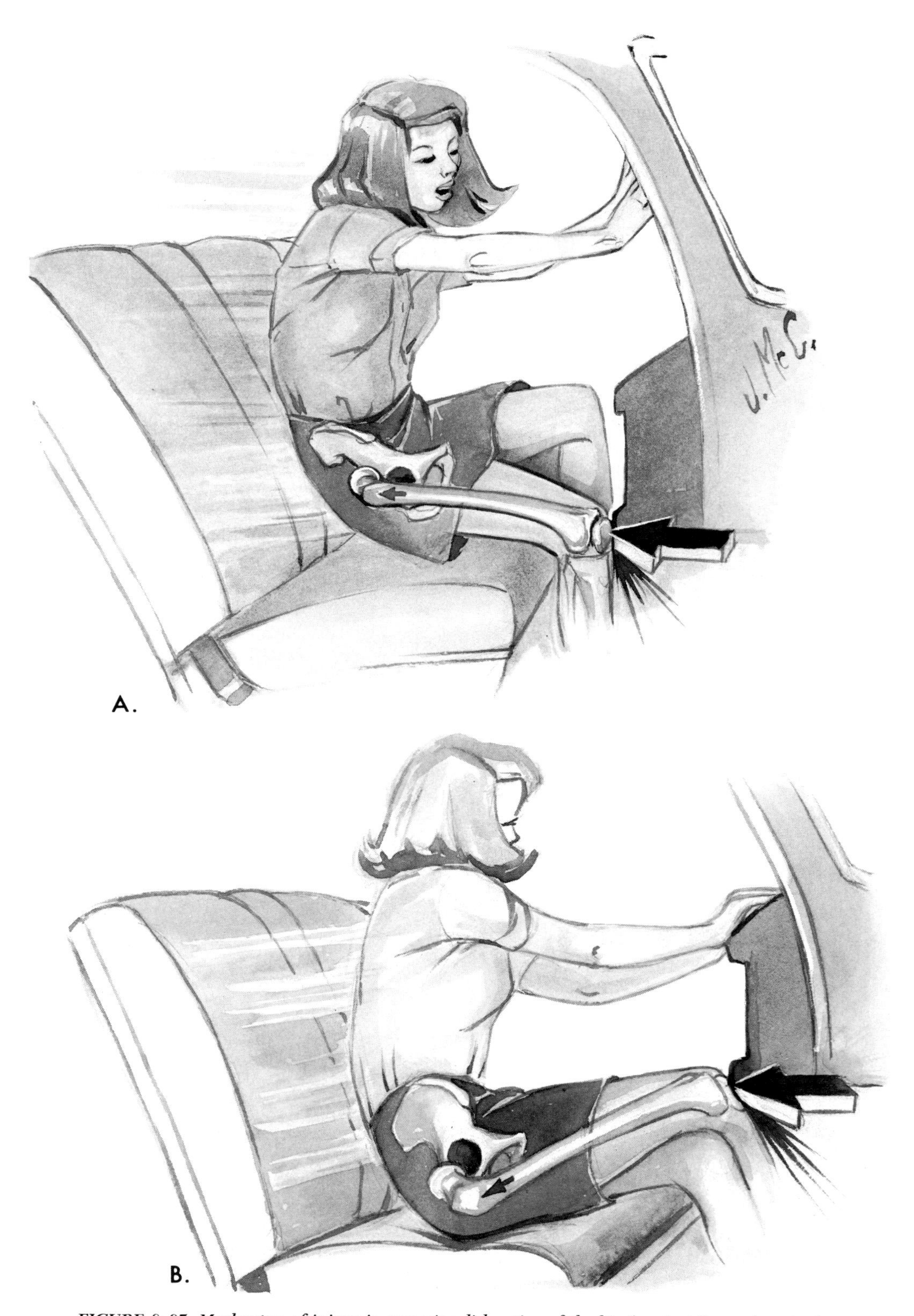

FIGURE 8–97. Mechanism of injury in posterior dislocation of the hip (see text for explanation).

A. The displacement of the femoral head is posterosuperior when the hip is semiflexed. **B**. The dislocation is posteroinferior when the hip is hyperflexed.

taining less damage (Fig. 8–97 B). In this type of injury, often there may be associated fracture of the patella, the upper end of the tibia, the femoral shaft, or the head and neck of the femur.

Anterior dislocation is usually sustained in a fall from a height, whose impact inflicts a direct blow on the posterior aspect of the abducted and laterally rotated thigh (Fig. 8–98 A). The femoral head is displaced forward, commonly lying external to the obturator foramen; greater force will displace the femoral head forward and upward in the region of the pubic crest.

Central dislocations with fractures of the acetabulum are frequently caused by a direct blow to the greater trochanter, such as that which results from the impact of a falling object or a fall from a height (Fig. 8–98 B). It may also be produced in "dashboard injuries," when the hip is in an extended and abducted position at the time of the direct blow on the flexed knee.

Pathologic Anatomy

In *posterior dislocation,* the ligamentum teres is ruptured and the capsule is torn in its posterior aspect. The tear in the capsule may be at its pelvic attachment or femoral insertion, or may run irregularly between the two. Upon departing from the acetabular socket, the femoral head migrates and enlarges the rent in the capsule. The iliofemoral ligament (the Y-ligament of Bigelow) is usually taut, with the hip in extended position, or it may be torn (Fig. 8–99 D and E). The short lateral rotator muscles—obturator internus, pyriformis, obturator externus, and quadratus muscles—are either partially or completely torn with the posterior part of the capsule. Occasionally, the femoral head may push its way between the short lateral rotators without causing them to tear. The gluteus maximus, medius, and minimus muscles are stretched and pushed backward by the femoral head, which lies deep to or within the fibers of these muscles. The hip adductors are stretched or partially torn by the indirect force and pull of the displaced femoral head.

In *anterior dislocations,* the anterior part of the capsule and the ligamentum teres are ruptured. The iliofemoral ligament is usually intact (Fig. 8–99 C). Muscles in the direct path of the femoral head are stretched or may be partially torn. In the pubic type of luxation the femoral nerve may be damaged. Very occasionally femoral vessels may be injured, particularly when the femoral head is dislocated anteriorly by hyperextension of the hip.

In *central dislocations,* the femoral head splits the acetabulum and displaces to a varying degree inside the pelvis. The pelvic fascia is strong, but injury to viscera in the pelvis or to the obturator nerve may occur.

Diagnostic Features

In *posterior dislocations* the deformity has a typical appearance (see Fig. 8–96 A and B). The involved lower limb is held in flexion, adduction, and medial rotation at the hip with the knee or foot resting on the normal leg. There is both apparent and actual shortening of the limb. The femoral head cannot be palpated in its normal location deep to the femoral vessels below the inguinal ligament; occasionally, it may be palpable posteriorly in the gluteal region. The patient is in excruciating pain and is unable to stand or walk on the affected limb. Any motion of the hip is painful and guarded by muscle spasm. Extension, abduction, and lateral rotation of the hip are markedly restricted. Flexion and medial rotation contracture of the hip are primarily produced by tension on the Y-ligament of Bigelow; they are directly proportionate to the amount the femoral head is displaced out of the acetabular socket. When the Y-ligament is torn (referred to as the "irregular type of hip dislocation" by Bigelow), the limb lies in lateral rotation, with no restriction of hip extension and lateral rotation (Fig. 8–99 E).

Posterior dislocations are commonly of the iliac type, with the femoral head lying between the sciatic notch and the acetabulum. High iliac luxations with the femoral head up, behind, and definitely on the lateral surface of the ilium are rare. Ischial posterior luxations are also uncommon.

In *anterior dislocations,* the hip is held in abduction, lateral rotation, and some flexion. There is fullness in the region of the obturator foramen, where the femoral head may be palpable. Because of its abducted position, there is apparent lengthening of the limb. Motion of the hip is markedly restricted, with almost no adduction and lateral rotation. In pubic luxations, the femoral head is displaced upward and forward, lying inferior to the pubic ramus or riding on it, in which case it can be easily palpated. There is loss of prominence of the greater trochanter (see Fig. 8–96 C and D).

In *central dislocations* with fractures of the acetabulum, all motions of the hip are markedly restricted by muscle spasm. The limb is not maintained in any characteristic deformed pos-

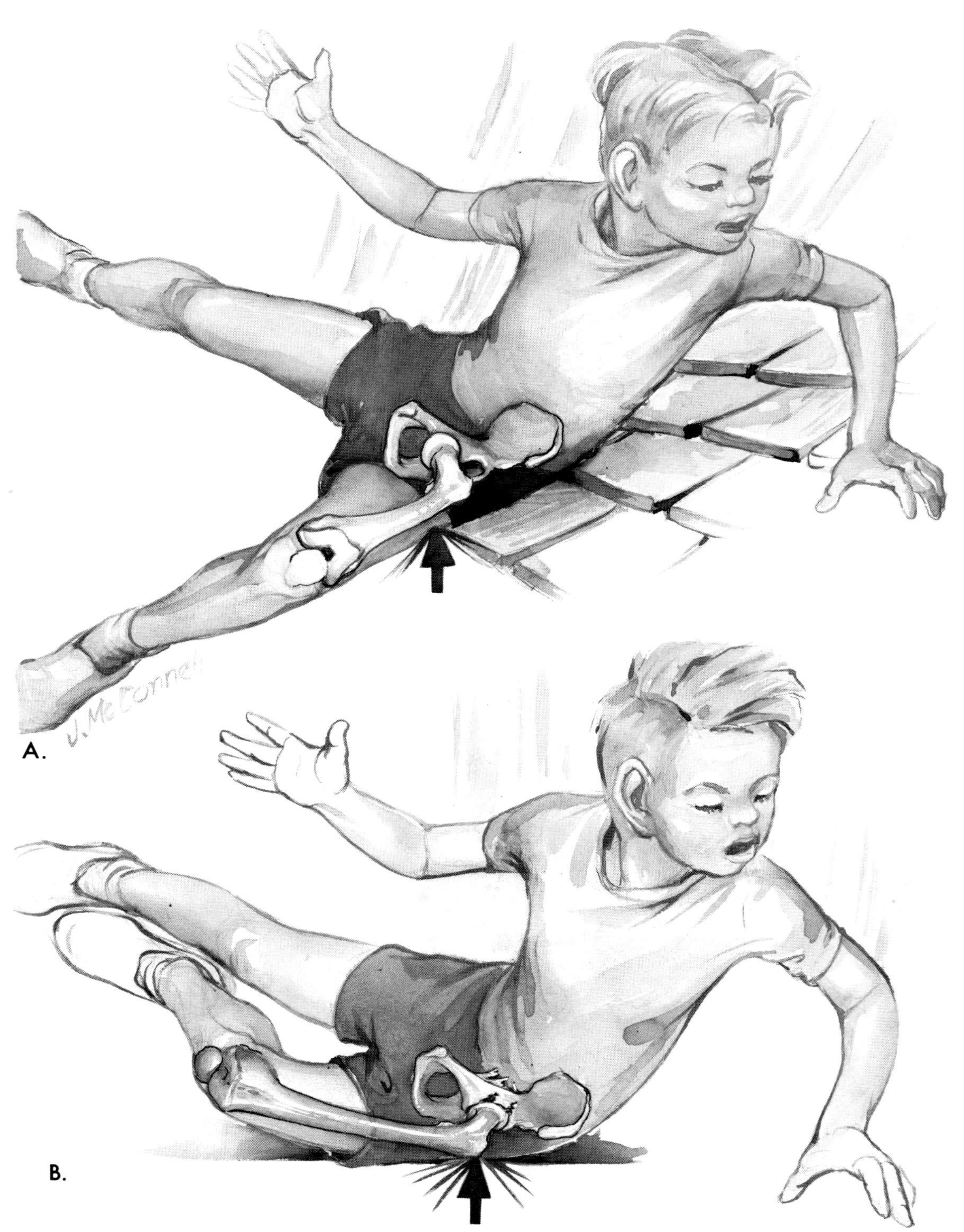

FIGURE 8–98. Mechanism of injury in dislocation of the hip.

A. Anterior dislocation. **B.** Central dislocation (see text for explanation).

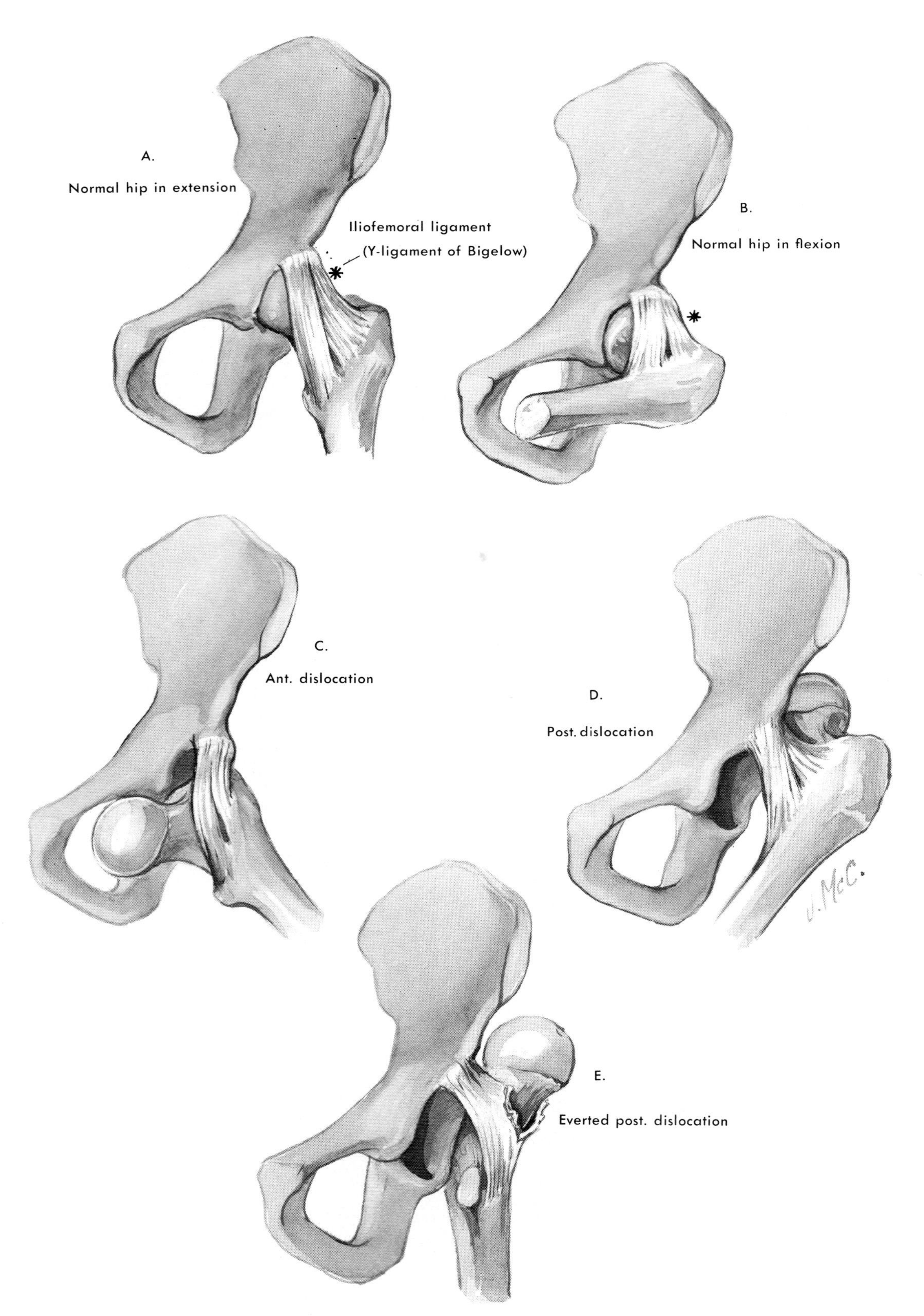

FIGURE 8–99. The iliofemoral ligament (or Y-ligament of Bigelow).

A. Normal ligament with the hip in extension. **B.** With hip in flexion it is relaxed. **C.** Anterior dislocation. **D.** Posterior dislocation. **E.** In everted posterior dislocation it is partially torn.

ture. Shortening is minimal. The lateral aspect of the hip is flattened because of inward displacement of the greater trochanter. Intrapelvic hemorrhage is common, as evidenced by the finding of suprapubic dullness on percussion of the abdomen. On rectal examination, a tender mass may be palpated deep to the fractured acetabulum, and the femoral head may be felt.

Radiograms will disclose the specific type of dislocation (Figs. 8–100 and 8–101). It is imperative that adequate films be made and associated fractures be ruled out.

In the severely injured patient, failure to examine and x-ray the hip joint adequately is a common pitfall, and fracture-dislocations of the hip have often been overlooked.

Treatment

Reduction of traumatic dislocation of the hip should be immediate; the longer it is delayed, the more difficult is the reduction and the poorer the prognosis.

Forceful manipulations must be avoided. It is best to administer a general anesthetic to obtain complete muscle relaxation.

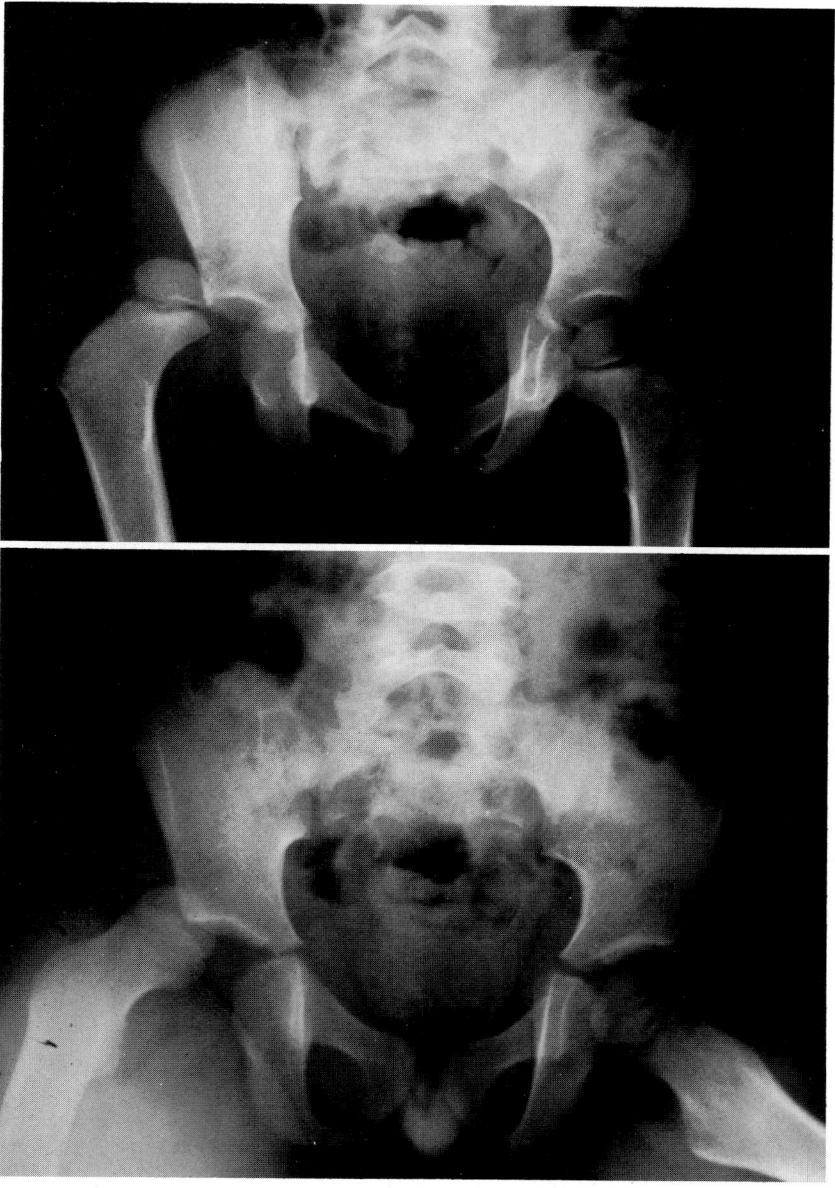

FIGURE 8–100. Traumatic posterior dislocation of right hip—iliac type.

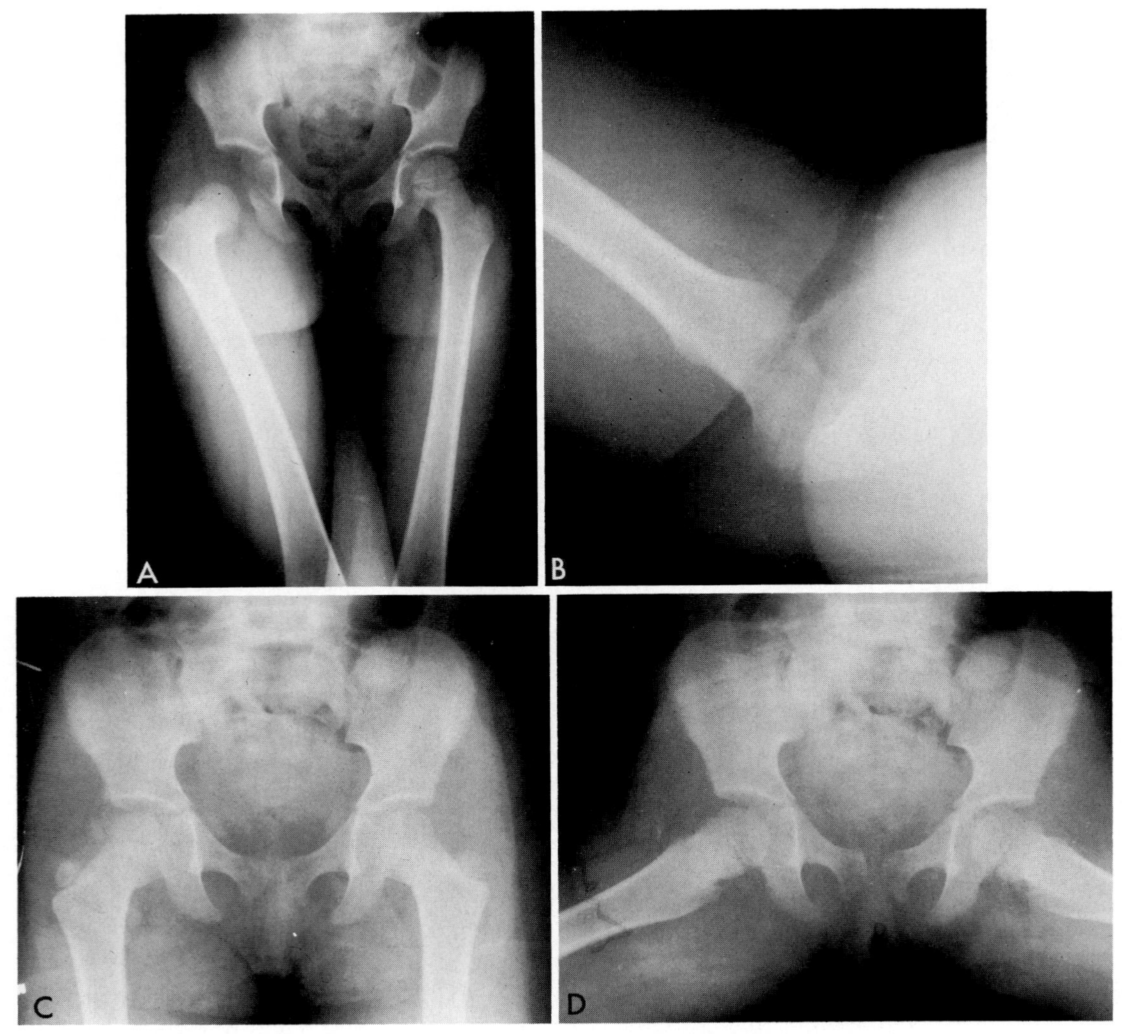

FIGURE 8–101. Traumatic posterior dislocation of right hip—ischial type.

A and **B.** Initial radiograms. **C** and **D.** Postreduction views. It is imperative that adequate films be obtained to rule out the presence of associated fractures.

The chief obstacle to reduction in posterior hip dislocation is the iliofemoral ligament, which is perhaps the strongest ligament in the body. Its somewhat triangular shape resembles an inverted Y, and it is often referred to as the Y-ligament of Bigelow. The apex of the ligament is in the markedly thickened fibers of the longitudinal fibers of the capsule, originating in the anteroinferior iliac spine and extending downward across the anterior aspect of the hip joint to be attached to the anterior intertrochanteric line. As it passes distally, it becomes broad and tends to separate into two bands; for this reason, its base may be considered to have a bifid attachment (see Fig. 8–92).

Normally, the iliofemoral ligament limits hyperextension and lateral rotation of the hip joint—an important function, because in stance the weight of the body tends to rotate the pelvis posteriorly upon the two femoral heads.

CLOSED REDUCTION OF POSTERIOR DISLOCATION

The three methods of closed reduction of posterior dislocation are those of Bigelow, Allis, and Stimson, all of which utilize the principle of hip flexion, causing the Y-ligament to relax, and bringing the femoral head adjacent to the acetabular margin near the rent in the capsule.

Gravity Method of Stimson (Fig. 8–102).[172] The patient is placed in prone position with his lower limbs hanging free from the end of the table. His pelvis is immobilized by an assistant who presses down on the sacrum. With his left

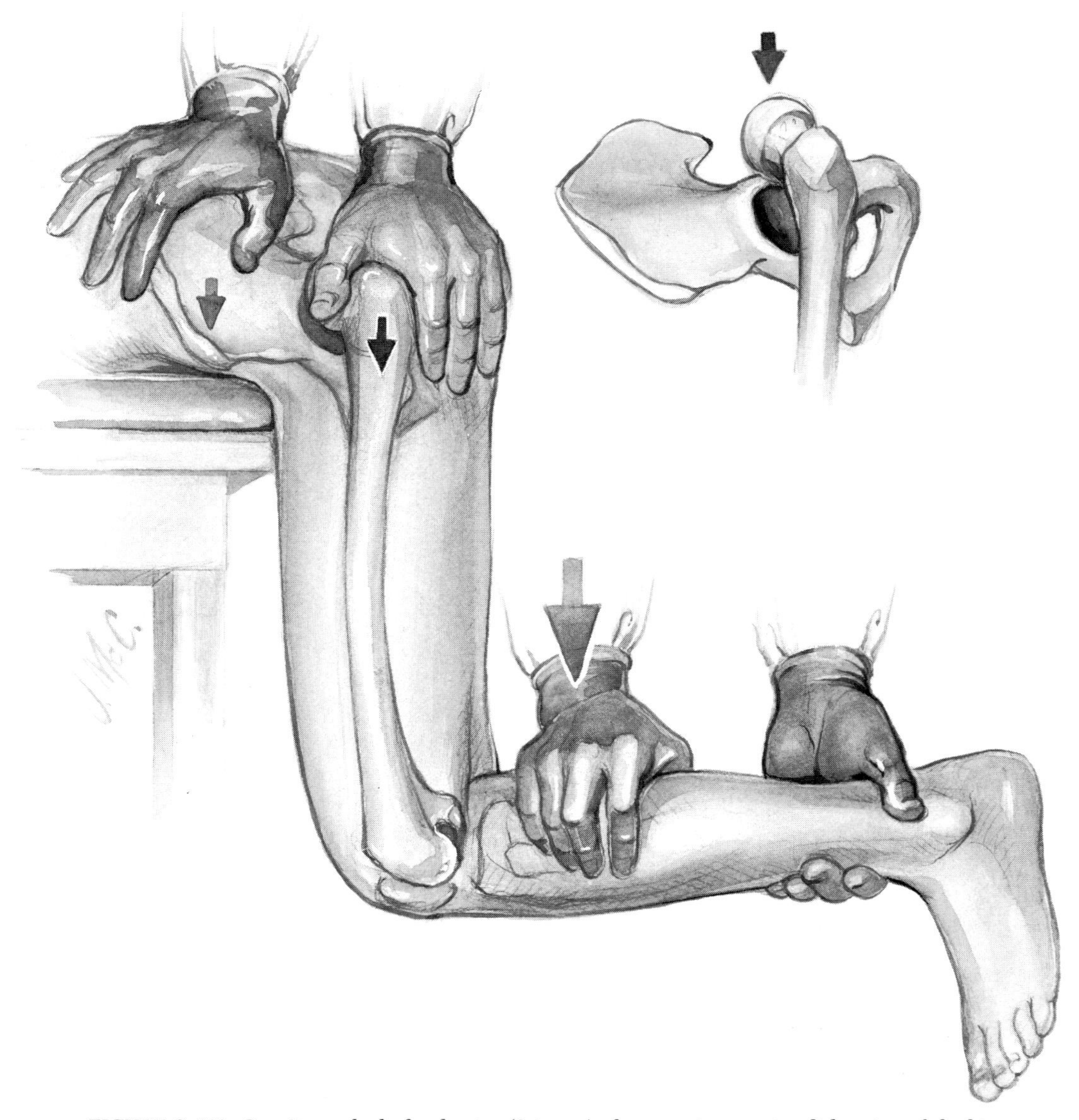

FIGURE 8–102. Gravity method of reduction (Stimson) of traumatic posterior dislocation of the hip (see text for explanation).

hand, the surgeon holds the ankle and flexes the knee of the injured limb to 90 degrees, and with his right hand, applies downward pressure to the leg just below the bent knee. Gentle rocking or rotatory motions of the limb and direct pressure over the femoral head may assist in the reduction. This method is the least forcible and most desirable, as it utilizes the weight of the limb to help the reduction. If necessary, a sandbag may be strapped to the leg to relax the taut muscles.

"Direct Method" of Allis (Fig. 8–103).[2] The patient is placed in supine position on the floor and his pelvis is immobilized by an assistant or by the surgeon's foot pressing on the anterior superior iliac spine. The hip and knee of the affected hip are flexed to 90 degrees, with the thigh in slight adduction and medial rotation. Then, with his forearm behind the knee, the surgeon applies vertical traction, and the femoral head is lifted over the posterior rim of the acetabulum, through the hole in the capsule, into the acetabular socket. The hip and knee are then gently extended. Occasionally one encounters soft-tissue resistance when lifting the femoral head; in such an instance, the capsule is first relaxed by increasing the degree of hip adduction and medial rotation, and reduction is again attempted by lifting the femoral head anteriorly and extending the hip. If this is unsuccessful, excessive force should be avoided because the femoral head may be caught by the short rotator muscles or by the sciatic nerve. Reduction is again initiated from the first step; however, this time, after the hip is flexed, it is gently rotated laterally to disengage the femoral head from the soft tissues. Direct pressure may be applied over the femoral head to assist it to slip back into place.

Circumduction Method of Bigelow (Fig. 8–104).[15, 16] The fully anesthetized patient is placed supine. An assistant applies countertraction by pressing downward on the anterior superior iliac spines and the ilia. If an assistant is not available, an alternate method is for the surgeon to apply pressure with his foot over the anterior superior iliac spine. The surgeon then grasps the affected limb at the ankle with one hand and places his opposite forearm behind the knee. First, the adducted and medially rotated thigh is flexed 90 degrees or more on the abdomen and longitudinal traction is applied in the line of the deformity. This maneuver will relax the Y-ligament and bring the femoral head near the posterior rim of the acetabulum. The femoral head is then freed from the rotator muscles by gently rotating and "rocking" the thigh forward and backward. Next, while traction is maintained, the femoral head is levered into the acetabulum by gentle

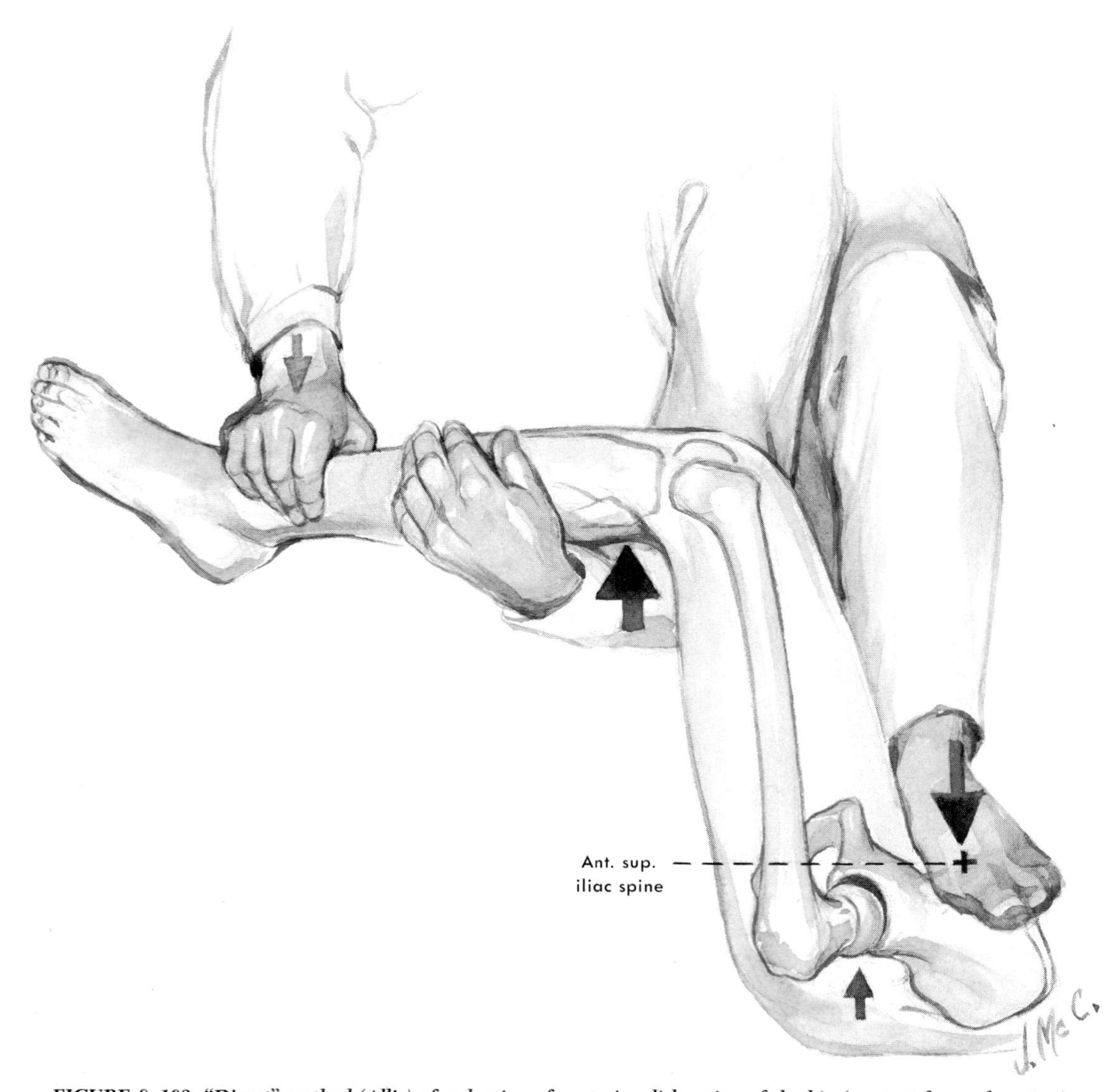

FIGURE 8–103. "Direct" method (Allis) of reduction of posterior dislocation of the hip (see text for explanation).

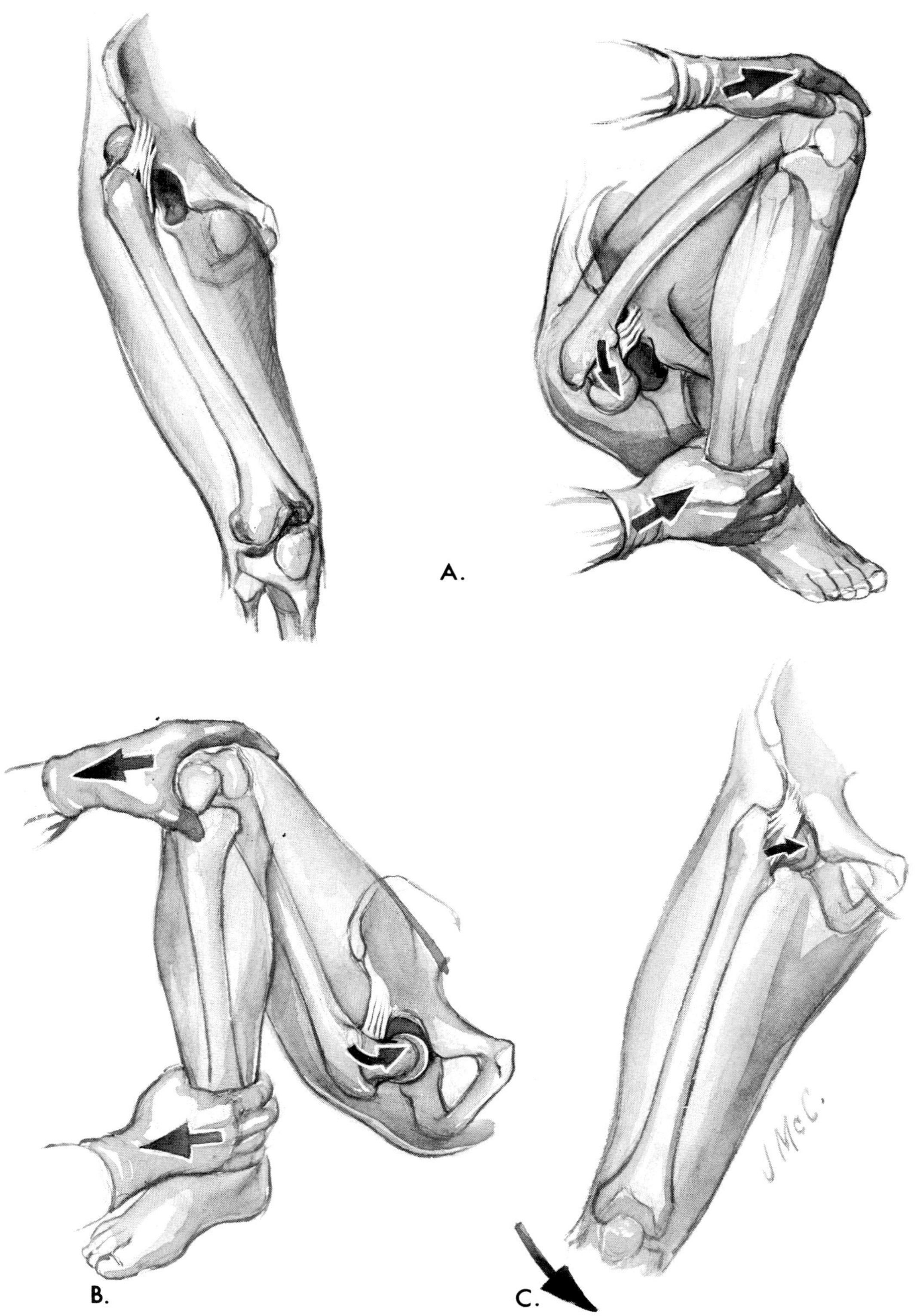

FIGURE 8–104. Circumduction method (Bigelow) of reduction of posterior dislocation of the hip (see text for explanation).

abduction, lateral rotation, and extension of the hip. During extension, the iliofemoral ligament is used as a fulcrum to force the femoral head into the acetabular socket. One must avoid excessive force in order to prevent rupture of the Y-ligament or damage to the sciatic nerve.

CLOSED REDUCTION OF ANTERIOR DISLOCATION

With anterior and medial displacement of the femoral head, no bony fulcrum is available to be used for reduction. The iliofemoral ligament lies across the femoral neck. During manipulation the femoral head is dislodged and brought opposite the tear in the capsule through which it is levered into the acetabular socket. The simplest and safest method is that of *Allis' reduction.* With the anesthetized patient in supine position on the floor, the following maneuver is carried out: (1) Flex the knee to relax the hamstrings. (2) Fully abduct the hip and bring it into flexion, the exact degree depending upon whether the femoral head is in the obturator or pubic location (Fig. 8–105 A). (3) Apply longitudinal traction in line with the longitudinal axis of the femur. (4) An assistant should fix the femoral head with the palm of his hand. Then, using the patient's thigh as the lever and the assistant's hand as the fulcrum while maintaining moderate traction, the surgeon gently adducts the hip and replaces the femoral head in the acetabulum (Fig. 8–105 B and C). The hip may be medially rotated as it is adducted to achieve reduction. Occasionally it is necessary to utilize a reverse Bigelow maneuver in which the hip is partially flexed and abducted; then, with moderate traction applied in line with the longitudinal axis of the femur, the hip is adducted in flexion, sharply medially rotated, and extended. Circumduction is in a clockwise direction.

Postoperative Care

Following reduction, radiograms are made to confirm its completeness. Again, x-rays are carefully scrutinized to rule out the possibility of any associated fractures. If the femoral head is displaced laterally a computed tomography scan and/or nuclear magnetic resonance imaging is performed to rule out intra-articular loose fracture fragments.[77, 133] Magnetic resonance imaging will depict cartilaginous loose bodies in the joint. Reduction is maintained in a one and one half hip spica cast with the affected hip in neutral extension and some abduction. In simple dislocations, the period of immobilization is four weeks in young children and six weeks in adolescents—this period should be sufficient for healing of capsular and soft-tissue structures. Following removal of the cast, the hip is partially protected with a three-point crutch gait. As soon as pain-free full range of motion of the hip is obtained, the patient is allowed to bear full weight with no protection, as the consensus of various authors is that a prolonged period without weight-bearing neither prevents aseptic necrosis nor does it affect the prognosis. A bone scan with technetium-99m is performed in order to rule out avascular necrosis of the femoral head. Radiographic follow-up should be at least for two years, with radiograms made at three-month intervals.

Treatment of Fracture-Dislocations of the Hip*

The method of treatment depends upon the severity of associated fracture of the acetabulum or the femoral head. Grade I and Grade II fracture-dislocations are treated by closed reduction and immobilization in a hip spica cast for six weeks. Grades III and IV fracture-dislocations always require open reduction and internal fixation of the acetabular fragments with screws. These injuries are very rare in children; the reader is referred to King and Richards for a description of operative technique.[95]

Central Dislocations of the Hip

These are essentially comminuted fractures of the central portion of the acetabulum with displacement of the fragments and the femoral head into the pelvis.[147] Associated injury to the pelvic viscera should be ruled out.

Reduction is achieved by skeletal traction applied through a Kirschner wire or a large threaded Steinmann pin inserted into the distal femoral metaphysis. In moderate inward displacements, it is best to also apply direct lateral traction through a large screw or a heavy threaded Steinmann pin (inserted in an anteroposterior plane) through the greater trochanter. After two or three weeks, the lateral traction is discontinued and distal traction is increased to correct upward displacement and to maintain the reduction. Active exercises are performed while the patient is in traction to mold the acetabulum.

*See references 47, 62, 75, 77, 87, 94, 95, 104, 109, 150, 171, 176, 178, and 183.

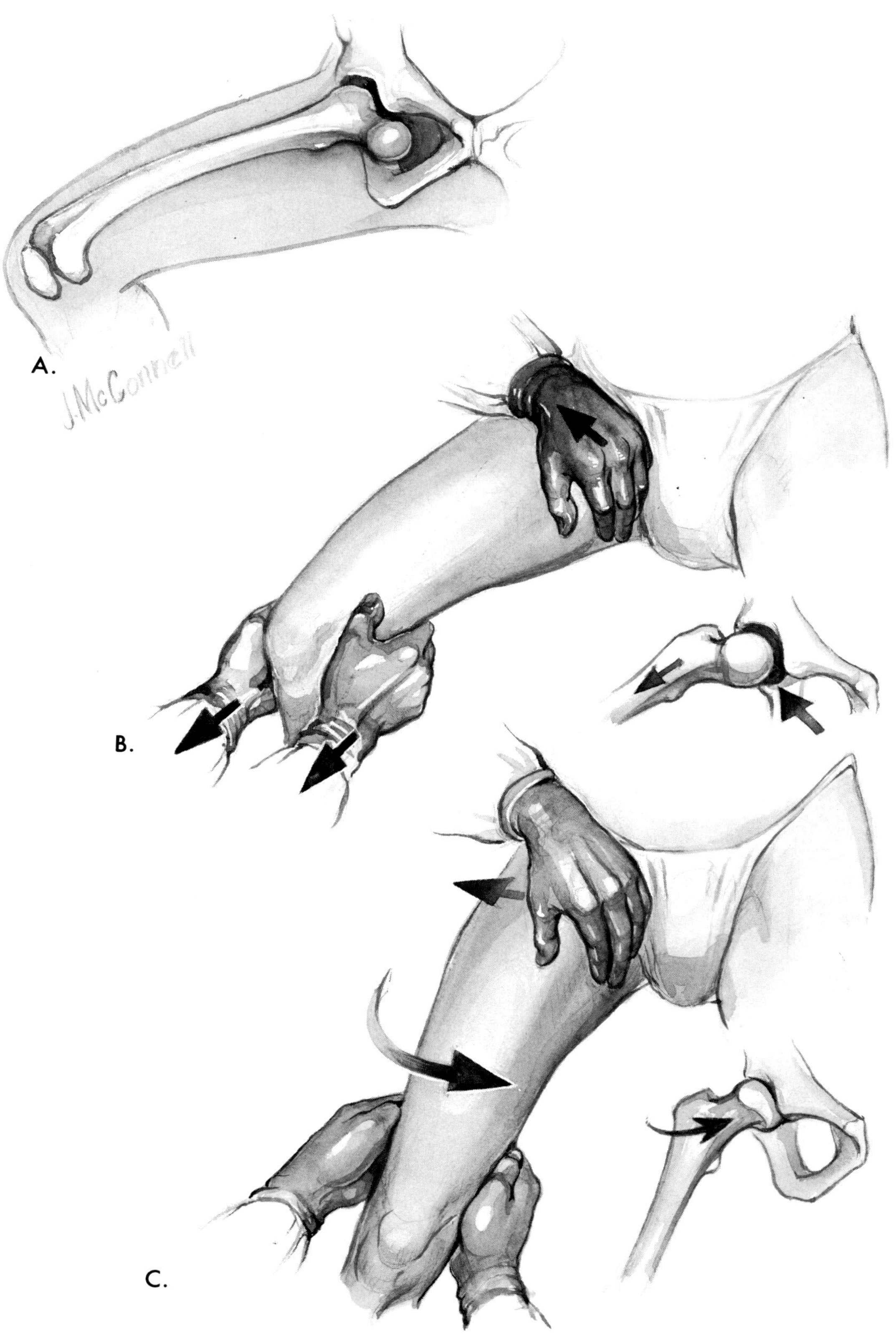

***FIGURE 8–105.** Closed reduction of anterior dislocation of the hip by the method of Allis (see text for explanation).*

Complications and Problems

These may be aseptic necrosis, sciatic nerve palsy, occlusion or tearing of femoral vessels in anterior dislocation, nonconcentric reduction due to trapped intra-articular fragment, degenerative arthritis of the hip, myositis ossificans, and recurrence of hip dislocation.

*ASEPTIC NECROSIS**

This complication occurs in 10 per cent of the cases. Factors that influence the incidence of avascular necrosis are a delay in reduction over 24 hours and severe trauma to the hip joint. In the very young patient, there appears to be some protection against aseptic necrosis. According to the Pennsylvania Orthopedic Society study, the zero to five year age group had the lowest incidence of this complication.[138] Diagnosis of aseptic necrosis can be made by bone scan with technetium-99m—it will show total or partial lack of uptake of the nucleotide. It is recommended that if the bone scan shows a "cold" femoral head, nuclear magnetic resonance imaging be performed for more accurate delineation of the pathologic anatomy. Treatment of avascular necrosis of the femoral head follows the same principles as those described for treatment of Legg-Perthes disease. Vascularized iliac or fibular bone grafting may be tried, but at present the results in the experience of this author have not been satisfactory.[37]

SCIATIC NERVE PALSY

Fortunately this is rare in children because of the low incidence of associated fracture.[93] When sciatic nerve palsy fails to show evidence of improvement in four to eight weeks, exploration is warranted after appropriate neurodiagnostic studies.

VASCULAR INJURY

In anterior dislocations the femoral vessels are at risk for occlusion or partial or complete tear. There are several case reports in the literature.[20, 76, 128, 130, 164] Always assess the circulatory status in the affected lower limb! Use Doppler studies if in doubt. Injury to femoral vessels is an acute emergency. Vascular surgical consultation should be obtained immediately for appropriate measures to be taken.

INCOMPLETE NONCONCENTRIC REDUCTION

This may be due to interposition by infolded capsule, inverted limbus, or entrapment by an osteocartilaginous fracture fragment. In the series of 26 cases of hip dislocation, Barquet reported two cases of intra-articular fragment entrapment.[7] Acetabular labrum tears and nonconcentric reduction will lead to early degenerative arthritis.[2] A computed tomography scan, with or without arthrogram, and nuclear magnetic resonance imaging will disclose the cause of nonconcentricity of reduction. Entrapped intra-articular loose body or the inverted labrum should be removed by open surgery.

DEGENERATIVE ARTHRITIS

This complication develops much less frequently in a child than in an adult following traumatic dislocation of the hip. The causes of degenerative arthritis are avascular necrosis or cartilage necrosis of the hip due to severe trauma or the presence of cartilaginous loose bodies in the joint, acetabular labrum tears, and nonconcentric reduction due to trapped osteocartilaginous fracture fragment or inverted limbus. Prevention is important—nonconcentric reduction should not be accepted. Every effort should be made to prevent avascular necrosis.

RECURRENT POST-TRAUMATIC DISLOCATION OF THE HIP

Recurrent dislocation of the hip due to marked ligamentous laxity is not uncommon in children, particularly in those with Down's syndrome. Recurrent post-traumatic dislocation of the hip is rare, however. Sullivan, Bickel, and Lipscomb reported one such case and traced several others of recurrent dislocation of the hip unassociated with fracture, acetabular dysplasia, sepsis, or paralysis.[174] Brav reported four cases of redislocation in 264 traumatic dislocations of the hip (1.5 per cent); however, only one of his cases was not associated with fracture of the acetabulum or the femoral head.[22] In the literature there are numerous reports of recurrent post-traumatic dislocation of the hip.* In the majority of these cases, there were aseptic necrotic changes in the femoral head.

Insufficiency of the capsule of the hip joint may be caused by a tear or defect of the capsule or a postinjury attenuation and elongation of the capsule without a tear. A tear in the capsule may be eliminated by arthrography.[7] Inadequate immobilization of the hip following reduction will result in incomplete healing of the capsule. Liebenberg and Dommisse, in their report of two cases of recurrent post-traumatic

---

*See references 6, 8, 35, 37, 42, 43, 48, 68, 73, 90, 92, 99, 102, 121, 146, and 155.

*See references 4, 18, 36, 41, 63, 71, 83, 84, 105, 127, 167, 174, and 177.

dislocation in adults, noted that the initial dislocation was caused by major trauma; often there was a significant delay in reduction. Subsequent dislocations followed slight injury. At operation, they found a large synovium-lined pouch or false joint cavity communicating with the true joint cavity through a broad defect in the posterior capsule. The ligamentum teres was ruptured and could not be found at operation. The hips could not be dislocated by applying moderate force unless intra-articular levers were used. On the basis of these anatomic findings, Liebenberg and Dommisse proposed the following theory:

The synovial fluid flows freely through the capsular defect between the hip joint space and the pseudocavity. During normal locomotion and movement of the lower limb, changes of volume within the two cavities occur, and the flow of fluid from one cavity to the other represents a normal adjustment of unequal hydrostatic pressures. Under certain circumstances consequent to temporary closure of the valve-like posterior defect, an increase of hydrostatic pressure of the fluid within the true cavity of the hip joint could develop. This pressure differential could be of such magnitude that it could force the femoral head across the acetabular rim, through the capsular defect, and into the pseudocavity. They believe the most important factor in development of the pseudocavity is probably a delay in reduction of the dislocation.[105]

Treatment consists of excision of the posterior pouch and repair of the capsular defect. If there is a defect or erosion of the fibrocartilaginous labrum, it is reinforced by appropriate acetabuloplasty.[69, 83, 127, 167, 174]

Failure to detect associated traumatic fractures of the femoral shaft, the patella, or the tibial plateau is a common pitfall. Conversely, in femoral shaft fractures, traumatic dislocation of the hip should always be ruled out. Ipsilateral femoral shaft fracture and hip dislocation are particularly difficult to treat. One gentle attempt of closed reduction by the Stimson maneuver may be made; however, often this is unsuccessful and the fractured femoral segments cause further soft tissue damage and serious bleeding. It is more expedient to apply skeletal traction through the trochanteric region and reduce the hip dislocation and then treat the femoral shaft fracture by skeletal traction or internal fixation with an intramedullary nail.*

Traumatic separation of the capital femoral epiphysis may be associated with hip dislocation.[11, 21, 51, 97, 101, 119] This requires open reduction. Avascular necrosis and poor result are very common in this double injury.

*See references 11, 39, 42, 79, 82, 89, 110, 116, 152, 155, 184, 185, and 189.

References

1. Aggarwall, N. D., and Singh, H.: Unreduced anterior dislocation of the hip. J. Bone Joint Surg., *49-B*:288, 1967.
2. Allis, O. A.: An Inquiry into the Difficulties Encountered in the Reduction of Dislocation of the Hip. Philadelphia, 1896.
3. Armstrong, J. R.: Traumatic dislocation of the hip joint. J. Bone Joint Surg., *30-B*:430, 1948.
4. Aufranc, O. E., Jones, W. N., and Harris, W. H.: Recurrent traumatic dislocation of the hip in a child. J.A.M.A., *90*:291, 1964.
5. Badgley, G. E.: Orthopedic correspondence club letter. As cited in personal communication, Liebenberg and Dommisse, 1968.
6. Banks, S. W.: Aseptic necrosis of the femoral head following traumatic dislocation of the hip. J. Bone Joint Surg., *23*:753, 1941.
7. Barquet, A.: Traumatic hip dislocation in children. Acta Orthop. Scand., *50*:549, 1979.
8. Barquet, A.: Recurrent traumatic dislocation of the hip in childhood. J. Trauma, *20*:1003, 1980.
9. Barquet, A.: Traumatic hip dislocation with fracture of the ipsilateral femoral shaft in childhood. Report of a case and review of the literature. Arch. Orthop. Trauma. Surg., *98*:69, 1981.
10. Barquet, A.: Traumatic anterior dislocation of the hip in childhood. Injury, *13*:435, 1982.
11. Barquet, A., and Vecsei, V.: Traumatic dislocation of the hip with separation of the proximal femoral epiphysis. Report of two cases and review of the literature. Arch. Orthop. Trauma. Surg., *103*:219, 1984.
12. Bassett, L. W., Gold, R. H., and Epstein, H. C.: Anterior hip dislocation: Atypical superolateral displacement of the femoral head. A.J.R., *141*:385, 1983.
13. Bennett, J. T., Alexander, H. H., and Morrissy, R. T.: Parathyroid adenoma presenting as a pathologic fracture of the femoral neck in an adolescent. Case report. J. Pediatr. Orthop., *6*:473, 1986.
14. Bernhang, A. M.: Simultaneous bilateral traumatic dislocation of the hip in a child. J. Bone Joint Surg., *52-A*:365, 1970.
15. Bigelow, H. J.: The Mechanism of Dislocation and Fracture of the Hip with the Reduction of the Dislocations by the Flexion Method. Philadelphia, Henry C. Lea & Co., 1869.
16. Bigelow, H. J.: The Mechanism of Dislocations and Fractures of the Hip. Boston, Little, Brown & Co., 1900.
17. Bjerkreim, I., Ronglan, E., and Russwurm, H.: Late diagnosed traumatic hip dislocation. Tidsskr. Nor. Laegeforen., *97*:180, 1977.
18. Body, J.: Luxation recidivante de la hanche chez un garcon de 7 ans. Rev. Chir. Orthop., *55*:65, 1969.
19. Böhler, J.: Die sogenannten Schenkelkopfnekrosen nach traumatischen Hüftverrenkungen. Wiederherstellungschir. Traum., *4*:75, 1957.
20. Bonnemaison, M. F. E., and Henderson, E. D.: Traumatic anterior dislocation of the hip with acute common femoral occlusion in a child. J. Bone Joint Surg., *50-A*:753, 1968.
21. Bonvallet, J. M.: On a rare case of traumatic dislocation of the hip in a child associated with a complete epiphyseal detachment and a fracture of the femoral head nucleus. Rev. Chir. Orthop., *51*:723, 1965.

22. Brav, E. A.: Traumatic dislocation of the hip joint. J. Bone Joint Surg., *44-A*:1115, 1962.
23. Byram, G., and Wickstrom, J.: Traumatic dislocation of the hip in children. South. Med. J., *60*:805, 1967.
24. Caamaño, A.: Luxaciones Traumáticas de la carderna en el niño. Semana Med., *1*:450, 1941.
25. Canale, S. T.: Traumatic dislocations and fracture-dislocations of the hip in children. Hip, *219*:45, 1981.
26. Canale, S. T., and Manugian, A. H.: Irreducible traumatic dislocation of the hip. J. Bone Joint Surg., *61-A*:7, 1979.
27. Charry, V.: Luxation traumatique invérterée de la hanche chez un enfant de sept ans et demi réduite par voie sanglante duex mois après l'accident. Rev. Orthop., *23*:147, 1936.
28. Charry, V.: Résultat éloigné d'une luxation traumatique de la hanche d'avant de deux mois et réduite par voie sanglante chez un enfant. Bull. Soc. Chir. Paris, *29*:160, 1937.
29. Chavette, J.: Luxation traumatique de la hanche chez l'enfant. Thesis, University of Lyon, 1968.
30. Chotigavanichaya, C.: Traumatic dislocation of the hip joint in childhood. J. Med. Assoc. Thai., *58*:329, 1975.
31. Choyce, C. C.: Traumatic dislocation of the hip in childhood and relation of trauma to pseudocoxalgia. Br. J. Surg., *12*:52, 1924.
32. Cinats, J. G., Moreau, M. J., and Swersky, J. F.: Traumatic dislocation of the hip caused by capsular interposition in a child. A case report. J. Bone Joint Surg., *70-A*:130, 1988.
33. Clarke, H. O.: Traumatic dislocation of the hip joint in a child. Br. J. Surg., *16*:690, 1929.
34. Craig, C. L.: Hip injuries in children and adolescents. Orthop. Clin. North Am., *11*:743, 1980.
35. Cros, J. A.: Osteochondrosis of the upper femoral epiphysis following traumatic dislocation of the hip joint. J. Bone Joint Surg., *41-A*:1335, 1959.
36. Dall, D., MacNab, I., and Gross, A.: Recurrent anterior dislocation of the hip. J. Bone Joint Surg., *52-A*:574, 1970.
37. Day, B., Shim, S. S., and Leung, G.: The iliopsoas muscle pedicle bone graft: An experimental study of femoral head vascularity after subcapital fractures and hip dislocations. Clin. Orthop., *191*:262, 1984.
38. De Guidi, G., Grassi, E., and Nicosia, U.: Traumatic dislocation of the hip in childhood. Minerva Pediatr., *19*:129, 1967.
39. Dehne, E., and Innerman, E. W.: Dislocation of the hip combined with fracture of the shaft of the femur on the same side. J. Bone Joint Surg., *33-A*:731, 1951.
40. Drejack, D.: Über Apophysenlosungen und Ossifikationsstörungen der Sitzbeinapophyse. Arch. Orthop. Unfallchir., *68*:370, 1970.
41. Duytjes, F.: Recurrent dislocation of the hip joint in a boy. J. Bone Joint Surg., *45-B*:432, 1963.
42. Elizalde, E. A.: Obstetrical dislocation of the hip associated with fracture of the femur. J. Bone Joint Surg., *28*:838, 1946.
43. Elmslie, R. C.: Pseudocoxalgia following traumatic dislocation of the hip in a boy aged four years. J. Orthop. Surg., *1*:109, 1919.
44. Elmslie, R. C.: Traumatic dislocation of the hip in a child aged seven with subsequent development of coxa plana. Proc. R. Soc. Med., *25*:1100, 1932.
45. Epstein, H. C.: Traumatic dislocations of the hip. Clin. Orthop., *92*:116, 1973.
46. Epstein, H. C.: Traumatic Dislocation of the Hip. Baltimore, Williams & Wilkins, 1980.
47. Epstein, H. C., Wiss, D. A., and Cozen, L.: Posterior fracture-dislocation of the hip with fractures of the femoral head. Clin. Orthop., *201*:9, 1985.
48. Fairbank, H. A. T.: Case of pseudo-coxalgia following traumatic dislocation in a boy. Proc. R. Soc. Med., *17*:40, 1924.
49. Fernandez-Herrera, E.: Luxacion traumatica anterior de la casera en la infancia. Bol. Med. Hosp. Infant. Mex., *22*:95, 1965.
50. Fettweis, E.: Prevention of hip dislocation in children. Z. Orthop., *109*:905, 1971.
51. Fiddian, N. J., and Grace, D. L.: Traumatic dislocation of the hip in adolescence with separation of the capital epiphysis. Two case reports. J. Bone Joint Surg., *65-B*:148, 1983.
52. Fineschi, G.: Die traumatische Huftverrenkung bei Kindern, Literaturübersicht und statistischer Beitrag von 7 Fallen. Arch. Orthop., *48*:225, 1956.
53. Fischer, L., and Inbert, J. C.: Simple retrocondyloid traumatic luxation of the hip in children without upward displacement: Necessity for profile picture. Lyon Med., *222*:825, 1969.
54. Fischer, L., Imbert, J. C., David, M., Comtet, J. J., Korkmaz, G., and Chavette, J. P.: Traumatic luxation successively affecting both hips in a child: Predisposing factors. Lyon Med., *222*:263, 1969.
55. Fordyce, A. J. W.: Open reduction of traumatic dislocation of the hip in a child. Case report and review of the literature. Br. J. Surg., *58*:705, 1971.
56. Freeman, G. E., Jr.: Traumatic dislocation of the hip in children. J. Bone Joint Surg., *43-A*:401, 1961.
57. Fregani, L., and Dorghetti, I.: Removal results of traumatic dislocation of the hip in the juvenile age. Arcisp. S. Anna Ferrara, *23*(4):261, 1970.
58. Fries, G.: On the treatment of old traumatic dislocations of the hip and dislocation fractures in childhood. Arch. Orthop. Unfallchir., *59*:229, 1966.
59. Fulkerson, J. P.: Arthrodesis for disabling hip pain in children and adolescents. Clin. Orthop., *128*:296, 1977.
60. Funk, F. J., Jr.: Traumatic dislocation of the hip in children. Factors influencing prognosis and treatment. J. Bone Joint Surg., *44-A*:1135, 1962.
61. Gartland, J. J., and Benner, J. H.: Traumatic dislocation in the lower extremity in children. Orthop. Clin. North Am., *7*:687, 1976.
62. Garvan, J. D.: Delayed presentation of posterior fracture dislocation of the hip in a child. Aust. N.Z. J. Surg., *53*:493, 1983.
63. Gaul, R. W.: Recurrent traumatic dislocation of the hip in children. Clin. Orthop., *90*:107, 1973.
64. Giraud, D. E. A.: Contribution à létude de la luxation traumatique de la hanche chez l'enfant. Thèses de Bordeaux, Geof-Josp., 1927.
65. Glass, A., and Powell, H. D. W.: Traumatic dislocation of the hip in children. Analysis of 47 patients. J. Bone Joint Surg., *43-B*:29, 1961.
66. Glynn, P.: Two cases of traumatic dislocation of the hip in children. Lancet, *1*:1093, 1932.
67. Godshall, R. W., and Hansen, C. A.: Incomplete avulsion of a portion of the iliac epiphysis. An injury of young athletes. J. Bone Joint Surg., *55-A*:1301, 1973.
68. Goldenberg, R. R.: Traumatic dislocation of the hip followed by Perthes' disease. J. Bone Joint Surg., *20*:770, 1938.
69. Gula, D. L.: Recurrent traumatic dislocation of the hip in children. J. Am. Osteopath. Assoc., *72*:32, 1972.
70. Gupta, R. C., and Shravat, B. P.: Reduction of neglected traumatic dislocation of the hip by heavy traction. J. Bone Joint Surg., *59-A*:249, 1977.
71. Guyer, B., and Levinsohn, E. M.: Recurrent anterior dislocation of the hip: Case report with arthrographic findings. Skeletal Radiol., *10*:262, 1983.
72. Haines, C.: Traumatic dislocation of the head of the femur in a child. J. Bone Joint Surg., *19*:1126, 1937.
73. Haliburton, R. A., Brockenshire, F. A., and Barber, J. R.: Avascular necrosis of the femoral capital epiph-

ysis after traumatic dislocation of the hip in children. J. Bone Joint Surg., *43-B*:43, 1961.

74. Hamada, G.: Unreduced anterior dislocation of the hip. J. Bone Joint Surg., *39-B*:471, 1957.
75. Hammond, G.: Posterior dislocation of the hip associated with fracture. Proc. R. Soc. Med., *37*:281, 1944.
76. Hampson, W. G. J.: Venous obstruction by anterior dislocation of the hip joint. Injury, *4*:69, 1972.
77. Harder, J. A., Bobechko, W. P., Sullivan, R., and Danerman, A.: Computerized axial tomography to demonstrate occult fractures of the acetabulum in children. Can. J. Surg., *24*:409, 1981.
78. Harper, M. C., and Henstorf, J.: Fractures of the femoral neck associated with technical errors in closed intramedullary nailing of the femur. Report of two cases. J. Bone Joint Surg., *68-A*:624, 1986.
79. Helal, B., and Skevis, X.: Unrecognized dislocations of the hip in fractures of the femoral shaft. J. Bone Joint Surg., *49-B*:293, 1967.
80. Hemmelbo, T.: Traumatic hip dislocation in childhood. Acta Orthop. Scand., *47*:546, 1976.
81. Henderson, R. S.: Traumatic anterior dislocation of the hip. J. Bone Joint Surg., *33-B*:602, 1951.
82. Henry, A. K., and Bayumi, M.: Fracture of the femur with luxation of the ipsilateral hip. Br. J. Surg., *22*:204, 1934.
83. Hensley, C. D., and Schofield, G. W.: Recurrent dislocation of the hip. A case report. J. Bone Joint Surg., *51-A*:573, 1969.
84. Hohmann, D.: Rezidivierende traumatische Hüftluxation beim Kind nach fehlerhafter Gipsfixation. Monatsschr. Unfallheilkd., *67*:352, 1964.
85. Hougaard, K., and Thomsen, P. B.: Traumatic posterior fracture-dislocation of the hip with fracture of the femoral head or neck, or both. J. Bone Joint Surg., *70-A*:233, 1988.
86. Hovelius, L.: Traumatic dislocation of the hip in children. Report of two cases. Acta Orthop. Scand., *45*:746, 1974.
87. Hunter, G. A.: Posterior dislocation of fracture dislocation of the hip. J. Bone Joint Surg., *51-B*:38, 1969.
88. Ingram, A., and Bachynski, B.: Fractures of the hip in children. J. Bone Joint Surg., *35-A*:867, 1953.
89. Ingram, A. J., and Turner, T. C.: Bilateral traumatic posterior dislocation of the hip complicated by bilateral fracture of the femoral shaft. J. Bone Joint Surg., *36-A*:1249, 1954.
90. Jaberg, H., and Ganz, R.: Complications of traumatic hip dislocation in children. Ther. Umsch., *40*:956, 1983.
91. Johner, R., and Ganz, R.: Traumatic disorders of the hip in children (author's transl.). Ther. Umsch., *34*:305, 1977.
92. Juan, A. C.: Osteochondrosis of the upper femoral epiphysis following traumatic dislocation of the hip joint. J. Bone Joint Surg., *41-A*:1335, 1959.
93. Katznelson, A. M.: Traumatic dislocation of the hip. J. Bone Joint Surg., *44-B*:129, 1962.
94. Kelly, R. P., and Yarbrough, S. H., III: Posterior fracture-dislocation of the femoral head with retained head fragment. J. Trauma, *11*:97, 1971.
95. King, D., and Richards, V.: Fracture-dislocation of the hip joint. J. Bone Joint Surg., *23*:533, 1941.
96. King, S. J., Seale, W. A., and Ametewee, K.: A new sign in anterior dislocation of the hip joint. Injury, *16*:51, 1984.
97. Klasen, H. J., and Binnendijk, B.: Fracture of the neck of the femur associated with posterior dislocation of the hip. J. Bone Joint Surg., *66-B*:45, 1984.
98. Kleiman, S. G., Stevens, J., Kolb, L., and Pankovich, A.: Late sciatic nerve palsy following posterior fracture-dislocation of the hip. J. Bone Joint Surg., *53-A*:781, 1971.
99. Kleinberg, S.: Aseptic necrosis of the femoral head following traumatic dislocation. Report of two cases. Arch. Surg., *39*:637, 1939.
100. Klems, H.: Traumatic dislocation of the hip in childhood. Z. Orthop., *110*:579, 1972.
101. Kumar, S., and James, R.: Dislocation of the hip with associated subcapital fracture—a successfully treated case. Injury, *16*:539, 1985.
102. Labaziewicz, L.: Inveterate traumatic dislocation of the hip with necrosis of the femoral head in a child. Chir. Narzadow Ruchu Ortop. Pol., *41*:5, 1976.
103. Laskowski, M., and Mazurkiewicz, S.: Traumatic hip dislocation in children. Chir. Narzadow Ruchu Ortop. Pol., *38*:23, 1973.
104. Lesourd, G.: Traumatic luxation of the right hip with epiphyseal detachment of the femoral head and fracture of the posterior cotyloid elevation in a 15-year-old child. Rev. Chir. Orthop., *55*:61, 1969.
105. Liebenberg, F., and Dommisse, G. F.: Recurrent post-traumatic dislocation of the hip. J. Bone Joint Surg., *51-B*:632, 1969.
106. Litton, L. O.: Traumatic anterior dislocation of the hip in children. J. Bone Joint Surg., *40-B*:1419, 1958.
107. Litton, L. O., and Workman, D.: Traumatic anterior dislocation of the hip in children. J. Bone Joint Surg., *40-A*:419, 1958.
108. Lugger, L. J.: Traumatische Huftverrenkung und gleichzeitiger Oberschenkelschaftbruch im Kindesalter. Zentralbl. Chir., *99*:340, 1974.
109. Lujubo Sic, N. A.: Acetabular injuries in childhood. Acta Chir. Orthop. Traumatol. Cech., *34*:393, 1967.
110. Lyddon, D. W., and Hartman, J. T.: Traumatic dislocation of the hip with ipsilateral femoral fracture. J. Bone Joint Surg., *53-A*:1012, 1971.
111. McFarland, J. A.: Anterior dislocation of the hip. Br. J. Surg., *23*:607, 1935.
112. MacFarlane, I. J. A.: Survey of traumatic dislocation of the hip in children. J. Bone Joint Surg., *58-B*:267, 1976.
113. MacFarlane, I., and King, D.: Traumatic dislocation of the hip joint in children. Aust. N.Z. J. Surg., *46*(3):227, 1976.
114. Maffei, F.: Contributo allo studio della lussazione traumatic dell'anca nell infanzia. Chir. Organi Mov., *6*:604, 1922.
115. Malimson, P. D.: Triple fracture-dislocation of the lower limb. Injury, *16*:11, 1984.
116. Malkawi, H.: Traumatic anterior dislocation of the hip with fracture of the shaft of the ipsilateral femur in children: Case report and review of the literature. J. Pediatr. Orthop., *2*:307, 1982.
117. Marsh, H. O.: Intertrochanteric and femoral neck fractures in children. J. Bone Joint Surg., *49-A*:1024, 1967.
118. Mason, M. L.: Traumatic dislocation of the hip in childhood. J. Bone Joint Surg., *36-B*:630, 1954.
119. Mass, D. P., Spiegel, P. G., and Laros, G. S.: Dislocation of the hip with traumatic separation of the capital femoral epiphysis: Report of a case with successful outcome. Clin. Orthop., *146*:184, 1980.
120. Meng, C. I.: Traumatic dislocation of the hip in childhood. Chinese Med. J., *48*:736, 1954.
121. Merle D'Aubigné, R., and Cormier: Nécrose traumatique de la tête due fémur en dehors des pseudarthroses. Rev. Chir. Orthop., *42*:246, 1956.
122. Miglietta, P.: A case of traumatic dislocation of the hip in a 23-month-old girl. Arch. Putti Chir. Organi Mov., *24*:383, 1969.
123. Morton, K. S.: Traumatic dislocation of the hip in children. Can. J. Surg., *3*:67, 1959.
124. Morton, K. S.: Traumatic dislocation of the hip in children. J.A.M.A., *47*:223, 1959.
125. Murphy, D. P.: Traumatic luxation of the hip in childhood. J.A.M.A., *80*:549, 1923.

126. Mutschler, H. M.: Sekundäre Oberschenkelkopf-necrose nach traumatischer Ausrenkung des Hüftgelenkes bei einem 14 Jahrigen. Munchen Med. Wschr., *86*:258, 1939.
127. Nelson, C. L.: Traumatic recurrent dislocation of the hip. Report of a case. J. Bone Joint Surg., *52-A*:128, 1970.
128. Nerubay, J.: Traumatic anterior dislocation of the hip joint with vascular damage. Clin. Orthop., *116*:129, 1976.
129. Nicoll, E. A.: Traumatic dislocation of the hip joint. J. Bone Joint Surg., *34-B*:503, 1952.
130. Niloff, R., and Petrie, J. G.: Traumatic anterior dislocation of the hip. Can. Med. Assoc. J., *62*:574, 1950.
131. Obel, W., and Debowskawojcik, D.: Traumatic hip luxation in children in the light of clinical observations. Pediatr. Pol., *51*:689, 1976.
132. Oni, O. O., Orhewere, F. A., and Kesawani, H.: The treatment of old unreduced traumatic dislocation of the hip. Injury, *15*:219, 1984.
133. Ordway, C. B., and Xeller, C. F.: Transverse computerized axial tomography of patients with posterior dislocation of the hip. J. Trauma, *24*:76, 1984.
134. Ostapowicz, G.: Traumatic hip dislocation in a 4-year-old boy. Monatsschr. Unfallheilkd., *71*:207, 1968.
135. Paus, B.: Traumatic dislocation of the hip. Acta Orthop. Scand., *21*:99, 1951.
136. Pearson, D. E., and Mann, R. J.: Traumatic hip dislocation in children. Clin. Orthop., *92*:189, 1973.
137. Pennsylvania Orthopedic Society: Traumatic dislocation of the hip joint in children. J. Bone Joint Surg., *42-A*:705, 1960.
138. Pennsylvania Orthopedic Society: Traumatic dislocation of the hip joint in children. Final Report. J. Bone Joint Surg., *50-A*:79, 1968.
139. Perry, B. F.: Traumatic dislocation of the hip in the child: Case report. Am. Surg., *32*:419, 1966.
140. Petrini, A., and Grassi, G.: Long term results in traumatic dislocation of the hip in children. Ital. J. Orthop. Traumatol., *9*:225, 1983.
141. Pietrafesa, C. A., and Hoffman, J. R.: Traumatic dislocation of the hip. J.A.M.A., *249*:3342, 1983.
142. Piggot, J.: Traumatic dislocation of the hip in childhood. J. Bone Joint Surg., *41-B*:209, 1959.
143. Piggot, J.: Traumatic dislocation of the hip in childhood. J. Bone Joint Surg., *43-B*:38, 1961.
144. Platt, H.: Traumatic dislocation of the hip joint in a child. Lancet, *1*:80, 1916.
145. Quinby, W. C., Jr.: Fractures of the pelvis and associated injuries in children. J. Pediatr. Surg., *1*:353, 1966.
146. Quist-Hanssen, S.: Caput necrosis after traumatic dislocation of the hip in a 4-year-old boy. Acta Chir. Scand., *95*:344, 1945.
147. Rao, J. P., and Read, R. B.: Luxatio erecta of the hip. A case report. Clin. Orthop., *110*:137, 1975.
148. Reed, M. H.: Pelvic fractures in children. J. Can. Assoc. Radiol., *27*:255, 1976.
149. Remec, P. T., and Evarts, C. M.: Bilateral central dislocation of the hip. A case report. Clin. Orthop., *181*:118, 1983.
150. Rigault, P., Hannouche, D., and Judet, J.: Traumatic dislocations of the hip and fractures of the acetabulum in children. Rev. Chir. Orthop., *54*:361, 1968.
151. Ring, P. A.: Hip fractures up to date. Br. Med. J. *2*:1429, 1976.
152. Rinke, W., and Protze, J.: Open traumatic hip-joint dislocation and simultaneous femoral fracture in childhood. Zentralbl. Chir., *101*:177, 1976.
153. Robertson, R. C., and Peterson, H. A.: Traumatic dislocation of the hip in children: Review of Mayo Clinic series. *In* The Hip. Vol. 2. St. Louis, Mosby, 1974.
154. Rocher, H. L., Rocher, C., and Cuzard, M.: Luxation traumatique de la hanche chez l'enfant. Bordeaux Chir., *8*:255, 1937.
155. Rogala, P., and Labaziewicz, L.: Inveterate traumatic hip dislocation associated with fracture of the femoral diaphysis in a child complicated by avascular femur head necrosis. Chir. Narzadow Ruchu Ortop. Pol., *42*:265, 1977.
156. Sadler, A. H., and DiStefano, M.: Anterior dislocation of the hip with ipsilateral basicervical fracture. A case report. J. Bone Joint Surg., *67-A*:326, 1985.
157. Saito, S., Takaoka, K., and Ono, K.: Tectoplasty for painful dislocation and subluxation of the hip. J. Bone Joint Surg., *68-B*:55, 1986.
158. Sakar, S. D.: Delayed open reduction of traumatic dislocation of the hip. A case report and historical review. Clin. Orthop., *186*:38, 1984.
159. Salai, M., Amit, Y., Blankstein, A., Chechik, A., and Horoszowski, H.: Isolated anterior inguinal dislocation of the hip joint. J. Trauma, *25*:563, 1985.
160. Sankarankutty, M.: Traumatic inferior dislocation of the hip (Luxatio Erecta) in a child. J. Bone Joint Surg., *49-B*:145, 1967.
161. Sarungi, P. M.: Traumatic posterior dislocation of the hip in a child. A case report. East Afr. Med. J., *51*:364, 1974.
162. Schlonsky, J., and Miller, P. R.: Traumatic hip dislocations in children. J. Bone Joint Surg., *55-A*:1057, 1973.
163. Schlonsky, J., and Olix, M. L.: Functional disability following avulsion fracture of the ischial epiphysis. Report of two cases. J. Bone Joint Surg., *54-A*:641, 1972.
164. Schwartz, D. L., and Haller, J. A., Jr.: Open anterior hip dislocation with femoral vessel transection in a child. J. Trauma, *14*:1054, 1974.
165. Scudese, V. A.: Traumatic anterior hip redislocation. Clin. Orthop., *88*:60, 1972.
166. Sibrandij, S.: Hip dislocations in children are easily overlooked. Ned. Tijdschr. Geneeskd., *118*:1145, 1974.
167. Simmons, R. L., and Elder, J. D.: Recurrent post-traumatic dislocation of the hip in children. South. Med. J., *65*:1463, 1972.
168. Sinha, S. N.: Simultaneous anterior and posterior dislocation of the hip joints. J. Trauma, *25*:269, 1985.
169. Soltanpur, A.: Bilateral traumatic dislocation of the hip. Injury, *14*:349, 1983.
170. Spissak, L., Kirnak, J., and Stojkovi, C. J.: Traumatic hip dislocation in children. Bratisl. Lek. Listy., *52*:464, 1969.
171. Stewart, M. J., and Milford, L. W.: Fracture dislocation of the hip. An end result study. J. Bone Joint Surg., *36-A*:315, 1954.
172. Strange, F. G. St. C.: The Hip. London, William Heinemann, 1965.
173. Stimson, L. A.: Treatise on Dislocation. Philadelphia, Lea Brothers and Co., 1888, pp. 397–463.
174. Sullivan, C. R., Bickel, W. H., and Lipscomb, P. R.: Recurrent dislocation of the hip. J. Bone Joint Surg., *37-A*:1266, 1955.
175. Thompson, V. P., and Epstein, H. C.: Traumatic dislocation of the hip. J. Bone Joint Surg., *33-A*:746, 1951.
176. Toni, A., Gulino, G., Baldini, N., and Gulino, F.: Clinical and radiographic long term results of acetabular fractures associated with dislocations of the hip. Ital. J. Orthop. Traumatol., *11*:443, 1985.
177. Townsend, R. G., Edwards, G. E., and Bazant, F. J.: Posttraumatic recurrent dislocation of the hip without fracture. J. Bone Joint Surg., *51-B*:194, 1969.
178. Trillat, A., and Ringot, A.: Erreurs d'interpretation radiographique dans les fractures du cotyle avec luxation de la tête femorale. Lyon Chir., *46*:472, 1951.

179. Trojan, E.: Traumatic dislocation and fracture-dislocations of the hip. Rev. Chir. Orthop., *45*:469, 1959.
180. Tronzo, R. G.: Traumatic dislocation of the hip in children. A problem in anesthetic management. J.A.M.A., *176*:526, 1961.
181. Upahyay, S. S., Moulton, A., and Burwell, R. G.: Biological factors predisposing to traumatic posterior dislocation of the hip. J. Bone Joint Surg., *67-B*:232, 1985.
182. Upahyay, S. S., Moulton, A., and Srikrishnamurthy, K.: An analysis of the late effects of traumatic posterior dislocation of the hip without fractures. J. Bone Joint Surg., *65-B*:150, 1983.
183. Urist, M. R.: Fracture-dislocation of the hip joint. J. Bone Joint Surg., *30-A*:1699, 1948.
184. Verdonk, R., and de Smet, L.: Hip dislocation combined with femoral shaft fracture. Two cases treated with the Lardennois hoop. Acta Orthop. Scand., *55*:185, 1984.
185. Wadsworth, T. G.: Traumatic dislocation of the hip with fracture of the shaft of the ipsilateral femur. J. Bone Joint Surg., *43-B*:47, 1961.
186. Weber, B. G.: Verletzungen des Hüftgelenkes. Chirurgie der Gegenwart, Band IV, 1975.
187. Wilchinsky, M. E., and Pappas, A. M.: Unusual complications in traumatic dislocation of the hip in children. J. Pediatr. Orthop., *5*:534, 1985.
188. Wilson, D. W.: Traumatic dislocation of the hip in children. A report of four cases. J. Trauma, *6*:739, 1966.
189. Wiltberger, B. R., Mitchell, C. L., and Hedrick, D. W.: Fracture of the femoral shaft complicated by hip dislocation. J. Bone Joint Surg., *30-A*:255, 1948.

FRACTURES OF THE NECK OF THE FEMUR

Fractures of the femoral neck are rare in children and indeed were hardly known to exist until the latter part of the nineteenth century. The initial case reports in the English literature were those of Barber, in 1871, and Cromwell, in 1885.[7, 24] Whitman, in 1891, described a fracture of the femoral neck in a child, and subsequently, in a series of papers (the last of which appeared in 1909), reported a total of 31 cases.[102–106] Most of Whitman's cases were encountered prior to the discovery of x-rays, and were recognized late because of the presence of coxa vara. Russell, in 1898, in his report of two femoral neck fractures in children, stressed the importance of distinguishing this rare injury from various diseases of the hip joint.[82] In 1917, Taylor reported six cases; and Bland-Sutton, in 1918, described the pathologic features of an anatomic specimen, dated 1893, of an intracapsular fracture of the neck of a child's femur found in the museum of Middlesex Hospital.[10, 92]

The rarity of this injury is indicated by the scanty literature with few case reports on the subject: 12 cases by Colonna, 10 cases by Wilson, 10 cases by Carrell and Carrell, 8 cases by Allende and Lezama, and 24 cases by McDougall.[2, 15, 23, 60, 107]

Detailed studies of a large series of cases were recently reported by Ratliff, Lam, and Boitzy.[12, 54, 55, 73–78]

The injury is more common in boys, with the male-to-female ratio being approximately 3:2. Lam, however, reports 57 of the 75 fractures in boys, or approximately 75 per cent.[54] The fracture may occur at any age, with the highest incidence between 11 and 12 years.

Classification

Fractures of the hip in children are classified according to anatomic location into four types (originally developed by Delbert and subsequently popularized by Colonna).[22, 23, 25]

Type I, or transepiphyseal—an acute traumatic separation of a previously normal epiphysis. It should not be confused with an acute slip of the upper femoral epiphysis. Anatomically, it is similar to the Type I physeal injury of Salter and Harris.

Type II, or transcervical—the mid-portion of the femoral neck.

Type III, or cervicotrochanteric—the base of the femoral neck.

Type IV, or pertrochanteric—between the base of the femoral neck and the lesser trochanter. The incidence of various types of fractures is shown in Table 8–5.

In the newborn there is another type of injury to the hip, namely, birth fracture of the metaphysis of the femoral neck (Fig. 8–106). As the capital femoral and greater trochanteric epiphyses are not yet ossified, these fractures are often mistaken for dislocation of the hip. Metaphyseal birth fractures and pathologic fractures of the femoral neck are considered elsewhere.

Mechanism of Injury

In children the femoral neck and head are hard and the force required to break them is considerable—such as that of a fall from a height, an automobile accident, or a fall off a bicycle. (In the latter the saddle of the bicycle is wedged against the perineum and acts as a fulcrum over which the femoral neck fractures.) This is in contrast to the fractures of the femoral neck in the elderly adult, in whom the osteoporotic bone breaks because of such minimal trauma as tripping over a carpet.

Because of the nature of severe violence producing the hip injury, in children there is often associated major trauma such as fractures of the skull, pelvis, and femoral shaft; visceral rupture; and soft-tissue loss over the affected

Table 8–5. Incidence of Various Types of Femoral Neck Fractures in Children

Author	Total No. of Cases	Transepiphyseal	Transcervical	Cervicotrochanteric (or Basal neck)	Pertrochanteric
Lam (1971)	75	2	37 (9 seen late)	23 (5 seen late)	13 (1 seen late)
Ratliff (1962)	70	2	38	26	4
McDougall (1961)	24	2	11	8	3
Ingram and Bachynski (1953)	24	6	11	5	2
Allende and Lezama (1951)	8	1	5	1	1
Carrell and Carrell (1941)	12	—	4	8	—
Total	213	13 (6%)	106 (50%)	71 (33%)	23 (11%)

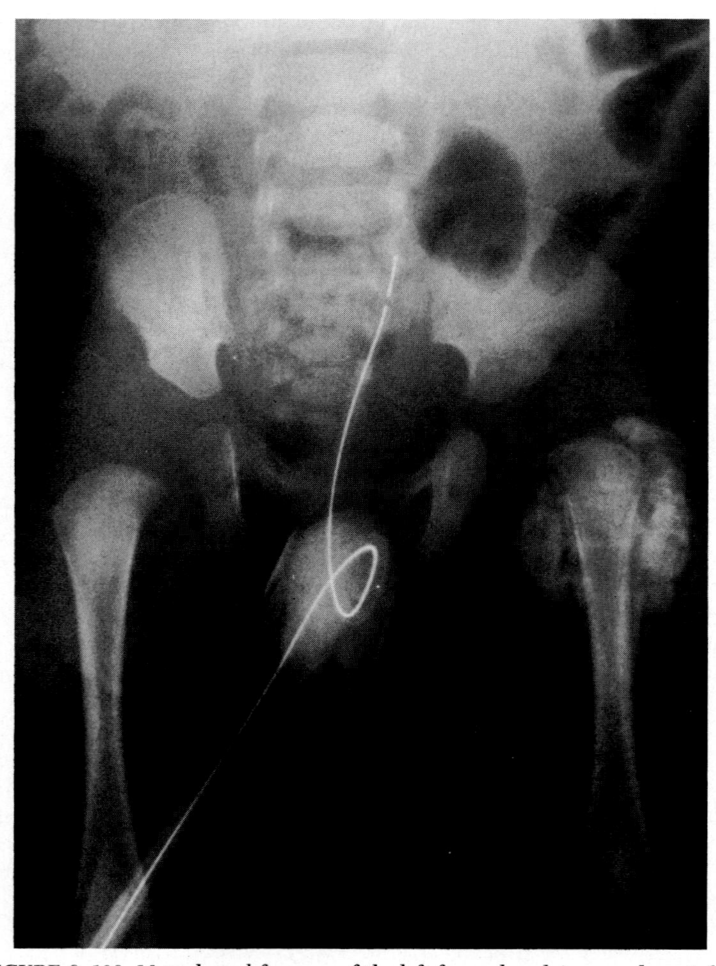

FIGURE 8–106. Metaphyseal fracture of the left femoral neck in a newborn infant.

limb. It is imperative to rule out multiple injury; conversely, when the fracture is caused by trivial injury, it is necessary to eliminate the possibility of pathologic fracture.

Diagnosis

The diagnosis is not difficult. There is a history of severe injury following which the patient complains of sudden pain in the hip. He is usually unable to stand or walk; however, if the fracture is of the greenstick or impacted type, he may be able to bear weight on the affected limb.

On physical examination, the injured limb is held rigidly in a varying degree of lateral rotation and slight adduction. In displaced fractures, the patient is unable to move the injured hip actively. Actual shortening of 1 to 2 cm. is present. On palpation, local tenderness is elicited and is most marked posteriorly where the femoral neck is superficially located. Some swelling in Scarpa's triangle may be noted. There is marked restriction of passive motions of the hip, particularly those of flexion, abduction, and medial rotation.

The diagnosis is confirmed by the use of radiograms, which should be made in the anteroposterior and lateral views. The direction of the fracture line and the degree of coxa vara are noted. The femoral head is retained in the acetabulum in its normal location, but the distal fragment of the femoral neck is displaced upward, anteriorly, and into slight lateral rotation.

Treatment

In the literature, various methods of treatment of femoral neck fractures in children have been advocated, and because this is a particularly difficult fracture, they are briefly reviewed here.

Traction was the method chosen by Barber, in 1871.[7] Forced manipulative reduction and immobilization in a hip spica cast were advocated by Whitman, who felt that it is imperative to restore normal anatomic alignment to prevent future deformity. He achieved forced reduction as follows: (1) The anesthetized patient is placed on the fracture table with the pelvis resting on a sacral support and the extended lower limbs held by assistants (or secured on a foot plate of the fracture table in the older child). (2) The normal hip is fully abducted to determine its range and to fix the pelvis. (3) Then, under longitudinal traction, the fractured hip is slowly abducted to its full limit. (4) With his hands, the surgeon presses the greater trochanter downward, utilizing the upper border of the acetabular rim as a fulcrum, to restore the normal relationship between the head-neck and shaft of the femur (Fig. 8–107). The extended hip is rotated medially to 20 degrees beyond neutral position, and the hip is then immobilized in this position in a one and one half hip spica cast.[102–106]

Russell recommended traction for a period of three weeks to allow "soft union" to occur prior to forced abduction and immobilization in a hip spica cast.[82] Taylor and Colonna followed Whitman's method of early forced manipulative reduction.[22, 23, 92] Böhler advocated continuous traction for three months, stating that femoral neck fractures in children should be treated like any other fracture of the femur in a child.[11]

Mitchell, in 1936, reported a series of ten fractures of the hip in children, of which only three were seen within two weeks of the initial trauma and were, therefore, classified as recent. Of these three, two were treated by the Whitman forced abduction method, the result being good in one and poor in the other. The third fracture was treated by manipulative reduction, followed by continuous well-leg traction with the hip immobilized in abduction in a plaster of Paris cast; the latter method showed a good result. Thus, Mitchell concluded that the method of choice in treatment of recent fractures of the femoral neck is continuous well-leg traction combined with immobilization in abduction in a hip spica cast.[65]

Wilson analyzed eight of his own cases of femoral neck fractures, four of which were treated initially by the Whitman method, with good results in some. He pointed out the difficulties involved in maintaining reduction by the Whitman method and recommended internal fixation with a nail, provided the physis is not damaged.[107]

Carrell and Carrell found it difficult to maintain reduction with the Whitman method, as alignment was retained in only one of their five patients treated in this manner. Three of their patients with four fractures were treated by closed reduction and immobilization in a Hoke type plaster cast with leg countertraction. As reduction was maintained in all three cases, they concluded that this is the best method of immobilization, particularly in the cervicotrochanteric type of fracture. Adductor myotomy was performed as necessary.[15]

The importance of the plane or the angle of the fracture line was pointed out by Allende and Lezama. When Pauwel's angle is less than

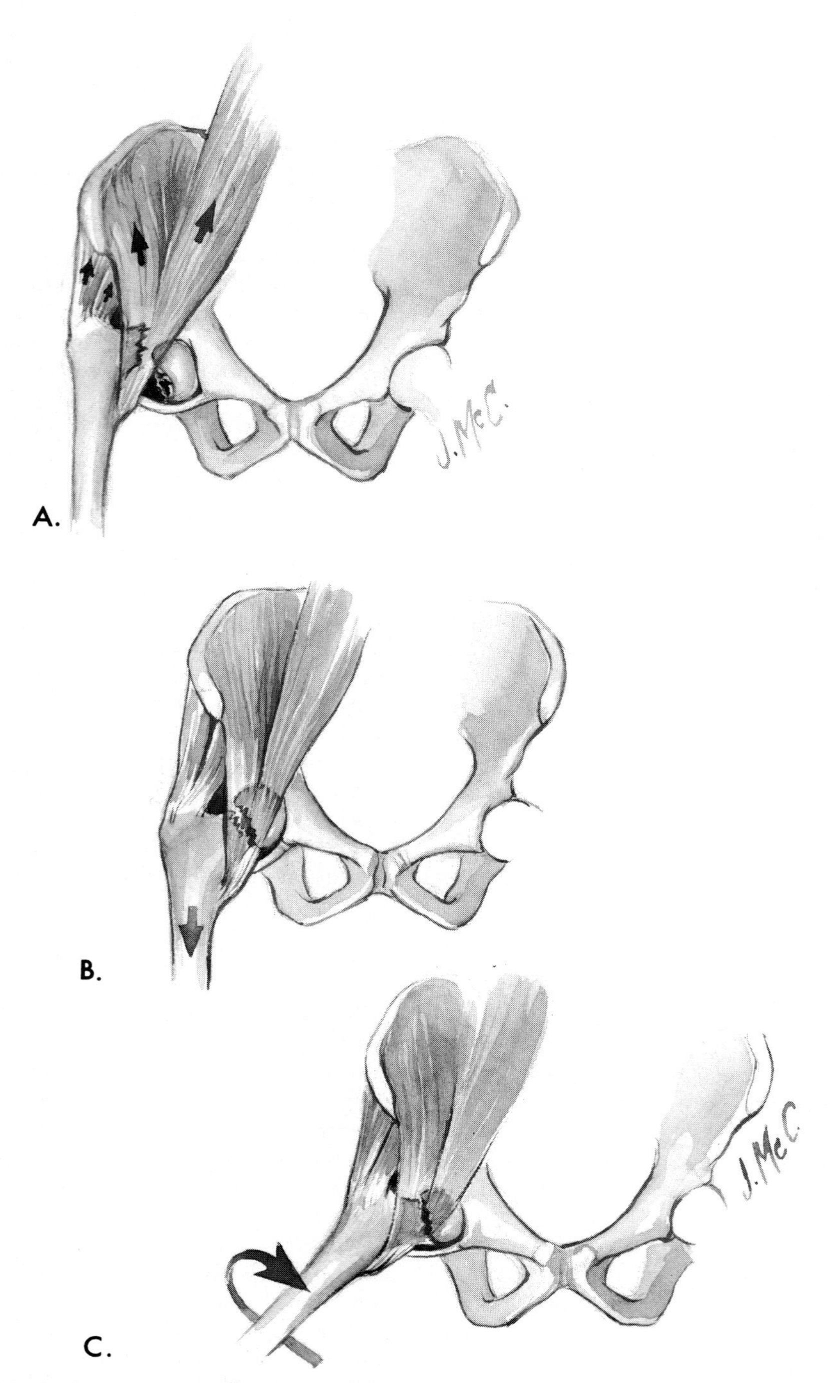

FIGURE 8–107. Diagram illustrating Whitman's method of reduction of femoral neck fractures.

A. The deformity is increased by the pull of the iliopsoas and gluteal muscles. **B.** Longitudinal traction is applied to pull the lower fragment distally. **C.** Gradual abduction of the hip and utilization of the upper border of the acetabular rim as a fulcrum reduce the fracture. The extended and abducted hip is rotated medially to 20 degrees beyond neutral position.

50 degrees, the fracture is considered stable and reduction can be maintained by the Whitman method; if the angle is greater than 50 degrees, the fracture is unstable and cannot be held by the Whitman method. In such cases, they recommended an intertrochanteric osteotomy to modify the angle of the fracture, and also advised a fibular bone graft at the time of osteotomy to promote union.[2]

Ingram and Bachynski recommended routine use of internal fixation preceded by closed reduction in all femoral neck fractures in children, except in the undisplaced cervicotrochanteric type. Knowles pins were used for internal fixation. They cautioned against the use of the Smith-Peterson nail because of its tendency to distract the fracture fragments. In cases of intertrochanteric fractures, treatment by closed manipulative reduction and immobilization in a Hoke-Martin traction cast was advised.[43] Green, in discussing the foregoing paper, cautioned against the use of threaded pins or screws of wood type for internal fixation, as they firmly hold the femoral head and arrest growth by compression of the epiphysis. On the other hand, a smooth nail or pin of a reasonable size will not do this. Green recommended the use of one or two pins or nails of small caliber in most fractures, with accessory protection as needed. In fractures of the distal portion of the femoral neck, he advised that the pins be stopped short of the physis, thereby decreasing the possibility of growth arrest. This is feasible because of the dense nature of the cancellous bone in the proximal portion of the child's femoral neck.[34] Sullivan, in his discussion of Ingram and Bachynski's paper, emphasized the difficulties in the technique of nailing because of the smaller target in the neck of the child's femur, the firm and springy cancellous bone, and the tendency of the fragments to separate as the nail is driven across the fracture line. He also agreed that use of a cast without internal fixation is not adequate to maintain reduction. Sullivan recommended immediate open reduction, drilling with a large-sized drill into the neck under radiographic visualization, and insertion of a graft of cancellous bone. He had done this in one case, in which x-rays subsequently showed healing of the fracture and solid union.[89]

In 1955, Blount advocated accurate reduction and internal fixation with ⅛-inch adjustable nails for treatment of displaced femoral neck fractures. McDougall, in 1961, in his end-result study of 24 femoral neck fractures, observed equally good or bad results from either conservative or operative methods.[60] It should be noted, however, that all his cervicotrochanteric fractures were treated conservatively by plaster cast, splint, or traction; whereas the transcervical fractures were, for the most part, treated by internal fixation. The duration of follow-up was 14 months to 16 years. In the cervicotrochanteric fractures, excellent or good results were obtained in only three of the eight cases (37.5 per cent), with the remainder (62.5 per cent—five patients) requiring secondary operative procedures. Excellent or good results were obtained in five of the eight transcervical fractures treated with internal fixation (62.5 per cent). Of the three transcervical fractures treated conservatively, the one treated by a plaster cast did poorly; however, the two treated by traction and a splint did well. It would seem that the evidence is in favor of internal fixation.

Ratliff, in his review of 71 cases, stressed the importance of the distinction between displaced and undisplaced fractures. The management of an undisplaced fracture did not present a problem; the results were good with immobilization in a hip spica cast. Occasionally avascular necrosis developed.[76] Treatment of displaced fractures (49 cases), however, was fraught with complications.[76]

Manipulative reduction and immobilization in a plaster hip spica cast was employed by Ratliff in 19 patients. The fracture was either not reduced or it became displaced following reduction in 15 out of 19 patients (79 per cent). In two patients, good position was maintained, but avascular necrosis developed, with consequent poor results, and in only two patients was the result good. *Manipulative reduction and internal fixation* was employed in 19 patients (transcervical fractures in 15 cases and basal neck fractures in 4 cases). Only one patient was under 11 years of age at the time of injury. Various types of internal fixation were used. The results were good in nine (about 50 per cent), fair in five, and poor in five. *Manipulative reduction and Thomas splint* was used in three patients, with poor results in two, and good in one. He did not recommend this method, as the Thomas splint is not designed to maintain the reduction of a femoral neck fracture. *Primary subtrochanteric osteotomy* was performed in four patients, in three because of failure of manipulative reduction; the results were good in two, and fair in the remaining two. Ratliff gave two indications for primary osteotomy: first, in a displaced fracture in a child under ten years of age (because of the great difficulty of internal fixation in this age group without disturbing the growth plate); and second, in a displaced fracture of the femoral neck in an older child in whom adequate manipulative reduction cannot be achieved.[76]

Lam reached the following conclusions in his study of 75 fractures of the femoral neck: (1) Undisplaced transcervical and cervicotrochanteric fractures can be adequately treated by simple immobilization in a plaster of Paris cast. (2) All pertrochanteric fractures can be satisfactorily treated by conservative means. (3) Minimally displaced transcervical and cervicotrochanteric fractures with considerable bony contact are best treated by closed reduction and immobilization in a plaster of Paris cast. (4) Displaced transcervical and cervicotrochanteric fractures with loss of all bony contact present a difficult problem. Lam could not give any firm advice based on his experience. Closed reduction should be attempted, and if successful, the hip immobilized in a one and one half plaster spica cast or well-leg traction in a younger child, or by the insertion of two or more threaded pins reinforced by a plaster spica in the older child. If closed reduction fails, open reduction is performed. In Lam's series, primary subtrochanteric osteotomy was not employed.[54] The various methods of treatment of femoral neck fractures in children are summarized in Table 8–6.

A categorical statement cannot be made as to the best method of treatment. Factors to consider are the type of fracture, the plane or angle of the fracture line, the degree of displacement, and the age of the patient. It is imperative to preserve the blood supply to the femoral head and neck. The vessels are most vulnerable to injury at the cervicotrochanteric area and at the capital femoral physis when they are in close proximity to bone and are quite rigidly fixed. Ordinarily circulation is disturbed as a result of the original trauma; however, the surgeon must take all precautions that his treatment does not aggravate the original injury. *Closed reductions must be performed very gently.*

Another important factor to consider is that growth of the capital femoral epiphysis should not be disturbed. In children, the cancellous bone of the femoral neck is dense, and whenever possible, the pins should stop short of the physis. Added protection and immobilization are provided by the hip spica cast. If the fracture is transepiphyseal or high cervical in location, and it is necessary to penetrate the capital epiphysis, only one or two smooth sharp pins of adequate size should be used. Wood screws or threaded pins that firmly hold the head will stop growth by compression of the physis. Under no circumstances should the Smith-Peterson nail or any other type of three-flanged nail be used because it will distract the fracture fragments.

Table 8–6. *Methods of Primary Treatment of Femoral Neck Fractures in Children*

Traction (Barber, Böhler)
Manipulative closed reduction and plaster hip spica cast (Whitman)
Manipulative closed reduction and immobilization in bilateral hip spica cast with well-leg countertraction
Manipulative closed reduction and Thomas splint
Gradual reduction by skeletal or skin traction and later plaster of Paris hip spica cast
Manipulative closed reduction, primary subtrochanteric osteotomy, internal fixation, and hip spica cast
Open reduction and internal fixation
Open reduction, bone grafting, and internal fixation
Open reduction with primary subtrochanteric abduction osteotomy

The author recommends the following plan of treatment, based upon his experience with 32 femoral neck fractures in children at the Children's Memorial Hospital, Chicago, and at the Children's Hospital Medical Center, Boston. First, all children with fractured hips are placed *immediately* in bilateral split Russell traction with medial rotation straps on both the thigh and leg of the affected limb. This measure will relieve muscle spasm, prevent further displacement, and may achieve gentle reduction. Rough handling of the limb should be avoided during physical examination and transport of the patient.

TRANSEPIPHYSEAL FRACTURES

If the fracture is undisplaced or minimally displaced (less than one fourth), immobilize the hip in a one and one half hip spica cast with the affected hip in moderate abduction, neutral extension, and 10 degrees of medial rotation. If displaced (more than one fourth), perform gentle closed manipulative reduction under general anesthesia; fix internally with two sharp smooth pins, which should penetrate the epiphysis; and immobilize in a one and one half hip spica cast. Ordinarily, eight to ten weeks is required to achieve bony union. Prognosis is poor. The patient should be carefully followed by periodic radiograms for possible development of the complications of avascular necrosis, coxa vara, or premature fusion of the physis. Early treatment of these complications by appropriate measures will salvage the hip.

UNDISPLACED TRANSCERVICAL OR CERVICOTROCHANTERIC FRACTURES

There is a great temptation to treat these conservatively by immobilization in a one and one half hip spica cast; however, anatomic alignment may be lost, leading to displacement and greater incidence of complications. As a general rule, if Pauwel's angle is less than 40 degrees, these fractures can be adequately treated by a one and one half hip spica cast. Absolutely no weight-bearing should be permitted. In an especially active child, a double hip spica cast is preferable. Frequent radiograms are made. If loss of position occurs, the fracture is internally fixed. If Pauwel's angle is more than 40 degrees, anatomic alignment is maintained by internal fixation with two small threaded pins, which should stop short of the capital femoral physis (Fig. 8–108). Again, a one and one half hip spica cast is applied to provide adequate immobilization. One cannot overemphasize the importance of internal fixation in maintaining reduction when Pauwel's angle is greater than 40 degrees. In personal experience with five such cases, the author lost position in four treated by simple immobilization in a hip spica cast. Some surgeons may prefer to treat these by a double hip spica cast with well-leg countertraction. The author recommends this only when a transcervical fracture is too close to the capital femoral physis.

DISPLACED TRANSCERVICAL AND CERVICOTROCHANTERIC FRACTURES

These should be treated by gentle closed reduction and internal fixation with two or three threaded pins or two cannulated hip screws. Age is not a factor. With modern image-intensifier radiographic control, the author finds it is feasible to pin the femoral neck accurately in a child under ten years of age. Again, the pins or compression hip screws should stop short of the capital femoral physis and a one and one half hip spica cast should be applied for added protection (Fig. 8–109). If adequate reduction cannot be achieved, or if, following reduction (particularly in transcervical fractures), Pauwel's angle is greater than 50 to 60 degrees with consequent high shearing stress, a primary subtrochanteric valgus osteotomy is recommended.

If closed reduction cannot be achieved, open reduction is performed; it is combined with a primary subtrochanteric abduction osteotomy if Pauwel's angle is greater than 50 to 60 degrees. One cannot overemphasize the importance of *not* using a Smith-Peterson or a trifin nail or a nail plate for internal fixation as it is difficult for the nail to penetrate the hard femoral head and neck; when it is being driven in the fracture fragments will become distracted.

Intertrochanteric fractures of the hip can be effectively treated by traction followed by immobilization in a hip spica cast (Figs. 8–110 and 8–111).

Complications

Treatment of fractures of the femoral neck is fraught with complications. Even with the most masterful reduction and adequate fixation, a normal hip cannot be assured; avascular necrosis, coxa vara, premature closure of the physis and nonunion may occur. Of the 189 cases reported in five large series in the literature, 110 (60 per cent) developed one or more of these complications. The displaced fracture of the femoral neck in children still remains an unsolved problem and a challenge to the orthopedic surgeon.

ASEPTIC NECROSIS

The great hazard of femoral neck fractures in children is aseptic necrosis. The blood supply to the femoral head and neck has been studied by Wolcott, Tucker, and Trueta.[95, 96, 108] The artery of the ligamentum teres from the acetabular branch of the obturator artery contributes little to the growing capital femoral epiphysis until about eight or nine years of age. The principal source of blood supply is through the lateral epiphyseal and superior and inferior metaphyseal vessels—all branches of the medial femoral circumflex artery. These vessels enter the capsule at its distal attachment posteriorly at the distal third of the femoral neck and traverse proximally in close proximity to the bone within the synovium. The physis in children acts as a barrier, precluding any significant anastomosis between those blood vessels that supply the epiphysis and those that supply the metaphysis. A fracture divides the vascular supply from the intraosseous nutrient vessels; it also produces a tear of the synovium, and therefore readily lacerates the posterior circumflex artery or its metaphyseal and lateral epiphyseal branches.

Ratliff has described three patterns of avascular necrosis following fractures of the femoral neck in children (Fig. 8–112). In *Type I* there

Text continued on page 3242

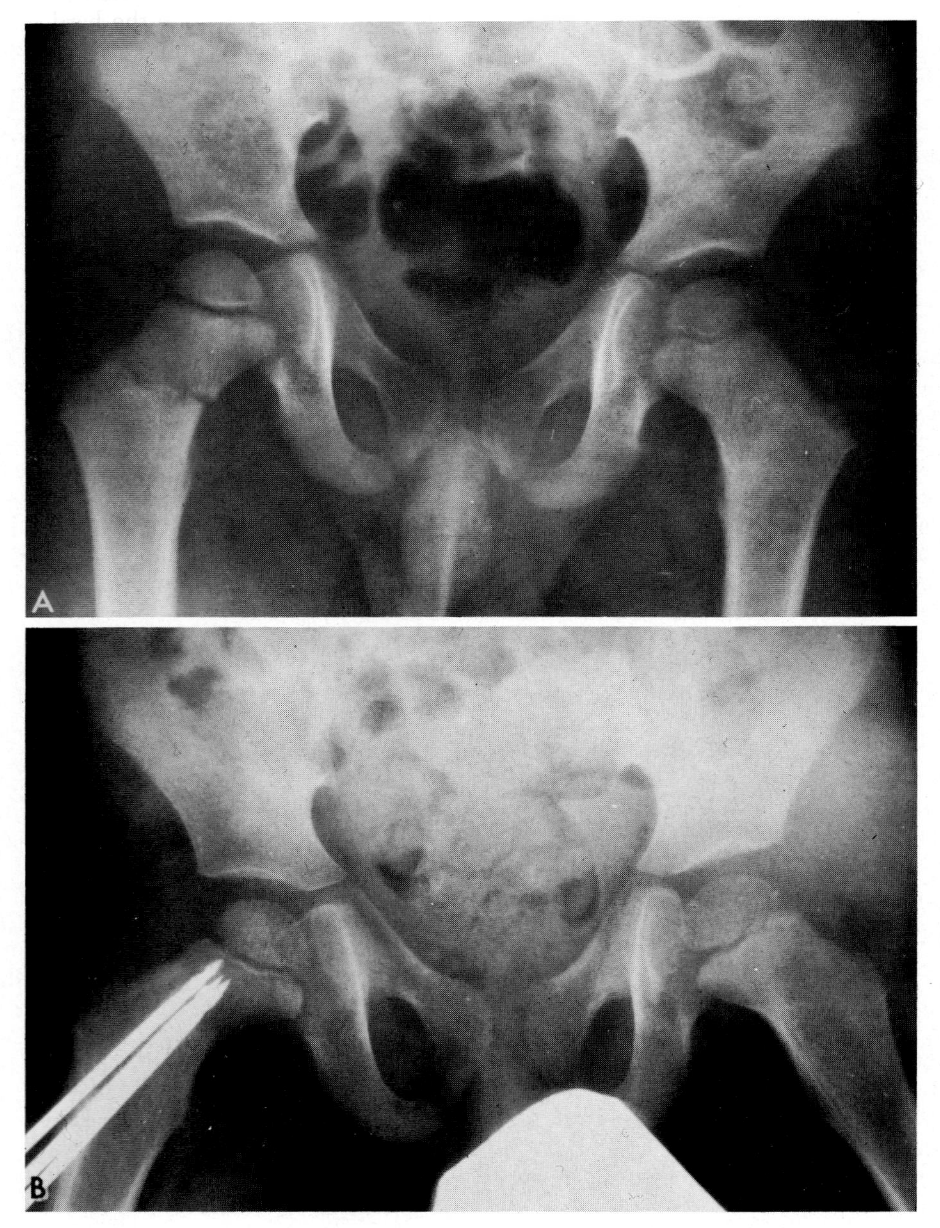

FIGURE 8–108. Minimally displaced cervicotrochanteric fracture of the left hip treated by percutaneous pinning and hip spica cast.

A. Preoperative radiogram. **B.** Postoperative radiogram showing that the pins have stopped short of the growth plate. (At present, this author recommends only two pins for internal fixation.)

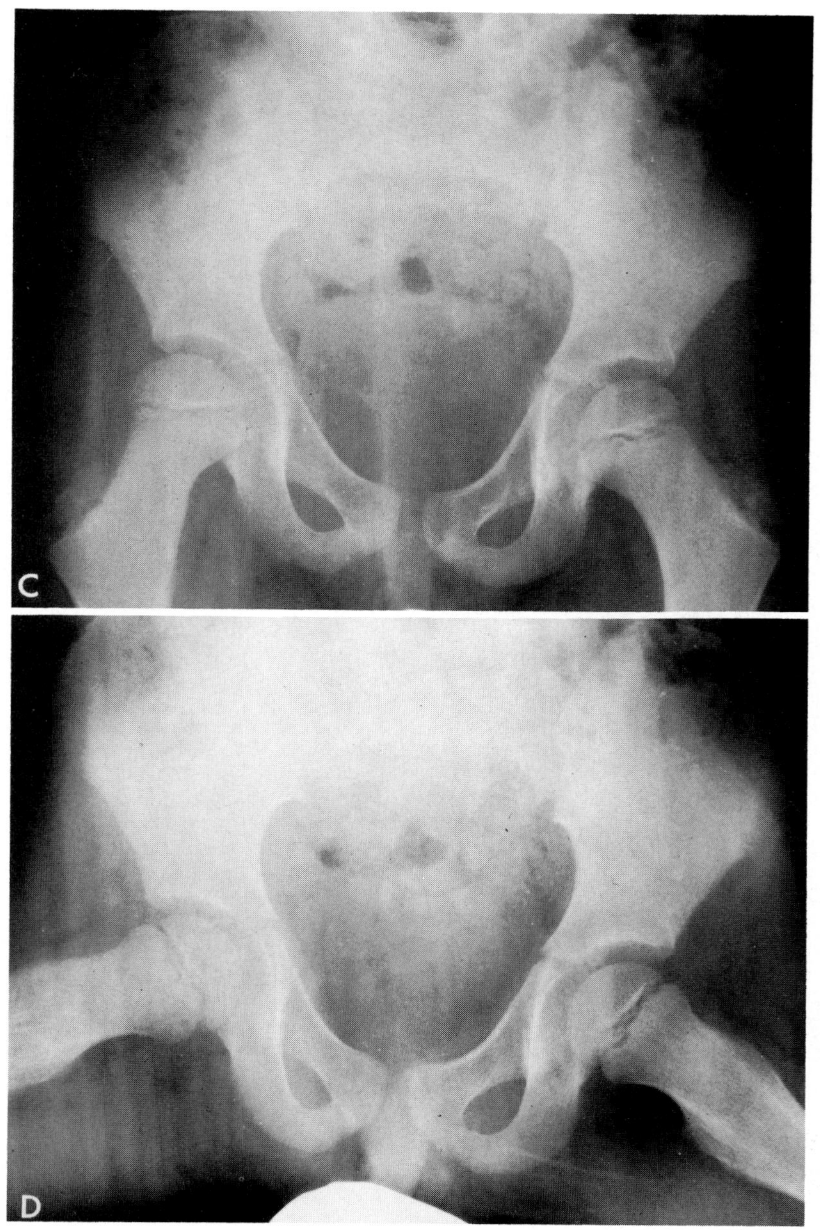

FIGURE 8–108 Continued. Minimally displaced cervicotrochanteric fracture of the left hip treated by percutaneous pinning and hip spica cast.

C and **D.** Radiograms two and one half years later, showing the healed fracture.

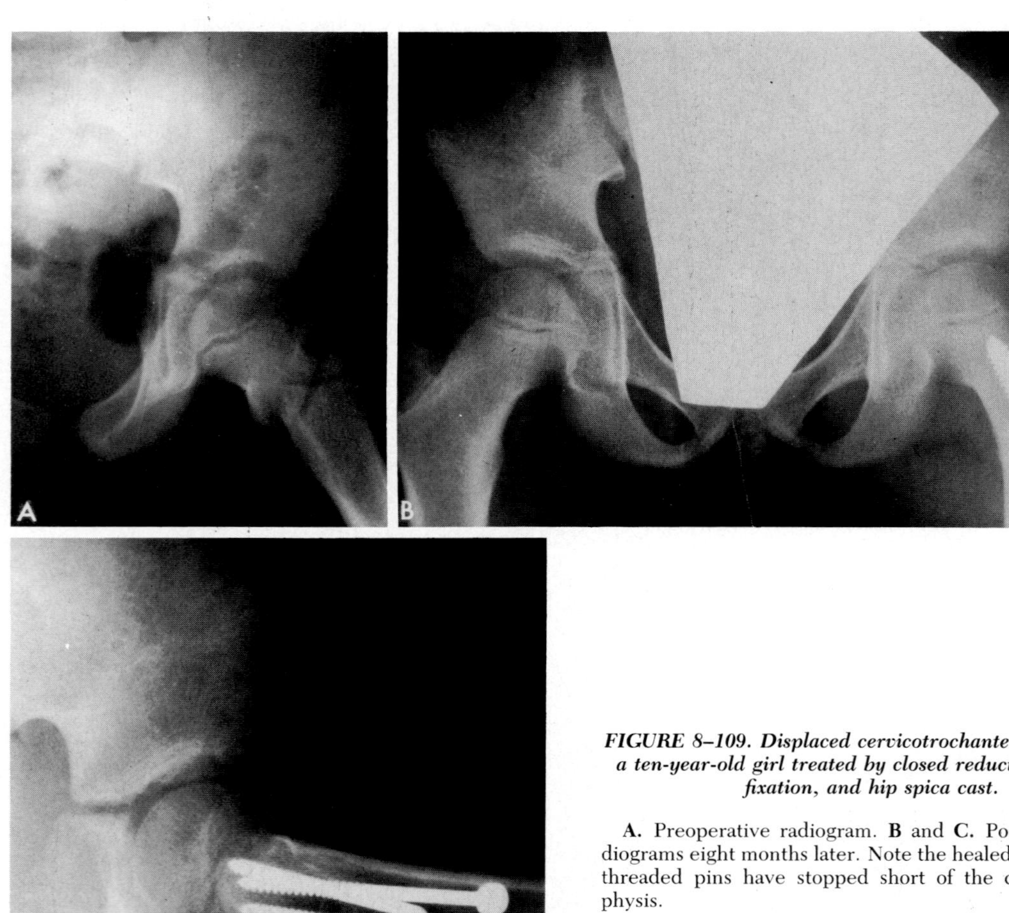

FIGURE 8–109. Displaced cervicotrochanteric fracture in a ten-year-old girl treated by closed reduction, internal fixation, and hip spica cast.

A. Preoperative radiogram. **B** and **C.** Postoperative radiograms eight months later. Note the healed fracture. Thin threaded pins have stopped short of the capital femoral physis.

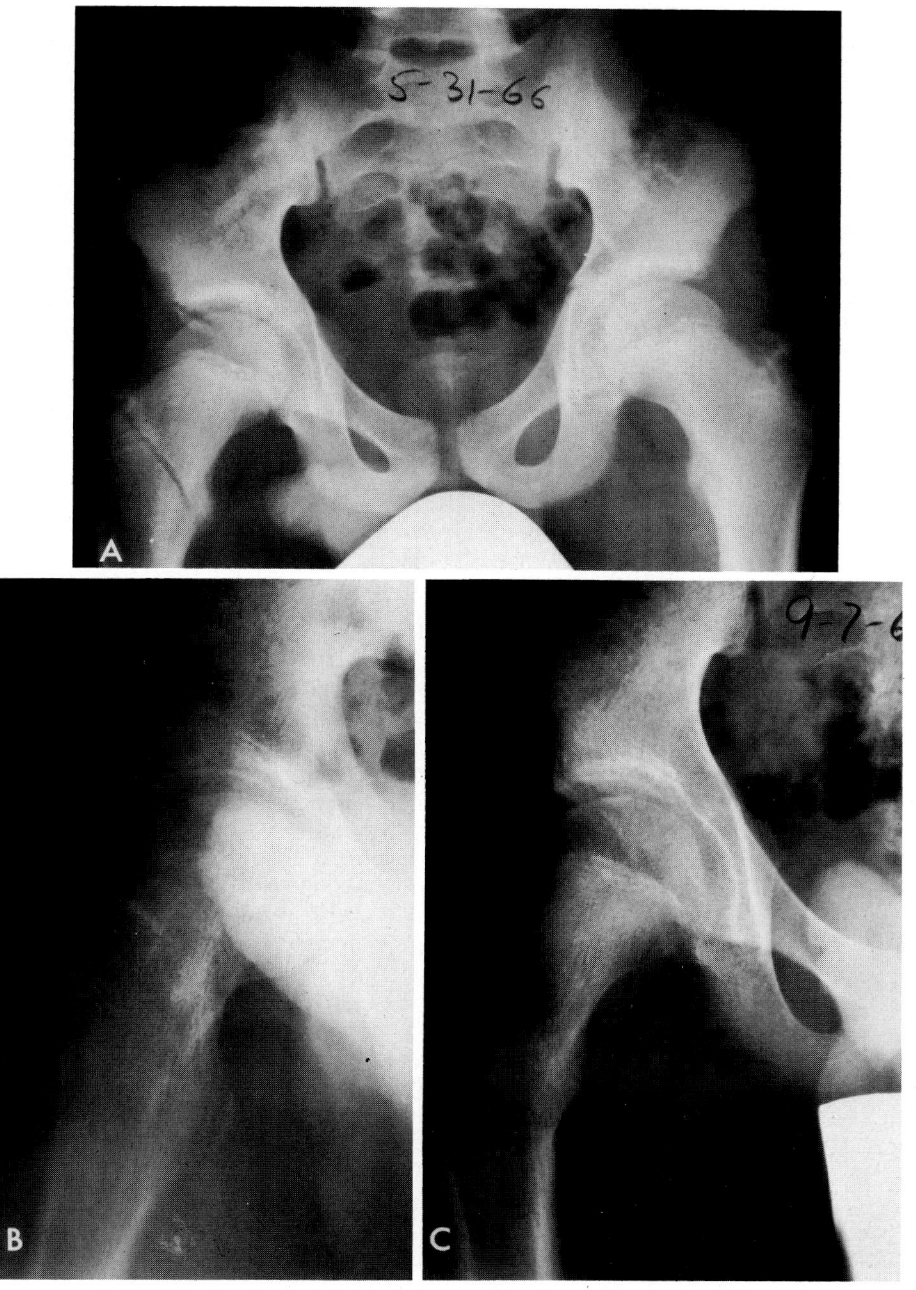

FIGURE 8–110. Intertrochanteric fracture of right hip in a 15-year-old boy.

Fracture was treated by traction for three weeks, followed by immobilization in a hip spica cast for five more weeks. **A.** Preoperative radiogram. **B** and **C.** Four months later. Note the healed fracture.

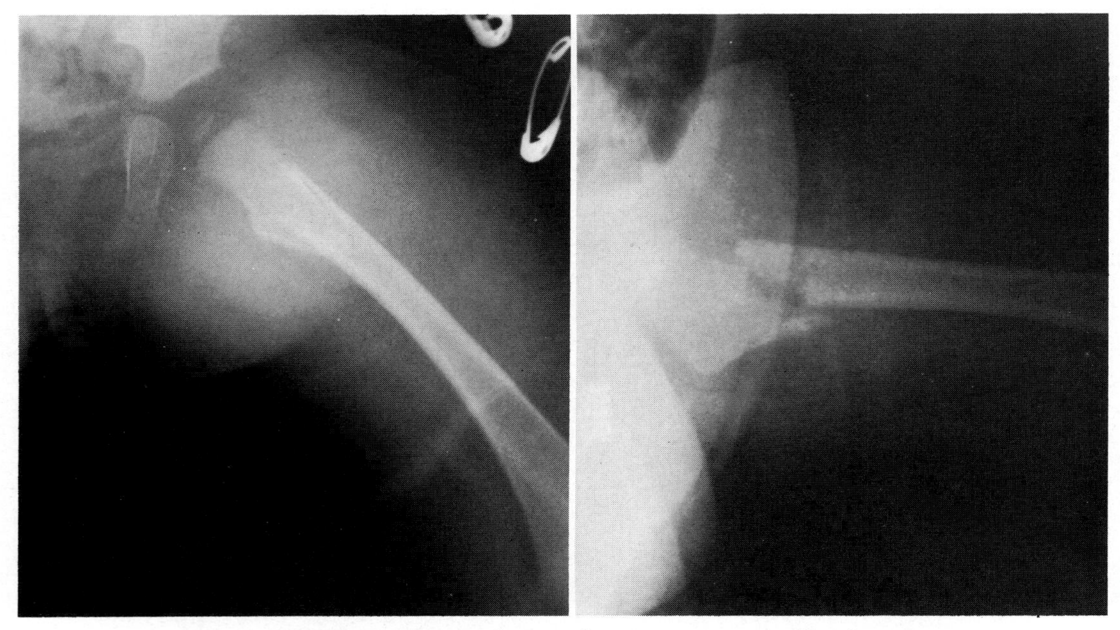

FIGURE 8–111. Pertrochanteric fracture in a one-year-old girl.

is severe diffuse necrosis of the femoral head and of the proximal fragment of the femoral neck, produced by interruption of the blood supply to the lateral epiphyseal vessels, metaphyseal vessels, and nutrient vessels (Fig. 8–112 A). This is the most common pattern, and occurs in approximately 50 per cent of those with necrosis; also, it has the poorest prognosis, with total collapse of the femoral head; none of the patients has attained a good end-result. In *Type II*, the necrotic changes are more localized (usually in the anterosuperior half of the femoral head), and are accompanied by minimal collapse of the bony epiphysis. It is caused by damage to only the lateral epiphyseal vessels before they enter the epiphysis (Fig. 8–112 C). Collapse occurs in 25 per cent of cases with this type of necrosis, but it has a good prognosis. In *Type III* the area of necrosis is confined to the femoral neck, delimited proximally by the fracture line. This occurred in the remaining 25 per cent of cases of avascular necrosis (Fig. 8–112 B). Ratliff proposes the cause of isolated necrosis of the femoral neck to be damage to only the superior metaphyseal vessels, with the lateral epiphyseal vessels remaining intact. It is noteworthy that almost all patients with Type III avascular necrosis were under 12 years of age, and that in 85 per cent of the cases, premature fusion of the upper femoral physis took place. In Type III avascular necrosis, the prognosis is fair, as the femoral head does not fragment or collapse.[73]

Approximately one third of children with femoral neck fractures develop avascular necrosis. On critical analysis of the cases reported in the literature, including the author's, it is obvious that transcervical fractures are somewhat more likely to undergo necrosis than are cervicotrochanteric fractures (34 per cent versus 27 per cent, respectively). Displaced transepiphyseal fractures have the poorest prognosis, with development of aseptic necrosis in 80 per cent of cases. The incidence of aseptic necrosis in those who are ten years of age or younger is 21 per cent, whereas in those over ten years of age it is 47 per cent.

The method of treatment seems to be a factor in the development of aseptic necrosis; 35 per cent of those fractures treated conservatively were complicated by necrosis, as opposed to only 27 per cent of those treated by internal fixation. That extreme abduction of the hip in the treatment of congenital dislocation of the hip decreases circulation to the femoral head has been well demonstrated and the practice is condemned. It is noteworthy that in Whitman's conservative method of treatment the fractured hip is *forced into extreme abduction* to reduce the fracture and then is immobilized in that position. The principle of reduction by Whitman's method is mechanically sound; however, following reduction, the affected hip should be brought into 30 to 40 degrees of abduction and moderate flexion, and then immobilized in that position. Likewise, following internal fixation,

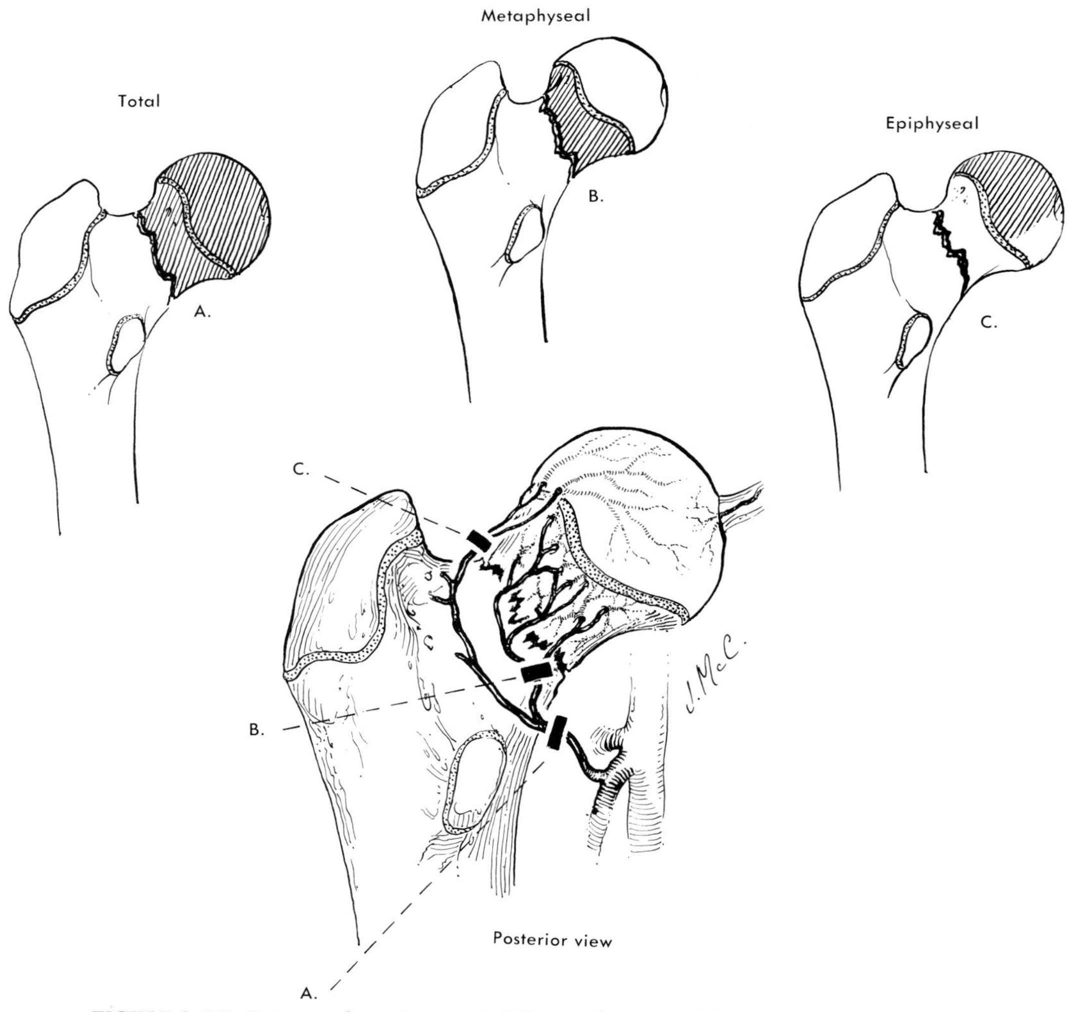

FIGURE 8–112. Patterns of aseptic necrosis following fractures of the femoral neck in children.

Type A or *total*. There is severe diffuse necrosis of the entire capital epiphysis and proximal fragment of the femoral neck. It is produced by interruption of blood supply from the lateral epiphyseal, metaphyseal, and nutrient vessels. (Contribution to circulation of the femoral head from the vessels along the ligamentum teres is minimal. The epiphyseal plate acts as a barrier to anastomosis between vessels supplying the epiphysis and those supplying the metaphysis.)

Type B or *metaphyseal*. The avascular necrosis is confined to the femoral neck, being outlined proximally by the epiphyseal plate and distally by the fracture line. The femoral head does not collapse or fragment. Necrosis is caused by interruption of blood supply from superior metaphyseal vessels with the lateral epiphyseal vessels remaining intact.

Type C or *partial epiphyseal*. The avascular necrotic changes are confined to the femoral head, usually in its superior half. This type is produced by interruption of lateral epiphyseal vessels before they enter the capital epiphysis. (Redrawn after Ratliff.)

the hip should not be immobilized in extreme abduction. One cannot overemphasize the importance of not further decreasing an already precarious circulation to the femoral head. Durbin has pointed out that aseptic necrosis may occur following undisplaced as well as displaced fractures of the femoral neck in children.[29]

Bone imaging with technetium-99m will show decreased uptake at the site of aseptic necrosis. Nuclear magnetic resonance imaging will show the extent of necrosis in detail.

Radiologic evidence of aseptic necrosis is usually apparent within 6 to 12 months after injury. Occasionally it is heralded by premature closure of the physis.

Treatment follows the same principles as those outlined in the section on management of Legg-Perthes disease. Congruity of the femoral head in the acetabulum should be achieved and maintained.

Goals of treatment are (1) provision and maintenance of functional range of hip motion, by traction, active and passive exercises, and continuous passive hip motion machine, as necessary; (2) concentric containment of the femoral head in the acetabulum by orthotic devices; and (3) provision of congruity of the joint. Ordinarily, orthotic containment is not well tolerated in the adolescent with post-traumatic necrosis of the femoral head; compliance is poor. Often, this author finds that protection of the affected hip with a three-point partial weight-bearing crutch is more pragmatic. Strenuous physical activities and contact sports are not allowed. Vascularized live bone grafting is an option; long-term results are not available at present. In partial aseptic necrosis, derotation-abduction-flexion or extension intertrochanteric osteotomy is another modality of management. This author has had greater success with osteotomy than with vascularized bone grafting.

COXA VARA

This is a common complication. Lam reported 23 instances of this deformity in 75 femoral neck fractures in children (32 per cent); it developed in 18 fresh fractures (30 per cent), and in 5 of the 15 late fractures.[54]

Coxa vara may be caused by several factors: (1) failure to reduce the fracture; (2) loss of alignment in a hip spica cast, either because of inadequate immobilization or delayed union; or (3) aseptic necrosis and premature fusion of the capital femoral physis, in which instance relative discrepancy of growth between the capital femoral epiphysis and the greater trochanteric apophysis will result in relative overgrowth of the greater trochanter and a short femoral neck (coxa breva).

In the series of Lam, 3 of the 18 cases of coxa vara in fresh fractures were associated with avascular necrosis of the proximal fragment in whole or in part with premature epiphyseal fusion: two with avascular necrosis alone; and two with premature fusion of the physis in the absence of avascular necrosis. In the remaining 11 cases, coxa vara occurred alone.[54]

Ratliff noted that coxa vara was associated with delayed union in 14 of his 71 cases.[73] Undoubtedly, this is an important predisposing factor.

Allende and Lezama, to reiterate, emphasized the importance of the obliquity of the fracture line. Fractures with a Pauwel's angle of less than 50 degrees responded well to treatment with a plaster cast; whereas those with an angle greater than 50 degrees did poorly, with coxa vara being the end-result. Mitchell, Wilson, and Ingram and Bachynski stressed the importance of internal fixation in prevention of coxa vara.[43, 65, 107] Of the 11 patients in whom Ingram and Bachynski used internal fixation, not one developed coxa vara.[43] McDougall, however, reported four cases of coxa vara in the seven transcervical fractures treated by internal fixation that went on to union. It is of interest to note, also, that all eight of his cervicotrochanteric fractures were treated conservatively and that five of them developed coxa vara. McDougall proposed that "in these fractures there is a degree of plasticity at the fracture site for a long time after union appears adequate, with a tendency to bending of the neck of the femur."[60]

The clinical signs of coxa vara—prominence and elevation of the greater trochanter, shortening of the limb, decreased hip abduction, and a gluteus medius limp—are well known. Treatment consists of subtrochanteric abduction osteotomy. If the capital femoral physis has prematurely fused, the varus deformity will recur with growth, necessitating repeat osteotomy after several years.

Relative overgrowth of the greater trochanter with gluteus medius limp and Trendelenburg lurch is treated by distal and lateral transfer of the greater trochanter (See Chapter 2 under Congenital Dislocation of the Hip).

PREMATURE FUSION OF CAPITAL FEMORAL PHYSIS

This will result in total shortening of the femoral neck, shortening of the lower limb and in coxa vara. When physeal closure is asymmetrical with the lateral part fused and medial part open, the femoral head will tilt progressively out of the acetabulum. In the literature, attention was drawn to this complication by Ratliff, who reported 11 patients with premature fusion of the upper femoral physis; in 6 of these, it followed avascular necrosis of the femoral head.[73] In the series of Lam, premature fusion of the upper femoral physis occurred in nine fresh and in six late fractures. He postulated long continued trauma to the capital femoral physis because of lack of immobilization to be the cause in the late cases.[54]

DELAYED UNION AND NONUNION

This complication usually develops in transcervical fractures (about 85 per cent of cases) with a Pauwel's angle greater than 60 degrees that are treated conservatively by plaster cast immobilization (about 70 per cent of cases). In those treated by internal fixation, the fracture fragments may be separated during insertion of trifin nails or held apart by the threaded portion of a large pin such as the Knowles pin. Aseptic necrosis is another important etiologic factor in delayed union.

Nonunion is treated by bone grafting and subtrochanteric abduction osteotomy aimed at converting the fracture angle from one of shearing stress to one of compression. In delayed union, abduction osteotomy alone is adequate; it is not necessary to bone graft.

References

1. Allegreni, R., and Duse, G.: Fractures of the neck of the femur in children and adolescents. Arch. Ortop., *78*:455, 1965.
2. Allende, G., and Lezama, L. G.: Fractures of the neck of the femur in children, a clinical study. J. Bone Joint Surg., *33-A*:387, 1951.
3. Ansorg, P., and Graner, G.: Valgus deformity of the femoral neck after nailing of infantile femoral shaft fractures. Zentralbl. Chir., *101*:968, 1976.
4. Ansorg, P., and Graner, G.: Femoral neck fractures in children and adolescents. Zentralbl. Chir., *105*:721, 1980.
5. Arct, W. A., and Oblonczek, G.: Modified tubular nail for fixation of fractures and osteotomies of the trochanteric region and supracondylar fractures of the femur. Chir. Narzadow Ruchu Ortop. Pol., *35*:113, 1970.
6. Arnold, W. D.: The effect of early weight-bearing on the stability of the femoral neck fractures treated with Knowles pins. J. Bone Joint Surg., *66-A*:847, 1984.
7. Barber, E. T.: Fracture of the neck of the femur in a child seven years of age—suit for malpractice. Pacific Med. Surg. J., N.S., *5*:61, 1871.
8. Berger, D., and Steinhauslin, C.: Fractures of the femur neck in children. Ther. Umsch., *40*:960, 1983.
9. Bernardczyk, K.: Fractures of the neck of femur in children. Chir. Narzadow Ruchu Ortop. Pol., *41*:1, 1976.
10. Bland-Sutton, J.: Spolia Opima—Presidential Address to the Surgical Section. Royal Society of Medicine. Br. Med. J., *2*:595, 1918.
11. Böhler, L.: The Treatment of Fractures. 4th English Ed. (Trans. from 4th German edition by E. W. Hey Groves.) Baltimore, William Wood & Co., 1935.
12. Boitzy, A.: La fracture du col du femur chez l'enfant et adolescent. Paris, Masson, 1971.
13. Butler, J. E., and Cary, J. M.: Fracture of the femoral neck in a child. J.A.M.A., *218*:398, 1971.
14. Canale, S. T., and Bourland, R. A.: Fracture of the neck and intertrochanteric region of the femur in children. J. Bone Joint Surg., *59-A*:431, 1977.

14a. Canale, S. T., and King, R. E.: Fractures of the hip. *In* Rockwood, C. A., Wilkins, K., and King, R. E. (eds.): Fractures in Children. Philadelphia, J. B. Lippincott, 1984, pp. 782–821.

15. Carrell, B., and Carrell, W. B.: Fractures in the neck of the femur in children, with particular reference to aseptic necrosis. J. Bone Joint Surg., *23*:225, 1941.
16. Cervenansk, Y. J.: Need for osteosynthesis of fractures of the proximal end of the femur in childhood. Acta Chir. Orthop. Traumatol. Cech., *36*:48, 1969.
17. Chigot, P. L., and Vialas, M.: Fracture du col du femur chez l'enfant. Ann. Chir. Infant., *4*:209, 1963.
18. Chong, K. C., Chacha, P. B., and Lee, B. T.: Fractures of the neck of the femur in childhood and adolescence. Injury, *7*:111, 1975.
19. Chrestian, P., Bollini, G., Jacquemier, M., and Ramaherison, P.: Femoral neck fractures in children. Chir. Pediatr., *22*:397, 1981.
20. Chung, S. M. K.: The arterial supply of the developing proximal end of the human femur. J. Bone Joint Surg., *58-A*:961, 1976.
21. Chung, S. M. K., Batterman, S. C., and Brighton, C. T.: Shear strength of the human femoral capital epiphyseal plate. J. Bone Joint Surg., *58-A*:94, 1976.
22. Colonna, P. C.: Fracture of the neck of the femur in childhood. Ann. Surg., *88*:902, 1928.
23. Colonna, P. C.: Fracture of the neck of the femur in children. Am. J. Surg., *6*:793, 1929.
24. Cromwell, B. M.: A case of intra-capsular fracture of the neck of the femur in a young subject. N.C. Med. J., *15*:309, 1885.
25. Delbert, P.: Quoted by Colonna, P. C.: Fractures of the neck of the femur in children. Am. J. Surg., *6*:793, 1929.
26. DeLuca, F. N., and Keck, C.: Traumatic coxa vara—a case report of spontaneous correction in a child. Clin. Orthop., *116*:125, 1976.
27. Descamps, L., Kerner, Y., and Lebras, A.: Synthese par clou-plaque desosteotomies de l'extremite superieure de femur de l'enfant. Rev. Chir. Orthop., *54*:671, 1968.
28. Drake, J. K., and Meyers, M. H.: Intracapsular pressure and hemarthrosis following femoral neck fracture. Clin. Orthop., *182*:172, 1984.
29. Durbin, F. C.: Avascular necrosis complicating undisplaced fractures of the neck of the femur in children. J. Bone Joint Surg., *41-B*:658, 1959.
30. Fardon, D. P.: Fracture of the neck and shaft of same femur—report of a case in a child. J. Bone Joint Surg., *52-A*:797, 1970.
31. Feigenberg, Z., Pauker, M., Levy, M., Seelenfreund, M., and Fried, A.: Fractures of the femoral neck in childhood. Results of conservative treatment. J. Trauma, *17*:937, 1977.
32. Fornaro, E., Brunner, C., and Weber, B. G.: Treatment of femoral neck fracture in childhood—emergency arthrotomy, reposition and screw insertion. Hefte Unfallheilkd., *158*:247, 1982.
33. Grassi, G., and Nigrisoli, P.: Traumatic separation of the upper femoral epiphysis in a child aged two. Ital. J. Orthop. Traumatol., *2*:135, 1976.
34. Green, W. T.: Discussion on fractures of the hip in children. J. Bone Joint Surg., *35-A*:886, 1953.
35. Greene, W. B., and Torre, B. A.: Femoral neck fracture in a child with autosomal dominant osteopetrosis. J. Pediatr. Orthop., *5*:483, 1985.
36. Greig, D. M.: Fracture of the cervix femoris in children. Edinburgh Med. J., *22*:75, 1919.
37. Gruber, U. F.: Prevention of fatal pulmonary embolism in patients with fractures of the neck of the femur. Surg. Gynecol. Obstet., *161*:37, 1985.
38. Heiser, J. M., and Oppenheim, W. L.: Fractures of the hip in children: A review of forty cases. Clin. Orthop., *149*:177, 1980.
39. Henriksson, L.: Measurement of femoral neck anteversion and inclination. A radiographic study in children. Acta Orthop. Scand. (Suppl.), *186*:1, 1980.
40. Herczegh, M.: Femoral neck and diaphyseal fracture on the same side in childhood. Magy. Traumatol. Orthop., *15*:18, 1972.
41. Hoeksema, H. D., Olsen, C., and Rudy, R.: Fracture of femoral neck and shaft and repeat neck fracture in a child, case report. J. Bone Joint Surg., *57*:271, 1975.
42. Hullin, L., and Schmidt, E.: Contribution to femur

neck fractures in children. Dtsch. Gesundheitsw., *21*:1494, 1966.
43. Ingram, A. J., and Bachynski, B.: Fractures of the hip in children—treatment and results. J. Bone Joint Surg., *35-A*:867, 1953.
44. Johansson, S.: Über Epiphysennekrose bei geheilten Collumfrakturen. Zentralbl. Chir., *54*:2214, 1927.
45. Jonasch, E.: Impacted fracture of the femoral neck in children. Unfallheilkunde, *85*:319, 1982.
46. Jungbluth, K. H., Daum, R., and Metzger, E.: Schenkelhalsfrakturen im Kindesalter. Z. Kinderchir., *6*:392, 1968.
47. Karr, R. K., and Schwab, J. P.: Subtrochanteric fracture as a complication of proximal femoral pinning. Clin. Orthop., *194*:214, 1985.
48. Kassur, T.: Femoral neck fractures in children. Pol. Tyg. Lek., *25*:1941, 1970.
49. Kay, S. P., and Hall, J. E.: Fracture of the femoral neck in children and its complications. Clin. Orthop., *80*:53, 1971.
50. Khattab, A. S.: Fractures of the neck of the femur in children. Egyptian Orthop., *3*:68, 1968.
51. King, R. E.: Special problems of femoral neck fractures in adolescents and young adults. J. Pediatr. Orthop., *3*:623, 1983.
52. Klasen, H. J., and Binnendijk, K. B.: Fracture of the neck of the femur associated with posterior dislocation of the hip. J. Bone Joint Surg., *66-B*:45, 1984.
53. Kohli, S. B.: Fracture of the neck of the femur in children. J. Bone Joint Surg., *56-B*:776, 1974.
54. Lam, S. F.: Fractures of the neck of the femur in children. J. Bone Joint Surg., *53-A*:1165, 1971.
55. Lam, S. F.: Fractures of the neck of the femur in children. Orthop. Clin. North Am., *7*:625, 1976.
56. Lambiris, E., Zapfe, E., and Gaudin, B.: Fractures of the femoral neck in children. Z. Orthop., *117*:825, 1979.
57. Leadbetter, G. W.: A treatment for fracture of the neck of the femur. J. Bone Joint Surg., *15*:931, 1933.
58. Lenart, G., and Kullmann, L.: An unusual case of bilateral fracture of the femoral neck in childhood. Arch. Orthop. Unfallchir., *70*:83, 1971.
59. Liuboshits, N. A.: Medial fractures of the femoral neck in children. Vestn. Khir., *103*:67, 1969.
60. McDougall, A.: Fracture of the neck of the femur in childhood. J. Bone Joint Surg., *43-B*:16, 1961.
61. Maroske, D., and Thon, K.: Fractures of the neck of the femur in children. Unfallheilkunde, *84*:186, 1981.
62. Meershoek, P. E. M.: Fractures of the femoral neck in children. Arch. Chir. Neerl., *20*:65, 1968.
63. Miller, F., and Wenger, D. R.: Femoral neck stress fracture in a hyperactive child. A case report. J. Bone Joint Surg., *61-A*:435, 1979.
64. Minikel, J., Sty, J., and Simons, G.: Sequential radionuclide bone imaging in avascular pediatric hip conditions. Clin. Orthop., *175*:202, 1983.
65. Mitchell, J. I.: Fracture of the neck of the femur in children. J.A.M.A., *107*:1603, 1936.
66. Naeraa, A.: On secondary epiphyseal necrosis after collum femoris fracture in young persons. Report of two cases. Acta Chir. Scand., *80*:238, 1937.
67. Niethard, F. U.: Physiopathology and prognosis of femoral neck fractures in childhood. Hefte Unfallheilkd., *158*:221, 1982.
68. Ogden, J.: Changing patterns of proximal femoral vascularity. J. Bone Joint Surg., *56-A*:941, 1974.
69. O'Reilly, D. E.: Acute traumatic separation of the capital femoral epiphysis. South. Med. J., *64*:847, 1971.
70. Peltokallio, P., and Kurkipaa, M.: Fractures of the femoral neck in children. Ann. Chir. Gynaecol. Fenn. (Suppl.), *48*:151, 1959.
71. Pforringer, W., and Rosemeyer, B.: Fractures of the hip in children and adolescents. Acta Orthop. Scand., *51*:91, 1980.
72. Quinlan, W. R., Brady, P. G., and Regan, B. F.: Fracture of the neck of the femur in childhood. Injury, *11*:242, 1980.
73. Ratliff, A. H. C.: Fractures of the neck of the femur in children. J. Bone Joint Surg., *44-B*:528, 1962.
74. Ratliff, A. H. C.: Traumatic separation of the upper femoral epiphysis in young children. J. Bone Joint Surg., *50-B*:757, 1968.
75. Ratliff, A. H. C.: Complications after fracture of the femoral neck in children and their treatment. J. Bone Joint Surg., *52-B*:175, 1970.
76. Ratliff, A. H. C.: Fractures of the neck of the femur in children. Orthop. Clin. North Am., *5*:903, 1974.
77. Ratliff, A. H. C.: Traumatic separation of the upper femoral epiphysis in young children. Orthop. Clin. North Am., *5*:925, 1974.
78. Ratliff, A. H. C.: Fracture of the neck of the femur in children. Hip, 1981, p. 188.
79. Rea, E.: Fracture of the neck of the femur in childhood. Med. J. Zambia, *14*:89, 1980.
80. Rettig, H.: The femoral neck fracture in childhood and its sequelae. Hefte Unfallheilkd., *91*:70, 1967.
81. Rigault, P., Iselin, F., Moreau, J., and Judet, J.: Fractures of the femur neck in children (study of 25 cases). Rev. Chir. Orthop., *52*:325, 1966.
82. Russell, R. H.: A clinical lecture on fracture of the neck of the femur in childhood. Lancet, *2*:125, 1898.
83. Ruter, A., and Kreuzer, U.: Femoral neck fractures in the child—therapy and results. Hefte Unfallheilkd., *158*:233, 1982.
84. Schmorl, G.: Die pathologische Anatomie der Schenkelhals Frakturen. Munchen. Med. Wschr., *71*:1381, 1924.
85. Sebastiani, C., and Bardelli, M.: Treatment of recent fractures of the femoral neck and their sequelae in childhood and adolescence. Arch. Putti Chir. Organi Mov., *27*:93, 1976.
86. Seddon, H. J.: Necrosis of the head of the femur following fracture of the neck in a child. Proc. R. Soc. Med., *30*:210, 1936.
87. Sonheim, K.: Fracture of the femoral neck in children. Acta Orthop. Scand., *43*:523, 1972.
88. Spissak, L.: Femur neck fractures in childhood. Acta Chir. Orthop. Traumatol. Cech., *46*:29, 1979.
89. Sullivan, R. H.: Discussions on fractures of the hip in children. J. Bone Joint Surg., *35-A*:887, 1953.
90. Swiontkowski, M. F., Hansen, S. T., Jr., and Kellam, J.: Ipsilateral fractures of the femoral neck and shaft. A treatment protocol. J. Bone Joint Surg., *66-A*:260, 1984.
91. Swiontkowski, M. F., Winquist, R. A., and Hansen, S. T., Jr.: Fractures of the femoral neck in patients between the ages of twelve and forty-nine years. J. Bone Joint Surg., *66-A*:837, 1984.
92. Taylor, H. L.: Fractures of the neck of the femur in children. N.Y. J. Med., *17*:508, 1917.
93. Tokmakov, P.: Fractures of the femur neck in children. Ortop. Travmatol. Protez., *30*:22, 1969.
94. Touzet, P., Rigault, P., Padovani, J. P., Pouliquen, J. C., Mallet, J. F., and Guyonvarch, G.: Fractures of the neck of the femur in children. Rev. Chir. Orthop., *65*:341, 1979.
95. Trueta, J.: The normal vascular anatomy of the human femoral head during growth. J. Bone Joint Surg., *39-B*:358, 1957.
96. Tucker, F. R.: Arterial supply to the femoral head and its clinical importance. J. Bone Joint Surg., *31-B*:82, 1949.
97. Vosmer, A. M., and Van Linge, B.: Surgical exposure of the lesser trochanter and the medial proximal part of the femur. Acta Orthop. Scand., *47*:214, 1976.

98. Wagner, H.: Orthopedic problems after femoral neck fractures in childhood. Hefte Unfallheilkd., *158*:141, 1982.
99. Wedlikowski, A., and Dymala, L.: Fractures of the femoral neck in children. Chir. Narzadow Ruchu Ortop. Pol., *30*:459, 1965.
100. Weiner, D. S., and O'Dell, H. W.: Fractures of the hip in children. J. Trauma, *9*:62, 1969.
101. Werkman, D. M.: The transepiphyseal fracture of the femoral neck. Injury, *12*:50, 1980.
102. Whitman, R.: Fracture of the neck of the femur in a child. Med. Rec., *39*:165, 1891.
103. Whitman, R.: Observations on fracture of the neck of the femur in childhood with especial reference to treatment and differential diagnosis from separation of the epiphysis. Med. Rec., *43*:227, 1893.
104. Whitman, R.: Further observations on fracture of the neck of the femur in childhood with especial reference to its diagnosis and to its more remote results. Ann. Surg., *25*:673, 1897.
105. Whitman, R.: Further observations on depression of the neck of the femur in early life, including fracture of the neck of the femur, separation of the epiphysis and simple coxa vara. Ann. Surg., *31*:145, 1900.
106. Whitman, R.: Further observations on injuries of the neck of the femur in early life with reference to the distinction between fracture of the neck and epiphyseal disjunction as influencing positive treatment. Med. Rec., *75*:1, 1909.
107. Wilson, J. C.: Fracture of the neck of the femur in childhood. J. Bone Joint Surg., *22*:531, 1940.
108. Wolcott, W. E.: The evolution of the circulation in the developing femoral head and neck. Surg. Gynecol. Obstet., *77*:61, 1943.
109. Zinghi, G. F., Specchia, L., Ruggieri, N., and Galli, G.: The role of osteotomy in the treatment of pseudarthrosis of the neck of the femur in younger patients. Ital. J. Orthop. Traumatol., *11*:341, 1985.
110. Zolczer, L., Kazar, G., Manoringer, J., and Nagy, E.: Fracture of the femoral neck in adolescents. Injury, *4*:41, 1973.
111. Zur Verth, M.: Sekundare Nekrose des Schenkelkopfes nach Schenkelhalsbruchen Jungendlicher. Zentralbl. Chir., *62*:2549, 1935.

AVULSION FRACTURES OF THE GREATER AND LESSER TROCHANTERS[1, 2]

These injuries occur as a result of muscular violence. The ossification center of the greater trochanter appears during the fourth year and that of the lesser trochanter, between the thirteenth and fourteenth years. They fuse with the femoral shaft between 18 and 19 years of age.

The *greater trochanter* is avulsed by sudden contraction of the gluteus medius and minimus muscles against resistance. The bone fragment is retracted proximally. When displacement is minimal, treatment consists of immobilization of the hip in a spica cast with the hip in abduction, bringing the greater trochanter into apposition with the upper end of the femoral shaft. The fracture will be healed in about six weeks. Moderately displaced fractures require open reduction and internal fixation with staples in the young child and cancellous screws in the adolescent.

The *lesser trochanter* is avulsed by the powerful contraction of the iliopsoas muscle against resistance, such as that which occurs during a football tackle or in an attempt to stop suddenly while running (Fig. 8–113). The displaced frac-

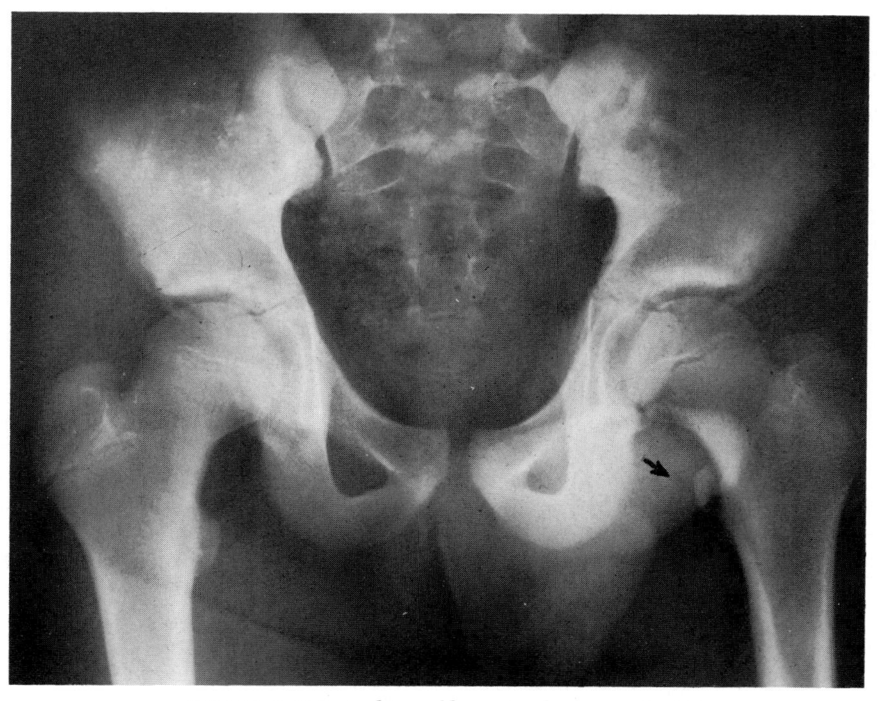

FIGURE 8–113. Avulsion of lesser trochanter on the left.

ture heals, with little or no disability. Open reduction is not indicated. The patient is kept in bed with the hips in flexion until he is comfortable and then he is allowed to ambulate with crutches—three-point partial weight-bearing gait. Immobilization in a hip spica cast is not necessary.

References

1. Fernbach, S. K., and Wilkinson, R. H.: Avulsion injuries of the pelvis and proximal femur. A.J.R., *137*:581, 1981.
2. Jones, J. B.: Screw fixation of the lesser trochanteric fragment. Clin. Orthop., *123*:107, 1977.

FRACTURES OF THE FEMORAL SHAFT

Fractures of the shaft of the femur are relatively frequent in children and should be considered serious injuries because of the blood loss and potential shock that may accompany the primary trauma.

The largest bone in the body, the femur is a long cylinder of heavy compact bone that is bowed anteriorly and laterally. The linea aspera, a sturdy elevated ridge extending along the middle of the posterior surface of the femoral shaft, acts as a thickened buttress, providing strength and serving as an attachment for muscles.

In normal stance, the femoral shaft inclines medially at an angle varying from 3 to 15 degrees with an average of 9.56 degrees. This tends to partially overcome the effect of the angle of inclination of the femoral neck by bringing the weight-bearing articular surfaces of the knee closer to the center of gravity.[201]

The femoral shaft can be broken only by tremendous force. The majority of these fractures occur as a result of major violence, either direct or indirect, such as that sustained in automobile accidents and falls from a height.

Pathologic Anatomy

The most common site of fracture of the femoral shaft is in its middle third, where the normal anterolateral bowing of the diaphysis is at its maximum; this is also the area most commonly subjected to severe direct violence. Of 250 cases of fracture of the femoral shaft admitted to the Children's Memorial Hospital, Chicago, 66 per cent were in the middle third, 17 per cent in the proximal third, 12 per cent in the distal third, and 5 per cent in the subtrochanteric region. Griffin, Green, and Anderson reported 70 per cent of the fractures in the middle third, 22 per cent in the proximal third, and 8 per cent in the distal third.[96] A similar distribution is reported by Blount, LeMesurier, Neer and Cadman, and Staheli.[26, 146, 179, 242]

The torsional force produced by indirect violence results in a long spiral or oblique fracture, whereas a transverse fracture is caused by direct trauma (Figs. 8–114 to 8–116). When the direct force is very severe, there may be comminution, or the fracture may be segmental, or both. Greenstick fractures may occur and are more common in the distal third.

Birth fractures, resulting from obstetrical trauma, usually occur in the middle third of the shaft and are transverse. Occasionally, however, they are metaphyseal in location (Fig. 8–117).

The displacement of the fragments in fracture of the femur depends upon the breaking force, the pull of the attached muscles, and the force of gravity acting upon the limb. As a rule, the distal fragment is laterally rotated consequent to outward rotation of the leg by the force of gravity. The severity of violence and the strong pull of the muscles will cause the fracture fragments to be completely displaced with variable amounts of overriding.

In fractures of the upper third of the femoral shaft, the proximal fragment is pulled into flexion by the iliopsoas muscle, into abduction by the gluteus medius and minimus, and into external rotation by the short external rotators and gluteus maximus. The shorter the proximal fragment, the greater is the degree of displacement. The distal fragment is drawn proximally by the hamstrings and quadriceps femoris muscles and into adduction by the adductors of the thigh. The distal fragment also falls posteriorly because of the force of gravity. Thus, the upper end of the distal fragment tends to lie posterior and medial to the proximal fragment, which is in flexion, abduction, and lateral rotation (Fig. 8–118).

Displacement of the fragments in the middle third does not follow any regular pattern. The tendency is for the proximal fragment to be in flexion and the distal fragment to be displaced backward; when the fracture level is in the upper half of the middle third, the proximal half is abducted; when the break is in the lower half, it is adducted (Fig. 8–119). However, displacements are not necessarily constant.

In fractures of the lower third, the fracture line may be transverse or oblique, or the break may be of the greenstick type. The gastrocnemius muscle is a chief deforming force. It arises

Text continued on page 3255

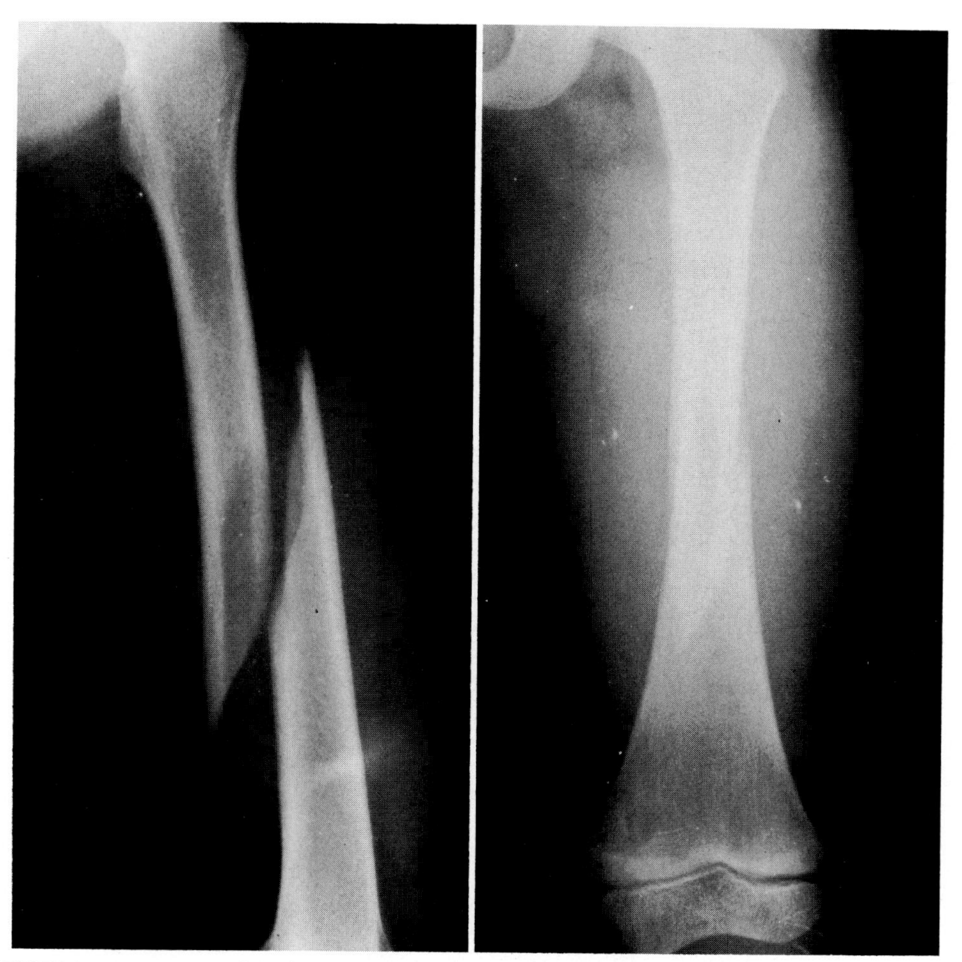

FIGURE 8–114. Long spiral fracture of the femoral shaft produced by torsional force of indirect violence.

The commonest site of fracture of the femoral shaft is in its middle third.

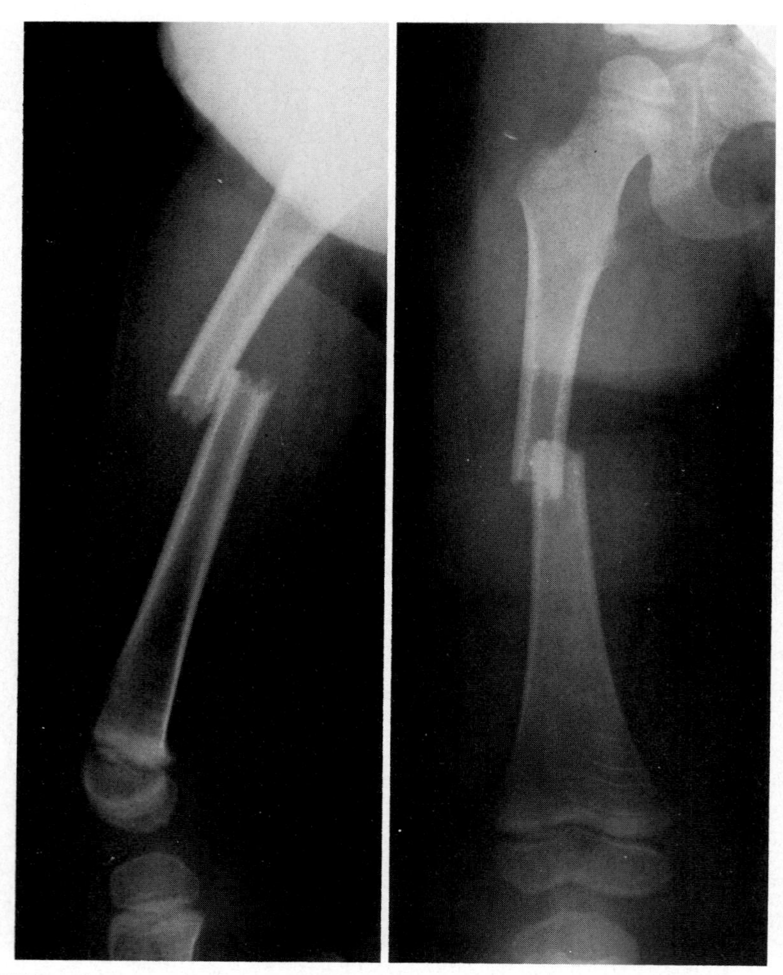

FIGURE 8–115. Transverse fracture of the femoral shaft—it is usually caused by direct trauma.

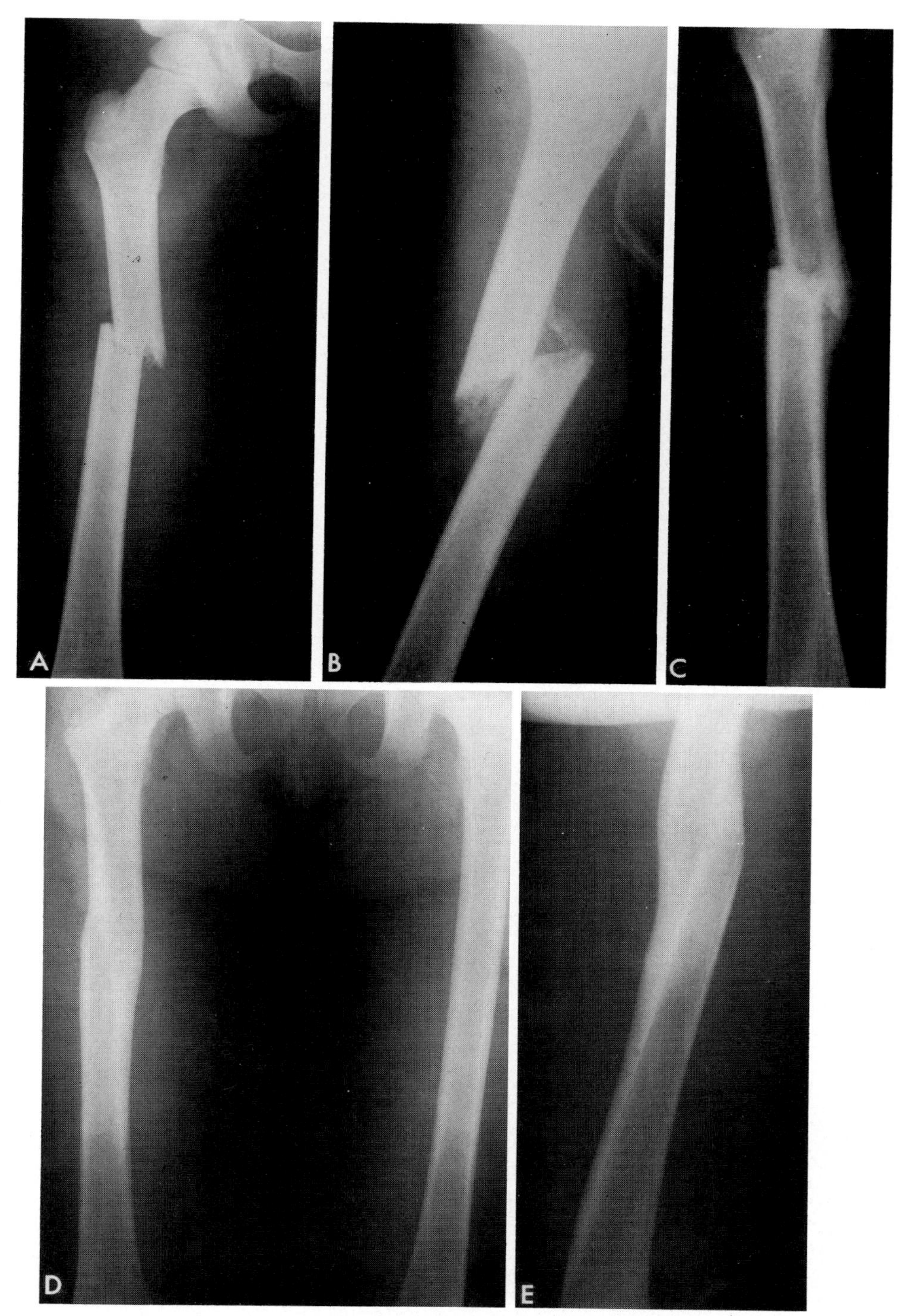

FIGURE 8–116. Short oblique fracture of the femoral shaft at the junction of its middle and proximal thirds in a six-year-old child.

A and **B.** Initial radiograms. Treated by 90°–90° skeletal traction followed by immobilization in a one and one half hip spica cast. **C.** Anteroposterior radiogram made when traction was discontinued. Note the 1 cm. overriding of the fragments, which is desirable in this age group. **D** and **E.** Ten months later—note the remodeling.

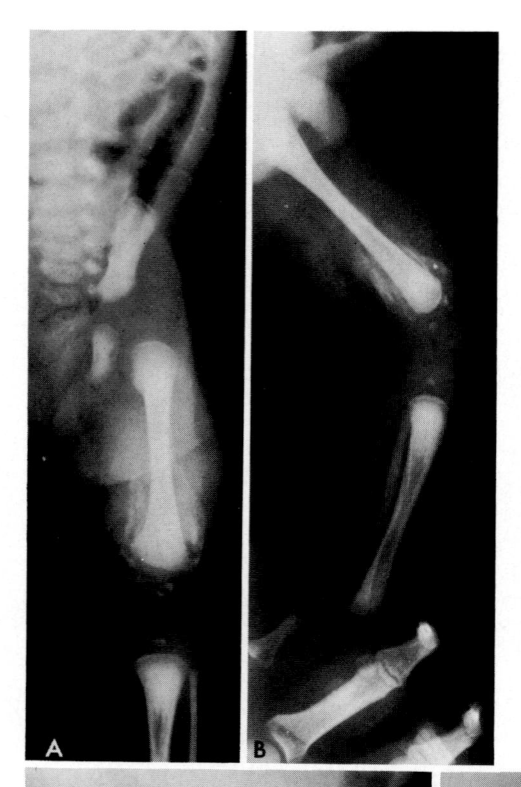

FIGURE 8–117. Birth fracture through metaphyseal region of distal left femur.

A and **B.** Initial radiograms showing excessive subperiosteal calcification. A diagnostic feature is the extension of new bone formation distal to the area of bone density of the diaphysis. The condition should not be mistaken for osteomyelitis. There is no area of radiolucency in the metaphysis. Syphilis, tuberculosis, and scurvy are other entities to consider in the differential diagnosis. No treatment is necessary. **C** and **D.** These are radiograms made three months later. Note the remodeling of the callus. **E.** An anteroposterior radiogram taken a year later.

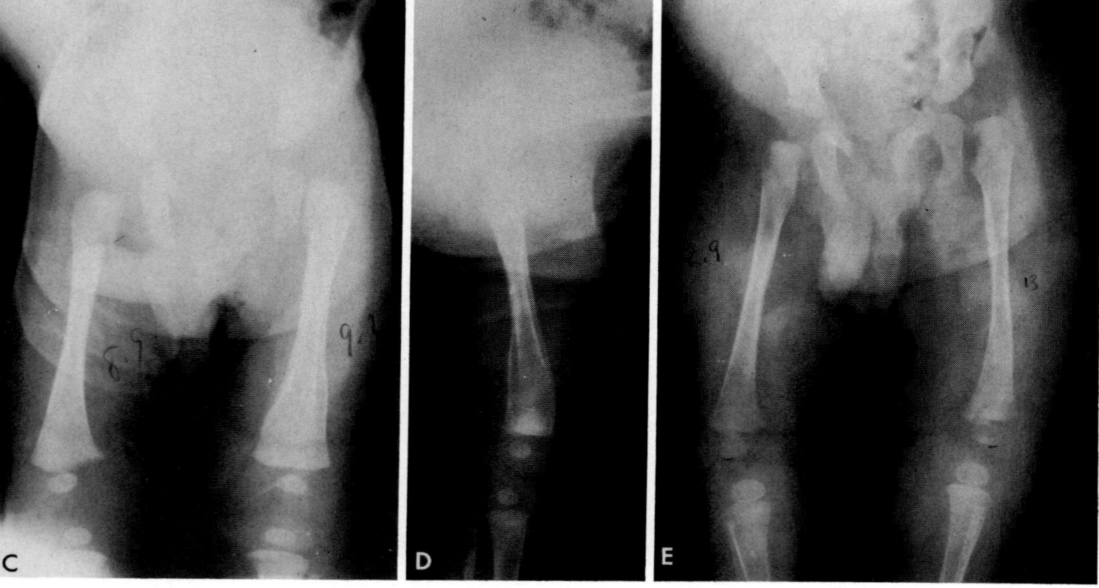

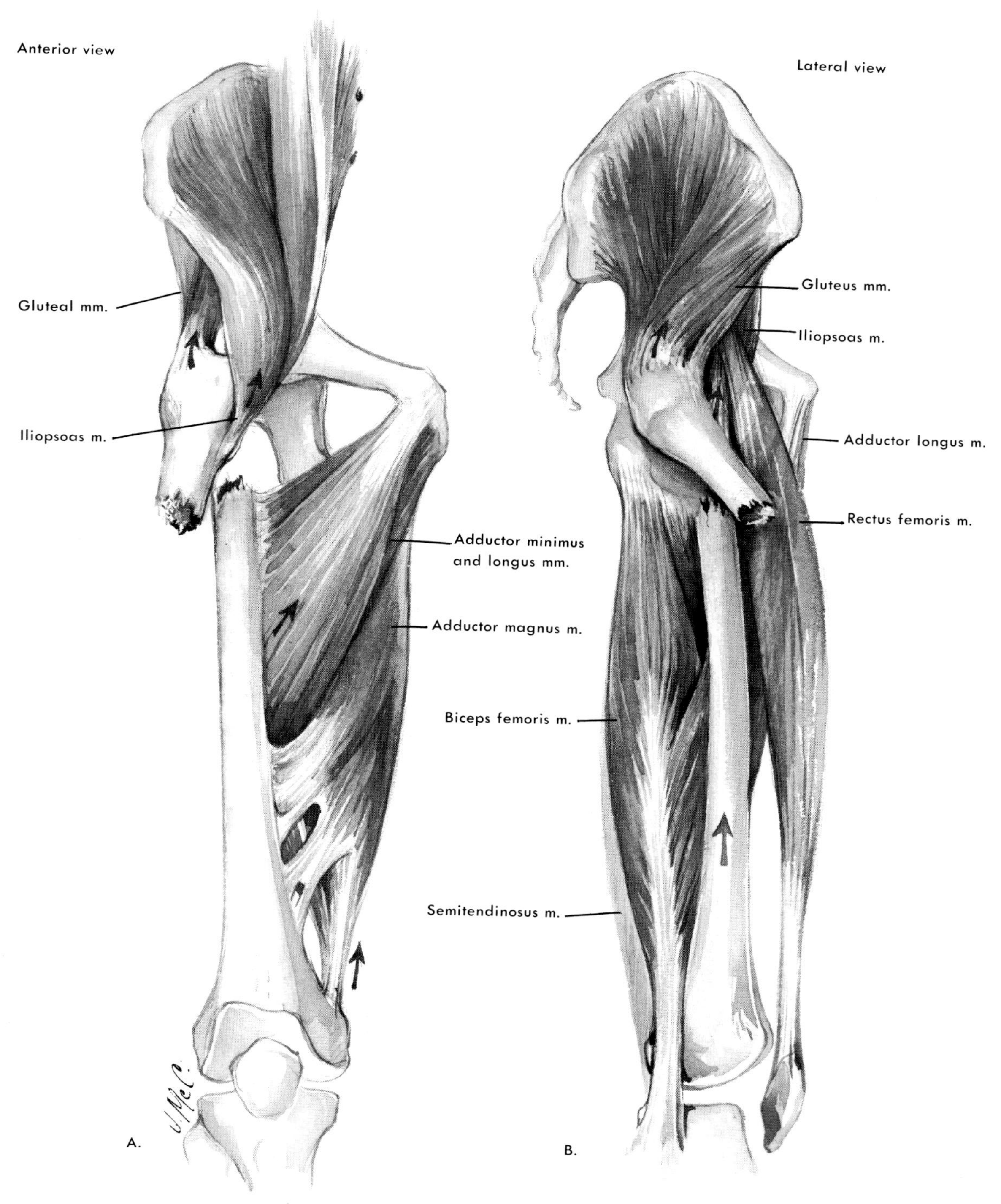

FIGURE 8–118. Displacement of fragments in fractures of the upper third of the femoral shaft.

Note the upper end of the distal fragment tends to lie posterior and medial to the proximal fragment, which is displaced into flexion, abduction, and external rotation by the pull of the iliopsoas, gluteal muscles, and short external rotators.

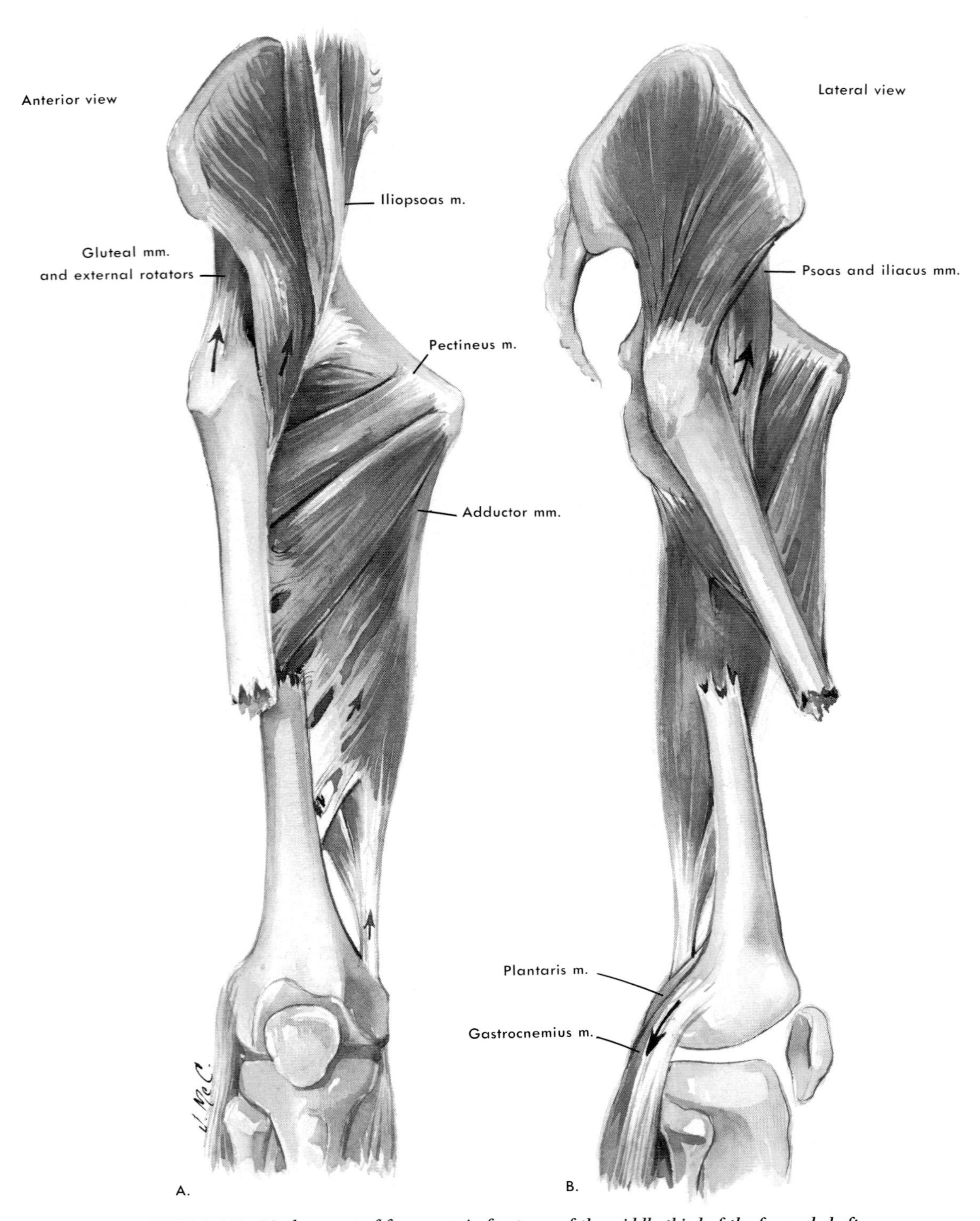

FIGURE 8–119. *Displacement of fragments in fractures of the middle third of the femoral shaft.*

from the posterior surface of the lower femur and pulls the distal fragment posteriorly into the popliteal space where it may cause damage to vessels and nerves. The lower end of the proximal fragment is driven forward and distally into the quadriceps femoris muscle.

Soft-tissue injury inevitably accompanies a femoral shaft fracture. Excessive hemorrhage with blood loss of 500 ml. or more is not uncommon. The source of bleeding may be either one or several branches of the profunda femoris artery (which courses around the posterior and lateral surfaces of the femoral shaft), the vessels of the richly vascular muscles that envelop the femur, or the vessels in the bone itself. Occasionally, the femoral artery itself may be torn.

Diagnosis

A history of injury, with the resultant local pain, tenderness, and swelling, inability to move the affected limb, deformity, shortening, abnormal mobility, lateral rolling of the limb distal to the level of the fracture, and crepitus render the diagnosis self-evident.

Examination of the patient should be very gentle, with great care exercised not to inflict unnecessary pain that might add to the possibly already present shock. The soft parts should not be damaged further. The fracture is distinguished as being either open or closed. Neurovascular status in the lower limb should be carefully assessed and recorded because injury to the femoral or popliteal vessels or to the sciatic nerve, or both, may occur, especially from posterior displacement of the distal fragment in fractures of the lower third of the shaft.

Because femoral shaft fractures usually result from major violence, it is imperative to evaluate the general condition of the patient meticulously. The sensorium, blood pressure, and pulse should be observed, and careful examination performed to detect any visceral damage in the intra-abdominal and genitourinary areas, cranial injury, other fractures, or hip dislocation.

Radiograms are taken to determine the exact level and nature of the fracture; however, this should not be done prior to proper splinting of the limb.

Treatment

Proper emergency care, i.e., initial gentle handling and adequate splinting of the fracture, is extremely important to prevent shock and further injury to the soft parts. Any movement of the injured limb will be quite painful, and one should *not* attempt to remove the patient's clothing or shoes.

An efficient means of immobilization is the Thomas splint or the Blake modification, in which there is only half of the ring. The size of the splint should be suitable for the child. The person applying the splint places his arm through the ring of the splint, grasps the patient's foot, and applies gentle and steady traction. Then, without releasing the traction on the foot, the splint is pushed proximally against the ischial tuberosity and traction is applied by a twisted rope or a strap sling that extends from the well-padded ankle to the end of the splint. The thigh and leg are supported on slings tightened under them or by encircling strips of cloth.

If a Thomas splint is not available, a splint may be improvised by using long boards or sticks, which should be padded to prevent pressure over bony prominences. The lateral splint extends from near the axilla to below the foot, and the medial one extends distally from the groin. Both splints are secured to the limb and the lateral one also to the trunk by means of an elastic bandage.

Another fairly satisfactory method of immobilization is to bandage the two lower limbs together. It is best to place some form of padding such as a folded blanket or clothing between the legs, and bind the feet together in order to control rotation. A pressure dressing over the fracture site will minimize bleeding into the soft tissues of the thigh. The author does not recommend the use of airsplints when transporting children with femoral shaft fractures, because of potential circulatory embarrassment.

In the definitive care of femoral shaft fractures in children, various factors determine the method chosen, namely: (1) the age of the patient; (2) the preference of the surgeon, based on past experience; (3) the condition of the skin and soft tissues; and (4) the level and degree of displacement or comminution of the fracture.

INFANTS AND CHILDREN UP TO TWO YEARS OF AGE

In infants and children, immediate reduction and cast immobilization has become the treatment of choice, provided that meticulous postcast care can be assured. Initially, it is best to admit these children to the hospital, place them in counterpoised traction, and rule out the possibility of child abuse. If the fracture was sustained in a violent accident such as being hit by a car, other associated injuries should be ruled out. If the fracture is displaced and closed reduction is required, it is best to take the child to the operating room and reduce the fracture under general anesthesia. The parents are instructed in hip spica cast care, and the child is discharged within a day or two. It is vital to make radiograms of the femur in anteroposterior and lateral projections (the tendency is to obtain inadequate lateral radiograms because of the difficulties involved with a spica cast). If there is any loss of alignment that is not acceptable, wedging of the cast should not be performed. Instead, the child should be taken back to the operating room, the loose cast removed, the fracture manipulated, and a snug hip spica cast applied.

A pitfall to avoid is immobilization of the affected femur in abduction. The pull of the hip adductors will angulate the fracture laterally. Place the hip in neutral or only 15 degrees of abduction. Another pitfall is to place the hip in extension. The pull of the iliopsoas muscle will anteriorly angulate the fracture. Immobilize the hip in semiflexion (Fig. 8–120). The possibility of changing the cast and potential problems of shortening and angular deformity should be explained to the parents initially to avoid later misunderstanding.

In the past, it was customary to place infants and children up to two years of age in Bryant's traction; it is still an effective and satisfactory method of maintaining reduction, provided there is no spasticity and contracture of the hamstrings. At present the only indication for Bryant's traction is the occasional case in which satisfactory alignment cannot be obtained and maintained by closed manipulative immobilization in cast.

Bryant's Traction. An overhead frame is placed over the crib—the type used varies in different hospitals. The child is placed on a Bradford frame to facilitate nursing care and to

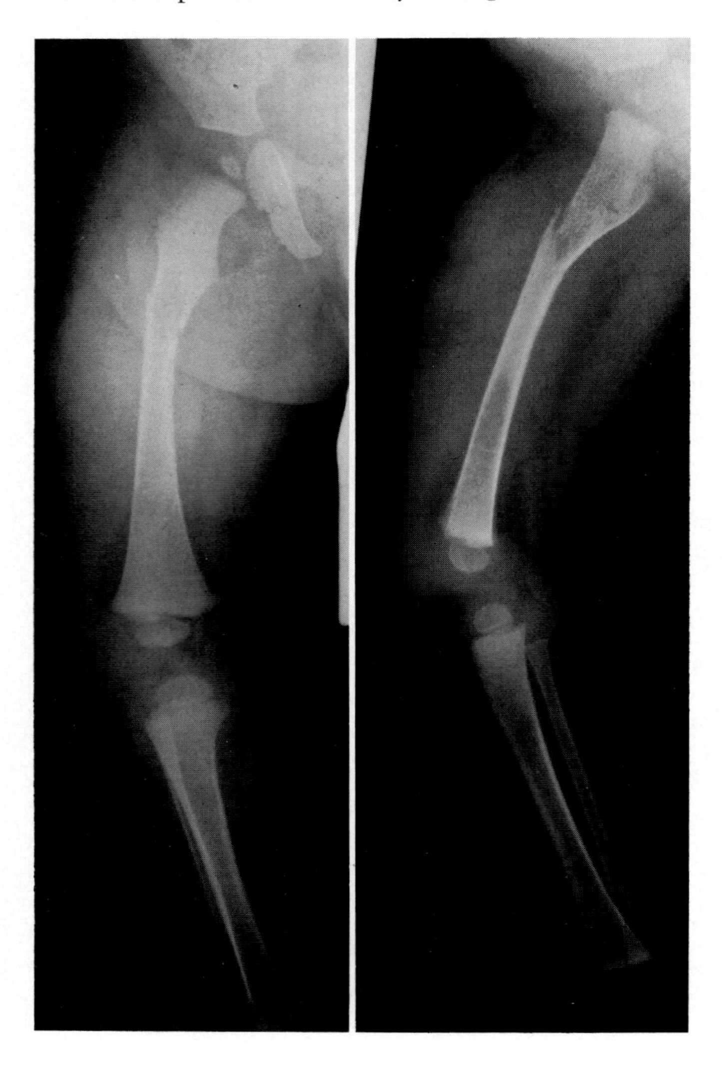

FIGURE 8–120. Fracture of the femoral shaft at its proximal third in a nine-month-old infant.

maintain the hip joint in a position directly underneath the overhead pulleys. A chest restraint is used to secure the patient on the frame (Figs. 8–121 and 8–122). Bryant originally put only the fractured femur in direct overhead vertical traction. Some surgeons still prefer to apply traction to the involved legs only, claiming that more traction force can be achieved in this way. The author, however, believes that traction on both legs provides more effective control of the pelvis and also prevents rotatory movements. Pressure on the malleoli is precluded by placing padding over them—a rolled short piece of stockinette or sheath wadding. Adhesive traction strips of proper length are smoothly applied, beginning proximally at the upper third of the thighs, and attached distally by straps to a spreader foot piece. Elastic bandages encircle the traction strips, beginning above the ankle and extending proximally; these should not be tight. The ropes extend from the foot piece and pass through pulleys located directly over the hip joints. The same amount of weight is applied on each leg and should be sufficient to lift the infant's pelvis by suspension until no weight is borne on the back of the sacrum. One should be cautious not to overpull the small infant and suspend him in the air. Adhesive tape applied between the foot pieces will control rotational alignment of the lower limbs.

The position of the fracture is checked by periodic radiograms. Distraction of the fragments should be avoided. Medial bowing caused by excessive pull of the hip adductors is corrected by decreasing the amount of weight on the affected limb and increasing traction on the contralateral normal limb. By tilting the

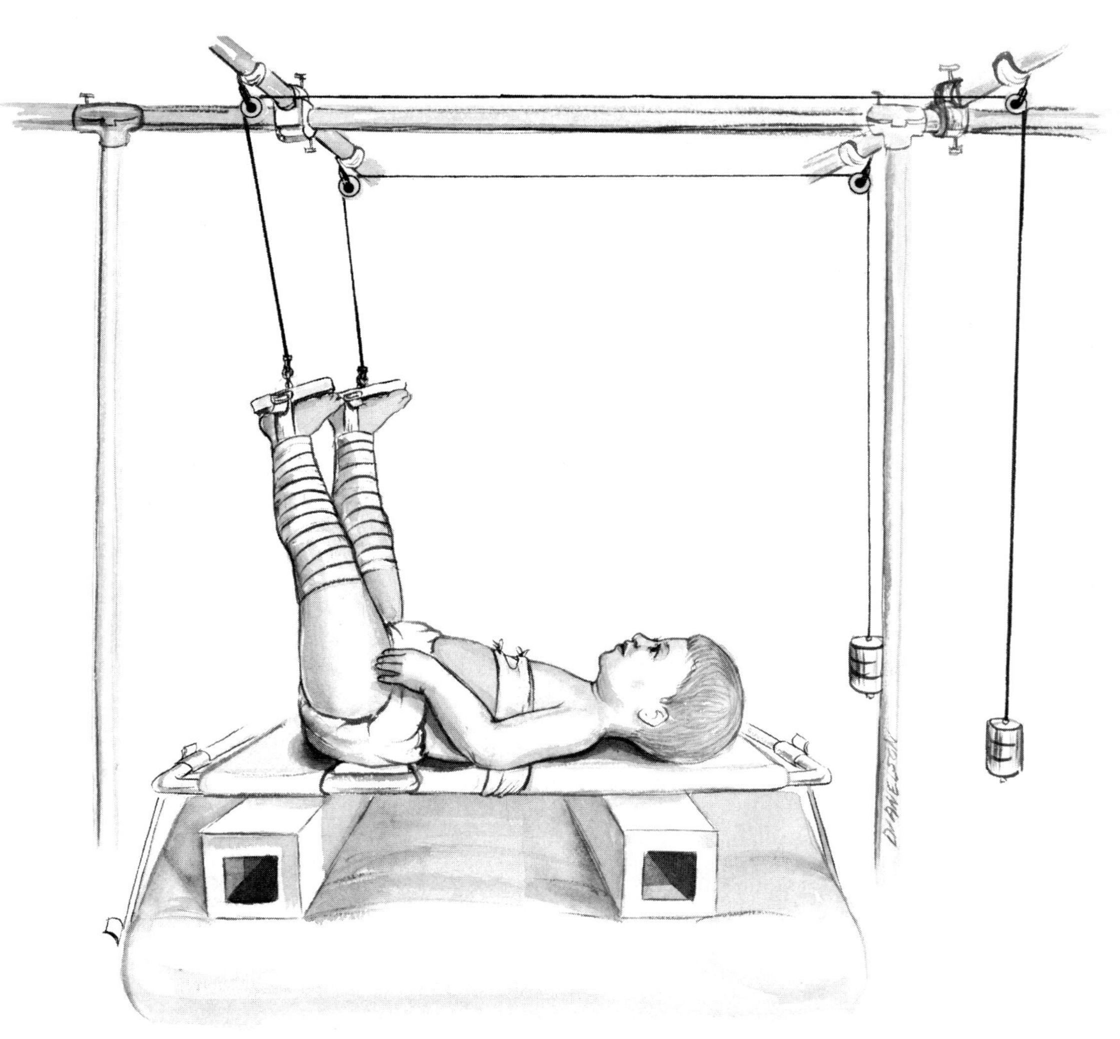

FIGURE 8–121. Bryant's direct overhead traction (see text for explanation).

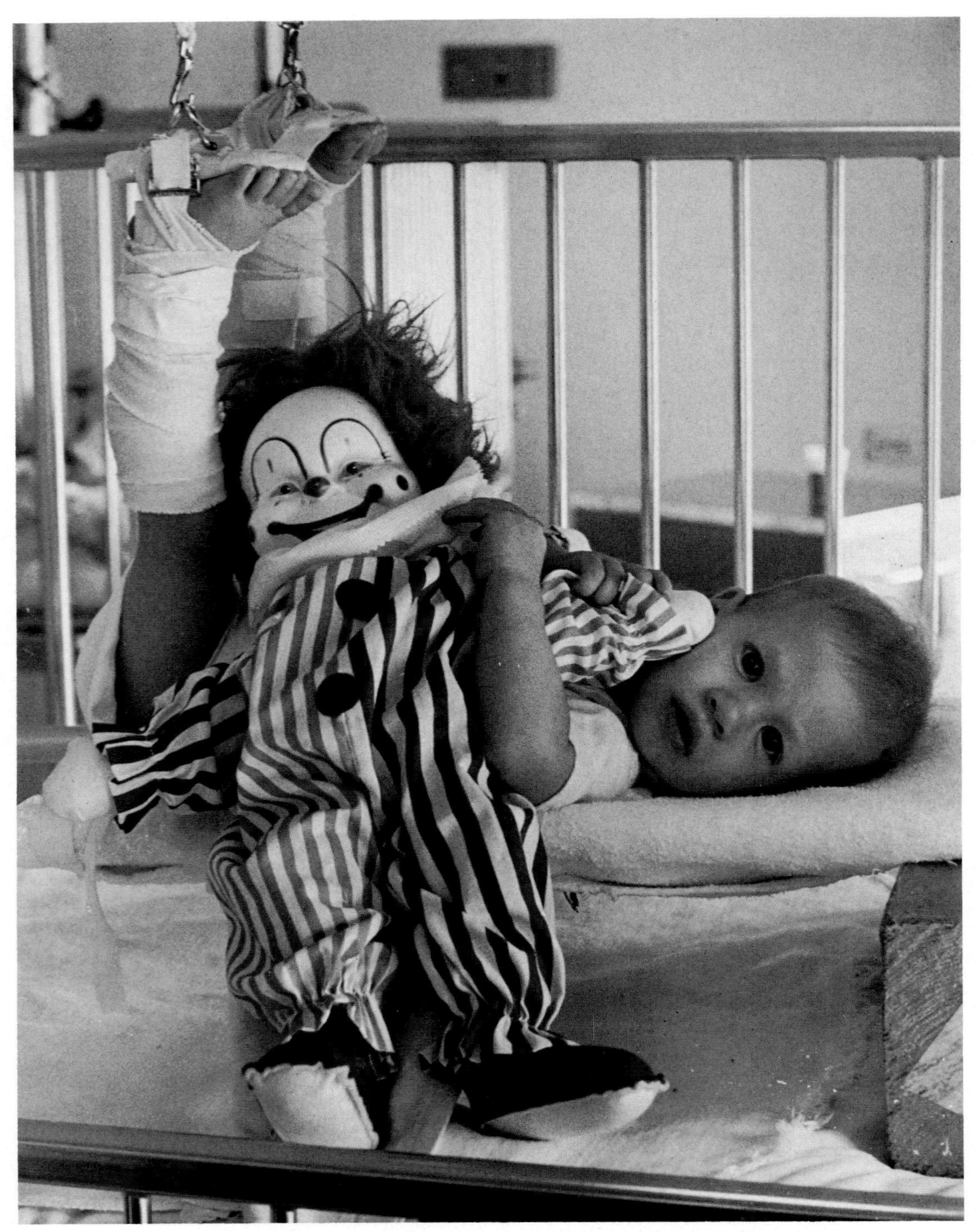

FIGURE 8–122. An infant with fractured femoral shaft treated in Bryant's traction.

pelvis distally on the contralateral side, the pull of the hip adductors will be released (Fig. 8–123).

The expectation that a bony deformity in childhood will correct itself spontaneously with growth and remodeling is not an excuse for ignoring it, if correction can be obtained by simple means. At the same time, a child should not be subjected to too frequent manipulations or unjustified trauma to correct mere minor displacements.

Callus forms rapidly in infants. Two to three weeks from the time of trauma, the tenderness of the callus will have disappeared and the fracture will usually be stable enough to remove the traction and continue immobilization in a one and one half hip spica cast without the risk of losing the position of the fragments. The normal hip and thigh are included in the cast to stabilize the pelvis. The patient can then be discharged from the hospital. Immobilization in the hip spica cast is continued at home until

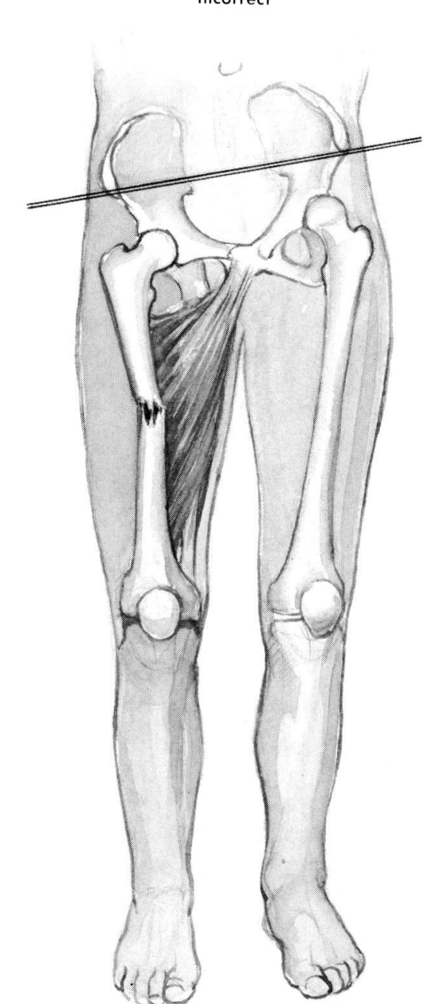

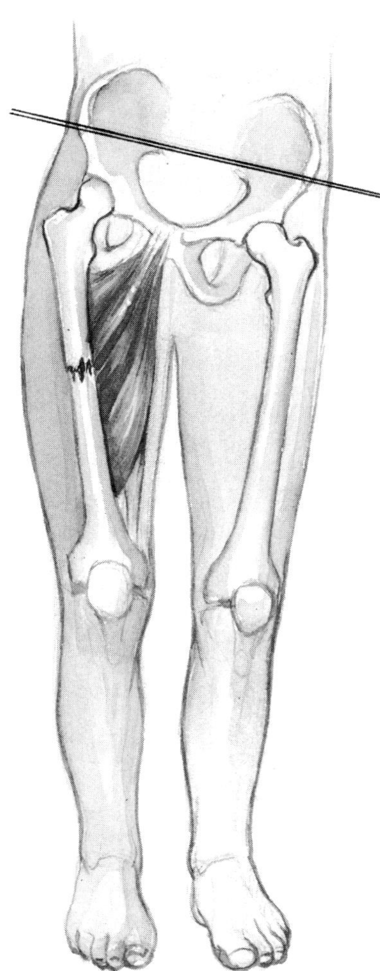

FIGURE 8–123. The wrong and right ways of correcting medial bowing of fracture of the femoral shaft caused by pull of the hip adductors.

A. *Wrong way.* Increasing weight on the fractured limb will tilt the pelvis distally, exaggerate functionally the degree of hip abduction, and increase the pull of the hip adductors; thus, the deformity is aggravated.

B. *Right way.* Increase the weights on the contralateral normal hip and tilt the pelvis distally on the normal side. Thus, the hip on the affected side is functionally in adducted position and the medial bowing is corrected by relaxing the pull of the hip adductors. (Redrawn after Blount.)

there is solid union of the fracture. In birth fractures, this usually occurs in three weeks, and in infants and young children, from four to six weeks from the day of original injury. The immobile joints spontaneously regain their full range of motion within a few weeks.

Complications of Overhead Traction. Bryant's traction does have its drawbacks, nevertheless, and its apparent simplicity should not lull the surgeon into a false sense of security. It should *not* be used in children over two years of age or in those weighing over 25 lb. Constant vigil should be kept for the possible development of any vascular, neurologic, or skin complications. Of these, circulatory embarrassment is the most serious and one that may assume tragic proportions.

Treatment of fractured femora by direct overhead traction may result in three degrees of circulatory insufficiency. The first is ischemic fibrosis of the muscles of the lower leg, with patches of sensory loss. There is almost complete paralysis of the muscles distal to the knee, except in the short toe flexors. The foot and ankle are usually deformed in rigid equinovarus position. The second degree of involvement is characterized both by the changes described in the first degree and by the presence of circumferential necrosis of the skin and underlying muscles in the calf. The third degree is the most severe form of circulatory insufficiency in which, in addition to the circumferential necrosis in the calf, the foot and ankle have become gangrenous.[181]

The first report of ischemic contracture in the lower limb in children was given in 1951 by Thompson and Mahoney, who described its occurrence following fractures of the femur in 13 children, one of whom had been treated by Bryant's traction.[252] Previously, Jones and Cotton had reported Volkmann's ischemia in the lower limb in two adults who had sustained crush injuries in the popliteal area.[127] Miller, Markin, and Grossman, in 1952, reported ischemic fibrosis of the lower limbs of seven children being treated for fractured femur, with six of the seven being treated in Bryant's traction. In all six, the ischemia manifested itself within the first two days. In three of the seven children, ischemia developed in the normal leg.[163] Nicholson, Foster, and Heath, in 1955, reported circulatory insufficiency in the legs of six children treated with Bryant's traction for simple fracture of the femur. In five of the six children, circulatory impairment developed in the uninjured leg.[181]

Impairment of circulation may be caused by several factors: (1) *The reduced hydrostatic pressure in the lower limbs* when they are held in vertical position makes it difficult for the blood to reach the foot and maintain adequate circulation. Nicholson, Foster, and Heath found an inversely proportionate ratio between the blood pressure of the ankle and the height of the ankle above the heart. When the leg was dependent over the side of the bed, blood pressure at the ankle was raised; when the leg was in horizontal position, it returned to normal; and with the leg in the elevated, or Bryant's, position the blood pressure was lowered. They further demonstrated, by making repeated oscillometric readings over a period of time, that with the leg maintained in Bryant's traction, the lowered blood pressure at the ankle remained constant and was not compensated.[181] (2) *Tautly applied circular bandages on the leg* can alter the level of blood pressure at the ankle. The pressure did not alter when the bandages were loosely applied; but when the bandages were tightly wrapped, particularly in children over two years of age, it could be reduced to zero.[181] (3) *Shock* is an important factor. The lowered systemic blood pressure may produce ischemia in legs held by Bryant's traction. (4) *Traction* and stretching of the vascular tree from its normal resting state in one lower limb produce a variable degree of spasm in both main and collateral arteries in both limbs. This was shown experimentally in dogs by Mustard and Simmon.[175] Allowing a fractured femur to maintain the vessels in a shortened state for 24 hours and then distracting them will result in diffuse arterial spasm. (5) *Hyperextension of the knee* can impair circulation. Nicholson and associates investigated the effect of knee position on the vascular supply to the lower leg. They made oscillometric readings at the ankle with the traction and bandages on the leg, with the knee held in hyperextension, with the limb both in the horizontal and in the vertical position. In children under two years of age, reasonable snugness and extent of the bandage made no appreciable difference; whereas in children over four years of age, the oscillometric readings at the ankle with the limb vertical and the knee hyperextended were invariably zero. Nicholson and coworkers demonstrated that one significant factor that interferes with circulation in the vertically held leg, with or without the use of traction, is knee hyperextension. Its effect is apparent in patients more than two years of age and is constant in patients more than four years old. They emphasized the dangers of using

Bryant's traction in patients over two years of age. Elevation of the leg to a vertical position with the knee hyperextended or fully extended may result in circulatory impairment.[181]

Peroneal nerve paralysis can occur. It is important that circulation, the degree of sensation in both feet, and the ability to move the toes be checked at frequent intervals. The circular turns of the elastic bandage may be displaced distally and cause pressure sores on the heel in children over four years of age. Careful inspection of the skin and rewrapping of the elastic bandages will prevent pressure necrosis of the skin.

Modification of Bryant's Traction. Ferry and Edgar modified Bryant's traction by utilizing the principles of Russell's traction (Fig. 8–124). This method is as follows: (1) The skin is painted with tincture of benzoin from the ankle to the midthigh. The painted area is then covered with stockinette that is smooth and not wrinkled. The malleoli are padded with a cotton-roll bandage. Traction strips are applied longitudinally on the medial and lateral aspects of the prepared area and are held in place by elastic bandage wrapped from the toes to the upper margin of the traction straps. The traction straps are then connected to a footplate that has a pulley on its bottom surface; it should be of adequate size to prevent pressure on the malleoli. A well-padded sling is secured on the back of the proximal part of the calf and distal to the popliteal fossa; the traction rope connected to the anterior end of the sling is passed to an overhead pulley A, through overhead pulley B, then through the pulley on the foot piece, and finally through overhead pulley C. Traction is applied on both lower limbs with sufficient weight on each limb to raise the buttocks slightly off the bed. Ordinarily 2 to 4 lb. of weight is sufficient. With this method, longitudinal traction force is applied in the direction of the long axis of the femur, raising the buttocks from the bed, but also maintaining the knees in a partially flexed position. In this position, the hydrostatic force working against the pulse pressure is less because the heart-to-toe height is less than in the vertical position maintained in Bryant's traction. It is not necessary to wrap the circular bandages tightly, as part of the traction force is exerted through the calf sling. With the knees maintained in flexion, the likelihood of vascular and neurologic complications is minimized.[79]

The author recommends the use of the Ferry and Edgar modification of Bryant's traction for

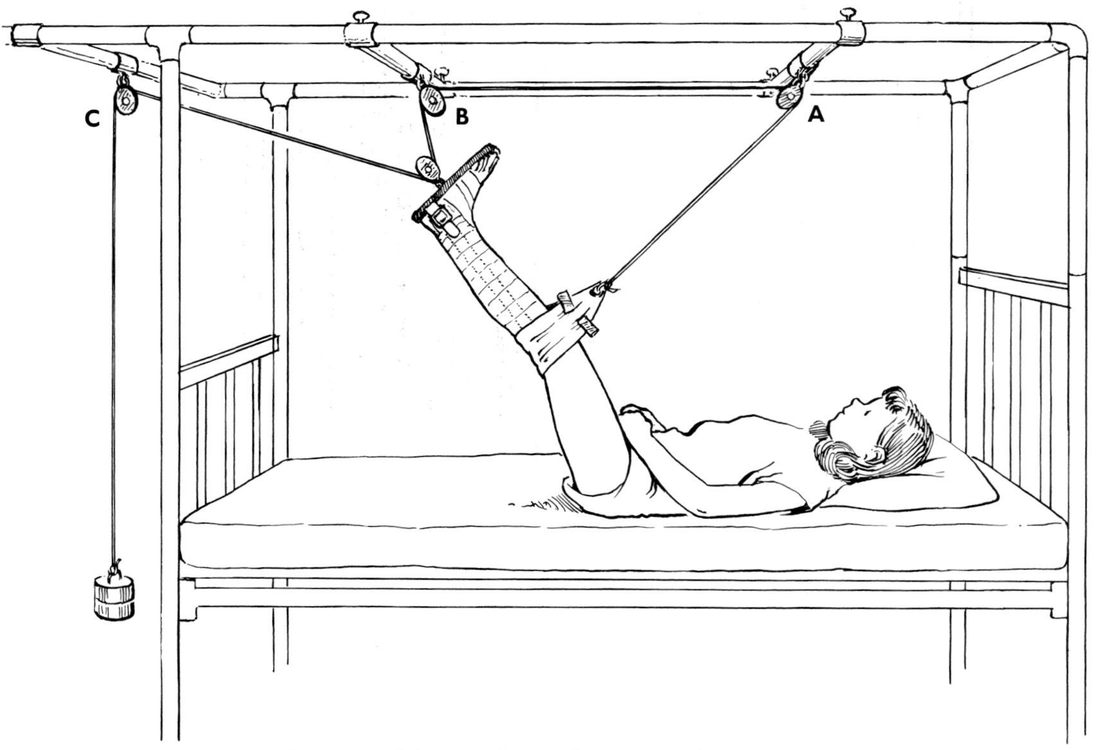

FIGURE 8–124. Ferry and Edgar modification of Bryant's traction utilizing the principle of Russell (see text for explanation).

children over two years of age in whom insertion of a pin through the distal femur for skeletal traction is undesirable, such as in pathologic fractures in osteogenesis imperfecta or in cases of children with myelomeningocele who have markedly osteoporotic bones.

CHILDREN BETWEEN THREE AND TEN YEARS OF AGE

If the fracture is undisplaced or minimally displaced, it is treated only with immobilization in a double or one and one-half hip spica cast. If it is displaced, several choices of treatment are available: immediate reduction and immobilization in a plaster of Paris cast, with or without traction being incorporated into the cast; or reduction and some type of traction until callus is formed and then immobilization in a spica cast until bony union is firm. In children, open reduction and internal fixation of femoral shaft fractures should not be performed under general anesthesia. During reduction, if alignment is satisfactory and the fracture is stable, a double or one and one-half hip spica cast is applied.

Treatment by Closed Reduction and Early Immobilization in Double Hip Spica Cast. The chief advantage of closed reduction and early immobilization in cast is that it decreases the duration of the hospital stay, which has obvious financial advantages. However, to maintain reduction is difficult, requiring close supervision by repeated radiograms. The cast is changed and the fracture remanipulated. Wedging of the cast is not recommended by this author because of the potential risk of skin, soft-tissue, and neurovascular complications.

Dameron and Thompson, in 1959, presented the end results in 53 patients treated by closed reduction and immobilization in a double hip spica cast. They incorporated the Kirschner wire bow in the cast. The average duration of follow-up was 6.9 years. In no patient could they find any deformity, abnormality of gait, or limitation of hip and knee motion. At the follow-up examination, the fractured limb was, on the average, 1/16 inch longer than the opposite normal limb. In only a few patients was the broken limb more than 1/4 inch shorter than the normal limb, and in five patients the affected limb was more than 1/4 inch longer. Complications of malunion, delayed union, nonunion, and Volkmann's contracture and gangrene were not encountered in any of their patients. These investigators recommended this method of treatment of femoral shaft fractures as safe, certain, comfortable, and economical.[59]

In the literature, there are numerous reports of results by closed reduction and early cast immobilization.[5, 6, 106, 121, 132, 138, 154, 168, 220, 234, 240, 241, 243, 247] Angular and rotational malalignment and limb length disparity occur in most series; they develop more frequently in the older child and when fracture displacement is severe. The parents should be forewarned of these complications and that a secondary procedure may be required for correction.

Regardless of the type of treatment used, if the fracture is displaced, it is best to perform a closed manipulative reduction initially.

This author prefers to employ traction to maintain alignment until there is adequate callus for stability (i.e., the callus is no longer tender and the femur moves as a unit on manipulation) and then immobilize in a one and one half hip spica cast. There are several types of traction available, namely: (1) skin traction—Russell or split Russell, (2) suspension skeletal or skin traction with a Thomas splint and Pearson attachment, and (3) "90°–90°" skeletal traction with a pin through the distal femur or the proximal tibia.

90°–90° Skeletal Traction. The author prefers 90°–90° skeletal traction with a pin through the distal femur because of its effectiveness and simplicity. Alignment of the fracture is easily achieved and maintained, as there is one line of traction and the pin through the distal femur provides good control of the fracture fragments. The gastrocnemius, hamstring, and iliopsoas muscles are relaxed by the flexed position of the hip and knee, making alignment of the fracture fragments relatively easy. Other advantages of 90°–90° traction are that it promotes dependent drainage; the thigh is readily accessible for clinical inspection of alignment without the use of portable x-ray equipment, and it facilitates change of dressings and wound inspection in infected open fractures. Preferably under general anesthesia, a heavy threaded Steinmann pin or a large Kirschner wire is inserted 2 cm. proximal to the adductor tubercle at the junction of the posterior third and anterior two thirds of the femoral shaft; using this site, one avoids injuring the physis and puncturing the suprapatellar pouch and knee joint. Small stab incisions in the skin are desirable. The pin is introduced at right angles to the longitudinal axis of the thigh. Pushing the skin slightly upward while drilling the wire through it will prevent undue pressure on the skin while traction is applied. Sterile dressings are placed over the skin wounds and a traction bow of correct size is applied with the pin under tension. A light below-knee cast is ap-

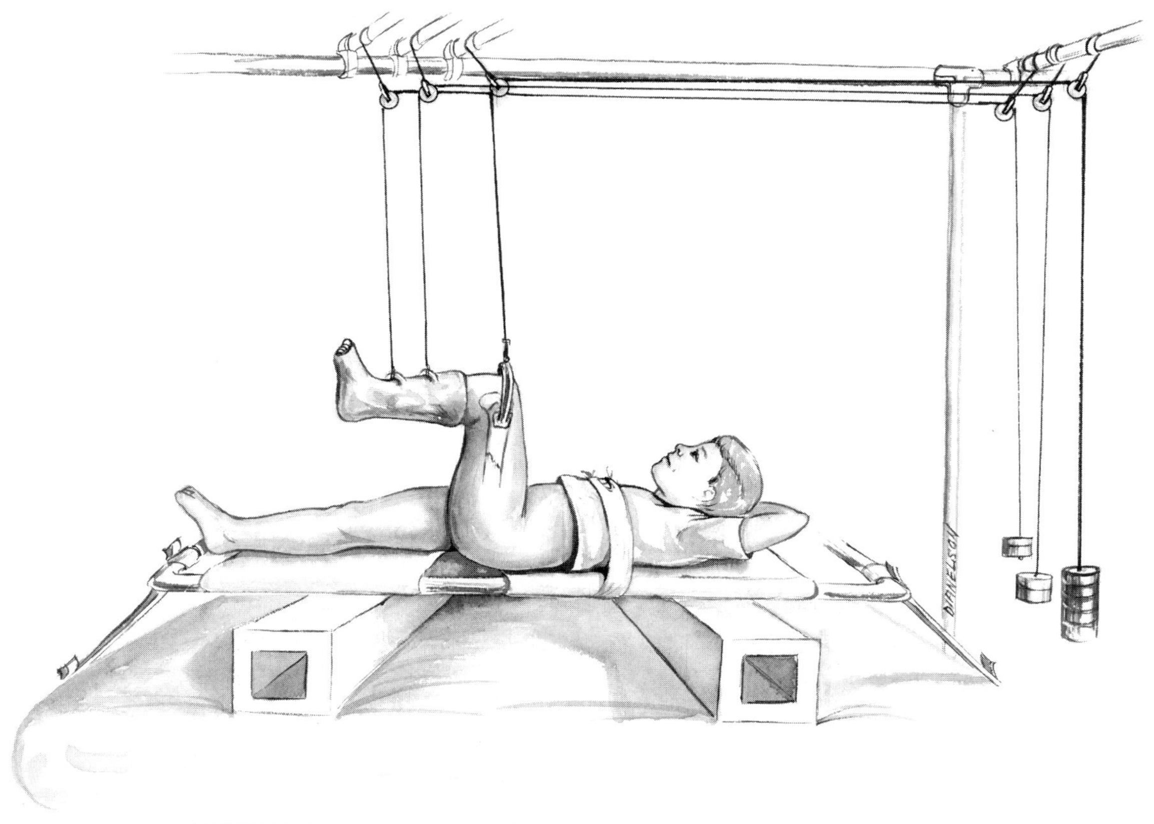

FIGURE 8–125. Ninety–ninety skeletal traction with wire through the distal femur.

It is used in children over two years of age for treatment of fractures of the femoral shaft.

plied with the ankle in neutral position. This should be well padded in the popliteal area and the dorsum of the foot and ankle to prevent pressure sores. Through two metal rings or plaster of Paris cast loops, one distal, the other proximal in position, traction ropes are extended to pulleys on the overhead frame to suspend the lower leg in horizontal position with the knee in 90 degrees of flexion. The weights are adjusted to counterbalance the weight of the leg plus that of the plaster boot, thus merely suspending the lower leg. A closed reduction of the fracture is performed next. Weights are placed via a rope on the traction bow with the hip in 90 degrees of flexion, the traction forces acting vertically in line with the longitudinal axis of the femoral shaft. The pelvis should be slightly lifted from the bed (Figs. 8–125 and 8–126).

Angulation and rotation can be easily corrected by shifting the overhead traction in the appropriate direction. If additional external support is necessary in an unstable fracture, coaptation splints may be employed; these are made of strips of balsa wood 2.5 cm. in width cut to the desired lengths and laid side-by-side between two pieces of moleskin. The splint is applied circumferentially around the thigh and held in place with buckled webbing straps over thin felt. Slings with 1 or 2 lb. of weight can be applied over the fracture site to control lateral or anteroposterior angulation. Small children are usually placed on a Bradford frame with split Russell traction on the normal leg for immobilization. A chest restraint is advisable if the child is very active.

The position and alignment of the fracture fragments are checked by periodic radiograms. Under no circumstances should one allow distraction of the fragments to take place. In children between two and ten years of age, side-to-side apposition with 0.5 to 1 cm. overriding is the ideal position (but it should not exceed 1.5 cm.). In infants and adolescents, however, end-to-end apposition is desirable.

Traction is continued for two to four weeks, until the callus is no longer tender on palpation and the femur moves in one piece. Adequate callus should also be visible on the radiograms. The patient is then placed in a one and one half hip spica cast. The affected thigh should be in 10 degrees of abduction or in neutral position with the opposite hip in moderate abduction to facilitate perineal hygiene. A common pitfall is to place the fractured thigh in marked abduction with resultant lateral bowing due to the pull of the strong adductors. It is always wise to extend the hip and knee gradually to 45 degrees of flexion before applying the hip spica cast. The pin in the femur is removed and is not incorporated in the cast.

Complications of this method of 90°–90° skeletal traction have been negligible in 280 fractures of the femoral shaft treated at the Children's Memorial Hospital, Chicago.

Humberger and Eyring have described a method of 90°–90° skeletal traction with the Kirschner wire inserted through the proximal tibia.[118] The author does not recommend their method because the Kirschner wire may injure the apophysis of the proximal tibial tubercle, either at the time of insertion or if it should migrate. Also, the wire in the proximal tibia does not provide direct control over the femur as does a wire through the distal femur. The only instance in which the author uses a wire through the proximal tibia is when the fracture is open and local skin lacerations preclude the use of a wire through the distal femur.

Suspension Traction. This method is preferred by many orthopedic surgeons for use in older children and adolescents.

The author does not use suspension traction because of the advantages listed previously for 90°–90° traction in which there are no shifting splints with multiple suspension ropes to be adjusted.

Russell Skin Traction.[222] This is preferred by some as an ideal method for treatment of femoral shaft fractures in older children. The medial and lateral adhesive traction strips extend from the ankle to a point just below the knee and are attached with straps to a footplate with a pulley on its inferior surface. There should be

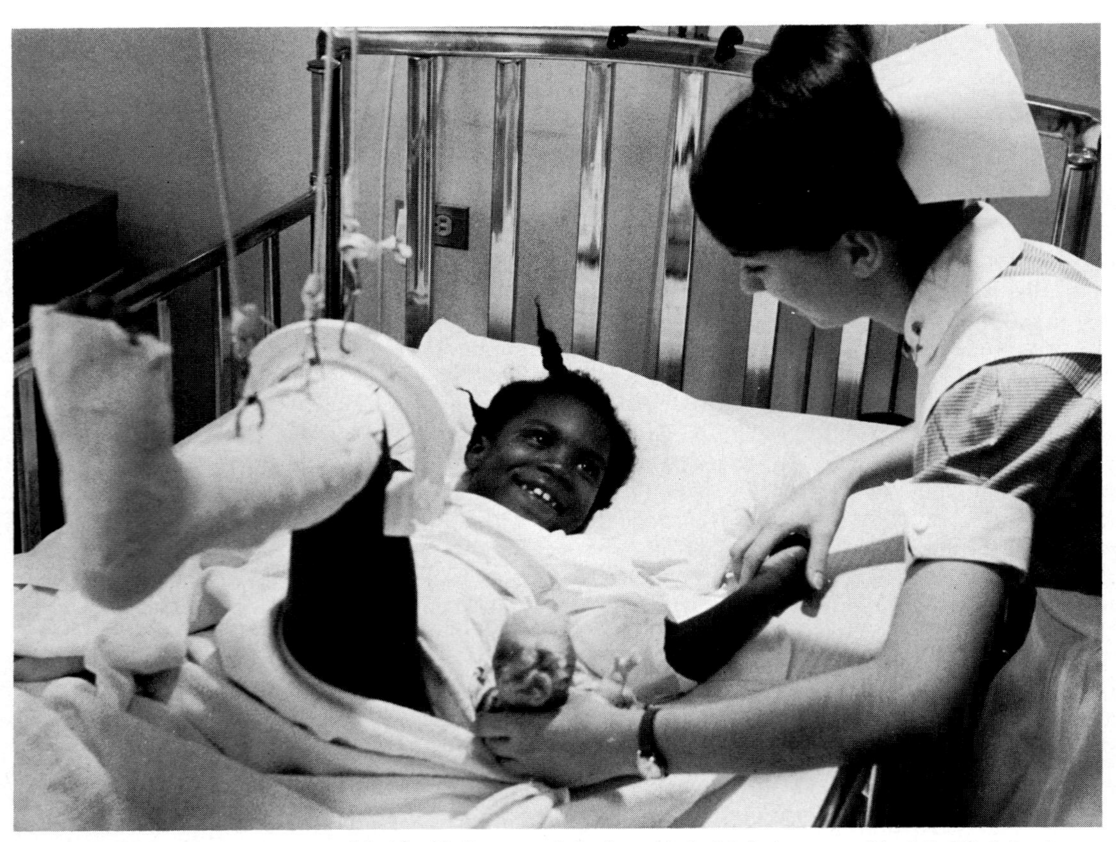

FIGURE 8–126. A seven-year-old girl with fracture of the femoral shaft is being treated by 90°–90° skeletal traction with a wire through the distal femur.

This is a very effective and simple method. The child is pain-free while in traction.

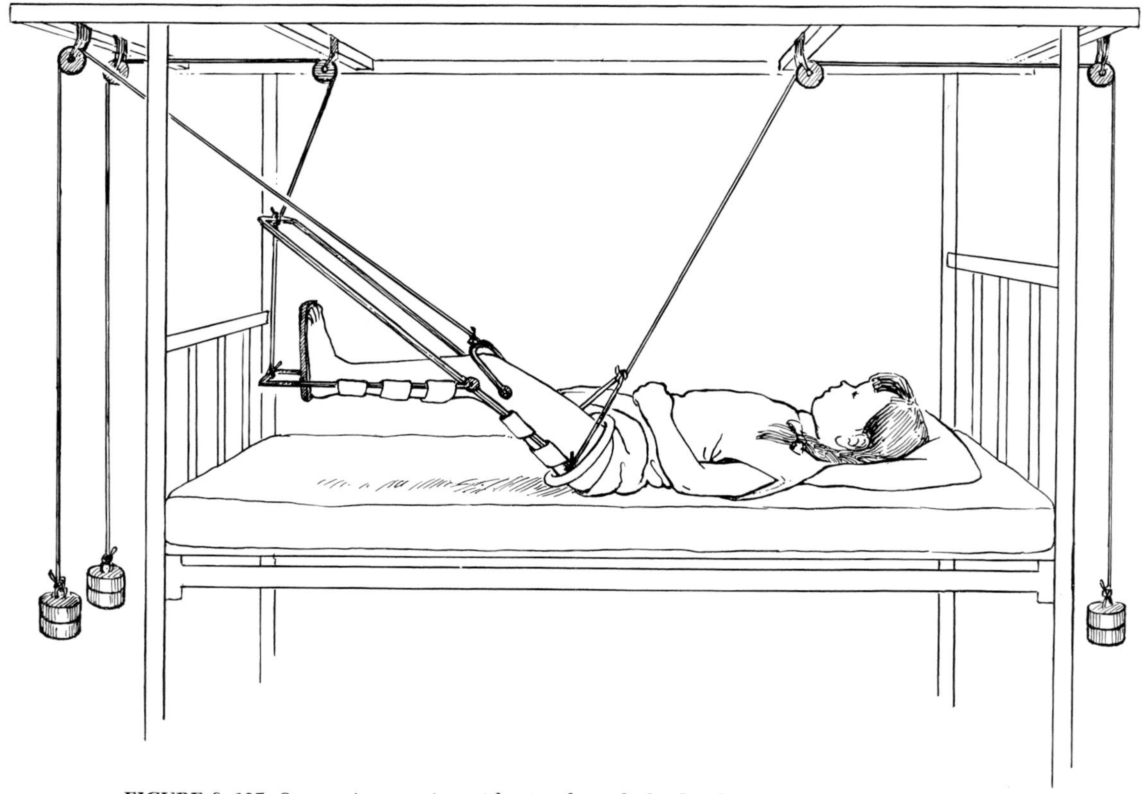

FIGURE 8–127. Suspension traction with wire through the distal femur with Thomas splint and Pearson attachment.

two pulleys at the foot of the bed and one overhead. A well-padded sling is placed beneath the knee. The traction rope extends from the sling to the overhead pulley, which is distal to the knee joint, so that the rope is directed upward and distally at an angle of 25 degrees, passing over the superior pulley attached to the end of the bed to which the skin traction straps are fixed and back again over the inferior pulley at the foot of the bed, where 5 to 8 lb. of weight is suspended. The lower limb rests on two pillows arranged so that the knee is in 30 degrees of flexion, the thigh is supported, and the foot just clears the mattress. The foot of the bed is raised 10 to 20 cm. to provide countertraction. The vertical traction force is roughly equal to the amount of weight used; whereas the horizontal traction force, because of the double pull from the footplate to the foot of the bed, is equal to approximately twice the amount of weight. The vertical and horizontal forces create a parallelogram of forces, with the resultant force in line with the long axis of the shaft of the femur (Fig. 8–128 A).

Advocates of Russell traction prefer it because of the ease with which it may be applied. The muscles are kept in balance, relatively less traction weight is required to overcome shortening and deformity, and the need for skeletal traction with its possible complications is eliminated. The disadvantages of this technique are: (1) the possible serious complication of peroneal nerve palsy with the resultant foot drop due to pressure by the knee sling in the region of the common peroneal nerve; (2) the potential for development of posterior bowing at the fracture site due to lack of effective external support under the thigh (often it is necessary to apply an additional sling beneath the thigh with vertical traction to restore the normal anterior bowing of the femur); (3) the difficulty of nursing care and the necessity for careful vigilance to ensure that correction traction is maintained; and (4) the child is initially in more pain than in 90°–90° traction.

The author employs split Russell traction instead of the original Russell traction with its 2:1 ratio of forces. In split Russell traction, skin traction is applied in the longitudinal axis of the limb and a balanced sling with a vertical force is placed under the distal femur or knee and suspended by weights to support the part and supply the necessary resolution of forces (Fig. 8–128 B). External rotation of the leg is controlled with medial rotation traction straps.

As stated previously, open reduction is not justified in femoral shaft fractures in children. Perfect anatomic reduction of fracture fragments is of less importance in the child than in the adult, as with growth and remodeling, malunion will correct itself.

When there is an open fracture of the femur, the wound is thoroughly debrided of all foreign material, and any contused dead tissue is excised. After copious irrigation with normal saline solution, suction catheters are inserted through separate stab wounds in the skin and the wound is primarily closed. The limb is placed in 90°–90° skeletal traction, as already described. Appropriate antibiotics and tetanus antitoxin are administered. There is no justification for immediate internal fixation because the fracture is open and the bone ends are exposed. The suction catheters connected to the Hemovac are removed in two to three days. An open fracture ordinarily requires a longer period of time to consolidate.

PREADOLESCENT AND ADOLESCENT AGE GROUP

In patients 11 years of age and older, this author recommends primary treatment by closed reduction and maintenance of reduction by 90°–90° skeletal traction with a pin through the distal femur followed by immobilization in a one and one-half hip spica cast. This is the safest, simplest, and best method of management in the experience of this author; the results are excellent.

In the adolescent age group, closed or open reduction and internal fixation with intramedullary nailing is an alternative method of management that is favored by some authors.[15, 110, 132, 158, 195, 217, 245, 261, 280]

The use of external fixator (Orthofix or Ilizarov) is another way to immobilize the fractured femur in the adolescent and allow the patient to be ambulatory.[57, 231] The use of an external fixator is also indicated when there is associated head injury and the patient is comatose and difficult to control in traction.[84, 91]

Subtrochanteric fractures are best treated by 90°–90° skeletal traction with a pin through the distal femur. When callus forms and the fracture is relatively stable, the hip is gently extended to 45 degrees of flexion and the fracture is immobilized with the hip and knee in 45 degrees of flexion.[53, 122]

Complications

DISCREPANCY IN LIMB LENGTH

Inequality in limb length following femoral shaft fractures in children may result from excessive overriding or distraction of the fragments or from stimulation of linear growth. In the literature there are several "late follow-up" observations.* Aitken, in a study of the end-results in 71 cases of femoral shaft fractures in children, concluded that in children under 13 years of age, one should expect an average overgrowth of 1 cm. from the position at the time of discharge regardless of the method of treatment.[2] In a meticulous analysis of femoral shaft fractures in children, Greville and Ivins observed that, between the ages of four and eight years, an average overgrowth of 0.6 cm. can be expected in midshaft fractures; they also noted some added growth in the unbroken tibia on the same side as the fractured femur.[93]

Anderson, Griffin, and Green arrived at the following conclusions based upon serial data collected from the Growth Study of Children's Hospital Medical Center in Boston. A total of 107 patients were included in their study. (1) Between two and ten years of age, it is desirable for the fracture to heal with some overriding, but this should not exceed 1.5 cm. All children in this age group with displaced femoral fractures showed some stimulation of growth of the affected limb as compared with that of the normal side. (2) In children under two years of age and in adolescents, a similar degree of growth stimulation was not noted. This might be explained by the fact that in infants the fracture heals rapidly and there is a shorter period of hyperemia, and that in adolescents there are only a few years of growth remaining with a shorter period for relative acceleration of growth to operate on epiphyses that are less responsive to growth. Thus, in children under two years of age and in adolescents, they recommend end-to-end reduction and no overriding, since the degree of stimulation in these two age groups is usually small.[7]

Leg lengths should be carefully checked at periodic intervals following femoral shaft fractures to detect any significant discrepancy.

---

*See references 2, 3, 18, 21, 49, 51, 64, 70, 89, 93, 100, 104, 108, 119, 136, 141, 142, 148, 152, 159, 172, 209, 227, 236, 242, 254, and 263.

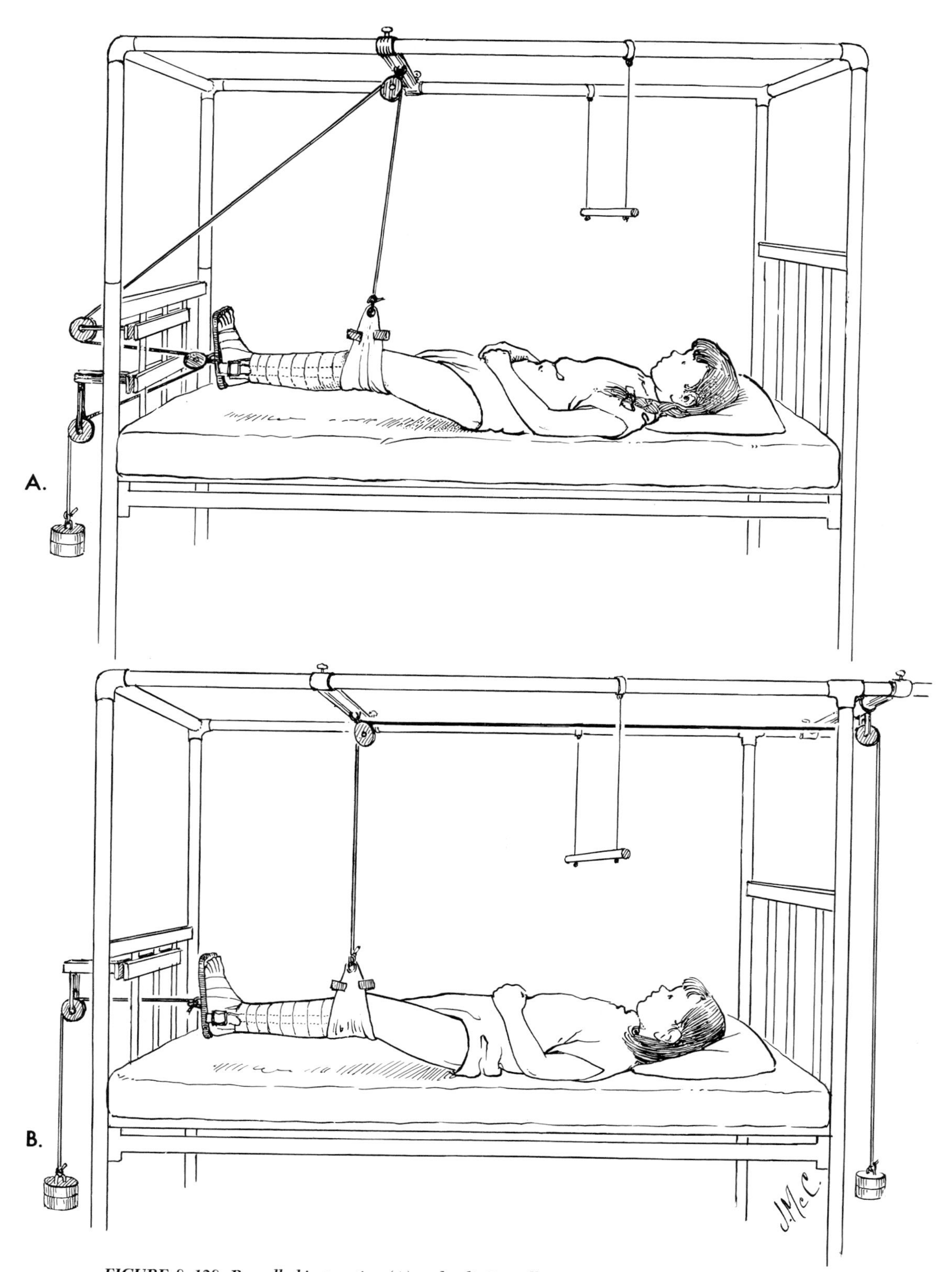

FIGURE 8–128. Russell skin traction (A) and split Russell traction (B). (See text for explanation.)

ANGULAR DEFORMITIES OF FEMORAL SHAFT

Linear growth of long bones takes place at the physis and epiphysis with the addition of new bone. Growth displaces angulation away from the end of the bone, instead of decreasing the angle. The remodeling of angular deformity is primarily a response to functional stresses on the femur by muscle pull and the force of gravity. Remodeling and changes in alignment occur slowly; this is in contrast to stimulation in rate of growth of the fractured femur, which occurs mostly during the first two years after injury.

Angular deformities occur more frequently in fractures of the proximal third of the femoral shaft, often with medial angulation, and correct themselves more slowly in the proximal third than in the distal two thirds.

Anderson, Griffin, and Green noted the rate of reduction of an angular deformity to be dependent upon the direction of angulation. In their series of cases within a five-year period, the average reduction of anterior bowing was 26 per cent, medial bowing 30 per cent, lateral bowing 46 per cent; and in 8 of the 11 who showed zero to 6 degrees of posterior bowing, it was more resistant to diminution through remodeling. They were unable to delineate the extremes of malalignment that will spontaneously correct themselves, as the patients in their series did not have severe angular deformities after reduction.[7]

Barford and Christiansen, in a follow-up study of 114 children with femoral shaft fractures 2 to 12 years following the original trauma, concluded that angulation of 25 degrees or less in the diaphyses of the femora can be expected to undergo sufficient correction with remodeling and growth so that a residual deformity is not apparent clinically, but may still be beyond normal limits when measured on the radiogram.[7, 18]

It is recommended that fracture fragments be aligned in as near normal a relationship as is possible and that angles that exceed the normal range by more than 15 degrees not be accepted. The surgeon should aim at complete absence of rotational deformity, and should strive to achieve angular deformities that do not exceed 10 degrees in the mediolateral direction, 15 degrees anteriorly, and 5 degrees posteriorly. These borderlines are easily obtainable with closed manipulative reduction, adequate supervised traction, and immobilization in hip spica cast.

References

1. Abbott, L. C.: Fractures of the femur: With special reference to the treatment of ununited and malunited cases by manipulation and caliper extension. Arch. Surg., *9*:413, 1924.
2. Aitken, A. P.: Overgrowth of the femoral shaft following fracture in children. Am. J. Surg., *49*:147, 1940.
3. Aitken, A. P., Blackett, C. W., and Cincotti, J. J.: Overgrowth of the femoral shaft fractures in children. J. Bone Joint Surg., *21*:334, 1939.
4. Alawneh, I.: Early fixation of femoral diaphysis fractures in multiple injuries in childhood. Med. Welt, *27*:1895, 1976.
5. Allen, B. L., Jr., Kant, P., and Emery, F. E.: Displaced fractures of the femoral diaphysis in children. Definitive treatment in a double spica cast. J. Trauma, *17*:8, 1977.
6. Allen, B. L., Jr., Schoch, E. P., and Emery, F. E.: Immediate spica cast system for femoral shaft fractures in infants and children. South. Med. J., *71*:18, 1978.
7. Anderson, M., Griffin, P. P., and Green, W. T.: Femoral shaft fractures in childhood. A report of later changes in growth and angulation of the injured bone. Personal communication.
8. Anderson, R. L.: Conservative treatment of fractures of the femur. J. Bone Joint Surg., *49-A*:1371, 1967.
9. Anderson, W. A.: The significance of femoral fractures in children. Ann. Emerg. Med., *11*:174, 1982.
10. Anischenko, S. M., Sultanskaia, E. A., and Oleksiuk, D. I.: Results of treatment of fractures of the long tubular bones in children. Vestn. Khir., *112*:84, 1974.
11. Aronson, D. D., Singer, R. M., and Higgins, R. F.: Skeletal traction for fractures of the femoral shaft in children. A long-term study. J. Bone Joint Surg., *69-A*:1435, 1987.
12. Asher, A., Tippett, W., Rockwood, A., Jr., and Zilber, S.: Compression fixation of subtrochanteric fractures. Clin. Orthop., *117*:202, 1976.
13. Ashhurst, A. C., and Newell, W. A.: Conservative treatment of fractures of the femur. Ann. Surg., *48*:749, 1908.
14. Axton, J. H., Bhagat, B. B., Rittey, D. A., Davies, J. C., and Dube, A.: Domiciliary management of simple femoral fractures in children. S. Afr. Med. J., *52*:27, 1977.
15. Baijal, E.: Instances in which intramedullary nailing of child's fracture is justifiable. Injury, *7*:181, 1976.
16. Barba, L., Augereau, B., and Apoil, A.: False aneurysm of the profunda femoris artery after external fixation for an open femoral fracture. Ann. Chir., *35*:48, 1981.
17. Barfield, G. A., Versfeld, G. A., and Schepeo, A.: Overgrowth following femoral fractures in children. J. Bone Joint Surg., *61-B*:256, 1979.
18. Barford, B., and Christiansen, J.: Fractures of the femoral shaft in children with special reference to subsequent overgrowth. Acta Chir. Scand., *116*:235, 1958–1959.
19. Benum, P., Ertresvag, K., and Hoiseth, K.: Torsion deformities after traction treatment of femoral fractures in children. Acta Orthop. Scand., *50*:87, 1979.
20. Berbeek, H. O., Bender, J., and Sawidis, K.: Rotational deformities after fractures of the femoral shaft in childhood. Injury, *8*:43, 1976.
21. Bisgard, J. D.: Longitudinal overgrowth of long bones with special reference to fractures. Surg. Gynecol. Obstet., *62*:823, 1936.
22. Bjerkreim, I., and Benum, P.: Genu recurvatum: A late complication of tibial wire traction in fractures of the femur in children. Acta Orthop. Scand., *46*:1012, 1975.

23. Bloch, R.: Les fractures de cuisse chez l'enfant. Rev. Orthop., *9*:447, 1922.
24. Blomquist, E., and Rudstrom, P.: Über Femurfrakturen bei Kindern unter besondere Beruchsichtigung des gesteigerten Langenwachstums. Acta Chir. Scand., *88*:267, 1943.
25. Blount, W. P.: Fractures in Children. Baltimore, Williams & Wilkins, 1955.
26. Blount, W. P., Schaefer, A. A., and Fox, G. W.: Fractures of the femur in children. South. Med. J., *37*:481, 1944.
27. Bombelli, R.: Risultati anatomo-funzionali della frattura dia fisaria del femore nei bambini. Minerva Orthop., *6*:125, 1955.
28. Bowker, P., Pratt, D. J., McLauchlan, J., and Wardlaw, D.: Early weight-bearing treatment of femoral shaft fractures using a cast-brace: A preliminary biomechanical study. J. Bioeng., *2*:463, 1978.
29. Breck, L.: Treatment of femoral shaft fractures in children. Clin. Orthop., *1*:109, 1953.
30. Broca, A.: Fractures du fémur chez les enfants. Bull. Soc. Chir. Paris, *47*:973, 1921.
31. Brouwer, K. J., Molenaar, J., and Vanlinge, B.: Rotational deformities after femoral shaft fractures in children. A retrospective study 27–32 years after the accident. Acta Orthop. Scand., *52*:81, 1981.
32. Brown, P. E., and Preston, E. T.: Ambulatory treatment of femoral shaft fractures with a cast brace. J. Trauma, *15*:860, 1975.
33. Brug, E., Beck, H., and Kraus, G.: Surgery of long-bone fractures in children using Hackethal's bundle nail. Zentralbl. Chir., *100*:466, 1975.
34. Bryant, J. D.: Operative Surgery. New York, Appleton, 1901.
35. Bryant, T.: The Practice of Surgery. London, J. & A. Churchill, 1876, Vol. 2, p. 405.
36. Buck, G.: An improved method of treating fractures of the thigh illustrated by cases and a drawing. Trans. N.Y. Acad. Sci., *2*:232, 1861.
37. Burdick, C. G., and Siris, I. E.: Fractures of the femur in children. Treatment and end result in 286 cases. Ann. Surg., *77*:736, 1923.
38. Burks, R. T., and Sutherland, D. H.: Stress fracture of the femoral shaft in children: Report of two cases and discussion. J. Pediatr. Orthop., *4*:614, 1984.
39. Burton, V. W., and Fordyce, A. J.: Immobilization of femoral shaft fractures in children aged 2–10 years. Injury, *4*:47, 1972.
40. Burwell, H. N.: Fractures of the femoral shaft in children. Postgrad. Med. J., *45*:617, 1969.
41. Bush, L.: Treatment of the fractured femur in children. Am. J. Surg., *64*:375, 1944.
42. Cail, W. S., Keats, T. E., and Sussman, M. D.: Plastic bowing fracture of the femur in a child. A.J.R., *130*:780, 1978.
43. Campden, K.: Concerning the treatment of fractures of the femur in children. Arch. Orthop. Trauma. Surg., *96*:305, 1980.
44. Cannon, S. R., and Pool, C. J.: Traumatic separation of the proximal femoral epiphysis and fracture of the mid-shaft of the ipsilateral femur in a child. A case report and review of the literature. Injury, *15*:156, 1983.
45. Carr, B. W.: The management of fractures of the shaft of the femur. Surg. Clin. North Am., *45*:53, 1965.
46. Childress, H. M.: Distal femoral 90-90 traction for shaft fractures of the femur in children. Orthop. Rev., *8*:45, 1979.
47. Christensen, E. E., and Dietz, G. W.: A radiographically documented intra-uterine femoral fracture. Br. J. Radiol., *51*:830, 1978.
48. Clark, W. A.: Fractures of the femur in children. J. Bone Joint Surg., *8*:273, 1926.
49. Clement, D. A., and Colton, C. L.: Overgrowth of the femur after fracture in childhood. J. Bone Joint Surg., *68-B*:534, 1986.
50. Cole, W. H.: Results of treatment of fractured femurs in children with especial reference to Bryant's overhead traction. Arch. Surg., *5*:702, 1922.
51. Cole, W. H.: Compensatory lengthening of the femur in children after fracture. Ann. Surg., *32*:609, 1925.
52. Colley, J. D., and Roper, H. A.: Experience in the treatment of femoral shaft fractures using a Vitrathene cast brace. Prosthet. Orthot. Int., *2*:76, 1978.
53. Colley, J. D., and Tachdjian, M. O.: Fractures of the proximal one-third of the femur in children: Efficacy of 90–90 traction. Personal communication from the Department of Orthopedic Surgery, The Children's Memorial Hospital, Chicago, Illinois.
54. Connolly, F., Dehne, E., and Lafollette, B.: Closed reduction and early cast-brace ambulation in the treatment of femoral fractures. Part II: Results in one hundred and forty-three fractures. J. Bone Joint Surg., *55-A*:1581, 1973.
55. Conwell, H. E.: Acute fractures of the shaft of the femur in children. J. Bone Joint Surg., *11*:593, 1929.
56. Crotwell, W.: The thigh-lacer: Ambulatory non-operative treatment of femoral shaft fractures. J. Bone Joint Surg., *60-A*:112, 1978.
57. Dabezies, E. J., D'Ambrosia, R., Shoji, H., Norris, R., and Murphy, G.: Fractures of the femoral shaft treated by external fixation with the Wagner device. J. Bone Joint Surg., *66-A*:360, 1984.
58. Dame, N. G., Ter-Egiazarov, G. M., and Osmanov, R.: Comparative evaluation of methods of treating diaphyseal fractures of the femur in children. Ortop. Travmatol. Protez., *32*:1, 1971.
59. Dameron, T. B., Jr., and Thompson, H. A.: Femoral shaft fractures in children. Treatment by closed reduction and double spica cast immobilization. J. Bone Joint Surg., *41-A*:1201, 1959.
60. Damholt, V., and Zdravkovic, D.: Quadriceps function following fractures of the femoral shaft in children. Acta Orthop. Scand., *45*:756, 1974.
61. Dashevski, I. F.: Treatment of open fractures of the femoral diaphysis. Ortop. Travmatol. Protez., *34*:79, 1974.
62. Daum, R., Jungbluth, K. H., Metzger, E., and Hecker, W. C.: Results of treatment of subtrochanteric and supracondylar femoral fractures in children. Chirurgie, *40*:217, 1969.
63. Daum, R., Metzger, E., Kurschner, J., and Hecker, W. C.: Analysis and late results of femur shaft fractures in children. Comparison of conservative and surgical therapy. Arch. Orthop. Unfallchir., *66*:18, 1969.
64. David, V. C.: Shortening and compensatory overgrowth following fractures of the femur in children. Arch. Surg., *9*:438, 1924.
65. Dehne, E., and Immermann, E.: Dislocation of the hip combined with fracture of the shaft of the femur on the same side. J. Bone Joint Surg., *33-A*:731, 1951.
66. Denton, J. S., and Manning, M. P. R. A.: Femoral nerve block for femoral shaft fractures in children. J. Bone Joint Surg., *70-B*:84, 1988.
67. Desault, P. J.: A Treatise on Fractures, Luxations, and Other Affections of the Bones. Philadelphia, Kimber & Conrad, 1811.
68. Deubelle, A., Vanneuville, G., Tanguy, A., and Levai, J. P.: Fractures of the femoral shaft in children. Apropos of a homogeneous series of 97 fractures. Rev. Chir. Orthop., *69*:513, 1983.

69. Dorrance, G. M.: Fracture of the femur in children. Ann. Surg., *105*:584, 1937.
70. Edvardsen, P., and Syversen, S. M.: Overgrowth of the femur fracture of the shaft in childhood. J. Bone Joint Surg., *58-B*:339, 1976.
71. Eikenbary, C. F., and LeCocq, J. F.: Fractures of the femur in children. J. Bone Joint Surg., *14*:801, 1932.
72. Eliason, E. L.: Results of treatment of 115 cases of fracture of the shaft of the femur at the University of Pennsylvania Hospital. Ann. Surg., *74*:206, 1921.
73. Engels, M., Lassnig, I., and Menzl, M.: Die konservative Behandlung der Oberschenkelfrakturen. Z. Kinderchir., *20*:79, 1977.
74. Estes, W. L.: Fractures of the femur. Ann. Surg., *64*:74, 1916.
75. Fardon, D. F.: Fracture of the neck and shaft of same femur. J. Bone Joint Surg., *52-A*:797, 1970.
76. Fardon, D. F.: Femoral shaft fractures with ipsilateral hip dislocation in a child. J.A.C.E.P., *7*:159, 1978.
77. Farkas, B., Bak, Z., and Fazekas, I.: Femoral fractures in childhood. Beitr. Orthop. Traumatol., *30*:143, 1983.
78. Fedoseeva, M. A., Makhmudova, K. M., Tukhtaev, Z. T., and Fuzailov, V.: Late treatment results in closed femoral fracture in children. Ortop. Travmatol. Protez., *12*:59, 1982.
79. Ferry, A. M., and Edgar, M. S.: Modified Bryant's traction. J. Bone Joint Surg., *48-A*:533, 1966.
80. Festge, O. A., Tischer, W., and Reding, R.: Operative and conservative treatment of femoral fractures in children. Zentralbl. Chir., *100*:473, 1975.
81. Firor, W. M.: The use of plaster in the treatment of fractured femurs. Bull. Johns Hopkins Hosp., *35*:412, 1924.
82. Fraser, R. D., Hunter, G. A., and Waddell, J. P.: Ipsilateral fracture of the femur and tibia. J. Bone Joint Surg., *60-B*:510, 1978.
83. Freuler, F., Wiedmer, U., and Bianchini, D.: Cast Manual for Adults and Children. New York, Springer, 1979.
84. Fry, K., Hoffer, M. M., and Brink, J.: Femoral shaft fractures in brain-injured children. J. Trauma, *16*:371, 1976.
85. Gallant, A. E.: Van Arsdale's triangular splint in thirty-three cases of fracture of the femur in infants and children under six years. J.A.M.A., *29*:1239, 1897.
86. Gatti, G.: Le fratture del femore nell' Infanzia. Arch. Atti. Soc. Ital. Chir., *27*:359, 1921.
87. Generowicz, Z., and Prezerwa-Tetmajer, A.: Our modification of skeletal traction in the treatment of femoral shaft fractures in children. Chir. Narzadow Ruchu Ortop. Pol., *40*:409, 1975.
88. Gibson, J.: Multiple injuries: The management of the patient with a fractured femur and a head injury. J. Bone Joint Surg., *42-B*:425, 1960.
89. Gibson, P. H., Papaioannou, T., and Kenwright, J.: The influence on the spine of leg-length discrepancy after femoral fractures. J. Bone Joint Surg., *65-B*:584, 1983.
90. Gillquist, J., Reiger, A., Sjodahl, R., and Bylund, P.: Multiple fractures of a single leg. Acta Chir. Scand., *139*:167, 1973.
91. Glenn, N., Miner, E., and Peltier, F.: The treatment of fractures of the femur in patients with head injuries. J. Trauma, *13*:348, 1973.
92. Gottschalk, E., and Ackermann, A.: Rush pin and pelvis-leg splint in pediatric femoral fractures. Zentralbl. Chir., *102*:1449, 1977.
93. Greville, N., and Ivins, J.: Fractures of the femur in children: An analysis of their effect on the subsequent length of both bones in the lower unit. Am. J. Surg., *93*:376, 1957.
94. Greville, N. R., and Jones, J. M.: An experimental study of overgrowth after fractures. Surg. Gynecol. Obstet., *105*:717, 1957.
95. Griffin, P.: Fractures of the femoral diaphysis in children. Orthop. Clin. North Am., *7*:633, 1976.
96. Griffin, P. P., Anderson, M., and Green, W. T.: Fractures of the shaft of the femur. Orthop. Clin. North Am., *3*:213, 1972.
97. Gross, R. H., and Stranger, M.: Causative factors responsible for femoral fractures in infants and young children. J. Pediatr. Orthop., *3*:341, 1983.
98. Gross, R. H., Davidson, R., Sullivan, J., Peeples, R. E., and Hufft, R.: Cast brace management of the femoral shaft fracture in children and young adults. J. Pediatr. Orthop., *3*:572, 1983.
99. Grossbard, G. D., and Love, B. R.: Femoral nerve block: A simple and safe method of instant analgesia for femoral shaft fractures in children. Aust. N.Z. J. Surg., *49*:592, 1979.
100. Hagglund, G., Hansson, K. I., and Norman, O.: Correction by growth of rotational deformity after femoral fracture in children. Acta Orthop. Scand., *54*:858, 1983.
101. Hamilton, F. H.: A Practical Treatise on Fractures and Dislocations. 8th Ed. Philadelphia, Lea Brothers, 1891.
102. Hedberg, E.: Femoral fractures in children. Acta Chir. Scand., *90*:568, 1945.
103. Hedlung, R., and Lindgren, U.: The incidence of femoral shaft fractures in children and adolescents. J. Pediatr. Orthop., *6*:47, 1986.
104. Hedstrom, O.: Growth stimulation of long bones after fracture or similar trauma. A clinical and experimental study. Acta Orthop. Scand. (Suppl.), *122*:1, 1969.
105. Helal, B., and Skevis, X.: Unrecognised dislocation of the hip in fractures of the femoral shaft. J. Bone Joint Surg., *49-B*:293, 1967.
106. Henderson, O. L., Morrissy, R. T., Gerdes, M. H., and McCarthy, R. E.: Early casting of femoral shaft fractures in children. J. Pediatr. Orthop., *4*:16, 1984.
107. Henriksson, L., Henrikson, B., and Blomberg, T.: Torsion in femoral fractures in childhood. A longitudinal investigation. Acta Radiol. [Diagn.] (Stockh.), *24*:213, 1983.
108. Henry, A. N.: Overgrowth after femoral shaft fractures in children. J. Bone Joint Surg., *45-B*:222, 1963.
109. Herzog, B., Affolter, P., and Jani, L.: Spätbefunde nach Marknagelung kindlicher Femurfrakturen. Z. Kinderchir., *19*:74, 1976.
110. Hiemer, W., Gerstner, C., Hopf, G., Aleksic, D., and Jaschke, W.: Operative treatment of femoral shaft fractures in infancy by Kuntscher nailing. Zentralbl. Chir., *105*:1503, 1980.
111. Hildebrandt, G.: Late results of conservatively treated thigh fractures in children. Dtsch. Gesundheitsw., *20*:1528, 1965.
112. Hinz, R.: X-ray studies of fractures healed with deformity. Arch. Klin. Chir., *161*:49, 1930.
113. Hirsch, C., and Evans, F.: Studies on some physical properties of infant compact bone. Acta Orthop. Scand., *35*:300, 1965.
114. Hoeksema, H., Olsen, C., and Rudy, R.: Fracture of femoral neck and shaft and repeat neck fracture in a child. J. Bone Joint Surg., *57-A*:271, 1975.
115. Holmes, S. J., Sedgwick, D. M., and Scobie, W. G.: Domiciliary gallows traction for femoral shaft fractures in young children. Feasibility, safety and advantages. J. Bone Joint Surg., *65-B*:288, 1983.
116. Horst, J. M.: The prognosis of defective callus in fractures of the lower extremity in the child. Acta Chir. Belg., *60*:27, 1961.
117. Hsu, J. D., and Garcia-Ariz, M.: Fracture of the

femur in the Duchenne muscular dystrophy patient. J. Pediatr. Orthop., *1*:203, 1981.
118. Humberger, F. W., and Eyring, E. J.: Proximal tibial 90–90 traction in treatment of children with femoral shaft fractures. J. Bone Joint Surg., *51-A*:499, 1969.
119. Hunter, Y., and Hensinger, R.: Premature monomelic growth arrest following fracture of the femoral shaft. A case report. J. Bone Joint Surg., *60-A*:850, 1978.
120. Hupfauer, W., and Balan, J.: Die konservative Behandlung kindlicher Oberschenkelfrakturen und ihre Ergebnisse. Monatsschr. Unfallheilkd., *74*:441, 1971.
121. Irani, R., Nicholson, T., and Chung, S. M. K.: Long-term results in the treatment of femoral-shaft fractures in young children by immediate spica immobilization. J. Bone Joint Surg., *58-A*:945, 1976.
122. Ireland, C. R., and Fisher, R. L.: Subtrochanteric fractures of the femur in children. Clin. Orthop., *110*:157, 1975.
123. Jani, L., and Morscher, E.: Prinzipien der Behandlung von posttraumatischen Wachstumsstörungen. 63. Kongress der Deutschen Gesellschaft für Orthopädie und Traumatologie. Z. Orthop., *115*:586, 1977.
124. Johnson, K. D., Johnston, D. W. C., and Parker, B.: Comminuted femoral-shaft fractures: Treatment by roller traction, cerclage wires and an intramedullary nail, or an interlocking intramedullary nail. J. Bone Joint Surg., *66-A*:1222, 1984.
125. Johnston, L. B.: The treatment of fractures of the shaft of the femur in children. Arch. Surg., *10*:730, 1925.
126. Jones, J. P.: The treatment of fractures of the femur from an orthopaedic point of view. J. Orthop. Surg., *2*:13, 1920.
127. Jones, S. G., and Cotton, F. J.: Ischaemic paralysis of leg simulating Volkmann's contracture. J. Bone Joint Surg., *17*:659, 1935.
128. Judet, J., and Judet, R.: Traitement des fractures de cuisse chez l'enfant. Rev. Chir. Orthop. Paris, *39*:658, 1953.
129. Katz, J.: Spontaneous fractures in paraplegic children. J. Bone Joint Surg., *35-A*:220, 1953.
130. Kavanaugh, H.: Occult infected fracture of the femur: Report of two cases with long-term followup. J. Trauma, *18*:813, 1978.
131. Kidner, F. C., and Laxoff, C. B.: Muscle interposition: A cause of delayed union in fracture of the femur. J.A.M.A., *79*:200, 1922.
132. Kirby, R. M., Winquist, R. A., and Hansen, S. T., Jr.: Femoral shaft fractures in adolescents: A comparison between traction plus cast treatment and closed intramedullary nailing. J. Pediatr. Orthop., *1*:193, 1981.
133. Kirmisson, E.: Des fractures du femur au cours de ankyloses du genou chez l'enfant. Bull. Med., *24*:767, 1910.
134. Klems, H., and Weigert, M.: Stable osteosynthesis of femoral fractures in childhood. Indications and method. Chirurg, *44*:511, 1973.
135. Knenn, R., and Graf, R.: Results of internal fixation of femoral shaft fractures in children. Acta Chir. Austriaca, *9*:1, 1977.
136. Kohan, L., and Cumming, W. J.: Femoral shaft fractures in children: The effect of initial shortening on subsequent limb overgrowth. Aust. N.Z. J. Surg., *52*:141, 1982.
137. Kristensen, A. E.: Femoral and tibial fractures of the same leg. Resident Staff Physician, *136*:1, 1977.
138. Kumar, R.: Treatment of fracture of femur in children by a "cast-brace." Int. Surg., *67*:551, 1982.
139. Kunze, K., and Grohs, M.: Follow-up study of 124 juvenile femoral shaft fractures. Hefte Unfallheilkd., *158*:150, 1982.
140. LaDuca, J. N., Bone, L. L., Seibel, R. W., and Border, J. R.: Primary open reduction and internal fixation of open fractures. J. Trauma, *20*:580, 1980.
141. von Laer, L.: Overgrowth of the femoral shaft and rotation deformities following femoral shaft fractures in childhood. Arch. Orthop. Unfallchir., *89*:121, 1977.
142. von Laer, L., and Herzog, B.: Leg length differences and rotation defects after femoral shaft fractures in childhood. Therapeutic influence and spontaneous correction. Helv. Chir. Acta, *45*:17, 1978.
143. Lansche, W. E., Mishkin, M. R., and Stamp, W. G.: The management of complications of femoral shaft fractures in children. South. Med. J., *56*:1001, 1963.
144. Lee, W., and Veal, J.: The Russell extension method in the treatment of fractures of the femur. Surg. Gynecol. Obstet., *56*:492, 1933.
145. Lefort, J.: Fractures of the femoral shaft in children. Ann. Chir., *35*:51, 1981.
146. LeMesurier, A. B.: The treatment of fractures of the shaft of the femur in children. Am. J. Surg., *49*:140, 1940.
147. Lennert, K. A., and Lucic, J.: Experience with proximal fractures of the femur in childhood. Bruns. Beitr. Klin. Chir., *220*:620, 1973.
148. Levander, G.: Increased growth of long bones of the lower extremities after they have been fractured. Acta Chir. Scand., *65*:5, 1929.
149. Lidge, R. T.: Complications following Bryant's traction. J. Bone Joint Surg., *41-A*:1540, 1959.
150. Ligier, J. N., Metaizeau, J. P., Prevot, J., and Lascombes, P.: Elastic stable intramedullary nailing of femoral shaft fractures in children. J. Bone Joint Surg., *70-B*:74, 1988.
151. Litchman, H. M., and Duffy, J.: Lower-extremity balanced traction. A modification of Russell traction. Clin. Orthop., *66*:144, 1969.
152. Lorenz, G. L., Rossi, P., Quaglia, F., Parenti, G., DeGuidi, G., and Pelilli, E.: Growth disturbances following fractures of femur and tibia in children. Ital. J. Orthop. Traumatol., *11*:133, 1985.
153. Louis, D. L., and Eyring, E. J.: Supplemental phosphate in children with femoral fractures. Clin. Orthop., *68*:149, 1970.
154. McCarthy, R. E.: A method for early spica cast application in treatment of pediatric femoral shaft fractures. J. Pediatr. Orthop., *6*:89, 1986.
155. McCollough, N. C., Vinsant, J. E., Jr., and Sarmiento, A.: Functional fracture-bracing of long-bone fractures of the lower extremity in children. J. Bone Joint Surg., *60-A*:314, 1978.
156. McMurray, T. P.: Thomas and his splint. Br. Med. J., *1*:872, 1946.
157. Malkawi, H., Shannak, A., and Hadidi, S.: Remodeling after femoral shaft fracture in children treated by the modified Blount method. J. Pediatr. Orthop., *6*:421, 1986.
158. Mann, D. C., Weddington, J., and Davenport, K.: Closed Ender nailing of femoral shaft fractures in adolescents. J. Pediatr. Orthop., *6*:651, 1986.
159. Meals, R.: Overgrowth of the femur following fractures in children: Influence of handedness. J. Bone Joint Surg., *61-A*:381, 1979.
160. Mesko, J. W., DeRosa, G. P., and Lindseth, R. E.: Segmental femur loss in children. J. Pediatr. Orthop., *5*:471, 1985.
161. Mikulicz, J.: Ueber individuelle Formdifferenzen am Femur und an der Tibia des Menschen. Arch. Anat. Physiol., *1*:351, 1878.
162. Metaizeau, J-P.: Osteosynthese Chez L'Infant. Montpellier, Sauramps Medicale, 1988.
163. Miller, D. S., Markin, L., and Grossman, E.: Ischemic fibrosis of the lower extremity in children. Am. J. Surg., *84*:317, 1952.

164. Miller, M. E., Bramlett, K. W., Kisell, E. U., and Niemann, K. M. W.: Improved treatment of femoral shaft fractures in children. The "pontoon" 90–90 spica cast. Clin. Orthop., *219*:140, 1987.
165. Mital, M. A., and Cashman, W. A.: Fresh ambulatory approach to treatment of femoral shaft fractures in children—a comparison with traditional conservative methods. J. Bone Joint Surg., *58-A*:285, 1976.
166. Moen, H., and Solheim, K.: Femoral shaft fractures in children. Tidsskr. Nor. Laegeforen., *96*:939, 1976.
167. Mohan, K.: Fracture of the shaft of the femur in children. Int. Surg., *60*:282, 1975.
168. Moore, R. A., and Schafer, E. W.: Treatment of simple fracture of the shaft of the femur by a fixed traction spica. A preliminary report. N.C. Med. J., 9:514, 1948.
169. Moorhead, E. L.: Fracture of the femur in a boy five years of age; open treatment following failure of nonoperative methods. Surg. Clin. Chicago, *3*:1215, 1919.
170. Moorhead, J. J.: Transfixation method of treatment of fractured femur in children. Med. Rec., *85*:1098, 1918.
171. Morita, S.: Surgical treatment of femur shaft fractures in children. Arch. Jpn. Chir., *36*:627, 1967.
172. Morita, S., and Oda, H.: Surgical treatment of femoral-shaft fractures in children. Nippon Geka Hokan, *36*:627, 1967.
173. Mrzena, V.: Fractures of the proximal femoral end in childhood. Acta Chir. Orthop. Traumatol. Cech., *43*:82, 1976.
174. Muller, M. E., Allgower, M., Schneider, R., and Willenegger, H.: Manual of Internal Fixation. 2nd Ed. New York, Springer, 1979.
175. Mustard, W. T., and Simmons, E. H.: Experimental arterial spasm in the lower extremities produced by traction. J. Bone Joint Surg., *35-B*:437, 1953.
176. Myrwold, H., Andersson, T., and Christoffersson, E.: Femoral fractures in children. Nord. Med., *86*:1595, 1971.
177. Nahoda, J., and Stryhal, F.: The problem of spontaneous overgrowth of the femur after childhood fracture. Acta Chir. Orthop. Traumatol. Cech., *36*:211, 1969.
178. Neer, C., Grantham, S., and Foster, R.: Femoral shaft fracture with sciatic nerve palsy. J.A.M.A., *214*:2307, 1970.
179. Neer, C. S., II, and Cadman, E. F.: Treatment of fractures of the femoral shaft in children. J.A.M.A., *163*:634, 1957.
180. Nemsadze, V. P.: Surgical treatment of tubular bone fractures in children. Vestn. Khir., *94*:73, 1965.
181. Nicholson, J. T., Foster, R. M., and Heath, R. D.: Bryant's traction: A provocative cause of circulation complications. J.A.M.A., *157*:415, 1955.
182. Niemann, F., Gunther, D., and Sykosch, H. J.: Conservative therapy for intraosseous fixation of femoral and tibial fractures. Zentralbl. Chir., *92*:701, 1967.
183. Nilsson, B., and Westlin, N.: Restoration of bone mass after fracture of the lower limb in children. Acta Orthop. Scand., *42*:78, 1971.
184. Nogi, J.: Non-union of a closed fracture in a child's femoral shaft. Va. Med., *107*:568, 1980.
185. Norman, O.: Roentgenographic determination of rotational displacement in fractures of the femur. Acta Orthop. Scand., *50*:353, 1979.
186. Oberhammer, J.: Degree and frequency of rotational deformities after infant femoral fractures and their spontaneous correction. Arch. Orthop. Trauma. Surg., 97:249, 1980.
187. Obletz, B. E.: Vertical traction in the early management of certain compound fractures of the femur. J. Bone Joint Surg., *28*:113, 1946.
188. Oeconomas, N.: Follow-up results of fractures of the femoral shaft in children. Rev. Orthop., *34*:375, 1948.
189. Ogden, J. A.: Skeletal Injury in the Child. Philadelphia, Lea & Febiger, 1982, pp. 488–505.
190. Ogden, J. A., Gossling, H. R., and Southwick, W. O.: Slipped capital femoral epiphysis following ipsilateral femoral fracture. Clin. Orthop., *110*:167, 1975.
191. Olesen, A.: Blockade of the femoral nerve in femoral shaft fractures. Ugeskr. Laeger, *141*:2613, 1979.
192. Omer, H., and Penndorf, K.: Femoral fractures in childhood. Results of a several-years-long follow-up. Chirurg, *38*:284, 1967.
193. Orr, T. G.: Conservative treatment of fractures of the femur in children. J. Kans. Med. Soc., *26*:55, 1926.
194. Osterwalder, A., Beeler, C., Huggler, A., and Matter, P.: Lengthwise growth of the lower extremities after shaft fractures in children. Helv. Chir. Acta, *45*:23, 1978.
195. Pankovich, A. M., Goldflies, M. L., and Pearson, R. L.: Closed Ender nailing of femoral-shaft fractures. J. Bone Joint Surg., *61-A*:222, 1979.
196. Parvinen, T., Viljanto, J., Paananen, M., and Vilkki, P.: Torsion deformity after femoral fracture in children. Ann. Chir. Gynaecol. Fenn., *62*:25, 1973.
197. Patterson, H., and Scott, W.: Ten years' experience with femoral shaft fractures. J. Trauma, *15*:958, 1975.
198. Pavlik, A.: Treatment of obstetrical fractures of the femur. J. Bone Joint Surg., *21*:939, 1939.
199. Pazolt, H. J., and Thomas, E.: Surgical treatment of the femoral fracture in childhood. Beitr. Orthop. Traumatol., *21*:472, 1974.
200. Pease, C. N.: Fractures of the femur in children. Surg. Clin. North Am., *37*:213, 1957.
201. Pick, J. W., Stack, J. K., and Anson, B. J.: Measurements on the human femur: I. Lengths, diameters and angles. Quart. Bull. Northwest. Univ. Med. School, *15*:281, 1941; *17*:121, 1943.
202. Piroth, P., and Bliesner, J. A.: Rotationsfehlstellung nach konservativer Behandlung kindlicher Oberschenkelschaft-Frakturen. Z. Kinderchir., *20*:172, 1977.
203. Pochon, J. P., and Schwobel, M.: Femoral shaft fractures. Ther. Umsch., *40*:965, 1983.
204. Potts, F., and Dunham, W.: Fractures of the femur in children. N.Y. State J. Med., *49*:2541, 1949.
205. Powell, H. D.: Domiciliary gallows traction for femoral shaft fractures in young children. Br. Med. J., 3:108, 1972.
206. Prey, D., and Foster, J.: Fracture of the femoral shaft: Comparative study of the present methods of treatment. Am. J. Surg., 25:116, 1934.
207. Probst, J.: Juvenile femoral shaft fracture and the physician's responsibility for care. Hefte Unfallheilkd., *158*:162, 1982.
208. Rang, M.: Children's Fractures. Philadelphia, Lippincott, 1983.
209. Raugstad, T. S., Alho, A., and Hvidsten, K.: Growth correction of misalignment following femoral shaft fractures in children. Tidsskr. Nor. Laegeforen., *99*:1460, 1979.
210. Reding, R.: On the treatment of femoral fractures in children. Dtsch. Gesundheitsw., *21*:87, 1966.
211. Reynolds, D. A.: Growth changes in fractured long bones. A study of 126 children. J. Bone Joint Surg., *63-B*:83, 1981.
212. Rice, J. D.: A new method of treating femoral fractures in the infant. Lancet, *2*:1130, 1900.
213. Richard, A.: Vertical extension therapy in femoral shaft fractures in children. Med. Welt, *12*:673, 1969.

214. Rippstein, J.: Zur Bestimmung der Antetorsion des Schenkelhalses mittels zweier Röntgenaufnahmen. Z. Orthop., *86*:345, 1955.
215. Roberts, B.: Management of fractures and fracture complications of the femoral shaft using the ASIF compression plate. J. Trauma, *17*:20, 1977.
216. Robinson, W.: Treatment of birth fractures of the femur. J. Bone Joint Surg., *20*:778, 1938.
217. Romer, K. H., and Reppin, G.: Medullary nailing of femoral fractures in childhood. Zentralbl. Chir., *98*:170, 1973.
218. Rosenberg, N. M., Vranesich, P., and Bottenfield, G.: Fractured femurs in pediatric patients. Ann. Emerg. Med., *11*:84, 1982.
219. Rosental, J., Gasper, M., Gjerdrum, T., and Newman, J.: Vascular injuries associated with fractures of the femur. Arch. Surg., *110*:494, 1975.
220. Roser, L. A.: Initial spica cast for femoral shaft fractures in children. Northwest Med., *68*:1012, 1969.
221. Russell, R.: Theory and method in extension of the thigh. Br. Med. J., *2*:637, 1921.
222. Russell, R. H.: Fractures of the femur. Br. J. Surg., *11*:491, 1924.
223. Ryan, J. R.: 90–90 skeletal femoral traction for femoral shaft fractures in children. J. Trauma, *21*:46, 1981.
224. Saimon, L. P.: Refracture of the shaft of the femur. J. Bone Joint Surg., *46-B*:32, 1964.
225. Saxier, U.: The treatment of femoral shaft fractures in children with Weber's vertical extension. Helv. Chir. Acta, *41*:271, 1974.
226. Schedl, R., and Fasol, P.: Follow-up study of femoral shaft fractures in children. Unfallchirurgie, *7*:249, 1981.
227. Schenk, K. M.: Der Femurschaftbruch beim Kind: Spätergebnisse. Arch. Klin. Chir., *286*:144, 1957.
228. Schonk, J. W.: Comparative follow-up study of conservative and surgical treatment of femoral shaft fractures in children. Arch. Chir. Neerl., *30*:231, 1978.
229. Schoppmeier, K.: Treatment of femoral fractures of children with the "Weber-Bock." A possibility of avoiding torsion displacement and resultant complication. Chirurg, *48*:348, 1977.
230. Schvingt, E., Jacquemaire, B., Babin, S., and Katzner, M.: L'enclouage d'alignement des fractures diaphysaires du femur. Rev. Chir. Orthop., *62*:1371, 1976.
231. Schwarz, N.: External fixation as the treatment method of femoral fracture in the child. Unfallheilkunde, *86*:359, 1983.
232. Schwemmle, K.: Traction therapy of femoral shaft fractures in infants. Chirurg, *40*:425, 1969.
233. Schwemmle, K.: Treatment of femoral shaft fractures in children. Zentralbl. Chir., *94*:1226, 1969.
234. Scott, J., Wardlaw, D., and McLauchlan, J.: Cast bracing of femoral shaft fractures in children: A preliminary report. J. Pediatr. Orthop., *1*:199, 1981.
235. Seimon, L.: Re-fracture of the shaft of the femur. J. Bone Joint Surg., *46-B*:32, 1964.
236. Shapiro, F.: Fractures of the femoral shaft in children. The overgrowth phenomenon. Acta Orthop. Scand., 52:649, 1981.
237. Silver, D.: A modification of the Bradford frame for the treatment by suspension of the fracture of the femur in young children. Ann. Surg., *49*:105, 1909.
238. Sokolova, V. N.: Fractures of the femoral diaphysis in children. Ortop. Travmatol. Protez., *28*:56, 1967.
239. Speed, K.: Analysis of the results of treatment of fractures of the femoral diaphysis in children under twelve years of age. Surg. Gynecol. Obstet., *32*:527, 1921.
240. Spinner, M., Freundlich, B. D., and Miller, I. J.: Double-spica technic for primary treatment of fractures of the shaft of the femur in children and adolescents. Clin. Orthop., *53*:109, 1967.
241. Splain, S. H., and Denno, J. J.: Immediate double hip spica immobilization as the treatment for femoral shaft fractures in children. J. Trauma, *25*:994, 1985.
242. Staheli, L. T.: Femoral and tibial growth following femoral shaft fractures in childhood. Clin. Orthop., *55*:159, 1967.
243. Staheli, L. T., and Sheridan, G. W.: Early spica cast management of femoral shaft fractures in young children. Clin. Orthop., *126*:162, 1977.
244. Stern, W. O.: Successful method of treating fracture of the femur in infancy. N.Y. Med. J., *81*:992, 1905.
245. Stock, H. J.: Intramedullary nailing of childhood femoral-shaft fractures while protecting the growth zones. Zentralbl. Chir., *103*:1072, 1978.
246. Stryker, H. H.: Safe traction in children with fractured femurs. J.A.M.A., *160*:388, 1956.
247. Sugi, M., and Cole, W. G.: Early plaster treatment for fractures of the femoral shaft in childhood. J. Bone Joint Surg., *69-B*:743, 1987.
248. Swiontkowski, M. F., Hansen, S. T., Jr., and Kellam, J.: Ipsilateral fractures of the femoral neck and shaft. A treatment protocol. J. Bone Joint Surg., *66-A*:260, 1984.
249. Szentpetery, J., and Papp, L.: The treatment of femoral shaft fractures in childhood. Arch. Orthop. Unfallchir., *61*:19, 1967.
250. Tessore, A., and Koszla, M. M.: The treatment of fractures of the femur in children. Minerva Ortop., *16*:651, 1965.
251. Teutsch, W.: Nachuntersuchungsergebnisse kindlicher Femur-schaftfrakturen. Zentralbl. Chir., *94*:1761, 1969.
252. Thompson, S. A., and Mahoney, L. J.: Volkmann's ischemic contracture: Relationship to fracture of the femur. J. Bone Joint Surg., *33-B*:336, 1951.
253. Tittel, K., Tittel, M., Gerhard, R., and Schauwecker, F.: Treatment of femoral shaft fractures in the growing skeleton. Beitr. Orthop. Traumatol., *27*:559, 1980.
254. Truesdell, E. D.: Inequality of lower extremity following fracture of the shaft of the femur in children. Ann. Surg., *74*:498, 1921.
255. VanEden, P. H.: Results in the treatment of fractures of the shaft of the femur. Acta Chir. Scand., *67*:320, 1930.
256. Velasco, R. U., and Comfort, T. H.: Analysis of treatment problems in subtrochanteric fractures of the femur. J. Trauma, *18*:513, 1978.
257. Vengerovski, I. S.: On the technic of skeletal traction in fracture of the femoral bone in children. Khirurgiia (Mosk.), *42*:115, 1966.
258. Verbeek, H. O. F., Bender, J., and Sawidis, K.: Rotational deformities after fractures of the femoral shaft in childhood. Injury, *8*:43, 1976.
259. Viljanto, J., Kiviluoto, H., and Paananen, M.: Remodelling after femoral shaft fracture in children. Acta Chir. Scand., *141*:360, 1975.
260. Viljanto, J., Linna, M. I., Kiviluoto, H., and Paananen, M.: Indications and results of operative treatment of femoral shaft fractures in children. Acta Chir. Scand., *141*:366, 1975.
261. Vinz, H.: Intermedullary nailing of femoral shaft fractures in childhood. Zentralbl. Chir., *97*:90, 1972.
262. Vontobel, V., Genton, N., and Schmid, R.: Die Spätergebnisse der lindlichen dislozierten Femurschaftfraktur. Helv. Chir. Acta, *28*:655, 1961.
263. Walsh, M. G.: Limb lengths following femoral shaft fracture in children. J. Ir. Med. Assoc., *66*:447, 1973.
264. Wardlaw, D.: The cast-brace treatment of femoral shaft fractures. J. Bone Joint Surg., *59-B*:411, 1977.

265. Warmbrod, G., Yelton, L., and Weiss, B.: Intramedullary nailing of femoral shaft fractures. Clin. Orthop., *114*:282, 1976.
266. Weber, B. G.: Inwieweit sind isolierte extreme Torsionsvarianten der unteren Extremitat als Deformitaten aufzufassen und welche klinische Bedeutung kommt ihnen zu? Z. Orthop., *94*:287, 1961.
267. Weber, B. G.: Zur Behandlung kindlicher Femurschaftbruche. Arch. Orthop. Unfallchir., *54*:713, 1963.
268. Weber, B. G.: Prophylaxe Achsenfehlstellungen bei der Behandlung kindlicher Frakturen. Z. Unfallmed. Berufskr., *1*:80, 1966.
269. Weber, B. G.: Fractures of the femoral shaft in childhood. Injury, *1*:65, 1969.
270. Weicz, G. M., Rang, M., and Salter, R. B.: Posttraumatic fat embolism in children. J. Trauma, *13*:529, 1973.
271. West, W.: Treatment of fractures in children by the use of skeletal traction. South. Med. J., *26*:644, 1933.
272. Widenhorn, H., and Faller, A.: The treatment of fractures of the femur in children—the results in eighty-eight cases. Int. Clin., *4*:168, 1934.
273. Wilder, M. C., and Evans, E. B.: Fractures of the femoral shaft treated surgically. Comparative results of early and delayed operative stabilization. J. Bone Joint Surg., *60-A*:489, 1978.
274. Winant, E. M.: The use of skeletal traction in the treatment of fractures of the femur. J. Bone Joint Surg., *31-A*:87, 1949.
275. Winquist, R. A., Hansen, S. T., and Clawson, D. K.: Closed intramedullary nailing of femoral shaft: A report of five hundred and twenty cases. J. Bone Joint Surg., *66-A*:529, 1984.
276. Wondr, A. E., and Doubravsk, Y. J.: Femoral fractures in children and their treatment. Rozhl. Chir., *44*:681, 1965.
277. Yano, S., and Sawada, M.: Rotationsfehler nach kindlichen Femurschaftfrakturen. Z. Orthop., *113*:119, 1975.
278. Yruegas, F.: Treatment of fractures of the femur in children. Medicina (Madr.), *33*:415, 1965.
279. Ziv, I., and Rang, M.: Treatment of femoral fracture in the child with head injury. J. Bone Joint Surg., *65-B*:276, 1983.
280. Ziv, I., Blackburn, N., and Rang, M.: Femoral intramedullary nailing in the growing child. J. Trauma, *24*:432, 1984.

FRACTURES INVOLVING THE DISTAL FEMORAL EPIPHYSIS

The ossification center of the distal femoral epiphysis is present at birth and becomes fused with the diaphysis between the eighteenth and nineteenth years. The largest and most actively growing epiphysis in the body, it contributes to 70 per cent of the length of the femur and 40 per cent of that of the entire lower limb.

The distal femoral epiphysis includes the entire articular surface of the lower end of the femur. The points of origin of the two heads of the gastrocnemius muscle and of the plantaris muscle are from the posterior surface of the distal diaphysis; the ligaments are attached to the medial and lateral femoral condyles. The bony configuration of the knee joint is such that in no position are the bones in more than partial contact. Thus, the strength of the knee joint is derived from the ligaments that surround it and not from the contour of the bones. An excessive force applied on the knee joint will put tension on the ligaments; when this strain is of sufficient degree, the epiphysis will separate from the diaphysis.

Fractures involving the distal femoral physis are rare, constituting 1 per cent of all physeal injuries. They may occur at any age before 17 years, the greatest incidence being between 11 and 15 years.

In the pre-automobile era when horse-drawn vehicles were the means of transportation, this injury was of common occurrence and was known as the "cartwheel" fracture. Boys stealing rides, while trying to board moving wagons from the rear, would get a leg or foot caught in the spokes of the rear wheel. Forced hyperextension of the knee was produced by the traction imparted by the rotatory force of the revolving rear wheel. The distal femoral epiphysis was displaced anteriorly, while the distal end of the diaphysis was forced into the popliteal space, lacerating or contusing the popliteal vessels or tibial nerve. These fractures were often open and were later complicated by gas-bacillus or tetanus infection. The extremely serious nature of this injury at that time is reflected by the report of Hutchinson, in 1894, who presented the end-results of 58 cases; among the 30 patients with open fractures, there were 10 deaths; and of the remaining 20, 17 required amputation. Of the 28 closed fractures, reduction could not be obtained in 12 cases, 6 of which developed sloughs, necessitating amputation in 4. Only 16 of the 28 closed fractures could be reduced with good end-results.[26] Fortunately, this gloomy picture has altered today; however, trauma to the distal femoral physis is still a serious problem and may be the source of troublesome complications. For a critical review of the early literature, which is particularly voluminous in the latter part of the nineteenth century, the reader is referred to Poland.[44]

Mechanism of Injury and Pathologic Anatomy

Separation of the distal femoral epiphysis is caused by a sudden severe force applied in the region of the knee joint. With changes in the means of transportation, the scene of injury has moved to the highway, the football field, and the farm. About 50 per cent of the cases are caused by automobile accidents, 20 per cent by football injuries, 15 per cent by falls from a height, and the remaining 15 per cent by miscellaneous accidents such as stepping in a hole, catching the foot in a moving wheel, or being dragged by a horse. Fractures involving the distal femoral physis can be divided into the following types according to the direction of the force causing the injury:

Abduction (Valgus) Type. This is caused by a blow to the lateral side of the distal femur, usually occurring on the high school football field (the adult who receives the same kind of trauma will sustain tears of the medial collateral ligament, medial meniscus, and cruciate ligament). The result is a Type II (Salter-Harris) physeal injury. The periosteum is ruptured on the medial side and the distal femoral epiphysis is displaced laterally with a lateral fragment of the metaphysis. It is usually associated with some rotation. This fracture may reduce itself spontaneously and may be missed if the triangular piece of metaphyseal bone is small. One should carefully scrutinize the radiogram and take special abduction stress views to detect the lesion, if indicated. Caution! Abduction type injuries often masquerade as strain or tear of the medial collateral ligament.

Hyperextension Type. This was the common variety in the wagon wheel injury of old times. The distal femoral epiphysis is displaced anteriorly by the hyperextension force and by the pull of the contraction of the quadriceps muscle. The periosteum on the posterior aspect is torn and the fibers of the gastrocnemius muscle are stretched or partially torn. The triangular metaphyseal bone fragment and the intact periosteal hinge are anterior in location. The distal end of the femoral shaft is driven posteriorly into the soft tissues of the popliteal fossa, where it may injure the popliteal vessels as well as the common peroneal or posterior tibial nerves.

Hyperflexion Type. Posterior displacement of the distal femoral epiphysis is extremely rare. It results from a forceful flexion injury caused by a direct blow on the distal femur.

Type IV (Salter-Harris) Physeal Injury. In a fourth variety, the fracture line traverses the joint surface as well as the physis. It is usually sustained as a result of an automobile accident or a fall from a height, and results from longitudinal thrust and lateral compressional forces. The fracture may be comminuted. In this injury, the prognosis for subsequent growth is very poor; often it is associated with Salter-Harris Type V growth plate injury.

A fifth type of distal femoral physeal trauma *(injury to the perichondrial ring)* occurs when the upper attachment of the collateral ligament is avulsed with a small part of the perichondrium and underlying bone. Injuries to the perichondrial ring will result in bony bridging between the epiphysis and metaphysis. The localized asymmetrical premature growth arrest will lead to progressive angular deformity. Occasionally, displacement of the perichondrial ring will produce a traumatic exostosis. Injuries to the perichondrial ring of the distal femoral physis are very rare.

Diagnosis

The child is presented in the emergency room with a history of violent injury to the lower limb. He is in severe pain and unable to bear weight on the affected leg. The knee is markedly swollen, tense, and held in partial flexion. Any attempt at passive extension of the joint is restricted and guarded by muscle spasm. There may be obvious deformity, with genu valgum in lateral displacements. In anterior displacements the femoral condyles may be palpable anterior to the distal diaphysis. The lower end of the femoral shaft or a large hematoma may be felt in the popliteal fossa. The pulsations of the posterior tibial and dorsalis pedis arteries may be absent, and the leg and foot may be cold and cyanotic.

Radiograms will disclose the fracture (Figs. 8–129 and 8–130). As stated previously, in abduction fractures the radiograms may be misinterpreted as normal unless one meticulously looks for the triangular piece of metaphyseal bone or takes special abduction strain views.

Treatment

The method of reduction depends upon the type of fracture. Ordinarily a general anesthetic is required to obtain adequate relaxation of the limb and the patient. The markedly swollen joint is aspirated to facilitate reduction.

ABDUCTION TYPE FRACTURES

These are simple to treat. There are no special problems of vascular injury or growth disturbance. The technique of reduction is as

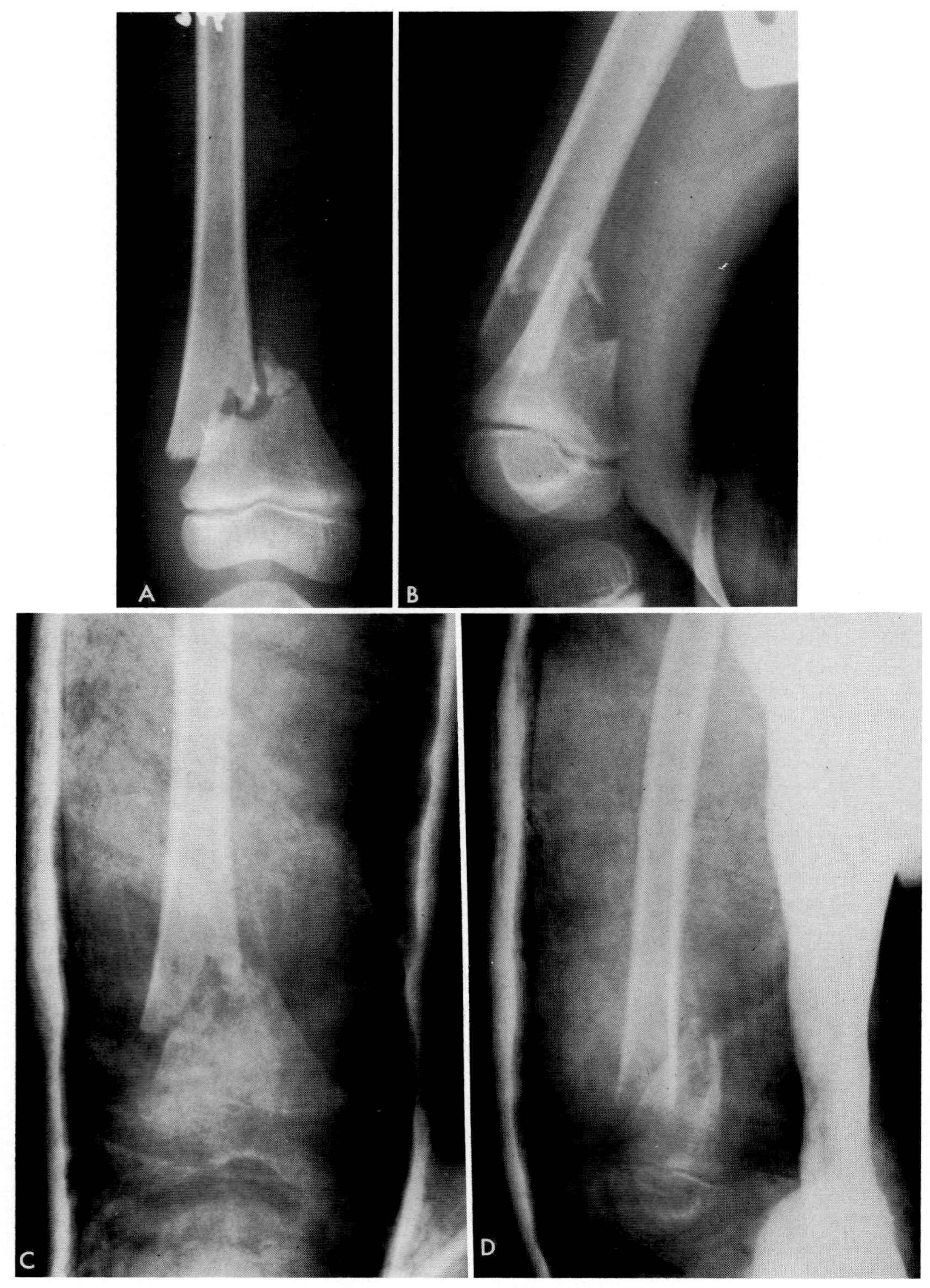

FIGURE 8–129. Remodeling of supracondylar fracture of distal femur.

A and **B.** Initial radiograms. **C** and **D.** In cast. Note posterior angulation of distal fragment.

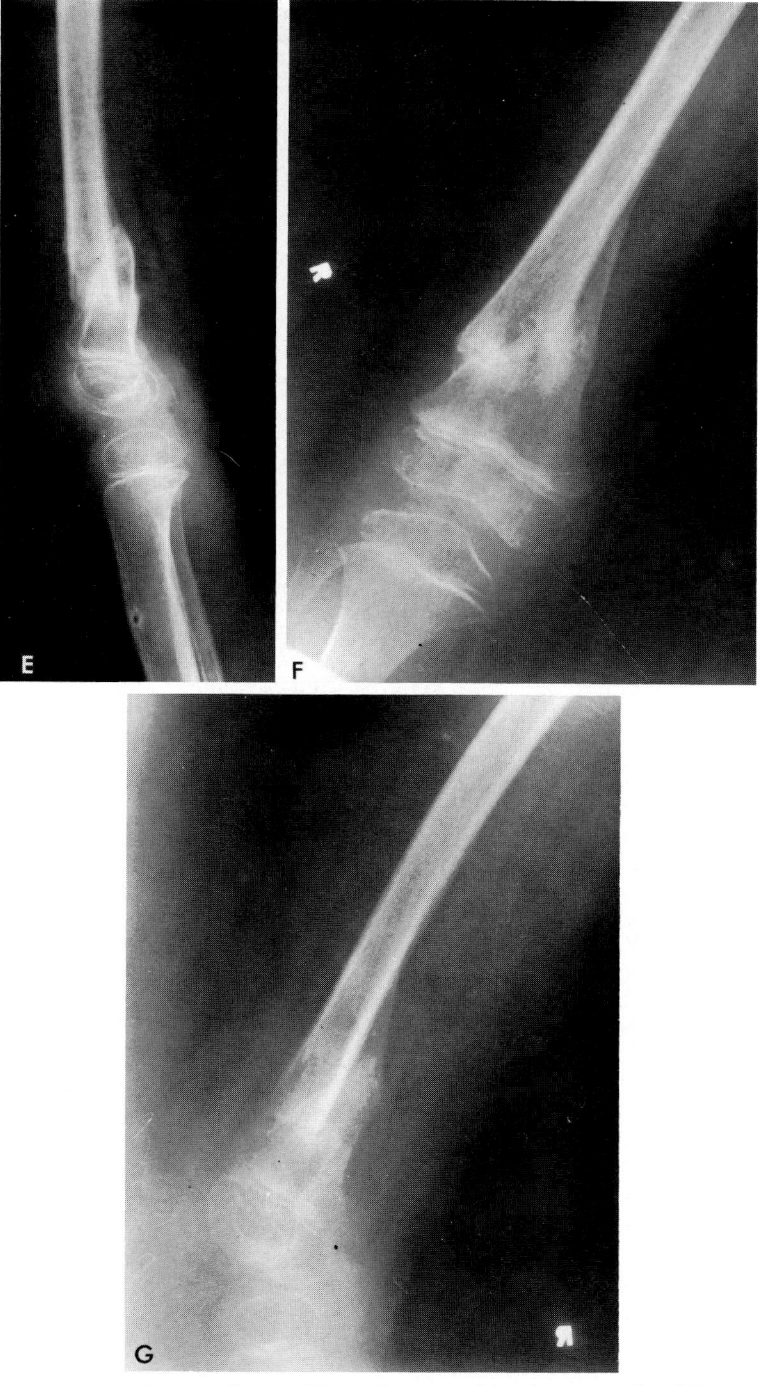

FIGURE 8–129 Continued. Remodeling of supracondylar fracture of distal femur.

E to **G.** Remodeling of angular deformity in the plane of knee motion.

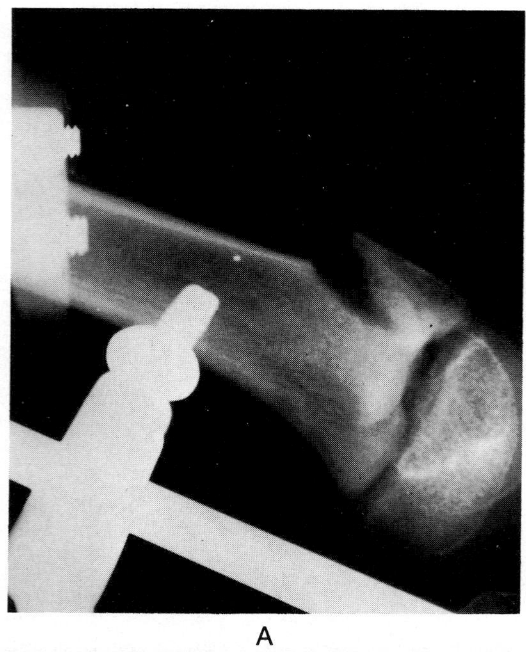

A

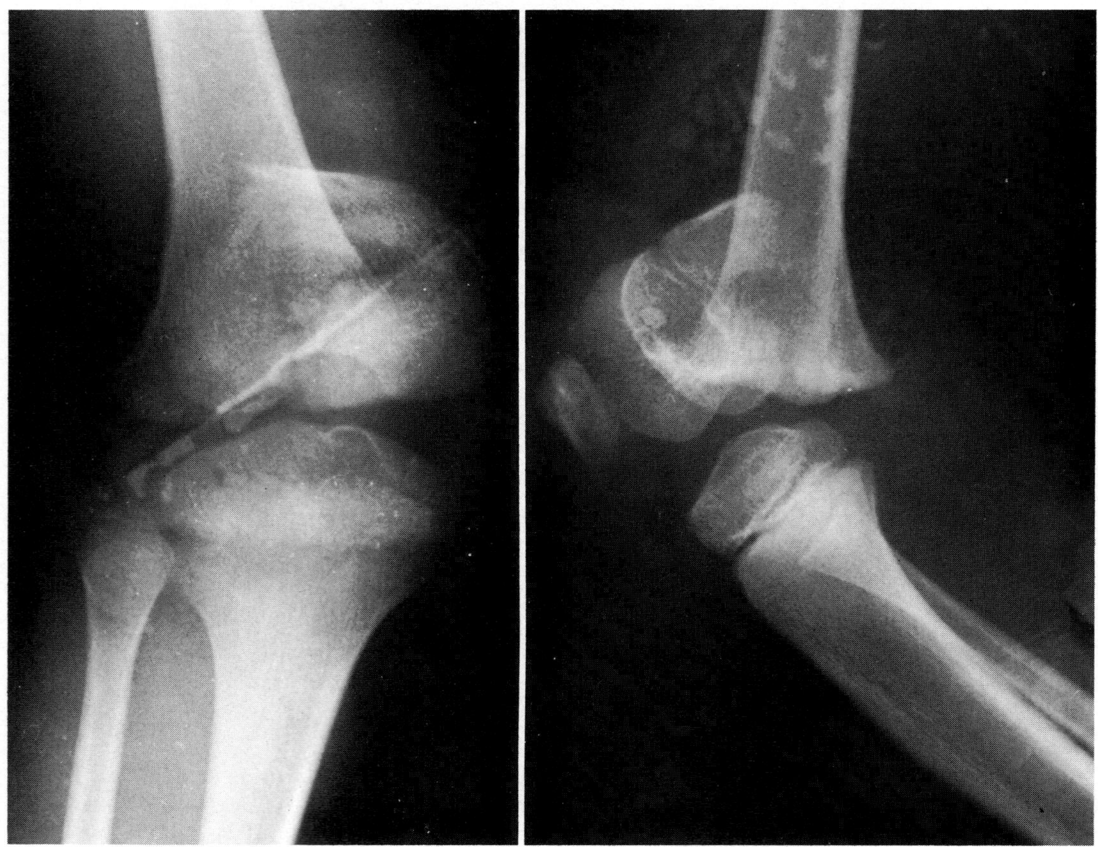

B

FIGURE 8–130. ***Type II (Salter and Harris) fracture involving the distal femoral physis.***

A. Minimally displaced. **B.** Markedly displaced.

follows: The anesthetized patient is placed on the fracture table with both feet strapped on the footplates. Longitudinal traction is applied on the extended knee. Reduction is accomplished by direct manual pressure, pushing the laterally displaced distal epiphysis medially and the lower end of the femoral shaft laterally. The fracture is held in a single hip spica cast. The knee is immobilized in extension. The three points of fixation—laterally at the ankle and the greater trochanter, and medially at the knee—are well padded. If only an above-knee cast is applied, the fracture may become displaced. Plaster immobilization is maintained for from four to six weeks.

HYPEREXTENSION TYPE FRACTURES

The hyperextension type of fracture presents several problems of management: first, the potential injury to the popliteal vessels, and second, the difficulty of achieving and maintaining reduction. Since the plane of displacement and the plane of the knee joint motion are in the same direction, there is lack of an adequate lever arm to grasp the distal fragment effectively. A closed reduction should be attempted first. The technique is as follows: The anesthetized patient is placed on the fracture table and the foot on the normal side is fastened to the footplate. The hip is flexed to relax the quadriceps muscle and the knee is flexed to relax the gastrocnemius and hamstring muscles. An assistant applies longitudinal traction on the lower leg, gradually increasing flexion of the knee; with his thumbs, the surgeon exerts direct pressure on the femoral epiphyses, pushing it first distally and then downward and posteriorly, while, with his other fingers, he pulls the lower femoral shaft anteriorly. Reduction is completed by acute flexion of the knee. Post-reduction radiograms are made to check restoration of the epiphysis to its normal anatomic position.

An alternative method of reduction (recommended by Rang) is to place the patient in prone position, apply distal traction, and while maintaining traction, lift the leg and foot to the ceiling and acutely flex the knee. Gravity, and if necessary, an assistant force the femoral shaft anteriorly. If reduction is successful, a single hip spica cast is applied, holding the knee in 60 to 90 degrees of flexion. The angle at which the knee is immobilized is of great importance in maintaining anatomic reduction. As pointed out by Aitken and Magill, recurrence of anterior displacement usually is caused by immobilization of the knee in insufficient flexion.[2]

In complete anterior displacements, a position of acute knee flexion may be necessary to maintain reduction (similar to supracondylar fracture of the humerus); however, immobilization of the knee in such a position may cause marked difficulty in regaining extension. In complete anterior displacements, it is best to insert heavy threaded Steinmann pins transversely in the distal femoral shaft well above the fracture site, and another pin in the proximal third of the tibia well distal to the physis and avoiding the apophysis of the proximal tibial tubercle. Assistants apply gentle skeletal traction to disengage the bone fragments as the surgeon reduces anterior displacement by manual pressure on the epiphysis. In the past this author incorporated the Steinmann pins in the cast. At present this author recommends to insert two smooth Steinmann pins, one through each femoral condyle into the diaphysis (similar to pinning a supracondylar fracture of the humerus). The use of image intensifier x-ray control makes percutaneous pinning simple. A hip spica cast is applied with the knee in 45 to 60 degrees of flexion. In three to four weeks, the cast and pins are removed and an above-knee cast is applied with the knee in 30 degrees of flexion. After two to three weeks, the second cast is removed, and active flexion-extension exercises are instituted to restore motor strength of the quadriceps muscle and joint motion. During this period the affected limb is protected by a three-point crutch gait. When the quadriceps muscle is of fair motor strength and the knee joint has attained complete extension, the crutches are discarded and full weight-bearing is allowed. Sometimes when knee motion is slow to return, a continuous passive knee motion machine is used to regain knee extension.

An alternative method of immobilization is by external fixator (Orthofix or Ilizarov). Open reduction of Type II (Salter-Harris) fractures is ordinarily not indicated. In anterior displacements of distal femoral epiphyses, angulation is in the plane of motion of the knee, and any deformity will be spontaneously corrected by remodeling.

If the patient is seen late and the interval between the injury and the initial manipulation is such that some healing has occurred, it is best to reduce the fracture by 90°–90° skeletal traction with a pin through the proximal tibia (cf. Fig. 8–125).

HYPERFLEXION TYPE FRACTURES

The posteriorly displaced distal femoral epiphysis is reduced as follows: The patient is placed on a fracture table with the normal limb fastened on the footplate. An assistant applies straight longitudinal traction on the injured side by pulling on the lower leg with the knee in complete extension. As the fragments are disengaged, the surgeon pulls the distal epiphyses anteriorly with one hand while pushing posteriorly on the lower end of the femoral shaft with the other. The reduced fracture is immobilized in a single hip spica cast with the knee in *complete extension.* To re-emphasize: At no time should the knee be immobilized in a position of semiflexion. Supracondylar fracture of the femur requires a position of knee flexion to relax the pull of the gastrocnemius muscle; since the fracture site is proximal to the origin of the heads of the gastrocnemius, the unopposed pull of this muscle results in a posterior displacement of the femoral condyle in relation to the diaphysis, and also flexion of the condyles in relation to the tibia (Fig. 8–131). Aitken and Magill have pointed out that in fractures involving the distal femoral physis, the fracture line is distal to the origin of the medial head of the gastrocnemius. Consequently, the distal femoral epiphysis may be posteriorly displaced, but does not become flexed on the tibia. With the knee fully extended, the medial head of the gastrocnemius is taut and provides a posterior dynamic splint, preventing posterior displacement of the reduced lower femoral epiphysis. When the knee joint is immobilized in flexion,

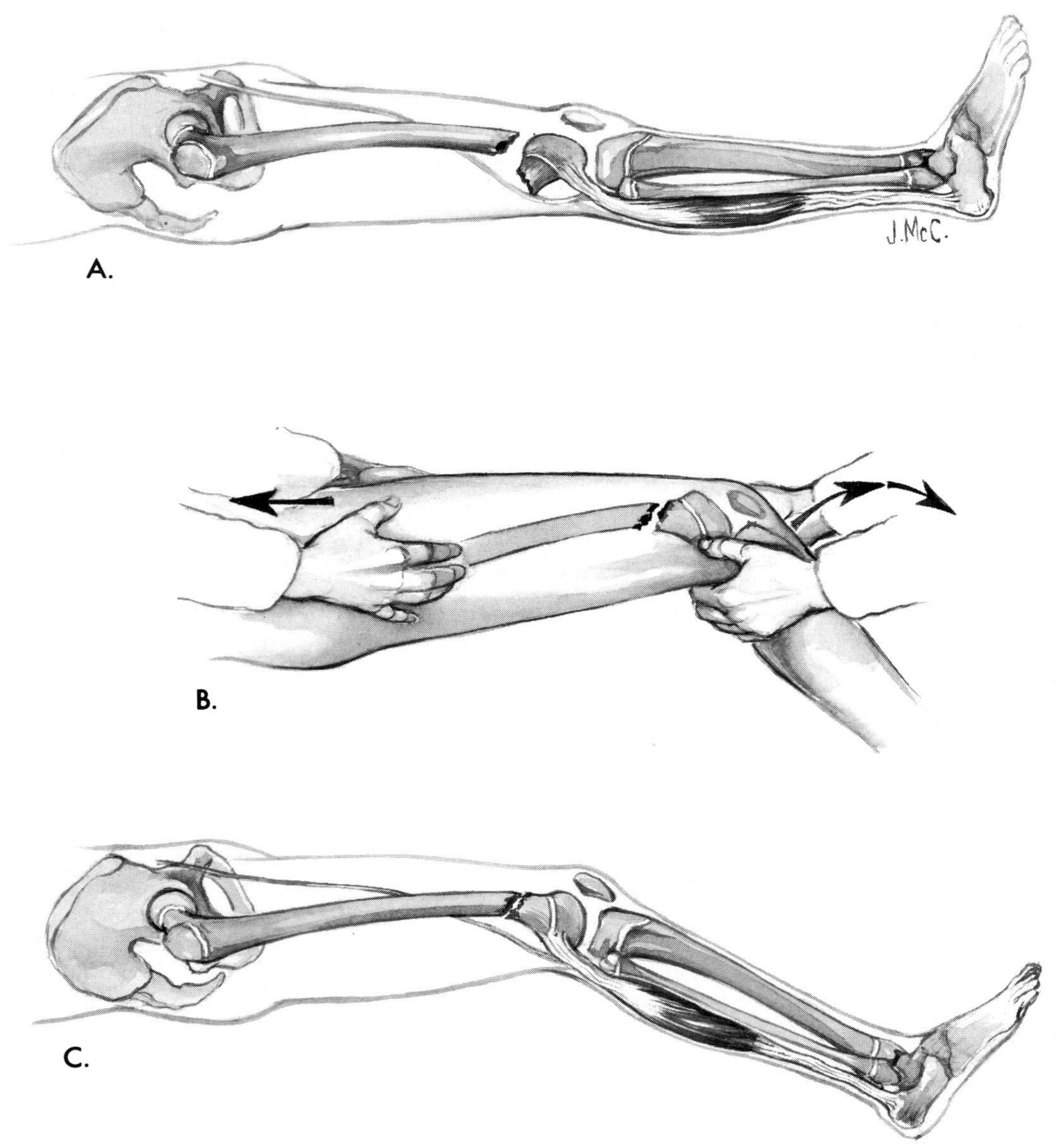

FIGURE 8–131. Technique of reduction of supracondylar fracture of distal femur.

the medial head of the gastrocnemius is relaxed and enhances posterior displacement of the femoral epiphysis.[2]

Type IV (Salter-Harris) fractures involving the distal femoral epiphysis often require open reduction and internal fixation with smooth Kirschner wires. During surgery, care should be taken that the blood supply to the epiphysis is preserved.

Injuries to the perichondrial ring are difficult to treat. Initial treatment consists of anatomic replacement of the ring. Later, when a bony bridge forms, it is excised and fat interposed at the site of the defect to prevent recurrence of bone bridging.

Problems and Complications

Loss of Alignment. This occurs because of instability of the fracture and a loose cast when swelling subsides. An unstable fracture may require open reduction if repeated manipulations are unsuccessful.

Vascular Injury. This occurs in less than 2 per cent of the fractures involving the distal femoral physis. It may be due to pressure, compression, or intimal tear or thrombosis. When the patient complains of pain with a cool and pale foot, it is important that vascular consultation be obtained and a femoral arteriogram performed.

Peroneal Nerve Paresis. This may occur because of stretching of the nerve by the anteriorly and medially displaced distal femoral epiphysis, or it may be iatrogenic during the rough manipulation of the injured limb at the time of closed reduction. If the nerve paresis persists for three months, nerve conduction and electromyographic studies are performed and repeated at six months post injury. If fibrillation of denervation and delayed nerve conduction persist, surgical exploration is indicated.

Growth Disturbance. Asymmetrical growth arrest will lead to progressive angular deformity. Linear and computed axial tomographic studies should be performed to protect the bony bridge and determine its size. If less than 50 per cent, the bony bridge is resected to prevent and correct progressive angular deformation.

Symmetrical growth arrest will cause progressive shortening. This is treated by equalization of limb lengths either by epiphysiodesis of the contralateral distal femur or by femoral lengthening, depending upon the severity of limb length disparity.

References

1. Abbott, L., and Gill, G.: Valgus deformity of the knee resulting from injury to the lower femoral epiphysis. J. Bone Joint Surg., *24*:97, 1942.
2. Aitken, A. P., and Magill, H. K.: Fractures involving the distal femoral epiphyseal cartilage. J. Bone Joint Surg., *34-A*:96, 1952.
3. Ansorg, P., and Graner, G.: The treatment of distal femoral fractures in childhood. Beitr. Orthop. Traumatol., *23*:359, 1976.
4. Bassett, F. H., III, and Goldner, L.: Fractures involving the distal femoral epiphyseal growth line. South. Med. J., *5*:545, 1962.
5. Bellin, H.: Traumatic separation of epiphysis of lower end of femur. Am. J. Surg., *37*:306, 1937.
6. Bertin, K. C., and Goble, E. M.: Ligament injuries associated with physeal fractures about the knee. Clin. Orthop., *177*:188, 1983.
7. Brashear, J. R., Jr.: Epiphyseal fractures of the lower extremities. South. Med. J., *51*:845, 1958.
8. Brashear, J. R., Jr.: Discussion of paper by Bassett, F., III, and Goldner, J. L.: Fractures involving the distal femoral epiphyseal growth line. South. Med. J., *55*:545, 1962.
9. Bright, R.: Operative correction of partial epiphyseal plate osseous bridge resection and silicone-rubber implant. J. Bone Joint Surg., *56-A*:655, 1974.
10. Burkus, J. K., and Ogden, J. A.: Development of the distal femoral epiphysis: A microscopic, morphological investigation of the zone of Ranvier. J. Pediatr. Orthop., *4*:661, 1984.
11. Burman, M. S., and Langsam, M. J.: Posterior dislocation of the lower femoral epiphysis in breech delivery. Arch. Surg., *38*:250, 1939.
12. Butler, J. E., Criswell, A. R., and Hand, W. I.: Abduction injuries of the distal femoral epiphysis. Clin. Orthop., *115*:189, 1976.
13. Bylander, B., Aronson, S., Egund, N., Hansson, L. I., and Selvik, G.: Growth disturbance after physeal injury of distal femur and proximal tibia studied by roentgen stereophotometry. Arch. Orthop. Trauma. Surg., *98*:225, 1981.
14. Caffey, J., Madell, S. H., Royer, C., and Morales, P.: Ossification of the distal femoral epiphysis. J. Bone Joint Surg., *40-A*:647, 1958.
15. Carlson, W. O., and Wenger, D. R.: A mapping method to prepare for surgical excision of a partial physeal arrest. J. Pediatr. Orthop., *4*:232, 1984.
16. Cassebaum, W. H., and Patterson, A. H.: Fractures of the distal femoral epiphysis. Clin. Orthop., *41*:79, 1965.
17. Cigala, F., Rega, A. N., and Lotito, F. M.: Growth disturbances following fracture of the femur and tibia in children. Ital. J. Orthop. Traumatol., *11*:121, 1985.
18. Criswell, A. R., Hand, W. L., and Butler, J. E.: Abduction injuries of the distal femoral epiphysis. Clin. Orthop., *115*:189, 1976.
19. DiLeo, P., Lispi, A., and Marciano, R.: Growth disturbances following fracture of the femur and tibia in children. Ital. J. Orthop. Traumatol., *11*:127, 1985.
20. Friedman, M. J., and Blevins, F.: Slipped distal femoral epiphyseal plate following closed manipulation of the knee. A case report. Am. J. Sports Med., *13*:201, 1985.
21. Griswold, A. S.: Early motion in the treatment of separation of the lower femoral epiphysis. J. Bone Joint Surg., *10*:75, 1928.
22. Grogan, D. P., and Bobechko, W. P.: Pathogenesis of a fracture of the distal femoral epiphysis. A case report. J. Bone Joint Surg., *66-A*:621, 1984.
23. Hagglund, G., Hansson, L. I., and Norman, O.: Correction by growth or rotational deformity after femoral fracture in children. Acta Orthop. Scand., *54*:858, 1983.
24. Healy, W. L., and Brooker, A. F., Jr.: Distal femoral fractures. Comparison of open and closed methods of treatment. Clin. Orthop., *174*:166, 1983.
25. Heller, E. P.: Fracture separation ("slipping") of the lower femoral epiphysis. J. Bone Joint Surg., *15*:474, 1933.

26. Hutchinson, J., Jr.: Lectures on injuries to the epiphysis and their results. Br. Med. J., *1*:669, 1894.
27. Kaplan, J. A., Sprague, S. B., and Benjamin, H. C.: Traumatic bilateral separation of the lower femoral epiphyses. J. Bone Joint Surg., *24*:200, 1942.
28. Kurlander, J. J.: Slipping of the lower femoral epiphysis. J.A.M.A., *96*:513, 1931.
29. Kusswetter, W., and Beck, E.: Therapeutic results in distal femoral injuries in childhood. Monatsschr. Unfallheilkd., *76*:245, 1973.
30. Langenskiöld, A.: An operation for partial closure of an epiphysial plate in children, and its experimental basis. J. Bone Joint Surg., *57-B*:325, 1975.
31. Lasi, C.: Etiopathogenetic considerations on an unusual case of intra-epiphyseal fracture of the distal end of the femur. Minerva Ortop., *17*:587, 1966.
32. Leavitt, P. H.: Traumatic separation of the lower femoral epiphysis. N. Engl. J. Med., *245*:565, 1951.
33. Lee, C. L., Pederson, H. E., and LaMont, R. L.: Fractures of the distal femoral epiphysis. Presented at the 44th meeting, A.A.O.S., February, 1977.
34. Levinthal, D. H.: Old traumatic displacement of the distal femoral epiphysis. J. Bone Joint Surg., *18*:199, 1936.
35. Lombardo, S. J., and Harvey, J. P.: Fractures of the distal femoral epiphyses. Factors influencing prognosis: A review of thirty-four cases. J. Bone Joint Surg., *59-A*:742, 1977.
36. Lorenzi, G. L., Rossi, P., Quaglia, F., Parenti, G., DeGuidi, G., and Pelilli, E.: Growth disturbances following fracture of the femur and tibia in children. Ital. J. Orthop. Traumatol., *11*:133, 1985.
37. Mize, R. D., Buchholz, R. W., and Grogan, D. P.: Surgical treatment of displaced, comminuted fractures of the distal end of the femur. J. Bone Joint Surg., *64-A*:871, 1982.
38. Neer, C. S.: Separation of the lower femoral epiphysis. Am. J. Surg., *99*:756, 1960.
39. Nerubay, J., and Pilderwasser, D.: Spontaneous bilateral distal femoral physiolysis due to scurvy. Acta Orthop. Scand., *55*:18, 1984.
40. Nicholson, J. T.: Epiphyseal fractures about the knee. A.A.O.S. Instr. Course Lect., *18*:74, 1961.
41. Padovani, J. P., Rigault, P., Raux, P., Liganc, F., and Guyonvarch, G.: Decollements epiphysaires traumatiques de l'extrémité inferieure du femur. Rev. Chir. Orthop., *62*:211, 1976.
42. Parrini, L., Paleari, M., and Biggi, F.: Growth disturbances following fracture of the femur and tibia in children. Ital. J. Orthop. Traumatol., *11*:139, 1985.
43. Patterson, W. J.: Separation of the lower femoral epiphysis. Can. Med. Assoc. J., *21*:301, 1929.
44. Poland, J.: Traumatic Separation of the Epiphyses. London, Smith, Elder & Co., 1898.
44a. Rang, M.: Children's Fractures. 2nd ed. Philadelphia, J. B. Lippincott, 1983, p. 279.
45. Rees, D.: Fracture-separation of the lower femoral epiphysis as a complication of the Sarmiento below-knee functional cast: A case report. Injury, *16*:117, 1984.
46. Riseborough, E. J., Barrett, I. R., and Shapiro, F.: Growth disturbances following distal femoral physeal fracture-separation. J. Bone Joint Surg., *65-A*:885, 1983.
47. Rumlova, E., Vogel, E., and Scharli, A. F.: Fractures of the distal femur in children. Ther. Umsch., *40*:969, 1983.
48. Schlesinger, A. E.: Distal femoral epiphysis: Normal standards for thickness and application to bone dysplasias. Radiology, *159*:515, 1986.
49. Seinsheimer, F., III: Fractures of the distal femur. Clin. Orthop., *153*:169, 1980.
50. Sideman, S.: Traumatic separation of the lower femoral epiphysis. J. Bone Joint Surg., *25*:913, 1943.
51. Simpson, W. C., Jr., and Fardon, D. F.: Obscure distal femoral epiphyseal injury. South. Med. J., *69*:1338, 1976.
52. Stephens, D. C., and Louis, D. S.: Traumatic separation of the distal femoral epiphyseal cartilage plate. J. Bone Joint Surg., *56-A*:1383, 1974.
53. Truesdell, E. D.: Birth Fractures and Epiphyseal Dislocations. New York, Paul B. Hoeber, 1917.
54. Weber, B. G., Brunner, C., and Freuler, F.: Treatment of Fractures in Children and Adolescents. New York, Springer-Verlag, 1980.
55. van der Werken, C., Marti, R. K., and Raaymakers, E. L.: Distal femoral fractures, results of operative treatment. Neth. J. Surg., *33*:230, 1981.

TRAUMATIC DISLOCATION OF THE PATELLA AND OSTEOCHONDRAL FRACTURES OF THE KNEE

In children, dislocation of the patella in a normal knee is a rather uncommon injury. It is usually a lateral dislocation caused by a direct blow in the inner side of the patella; occasionally it may result from violent muscle contraction when the knee is in adduction and flexion. Dislocation may be complete, especially when the quadriceps muscle is relaxed, the patella slipping over the lateral edge of the femoral condyle and resting on its lateral surface; or it may be incomplete, the patella riding on the lateral edge of the condyle.

The patellar displacement is accompanied by a variable degree of injury and tearing of the soft tissues on the inner side of the knee, namely the patellar retinaculum, the vastus medialis, the capsule, and the synovial membrane. Usually there is also hemorrhage into the joint. In incomplete dislocations the soft-tissue injury may be minimal, but in complete dislocations, there may be wide longitudinal tears.

When lateral dislocation of the patella is produced by muscle action only, and especially when it recurs, genu valgum, deficient development of the lateral femoral condyle, and contracture of the iliotibial band or a high-riding patella are additional pathogenetic factors.

In rare instances, the patella is displaced medially, or it may be rotated upon its longitudinal axis so that its articular surface faces forward.

Diagnosis

Often the patella reduces itself spontaneously on extension of the knee, or a bystander may push it back into its normal position. Only rarely does the orthopedic surgeon see the patella in a dislocated state in which the injured limb is completely useless, with pain and swelling in the knee. The knee is maintained in flexion, with definite limitation of further flexion. Active extension of the knee is impossible; it can, however, be extended passively in its abnormal position. The smooth anterior surface of the femoral condyles can be easily identified beneath the skin and subcutaneous tissues. Occasionally one may be able to palpate a longitudinal tear on the medial side of the joint capsule and patellar retinaculum. The knee joint is distended with fluid.

Diagnosis of a recently reduced dislocation of the patella is difficult. It is based on the history and clinical findings of hemarthrosis and tenderness on the medial aspect of the patella, which has abnormal lateral mobility.

Treatment

Ordinarily reduction is very easy. The hip is flexed to relax the rectus femoris, the knee is extended, and the patella is pushed forward and medially into its normal position. Occasionally, in a hypersensitive adolescent patient, general anesthesia may be necessary to perform the reduction. After reduction there is, of course, some effusion in the knee joint, but as a rule, aspiration of the joint is not necessary. The limb is immobilized in an above-knee walking cylinder cast with the knee in full extension for a period of three weeks. This provides adequate time for the torn soft tissues to heal.

Surgical intervention is indicated in the very rare case in which a definite wide rent in the medial capsule can be palpated. A medial parapatellar incision is employed for the exposure. The capsule is repaired and imbricated by sutures to prevent recurrence, and the limb is immobilized in a cast, as just described. After removal of the cast, muscle power is restored by progressive quadriceps exercises.

Treatment of the rare medial and rotatory dislocations is similar to that described for lateral dislocations, except that reduction is accomplished by pushing outward in a medial dislocation and derotating in rotatory dislocation.

Osteochondral fractures of the lateral femoral condyle or of the posterior articular surface of the patella may be caused by rapid lateral dislocation and spontaneous reduction of the patella. Sporadic cases have been reported in the literature; Rosenberg reported 15 such fractures and Ahstrom, 18 cases.[1, 43]

The injury usually occurs in an adolescent patient who twists his flexed knee into a valgus position; he then falls down, his knee giving way because of the severe pain. On examination, the knee is markedly distended with effusion; there is loss of full active knee extension, local tenderness over the lateral femoral condyle, and over the medial capsule and patellar retinaculum.

On pressing the patella against the femur, local pain is elicited. The fracture fragment may be seen as a loose body; however, it is often very thin and difficult to visualize in the initial x-ray films. If clinical findings suggest the knee should be aspirated, the joint fluid is usually found to be bloody; the presence of fat globules indicates an intra-articular fracture. An arthrogram will assist in making the diagnosis.

Treatment consists of removal of the loose fragment, and shaving down and drilling its site of origin. The procedure is performed by arthroscopy, if possible. When open arthrotomy is required to remove the loose fragment, the medial capsular tissues are imbricated. The knee is immobilized in a cast for four weeks.

References

1. Ahstrom, J. P.: Osteochondral fracture in the knee joint associated with hypermobility and dislocation of the patella. J. Bone Joint Surg., *47-A*:1491, 1965.
2. Blitzer, C. M., Johnson, R. J., Ettlinger, C. F., and Aggeborn, K.: Downhill skiing injuries in children. Am. J. Sports Med., *12*:142, 1984.
3. Cavlak, Y., and Rucker, P.: Overlooked osteochondral fractures of the knee-joint area among juveniles. Med. Klin., *73*:1555, 1978.
4. Chaklin, V. D.: Injuries to the cartilage of the patella and femoral condyles. J. Bone Joint Surg., *21*:133, 1939.
5. Cofield, H., and Bryan, S.: Acute dislocation of the patella: Results of conservative treatment. J. Trauma, *17*:526, 1977.
6. Coleman, H. M.: Recurrent osteochondral fracture of the patella. J. Bone Joint Surg., *30-B*:153, 1948.
7. Critchley, I. J., and Bracey, D. J.: The acutely locked knee—is a manipulation worthwhile? Injury, *16*:281, 1985.
8. Crawford, A. H.: Fractures about the knee in children. Orthop. Clin. North Am., *7*:639, 1976.
9. DeLee, J. C.: Complete dislocation of the knee in a nine-year-old. Contemp. Orthop., *1*:29, 1979.
10. Fairbank, H. A. T.: Internal derangement of the knee in children and adolescents. Proc. R. Soc. Med., *30*:427, 1936.
11. Frandsen, P. A., and Kristensen, H.: Osteochondral fracture associated with dislocation of the patella: Another mechanism of injury. J. Trauma, *19*:195, 1979.
12. Frangakis, E. K.: Intra-articular dislocation of the patella: A case report. J. Bone Joint Surg., *56-A*:423, 1974.
13. Gerard, Y., Segal, P., and Henry, C.: Lesions traumatiques cartilagineuses pures de condyle interne du genou en pratique sportive. Rev. Chir. Orthop., *62*:245, 1976.
14. Gore, D. R.: Horizontal dislocation of the patella. J.A.M.A., *214*:1119, 1970.

15. Gross, R. M.: Acute dislocation of the patella: The Mudville mystery. Report of five cases. J. Bone Joint Surg., *68-A*:780, 1986.
16. Hanspal, R. S.: Superior dislocation of the patella. Injury, *16*:487, 1985.
17. Harmon, P. H.: Intra-articular osteochondral fracture as a cause for internal derangement of the knee in adolescents. J. Bone Joint Surg., *27*:703, 1945.
18. Helfet, A. J., Manley, M. T., and Vaughan, C. L.: The helicoid knee brace: A lightweight but effective support for the damaged knee. Injury, *15*:189, 1983.
19. Hopkinson, W. J., Mitchell, W. A., and Curl, W. W.: Chondral fractures of the knee. Cause for confusion. Am. J. Sports Med., *13*:309, 1985.
20. Jacobsen, K.: Stress radiographical measurements of post-traumatic knee instability. Acta Orthop. Scand., *48*:301, 1977.
21. Jensen, C. M., and Roosen, J. U.: Acute traumatic dislocation of the patella. J. Trauma, *25*:160, 1985.
22. Kaufman, I., and Habermann, E. T.: Intercondylar vertical dislocation of the patella. Bull. Hosp. J. Dis., *34*:222, 1973.
23. Keller, J., Andreassen, T. T., Joyce, F., Knudsen, V. E., Jorgensen, P. H., and Lucht, U.: Fixation of osteochondral fractures. Fibrin sealant tested in dogs. Acta Orthop. Scand., *56*:323, 1985.
24. Kennedy, J. C. (ed.): The Injured Adolescent Knee. Baltimore, Williams & Wilkins, 1979.
25. Kleinberg, S.: Vertical fracture of the articular surface of the patella. J.A.M.A., *81*:1205, 1923.
26. Kleinberg, S.: Traumatic lateral dislocation of the patella. Ann. Surg., *95*:635, 1932.
27. Krida, A.: Osteochondral fractures of the knee joint. Surg. Gynecol. Obstet., *39*:791, 1924.
28. Lancourt, E., and Christini, A.: Patella alta and patella infera. Their etiological role in patellar dislocation, chondromalacia and apophysitis of the tibial tubercle. J. Bone Joint Surg., *57-A*:1112, 1975.
29. Lemon, R. A., and Bartlett, D. H.: Arthroscopic assisted internal fixation of certain fractures about the knee. J. Trauma, *25*:355, 1985.
30. McManus, F., Rang, M., and Heslin, D. J.: Acute dislocation of the patella in children. A natural history. Clin. Orthop., *139*:88, 1979.
31. Makin, M.: Osteochondral fracture of the lateral femoral condyle. J. Bone Joint Surg., *33-A*:262, 1951.
32. Matthewson, M. H., and Dandy, D. J.: Osteochondral fractures of the lateral femoral condyle—a result of indirect violence to the knee. J. Bone Joint Surg., *60-B*:199, 1978.
33. Mayer, P. J., and Micheli, L. J.: Avulsion of the femoral attachment of the posterior cruciate ligament in an eleven-year-old boy. J. Bone Joint Surg., *61-A*:431, 1979.
34. Milgram, J. E.: Tangential osteochondral fracture of the patella. J. Bone Joint Surg., *25*:271, 1943.
35. Milgram, J. W.: Case report 333: Osteochondral fracture of the right patella without an osteochondral defect. Skeletal Radiol., *14*:231, 1985.
36. Milgram, J. W.: Injury to articular cartilage joint surfaces. I. Chondral injury produced by patellar shaving: A histopathologic study of human tissue specimens. Clin. Orthop., *192*:168, 1985.
37. Millard, D. G., and Lee, T. H.: "The twist" fracture dislocation of the patella. N. Engl. J. Med., *267*:246, 1962.
38. Naver, L., and Aalberg, J. R.: Avulsion of the popliteus tendon. A rare cause of chondral fracture and hemarthrosis. Am. J. Sports Med., *13*:423, 1985.
39. Rennutte, A.: Rotolar subluxation. Rev. Med. Liege, *25*(22):743, 1970.
40. Robinson, S. C., and Driscoll, S. E.: Simultaneous osteochondral avulsion of the femoral and tibial insertions of the anterior cruciate ligament. Report of a case in a thirteen-year-old boy. J. Bone Joint Surg., *63-A*:1342, 1981.
41. Rogers, L. F., Jones, S., Davis, A. R., and Dietz, G.: "Clipping injury" fracture of the epiphysis in the adolescent football player: An occult lesion of the knee. A.J.R., *121*:69, 1974.
42. Rorabeck, C. H., and Bobechko, W. P.: Acute dislocation of the patella with osteochondral fracture. A review of eighteen cases. J. Bone Joint Surg., *58-B*:237, 1976.
43. Rosenberg, N. J.: Osteochondral fracture of the lateral femoral condyle. J. Bone Joint Surg., *46-A*:1013, 1964.
44. Rutt, A.: Zur Pathogenese der Patellaluxation. Arch. Orthop. Unfallchir., *61*:353, 1967.
45. Saxena, P. S., and Sharma, K. K.: Compound complicated intra-articular horizontal dislocation of patella. Indian J. Med. Sci., *29*:19, 1975.
46. Slocum, D. B., James, S. L., Larson, R. L., and Singer, K. M.: Clinical test for anterolateral rotatory instability of the knee. Clin. Orthop., *118*:63, 1976.
47. Smith, J. B.: Knee problems in children. Pediatr. Clin. North Am., *24*:841, 1977.
48. Suman, R. K., Stother, I. G., and Illingworth, G.: Diagnostic arthroscopy of the knee in children. J. Bone Joint Surg., *66-B*:535, 1984.
49. Thomsen, P. B., Rud, B., and Jensen, U. H.: Stability and motion after traumatic dislocation of the knee. Acta Orthop. Scand., *55*:278, 1984.
50. Tischer, W.: Injuries of the knee-joint in infancy (author's transl.). Zentralbl. Chir., *102*:988, 1977.
51. Titze, A.: Intra-articular fractures of the knee joint. Reconstr. Surg. Traumatol., *12*:64, 1971.
52. Verhelst, P., Spaas, F. M., and Fabry, G.: Progressive valgus deformity of the knee after resection of an exostosis at the proximal medial tibial metaphysis. Acta Orthop. Belg., *41*:689, 1975.
53. Waldrop, J. I., and Broussard, T. S.: Disruption of the anterior cruciate ligament in a three-year-old child. A case report. J. Bone Joint Surg., *66-A*:1113, 1984.

FRACTURES OF THE PATELLA

The patella, embedded in the quadriceps tendon, is the largest sesamoid bone in the body. It usually has one center of ossification, which appears at two or three years of age but may, at times, be delayed until the sixth year. In approximately 2 to 3 per cent of patellae, a separate center of ossification is present in the upper lateral angle, where it may be unfused or incompletely fused to the main patella. These bipartite patellae are usually bilateral and should not be confused with fractures.[10, 24]

Fractures of the patella are rare in children. A direct blow will crush the patella against the femoral condyles and result in a stellate, comminuted fracture. Lateral marginal fracture is produced when the direct blow is applied to the periphery rather than to the center of the bone. A sudden powerful contraction of the quadriceps muscle with the knee flexed will cause a transverse avulsion type of fracture of the patella and a transverse tear in the quadriceps expansion.

Clinically, there is local pain, swelling, and effusion into the knee joint. If there is discon-

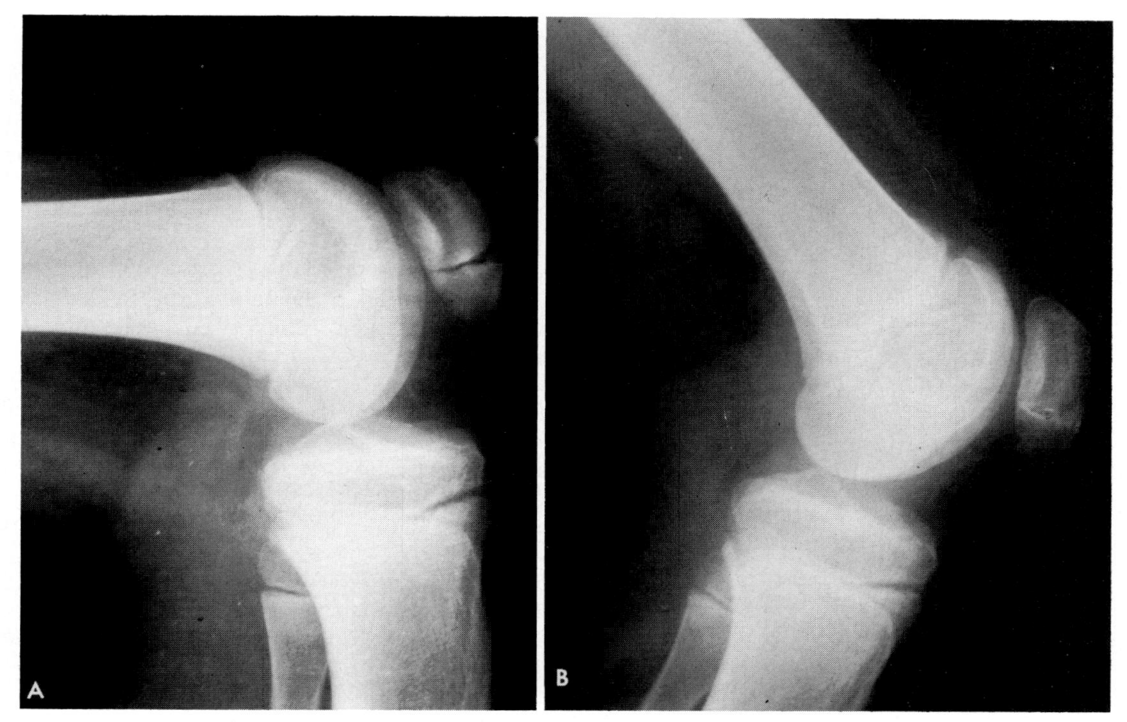

FIGURE 8–132. Fracture of the patella—transverse, minimally displaced.

Fracture was treated by immobilization in a long leg cast with the knee in extension. **A.** Initial lateral radiogram. **B.** Six weeks later.

tinuity of the quadriceps mechanism, the patient will be unable to extend the knee against gravity. The gap between the separated fragments may be palpable.

Radiograms will best disclose the fracture in the lateral projection (Fig. 8–132). If there is doubt, radiograms of the normal knee should be made for comparison.

Treatment of the fractured patella in a child follows the same principles as its treatment in an adult. Undisplaced or minimally displaced fractures are treated by immobilization of the knee in extension in an above-knee cylinder walking cast. Avulsion fractures with separation of the fragments require open reduction, repair of the torn medial and lateral quadriceps expansions, and internal fixation by tension band wiring. Undisplaced crush fractures are treated by immobilization in a long-leg cylinder walking cast; the hemarthrosis is aspirated if the joint is markedly swollen. Displaced comminuted fractures are treated by excision of all bone fragments and repair of the quadriceps expansion.

References

1. Belman, D. A., and Neviaser, R. J.: Transverse fracture of the patella in a child. J. Trauma, *13*:917, 1973.
2. Bensahel, H., and Sprung, R.: Fractures of the patella in children. J. Chir. (Paris), *99*:45, 1970.
3. Cahuzac, J. P., Labarbier, P., Picard, P., and Pasquie, M.: Partial fractures of the patella (author's transl.). Chir. Pediatr., *20*:403, 1979.
4. Cahuzac, M., Nichil, J., Olle, R., Touchard, A., and Cahuzac, J. P.: Fatigue fracture of the patella in cerebral palsy (author's transl.). Rev. Chir. Orthop., *65*:87, 1979.
5. Coleman, H. M.: Recurrent osteochondral fracture of the patella. J. Bone Joint Surg., *30-B*:153, 1948.
6. Crawford, A. H.: Fractures about the knee in children. Orthop. Clin. North Am., *7*:639, 1976.
7. Da Silva, O. L., and Brat, J. F.: Stress trajectories in the patella. Study by the photoelastic method. Acta Orthop. Scand., *41*:608, 1970.
8. Devas, M. B.: Stress fractures of the patella. J. Bone Joint Surg., *42-B*:71, 1960.
9. Dickason, J. M., and Fox, J. M.: Fracture of the patella due to overuse syndrome in a child. A case report. Am. J. Sports Med., *10*:248, 1982.
10. George, R.: Bilateral bipartite patellae. Br. J. Surg., *22*:555, 1935.
11. Goodfellow, J., Hungerford, D. S., and Woods, C.: Patello-femoral joint mechanics and pathology. J. Bone Joint Surg., *58-B*:291, 1976.
12. Green, W. T., Jr.: Painful bipartite patellae. A report of three cases. Clin. Orthop., *110*:197, 1975.
13. Hanel, D. P., and Burdge, R. E.: Consecutive indirect patella fractures in an adolescent basketball player. A case report. Am. J. Sports Med., *9*:327, 1981.
14. Houghton, G. R., and Ackroyd, C. E.: Sleeve fractures of the patella in children: A report of three cases. J. Bone Joint Surg., *61-B*:165, 1979.
15. Hung, L. K., Chan, K. M., Chan, Y. N., and Leung,

P. C.: Fractured patella: Operative treatment using tension band principle. Injury, *16*:343, 1985.
16. Insall, J.: Patella position in the normal knee joint. Radiology, *101*:101, 1971.
17. Iwaya, T., and Takatori, Y.: Lateral longitudinal stress fracture of the patella: Report of three cases. J. Pediatr. Orthop., *5*:73, 1985.
18. Jacquemier, H., Chrestian, P., Guys, J. M., Mailaender, C., Billet, P., and Bouyala, J. M.: Fracture-avulsions of the patella in children. Apropos of 3 cases. Chir. Pediatr., *24*:201, 1983.
19. Kleinberg, S.: Vertical fracture of the articular surface of the patella. J.A.M.A., *81*:1205, 1923.
20. Leung, P. C., Mak, K. H., and Lee, S. Y.: Percutaneous tension band wiring: A new method of internal fixation for mildly displaced patella fracture. J. Trauma, 23:62, 1983.
21. Levack, B., Flannagan, J. P., and Hobbs, S.: Results of surgical treatment of patellar fractures. J. Bone Joint Surg., *67-B*:416, 1985.
22. Ma, Y. Z., Zhang, Y. F., Qu, K. F., and Yeh, Y. C.: Treatment of fractures of the patella with percutaneous suture. Clin. Orthop., *191*:235, 1984.
23. Mayba, I. I.: Avulsion fracture of the tibial tubercle apophysis with avulsion of the patellar ligament. J. Pediatr. Orthop., *2*:303, 1982.
24. Oetteking, B.: Anomalous patellae. Anat. Rec., *23*:269, 1922.
25. Peterson, L., and Stener, B.: Distal disinsertion of the patellar ligament combined with avulsion fractures at the medial and lateral margins of the patella. A case report and an experimental study. Acta Orthop. Scand., *47*:680, 1976.
26. Quang-Li, L., and Jia-Wen, W.: Fracture of the patella treated by open reduction and external compression skeletal fixation. J. Bone Joint Surg., *69-A*:83, 1987.
27. Spalding, C. B.: Patellar fracture in child two years old. Int. Clin., *4*:245, 1918.
28. Stewart, S. F.: Frontal fractures of the patella. Ann. Surg., *81*:536, 1925.
29. Sugiura, Y., and Kaneko, F.: Rupture of the patella ligament with avulsion fracture of the lower pole of the patella—a case report. Orthop. Surg. (Tokyo), *23*:384, 1972.
30. Titze, A.: Intra-articular fractures of the knee joint. Reconstr. Surg. Traumatol., *12*:64, 1971.
31. Villiger, K. J.: Fractures of the patella. Praxis, *71*:1708, 1982.

FRACTURES OF THE INTERCONDYLAR EMINENCE OF THE TIBIA

The intercondylar eminence (tibial spine) is located between the medial and lateral articular facets on the superior surface of the upper end of the tibia. In front of and behind the intercondylar eminence are rough depressions for the attachments of the menisci and the anterior and posterior cruciate ligaments. The intercondylar eminence is located directly beneath the hollow of the intercondyloid fossa of the femur, and does not articulate with the gliding articular surface of either femoral condyle.

Fractures of the intercondylar eminence of the tibia occur most frequently between the ages of 8 and 13 years; they are not found in children before the age of 7 years.

Mechanism of Injury

Fractures of the intercondylar eminence are essentially avulsions of either the anterior or posterior cruciate ligaments with an attached piece of bone. In children, the ligamentous tissues are resilient and seldom are avulsions of the tibial spine associated with tears of the menisci or of the ligaments. A blow to the front of the flexed knee will drive the femur posteriorly on the fixed tibia and result in avulsions of the anterior part of the tibial spine; a common incident is a bicycle injury in which a child falls and lands on the front of the flexed knee. In Meyers and McKeever's series of 35 fractures of the intercondylar eminence of the tibia in children, 17 patients sustained the injury in a fall from a bicycle. Meyers and McKeever pointed out that the anterior cruciate ligament serves as a deterrent to excessive medial rotation of the tibia on the femoral condyles; they proposed that during the fall on the bent knee there is a violent forced medial rotation of the tibia on the femur, which places a severe strain on the anterior cruciate ligament.[21]

Avulsion of the posterior part of the tibial spine is very rare. Roberts and Lovell reported a 10 : 1 ratio of the fracture of the anterior eminence to fracture of the posterior eminence.[25] It is caused by a direct force that strikes the proximal part of the flexed tibia and drives it posteriorly. Most of the injuries occur in motorcycle accidents. Occasionally the same injury results from hyperextension injury of the knee joint; in such an instance, an associated tear of the posterior part of the capsule will almost invariably occur. In the report of Torisu of 21 cases, the youngest patient was 15 years old.[31] Avulsion of the posterior intercondylar eminence is an injury in the skeletally mature patient. Fractures of the anterior intercondylar eminence will be discussed in this text.

Classification

Meyers and McKeever subdivided fractures of the intercondylar eminence of the tibia into three types based upon the degree of displacement of the avulsed fragment (Fig. 8–133).[20]

In *Type I*, the avulsed fragment of bone is minimally displaced, with only slight elevation of its anterior margin. In *Type II*, there is greater displacement, with the anterior third to half of the avulsed fragment being elevated from its bone bed. This produces a beaklike deformity on the lateral radiogram. In a *Type III* fracture, the avulsed fragment is completely elevated from its bed on the tibia. There is total

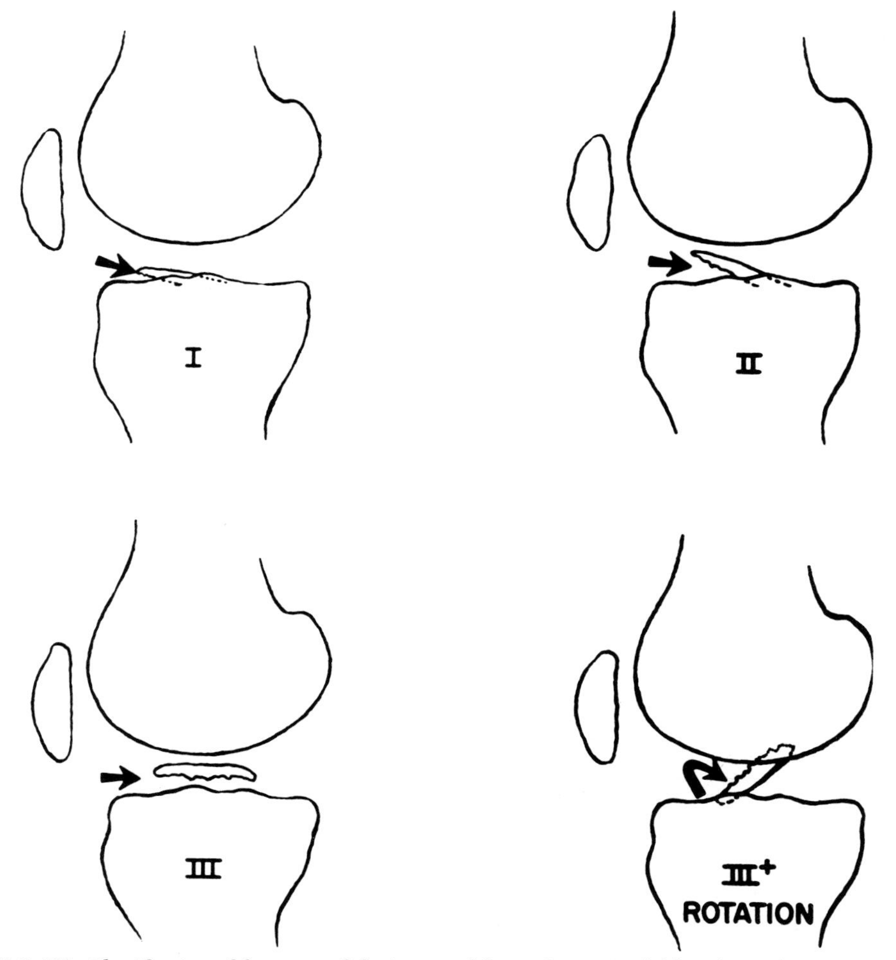

FIGURE 8–133. Classification of fractures of the intercondylar eminence in children (according to Meyers and McKeever).

Type I. No dislodgement of the fragment from its bed. There is minimal displacement and slight elevation of its anterior margin. *Type II.* Anterior third to half of the avulsed fragment is elevated from its bone bed. It has a beaklike appearance in the lateral radiogram. *Type III.* The avulsed fragment is completely dislodged from its bone bed. It may be rotated so that its cartilaginous surface faces the raw bone of the bone bed, making union impossible.

Type I and Type II fractures are treated by simple immobilization in a long leg cast with the knee in comfortable flexion. (The anterior cruciate ligament is taut in extension or hyperextension of the knee; it is relaxed in the first arc of flexion.) Type III fractures require open reduction, internal fixation (with simple catgut suturing to the adjacent meniscus), and immobilization. (From Meyers, M. H., and McKeever, F. M.: Fracture of the intercondylar eminence of the tibia. J. Bone Joint Surg., *41-A*:214, 1959.)

lack of bone apposition. In some instances, the avulsed fragment is rotated so that its cartilaginous surface faces the bare bone of the intercondylar eminence, making union impossible.

Clinical Picture

Rapid development of hemarthrosis of the knee following an injury is a sign suggestive of fracture of the intercondylar eminence. The knee is held in partial flexion, and any attempt at passive extension of the knee is painful. From the position of fixed flexion deformity of 10 to 30 degrees, the knee can be further flexed to 60 to 100 degrees. Restriction of joint motion is caused by muscle spasm and not by the avulsed fragment; the latter lies below the hollow of the intercondylar notch of the femur and does not lock the knee by being trapped between the femur and tibia. On palpation, the local tenderness is in the central region of the anterior aspect of the joint line, and not on the medial or lateral side. Anteroposterior instability (drawer sign) is usually absent; when present, it is minimal. Positive drawer sign suggests an associated tear of the medial collateral ligament. In children, even under the relaxation of a general anesthetic, mediolateral instability of the knee cannot be demonstrated unless there is concomitant tear of the medial collateral ligament.

Radiographic Findings

Radiograms will disclose the avulsed bone fragment, which can best be visualized in the lateral projection (Fig. 8–134). When displacement is minor, the fracture may be completely overlooked in the anteroposterior film. It is extremely important to obtain adequate radiograms and to determine the type of fracture. Computed tomography is valuable in depicting the avulsed fragment in dubious cases. In the differential diagnosis, one should consider osteochondral fractures of the femoral condyles and osteochondritis dissecans.

Treatment

This depends upon the type of fracture. When the joint is markedly swollen and tense, the hemarthrosis is aspirated first. *Type I* and *Type II* fractures require simple immobilization in an above-knee cylinder cast, as there is still some apposition between the avulsed fragment and its bed of origin. The position of the knee is 20 to 30 degrees of flexion; this is because the anterior cruciate ligament is taut when the knee is in extension and hyperextension, relaxed in the first portion of the arc of flexion, and becomes taut again as complete flexion is reached. General anesthesia is not necessary during application of the cast. Manipulating the knee into hyperextension with the patient anesthetized serves no useful purpose and may, in fact, further displace the avulsed fragment attached to the distal end of the anterior cruciate ligament. When the degree of knee extension is symmetrical to that of the contralateral normal knee it is a good clinical sign of satisfac-

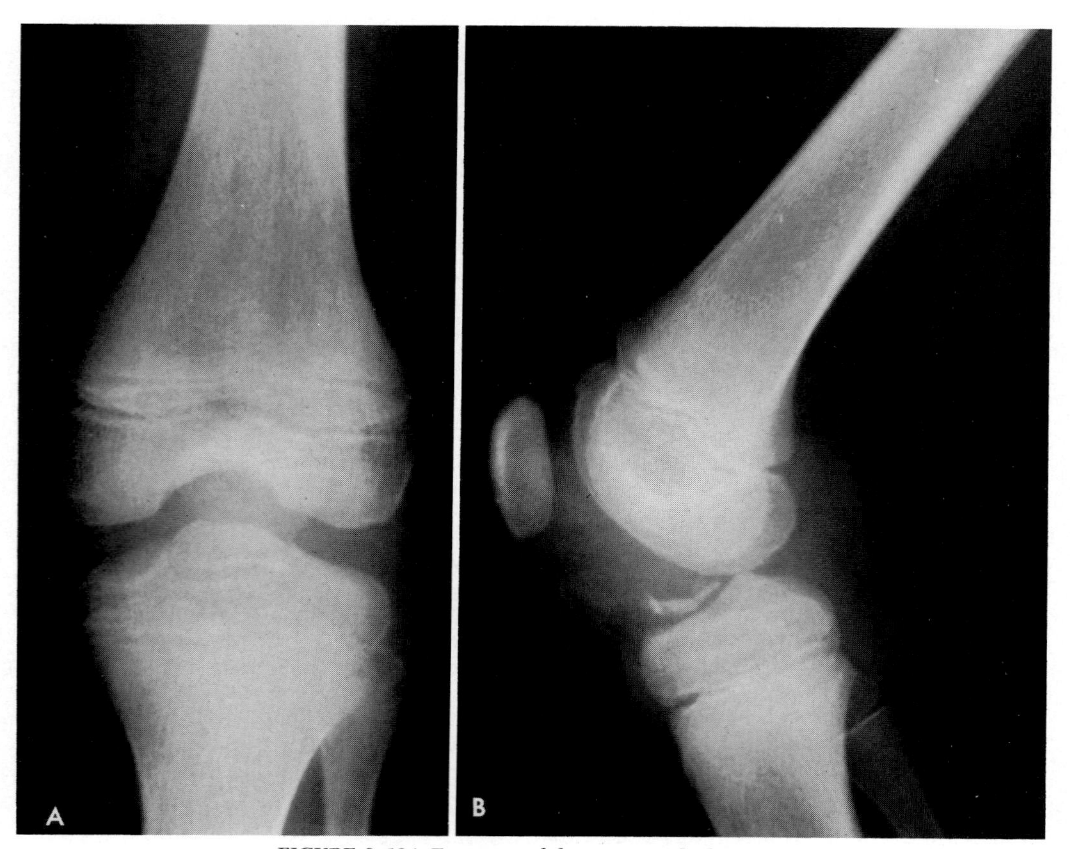

FIGURE 8–134. Fractures of the anterior tibial spine.

A and **B.** Minimally displaced fracture of anterior tibial spine was treated conservatively by an above-knee cast with the knee in extension.

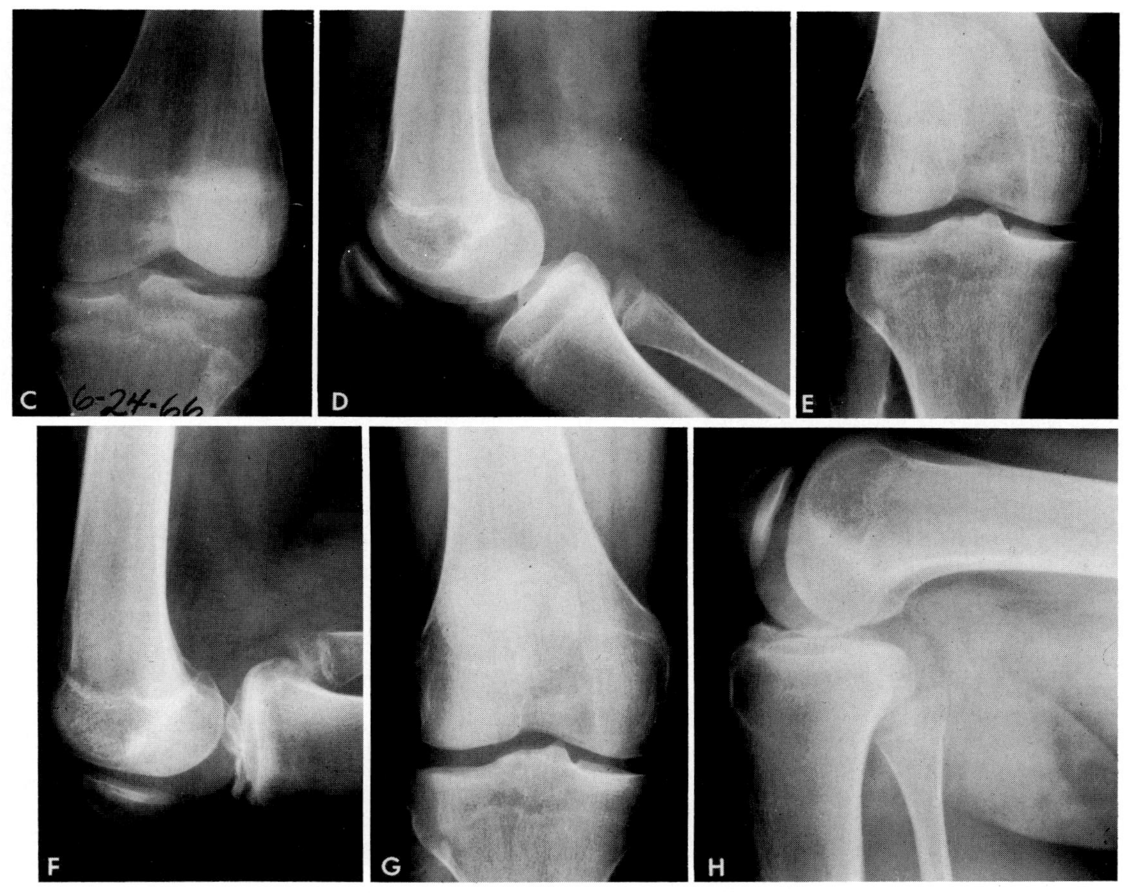

FIGURE 8–134 Continued. Fractures of the anterior tibial spine.

C to **H.** Markedly displaced fracture of the anterior tibial spine. This is treated by arthrotomy, open reduction, and internal fixation with simple catgut suture to the meniscus. **C** and **D.** Initial radiograms. **E** and **F.** Three months later. Note the slight separation of anterior tibial spine. **G** and **H.** Six months later; the fractured spine is well incorporated into the tibial plateau.

tory reduction. Immobilization is maintained for six to eight weeks or until union of the bone fragment to its bed on the tibia is demonstrated on the radiogram. In the older adolescent it may take longer, up to 12 weeks. After removal of the cast, active knee exercises and gradual weight-bearing are instituted. In a child, a period of two to three months is usually required to restore normal motion and strength to the knee.

Type III fractures require open reduction. This author recommends reduction and internal fixation through the arthroscope.

Failure of closed reduction usually is due to interposition of the anterior pole of the lateral meniscus between the fragment and its bed. After aspiration and irrigation of the knee joint, the detached fragment is visualized through the arthroscope; the entrapped pole of the lateral meniscus is liberated with a hook. The fragment is pushed down toward its bed and anatomic reduction is obtained. The knee is extended and stability of reduction is assessed. If stable, an above-knee cylinder cast is applied with the knee in extension but not hyperextension. With the knee in extension the apposed distal femur maintains reduction. If unstable, it should be internally fixed.

Meyers and McKeever have demonstrated that it is not necessary to transfix the fragment with a screw or nail, nor to drill a hole through the upper end of the tibia and pass removable retention sutures around the avulsed fragment. They recommend internal fixation with a simple absorbable catgut suture passed, with a cutting needle, through the thin edge of the avulsed fragment and through the meniscus near its sharp margin. They report excellent results in six patients treated by open reduction and suturing done in this fashion. Following open reduction, the knee is immobilized in an above-knee cylinder cast in partially flexed position. Immobilization is continued until there is radiographic evidence of healing—usually about eight weeks.[20, 21]

Other methods of fixation are with small threaded pins or screws transfixing the fragment into the epiphysis. A loop may be passed over the superior surface of the fragment behind the anterior cruciate ligament and through drill holes in the proximal tibial epiphysis, exiting anteriorly. The proximal tibial physis should not be crossed. This author prefers to use simple suture for internal fixation. The use of pins, screws, or wire loops is not required for stability of reduction.

When visualization and reduction-fixation of the fracture are difficult and open arthrotomy of the knee is required, use the anterolateral approach, as the pathology is lateral.

References

1. Apley, A.: Fractures of the tibial plateau. Orthop. Clin. North Am., *10*:61, 1979.
2. Bakalim, G., and Wilppula, E.: Closed treatment of fracture of the tibial spines. Injury, 5:210, 1974.
3. Borch-Madsen, P.: On symmetrical bilateral fracture of the tuberosities tibiae and eminentia intercondyloidea. Acta Orthop. Scand., *24*:44, 1954.
4. Cigit, I., and Vrtar, Z.: Injuries to the intercondylar tibial eminence in childhood. Acta Chir. Iugosl., *24*:309, 1977.
5. Falstie-Jensen, S., and Sondergard Petersen, P. E.: Incarceration of the meniscus in fractures of the intercondylar eminence of the tibia in children. Injury, *15*:236, 1984.
6. Fyfe, I. S., and Jackson, J. P.: Tibial intercondylar fractures in children: A review of the classification and the treatment of mal-union. Injury, *13*:165, 1981.
7. Garcia, A., and Neer, C. S., II: Isolated fractures of the intercondylar eminence of the tibia. Am. J. Surg., *95*:593, 1958.
8. Germaneau, J., Cahuzac, J. P., Lebardier, P., Pasquie, M., and Bondonny, J. M.: Fractures of intercondylar eminence of the tibia in childhood (author's transl.). Chir. Pediatr., *21*:161, 1980.
9. Gossling, H. R., and Peterson, C. A.: A new surgical approach in the treatment of depressed lateral condylar fractures of the tibia. Clin. Orthop., *140*:96, 1979.
10. Gronkvist, H., Hirsch, G., and Johansson, L.: Fracture of the anterior tibial spine in children. J. Pediatr. Orthop., *4*:465, 1984.
11. Hansson, L. I., Hybbinette, C. H., and Sjostrano, L. O.: Reimplantation of a traumatically expelled tibial diaphysis. Acta Orthop. Scand., *48*:108, 1977.
12. Hansson, L. I., Hybbinette, C. H., and Sjostrano, L. O.: Reimplantation of a tibial diaphysis. Mod. Med., p. 129, 1978.
13. Hayes, J. M., and Masear, V. R.: Avulsion fracture of the tibial eminence associated with severe medial ligamentous injury in an adolescent. A case report and literature review. Am. J. Sports Med., *12*:330, 1984.
14. Holz, U.: Forms and classification of tibial-head fractures. Chirurg, *46*:341, 1975.
15. Jones, R., and Smith, S. A.: On rupture of the crucial ligaments of the knee, and on fractures of the spine of the tibia. Br. J. Surg., *1*:70, 1913.
16. Lansinger, O., Bergman, B., Korner, L., and Andersson, G. B. J.: Tibial condylar fractures. A twenty year follow-up. J. Bone Joint Surg., *68-A*:13, 1986.
17. Lee, H. G.: Avulsion fracture of the tibial attachments of the crucial ligaments. Treatment by operative reduction. J. Bone Joint Surg., *19*:460, 1937.
18. Lipscomb, A. B., and Anderson, A. F.: Open reduction of a malunited tibial spine fracture in a 12-year-old male. A case report. Am. J. Sports Med., *13*:419, 1985.
19. Losee, E., Johnson, R., and Southwick, W. O.: Anterior subluxation of the lateral tibial plateau. A diagnostic test and operative repair. J. Bone Joint Surg., *60-A*:1015, 1978.
20. Meyers, M. H., and McKeever, F. M.: Fracture of the intercondylar eminence of the tibia. J. Bone Joint Surg., *41-A*:209, 1959.
21. Meyers, M. H., and McKeever, F. M.: Fracture of the intercondylar eminence of the tibia. J. Bone Joint Surg., *52-A*:1677, 1970.
22. Molander, M. L., Wallin, G., and Wilkstad, I.: Fracture of the intercondylar eminence of the tibia: A review of 35 patients. J. Bone Joint Surg., *63-B*:89, 1981.
23. Nevelos, A. B., and Colton, C. L.: Rotational displacement of the lower tibial epiphysis due to trauma. J. Bone Joint Surg., *59-B*:331, 1977.
24. Pringle, J. A.: Avulsion of the spine of the tibia. Ann. Surg., *46*:169, 1907.
25. Roberts, J. M., and Lovell, W. W.: Fractures of the intercondylar eminence of tibia. *In* Proceedings of the American Academy of Orthopedic Surgeons. J. Bone Joint Surg., *52-A*:827, 1970.
26. Rondhuis, J. J.: Avulsion fracture of the intercondylar tibial eminence. Ned. Tijdschr. Geneeskd., *127*:1668, 1983.
27. Roth, P.: Fracture of the spine of the tibia. J. Bone Joint Surg., *29*:509, 1928.
28. Salenius, P., and Vankka, E.: The development of the tibiofemoral angle in children. J. Bone Joint Surg., *57-A*:259, 1975.
29. Silberman, W. W., and Murphy, J. L.: Avulsion fracture of the proximal tibial epiphysis. J. Trauma, *6*:592, 1966.
30. Smith, J. B.: Knee instability after fractures of the intercondylar eminence of the tibia. J. Pediatr. Orthop., *4*:462, 1984.
31. Torisu, T.: Isolated avulsion fracture of the tibial attachment of the posterior cruciate ligament. J. Bone Joint Surg., *59-A*:68, 1977.
32. Williams, A. T.: An unusual fracture of the tibial plateau. Med. Biol. Illus., *15*:266, 1965.
33. Zaricznyj, B.: Avulsion fracture of the tibial eminence: Treatment by open reduction and pinning. J. Bone Joint Surg., *50-A*:111, 1977.

FRACTURES INVOLVING THE PROXIMAL TIBIAL PHYSIS AND THE APOPHYSIS OF THE TIBIAL TUBERCLE AND AVULSION FRACTURES OF THE APOPHYSIS OF THE TIBIAL TUBERCLE

Fractures Involving the Proximal Tibial Physis

Injuries to the proximal tibial physis are rare, constituting only 0.8 per cent of all physeal injuries. This immunity from fractures is due to the relative lack of ligamentous attachments to the proximal tibial epiphysis; the lateral collateral ligament inserts to the fibular head, and the principal part of the medial collateral ligament is attached to the metaphyseal region, well distal to the physis. Thus, abduction or adduction strain is transmitted to the distal femur instead of to the proximal tibial epiphysis.

As stated, normally only a small part of the medial collateral ligament is inserted into the epiphysis. Occasionally this attachment is large, and upon exertion of a valgus strain, Type II (Salter-Harris) physeal injury is produced. This is the most common type of physeal injury involving the proximal tibial epiphysis (9 of 14 cases in the series of Aitken).[1] The distal fragment is usually displaced posterolaterally; circulatory embarrassment may result if the sharp upper end of the distal fragment impinges on the popliteal vessels (Fig. 8–135). A Type II (Salter-Harris) fracture with anteromedial displacement of the distal fragment has been reported by Aitken and Ingersoll.[2]

Type III (Salter-Harris) physeal injury can occur (2 of Aitken's 14 cases).[1] The detached epiphyseal fragment is usually unstable and becomes displaced either medially, anteriorly, posteriorly, or proximally.

Direct crushing injury may cause Type IV (Salter-Harris) fracture; this is usually associated with crushing of the physis and avulsion fracture of the tibial spine.

TREATMENT

Closed reduction is performed in all Type II fractures and the lower limb is immobilized in an above-knee cast for a period of four to six weeks. In Aitken's series of nine patients, despite some persistent displacement, complete spontaneous correction occurred without deformity or clinical shortening in all cases.

Type III (Salter-Harris) fractures require open reduction and internal fixation with screws. Open surgery is indicated also in Type IV fractures when fragments are displaced and cannot be anatomically reduced by closed methods. Premature growth arrest with resultant varus, valgus, or recurvatus deformity almost always occurs with Type IV fractures; these require excision of bony bridge and fat interposition (Langenskiöld procedure) and/or osteotomy for correction of deformity.

Avulsion Fractures of Apophysis of the Tibial Tubercle

Avulsion fracture of the tibial tubercle is a traumatic separation through the physis deep to the ossific nucleus of the tubercle. It should be distinguished from Osgood-Schlatter lesion, in which there is an avulsion of the anterior surface of the apophysis without displacement between the ossific nucleus of the apophysis and the subjacent tibial metaphysis.[33]

It commonly occurs in boys between the ages of 14 and 16 years. The distal ligamentous expansion of the insertion of the quadriceps mechanism spreads out like a fan as it attaches to the proximal tibial surface. The apophysis of the tibial tubercle is located in the middle of this tendinous expansion. Because of the diffuse insertion of the quadriceps mechanism, it is rare for the tibial tubercle to be completely avulsed; however, partial avulsion is a frequent occurrence.

The tibial tubercle may develop in two different forms, according to Smillie: as a tongue-shaped downward protrusion of the proximal tibial epiphysis on the anterior proximal tibial surface, which fuses with the proximal tibia at the age of 18 years; or in the second form, as a separate center of ossification that fuses with the main body of the epiphysis at the age of 16 and, together with the main body of the epiphysis, fuses to the tibial diaphysis at the age of 18. In both complete and partial avulsions of the epiphysis of the tibial tubercle, injury occurs before the epiphysis fuses to the tibia at the age of 18.[46]

MECHANISM OF INJURY

When complete avulsion occurs, it is usually the result of the knee's being forcibly flexed against the resistance of the strongly contracting quadriceps muscle. These injuries are usually sustained in athletic activities, such as high jumping or football.

If the first of Smillie's two types of tibial tubercle apophysis is present, a projecting tongue-like flap may either be raised from the anterior tibial surface and not detached from the main body of the epiphysis, or it may be raised from the tibial surface and fractured from the main body of the epiphysis at its base. In the second of Smillie's two types, in which the injury occurs in a knee in which the tibial tubercle is developing as a separate center of ossification, this small fragment is avulsed from its bed.

CLASSIFICATION

Watson-Jones has classified these fractures into three types (Fig. 8–136): *Type I* fractures are those in which the tongue-like projection of the epiphysis has been lifted upward without displacement at its proximal base. *Type II* frac-

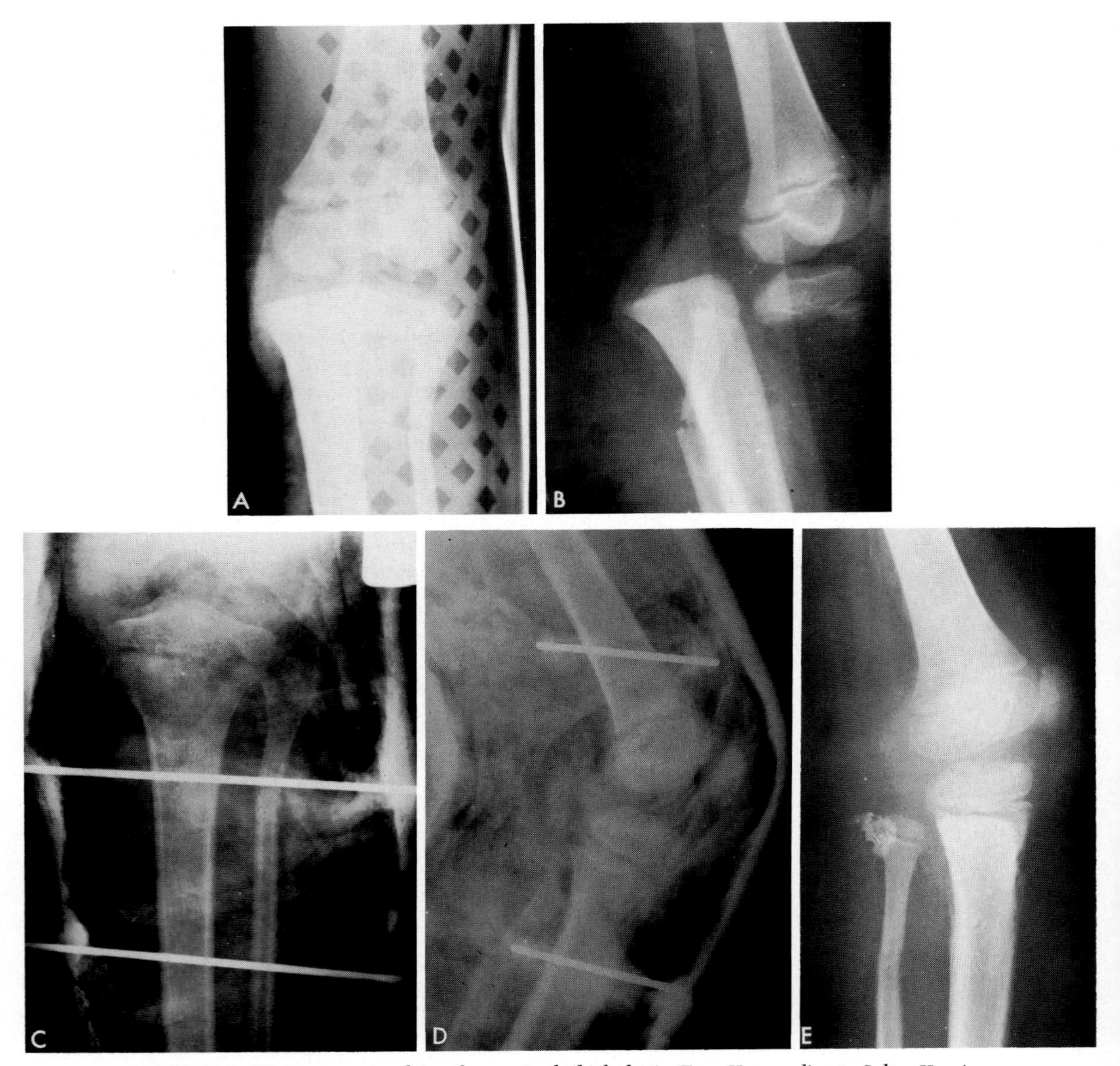

FIGURE 8–135. Fracture involving the proximal tibial physis, Type II according to Salter-Harris.

A and **B.** Initial radiograms. Note the complete separation with posterior and superior displacement of distal fragment. Anterior metaphyseal fragment is small; there is associated fracture of the proximal fibula. Posterior tibial and dorsalis pedis pulsations were absent and the foot and leg were cold. Immediate closed reduction was carried out with two pins in the tibia and one pin in the distal femur to secure maintenance of reduction. An above-knee cast was applied. **C** and **D.** Immediate postreduction radiograms. Note the anatomic alignment. **E.** Oblique-lateral radiogram four months later, showing healing.

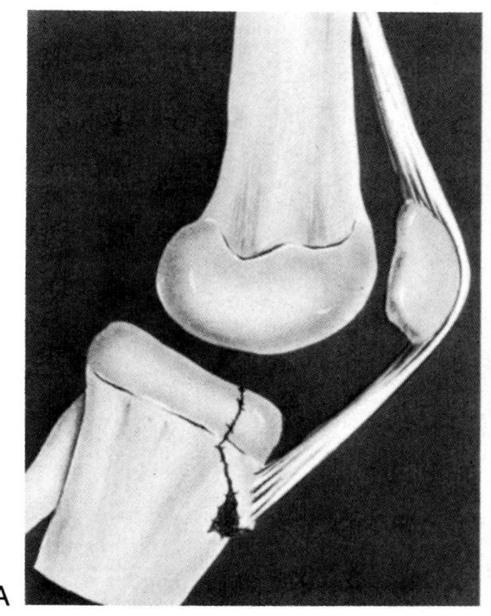

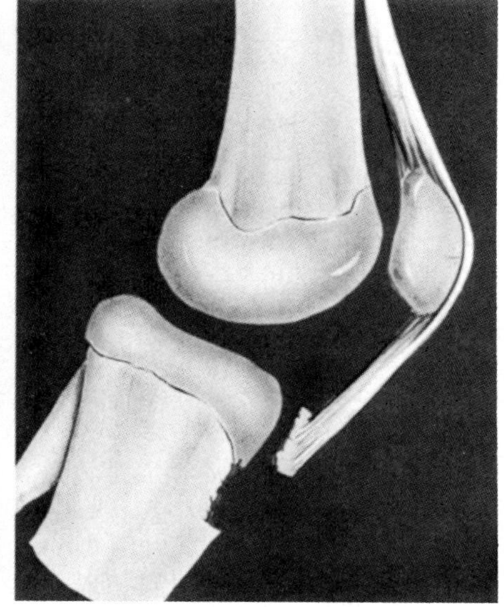

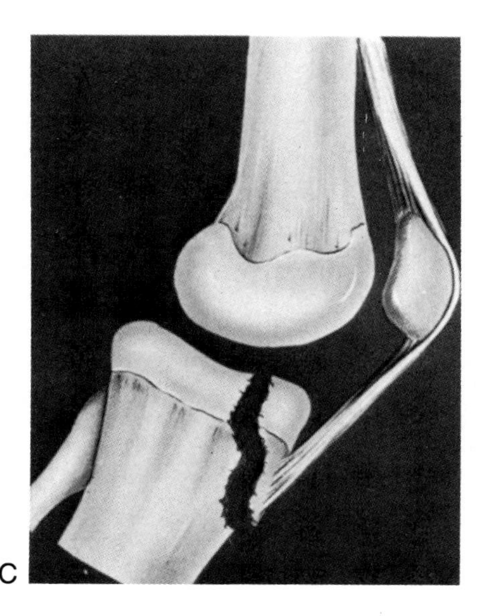

FIGURE 8–136. Three types of fracture of the proximal tibial tubercle (according to Watson-Jones).

A. *Type I injury.* The tubercle is hinged upward without displacement at its proximal base. **B.** *Type II injury.* A small portion of the tubercle is avulsed and retracted proximally. **C.** *Type III injury.* This is the more severe form of Type I with fracture line extending across the articular surface. (From Hand, W. L., Hand, C. R., and Dunn, A. W.: Avulsion fractures of the tibial tubercle. J. Bone Joint Surg., 53-A:1150, 1971.)

tures correspond to injuries of the second of Smillie's two forms of epiphysis, in which the separate center of ossification, not having fused with the main body of the epiphysis, has been completely avulsed from its bed. *Type III* is the most severe injury and is actually an extension of the Type I fracture with extension across the articular surface.[49]

Ogden and associates gave the following classification, depending upon the distance of the separation from the distal tip. The degree of displacement is determined by the severity of injury. In *Type I,* the fracture-separation takes place across the secondary ossification center of the tubercle distal to the proximal tibial physis at a level with the posterior border of the insertion of the patellar tendon. In *Type II,* the fracture-separation occurs at the junction of the primary and secondary ossification centers of the proximal tibial epiphysis—between the tubercle and epiphysis. In *Type III,* the fracture is a Salter-Harris Type III with the fracture line extending upward across the primary ossification center of the proximal tibial epiphysis into the knee joint. In Type III, the posterior part of the proximal tibial physis is closing and the fracture is similar to the fracture of Tillaux at the ankle.[33]

TREATMENT

In complete avulsion treatment depends upon whether or not the tongue-shaped epiphysis has been completely detached from the main body of the epiphysis. If it is still attached, it may often be replaced by manipulative reduction and held by an above-knee cast with the knee in extension. However, if it has fractured from the main body of the epiphysis, or if a separate center of ossification (Type II) has been avulsed, open reduction is indicated. An infolded flap of periosteum may prevent closed reduction. The best means of maintaining anatomic repositioning is by suturing the epiphysis to the surrounding fibrous attachments of the quadriceps mechanism and immobilizing it in an above-knee cast with the knee in extension. Sometimes internal fixation with a cancellous screw or several threaded Steinmann pins is indicated in unstable fractures. The fracture heals by epiphysiodesis, but genu recurvatum does not develop because of the skeletal maturity and little growth remaining from the proximal tibial physis.

References

1. Aitken, A. P.: Fractures of the proximal tibial epiphyseal cartilage. Clin. Orthop., *41*:92, 1965.
2. Aitken, A. P., and Ingersoll, R. E.: Fractures of proximal tibial epiphyseal cartilage. J. Bone Joint Surg., *38-A*:787, 1956.
3. Barnhart, J.: Premature closure of the proximal tibial epiphysis following fracture of the tibial shaft. South. Med. J., *60*:317, 1967.
4. Bertin, K. C., and Goble, E. M.: Ligament injuries associated with physeal fractures about the knee. Clin. Orthop., *177*:188, 1983.
5. Blokker, C. P., Rorabeck, C. H., and Bourne, R. B.: Tibial plateau fractures. An analysis of the results of treatment in 60 patients. Clin. Orthop., *182*:193, 1984.
6. Borch-Madsen, P.: On symmetrical bilateral fractures of the tuberosities tibiae and eminentia intercondyloidea. Acta Orthop. Scand., *24*:44, 1954.
7. Burkhart, S. S., and Peterson, H. A.: Fractures of the proximal tibial epiphysis. J. Bone Joint Surg., *61-A*:996, 1979.
8. Cahill, B. R.: Stress fracture of the proximal tibial epiphysis. Am. J. Sports Med., *5*:86, 1977.
9. Christie, M. J., and Dvonch, V. M.: Tibial tuberosity avulsion fracture in adolescents. J. Pediatr. Orthop., *1*:391, 1981.
10. Cozen, L.: Fracture of the proximal portion of the tibia in children followed by valgus deformity. Surg. Gynecol. Obstet., *72*:183, 1953.
11. Currarino, G., and Pinckney, L. E.: Genu valgum after proximal tibial fractures in children. A.J.R., *136*:915, 1981.
12. Dias, J. J., Stirling, A. J., Finlay, D. B. L., and Gregg, P. J.: Computerized and axial tomography for tibial plateau fractures. J. Bone Joint Surg., *69-B*:84, 1987.
13. Deliyannis, S. N.: Avulsion of the tibial tuberosity: Report of two cases. Injury, *4*:341, 1973.
14. Driessnack, R. P., and Marcus, N. W.: Fracture of an unossified tibial tubercle. J. Pediatr. Orthop., *5*:728, 1985.
15. Dvonch, V. M., and Bunch, W. H.: Pattern of closure of the proximal femoral and tibial epiphyses in man. J. Pediatr. Orthop., *3*:498, 1983.
16. Gibson, A.: Separation of the upper epiphysis of the tibia. Ann. Surg., *77*:485, 1923.
17. Gill, J. G., Chakrabarti, H. P., and Becker, S. J.: Fractures of the proximal tibial epiphysis. Injury, *14*:324, 1983.
18. Gill, J. G., Chakrabarti, H. P., and Becker, S. J.: Fractures of the proximal tibial epiphysis. Injury, *14*:324, 1983.
19. Hand, W. H., Hand, C. R., and Dunn, A. W.: Avulsion fractures of the tibial tubercle. J. Bone Joint Surg., *53-A*:1579, 1971.
20. Harries, T. J., Lichtman, D. M., and Lonon, W. D.: Irreducible Salter-Harris II fracture of the proximal tibia. J. Pediatr. Orthop., *3*:92, 1983.
21. Harris, H. A.: The growth of long bones in childhood with special reference to certain bony striations of the metaphysis and to the role of vitamins. Arch. Intern. Med., *38*:785, 1926.
22. Henard, D. C., and Bobo, R. T.: Avulsion fractures of the tibial tubercle in adolescents. A report of bilateral fractures and a review of the literature. Clin. Orthop., *177*:182, 1983.
23. Kaplan, E. B.: Avulsion fracture of proximal tibial epiphysis. Bull. Hosp. J. Dis., *24*:119, 1963.
24. Lehner, A., and Dubas, J.: Sekundare Deformierungen nach Epiphysenlosungen und epiphysenliniennahen Frakturen. Helv. Chir. Acta, *21*:388, 1954.
25. Levi, J. H., and Coleman, C. R.: Fracture of the tibial tubercle. Am. J. Sports Med., *6*:254, 1976.
26. Lipscomb, A. B., Gilbert, P. P., Johnston, R. K., Anderson, A. F., and Snyder, R. B.: Fracture of the tibial tuberosity with associated ligamentous and meniscal tears. A case report. J. Bone Joint Surg., *66-A*:790, 1984.
27. McGuigan, J. A., O'Reilly, M. J., and Nixon, J. R.: Popliteal artery thrombosis resulting from disruption of the upper tibial epiphysis. Injury, *16*:49, 1984.
28. Mayba, I. I.: Avulsion fracture of the tibial tubercle apophysis with avulsion of patellar ligament. J. Pediatr. Orthop., *2*:303, 1982.
29. Mayer, V., and Marchisello, P. J.: Traumatic partial arrest of tibial physis. Clin. Orthop., *183*:99, 1984.
30. Morton, K. S., and Starr, D. E.: Closure of the anterior portion of the upper tibial epiphysis as a complication of tibial-shaft fracture. J. Bone Joint Surg., *46-A*:570, 1964.
31. Nicholson, J. T.: Epiphyseal fractures about the knee. A.A.O.S. Instr. Course Lect., *18*:74, 1967.
32. Ogden, J. A., Hempton, R., and Southwick, W.: Development of the tibial tuberosity. Anat. Rec., *182*:431, 1975.
33. Ogden, J. A., Tross, R. B., and Murphy, M. J.: Fractures of the tibial tuberosity in adolescents. J. Bone Joint Surg., *62-A*:205, 1980.
34. Pappas, A. M., Anas, P., and Toczylowski, H. M., Jr.: Asymmetrical arrest of the proximal tibial physis and genu recurvatum deformity. J. Bone Joint Surg., *66-A*:575, 1984.
35. Parrini, L., Paleari, M., and Biggi, F.: Growth disturbances following fractures of the femur and tibia in children. Ital. J. Orthop. Traumatol., *11*:139, 1985.
36. Peterson, H. A.: Partial growth plate arrest and its treatment. J. Pediatr. Orthop., *4*:246, 1984.
37. Peters, W., and Steinert, V.: Injuries of proximal tibial epiphysis. Zentralbl. Chir., *97*:1791, 1972.
38. Polakoff, D. R., Bucholz, R. W., and Ogden, J. A.: Torsion band wiring of displaced tibial tuberosity fractures in adolescents. Clin. Orthop., *209*:161, 1986.
39. Rivero, H., Bolden, R., and Young, L. W.: Proximal tibial physis fracture and popliteal artery injury. Radiology, *150*:390, 1984.

40. Roberts, J. M.: Avulsion fractures of the proximal tibial epiphysis. *In* Kennedy, J. C. (ed.): Injured Adolescent Knee. Baltimore, Williams & Wilkins, 1979.
41. Roberts, J. M.: Fractures and dislocations of the knee. *In* Rockwood, C. A., Jr., Wilkins, K. E., and King, R. E.: Fractures in Children. Philadelphia, Lippincott, 1984, pp. 891–982.
42. Ryu, R. K., and Debenham, J. O.: An unusual avulsion fracture of the proximal tibial epiphysis. Case report and proposed addition to the Watson-Jones classification. Clin. Orthop., *194*:181, 1985.
43. Sarcev, V., Mikic, Z., and Ercegan, G.: Traumatic epiphysiolysis of the proximal part of the tibia (2 case reports). Med. Pregl., *36*:217, 1983.
44. Shelton, W. R., and Canale, S. T.: Fractures of the tibia through the proximal tibial epiphyseal cartilage. J. Bone Joint Surg., *61-A*:167, 1979.
45. Silberman, W. W., and Murphy, J. L.: Avulsion fracture of the proximal tibial epiphysis. J. Trauma, *6*:592, 1966.
46. Smillie, I. S.: Injuries to the Knee Joint. 4th Ed. Baltimore, Williams & Wilkins, 1970.
47. Thompson, G. H., and Gesler, J. W.: Proximal tibial epiphyseal fracture in an infant. J. Pediatr. Orthop., *4*:114, 1984.
48. Vainionpaa, S., Bostman, O., Patiala, H., and Rokkanen, P.: Fracture of the tibial tuberosity in adolescents. Arch. Orthop. Trauma. Surg., *104*:20, 1985.
49. Watson-Jones, R.: Fractures and Joint Injuries. 4th Ed. Edinburgh, E. & S. Livingstone, 1955–1956.
50. Welch, P. H., and Wynne, G. H.: Proximal tibial epiphyseal fracture separation. J. Bone Joint Surg., *45-A*:782, 1963.

FRACTURES OF THE SHAFT OF THE TIBIA AND FIBULA

The type of fracture sustained by the tibia varies with the age of the child and is dependent upon the nature of the violence—whether it is an indirect rotational twisting force or a direct blow.

In infants and young children, the typical injury is a spiral fracture of the tibia with an intact fibula. Between three and six years of age, a torsional stress applied on the medial aspect of the leg will result in a greenstick fracture of the proximal metaphysis or upper diaphysis of the tibia with an intact fibula, or it will cause a spiral fracture of the tibia, with or without a break of the fibula (Figs. 8–137 and 8–138). In the five- to ten-year age group, the common injury is a simple transverse fracture with or without displacement due to direct trauma (Fig. 8–139). In adolescents, athletic injuries cause comminuted fracture of the middle third of the tibia and fibula with a butterfly fragment (Fig. 8–140).

Ordinarily, fracture fragments are held to-

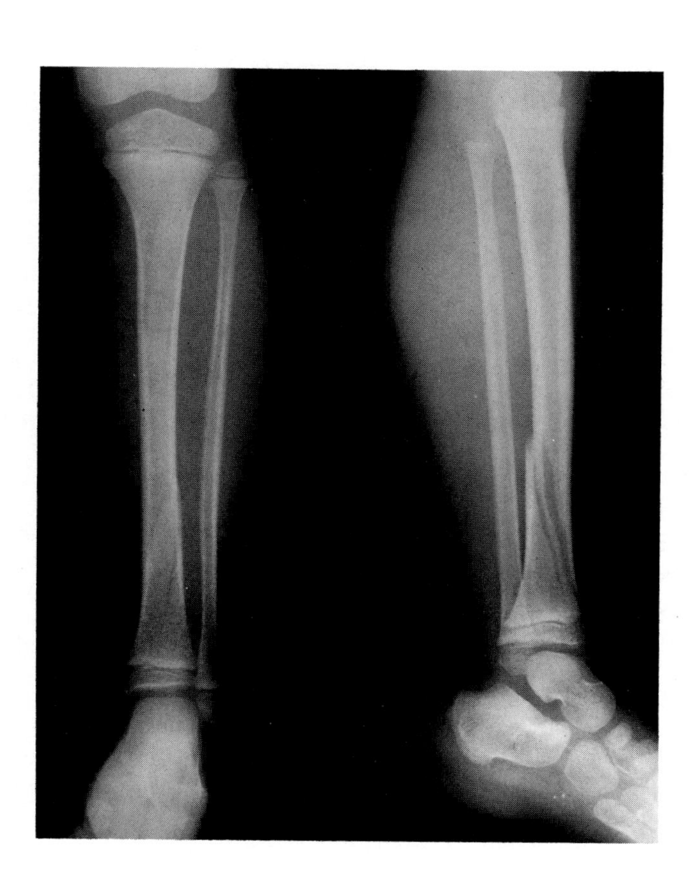

FIGURE 8–137. Spiral fracture of distal third of tibia with the fibula intact results from torsional stress on the leg.

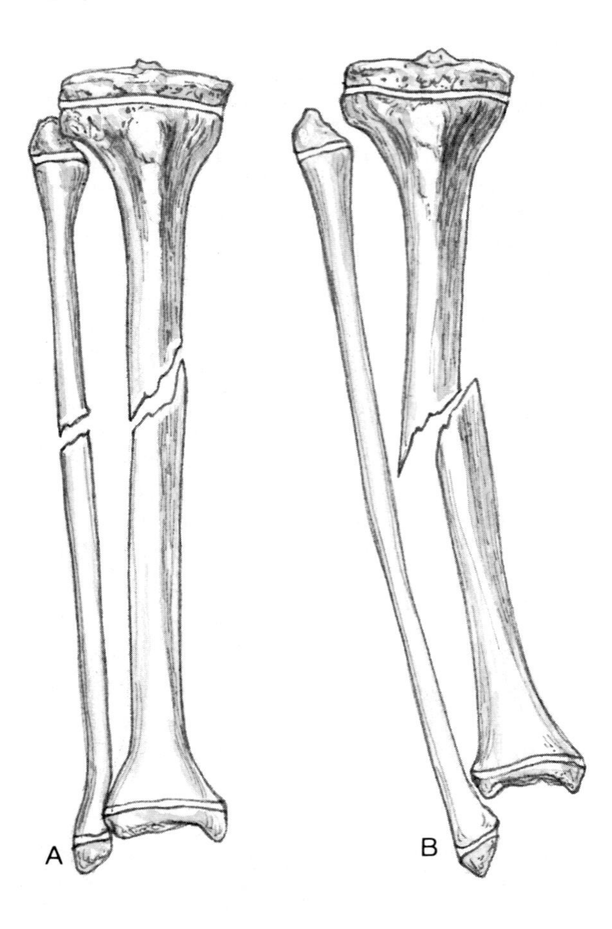

FIGURE 8–138. Spiral fracture of the tibia.

A. With spiral fracture of the fibula. This is usually stable owing to the thick periosteum. **B.** With the fibula intact. Note the varus drift of the distal fragment of the tibia.

gether by a thick periosteal sleeve and displacement of the fragments is minimal. Consequently, they are stable and can be adequately managed by closed methods; open surgical reduction is contraindicated in the treatment of closed fractures in infants and children. In automobile accidents, open fractures of the tibia and fibula with marked displacement of the fragments can occur.

Spiral Fracture of Tibia with Intact Fibula in Infancy and Early Childhood

This is produced by a torsional force on the leg when a child falls from his crib or twists his leg and falls down when attempting to pry his foot loose from the playpen. Because of its resiliency in infants, the fibula is usually not broken.

The child refuses to walk or bear weight on the affected lower limb, or he walks with an antalgic limp. He is unusually irritable and is constantly crying with pain. On examination, there is no obvious deformity; however, by careful palpation and by paying attention to the intensity of the cry, one should be able to localize the area of tenderness on the tibia. A common error is to suspect an injured foot and, on obtaining radiograms, to find that it is normal. Frequently spiral fractures of the tibia in an infant remain undiagnosed at the time of injury. Then, a week or ten days later, because of persistence of the limp and irritability, the parents bring the child for another consultation. At this time, a tender thickening on the subcutaneous surface of the tibia is palpable. Radiograms will disclose subperiosteal new bone formation. A hairline fracture may or may not be visualized—the fracture line may not be demonstrated because the fracture has consolidated, leaving only the periosteal reaction as evidence of the healing fracture. This may be mistaken for osteomyelitis, eosinophilic granuloma, acute leukemia, or some other neoplastic lesion. However, the true diagnosis will be established by repeating the radiograms of the tibia in six to eight weeks, when, in a fracture, they will be normal and all periosteal reaction will have disappeared.

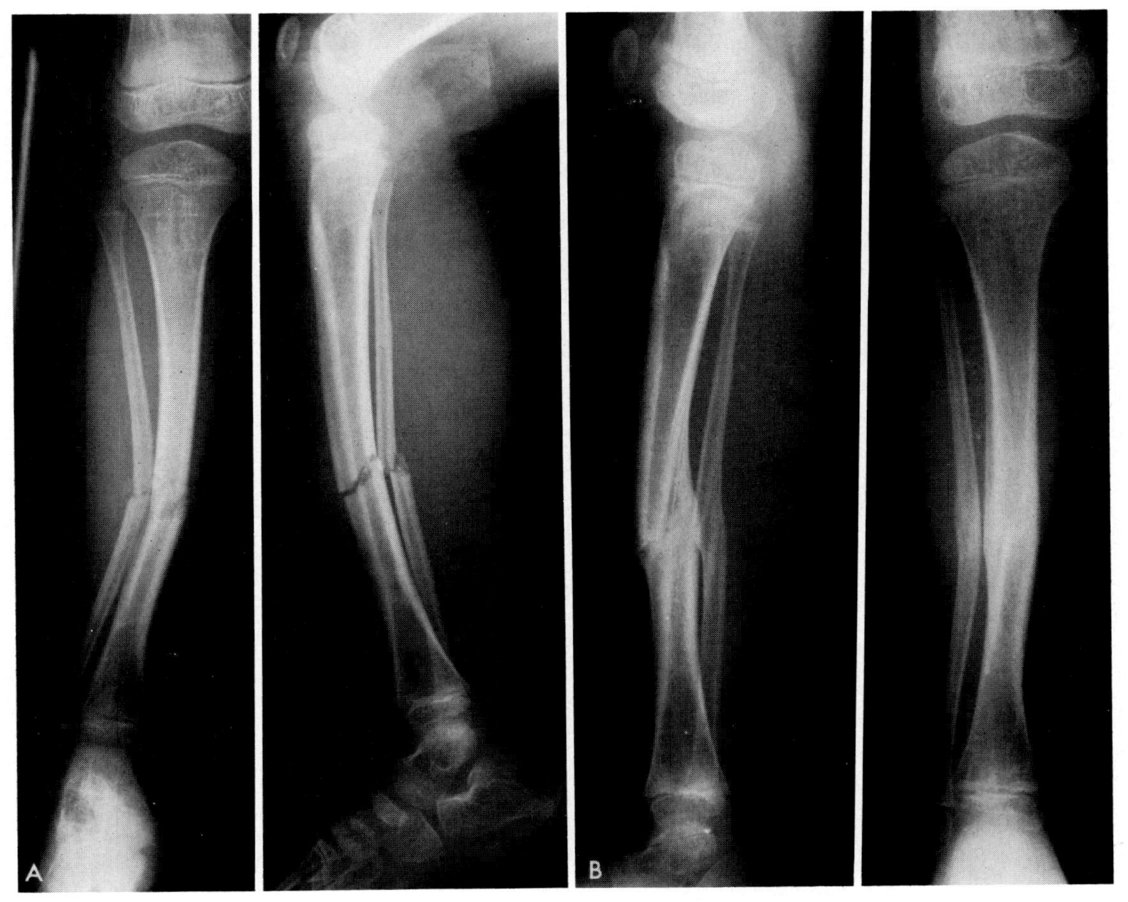

FIGURE 8–139. Fracture of tibia and fibula in its middle third resulting from direct injury.

A. Initial radiogram. **B.** Six weeks following closed manipulative reduction and immobilization in a long leg cast.

When the diagnosis is made at the time of initial injury, treatment consists of immobilization of the limb in an above-knee cast for a period of three weeks.

A spiral fracture of the tibia with intact fibula in the older child may become displaced with varus drift of the distal segment. When both bones are broken, the fracture will not drift into varus (Fig. 8–138).

Greenstick Fracture of Proximal Metaphysis or Upper Shaft of Tibia

An undisplaced or greenstick fracture of the proximal metaphysis or upper part of the diaphysis of the tibia is not uncommon in children. They usually occur between the ages of three and six years, although they may be encountered in the older child.

The mechanism of injury is usually a torsional stress applied from the medial aspect of the leg or, occasionally, direct violence. The distal fragment is angulated laterally, but there is no loss of apposition and the fragments do not override. The fibula ordinarily escapes injury, though occasionally it may sustain a greenstick fracture.

Treatment consists of correction of lateral angulation by manipulative reduction and immobilization in a long leg cast for a period of four to six weeks. An angulated greenstick fracture of the proximal tibia should be broken through by bending the leg toward the angulation, then slightly overcorrecting the deformity and applying a long leg cast. A common pitfall is failure to complete the fracture. The deformity will recur if the fracture is reduced by simple straightening of the leg prior to application of the cast.

The proximal metaphyseal fracture of the

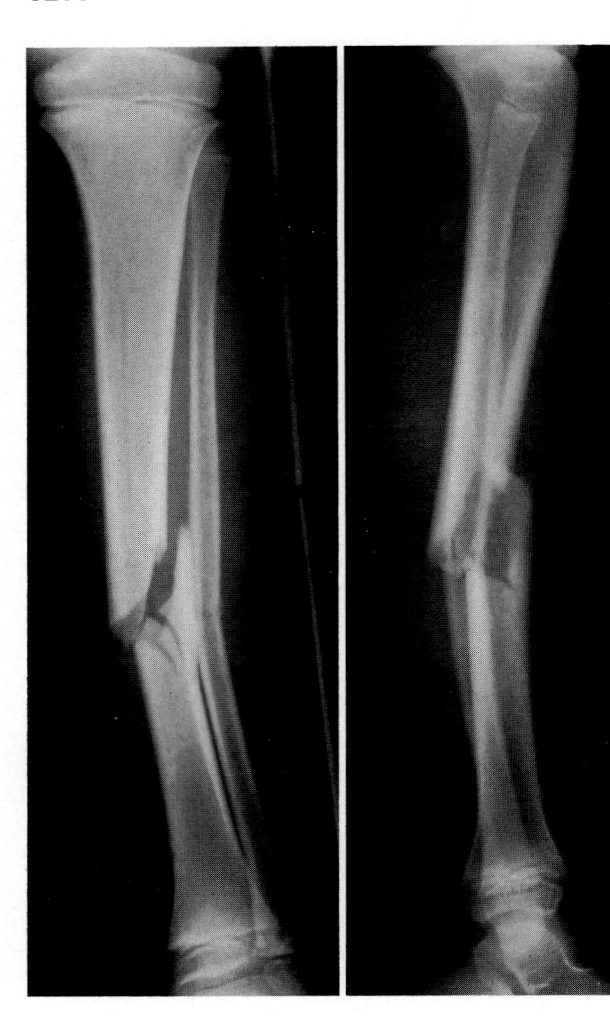

FIGURE 8–140. Comminuted fracture of middle third of tibia and fibula with butterfly fragment.

tibia is considered to be an innocuous injury. However, a common potential complication is asymmetrical tibial overgrowth and genu valgum (Fig. 8–141). Tibial leg length studies by orthoroentgenography or CAT scan will disclose the increased length of the tibia, which is longer on its medial than on its lateral aspect. Another factor to consider is a discrepancy of growth between the tibia and fibula, with the fibula exerting a tethering effect.[11, 12]

Treatment consists of observation, as some of the cases will correct spontaneously with growth and remodeling. If the tibial valgus deformity exceeds 20 degrees, a knock-knee long leg orthosis may be given to accelerate correction; however, there are no hard scientific data to document this. If the valgus deformity is severe and persistent, corrective osteotomy may be necessary. An osteotomy of the fibula is performed simultaneously to prevent recurrence of deformity.

Fractures of Tibia and Fibula in Older Children and Adolescents

These are treated by closed reduction, correcting both angular and rotational malalignment (Fig. 8–142). The limb is immobilized in a long leg cast, with the knee flexed to 90 degrees in order to control rotation and to prevent the child from bearing weight. In children, bayonet apposition of the fracture fragments and 1 cm. of overriding can be accepted. Immobilization is maintained for six weeks; during the last two weeks, the fracture may be sufficiently healed to permit partial weight-bearing in a walking cast.

In adolescents, comminuted unstable fractures of the tibia may be difficult to hold in a cast; in such an instance, pins are inserted above and below the fracture site and are incorporated in the cast to maintain reduction. Open reduction and internal fixation are not warranted.

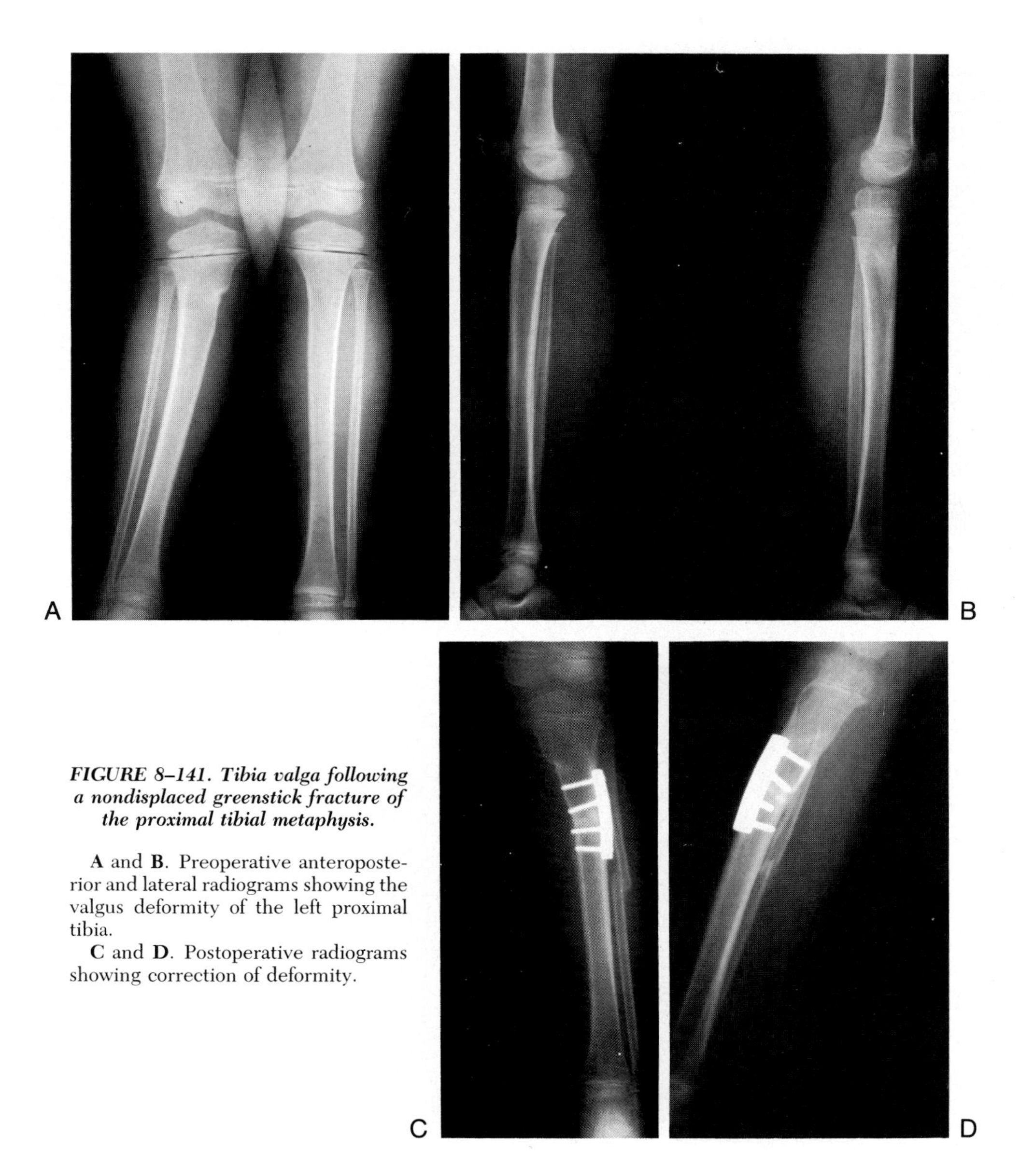

FIGURE 8–141. Tibia valga following a nondisplaced greenstick fracture of the proximal tibial metaphysis.

A and **B**. Preoperative anteroposterior and lateral radiograms showing the valgus deformity of the left proximal tibia.

C and **D**. Postoperative radiograms showing correction of deformity.

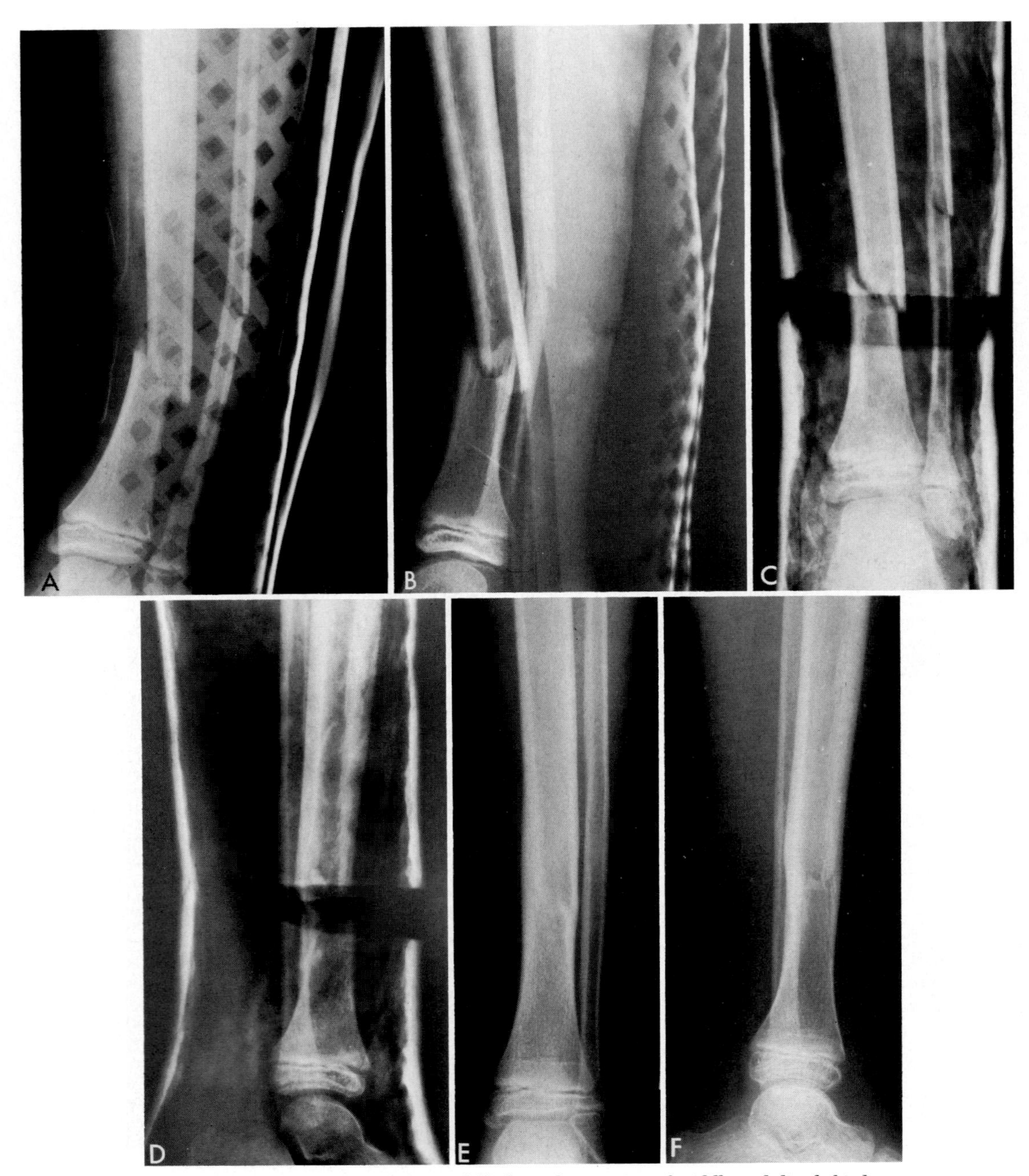

FIGURE 8–142. Fracture of tibia and fibula at the junction of middle and distal thirds.

A and **B.** Initial radiograms. **C** and **D.** Following closed reduction and wedging of the cast, accurate alignment was obtained. **E** and **F.** Four months later, radiograms show excellent alignment and healing.

References

1. Ahl, T., Andersson, G., Herberts, P., and Kalen, R.: Electrical treatment of non-united fractures. Acta Orthop. Scand., *55*:585, 1984.
2. Ansorg, P., and Graner, G.: Management of multiple fractures of the lower extremity in childhood. Beitr. Orthop. Traumatol., *25*:339, 1978.
3. Bahnson, D. H., and Lovell, W. W.: Genu valgum following fractures of the proximal tibial metaphysis in children. Orthop. Trans., *4*:306, 1980.
4. Beekman, F., and Sullivan, J. E.: Some observations on fractures of the long bones in children. J. Surg., *51*:736, 1941.
5. Borowski, M., and Rodziewicz, H.: Regeneration of posttraumatic loss of tibial shaft in a child. Chir. Narzadow Ruchu Ortop. Pol., *36*:459, 1971.
6. Boruch, Z., Zaluska-Matuszewska, M., and Wnuk-Katynska, U.: Slowly developing fracture of the tibia in children. Pol. Przegl. Chir., *39*:618, 1967.
7. Bostman, O. M.: Spiral fractures of the shaft of the tibia. Initial displacement and stability of reduction. J. Bone Joint Surg., *68-B*:462, 1986.
8. Chan, K. M., Leung, Y. K., Cheng, J. C., and Leung, P. C.: The management of type III open tibial fractures. Injury, *16*:157, 1984.
9. Clancey, G. J., and Hansen, S. T., Jr.: Open fractures of the tibia. A review of one hundred and two cases. J. Bone Joint Surg., *60-A*:118, 1978.
10. Coates, R.: Knock-knee deformity following upper tibial "greenstick" fractures. J. Bone Joint Surg., *59-B*:516, 1977.
11. Cozen, L.: Fracture of the proximal portion of the tibia in children followed by valgus deformity. Surg. Gynecol. Obstet., *97*:183, 1953.
12. Cozen, L.: Knock knee deformity after fracture of the proximal tibia in children. Orthopaedics, *1*:230, 1959.
13. Currarino, G., and Pinckney, L. E.: Genu valgum after proximal tibial fractures in children. A.J.R., *136*:915, 1981.
14. Dias, L. S.: Fractures of the tibia and fibula. *In* Rockwood, C. A., Jr., Wilkins, K. E., and King, R. E.: Fractures in Children. Philadelphia, Lippincott, 1984, pp. 983–1042.
15. Dunbar, J. S., Owen, H. F., Nogrady, M. B., and McLesse, R.: Obscure tibial fractures of infants—the toddler's fracture. J. Can. Assoc. Radiol., *25*:136, 1964.
16. Evans, P. E., and Thomas, W. G.: Tibial fractures through a traction-pin site. A report of two cases. J. Bone Joint Surg., *66-A*:1475, 1984.
17. Feldkamp, G., Hausler, U., and Daum, R.: Observations of the course of tibia-shaft-fractures in children. Unfallheilkunde, *80*:139, 1977.
18. Feldkamp, G., Krastel, A., and Braus, T.: Which factors influence growth phenomena after childhood tibial shaft fractures? (author's transl.). Unfallheilkunde, *81*:96, 1978.
19. Felman, A. H.: Bicycle spoke fractures. J. Pediatr., *82*:302, 1973.
20. Garrick, J. G., Riggins, R. S., Regua, R. K., and Lipscomb, P. R.: Fracture of the mid-shaft of the tibia and fibula. A survey of treatment. Clin. Orthop., *88*:131, 1972.
21. Golimbu, C., Firooznia, H., Rafii, M., and Waugh, T.: Acute traumatic fibular bowing associated with tibial fractures. Clin. Orthop., *182*:211, 1984.
22. Green, N. E.: Tibia valga caused by asymmetrical overgrowth following a nondisplaced fracture of the proximal tibial metaphysis. J. Pediatr. Orthop., *3*:235, 1983.
23. Greiff, J., and Bergman, F.: Growth disturbance following fracture of the tibia in children. Acta Orthop. Scand., *51*:315, 1980.
24. Greinemann, H.: Fractures of the lower leg in childhood. Hefte Unfallheilkd., *117*:50, 1974.
25. Gushchanskii, S. I.: Late results of the treatment of closed diaphyseal fractures of the leg bones in children. Ortop. Travmatol. Protez., *34*:79, 1973.
26. Haas, L. M., and Staple, T. W.: Arterial injuries associated with fractures of the proximal tibia following blunt trauma. South. Med. J., *62*:1439, 1969.
27. Halloran, W. X., Thomassen, J. P., Kiernan, E. R., and Young, S.: Bumper fracture of the tibia with severed posterior tibial artery. Orthop. Rev., *6*:41, 1975.
28. Hammer, R.: External fixation of tibial shaft fractures. A review of 42 fractures by the Hoffman-Vidal-Adrey external fixation system. Arch. Orthop. Trauma. Surg., *104*:271, 1985.
29. Hansen, B., Greiff, J., and Bergmann, F.: Fractures of the tibia in children. Acta Orthop. Scand., *47*:448, 1976.
30. Hansson, L. I., Hybbinette, C. H., and Sjostrand, L. O.: Re-implantation of a traumatically expelled tibial diaphysis. Acta Orthop. Scand., *48*:108, 1977.
31. Harley, J. M., Campbell, M. J., and Jackson, R. K.: A comparison of plating and traction in the treatment of tibial shaft fractures. Injury, *17*:91, 1986.
32. Hasenhuttl, K.: The treatment of unstable fractures of the tibia and fibula with flexible medullary wires. A review of two hundred and thirty-five fractures. J. Bone Joint Surg., *63-A*:921, 1981.
33. Hoover, N. W.: Injuries of the popliteal artery associated with fractures and dislocations. Surg. Clin. North Am., *41*:1099, 1961.
34. Ippolito, E., and Pentimalli, G.: Post-traumatic valgus deformity of the knee in proximal tibial metaphyseal fractures in children. Ital. J. Orthop. Traumatol., *10*:103, 1984.
35. Izant, R. J., Rothman, B. F., and Frankel, V.: Bicycle spoke injuries of the foot and ankle in children: An underestimated "minor" injury. J. Pediatr. Surg., *4*:654, 1969.
36. Jackson, D. W., and Cozen, L.: Genu valgum as a complication of proximal tibial metaphyseal fractures in children. J. Bone Joint Surg., *53-A*:1571, 1971.
37. Karlstrom, G., and Olerud, S.: Percutaneous pin fixation of open tibial fractures. Double-frame anchorage using the Vidal-Adrey method. J. Bone Joint Surg., *57-A*:915, 1975.
38. Karlstrom, G., and Olerud, S.: Stable external fixation of open tibial fractures. Orthop. Rev., *6*:25, 1977.
39. Karlstrom, G., Lonnerholm, T., and Olerud, S.: Cavus deformity of the foot after fracture to the tibial shaft. J. Bone Joint Surg., *57-A*:893, 1975.
40. Karrholm, J., Hansson, L. I., and Svensson, K.: Incidence of tibio-fibular shaft and ankle fractures in children. J. Pediatr. Orthop., *2*:386, 1982.
41. Kay, L., Hansen, B. A., and Raaschou, H. O.: Fractures of the tibial shaft conservatively treated. Injury, *17*:5, 1986.
42. Koch, A., Kehrer, B., and Tschappeler, H.: Fractures of the proximal tibial metaphysis. Ther. Umsch., *40*:978, 1983.
43. Korisek, G.: The supramalleolar fracture of the tibia and lower leg in children and juveniles (author's transl.). Unfallheilkunde, *80*:369, 1977.
44. Kurz, W., and Vinz, H.: Tibial fractures in children (author's transl.). Zentralbl. Chir., *104*:1402, 1979.
45. Leach, R. E., Hammond, G., and Stryker, W. S.: Anterior tibial compartment syndrome. J. Bone Joint Surg., *49-A*:451, 1967.
46. Light, T. R., Ogden, D. A., and Ogden, J. A.: The anatomy of metaphyseal torus fractures. Clin. Orthop., *188*:103, 1984.
47. Manoli, A., II: Traumatic fibular bowing with tibial fracture: Report of two cases. Orthopedics, *1*:145, 1978.
48. Matin, P.: The appearance on bone scans following fractures, including immediate and long-term studies. J. Nucl. Med., *20*:1227, 1979.

49. Matsen, F. A., III, and Cawson, D. K.: The deep posterior compartmental syndrome of the leg. J. Bone Joint Surg., *57-A*:34, 1975.
50. Matsen, F. A., and Staheli, L. T.: Neurovascular complications following tibial osteotomy in children. Clin. Orthop., *110*:210, 1975.
51. Mollica, Q., Gangitano, R., and Longo, G.: Elastic intramedullary nailing in shaft fractures of the femur and tibia. Orthopedics, 9:1065, 1986.
52. Morton, K. S., and Starr, D. E.: Closure of the anterior portion of the upper tibial epiphysis as a complication of tibial-shaft fracture. J. Bone Joint Surg., *46-A*:570, 1964.
53. Nilsson, B. E., and Westlin, N. E.: Restoration of bone mass after fracture of the lower limb in children. Acta Orthop. Scand., *42*:78, 1971.
54. Olerud, C.: The pronation capacity of the foot—its consequences for axial deformity after tibial shaft fractures. Arch. Orthop. Trauma. Surg., *104*:303, 1985.
55. Parsch, K., Manner, G., and Dippe, K.: Genu valgum after proximal tibial fracture in children (author's transl.). Arch. Orthop. Unfallchir., *90*:289, 1977.
56. Perry, C. R., Rice, S., Rao, A., and Burdge, R.: Posterior fracture-dislocation of the distal part of the fibula. Mechanism and staging of injury. J. Bone Joint Surg., *65-A*:1149, 1983.
57. Poell, J., and Lehner, M.: Results of conservative treatment of transverse fracture of the distal tibia and fibula in children. Helv. Chir. Acta, *44*:211, 1977.
58. Pollen, A. G.: Fractures and Dislocations in Children. Baltimore, Williams & Wilkins, 1973.
59. Puno, R. M., Teynor, J. T., Nagano, J., and Gustilo, R. B.: Critical analysis of results of treatment of 201 tibial shaft fractures. Clin. Orthop., *212*:113, 1986.
60. Rang, M.: Children's Fractures. Philadelphia, Lippincott, 1983.
61. Reynolds, D. A.: Growth changes in fractured long bones. J. Bone Joint Surg., *63-B*:83, 1981.
62. Ricciardi, L., Perissinotto, A., and Visentin, E.: Ultrasonography in the evaluation of osteogenesis in fractures treated with Hoffman external fixation. Ital. J. Orthop. Traumatol., *12*:185, 1986.
63. Rommens, P., Broos, P., and Gruwez, J. A.: External fixation of tibial shaft fractures with severe soft tissue injuries by Hoffman-Vidal-Adrey osteotaxis. Arch. Orthop. Trauma. Surg., *105*:170, 1986.
64. Rorabeck, C. H.: Anterior tibial compartment syndrome complicating fractures of the shaft of the tibia. J. Bone Joint Surg., *58-A*:549, 1976.
65. Salter, R. B., and Best, T.: The pathogenesis and prevention of valgus deformity following fractures of the proximal metaphyseal region of the tibia in children. J. Bone Joint Surg., *55-A*:1324, 1973.
66. Sarmiento, A.: A functional below-the-knee cast for tibial fractures. J. Bone Joint Surg., *49-A*:855, 1967.
67. Sarmiento, A., Latta, L., Zilioli, A., and Sinclair, W.: The role of soft tissue in the stabilization of tibial fractures. Clin. Orthop., *105*:116, 1974.
68. Schroder, H. A., Christoffersen, H., and Sorensen, T. S.: Fractures of the shaft of the tibia treated with Hoffman external fixation. Arch. Orthop. Trauma. Surg., *105*:28, 1986.
69. Shannak, A. O.: Tibial fractures in children. Follow-up study. J. Pediatr. Orthop., *8*:306, 1988.
70. Skak, S. V.: Valgus deformity following proximal tibial metaphyseal fracture in children. Acta Orthop. Scand., *53*:141, 1982.
71. Stanford, J. C., Rodriquez, R. P., and Hayes, J. T.: Tibial shaft fractures in adults and children. J.A.M.A., *195*:1111, 1966.
72. Steinert, V.: Indications for corrective osteotomy following fractures of the lower leg in childhood. Beitr. Orthop. Traumatol., *14*:747, 1967.
73. Steinert, V., and Bennek, J.: Tibial fractures in children. Zentralbl. Chir., *91*:1387, 1966.
74. Stenstrom, R., Gripenberg, L., and Bergius, A. R.: Traumatic bowing of forearm and lower leg in children. Acta Radiol. [Diagn.] (Stockh.), *19*(1B):243, 1978.
75. Taylor, S. L.: Tibial overgrowth: A cause of genu valgum. J. Bone Joint Surg., *45-A*:659, 1963.
76. Teitz, C. C., Carter, D. R., and Frankel, V. H.: Problems associated with tibial fractures with intact fibulae. J. Bone Joint Surg., *62-A*:770, 1980.
77. Veith, R. G., Winquist, R. A., and Hansen, S. T., Jr.: Ipsilateral fractures of the femur and tibia. A report of fifty-seven consecutive cases. J. Bone Joint Surg., *66-A*:1002, 1984.
78. Viljanto, J.: Bicycle and Moped spoke injuries in children. Analysis of 103 consecutive cases. Ann. Chir. Gynaecol. Fenn., *64*:100, 1975.
79. Visser, J. D., and Veldhuizen, A. G.: Valgus deformity after fracture of the proximal tibial metaphysis in childhood. Acta Orthop. Scand., *53*:663, 1982.
80. Walker, A. P.: Bilateral fracture of the upper third of the fibula caused by indirect trauma. Orthopedics, 9:1081, 1986.
81. Weber, B. G.: Fibrous interposition causing valgus deformity after fracture of the upper tibial metaphysis in children. J. Bone Joint Surg., *59-B*:290, 1977.
82. Weber, B. G., Brunner, C., and Freuier, F. (eds.): Treatment of Fractures in Children and Adolescents. Berlin, Springer-Verlag, 1980.
83. Wiss, D. A., Segal, D., and Gumbs, V. L.: Flexible medullary nailing of acute tibial shaft fractures. Clin. Orthop., *212*:122, 1986.
84. Wiss, D. A., Segal, D., and Gumbs, V. L.: Flexible medullary nailing of tibial shaft fractures. J. Trauma, *26*:1106, 1986.
85. Wood, D., and Hoffer, M. M.: Tibial fractures in head-injured children. J. Trauma, 27:65, 1987.

FRACTURES OF THE ANKLE

The ossific nucleus of the distal tibial epiphysis appears between six and ten months of life. The medial malleolus ossifies as a downward prolongation from the main nucleus, appearing at the age of seven years in girls and eight years in boys (Fig. 8–143). Occasionally the medial malleolus develops from a separate center of ossification; this should not be mistaken for a fracture. By 14 or 15 years of age, the entire lower end of the tibia (including the medial malleolus) is completely ossified; it unites with the diaphysis at about the eighteenth year. The lower epiphysis contributes 45 per cent of the growth of the tibia.

The distal epiphysis of the fibula begins to ossify during the second year of life, usually between the ages of 18 and 20 months. Occasionally its ossification may be delayed until the end of the third year. Union with the diaphysis occurs around the twentieth year.

Fractures involving the lower tibial physis constitute 11 per cent of all physeal injuries. They are more common in boys, who account for about 80 per cent of the cases. The common age of incidence ranges from 11 to 15 years, the median ages being 14 years in males and 12 years in females.

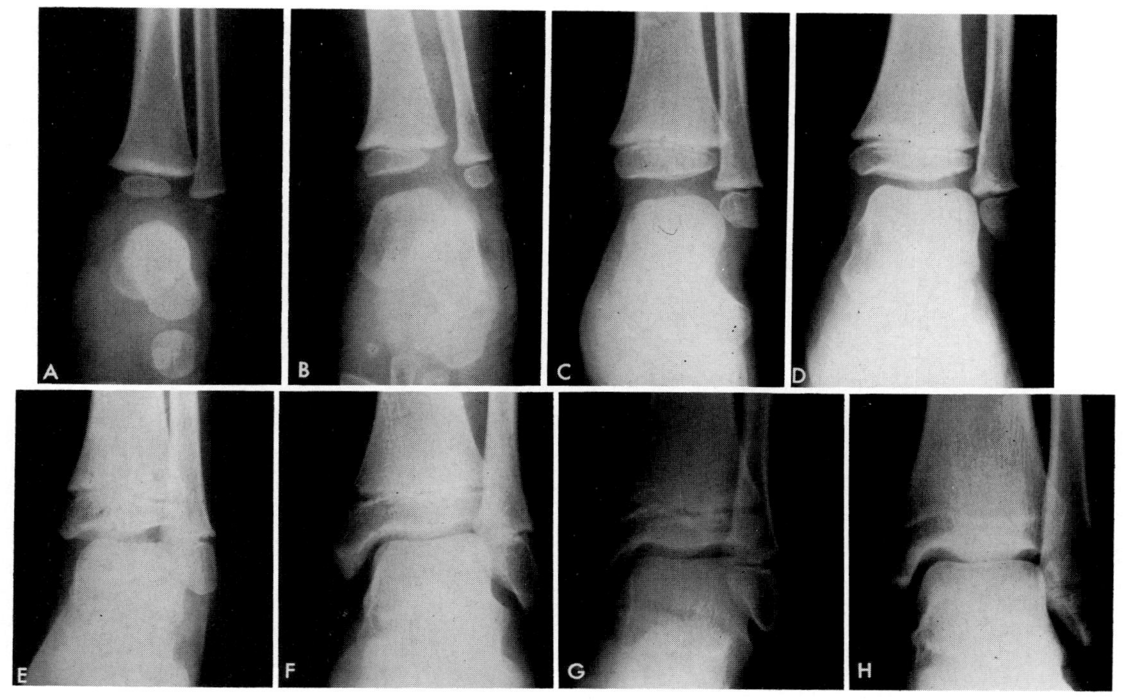

FIGURE 8–143. Ossification of distal epiphyses of tibia and fibula.

A. One year of age. **B.** Two years. **C.** Four years. **D.** Six years. **E.** Seven years. **F.** Ten years. **G.** Twelve years. **H.** Adult.

Fractures involving the distal fibular physis may occur alone or in association with those of the distal tibial physis. They usually take place in the age range of 8 to 15 years.

Classification and Mechanism of Injury

The ankle is a true mortise joint that moves in only one plane—into plantar flexion and dorsiflexion—and is stable and distinctly limited in all other planes. This shape of the ankle joint renders the distal tibial epiphysis particularly vulnerable to crushing injuries.

All the ligaments of the ankle are attached to the distal epiphyses of the tibia and fibula. Ligamentous injuries are rare in children because the ligaments are stronger than the growth plate, and tension on them will cause fracture-separation of the physis.

The tibia and fibula are bound together by the interosseous membrane. In adduction-inversion injuries, fracture through both physes may take place and the distal epiphyses of the tibia and fibula will move as a unit, as shown in Figure 8–144; or only the distal fibular physis may separate, and the talus will shift medially to impinge on the medial malleolus and the medial corner of the weight-bearing articular surface of the tibia, resulting in the intra-articular fracture (Fig. 8–144 B). The lower fibular physis lies farther distal than that of the tibia. When the distal tibial epiphysis moves laterally it impinges on the metaphysis of the fibula and causes a fracture of the fibula at a higher level. Occasionally the interosseous membrane will rupture (Fig. 8–144 C).

ANATOMIC CLASSIFICATION

Fractures involving the distal tibial physis and fibula can be classified anatomically according to the Salter-Harris classification.

MECHANISTIC CLASSIFICATIONS

Ankle fractures are usually caused by indirect violence; the fixed foot is forced into either abduction, adduction, lateral or medial rotation, eversion or inversion, or plantar flexion or dorsiflexion. Pronation and supination are the positions of the foot attained by rotational movement around the axis of the talocalcaneonavicular joint. Medial and lateral rotational movements of the talus take place around the sagittal axis of the weight-bearing articular surface of the tibia. These forces are

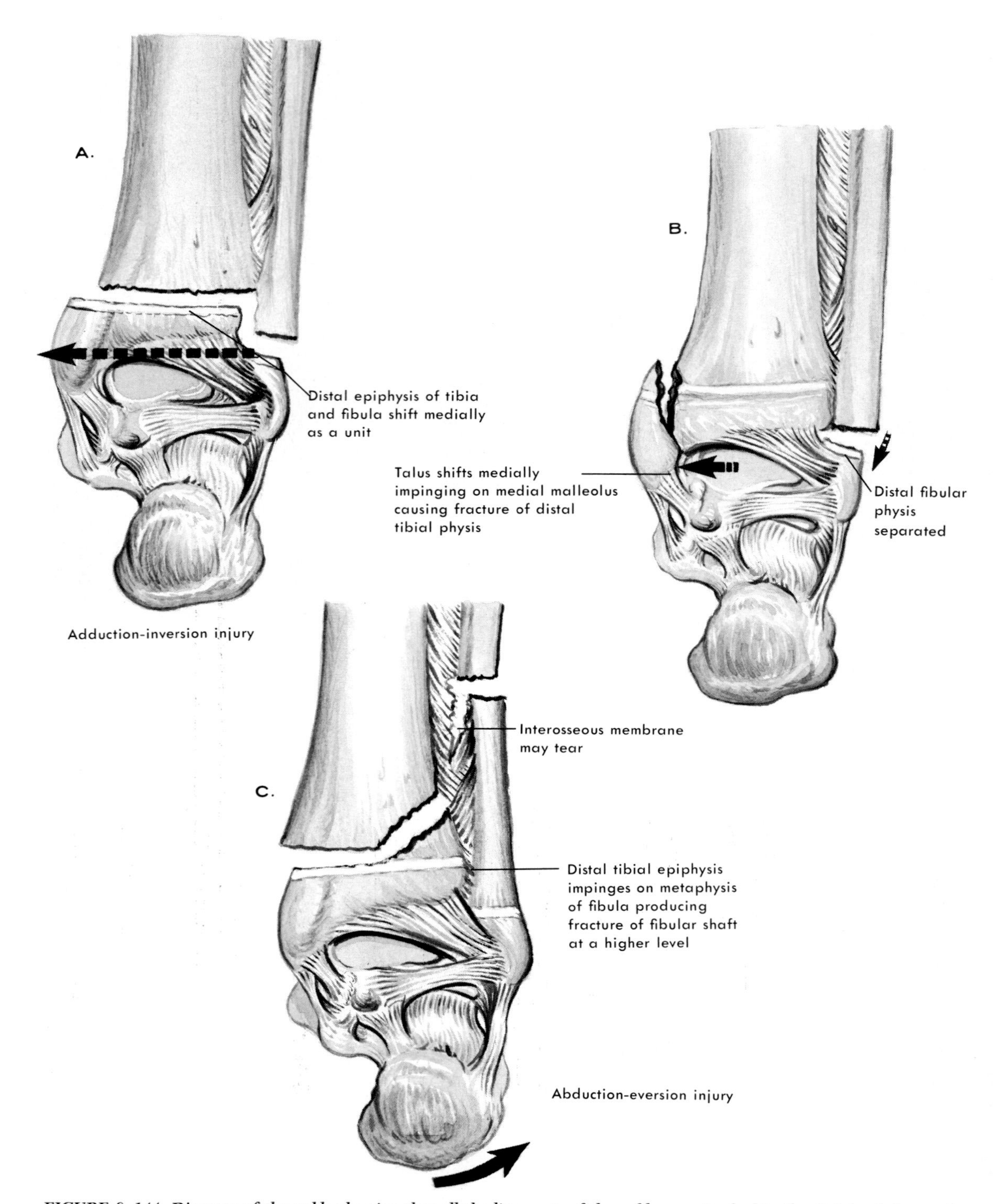

FIGURE 8–144. Diagram of the ankle showing that all the ligaments of the ankle are attached to the distal epiphyses of the tibia and fibula.

The lower physis of the fibula lies more distal than that of the tibia. The fibula and tibia are bound together by the interosseous membrane. **A** and **B.** On adduction-inversion injury, the distal epiphyses of the tibia and fibula may shift medially as a unit or the distal fibular physis may separate and the talus shift medially, impinging on the medial malleolus or the medial corner of the weight-bearing articular surface of the tibia and causing a Salter-Harris Type III or IV fracture of the distal tibial epiphysis. **C.** On abduction-eversion injuries the distal epiphysis of the tibia impinges on the metaphysis of the fibula, producing a fracture of the fibular shaft at a higher level; occasionally the interosseous membrane may tear.

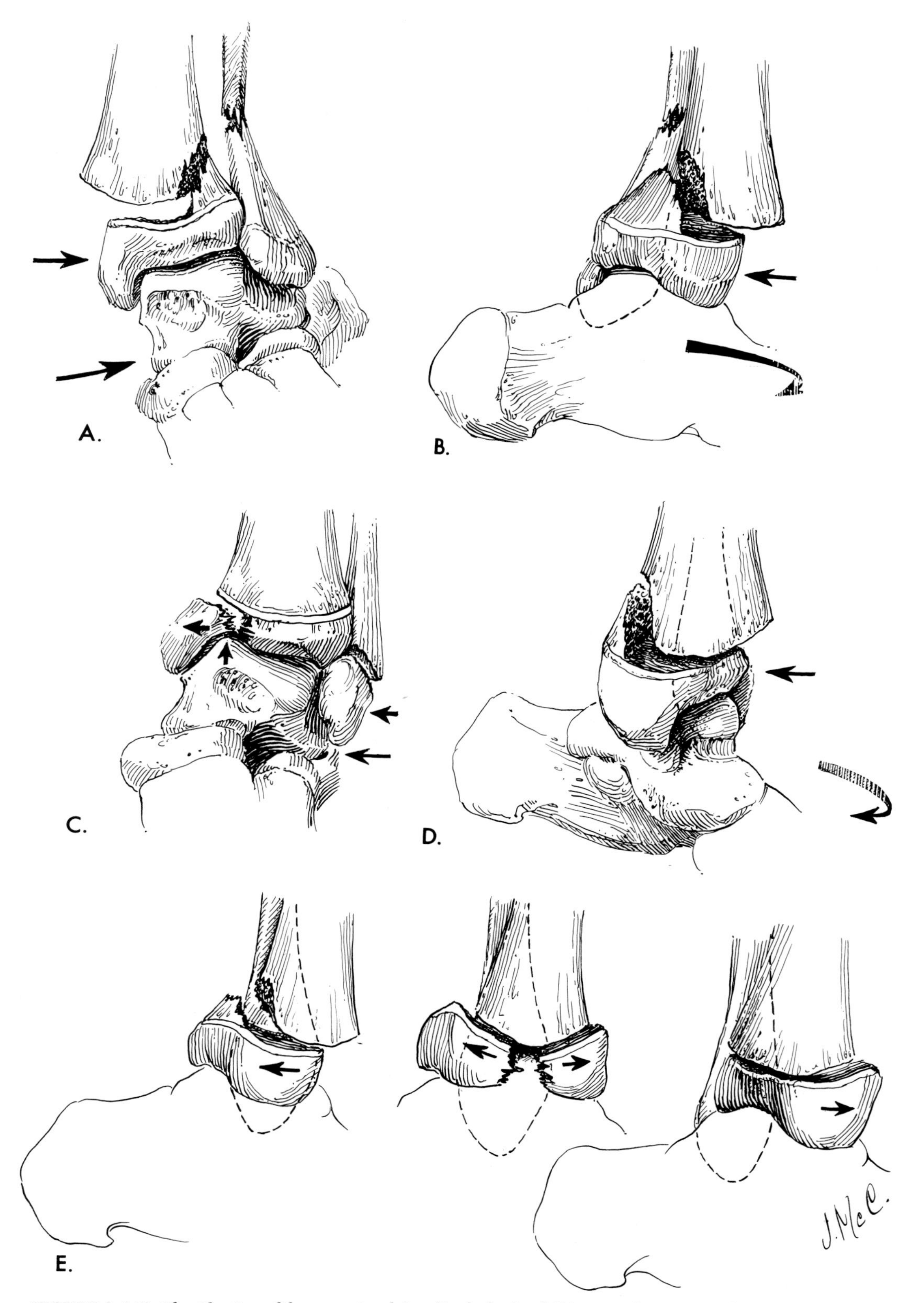

FIGURE 8–145. ***Classification of fractures involving distal physis of tibia according to Carothers and Crenshaw.***

A. Abduction injury. **B.** External rotation injury. **C.** Adduction injury. **D.** Plantar flexion injury. **E.** Axial compression injury and injury caused by direct violence.

transmitted by the deltoid and lateral collateral ligaments to the epiphyses of the distal tibia and fibula, exerting tension at the physes. Ankle fractures may also be caused by direct violence, as in an automobile accident or a fall. In direct crush injuries, the fractures may be open.

In 1932, Bishop modified the Ashhurst-Bromer classification of ankle fractures and subdivided ankle injuries in children on a mechanical basis.[10] Carothers and Crenshaw considered the direction of the injuring force and, in 1955, further modified the classification, listing (1) abduction injuries; (2) external rotation injuries; (3) adduction injuries; (4) plantar flexion injuries; and (5) axial compression injuries and injuries caused by direct violence (Fig. 8–145).[19]

Lauge-Hansen showed that in the study of the mechanism of ankle fractures in the adult three factors should be considered: the axial load, the position of the foot at the moment of trauma, and the direction of the abnormal force.[70–74] In children, an additional factor determining the pattern of fracture is the state of maturity of the physis.

Dias and Tachdjian devised a classification of physeal injuries of the ankle in children that utilizes Lauge-Hansen's categories of foot position and direction of abnormal force in correlation with the Salter-Harris classification. Four mechanisms are proposed; in each, the first term refers to the position of the foot at the time of injury and the second, to the direction of injuring force on the ankle joint. Grades of injury are described in a progressively increasing order of severity (Table 8–7).[34] The fracture patterns and displacement of fragments are quite characteristic for each mechanism. In classifying an ankle fracture, one should study the radiograms carefully to determine the type of Salter-Harris physeal injury, the direction of the fracture line, and the direction of displacement of the epiphyseal-metaphyseal fracture fragment in relation to localized swelling and tenderness.

Supination-Inversion Injury. In this type of ankle fracture an inversion force is exerted on a foot that is fixed in supination.

In *grade 1* supination-inversion injury, traction by the lateral ligaments of the ankle will produce a Salter-Harris Type I or II fracture separation of the distal fibular physis (Fig. 8–146 A and B, and Fig. 8–147). Occasionally the calcaneofibular and talofibular ligaments may rupture, as shown in Figure 8–146 C, or a fracture of the distal tip of the lateral malleolus may take place (Figs. 8–146 D and 8–148). In almost all cases the displacement of the distal fibular epiphysis is medial and minimal. Injury to the distal fibular physis usually goes undiagnosed because the displacement of the epiphysis is slight. After twisting the ankle, the patient walks with an antalgic limp and complains of pain. There is local tenderness and swelling. In the routine anteroposterior and lateral radiograms of the ankle, this physeal injury is usually not visualized; oblique views are required to depict the minimal displacement (Fig. 8–149).

In *grade 2* supination-inversion injury, following fracture of the distal fibular epiphysis, the inversion force will medially displace the talus against the medial malleolus. The medial border of the upper surface of the talus impinges on the medial half of the lower end of the tibia and exerts a crushing force at this point. The intra-articular shearing force causes either a Type IV Salter-Harris physeal injury (in which the epiphysis, physis, and a portion of the metaphysis are completely split and there is upward and medial displacement of the medial fragment, as shown in Figures 8–150 and 8–151) or a Type III Salter-Harris physeal injury (in which the fracture extends from the articular surface to the zone of the hypertrophic cartilage cells of the physis and then along the plate to its medial border, as seen in Figures 8–150 B and 8–152 to 8–156). Occasionally the inversion-adduction force will displace the entire distal tibial epiphysis medially with a medial metaphyseal tibial fragment attached to it (Type II physeal injury, shown in Figure 8–150 C) or without a metaphyseal fragment (Type I physeal injury). The displacement of the fracture fragments is usually medial, occasionally posteromedial.

Supination–Plantar Flexion Fracture. With the foot fixed in full supination, a plantar flexion force exerted on the ankle causes this type of injury.

The common pattern (grade 1) is a Salter-Harris Type II physeal injury of the distal tibial epiphysis with posterior displacement of the epiphyseal-metaphyseal fracture fragment. The metaphyseal fragment is posterior. The fracture is best visualized in the lateral projection. There is no associated fibular fracture (Figs. 8–157 and 8–158).

Supination–Lateral Rotation Fracture. This type of fracture occurs when, with the foot in full supination, a lateral rotation force is exerted on the ankle joint. The fracture caused by this mechanism may fall into one of two grades. In the *grade 1* injury a Salter-Harris Type II fracture of the distal tibial epiphysis occurs with a long spiral fracture of the distal tibia beginning at the lateral (fibular) end of the distal tibial

Text continued on page 3316

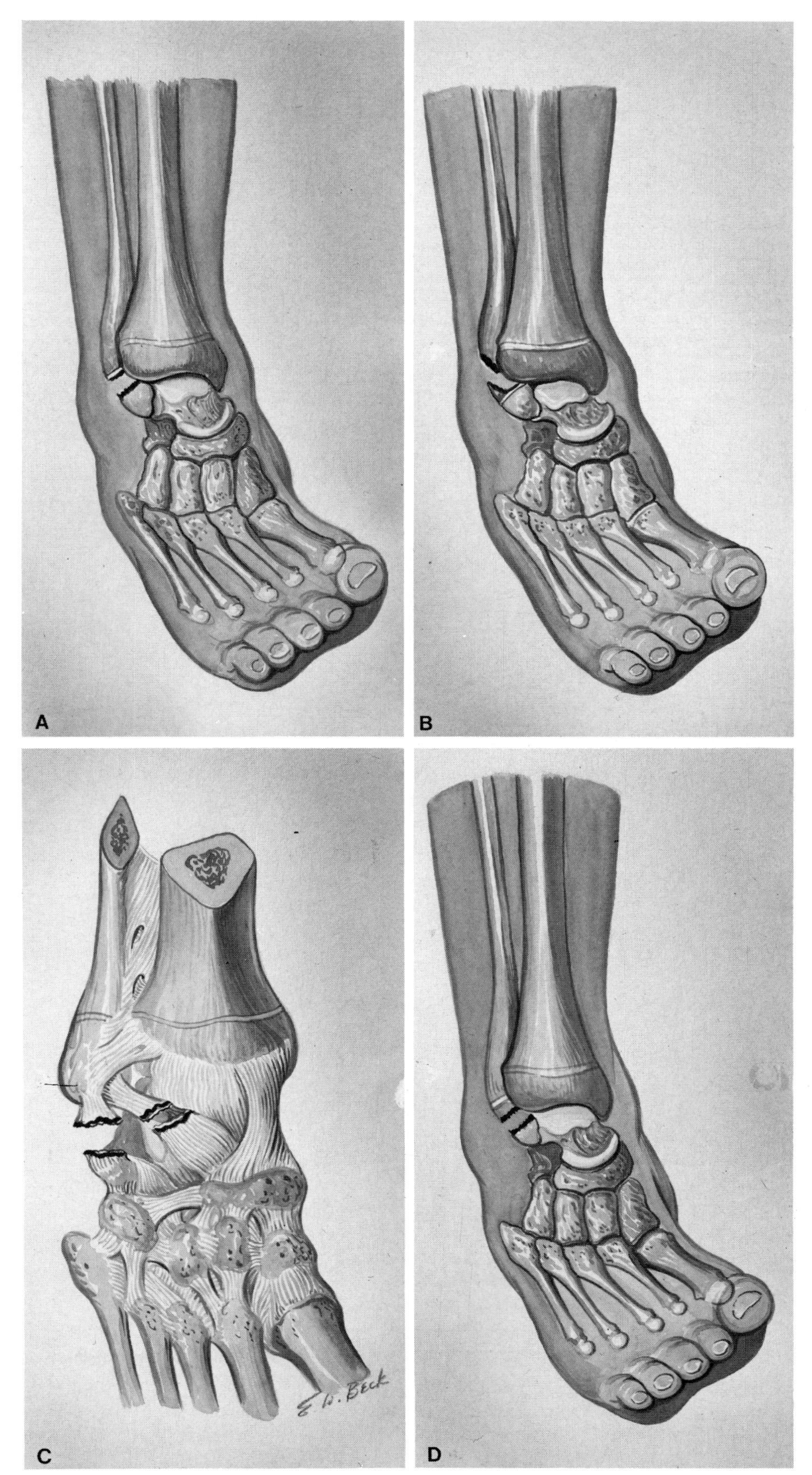

FIGURE 8–146 *See legend on following page*

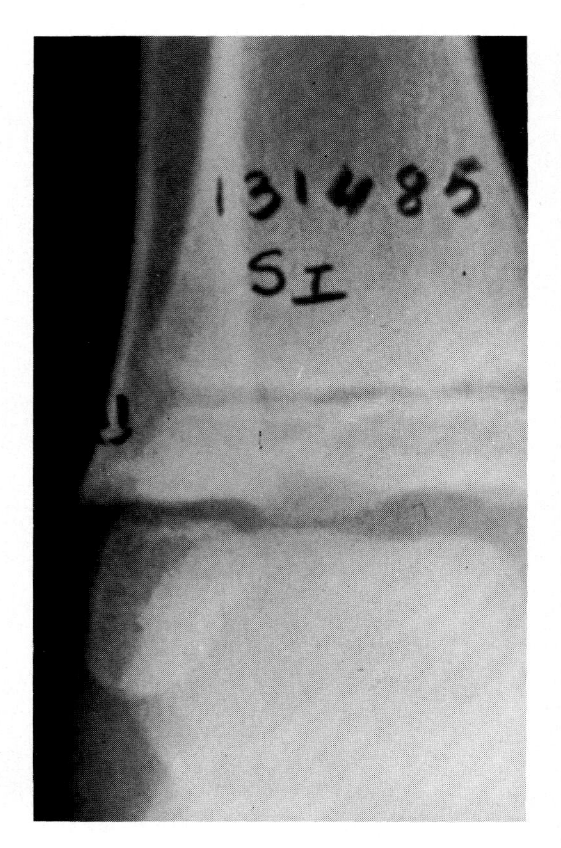

FIGURE 8–147. Fracture-separation of distal fibular epiphysis with minimal displacement (supination-inversion grade 1 physeal injury of the ankle).

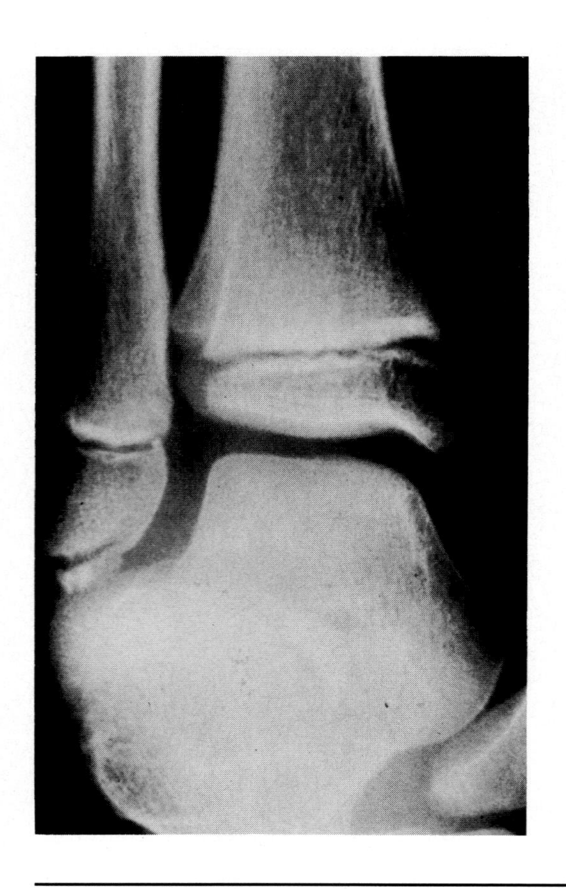

FIGURE 8–148. Fracture of distal tip of lower fibular epiphysis (supination-inversion grade 1 injury of the ankle).

FIGURE 8–146. Supination-inversion physeal injury of the ankle in children—grade 1.

An inversion force exerted with the foot fixed in supinated position will produce: **A** and **B.** Salter-Harris Type I or II physeal injury of the distal fibular physis. **C.** Occasionally rupture of the calcaneofibular or talofibular ligaments may result. **D.** The distal tip of the lateral malleolus may be fractured. Note that the displacement of the distal fibular epiphysis is medial and not marked.

Table [illegible]. Classification of Physeal Injuries of the Ankle in Children (Modified from Lauge-Hansen)

Type	Grade	Position of Foot	Injuring Force	Pattern of Fracture	Comment
Supination–inversion	1	Supinated	Inversion	Usually Salter-Harris I or II fracture separation of distal fibular physis Occasionally rupture of lateral ligament or fracture of tip of lateral malleolus	Displacement minimal and almost always medial
	2	Supinated	Inversion	Usually Salter-Harris III or IV of medial part of tibial epiphysis Rarely Salter-Harris I or II with medial displacement of entire tibial epiphysis	Caution! Asymmetrical growth arrest causes varus ankle
Supination–plantar flexion	1	Supinated	Plantar flexion	Commonly Salter-Harris II of tibial epiphysis Rarely Salter-Harris I of tibial physis No associated fracture of fibula Metaphyseal fragment and displacement posterior Fracture line best seen in lateral x-ray	Prognosis good Caution! Do not damage growth plate by forced manipulation. Posterior displacement will remodel
Supination–lateral rotation	1	Supinated	Lateral rotation	Salter-Harris II of distal tibial epiphysis with long spiral fracture of distal tibia starting laterally at distal tibial growth plate	Distinguishing feature is direction of fracture line starting laterally and running medially and proximally
	2	Supinated	Lateral rotation	Grade 1 plus spiral fracture of distal fibular shaft	—
Pronation–eversion–lateral rotation	1	Pronated	Eversion–lateral rotation	Salter-Harris II of distal tibial epiphysis Metaphyseal fragment lateral or posterolateral Displacement lateral or posterolateral Fibular fracture short, oblique, 4 to 7 cm. from tip of lateral malleolus	—
Miscellaneous					
Adolescent Tillaux	–	? Neutral?	Lateral rotation	Salter-Harris III of lateral part of distal tibial epiphysis Should not be any metaphyseal fragment Displacement anterolateral	Medial part of distal tibial physis closed
Triplane three-fragment	–	?	Lateral rotation	Fracture in three planes—coronal, sagittal, and transverse Combination of Salter-Harris II and III Fracture produces three fragments	Medial part of distal tibial physis open
Triplane two-fragment	–	?	Lateral rotation	Fracture in three planes—coronal, sagittal, and transverse Combination of Salter-Harris II and III Fracture creates two fragments	Medial part of distal tibial physis usually closed
Comminuted fracture of distal end of tibia	–	?	Crushing injuries Direct violence	Comminuted fracture involving distal tibial epiphysis Physis often damaged Fibular fracture at various levels	Poor prognosis

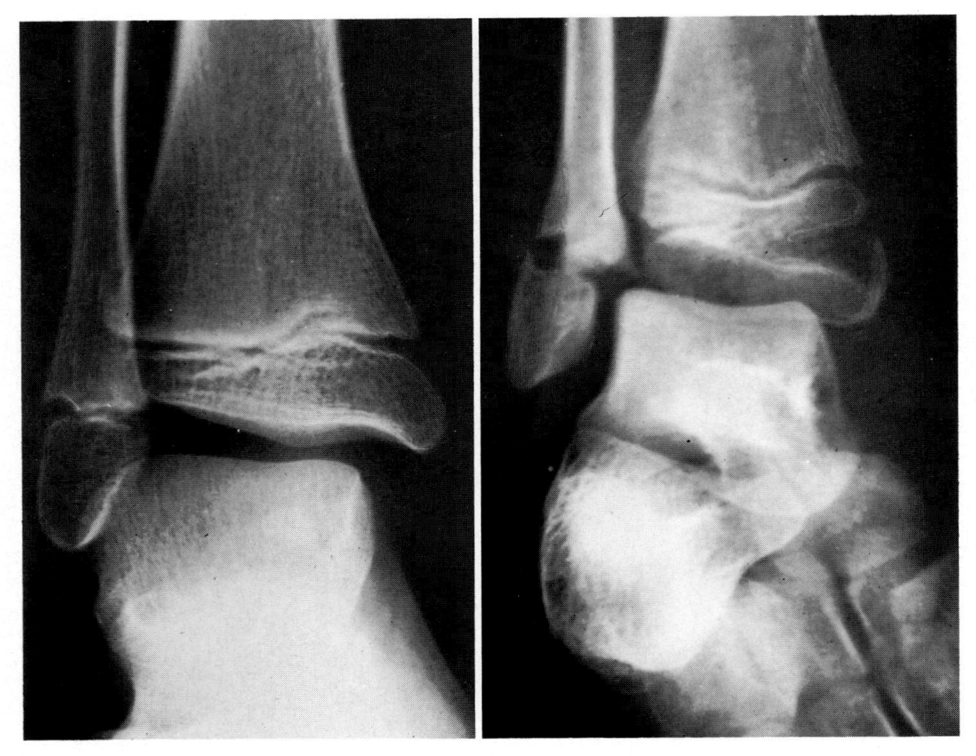

FIGURE 8–149. Anteroposterior and lateral radiograms of the ankle showing fracture-separation of the distal fibular epiphysis.

The importance of taking oblique views is obvious.

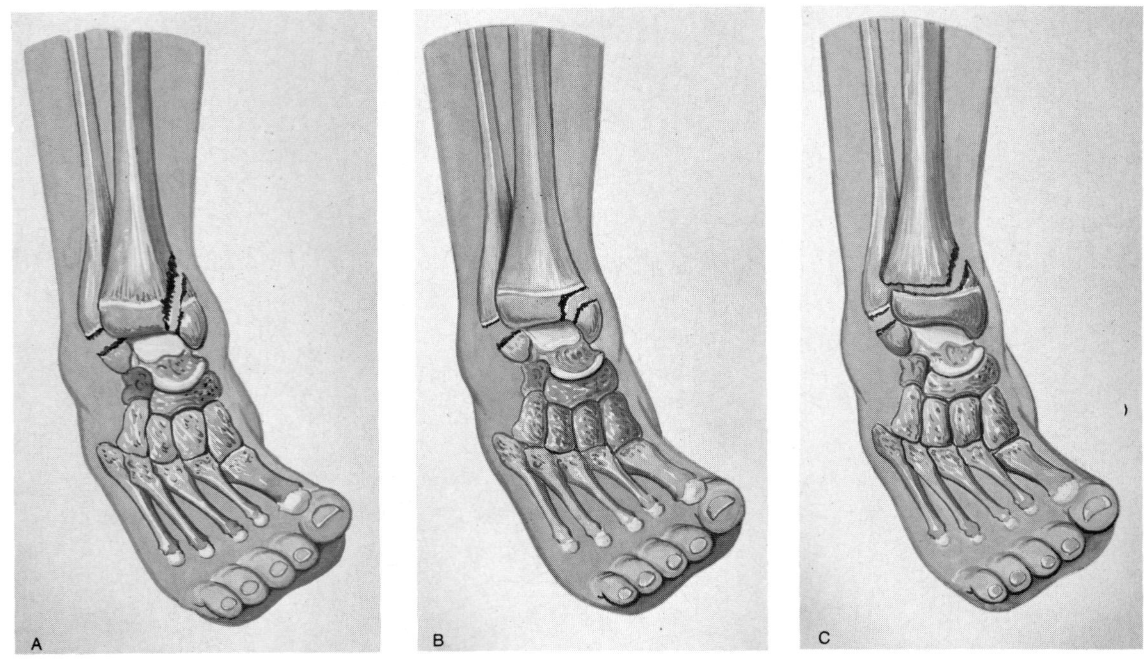

FIGURE 8–150. Supination-inversion fracture of the ankle—grade 2.

After separation of the distal fibular epiphysis the inversion-adduction force against the medial malleolus will produce: **A.** Type IV Salter-Harris physeal injury. **B.** Type III Salter-Harris physeal injury. **C.** Occasionally, a Type II Salter-Harris physeal injury.

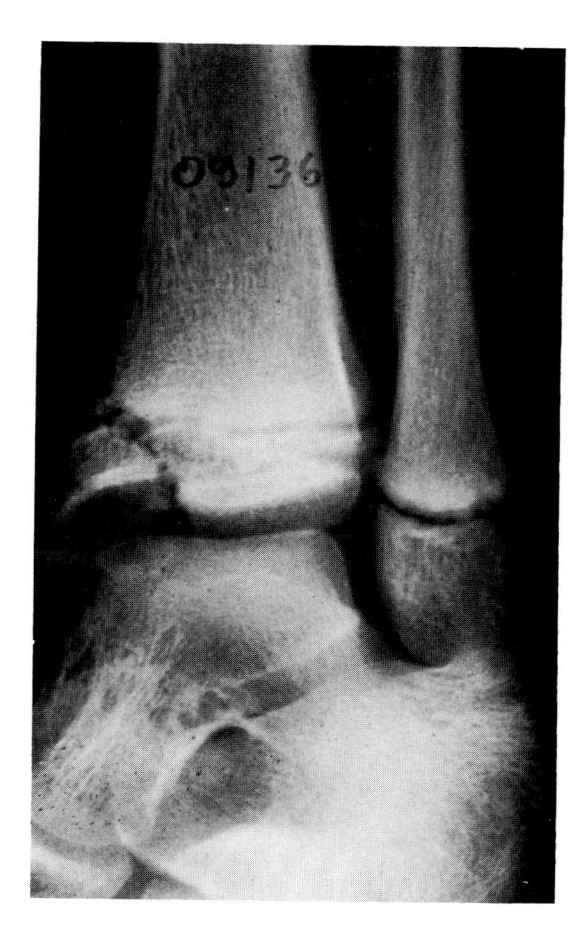

***FIGURE 8–151.** Oblique radiogram of the ankle showing Type III Salter-Harris physeal injury of the distal tibial epiphysis and Type I physeal injury of the distal fibular epiphysis (grade 2 supination-inversion ankle fracture).*

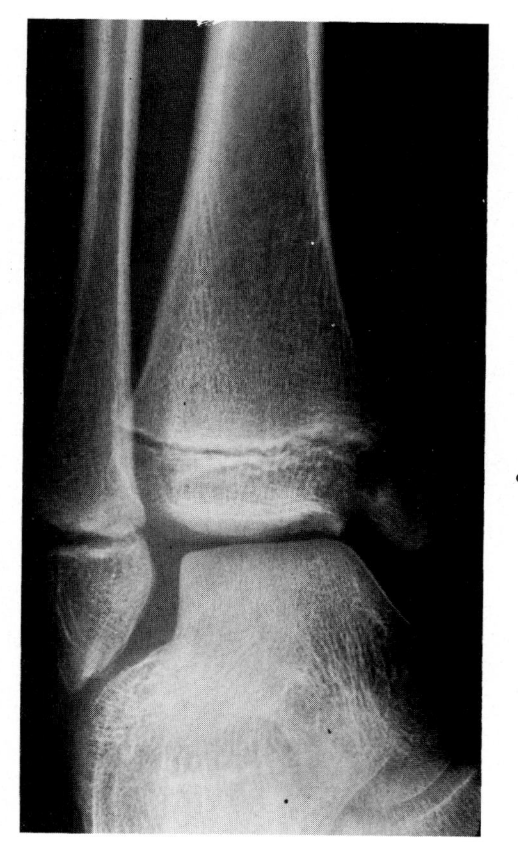

***FIGURE 8–152.** Oblique radiogram of the ankle showing grade 2 supination-inversion fracture of the ankle.*

Note the Type III Salter-Harris physeal injury of the distal tibial epiphysis and Type I Salter-Harris injury of the distal fibular epiphysis.

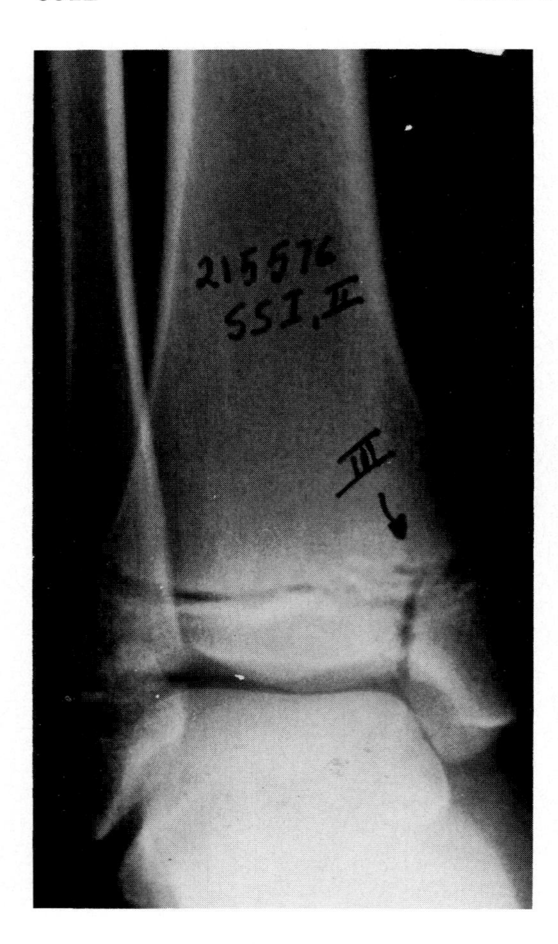

FIGURE 8–153. Supination-inversion grade 2 fracture of the ankle with Salter-Harris Type I injury of the distal fibula and Type III injury of the medial part of the distal tibial epiphysis.

The displacement is less than 2 mm.

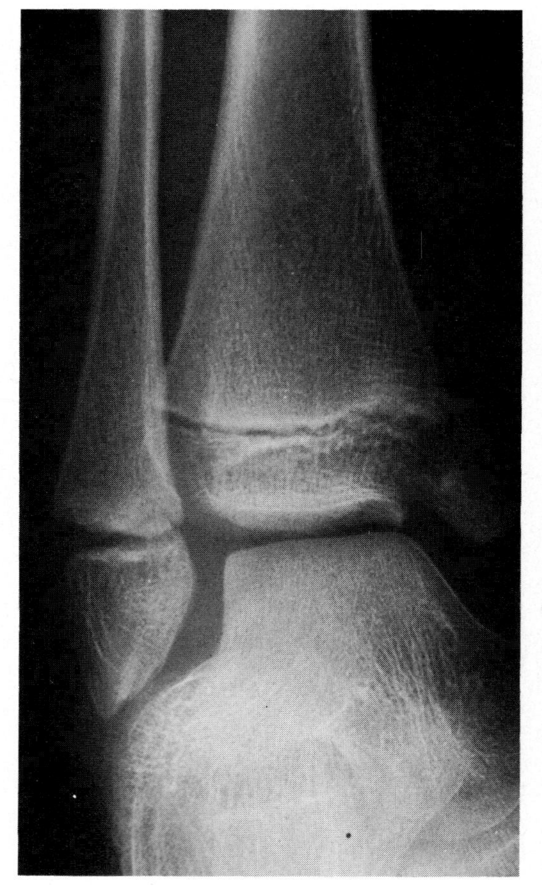

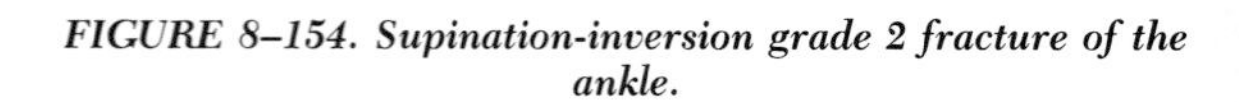

FIGURE 8–154. Supination-inversion grade 2 fracture of the ankle.

Note the Salter-Harris Type I injury of the distal fibula and the marked displacement of the Salter-Harris Type III injury of the medial part of the distal tibia. Open reduction and anatomic alignment are mandatory.

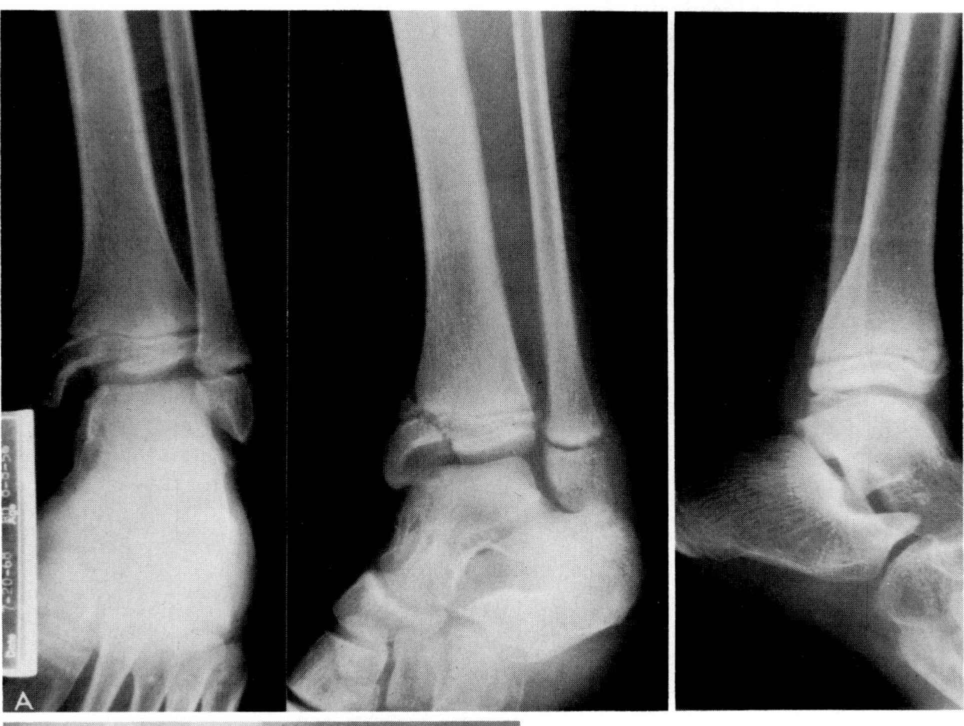

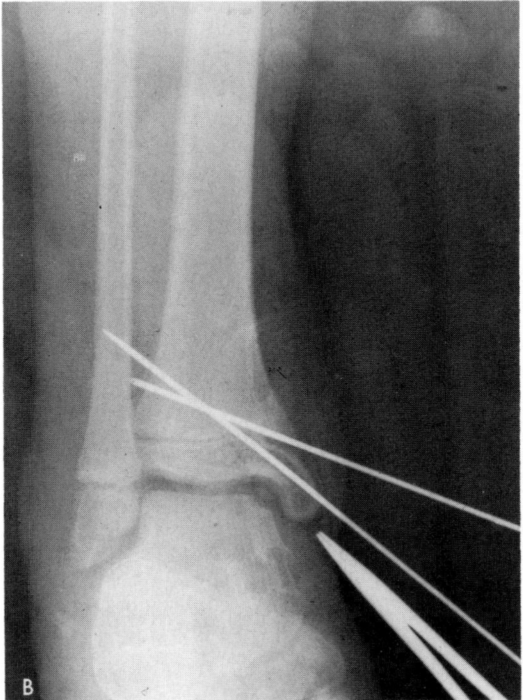

FIGURE 8–155. Supination-inversion grade 2 fracture of the ankle—Salter-Harris Type III physeal injury of the distal tibial epiphysis and Salter-Harris Type I injury of the distal fibular epiphysis.

A. Anteroposterior, oblique, and lateral radiograms. Note the superior and medial displacement of the tibial fracture fragment. Anatomic reduction is vital. **B.** Radiogram made in the operating room. Open reduction and internal fixation with two smooth Kirschner wires was carried out.

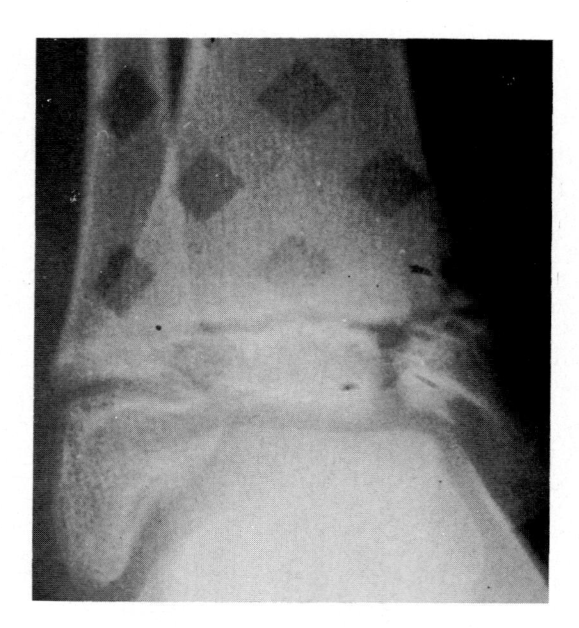

FIGURE 8–156. Supination-inversion grade 2 fracture of the ankle.

Note the Salter-Harris Type IV physeal injury of the medial part of the distal tibial epiphysis. The prognosis is poor because of the asymmetrical growth arrest. This fracture should be treated by open reduction and internal fixation. There is also a Salter-Harris Type I fracture of the distal fibular physis.

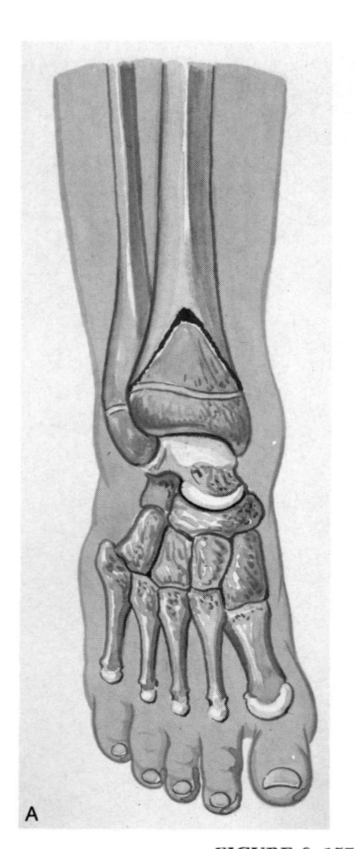

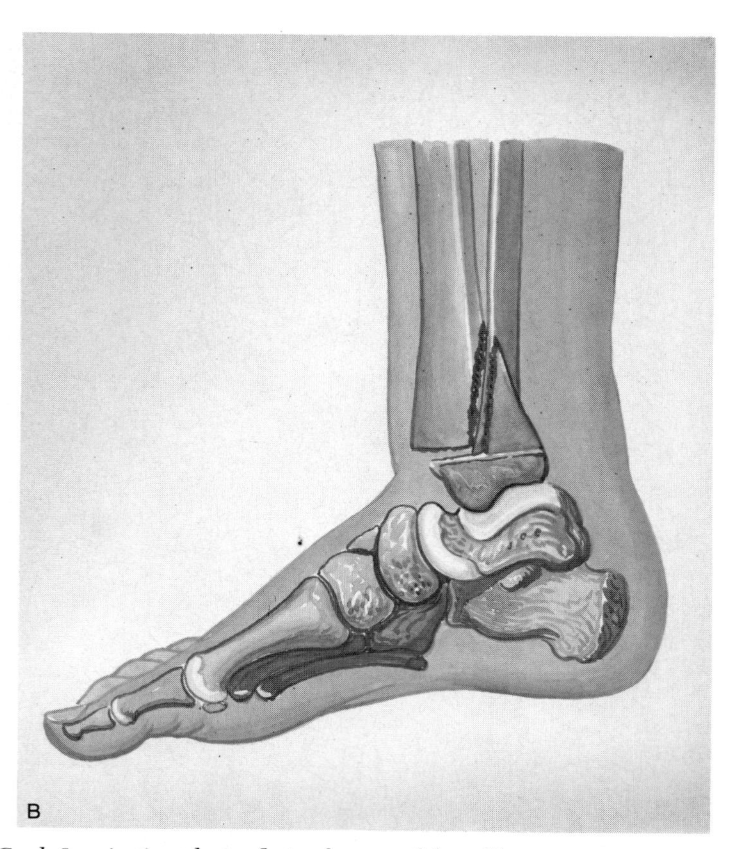

FIGURE 8–157. Grade I supination–plantar flexion fracture of the ankle.

Note the Salter-Harris Type II physeal injury of the distal tibial epiphysis. There is no associated fracture of the fibula. The metaphyseal fragment is posterior and the fracture fragment is displaced posteriorly. The fracture line is best visualized in the lateral projection.

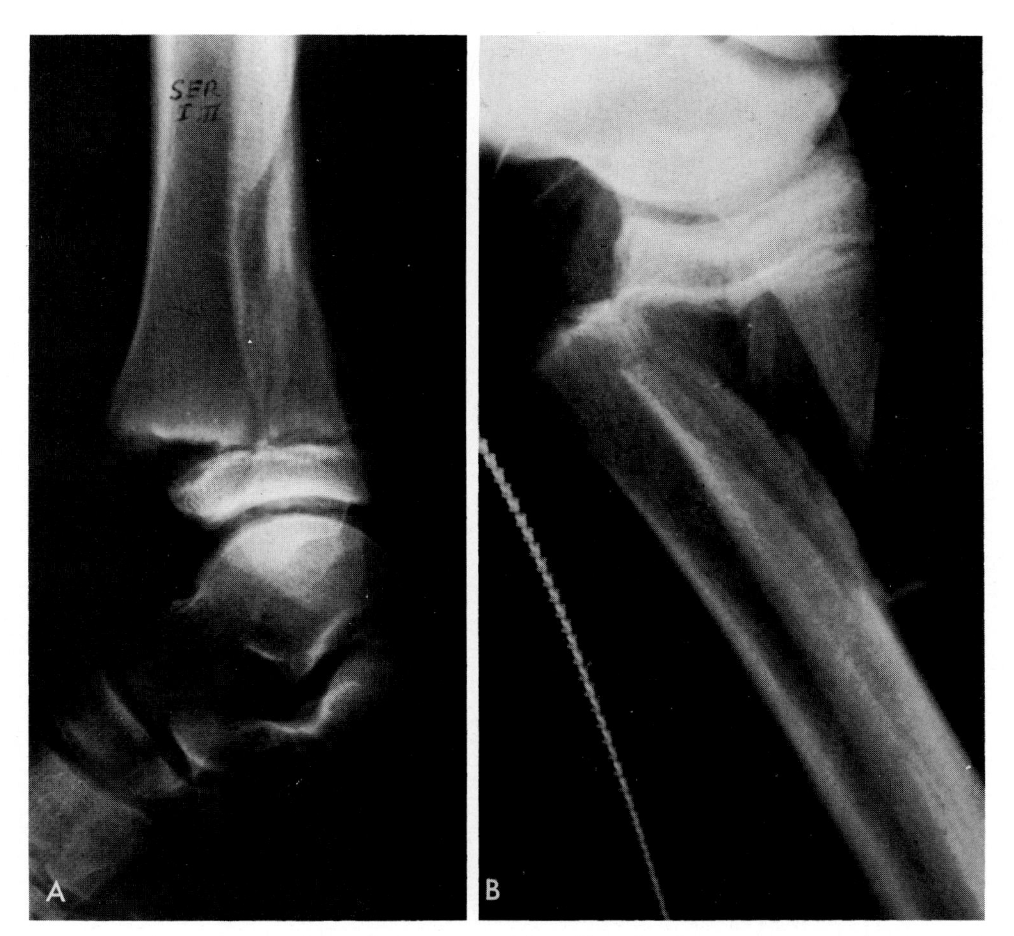

FIGURE 8–158. Supination–plantar flexion injury of the ankle with Salter-Harris Type II fracture of the distal tibial physis.

A. The posterior metaphyseal fragment is partially displaced backward. **B.** It is markedly displaced backward.

physis and extending proximally and medially. The metaphyseal-diaphyseal segment is posteriorly located, and the displacement of the fracture segment is posterior. The fibula is intact (Figs. 8–159 and 8–160). In the lateral projection the grade 1 supination–lateral rotation fracture is very similar to supination–plantar flexion fracture; on careful analysis of the anteroposterior view, however, the characteristic feature of supination–lateral rotation type is that the fracture line starts laterally and runs medially and proximally. In *grade 2* supination–lateral rotation fracture of the ankle, continuation of the lateral rotation force produces in addition a spiral fracture of the fibula; the fracture line of the fibula begins medially and runs superiorly and posteriorly. There is no injury to the distal fibular physis (Fig. 8–161).

Pronation–Eversion–Lateral Rotation Fracture. In this type of injury an eversion and lateral rotation force is applied on the distal tibial epiphysis while the foot is pronated. The metaphyseal fragment is characteristically located *laterally* and posteriorly. The displacement of the fracture fragment is posterior and lateral. There is a short oblique fracture of the lower fibular shaft, located approximately 4 to 7 cm. proximal to the tip of the lateral malleolus (Figs. 8–162 and 8–163).

MISCELLANEOUS FRACTURES

Fracture of Tillaux in the Adolescent. Fracture of the lateral portion of the distal end of the tibia in the adult was first described by Sir Astley Cooper; in the literature, however, it is referred to as the fracture of Tillaux.[28, 59]

The distal physis of the tibia closes first on its medial half at the age of 13 or 14 years; the lateral part closes at 14½ to 16 years. Thus there is a period of 18 months during which the lateral part of the distal tibial growth plate is open while the medial half is closed. The lower metaphysis of the fibula is connected with the anterolateral part of the tibial epiphysis by the

Text continued on page 3321

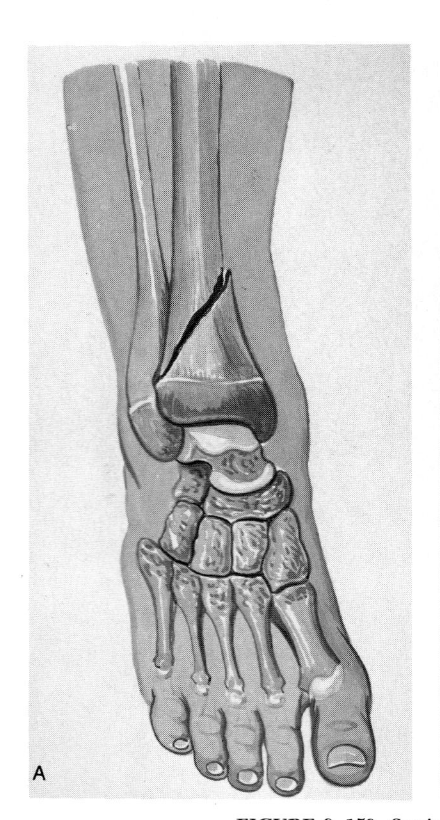

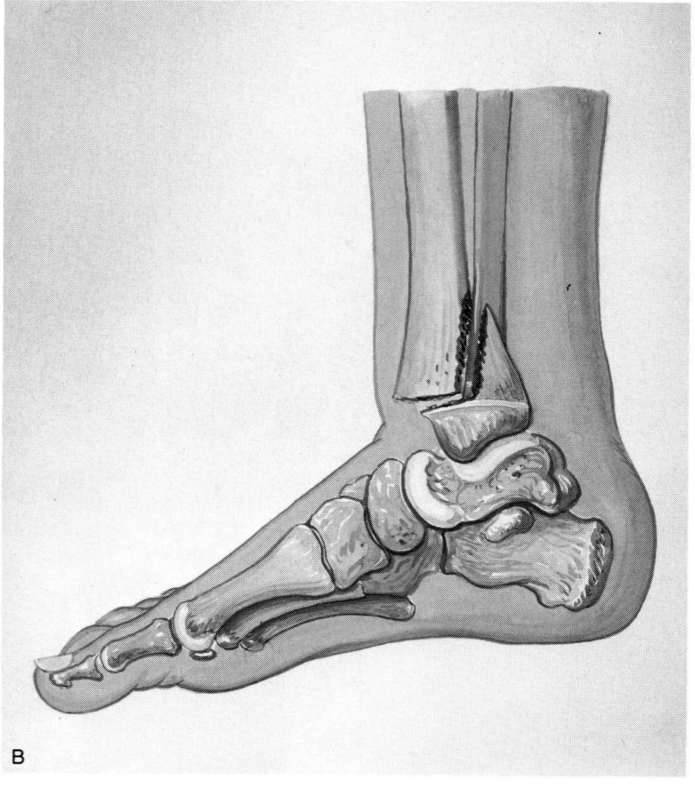

FIGURE 8–159. Supination–lateral rotation fracture of the ankle, grade 1.

A. Anteroposterior view. **B.** Lateral view. Note the Salter-Harris Type II physeal injury of the distal tibial epiphysis. The metaphyseal-diaphyseal segment is posteriorly located. Displacement of the fracture fragment is posterior. The fibula is intact. The fracture line starts laterally at the physis and extends proximally and medially. This is a characteristic feature of supination–lateral rotation fracture of the ankle, distinguishing it from supination–plantar flexion fracture.

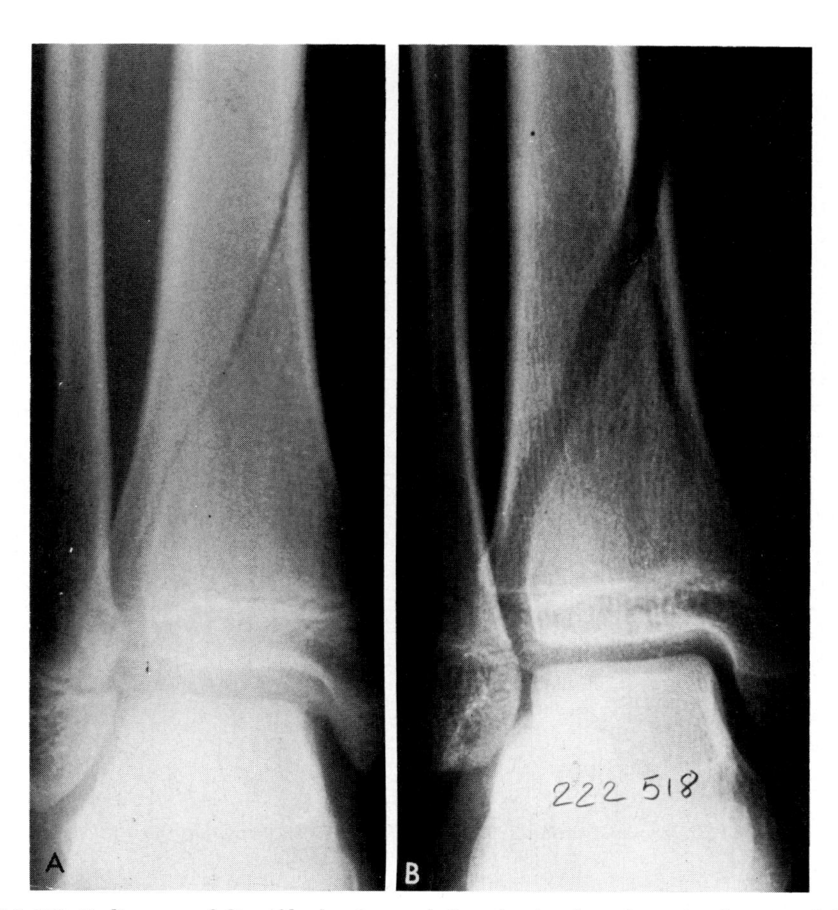

FIGURE 8–160. Radiograms of the ankle showing grade 1 supination–lateral rotation fracture of the ankle.

In this Salter-Harris Type II fracture of the distal tibial epiphysis, the fracture line starts laterally at the physis and extends proximally and medially. The fibula is intact. **A.** The fracture is minimally displaced. **B.** The displacement is marked.

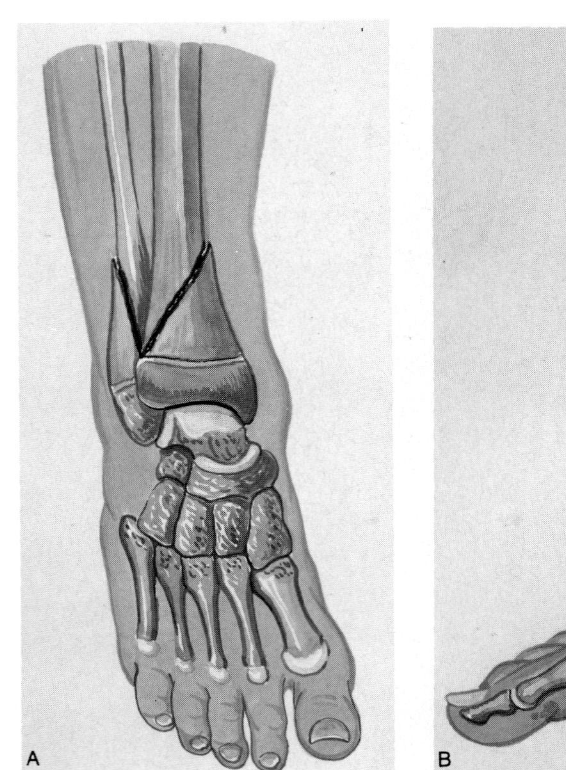

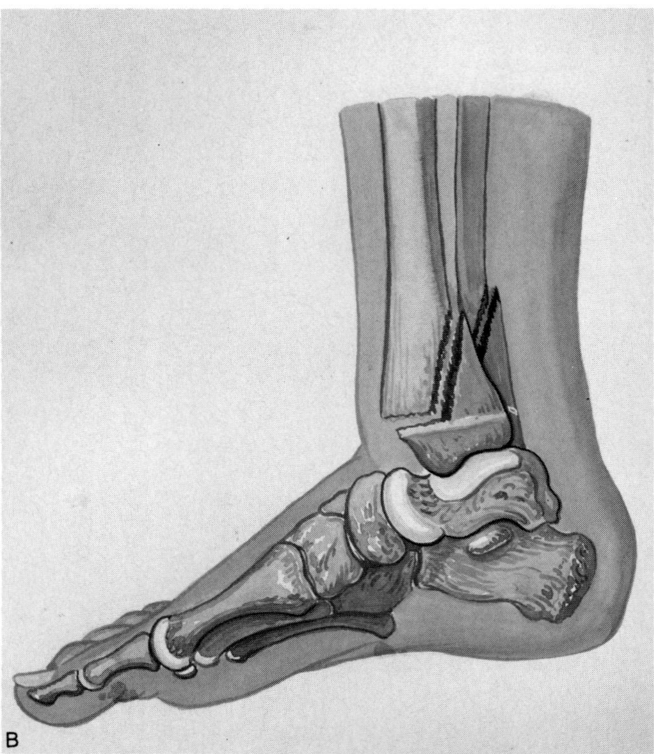

FIGURE 8–161. Diagrams illustrating grade 2 supination–lateral rotation fracture of the ankle.

In addition to the Salter-Harris Type II physeal injury of the distal tibial epiphysis there is a spiral fracture of the lower fibular shaft that starts medially and runs superiorly and laterally. Displacement is lateral or posterolateral. **A.** Anteroposterior view. **B.** Lateral view.

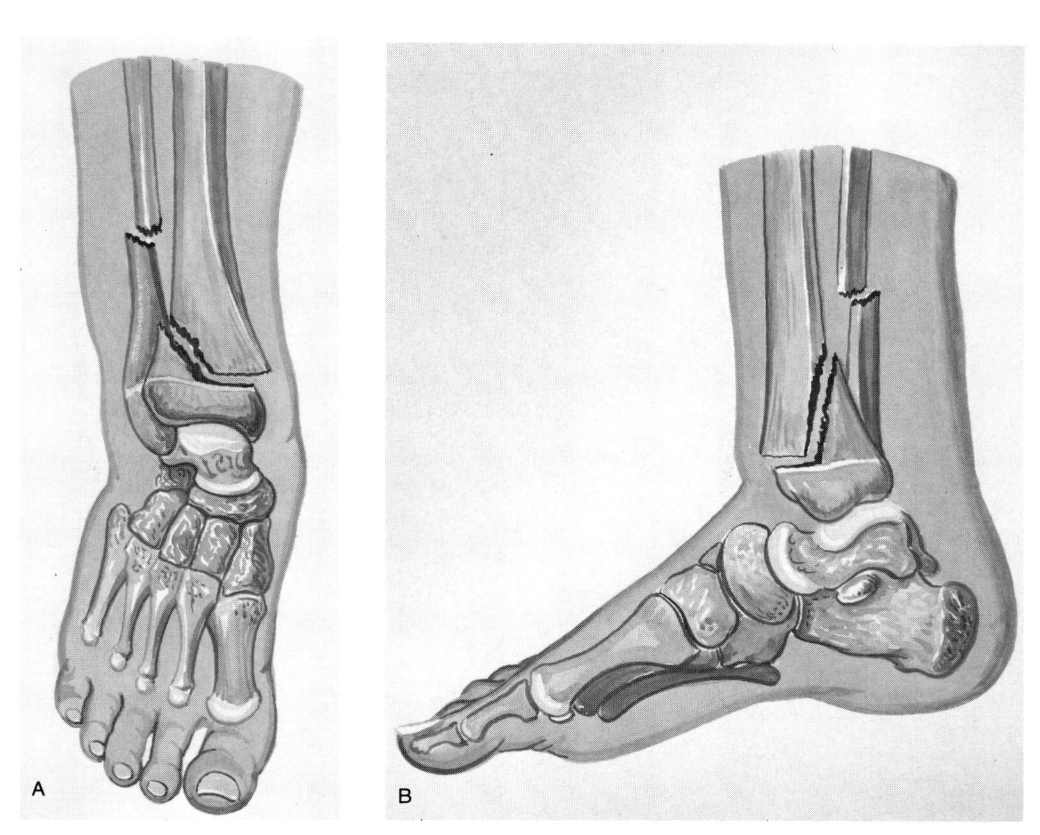

FIGURE 8–162. Diagrams illustrating grade 1 pronation–eversion–lateral rotation fracture of the ankle.

Note the Salter-Harris Type II physeal injury of the distal tibial epiphysis; the metaphyseal segment is located laterally and posteriorly. The displacement of the fracture fragment is posterolateral. Also note the fracture of the lower diaphysis of the fibula, running a short oblique course and located 4 to 7 cm. proximal to the tip of the lateral malleolus.

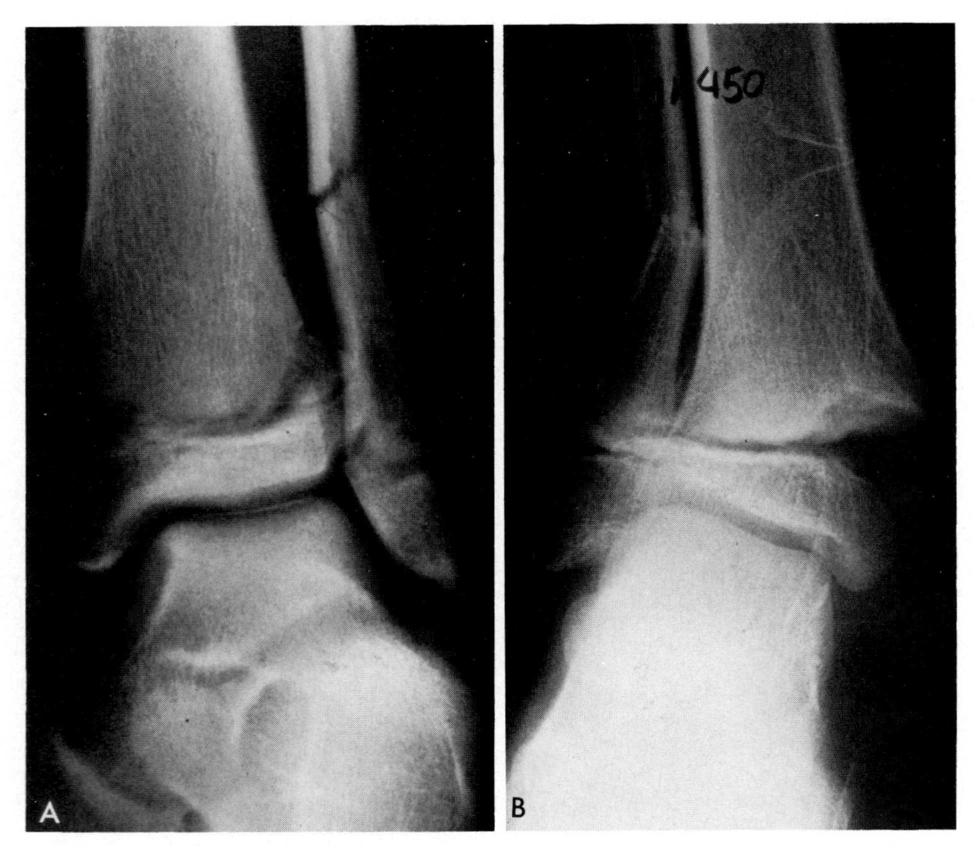

FIGURE 8–163. Radiograms of the ankle showing pronation–eversion–lateral rotation fracture of the ankle.

A. The laterally and posteriorly placed metaphyseal fragment is clearly seen. **B.** The metaphyseal fragment is very small.

anterior talofibular ligament. A lateral rotatory force may fracture the tibial epiphysis at the junction of the open and closed portions of the physis. The fracture line is vertical, extending from the articular surface proximally and then laterally to exit on the lateral cortex of the tibia. The more skeletally mature the child, the more lateral is the vertical fracture line. The physeal injury is Salter-Harris Type III of the lateral part of the distal tibial epiphysis (Figs. 8–164 and 8–165). The anterolateral and posterolateral tibiofibular ligaments are intact, and the fractured fragment rotates anterolaterally; the displacement is usually minimal, but occasionally it may be marked.

On clinical examination there is local tenderness and swelling over the anterolateral part of the distal tibial epiphysis. When displacement of the fragment is minimal, the vertical and horizontal fracture lines may be difficult to visualize on the anteroposterior and lateral radiograms of the ankle. Oblique views are essential, and computed tomography will clearly depict the fracture.

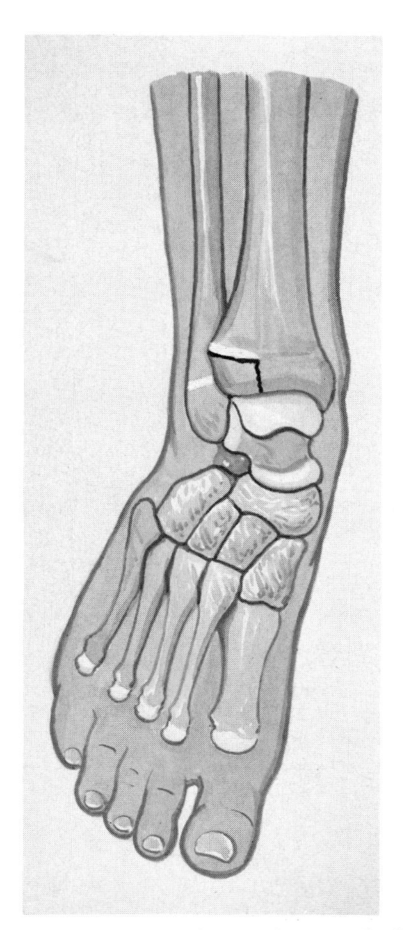

FIGURE 8–164. Diagram showing fracture of Tillaux in the adolescent.

Note the Salter-Harris Type III fracture of the lateral part of the distal tibial physis. The medial part of the physis is closed. There is no metaphyseal fragment.

Triplane Fracture of the Distal End of the Tibia. This unusual fracture was first reported by Marmor, in 1970.[85] Lynn, in 1972, described two additional cases and gave it the name *triplane fracture*.[79] Torg and Ruggiero reported a similar fracture in 1975.[116] Cooperman, Spiegel, and Laros, in 1978, reported 15 cases of triplane fracture of the distal end of the tibia, representing 6 per cent of 237 consecutive physeal injuries of the ankle.[29]

The fracture usually occurs in adolescents near skeletal maturity, the average age being 13½ years and the age range 10 to 16 years. It seems a maturing or partially fused physis is particularly susceptible to this injury.

In the triplane fracture of the distal end of the tibia the fracture occurs in three planes—sagittal, transverse, and coronal—giving the radiographic appearance of a combination of Salter-Harris Types II and III physeal injuries (Fig. 8–166). In the lateral projection there is a vertical fracture line that separates the posterior metaphyseal triangular fragment from the distal tibial diaphysis. This fracture line becomes indistinct as one traces it distally into the epiphysis; i.e., the fracture line does not cross the epiphysis but runs along the physis for a varying distance, depending upon the stage of fusion of the growth plate in its different parts. The size of the posterior metaphyseal segment also varies, its vertical height measuring from 1 to 6 cm. above the physis and its width (measured along the physis from the fracture line to the posterior tibial cortex) between one tenth and one half that of the metaphysis.

In the anteroposterior projection there is a vertical fracture line in the bony epiphysis that extends proximally from the articular surface of the ankle to the physis and then courses along the growth plate (Salter-Harris Type III). This vertical fracture line in the sagittal plane is usually at or close to the center of the width of the physis or occasionally medial to the center. The degree of displacement of the fracture fragments on the anteroposterior radiogram varies; in the series of 15 cases of Cooperman and associates it measured more than 2 mm. in four, 2 mm. in seven, and less than 2 mm. in four.[29]

There is disagreement in the literature as to whether the triplane fracture gives rise to three or two major fragments. According to both Lynn and Rang, it produces three major fragments:

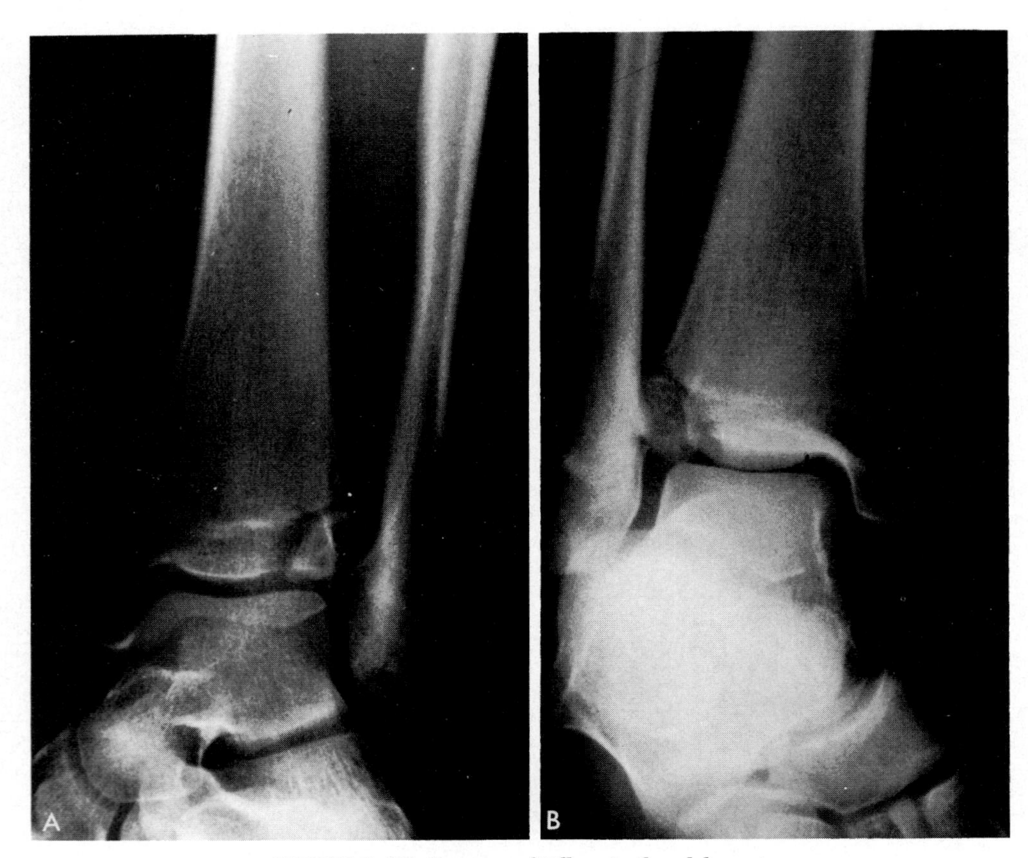

FIGURE 8–165. Fracture of Tillaux in the adolescent.

A. The growth plate of the medial part of the distal tibia is closed. The fracture is a Salter-Harris Type III physeal injury of the lateral part of the distal tibia. The displacement is anterolateral. **B.** Fracture of Tillaux in the more skeletally mature adolescent. The lateral part of the physis of the distal tibia is almost completely closed.

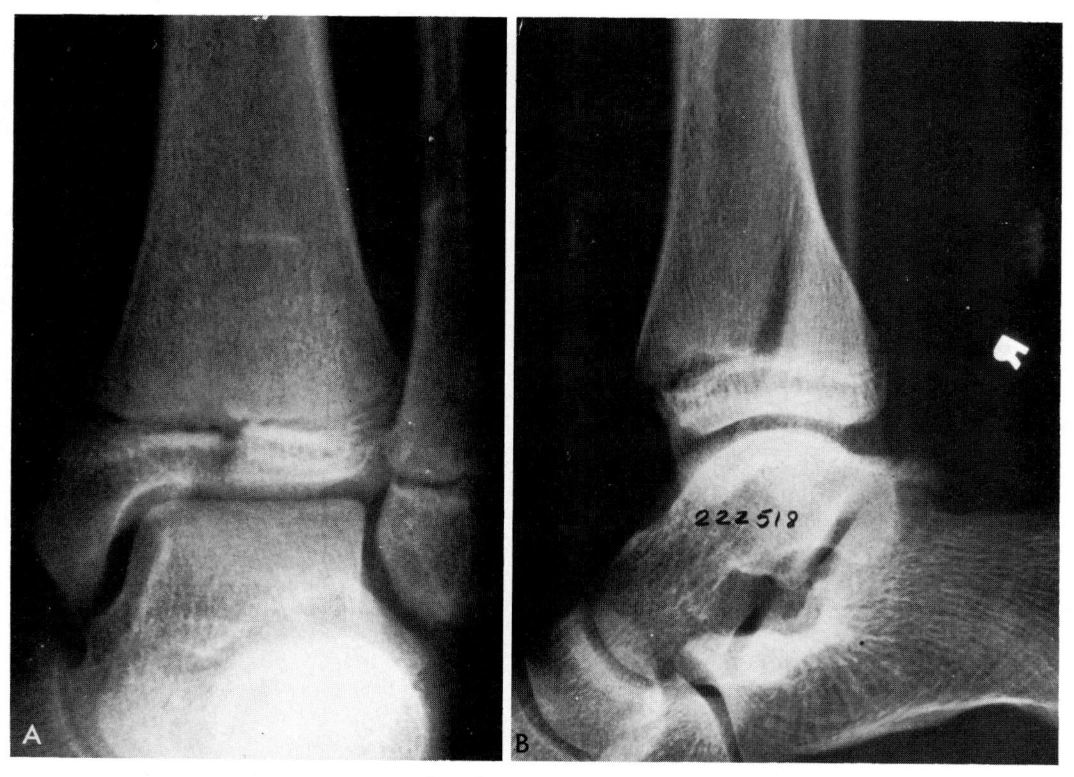

FIGURE 8–166. Triplane fracture of the ankle—three fragments.

The medial and lateral parts of the distal tibial physis are open. **A.** Anteroposterior view showing the Salter-Harris Type III physeal injury. **B.** Lateral projection showing Salter-Harris Type II injury.

(1) a rectangular fragment representing the anterolateral quadrant of the distal tibial epiphysis, (2) a posterior triangular metaphyseal segment along with the medial and posterior portion of the epiphysis, and (3) the distal tibial metaphysis (Fig. 8–167 A and B). The triplane fracture separates fragments 2 and 3 in the coronal plane, and fragments 1 and 2 in the sagittal plane, and courses through the physis in the transverse plane.[79, 98]

Cooperman, Spiegel, and Laros studied the three-dimensional configuration of the triplane fracture by tomography in five cases. In all of them the triplane fracture produced *two* and not three fragments; the anteromedial fragment consisted of the major part of the tibial shaft, the attached medial malleolus, and the anteromedial part of the distal tibial epiphysis; the posterolateral fragment consisted of the remainder of the distal tibial epiphysis, the posterior tibial metaphyseal fragment, and the fibula connected with strong interosseous ligaments (Figs. 8–167 C to E and 8–168).[28] In a triplane fracture studied by computed tomography, the two-fragment configuration of the fracture was also noted (Fig. 8–168 H).

The pattern of fracture varies not only with the direction and degree of severity of the axial lateral rotation load and the position of the foot but also with the degree of skeletal maturity of the distal tibial physis. This author has found that the triplane fracture may produce a three-fragment fracture when the medial part of the distal tibial physis is open and will result in a two-fragment fracture when the medial part of the distal tibial physis is closed.

Comminuted fracture of the distal end of the tibia is usually caused by axial compression injury or direct violence. The distal tibial epiphysis is shattered, involving the joint (Fig. 8–169). The crushing often damages the physis, and the prognosis is poor.

Treatment

Principles of management of fractures involving the physis are well delineated by Salter and Harris.[102]

All reductions, whether closed or open, should be performed with the utmost gentleness in order to avoid damage to the delicate cartilage of the physis. Forceful manipulations

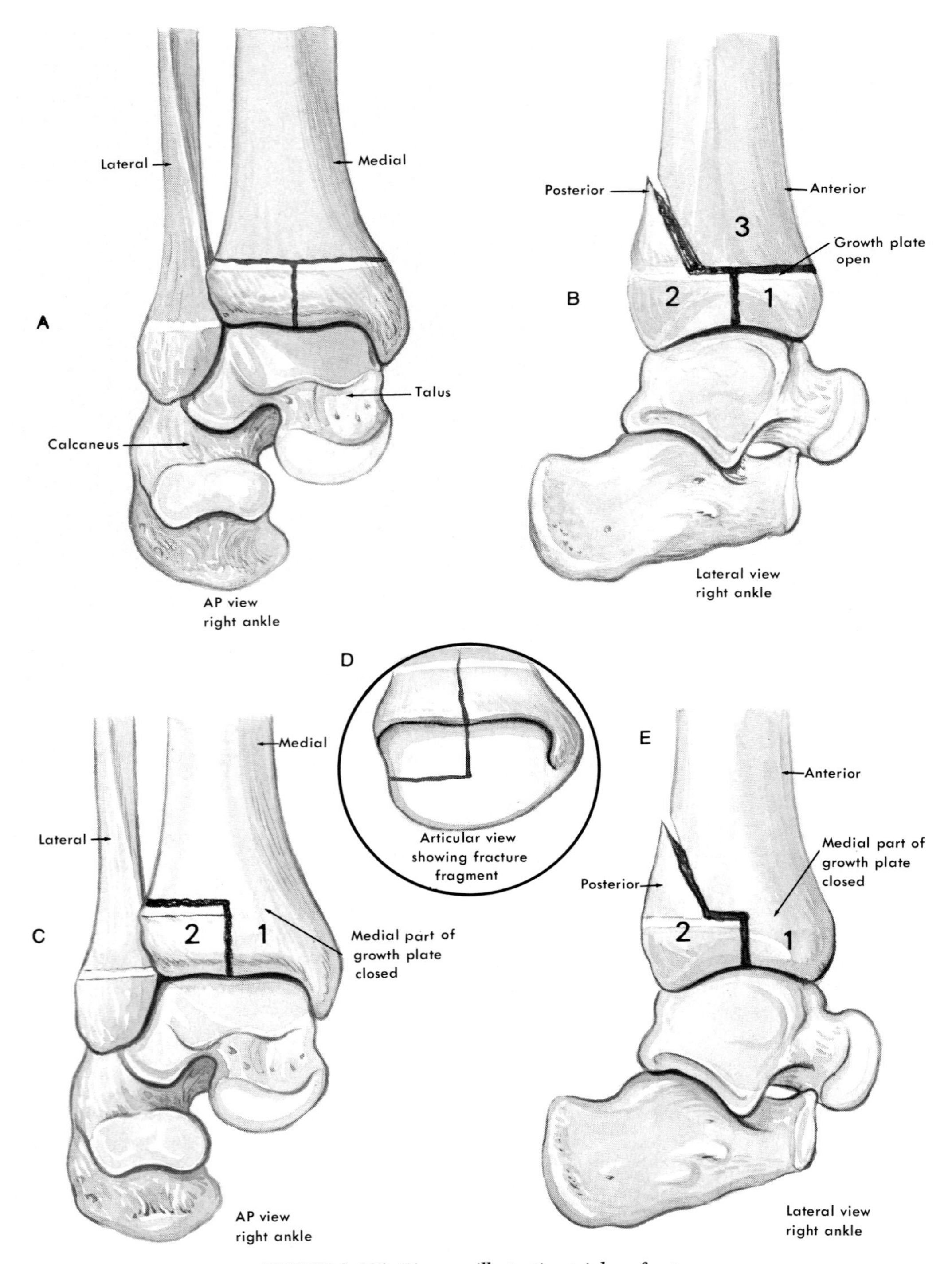

FIGURE 8–167. Diagram illustrating triplane fracture.

A and **B.** *Three-fragment type.* The medial part of the distal tibial physis is open. The fragments are (1) a rectangular one representing the anterolateral quadrant of the distal tibial epiphysis; (2) a posterior triangular metaphyseal segment along with the medial and posterior portion of the tibial metaphysis; and (3) the distal tibial metaphysis. The fracture through the physis is in the transverse plane; fragments 1 and 2 are separated in the sagittal plane, and fragments 2 and 3 in the coronal plane. **C** to **E.** *Two-fragment type.* The medial part of the distal tibial physis is closed. (1) The anteromedial fragment consists of the major part of the tibial diaphysis and the attached medial malleolus; (2) the posterolateral fragment consists of the remainder of the distal tibial epiphysis—the posterior tibial metaphyseal fragment and the fibula connected with strong interosseous ligaments.

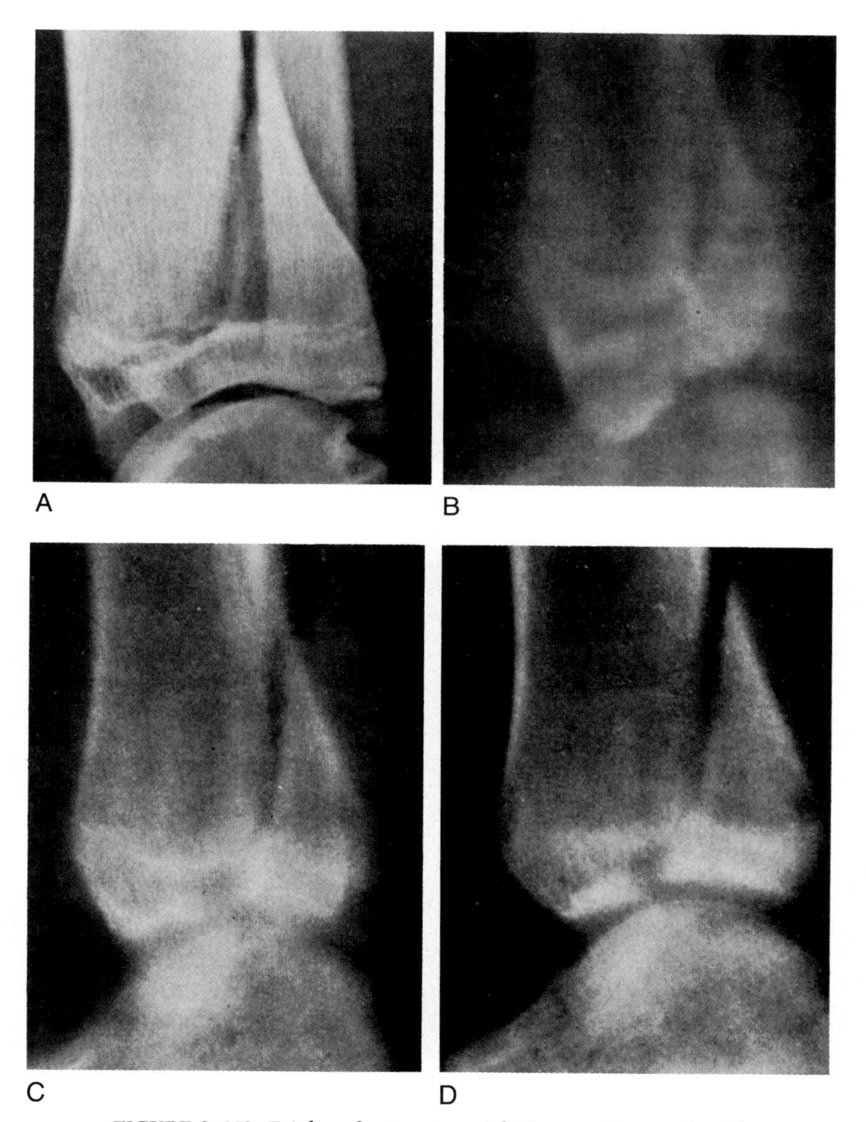

FIGURE 8–168. Triplane fracture in a girl 12 years nine months old.

A. The routine lateral x-ray shows a coronal fracture with the medial malleolus and tibial diaphysis displaced forward as a unit. **B** to **E.** Lateral tomograms. In **B** the cut is at 9.0 cm. and shows the fracture line in the coronal plane along the posterior border of the medial malleolus; in **C** (8.5 cm. cut) and **D** (8.0 cm. cut), the continuity of the medial malleolus and tibial shaft is obvious. Note the articular step-off in **D**.

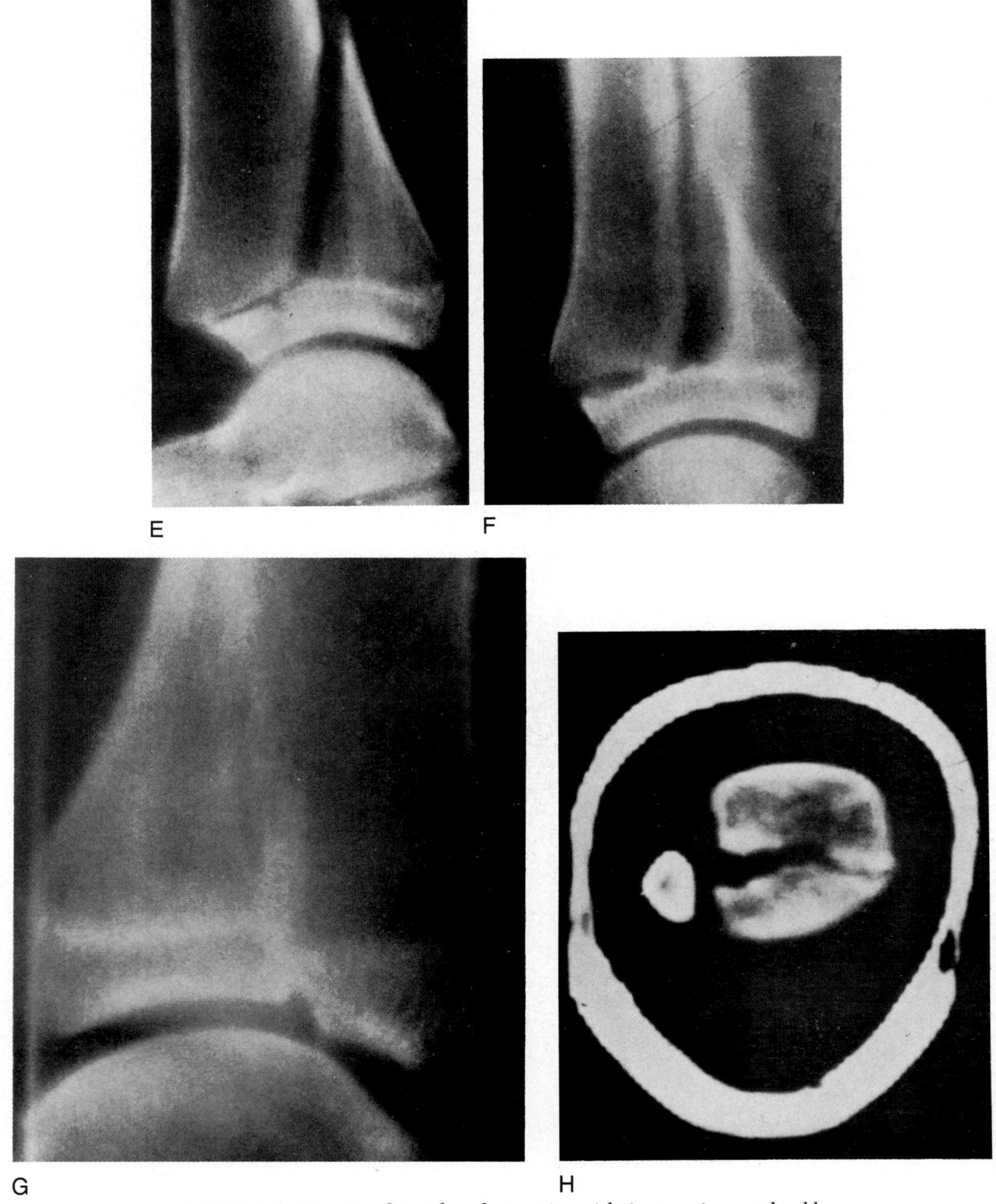

FIGURE 8–168 Continued. Triplane fracture in a girl 12 years nine months old.

E and **F.** Tomographic cuts at 7.0 and 6.0 cm. show that the posterior epiphysis and metaphyseal fragment are continuous with the lateral epiphysis as a unit. **G.** A lateral tomogram, six months post fracture; note the persistence of articular incongruity. **H.** Computed tomography, one month post injury, at a level 4 mm. superior to the epiphysis. Note the fracture line in the tibia; the fragments are not displaced medially but are widely separated laterally. (From Cooperman, D. R., Spiegel, P. G., and Laros, G. S.: Tibial fracture involving the ankle in children—the so-called triplane fracture. J. Bone Joint Surg., *60-A*:1042–1043, 1978. Reprinted by permission.)

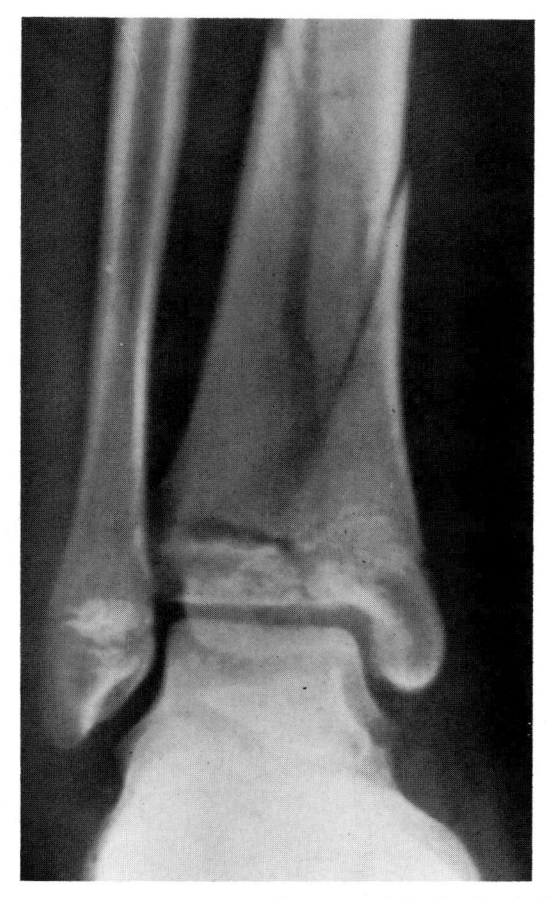

FIGURE 8–169. Comminuted fracture of the distal end of the tibia, involving the ankle joint.

are condemned. During open reduction, direct pressure on the physis by blunt instruments should be avoided.

Epiphyseal separations should be reduced immediately; each day of delay will make it progressively more difficult. In fact, after ten days, physeal injuries of Types I and II cannot be reduced without exerting undue force and damaging the cartilaginous growth plate. When such a fracture is seen late (i.e., after seven to ten days), it is better to accept malunion than to cause growth arrest by forceful manipulation or open surgery. In Type III or IV physeal injuries, congruity of articular surfaces is essential; in such cases, delayed reduction is performed, if indicated.

As stated earlier, reduction of Type I and Type II fractures involving the physis can be readily obtained and maintained. In Type III physeal injuries, open reduction may be indicated to restore a congruous articular surface, particularly in weight-bearing joints. Open reduction is required in almost all cases of Type IV fractures of the physis. Care must be taken not to compromise circulation of the epiphysis. Only smooth Kirschner wires must be used for internal fixation, and under no circumstances should screws or threaded wires be inserted across the physis. The internal fixation device is removed when the fracture has healed.

Type III and Type IV physeal injuries require accurate anatomic reduction. In Type I and Type II fractures of the physis, perfect reduction is desirable but not mandatory; bone remodeling will correct moderate residual deformities. In general, one can accept a greater degree of deformity in multiplane joints (such as the shoulder) than in single plane joints (such as the knee and ankle).

Types I, II, and III injuries consolidate very rapidly, usually in about half the time required for a fracture through the metaphysis of the same bone. Type IV injuries require the same period for union as metaphyseal fractures.

Fractures involving the physis should be closely followed for possible development of growth disturbance. Parents should be warned of potential complications, but without causing much anxiety. As already indicated, the factors that determine the prognosis are the type of physeal injury, the age of the child at the time of fracture, the integrity of the blood supply to the epiphysis, the method of reduction, and whether the fracture is open or closed.

Treatment varies according to the type of fracture. Post-traumatic reactive swelling is prevented by the immediate application of a well-padded compression dressing and a posterior splint. The routine radiograms should include anteroposterior, lateral, and oblique views. In difficult cases, such as triplane fracture, plain tomography or computed tomography may be indicated. Closed reduction should be performed as soon as possible; each day of delay will make reduction much more difficult. Time is of the essence.

The reverse of the mechanism of injury will reduce the fracture. The golden rule is *be gentle*. A major manipulation, especially in an uncooperative child, is best performed under general anesthesia. Relaxation of muscles and absence of pain will make the manipulation easy and least traumatic. The knee is flexed 90 degrees and the foot is plantar-flexed to relax the triceps surae muscle. An assistant applies countertraction by pulling up on the leg. With one hand, the surgeon grasps the foot by the heel while steadying the anterior aspect of the lower fourth of the tibia with the palm of his other hand. First, distal traction is applied in the line of deformity and then in the direction opposite to the injuring force to reduce the fracture.

In *supination-inversion injuries,* first longitudinal distal traction is applied medially, and then the hindfoot is everted (Fig. 8–170). The foot is immobilized in slight pronation with the ankle in neutral dorsiflexion. In Salter-Harris Type I or II fractures of the distal physis of the fibula the cast is worn for three to four weeks. The prognosis is excellent. The rare fracture of the tip of the lateral malleolus and rupture of the lateral collateral ligament is treated by a below-knee walking cast for three weeks. In *grade 2* supination-inversion injuries there is Salter-Harris Type III or IV physeal fracture of the distal tibial epiphysis. Anatomic reduction is mandatory. Separation of fracture fragments should be less than 2 mm. If one is unable to reduce and maintain anatomic reduction by closed method, open surgical reduction is performed. Smooth Kirschner wires or a cancellous screw is used for internal fixation (see Fig. 8–155). After closed or open reduction an above-knee cast is applied with the knee in 45 degrees of flexion. The palms of the hands are used to mold the plaster carefully over the malleoli and the heel of the foot. The cast is extended above the flexed knee to relax the pull of the tendo Achillis and to prevent weight-bearing. Immobilization is continued for six to eight weeks, and then gradual weight-bearing is allowed. Restraint from weight-bearing for longer periods is of no value in preventing deformity once the physis has been injured. The risk of growth arrest of the medial part of the distal tibial physis is great. With asymmetrical growth, varus deformity of the ankle and shortening of the leg will gradually develop.

In *supination–plantar flexion fracture,* first longitudinal traction is applied in plantar flexion, and then, while the downward traction is maintained, the ankle is gently dorsiflexed (Fig. 8–171). The limb is immobilized for four to six weeks in an above-knee cast with the ankle in

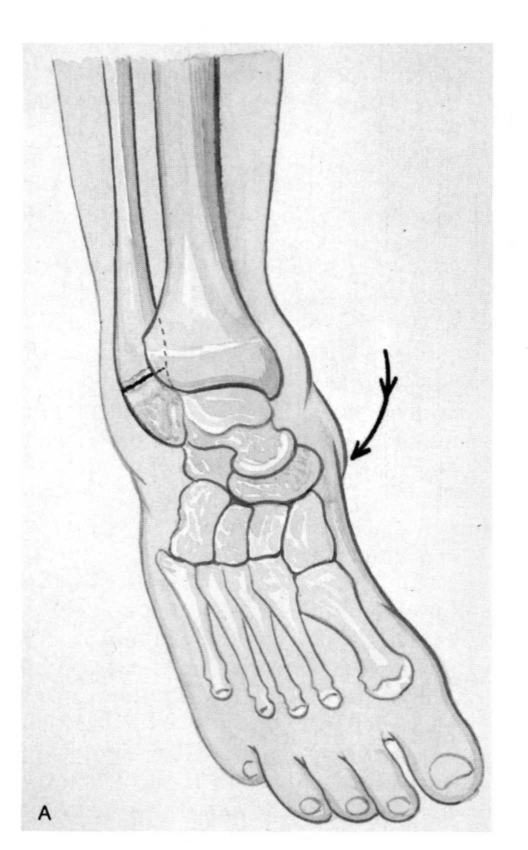

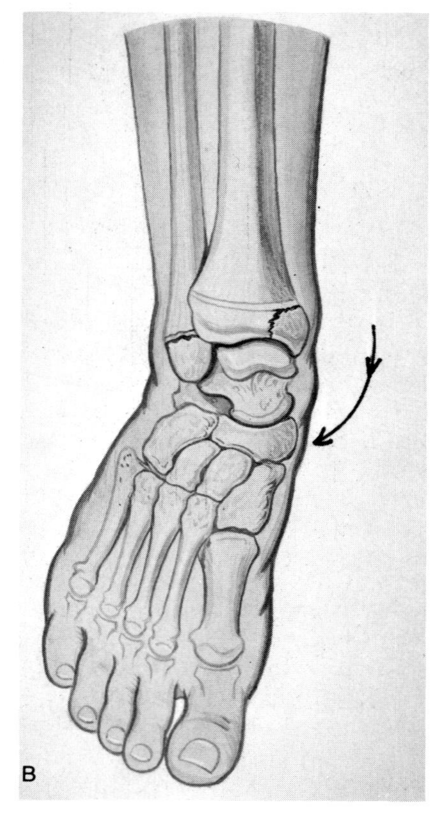

FIGURE 8–170. Method of reduction of supination-inversion injury.

A. Apply longitudinal traction distally in the line of deformity, i.e., in inversion. **B.** Then *evert* the hindfoot and apply cast with the foot in slight pronation and the ankle in neutral dorsiflexion. In Salter-Harris Type III physeal injuries anatomic reduction is imperative. Open reduction is required if separation of fracture fragments of the tibial epiphysis is greater than 2 mm.

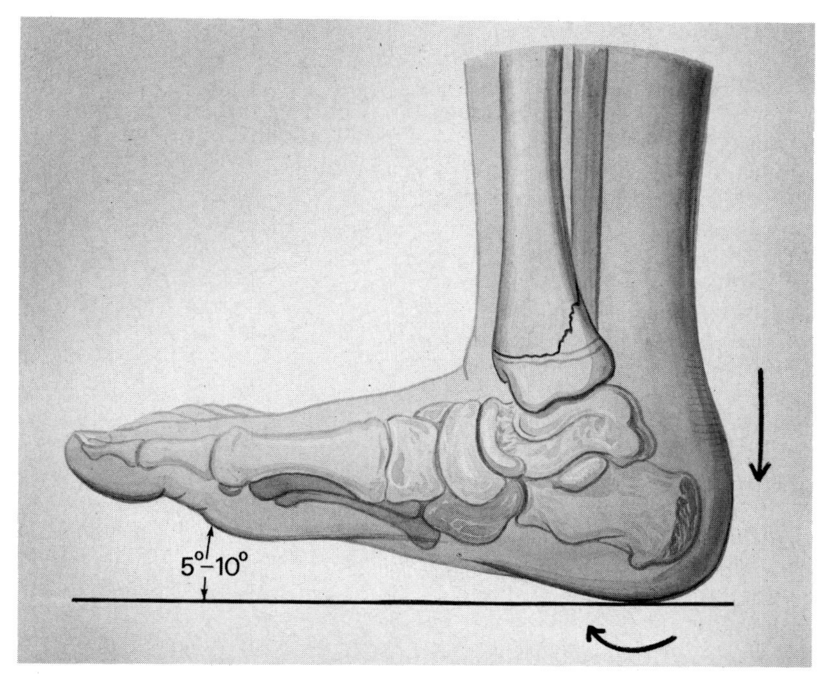

FIGURE 8–171. Method of reduction of supination–plantar flexion fracture of the ankle.

First, longitudinal traction is applied distally and in plantar flexion; then, the ankle is gently dorsiflexed. The limb is immobilized in an above-knee cast with ankle in 5 to 10 degrees of dorsiflexion and the foot in slight pronation.

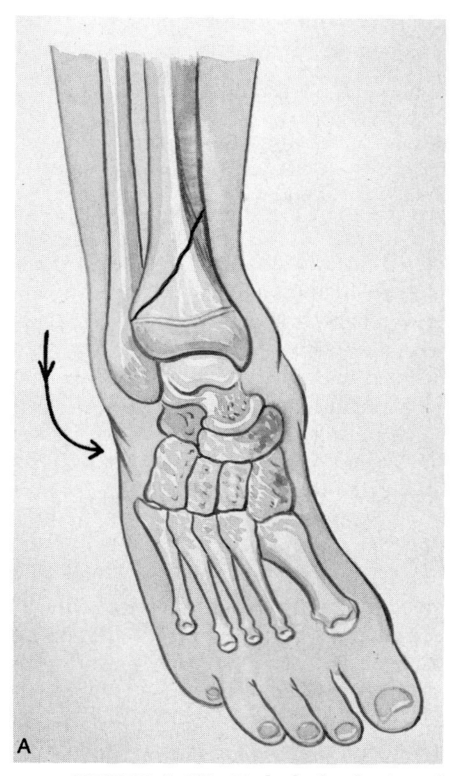

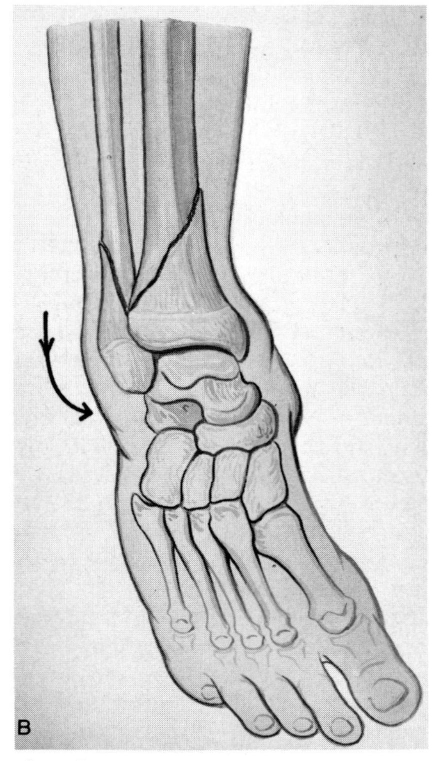

FIGURE 8–172. Method of reduction of supination–lateral rotation fracture of the ankle.

A. Grade 1. **B.** Grade 2. Longitudinal axial traction is applied, and while distal traction is maintained, the foot is medially rotated. An above-knee cast is applied with the foot in slight inversion. The period of immobilization in the cast is eight weeks.

5 to 10 degrees of dorsiflexion. The common physeal injury is a Salter-Harris Type II fracture of the distal tibial epiphysis with a posterior metaphyseal fragment and posterior displacement. Moderate residual deformity tends to disappear spontaneously with subsequent growth and remodeling. Posterior displacement corrects itself readily, as it is in the plane of ankle motion. The danger in management of supination–plantar flexion injury of the ankle is iatrogenic trauma by repeated forceful manipulation. If after two attempts accurate reduction cannot be achieved, it is wise to accept the deformed position.

Supination–lateral rotation fractures of the ankle, both grade 1 and grade 2, are reduced by longitudinal axial traction and medial rotation of the foot (Fig. 8–172). An above-knee cast is applied with the foot and ankle in slight inversion. The period of immobilization is eight weeks. The prognosis is excellent for complete healing with no deformity or disability.

Pronation–eversion–lateral rotation fracture of the ankle is reduced first by longitudinal axial traction in the line of deformity (i.e., in lateral rotation and with the hindfoot everted), and distal traction is maintained on the hindfoot, which is then *inverted and medially rotated* (Fig. 8–173). An above-knee cast is applied with the foot and ankle in inversion and medial rotation. The physeal injury is a Salter-Harris Type II fracture of the distal tibial epiphysis with the metaphyseal fragment located on the lateral or posterolateral side. The displacement is lateral, producing a valgus lateral rotation deformity of the ankle. A valgus tilt of the ankle up to 15 degrees can be accepted. In the report of Crenshaw, radiograms made soon after the reduction showed a valgus tilt of the ankle in 6 of the 20 abduction fractures, and by the time of skeletal maturity, this tilt had disappeared spontaneously in every instance. The most severe tilt measured 12 degrees (in a 13½-year-old patient) and the least severe was 4 degrees (in a 10-year-old child). One patient with a lateral rotation fracture had a valgus tilt at the ankle of 10 degrees immediately following treatment, but the deformity disappeared completely during later growth.[30]

If a valgus tilt of more than 15 degrees is present at the ankle, a well-padded below-knee cast is applied, and after three or four days, gentle closed reduction is reattempted under general anesthesia; by then the reactive swelling will have subsided under the compression from the cast and the elevation of the leg. If reduction fails and more than 15 degrees of lateral angulation of the ankle mortise persists, open reduction should not be performed. The fracture is allowed to heal, and if, after two or three years, the deformity still persists, a supramalleolar osteotomy is performed to correct the valgus deformity at the ankle.

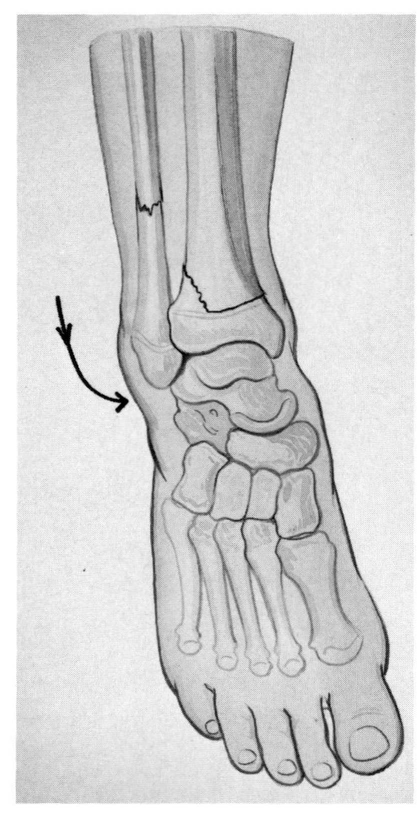

FIGURE 8–173. Method of reduction of pronation–eversion–lateral rotation fracture of the ankle.

First, apply longitudinal traction in the line of deformity—in lateral rotation and with the hindfoot everted, and then, while maintaining distal traction, *invert* and medially rotate the hindfoot.

The *adolescent fracture of Tillaux* is reduced by applying longitudinal axial traction and, while traction is maintained, medially rotating the hindfoot on the leg. The limb is immobilized in an above-knee cast for six to eight weeks (Fig. 8–174). The physeal injury is Salter-Harris Type III, involving the lateral part of the distal tibial epiphysis. Anatomic reduction is mandatory. If the fracture fragments are displaced more than 2 mm., open reduction and internal fixation with a cancellous screw or smooth Kirschner wires is required through an anterolateral approach. With accurate reduction the prognosis is excellent. Deformity due to asymmetrical growth from physeal injury does not follow this fracture. Joint incongruity can be prevented by anatomic reduction. The only

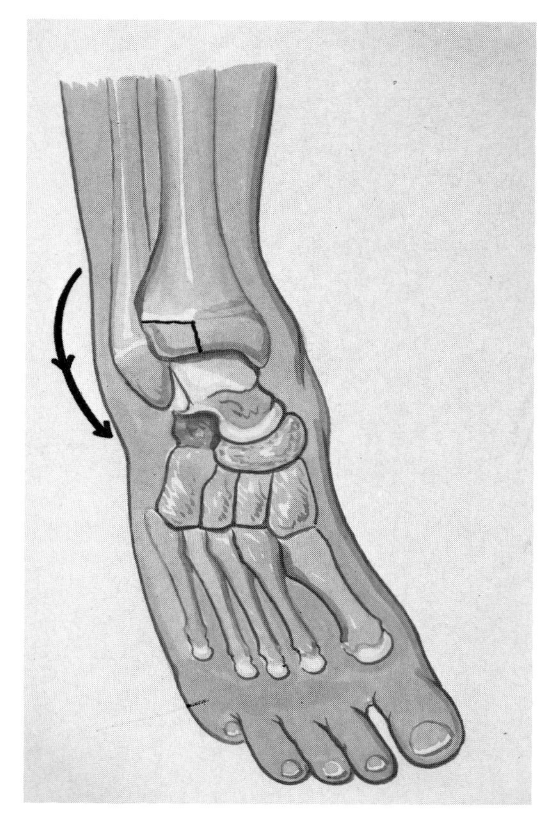

FIGURE 8–174. Method of reduction of adolescent Tillaux fracture.

While longitudinal axial traction is applied, the hindfoot is medially rotated. Caution! This is a Salter-Harris Type III fracture of the lateral part of the distal tibial epiphysis. If the fragments are separated by 2 mm. or more, open reduction and internal fixation are required.

significant problem of Tillaux fracture in the adolescent is tendon adhesions.

The undisplaced or minimally displaced (less than 2 mm.) *triplane fracture* is reduced by medial rotation of the hindpart of the foot on the tibia. The limb is immobilized in an above-knee non-weight-bearing cast for four weeks, then by a below-knee non-weight-bearing cast for an additional two to four weeks. In the cast the hindpart of the foot should be in medial rotation.

If on the routine anteroposterior and lateral radiograms the fracture is displaced more than 2 mm. and the fibula is intact, closed reduction under general anesthesia is ordinarily required. Medial rotation of the heel on the leg will usually be successful in reducing the fracture. Tomograms are made, if necessary, to delineate the accuracy of anatomic reduction. An associated greenstick or displaced fracture of the fibula may prevent reduction of the triplane fracture of the distal end of the tibia; the strong ligmentous attachments to the fibula and the lateral part of the tibia will maintain its angular deformity and the resultant shortening of the attached tibial fragment. Reduction of the triplane fracture cannot be accomplished until the fibular fracture is reduced.

If closed reduction is unsuccesful, open reduction and internal fixation with pins or cancellous screws is performed. In the reported cases of Marmor, Lynn, and Torg and Ruggiero, the triplane fracture of the distal end of the tibia was found to be unstable, requiring open reduction and internal fixation.[79, 85, 116] In the series of Cooperman and co-workers, however, only 2 of the 15 triplane fractures were treated by open surgical reduction.[29] First, the posterior fragment is reduced through a posteromedial approach and fixed internally with two cancellous screws. If on the anteroposterior radiogram the vertical fracture line through the sagittal plane is 2 mm. or more in width, an anterior approach is used to visualize the fracture; it is anatomically reduced and fixed securely with a transverse cancellous screw inserted immediately above the medial malleolus. Injury to the growth plate or penetration of the articular surface by the screw should be avoided. The limb is immobilized in an above-knee cast for six to eight weeks.

Complications

Premature Closure of Physis. Asymmetrical and symmetrical growth arrest results from crushing of the germinal layer of the physis. It may be complete, causing leg length inequality, or partial and asymmetrical, causing angular deformity.

In grade 2 supination-inversion injury of the ankle with Salter-Harris Type IV or V fracture the medial part of the tibial physis will fuse, whereas the lateral portion of the tibial physis and the distal fibular physis will remain open and continue to grow, causing progressive varus deformity of the ankle (Figs. 8–175 and 8–176). The younger the patient, the greater will be the deformity.

The extent of fusion of the growth plate is determined by anteroposterior and lateral tomography of the ankle joint. If less than 40 per cent of the growth plate is fused, the bone bridge is resected and replaced with adipose tissue from the gluteal region (Figs. 8–177 and 8–178). The excision of the bony bridge should be complete; it is performed with a dental drill and image-intensifier control. Langenskiöld has demonstrated that interposition of fatty tissue

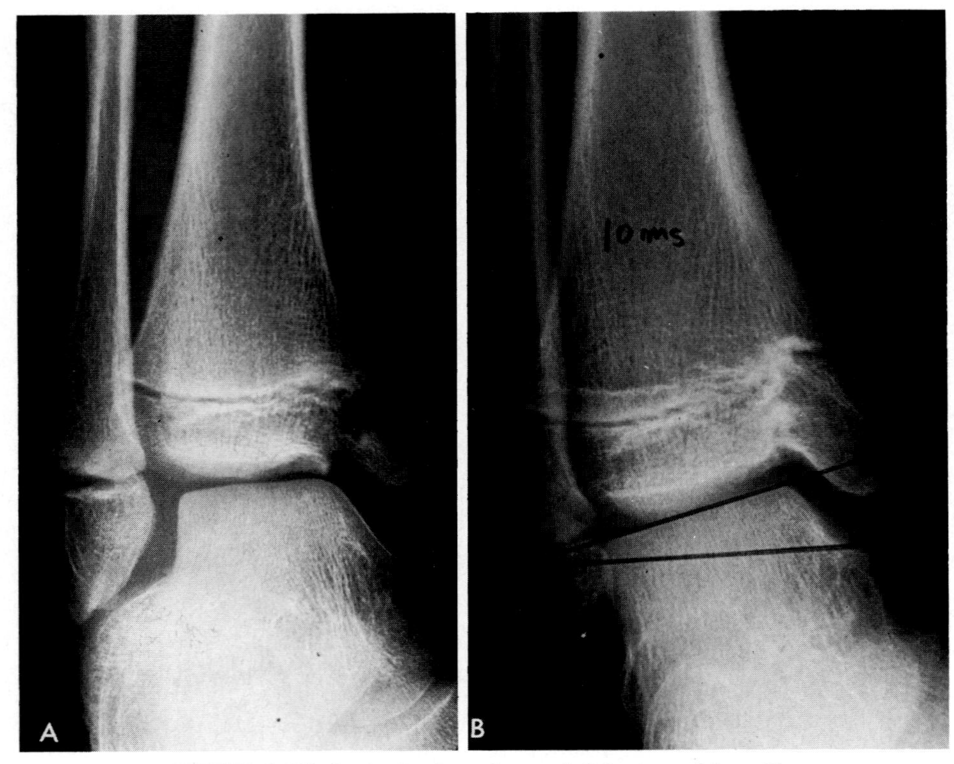

FIGURE 8–175. Supination-inversion grade 2 fracture of the ankle.

A. Note the Salter-Harris Type I fracture separation of the distal fibular physis and the Type IV fracture of the medial part of the distal tibial physis. **B.** Ten months later, there is varus ankle deformity secondary to asymmetrical growth arrest of the medial part of the distal tibial physis and continued growth of the lateral part of the distal tibial physis and the lower fibular physis.

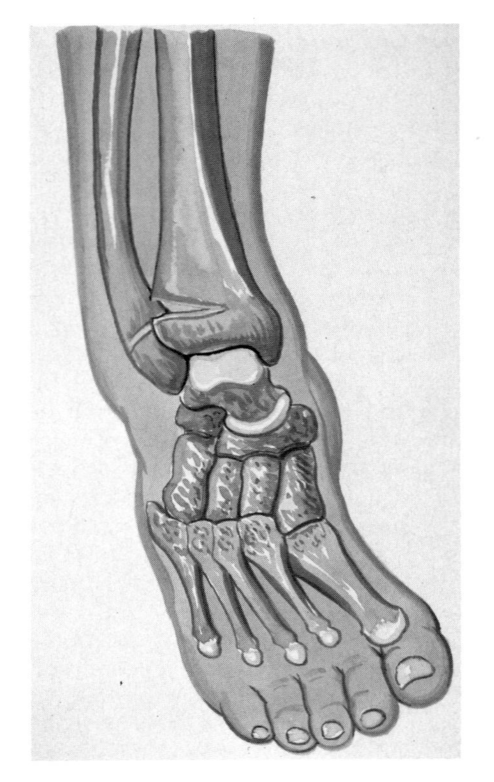

FIGURE 8–176. Diagram showing ankle varus deformity secondary to grade 2 supination-inversion fracture of the ankle.

Note the closure of the medial part of the distal tibial physis; the lateral part of the distal tibial physis and the fibular physis are open and continue to grow.

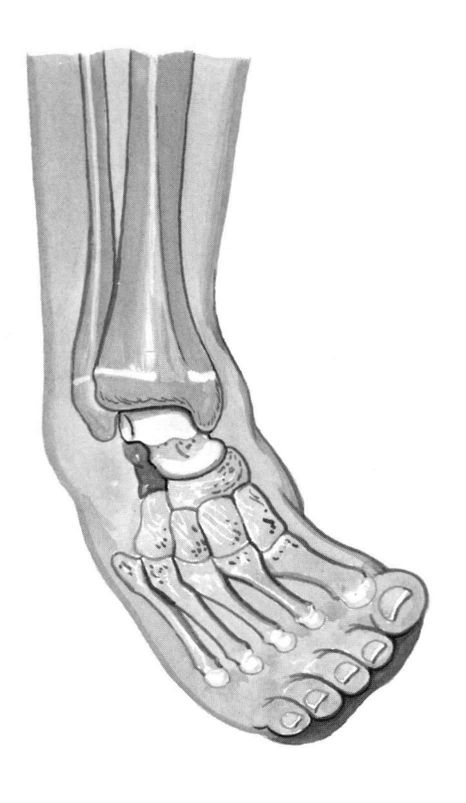

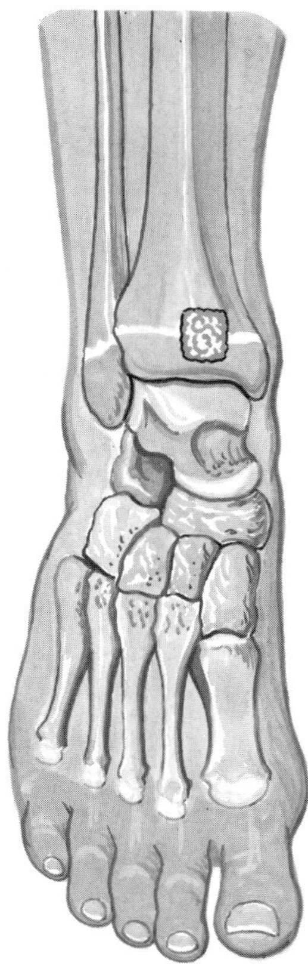

FIGURE 8–177. Diagram showing treatment of asymmetrical growth arrest of the medial part of the distal tibial physis.

The bony bridge across the growth plate is resected and replaced with adipose tissue from the gluteal region. Interposition of fatty tissue will prevent regeneration of bone.

will prevent regeneration of bone and fusion across the physis.[69]

If the size of the bony bridge across it is greater than 50 per cent of the width of the physis, the varus deformity at the ankle joint may be corrected by either "close-up" or "open-up" supramalleolar osteotomy of the tibia. The age of the patient and the amount of shortening will determine the operative procedure chosen. If surgery is postponed until ossification of the physis is complete in children and young adolescents (under 12 years of age for girls and under 14 years for boys), structural changes due to walking in inversion may take place in the ankle mortise. Also, resultant shortening of the leg and overgrowth of the fibula may be of considerable magnitude. Thus, it is best to perform an open-up osteotomy without disturbing the lateral portion of the distal tibial physis. With growth, the varus deformity will recur, and a second osteotomy will be required for correction; this should be explained to the parents.

The technique of open-up supramalleolar wedge osteotomy is as follows: A 3-cm. linear incision is made over the lateral aspect of the distal diaphysis of the fibula. The peroneal tendons are retracted posteriorly, the periosteum is divided, and the fibula is osteotomized obliquely at a level 2 cm. proximal to its distal physis. Then a 5-cm. linear incision is made over the medial aspect of the tibia, beginning at the distal tibial physis and extending proximally. The subcutaneous tissue is divided, exposing the periosteum. The level of osteotomy is 1 cm. proximal to the distal tibial physis. A smooth Kirschner wire is drilled into the tibia, and an anteroposterior radiogram is made to ascertain its site. Next, with starters and a drill, holes are made through the medial four fifths of the tibia, which is divided transversely with sharp osteotomes, leaving the lateral cortex intact. An alternative method is the use of an oscillating electric saw. The distal fragment of the tibia and the foot are angulated laterally, opening up the osteotomy site. Wedges of iliac

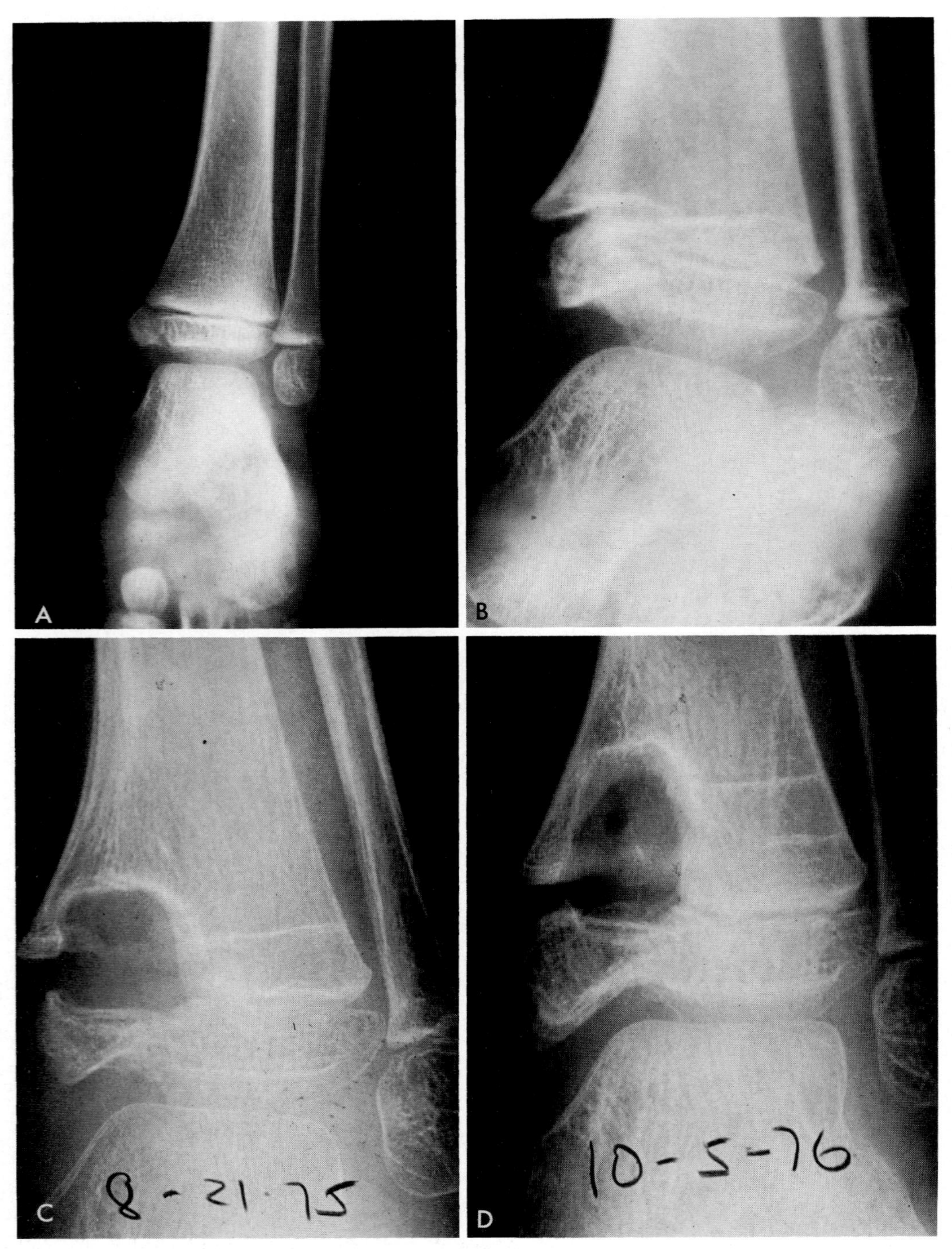

FIGURE 8–178. Radiograms of the ankle showing varus deformity due to asymmetrical growth arrest of medial part of the distal tibial physis.

The deformity was treated by excision of the bony bridge across the physis and its replacement in the defect with adipose tissue from the gluteal region to prevent regeneration of bone. Note in the follow-up radiograms the continued growth of the medial part of the tibial physis and correction of varus deformity.

bone of appropriate width are obtained and inserted into the gap on the medial side of the tibia (a laminectomy spreader may be used to keep the tibial bone fragments apart while the iliac bone grafts are being inserted). Radiograms are made to determine the degree of correction obtained. The osteotomy is fixed internally with either two wide staples or criss-cross Kirschner wires. Caution is exercised to avoid overstretching of the tibial vessels and ischemia of the foot. The tourniquet is released, and after complete hemostasis and return of normal circulation in the limb, the wound is closed and an above-knee plaster cast is applied. The osteotomy will heal and the bone graft will be incorporated in about two to three months.

In the author's experience, in the young child supramalleolar open-up wedge osteotomy has been a satisfactory procedure. It is important to correct overgrowth of the fibula by wedge resection of the lower fibular diaphysis or by epiphysiodesis of the distal fibula at the appropriate age.

The author does not recommend "close-up" supramalleolar osteotomy to correct varus deformity of the ankle joint because it will aggravate the leg length discrepancy.

In an older patient (girls over 12 years and boys over 14 years) epiphysiodesis of the distal fibula and of the lateral half of the distal tibial physis is performed to prevent the development of varus deformity of the ankle. If significant ankle varus deformity has already occurred, the procedure is combined with an open-up wedge osteotomy of the medial aspect of the distal tibia.

Premature growth arrest of the entire distal tibial epiphysis will result in shortening of the tibia. In the older patient, this is inconsequential clinically because of the proximity to termination of skeletal growth, whereas in the younger child, leg length discrepancy may be so marked that an epiphyseal arrest of the contralateral leg will be indicated. An epiphysiodesis of the distal fibula on the affected side is performed to prevent its overgrowth.

Lateral Rotation Deformity. This complication is caused by inadequate reduction. It occurred in 3 of the 15 cases of triplane fracture of Cooperman, Spiegel, and Laros, who, by computed tomography, demonstrated the fracture gap to be wider laterally than medially. This was verified by lateral tomography, which showed the persistent posterior position of the fibula and its attached tibial fragment. In another case Cooperman and his associates studied the mechanism of reduction by premanipulation and postmanipulation tomography; medial rotation of the foot in relation to the tibia closed the fracture gap.[29]

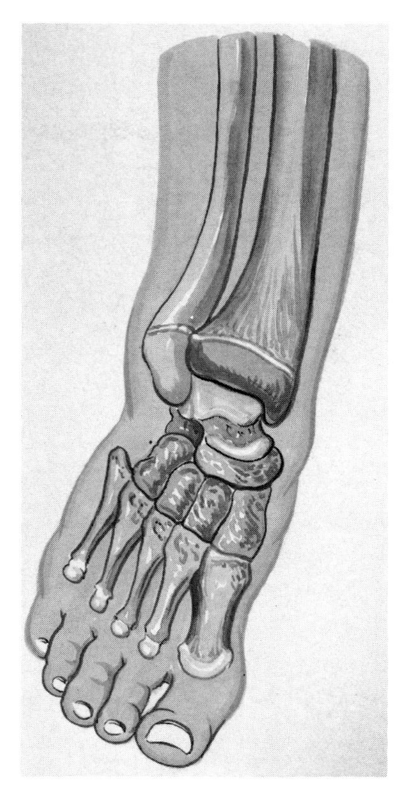

FIGURE 8–179. Valgus deformity of the ankle results from inadequate reduction of pronation–eversion–lateral rotation fracture of the ankle.

Valgus Deformity. Ankle valgus deformity usually results from inadequate reduction of pronation–eversion–lateral rotation fracture of the ankle (Figs. 8–179 and 8–180). A valgus tilt of the ankle greater than 15 to 20 degrees will not correct itself by remodeling with skeletal growth and cannot be accepted. It should be corrected surgically. If sufficient growth potential of the distal tibial epiphysis is present, the deformity may be corrected by epiphyseal arrest of the medial side of the distal tibia. Stapling of the medial side of the physis may be performed if it is difficult to calculate the exact skeletal age of the child. Growth arrest will cause further shortening of the limb.

If skeletal growth is complete, osteotomy of the distal tibia and fibula is performed to correct the deformity. A simple close-up wedge osteotomy of the distal tibia will cause unsightly prominence of the medial malleolus and shortening of the limbs (Fig. 8–181). Wiltse has designed a technique of tibial osteotomy in which a triangular segment of bone from the tibia is resected with its apex pointing proxi-

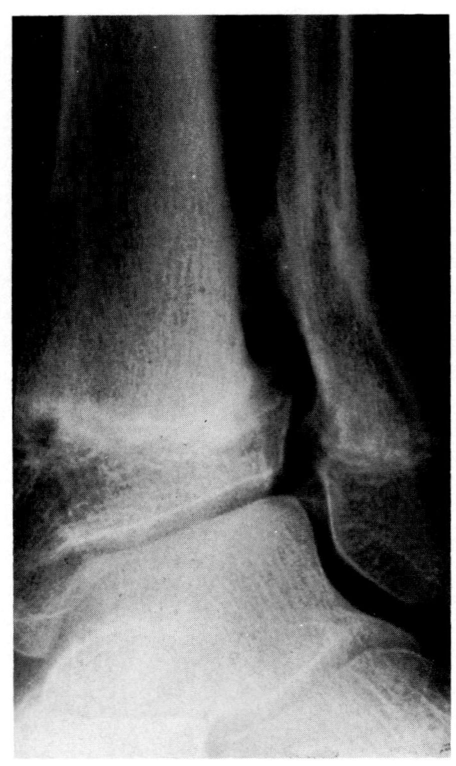

FIGURE 8–180. Anteroposterior radiogram showing valgus ankle due to poor reduction of pronation–eversion–lateral rotation fracture of the ankle.

A valgus tilt of greater than 15 degrees will usually not be remodeled.

mally and the fibula is cut obliquely (from distal-lateral to proximal-medial). The distal fragments of tibia and fibula are rotated medially and shifted laterally, thereby producing normal alignment of the ankle without an unsightly appearance of the medial malleolus. The limb will be shortened less than by a simple closing wedge osteotomy. Osteosynthesis is achieved by staples in a three- or four-hole plate.[122]

Joint Incongruity. A potentially serious complication, joint incongruity may cause early degenerative arthritis. Separation of fracture fragments greater than 2 mm. should not be accepted.

Johnson and Fahl reported three additional complications, each of which occurred once following significant displacement of Salter-Harris Type II abduction fractures. In the first case, circulation in the distal part of the foot was decreased, but it quickly returned following reduction of the fracture. With the second (abduction injury), the anterior tibial tendon and periosteum were interposed between the epiphysis and the tibia. Open reduction was necessary to remove the tendon and periosteum before accurate repositioning of the epiphysis could be carried out. In the third case, adhesions developed about the extensor hallucis longus tendon. Following operative lysis of these adhesions, full function was restored.[52]

References

1. Aitken, A. P.: The end results of the fractured distal tibial epiphysis. J. Bone Joint Surg., *18*:685, 1936.
2. Apley, A. G.: The ankle. *In* Apley, A. G. (ed.): A System of Orthopaedics and Fractures. 4th Ed. London, Butterworth, 1973, pp. 503–511.
3. Ashhurst, A. P. C., and Bromer, R. S.: Classification and mechanism of fractures of the leg bones involving the ankle. Arch. Surg., *4*:51, 1922.
4. Bartl, R.: Die traumatische Epiphysenlosung am distalen Ende des Schienbeines und des Wadenbeines. Hefte Unfallheilkd., *54*:228, 1956.

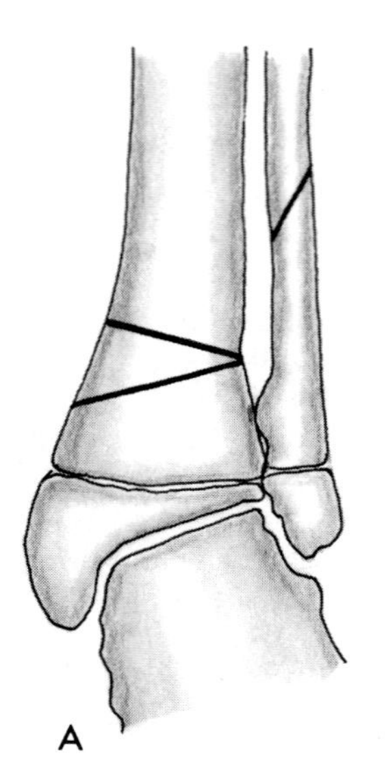

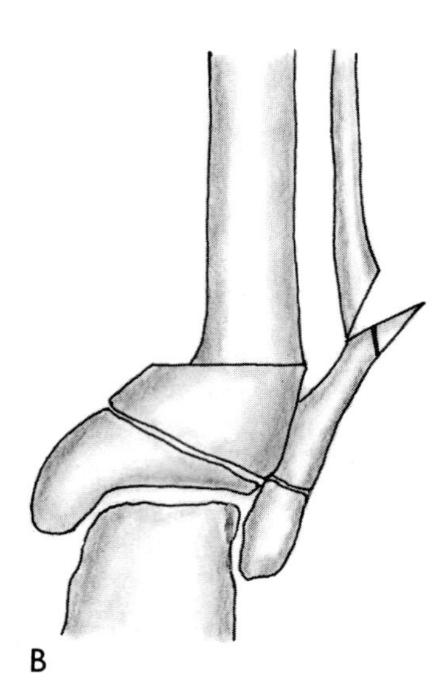

FIGURE 8–181. Close-up wedge osteotomy to correct valgus ankle.

This procedure will shorten the limb and cause an unsightly prominence of the medial malleolus.

5. Bauer, M., Jonsson, K., and Nilsson, B.: Thirty-year follow-up of ankle fractures. Acta Orthop. Scand., *56*:103, 1985.
6. Beck, E., and Engler, I.: Zur Prognose der Epiphysenverletzungen an distalen Schienbeinende. Arch. Orthop. Unfallchir., *65*:47, 1969.
7. Bergenfeldt, E.: Beitrage zur Kenntnis der traumatischen Epiphysenlosungen an den langen Rohrenknochen der Extremitaten. Eine klinisch-röntgenologische Studie. Acta Chir. Scand. (Suppl.), *28*, 1933.
8. Berridge, F. R., and Bonnin, J. G.: The radiographic examination of the ankle joint including arthrography. Surg. Gynecol. Obstet., *79*:383, 1944.
9. Birch, J. G., Herring, J. A., and Wenger, D. R.: Surgical anatomy of selected physes. J. Pediatr. Orthop., *4*:224, 1984.
10. Bishop, P. A.: Fractures and epiphyseal separation fractures of the ankle—a classification of 332 cases according to the mechanism of their production. A.J.R., *28*:49, 1932.
11. Blount, W. P.: Injuries of the leg and ankle. *In* Blount, W. P. (ed.): Fractures in Children. Huntington, N.Y., R. E. Krieger, 1977, pp. 183–193.
12. Bonnin, J. G.: Injuries to the Ankle. London, William Heinemann, 1950.
13. Bourne, R. B., Rorabeck, C. H., and Macnab, J.: Intra-articular fractures of the distal tibia: The pilon fracture. J. Trauma, *23*:591, 1983.
14. Brashear, H. R.: Epiphyseal fractures of the lower extremity. South. Med. J., *51*:845, 1958.
15. Bright, R. W.: Surgical correction of partial epiphyseal plate closure in dogs by bone bridge resection and use of silicone rubber implants. J. Bone Joint Surg., *54-A*:1133, 1972.
16. Bright, R. W., Burstein, A. H., and Elmore, S.: Epiphyseal plate cartilage. A biomechanical and histological analysis of failure modes. J. Bone Joint Surg., *56-A*:688, 1974.
17. Broock, G. J., and Greer, R. B.: Traumatic rotational displacements of the distal tibial growth plate. A case report. J. Bone Joint Surg., *52-A*:1666, 1970.
18. Cameron, H. U.: A radiologic sign of lateral subluxation of the distal tibial epiphysis. J. Trauma, *15*:1030, 1975.
19. Carothers, C. O., and Crenshaw, A. H.: Clinical significance of a classification of epiphyseal injuries of the ankle. Am. J. Surg., *89*:879, 1953.
20. Cass, J. R., and Peterson, H. A.: Salter-Harris type-IV injuries of the distal tibial epiphyseal growth plate, with emphasis on those involving the medial malleolus. J. Bone Joint Surg., *65-A*:1059, 1983.
21. Cassidy, R. H.: Epiphyseal injuries of the lower extremities. Surg. Clin. North Am., *38*:125, 1958.
22. Cedell, C. A.: Editorial: Is closed treatment of ankle fractures advisable? Acta Orthop. Scand., *56*:101, 1985.
23. Chigot, P. L., and Esteve, P.: Traumatologie Infantile. 2nd Ed. Paris, Expansion Scientifique Francaise, 1967, pp. 299–311.
24. Chigot, P. L., and Thuilleux, G.: Traitement des fractures-decollement epiphysaire de la malleole interne, dites de MacFarland. Chirurgie, *98*:229, 1972.
25. Chironi, P.: Considerazioni sulla frattura isolata de margine esterno dell epifisi tibiale inferiore. Minerva Ortop., *6*:123, 1955.
26. Clement, D. A., and Worlock, D. H.: Triplane fracture of the distal tibia. J. Bone Joint Surg., *69-B*:412, 1987.
27. Cone, R. O., III, et al.: Triplane fracture of the distal tibial epiphysis: Radiographic and CT studies. Radiology, *153*:763, 1984.
28. Cooper, A.: A Treatise on Dislocations and Fractures of the Joints. London, Longman, Hurst, Orme and Brown; E. Cox & Sons, 1822, pp. 238–240.
29. Cooperman, D. R., Spiegel, P. G., and Laros, G. S.: Tibial fractures involving the ankle in children. The so-called triplane epiphyseal fracture. J. Bone Joint Surg., *60-A*:1040, 1978.
30. Crenshaw, A.: Injuries to the distal tibial epiphysis. Clin. Orthop., *41*:98, 1965.
31. Dias, L. S.: Valgus deformity of the ankle joint: Pathogenesis of fibular shortening. J. Pediatr. Orthop., *5*:176, 1985.
32. Dias, L. S., and Foerster, T. P.: Traumatic lesions of the ankle joint. The supination-external rotation mechanism. Clin. Orthop., *100*:219, 1974.
33. Dias, L. S., and Giegerich, C. R.: Fractures of the distal tibial epiphysis in adolescence. J. Bone Joint Surg., *65-A*:438, 1983.
34. Dias, L. S., and Tachdjian, M. O.: Physeal injuries of the ankle in children. Clin. Orthop., *136*:230, 1978.
35. Dias, L. S., Guise, E. R., and Foerster, T.: Classification of Ankle Fracture. A Mechanistic Approach. Scientific Exhibit, A.A.O.S., October, 1974. Detroit, Henry Ford Hospital, 1974.
36. Dingeman, R. D., and Shaver, G. B., Jr.: Operative treatment of displaced Salter-Harris III distal tibial fractures. Clin. Orthop., *135*:101, 1978.
37. Dosa, G., Endrodi, J., Jokai, I., and Sandor, L.: The treatment of the distal epiphyseal fracture of the tibia (author's transl.). Magy. Traumatol. Orthop. Helyreallito Sebesz., *24*(4):241, 1981.
38. Duhaime, M., Gauthier, B., Labelle, P., and Simoneau, R.: Traumatismes epiphysaires de l'extremité distale du tibia. Union Med. Can., *101*:1827, 1972.
39. Ehlers, P. N., and Eberlein, H.: Epiphysenfrakturen: Klinischer Beitrag zur Frage der Spatfolgen. Langenbecks Arch. Klin. Chir., *305*:213, 1964.
40. Frain, P.: Epiphysial dislocations of the lower end of the tibia. J. Chir. (Paris), *91*:113, 1966.
41. Gall, F.: Nachuntersuchungen von Epiphysenfugenbruchen. Langenbecks Arch. Klin. Chir., *289*:372, 1958.
42. Gill, G., and Abbot, L.: Varus deformity of ankle following injury to the distal epiphyseal cartilage of the tibia in growing children. Surg. Gynecol. Obstet., *72*:659, 1941.
43. Gille, P., Aubert, D., Toulouse, J., Francois, J. Y., and Leclerc, D.: Fractures of the anterolateral tubercle of the distal tibial epiphysis in adolescence (author's transl.). Rev. Chir. Orthop., *67*:675, 1981.
44. Giuliani, K.: Spätzustande nach traumatischmechanischen Schadigungen der Epiphyse am distalen Tibiaende. Arch. Orthop. Unfallchir., *45*:386, 1952.
45. Goldberg, W. M., and Aadalen, R.: Distal tibial epiphyseal injuries: The role of athletics in 53 cases. Am. J. Sports Med., *6*:263, 1978.
46. Grace, D. L.: Irreducible fracture-separation of the distal tibial epiphysis. J. Bone Joint Surg., *65*:160, 1983.
47. Harper, M. C.: An anatomic study of the short oblique fracture of the distal fibula and ankle stability. Foot Ankle, *4*:23, 1983.
48. Henke, J. A., and Kiple, D. L.: Rotational displacement of the distal tibial epiphysis without fibular fracture. J. Trauma, *19*:64, 1979.
49. Hohmann, G.: Zur Korrektur frischer und veratteter Falle von Verletzung der distalen Tibiaepiphyse. Arch. Orthop. Unfallchir., *45*:395, 1952.
50. Horne, G.: Pes cavovarus following ankle fracture. A case report. Clin. Orthop., *184*:249, 1984.
51. Jani, L., and Hertel, E.: Correction of late sequelae of fractures with injuries of the distal tibial epiphysis. Beitr. Orthop. Traumatol., *14*:745, 1967.
52. Johnson, E. W., and Fahl, J. C.: Fractures involving the distal tibial epiphysis of the tibia and fibula in children. Am. J. Surg., *93*:778, 1957.
53. Judet, J., and Judet, R.: Fractures et Orthopaedie de l'Enfant. Paris, Librairie Maloine, 1974.
54. Judet, R., Judet, J., and LaGrange, J.: Les Fractures

des Membres chez l'Enfant. Paris, Librairie Maloine, 1958, pp. 235–238.
55. Kaplan, L.: Epiphyseal injuries in children. Surg. Clin. North Am., *17*:1637, 1937.
56. Karrholm, J., Hansson, L. I., and Selvik, G.: Changes in tibiofibular relationships due to growth disturbances after ankle fractures in children. J. Bone Joint Surg., *66-A*:1198, 1984.
57. Kleiger, B.: The mechanism of ankle injuries. J. Bone Joint Surg., *38-A*:59, 1956.
58. Kleiger, B., and Barton, J.: Epiphyseal ankle fractures. Bull. Hosp. J. Dis., *25*:240, 1964.
59. Kleiger, B., and Mankin, H. J.: Fracture of the lateral portion of the distal tibial epiphysis. J. Bone Joint Surg., *46-A*:25, 1964.
60. Kling, T. F., Jr., Bright, R. W., and Hensinger, R. N.: Distal tibial physeal fractures in children that may require open reduction. J. Bone Joint Surg., *66-A*:647, 1984.
61. Kristensen, T. B.: Treatment of malleolar fractures according to Lauge-Hansen's method. Preliminary results. Acta Chir. Scand., *97*:362, 1949.
62. Kristensen, T. B.: Fractures of the ankle. VI. Follow-up studies. Arch. Surg. (Chicago), *73*:112, 1956.
63. Kump, W. L.: Vertical fractures of the distal tibial epiphysis. A.J.R., *97*:676, 1966.
64. von Laer, L.: The "uncompleted" in growth: The transitional fracture of the distal tibia (author's transl.). Unfallheilkunde, *84*:373, 1981.
65. von Laer, L.: Post-traumatic partial closure of the distal tibial epiphyseal groove. Etiology, prognosis and prophylaxis? I: Case load, method and results. Unfallheilkunde, *85*:445, 1982.
66. von Laer, L., Gerber, B., and Jehle, B.: Epiphyseal fractures and epiphysiolyses of the distal tibia. Z. Kinderchir., *36*:125, 1982.
67. Landin, L. A., Danielsson, L. G., Jonsson, K., and Pettersson, H.: Late results in 65 physeal ankle fractures. Acta Orthop. Scand., *57*:530, 1986.
68. Langenskiöld, A.: Traumatic premature closure of the distal tibial epiphyseal plate. Acta Orthop. Scand., *38*:520, 1967.
69. Langenskiöld, A.: An operation for partial closure of an epiphyseal plate in children and its experimental basis. J. Bone Joint Surg., *57-B*:325, 1975.
70. Lauge-Hansen, N.: Fractures of the ankle: I. Analytic historic survey as basis of new experimental, roentgenologic, and clinical investigations. Arch. Surg., *56*:259, 1948.
71. Lauge-Hansen, N.: Fractures of the ankle: II. Combined experimental-surgical and experimental-roentgenologic investigations. Arch. Surg. (Chicago), *60*:957, 1950.
72. Lauge-Hansen, N.: Fractures of the ankle: IV. Clinical use of genetic roentgen diagnosis and genetic reduction. Arch. Surg. (Chicago), *64*:488, 1952.
73. Lauge-Hansen, N.: Fractures of the ankle: V. Pronation-dorsiflexion fracture. Arch. Surg. (Chicago), *67*:813, 1953.
74. Lauge-Hansen, N.: Fractures of the ankle: III. Genetic roentgenologic diagnosis of fractures of the ankle. A.J.R., *71*:456, 1954.
75. Laurin, C., and Mathieu, J.: Sagittal mobility of the normal ankle. Clin. Orthop., *108*:99, 1975.
76. Lechner, F., and Primbs, P.: Ski injuries during growth. Fortschr. Med., *93*:107, 1975.
77. Linhart, W., Hollwarth, M., and Schimpl, G.: Fractures of the distal tibial epiphysis. Unfallheilkunde, *86*:510, 1983.
78. Lovell, E. S.: An unusual rotatory injury of the ankle. J. Bone Joint Surg., *50-A*:163, 1968.
79. Lynn, M. D.: The triplane distal tibial epiphyseal fracture. Clin. Orthop., *86*:187, 1972.
80. McFarland, B.: Traumatic arrest of epiphyseal growth at the lower end of the tibia. Br. J. Surg., *19*:1931, 1932.
81. MacNealy, G. A., Roger, L. F., Hernandez, R., and Poznanski, A. K.: Injuries of the distal tibial epiphysis: Systematic radiographic evaluation. A.J.R., *138*:683, 1982.
82. McWilliams, D. J.: Fracture of fibular aspect of lower tibial epiphysis. Ulster Med. J., *31*:185, 1962.
83. Mallet, J.: Partial traumatic epiphysiodesis of the lower end of the tibia in children. Treatment with disepiphysiodesis. Rev. Chir. Orthop., *61*:5, 1975.
84. Mandell, J.: Isolated fractures of the posterior tibial lip at the ankle as demonstrated by an additional projection, the "poor" lateral view. Radiology, *101*:319, 1971.
85. Marmor, L.: An unusual fracture of the tibial epiphysis. Clin. Orthop., *73*:132, 1970.
86. Maylahn, D. J., Zemel, N. P., and Fahey, J. J.: Fractures involving the epiphyseal cartilage plate of the distal tibia. Personal communication, 1976.
87. Molster, A., Soreide, O., Solhaug, J. H., and Raugstad, T. S.: Fractures of the lateral part of the distal tibial epiphysis (Tillaux or Kleiger fracture). Injury, *8*:260, 1977.
88. Nevelos, A. B., and Colton, C. L.: Rotational displacement of the lower tibial epiphysis due to trauma. J. Bone Joint Surg., *59-B*:331, 1977.
89. Paleari, G. L.: Sul meccanismo di poduzione dei distacchi antero-esterni dell' epifisi distale della tibia. Arch. Orthop., *73*:1146, 1960.
90. Pankovich, A. M.: Fractures of the fibula proximal to the distal tibiofibular syndesmosis. J. Bone Joint Surg., *60-A*:221, 1978.
91. Peiro, A., Aracil, J., Martos, F., and Mut, T.: Triplane distal tibial epiphyseal fracture. Clin. Orthop., *160*:196, 1981.
92. Peiro, A., Aracil, J., Martos, F., and Mut, T.: Fractures of the distal tibial epiphysis in adolescence (letter). J. Bone Joint Surg., *65-A*:1208, 1983.
93. Perry, C. R., Rice, S., Rao, A., and Burdge, R.: Posterior fracture-dislocation of the distal part of the fibula. Mechanism and staging of injury. J. Bone Joint Surg., *65-A*:1149, 1983.
94. Peterson, H. A., Brewster, R. C., and Johnson, K. A.: Epiphyseal growth plate injuries of the distal tibia. Minn. Med., *60*:44, 1977.
95. Poland, J.: Traumatic Separation of the Epiphyses. London, Smith, Elder & Co., 1898.
96. Pollen, A. G.: Ankle and foot. *In* Fractures and Dislocations in Children. Baltimore, Williams & Wilkins, 1973, pp. 198–215.
97. Quigley, T. B.: Analysis and treatment of ankle injuries produced by rotatory, abduction, and adduction forces. A.A.O.S. Instr. Course Lect., *19*:172, 1970.
98. Rang, M.: Children's Fractures. Philadelphia, Lippincott, 1974, pp. 198–209.
99. Robertson, D. E.: Post-traumatic osteochondritis of the lower tibial epiphysis. J. Bone Joint Surg., *46-B*:212, 1964.
100. Robichon, J., Pegington, J., Mooje, V. B., and Des Jardins, J. P.: Functional anatomy of the ankle joint and its relationship to ankle injuries. Can. J. Surg., *15*:145, 1972.
101. Salter, R. B.: Injuries of the ankle in children. Orthop. Clin. North Am., *5*:147, 1974.
102. Salter, R. B., and Harris, W. R.: Injuries involving the epiphyseal plate. J. Bone Joint Surg., *45-A*:587, 1963.
103. Sammarco, G. J., Burstein, A. H., and Frankel, V. H.: Biomechanics of the ankle: A kinetic study. Orthop. Clin. North Am., *4*:75, 1973.
104. Schatzker, J., and Johnson, R. G.: Fracture dislocation of the ankle with anterior dislocation of the fibula. J. Trauma, *23*:420, 1983.

105. Schenk, R. K., Spiro, D., and Weiner, J.: Cartilage resorption in the tibial epiphyseal plate of growing rats. J. Cell. Biol., *34*:275, 1967.
106. Schweitzer, G.: Injuries to the distal tibial epiphysis. S. Afr. Med. J., *43*:1258, 1969.
107. Seitz, W. H., Jr., and LaPorte, J.: Medial triplane fracture delineated by computerized axial tomography. J. Pediatr. Orthop., *8*:65, 1988.
108. Seitz, W. H., Andrews, D. L., Shelton, M. L., and Feldman, F.: Triplane fractures of the adolescent ankle—a report of three cases. Injury, *16*:547, 1985.
109. Siffert, R. S., and Arkin, A. M.: Post-traumatic aseptic necrosis of the distal tibial epiphysis. J. Bone Joint Surg., *32-A*:691, 1950.
110. Spiegel, P. G., Cooperman, D. R., and Laros, G. S.: Epiphyseal fractures of the distal ends of the tibia and fibula—a retrospective study of two hundred and thirty-seven cases in children. J. Bone Joint Surg., *60-A*:1046, 1978.
111. Spiegel, P. G., Mast, J. W., Cooperman, D. R., and Laros, G. S.: Triplane fractures of the distal tibial epiphysis. Clin. Orthop., *188*:74, 1984.
112. Stampfel, O., Zoch, G., Scholz, R., and Ferlic, P.: Ergbnisse der operativen Behandlung von Verletzunger der distalen Tibia epiphyse. Arch. Orthop. Unfallchir., *84*:211, 1976.
113. Stern, M. B., Grant, S. S., and Isaacson, A. S.: Bilateral distal tibial and fibular epiphyseal separation associated with spina bifida. Clin. Orthop., *50*:191, 1967.
114. Sussenbach, F., and Weber, B. G.: Epiphysenfugenletzungen am distalen Unterschenkel. Stuttgart, Huber, 1970.
115. Tinnemans, J. G., and Severijnen, R. S.: The triplane fracture of the distal tibial epiphysis in children. Injury, *12*:393, 1981.
116. Torg, J., and Ruggiero, R.: Comminuted epiphyseal fracture of the distal tibia. Clin. Orthop., *110*:215, 1975.
117. Weber, B. G.: Prophylaxe der Achsenfehlstellungen bei der Behandlung kindlicher Frakturen. *In* Muller, M. E. (ed.): Posttraumatische Achsenfehlstellungen an den unteren Extremitaten. Stuttgart, Huber, 1967.
118. Wehner, W., and Hasek, P.: Osteosynthesis of the child's malleolus. Beitr. Orthop. Traumatol., *24*:37, 1977.
119. Wicky, B., and Stauffer, U. G.: Epiphyseal fractures of the distal tibia. Treatment and results. Chirurg, *53*:697, 1982.
120. Wicky, B., and Stauffer, U. G.: Triplane fractures of the distal tibia. Z. Kinderchir., *38*:Suppl.:51, 1983.
121. Wilson, F. C.: Fractures and dislocations of the ankle. *In* Rockwood, C. A. (ed.): Fractures. Philadelphia, Lippincott, 1975, pp. 1361–1399.
122. Wiltse, L. L.: Valgus deformity of the ankle as a sequel to acquired or congenital anomalies of the fibula. J. Bone Joint Surg., *54-A*:595, 1972.
123. Witt, A. N.: Die Therapie der Epiphysenfugenschadigungen. Langenbecks Arch. Klin. Chir., *289*:361, 1958.
124. Witt, A. N., and Mittelmeier, H.: Epiphysenverletzungen des Unterschenkels. *In* d. Orthopädie, Bd. IV, S. 1174. Stuttgart, Thieme, 1961.
125. Yao, J., and Huurman, W. W.: Tomography in juvenile Tillaux fracture. J. Pediatr. Orthop., *6*:349, 1986.

FRACTURES OF THE FOOT

The flexibility and resiliency of a child's foot make it relatively immune to injury. The forces of indirect violence are transmitted proximally, causing fractures of the tibia or fibula.

In children fractures of the foot are usually produced by direct violence in a crushing injury, such as is caused by a heavy object being dropped on the foot, by being run over by the wheels of an automobile, or by falling from a height and landing on the heels. The crushing force may not break the skin, but it will cause marked soft-tissue injury to the child's foot.

In treatment, the first step is to decrease the soft-tissue swelling by application of a Jones compression dressing and elevation of the foot and leg. Often it is wise to admit the child to the hospital for observation and treatment. During the first few days following trauma the neurovascular and muscular status and the skin are thoroughly assessed. Management of soft-tissue injury takes priority over that of the fracture. When the soft-tissue swelling has subsided and the vascular and skin status permits, the fracture is reduced and immobilized in a plaster of Paris cast. Fractures of the individual bones of the foot are briefly discussed next.

Fractures of the talus are rare in children.[20, 25, 33, 43, 45, 56, 57] They usually occur in the adolescent. In general they heal adequately without serious complications, such as aseptic necrosis. A vertical fracture through the *neck of the talus* is the most common injury. If not displaced or minimally displaced, it is treated by immobilization in a below-knee cast for four to six weeks. Weight-bearing is not permitted.

When the talar neck fracture is displaced, the head of the talus is usually displaced dorsally. The fracture is reduced by closed manipulation and immobilized with the foot in 30 degrees of plantar flexion in a non-weight-bearing below-knee cast for six to eight weeks. Malunion should be avoided. If closed reduction is unsuccessful, open reduction and internal fixation with two Kirschner wires are carried out. It is best to utilize a lateral approach and dissect minimally to prevent further injury to the medial artery to the body of the talus. The reduced but unstable fracture may be fixed by percutaneous pinning under an image intensifier.

Talar neck fracture may be associated with subtalar dislocation. The distal talar fragment and the foot are medially luxated, and the talar body is rotated posteromedially. If the distal fragment is displaced anteriorly, the risk of aseptic necrosis to the body of the talus is very great. The dislocation usually can be reduced by closed manipulation; occasionally, however, open reduction may be required.

Fractures of the *body of the talus* result from violent trauma, as in a fall from a height or an automobile accident (Fig. 8–182). The fracture

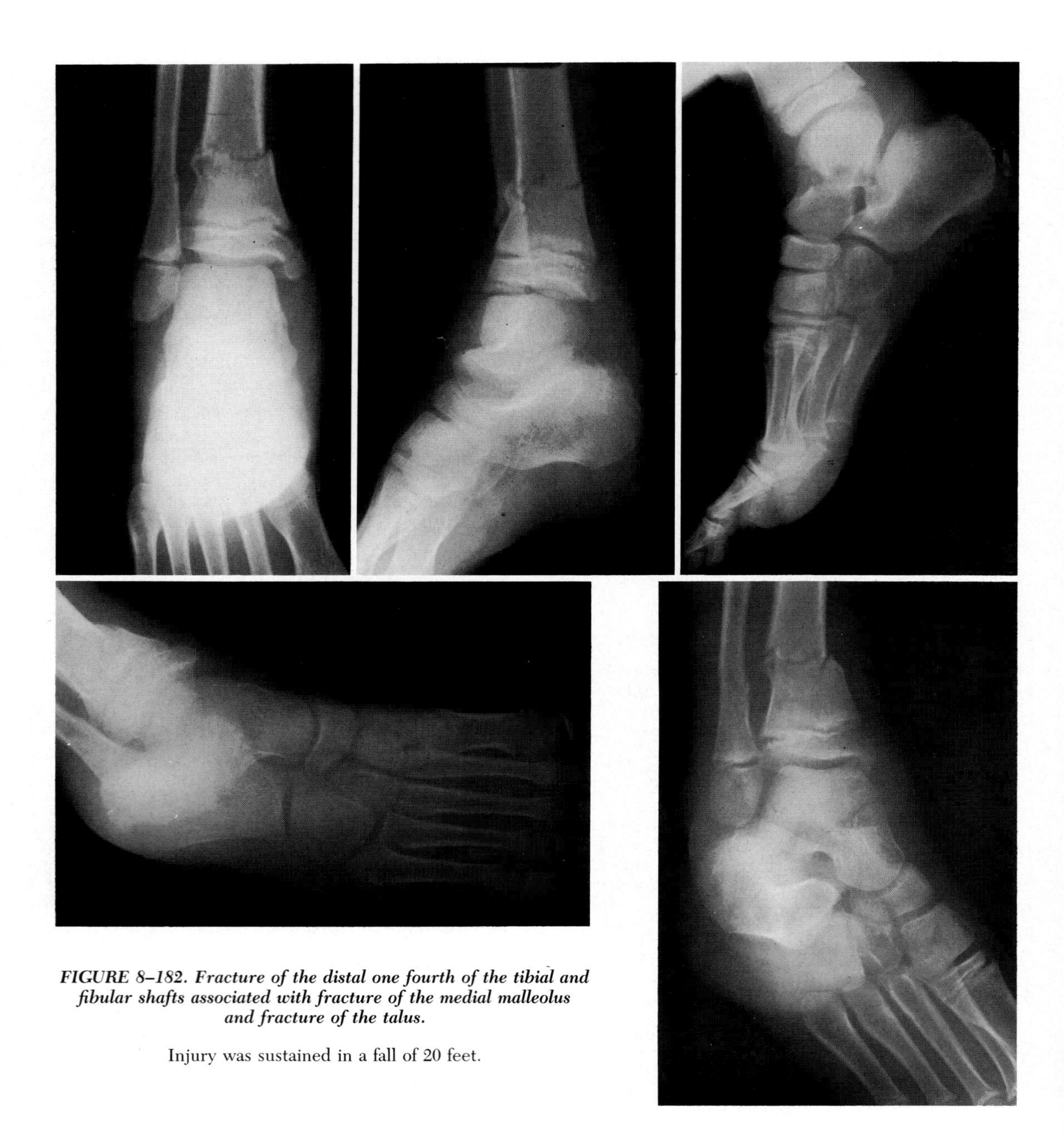

FIGURE 8–182. Fracture of the distal one fourth of the tibial and fibular shafts associated with fracture of the medial malleolus and fracture of the talus.

Injury was sustained in a fall of 20 feet.

usually consists of compression of the dome of the talus with varying degrees of comminution and collapse. A conservative approach is recommended in such cases. A below-knee cast is applied for eight weeks and is followed by protection in a patellar tendon–bearing foot-ankle orthosis for one or two years. It is surprising how well the fracture is remodeled and how much functional range of ankle motion is achieved. Primary ankle fusion should not be performed; it is reserved as a salvage procedure for relief of pain, later on in adult life, if necessary.

Indirect violence, such as is sustained in a fall with the foot caught in the spokes of a bicycle, may cause a transverse oblique fracture through the body of the talus. Undisplaced fractures are treated by immobilization in a below-knee cast for two months. Displaced fractures require restoration of anatomic alignment, often by open reduction and internal fixation with Kirschner wires.

Fracture of the *lateral process of the talus* is usually caused by a twisting injury of the ankle; the process is avulsed by the pull of the anterior talofibular ligament.[33] Careful palpation reveals point tenderness immediately anterior to the lateral malleolus. Oblique radiograms of the ankle in 10 to 20 degrees of medial rotation will demonstrate the fractured fragment. Sometimes tomography is indicated. Persistent and disabling pain may require excision of the loose fragment.

Osteochondral fracture fragments of the dome of the talus, if displaced, are best removed by arthrotomy (see section on osteochondritis dissecans).

Fractures of the calcaneus are very infrequent in children and usually do not involve the subtalar joint. Treatment consists of application of a Robert Jones compression dressing and elevation of the foot and leg for several days. It is best to admit the child to the hospital. Then the limb is immobilized in a below-knee cast for three to four weeks.[24, 44, 56, 59] Open surgical reduction of displaced os calcis fractures is contraindicated. Malunions will undergo marked remodeling with restoration of normal structure. The occasional persistent varus deviation of the heel may be corrected by Dwyer's osteotomy of the calcaneus.

Lisfranc's *tarsometatarsal fracture-disloca-*

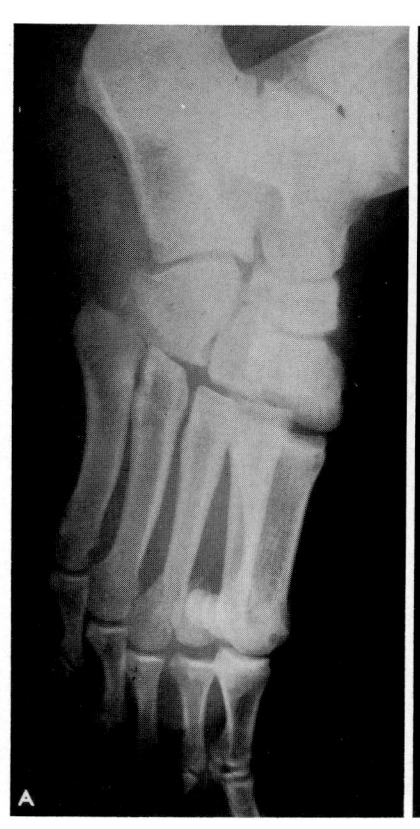

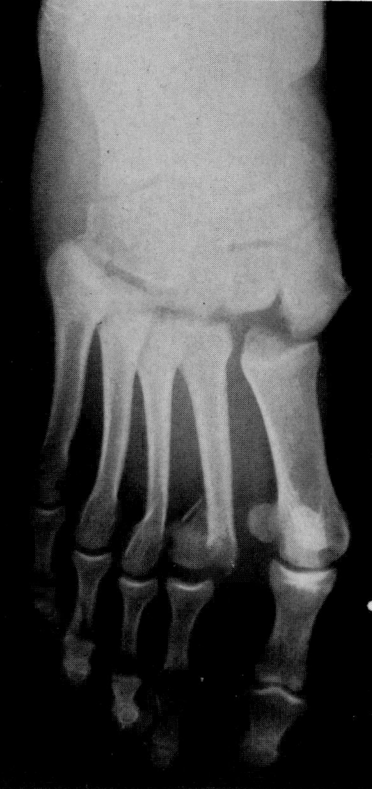

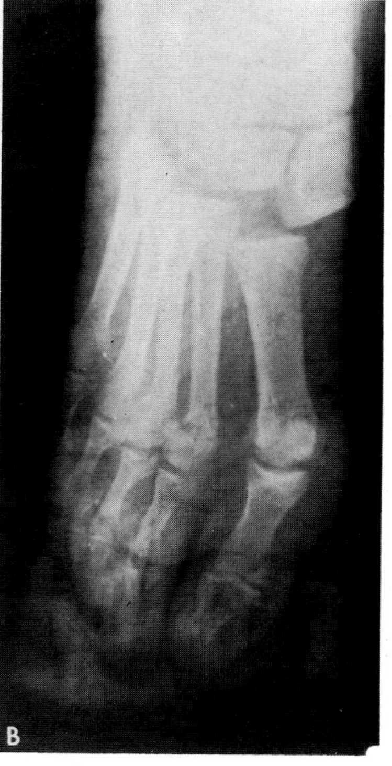

FIGURE 8–183. Lisfranc's tarsometatarsal dislocation with fracture of the second metatarsal neck.

A and **B.** Initial radiograms.

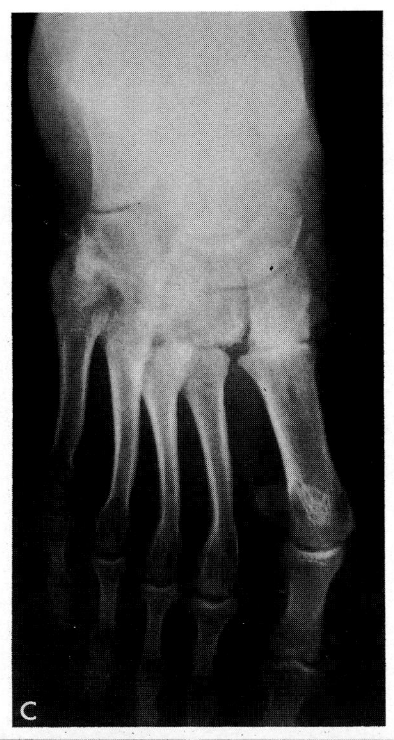

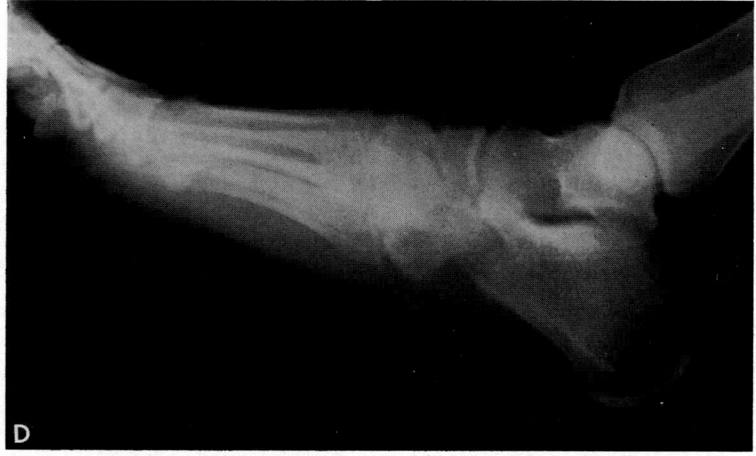

FIGURE 8–183 Continued. Lisfranc's tarsometatarsal dislocation with fracture of the second metatarsal neck.

C and **D.** Two years after closed reduction. Note the degenerative changes in the midtarsal joints.

tions are treated by closed manipulation; if adequate reduction cannot be achieved, open surgery is indicated (Fig. 8–183).[43, 63]

Fractures of the navicular, cuboid, and cuneiforms are caused by crushing injury.[23] Primary treatment is directed toward control of soft-tissue swelling with a Robert Jones compression dressing and elevation of the foot. After soft-tissue swelling has subsided a below-knee walking cast is applied and worn for four weeks.

Metatarsal fractures are produced by direct compression force, and usually more than one metatarsal bone is involved (Fig. 8–184).[37] Treatment consists of simple immobilization of the foot in a below-knee cast for four weeks. Markedly displaced fractures may require open reduction and internal fixation with Kirschner wires. Nonunions and malunions may result in shortened rays and metatarsalgia due to depression of the metatarsal heads.

Fractures of the proximal end of the fifth metatarsal are of two distinct types: a fracture through the tuberosity (known as Jones's fracture, since Sir Robert Jones first described it in

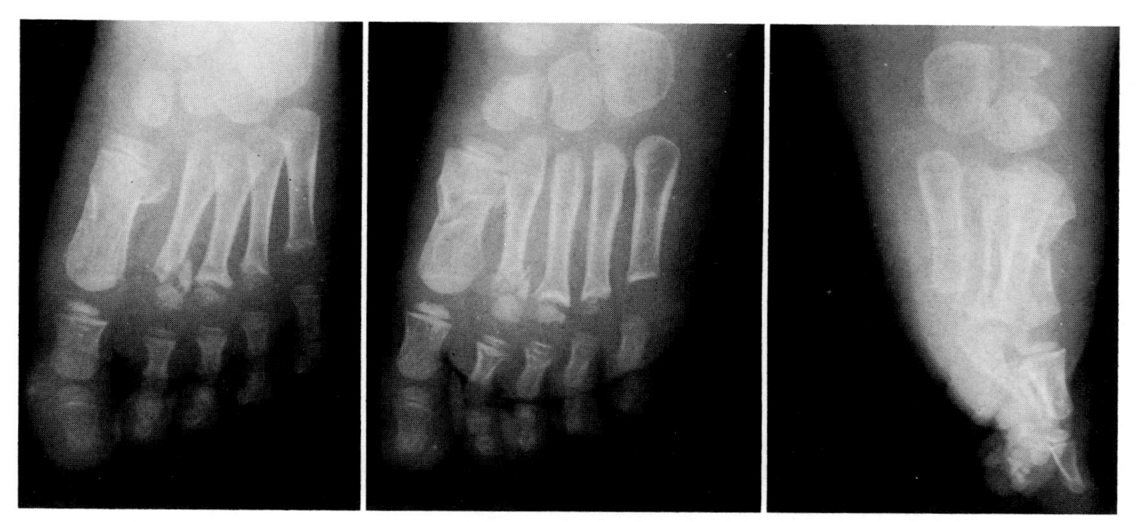

FIGURE 8–184. Fracture of first metatarsal shaft and neck of second metatarsal caused by direct crushing injury.

1902), and a fracture through the proximal part of the diaphysis within a distance of 1.5 cm. from the tuberosity.[17, 38, 57]

Fractures through the tuberosity of the fifth metatarsal are caused by forced inversion of the plantar-flexed foot. Treatment is symptomatic. An elastic bandage and partial weight-bearing with crutches are used for about three weeks. If symptoms are severe, for the greater comfort of the patient and convenience of the surgeon, a below-knee cast is applied. Radiographic osseous union takes place almost uniformly in less than two months.

The problem with fractures of the tuberosity of the fifth metatarsal is erroneous diagnosis. Dameron has clearly described the anatomic variations of the proximal portion of the fifth metatarsal, where the secondary center of ossification in the tuberosity may be mistaken for a fracture line. Study of the radiograms of one foot of 164 unselected children (56 girls and 108 boys) ranging in age from 7 to 16 years disclosed no radiographic evidence of this secondary ossification center before the age of 8 years. It became visible on the radiogram between 9 and 11 years in girls and between 11 and 14 years in boys. The apophysis was seen to be united to the shaft before the age of 12 in all the girls and before the age of 15 in all the boys.[17]

The secondary center of ossification appears as a fleck of bone located within the plantar and lateral parts of the cartilaginous flare and obliquely oriented with respect to the metatarsal shaft. At this stage of maturation it can closely resemble a fracture.

Other structures that may cause difficulty in diagnosis are the *os peroneum* (located in the peroneus longus tendon and present on 15 per cent of radiograms of the foot) and *os vesalianum* (which is thought to be either an ossicle in the peroneus brevis tendon or part of the tuberosity of the fifth metatarsal and present on 0.1 per cent of radiograms of the feet). Both ossicles have smooth, sclerotic opposing surfaces that are easily differentiated from the jagged margin of a recent fracture. A transverse radiolucent line in the proximal end of the fifth metatarsal is another anomaly that may cause confusion. This apophyseal line does not extend proximally to the cuboid–fifth metatarsal joint or medially into the articulation between the fourth and fifth metatarsals, and its line of orientation is oblique (almost parallel) to the long axis of the shaft. In contrast, a fracture is perpendicular to the fifth metatarsal shaft, and usually the fracture line extends into one or both articulations between the fourth and fifth metatarsals and between the fifth metatarsal and the cuboid bone.

Fractures through the proximal part of the fifth metatarsal usually take place 1.5 cm. distal to the tuberosity. They are notorious for slow healing. It is best to treat them by immobilization in a below-knee cast for six weeks. In case of delayed healing, Dameron recommends consideration of early bone grafting in professional athletes and symptomatic treatment in sedentary persons.[17]

References

1. Aitken, A. P., and Poulson, D.: Dislocation of the tarsometatarsal joint. J. Bone Joint Surg., *45-A*:246, 1963.
2. Anderson, L. D.: Injuries of the forefoot. Clin. Orthop., *122*:18, 1977.
3. Arangio, G. A.: Proximal diaphyseal fractures of the

fifth metatarsal (Jones' fracture): Two cases treated by cross-pinning with review of 106 cases. Foot Ankle, *3*:293, 1983.
4. Arntz, C. T., Veith, R. G., and Hansen, S. T.: Fractures and fracture-dislocations of the tarsometatarsal joint. J. Bone Joint Surg., *70-A*:173, 1988.
5. Bauer, J., Blaske, V., and Franclik, J.: Results of treatment procedures in fractures of the talus. Hefte Unfallheilkd., *133*:63, 1979.
6. Bensahel, H., and Huguenin, P.: Fractures of the ankle and foot in children (author's transl.). Ann. Chir., *35*:114, 1981.
7. Bensahel, H., and Huguenin, P.: Fractures of the ankle and foot in children (author's transl.). Ann. Paediatr. (Paris), *28*:437, 1981.
8. Blount, W. P.: Injuries of the foot. *In* Blount, W. P. (ed.): Fractures in Children. Huntington, N.Y., E. Krieger, 1977, pp. 195–201.
9. Bovill, E. G., Jr., and Inman, V. T.: Fractures and fracture-dislocations of the foot and ankle. *In* Inman, V. T. (ed.): DuVries' Surgery of the Foot. St. Louis, Mosby, 1973, pp. 119–167.
10. Brown, D. C., and McFarland, G. B.: Dislocation of the medial cuneiform bone in tarsometatarsal fracture-dislocation. J. Bone Joint Surg., *57-A*:858, 1975.
11. Brunet, J. A., and Wiley, J. J.: The late results of tarsometatarsal joint injuries. J. Bone Joint Surg., *69-B*:437, 1987.
12. Buchanan, J., and Greer, R. B., III: Stress fractures in the calcaneus of a child. Clin. Orthop., *135*:119, 1978.
13. Burkus, J. K., Sella, E. J., and Southwick, W. O.: Occult injuries of the talus diagnosed by bone scan and tomography. Foot Ankle, *4*:316, 1984.
14. Canale, S. T., and Belding, R. H.: Osteochondral lesions of the talus. J. Bone Joint Surg., *62-A*:97, 1980.
15. Chiari, K.: Die traumatische Talusrollennekrose. Wien Med. Wochenschr., *99*:119, 1949.
16. Comfort, T. H., Behrens, F., Gaither, D. W., Denis, F., and Sigmond, M.: Long-term results of displaced talar neck fractures. Clin. Orthop., *199*:81, 1985.
17. Dameron, T. B.: Fractures and anatomical variation of the proximal portion of the fifth metatarsal. J. Bone Joint Surg., *57-A*:788, 1975.
18. Davidson, A. M., Steele, H. D., MacKenzie, D. A., and Penny, J. A.: A review of twenty-one cases of transchondral fracture of the talus. J. Trauma, *7*:378, 1967.
19. Dolling, D., and Franke, D.: Fracture of the navicular bone in childhood and its peculiarities. Bruns. Beitr. Klin. Chir., *219*:462, 1972.
20. Dunn, A. R., Jacobs, B., and Campbell, R. D.: Fractures of the talus. J. Trauma, *6*:443, 1966.
21. Dworczynski, W., and Pomierna, I.: Fracture of the calcaneus in a 32-month-old child. Chir. Narzadow Ruchu Orthop. Pol., *46*:107, 1981.
22. Ehrensperger, J.: Fractures of the foot in children and adolescents. Ther. Umsch., *40*:996, 1983.
23. Elghawabi, M. H.: Fractures of the cuneiform bones. Classification and treatment. Egypt. Orthop. J., *7*:206, 1972.
24. Essex-Lopresti, P.: The mechanism, reduction, technique and results of fractures of the os calcis. Br. J. Surg., *39*:395, 1952.
25. Fahey, J. J., and Murphy, J. L.: Dislocations and fractures of the talus. Surg. Clin. North Am., *45*:79, 1965.
26. Giannestras, N. J., and Sammarco, G. J.: Fractures and dislocations in the foot. *In* Rockwood, C. A., and Green, D. P. (eds.): Fractures. Philadelphia, Lippincott, 1975, Vol. 2, pp. 1400–1495.
27. Goiney, R. C., Connell, D. G., and Nichols, D. M.: CT evaluation of tarsometatarsal fracture-dislocation injuries. A.J.R., *144*:985, 1985.
28. Goossens, M., and DeStoop, N.: Lisfranc's fracture-dislocation: Etiology, radiology and results of treatment. A review of 20 cases. Clin. Orthop., *176*:154, 1983.
29. Gregg, J. R., and Das, M.: Foot and ankle problems in the preadolescent and adolescent. Clin. Sports Med., *1*:131, 1982.
30. Grob, D., Simpson, L. A., Weber, B. G., and Bray, T.: Operative treatment of displaced talus fractures. Clin. Orthop., *199*:88, 1985.
31. Guyer, B. H., Levinsohn, E. M., Fredrickson, B. E., Bailey, G. L., and Formikell, M.: Computed tomography of calcaneal fractures: Anatomy, pathology, dosimetry and clinical relevance. A.J.R., *145*:911, 1985.
32. Hainbock, R.: Calcaneus fractures in childhood. Hefte Unfallheilkd., *134*:169, 1979.
33. Hawkins, L. G.: Fractures of the lateral process of the talus. J. Bone Joint Surg., *47-A*:1170, 1965.
34. Heckman, J. D., and McLlean, M. R.: Fractures of the lateral process of the talus. Clin. Orthop., *199*:108, 1985.
35. Heger, L., Wulff, K., and Seddiqi, M. S.: Computed tomography of calcaneal fractures. A.J.R., *145*:131, 1985.
36. Hesp, W. L., van der Werken, C., and Goris, R. J.: Lisfranc dislocations: Fractures and/or dislocations through the tarso-metatarsal joints. Injury, *15*:261, 1984.
37. Jaffe, A. C., and Lasser, D. H.: Multiple metatarsal fractures in child abuse. Pediatrics, *60*:642, 1977.
38. Jonasch, E.: Calcaneus fractures in children. Hefte Unfallheilkd., *134*:170, 1979.
39. Jones, R.: Fracture of the base of the fifth metatarsal bone by indirect violence. Ann. Surg., *35*:697, 1902.
40. Joplin, R. J.: Injuries of the foot. *In* Cave, E. F., Burke, J. F., and Boyd, R. J. (eds.): Trauma Management. Chicago, Year Book, 1974, pp. 837–868.
41. Kenwright, J., and Taylor, R. G.: Major injuries of the talus. J. Bone Joint Surg., *52-B*:36, 1970.
42. Letts, R. M., and Gibeault, D.: Fractures of the neck of the talus in children. Foot Ankle, *1*:74, 1980.
43. Main, B. J., and Josett, R. L.: Injuries of the midtarsal joint. J. Bone Joint Surg., *57-B*:89, 1975.
44. Matter, R. E., and Frymoyer, J. W.: Fracture of the calcaneus in young children. Report of three cases. J. Bone Joint Surg., *55-A*:1091, 1973.
45. Mukherjee, S. K., and Young, A. B.: Dome fracture of the talus. A report of ten cases. J. Bone Joint Surg., *55-B*:319, 1973.
46. Ogden, J. A.: Skeletal Injury in the Child. Philadelphia, Lea & Febiger, 1982, pp. 621–641.
47. Omoto, H., Sakurda, K., Sugi, M., and Nakamura, K.: A new method of manual reduction for intra-articular fracture of the calcaneus. Clin. Orthop., *177*:104, 1983.
48. Pablot, S. M., Daneman, A., Stringer, D. A., and Carroll, N.: The value of computed tomography in the early assessment of comminuted fractures of the calcaneus: A review of three patients. J. Pediatr. Orthop., *5*:435, 1985.
49. Pathi, K.: Fracture of the neck of the talus in children. J. Indian Med. Assoc., *63*:157, 1974.
50. Pollen, A. G.: Ankle and foot. *In* Pollen, A. G. (ed.): Fractures and Dislocations in Children. Baltimore, Williams & Wilkins, 1973, pp. 198–215.
51. Renfrew, D. L., and el-Khoury, G. Y.: Anterior process fractures of the calcaneus. Skeletal Radiol., *14*:121, 1985.
52. Richli, W. R., and Rosenthal, D. I.: Avulsion fracture of the fifth metatarsal: Experimental study of pathomechanics. A.J.R., *143*:889, 1984.
53. Schantz, K., and Rasmussen, F.: Calcaneus fractures in the child. Acta Orthop. Scand., *58*:507, 1987.
54. Schellenberg, P., and Mebold, A.: Juvenile fracture of the calcaneus (author's transl.). Aktuel. Traumatol., *10*:251, 1980.

55. Schwarz, N., and Gebauer, M.: Fractures of the talus in children. Unfallheilkunde, *86*:212, 1983.
56. Spak, I.: Fractures of the talus in children. Acta Chir. Scand., *107*:553, 1966.
57. Stephens, N. A.: Fracture dislocation of the talus in childhood, a report of two cases. Br. J. Surg., *43*:600, 1956.
58. Stewart, I. M.: Jones fracture: Fracture of base of fifth metatarsal. Clin. Orthop., *16*:190, 1960.
59. Thomas, H. M.: Calcaneal fracture in childhood. Br. J. Surg., *56*:664, 1969.
60. Torg, J. S., Balduini, F. C., Zelko, R. R., Pavlov, H., Peff, T. C., and Das, M.: Fractures of the base of the fifth metatarsal distal to the tuberosity. Classification and guidelines for non-surgical and surgical management. J. Bone Joint Surg., *66-A*:209, 1984.
61. Trafton, P. G.: Epiphyseal fracture of the base of the first metatarsal: A case report. Orthopedics, *2*:256, 1979.
62. Wiley, J. J., and Profitt, A.: Fractures of the os calcis in children. Clin. Orthop., *188*:131, 1984.
63. Wilson, D. W.: Injuries of the tarso-metatarsal joints. J. Bone Joint Surg., *54-B*:677, 1972.

Injuries to the Spine and Pelvis

INJURIES TO THE SPINE

Fracture-dislocations of the vertebral column are very rare in children; they usually are sustained by adolescents. For a detailed discussion of these injuries, the reader is referred to general textbooks on fractures.

Rotatory Subluxation of Atlantoaxial Joint

This is a relatively common injury in a child, particularly if he has an upper respiratory infection; the associated hyperemia softens the ligaments that support the upper cervical spine and make the atlantoaxial joint unstable. The subluxation is produced by suddenly twisting the neck, rotating it beyond its normal range.

The child is presented with painful torticollis accompanied by marked spasm of the sternocleidomastoid muscle. He may support his head with his hands or prefer to be recumbent. On palpation of the posterior aspect of the neck, there is local tenderness over the atlantoaxial joint. A neurologic examination is performed to rule out intraspinal lesions, such as tumors of the spinal cord (see page 1887 in Chapter 5).

Radiograms will disclose persistent asymmetry at the atlantoaxial joint in the open mouth view. Partial anterior subluxation of the second or third cervical vertebra is a normal variant in the appearance of lateral radiograms of the flexed cervical spine. Dunlop, Morris, and Thompson surveyed 47 *normal* children and found that 5 had marked subluxation of the second or the third cervical vertebra, and that 3 had borderline dislocations.[34] The width of the intraspinal canal should always be measured to detect the presence of slowly growing neoplasms of the cord.

Treatment consists of continuous traction with a head halter. The subluxation will be reduced within a few days and muscle spasm will subside. The neck is then supported in a soft cervical collar (stockinette filled with white orthopedic felt) for two or three weeks.

Fracture of Odontoid Process with Anterior Dislocation of Atlas

This is an extremely rare injury caused by a direct blow on the side or top of the head. It is incurred when a child is thrown out of an automobile and lands on his head, dives into shallow water, or is injured during body contact sports. Spinal cord injury is common in this fracture-dislocation. Treatment consists of reduction by continuous traction through skull tongs followed by immobilization in a halo fixation apparatus.[40] The fracture usually heals in three months. If it fails to unite, the joint should be stabilized by a posterior arthrodesis.

Compression Fractures of Vertebrae in Thoracic and Lumbar Spine

These are rare in childhood because of the flexibility of the spinal column. The injury is sustained when a child falls from a height and lands on his feet (Fig. 8–185). Rupture of the posterior longitudinal ligament and injury to the spinal cord or cauda equina usually do not occur. Treatment consists of immobilization of the spine in a body cast for two months. The prognosis is excellent for full recovery. Occasionally in fracture-dislocations of the lumbar spine, some residual instability may persist and spinal fusion will be required.

FRACTURES OF THE PELVIS

The pelvic ring is formed by the combination of the two innominate bones, which are united anteriorly at the symphysis and the sacrum, which closes the ring posteriorly by its articulations with the innominate bones at the sacroiliac joints. The pelvis supports the spine and

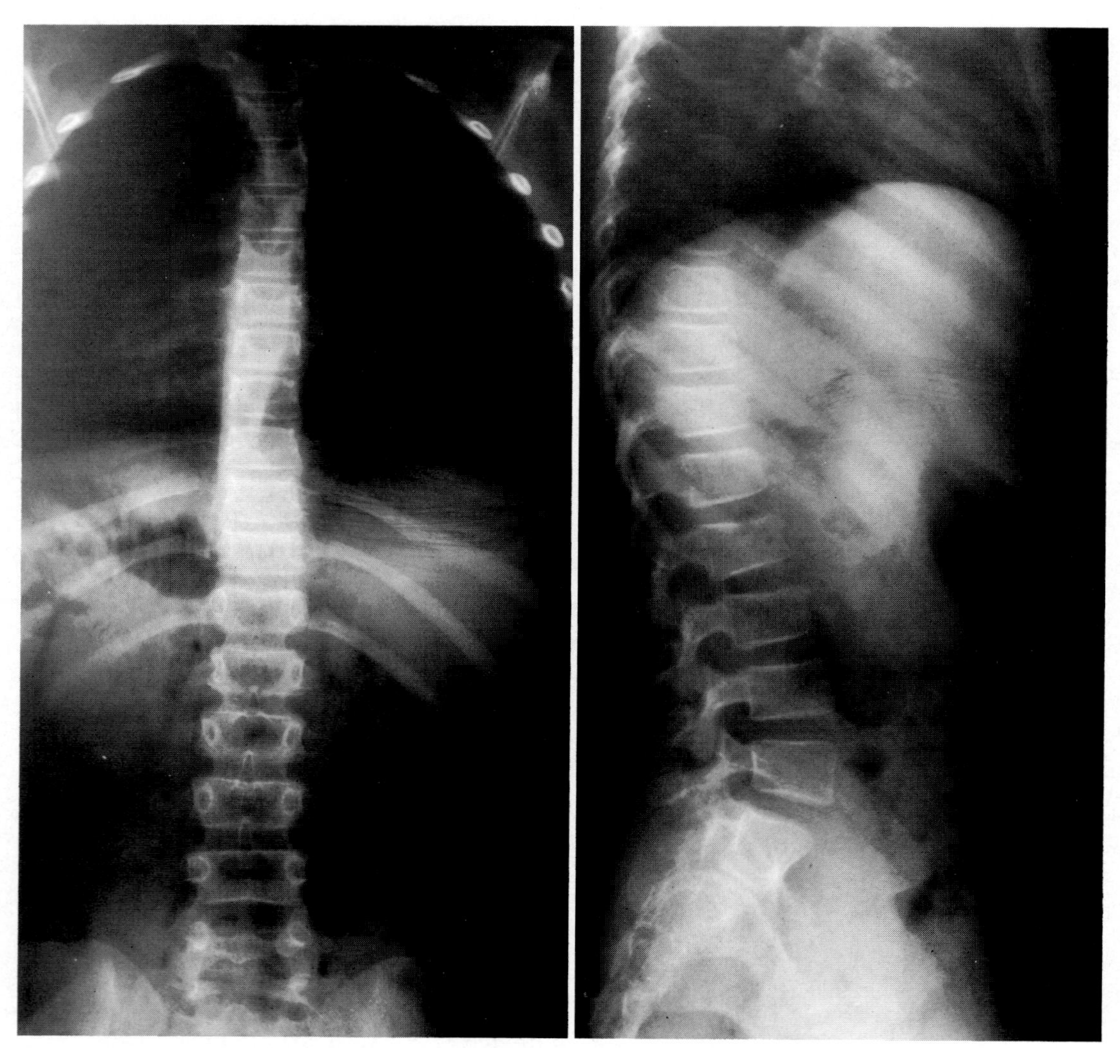

FIGURE 8–185. Compression fracture of first, second, and third lumbar vertebrae.

In children, collapse of cancellous bone will increase the height of intervertebral disc interspace.

transmits the body weight to the lower limbs; it also contains and protects the intrapelvic viscera.

In children, serious fractures of the pelvis usually do not occur, as its cartilaginous components—that at the symphysis pubis, the triradiate cartilage, and that of the sacroiliac joints—give a certain flexibility and elasticity to a child's pelvis.

Fractures of the pelvis may be divided into four groups: (1) unstable fractures with disruption of the pelvic ring; (2) intra-articular fractures of the acetabulum; (3) isolated fractures with continuity of the pelvic ring; (4) avulsion fractures resulting from muscular violence. The clinical picture and treatment vary according to the type of fracture. Fractures of the acetabulum are described in the section on central dislocation of the hip.

Unstable Fractures with Disruption of the Pelvic Ring

These are caused by direct crushing or compression violence, such as the wheels of an automobile running over the pelvis. Symptoms consist of severe local pain and inability to stand or walk. On examination, there is local swelling and tenderness. Frequently there is associated injury to the bladder or urethra. This possibility should be ruled out immediately by inserting a catheter into the bladder. If it cannot be introduced into the bladder, the urethra is crushed; if the catheter can be passed into the bladder and bloody urine is obtained, the bladder has been lacerated; if no fluid is obtained, most probably the bladder has been ruptured and the urine has extravasated into the peritoneal cavity. A definite diagnosis is established by a cystogram.

Severe shock due to massive intrapelvic hemorrhage is of common occurrence in fractures of the pelvis. The source of bleeding may be the cancellous bone or a torn major vessel. These require immediate attention by transfusion. Over 50 per cent of the circulating blood volume may be lost by a child with a major fracture of the pelvis. The ensuing resultant hematoma will cause paralytic ileus. Sciatic nerve palsy may develop, but it is usually incomplete and transient. The intrapelvic visceral complications and the severe hemorrhagic shock require more immediate care than the fracture itself.

Adequate radiograms are essential to delineate the nature and extent of the fractures; these should include an anteroposterior projection, a tangential projection with the x-ray tube directed 50 degrees cephalad, and a pelvic inlet view with the x-ray tube directed inferiorly 60 degrees.

Treatment depends upon the type of the fracture. Anteroposterior compression of the pelvis will produce combined fractures of the pubic and iliac segments of the pelvic ring; this may result in either fractures of both pubic rami with luxation of the sacroiliac joint, a dislocation of the symphysis pubis with fracture of the ilium near the sacroiliac joint (Fig. 8–186), or a dislocation of the symphysis pubis with luxation of the sacroiliac joint. These fracture-dislocations are reduced in lateral recumbency (the patient lying on his normal side) according to the technique of Watson-Jones. The reduction is maintained in a well-molded bilateral hip spica cast with the hips in internal rotation. The pelvic bones have abundant blood supply and unite within four weeks. Any malunion will be remodeled with growth.

Lateral compression of the pelvis will result in either a bilateral fracture of both pubic rami or a unilateral fracture of the pubic ramus with separation of the symphysis pubis. Inequality of limb length or malalignment of weight-bearing joints does not occur in these fractures. Treatment consists of simple bed rest in supine posture—the child should not be allowed to lie on his side. These fractures consolidate in three to four weeks.

Isolated Fractures with Stable Pelvic Ring

These include a unilateral fracture of one or both pubic rami and fractures of the ilium, sacrum, or coccyx. Displacement of fragments is minimal, usually resulting from direct violence. Treatment consists of bed rest until the patient is comfortable; he is then allowed to begin walking with a three-point crutch gait, protecting the injured side. Within three to four weeks, full weight-bearing is permitted. The prognosis for complete recovery is excellent.

Avulsion Fractures of the Pelvis

These result from sudden and severe contraction of muscles attached to the pelvis. The ischial apophysis is avulsed by the action of the hamstrings; forceful contraction of the sartorius detaches the anterior superior iliac spine, and the anterior inferior iliac spine is avulsed by the action of the rectus femoris muscle (Fig. 8–187). Treatment is by simple bed rest until the patient is comfortable; he is then allowed to

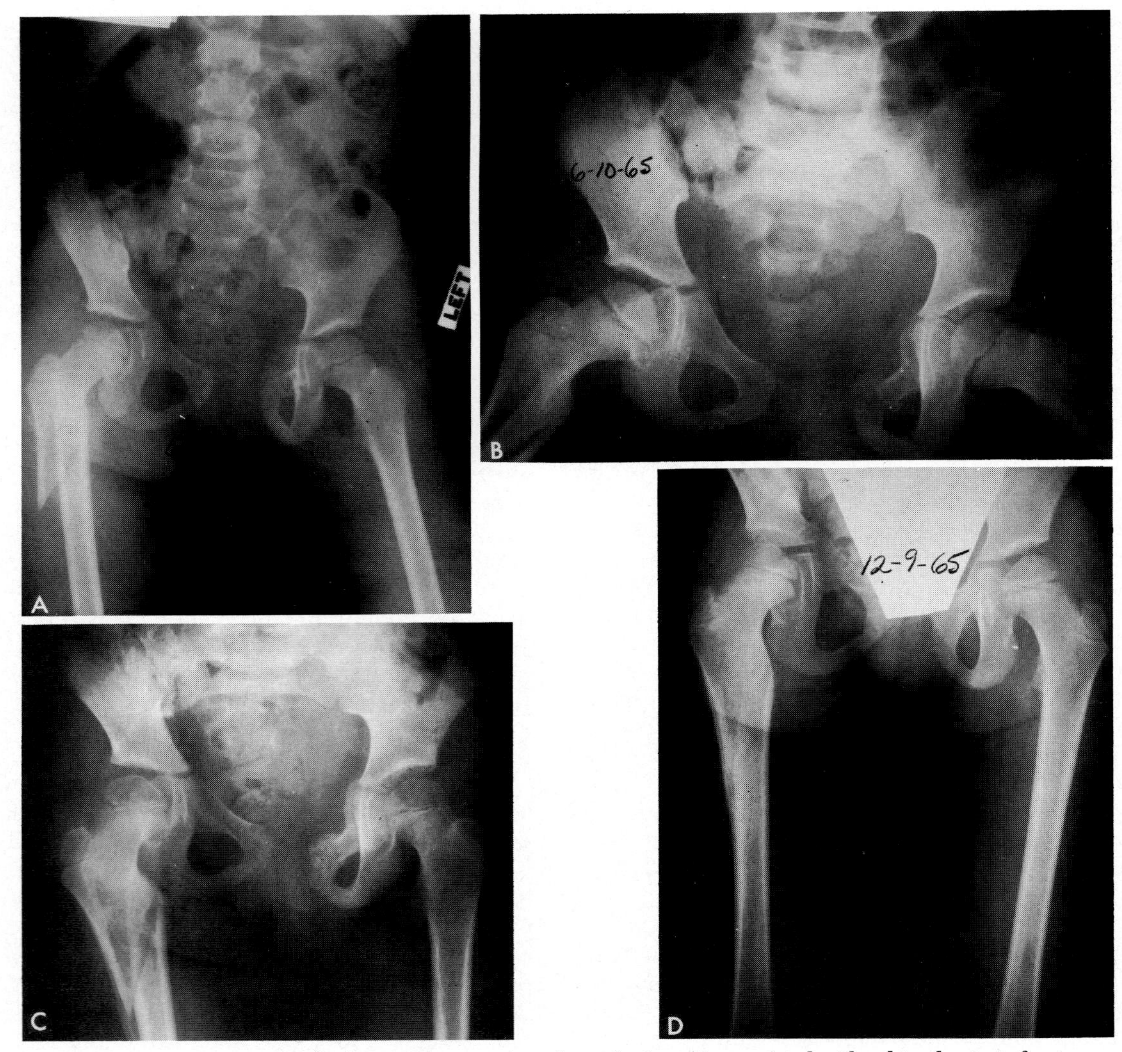

FIGURE 8–186. Fracture of right ilium with separation of symphysis pubis associated with subtrochanteric fracture treated by skeletal traction through the distal femur.

A and **B.** Initial radiograms. **C.** Six weeks later showing healing. **D.** Four months thereafter there is solid union of subtrochanteric fracture.

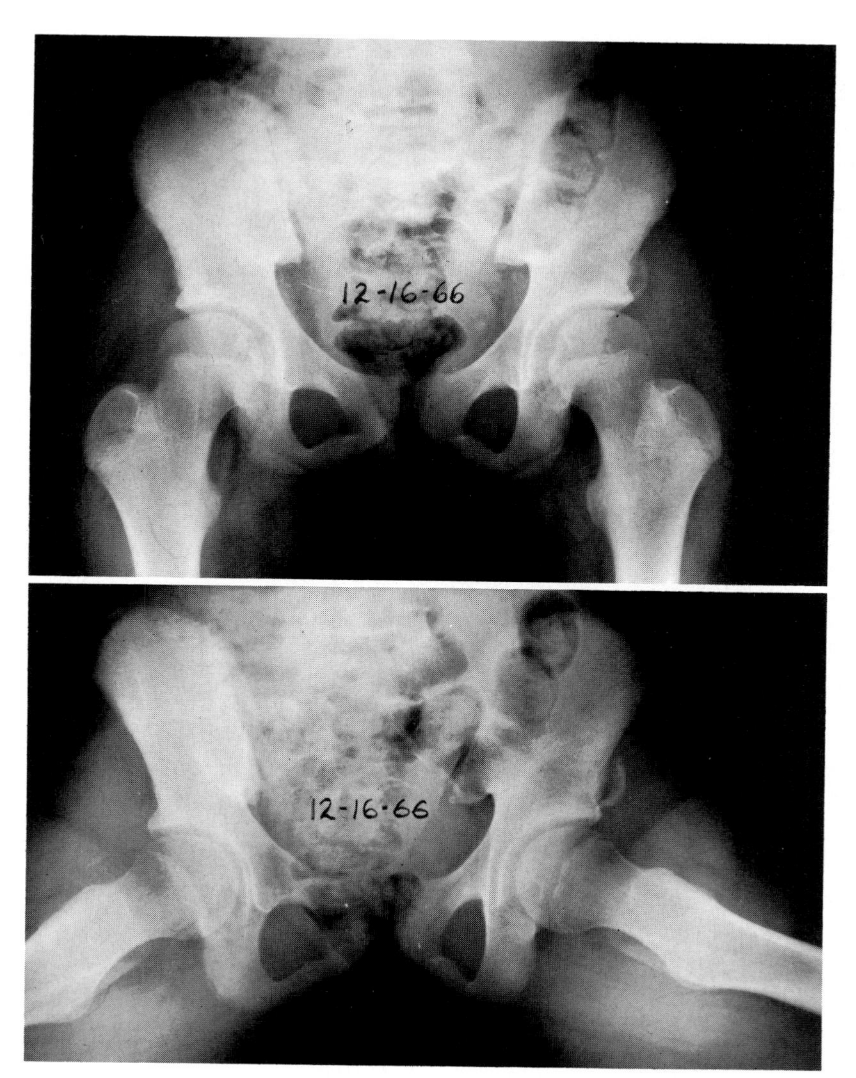

FIGURE 8–187. Avulsion of anterior inferior iliac spine.

ambulate. *Os acetabuli* should not be misdiagnosed as a fracture.

References

1. Ahmann, P. A., Smith, S. A., Schwartz, J. J., and Clark, D. D.: Spinal cord infarction due to minor trauma in children. Neurology, *25*:301, 1975.
2. Alexander, E., Jr.: Decompression and fixation in cervical spine fractures: Indications and techniques. Clin. Neurosurg., *27*:401, 1980.
3. Allen, B. L., Jr., Ferguson, R. L., Lehman, T. R., and O'Brien, R. P.: A mechanistic classification of closed, indirect fractures and dislocations of the lower cervical spine. Spine, *7*:1, 1982.
4. Allen, J. P., Myers, G. G., and Condon, V. R.: Laceration of the spinal cord related to breech delivery. J.A.M.A., *208*:1019, 1969.
5. Anderson, J. M., and Schutt, A. H.: Spinal injury in children: A review of 156 cases seen from 1950 through 1978. Mayo Clin. Proc., *55*:499, 1980.
6. Anderson, L. D., and D'Alonzo, R. T.: Fractures of the odontoid process of the axis. J. Bone Joint Surg., *56-A*:1663, 1974.
7. Aufdermaur, M.: Spinal injuries in juveniles. Necropsy findings in twelve cases. J. Bone Joint Surg., *56-B*:513, 1974.
8. Bailey, D. K.: The normal cervical spine in infants and children. Radiology, *59*:712, 1952.
9. Balau, J., and Hupfauer, W.: The differential diagnosis of injuries of the atlanto-axial joint in childhood (author's transl.). Arch. Orthop. Unfallchir., *78*:343, 1974.
10. Benner, B., Moiel, R., Dickson, J., and Harrington, P.: Instrumentation of the spine for fracture dislocations in children. Childs Brain, *3*:249, 1977.
11. Berkheiser, E. J., and Seidler, F.: Nontraumatic dislocations of the atlanto-axial joint. J.A.M.A., *96*:517, 1931.
12. Bhattacharyya, S. K.: Fracture and displacement of the odontoid process in a child. J. Bone Joint Surg., *56A*:1071, 1974.
13. Blockey, N. J., and Purser, D. W.: Fractures of the odontoid process of the axis. J. Bone Joint Surg., *38-B*:794, 1956.
14. Bondarenko, N. S., Kazitskii, V. M., Dovgan, B. L., and Beda, I. F.: Closed spinal fractures in children. Vestn. Khir., *130*:107, 1983.
15. Braakman, R., and Penning, L.: Injuries of the Cervical Spine. Amsterdam, Excerpta Medica, 1971, pp. 53–76.
16. Bresnan, M. J., and Abrams, I. F.: Neonatal spinal cord transection secondary to intrauterine hyperextension of the neck in breech position. J. Pediatr., *84*:734, 1974.
17. Broger, E.: Unusual fracture of the cervical spine in infancy. Chir. Organi Mov., *57*:70, 1968.
18. Bucholz, R. W., and Burkhead, W. Z.: The pathological anatomy of fatal atlanto-occipital dislocations. J. Bone Joint Surg., *61-A*:248, 1979.
19. Burke, D. C.: Spinal cord trauma in children. Paraplegia, *9*:1, 1971.
20. Burke, D. C., and Murray, D. D.: The management of thoracic and thoracolumbar injuries of the spine with neurological involvement. J. Bone Joint Surg., *58-B*:72, 1976.
21. Caffey, J.: The whiplash shaken infant syndrome. Pediatrics, *54*:396, 1974.
22. Campbell, J., and Bonnett, C.: Spinal cord injury in children. Clin. Orthop., *112*:114, 1975.
23. Carlioz, H., and Dubousset, J.: Les instabilites entre l'atlas et l'axis chez l'enfant. Rev. Chir. Orthop., *59*:291, 1973.
24. Cattell, H. S., and Filtzer, D. L.: Pseudosubluxation and other normal variations in the cervical spine in children. J. Bone Joint Surg., *47-A*:1295, 1965.
25. Chaplinski, V. V., Iatskevich, A. E., and Chaploutsi, V. D.: Characteristics of spinal fractures in children. Ortop. Travmatol. Protez., *7*:67, 1976.
26. Chaplinski, V. V., Iunko, M. A., and Boichuk, P. F.: Therapeutic results of cervical fractures in children. Ortop. Travmatol. Protez, *9*:75, 1977.
27. Crothers, B., and Putnam, M. C.: Obstetrical injuries of the spinal cord. Medicine, *6*:41, 1927.
28. Dalinka, M. K.: CT in pelvic trauma. Orthop. Clin. North Am., *16*:471, 1985.
29. Dawson, E. G., and Smith, L.: Atlanto-axial subluxation in children due to vertebral anomalies. J. Bone Joint Surg., *61-A*:582, 1979.
30. Denis, F.: The three column spine and its significance in the classification of acute thoraco-lumbar spinal injuries. Spine, *8*:817, 1983.
31. Denis, F.: Spinal instability as defined by the three-column spine concept in acute spinal trauma. Clin. Orthop., *189*:65, 1984.
32. Desgrippes, Y., and Bensahel, H.: Fractures of the spine in children without permanent neurological injuries. J. Chir., *112*:329, 1976.
33. Donaldson, J. S.: Acquired torticollis in children and young adults. J.A.M.A., *160*:458, 1956.
34. Dunlap, J. P., Morris, M., and Thompson, R. G.: Cervical spine injuries in children. J. Bone Joint Surg., *40-A*:681, 1958.
35. Emminger, E.: Die Wirbelgelenksluxation. Monatsschr. Unfallheilkd., *71*:81, 1968.
36. Erlacher, G., and Povacz, F.: Vertebral fractures in children. Hefte Unfallheilkd., *108*:124, 1971.
37. Esposito, P. W., *et al.*: Delayed overdistraction of a surgically treated unstable thoracolumbar fracture. A case report. Spine, *10*:393, 1985.
38. Evans, D. K.: Anterior cervical subluxation. J. Bone Joint Surg., *58-B*:318, 1976.
39. Evarts, C. M.: Fracture of the odontoid process in a seventeen-month old infant treated with a halo. J. Bone Joint Surg., *53-A*:1636, 1971.
40. Ewald, F. C.: Fracture of the odontoid process in a 17-month old infant treated with a halo. J. Bone Joint Surg., *53-A*:1636, 1971.
41. Festge, O. A., and Tischer, W.: Injuries of shoulder girdle and neck in infancy and childhood. Kinderarztl. Prax., *46*:465, 1978.
42. Fielding, J. W.: Disappearance of the central portion of the odontoid process, a case report. J. Bone Joint Surg., *47-A*:1228, 1965.
43. Fielding, J. W.: Cervical spine injuries in children. *In* The Cervical Spine. Philadelphia, Lippincott, 1983, pp. 268–281.
44. Fielding, J. W., and Hawkins, R. J.: Atlanto-axial rotatory fixation (fixed rotatory subluxation of the atlanto-axial joint). J. Bone Joint Surg., *59-A*:37, 1977.
45. Fielding, J. W., Hawkins, R. J., and Ratzan, S. A.: Spine fusion for atlanto-axial instability. J. Bone Joint Surg., *58-A*:400, 1976.
46. Fielding, J. W., Hensinger, R. N., and Hawkins, R. J.: Os odontoideum. J. Bone Joint Surg., *62-A*:376, 1980.
47. Fielding, J. W., Cochran, G. V. B., Lawsing, J. F., III, and Hohl, M.: Tears of the transverse ligament of the atlas: A clinical and biomechanical study. J. Bone Joint Surg., *56-A*:1683, 1974.
48. Finerman, G. A. M., Sakai, D., and Weingarten, S.: Atlanto-axial dislocation with spinal cord compression in a Mongoloid child: A case report. J. Bone Joint Surg., *58-A*:408, 1976.
49. Freiburger, R. H., Wilson, P. D., and Nicholas, J. A.: Acquired absence of the odontoid process. J. Bone Joint Surg., *47-A*:1231, 1965.

50. Gabrielson, T. O., and Maxwell, J. A.: Traumatic atlanto-occipital dislocation. A.J.R., *97*:624, 1966.
51. Gaufin, L. M., and Goodman, S. J.: Cervical spine injuries in infants; problems in management. J. Neurosurg., *42*:179, 1975.
52. Geehr, R. B., Rothman, S. L. G., and Kier, E. L.: The role of computer tomography in the evaluation of upper cervical spine pathology. Comput. Tomogr., *2*:79, 1978.
53. Giammattei, F. P.: Diagnosis of vertebral fractures (letter). J. Bone Joint Surg., *65-A*:135, 1983.
54. Gill, K.: The role of computerized tomographic scanning in the evaluation of major pelvic fractures. J. Bone Joint Surg., *66-A*:34, 1984.
55. Graner, G., and Ansorg, P.: Spinal column injuries in childhood (author's transl.). Zentralbl. Chir., *106*:588, 1981.
56. Griffiths, H. J.: Computed tomography in the management of acetabular fractures. Skeletal Radiol., *11*:22, 1984.
57. Griffiths, S. C.: Fracture of the odontoid process in children. J. Pediatr. Surg., *7*:680, 1972.
58. Grogono, B. J. S.: Injuries of the atlas and axis. J. Bone Joint Surg., *36-B*:397, 1954.
59. Hamacher, P., and Pingel, P.: Injuries of growing symphyses. Z. Allgemeinmed., *47*:176, 1971.
60. Hamilton, A. R.: Injuries of the atlanto-axial joint. J. Bone Joint Surg., *33-B*:434, 1951.
61. Hasue, M., Hoshino, R., Omata, S., Kuramochi, E., Furukawa, K., and Nakamura, T.: Cervical spine injuries in children. Fukushima J. Med. Sci., *20*:115, 1974.
62. Hawkins, R. J., Fielding, J. W., and Thompson, W. J.: Os odontoideum: Congenital or acquired. J. Bone Joint Surg., *58-A*:413, 1976.
63. Hegenbarth, R., and Ebel, K. D.: Roentgen findings in fractures of the vertebral column in childhood examination of 35 patients and its results. Pediatr. Radiol., *5*:34, 1976.
64. Hellstrom, B., and Sallmander, V.: Prevention of spinal cord injury in hyperextension of the fetal head. J.A.M.A., *204*:1041, 1968.
65. Henrys, P., Lyne, E. D., Lifton, C., and Salciccioli, G.: Clinical review of cervical spine injuries in children. Clin. Orthop., *129*:172, 1977.
66. Herkowitz, H. N., and Samberg, L. C.: Vertebral column injuries associated with tobogganing. J. Trauma, *18*:806, 1978.
67. Hess, J. H., Bronstein, I. P., and Abelson, S. M.: Atlanto-axial dislocation unassociated with trauma and secondary to inflammatory foci of the neck. Am. J. Dis. Child., *49*:1137, 1935.
68. Holdsworth, F.: Fractures, dislocations and fracture-dislocations of the spine. J. Bone Joint Surg., *52-A*:1534, 1970.
69. Holtgrave, E., Rosli, A., and Spiessl, B.: The treatment of column fractures in children, clinical and radiographic results. Dtsch. Zahnarztl. Z., *30*:213, 1975.
70. Horal, J., Nachemson, A., and Scheller, S.: Clinical and radiological long-term follow-up of vertebral fractures in children. Acta Orthop. Scand., *43*:491, 1972.
71. Hubbard, D. D.: Injuries of the spine in children and adolescents. Clin. Orthop., *100*:56, 1974.
72. Hubbard, D. D.: Fractures of the dorsal and lumbar spine. Orthop. Clin. North Am., *7*:605, 1976.
73. Huelke, D. F., Mendelsohn, R. A., States, J. D., and Melvin, J. W.: Cervical fractures and fracture-dislocations sustained without head impact. J. Trauma, *18*:533, 1978.
74. Husby, J., and Sorensen, K. H.: Fracture of the odontoid process of the axis. Acta Orthop. Scand., *45*:182, 1974.
75. Jacobs, B.: Cervical fractures and dislocations (C3-7). Clin. Orthop., *109*:18, 1975.
76. Jacobson, G., and Bleeker, H. H.: Pseudosubluxation of the axis in children. A.J.R., *82*:472, 1959.
77. Jones, E. L.: Birth trauma and the cervical spine. Arch. Dis. Child., *45*:147, 1970.
78. Kilfovle, R. M., Foley, J. J., and Norton, P. L.: Spine and pelvic deformity in childhood and adolescent paraplegia. A study of 104 cases. J. Bone Joint Surg., *47-A*:659, 1965.
79. King, H. A., and Bradford, D. S.: Fracture-dislocation of the spine after spine fusion and Harrington instrumentation for idiopathic scoliosis. A case report. J. Bone Joint Surg., *62*:1374, 1980.
80. Kopits, S. E., and Steingass, M. H.: Experience with the "halo-cast" in small children. Surg. Clin. North Am., *50*:935, 1970.
81. La Follette, B. F., Levine, M. I., and McNiech, L. M.: Bilateral fracture-dislocation of the sacrum. A case report. J. Bone Joint Surg., *68-A*:1099, 1986.
82. Lipkowitz, G.: Hemipelvectomy, a lifesaving operation in severe open pelvic injury in childhood. J. Trauma, *25*:823, 1985.
83. Lippitt, A. B.: Fracture of a vertebral body end plate and disk protrusion causing subarachnoid block in an adolescent. Clin. Orthop., *116*:112, 1976.
84. Lipscomb, P. R.: Cervico-occipital fusion for congenital and post-traumatic anomalies of the atlas and axis. J. Bone Joint Surg., *39-A*:1289, 1957.
85. Lipson, S. J., and Mazur, J.: Anteroposterior spondyloschisis of the atlas revealed by computerized tomography scanning. J. Bone Joint Surg., *60-A*:1104, 1978.
86. Lob, A.: Die Ausheilungsvorgänge am Wirbelbruch. Dtsch. Z. Chir., *248*:452, 1937.
87. Lob, A.: Die Wirbelsaulenverletzung und ihre Ausheilung. Stuttgart, Thieme, 1950.
88. Locke, G. R., Gardner, J. I., and VanEpps, E. F.: Atlas-dens interval (ADI) in children. A study based on 200 normal cervical spines. A.J.R., *97*:135, 1966.
89. London, P. S.: Unsuspected injury of the caecum accompanying fracture of the pelvis. Injury, *16*:324, 1985.
90. McCoy, S. H., and Johnson, K. A.: Sagittal fracture of the cervical spine. J. Trauma, *16*:310, 1976.
91. McPhee, I. B.: Spinal fractures and dislocations in children and adolescents. Spine, *6*:533, 1981.
92. McWhorter, J. M., Alexander, E., Davis, C. H., and Kelly, L.: Posterior cervical fusion in children. J. Neurosurg., *45*:211, 1976.
93. Malek, R. S., O'Dea, M. J., and Kelalis, P. P.: Management of ruptured posterior urethra in childhood. J. Urol., *117*:105, 1977.
94. Marar, B. C., and Balachandran, N.: Non-traumatic atlanto-axial dislocation in children. Clin. Orthop., *92*:220, 1973.
95. Martel, W., Uyham, R., and Stimson, C. W.: Subluxation of the atlas causing spinal cord compression in a case of Down's syndrome with a manifestation of an occipital vertebra. Radiology, *93*:839, 1969.
96. Mazo, I. S., and Beilin, L. G.: X-ray diagnosis of compression fractures of the vertebrae in children. Vestn. Rentgenol. Radiol., *47*:91, 1972.
97. Miller, W. E.: Fractures of the hip in children from birth to adolescence. Clin. Orthop., *92*:155, 1973.
98. deMourgues, G., Fischer, L., Comtet, J. J., Schnepp, J., and Caltran, M.: Fractures de l'apophyse odontoide de l'axis; á propos d'une serie de 80 fractures. Acta Orthop. Belg., *38*:137, 1972.
99. Naik, D. R.: Cervical spinal canal in normal infants. Clin. Radiol., *21*:323, 1970.
100. Nicoll, A. E.: Fractures and dislocations of the spine. *In* Apley, A. G. (ed.): Modern Trends in Orthopaedics. London, Butterworth, 1962.
101. Norton, W. L.: Fractures and dislocations of the cervical spine. J. Bone Joint Surg., *44-A*:115, 1962.
102. Palomo, J. A.: Fracture luxation of the cervical spine.

Different treatments. Acta Neurol. Latinoam., *22*:168, 1976.
103. Pennecot, G. F., Chadoutaud, F., and Pouliquen, J. C.: Severe spinal trauma in children (author's transl.). Ann. Pediatr. (Paris), *29*:311, 1982.
104. Pouliquen, J. C., and Pennecot, G. F.: Fractures of the spine in children. Rev. Chir. Orthop., *63*:440, 1977.
105. Pouliquen, J. C., Beneux, J., and Pennecot, G. F.: The incidence of progressive scoliosis and kyphosis after fractures and dislocations of the spine in children. Rev. Chir. Orthop., *64*:487, 1978.
106. Rabenseifner, L.: Prognosis and treatment of spinal fractures in children (author's transl.). Unfallheilkunde, *84*:309, 1981.
107. Reff, R. B., *et al.*: The use of external fixation devices in the management of severe lower-extremity trauma and pelvic injuries in children. Clin. Orthop., *188*:21, 1984.
108. Resjo, M., Harwood-Nash, D. C., and Fitz, C. R.: Normal cord in infants and children examined with computed tomographic metrizamide myelography. Radiology, *130*:691, 1979.
109. Ricciardi, J. E., Kaufer, H., and Louis, D. S.: Acquired os odontoideum following acute ligament injury. J. Bone Joint Surg., *58-A*:410, 1976.
110. Rolander, S. D., and Blair, W. E.: Deformation and fracture of the lumbar vertebral end plate. Orthop. Clin. North Am., *6*:75, 1975.
111. Ruckstuhl, J., Morscher, E., and Jani, L.: Treatment and prognosis in vertebral fractures in children and adolescents. Chirurg, *47*:458, 1976.
112. Sammarco, G. J.: Diagnosis and treatment in dancers. Clin. Orthop., *187*:176, 1984.
113. Scripcaru, G., Ianovici, N., and Anghel, M.: Fetal cervical spine injuries. Rev. Med. Chir. Soc. Med. Nat. Iasi, *81*:47, 1977.
114. Seimon, L. P.: Fracture of the odontoid process in young children. J. Bone Joint Surg., *59*:943, 1977.
115. Semine, A. A., Ertel, A. N., Goldberg, M. J., and Bull, M. J.: Cervical-spine instability in children with Down's syndrome (trisomy 21). J. Bone Joint Surg., *60-A*:649, 1978.
116. Shacked, I., Rappaport, Z. H., Barzilay, Z., and Ohri, A.: Two-level fracture of the cervical spine in a young child. A case report with operative treatment. J. Bone Joint Surg., *65A*:119, 1983.
117. Sherk, H. H., and Nicholson, J. T.: Fractures of the atlas. J. Bone Joint Surg., *52-A*:1017, 1970.
118. Sherk, H. H., Nicholson, J. T., and Chung, S. M.: Fractures of the odontoid process in young children. J. Bone Joint Surg., *60*:921, 1978.
119. Sherk, H. H., Schut, L., and Lane, J. M.: Fractures and dislocations of the cervical spine in children. Orthop. Clin. North Am., *7*:593, 1976.
120. Shulman, S. T., Madden, J. D, Esterly, J. R., and Shanklin, D. R.: Transection of spinal cord. A rare obstetrical complication of cephalic delivery. Arch. Dis. Child., *46*:291, 1971.
121. Stauffer, E. S., and Kelly, E. G.: Fracture-dislocation of the cervical spine. Instability and recurrent deformity following treatment by anterior interbody fusion. J. Bone Joint Surg., *59*:45, 1977.
122. Stauffer, E. S., and Mazur, J. M.: Cervical spine injuries in children. Pediatr. Ann., *11*:502, 1982.
123. Steel, H. H.: Anatomical and mechanical considerations of the atlantoaxial articulations. J. Bone Joint Surg., *50-A*:1481, 1968.
124. Stern, W. E., and Rand, R. W.: Birth injuries to the spinal cord: Report of 2 cases and review of the literature. Am. J. Obstet. Gynecol., *78*:498, 1959.
125. Stillwell, W. T., and Fielding, J. W.: Acquired os odontoideum. Clin. Orthop., *135*:71, 1978.
126. Sullivan, C. R., Bruwer, A. J., and Harris, L. E.: Hypermobility of the cervical spine in children: A pitfall in the diagnosis of cervical dislocation. Am. J. Surg., *95*:636, 1958.
127. Swischuk, L. E.: Spine and spinal cord trauma in the battered child syndrome. Radiology, *92*:733, 1969.
128. Swischuk, L. E.: Anterior displacement of C2 in children: Physiologic or pathologic. Radiology, *122*:759, 1977.
129. Taylor, A. S.: Fracture-dislocation of the cervical spine. Ann. Surg., *90*:321, 1929.
130. Teng, P., and Papatheodorou, C.: Traumatic subluxation of C2 in young children. Bull. Los Angeles Neurol. Soc., *32*:197, 1967.
131. Ter-Egiazarov, G. M., Sanakoeva, I. I., and Belenkii, V. E.: Clinical and biomechanical analysis of the efficacy of using a corset in the treatment of children with compression fractures of the spine. Ortop. Travmatol. Protez., *4*:28, 1982.
132. Torg, J. S., *et al.*: Trampoline-related quadriplegia: Review of the literature and reflections on the American Academy of Pediatrics' position statement. Pediatrics, *74*:804, 1984.
133. Torode, I.: Pelvic fractures in children. J. Pediatr. Orthop., *5*:76, 1985.
134. Webb, J. K., Broughton, R. B. K., McSweeney, T., and Park, W. M.: Hidden flexion injury of the cervical spine. J. Bone Joint Surg., *58-B*:322, 1976.
135. Weber, B. G.: Wirbelsaulenverletzunger und ihre Spätfolgen. *In* Rheumatismus in Forschung und Praxis, Bd. II: Die Funktionsstörunger der Wirbelsaule, 102. Bern-Stuttgart, Huber, 1963.
136. Weber, B. G.: Operative Frühbehandlung bei traumatischer Paraplegie. *In* Rehabilitation der Para- und Tetraplegiker, Fortbildungskurs Schweiz. Bern, Rehabilitationskomission, 1966.
137. Weiss, M. H.: Hangman's fracture in an infant. Am. J. Dis. Child., *126*:268, 1973.
138. Yates, P. O.: Birth trauma to vertebral arteries. Arch. Dis. Child., *34*:436, 1959.

Miscellaneous Fractures

OBSTETRICAL OR BIRTH INJURIES

Trauma to long bones in the newly born is sustained during a difficult delivery, particularly when the baby is especially large and the presentation is breech. Fetal anoxia and urgency of delivery often necessitate forceful extraction. These injuries are of special concern to the obstetrician, pediatrician, radiologist, and orthopedic surgeon. The skeletal injuries in order of decreasing frequency are fractures of the clavicle, fractures of the humeral shaft, fractures of the femoral shaft, traumatic fracture-separation of the upper humeral and lower humeral epiphysis, and displacement of the upper and lower femoral epiphyses. Fractures distal to the elbow and knee are very rare. In fact, fracture of the tibia in a newborn is almost always pathologic, and congenital pseudarthrosis of the tibia should be ruled out. When multiple fractures are present, they are most probably pathologic, osteogenesis imperfecta being the most common cause. Multiple birth fractures also occur in arthrogryposis multiplex congenita, particularly when the knees and elbows are rigidly fixed in extension. Traumatic dislocation of a previously normal joint rarely, if ever, occurs. Epiphyseal separations at birth were frequently misdiagnosed in the past as acute traumatic dislocation.

Birth Fractures of Shafts of Long Bones

Fracture of the diaphysis of the humerus usually occurs in its middle third; it is either transverse or oblique and angulated laterally by the pull of the deltoid muscle. Often it is associated with radial nerve palsy, which resolves completely within six to eight weeks. Diagnosis is readily made by the obstetrician, who feels and often hears the bone break. The infant's arm dangles by his side without active motion. Radiograms disclose the fracture. Treatment consists of immobilizing the arm, with the elbow acutely flexed across the chest, with an Ace bandage. Soft pads are placed in the axilla to maintain the arm in abduction. The fracture will heal within two weeks, and angular deformities will be spontaneously corrected with growth.

Birth fractures of the shafts of the clavicle and femur are discussed in the treatment of fractures of the individual bones.

Birth Fractures Involving Physes of Long Bones

Epiphyseal fracture-displacement or traumatic separation of the *upper femoral epiphysis* is a rare injury and is often confused with congenital dislocation of the hip.[17, 18, 33, 46, 47, 57, 70, 79, 82] The term *pseudodislocation* of the hip has been used to describe it.[46, 47] Presentation in the birth canal is frequently abnormal, the baby being delivered by version and extraction. The mechanism of injury is one of hyperextension, abduction, and rotation by forceful traction in the leg as it is brought forward.

The line of separation is distal to the combined upper growth cartilage, extending in a crescentic line from the greater to the lesser trochanter. The "snap" is usually not felt by the obstetrician as the epiphysis slides off the metaphysis. On closer examination, however, there is obvious shortening of the involved lower limb, which is held in flexion, abduction, and external rotation at the hip. Acute injury is suggested by pseudoparalysis—the infant holds the leg still, avoiding active movements.

Since, at birth, the femoral head, neck, and greater trochanter are entirely cartilaginous, radiographic diagnosis may be difficult. The upper end of the femoral diaphysis is displaced upward and laterally. Because the femoral head is in its normal position, the acetabula are symmetrically developed. As was stated earlier, this injury is often misdiagnosed as congenital dislocation of the hip; however, in traumatic separation of the upper femoral epiphysis, the hip appears reduced when held in abduction, medial rotation, and extension, but is grossly displaced when maintained in flexion, abduction, and external rotation (the so-called "frog-leg" position). Arthrography of the hip will establish the diagnosis. Commonly, the injury is not detected until fracture callus appears on the radiogram (cf. Fig. 8–106).

If the diagnosis is made at birth, treatment consists of immobilization of the hip in abduction, partial flexion, and medial rotation in a spica cast for two to three weeks. However, diagnosis is frequently delayed until the healing phase, when the coxa vara has become fixed and irreducible. Though there is a high potential for remodeling and spontaneous correction in infants, it should be pointed out that there are several case reports of coxa vara persisting until four years of age.[57, 82] Avascular necrosis is not a complication, as the entire cartilaginous proximal femur (head, neck, and greater trochanter) is displaced, and the blood supply is not disturbed. The ossification center of the femoral head appears first and is larger than on the normal side. Michael and associates reported a case in which the ossification center of the femoral head appeared at the exceptionally early age of 15 days.[79]

Traumatic Separation of Distal Femoral Epiphysis

This presents no problem in radiographic diagnosis, since the ossification center of the distal femoral epiphysis is present at birth.[14] However, the injury is not suspected until the knee becomes enlarged by ossification of the massive subperiosteal hematoma. The lower femoral epiphysis is almost always displaced posteriorly, with extensive stripping of the periosteum from the back of the lower femoral shaft. The fracture is a Type I physeal injury (Salter-Harris) with an excellent prognosis for subsequent growth. Care must be taken to avoid injury to the popliteal vessels by manipulative reduction of the posteriorly displaced epiphysis. If the degree of separation of the epiphysis is minimal or moderate, a single hip spica is applied for two weeks with the knee in partial flexion. Any residual angular deformity will spontaneously correct itself with growth. Markedly displaced lower femoral epiphyses are treated by split Russell traction with a proximal sling behind the knee for two weeks. Bryant's traction should not be employed because of the possible danger of compressing the popliteal vessels and causing ischemia of the foot.

Traumatic Displacement of Distal Humeral Epiphysis

Displacement of the distal humeral epiphysis at birth is a very rare injury. Siffert reported three cases and described its characteristic diagnostic features.[113] The infants are the product of a difficult delivery, either total breech or vertex presentation with shoulder dystocia. The involved elbow is swollen, and on flexion-extension, definite crepitus can be palpated. The medial and lateral epicondyles and the tip of the olecranon are in a normal relationship to one another as the elbow is manipulated—a finding that distinguishes displacement of the distal humeral epiphysis from dislocation of the elbow. Radiographic diagnosis is difficult because the distal humeral epiphysis is entirely cartilaginous. In the lateral projection, the upper parts of the radius and ulna are posteriorly displaced in relation to the long axis of the humerus; in the anteroposterior projection, the distance between the ossified lower end of the humeral diaphysis and the upper end of both bones of the forearm is foreshortened, as compared with the normal side. When the diagnosis is made at birth, treatment consists of gentle traction and forward manipulation of the olecranon. The elbow is immobilized in a posterior plaster splint for two to three weeks. Often the diagnosis is delayed until the appearance of callus of the healing fracture on the radiogram; in such an instance, immobilization of the elbow is not indicated (Fig. 8–188). Siffert points out that the condition is not altogether innocuous; in one child, there was residual limitation of flexion and cubitus varus at the end of two years, and in a second child, a follow-up examination after nine months disclosed persistent slight limitation of flexion and angulation of the distal end of the humerus.[113]

Birth fracture involving the *proximal humeral physis* may occur alone or in association with brachial plexus paralysis.[80, 103, 120] The shoulder will be markedly swollen. Often the condition is mistaken for suppurative arthritis of the shoulder with secondary dislocation. Diagnosis is again initially difficult because of the cartilaginous state of the humeral head. If doubt exists, aspiration of the joint and arthrography may be indicated. The diagnosis is established with the appearance of callus of the healing fracture (Fig. 8–189). Treatment consists of simply bandaging the arm across the chest. The prognosis is excellent.

Other Obstetrical Injuries

Nerve palsies are not rare at birth; obstetrical brachial plexus palsy and sciatic nerve palsy have been discussed in the chapter on the neuromuscular system. Trauma to the spinal cord may occur at birth with breech delivery.[15, 24, 36] If the level of transection is above the fifth cervical segment, it results in sudden death due to respiratory paralysis; if it is distal to the fifth cervical segment, diaphragmatic function is preserved and respiration can be maintained by the infant with adequate assistance. Initially there is complete flaccid paralysis of the trunk and both upper and lower limbs. Anesthesia in all modalities is present distal to the level of injury. Sphincter control is lost. Within a few days, or a few weeks, with gradual recovery from spinal shock, muscle tone and reflex activity return, the degree of functional return being dependent on the extent of cord damage. Meticulous nursing care will keep these infants alive. Later orthopedic management will follow the principles outlined in the discussion of cerebral palsy.

Depressed fracture of the skull at birth is extremely rare because of the pliability of the skull with wide open sutures. The parietal bones are usually involved, injury arising either from forceps pressure or from compression by the walls of a contracted pelvis. Spontaneous recovery is the rule.

Intrauterine fractures of normal bones are of extremely rare occurrence.[14, 60] They may result from indirect violence to the fetus during pregnancy when the mother sustains a direct blow to her abdomen, as in an automobile accident. The diagnosis of intrauterine fracture is established when radiograms obtained immediately

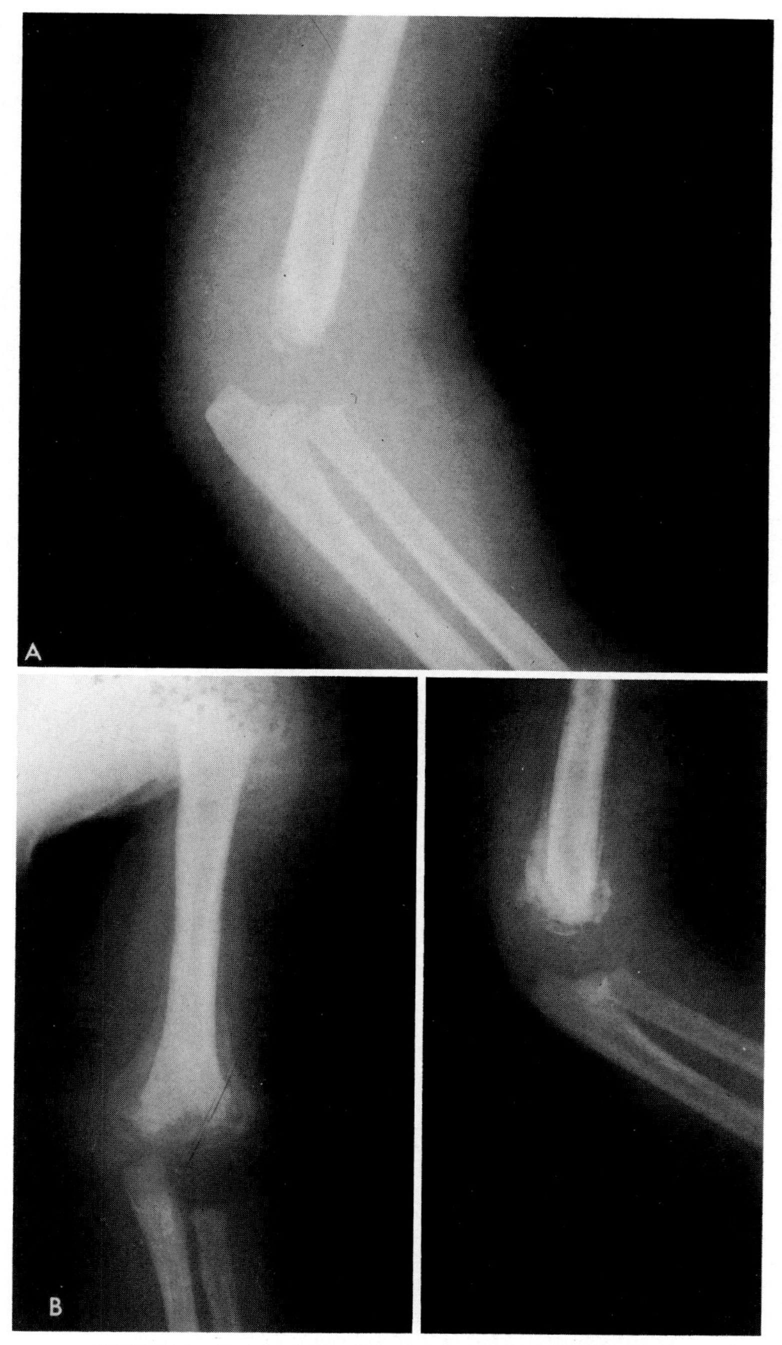

FIGURE 8–188. Metaphyseal birth fracture of distal humerus.

A. Initial radiogram; note the distal metaphyseal fragment. **B.** Three weeks after, extensive subperiosteal new bone formation extends beyond the ossified lower end of the diaphysis.

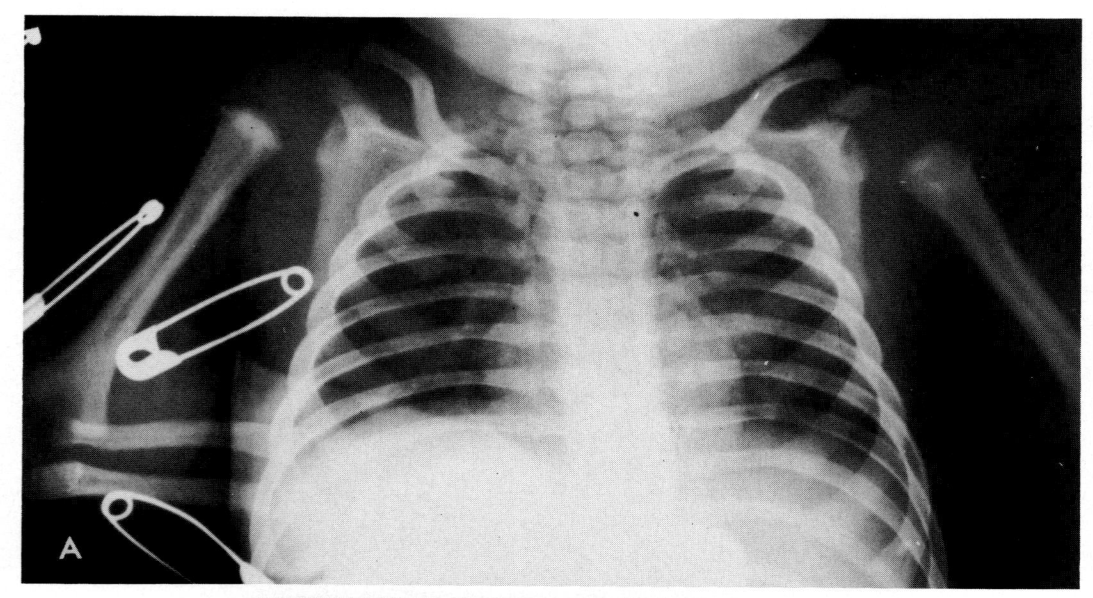

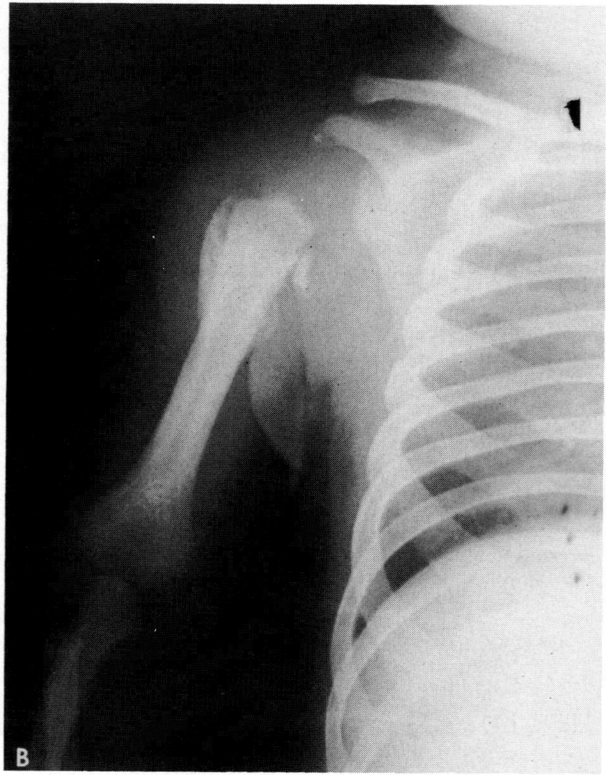

FIGURE 8–189. Metaphyseal fracture of proximal left humerus.

A. Initial radiograms. **B.** Three weeks later.

after birth show evidence of fracture callus in normal bone. (A delay of one week would not rule out a birth fracture.) Pathologic intrauterine fractures are common, particularly in osteogenesis imperfecta.

References

1. Amiel-Tison, C.: A method for neurological evaluation within the first year of life: Experience with full-term newborn infants with birth injury. Ciba Found. Symp., *59*:107, 1978.
2. Amir, J., Katz, K., Grunebaum, M., Yosipovich, Z., Wielunsky, E., and Reisner, S. H.: Fractures in premature infants. J. Pediatr. Orthop., *8*:41, 1988.
3. Babbitt, D. P., and Cassidy, R. H.: Obstetrical paralysis and dislocation of the shoulder in infancy. J. Bone Joint Surg., *50-A*:1447, 1968.
4. Bairov, G. A., Popov, A. A., Bairov, V. G., and Pisareva, O. K.: Treatment of injuries of the cervical spine in newborn infants. Vestn. Khir., *131*:73, 1983.
5. Banagale, R. C., and Kuhns, L. R.: Traumatic separation of the distal femoral epiphysis in the newborn. J. Pediatr. Orthop., *3*:396, 1983.
6. Barbieri, E., Ghiringhelli, C., and Fossati, E.: On obstetrical fractures and humeral diaphysis. Minerva Ortop., *22*:292, 1971.
7. Barkova, L. A., Barkova, M. K., and Kreminsky, I. M.: Birth injury to term infants as a cause of early infant mortality. Peditr. Akush. Ginekol., *4*:48, 1979.
8. Bauer, O., Weidenbach, A., and Thieme, R.: Skeletal birth injuries in the newborn. Munch. Med. Wochenschr., *109*:998, 1967.
9. Bayne, O., and Rang, M.: Medial dislocation of the radial head following breech delivery: A case report and review of the literature. J. Pediatr. Orthop., *4*:485, 1984.
10. Bianco, A. J., Schlein, A. P., Kruse, R. L., and Johnson, E. W., Jr.: Birth fractures. Minn. Med., *55*:471, 1972.
11. Brandesky, G.: Die wachsende Schadelfraktur im Sauglings- und Kelinkinsesalter. Z. Kinderchir., *11*:Suppl.:381, 1972.
12. Bucher, H. U., Boltshauser, E., Friderich, J., and Isler, W.: Birth injury to the spinal cord. Acta Paediatr. Helv., *34*:517, 1979.
13. Burke, S. W., Jameson, V. P., Roberts, J. M., Johnston, C. E., and Willis, J.: Birth fractures in spinal muscular atrophy. J. Pediatr. Orthop., *6*:34, 1986.
14. Burman, M. S., and Langsam, M. J.: Posterior dislocation of the lower femoral epiphysis in breech delivery. Arch. Surg., *38*:250, 1939.
15. Byers, R. K.: Transection of the spinal cord in the newborn. Arch. Neurol. Psychiatr., *23*:585, 1923.
16. Byers, R. K.: Spinal-cord injuries during birth. Dev. Med. Child Neurol., 1975.
17. Camera, R.: Il distacco epifisario ostetrico dell'estremita prossimale del femore. Chir. Organi Mov., *33*:331, 1949.
18. Caritat, R. J., and Peluffo, E.: El decolamiento de la epifisis superior del humero por traumatismo obstetrico. Arch. Pediatr. Uruguay, *12*:785, 1941.
19. Carletti, B., Rosti, D., and Barbaccia, P.: Anterior sternoclavicular luxation in a newborn infant. Minerva Pediatr., *30*:1091, 1978.
20. Cesarisca, D. E.: Considerations on bilateral obstetrical clavicular fractures. Orizz. Ortop. Odie. Riabil., *11*:147, 1966.
21. Chung, S. M. K., and Nissenbaum, N. M.: Obstetrical paralysis. Orthop. Clin. North Am., *6*:393, 1975.
22. Cohen, A. W., and Otto, S. R.: Obstetric clavicular fractures. A three-year analysis. J. Reprod. Med., *25*:119, 1980.
23. Crothers, B.: Injury of the spinal cord in breech extractions as an important cause of fetal death and paraplegia in childhood. Am. J. Med. Sci., *165*:94, 1923.
24. Crothers, B., and Putnam, M. C.: Obstetrical injuries of the spinal cord. Medicine, *6*:41, 1927.
25. Cumming, W. A.: Neonatal skeletal fractures. Birth trauma or child abuse? J. Can. Assoc. Radiol., *30*:30, 1979.
26. Curran, J. S.: Birth associated injury. Clin. Perinatol., *8*:111, 1981.
27. Danielsson, L. G., and Theander, G.: Traumatic dislocation of the radial head at birth. Acta Radiol. [Diagn.] (Stockh.), *22*:379, 1981.
28. Dogonadze, M. A.: Fractures of the proximal section of the femur in the newborn. Ortop. Travmatol. Protez., *28*:67, 1967.
29. Domanski, B. V.: On the problem of injuries of the neck and head of the femur in newborn infants. Khirurgiia (Mosk.), *41*:124, 1965.
30. Donn, S. M., and Faix, R. G.: Long-term prognosis for the infant with severe birth trauma. Clin. Perinatol., *10*:507, 1983.
31. Downs, D. M., and Wirth, C. R.: Fracture of the distal humeral chondroepiphysis in the neonate. A case report. Clin. Orthop., *169*:155, 1982.
32. Ekengren, K., Berghahl, S., and Ekstrom, G.: Birth injuries to the epiphyseal cartilage. Acta Radiol. [Diagn.] (Stockh.), *19*:197, 1978.
33. Elizalde, E. A.: Obstetrical dislocation of the hip associated with fracture of the femur. J. Bone Joint Surg., *28-A*:838, 1946.
34. Faix, R. G., and Donn, S. M.: Immediate management of the traumatized infant. Clin. Perinatol., *10*:487, 1983.
35. Fontanesi, F., and Costa, P.: Outcome of obstetrical lesions of the femur. Chir. Organi Mov., *62*:555, 1975.
36. Ford, F. R.: Breech delivery with special reference to infantile paraplegia. Arch. Neurol. Psychiatr., *14*:742, 1925.
37. Forster, A.: Neonatal metaphyseal injuries: Typical changes and unusual site. Ann. Radiol. (Paris), *14*:315, 1971.
38. Friedrich, I., Junge, W. D., and Fischer, B.: Causes of clavicular fracture in newborns (author's transl.). Zentralbl. Gynakol., *101*:1528, 1979.
39. Gagnaire, J. C., Thoulon, J. M., Chappuis, J. P., Varnier, C. H., and Mered, B.: Injuries to the upper extremities in the newborn diagnosed at birth. J. Gynecol. Obstet. Biol. Reprod. (Paris), *4*:245, 1975.
40. Gavinelli, R.: On clavicular fracture in the newborn. Clinico-statistical study. Minerva Pediatr., *20*:41, 1968.
41. Giorgi, B., and Scoccianti, P.: Obstetric fractures. Arch. Putti Chir. Organi Mov., *21*:1, 1966.
42. Grcic, R.: Prevention of birth injuries. Nar. Zdrav., *32*:156, 1976.
43. Gresham, E. L.: Birth trauma. Pediatr. Clin. North Am., *22*:317, 1975.
44. Grosfeld, O., Kretowiccz, J., and Brokowski, J.: The temporomandibular joint in children after breech delivery. J. Oral Rehabil., *7*:65, 1980.
45. Haidvogl, M., Borkenstein, M., Stix, H., and Fritsch, G.: Spinal cord lesions due to birth injuries. Wien. Med. Wochenschr., *128*:63, 1978.
46. Halliburton, R. A., Barber, J. R., and Fraser, R. L.: Pseudodislocation—an unusual birth injury. J. Bone Joint Surg., *50-B*:437, 1968.
47. Harrenstein, R. J.: Pseudoluxatio coxae durch Abreissen der Femur Epiphyse bei der Geburt. Bruns. Beitr. Klin. Chir., *146*:593, 1929.
48. Herberts, P.: Birth injuries of the locomotor apparatus. Lakartidningen, *69*:4505, 1972.

49. Herold, G.: Femoral fracture in a newborn infant. Z. Allg. Med., *48*:63, 1972.
50. Iakunin, I. A., Iampolskaia, E. I., Kipnis, S. L., and Burkova, A. S.: Syndromological characteristics and therapy of perinatal lesions of the central nervous system during recovery period. Pediatriia, *5*:61, 1977.
51. Ismagilov, M. F., Kozina, E. V., Tretiakov, V. P., Mugerman, B. I., and Ryzvanov, A. A.: Clinico-electrophysiologic and pathomorphologic characteristics of congenital paralysis of the arms. Zh. Nevropatol. Psikhiatr., *80*:1491, 1980.
52. Iukhnova, O. M., and Durov, M. F.: Diagnosis and treatment of birth spinal and spinal cord injuries in children. Ortop. Travmatol. Protez., *7*:15, 1983.
53. Jacobs, H. J., vanZaane, D. J., and Fleury, P.: Paraplegia as a result of birth trauma. Ned. Tijdschr. Geneeskd., *125*:2094, 1981.
54. Jacquemain, B.: Significance of separation of the proximal femoral epiphysis as a result of birth injury. Geburtshilfe Fraunheilkd., *27*:690, 1967.
55. Jones, R.: Treatment of fractures of the femur in the newly born. Br. Med. J., *1*:1358, 1908.
56. Kavouksorian, C. A., and Noone, R. B.: Flexor tendon repair in the neonate. Ann. Plast. Surg., *9*:415, 1982.
57. Kennedy, P. C.: Traumatic separation of the upper femoral epiphysis. A birth injury. A.J.R., *51*:707, 1944.
58. Khaibullina, F. G.: Cerebral hemodynamic disorders in children who have had a birth injury to the cervical portion of the spinal cord and their dynamics in the pathogenetic therapy process. Pediatriia, *3*:51, 1980.
59. Khaibullina, F. G.: Effect of functional loads for detecting latent cerebral hemodynamic disorders in children with birth injuries to the cervical spine and spinal cord. Vopr. Okhr. Materin. Det., *25*:47, 1980.
60. Koch, B. M., and Eng, G. M.: Neonatal spinal cord injury. Arch. Phys. Med. Rehabil., *60*:378, 1979.
61. Kolber, S., Anderson, R. M., Campbell, P. E., and Roy, R. N.: Birth injury with unusual clinical features simulating Werdnig Hoffmann disease. Aust. Paediatr. J., *15*:47, 1979.
62. Kolontai, I. I., and Kolodko, E. D.: Birth injuries. Ortop. Travmatol. Protez., *10*:61, 1982.
63. Kuhn, D., and Rosman, M.: Traumatic, nonparalytic dislocation of the shoulder in a newborn infant. J. Pediatr. Orthop., *4*:121, 1984.
64. Kyle, J. W., and Jenkinson, D.: Depressed fracture in the newborn (letter). Br. Med. J., *3*:698, 1973.
65. Lasi, C., and Fiorio, E.: Clinico-statistical and therapeutic considerations on obstetrical fractures of the clavicle. Minerva Ortop., *17*:664, 1966.
66. Lehman, M. A., and Wiese, F. W.: Nonunion of an olecranon fracture following birth injury. Bull. Hosp. J. Dis., *26*:187, 1965.
67. Leonova, P. T.: Fracture of the acromion scapulae in the newborn. Vopr. Okhr. Materin. Det., *18*:86, 1973.
68. Lichtblau, P. D.: Shoulder dislocation in the infant. Case report and discussion. J. Fla. Med. Assoc., *64*:313, 1977.
69. Liebolt, F. D., and Furey, J. C.: Obstetrical paralysis with dislocation of the shoulder. J. Bone Joint Surg., *36-A*:227, 1953.
70. Lindseth, R. E., and Rosene, H. A.: Traumatic separation of the upper femoral epiphysis in a newborn infant. J. Bone Joint Surg., *53-A*:1641, 1971.
71. Longo, R., and Ruggiero, L.: Left pneumothorax with subcutaneous emphysema secondary to left clavicular fracture and homolateral obstetrical paralysis of the arm. Minerva Pediatr., *31*:273, 1982.
72. Lubrano di Diego, J. G., Chappuis, J. P., Montsegur, P., Kohler, R., Dodat, H., Bertrix, L., Eulry, M. L., and Daudet, M.: Eighty-two obstetrical astro-articular injuries of the newborn (excepting brachial plexus palsies). Limits of initial therapeutic aggression and follow-up of evolution, particularly concerning traumatic separation of upper femoral epiphysis (author's transl.). Chir. Pediatr., *19*:219, 1978.
73. Lukac, R., Bumbic, S., Najdanovic, Z., and Maksimovic, L.: Proximal and distal femoral epiphyseolysis occurring during delivery. Srp. Arh. Celok. Lek., *108*:1067, 1980.
74. Madsen, E. T.: Fractures of the extremities in the newborn. Acta Obstet. Gynecol. Scand., *34*:41, 1955.
75. Maszkiewicz, W., and Irzynska, D.: Perinatal mandibular injury in a premature infant. Wiad. Lek., *36*:1217, 1983.
76. Menon, T. J.: Fracture separation of the lower humeral epiphysis due to birth injury: A case report. Injury, *14*:168, 1982.
77. Menzel, K., Genssler, W., Gottschlak, E., Linke, M., and Topke, B.: Paralysis of phrenic nerve due to birth injury. Acta Paediatr. Acad. Sci. Hung., *18*:69, 1977.
78. Meyenberg, H.: Clavicle fracture of the newborn. Zentralbl. Gynakol., *93*:1093, 1971.
79. Michael, J. P., Theodorou, S., Houlizras, K., and Siatis, N.: Two cases of obstetrical separation (epiphyseolysis) of the upper femoral epiphysis. J. Bone Joint Surg., *40-B*:477, 1958.
80. Michel, L.: Obstetrical dislocation of the upper humeral epiphysis. Rev. Chir. Orthop., *24*:201, 1973.
81. Mikhailov, M. K., and Saidova, M. V.: Roentgenological characteristics of the respiratory organs in children with birth injuries of the spine and spinal cord. Vestn. Rentgenol. Radiol., *4*:57, 1983.
82. Mortens, J., and Christensen, P.: Traumatic separation of the upper femoral epiphysis as an obstetrical lesion. Acta Orthop. Scand., *34*:239, 1964.
83. Nikolic, C. J., Marjanovi, C. M., Palic, D., and Popovic, L.: Obstetrical fractures of collar bones in newborn infants. Med. Pregl., *24*:217, 1971.
84. Ogden, J. A., Lee, K. E., Rudicel, S. A., and Pelker, R. R.: Proximal femoral epiphysiolysis in the neonate. J. Pediatr. Orthop., *4*:285, 1984.
85. Okura, T., Kawagishi, R., and Fujii, M.: Six cases of clavicular fracture in newborn infants. Sanfujinka Jissai, *17*:1112, 1968.
86. Osna, A. I., Brodskaia, Z. L., and Kholkina, G. F.: Diagnosis and treatment of birth injuries of the cervical portion of spine and spinal cord in newborn infants. Zh. Vopr. Neirokhir., *6*:33, 1979.
87. Owens, W. F., Jr.: Orthopaedic evaluation of the newborn. J. Miss. State Med. Assoc., *12*:247, 1971.
88. Page, M. L., *et al.*: Separation of the distal humeral epiphysis in the neonate. A continued clinical and roentgenographic diagnosis. Am. J. Dis. Child., *139*:1203, 1985.
89. Painter, M. J., and Bergman, I.: Obstetrical trauma to the neonatal central and peripheral nervous system. Semin. Perinatol., *6*:89, 1982.
90. Paribelli, E., and Zangrando, A.: Outcome of an obstetrical fracture of the forearm. Chir. Organi Mov., *63*:669, 1977.
91. Perricone, G.: Rib fractures in the newborn infant. Chir. Organi Mov., *55*:512, 1967.
92. Perricone, G.: So-called obstetrical fractures of the forearm. Chir. Organi Mov., *66*:531, 1980.
93. Prantskiavichius, S. V.: Some suggestions concerning treatment of birth injuries of the musculoskeletal system in the newborn. Ortop. Travmatol. Protez., *30*:79, 1969.
94. Prantskiavichius, S. V.: Birth injuries of the musculoskeletal system in the newborn. Ortop. Travmatol. Protez., *31*:45, 1970.
95. Purwar, M. B., and Deshpande, A. S.: Fracture of parietal bone in a neonate (letter). Indian J. Pediatr., *18*:355, 1981.
96. Ratner, A. I.: Birth injury of the spinal cord in children. Pediatriia, *5*:68, 1977.

97. Ratner, A. I.: Spinal and spinal cord lesions in infants at birth. Akush. Ginekol. (Mosk.), *4*:56, 1978.
98. Ratner, A. I., and Marulina, V. I.: Clinical picture and diagnosis of a myotonic syndrome in children resulting from birth injury. Zh. Nevropatol. Psikhiatr., *81*:1461, 1981.
99. Reid, H.: Birth injury to the cervical spine and spinal cord. Acta Neurochir. (Suppl.) (Wien), *32*:87, 1983.
100. Roasenda, F.: Osteoarticular obstetrical injuries. Minerva Ginecol., *20*:1413, 1968.
101. Robinson, W. H.: Treatment of birth fractures of the femur. J. Bone Joint Surg., *20*:778, 1938.
102. Rosa, G., Chianca, I., Savarese, A., and Copolla, D.: Surgical treatment in sequelae of obstetrical lesions of the shoulder. Chir. Organi Mov., *64*:65, 1978.
103. Ruiz Moreno, M.: Obstetrical fractures of the humerus and femur. Prensa Med. Argent., *25*:321, 1938.
104. Rutherford, Y., Fomufod, A. K., Gopalakrishnan, L. J., and Beeks, E. C.: Traumatic distal femoral periostitis of the newborn: A breech delivery birth injury. J. Natl. Med. Assoc., *75*:933, 1983.
105. Sadurny, G., Figliolini, M., and Policicchio, A.: Considerations on 162 cases of fracture of the clavicle by obstetric causes. Quad. Clin. Obstet. Ginecol., *227*:453, 1967.
106. Saidova, M. V.: Respiratory disorders in children with birth injuries to the cervical spine and spinal cord. Pediatriia, *5*:35, 1983.
107. Samojlowicz, J.: Case of post-traumatic paralysis of the peroneal nerve in a newborn infant. Wiad. Lek., *15*:867, 1983.
108. Scaglietti, O.: The obstetrical shoulder trauma. Surg. Gynecol. Obstet., *66*:868, 1938.
109. Schuldt, M. W.: Femoral fracture in the newborn. Rocky Mt. Med. J., *70*:45, 1973.
110. Shimada, N.: Clavicular fracture of the newborn infant. Jissai, *19*:1163, 1970.
111. Shirokova, S. A.: Value and feasibility of electromyographic studies in the diagnosis of birth injuries to the cervical portion of the spinal cord. Zh. Nevropatol. Psikhiatr., *78*:1454, 1978.
112. Shirokova, S. A., and Marulina, V. I.: Role of electromyography in diagnosing birth-caused myotonic syndrome in infants. Pediatriia, *11*:39, 1982.
113. Siffert, R. S.: Displacement of distal humeral epiphysis in the newborn infant. J. Bone Joint Surg., *45-A*:105, 1963.
114. Slesarev, S. P.: Dysplasia and birth injury of the shoulder joint. Ortop. Travmatol. Protez., *1*:32, 1983.
115. Snedecor, S. T., and Wilson, H. B.: Some obstetrical injuries in the long bones. J. Bone Joint Surg., *31-A*:378, 1949.
116. Spies, H., and Wittscheck, R.: Late sequelae of clavicular fractures due to birth trauma. Beitr. Orthop. Traumatol., *21*:143, 1974.
117. Stanley, P., Duncan, A. W., Isaacson, J., and Isaacson, A. S.: Radiology of fracture dislocation of the cervical spine during delivery. A.J.R., *145*:621, 1985.
118. Taffel, S.: Congenital anomalies and birth injuries among live births: United States, 1973–74. Vital Health Stat., *31*:1, 1978.
119. Taricco, G., and Pansecchi, V.: Obstetrical fractures of the clavicle. Arch. Sci. Med. (Torino), *125*:106, 1968.
120. Tavernier: Sequelle d'un décollement épiphysaire obstetrical de l'extrémité superiure de l'humerus. Lyon Chir., *32*:465, 1935.
121. Theodorou, S. D., Ierodiaconou, M. N., and Mitsou, A.: Obstetrical fracture-separation of the upper femoral epiphysis. Acta Orthop. Scand., *53*:239, 1982.
122. Tischer, W., and Jahrig, K.: Perinatal injuries of skeletal system. Zentralbl. Gynakol., *104*:1169, 1982.
123. Towbin, R., and Crawford, A. H.: Neonatal traumatic proximal femoral epiphysiolysis. Pediatrics, *63*:456, 1979.
124. Valdiserri, L., and Kelescian, G.: On a case of obstetrical epiphyseal detachment of the distal extremity of the humerus. Osp. Ital. Chir., *13*:407, 1965.
125. Valman, H. B.: Birth trauma. Br. Med. J., *15*:1566, 1979.
126. Venbrocks, H. P.: Birth injuries in the shoulder region. Med. Klin., *68*:521, 1973.
127. Vijaya, S.: Treatment of fracture of the shaft of the femur in the newborn. J. Singapore Paediatr. Soc., *8*:66, 1966.
128. Weiss, M. H., and Kaufman, B.: Hangman's fracture in an infant. Am. J. Dis. Child., *126*:268, 1973.
129. Wendling, P., and Hofmann, S.: Birth fractures of the femur. Prog. Pediatr. Surg., *10*:247, 1977.
130. Weston, W. J.: Metaphyseal fractures in infancy. J. Bone Joint Surg., *39-B*:694, 1957.
131. Wiaczek, M.: Perinatal fetal injuries. Pieleg. Polozna., *3*:5, 1981.
132. Wojtowycz, M., Starshak, R. J., and Sty, J. R.: Neonatal proximal femoral epiphyseolysis. Radiology, *136*:647, 1980.
133. Zlanabitnig, H. P., Landschek, P., and Kock, H. J.: Delivery-related humeral shaft fractures in the newborn infant. Zentralbl. Gynakol., *100*:1075, 1978.
134. Zionts, L. E., Leffers, D., Oberto, M. R., and Harvey, J. P., Jr.: Plastic bowing of the femur in a neonate. J. Pediatr. Orthop., *4*:749, 1984.

STRESS FRACTURES

Stress (or fatigue) fracture is a gradual localized dissolution of bone caused by prolonged repetitive muscular action on a bone in a limb that is not accustomed to it. The break takes place in a bone with normal elastic resistance and occurs in individuals who engage in physical activities such as jogging or cross-country skiing.

The fatigue type of stress fracture should be distinguished from the *insufficiency* fracture, which occurs in a bone with deficient elastic resistance.[114] In insufficiency fracture, the stress exerted on the bone is physiologic and not strenuous. Conditions predisposing to insufficiency fractures may be classified as *those due to developmental affections* (such as osteogenesis imperfecta, osteopetrosis [marble bone disease], arachnodactyly); *those due to vitamin deficiency and endocrine disorders* (such as rickets, scurvy, primary or secondary hyperparathyroidism, hyperpituitarism [Cushing's syndrome], cortisone treatment); *those due to disuse atrophy* (such as immobilization, paralytic diseases such as myelomeningocele, cerebral palsy, and arthrogryposis multiplex congenita); and *those due to inflammatory conditions* (such as rheumatoid arthritis).

The term *pathologic fracture* should be restricted to fractures that are caused by trivial trauma in bones that are weakened by preexisting local lesions such as benign or malignant tumors, osteomyelitis, or postirradiation local osteoporosis.

Sites of Involvement

Historically "stress fracture" was synonymous with the "march fracture" of the metatarsals seen in military recruits.* During the past three decades, however, it has been recognized that stress fractures occur in many bones. Their sites are often predictable, depending upon the activity causing them. For example, stress fracture of the sesamoids of the first metatarsal is produced by prolonged standing; that of the metatarsal shafts by marching, prolonged standing, or ballet; of the tarsal navicular by long-distance running or stamping on the ground as in aerobic exercise; of the calcaneus by prolonged standing (especially on a recently immobilized limb); of the distal shaft of the fibula and proximal diaphysis of the tibia by long-distance running; of the patella by hurdling; of the femur (shaft and neck) by ballet, gymnastics, and long-distance running; of the ischial pubic rami of the pelvis by bowling, stooping, and gymnastics; of the pars interarticularis of the lumbar vertebrae by heavy lifting and ballet; of the ribs by golf, carrying heavy packs, and coughing; of the ulnar shaft by propelling a wheelchair, and of the coronoid process of the ulna and the distal humeral shaft by pitching a ball.†

In children the tibia and fibula are frequent sites of stress fractures; they differ from similar fractures in the adult because in children bone has a richer blood supply and greater biologic plasticity.

Pathogenesis

Stress fractures are produced by muscular activity on bone and not from direct impact upon a bone. For example, during running, contraction of the triceps surae muscle plantarflexes the ankle, dorsiflexion of the foot is restricted, and the tibia and fibula are pulled together maximally at a point immediately above the lateral malleolus. This is a common site of stress fracture in runners, especially children.

Resorption of cortical bone is a normal process that takes place in childhood, adolescence, and early adult life. Osteoclastic activity produces many microscopic channels in the cortex. Eventually these resorption cavities are filled by mature haversian systems, and the circumferential lamellar bone is gradually replaced by the structurally sounder osteomal bone of the adult.

Bone responds to excessive stress and strain by acceleration of the normal process of cortical resorption. The bony cortex is weakened by the formation of numerous resorption channels. In an attempt to splint the cortex, the endosteal and periosteal tissues respond by forming new bone adjacent to the areas of cortical resorption. If the buttressing process is adequate, the periosteal and endosteal new bone will mature, and the cortical resorption cavities will fill in and eventually become osteomal bone. If this buttressing process does not take place rapidly enough, and if continued excessive stress is applied to the bone, fracture will occur. Stress fracture begins as a small cortical crack.[164] With increase and continuation of stress, the crack progresses by initiation of subcortical infraction ahead of the main crack.

Clinical Findings

When the bones in the lower limb are affected, the child has an antalgic limp, usually of gradual but occasionally of sudden onset. There is no history of acute trauma, although it may be ascertained that the child has recently taken part in some vigorous activity to which he has previously been unaccustomed.

Local pain is frequently present; it is aggravated by activity and relieved by rest.

On palpation, there is a varying degree of local swelling and tenderness. The adjacent joints have full range of motion, but when the ischiopubic ramus or the femoral neck is involved, the hip joint is restricted in abduction and rotation (medial rotation with femoral neck fracture and lateral rotation with ischiopubic ramus fracture).

Radiographic Findings

Factors that determine the appearance of a fracture on the radiogram are the location of the fracture and the time between injury and the initial radiographic examination. In the early phase a stress fracture in a long bone will manifest itself as a radiolucent zone through the cortical surface without periosteal reaction or callus. With repeated injury and healing, solid or thick laminar periosteal reaction may be seen (Figs. 8–190 and 8–191). In a cancellous bone

---

*See references 8, 12, 20, 23, 28, 48, and 80.

†See references: tarsal navicular, 151; calcaneus, 15, 31, 66, 78, 143, 161; fibula, 16, 17, 58, 74, 83, 86, 100, 127; proximal diaphysis of tibia, 6, 7, 18, 33, 50, 69, 70, 72, 74, 75, 84, 92, 129, 132, 142, 144; patella, 34; femur (shaft and neck), 10, 37, 44, 95, 101, 122, 163; ischial ramus, 156; lumbar vertebrae, 29, 47, 58, 138, 160; ribs, 125; coronoid process of ulna and distal humeral shaft, 45, 149, 152.

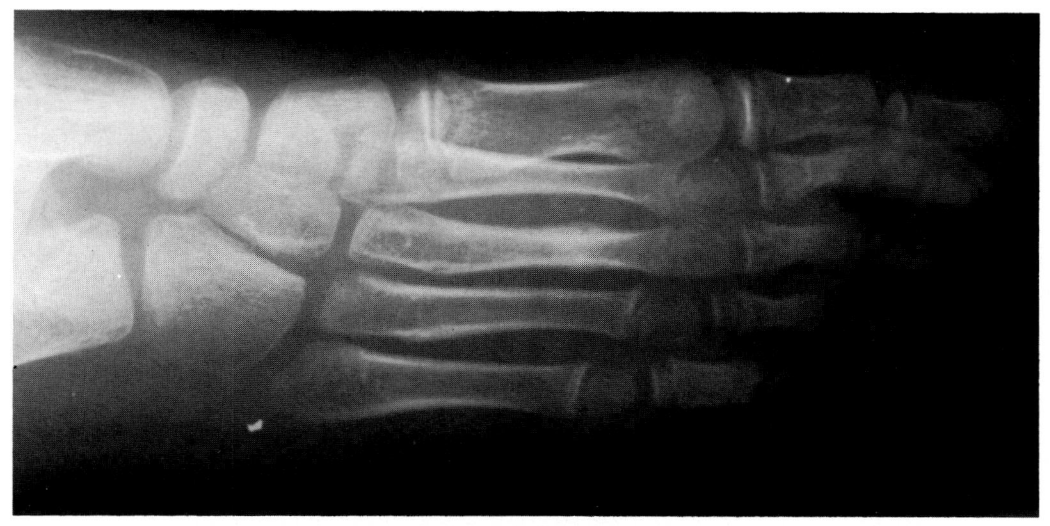

FIGURE 8–190. Stress fracture of the third metatarsal (March fracture).

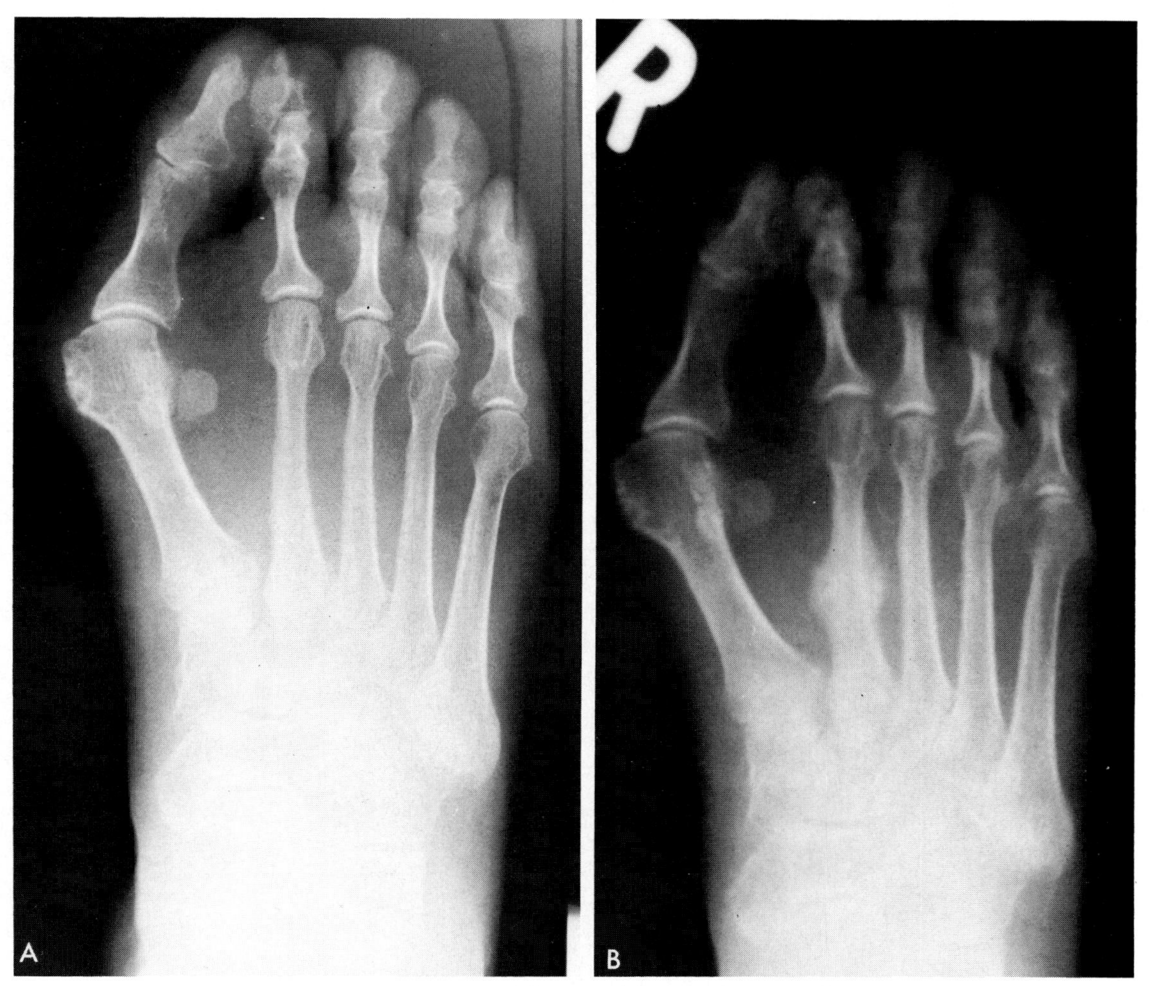

FIGURE 8–191. Stress fracture of the second metatarsal.

A. Initial radiogram. Note the periosteal thickening and the absence of a fracture line. **B.** Two weeks later anteroposterior radiogram of the foot shows rapid consolidation of subperiosteal callus and fracture line.

such as the calcaneus or in the metaphyseal region of a long bone, a stress fracture may appear as an area of focal sclerosis.

Two types of stress fractures have been described by Devas: a *compression type*, common in children, is seen in the calcaneus or the femoral neck, and a *distraction type* begins in one cortex and may be oblique (the most frequent), transverse, or longitudinal.[38] Oblique radiographic views and tomography (linear or computed axial) will assist in delineating osseous detail.

In the *tibia* the site of stress fracture is nearly always in its proximal third, involving the posteromedial or posterolateral cortex; it rarely occurs on the anterior aspect of the tibia (Fig. 8–192).[144] There are a haze of internal callus across the diaphysis, subperiosteal new bone formation, and slight disruption of the cortex. An actual linear fracture across the shaft is not seen.

In the *fibula* the earliest radiographic sign is the presence of thin layers of "eggshell" callus along the diaphysis. The fracture itself cannot be visualized because it is obscured by the exuberant callus that extends up and down the shaft.

Radioisotope scanning with technetium-99m

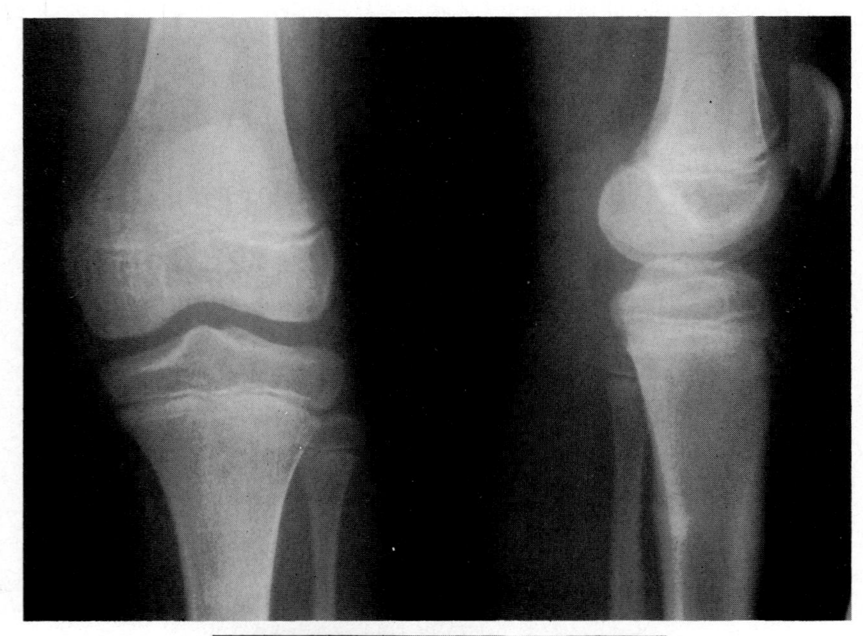

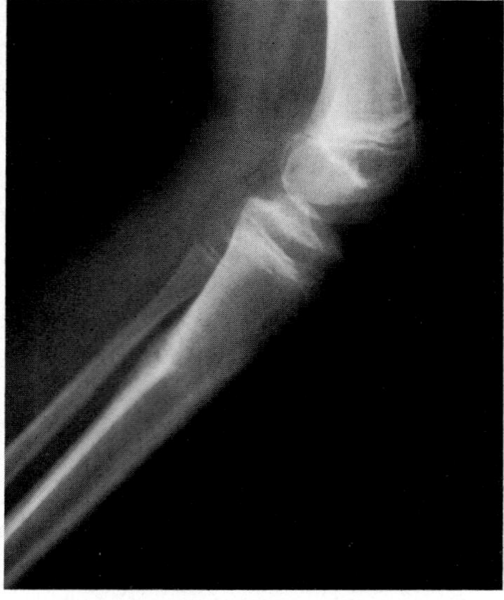

FIGURE 8–192. Stress fracture of proximal tibial diaphysis.

will show increased isotope uptake due to osteoblastic new bone formation. The bone scan will be positive before plain radiograms show any changes.[53, 85, 111, 121, 158]

The diagnosis of stress fracture is made in the great majority of cases by clinical information, plain radiograms, and bone scan with technetium-99m. If in doubt, simple tomography is of great value. Occasionally one may have to resort to computed tomography (CT). CT scan will demonstrate lucent fracture lines in the cortex and periosteal reaction.[30, 99]

In the differential diagnosis, one should rule out osteoid osteoma, acute osteomyelitis, chronic sclerosing osteomyelitis, osteogenic sarcoma, Ewing's sarcoma, acute leukemia, and osteomalacia.[92]

In *osteoid osteoma*, a benign lesion, there is a history of pain at night that is relieved by aspirin. In stress fracture the pain occurs on strenuous physical activity and is relieved by rest. On the radiogram there is a lucent nidus surrounded by a dense area of sclerosis. The appearance of osteoid osteoma in the bone scan and CT scan is quite characteristic. *Osteogenic sarcoma* is usually a metaphyseal lesion with moth-eaten pattern of lysis in the medulla, tumor bone formation, and periosteal reaction that is aggressive, showing spiculation, thin lamination, coarse deposition, and sometimes Codman's triangle. In osteogenic sarcoma there is progressive destruction of bone. In time, it no longer resembles a healing fracture. The diagnosis of *acute osteomyelitis* is simple by thorough clinical examination. In *chronic sclerosing osteomyelitis* there is diffuse cortical sclerosis with no apparent radiolucency. There is absence of the linear sclerotic pattern of a healing fracture.

If stress fracture is suspected the limb is put to rest. Within 10 to 14 days radiograms are repeated; during this time there should be evidence of healing. Biopsy should not be performed unless there is clear-cut radiographic evidence that no healing is taking place and there is a suggestion of malignancy or infection.

Treatment

Treatment consists of rest of the affected part. The type of rest depends on the location of the fracture and whether the break involves one cortex or extends to be a complete fracture. In general, complete fractures are best treated in a plaster of Paris walking cast, whereas infractions are treated by abstinence from strenuous physical activity and use of crutches if necessary.

References

1. Adams, J.: Bone injuries in very young athletes. Clin. Orthop., *58*:129, 1968.
2. Annan, I. H., and Buxton, R. A.: Bilateral stress fractures of the femoral neck associated with abnormal anatomy—a case report. Injury, *17*:164, 1986.
3. Aro, H., and Dahlstrom, S.: Conservative management of distraction-type stress fractures of the femoral neck. J. Bone Joint Surg., *68-B*:65, 1986.
4. Bargren, J. H., Tilson, D. H., Jr., and Bridgeford, O. E.: Prevention of displaced fatigue fracture of the femur. J. Bone Joint Surg., *53-A*:1115, 1972.
5. Bell, R. H., and Hawkins, R. J.: Stress fracture of the distal ulna. A case report. Clin. Orthop., *209*:169, 1986.
6. Benedict, J. S.: Stress fractures of tibia; analysis of thirty-five cases. J. Int. Coll. Surg., *32*:174, 1959.
7. Berkebile, R. D.: Stress fracture of the tibia in children. A.J.R., *91*:588, 1964.
8. Bernstein, A., and Stone, J. R.: March fracture. A report of three hundred seven cases and a new method of treatment. J. Bone Joint Surg., *26*:743, 1944.
9. Bjelland, J. C., Pitt, J. J., and Capp, M. P.: Acute bowing fractures of the extremities: A frequently missed roentgen diagnosis. Medical Imaging, *3*:13, 1978.
10. Blickenstaff, L. D., and Morris, J. M.: Fatigue fractures of the femoral neck. J. Bone Joint Surg., *48-A*:1031, 1966.
11. Bosman, J., and Tondeur, G.: Spontaneous fractures in children. Acta Paediatr. Belg., *21*:113, 1967.
12. Branch, H. E.: March fractures of the femur. J. Bone Joint Surg., *26*:387, 1944.
13. Bretagne, M. C., Mouton, J. N., Pierson, M., Prevot, J., Olive, D., and Treheux, A.: Periosteal appositions in paediatrics (author's transl.). J. Radiol. Electr., *58*:119, 1977.
14. Brubacker, C. E., and James, S. L.: Injuries to runners. Am. J. Sports Med., *2*:189, 1974.
15. Buchanan, J., and Greer, R. B.: Stress fractures in the calcaneus of a child. A case report. Clin. Orthop., *135*:119, 1978.
16. Burrows, H. J.: Spontaneous fracture of the apparently normal fibula in its lowest third. Br. J. Surg., *28*:82, 1940.
17. Burrows, H. J.: Fatigue fractures of the fibula. J. Bone Joint Surg., *30-B*:266, 1948.
18. Burrows, H. J.: Fatigue infraction of the middle of the tibia in ballet dancers. J. Bone Joint Surg., *38-B*:83, 1956.
19. Cail, W. S., Keats, T. E., and Sussman, M. D.: Plastic bowing fracture of the femur in a child. A.J.R., *130*:780, 1978.
20. Carlson, G. D., and Wertz, R. F.: March fracture, including others than those of the foot. Radiology, *43*:48, 1944.
21. Chamay, A.: Mechanical and morphological aspects of experimental overload and fatigue in bone. J. Biomech., *3*:263, 1970.
22. Chamay, A., and Tschants, P.: Mechanical influence in bone remodeling. Experimental research of Wolff's law. J. Biomech., *5*:173, 1972.
23. Childress, H. M.: March foot in a seven-year-old child. J. Bone Joint Surg., *28*:877, 1946.
24. Clement, D.: Tibial stress syndrome in athletes. Am. J. Sports Med., *2*:81, 1974.
25. Collins, H. R., and Evarts, C. M.: Injuries to the adolescent athlete. Postgrad. Med., *49*:72, 1971.
26. Crass, J. R., and L'Heureux, P.: Bone scan appearance of stress fractures. Differentiation from osteosarcoma. Minn. Med., *645*:535, 1981.
27. Cullen, R. J., Jr., and Page, L. K.: Growing fractures in children. J.A.M.A., *60*:21, 1973.
28. Cwiklicki, Z.: Stress fracture of the third metatarsal

bone in a child. Chir. Narzadow Ruchu Ortop. Pol., *30*:333, 1965.
29. Cyron, B. M., Hutton, W. C., and Troup, J. D. G.: Spondylolytic fracture. J. Bone Joint Surg., *58-B*:462, 1976.
30. Daffner, R. H.: Stress fractures. Current concepts. Skeletal Radiol., *2*:221, 1978.
31. Darby, R. E.: Stress fractures of the os calcis. J.A.M.A., *200*:1183, 1967.
32. DeLee, J. C., Evans, J. P., and Julian, J.: Stress fracture of the fifth metatarsal. Am. J. Sports Med., *11*:349, 1983.
33. Devas, M.: Stress fracture of the tibia in athletes or "shin soreness." J. Bone Joint Surg., *40-B*:227, 1958.
34. Devas, M. B.: Stress fractures of the patella. J. Bone Joint Surg., *42-B*:71, 1960.
35. Devas, M. B.: Compression stress fractures in man and the greyhound. J. Bone Joint Surg., *43-B*:540, 1961.
36. Devas, M. B.: Stress fractures in children. J. Bone Joint Surg., *45-B*:528, 1963.
37. Devas, M. B.: Stress fractures of the femoral neck. J. Bone Joint Surg., *47-B*:728, 1965.
38. Devas, M. B.: Stress Fractures. New York, Churchill-Livingstone, 1975.
39. Devas, M. B., and Sweetnam, R.: Stress fractures of the fibula. J. Bone Joint Surg., *38-B*:818, 1956.
40. Devereaux, M. D., Parr, G. R., Lachmann, S. M., Page-Thomas, P., and Hazelman, B. L.: The diagnosis of stress fractures in athletes. J.A.M.A., *252*:531, 1984.
41. Dugan, R. C., and D'Ambrosia, R.: Fibular stress fractures in runners. J. Fam. Pract., *17*:415, 1983.
42. Elton, R. C., and Abbott, H. G.: An unusual case of multiple stress fractures. Milit. Med., *130*:1207, 1965.
43. Engh, C. A., Robinson, R. A., and Milgram, J.: Stress fractures in children. J. Trauma, *10*:532, 1970.
44. Ernst, J.: Stress fractures of the femoral neck. J. Trauma, *4*:71, 1964.
45. Evans, D. L.: Fatigue fracture of the ulna. J. Bone Joint Surg., *37-B*:618, 1955.
46. Evans, F. G., and Riolo, M. L.: Relations between the fatigue life and histology of adult cortical bone. J. Bone Joint Surg., *52-A*:1579, 1970.
47. Farfan, H. F., Osteria, V., and Lamy, C.: The mechanical etiology of spondylosis and spondylolisthesis. Clin. Orthop., *117*:40, 1976.
48. Ford, L. T., and Gilula, L. A.: Stress fractures of the middle metatarsals following the Keller operation. J. Bone Joint Surg., *59-A*:117, 1977.
49. Friberg, O.: Leg length asymmetry in stress fractures. A clinical and radiological study. J. Sports Med. Phys. Fitness, *22*:485, 1982.
50. Fructer, Z., and Enachesco, L.: Radiodiagnosis of tibial stress fractures in children. J. Radiol. Electr., *51*:155, 1970.
51. Fuchs, G.: Diagnosis and therapy of spontaneous fractures in childhood and adolescence. Hefte Unfallheilkd., *102*:76, 1970.
52. Ganz, R., *et al.*: Parasymphyseal insufficiency fractures of the os pubis. A.J.R., *142*:581, 1984.
53. Geslein, G. E., Thrall, J. H., Espinosa, J. L., and Older, R. A.: Early detection of stress fractures using 99mTc-polyphosphate. Radiology, *121*:683, 1976.
54. Gilbert, R. S., and Johnson, H. A.: Stress fracture in military recruits—a review of twelve years' experience. Milit. Med., *8*:716, 1966.
55. Goergen, T. G., Venn-Watson, E. A., Rossman, D. J., Resnick, D., and Gerber, K. H.: Tarsal navicular stress fractures in runners. A.J.R., *136*:201, 1981.
56. Goldman, A. B., and Jacobs, B.: Femoral neck fractures complicating Gaucher's disease in children. Skeletal Radiol., *12*:162, 1984.
57. Green, N. E., Rogers, R. A., and Lipscomb, A. B.: Nonunions of stress fractures of the tibia. Am. J. Sports Med., *13*:171, 1985.
58. Griffiths, A. L.: Fatigue fracture of the fibula in childhood. Arch. Dis. Child., *27*:552, 1952.
59. Hadley, L. A.: Stress fracture with spondylolysis. A.J.R., *90*:1258, 1963.
60. Haluzicky, M., and Szabad, F.: Fracture of long bones from fatigue in sportsmen. Acta Chir. Orthop. Traumatol. Cech., *42*:72, 1975.
61. Hamilton, A. S., and Finklestein, H. E.: March fracture: Report of a case involving both fibulae. J. Bone Joint Surg., *26*:146, 1944.
62. Hartley, J. B.: Fatigue fracture of the tibia. Br. J. Surg., *30*:9, 1942.
63. Hartley, J. B.: "Stress" or "fatigue" fractures. Br. J. Radiol., *16*:255, 1943.
64. Hulkko, A., Orava, S., Pellinen, P., and Puranen, J.: Stress fractures of the sesamoid bones of the first metatarsophalangeal joint in athletes. Arch. Orthop. Trauma. Surg., *104*:113, 1985.
65. Hulkko, A., Orava, S., Peltokallio, P., Tulikoura, I., and Walden, M.: Stress fractures of the navicular bone. Nine cases in athletes. Acta Orthop. Scand., *56*:503, 1985.
66. Hullinger, C. W.: Insufficiency fracture of the calcaneus—similar to march fracture of the metatarsal. J. Bone Joint Surg., *26*:751, 1944.
67. Ingersoll, C. F.: Ice skater's fracture. A.J.R., *50*:469, 1943.
68. Jones, H. H., Priest, J. D., Hayes, W. C., Tichenor, C. C., and Nagel, D. A.: Humeral hypertrophy in response to exercise. J. Bone Joint Surg., *59-A*:204, 1977.
69. Kelly, R. P., and Murphy, F. E.: Fatigue fractures of the tibia. South. Med. J., *44*:290, 1951.
70. Kimball, P. R., and Savastano, A. A.: Fatigue fractures of the proximal tibia. Clin. Orthop., *70*:170, 1970.
71. Kitchin, I. D.: Fatigue fracture of the ulna. J. Bone Joint Surg., *30-B*:622, 1948.
72. Kochhar, V. S., and Srivastava, K. K.: Stress fracture of the tibia: Report of a case. Aust. N.Z. J. Surg., *43*:266, 1973.
73. Kolisch, P. D.: Stress fractures in children (letter). J.A.M.A., *237*:2038, 1977.
74. Kozlowski, K., Pietron, K., and Puk, E.: Stress fracture of the tibia in children. Ann. Radiol. (Paris), *11*:679, 1968.
75. Krause, G. R., and Thompson, J. R. G.: March fracture of tibia. Radiology, *41*:580, 1943.
76. Kroenig, P. M., and Shelton, M. L.: Stress fractures. A.J.R., *89*:1281, 1963.
77. Laferty, J. F., Winter, W. G., and Gambaro, S. A.: Fatigue characteristics of posterior elements of vertebrae. J. Bone Joint Surg., *59-A*:54, 1977.
78. Leabhart, J. W.: Stress fractures of the calcaneus. J. Bone Joint Surg., *41-A*:1285, 1959.
79. Leveton, A. L.: March (fatigue) fractures of the long bones of the lower extremity and pelvis. Am. J. Surg., *71*:222, 1946.
80. Levine, D. C., Blazina, M. E., and Levine, E.: Fatigue fractures of the shaft of the femur. Simulation of malignant tumor. Radiology, *89*:883, 1967.
81. Li, G. P., Zhang, S. D., Chen, G., Chen, H., and Wang, A. M.: Radiographic and histologic analyses of stress fracture in rabbit tibias. Am. J. Sports Med., *13*:285, 1985.
82. McBryde, A. M.: Stress fractures in athletes. Am. J. Sports Med., *3*:212, 1975.
83. McPhee, H. R., and Franklin, C. M.: March fracture of the fibula in athletes. J.A.M.A., *131*:574, 1946.
84. Manoli, A.: Traumatic fibular bowing with tibial fracture. Orthopedics, *1*:145, 1978.

85. Marta, J. B., Williams, H. J., and Smookler, R. A.: Gallium-67 uptake in a stress fracture (letter). J. Nucl. Med., *23*:271, 1982.
86. Martin, W., and Riddervold, H. D.: Acute plastic bowing fractures of the fibula. Radiology, *131*:639, 1979.
87. Meurman, K. O., and Elfving, S.: Stress fracture of the cuneiform bones. Br. J. Radiol., *53*:157, 1980.
88. Micheli, L. J.: Stress fractures of the second metatarsal involving Lisfranc's joint in ballet dancers. A new overuse injury of the foot. J. Bone Joint Surg., *67-A*:1372, 1985.
89. Micheli, L. J., and Gerbino, P. G.: Etiologic assessment of stress fractures of the lower extremities in young athletes. Orthop. Trans., *4*:51, 1980.
90. Michetti, M. L.: March fracture following a McBride bunionectomy. A case report. J. Am. Podiatry Assoc., *60*:286, 1970.
91. Milgrom, C., Chisin, R., Margulies, J., Giladi, M., Stein, M., Kashtan, H., and Atlan, H.: Stress fractures of the medial femoral condyle. J. Trauma, *26*:199, 1986.
92. Milkman, L. A.: Pseudofractures (hunger osteopathy, late rickets, osteomalacia). Report of a case. A.J.R., *32*:622, 1934.
93. Miller, B., Markheim, H. R., and Towbin, M. N.: Multiple stress fractures in rheumatoid arthritis. J. Bone Joint Surg., *49-A*:1408, 1967.
94. Miller, E. H., Schneider, J. H., Bronson, J. L., and McLain, D.: A new consideration in athletic injuries. The classical ballet dancer. Clin. Orthop., *111*:181, 1975.
95. Miller, F., and Wenger, D. R.: Femoral neck stress fracture in a hyperactive child. J. Bone Joint Surg., *61-A*:435, 1979.
96. Morris, J. M., and Blickenstaff, L. D.: Fatigue Fractures. Clinical Study. Springfield, Ill., Charles C Thomas, 1967.
97. Moss, A., and Mowat, A. G.: Ultrasonic assessment of stress fractures. Br. Med. J. (Clin. Res.), *286*:1479, 1983.
98. Mowat, A. G., and Kay, V. J.: Ischial stress fracture. Br. J. Sports Med., *17*:94, 1983.
99. Murcia, M., Brennan, R. E., and Edeiken, J.: Computed tomography of stress fracture. Skeletal Radiol., *8*:193, 1982.
100. Murray, D. S.: Fatigue fractures of the lower tibia and fibula in the same leg. J. Bone Joint Surg., *39-B*:302, 1957.
101. Nand, S., and Shukla, R. K.: Fatigue fractures of the femoral neck. Int. Surg., *61*:31, 1976.
102. Nicastro, J. F., and Haupt, H. A.: Probable stress fracture of the cuboid in an infant. A case report. J. Bone Joint Surg., *66-A*:1106, 1984.
103. Nix, R. A.: Stress fractures in the lower extremity. J. Arkansas Med. Soc., *80*:10, 1983.
104. Noakes, T. D.: Diagnosis of stress fracture in athletes (letter). J.A.M.A., *254*:3422, 1985.
105. North, K. A.: Multiple stress fractures simulating osteomalacia. A.J.R., *97*:672, 1966.
106. O'Boyle, C. M.: Sports injuries in adolescents: Emergency care. Am. J. Nurs., *75*:1732, 1975.
107. Ollenquist, I. J.: Osteopathia itineraria tibiae. Acta Radiol., *18*:526, 1937.
108. Orava, S.: Stress fractures. Br. J. Sports Med., *14*:40, 1980.
109. Orava, S., Jormakka, E., and Hulkko, A.: Stress fractures in young athletes. Arch. Orthop. Trauma. Surg., *98*:271, 1981.
110. Orava, S., Puranen, J., and Ala-Ketola, L.: Stress fractures caused by physical exercise. Acta Orthop. Scand., *49*:19, 1978.
111. Park, C. H., Kapadia, D., and O'Hara, A. E.: Three phase bone scan findings in stress fracture. Clin. Nucl. Med., *6*:587, 1981.
112. Patel, M. R., Irizarry, J., and Stricevic, M.: Stress fracture of the ulnar diaphysis: Review of the literature and report of a case. J. Hand Surg., *11-A*:443, 1986.
113. Pavlos, H., et al.: Tarsal navicular stress fractures: Radiographic evaluation. Radiology, *148*:641, 1983.
114. Pentecost, R. L., Murray, R. A., and Brindley, H. H.: Fatigue, insufficiency, and pathologic fractures. J.A.M.A., *187*:1001, 1964.
115. Percy, E. C., and Gamble, F. O.: An epiphyseal stress fracture of the foot and shin splints in an anomalous calf muscle in a runner. Br. J. Sports Med., *14*:110, 1980.
116. Perl, T., and Carsky, E. W.: Stress fractures in children. N.Y. J. Med., *66*:391, 1966.
117. Perry, C. R., Perry, H. M., III, and Burdge, R. E.: Stress fracture of the radius following a fracture of the ulnar diaphysis. Clin. Orthop., *187*:193, 1984.
118. Pietron, K., Kozlowski, K., and Boruch, Z.: Stress fractures of the metatarsals in children. Ann. Radiol. (Paris), *15*:149, 1972.
119. Pilgaard, S., Poulsen, J. O., and Christensen, J. H.: Stress fractures. Acta Orthop. Scand., *47*:167, 1976.
120. Podlaha, M., and Podlahov, A. J.: Creeping fatigue fractures in children. Cesk. Radiol., *22*:57, 1968.
121. Prather, J. L., Nusynowitz, M. L., Snowdy, H. A., Hughes, A. D., McCartney, W. H., and Bagg, R. J.: Scintigraphic findings in stress fractures. J. Bone Joint Surg., *59-A*:839, 1977.
122. Provost, R. A., and Morris, J. M.: Fatigue fracture of the femoral shaft. J. Bone Joint Surg., *51-A*:487, 1969.
123. Rafii, M., Firooznia, H., Golimbu, C., and Sokolow, J.: Bilateral acetabular stress fractures in a paraplegic patient. Arch. Phys. Med. Rehabil., *63*:240, 1982.
124. Rappoport, A. S., Sosman, J. L., and Weissman, B. N.: Spontaneous fractures of the olecranon process in rheumatoid arthritis. Radiology, *119*:83, 1976.
125. Rasad, S.: Golfer's fractures of the ribs. Report of 3 cases. A.J.R., *120*:901, 1974.
126. Rettig, A. C.: Stress fracture of the ulna in an adolescent tournament tennis player. Am. J. Sports Med., *11*:103, 1983.
127. Richmond, D. A.: Fatigue fracture of the fibula: Report on two cases. Lancet, *1*:273, 1945.
128. Rivera, J. J., Mason, B. E., and Anderson, P. J.: Diagnostic imaging in stress fracture. Bol. Assoc. Med. P.R., *74*:22, 1982.
129. Roberts, S. M., and Vogt, E. C.: Pseudofracture of the tibia. J. Bone Joint Surg., *21*:891, 1939.
130. Robin, P. A., and Thompson, S. B.: Fatigue fractures. J. Bone Joint Surg., *26*:557, 1944.
131. Ross, D. G., *et al.*: Tibial stress fracture in pyrophosphate arthropathy. J. Bone Joint Surg., *65-B*:474, 1983.
132. Samuel, E.: Fatigue (insufficiency) fracture of the tibia. S. Afr. Med. J., *29*:89, 1955.
133. Sandrock, A. R.: Another sports fatigue fracture. Stress fracture of the coracoid process of the scapula. Radiology, *117*:274, 1975.
134. Savoca, C. J.: Stress fractures. A classification of the earliest radiographic signs. Radiology, *100*:519, 1971.
135. Sawmiller, S., Michener, W. M., and Hartman, J. T.: Stress fracture in childhood. Cleve. Clin. Q., *32*:119, 1965.
136. Schneider, H. J., King, A. Y., Bronson, J. L., and Miller, E. H.: Stress injuries and developmental changes of lower extremities in ballet dancers. Radiology, *113*:627, 1974.
137. Schneider, R., and Kaye, J. J.: Insufficiency and stress fractures of the long bones occurring in patients with rheumatoid arthritis. Radiology, *116*:595, 1975.
138. Sherman, F. C., Wilkinson, R. H., and Hall, J. E.:

Reactive sclerosis of a pedicle and spondylolysis in the lumbar spine. J. Bone Joint Surg., *59-A*:49, 1977.
139. Siffert, R. S., and Levy, R. N.: Athletic injuries in children. Pediatr. Clin. North Am., *12*:1027, 1965.
140. Singer, M., and Maudsley, R. H.: Fatigue fractures of lower tibia: Report of five cases. J. Bone Joint Surg., *36-B*:647, 1954.
141. Stanitski, C. L., McMaster, J. H., and Scranton, P. E.: On the nature of stress fractures. Am. J. Sports Med., *6*:391, 1978.
142. Stark, H. H., Jobe, F. W., Boyes, J. H., and Ashworth, C. R.: Fracture of the hook of the hamate in athletes. J. Bone Joint Surg., *59-A*:575, 1977.
143. Stein, R. E., and Stelling, F. H.: Stress fracture of the calcaneus in a child with cerebral palsy. J. Bone Joint Surg., *59A*:131, 1977.
144. Subbarao, K.: Radiologic problem of the month. Stress fractures involving anterior tibial cortex. N.Y. J. Med., *80*:1419, 1980.
145. Symeonides, P. P.: High stress fractures of the fibula. J. Bone Joint Surg., *62-B*:192, 1980.
146. Taunton, J. E., Clement, D. B., and Webber, D.: Lower extremity stress fractures in athletes. Phys. Sports Med., *9*:77, 1981.
147. Tondeur, G., and Bosman, J.: Spontaneous fractures in the child. Acta Orthop. Belg., *32*:825, 1966.
148. Torg, J. S., and Moyer, R. A.: Non-union of a stress fracture through the olecranon epiphyseal plate observed in an adolescent baseball pitcher. J. Bone Joint Surg., *52-A*:376, 1970.
149. Torg, J. S., Pollack, H., and Sweterlitsch, P.: The effect of competitive pitching on the shoulders and elbows of preadolescent baseball players. Pediatrics, *49*:267, 1972.
150. Tountas, A. A., and Waddell, J. P.: Stress fractures of the femoral neck. A report of seven cases. Clin. Orthop., *210*:160, 1986.
151. Towne, L. C., Blazina, M. E., and Cozen, L. N.: Fatigue fracture of the tarsal navicular. J. Bone Joint Surg., *52-A*:376, 1970.
152. Tullos, H. S., and Fain, R. H.: Little League shoulder: Rotational stress fracture of proximal epiphysis. J. Sports Med., *2*:152, 1974.
153. Van Hal, M. E., Keene, J. S., Lange, T. A., and Clancy, W. G., Jr.: Stress fractures of the great toe sesamoids. Am. J. Sports Med., *10*:122, 1982.
154. Volder, J. G.: A case of a stress fracture in a child. Arch. Chir. Nedrl., *24*:43, 1972.
155. Walter, N. E., and Wolf, M. D.: Stress fractures in young athletes. Am. J. Sports Med., *5*:165, 1977.
156. Wang, C. C., Lowrey, C. W., and Severance, R. L.: Fatigue fracture of pelvis and lower extremity. N. Engl. J. Med., *260*:958, 1959.
157. Weaver, J. B., and Francisco, C. B.: Pseudofractures: A manifestation of non-suppurative osteomyelitis. J. Bone Joint Surg., *22*:610, 1940.
158. Wilcox, J. R., Jr., Moniot, A. L., and Green, J. P.: Bone scanning in the evaluation of exercise-related stress injuries. Radiology, *123*:699, 1977.
159. Wilson, E. S., and Katz, F. N.: Stress fractures. Radiology, *92*:481, 1969.
160. Wiltse, L. L., Widell, E. H., Jr., and Jackson, D. W.: Fatigue fracture: The basic lesion of isthmic spondylolisthesis. J. Bone Joint Surg., *57-A*:17, 1975.
161. Winfield, A. C., and Dennis, J. M.: Stress fracture of the calcaneus. Radiology, *72*:415, 1959.
162. Wolfe, H. R. I., and Robertson, J. M.: Fatigue fracture of femur and tibia. Lancet, *2*:11, 1945.
163. Wolfgang, G. L.: Stress fracture of the femoral neck in a patient with open capital femoral epiphyses. A case report. J. Bone Joint Surg., *59-A*:680, 1977.
164. Wright, T. M., and Hayes, W. C.: The fracture mechanics of fatigue crack propagation in compact bone. J. Biomed. Mater. Res., *7*:637, 1976.

PATHOLOGIC FRACTURES

Pathologic fractures are those that are caused by minimal trauma in bones that have been weakened by some generalized abnormality or local disease. Pathologic fractures may be classified as follows:

Those due to generalized abnormalities of the skeleton

- Developmental affections
  - Osteogenesis imperfecta
  - Osteopetrosis or marble bone disease
  - Arachnodactyly
- Vitamin deficiency and endocrine disorders
  - Scurvy
  - Rickets
  - Hyperparathyroidism—primary and secondary
  - Hyperpituitarism or Cushing's syndrome
  - From cortisone treatment
- Disuse atrophy
  - Due to immobilization
  - Paralytic diseases of neuromuscular system—myelomeningocele, poliomyelitis, cerebral palsy, arthrogryposis multiplex congenita

Those due to local causes

- Inflammatory conditions
  - Osteomyelitis
  - Rheumatoid arthritis
- Postirradiation local osteoporosis
- Benign tumors or tumorous lesions
  - Nonossifying fibroma (Fig. 8–193)
  - Fibrous dysplasia
  - Unicameral bone cyst
  - Enchondroma
  - Aneurysmal bone cyst
  - Neurofibromatosis
- Malignant bone tumors
  - Primary—such as osteogenic sarcoma
  - Metastatic—such as Wilms' tumor or neuroblastoma

The possibility that a fracture is pathologic should be suspected whenever it is produced by trivial injury. The radiograms should be carefully studied to rule out the presence of local or generalized bone disease. The diagnosis and treatment of the foregoing entities have been described under the individual lesions elsewhere in the textbook.

THE BATTERED CHILD

A battered child is one who is a victim of deliberate nonaccidental physical trauma that has been inflicted by a person or persons responsible for his care.

Although reports of physical abuse of children

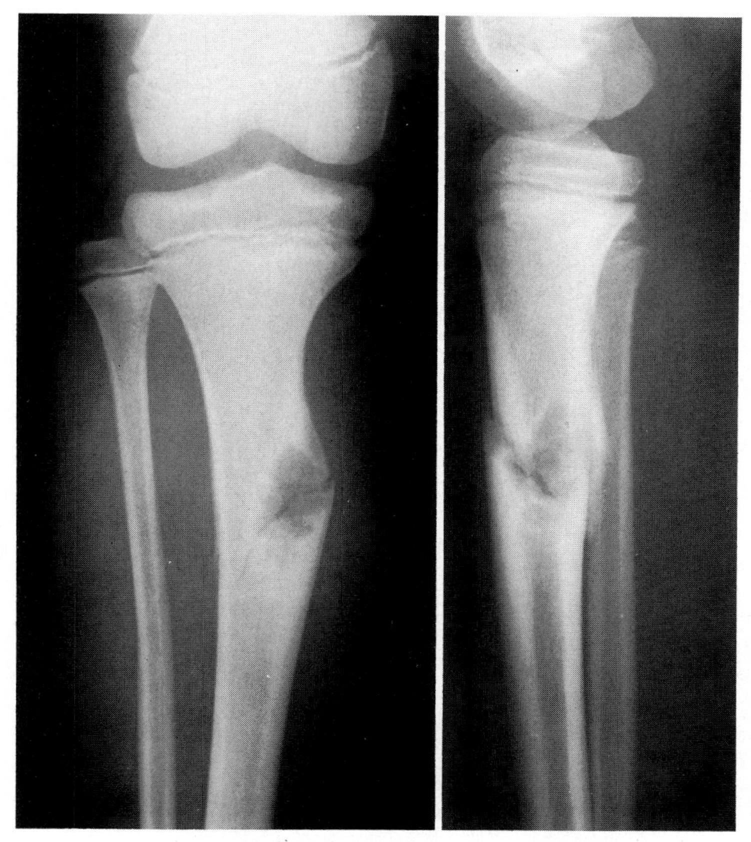

FIGURE 8–193. Pathologic fracture through a nonossifying fibroma.

antedate the discovery of roentgen rays, the syndrome of the battered child was not recognized until the signs of bone injury and repair were depicted in the roentgenograms. Caffey, in 1946, first drew attention to the association of multiple fractures of long bones with a significant number of cases of subdural hematoma.[22] Initially, these fractures were thought to be pathologic, occurring spontaneously in bones with some structural abnormality. In 1953, Silverman presented a report on multiple long bone fractures without subdural hematoma in three children, and established their traumatic basis.[103] The condition is sometimes referred to as Silverman's syndrome. Woolley emphasized that the radiographic manifestations of injury and its repair were identical, whether a history of injury was or was not obtained and regardless of the presence or absence of subdural hematoma. He also reviewed the undesirable environmental factors and family circumstances that led to physical attack on these children.[127] Since then, numerous reports have appeared in the literature, which lucidly delineate the syndrome of the battered child. The problem is complex, with many psychopathologic, social, and legal aspects; for a discussion of these, the reader is referred to the monograph on the subject by Helfer and Kempe.[54]

Battered children tend to be very young, about two thirds of them being under three years and one third under six months of age. Boys are slightly more subject to parent-induced trauma than girls. The abused child is usually in poor general health, underweight, malnourished, and retarded in development.

Suspicion is usually aroused when, on presentation of the child at the emergency room, the history of injury as given by the parents is obviously unsatisfactory or too facile. The parents of these children are usually in their mid-twenties and are emotionally maladjusted. Multiple fractures, evidence of repeated trauma, and bruises and lacerations should make the condition further suspect. The deformity of gross fractures is obvious.

The characteristic features of skeletal lesions in the battered child syndrome are well described by Silverman; there is predilection for the metaphysis, exaggerated periosteal reaction, and multiplicity of lesions in various stages of healing and repair (Figs. 8–194 and 8–195).[103]

Trauma is inflicted by vigorous pulling on the

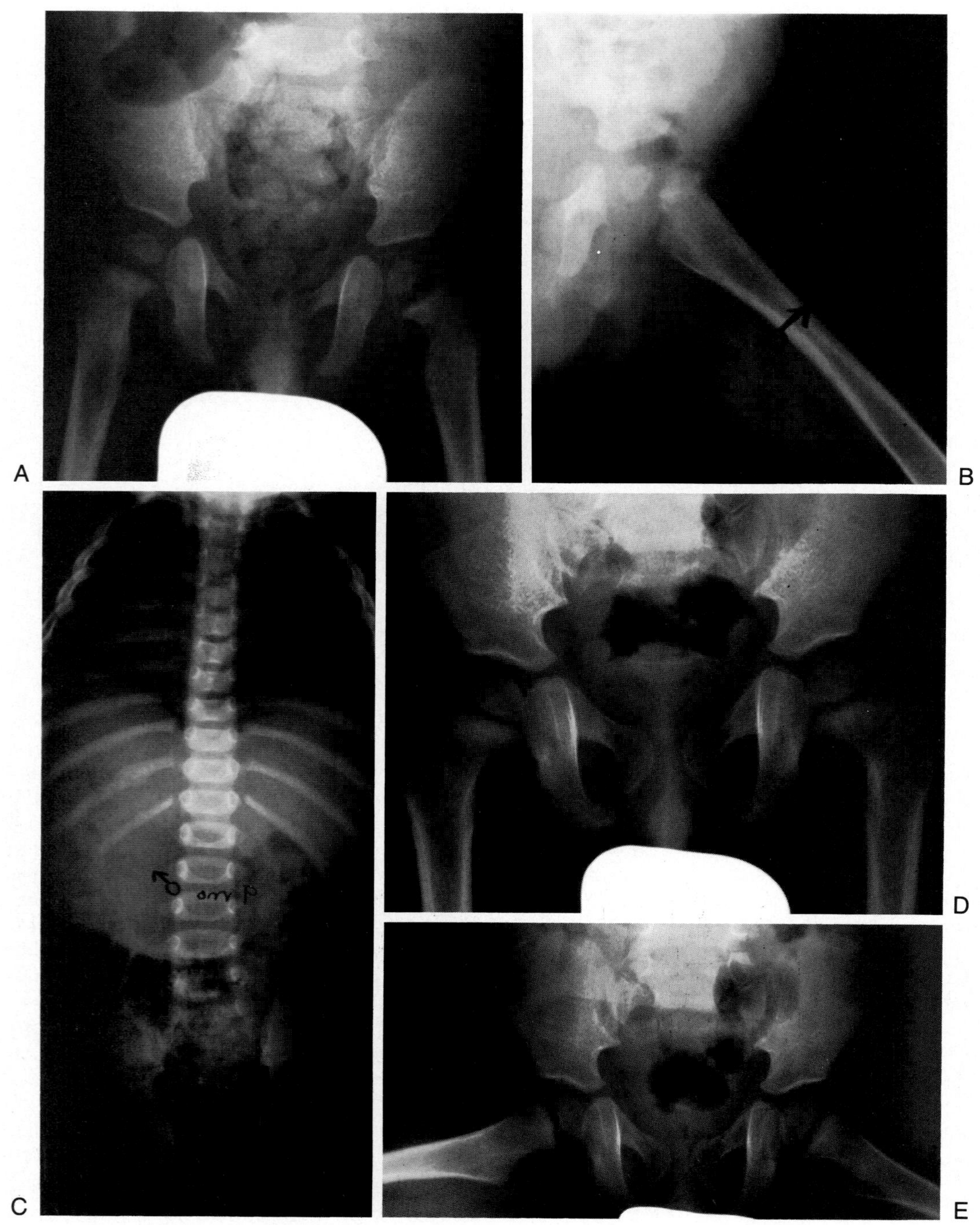

FIGURE 8–194. A six-month-old battered child with Slater-Harris Type I physeal fracture of the left capital femoral epiphysis and fracture of the eleventh rib.

A and **B.** Initial anteroposterior and true lateral radiograms of the left hip. Note the displaced capital femoral epiphysis on the left. **C.** Anteroposterior radiogram of the spine and the thoracic cage. Note the healing fracture of the eleventh rib on the left. The fractured hip was treated by immobilization in a spica cast for six weeks. **D** and **E.** Two years later showing the healed fracture with no residual deformity.

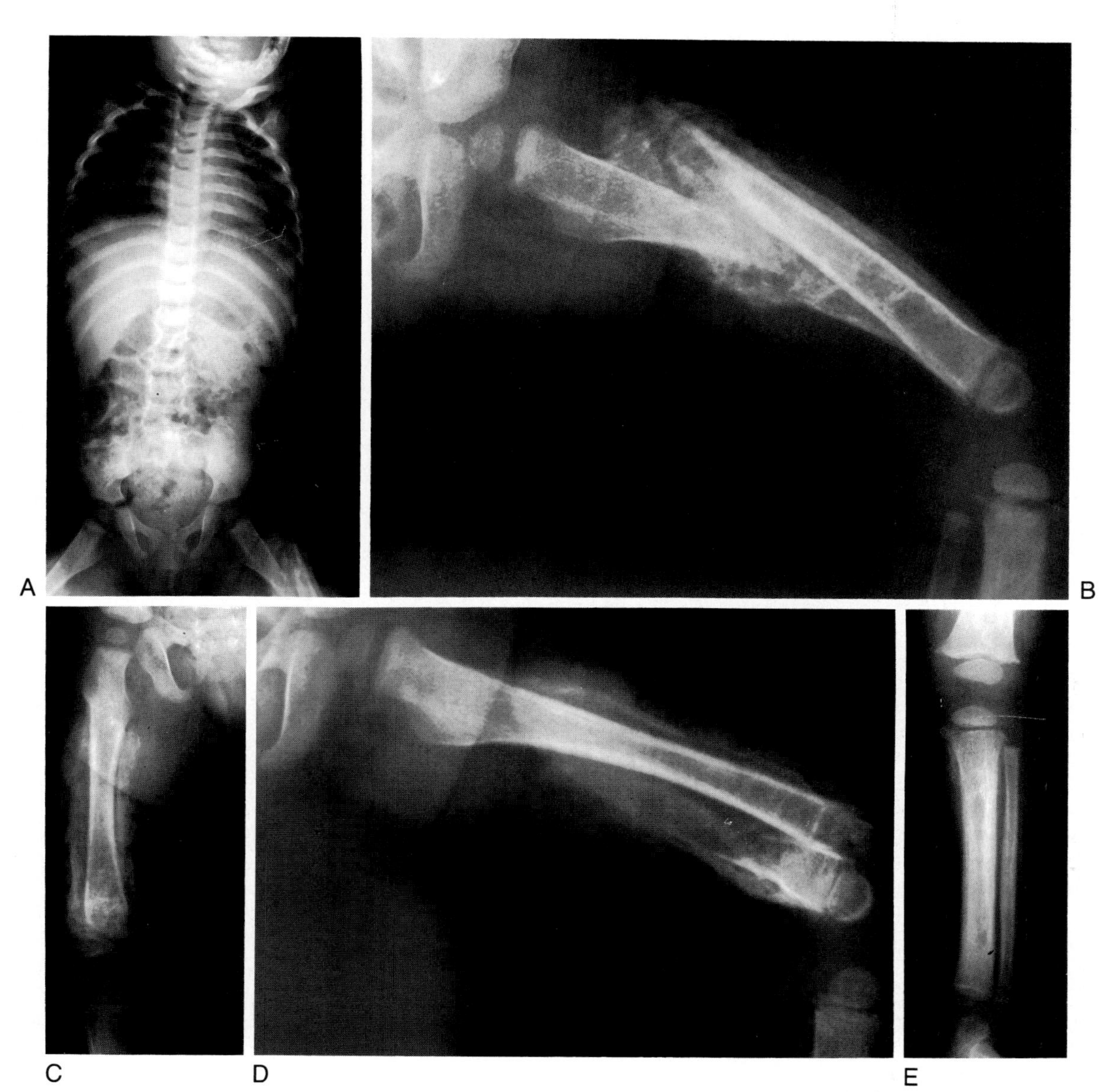

FIGURE 8–195. Battered child with multiple fractures in various stages of healing.

A. Anteroposterior radiogram of the spine and hips showing the fractured femur on the left with marked angulation and healing callus. **B.** Lateral radiogram of the left femur showing the marked anterior angulation. **C** and **D.** Anteroposterior radiogram of the right femur showing the distal femoral physeal fracture with extensive subperiosteal new bone formation. **E.** Anteroposterior view of the right tibia showing the proximal physeal fracture separation with subperiosteal new bone formation.

Illustration continued on following page

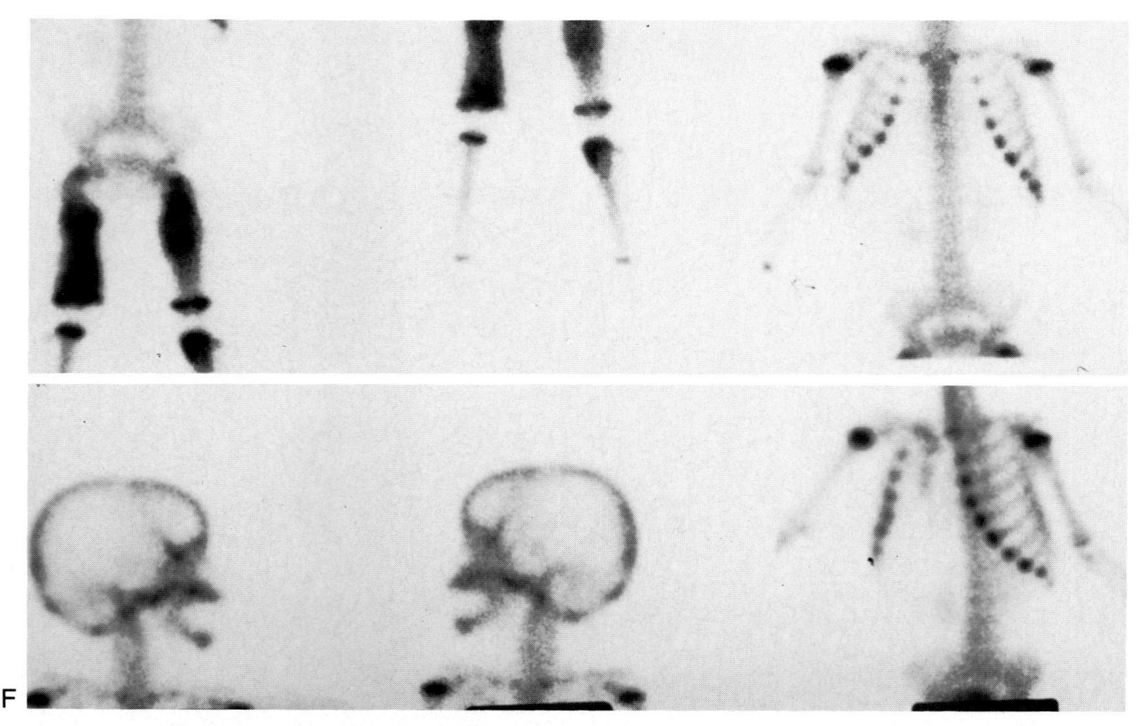

FIGURE 8–195 Continued. Battered child with multiple fractures in various stages of healing.

F. Bone scan with technetium-99m showing increased uptake at the fracture sites.

limbs, direct blows, or throwing the child around. Since the victim is usually an infant or a young child, physeal injuries with gross or minimal displacement of the epiphysis are common. Recent injury may show only soft-tissue swelling in the radiograms; the older injury will be evident by abundant subperiosteal new bone formation and later by the relatively thick, dense cortex. The repetitive nature of the injury is hallmarked by the presence of various stages of bone repair. In the diagnostic work-up of a battered child, a bone scan with technetium-99m and radiograms of suspect areas are essential. The possibility of subdural hematoma must always be considered. Injuries to visceral organs can occur; rupture of the small intestine, laceration of the liver, perforation of the stomach, laceration of the lung, and subpleural hemorrhage have been reported.[78]

In the differential diagnosis, one should rule out osteogenesis imperfecta, congenital insensitivity to pain, scurvy, congenital lues, and infantile cortical hyperostosis.

Management of various skeletal injuries is described in the sections on treatment of fractures of the specific bones.

It is the duty of physicians to report their suspicions to appropriate authorities, with the understanding that the reporter is granted immunity from legal liability that might follow from making such a report.

In the United States, protective child legislation requires that a welfare department investigate and offer social services to families in cases of alleged child abuse. If this is refused, the case is brought to the attention of the juvenile court.

The battered child should be placed in a foster home and should not be returned to his original environment. The probability of abuse of other children in the same family should be investigated, as well as the possibility of a neighbor or sibling's being the person who inflicted the trauma.

References

1. Akbarnia, B. A., and Akbarnia, N. O.: The role of orthopedist in child abuse and neglect. Orthop. Clin. North Am., 7:733, 1976.
2. Akbarnia, B., Torg, J. S., Kirkpatrick, J., and Sussman, S.: Manifestations of the battered child syndrome. J. Bone Joint Surg., 56-A:1159, 1974.

3. Altman, D. H., and Smith, R. L.: Unrecognized trauma in infants and children. J. Bone Joint Surg., *42-A*:407, 1960.
4. Amacher, A. L.: Child-battering and the social order. Indian J. Pediatr., *44*:212, 1977.
5. Armanda Torrelio, E., and Casanovas Vargas, M. C.: The battered child syndrome. Preliminary review in a Bolivian pediatric hospital. Bol. Med. Hosp. Infant. Mex., *36*:923, 1979.
6. Astley, R.: Multiple metaphyseal fractures in small children. Br. J. Radiol., *26*:577, 1953.
7. Baetz, K., Sledziewski, W., Margetts, D., Koren, L., Levy, M., and Pepper, R.: Recognition and management of the battered child syndrome. J. Dent. Assoc. S. Afr., *32*:13, 1977.
8. Bakwin, H.: Multiple skeletal lesions in young children due to trauma. J. Pediatr., *49*:7, 1956.
9. Balaban, I., Ciofu, E., Viasceanu, S., Diaconu, T., and Popescu, V.: The Caffey-Kempe syndrome (battered children syndrome). Diagnostic problems. Rev. Pediatr. Obstet. Ginecol., *26*:321, 1977.
10. Baron, M. A., Bejar, R. L., and Sheaff, P. J.: Neurologic manifestations of the battered child syndrome. Pediatrics, *45*:1003, 1970.
11. Barrett, I. R., and Kozlowski, K.: The battered child syndrome. Australas. Radiol., *23*:72, 1979.
12. Beals, R. K., and Rufts, E.: Fractured femur in infancy: The role of child abuse. J. Pediatr. Orthop., *3*:583, 1983.
13. Ben-Youssef, L., and Schmidt, T. L.: Battered child syndrome simulating myositis. J. Pediatr. Orthop., *3*:392, 1983.
14. Biermann, G.: Kinderzuchtigung und Kindesmisshandlung, eine Dokumentation. Munich, 1969.
15. Birrell, R. G., and Birrell, J. H.: The maltreatment syndrome in children: A hospital survey. Med. J. Aust., *2*:1023, 1968.
16. Blount, J. G.: Radiologic seminar 138: The battered child. J. Miss. State Med. Assoc., *15*:136, 1974.
17. Bornstein, S., Martel, J., Ruat, A., and Harlay, A.: Perpetrators of child abuse. Ann. Med. Psychol., *138*:939, 1980.
18. Boshoff, E.: Battered child syndrome. Nurs. J., *44*:12, 1977.
19. Brailsford, J. F.: Ossifying hematoma and other simple lesions mistaken for sarcomata. Br. J. Radiol., *21*:157, 1948.
20. British Paediatric Association: The battered baby. Br. Med. J., *1*:601, 1966.
21. Brosseau, B. E.: Battered child and unwanted pregnancy (letter). Can. Med. Assoc. J., *112*:1039, 1975.
22. Caffey, J.: Multiple fractures in the long bones of infants suffering from chronic subdural hematoma. A.J.R., *56*:163, 1946.
23. Caffey, J.: Significance of the history in the diagnosis of traumatic injury to children. J. Pediatr., *67*:1008, 1965.
24. Caffey, J.: The parent-infant traumatic stress syndrome (Caffey-Kempe syndrome). Battered baby syndrome. The First Annual Neuhauser Presidential Address of the Society for Pediatric Radiology. A.J.R., *114*:217, 1972.
25. Cameron, J. M.: The battered baby syndrome. Practitioner, *209*:302, 1972.
26. Child abuse editorial. Lancet, 2:929, 1978.
27. Cohen, S. J., and Sussman, A.: The incidence of child abuse in the United States. Child Welfare, *54*:432, 1975.
28. Cremin, B. J.: Battered baby syndrome. S. Afr. Med. J., *44*:1044, 1970.
29. Cullen, J. C.: Spinal lesions in battered babies. J. Bone Joint Surg., *57-B*:364, 1975.
30. Curran, W. J.: Failure to diagnose battered-child syndrome. N. Engl. J. Med., *296*:795, 1977.
31. Dickson, R. A., and Leatherman, K. D.: Spinal injuries in child abuse: Case report. J. Trauma, *18*:811, 1978.
32. Donna, S. P., and Duckworth, P. M.: Suspected child abuse: Experience in Guy's Hospital Accident & Emergency Department. Guy's Hosp. Rep., *121*:295, 1972.
33. Duke, R. F.: Battered babies (letter). Br. Med. J., *2*:194, 1975.
34. Ebbin, A. J., Gollub, M. H., Stein, A. M., and Wilson, M. G.: Battered child syndrome at the Los Angeles County General Hospital. Am. J. Dis. Child., *118*:660, 1969.
35. Ellerstein, N. W.: Maltreated children requiring hospitalization, thirteen-year study. N.Y. State J. Med., *78*:1704, 1978.
36. Farn, K. T.: Deaths from non-accidental injury in children. Br. Med. J., *3*:1145, 1980.
37. Fiser, R. H., Kaplan, J., and Holder, J. C.: Congenital syphilis mimicking the battered child syndrome. How does one tell them apart? Clin. Pediatr., *11*:305, 1975.
38. Fisher, S. H.: Skeletal manifestations of parent-induced trauma in infants and children. South. Med. J., *51*:956, 1985.
39. Friedman, M. S.: Traumatic periostitis in infants and children. J.A.M.A., *166*:1840, 1958.
40. Friedman, S. B., and Morse, C. W.: Child abuse: A five year follow-up of early case findings in the emergency department. Pediatrics, *54*:404, 1974.
41. Friedrich, W. N., Einbender, A. J., and Luecke, W. J.: Cognitive and behavioral characteristics of physically abused children. J. Consult. Clin. Psychol., *51*:313, 1983.
42. Fritch, C. D.: Battered baby syndrome in an infant with severe retinopathy of prematurity. Ann. Ophthalmol., *15*:132, 1983.
43. Galleno, H., and Oppenheim, W. L.: The battered child syndrome revisited. Clin. Orthop., *162*:11, 1982.
44. Gelles, R. J.: Violence toward children in the United States. Am. J. Orthopsychiatry, *48*:580, 1978.
45. Gille, P., Bonneville, J. F., Francois, J. Y., Aubert, D., Peltre, G., and Canal, J. P.: Fractures of axis pedicles in battered infant. Chir. Pediatr., *21*:343, 1980.
46. Gray, D. R., and Leaverton, D. R.: Physical child abuse: A review of all cases seen at Sacramento Medical Center in 1975. West. J. Med., *129*:461, 1978.
47. Green, A. H.: Self-destructive behavior in battered children. Am. J. Psychiatry, *135*:579, 1978.
48. Greinacher, I., and Troger, J.: The so-called "battered child syndrome" from the viewpoint of the pediatric radiologist. Radiologe, *22*:342, 1982.
49. Griffiths, D. L., and Moynihan, F. J.: Multiple epiphyseal injuries in babies ("battered baby syndrome"). Br. Med. J., *2*:1, 1963.
50. Grossman, M.: Editorial: Physical child abuse. West. J. Med., *129*:493, 1978.
51. Gwinn, J. L., Lewin, K. W., and Peterson, H. G., Jr.: Roentgenographic manifestations of unsuspected trauma in infancy. J.A.M.A., *176*:926, 1962.
52. Harcke, H. T., Jr.: Bone imaging in infants and children, a review. J. Nucl. Med., *19*:324, 1978.
53. Hardy, M., McElroy, E., and Patchett, D. R.: Prevention of baby battering. Practitioner, *222*:243, 1979.
54. Helfer, R. E., and Kempe, C. H. (eds.): The Battered Child. Chicago, University of Chicago Press, 1968.
55. Herndon, W. A.: Child abuse in a military population. J. Pediatr. Orthop., *3*:73, 1983.
56. High, D. W., Bakalar, H. R., and Lloyd, J. R.: Inflicted burns in children. Recognition and treatment. J.A.M.A., *242*:517, 1979.
57. Hiller, H. G.: Battered or not—a reappraisal of metaphyseal fragility. A.J.R., *114*:241, 1972.

58. Hilton, J. E.: Battered babies. Practitioner, *221*:607, 1978.
59. Horodniceanu, C., Grunebaum, M., Volovitz, B., and Nitzan, M.: Unusual bone involvement in congenital syphilis mimicking the battered child syndrome. Pediatr. Radiol., *7*:232, 1978.
60. Iida, Y.: Battered child syndrome. Nippon Rinsho, *1*:1158, 1977.
61. Jenkins, J., and Gray, O. P.: Changing clinical picture of non-accidental injury to children. Br. Med. J., *10*:1767, 1983.
62. Kempe, C. H., and Helfer, R. E.: Helping the Battered Child and His Family. Philadelphia, Lippincott, 1972.
63. Kempe, C. H., Silverman, F. N., Steele, B. F., Droegemueller, W., and Silver, H. K.: The battered child syndrome. J.A.M.A., *181*:17, 1962.
64. Kimmel, R. L., and Sty, J. R.: 99mTc-methylene diphosphonate renal images in a battered child. Clin. Nucl. Med., *4*:166, 1979.
65. Kirks, D. R.: Radiological evaluation of visceral injuries in the battered child syndrome. Pediatr. Ann., *12*:888, 1983.
66. Kleinman, P. K., Marks, S. C., and Blackbourne, B.: The metaphyseal lesion in abused infants: A radiologic-histopathologic study. A.J.R., *146*:895, 1986.
67. Kleinman, P. K., Raptopoulos, V. D., and Brill, P. W.: Occult nonskeletal trauma in the battered-child syndrome. Radiology, *141*:393, 1981.
68. Kogutt, M. S., Swischuk, L. E., and Fagan, C. J.: Patterns of injury and significance of uncommon fractures in the battered child syndrome. Am. J. Roentgenol. Radium Ther. Nucl. Med., *121*:143, 1974.
69. Krige, H. N.: The abused child complex and its characteristic x-ray findings. S. Afr. Med. J., *40*:490, 1966.
70. Kumar, K., Khan, A. J., Flicker, S., Soborio, J., Schaeffer, H. A., and Evans, H. E.: Acute renal failure in battered child syndrome. J. Natl. Med. Assoc., *72*:27, 1980.
71. Kurland, R. L., Bianco, A. J., Jr., Hick, J. F., Hoffman, A. D., and Duffney, V.: Child abuse. Minn. Med., *65*:477, 1982.
72. Lagerberg, D.: Child abuse; a literature review. Acta Paediatr. Scand., *67*:683, 1978.
73. Laing, S. A.: Bilateral injuries in childhood, an altering sign? (letter). Br. Med. J., *2*:1355, 1977.
74. Lascari, A. D.: The abused child. J. Iowa Med. Soc., *62*:229, 1972.
75. Leonidas, J. C.: Skeletal trauma in the child abuse syndrome. Pediatr. Ann., *12*:875, 1983.
76. Lis, E. F., and Frauenberger, G. S.: Multiple fractures associated with subdural hematoma in infancy. Pediatrics, *6*:890, 1950.
77. McAnarney, E.: The older abused child (letter). Pediatrics, *55*:298, 1975.
78. McCort, J., and Vandagua, J.: Visceral injuries in battered children. Radiology, *82*:424, 1964.
79. MacFarlane, I. J.: Hip problems in a battered child: A case report. Aust. N.Z. J. Surg., *49*:107, 1979.
80. McHenry, T., Girdany, B. R., and Elmer, E.: Unsuspected trauma with multiple skeletal injuries during infancy and childhood. Pediatrics, *31*:903, 1963.
81. Margrain, S. A.: Review: Battered children, their parents, treatment and prevention. Child Care Health Dev., *3*:49, 1977.
82. Marten, D. F.: Introduction. The battered child syndrome: The role of radiological imaging. Pediatr. Ann., *12*:867, 1983.
83. Marten, D. F., and Osborne, D. R.: Craniocerebral trauma in the child abuse syndrome. Pediatr. Ann., *12*:882, 1983.
84. Marten, D. F., Kirks, D. R., and Ruderman, R. J.: Occult humeral epiphyseal fracture in battered infants. Pediatr. Radiol., *10*:151, 1981.
85. Meeting of the Eastern and Northern Pediatric Societies. Round table on the battered child. Pediatrie, *35*:84, 1980.
86. Milowe, I., and Lourie, R.: The child's role in the battered child syndrome. J. Pediatr., *65*:1079, 1964.
87. Money, J.: Child abuse, growth failure, IQ deficit, and learning disability. J. Learn. Disabil., *15*:579, 1982.
88. Naumann, P.: Child abuse. Munch. Med. Wochenschr., *109*:1703, 1967.
89. O'Neill, J. A., Jr., Meacham, W. F., Griffin, J. P., and Sawyers, J. L.: Patterns of injury in the battered child syndrome. J. Trauma, *13*:332, 1973.
90. Paterson, C. R.: Vitamin D deficiency rickets simulating child abuse. J. Pediatr. Orthop., *1*:423, 1981.
91. Pickett, W. J., Faleski, E. J., Chacko, A., and Jarrett, R. V.: Comparison of radiographic and radionuclide skeletal surveys in battered children. South. Med. J., *76*:207, 1983.
92. Radkowski, M. A.: The battered child syndrome: Pitfalls in radiological diagnosis. Pediatr. Ann., *12*:894, 1983.
93. Rivara, F. P., Kamitsuka, M. D., and Quan, L.: Injuries to children younger than 1 year of age. Pediatrics, *81*:93, 1988.
94. Rose, C. B.: Unusual periostitis in children. Radiology, *27*:131, 1936.
95. Roussey, M., LeFrancois, M. C., LeMarec, B., Gandon, Y., Carsin, M., and Senecal, J.: Cranial CT in child abuse. Ann. Radiol. (Paris), *25*:237, 1982.
96. Roussey, M., LeFrancois, M. C., LeMarec, B., Gandon, Y., Carsin, M., and Senecal, J.: Cranial tomodensitometry in battered children. Ann. Pediatr. (Paris), *30*:95, 1983.
97. Salmon, M. A.: The spectrum of abuse in the battered child syndrome. Injury, *2*:211, 1971.
98. Sauer, H., Kurz, R., and Fink, M.: Thoraco-abdominal injuries and bone fractures in the battered child syndrome. Monatsschr. Unfallheilkd., *78*:533, 1975.
99. Schleberger, R., Schulze, H., and Kemperdick, F.: The battered child syndrome from the orthopedic point of view. Z. Orthop., *121*:23, 1983.
100. Schwokowksi, C. F.: Severe traumatic destruction of both knee joints and multiple face hematomas in an 8-month old infant, a contribution on the "battered child syndrome." Zentralbl. Chir., *92*:2484, 1967.
101. Scott, P. D.: Non-accidental injury in children. Memorandum of evidence to the Parliamentary Select Committee on Violence in the Family. Br. J. Psychiatry, *131*:366, 1977.
102. Shaw, A.: The surgeon and the battered child. Surg. Gynecol. Obstet., *119*:355, 1964.
103. Silverman, F. N.: The roentgen manifestations of unrecognized skeletal trauma in infants. A.J.R., *69*:413, 1953.
104. Silverman, F. N.: Unrecognized trauma in infants, the battered child syndrome, and the syndrome of Ambroise Tardieu. Radiology, *104*:337, 1972.
105. Silverman, F. N.: Problems in pediatric fractures. Semin. Roentgenol., *13*:167, 1978.
106. Simons, B., Downs, E. F., Hurster, M. N., and Archer, M.: Child abuse: Epidemiologic study of medically reported cases. N.Y. State J. Med., *66*:2783, 1966.
107. Smith, M. J.: Subdural hematoma with multiple fractures. A.J.R., *63*:342, 1950.
108. Solomons, G., and Young, H. A.: Malpractice and child abuse. J. Iowa Med. Soc., *68*:239, 1978.
109. Sopher, I. M.: The dentist and the battered child syndrome. Dent. Clin. North Am., *21*:113, 1977.
110. Sriram, K., Rathnavel, S., Papkumari, M., and So-

masundaram, O.: Battered baby syndrome: A review of eight cases. Ann. Acad. Med. Singapore, *10*:466, 1981.
111. Swischuk, L. E.: Spine and spinal cord trauma in the battered child syndrome. Radiology, *92*:733, 1969.
112. Tanous, H., and Vance, B.: Battered babies: Their screams of terror go unheard. Leg. Aspects Med. Pract., *6*:31, 1978.
113. Taylor, M. R., and Kevany, J. P.: Battered babies in hospital—pathways for their care. Ir. Med. J., *69*:79, 1977.
114. Trevisio, A., Colonna, F., Pepino, G., and DiCagno, L.: Battered children. Cases during a period of 7 years observed in the University Institutes of Pediatrics and the Regina Margherita Infantile Hospital of Turin. Minerva Pediatr., *30*:1643, 1978.
115. Troger, J.: The battered child. Radiologe, *18*:233, 1978.
116. Trube-Becker, E.: Die Kindesmisshandlung und ihre Folgen. Padiat. Praxis, *12*:389, 1973.
117. Trube-Becker, E.: Bite-marks on battered children. Z. Rechtsmed., *79*:73, 1977.
118. Vicuna, J. R.: The battered child: Epidemiological, clinical and juridico-social considerations. Rev. Chil. Pediatr., *52*:333, 1981.
119. Wahlgren, V., and Yngve, D. A · Child abuse. Orthopedics, *9*:275, 1986.
120. Weber, A.: Child abuse. Praxis, *57*:188, 1968.
121. Wecht, C. H., and Larkin, G. M.: The battered child syndrome, a forensic pathologist's viewpoint. Leg. Med., *31*, 1980.
122. Wecht, C. H., and Larkin, G. M.: The battered child syndrome—a forensic pathologist's viewpoint. Med. Trial. Tech. Q., *28*:1, 1981.
123. Wenger, D. R., and Rokicki, R. R.: Spinal deformity secondary to scar formation in a battered child. A case report. J. Bone Joint Surg., *60A*:847, 1978.
124. Wichlacz, C. R., Randall, D. H., Nelson, J. H., and Kempe, C. H.: The characteristics and management of child abuse in the U.S. Army, Europe. Clin. Pediatr., *14*:545, 1975.
125. Wong, C. S.: The battered child syndrome in Singapore. J. Singapore Paediatr. Soc., *21*:148, 1979.
126. Wong, C. S.: The battered child syndrome in Singapore. Nurs. J. Singapore, *20*:57, 1980.
127. Woolley, P. V., Jr.: The pediatrician and the young child subjected to repeated physical abuse. J. Pediatr., *62*:628, 1963.
128. Woolley, P. V., and Evans, W. A.: Significance of skeletal lesions in infants resembling those of traumatic origin. J.A.M.A., *158*:539, 1955.
129. Wurfel, L. J., and McCoy, W. T.: Radiographic features of the battered child syndrome. J. Coll. Radiol. Aust., *9*:220, 1965.

Index

Note: Page numbers in *italics* refer to illustrations; page numbers in boldface refer to surgical plates. Page numbers followed by the letter t refer to tables.

A

B

D

E

F

G

I

J

K

L

M

N

O

Q

R

S

T

U